MW01097531

Withrow & MacEwen's
Small Animal Clinical Oncology

Withrow & MacEwen's Small Animal Clinical Oncology

SIXTH EDITION

David M. Vail, DVM, MS, DACVIM (Oncology)

Professor and Barbara A. Suran Chair of Comparative Oncology
Department of Medical Sciences
School of Veterinary Medicine
University of Wisconsin–Madison
Madison, Wisconsin, United States

Douglas H. Thamm, VMD, DACVIM (Oncology)

Barbara Cox Anthony Professor of Oncology
Director of Clinical Research
Flint Animal Cancer Center
Department of Clinical Sciences
College of Veterinary Medicine and Biomedical Sciences
Colorado State University
Fort Collins, Colorado, United States

Julius M. Liptak, BVSc, MVetClinStud, FACVSc, DACVS-SA, DECVS, ACVS Founding Fellow, Surgical Oncology

Staff Small Animal Surgeon and Surgical Oncologist
VCA Canada - Alta Vista Animal Hospital
Ottawa, Ontario, Canada
Adjunct Professor
Ontario Veterinary College, University of Guelph
Guelph, Ontario, Canada

ELSEVIER   Edinburgh   London   New York   Oxford   Philadelphia   St Louis   Sydney   2020

3251 Riverport Lane
St. Louis, Missouri 63043

WITHROW AND MACEWEN'S SMALL ANIMAL CLINICAL ONCOLOGY,
6TH EDITION

ISBN: 978-0-323-59496-7

Library of Congress Control Number: 2019943582

Senior Content Strategist: Jennifer Catando
Senior Content Development Manager: Luke Held
Senior Content Development Specialist: Kelly Skelton
Publishing Services Manager: Shereen Jameel
Senior Project Manager: Karthikeyan Murthy
Design Direction: Amy Buxton

Printed in China

Last digit is the print number: 9 8 7 6 5 4 3 2 1

Working together
to grow libraries in
developing countries

www.elsevier.com • www.bookaid.org

Contributors

Pierre M. Amsellem, Doct. Vet., MS, DACVS, DECVS, ACVS Founding Fellow, Surgical Oncology
Associate Professor of Small Animal Surgery
Department of Veterinary Clinical Sciences
University of Minnesota
Saint Paul, Minnesota, United States
Cancer of the Gastrointestinal Tract: Esophageal Tumors

David J. Argyle, BVMS, PhD, DECVIM-CA (Oncology), FRSE, FRCVS
RCVS and European Recognised Specialist in Veterinary Oncology
William Dick Chair of Veterinary Clinical Studies
Dean of Veterinary Medicine and Head of School
Royal (Dick) School of Veterinary Studies
The University of Edinburgh
Roslin, Midlothian, United Kingdom
Tumor Biology and Metastasis
Molecular/Targeted Therapy of Cancer: Gene Therapy for Cancer; Novel and Emerging Therapeutic Agents

Anne C. Avery, VMD, PhD
Professor
Department of Microbiology, Immunology, and Pathology
Colorado State University
Fort Collins, Colorado, United States
Molecular Diagnostics

Nicholas J. Bacon, MA, VetMB, CertVR, CertSAS, DECVS, DACVS, FRCVS
Clincal Director
Fitzpatrick Referrals Oncology and Soft Tissue
Professor, Surgical Oncology
University of Surrey School of Veterinary Medicine
University of Surrey
Guildford, Surrey, United Kingdom
Tumors of the Respiratory System: Cancer of the Larynx and Trachea

Dennis B. Bailey, DVM, DACVIM (Oncology)
Staff Oncologist
Oradell Animal Hosptial
Paramus, New Jersey, United States
Paraneoplastic Syndromes
Cancer Chemotherapy

Philip J. Bergman, DVM, PhD, DACVIM (Oncology)
Director, Clinical Studies
VCA
Stamford, Connecticut,
Adjunct Associate,
Memorial Sloan-Kettering Cancer Center
New York, New York, United States
Melanoma

Barbara Biller, DVM, PhD, DACVIM (Oncology)
Medical Oncologist
Boulder Road Veterinary Specialists
Lafayette, Colorado, United States
Adjunct Professor of Oncology
Department of Clinical Sciences
Colorado State University
Fort Collins, Colorado, United States
Molecular/Targeted Therapy of Cancer: Antiangiogenic and Metronomic Therapy

Brenda N. Bonnett, DVM, PhD
CEO, B Bonnett Consulting
CEO, International Partnership for Dogs
Georgian Bluffs, Ontario, Canada
Epidemiology and the Evidence-Based Medicine Approach

Sarah E. Boston, DVM, DVSc, DACVS, ACVS Founding Fellow, Surgical Oncology, ACVS Founding Fellow, Oral and Maxillofacial Surgery
Staff Surgeon
VCA Canada, 404 Veterinary Emergency and Referral
Newmarket, Ontario, Canada
Cancer of the Gastrointestinal Tract: Salivary Gland Neoplasia
Tumors of the Endocrine System

Jenna H. Burton, DVM, MS, DACVIM (Oncology)
Associate Professor of Clinical Oncology
Director, Veterinary Center for Clinical Trials
Department of Surgical and Radiological Sciences
University of California, Davis
School of Veterinary Medicine
Davis, California, United States
Miscellaneous Tumors: Neoplasia of the Heart

Neil I. Christensen, BVSc, DACVR (Radiation Oncology), FANZCVS (Medical Oncology)
Staff Radiation Oncologist
Small Animal Specialist Hospital
Sydney, New South Wales, Australia
Soft Tissue Sarcomas
Tumors of the Skeletal System

Craig A. Clifford, DVM, MS, DACVIM (Oncology)
Director of Clinical Studies
Medical Oncology
Hope Veterinary Specialists
Malvern, Pennsylvania, United States
Miscellaneous Tumors: Hemangiosarcoma; Histiocytic Diseases

William T.N. Culp, VMD, DACVS, ACVS Founding Fellow, Surgical Oncology, ACVS Founding Fellow, Minimally Invasive Surgery
Professor
Department of Surgical and Radiological Sciences
University of California, Davis
Davis, California, United States
Interventional Oncology
Tumors of the Respiratory System: Cancer of the Nasal Planum; Pulmonary Neoplasia

Steven Dow, DVM, PhD, DACVIM (Internal Medicine)
Professor of Immunology
Department of Clinical Sciences
Flint Animal Cancer Center, Colorado State University
Fort Collins, Colorado, United States
Cancer Immunotherapy

Nicole P. Ehrhart, VMD, MS, DACVS, ACVS Founding Fellow, Surgical Oncology
Professor, Surgical Oncology
Department of Clinical Sciences
Colorado State University Flint Animal Cancer Center
Fort Collins, Colorado, United States
Biopsy and Sentinel Lymph Node Mapping Principles
Tumors of the Skeletal System

Timothy M. Fan, DVM, PhD, DACVIM (Oncology, Internal Medicine)
Professor
Department of Veterinary Clinical Medicine
University of Illinois at Urbana-Champaign
Urbana, Illinois, United States
Supportive Care for the Cancer Patient: Management of Chronic Cancer Pain
Tumors of the Skeletal System

James P. Farese, DVM, DACVS, ACVS Founding Fellow, Surgical Oncology
Staff Surgeon
North Bay Veterinary Surgical
Kentfield, California, United States
Surgical Oncology
Cancer of the Gastrointestinal Tract: Esophageal Tumors

Brian K. Flesner, DVM, MS, DACVIM (Oncology)
Assistant Professor
Department of Veterinary Medicine and Surgery
University of Missouri College of Veterinary Medicine
Columbia, Missouri, United States
The Etiology of Cancer: Chemical, Physical, and Hormonal Factors

Kristen R. Friedrichs, DVM, DACVP
Clinical Associate Professor of Clinical Pathology
Department of Pathobiological Sciences
University of Wisconsin School of Veterinary Medicine
Madison, Wisconsin, United States
Diagnostic Cytopathology in Clinical Oncology

Christopher M. Fulkerson, DVM, MS, DACVIM (Oncology)
Clinical Assistant Professor of Veterinary Medical Oncology
Department of Veterinary Clinical Sciences
Purdue University College of Veterinary Medicine
Purdue University Center for Cancer Research
West Lafayette, Indiana, United States
Tumors of the Urinary System

Laura D. Garrett, DVM, DACVIM (Oncology)
Clinical Professor, Oncology
Department of Veterinary Clinical Medicine
University of Illinois College of Veterinary Medicine
Urbana, Illinois, United States
Miscellaneous Tumors: Mesothelioma

Nicole Giancristofaro, DVM
Staff Veterinarian
The Oncology Service
Richmond, Virginia, United States
Tumor Biology and Metastasis

Ira K. Gordon, DVM, DACVR (Radiation Oncology)
Medical Director and Radiation Oncologist
The Oncology Service (TOS) by Ethos Veterinary Health
Leesburg, Virginia
XPrep Learning Solutions
San Diego, California
Radiation Oncology

Daniel L. Gustafson, PhD
Professor
Department of Clinical Sciences
Colorado State University
Fort Collins, Colorado, United States
Cancer Chemotherapy

Amanda Guth, PhD, DVM
Assistant Professor
Flint Animal Cancer Center, Department of Clinical Sciences
Colorado State University
Fort Collins, Colorado, United States
Cancer Immunotherapy

Marlene L. Hauck, DVM, PhD, DACVIM (Oncology)
Professor Emeritus
Department of Clinical Sciences
North Carolina State University
Raleigh, North Carolina, United States
Partner, Bear Creek Veterinary Services, PLLC
Victor, Montana, United States
Tumors of the Skin and Subcutaneous Tissues

Carolyn J. Henry, DVM, MS, DACVIM (Oncology)
Dean
College of Veterinary Medicine
University of Missouri
Columbia, Missouri, United States
The Etiology of Cancer: Chemical, Physical, and Hormonal Factors

Debra A. Kamstock, DVM, PhD, DACVP
Director and Chief of Pathology
KamPath Diagnostics & Investigation
Founding President, VCS/ACVP Oncology-Pathology Working
Group
Fort Collins, Colorado, United States
The Pathology of Neoplasia

Michael S. Kent, MAS, DVM, DACVIM (Oncology), DACVR (Radiation Oncology), DECVDI (Radiation Oncology)
Professor
Department of Surgical and Radiological Sciences
Director, Center for Companion Animal Health
University of California, Davis
Davis, California, United States
Melanoma

Chand Khanna, DVM, PhD, DACVP (HON), DACVIM (Oncology)
Chief Science Officer
Ethos Veterinary Health
President, Ethos Discovery
Woburn, Massachussetts, United States
Tumor Biology and Metastasis
Molecular Diagnostics

Jong Hyuk Kim, DVM, PhD
Assistant Professor
Department of Veterinary Clinical Sciences
University of Minnesota
St. Paul, Minnesota, United States
The Etiology of Cancer: The Genetic Basis of Cancer

Deborah W. Knapp, DVM, MS, DACVIM (Oncology)
Dolores L. McCall Professor of Comparative Oncology
Department of Veterinary Clinical Sciences
Purdue University Center for Cancer Research
Purdue University
West Lafayette, Indiana, United States
Tumors of the Urinary System

Susan E. Lana, DVM, MS, DACVIM (Oncology)
Professor and Stuart Chair in Oncology
Department of Clinical Sciences
Colorado State University
Fort Collins, Colorado, United States
Tumors of the Respiratory System: Nasal Cavity and Sinus Tumors

Susan M. LaRue, DVM, PhD, DACVS, DACVR (Radiation Oncology)
Professor
Department of Environmental and Radiological Health Sciences
Colorado State University Flint Animal Cancer Center
Fort Collins, Colorado, United States
Radiation Oncology

B. Duncan X. Lascelles, BSc, BVSc, PhD, MRCVS, CertVA, DSAS(ST), DECVS, DACVS
Professor
Translational Research in Pain Program, Comparative Pain
Research and Education Center
North Carolina State University
Raleigh, North Carolina, United States
Supportive Care for the Cancer Patient: Management of Chronic Cancer Pain

Jessica A. Lawrence, DVM, DACVIM (Oncology), DACVR (Radiation Oncology), DECVDI (Add On Radiation Oncology)
Associate Professor of Radiation Oncology
Department of Veterinary Clinical Sciences
University of Minnesota
St. Paul, Minnesota, United States
Tumors of the Female Reproductive System
Tumors of the Male Reproductive System

Amy K. LeBlanc, DVM, DACVIM (Oncology)
Director
Comparative Oncology Program
National Cancer Institute, National Institutes of Health
Bethesda, Maryland, United States
Clinical Trials and Developmental Therapeutics

Julius M. Liptak, BVSc, MVetClinStud, FACVSc, DACVS-SA, DECVS, ACVS Founding Fellow, Surgical Oncology
Staff Small Animal Surgeon and Surgical Oncologist
VCA Canada - Alta Vista Animal Hospital
Ottawa, Ontario, Canada
Adjunct Professor
Ontario Veterinary College, University of Guelph
Guelph, Ontario, Canada
Surgical Oncology
Soft Tissue Sarcomas
Cancer of the Gastrointestinal Tract: Oral Tumors; Hepatobiliary Tumors; Perianal Tumors

Cheryl A. London, DVM, PhD, DACVIM (Oncology)
Anne Engen and Dusty
Professor of Comparative Oncology
Department of Clinical Sciences
Cummings School of Veterinary Medicine, Tufts University
North Grafton, Massachusetts, United States
Research Professor, Department of Immunology
Tufts University School of Medicine
Boston, Massachusetts, United States
Molecular/Targeted Therapy of Cancer: Signal Transduction and Cancer
Mast Cell Tumors

Katharine F. Lunn, BVMS, MS, PhD, MRCVS, DACVIM (Internal Medicine)
Associate Professor
Department of Clinical Sciences
North Carolina State University College of Veterinary Medicine
Raleigh, North Carolina, United States
Tumors of the Endocrine System

Dennis W. Macy, DVM, MS, DACVIM (Internal Medicine/Oncology)
Professor Emeritus
Department of Clinical Sciences
Colorado State University
Fort Collins, Colorado, United States
Medical Oncologist, Paws and Claws Urgent Care and Advanced Imaging Center
Palm Desert, California, United States
Medical Oncologist, VCA Valley Animal Medical Center and Emergency Hospital
Indio, California, United States
Medical Oncologist, West Flamingo Animal Hospital
Las Vegas, Nevada, United States
The Etiology of Cancer: Cancer-Causing Viruses

Kara Magee, DVM
Resident in Medical Oncology
School of Veterinary Medicine
University of Wisconsin–Madison
Madison, Wisconsin, United States
Molecular Diagnostics

Carlos H. de Mello Souza, DVM, MS, DACVIM (Oncology), DACVS-SA, ACVS Fellow, Surgical Oncology
Assistant Professor of Surgical Oncology
Department of Small Animal Clinical Sciences
University of Florida College of Veterinary Medicine
Gainesville, Florida, United States
Miscellaneous Tumors: Thymoma

Constanza Meneses, DVM, MS
Graduate Research Assistant
Comparative Biomedical Sciences (Neuroscience)
Comparative Pain Research and Education center Translational Research in Pain (TRiP) Program
North Carolina State University
Raleigh, North Carolina, United States
Supportive Care for the Cancer Patient: Management of Chronic Cancer Pain

Paul E. Miller, DVM, DACVO
Clinical Professor of Comparative Ophthalmology
Department of Surgical Sciences
School of Veterinary Medicine, University of Wisconsin–Madison
Madison, Wisconsin, United States
Ocular Tumors

Jaime F. Modiano, VMD, PhD
Alvin and June Perlman Professor of Animal Oncology
Department of Veterinary Clinical Sciences, College of Veterinary Medicine
Director, Animal Cancer Care and Research Program
Professor and Full Member, Masonic Cancer Center
University of Minnesota
St. Paul, Minnesota, United States
The Etiology of Cancer: The Genetic Basis of Cancer

Peter F. Moore, BVSc, PhD, DACVP
Professor
Department of Pathology, Microbiology and Immunology
University of California, School of Veterinary Medicine
Davis, California, United States
Miscellaneous Tumors: Histiocytic Diseases

Christine Mullin, VMD, DACVIM (Oncology)
Medical Oncologist
Hope Veterinary Specialists
Malvern, Pennsylvania, United States
Miscellaneous Tumors: Hemangiosarcoma

Anthony J. Mutsaers, DVM, PhD, DACVIM (Oncology)
Associate Professor
Department of Clinical Studies; Biomedical Sciences
Ontario Veterinary College, University of Guelph
Guelph, Ontario, Canada
Molecular/Targeted Therapy of Cancer: Antiangiogenic and Metronomic Therapy

Michael W. Nolan, DVM, PhD, DACVR (Radiation Oncology)
Associate Professor, Radiation Oncology
Department of Clinical Sciences
North Carolina State University
Raleigh, North Carolina, United States
Supportive Care for the Cancer Patient: Management of Chronic Cancer Pain

Stephanie Nykamp, DVM, MSc, DACVR
Associate Professor
Department of Clinical Studies
Ontario Veterinary College, University of Guelph
Guelph, Ontario, Canada
Diagnostic Imaging in Oncology

Michelle L. Oblak, DVM, DVSc, DACVS-SA, ACVS Founding Fellow, Surgical Oncology
Associate Professor, Soft Tissue & Oncologic Surgery
Department of Clinical Studies
Ontario Veterinary College, University of Guelph
Guelph, Ontario, Canada
Tumors of the Skin and Subcutaneous Tissues

Rodney L. Page, DVM, DACVIM (Internal Medicine/Oncology)
Professor and Director, Flint Animal Cancer Center
Stephen Withrow Presidential Chair in Oncology
Department of Clinical Sciences
Colorado State University
Fort Collins, Colorado, United States
Epidemiology and the Evidence-Based Medicine Approach

Theresa E. Pancotto, DVM, MS, DACVIM (Neurology), CCRP
Associate Professor
Department of Small Animal Clinical Sciences
Virginia-Maryland College of Veterinary Medicine
Blacksburg, Virginia, United States
Tumors of the Nervous System

Melissa C. Paoloni, DVM, DACVIM (Oncology)
VP, Medical Affairs and Clinical Partnerships
Arcus Biosciences
Hayward, California
Molecular Diagnostics

Marie Pinkerton, DVM, DACVP
Clinical Associate Professor
Department of Pathobiological Sciences
University of Wisconsin–Madison
Madison, Wisconsin, United States
Hematopoietic Tumors: Canine Lymphoma and Lymphocytic Leukemias; Feline Lymphoma and Leukemia

Barbara E. Powers, DVM, PhD, DACVP
Diagnostic Anatomic Pathologist
Antech Diagnostics
Professor Emeritus, Colorado State University
Fort Collins, Colorado, United States
The Pathology of Neoplasia

Elissa Randall, DVM, MS, DACVR
Associate Professor, Diagnostic Imaging
Department of Environmental and Radiological Health Sciences
Colorado State University
Fort Collins, Colorado, United States
Diagnostic Imaging in Oncology

Jennifer K. Reagan, DVM, DACVS
Seattle Veterinary Specialists BluePearl Downtown
Seattle, Washington, United States
Cancer of the Gastrointestinal Tract: Intestinal Tumors

Robert B. Rebhun, DVM, PhD, DACVIM (Oncology)
Professor and Maxine Adler Endowed Chair in Oncology
Department of Veterinary Surgical and Radiological Sciences
University of California, Davis
Davis, California, United States
Tumors of the Respiratory System: Pulmonary Neoplasia

Narda G. Robinson, DO, DVM, MS
President and CEO
CuraCore Integrative Medicine & Education Center
Fort Collins, Colorado, United States
Integrative Oncology

John H. Rossmeisl Jr., DVM, MS, DACVIM (Internal Medicine/Neurology)
Dr. and Mrs. Dorothy Taylor Mahin Professor, Neurology/Neurosurgery
Department of Small Animal Clinical Sciences
Virginia-Maryland College of Veterinary Medicine
Blacksburg, Virginia, United States
Tumors of the Nervous System

Audrey Ruple, DVM, MS, PhD, DACVPM, MRCVS
Assistant Professor of One Health Epidemiology
Department of Comparative Pathobiology
Purdue University
West Lafayette, Indiana, United States
Epidemiology and the Evidence-Based Medicine Approach

Duncan S. Russell, BVMS (Hons), DACVP
Assistant Professor
Department of Biomedical Sciences, Carlson College of Veterinary Medicine
Oregon State University
Corvallis, Oregon, United States
The Pathology of Neoplasia

Corey F. Saba, DVM, DACVIM (Oncology)
Professor of Oncology
Department of Small Animal Medicine & Surgery
University of Georgia
Athens, Georgia, United States
Tumors of the Female Reproductive System
Tumors of the Male Reproductive System

Laura E. Selmic, BVetMed (Hons), MPH, DACVS-SA, DECVS, ACVS Founding Fellow, Surgical Oncology
Assistant Professor, Small Animal Surgical Oncology
Department of Veterinary Clinical Medicine
The Ohio State University
Columbus, Ohio, United States
Melanoma
Cancer of the Gastrointestinal Tract: Exocrine Pancreatic Cancer; Intestinal Tumors

Kim A. Selting, DVM, MS, DACVIM (Oncology), DACVR (Radiation Oncology)
Associate Professor
Department of Veterinary Clinical Medicine
University of Illinois at Urbana-Champaign
Urbana, Illinois, United States
Cancer of the Gastrointestinal Tract: Intestinal Tumors

Jane R. Shaw, DVM, PhD
Associate Professor
Department of Clinical Sciences
Colorado State University
Fort Collins, Colorado, United States
Supportive Care for the Cancer Patient: Relationship-Centered Approach to Cancer Communication

Owen T. Skinner, BVSc, DECVS, DACVS-SA, MRCVS, ACVS Fellow, Surgical Oncology
Assistant Professor of Small Animal Surgical Oncology
Department of Veterinary Medicine and Surgery
University of Missouri
Columbia, Missouri, United States
Cancer of the Gastrointestinal Tract: Gastric Cancer

Katherine A. Skorupski, DVM, DACVIM (Oncology)
Professor of Clinical Medical Oncology
Department of Surgical and Radiological Sciences
University of California, Davis
Davis, California, United States
Miscellaneous Tumors: Histiocytic Diseases

Karin U. Sorenmo, DVM, DACVIM (Oncology), DECVIM-CA (Oncology)
Professor of Oncology
Department of Biomedical Sciences
School of Veterinary Medicine, University of Pennsylvania
Philadelphia, Pennsylvania, United States
Tumors of the Mammary Gland

Joshua A. Stern, DVM, PhD, DACVIM (Cardiology)
Associate Professor of Cardiology
Department of Medicine and Epidemiology
School of Veterinary Medicine, University of California, Davis
Davis, California, United States
Miscellaneous Tumors: Neoplasia of the Heart

Leandro B.C. Teixeira, DVM, MSc, DACVP
Assistant Professor
Department of Pathobiological Sciences
University of Wisconsin–Madison
Madison, Wisconsin, United States
Ocular Tumors

Douglas H. Thamm, VMD, DACVIM (Oncology)
Barbara Cox Anthony Professor of Oncology
Director of Clinical Research
Flint Animal Cancer Center, Department of Clinical Sciences
College of Veterinary Medicine and Biomedical Sciences
Colorado State University
Fort Collins, Colorado, United States
Molecular/Targeted Therapy of Cancer: Novel and Emerging Therapeutic Agents
Clinical Trials and Developmental Therapeutics
Mast Cell Tumors

Michelle M. Turek, DVM, DACVIM (Oncology), DACVR (Radiation Oncology)
Clinical Assistant Professor
Department of Surgical Sciences
University of Wisconsin–Madison School of Veterinary Medicine
Madison, Wisconsin, United States
Cancer of the Gastrointestinal Tract: Perianal Tumors
Tumors of the Respiratory System: Nasal Cavity and Sinus Tumors

David M. Vail, DVM, MS, DACVIM (Oncology)
Professor and Barbara A. Suran Chair of Comparative Oncology
Department of Medical Sciences
School of Veterinary Medicine
University of Wisconsin–Madison
Madison, Wisconsin, United States
Clinical Trials and Developmental Therapeutics
Hematopoietic Tumors: Canine Lymphoma and Lymphocytic Leukemias; Feline Lymphoma and Leukemia; Canine Acute Myeloid Leukemia, Myeloproliferative Neoplasms, and Myelodysplasia; Myeloma-Related Disorders

Joseph Wakshlag, DVM, PhD, DACVN, DACVSMR
Professor
Department of Clinical Sciences
Cornell University College of Veterinary Medicine
Ithaca, New York, United States
Supportive Care for the Cancer Patient: Nutritional Management of the Cancer Patient

Stephen J. Withrow, DVM, DACVS, DACVIM (Oncology)
Founding Director
University Distinguished Professor
Stuart Chair in Oncology Emeritus
Flint Animal Cancer Center
Colorado State University
Fort Collins, Colorado, United States
Surgical Oncology

J. Paul Woods, DVM, MS, DACVIM (Internal Medicine, Oncology)
Professor of Oncology & Internal Medicine
Department of Clinical Studies
Ontario Veterinary College
Co-Director, Institute for Comparative Cancer Investigation
University of Guelph
Guelph, Ontario, Canada
Miscellaneous Tumors: Canine Transmissible Venereal Tumor

Deanna R. Worley, DVM, DACVS-SA, ACVS Founding Fellow, Surgical Oncology
Associate Professor, Surgical Oncology
Department of Clinical Sciences
Flint Animal Cancer Center
Colorado State University
Fort Collins, Colorado, United States
Tumors of the Mammary Gland

Karen M. Young, VMD, PhD
Professor of Clinical Pathology
Department of Pathobiological Sciences
School of Veterinary Medicine, University of Wisconsin–Madison
Madison, Wisconsin, United States
Diagnostic Cytopathology in Clinical Oncology
Hematopoietic Tumors: Canine Lymphoma and Lymphocytic Leukemias; Canine Acute Myeloid Leukemia, Myeloproliferative Neoplasms, and Myelodysplasia

Valentina Zappulli, DVM, MSc, PhD, DECVP
Professor
Department of Comparative Biomedicine and Food Science (BCA)
University of Padua
Legnaro, Padua, Italy
Tumors of the Mammary Gland

The sixth edition of *Small Animal Clinical Oncology* continues to chronicle significant advancement in the field of comparative clinical oncology. Since the first edition in 1989, this text has expanded all segments of the book to keep current with the profound changes in cancer biology and technology; in fact, each edition could be considered a milestone in the development of this specialty. The intent of this text continues to be production of a relevant summary of the field of comparative cancer biology and management for those engaged in all aspects of the veterinary profession. Approximately 20% of this edition has been substantially changed, with new authors and additions and deletions of entire chapters to reflect an appropriate emphasis on the current state of the profession.

This text, in all its editions, parallels the expansion and maturity of comparative oncology during the past 30 years. The Specialty of Oncology was formalized under the American College of Veterinary Internal Medicine (ACVIM) in 1989 and has grown steadily, particularly in the past 10 to 15 years. Likewise, the European College of Veterinary Internal Medicine (ECVIM)–Oncology Specialty is now a robust and dynamic organization providing important resources to students and practitioners in Europe. The American College of Veterinary Surgeons (ACVS) has formally authorized the Fellowship Training Programs in Veterinary Surgical Oncology, which will promote the expansion of new centers of surgical excellence in this field. Equally important has been the growth of the Veterinary Cancer Society (VCS) and the European Society of Veterinary Oncology (ESVONC), as well as other like-minded associations in Japan (JVCS), Brazil (ABROVET), and others to develop soon. The globalization of the interest and desire for high-quality cancer care for companion species is a remarkable and welcome occurrence.

During the past decade, the formalization of clinical trials in companion animals for investigation of animal and human health has matured significantly. The Comparative Oncology Program at the National Cancer Institute (NCI) continues to lead the effort to promote the benefits of companion animals in human cancer control and has currently completed or initiated more than 25 multicenter trials through the Comparative Oncology Trials Consortium. Other clinical trial organizations and centers, within both the public and private sector, have emerged and have established a more formal infrastructure for cooperative clinical research. No better evidence of this exists than the U.S. Food and Drug Administration (FDA) and U.S. Department of Agriculture (USDA) approvals for products licensed for use specifically in canine cancer that occurred due to a clinician–animal health industry partnership.

Examples of marked advances in the field of cancer biology, etiology, and staging reflected in this text include a complete rewrite of the role of genetics in cancer development (Chapter 1, Section A), cancer epidemiology (Chapter 4), tumor imaging technology (Chapter 6), and the reliance on more sophisticated molecular diagnostics (Chapter 8). All chapters devoted to specific cancer types have been updated, along with significant additions in sections on therapeutic options. Although consensus standards-of-care do not exist for most malignancies in veterinary species, available therapeutic options and published outcomes are presented that should allow the reader to choose the option best suited for his or her particular patient and client population.

There is still much to be done and future advances should continue to be a focus for expansion in subsequent editions of this text. Advancing the use and application of evidence-based medicine still remains a challenge in veterinary oncology. The desire to increase evidence-based decision-making in clinical practice is being considered throughout the veterinary profession as a whole, and appropriate reporting guidelines for manuscript submission have been implemented in the leading veterinary journals. Such guidelines permit sorting of levels of evidence and an opportunity to engage in formal post-publication data analysis for systematic reviews. We look forward to the next edition of the text that includes therapeutic recommendations based on strong evidence and consensus opinion from leading veterinary collaborative scientific organizations. We also continue to hope that the next edition will see a quantum leap in satisfying several critical needs in the field. We urgently need improved durable outcomes for canine lymphoma, hemangiosarcoma, and osteosarcoma, and validated biomarkers to assist with prognostic and predictive estimates for all cancers—but in particular, those highly lethal disease processes mentioned previously that have frustrated all of us for decades. Furthermore, advancements in supportive measures that can ensure the maintenance of quality of life and abrogation of adverse events are similarly in need of further development.

It is also important to consider potential operational effects and solutions to the continued development of comparative oncology. The inconsistent availability of certain chemotherapy drugs often now rises to levels of serious concern for continuity of care and will require innovative business solutions to ensure robust coverage of the expanding market need. It is obvious that the cost of care for companion animals will continue to rise, and the role that companion animal healthcare insurance will play in this dynamic could have far-reaching effects on the profession in the next decade. Likewise, the potential changes in the profession from increasing liability issues related to emotional pain and suffering litigation could create new operating paradigms.

The authors and editors have created the following text, which both describes the phenomenal strides made during the past 5 to 6 years and sets the standard to measure future growth and understanding of comparative oncology. We hope that it will be a useful resource for those engaged in animal and human oncology and for the ultimate improvement of the quality and length of life for our patients.

We dedicate this edition to these fine men, each of whom
pioneered his particular branch of veterinary oncology:

Dr. E. Gregory MacEwen
1943–2001
*The father of veterinary medical oncology, Greg was
personally responsible for educating and inspiring the current
generation of medical oncologists, both as clinicians and clinician scientists.*

Dr. Robert S. Brodey
1927–1979
*The father of veterinary surgical oncology, Bob will be remembered for
his tireless effort to advance the field of oncology, to teach
principles of surgery, and, most importantly, to preserve nature.*

Dr. Edward L. Gillette
1932–2006
*The father of veterinary radiation oncology, Ed was a leader in comparative oncology.
His vision and leadership have created a new and contemporary
breed of oncologists in all disciplines.*

Contents

Introduction

Why Worry About Cancer in Companion Animals?

Why should health care professionals in general, and veterinarians in particular, be concerned about cancer in companion animals? Several compelling motivations and opportunities exist for the profession as a whole to continue, and indeed expand on, the significant role we play in the understanding, prevention, and elimination or control of this devastating constellation of disease processes. Although, as veterinarians, our prime directive is to ensure the health and quality of life of the companions under our care, the needs of our client caregivers during the difficult times of cancer diagnosis, treatment, and outcome (whether optimistic or pessimistic) should be of nearly equal importance. Because cancer is a disease that knows no species boundaries, our profession has considerable opportunity to play a key role in comparative oncologic investigations, with the ultimate goal of effecting cure or, in the absence of cure, transforming cancer from an acute life-threatening disorder into a manageable chronic condition (much like diabetes) in all species; essentially the basis of the "One Medicine" approach to disease investigation.

The sheer numbers involved highlight the magnitude of the problem of cancer in companion species. The prevalence of cancer in companion animals continues to rise for a variety of reasons, not the least of which is related to animals living longer thanks to the increasing care offered by caregivers and the advanced veterinary care they seek. There are more than 165 million dogs and cats at risk in the United States,[1] and cancer remains a major cause of companion animal morbidity and mortality (see Chapter 4), with at least 4 million dogs and 4 million cats developing cancer each year.[2-6] Although the true incidence or prevalence of companion animal cancer is currently not known, based on necropsy surveys describing proportional mortality, 45% of dogs that live to 10 years or older die of cancer.[4] With no age adjustment, 23% of patients presenting for necropsy died of cancer. In a 1998 Morris Animal Foundation (MAF) Animal Health Survey, more than 2000 respondents stated that cancer was the leading cause of disease-related death in both dogs (47%) and cats (32%).[3] Another MAF survey performed in 2005 revealed that cancer was by far the largest health concern among dog owners (41%), with heart disease the number two concern at 7%. Regardless of the exact numbers, both the reality and the perception support the clients' point of view that cancer remains the number one concern in their minds with respect to the health and quality of life of their companions—the so called "emperor of all maladies".[7] Furthermore, breakthroughs in the management of human cancers have received a great deal of exposure through the Internet, news media, and popular press, which further serves to educate companion caregivers and raise the level of expectations as to therapeutic possibilities and promote an atmosphere of optimism and a demand for similar care for their animals. Increased longevity of companion animals, the increasing prevalence of cancer, and enhanced caregiver expectations require that the veterinary profession be prepared to meet these challenges and opportunities.

Because cancer is a common and serious disease for human beings, many owners have had or will have a personal experience with cancer in themselves, a family member, or a close friend. Realizing the importance of companion animals to our clients, it must be appreciated that they value the veterinarian's ability to care as much as his or her ability to cure. Keeping this in mind, the veterinarian should approach the patient with cancer in a positive, compassionate, and knowledgeable manner. Frequently, the veterinary profession has taken a pessimistic approach to cancer. This attitude is not only a detriment to the companion but may also negatively reinforce unfounded fears in the client about the disease in humans. We owe it to our companion animal patients and their caregivers to be well informed and up-to-date on current treatment methods to prevent imparting unnecessary feelings of hopelessness.

Perhaps the greatest opportunity presented to our profession, beyond the immediate care of our patients' and clients' needs, is the more global role (and responsibility) we play in advancing the understanding of cancer biology, prevention, and treatment from a comparative oncology standpoint. Companion animals with spontaneously developing cancer provide an excellent opportunity to investigate many aspects of cancer, from etiology to treatment. Indeed, the role of comparative oncology was highlighted at a National Cancer Policy Forum hosted by the National Academy of Sciences in 2015 entitled "The Role of Clinical Studies for Pets with Naturally Occurring Tumors in Translational Cancer Research".[8] One of the most exciting achievements in veterinary oncology over the past 15 years has been the development of successful and collaborative consortia groups that are purposed to perform multicenter clinical trials and prospective tumor biospecimen repository collections. These include the Comparative Oncology Trials Consortium (COTC; https://ccrod.cancer.gov/confluence/display/CCRCOPWeb/Comparative+Oncology+Trials+Consortium) and the Canine Comparative Oncology and Genomics Consortium (CCOGC, www.ccogc.net) centrally managed by the National Institutes of Health (NIH)-National Cancer Institute's Comparative Oncology Program (NCI-COP) and discussed in Chapter 18. Their infrastructure allows larger scale clinical trials and provides the voice for collective advocacy in veterinary and comparative oncology. Their success is an example of the growing importance of the study of comparative tumor biology and clinical investigations. Access to novel drugs and biologics will speed clinical applications for both veterinary species and humans. Ultimately, including companion animal populations in clinical trials assessing novel drugs and biologics of interest to the National Cancer Institute, the U.S. Food and Drug Administration, and the pharmaceutical industry will both advance veterinary-based practice and inform future human clinical trials that may follow. Some of the aspects of companion animal cancer that enable attractive comparative models include the following:

1. Companion dogs and cats are genetically outbred (like humans), as opposed to many experimental models of rodents and other animals.

2. The cancers seen in practice are spontaneously developing as opposed to experimentally induced and better recapitulate the natural human and veterinary condition.

3. Companion species share the same environment as their caregivers and may serve as epidemiologic or etiologic sentinels for the changing patterns of cancer development seen in humans.

4. Companion species have a higher incidence of some cancers (e.g., osteosarcoma, non-Hodgkin lymphoma) than humans.

5. Most animal cancers will progress at a more rapid rate than will the human counterparts. This permits more rapid and less costly outcome determinations such as time to metastasis, local recurrence, and survival.

6. Because fewer established "gold standard" treatments exist in veterinary medicine compared with human medicine, it is ethically acceptable to attempt new forms of therapy on an untreated cancer rather than wait to initiate new treatments until all "known" treatments have failed, as is common in the human condition. It is important to recognize that this latitude in clinical trials can be misused to permit diverse and poorly characterized or even unethical treatments to be attempted as well. We have an obligation to ensure that our patients are not denied known effective treatment while at the same time planning well-designed prospective clinical trials of newer, scientifically sound treatment methods.

7. Companion species' cancers are more akin to human cancers than are rodent tumors in terms of patient size and cell kinetics. Dogs and cats also share similar characteristics of physiology and metabolism for most organ systems and drugs. Such correspondence allows better and safer comparison of treatment modalities such as surgery, radiation, and chemotherapy between animals and humans to be made.

8. Dogs and cats have intact immune systems as opposed to many rodent model systems, which allows immunologic assays and treatment approaches to be explored. Furthermore, their cancers develop in a syngeneic tumor microenvironment and tumor–tumor microenvironment interactions are equally important to understand basic tumor biology and the development of novel therapeutic targets.

9. Companion animal trials are generally more economical to perform than human trials.

10. Companion animals live long enough to determine the potential late effects of treatment.

11. Regional referral centers exist to concentrate case accrual and facilitate clinical trials.

12. Clients are often willing to allow a necropsy, which is a crucial end point for not only tumor control but also treatment-related toxicity.

13. Dogs and cats are large enough for high-resolution imaging studies and multiple sampling opportunities, as well as for surgical interventions.

14. The elucidation of the canine genome and its resemblance and relevance to the human genome open unique and unparalleled opportunities to study comparative oncology from a genetic perspective.[9]

Clients who seek treatment for their companion animals with cancer are a devoted and compassionate subset of the population. Working with these caregivers can be a very satisfying aspect of a frequently frustrating specialty. Clients are almost always satisfied with an honest and aggressive attempt to cure, control, or palliate the disease of their companion, making the experience satisfying for the veterinarian, for the client, and, most important, for the companion.

Oncology also offers the inquisitive veterinarian a complex and challenging area for both clinical and basic research. The challenges and accomplishments in oncology have been and continue to be very impressive. Oncology offers unlimited opportunity for the pursuit of knowledge for the benefit of animals and humankind. "Cancer, unlike politics and religion, is not a topic of controversy. No one is for it. Cancer is not another word for death. Neither is it a single disease for which there is one cure. Instead, it takes many forms, and each form responds differently to treatment".[10]

Clinical and comparative oncology continues to be a rapidly advancing field of study. More training programs are developed each year that allow a wider distribution of experienced veterinarians into practice, research, industry, government, and the academic setting. Through the continued investigation of tumor biology and treatment and the inclusion of veterinary species in well-designed, rigorous, and humane clinical trials, the veterinary profession will play a key role in advancing the diagnosis, treatment, and prevention of cancer for all species.

David M. Vail, Douglas H. Thamm, and Julius M. Liptak

References

1. American Pet Products Association 2011-2012 National Pet Owners Survey. http://www.americanpetproducts.org/press_industrytrends.asp. Accessed December 28, 2011.
2. Dorn CR: Epidemiology of canine and feline tumors, *Compend Contin Educ Pract Vet* 12:307–312, 1976.
3. Animal Health Survey: In *Companion animal news*, Englewood, CO, 1998, Morris Animal Foundation, 2005.
4. Bronson RT: Variation in age at death of dogs of different sexes and breeds, *Am J Vet Res* 43:2057–2059, 1982.
5. Gobar GM, Case JT, Kass PH: Program for surveillance of causes of death of dogs, using the Internet to survey small animal veterinarians, *J Am Vet Med Assoc* 213:251–256, 1998.
6. Hansen K, Khanna C: Spontaneous and genetically engineered animal models: use in preclinical cancer drug development, *Eur J Cancer* 40:858–880, 2004.
7. Mukherjee S: *The emperor of all maladies: a biography of cancer*, New York, 2010, Scribner.
8. LeBlanc AK, Breen M, Choyke P, et al.: Perspectives from man's best friend: National Academy of Medicine's Workshop on Comparative Oncology, *Sci Transl Med* 8:324ps5, 2016.
9. Linblad-Toh K, Wade CM, Mikkelsen TS, et al.: Genome sequence, comparative analysis and haplotype structure of the domestic dog, *Nature* 438:803–819, 2005.
10. Mooney S: *A snowflake in my hand*, New York, 1989, Dell Publishing, Bantam Doubleday.

1

The Etiology of Cancer

SECTION A: THE GENETIC BASIS OF CANCER

JAIME F. MODIANO AND JONG HYUK KIM

Cancer is a powerful and fearsome word describing a group of diseases that have recently surpassed cardiovascular disease as the most common cause of death for humans in 12 European countries[1] and in 22 states in the United States.[2] Cancer is also believed to be the most common cause of disease-related death in companion and working dogs in the developed world.[3–6] The fear of cancer, however, is rooted in misunderstanding, misconception, and mysticism. Thus the goals of this chapter are to clarify why cancer happens and highlight advances have been made that allow many human and animal cancer patients to lead full and productive lives after diagnosis.

The seminal work of Nowell and Hungerford in the early 1960s describing the nonrandom translocation between two chromosomes in chronic myelogenous leukemia represents the first time a genetic event (the translocation) could be linked to a specific cancer.[7,8] These observations can be considered the start of the modern era of cancer genetics, and they still pose one of the best arguments for why a strong foundation in contemporary genetics is necessary to understand the etiology of cancer. This chapter provides context for the genetic basis of cancer, updating recent data from domestic animals, especially dogs, that highlights how the judicious application of comparative oncology studies can improve our understanding of cancer risk, progression, and therapy.

Cancer Risk

Cancer is neither a single nor simple disease. Rather, the term *cancer* describes a large number of diseases for which the only common feature is uncontrolled cell growth and proliferation. These only critical requirement for the manifestation of cancer is multicellularity, and neoplastic diseases have been described in representative species from every group in the animal kingdom and also in plants.[9]

An important concept that is now universally accepted is that cancer is a genetic disease, although it is not always heritable. Tumors arise from the accumulation of mutations that eliminate normal constraints of proliferation and genetic integrity in a somatic cell, promoting immortalization and the capacity to modify and maintain a supportive niche for survival and expansion. Among other causes, mutations can arise after exposure to environmental mutagens, such as cigarette smoke and ultraviolet irradiation. Changes in the cancer incidence in humans over the course of the 20th century underscore the significant influence the environment can exert on the genetic makeup of individuals. Some environmental effects reflect behavior patterns (e.g., lung cancer in smokers), infectious diseases (e.g., stomach cancer in people infected with *Helicobacter pylori*), or exposure to cultural factors, such as urbanization or changes in diet (e.g., increasing breast cancer rates in the second and subsequent generations of Asian American women). Nevertheless, it would be incorrect to assume that the environment is wholly responsible for most tumors, especially because the increased risk of cancer upon exposure to potential environmental carcinogens is relatively small, except for tobacco products, ultraviolet or gamma irradiation, and a small group of chemical mutagens.

Another important intrinsic "mutagen" is the inherent error rate of enzymes that control DNA replication, which introduces 1 in 10 million to 1 in 1 million mutations for each base that is replicated during each round of cell division. Mammalian genomes comprise approximately 2 billion to 3 billion (10^9) base pairs; therefore every time a cell divides, each daughter cell is likely to carry a few hundred to a few thousand mutations in its DNA. Most mutations, whether caused by extrinsic or intrinsic factors, are silent and do not hinder the cell's ability to function; however, others can disable tumor suppressor genes or activate proto-oncogenes, which respectively inhibit or promote cell division and survival. Thus it can be said that simply being alive is the single largest risk factor for cancer.

The concept of intrinsic mutagenicity describes cancer risk as a function of the number of stem cell divisions required to maintain structure and function for a given tissue; it also suggests that more than two-thirds of human cancers originate from mutations caused by errors in DNA replication and are stochastic (random) in nature.[10–12] Furthermore, this concept suggests that more than half of the mutational load present in cancer cells occurs before tumors ever form. This is actually a "good news" scenario, in that it makes it possible to envision the development of strategies for early cancer detection using genomic tools.

Normal tissues and organs contain different numbers of stem cells that maintain homeostasis. These stem cells self-renew and live longer than other tissue resident cells, which are replaced to maintain normal organ structure and function. Recent studies by Tomasetti and Vogelstein identified a strong correlation (r = 0.81) between the total number of stem cell divisions and the lifetime risk of cancer arising from 31 distinct tissues (Fig. 1.1A).[11] In contrast, no significant correlations were seen between the risk for these cancers and heritable or environmental and geographic factors.[10]

The take-home message from this work is that DNA replication (R) represents a major risk factor for cancer, joining heritable risk (H) and environmental risk (E) as the major causes of mutations that can lead to cancer (see Fig. 1.1B). Heritable risk arises from mutations in the germline, such as those in the genes *BRCA1* and *BRCA2, TP53,* and *CDKN2A* that are associated, respectively, with breast cancer risk, with Li-Fraumeni syndrome and susceptibility to many cancers, and with susceptibility to melanoma and pancreatic carcinoma. Only one heritable cancer syndrome has been identified in domestic dogs. A germline mutation of the *BHD* gene encoding folliculin was identified in a family of German shepherd dogs that showed susceptibility to a syndrome of renal cystadenoma and nodular dermatobibrosis[13]; however, controlled breeding practices make it difficult for heritable cancers associated with single gene mutations to be perpetuated in domestic animals outside a laboratory environment.

In animals, and specifically in dogs, in which the lifetime risk of cancer seems to be approximately equivalent to that of humans, the apparent increased prevalence of certain tumor types in certain breeds (closed gene pools) suggests that incompletely penetrant, heritable factors might contribute to cancer causation. Indeed, even relatively minor traits that do not considerably alter the phenotypic appearance have been found to be associated with risk. Perhaps this is most easily appreciated in greyhounds; registered racing greyhounds are at higher risk of developing osteosarcoma (OSA) than American Kennel Club (AKC) "show" greyhounds.[14] This suggests that different components of risk could have become established in the founders of the racing and show greyhound lineages. In the racing greyhounds, however, part of the risk could be due to concussive forces during training and performance racing, which have the potential to create microfractures and activate chronic repair processes.

Environmental risk factors include chronic exposures to genotoxic agents, including habitual use of tobacco products; high-energy radiation from the sun or from occupational hazards, such as uranium mining; workplace chemicals, such as vinyl chloride; and agents that promote chronic inflammation and activate tissue repair processes unremittingly, such as asbestos. Tobacco use and sun exposure account for a large portion of human cancers worldwide. The risk of cancer from these exposures has been compounded in the past century by the increased longevity of human populations, which allows more time for mutations to accumulate.[10] In animals, strong associations have been established between exposure to ultraviolet radiation from the sun and some skin cancers in dogs, cats, cows, and horses; however, these account for a small proportion of cancer in these populations. Likewise, exposure to environmental tobacco smoke seems to increase the risk for a small proportion of cancers of dogs (nasal carcinoma) and cats (possibly lymphoma). The association between risk for cancer and exposure to other chemicals in dogs, cats, and other domestic animals is a topic of controversy; such exposure is likely to account for a small fraction of cancers seen in these species, although, as in humans,

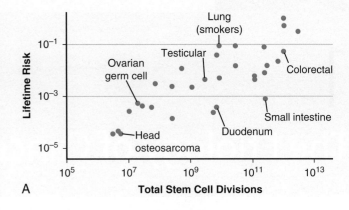

A

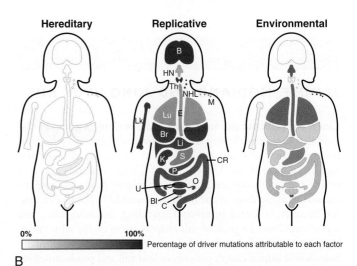

B

• **Fig. 1.1** (A) The relationship between the number of stem cell divisions in the lifetime of a given tissue and the lifetime risk of cancer in that tissue. (B) Etiology of driver gene mutations in women with cancer. For each of 18 representative cancer types, the schematic depicts the proportion of mutations that are inherited due to environmental factors or due to errors in DNA replication (i.e., not attributable either to heredity or to environment). The sum of these three proportions is 100%. The color codes for hereditary, replicative, and environmental factors are identical and span white (0%) to brightest red (100%). *B,* brain; *BI,* bladder; *Br,* breast; *C,* cervical; *CR,* colorectal; *E,* esophagus; *HN,* head and neck; *K,* kidney; *Li,* liver; *Lk,* leukemia; *Lu,* lung; *M,* melanoma; *NHL,* non–Hodgkin lymphoma; *O,* ovarian; *P,* pancreas; *S,* stomach; *Th,* thyroid; *U,* uterus. (Reproduced with permission. (A) From Couzin-Frankel J. Biomedicine: the bad luck of cancer. *Science.* 2015 Jan 2;347(6217):12. doi: 10.1126/science.347.6217.12.; Tomasetti C, Vogelstein B. Variation in cancer risk among tissues can be explained by the number of stem cell divisions. *Science.* 2015 Jan 2;347(6217):78-81. https://doi.org/10.1126/science.1260825. Fig. 1.1. (B) Illustration by Corinne Sandone © 2017 Johns Hopkins University. Used with permission.)

their effects might be compounded by the increased life span provided by modern veterinary care.

Replicative risk of cancer is ever present, and it increases inexorably with age. The stochastic nature of replicative risk is reflected in the molecular heterogeneity observed in histologically similar tumors, and the strong correlation between cancer and advanced age in dogs suggests that the replication-associated R factor likely is responsible for an even greater proportion of cancers in this species than it is in humans.

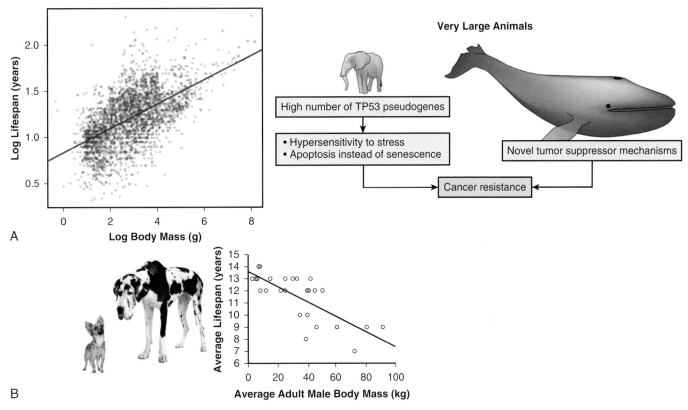

• **Fig. 1.2** Body size and life span. (A) Relationship between body mass (g) and life span (years) among 2556 vertebrates. In the left panel, the *blue line* shows the linear regression between log (body mass) and log (life span), R2 = 0.32. The right panel illustrates potential anticancer mechanisms in the largest mammals: elephants and whales. Elephants have evolved multiple copies of the *TP53* gene (pseudogenes) that are associated with an increased apoptotic response. Anticancer mechanisms in the largest mammals, whales, are not yet known, but they do not involve *TP53* duplications. (B) The relationship between body mass and life span across 32 different dog breeds. The diversity of size and life span among dog breeds is remarkable, but it is also well known that larger breeds tend to be short-lived relative to small breeds. (Reproduced with permission. (A) Redrawn from Sulak M, Fong L, Mika K, et al. *TP53* copy number expansion is associated with the evolution of increased body size and an enhanced DNA damage response in elephants. *eLife*. 2016 Sep 19;5:pii:e11994. https://doi.org/10.7554/eLife.11994. Fig. 1.1A. (B) Redrawn from Selman C, Nussey DH, Monaghan P. Ageing: it's a dog's life. *Curr Biol*. 2013 May 20;23(10):R451-R453. https://doi.org/10.1016/j.cub.2013.04.005. Fig. 1.1.) Photo of dogs © iStockphoto.com.

It should be noted that infectious agents can also be causally linked to cancer, by acting as direct mutagens or by increasing inflammation, replication, and repair, and consequently cancer risk.

Body Size and Cancer

The notion that mutations that accumulate stochastically during normal cell replication drive malignant transformation raises an important question: Why aren't bigger animals that have more cells more vulnerable to cancer? This question, originally posed by Sir Richard Peto,[15] is commonly referred to as Peto's paradox (at the species level, the incidence of cancer does not appear to correlate with the number of cells in an organism). The answer involves evolution and natural selection. Several cancer-protective mechanisms have been identified in mammals at the extremes of size. Elephants are the largest living land mammals; in the elephant lineage, cancer protection seems to be associated with enhanced activity of the *TP53* tumor suppressor gene, which underwent multiple duplication events after the split from a

common ancestor that gave rise to hyraxes and manatees but that preceded diversification into mastodons, mammoths, and modern elephants.[16,17] Whales include the largest living animals, and in the bowhead whale lineage, for example, variants or alterations of multiple genes seem to confer protection from cancer and aging.[18] However, in the common minke whale, an alternative adaptation has evolved that resulted in fewer microsatellites in genomic regions near proto-oncogenes and tumor suppressor genes, where cumulative mutations could lead to an increased cancer risk.[19] As these examples illustrate, adaptive solutions that enable large size and longevity likely are unique and specific to the evolutionary history of each species (Fig. 1.2A).

The norm for mammalian evolution is that large size is correlated with longevity. This is consistent with selective pressures that otherwise would disfavor the energy expenditure required to achieve large size. However, this trend is reversed in domestic dogs,[20] in which large body size is associated with shorter life spans and possibly with a higher rate of certain diseases, including cancer (see Fig. 1.2B). The precise reasons for this remain unclear, but dogs present a unique natural model to study associations between age, body mass, and disease risk under conditions in which artificial selection has superseded natural selection. Specifically, natural selective pressures in dogs were replaced by artificial selection since the initial domestication events approximately 10,000 to 25,000 years ago.[21] Changes in demand for form, instead of function, drove the creation of more than 400 breeds in the past 300 to 400 years. This artificial selection, usually for a single or a few phenotypic traits, gives little chance for adaptation across the rest of the genome. Consequently, the risks of mutation associated with normal processes of cell replication during development, growth, and maintenance into adulthood are enhanced in large dogs (more cells), making it possible to explain the disproportionate risk of certain cancers, such as appendicular OSA, by manipulation of their genomic plasticity with extreme selection for size. This is also consistent with the fact that the overall risk for axial OSA in dogs is similar to that observed in other species, accounting for the effects of size and functional/mechanical stresses on bone. The greater risk for large and giant dogs to develop appendicular OSA can be explained, at least in part, by the fact that more cell divisions are needed to create and maintain large bones, especially as bone tissues undergo continuous remodeling. Each round of replication for an osteoblast, in turn, contributes to its mutational burden and potential transformation. The late age of onset in dogs is consistent with chronic selection for cells that accumulate a critical complement of mutations. In humans, OSA is among the cancers in which the R factor can explain virtually all of the risk; also, an association has been recognized that shows OSA is more common in children in the higher percentiles of size for their age.[22–24]

Accounting for the risk of appendicular OSA (or other cancer types) stochastically as a function of replication risk leaves another important question unanswered: Why does the risk for some dog breeds seem to be higher (or lower) than expected based on their overall size? Partial answers to this question are available, and again, solid data is available for OSA. In terms of breed-specific risk, multiple heritable factors seem to influence the risk for OSA. Data from a genome-wide association study (GWAS) in three high-risk dog breeds indicates that the patterns of heritable risk for OSA are complex and incompletely penetrant.[14] However, selective breeding, especially for large size, seems to have enriched risk alleles that are now fixed in certain populations.[14,25,26] Fixed alleles associated with risk are not unique to OSA; they have also been associated with breed-specific risk for canine mammary cancer,[27] canine digital squamous cell carcinoma,[28] and other cancer types (discussed later in the chapter).

In humans a GWAS identified two loci associated with the presence of OSA[29] and a single, distinct locus in the *NFIB* gene associated with the presence of metastasis at diagnosis.[30] The risk alleles for humans and dogs are not located in orthologous regions of the genome. It appears, then, that achieving a large size relatively rapidly, and not breed-specific (or individual) traits in the germline, is the overwhelming contributor to OSA risk. It is thus reasonable to conclude that Peto's paradox arises as a result of barriers of natural selection, and that when such barriers are removed and the natural life span of an organism is extended, as is the case for dogs, the paradox disappears, revealing the overwhelming influence of DNA replication errors on individual cancer risk.

The examples provided underscore that cancer risk and progression have both shared and unique traits across species in the animal kingdom. This creates opportunities to study the natural history of cancer in a spontaneous setting. However, it is important to avoid the significant pitfalls that arise from assumptions of equivalence where none exists. The next section of this chapter reviews the hallmarks of cancer that are shared by virtually every cancer from every species. The final section of the chapter focuses on recent studies that elevate companion dogs as models for understanding the complex genetics of cancer through the use of contemporary technology and cautious, deliberate interpretation of data.

The Hallmarks of Cancer

Forty years of research culminated in an insightful and a thorough review paper by Douglas Hanahan and Robert Weinberg in 2011 that synthesized knowledge about cancer into 10 essential, acquired characteristics.[31]

In 2000 the same authors had described six characteristics necessary for cellular transformation, which comprised the abilities to (1) sustain proliferative signaling, (2) evade growth suppressors, (3) resist cell death, (4) enable replicative immortality, (5) induce angiogenesis, and (6) activate invasion and metastasis.[32] In this initial paper describing the hallmarks of cancer, Hanahan and Weinberg created a paradigm shift by providing the first ever comprehensive synthesis of the molecular events leading to cancer. The important concepts that were clarified included these: no single gene is universally responsible for transformation; five or six critical (driver) mutations are the minimum theoretical number required to endow the cancer phenotype (an observation that has since been confirmed experimentally)[33]; each step in the path toward transformation and cancer progression is regulated by multiple interactive biochemical pathways,[34] and thus, mutations of different genes along a pathway can result in equivalent phenotypes and, conversely, mutations of the same gene can result in different cancers with distinct biology; tumors behave as tissues; and the interactions between the tumor and its microenvironment are major drivers of cancer behavior.

The updated hallmarks of cancer added two "enabling" characteristics, (7) genome instability and mutation and (8) tumor-promoting inflammation, and two "emerging" hallmarks, (9) deregulating cellular energetics and (10) avoiding immune destruction.

The effect of this unifying conceptualization of cancer genetics and this level of understanding are clearly evident when one considers how they have influenced the design, development, implementation, and success of new cancer therapies (Fig. 1.3). A summary of the information with added refinements is provided later in the chapter.

Sustaining Proliferative Signaling

Arguably the most important event in neoplastic transformation is the capability of cells to proliferate in perpetuity. Under normal conditions, cells communicate with each other and integrate environmental signals by sensing cues and gradients. For example, migration, metabolism, and proliferation of mature hematopoietic cells are regulated in autocrine and paracrine fashions by locally secreted cytokines. The same cytokines may act systemically in an endocrine fashion. With the notable exception of steroid hormones that bind to intracellular receptors, growth-promoting cytokines work by binding transmembrane receptors, which in turn initiate signaling cascades that culminate in transcriptional changes. These transcriptional responses, in turn, allow cells to adapt their behavior to match

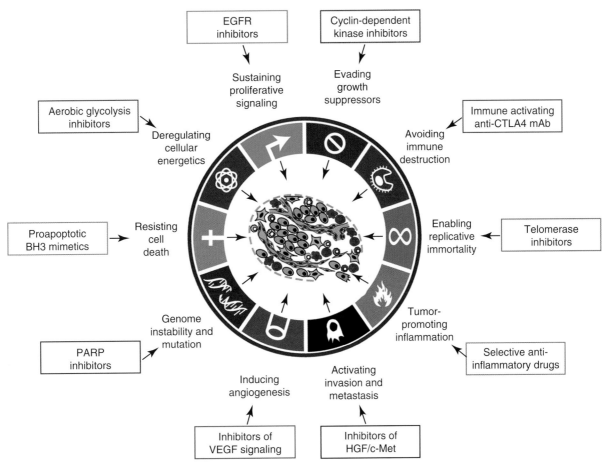

• **Fig. 1.3** Therapeutic targeting of the hallmarks of cancer. Drugs that interfere with each of the acquired capabilities necessary for tumor growth and progression have been developed and are in clinical trials, or in some cases have been approved for clinical use in treating certain forms of human cancer. Additionally, the investigational drugs are being developed to target each of the enabling characteristics and emerging hallmarks, which also hold promise as cancer therapeutics. The drugs listed are examples; a deep pipeline of candidate drugs with different molecular targets and modes of action is in development for most of these hallmarks. (Reproduced with permission from Hanahan D, Weinberg RA. Hallmarks of cancer: the next generation. *Cell.* 2011 Mar 4;144(5):646-674. https://doi.org/10.1016/j.cell.2011.02.013. Fig. 1.6.)

the environmental signals. The activity of cytokines, their receptors, and the corresponding signaling molecules are finely tuned. The system can be shut down when the concentration of the cytokine falls below a threshold that can stably bind the receptor, when the receptor ceases to be expressed, or when signaling molecules are downregulated or otherwise inactivated; however, mutations in even one of the molecules involved in regulating these pathways can provide sustained growth signals in the absence of the initiating cytokine. Among many examples is a translocation between chromosome 2 and chromosome 5 (t(2;5)) that is present in almost half of human anaplastic lymphomas. The translocation creates a fusion protein between the nucleophosmin gene *(NPM1)* and the anaplastic lymphoma kinase gene *(ALK);* this aberrantly activates the Jak2/STAT5 signaling pathway,[35] which normally is responsive to various interleukins (IL), including IL-2, IL-3, and IL-6. The genes that encode the normal growth-promoting proteins (e.g., ALK, Jak2, and STAT5) are called *proto-oncogenes;* the mutated versions that allow cells to gain self-sufficiency from the environmental signals are called *oncogenes.* It is important to note that not all growth-promoting genes have the capacity

to become oncogenes and that the outcomes of oncogenic activation are most commonly senescence or apoptosis, unless additional events promote stable transformation and survival.

Evading Growth Suppressors

In addition to the hallmark capability of inducing and sustaining positively acting growth-stimulatory signals, cancer cells must also circumvent powerful programs that negatively regulate cell proliferation; many of these programs depend on the actions of tumor suppressor genes. To maintain homeostasis, cells also must integrate antigrowth signals from the environment. Quiescence in nonhematopoietic cells is enforced by signals delivered by contact inhibition.[36] Hematopoietic cells, on the other hand, use cell-cell contacts to maintain interactions within the niche and to regulate the timing and intensity of hematopoiesis, inflammation, and immunity.[37]

"Stop" signals usually are delivered and integrated by the products of tumor suppressor genes, which derive their name largely from the observation that their inactivation facilitates tumor formation. Tumor suppressor genes balance the activity of growth-promoting proto-oncogenes and tend to act in tandem with these in most biochemical pathways. Loss of function of one or more tumor suppressor genes occurs in virtually every cancer; inactivation of *TP53, RB1, PTEN,* or *CDKN2A* is seen in more than 50% of all tumors. Inactivation of these pathways seems to contribute to the pathogenesis of companion animal tumors, and their dysfunction also may be predictive for outcomes in some of them (see for example refs.[38–42]).

Resisting Cell Death

Apoptosis, or programmed cell death, is the imprinted outcome for every cell in multicellular organisms. Survival requires support from extrinsic (environmental) factors, in addition to a precise balance of cellular energetics and metabolism. Bone marrow–derived cells (BMDCs) normally undergo apoptosis when concentrations of survival factors (e.g., stem cell factor, IL-3, IL-7) or nutrients are limiting or when cellular bioenergetics is severely disrupted.[43]

Evasion of apoptosis is an essential acquired feature of all cancers, and it can result from loss of proapoptotic tumor suppressor genes, such as *TP53* or *PTEN,* or by gain of function of antiapoptotic genes, such as *BCL2.* Gain of function of *BCL2* in humans generally is associated with indolent, follicular lymphomas that carry t(14:18) translocations that juxtapose *BCL2* and the immunoglobulin heavy enhancer locus *(IGH).* These tumors rarely are seen in domestic animals, but evasion of apoptosis may be an important mechanism in the pathogenesis of other indolent tumors seen more commonly in these species.

A more recent concept in the cell death field is autophagy—a process that tumor cells have efficiently co-opted as a means to survive under adverse conditions.[44] As part of the autophagy program, intracellular vesicles called *autophagosomes* surround intracellular organelles and fuse with lysosomes. There, the organelles are broken down and then channeled to form new molecules that support the energy-producing machinery of the cell, allowing it to survive in the stressed, nutrient-limited environment that defines most cancers.

Tumor cells also must avoid death by anoikis, or loss of integral cell-to-cell or cell-to-matrix contacts.[36] Absent these physiologic death pathways, the body often reacts to the anatomic and physiologic disruptions caused by cancer cells by targeting these cells for destruction through inflammatory pathways, leading to necrosis. The process of necrosis might also be regulated genetically, providing another mechanism that favors survival of the whole (organism or tumor) over survival of the one. New findings that lend further nuance to the perception of how evasion (or incitation) of these cell death mechanisms contributes to neoplastic transformation and tumor progression continue to be published almost daily, and readers are encouraged not to limit their investigation to this summary, but rather to seek recent updates to the literature in this field.

Enabling Replicative Immortality

Immortalization is another essential feature of cancer. The genetic program limits the number of times a cell is able to replicate (the so-called Hayflick limit), and when this limit is reached, replicative senescence is induced. Induction of replicative senescence does not induce death; cells maintain energetic homeostasis and remain functional, but they undergo significant genetic changes characterized by telomere erosion. Cells that are able to replicate must maintain the integrity of telomeres, which are "caps" made

of repetitive DNA sequence that protect chromosomes from destruction. Solid tumors acquire immortalization predominantly by activation of the telomerase enzyme system and the consequent maintenance of telomere integrity. In hematopoietic cells, telomerase activity seems to be retained longer than in other somatic cells, so this may facilitate immortalization in lymphoma and leukemia.[45] The role of immortalization and the importance of telomerase (both to maintain telomere length and to maintain other biochemical functions that are essential for cell survival) are well established; however, the role of replicative senescence has been questioned recently because improved technology has allowed researchers to circumvent this process in normal cells.[31] Mouse models complicate the story because of significant differences in telomere length between rodents and humans; therefore this is an area in which other models, such as companion animals, might provide clarity in the future.[46]

Inducing Angiogenesis

Folkman proposed a role for angiogenesis in cancer more than 30 years ago,[47,48] but this idea took time to gain traction in the scientific community. It is now apparent that angiogenesis not only is an important pathogenetic mechanism during tumor progression, but also a potential target for therapeutic intervention.

Angiogenesis is a complex, tightly regulated process that requires the coordinated action of a variety of growth factors and cell adhesion molecules in endothelial and stromal cells. So far, vascular endothelial growth factor (VEGF-A) and its receptors comprise the best-characterized signaling pathway in tumor angiogenesis.[49] VEGF binds several receptor tyrosine kinases, including VEGF receptor-1 (VEGFR-1 [also known as Flt-1]) and VEGFR-2 (KDR or Flk-1). Genetic polymorphisms of *VEGF* or of *FLT1* or *KDR* genes are associated with increased angiogenesis, and mutations of *KDR* are reported in human vascular tumors.[50,51] VEGF expression also is upregulated by hypoxia and inflammation. The transcription factor hypoxia-inducible factor-1α (HIF), which is part of a pathway that also includes regulation by the von Hippel-Lindau (VHL) tumor suppressor gene, is a major regulator of VEGF expression. Under conditions of normal oxygen tension, the VHL protein targets HIF for degradation; under low oxygen conditions, HIF increases as VHL-mediated degradation is reduced, allowing for upregulation of VEGF.

Other signaling molecules also contribute to angiogenesis, including platelet-derived growth factor-β (PDGF-β) and its receptor (PDGFR), and the angiopoietins Ang-1 and Ang-2 and their receptors Tie-1 and Tie-2. PDGF-β is required for recruitment of pericytes and maturation of new capillaries. Recent studies also document the importance of tumor-derived PDGF in the recruitment of stroma that produces VEGF and other angiogenic factors.

Tumors use multiple mechanisms to resist antiangiogenic therapy. For example, tumor cells cooperate with niche cells, such as endothelial cells, BMDCs, cancer-associated fibroblasts (CAFs), and pericytes, to create a microenvironment that abolishes the therapeutic benefits of VEGF blockade.[52] But overall, it is apparent that antiangiogenic therapies can benefit cancer patients by promoting vascular normalization, at least partially restoring the balance among blood vessel–forming and stromal cells, including pericytes, myeloid-derived cells, endothelial progenitors, and fibroblasts. This, in turn, can reverse the anatomic and hemodynamic dysfunction created by the tumor microenvironment, disabling some of the intrinsic advantages this dysfunction provides for cancer cells and allowing better penetration of drugs. (Chapter 15, Section C, provides additional information about antiangiogenic therapies.)

Angiogenesis takes center stage in malignant vascular tumors such as hemangiosarcoma (HSA), which occurs commonly in dogs.[53] Malformed, disorganized vascular structures composed of a mixture of malignant and nonmalignant cells are the defining feature of canine HSA and human angiosarcomas. Among other proangiogenic drivers, canine HSAs show elevated production of VEGF,[54–56] IL-8,[57] and sphingosine-1 phosphate (S1P) and its receptor, S1P1[58]. Furthermore, the magnitude of the angiogenic drive is associated with somatic mutations of angiopoietin, VEGF, and PI3K signaling pathways, in addition to the biologic behavior of the tumors.[42,59] This data suggests that canine HSA may provide a powerful, spontaneous model for unraveling critical events that control tumor angiogenesis.

Activating Invasion and Metastasis

The role of genetic events in invasion and metastasis is still incompletely understood. The classic model of metastasis proposed by Fidler suggests a stepwise acquisition of assets that enables cells to leave the primary tumor site, travel through the blood or lymph, invade stroma in favorable locations, and thus become reestablished at distant sites.[60] Other research suggests that most tumors have the ability to dislodge cells that travel to distant sites, and the ability of such cells to survive in capillary beds may be the most important step in the metastatic process.[61–65] A systematic assessment of metastasis reveals that it is a complicated process partly controlled by tumor heterogeneity and in which genetically distinct cells contribute to the dissemination of tumor cells from primary sites to metastatic sites (Fig. 1.4).[66]

BMDCs have intrinsic properties that allow them to travel throughout the body, traffic through all major organs, and home to areas of inflammation. Thus bone marrow–derived tumors are inherently metastatic. Nevertheless, hematopoietic tumors that are cytologically indistinguishable can have distinct and preferential tissue distribution. The events that make leukemic cells stay in the peripheral circulation are not yet fully understood, even though cells from corresponding lymphomas or myeloid sarcomas, with virtually identical molecular signatures, stay confined to lymphoid or visceral organs.

In epithelial neoplasms that account for most tumors in humans, the epithelial-to-mesenchymal transition (EMT) has received increasing attention for its role in metastasis. It remains unclear whether EMT is equally important in the sarcomas more commonly seen in domestic animals, in which the cells of origin seem to retain EMT capabilities to a greater extent. Increasing evidence indicates that interactions between cancer cells, including both the "initiating" population in the tumor (colloquially referred to as cancer stem cells, or CSCs), and the remainder (bulk) of tumor cells and other cells in the tumor microenvironment, including mesenchymal stem cells (MSCs), CAFs, inflammatory cells, and angiogenic cells, may be responsible for cancers' invasive behaviors and for their ability to survive in hostile environments at distant (metastatic) sites. One example is signaling through the CXCR4-CXCL12 axis, which contributes to the metastatic process through interactions between tumor cells and the tumor-permissive niche.[67] CXCR4 is upregulated recurrently in canine HSA and OSA,[68–70] where it is presumed to promote invasion and migration upon binding CXCL12.

Thus dogs with HSA and OSA provide an opportunity to test therapeutic inhibition of the CXCR4-CXCL12 axis as a means to delay or prevent metastasis. (Chapter 2 presents additional information about basic mechanisms and treatments to manage cancer metastasis.)

Genomic Instability and Mutation

The concept of genomic instability is not new, but it was incorporated as an "enabling hallmark" into the updated Hanahan and Weinberg model.[31] Traditionally, stepwise clonal evolution provided a satisfactory explanation of tumor progression because it could be correlated with discrete pathologic changes. This is especially true for epithelial tumors, in which such progression can be appreciated in lesions that go through stages of hyperplasia, atypical hyperplasia (dysplasia), adenoma, carcinoma in situ, invasive carcinoma, and metastatic carcinoma. However, analysis of tumor genomes, even in early stages, usually shows aneuploidy (an abnormal DNA copy number), in addition to chaotic changes indicative of multiple numeric and structural DNA abnormalities. Similar abnormalities, first noticed by Boveri more than 100 years ago in studies of sea urchin cells, led him to formulate the "aneuploidy theory" of cancer.[71] Aneuploidy now is known to be especially evident in solid tumors; based on this, Loeb proposed the existence of the "mutator phenotype," in which cells are predisposed to undergo multiple mutations, some of which inevitably lead to cancer.[72] Some tenets of his hypothesis appear to be correct, although perhaps through different mechanisms than those envisioned by Loeb, as they might relate to increased activity of polymerases with low fidelity under conditions in which the rate of DNA damage (and consequently mutations) is higher than the expected background from normal DNA replication (e.g., in lung epithelial cells from heavy smokers). However, direct measurements of mutation rates of sporadic tumors are much lower than those predicted if a "mutator phenotype" was operative in these tumors.[73] Indeed, the minimum number of "critical" or driver mutations required for the clinical onset of cancer in solid tumors, based on sequencing of solid tumor genomes, probably is on the order of 15 to 25.[74] However, this may apply mainly to tumors with chaotic karyotypes, because the number of mutations identified in a cytogenetically stable leukemia was significantly smaller.[33]

Still, genetic instability is a hallmark of most tumors, and although it can be partly explained by increased errors in DNA replication and chromosomal segregation in cells that are rapidly dividing, other mechanisms are clearly operative, involving telomeres and telomerase.[73,75–79] Although many of these changes are not "recurrent" and appear to be random products of instability, some may in fact contribute to a proliferative crisis.[80] This is consistent with Tomasetti and Vogelstein's observation that initiation events for many tumors occur early in life, during highly proliferative stages of tissue growth and remodeling, but they become evident later in life when one or a few critical mutations allow the transformed cell to reach this crisis stage.

Tumor-Promoting Inflammation

The role of inflammation in cancer has received considerable attention in the past 20 years. Although our understanding of this phenomenon remains incomplete, it clearly met the criteria for inclusion as an "enabling hallmark" in the updated Hanahan and Weinberg model.[31] The importance of inflammation was

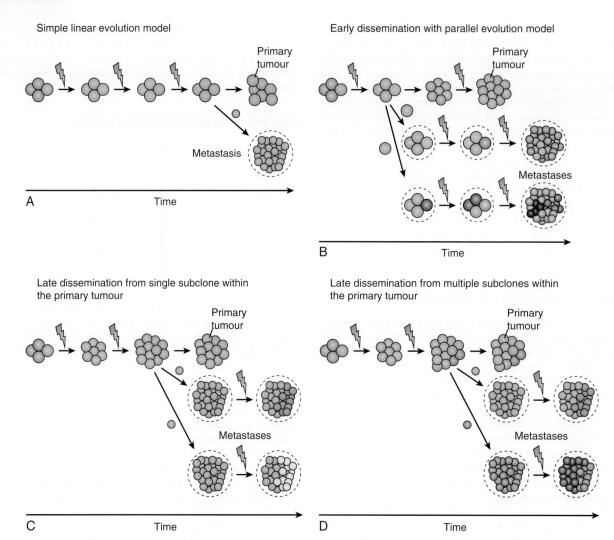

• **Fig. 1.4** Models of metastasis evolution and implications of genetic heterogeneity. (A) The classic simple linear model, in which clones sequentially arise that dominate the primary tumor owing to survival and proliferative advantages. (B) The early dissemination and parallel evolution model, in which tumor cells begin to disseminate early in the primary tumor life span and continue to evolve somatically in parallel with the primary tumor during clinical dormancy until they acquire metastatic capacity and proliferate into a clinically relevant lesion. (C) The late dissemination model, in which tumors evolve over time until a late-arising subclone is able to seed multiple metastases successfully. (D) Late dissemination from multiple metastatically competent subclones within the primary tumor. Metastases seeded by this mechanism share all the somatic events acquired by the tumor preceding the divergence of the different metastatically competent primary tumor subclones. The blizzard symbol indicates somatic genetic alterations. (Reproduced with permission from Hunter KW, Amin R, Deasy S, et al. Genetic insights into the morass of metastatic heterogeneity. *Nat Rev Cancer*. 2018 April;18(4):211-223. https://doi.org/10.1038/nrc.2017.126. Fig. 1.1.)

inferred from the earliest microscopic studies of cancer, but it was a seminal paper by Dvorak in 1986, in which he described tumors as "wounds that never heal,"[81] that provided synthesis for the recurrent observation that tumors often were infiltrated by inflammatory cells of the innate immune system (granulocytes, histiocytes, and macrophages) and the adaptive immune system (lymphocytes). Mechanistic distinctions between inflammation that favors tumor growth and inflammation that retards growth or eliminates the tumor remain to be defined[82–84]; however, it can be concluded confidently that inflammation contributes to tumor growth and survival by supplying factors that sustain proliferation; factors that limit cell death; proangiogenic factors; extracellular matrix-modifying enzymes that facilitate angiogenesis, invasion,

and metastasis; and other signals that lead to activation of EMT and other hallmark-facilitating programs.[31] Inflammatory cells also release reactive oxygen species that are actively mutagenic for nearby cancer cells, accelerating their genetic evolution toward states of heightened malignancy.[85]

Deregulating Cellular Energetics

In the early years of the 20th century, Otto Warburg observed that cancer cells preferentially used glycolytic (anaerobic) rather than oxidative (aerobic) pathways to generate, energy even under conditions of normal or high oxygen. This metabolic peculiarity of cancer cells, called the *Warburg effect*, seems to be driven by activated oncogenes and/or by loss of tumor suppressor genes, providing cancer cells with selective growth and survival advantages by conferring the hallmark capabilities of cell proliferation, avoidance of cytostatic controls, and attenuation of apoptosis. The reliance of cancer cells on glycolysis can be further accentuated under hypoxic conditions. In fact, Warburg-like metabolism seems to be present in rapidly dividing embryonic tissues, suggesting a role in supporting large-scale biosynthetic programs that are required for active cell proliferation.

Cancer cells do not seem to enable the Warburg effect universally. Rather, much like other cells with high energetic demands, they seem to sort out into lactate-secreting (Warburg) and lactate-consuming cells, providing an efficient, albeit homeostatically disturbed, energy environment. Furthermore, it seems that oxygenation is not static in tumors, but instead fluctuates temporally and regionally as a result of the instability and chaotic organization of tumor-associated neovasculature. Altered energy metabolism is proving to be as widespread in cancer cells as in many of the other cancer-associated traits that have been accepted as hallmarks of cancer. This realization raises the question of whether deregulating cellular energy metabolism is a core hallmark capability of cancer cells that is as fundamental as the six well-established core hallmarks. In fact, the redirection of energy metabolism is largely orchestrated by proteins that are involved in one way or another in programming the core hallmarks of cancer. When viewed in this way, aerobic glycolysis is simply another phenotype that is programmed by proliferation-inducing oncogenes, and the designation of reprogrammed energy metabolism as an emerging hallmark seems most appropriate.

It is worth noting that this characteristic of tumor cells provides at least one important diagnostic advantage. Upregulation of the major glucose transporter, GLUT-1, is seen in virtually all tumors, making the cells efficient glucose scavengers. This can be exploited to image tumor cells precisely and noninvasively by visualizing glucose uptake using positron emission tomography (PET) with a radiolabeled analog of glucose (^{18}F-fluorodeoxyglucose, or ^{18}F-FDG) as a reporter. The combination of PET with computed tomography (PET-CT) now is one of the most robust means to evaluate composition of tumors, minimal residual disease, and tumor-specific objective responses in patients receiving conventional and experimental therapies, and it increasingly is being applied to improve the diagnosis and staging of dogs with cancer.[86–88]

In addition, evidence is accumulating that deregulated cellular energetics contribute to tumor progression through immunomodulation. Our group has proposed a model in which cancer cells' self-renewal is causally related to reprogramming of fatty acid metabolism and immune signaling[89]; this supports the notion that fate decisions of tumor-initiating or stem cells rely on cellular metabolism and immunomodulation in the tumor microenvironment.

Avoiding Immune Destruction

Burnet and Thomas proposed the concept that the immune system can recognize and destroy incipient tumors (cancer immunosurveillance) in the 1950s.[90] Their hypothesis was far ahead of its time, and technologic obstacles impeded proof, so the theory fell into disfavor. In recent years the immunosurveillance theory has gained traction anew because data strongly suggest that the immune system helps to keep tumors at bay, and thus tumors must evade the immune response to survive. In its recent incarnation, the theory has been refined to incorporate the concept of

immunoediting, in which the immune system destroys strongly antigenic tumor cells, providing weakly antigenic cells a survival advantage.[90] Experimental evidence for this concept includes differences between tumors grown in immunocompetent mice (only weakly antigenic tumors survive) and immunocompromised mice (no selection against strongly antigenic tumors is observed), but evidence only now is emerging that will allow us to understand the importance of immunoediting in spontaneous cancers.

That the tumor microenvironment forms and maintains an immunosuppressive barrier provides more compelling evidence for the role of the immune system in limiting tumor growth and metastasis.[91,92] This immunosuppressive barrier includes cellular factors, such as regulatory T cells (T_{regs}), myeloid-derived suppressor cells (MDSCs), and MSCs. Soluble factors, including transforming growth factor-β (TGF-β) and immunoglobulins, also contribute to the immunosuppressive barrier directly and indirectly.[93] This is an active area of basic and clinical research in which companion animal oncology has been at the forefront; for example, through the generation and approval of the first active gene-based therapeutic cancer vaccine for canine melanoma.[94]

A transformational advance in cancer therapy has been the ability to block immune checkpoints that are engaged by a number of tumors—particularly those that have unstable genomes and tend to generate greater numbers of neoantigens (Fig. 1.5).[95,96] Antibodies against cytotoxic T lymphocyte-associated protein 4 (CTLA-4), and against programmed cell death protein 1 (PD-1) and its corresponding ligand, programmed death-ligand 1 (PD-L1), aim to reactivate tumor-specific T cells and cause a robust antitumor immune response.[97,98] The remarkable responses observed in patients receiving immune checkpoint blockade as adjunctive or first-line therapy have made this class of compounds part of the standard of care for several types of lung cancer, malignant melanoma, renal cell carcinoma, Hodgkin lymphoma, head and neck squamous cell carcinoma, urothelial carcinoma, certain colon cancers, and certain liver cancers.

Checkpoint inhibitors currently are being tested in canine clinical trials[99]; expression of canine PD-L1 has been detected in a number of canine tumor types, including mastocytoma, melanoma, renal cell carcinoma, and several others.[100] Canine CTLA-4 has been identified and cloned,[101] and although canine anti–CTLA-4 has not yet been developed, an agonistic recombinant canine CTLA-4 molecule has been successfully used to induce tolerance in a transplant model.[102] (Chapter 14 presents additional information about cancer immunotherapy.)

Adaptive Evolution and the Tumor Microenvironment

A bidirectional flow of information occurs between the tumor and the microenvironment, with each helping to mold the other into functional growing tissue that can evade or withstand attack by the host.[103] The previous reference to a "selective growth advantage" that is reminiscent of darwinian selection is not accidental. The clonal evolution theory[104] addresses the significance of sequential genetic changes providing growth and survival advantages; however, to this must be added the fact that, in addition to these self-sufficient events that influence growth and survival, tumor cells must also evade "predators" (e.g., inflammation and the immune system).[90,105] In essence, the interaction of the tumor

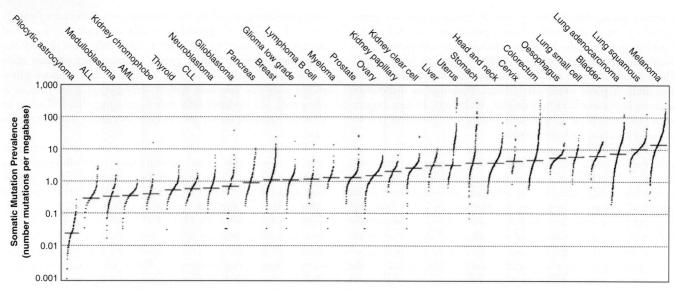

• **Fig. 1.5** The prevalence of somatic mutations across human cancer types. Every dot represents a sample, and the red horizontal lines are the median numbers of mutations in the respective cancer types. The vertical axis (log scaled) shows the number of mutations per megabase; the different cancer types are ordered on the horizontal axis based on their median numbers of somatic mutations. *ALL,* Acute lymphoblastic leukemia; *AML,* acute myeloid leukemia; *CLL,* chronic lymphocytic leukemia. (Reproduced with permission from Alexandrov LB, Nik-Zainal S, Wedge DC, et al. Signatures of mutational processes in human cancer. *Nature.* 2013 Aug 22;500(7463):415-421. https://doi.org/10.1038/nature12477. Fig. 1.1.)

with its microenvironment and ultimately with the host is in fact subject to darwinian laws of evolution, albeit in an accelerated time scale.[75] This is evident in the ability of tumors to modulate stromal cells to support their own growth by providing a suitable matrix and an abundance of nutrients while keeping antitumor responses at bay.

As is true for other selective environments, tumors that outgrow the capability of their immediate surroundings to support their growth must alter that environment to suit their needs or identify other favorable locations where they can become established. The tumor microenvironment recently was shown to exert a significant effect on the complement of genes expressed by incipient tumor cells.[106] Incipient sarcoma cells, in turn, can reside as quiescent inhabitants of distant microenvironments, themselves modulating growth, morphology, and behavior of microenvironment constituents in the process of metastatic dissemination.[53,57]

Epigenetic Events

Events leading to cancer need not necessarily be caused by mutational events, but instead can be caused by epigenetic changes, which can alter the phenotype without changing the genotype. Two well-characterized epigenetic mechanisms regulate gene expression; methylation of 5'—C—phosphate—G—3' (CpG) residues in promoter regions and histone deacetylation both result in gene silencing by interfering with the transcriptional machinery. The effects of global changes in methylation or deacetylation (e.g., by inactivation of DNA methylases or histone deacetylases) remain incompletely understood, but silencing of specific genes by methylation is implicated in numerous cancers of humans and animals.[107–110] One important observation is that most (or all) genes subject to silencing by methylation in specific cancers are inactivated by mutation or deletion in other cancers, and it is apparent that developmental programs that control chromatin

structure play a role in defining susceptibility to mutations[111] and thus presumably cancer risk. This area of research is likely to create the next giant leap in our understanding of cancer etiology.

As is true for mutations, gene regulation by epigenetic methylation can occur sporadically or it can be heritable. Silencing of some tumor suppressor genes in sporadic cancers occurs more frequently by epigenetic methylation than by mutation or deletion. These different mechanisms of gene silencing are not equivalent, because they each result in specific tumor phenotypes. For example, data from our laboratories indicates that loss of canine chromosome 11, with resultant deletion of the *INK4* tumor suppressor locus containing the *CDKN2A, CDKN2B,* and *ARF* genes, and methylation of *CDKN2A* are each associated with morphologically distinct types of T-cell lymphoma that have a different clinical presentation and prognosis.[39,40]

Genomic imprinting presents a unique example in which heritable epigenetic changes influence cancer predisposition. Genomic imprinting refers to a pattern of gene expression that is determined by the parental origin of the gene; in other words, unlike most genes in which both parental alleles are expressed, only one allele (specifically derived from the mother or from the father, depending on the gene) of an imprinted gene is expressed and the other one is permanently repressed. Epigenetic changes in Wilms tumor and in heritable colon cancer (among others) alter the expression of the imprinted allele, leading to loss of imprinting that causes overexpression of the insulin growth factor-2 *(IGF2)* gene.[107,112]

Cancer Stem Cells

The paradoxical nature of some cancers gave rise to the notion of a "cancer progenitor" or a CSC, as far back as the 1960s. The best illustration of this concept is chronic myelogenous leukemia (CML), in which the bulk of the tumor consists of terminally differentiated neutrophils incapable of recreating the malignancy.

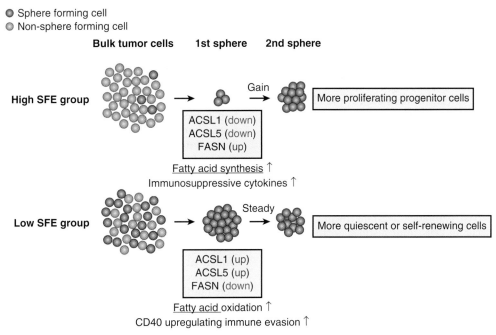

○ Sphere forming cell
○ Non-sphere forming cell

• **Fig. 1.6** A proposed model of cancer cells showing their distinct capacity to form and maintain spheres. (Reproduced with permission from Kim JH, Frantz AM, Sarver AL, et al. Modulation of fatty acid metabolism and immune suppression are features of in vitro tumor sphere formation in ontogenetically distinct dog cancers. *SFE*, sphere-forming efficiency. *Vet Comp Oncol*. 2018 March;16(1):E176-E184. https://doi.org/10.1111/vco.12368. Fig. 1.5.)

However, it was apparent that multipotent stem cells were present in this tumor population. In 1994 Dick's group proved conclusively that another type of leukemia, acute myelogenous leukemia (AML), was a hierarchically organized disease in which a small number of cells undetectable by conventional methods could be isolated from patients and made to recapitulate the full spectrum of the disease in an animal model.[113] This gave rise to the CSC, or "tumor-initiating cell," hypothesis, which is based on the concept that tumors are hierarchically organized into a subpopulation of cells that retain or acquire the capacity for self-renewal and are capable and responsible for initiating and maintaining the tumor.[114] Another subpopulation of cells that consists of the CSC progeny undergo partial to complete differentiation and lose the capability to support the tumor, albeit still contributing to the morbidity of cancer. This hypothesis fundamentally altered the way cancer is understood, but it also gave rise to a debate about how widely this model applies. In the competing hypothesis, commonly referred to as the stochastic model, all the cells in a tumor have an equal capacity for self-renewal. According to this model, the process of cancer is driven entirely (or almost entirely) by environmental selection of favorable mutations; this model necessarily would predict that cancer is an inevitable outcome for multicellular organisms, and few, if any, long-lived animals would reach reproductive age.[115] Thus, by necessity, this model must invoke the existence of protective mechanisms independent of the cancer risk (e.g., efficient DNA repair mechanisms and immune surveillance).

The two models may represent a continuum dependent on the extent to which CSCs undergo asymmetric versus symmetric divisions. Under conditions in which CSC divisions are primarily asymmetric, few CSCs would be apparent and the population would achieve a hierarchical organization; under conditions in which CSCs underwent symmetric divisions, virtually every cell in the tumor would have CSC-like properties and the organization

would be more consistent with a stochastic model. The prevailing opinion is that CSCs exist and are characterized both by peculiar phenotypes and defined sets of mutations of a small number of genes.[116–118] Other mutations then endow their progeny with a limited or an extensive capacity to undergo programmed differentiation, thus resulting in the distinct clinical phenotypes that characterize acute and chronic leukemias or high-grade and low-grade solid tumors.

In companion animals, progenitor cells with putative CSC or tumor-propagating properties have been identified in HSA, OSA, brain tumors, and possibly lymphoma.[119–122] These cells appear to rely on metabolic and immune reprogramming to regulate their self-renewal and differentiation programs (Fig. 1.6).[89]

As is true for the rest of cancer genetics, information in this field is rapidly evolving. Large-scale bioinformatics and conceptual advances are integrating the CSC theory into the mainstream of cancer research and biology, and also into the design for new diagnostic and therapeutic strategies. For example, it appears that much like hematopoietic stem cells, the CSC niche favors oligoclonality and some genetic diversity. Thus clonal competition can ensue, giving rise to heterogeneous tumors and maintaining a reservoir of cells that can reestablish the tumor when a therapy effectively kills the predominant CSC clone and its progeny. Similarly, clonal competition can facilitate distant spread by selection of cells with different capabilities. An extreme example may be the potential for a single tumor cell (or a small population of oligoclonal cells in a tumor) to give rise to histologically distinct tumors—an event that has been observed in xenotransplanted sarcomas.

Recent Advances in Canine Cancer Genetics

An important conceptual advance in canine cancer genetics was the identification of conserved (homologous) aberrations in spontaneous dog tumors that had been previously characterized in human tumors. The prototypical example was a structural aberration resulting from a balanced chromosomal translocation that creates a fusion gene composed of most of the *BCR* gene (located on chromosome 22 in humans and on chromosome 26 in dogs) and a truncated form of the *ABL* gene (coincidentally located on chromosome 9 in both humans and dogs) in CML.[123] Both translocations give rise to a derivative chromosome, the Philadelphia (Ph) chromosome in humans and the "Raleigh" chromosome in dogs. Certain numeric aberrations (changes in DNA copy number) are similarly conserved in both species in a variety of cancers, including lymphoma, soft tissue sarcomas, OSA, and brain tumors.[124–129]

The development of specific tumors from cells harboring such shared mutations is not surprising, but why would homologous, highly conserved pathologic rearrangements, deletions, or amplifications occur in cells from distinct organisms? One possibility is selection for phenotype; in other words, the genetic change "freezes" development at a particular stage for that cell lineage and enhances growth and survival compared with normal cells in the niche. But it is also possible that these mutations are evolutionarily related on a mechanistic basis. For example, rearrangements of the immunoglobulin heavy chain locus and the *MYC* locus are thought to be due to recognition of *MYC* flanking sequences by the recombinase enzyme system.[123] No such mechanism is known to be operative for other defined sites, so these other mutational events could occur stochastically, with their recurrent characterization across multiple species being the result of the selective advantage provided by the acquired gene to a cell of a highly specific lineage under highly specific conditions. Another possibility is that they are related to the nuclear anatomy of the cell and specifically caused by proximity of chromosomal regions, cellular stress, inappropriate DNA repair (or, as mentioned previously, recombination), and DNA sequence and chromatin features, such as reuse breakpoints.[130] A third intriguing possibility is that cellular genomes are reverting to a conformation that was found in a common ancestor (thus the high affinity and specificity between the rearranged chromosomal segments lead to the same recurrent event in many patients) but lost during the process of chromosomal reorganization in evolution, or that these sites represent targets for gene deletions or duplications that have been repeatedly advantageous to species under conditions of natural selection and so have become embedded in their contemporary descendants.

In dogs and other domestic animals, the coexistence of genetic isolates in closed populations we call "breeds," along with animals of mixed breeding, lends itself to the study of how a relatively homogeneous background influences cancer in outbred populations. Dogs were the first species in which genetic background was shown to mold tumor genomes and tumor gene expression profiles, highlighting the utility of comparative approaches to understanding cancer genetics.[55,128,131] Over the past decade, technologic advances in next-generation sequencing and bioinformatics have improved our understanding of these relationships; GWASs have identified disease-specific risk alleles in histiocytic sarcoma,[132] squamous cell carcinoma of the digit,[28] OSA,[14] canine mammary tumors,[27] B-cell lymphomas and HSA,[133,134] mast cell tumors,[135] and brain tumors[136] in susceptible dog breeds. In the case of OSA, the GWAS revealed 33 unique risk loci in three breeds, and although none obviously overlapped, the existence of shared risk alleles might have been masked because they reside within fixed regions in some breeds (Fig. 1.7).[14] Convergent data

from the GWAS suggested a role for *CDKN2* and the associated cycle regulatory processes in OSA risk; the significance of these pathways was independently confirmed as a key indicator of the prognosis in canine OSA using gene expression studies.[41,137,138] In the case of HSA and B-cell lymphomas, two histologically different tumors that occur commonly in golden retrievers, the GWAS identified two shared risk loci on chromosome 5.[133] This observation suggests that HSAs and B-cell lymphomas might originate from a common lineage of hematopoietic progenitor cells.[119,139] Such meticulous work has improved our understanding of how distinct heritable traits segregate with cancer phenotypes in dogs, although it remains to be seen if these traits will be shared between closely related breeds or whether they contribute to risk independently among different breeds.[127]

Next-generation sequencing of tumor and normal exomes has been completed for canine lymphoma (Fig. 1.8), HSA, and OSA.[41,59,140–142] In the case of B-cell lymphomas, 64 exomes were sequenced from golden retrievers and cocker spaniels. The tumors had an average of 500 somatic mutations each, of which about 20 were nonsilent coding mutations. The most common recurrently mutated genes were *TRAF3*, *FBXW7*, and *POT1*, which regulate signaling pathways of telomerase and autoimmunity. *FBXW7* mutations, in particular, were found in 15 of 54 (28%) golden retriever samples and in 1 in 10 (10%) cocker spaniel samples. The two most common, nonsilent mutations in *FBXW7* were mutually exclusive and created arginine to leucine amino acid substitution at positions 470 and 484, respectively. These residues are also hotspots of *FBXW7* mutation in human cancers.

The exomes in T-cell lymphomas were more heterogeneous; still, 7 of 16 peripheral T-cell lymphomas from boxers harbored mutations in the *PTEN*-mTOR pathways. The data, however, is not sufficient to distinguish whether this is due to a genetic propensity for mutations of *PTEN* and other functionally related genes in boxers, or to an association in which such mutations favor selection for ontogenetically related tumors. Because genes in the *PTEN*-mTOR axis are also common targets of mutation in human cancers, studies of canine T-cell lymphoma might help to unravel their contribution to the origin and progression of cancer in a vulnerable breed and provide a discovery platform to test the safety and efficacy of drugs that target these pathways.

In the case of HSA, independent reports by two groups documented recurrent somatic mutations of *TP53* and *PIK3CA* in more than 50% of tumors within a background of many "private" mutations (i.e., unique to individual tumors). And in the case of OSA, two independent reports identified somatic mutations of *TP53* as the most common genetic abnormality in this tumor. Exome sequencing also confirmed that chaotic OSA and HSA genomes had extensive, albeit minimally overlapping, copy number aberrations, which were far in excess of those found in lymphomas[124,125,128]; predictably, translocations resulting in de novo fusion genes also were more frequent in HSA and OSA than they were in lymphoma.[42]

Most of the coding mutations identified by exome sequencing were confirmed in RNAseq data sets from the same cases, allowing us to extend the observations to additional dogs and other breeds and then to conclude that common somatic mutations in lymphoma, HSA, and OSA are not associated with breed, age, sex, or hormonal status (intact or neutered).

Genomic studies, including GWAS, comparative genomic hybridization, and next-generation sequencing, are expected to proceed in cats with the advent of the feline genome sequence.[143,144]

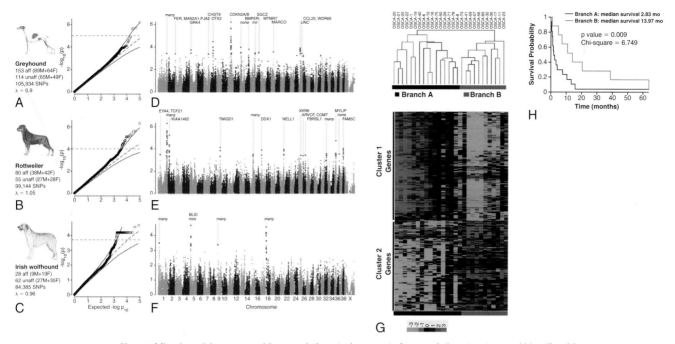

• **Fig. 1.7** Mixed model genome-wide association study corrects for population structure and identifies 33 osteosarcoma-associated loci, explaining a large fraction of phenotype variance. In each breed the QQ plots show no evidence of stratification relative to the expected distribution, identifying nominal significance at –log10p of 3.5 and the 95% empirically determined confidence intervals *(dashed gray line)* at –log10p of (A) 5 in greyhounds, (B) 4 in Rottweilers, and (C) 3.7 in Irish wolfhounds (IWHs). In IWHs a plateau of SNPs at P = 6.6 × 10 to 5 corresponds to a 1.65 Mb haplotype on chromosome 18, peaking at the gene *GRB10*. (D) In greyhounds 14 loci have p > 0.0005, with 1 locus, on chromosome 11, exceeding 95% confidence intervals *(dashed lines)*. (E) In Rottweilers 15 and 6 loci are identified, (F) whereas only 4 and 2 loci are identified in IWHs. (G) Unsupervised hierarchical clustering defines two osteosarcoma subtypes (Branch A and Branch B), characterized by two reciprocal gene clusters (Gene Cluster 1 and Gene Cluster 2). Heat map showing 282 differentially expressed transcripts (p ≤ 0.0068, mean average fold-change > 3). Heat map colors represent median-centered fold change expression after log2 transformation (a quantitative representation of the colors is provided in the scale at the bottom). Upregulated genes are shown in red, and down regulated genes are shown in green. (H) Kaplan-Meier survival (KM) and log rank analysis of 21 dogs in the cohort with known survival outcomes show two clinically significant groups in canine osteosarcoma. The toe bar defines groups for the KM analysis. The median survival time for dogs in Branch A was ~2.8 months, and the median survival time for dogs in Branch B was ~14 months. (Reproduced with permission. (A–F) from Karlsson EK, Sigurdsson S, Ivansson E, et al. Genome-wide analyses implicate 33 loci in heritable dog osteosarcoma, including regulatory variants near CDKN2A/B. *Genome Biol.* 2013 Dec 12;14(12):R132. https://doi.org/10.1186/gb-2013-14-12-r132. Fig. 1.2a–f. (G) and (H) from Scott MC, Sarver AL, Gavin KJ, et al. Molecular subtypes of osteosarcoma identified by reducing tumor heterogeneity through an interspecies comparative approach. *Bone.* 2011 Sep;49(3):356-367. https://doi.org/10.1016/j.bone.2011.05.008. Figs. 1.1 and 1.6B, respectively.)

Conclusion

The genetic basis of cancer is now beyond question. It is estimated that at least five to seven mutational events are required for overt malignant transformation. These events can occur through multiple mechanisms, including heritable factors, environmental elements, and/or stochastic DNA damage during cell replication. Genomic instability seems to be necessary to establish a pathogenic molecular program of convergent regulatory signaling pathways that cause clinical disease. Ultimately, a subpopulation endowed with metastatic properties that is drug resistant leads to death of the cancer patient. The rate and the flow of information are such that we predict the coming decade will see additional transformational changes in our perception of how genes interact with the macroenvironment at the organism level and with the microenvironment in tumors. Although it is possible that cancer in higher vertebrates is an inevitable consequence of evolution,[145] improvements in our understanding of fundamental mechanisms that account for malignant transformation and tumor progression will allow the design of strategies to improve quality of life and outcomes for cancer patients.

SECTION B: CHEMICAL, PHYSICAL, AND HORMONAL FACTORS

CAROLYN J. HENRY AND BRIAN K. FLESNER

In 1978 the US Congress ordered the development of the first Report on Carcinogens (RoC), a document designed to educate the public and health professionals on potential cancer hazards. The

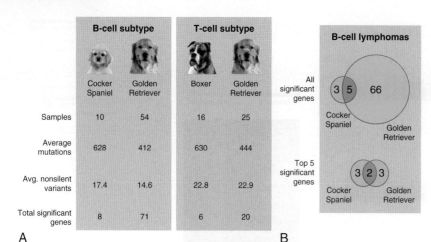
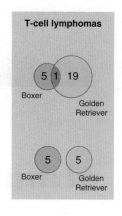
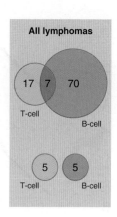

• **Fig. 1.8** Next generation sequencing of tumor and normal exomes for canine lymphoma in three breeds. (A) Sample numbers and average mutations per breed and immunophenotype. (B) Overlap of significantly mutated genes between lymphoma types. *Left panel,* The two B-cell lymphoma-predisposed breeds share some of their most significantly mutated genes. *Center panel,* The two T-cell lymphoma-predisposed breeds do not share any top significantly mutated genes. *Right panel,* Some overlap in significantly mutated genes can be seen between all the B-cell lymphomas and all the T-cell lymphomas. (Reproduced with permission from Elvers I, Turner-Maier J, Swofford R, et al. Exome sequencing of lymphomas from three dog breeds reveals somatic mutation patterns reflecting genetic background. *Genome Res.* 2015 Nov;25(11):1634-1645. https://doi.org/10.1101/gr.194449.115. Figs. 1.1A and 1.2.)

document is now required by law to be released every 2 years by the Secretary of the Department of Health and Human Services. The fourteenth edition of the RoC, released in 2016, lists 248 potential carcinogens, of which 61 are categorized as known to be human carcinogens, and 186 are categorized as reasonably anticipated to be human carcinogens.[146,147] Five of the seven additional carcinogens were viruses: Epstein-Barr virus, human immunodeficiency virus (HIV) type 1, human T-cell lymphotrophic virus type 1, Kaposi sarcoma–associated herpesvirus, and Merkel cell polyomavirus. Although no such report exists for companion animals, one could reasonably assume that there would be considerable overlap between such a list and the potential carcinogens found in the RoC. Although the list of carcinogens reportedly associated with cancer in companion animals is less extensive, this section addresses chemical, physical, and hormonal factors that have been linked to carcinogenesis in pet animals. Viral carcinogenesis is addressed in a separate section (see Section C later in the chapter). Additionally, more in-depth information regarding the epidemiology of cancer, and the strength of evidence for these factors, is addressed in Chapter 4 (see Tables 4.4 and 4.5, specifically).

Chemical Factors

Environmental Tobacco Smoke

In people tobacco use continues to be one of the leading causes of mortality worldwide; an estimated 1 billion deaths could be possible in the next century.[148] Cancers currently recognized by the US Surgeon General as being caused by smoking include lung, esophagus, bladder, pancreas, and other cancers.[149] Of course, animals are not likely to be primary smokers, but they do share our environment and can commonly be exposed to secondhand smoke. Despite ample evidence that secondhand smoke increases the risk of lung cancer in people,[150,151] the data for this effect in companion animals is less compelling. One case-control study involving dogs with lung cancer from two veterinary hospitals

showed only a weak relationship between living with a smoker and the development of lung cancer, and the risk did not increase with an increased smoke exposure index.[152] Additionally, a more recent case-control study found no association between secondhand smoke and primary lung cancer in dogs.[153] However, an association between environmental tobacco smoke (ETS) and nasal cancer in dogs, especially in dolichocephalic breeds, was supported in a case-control study that ran from 1986 to 1990.[154]

Based on human data suggesting that smoking may increase the risk of non–Hodgkin lymphoma,[155,156] Bertone et al examined the relationship between ETS exposure and the development of feline lymphoma.[157] In a case-control study of 80 cats with malignant lymphoma and 114 control cats with renal disease that presented between 1993 and 2000, the relative risk of lymphoma for cats with any household ETS exposure was 2.4. As reported for male smokers,[158] the risk of lymphoma increased with increases in either duration or quantity of exposure. More recently, an Italian study of waste management and cancer in companion animals demonstrated that ETS exposure significantly increased the risk of the development of lymphoma in dogs.[159]

Hypothesizing that inhalation and ingestion of carcinogens in ETS during grooming might predispose cats in smoking households to the development of oral squamous cell carcinoma (SCC), Bertone et al examined ETS and other environmental and lifestyle risk factors in cats with SCC.[160] Exposure to ETS was associated with a twofold, but statistically insignificant, increased risk of oral SCC.[160] In a separate report the investigators found positive associations between ETS and p53 overexpression; however, the findings again were not statistically significant.[161] Loss of wild type p53 and/or gain of mutant p53 function have been shown to be critical to carcinogenesis from tobacco exposure in human lung cancer.[162] The aforementioned suggestion that both ETS and p53 mutations might play a role in the etiology of feline oral SCC is intriguing. The study of other genetic mutations[163] and epigenetic aberrations[164] in tumor-bearing animals with ETS exposure is warranted.

Pesticides, Herbicides, and Insecticides

In 1991, investigators at the National Cancer Institute (NCI) completed a case-control study to examine the relationship between the exposure of dogs to the herbicide 2,4-dichlorophenoxyacetic acid (2,4-D), and the development of lymphoma.[165] Dogs with a histologically confirmed diagnosis of lymphoma during a 4-year period were identified through the computerized medical record information from three veterinary teaching hospitals. Each case animal was age matched with two control animals. The first control group consisted of dogs diagnosed with tumors other than lymphoma during the same time period, and the second control group was a nontumor group, selected from all other dogs presenting for conditions deemed unrelated to chemical exposure. Owners were questioned about household use of and potential pet exposure to commercial lawn care and owner-applied herbicides. A positive association was found between exposure to owner-applied 2,4-D or the use of commercial lawn care services and the development of lymphoma. The risk of lymphoma doubled when owners applied 2,4-D liquid or granules to the lawn four or more times a year. After these findings were reported, an independent review panel was convened to assess the validity of the NCI study.[166] The panel voiced concerns about the original study design, data analysis, and interpretation, concluding that a relationship between 2,4-D exposure and the development of canine lymphoma could not be established based on the reported data. In response, the original investigators reanalyzed their data, addressing many of the concerns raised by the scientific review panel.[167] A more stringent definition of exposure to 2,4-D was used, including only cases in which the owner applied 2,4-D as the sole herbicide and did not use other lawn chemicals or lawn care services. The second report did not show a statistically significant association between exposure to 2,4-D and the development of lymphoma[167]; however, it did indicate a dose-response relationship between disease incidence and the number of yearly 2,4-D applications by dog owners. In a subsequent study conducted by researchers at Michigan State University, the original 1991 data again were reanalyzed, using the more stringent definition of exposure, and a dose-response analysis was completed. The study, which was funded by a chemical industry task force, showed no dose-response relationship between the number of 2,4-D applications and the occurrence of canine lymphoma.[168] Although increased urinary excretion of 2,4-D has been demonstrated in dogs exposed to herbicide-treated lawns, a direct link between such exposure and development of lymphoma has not been shown.[169]

A 2011 case-control study conducted in Italy was designed to assess the effect of residential exposure to environmental pollutants on the risk of developing lymphoma.[170] The investigators were unable to demonstrate an association between exposure to pesticides (which by their definition included herbicides) and the development of lymphoma. However, they did find that living in industrial areas and owner use of chemicals such as paints and solvents were significantly and independently associated with lymphoma. A larger case-control study with more 260 cases of canine lymphoma and 240 and 230 cases of benign tumors and chronic diseases, respectively, was performed at a single veterinary teaching hospital.[171] In this questionnaire-based study, cases of canine lymphoma were more likely to come from a household with professionally applied pesticides (OR = 1.7) or self-applied insect growth regulators (OR = 2.7). Flea and tick control products were not associated with the risk of lymphoma.[171]

Canine transitional cell carcinoma (TCC) of the urinary bladder is another malignancy that has been linked to environmental carcinogens, including insecticides and herbicides. To further elucidate a mechanism for the carcinogenesis of canine urothelium exposed to lawn chemicals, 2,4-D and other herbicides were measured in the urine of dogs within a 50 mile radius of West Lafayette, Indiana.[172] Interestingly, chemicals were found in the urine of dogs from both treated and untreated yards. However, dogs in this study were not followed for the development of TCC.[172] In a case-control study of 59 dogs with TCC and 71 age-matched and breed size–matched control dogs with other neoplasms or chronic disease, investigators compared the two populations to assess the effect of obesity, exposure to sidestream cigarette smoke and chemicals, and the use of topical insecticides, on the risk of TCC.[173] They reported an increased risk of TCC in dogs treated with topical insecticides, with an enhancement of this risk in overweight or obese dogs. Scottish terriers, already at an increased risk of developing urothelial cancer because of a breed predisposition,[174] have been more extensively studied in regard to chemical exposure. Scottish terriers exposed to lawn and garden care products containing phenoxy herbicides, including 2,4-D, 4-chloro-2-methylphenoxy acetic acid (MCPA), and 2-(4-chloro-2-methylphenoxyl) propionic acid (MCPP), have an increased risk of developing TCC.[175] Newer topical spot-on flea and tick products have been evaluated in Scottish terrier populations and were not associated with an increased risk of TCC.[176]

In the aforementioned study of risk factors for oral SCC in cats, a significantly increased risk of oral SCC was seen in cats that wore flea collars.[160] Although links between phenoxy herbicides and the development of cancers such as SCC, lymphoma and TCC have been inconsistent, attempts to limit exposure of pets to these products is advised.

Cyclophosphamide

The cytotoxic alkylating agent cyclophosphamide (CYC) has been implicated in the development of urinary bladder cancer in people and dogs.[177–179] A known potential side effect of CYC therapy is sterile hemorrhagic cystitis, which develops from the generation of its metabolite, acrolein.[180] Acrolein causes a pyroptotic reaction in the urothelium, leading to ulceration; it also upregulates reactive oxygen species and nitric oxide production.[181] A recent review of CYC use for human rheumatic diseases listed several key conclusions. Daily oral CYC was associated with an increased risk of both hemorrhagic cystitis and bladder cancer, and patients who developed hemorrhagic cystitis had an increased risk of bladder cancer years later.[182] In dogs treated with metronomic chemotherapy,[183,184] the occurrence of hemorrhagic cystitis appears to be higher than in dogs receiving maximally tolerated dose CYC.[185,186] Although rare, bladder cancer development after CYC therapy has been reported in dogs.[187] Diligent monitoring of the urogenital tract seems warranted in patients receiving metronomic CYC.

Rural Versus Urban Environment

Several reports have identified differences in the cancer incidence between companion animals living in urban settings and those living in rural settings. The underlying cause for these differences is unclear. An increased incidence of some canine cancers, including lymphoma, tonsillar SCC, and nasal carcinoma,[154,170,173,188] has been reported in urban/industrial settings compared with rural settings. However, the coexistence of multiple environmental carcinogens in the same setting makes discerning the "smoking gun" a difficult task. Nonetheless, the study of animals as sentinels of environmental health hazards has been recommended and provides supportive evidence for carcinogenic risk assessment across species.[172,189–192] The results of a hospital-based case-control study conducted in Naples, Italy, and nearby cities with known high levels of illegal waste dumping suggest that living in these sites of waste emission increases the risk of cancer development in dogs, but not cats. This may relate to reduced exposure of cats to environmental carcinogens, because they are more often exclusively indoor pets.[159]

Physical Factors

Sunlight

The relationship between sunlight exposure or ultraviolet (UV) irradiation and the subsequent development of skin cancer is one of the better known examples of physical carcinogenesis. Recognized for its role in human SCC induction, sunlight also has been implicated as a cause of SCC in domestic animals and livestock.[193–196] In particular, light skin pigmentation and chronic sun exposure are associated with the development of facial, aural, and nasal planum SCC in white or partially white cats and may play a similar role in some cutaneous SCC lesions in dogs.[197–199] The portion of the UV spectrum most likely to be responsible for nonmelanotic skin lesions in people and animals is UV B (UV-B), which is in the range of 280 to 320 nm. Cumulative long-term exposure to UV-B may induce skin tumors directly through genetic mutations, including mutations in p53, and indirectly by impairing the response of the immune system to tumor antigens.[200–202] Pets are at greatest risk of exposure to UV-B during the midday hours and should be protected from this exposure, especially if they are a lightly pigmented breed.

Trauma/Chronic Inflammation

Tumor-promoting inflammation recently was deemed an enabling characteristic, because it allows cancer the ability to acquire core and emerging hallmarks necessary to continue uncontrolled propagation.[203] In four dogs with chronic pigmentary keratitis, neoplastic lesions of the cornea were reported, including three SCCs and one squamous papilloma.[204] Although the underlying etiology of the keratitis could not be confirmed, the neoplastic transformation likely was related to chronic inflammation. Earlier reports have linked feline eye tumors to ocular trauma that induces secondary uveitis and lens rupture (see Chapter 32).[205] Unlike the corneal tumors reported in dogs with pigmentary keratitis, the ocular lesions in cats were intraocular sarcomas. Despite the varied histology, the underlying etiology in all cases was thought to be related to inflammatory changes. Chronic inflammation also has been suggested as a cause of intraocular sarcoma in the domestic rabbit.[206] Another companion animal malignancy thought to be associated with inflammation is injection site sarcoma in the cat. This tumor type and its etiology are discussed in detail in Chapter 22.

Magnetic Fields

Nearly 40 years ago a potential link was proposed between chronic low-dose exposure to magnetic fields and the development of childhood cancer.[207] Since then multiple studies have been conducted in an attempt to discern links between magnetic fields and a variety of human cancers, ranging from hematopoietic malignancies to breast cancer. The extremely-low-frequency magnetic fields (<60 Hz) in question are ubiquitous in today's society and are generated by household appliances, industrial machinery, and electrical power lines. Because pets share our environment and have similar exposure to magnetic fields, a similar risk of cancer development has been presumed for companion animals. In a 1995 study the risk for the development of lymphoma was found to be highest in dogs from households with the highest measured exposure to magnetic fields.[208] The risk was related both to the duration and the intensity of exposure and was highest for dogs that spent more than 25% of the day outdoors. The next year, at the request of Congress, a report was published by the National Research Council (NRC) that reviewed more than 500 studies on the subject of cancer risk and exposure to electromagnetic fields.[209] The report concluded that, although a weak association has been shown between the development of childhood leukemia and exposure to electromagnetic fields, no clear evidence exists to suggest that exposure to electromagnetic fields is a true threat to human health. To the authors' knowledge, no reports on a possible link between magnetic fields and cancer in companion animals have been published since the 1995 report, although the magnetic field debate continues in the human literature. The NRC report suggested that other factors, including air quality and proximity to high traffic density, may be more likely environmental causes of cancer than low-frequency magnetic fields.

Radiation

The first report of cancer development after therapeutic irradiation in a dog dates back more than 30 years, when orthovoltage radiation was considered state of the art.[210] At that time the term *malignant transformation* was used to describe the development of epithelial malignancies at the site of prior irradiation for acanthomatous epulides in four dogs. After a review of more recent cases involving megavoltage irradiation, the author of the original report has suggested that the concept of malignant transformation should be discarded, because the occurrence of second tumors was not likely due to a true transformation of epulides into carcinomas.[211] Rather, the relatively high rate of carcinomas at previously irradiated sites for epulides is a result of less effective forms of irradiation or misclassification of the tumor type. Radiation carcinogenesis is considered the cause of secondary tumors arising in radiation fields. In human oncology most tumors occurring in heavily irradiated treatment fields are mesenchymal, rather than epithelial, in origin.[212–214] Several reports of sarcomas occurring in sites of prior irradiation also can be found in the veterinary literature.[215–217] A retrospective review of 57 dogs undergoing definitive megavoltage radiation therapy with [205]cobalt photons for acanthomatous epulides[211] described the development of a second tumor (one sarcoma and one OSA) in two dogs, occurring 5.2 and 8.7 years after the initial treatment, respectively. The overall incidence of second tumors (3.5%) was lower than in previous reports. The report suggests that the risk of second tumors at sites of radiation therapy is primarily of clinical concern for young dogs expected to enjoy long-term survival. Secondary tumors have been reported in at least 36 people who have undergone stereotactic radiosurgery; thus the risk for a secondary neoplasm is low but not zero.[218] As this radiation technique becomes more commonplace in veterinary medicine, the possibility of second tumors may need to be considered in companion animals undergoing stereotactic radiosurgery.

Surgery and Implanted Devices

The development of sarcomas at the site of metallic implants has been reported in people, dogs, and laboratory animal models[219–221]; however, it often is difficult to discern whether sarcoma development is related to implants or to other factors, including wound healing complications and osteomyelitis. Three large veterinary studies have examined the relationship between surgical implants and tumor development in dogs. The first reported on 222 dogs that developed tumors of any kind after fracture fixation, compared with 1635 dogs that underwent fracture fixation without subsequent tumor development.[220] The authors concluded that the use of metallic implants was not a risk factor for bone tumor development. A second case-control study, using the Veterinary Medical Databases (VMDB), included more than 19,000 dogs with fracture fixation; this study also found no increased risk of a case reappearing in the VMDB a minimum of 2 years later with a diagnosis of OSA.[222] This was compared with dogs undergoing open joint reduction. The second report was a bi-institutional cohort study that evaluated more than 2400 dogs undergoing tibial plateau leveling osteotomies (TPLO), with more than 1 year of follow-up.[223] The authors concluded that the incidence of OSA at TPLO sites is rare and did not find an increased association between infection or fracture and tumor development. The median time to occurrence of OSA after TPLO was approximately 4.5 years, longer than tumors occurring at sites distant to TPLO. The investigators postulate that the pathogenesis for implant-associated tumors was different from that of spontaneously developing tumors.[223]

Newer reports have tried to establish a cause and effect relationship between implants and secondary tumors[224,225]; however, the small number of cases and questionable controls prevent these studies from providing a definitive link. Other types of implants and foreign materials related to surgery sporadically are implicated in carcinogenesis in human and veterinary case reports. Published examples include dogs developing sarcomas associated with pacemakers, and multiple dogs with tumor formation caused by retained surgical swabs or gauze.[226–230] Although a true cause and effect relationship has yet to be determined, neoplasia at the site of a previous surgery should be a differential in animals with new pain or lameness.

Asbestos

Asbestos exposure is a known risk factor for the development of mesothelioma in people.[231] In fact, an estimated 60% to 88% of all cases of human mesothelioma are attributable to asbestos exposure.[231] A similar association has been found for dogs whose owners have an asbestos-related occupation or hobby.[232] This association was further supported by a study in which significantly more asbestos bodies were found in dogs with mesothelioma than in control dogs.[233] Pericardial mesothelioma was reported in five golden retrievers with histories of chronic idiopathic hemorrhagic pericardial effusion, suggesting that other factors, including breed predispositions and chronic inflammation unrelated to asbestos exposure, may be involved in the etiology of mesothelioma affecting the pericardium.[234]

Hormonal Factors

The debate about spaying and neutering pets has increased over the past decade. Although neutering may be protective against

TABLE 1.1	Tumors That May Be Influenced by Spay/Neuter Status	
Tumor Types Possibly Influenced	Concerning Breeds
Tumor with Increased Risk After Castration	
Cardiac tumors	All
Osteosarcoma	All, purebred dogs, rottweilers (<1 yr of age at castration)
Prostatic epithelial tumors (including transitional cell)	All
Urinary bladder transitional cell carcinoma	All
Lymphoma	All, golden retrievers (<1 yr of age at castration)
Tumors with Decreased Risk After Castration	
Testicular	All
Tumors with Increased Risk After Spay	
Cardiac tumors (including hemangiosarcoma)	All
Osteosarcoma	All, purebred dogs, rottweilers (<1 yr of age at spay)
Splenic hemangiosarcoma	All, Vizslas, golden retrievers (>1 yr of age at spay)
Mast cell tumors	All, Vizslas, golden retrievers
Lymphoma	All
Tumors with Decreased Risk After Spay	
Ovarian tumors	All
Uterine tumors	All
Canine mammary tumors (spay before third estrus)	All
Feline mammary tumors (spay before third estrus)	All

Reproduced with permission. Smith AN. The role of neutering in cancer development. *Vet Clin North Am Small Anim Pract.* 2014;44:965–975.

some cancers, recent breed-specific reports have shown a potential association between neutering and cancer development (Table 1.1).[235] In the next section, the authors discuss organ-specific relationships between gonad status, potential hormone-related pathogenesis, and tumor development. However, although spaying and neutering may be associated with an increased risk of cancer in some breeds, if we extrapolate that information to the entire pet population, the risk does not outweigh the issue of overpopulation and multiple, life-threatening diseases.

Canine Mammary Cancer

Canine mammary cancer is a well-established model of hormonal carcinogenesis in domestic animals (see Chapter 28). The most common neoplasm of female intact dogs,[235] mammary tumors affect approximately 260 in 100,000 dogs in the United States each year.[194,236] Dogs spayed before their first estrus cycle have a greatly reduced risk of developing breast cancer; the risk rises to

26% for dogs spayed after their second estrus.[237,238] Mammary tumors primarily affect late middle-aged (9 to 11 years) female intact dogs, and an increased incidence begins at approximately 6 years of age.[239] Despite the studies describing the protective effect of spaying on mammary tumor development, the highest level of evidence manuscript in veterinary medicine found only weak evidence of an association because of potential bias in almost all studies screened.[240] A systematic review retrieved more than 11,000 references, with only 13 studies published in peer-reviewed English language journals addressing the authors' research question. According to the Scottish Intercollegiate Guidelines Network (SIGN) level of evidence system, 9 of the 13 studies were judged to be at high risk of bias. The remaining four studies had mixed results, with some bias noted in all studies. The authors concluded that some evidence suggested that neutering female dogs before 2.5 years of age resulted in a considerable reduction in the risk of malignant mammary tumors, with further reduction possible if neutering occurred before the first estrus.[240] Randomized controlled clinical trials published after this systematic review have shown a protective effect. In dogs spayed at the time of mammary tumor excision, significantly fewer dogs subsequently developed nonmalignant tumors than if they were not spayed at the same time (hazard ratio 0.47).[241] The same group then looked at dogs with malignant tumors and found a subset of dogs, those with intermediate-grade and estrogen receptor–positive tumors, benefited from ovariohysterectomy.[242]

Sexual steroid hormones likely have their primary effect on target cells during the very early stages of mammary carcinogenesis in dogs; thus the protective effect of spaying is lost with time.[243–249] In addition to the influence of ovarian hormones on breast cancer development, the use of medroxyprogesterone acetate products (progestin and estrogen combination) to prevent estrus or to treat pseudopregnancy has been linked to an increased incidence of mammary tumor development in dogs.[250–252]

Progestin-induced growth hormone (GH) excess in dogs originates in the mammary gland. Within the mammary gland the gene encoding GH may act in an autocrine/paracrine fashion, effecting cyclic epithelial changes and, perhaps, carcinogenesis. Research to determine the mechanism of progestin-induced mammary GH expression in dogs has led to the cloning and cellular localization of the canine progesterone receptor (PR).[253] The investigators concluded that within the same mammary gland cell, the activated PR may transactivate GH expression and function as a prerequisite transcription factor; however, this regulation may be lost during malignant transformation. Mammary GH expression also has been reported in people, suggesting that evaluation of links between this hormone and mammary carcinogenesis may have implications for both species.[254,255]

Feline Mammary Cancer

Both estrogen and progesterone are thought to play important roles in feline mammary carcinogenesis, although the underlying mechanisms are less clear than for dogs. Prior studies have shown that intact female cats and cats exposed regularly to progestin are at an increased risk for mammary cancer development. The literature also suggests that, as is the case in dogs, ovariectomy may be protective against mammary tumor development in cats.[194,256–258] In one study, cats ovariectomized at 6 months of age had an approximate sevenfold reduction in risk of mammary tumor development compared with intact cats.[194] What has been lacking in the veterinary literature is an epidemiologic study of cats with age-matched

controls for comparison to specifically investigate the effects that spaying and age of spay have on the risk of feline mammary carcinoma development. Overley et al attempted to address these issues in a retrospective study that compared a population of 308 cats with biopsy-proven mammary carcinoma diagnosed between 2000 and 2001 and a control population of 400 female cats not diagnosed with mammary tumors but from the same biopsy service population as the affected cats. Cats from the two groups were frequency matched by age and year of diagnosis.[258] The study reported a 91% reduction in risk for those spayed before 6 months of age and an 86% reduction in risk for those spayed before 1 year of age, compared with intact cats. Although the study was retrospective in nature and relied on questionnaire data from a survey with a 58% response rate, the manuscript is the first published report attempting to age match controls and evaluate age at time of spay as a risk factor for mammary tumor development in cats. Although further epidemiologic evaluation and prospective assessment are needed to confirm these findings, the reported results provide some justification for recommending ovariohysterectomy before 1 year of age in cats.

Lymphoma

The National Cancer Institute's Surveillance, Epidemiology and End Results (SEER) data indicate that non–Hodgkin lymphoma is approximately 50% more common among men than women.[259] Although a similar male predisposition is reported for canine lymphoma, the underlying role of sex in lymphoma etiology remains elusive. The author and others undertook a population-based study using the VMDB to determine the relationship between sex and the development of canine lymphoma.[260] The VMDB included nearly 15,000 lymphoma cases in a population of more than 1.2 million dogs over a span of 20 years. Intact female dogs were about half as likely to develop lymphoma compared with spayed females and with males, whether neutered or intact.[260] In addition, two breed-specific studies have evaluated gonad status and lymphoma development.[261,262] Both studies concluded that spaying increases the risk of lymphoma in golden retrievers[261] and Vizslas.[262] A retrospective, single-institution medical record search involving more than 90,000 dogs evaluated at the University of California–Davis (UCD), assessed odds ratios (OR) and neuter status in multiple disease processes and neoplasms.[263] In this study spayed female dogs had more than double the risk (OR 2.25) of developing lymphoma compared with intact female dogs.[263] Male castrated dogs also were at an increased risk of lymphoma diagnosis compared with intact males. Further examination of the role of estrogen and neuter status in the development or prevention of canine lymphoma is warranted.

Osteosarcoma

Although historically reported to be a disease more common in male dogs, a review of all dogs with OSA presenting to Colorado State University over 27 years found an equal male-to-female relationship (see Chapter 25). A case-control study using the VMDB that evaluated gonad status and the development of OSA found a twofold excess risk of OSA development among neutered dogs.[264] Data collected through questionnaires from owners of 683 rottweiler dogs from North America showed that the age of spay or neuter had a significant influence on bone sarcoma incidence.[265] Both male and female dogs that underwent gonadectomy before 12 months of age were significantly more likely to develop a bone tumor than intact dogs. For each additional month of being intact, a 1.4% reduction in tumor risk was noted.[265] OSA also was evaluated in the aforementioned Davis study of more than 90,000 dogs.[263] Both spayed female and neutered male dogs had a significantly increased risk of having OSA, OR 2.53 and 1.62, respectively, compared with intact animals. The authors did theorize that this increased risk could be associated with greater longevity in neutered dogs.[263]

Hemangiosarcoma

A highly aggressive and almost uniformly fatal neoplasm, hemangiosarcoma (HSA) is diagnosed more frequently in dogs than in any other species, with breed predilections in retriever breeds (see Chapter 34). The aforementioned breed-specific studies[261,262] reported an increased risk for HSA development in spayed female dogs compared with intact female dogs. Female golden retrievers spayed after 1 year of age were diagnosed with HSA four times more frequently than intact female dogs, or dogs spayed "early."[261] Of note, only overall percentages of disease incidence were reported; statistical analysis of those percentages and subsequent p-values were not available. The authors did not report a difference in neuter status and HSA development in male golden retrievers.[261] Spayed Vizsla dogs were nine times more likely than intact females to develop HSA.[262] As in the golden retriever study, no difference in intact or neutered males was noted. In the large UCD retrospective study, neutered female and male dogs were at increased risk (ORs 3.18 and 1.39, respectively) of developing HSA compared with their intact counterparts.[263] Also at UCD, an association between age of cancer-related mortality and gonadectomy in golden retrievers was explored.[266] Goldens available for a necropsy examination from 1989 to 2016 were included. HSA was the most common cause of cancer-related death in this breed. Although a greater proportion of spayed female dogs died of cancer, their overall life span (9.83 years) was significantly longer than dogs that died of non–cancer-related causes (6.93 years).[266] The authors concluded that age had a larger effect on cancer-related mortality than reproductive status.

Mast Cell Tumors

Breed predilections for mast cell tumor (MCT) development have been reported, but a gender predilection in this neoplasm appears to be lacking (see Chapter 21). Again, in the retrospective study of 90,000 dogs at UCD, spayed female and neutered male dogs were at an increased risk for MCT development compared with intact dogs.[263] Mirroring the findings for previously described cancers, spayed female dogs seemed to have the highest risk of MCT development. This phenomenon is reflected in golden retrievers and Vizslas.[261,262] In a case-control study of 252 dogs with MCTs, an increased risk for development was found in spayed female dogs (OR 4.1).[267] Despite the repeatable finding of increased risk in spayed female dogs, the influence of hormones in canine MCTs remains unclear. Conflicting evidence exists on the presence of estrogen receptors in canine MCTs.[268,269]

Perianal Adenoma

Perianal adenoma is androgen dependent and occurs primarily in intact male dogs, whereas perianal adenocarcinoma occurs in both intact and castrated males. Perianal adenomas also may develop in female dogs secondary to androgenic hormone secretion from the adrenal gland.[270] Most of these tumors in male dogs resolve after castration, a fact that lends further support to the assertion that androgens are involved in the etiology of this tumor (see Chapter 23).[271]

Prostate Cancer

Although a well-established link exists between the presence of testosterone and the development of benign prostatic hyperplasia (BPH) in dogs and man, prostatic cancer risk is not higher in intact dogs compared with those that are castrated.[272] To the contrary, neutered dogs have been shown to be at increased risk. Castration is likely not an initiating event, but it is thought to favor tumor progression.[273–276] A clear relationship between age at castration and the risk of prostate cancer development has yet to be determined (see Chapter 29).

SECTION C: CANCER-CAUSING VIRUSES

DENNIS W. MACY

Both DNA- and RNA-containing viruses are known to cause cancer. An initial step in malignant transformation of normal cells by most tumor viruses is the integration of all or part of the viral DNA (or DNA copy of retroviral RNA) into the host cell genome. For some viruses specific viral genes (oncogenes) have been identified that lead to malignant transformation when expressed in normal cells. Other viruses, through the process of integration, enhance or repress the expression of normal cellular genes, resulting in cellular transformation or uncontrolled growth.[277]

Tumor-Causing Viruses of Dogs

Papillomaviruses

Papillomaviruses are potentially oncogenic, contagious, and infectious and have been described in wild and domestic animal species.[278] Papillomaviruses are considered relatively species specific, and isolates of humans, cattle, and dogs lack serologic cross-reactivity.[278] However, cross-infection with other species can occur. For example, the coyote can be infected with dog isolates, and bovine papillomaviruses type 1 and type 2 have been reported to infect horses.[279] In addition, bovine papillomaviruses have been isolated from tumors in cats, indicating a unique cross-species infection in a dead-end host.[280]

Sixteen papillomaviruses from three different genera infect dogs and are responsible for a wide spectrum of clinical syndromes— canine papillomavirus (CPV)-1, oral papillomas; CPV-2 and -6, cutaneous papillomas and cutaneous pigmented plaque. CPV-3, -4, -7, -8, -9, -10, -11, -14, -15, -16 are papillomaviruses of the family Papovaviridae; they produce benign, mucocutaneous and cutaneous canine papillomas and in rare cases transform into squamous cell carcinoma.[281,282,403]

The canine papillomaviruses are naked (e.g. non-enveloped) DNA viruses; they are larger than the canine parvoviruses but similar in structure. In vitro propagation methods are not used to identify the virus, but electron microscopy has been used to detect the virus in infected tissues. Other methodologies with varying sensitivity and specificity, such as Southern blot hybridization, dot blot, and reverse hybridization, have been used more recently to identify the virus. Although considered less sensitive, the polymerase chain reaction (PCR) most often is used to detect the virus in tissues.[403] Detection of the P16 protein in tissues by immunohistochemistry often is used to link papilloma infection to neoplastic transformation.[404,405] As are other papillomaviruses, canine papillomaviruses are resistant, acid stable, and relatively thermostable.[283] Only limited sequence homology exists between the DNA sequences of papillomaviruses of different species, but substantial sequence homology exists between isolates from any given species. Canine isolates have preferential tissue tropisms, but these tropisms have been shown to broaden with glucocorticoids and other immunosuppressive therapies.[403]

Pathogenesis

Papillomaviruses have a tropism for squamous epithelial tissues. After the introduction of the papillomavirus through breaks in the surface of the epithelium, replication of the virus is linked to the growth and differentiation of the cells in the stratified squamous epithelium. After the virus enters the basal layer keratinocytes, the virus undergoes disassembly and early (E) protein enters the nucleus and produces episomal copies of viral DNA. The ability of the papillomavirus to express the E gene forces the infected cell to divide, thus maintaining viral replication.[403] As these cells progress to the surface, they express the late gene (L), which forms the capsids of the virus, which then are released in the sloughing epithelial surfaces. A key feature of papillomaviruses in tumorigenesis is the E proteins, which prevent infected cells from leaving the cell cycle and are classified as oncoproteins. The amount of E protein produced and the interactions of these proteins with cellular regulatory systems, including p53, is believed to be responsible for lesion production and tumor risk.[403]

The tissue tropism for papillomaviruses may be expanded in immunosuppressed patients. The type of papillomavirus and the host's immune response after inoculation predict the risk for clinical disease; a good host response provides protection from the development of clinical disease, in which case the infection remains asymptomatic.[404,408] The presence and location of mature complete viruses on the surface of papillomas are believed to aid in their transmission to adjacent epithelial tissues and often are believed to be the cause of surgical treatment failure.[278] In contrast to other oncogenic or transforming DNA viruses, papillomaviruses rarely integrate into the cellular genome and remain episomal.[278]

Infection of epithelial cells results in a marked increase in cellular mitosis and hyperplasia of cells within the stratum spongiosum, with subsequent degeneration and hyperkeratinization.[286] Clinical evidence of hyperplasia and hyperkeratinization usually manifests 4 to 6 weeks after experimental infection.[286] Canine papillomas generally persist for 4 to 6 months in the mouth and 6 months to 1 year on the skin before undergoing spontaneous regression, and multiple papillomas generally regress simultaneously.[286] Although antibodies are produced against the papillomavirus, antibody levels do not appear to correlate with either growth or regression of the papilloma during infection; the mechanism of induction or regression remains unknown. Although vaccination has been shown to protect against infection, it is thought to be associated with induction of cell-mediated immunity.[287] The development of multiple papillomavirus-associated epidermal lesions and SCC in situ in a dog after treatment with prednisone and cyclosporine has been reported.[288,409]

Clinical Features

Papillomas may be referred to as warts, verruca vulgaris, squamous cell papillomas, or cutaneous papillomatosis. Papillomas caused by the papillomavirus usually are multiple and frequently involve

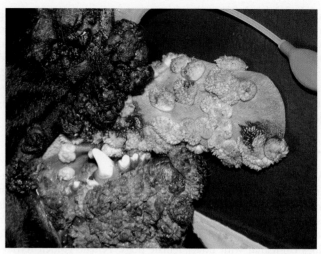

• **Fig. 1.9** Multiple papillomatosis in the oral cavity of the dog.

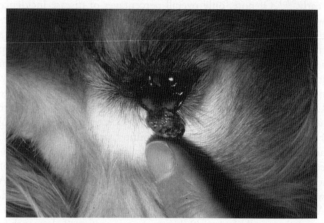

• **Fig. 1.10** Solitary ocular papilloma in a dog.

young dogs. In the dog multiple papillomatosis most frequently is seen in the oral cavity, involving the labial margins, tongue, pharyngeal mucosa, hard palate, and epiglottis (Fig. 1.9).[287] Four to 8 weeks after infection, small, pale, smooth, elevated lesions appear; these quickly develop a cauliflower-like appearance, with fine, white fronds extending from the surface of the lesions. Multiple sites of susceptible tissue in the oral cavity appear to be affected early in the course of the disease; as many as 50 to 100 tumors may be present at the time of diagnosis.[287] The primary complaints of owners of infected dogs are halitosis, ptyalism, hemorrhage, and dysphagia. Most oral cavity papillomas start regressing after 4 to 8 weeks; however, some oral lesions may show incomplete regression, and some have been known to persist up to 24 months.[287,406]

Canine cutaneous (exophytic) papillomas are most commonly found in older dogs. Certain breeds, such as Kerry blue terriers and cocker spaniels, appear to be predisposed. Most lesions appear on the head, eyelids (Fig. 1.10), and feet. Lesions may be single or multiple, pigmented and/or alopecic.

Cutaneous inverted papillomas are found most frequently in young dogs and are located on the ventral abdomen and inguinal regions. The lesions maybe single or multiple and are considered self-limiting (Fig. 1.11).[406]

Multiple pigmented plaques have been described in young miniature schnauzers and pugs. The plaques may progress to scaly, hyperkeratotic flat masses and then may progress to SCC.[289,406]

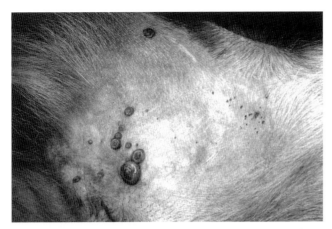

• **Fig. 1.11** Multiple cutaneous papillomatosis in the inguinal region of a dog.

Canine genital papillomas are considered uncommon but venereal in nature and are characterized by raised papillomatous plaques on the penis or vaginal mucosa.

Canine footpad papilloma was first noted in young greyhounds but now is recognized in adult dogs and other breeds. It may be present on multiple footpads, interdigital spaces, and on multiple limbs.[289,406]

Ocular papillomas, which are less numerous and less common than the oral type, appear on the conjunctiva, cornea, and eyelid margins (see Fig. 1.10).[287] Experimentally, viruses isolated from ocular lesions can produce oral papillomatosis, although whether this occurs in nature is unknown.[284] Ocular papillomatosis most frequently occurs in dogs 6 months to 4 years of age, but it occasionally is reported in older dogs.

Although papillomatosis generally should be considered a benign disease, in rare cases oral and corneal papillomas have transformed into SCC.[281,282]

Treatment

Most clinicians elect not to treat papillomatosis because of the lack of proven efficacy of recommended treatments and the expected spontaneous regression of these tumors; however, if the number of papillomas increases or if the animal has significant dysphagia, owners often request treatment. Surgical excision, cryotherapy, laser surgery, radiation therapy, electrocautery, or surgery for just a few lesions has resulted in regression of the remaining papillomas, presumably through immunologic mechanisms.[287,290,291]

If surgery is performed, seeding of the virus is a possible complication, resulting in lesion recurrence. The exact mechanism by which regression of papillomas occurs is unknown. Serum from dogs in which papillomas have undergone spontaneous regression not only fails to produce tumor regression when administered to infected animals, but may enhance existing tumor growth. This effect may be a result of induction of blocking antigen-antibody factors, which may impede cytotoxic lymphocyte action on target cells. CD4 T cells activate macrophages and have been shown to inhibit the virus in dogs, and administration of immune lymphocytes from dogs in which tumors have regressed has been shown to enhance regression.[283] Interferon-α also has been tried therapeutically, with some success (1–3 million IU/m^2 given subcutaneously three times a week [Monday-Wednesday-Friday]), and chemotherapy of resistant lesions has produced variable results.[292] Azithromycin (5–10 mg/kg PO every 12 to 48 hours) has been reported to be

beneficial, as has imiquimod cream (Aldara) applied topically every 24 to 48 hours.[406] A new recombinant canine oral papillomavirus vaccine (COPV) produced by Georgetown University Medical center has been reported effective. The vaccine presents the capsid protein L1 of CPV-1 and was given in six injections; after the initial vaccination, three booster vaccines were given every 2 weeks followed by two more boosters given monthly.[406] Corticosteroids should be avoided because they are thought to contribute to papilloma dissemination.[293,409]

Most systemic chemotherapeutic agents (e.g., bleomycin, vincristine, cyclophosphamide, and doxorubicin) have failed to cause regression of papillomas. However, the retinoid drug etretinate (1 mg/kg PO every 24 hours) has been effective in some dogs with persistent papillomas.[294] Topical or intralesional compounds containing 5-fluorouracil (5-FU) have been used in both humans and dogs to treat papillomas.[406] In the past, autologous wart vaccines have been recommended, but they have proved of little value in the treatment of resistant papillomatosis in the dog.[287] In at least one study papillomavirus vaccines have been shown to prevent the development of oral papillomas in the dog; however, cutaneous neoplasms at the injection sites have been attributed to administration of the vaccines.[285,295,296]

Tumor-Causing Viruses of the Cat

Papillomaviruses

Feline viral papillomatosis is a less commonly recognized clinical condition caused by a papillomavirus specific to the cat.[409] The virus is widespread in the cat population, and most infections are asymptomatic.[408] At least three papilloma viruses FcaPV-1, -2, -3, have been recently sequenced for the domestic cat and are responsible for cutaneous plaques, bowenoid in situ carcinoma (Bowen disease), and cutaneous SCC.[403] These viruses are thought to be genomically similar to the canine isolates but are considered species specific.[297] Bovine papillomavirus BPV-14 is thought to be responsible for feline sarcoid.[403] Papillomavirus-associated lesions have been reported in six species of felids besides the domestic cat: the mountain lion, Florida panther, bobcat, Asian lion, snow leopard, and clouded leopard.[298,299] Unlike in the domestic cat, in which the lesions commonly affect areas of haired skin, papillomas in exotic species most often are found in the oral cavity, similar to those in the dog.[298,302] Despite the clinical similarities, genetic and antigenic studies indicate that each species of felid is infected by a unique papillomavirus.

Pathogenesis

In cats, as in other species, papillomas are believed to develop after the virus is introduced through lesions or abrasions in the skin. Unlike in the dog most feline case reports involve older cats (6 to 13 years of age), although papillomavirus lesions have been reported in kittens as young as 6 to 7 months old.[300,301] As in other species, impaired T-cell function likely plays a significant role in lesion formation. Papillomas in cats that are receiving immunosuppressive therapy or are infected with the feline immunodeficiency virus (FIV) support this hypothesis.

Although papillomas most frequently are benign lesions, recent studies have associated the papillomavirus with SCCs and other malignant neoplasms in cats[302]; specifically, papillomavirus has been isolated from 30 of 63 SCC in situ skin lesions. Through the use of PCR techniques, papillomaviruses have been found in

17 of 19 and 9 of 12 fibropapillomas in cats.[303,304] Although a cause and effect relationship has yet to be proved for carcinoma in situ, Bowen disease, fibropapillomas, and papillomaviruses, the evidence is compelling.[302–304]

Bovine papillomaviruses may also play a role in the pathogenesis of feline cutaneous fibropapilloma (sarcoid). In a study of 20 cats with fibropapillomas, more than half were known to have exposure to cattle, and all were within an area with dairy farms.[303] In one isolate the nucleotide sequence was similar to that of the bovine papillomavirus. Injection of that isolate back into bovine skin resulted in asymptomatic infection.

Clinical Features

Lesions in the cat differ from those in the dog because they are more like plaques than warts.[406] The plaques are several millimeters in diameter, may be white or pigmented, and are scaly or greasy. Lesions in the cat usually affect haired skin. Thought to be associated with grooming activity, lesions on the ventral tongue surface that are sessile in character also occur.[298,302] Cutaneous viral plaques and bowenoid in situ carcinomas (BISCs) are caused by FcaPV-2; the former are a precursor to BISC. Some of these lesions progress to SCC, with spread to lymph nodes and lungs. Sarcoids occur in young cats and appear on the head, neck and digits.

Diagnosis

Definitive diagnosis depends on histopathologic, immunohistochemical (IHC), or electron microscopic (EM) examination of excised lesions. Histologic features include proliferation of all cell layers with little or no inflammation. Typically, epidermal hyperplasia is accompanied by acanthosis, hypergranulosis, hyperkeratosis, and ballooning degeneration of cells of the stratum spinosum and stratum granulosum. Amphiphilic cytoplasmic inclusion structures may be present in cells of the upper stratum granulosum. EM findings in the lesions include intranuclear particles within keratinized cells in the superficial epithelial strata of the plaques.[403] IHC can be performed on tissue sections using band-reactive, genus-specific antisera. Interestingly, the histologic features of the feline fibropapilloma are very similar to those of equine sarcoids, with characteristic fibroblastic proliferation, hyperplasia of epidermis, and rete ridges.[303] PCR also has demonstrated papillomavirus DNA in 40% of SCCs, but whether it is responsible for these tumors in all cases is unknown.[404]

Treatment

Surgical excision generally is used; however, parenteral human recombinant interferon-α-2a has been suggested as an alternative. Medications containing 5-FU that are used in humans and dogs should **not** be used in cats.[409] Imiquimod 5% cream is a novel immune-response modifier (IRM) that has been used in humans with Bowen disease and recently has been used in cats with the same disease. Although 41% of cats treated with imiquimod developed some level of toxicity, most adverse events were manageable.[305]

Retroviruses

Retroviral infections are considered the number one infectious cause of morbidity and mortality in the domestic cat. Before the vaccine was developed and routine testing and control measures became widespread, the feline leukemia virus (FeLV) was associated with one-third of deaths in cats.[306,307] Since the introduction

of the feline leukemia vaccine in 1985, the incidence of lymphoma in cats in the United States and Europe has markedly declined; however, along with the reduction in FeLV-related disease, there has been a rise in FeLV vaccine injection site tumors.[407] The cat is believed to be affected by the largest number of retroviruses of any companion animal, and these viruses produce a wide spectrum of diseases, including cancer.[308–310]

The cat has both endogenous and exogenous retroviruses. The endogenous retroviruses generally are considered nonpathogenic, are present in the host DNA, and are passed from generation to generation genetically, as are other chromosomal genes. The exogenous retroviruses include both pathogenic and nonpathogenic viruses and are passed horizontally and vertically between cats. Pathogenic exogenous retroviruses include FeLV and FIV.[311] The exogenous RNA sequences of FeLV play the most important role in tumorigenesis in the cat.[310] Another pathogenic retrovirus, the feline sarcoma virus (FeSV), arises from the recombination of exogenous FeLV and proto-oncogenes in the cat's genome.[312] Feline syncytium-forming virus (FeSFV), also called the feline foamy virus, is a nonpathogenic exogenous retrovirus.[306]

FeLV is believed to have been contracted from the ancestral rat approximately 10 million years ago.[313] The ancestral source of other retroviruses is unknown.

Feline Leukemia Virus

The retrovirus FeLV belongs to the subfamily Oncornavirinae, or tumor-producing RNA viruses. As do other retroviruses, it has a single strand of RNA and an enzyme, reverse transcriptase (RT), which synthesizes DNA from the virus RNA template. Nondomestic felids, including the cheetah and bobcat, can be infected by FeLV; however, it is considered enzootic in wild felids, and in European wild cats in France and Scotland. It has been reported in mountain lions in the United States.[314,315]

The basic FeLV proteins include the envelope proteins and the core proteins, several of which are important clinically. Two envelope proteins, the P15E and the GP70 glycoproteins, have particular clinical significance.[316–318] P15E is thought to be one of the mediators of immunosuppression in FeLV-infected cats.[319] The glycoprotein of the envelope GP70 may contain three subgroup antigens, A, B, and C.[320–321] An individual cat may have combinations of viruses with these subgroup viral antigens. Considerable antigenic variation exists within subgroups, which can affect the biologic properties of the individual isolates or strains of FeLV.[310,320] These subgroup antigens bind the virion to receptors on the surface of cells. The specific characters of these proteins also predict the pathogenicity, host range, infectivity, and other biologic properties of the virus.[310,320] Antibodies produced against envelope proteins can be neutralizing and thereby can prevent infection. Envelope proteins thus are important components of FeLV vaccines.

Core proteins (capsids) include P15C, P12, P10, and P27. P27 is quite soluble and can be found in large amounts in the cytoplasm of cells and bodily fluids, such as tears and serum.[316–318] P27 is the antigen that is detected in immunofluorescent assay (IFA) tests and enzyme-linked immunosorbent assays (ELISAs), which are commonly used in the diagnosis of FeLV infection.[321]

Transmission

FeLV is an enveloped virus and is considered very fragile. Desiccation rapidly reduces the amount of viable virus in saliva, and inactivation occurs in 1 to 2 hours. In exudates or blood the virus may be viable for only 48 hours (at 37°C) or 1 to 2 weeks (at 22°C).[322]

Like most retroviruses, FeLV is rapidly inactivated by heating and most disinfectants.[317] Given these characteristics, environmental contamination (e.g., examination tables, cages, and waiting rooms) is unlikely to be a potential source of FeLV infection.[310] Although saliva may contain up to 100,000 virus particles per milliliter, prolonged, intimate contact with infected cats usually is required for transmission. The factors most frequently incriminated in the transmission of FeLV are licking, biting, grooming, and sharing of litter pans, food bowls, and water dishes. Intimate contact is enhanced in catteries and multiple-cat households, where infection rates may be very high.[319]

Before vaccines and routine testing became available, the overall prevalence of FeLV infection in the United States was estimated at 1% to 3% of the cat population.[308,309] The prevalence of FeLV infection was less than 1% in single-cat households and as high as 30% in multiple-cat households.[327] The incidence of FeLV-positive test results in sick cats in the United States was approximately 11.5%.[328] Several studies have reported a decline in the prevalence of FeLV by as much as 50% over the past 20 years; this decrease may be attributed partially to the widespread use of FeLV vaccination.[307,329,330]

Although cats may be infected with FeLV subgroups A, B, or C or other recombinants, only subgroup A has been found in cell-free fluids and is thought to be associated with natural transmission of FeLV. Subgroups B and C and other recombinants are more cell associated and are not thought to be transmitted in nature.[323–326]

The FeLV subgroups are characterized by their cross-interference with homologous but not heterologous subgroups of FeLV and by their host range and other factors. All naturally infected FeLV cats have subgroup A, 50% of infected cats have a combination of subgroups A and B, and 1% of infected cats in nature have a mixture of subgroup C, either as AC or ABC.[308,328,331]

The relevance of subgroups in strains is essential to an understanding of the biodiversity of the clinical disease caused by FeLV infection. Although subgroups A, B, and C maintain 85% genomic homology, cats infected with various combinations of these subgroups may manifest vastly different diseases.

Subgroup A has a variety of strains that range from nonpathogenic to very pathogenic.[332] Although most strains of subgroup A have limited pathogenicity, their pathogenicity increases dramatically if they are present with other subgroups.

Subgroup B is created when subgroup A recombines with endogenous FeLV envelopes at sequences already in the feline genome.[333–335] Each recombination is unique, resulting in many strains of FeLV-B. The combination of subgroups A and B is more contagious and pathogenic than subgroup A alone.[328,331,332] Cats infected with subgroups A and B often develop thymic lymphoma and myeloproliferative disease.[333]

Subgroup C arises from the mutation of subgroup A.[336] Cats may be infected with a combination of C and other subgroups, although these combinations are uncommon and are found in only about 1% of naturally infected cats. FeLV-C is antigenically similar to the associated membrane antigen (feline oncornavirus-associated cell membrane antigen [FOCMA]); cats carrying FeLV-C have developed severe erythroid hypoplasia and anemia and usually die within 1 to 2 months.[323] Further complicating the biodiversity of subgroups and strains is the fact that subgroups A and B can recombine with proto-oncogenes, such as MYC or TCR, producing FeLV-MYC or FeLV-TCR.[306] Both of these recombinants are considered more potent tumor producers than their nonrecombinant FeLV parent. Another subgroup, T, is highly cytolytic for T lymphocytes and causes severe immunosuppression.[324–326]

The Rickard strain of FeLV (FeLV-R), although similar to MYC-containing recombinant strains in its ability to rapidly produce mediastinal lymphoma, does not recombine with the MYC gene.[306,337] Instead, it exerts some of the biologic effects by integrating adjacent to the MYC gene, causing its overexpression.[306]

Feline Oncornavirus-Associated Cell Membrane Antigen

FOCMA is a protein found on the surface of FeLV and FeLV-induced neoplasms but not on nonneoplastic feline cells.[338,339] FOCMA is detected serologically when cells expressing it react to immunoglobulins produced in cats that have regressed FeSV-induced fibrosarcoma or FeLV infection. The presence of the FOCMA antibody is determined by the ability of the serum to react with FL74 cells, a transformed infected feline lymphocyte line.[340] Antibodies to FOCMA protect against neoplastic and myeloproliferative disease. Some FeLV vaccines contain FOCMA and elicit an anti-FOCMA response.[341] The relative importance of this in preventing disease in vaccinates is unknown.

Neoplastic Diseases Caused by Feline Leukemia Virus

Much has yet to be learned about the genetic basis for the vast diversity of tumor types produced by FeLV and its recombinants. We now know that FeLV, through one or another of its recombinants, may cause virtually any hematopoietic neoplasm in the cat. The only hematopoietic neoplasms not yet associated with FeLV in nature are mast cell leukemia, eosinophilic leukemia, plasma cell tumors, and polycythemia vera.[306]

Although FeLV infection is considered the most significant infectious cause of morbidity and mortality in cats, only 20% of cats persistently infected with FeLV develop lymphoid cancer.[342,343] The cat has the highest incidence of hematopoietic neoplasms of domestic animals, and the prevalence of lymphoma ranges from 44 to 200 cases per 100,000 cats, six times the rate of this disease in humans.[306] Twenty years ago 70% of lymphomas in cats were believed to be caused by FeLV.

Some cancers are more commonly associated with FeLV infection than others. Large granular lymphoma and globular leukocyte tumors usually test negative for FeLV,[344–345] whereas 70% to 90% of cats with nonlymphoid hematopoietic neoplasia (myeloproliferative disease) test positive for FeLV.[306] The percentage of lymphomas that test positive for FeLV also varies, depending on the anatomic location of the tumor.[346–347] Cats with spinal, mediastinal, ocular, and renal lymphoma frequently tested positive for FeLV before routine vaccination (more than 70%).[349] Extranodal lymphomas, such as those of the nasal cavity and the alimentary tract, frequently test negative for FeLV infection.[306] Over the past 20 years, the multicentric FeLV-positive form has declined in young cats, and the FeLV-negative alimentary form in older cats has increased.[350,351] Although the alimentary form most often is FeLV negative, as assessed by IFA and ELISA testing, some of these lesions have been shown by PCR to be FeLV positive, which suggests that the disease may be related to previous FeLV exposure.

Although not all lymphomas are caused by FeLV, the relative risk of developing lymphoma is 62 times higher in FeLV-positive cats, and cats that are FeLV negative but that have had previous exposure to FeLV have a fortyfold increase in the risk of developing lymphoma.[352] Most spontaneous lymphomas of cats that test positive for FeLV arise from T cells, whereas FeLV-negative lymphoma frequently is of alimentary or B-cell origin.[353,354] The time from infection to tumor development varies and may depend on the age at which the cat is infected or on other factors, such as strain, anatomic location, and viral subgroup.[306] The range from the time of experimental infection to tumor production is 1 to 23 months (mean, 5.3 months).[355,356] The younger the cat when infected with FeLV, the shorter the time to the development of neoplastic disease. Some cats infected with FeLV die of immuno-suppressive disease before tumors have a chance to develop.

Treatment of Feline Leukemia Virus Infections

Although no effective treatment exists to eliminate established FeLV infection in cats, a variety of antiviral drugs and biologic response modifiers (BRMs) have been used to manage retroviral infections in cats and humans. The mainstay of therapy for cats infected with FeLV or other retroviruses is supportive care.[357–359] Maintaining hydration and nutritional status not only prolongs life, but also enhances quality of life. The cat should be kept in a humid environment to reduce the chance of water loss. Appetite stimulants and placement of gastrostomy tubes may facilitate nutritional therapy. The cat's requirement for B vitamins is eight times that of the dog, and dietary concentrations must be maintained to maintain appetite. Semimoist cat foods often contain propylene glycol, which can shorten red blood cell survival. These foods, although often quite palatable, should not be used for the nutritional management of cats infected with FeLV.[358] Many cats with FeLV are anemic, but administering erythropoietin is not helpful because endogenous erythropoietin levels usually are 20 times normal.[360]

Biologic Response Modifiers

A variety of BRMs have been used in cats infected with FeLV,[361–369] but none has shown benefit in controlled trials. A few of the most popular are discussed here.

Human recombinant, bovine, and feline interferons have been studied extensively for the management of FeLV infection, but the results have been mixed. However, some uncontrolled studies have shown improvement in the clinical status of cats treated with oral human recombinant interferon-α,[368] and one study in a limited number of cats using feline interferon subcutaneously showed improvement compared with placebo-treated controls.[410] Larger controlled trials are needed to establish the true efficacy of interferon products. Orally administered interferon probably is inactivated by gastric acid in the stomach. Parenterally administered interferons from other species (i.e., bovine and human) are likely to have only temporary activity because of the production of neutralizing antibodies.

Carrisyn (Acemannan) is a BRM designed to enhance macrophage phagocytosis and cell killing. Viremic cats treated with Carrisyn have been reported to improve clinically; however, the studies reporting these results have not been well controlled, and the observed benefit may be due to the natural waxing and waning of the clinical course commonly observed in FeLV-positive cats.[369]

A lymphocyte T-cell immunomodulator (LTCI) recently has become commercially available for the treatment of cats infected with FeLV and FIV. The true efficacy of this product, if any, awaits the results of controlled trials in cats.[370]

The apparent positive effect of many of the BRMs, which, in fact, may be due to the anabolic effect observed with some of these cytokines, is thought to be based on endorphin release rather than a direct effect on the viral infection.

Reverse Transcriptase Inhibitors

Drugs that inhibit RT and retrovirus integration into the host cell have been evaluated for their potential use in the treatment of FeLV-positive cats. The drugs evaluated include suramin (a polyionic dye used to treat filariasis in humans), nucleoside analogs (AZT, DDC, DDA, and PNEA), glucose homopolymers, dextran sulfate, phosphonate, and others.[371–374] More detailed descriptions of these therapies are provided elsewhere.[371,374] In general, most of these agents have shown efficacy *in vitro* against FeLV, the human immunodeficiency virus (HIV), and in some cases, FIV. Most of these drugs result in some reduction in viremia *in vivo*, but none are capable of reversing established viremia, although some may prevent viremia if administered prophylactically. Most of these drugs cause significant adverse effects at the dosages needed to produce antiviral effects and therefore have not gained popularity in clinical practice. Azidothymidine (AZT, zidovudine) is the most widely studied RT inhibitor.[375] AZT inhibits FeLV reverse transcriptase when administered at a dosage of 10 to 20 mg/kg in daily divided doses. AZT prevents viremia if given within 72 hours of exposure to FeLV. The antiviral effects of AZT appear to be synergistic with human recombinant interferon-α-2a.[376,377] Reversal of established experimental FeLV viremia through adoptive transfer of lectin/IL-2–activated lymphocytes, interferon-α, and AZT has been reported.

Prevention and Control

The most effective means of preventing FeLV infection is to eliminate contact with viremic cats. The "test and removal" program is the most effective means of controlling FeLV in multiple-cat households.[378] The program consists of closing the household or cattery to new cats, testing the remaining cats every 3 months, and removing all animals that test positive. When all cats test negative for two consecutive sessions, the facility is determined to be FeLV free. New cats may enter the household or facility only after a 3-month quarantine and two negative FeLV tests. The test and removal system has been shown to reduce the incidence of FeLV in a variety of settings and geographic locations.[378]

Prevention by Vaccination

Vaccinations help control or eliminate many infectious diseases in veterinary medicine. The first commercial FeLV vaccine was introduced in 1985. Since then many FeLV vaccine products have been licensed for sale to veterinarians in the United States. Despite the fact that FeLV vaccines have been available for decades, they come with the risk of injection site tumors. The frequency of use of FeLV vaccines continues to be debated, especially in adult cats, most of which develop age-acquired immunity. In addition to age-acquired immunity and the risk of injection site tumors, most currently available FeLV vaccines, although effective in preventing persistent viremia, fail to prevent latent infections of the bone marrow after challenge. Some studies of available vaccines have reported efficacies ranging from 0% to 100%.[379,380]

FeLV vaccination issues are discussed elsewhere.[341] However, several comments about FeLV vaccines should help practitioners decide whether to use FeLV vaccines in their practice. FeLV vaccines may contain two or three subgroup antigens. Because only subgroup A is transmitted contagiously between cats, vaccines need only to contain subgroup A. Their primary means of protecting against tumor development is preventing persistent viremia. If a vaccine protects against persistent FeLV infection, it need not contain FOCMA. The value of FOCMA in FeLV vaccines has yet to be proven. Vaccines should protect against a variety of strains of subgroup A, and none of the available vaccines contain more than one strain of subgroup A. Differences in published comparative studies of vaccine efficacy probably are related to differences in vaccine strains and to the challenge strains used. Vaccines that contain adjuvants enhance immunity but at the expense of producing local inflammatory reactions at the injection site.[381] These local reactions may lead to the development of soft tissue sarcomas; however, the development of soft tissue sarcomas after vaccination, either with rabies or FeLV vaccines, is thought to occur in only 1 in 1000 to 1 in 10,000 vaccinates.[380] Nonadjuvanted FeLV vaccines have shown little or no inflammatory reaction 21 days after administration.[381] A canarypox-vectored FeLV nonadjuvanted vaccine is available that stimulates both cellular and humoral immunity without significant injection site inflammation. Clinical discretion, considering the potential risk and benefit, should be used when recommending FeLV vaccines. The reader is advised to consider the current recommendations of the American Association of Feline Practitioners (AAFP) (www.catvets.com).

Feline Sarcoma Virus

FeSVs are true hybrids that result from the rare recombination of FeLV DNA provirus with cat proto-oncogenes. Cats have at least 30 proto-oncogenes.[306,382,383] Proto-oncogenes have many biologic functions; when they are altered and activated inappropriately, they are called *oncogenes*, which can play a key role in the development of cancerous phenotypes. Proto-oncogenes can be activated by mutations that produce chromosomal translocations, such as those that may be associated with inflammation and vaccine-associated sarcomas, or by incorporation into a retrovirus, such as FeLV.[382–384] When FeLV-derived DNA inserts near a proto-oncogene and takes up the proto-oncogene into the FeLV provirus, formation of FeSV results. In the process, part of the FeLV *GAG* gene, most of the FeLV envelope gene, and all of the pol genes are lost.[383] The loss of these vital components makes FeSV dependent on FeLV as a helper virus for replication. Cats that have FeSV always test FeLV positive. Because several different recombinations may recur with several different proto-oncogenes, each recombination is a unique event, and each isolate is distinct.[384] Despite this phenotypic heterogeneity, the recombinations transform fibroblasts, and all produce fibrosarcomas.

Natural transmission of FeSV between cats has not been described, and as with other FeLV recombinants (e.g., FeLV-B), transmission of the recombinant product is not thought to occur in nature. Some cats are capable of rejecting transformed cells and producing FOCMA antibody.[359,360] FOCMA is important in the experimental response of cats to FeSV because it has been associated with tumor regression and failure to develop tumors.[385] Cats that fail to develop antibodies against FOCMA die quickly of fast-growing sarcomas.[386]

Clinical Features of Feline Sarcoma Virus–Induced Fibrosarcomas

Only 2% of fibrosarcomas of cats are virally induced.[312] In contrast to the solitary, slow-growing, nonvirally induced sarcomas seen in older cats, FeSV-induced tumors are multicentric and are found most frequently in young cats.[387] They are characterized by rapid growth, including doubling times as short as 12 to 72 hours.[306] This rapid growth often is accompanied by superficial ulceration. Lesions frequently occur at sites of previous bite wounds.[306] Metastasis to the lungs or other organs occurs with approximately 30% of virally induced fibrosarcomas in cats. Hypercalcemia was observed in association with multicentric fibrosarcomas in one cat with FeSV.[306] Virally induced fibrosarcomas are always FeLV

positive; this helps differentiate them from vaccine-associated sarcomas, which may have growth characteristics similar to those of virally induced tumors. Cats with multicentric FeSV-induced tumors have a very poor prognosis.

Feline Immunodeficiency Virus

FIV, which is classified as a retrovirus in the subfamily Lentivirinae, is distinct from other retroviruses that infect cats. As are other retroviruses, FIV is an enveloped, single-stranded RNA virus in which the RNA is copied into the DNA in the infected host by RT in the virus.

The nucleotide sequence of several FIV isolates has been determined, and genetic homology falls between 36% and 97%. Despite this homology, significant differences in pathogenicity and infectivity exist between FIV strains.[389,390] Although lentiviruses are known to infect wild felids, they are antigenically distinct from domestic cat isolates; they also are well adapted to their host and seldom cause clinical disease.

Transmission

FIV is present in all bodily fluids of infected cats, similar to FeLV, but at much lower concentrations. FIV is mainly cell associated and is present in relatively low concentrations in the blood, although high amounts can be found in the saliva.[391,392] FIV is not thought to be highly infectious and is mainly transmitted through biting during cat fights.[393,394]

Feline Immunodeficiency Virus–Associated Neoplasms

The prevalence of neoplasms in FIV-positive cats ranges from 1% to 62%.[352,395,396] Lymphomas and myeloid tumors (myelogenous leukemia, myeloproliferative disease) and a few carcinomas and sarcomas are the neoplasms most commonly linked to FIV infection. One study found that cats infected with FIV and FeLV are 5.6 times more likely to develop lymphoma or leukemia than if they had been infected with either virus alone. Cats with combined infections had a 77% greater likelihood of developing lymphoma or leukemia than noninfected cats.[352] In contrast to FeLV-associated lymphomas, FIV-associated lymphomas most often develop in extranodal sites and occur in older cats (mean age, 8.7 years).[352] Myeloproliferative disease also has been observed in cats naturally and in cats experimentally infected with FIV.[352,397,398]

Although lentiviruses such as FIV have not been thought to be oncogenic in themselves, they are markedly immunosuppressive and affect normal immunosurveillance of neoplastic cells. FIV-positive cats with lymphoma have extremely low CD4 lymphocyte counts.[388] SCCs of the skin have been linked to FIV infection in two geographic areas, California and Colorado, but this association is believed to be due to a co-risk behavior (outdoor cats) rather than to any direct viral contribution to tumor development.[399,400] Other reports have linked FIV infection to oral SCC, mammary carcinoma, fibrosarcoma, myeloproliferative disease, Bowen disease and histiocytic mast cell disease.[395,401,402] The nature of these associations awaits further investigation.

Treatment

The same treatment considerations in the management of cats with FeLV can be applied to the treatment of FIV-positive cats. The most widely applied treatments have been the RT inhibitors and human recombinant interferon-α (see the earlier discussion on the treatment of FeLV). As in the treatment of FeLV,

FIV-positive cats remain positive despite these therapies. A single inactivated FIV vaccine has been licensed for use in domestic cats. However, this is an adjuvanted vaccine, and it may be associated with an increased risk of vaccine-associated sarcoma. The primary concern with the vaccine is that it generates antibodies that cross-react with the currently recommended antibody-based diagnostic test for FIV infection. PCR-based tests are not currently considered reliable for diagnosis of FIV, and antibody-based testing remains the gold standard.[409] It is important to note that the AAFP does not recommend the use of an FIV vaccine in domestic cats.

Comparative Aspects

The association between human viruses and certain cancers has been established on the basis of epidemiologic, clinical, and molecular studies.[277] Human T-cell leukemia virus (HTLV-1) has been linked to adult T-cell leukemia. More than 100 papillomaviruses occur in humans; these are believed to be responsible for cervical cancer; for 25% to 60% of SCCs of the oral cavity; and in rare cases some SCCs that occur on the skin surface.[33] The human papillomavirus (HPV) is associated with cervical cancer. The Epstein-Barr virus (EBV) is related to the development of Burkitt lymphoma and nasopharyngeal carcinoma, and the human hepatitis B and hepatitis C viruses are associated with hepatocellular carcinoma. The human herpes virus (HHV) is implicated in the development of Kaposi sarcoma.

References

1. Townsend N, Wilson L, Bhatnagar P, et al.: Cardiovascular disease in Europe: epidemiological update 2016, *Eur Heart J* 37:3232–3245, 2016.
2. Heron M, Anderson RN: Changes in the leading cause of death: recent patterns in heart disease and cancer mortality, *NCHS Data Brief* 1–8, 2016.
3. Adams VJ, Evans KM, Sampson J, et al.: Methods and mortality results of a health survey of purebred dogs in the UK, *J Small Anim Pract* 51:512–524, 2010.
4. Bonnett BN, Egenvall A, Hedhammar A, et al.: Mortality in over 350,000 insured Swedish dogs from 1995-2000: I. Breed-, gender-, age- and cause-specific rates, *Acta Vet Scand* 46:105–120, 2005.
5. Proschowsky HF, Rugbjerg H, Ersboll AK: Mortality of purebred and mixed-breed dogs in Denmark, *Prev Vet Med* 58:63–74, 2003.
6. Moore GE, Burkman KD, Carter MN, et al.: Causes of death or reasons for euthanasia in military working dogs: 927 cases (1993-1996), *J Am Vet Med Assoc* 219:209–214, 2001.
7. Nowell PC, Hungerford DA: A minute chromosome in human chronic granulocytic leukemia, *Science* 132:1497, 1960.
8. Nowell PC, Hungerford DA: Chromosome studies in human leukemia. II. Chronic granulocytic leukemia, *J Natl Cancer Inst* 27:1013–1035, 1961.
9. Albuquerque TAF, Drummond do Val L, Doherty A, et al.: From humans to hydra: patterns of cancer across the tree of life, *Biol Rev Camb Philos Soc* 93:1715–1734, 2018.
10. Tomasetti C, Li L, Vogelstein B: Stem cell divisions, somatic mutations, cancer etiology, and cancer prevention, *Science* 355:1330–1334, 2017.
11. Tomasetti C, Vogelstein B: Cancer etiology. Variation in cancer risk among tissues can be explained by the number of stem cell divisions, *Science* 347:78–81, 2015.
12. Tomasetti C, Vogelstein B, Parmigiani G: Half or more of the somatic mutations in cancers of self-renewing tissues originate prior to tumor initiation, *Proc Natl Acad Sci U S A* 110:1999–2004, 2013.
13. Lingaas F, Comstock KE, Kirkness EF, et al.: A mutation in the canine BHD gene is associated with hereditary multifocal renal cystadenocarcinoma and nodular dermatofibrosis in the German Shepherd dog, *Hum Mol Genet* 12:3043–3053, 2003.
14. Karlsson EK, Sigurdsson S, Ivansson E, et al.: Genome-wide analyses implicate 33 loci in heritable dog osteosarcoma, including regulatory variants near CDKN2A/B, *Genome Biol* 14:R132, 2013.
15. Peto R: Quantitative implications of the approximate irrelevance of mammalian body size and lifespan to lifelong cancer risk, *Philos Trans R Soc Lond B Biol Sci* 370, 2015.
16. Abegglen LM, Caulin AF, Chan A, et al.: Potential mechanisms for cancer resistance in elephants and comparative cellular response to DNA damage in humans, *JAMA* 314:1850–1860, 2015.
17. Sulak M, Fong L, Mika K, et al.: TP53 copy number expansion is associated with the evolution of increased body size and an enhanced DNA damage response in elephants, *Elife* 5, 2016.
18. Keane M, Semeiks J, Webb AE, et al.: Insights into the evolution of longevity from the bowhead whale genome, *Cell Rep* 10:112–122, 2015.
19. Park JY, An YR, An CM, et al.: Evolutionary constraints over microsatellite abundance in larger mammals as a potential mechanism against carcinogenic burden, *Sci Rep* 6:25246, 2016.
20. Selman C, Nussey DH, Monaghan P: Ageing: it's a dog's life, *Curr Biol* 23:R451–453, 2013.
21. Larson G, Karlsson EK, Perri A, et al.: Rethinking dog domestication by integrating genetics, archeology, and biogeography, *Proc Natl Acad Sci U S A* 109:8878–8883, 2012.
22. Longhi A, Pasini A, Cicognani A, et al.: Height as a risk factor for osteosarcoma, *J Pediatr Hematol Oncol* 27:314–318, 2005.
23. Mirabello L, Pfeiffer R, Murphy G, et al.: Height at diagnosis and birth-weight as risk factors for osteosarcoma, *Cancer Causes Control* 22:899–908, 2011.
24. Troisi R, Masters MN, Joshipura K, et al.: Perinatal factors, growth and development, and osteosarcoma risk, *Br J Cancer* 95:1603–1607, 2006.
25. Anfinsen KP, Grotmol T, Bruland OS, et al.: Breed-specific incidence rates of canine primary bone tumors—a population based survey of dogs in Norway, *Can J Vet Res* 75:209–215, 2011.
26. Phillips JC, Stephenson B, Hauck M, et al.: Heritability and segregation analysis of osteosarcoma in the Scottish deerhound, *Genomics* 90:354–363, 2007.
27. Melin M, Rivera P, Arendt M, et al.: Genome-wide analysis identifies germ-line risk factors associated with canine mammary tumours, *PLoS Genet* 12:e1006029, 2016.
28. Karyadi DM, Karlins E, Decker B, et al.: A copy number variant at the KITLG locus likely confers risk for canine squamous cell carcinoma of the digit, *PLoS Genet* 9:e1003409, 2013.
29. Savage SA, Mirabello L, Wang Z, et al.: Genome-wide association study identifies two susceptibility loci for osteosarcoma, *Nat Genet* 45:799–803, 2013.
30. Mirabello L, Koster R, Moriarity BS, et al.: A genome-wide scan identifies variants in NFIB associated with metastasis in patients with osteosarcoma, *Cancer Discov* 5:920–931, 2015.
31. Hanahan D, Weinberg RA: Hallmarks of cancer: the next generation, *Cell* 144:646–674, 2011.
32. Hanahan D, Weinberg RA: The hallmarks of cancer, *Cell* 100:57–70, 2000.
33. Ley TJ, Mardis ER, Ding L, et al.: DNA sequencing of a cytogenetically normal acute myeloid leukaemia genome, *Nature* 456:66–72, 2008.
34. Hahn WC, Weinberg RA: Modelling the molecular circuitry of cancer, *Nat Rev Cancer* 2:331–341, 2002.
35. Ruchatz H, Coluccia AM, Stano P, et al.: Constitutive activation of Jak2 contributes to proliferation and resistance to apoptosis in NPM/ALK-transformed cells, *Exp Hematol* 31:309–315, 2003.
36. Modiano JF, Ritt MG, Wojcieszyn J, et al.: Growth arrest of melanoma cells is differentially regulated by contact inhibition and serum deprivation, *DNA Cell Biol* 18:357–367, 1999.

37. Modiano JF, Johnson LD, Bellgrau D: Negative regulators in homeostasis of naive peripheral T cells, *Immunol Res* 41:137–153, 2008.

38. Scott MC, Temiz NA, Sarver AE, et al.: Comparative transcriptome analysis quantifies immune cell transcript levels, metastatic progression, and survival in osteosarcoma, *Cancer Res* 78:326–337, 2018.

39. Fosmire SP, Thomas R, Jubala CM, et al.: Inactivation of the p16 cyclin-dependent kinase inhibitor in high-grade canine non-Hodgkin's T-cell lymphoma, *Vet Pathol* 44:467–478, 2007.

40. Modiano JF, Breen M, Valli VE, et al.: Predictive value of p16 or Rb inactivation in a model of naturally occurring canine non-Hodgkin's lymphoma, *Leukemia* 21:184–187, 2007.

41. Sarver AL, Mills L, T'emiz N, et al.: Comparative genomic analyses of osteosarcoma etiology reveal a chromosomal structural rationale for the increased incidence of osteosarcoma in dogs, *Annual Meeting of the American Association for Cancer Research*, 2018; Asbtract #3399.

42. Kim JH, Megquier K, Sarver AL, et al.: Mutational and transcriptomic profiling identify distinct angiogenic and inflammatory subtypes of angiosarcoma, *Annual Meeting of the American Association for Cancer Research*, 2018; Asbtract #5357.

43. Hammerman PS, Fox CJ, Thompson CB: Beginnings of a signal-transduction pathway for bioenergetic control of cell survival, *Trends Biochem Sci* 29:586–592, 2004.

44. White E, DiPaola RS: The double-edged sword of autophagy modulation in cancer, *Clin Cancer Res* 15:5308–5316, 2009.

45. Ohyashiki JH, Sashida G, Tauchi T, et al.: Telomeres and telomerase in hematologic neoplasia, *Oncogene* 21:680–687, 2002.

46. Pang LY, Argyle DJ: Using naturally occurring tumours in dogs and cats to study telomerase and cancer stem cell biology, *Biochim Biophys Acta* 1792:380–391, 2009.

47. Folkman J: The role of angiogenesis in tumor growth, *Semin Cancer Biol* 3:65–71, 1992.

48. Folkman J: Tumor angiogenesis: therapeutic implications, *N Engl J Med* 285:1182–1186, 1971.

49. Ferrara N, Kerbel RS: Angiogenesis as a therapeutic target, *Nature* 438:967–974, 2005.

50. Buysschaert I, Schmidt T, Roncal C, et al.: Genetics, epigenetics and pharmaco-(epi)genomics in angiogenesis, *J Cell Mol Med* 12:2533–2551, 2008.

51. Jain RK, Duda DG, Willett CG, et al.: Biomarkers of response and resistance to antiangiogenic therapy, *Nat Rev Clin Oncol* 6:327–338, 2009.

52. Carmeliet P, Jain RK: Molecular mechanisms and clinical applications of angiogenesis, *Nature* 473:298–307, 2011.

53. Kim JH, Graef AJ, Dickerson EB, et al.: Pathobiology of hemangiosarcoma in dogs: research advances and future perspectives, *Vet Sci* 2:388–405, 2015.

54. Tamburini BA, Phang TL, Fosmire SP, et al.: Gene expression profiling identifies inflammation and angiogenesis as distinguishing features of canine hemangiosarcoma, *BMC Cancer* 10:619, 2010.

55. Tamburini BA, Trapp S, Phang TL, et al.: Gene expression profiles of sporadic canine hemangiosarcoma are uniquely associated with breed, *PLoS One* 4:e5549, 2009.

56. Clifford CA, Hughes D, Beal MW, et al.: Plasma vascular endothelial growth factor concentrations in healthy dogs and dogs with hemangiosarcoma, *J Vet Intern Med* 15:131–135, 2001.

57. Kim JH, Frantz AM, Anderson KL, et al.: Interleukin-8 promotes canine hemangiosarcoma growth by regulating the tumor microenvironment, *Exp Cell Res* 323:155–164, 2014.

58. Rodriguez AM, Graef AJ, LeVine DN, et al.: Association of sphingosine-1-phosphate (S1P)/S1P receptor-1 pathway with cell proliferation and survival in canine hemangiosarcoma, *J Vet Intern Med* 29:1088–1097, 2015.

59. Megquier K, Tonomura N, Fall T, et al.: *Connecting inherited risk factors, tumor mutation profiles and clinical outcomes in golden retriever hemangiosarcoma*, St. Paul, MN, 2017, International Conference on Advances in Canine and Feline Genomics and Inherited Diseases.

60. Fidler IJ: The pathogenesis of cancer metastasis: the 'seed and soil' hypothesis revisited, *Nat Rev Cancer* 3:453–458, 2003.

61. Kim JW, Wong CW, Goldsmith JD, et al.: Rapid apoptosis in the pulmonary vasculature distinguishes non-metastatic from metastatic melanoma cells, *Cancer Lett* 213:203–212, 2004.

62. Wong CW, Song C, Grimes MM, et al.: Intravascular location of breast cancer cells after spontaneous metastasis to the lung, *Am J Pathol* 161:749–753, 2002.

63. Wong CW, Lee A, Shientag L, et al.: Apoptosis: an early event in metastatic inefficiency, *Cancer Res* 61:333–338, 2001.

64. Koshkina NV, Khanna C, Mendoza A, et al.: Fas-negative osteosarcoma tumor cells are selected during metastasis to the lungs: the role of the Fas pathway in the metastatic process of osteosarcoma, *Mol Cancer Res* 5:991–999, 2007.

65. Krishnan K, Bruce B, Hewitt S, et al.: Ezrin mediates growth and survival in Ewing's sarcoma through the AKT/mTOR, but not the MAPK, signaling pathway, *Clin Exp Metastasis* 23:227–236, 2006.

66. Hunter KW, Amin R, Deasy S, et al.: Genetic insights into the morass of metastatic heterogeneity, *Nat Rev Cancer* 18:211–223, 2018.

67. Scala S: Molecular pathways: targeting the CXCR4-CXCL12 axis—untapped potential in the tumor microenvironment, *Clin Cancer Res* 21:4278–4285, 2015.

68. Im KS, Graef AJ, Breen M, et al.: Interactions between CXCR4 and CXCL12 promote cell migration and invasion of canine hemangiosarcoma, *Vet Comp Oncol* 15:315–327, 2017.

69. Byrum ML, Pondenis HC, Fredrickson RL, et al.: Downregulation of CXCR4 expression and functionality after zoledronate exposure in canine osteosarcoma, *J Vet Intern Med* 30:1187–1196, 2016.

70. Fan TM, Barger AM, Fredrickson RL, et al.: Investigating CXCR4 expression in canine appendicular osteosarcoma, *J Vet Intern Med* 22:602–608, 2008.

71. Boveri T: Concerning the origin of malignant tumours by Theodor Boveri. Translated and annotated by Henry Harris, *J Cell Sci* 121(Suppl 1):1–84, 2008.

72. Loeb LA: Mutator phenotype may be required for multistage carcinogenesis, *Cancer Res* 51:3075–3079, 1991.

73. Pihan G, Doxsey SJ: Mutations and aneuploidy: co-conspirators in cancer? *Cancer Cell* 4:89–94, 2003.

74. Sjoblom T, Jones S, Wood LD, et al.: The consensus coding sequences of human breast and colorectal cancers, *Science* 314:268–274, 2006.

75. Breivik J: The evolutionary origin of genetic instability in cancer development, *Semin Cancer Biol* 15:51–60, 2005.

76. Albertson DG, Collins C, McCormick F, et al.: Chromosome aberrations in solid tumors, *Nat Genet* 34:369–376, 2003.

77. Teixeira MR, Heim S: Multiple numerical chromosome aberrations in cancer: what are their causes and what are their consequences? *Semin Cancer Biol* 15:3–12, 2005.

78. Gollin SM: Mechanisms leading to chromosomal instability, *Semin Cancer Biol* 15:33–42, 2005.

79. Rajagopalan H, Lengauer C: Aneuploidy and cancer, *Nature* 432:338–341, 2004.

80. Maser RS, DePinho RA: Connecting chromosomes, crisis, and cancer, *Science* 297:565–569, 2002.

81. Dvorak HF: Tumors: wounds that do not heal. Similarities between tumor stroma generation and wound healing, *N Engl J Med* 315:1650–1659, 1986.

82. Lin WW, Karin M: A cytokine-mediated link between innate immunity, inflammation, and cancer, *J Clin Invest* 117:1175–1183, 2007.

83. Mantovani A, Allavena P, Sica A, et al.: Cancer-related inflammation, *Nature* 454:436–444, 2008.

84. Bhatia R, McGlave PB, Dewald GW, et al.: Abnormal function of the bone marrow microenvironment in chronic myelogenous leukemia: role of malignant stromal macrophages, *Blood* 85:3636–3645, 1995.

85. Grivennikov SI, Greten FR, Karin M: Immunity, inflammation, and cancer, *Cell* 140:883–899, 2010.

86. Borgatti A, Winter AL, Stuebner K, et al.: Evaluation of 18-F-fluoro-2-deoxyglucose (FDG) positron emission tomography/computed tomography (PET/CT) as a staging and monitoring tool for dogs with stage-2 splenic hemangiosarcoma - a pilot study, *PLoS One* 12:e0172651, 2017.

87. Griffin LR, Thamm DH, Selmic LE, et al.: Pilot study utilizing Fluorine-18 fluorodeoxyglucose-positron emission tomography/computed tomography for glycolytic phenotyping of canine mast cell tumors, *Vet Radiol Ultrasound* 59:461–468, 2018.

88. Leblanc AK, Miller AN, Galyon GD, et al.: Preliminary evaluation of serial (18) FDG-PET/CT to assess response to toceranib phosphate therapy in canine cancer, *Vet Radiol Ultrasound* 53:348–357, 2012.

89. Kim JH, Frantz AM, Sarver AL, et al.: Modulation of fatty acid metabolism and immune suppression are features of in vitro tumour sphere formation in ontogenetically distinct dog cancers, *Vet Comp Oncol* 16:E176–E184, 2018.

90. Dunn GP, Bruce AT, Ikeda H, et al.: Cancer immunoediting: from immunosurveillance to tumor escape, *Nat Immunol* 3:991–998, 2002.

91. Modiano JF, Lindborg BA, McElmurry RT, et al.: Mesenchymal stromal cells inhibit murine syngeneic anti-tumor immune responses by attenuating inflammation and reorganizing the tumor microenvironment, *Cancer Immunol Immunother* 64:1449–1460, 2015.

92. Anderson KL, Modiano JF: Progress in adaptive immunotherapy for cancer in companion animals: success on the path to a cure, *Vet Sci* 2:363–387, 2015.

93. Erez N, Truitt M, Olson P, et al.: Cancer-associated fibroblasts are activated in incipient neoplasia to orchestrate tumor-promoting inflammation in an NF-kappaB-dependent manner, *Cancer Cell* 17:135–147, 2010.

94. Bergman PJ: Anticancer vaccines, *Vet Clin North Am Small Anim Pract* 37:1111–1119, vi-ii, 2007.

95. Alexandrov LB, Stratton MR: Mutational signatures: the patterns of somatic mutations hidden in cancer genomes, *Curr Opin Genet Dev* 24:52–60, 2014.

96. Alexandrov LB, Nik-Zainal S, Wedge DC, et al.: Signatures of mutational processes in human cancer, *Nature* 500:415–421, 2013.

97. Sharma P, Allison JP: Immune checkpoint targeting in cancer therapy: toward combination strategies with curative potential, *Cell* 161:205–214, 2015.

98. Weintraub K: Drug development: Releasing the brakes, *Nature* 504:S6–S8, 2013.

99. Maekawa N, Konnai S, Takagi S, et al.: A canine chimeric monoclonal antibody targeting PD-L1 and its clinical efficacy in canine oral malignant melanoma or undifferentiated sarcoma, *Sci Rep* 7:8951, 2017.

100. Maekawa N, Konnai S, Ikebuchi R, et al.: Expression of PD-L1 on canine tumor cells and enhancement of IFN-gamma production from tumor-infiltrating cells by PD-L1 blockade, *PLoS One* 9:e98415, 2014.

101. Shin IS, Choi EW, Chung JY, et al.: Cloning, expression and bioassay of canine CTLA4Ig, *Vet Immunol Immunopathol* 118:12–18, 2007.

102. Graves SS, Stone D, Loretz C, et al.: Establishment of long-term tolerance to SRBC in dogs by recombinant canine CTLA4-Ig, *Transplantation* 88:317–322, 2009.

103. Mueller MM, Fusenig NE: Friends or foes - bipolar effects of the tumour stroma in cancer, *Nat Rev Cancer* 4:839–849, 2004.

104. Nowell PC: Mechanisms of tumor progression, *Cancer Res* 46:2203–2207, 1986.

105. Modiano JF, Lamerato-Kozicki AR, Jubala CM, et al.: Fas ligand gene transfer for cancer therapy, *Cancer Ther* 2:561–570, 2004.

106. Nguyen DH, Oketch-Rabah HA, Illa-Bochaca I, et al.: Radiation acts on the microenvironment to affect breast carcinogenesis by distinct mechanisms that decrease cancer latency and affect tumor type, *Cancer Cell* 19:640–651, 2011.

107. Ponder BA: Cancer genetics, *Nature* 411:336–341, 2001.

108. Wolffe AP, Matzke MA: Epigenetics: regulation through repression, *Science* 286:481–486, 1999.

109. Costello JF: Comparative epigenomics of leukemia, *Nat Genet* 37:211–212, 2005.

110. Yu L, Liu C, Vandeusen J, et al.: Global assessment of promoter methylation in a mouse model of cancer identifies ID4 as a putative tumor-suppressor gene in human leukemia, *Nat Genet* 37:265–274, 2005.

111. Rendeiro AF, Schmidl C, Strefford JC, et al.: Chromatin accessibility maps of chronic lymphocytic leukaemia identify subtype-specific epigenome signatures and transcription regulatory networks, *Nat Commun* 7:11938, 2016.

112. Cui H, Cruz-Correa M, Giardiello FM, et al.: Loss of IGF2 imprinting: a potential marker of colorectal cancer risk, *Science* 299:1753–1755, 2003.

113. Lapidot T, Sirard C, Vormoor J, et al.: A cell initiating human acute myeloid leukaemia after transplantation into SCID mice, *Nature* 367:645–648, 1994.

114. O'Brien CA, Kreso A, Jamieson CH: Cancer stem cells and self-renewal, *Clin Cancer Res* 16:3113–3120, 2010.

115. Clarke MF, Fuller M: Stem cells and cancer: two faces of eve, *Cell* 124:1111–1115, 2006.

116. Huntly BJ, Gilliland DG: Leukaemia stem cells and the evolution of cancer-stem-cell research, *Nat Rev Cancer* 5:311–321, 2005.

117. Singh SK, Hawkins C, Clarke ID, et al.: Identification of human brain tumour initiating cells, *Nature* 432:396–401, 2004.

118. Smith GH: Mammary cancer and epithelial stem cells: a problem or a solution? *Breast Cancer Res* 4:47–50, 2002.

119. Lamerato-Kozicki AR, Helm KM, Jubala CM, et al.: Canine hemangiosarcoma originates from hematopoietic precursors with potential for endothelial differentiation, *Exp Hematol* 34:870–878, 2006.

120. Wilson H, Huelsmeyer M, Chun R, et al.: Isolation and characterisation of cancer stem cells from canine osteosarcoma, *Vet J* 175:69–75, 2008.

121. Stoica G, Lungu G, Martini-Stoica H, et al.: Identification of cancer stem cells in dog glioblastoma, *Vet Pathol* 46:391–406, 2009.

122. Ito D, Endicott MM, Jubala CM, et al.: A tumor-related lymphoid progenitor population supports hierarchical tumor organization in canine B-cell lymphoma, *J Vet Intern Med* 25:890–896, 2011.

123. Breen M, Modiano JF: Evolutionarily conserved cytogenetic changes in hematological malignancies of dogs and humans—man and his best friend share more than companionship, *Chromosome Res* 16:145–154, 2008.

124. Thomas R, Seiser EL, Motsinger-Reif A, et al.: Refining tumor-associated aneuploidy through 'genomic recoding' of recurrent DNA copy number aberrations in 150 canine non-Hodgkin lymphomas, *Leuk Lymphoma* 52:1321–1335, 2011.

125. Thomas R, Borst L, Rotroff D, et al.: Genomic profiling reveals extensive heterogeneity in somatic DNA copy number aberrations of canine hemangiosarcoma, *Chromosome Res* 22:305–319, 2014.

126. Angstadt AY, Motsinger-Reif A, Thomas R, et al.: Characterization of canine osteosarcoma by array comparative genomic hybridization and RT-qPCR: signatures of genomic imbalance in canine osteosarcoma parallel the human counterpart, *Genes Chromosomes Cancer* 50:859–874, 2011.

127. Hedan B, Thomas R, Motsinger-Reif A, et al.: Molecular cytogenetic characterization of canine histiocytic sarcoma: a spontaneous model for human histiocytic cancer identifies deletion of tumor suppressor genes and highlights influence of genetic background on tumor behavior, *BMC Cancer* 11:201, 2011.

128. Thomas R, Wang HJ, Tsai PC, et al.: Influence of genetic background on tumor karyotypes: evidence for breed-associated cytogenetic aberrations in canine appendicular osteosarcoma, *Chromosome Res* 17:365–377, 2009.

129. Thomas R, Duke SE, Wang HJ, et al.: 'Putting our heads together': insights into genomic conservation between human and canine intracranial tumors, *J Neurooncol* 94:333–349, 2009.

130. Mani RS, Chinnaiyan AM: Triggers for genomic rearrangements: insights into genomic, cellular and environmental influences, *Nat Rev Genet* 11:819–829, 2010.

131. Modiano JF, Breen M, Burnett RC, et al.: Distinct B-cell and T-cell lymphoproliferative disease prevalence among dog breeds indicates heritable risk, *Cancer Res* 65:5654–5661, 2005.

132. Shearin AL, Hedan B, Cadieu E, et al.: The MTAP-CDKN2A locus confers susceptibility to a naturally occurring canine cancer, *Cancer Epidemiol Biomarkers Prev* 21:1019–1027, 2012.

133. Tonomura N, Elvers I, Thomas R, et al.: Genome-wide association study identifies shared risk loci common to two malignancies in golden retrievers, *PLoS Genet* 11:e1004922, 2015.

134. Megquier K, Tonomura N, Fall T, et al.: *Analyzing GWAS data for disease modifiers in 200 cases of hemangiosarcoma in the golden retriever*, Cambridge, U.K., 2015, International Conference on Advances in Canine and Feline Genomics and Inherited Diseases.

135. Arendt ML, Melin M, Tonomura N, et al.: Genome-wide association study of golden retrievers identifies germ-line risk factors predisposing to mast cell tumours, *PLoS Genet* 11:e1005647, 2015.

136. Truve K, Dickinson P, Xiong A, et al.: Utilizing the dog genome in the search for novel candidate genes involved in glioma development-genome wide association mapping followed by targeted massive parallel sequencing identifies a strongly associated locus, *PLoS Genet* 12:e1006000, 2016.

137. Scott MC, Sarver AL, Gavin KJ, et al.: Molecular subtypes of osteosarcoma identified by reducing tumor heterogeneity through an interspecies comparative approach, *Bone* 49:356–367, 2011.

138. Scott MC, Sarver AL, Tomiyasu H, et al.: Aberrant retinoblastoma (RB)-E2F transcriptional regulation defines molecular phenotypes of osteosarcoma, *J Biol Chem* 290:28070–28083, 2015.

139. Gorden BH, Kim JH, Sarver AL, et al.: Identification of three molecular and functional subtypes in canine hemangiosarcoma through gene expression profiling and progenitor cell characterization, *Am J Pathol* 184:985–995, 2014.

140. Elvers I, Turner-Maier J, Swofford R, et al.: Exome sequencing of lymphomas from three dog breeds reveals somatic mutation patterns reflecting genetic background, *Genome Res* 25:1634–1645, 2015.

141. Wang G, Wu M, Maloneyhuss MA, et al.: Actionable mutations in canine hemangiosarcoma, *PLoS One* 12:e0188667, 2017.

142. Sakthikumar S, Elvers I, Kim J, et al.: SETD2 is recurrently mutated in whole-exome sequenced canine osteosarcoma, *Cancer Res* 78:3421–3431, 2018.

143. JU Pontius, Mullikin JC, Smith DR, et al.: Initial sequence and comparative analysis of the cat genome, *Genome Res* 17:1675–1689, 2007.

144. Thomas R, Valli VE, Ellis P, et al.: Microarray-based cytogenetic profiling reveals recurrent and subtype-associated genomic copy number aberrations in feline sarcomas, *Chromosome Res* 17:987–1000, 2009.

145. Modiano JF, Breen M: Shared pathogenesis of human and canine tumors - an inextricable link between cancer and evolution, *Cancer Therapy* 6:239–246, 2008.

146. Carcinogens report adds seven agents, *Cancer Discov* 7(5), 2017.

147. NTP (National Toxicology Program): *Report on Carcinogens*, ed 14, Research Triangle Park, NC, 2016, U.S. Department of Health and Human Services, Public Health Service.

148. World Health Organization: *WHO Report on the Global Tobacco Epidemic, The MPOWER package*, Geneva, 2008, World Health Organization.

149. DeVita VT, Lawrence TS, Rosenberg SA: *Devita, Hellman, and Rosenberg's cancer: principles & practice of oncology*, ed 10, Philadelphia, 2015, Wolters Kluwer.

150. Leonard CT: Environmental tobacco smoke and lung cancer incidence, *Curr Opin Pulm Med* 5:189–193, 1999.

151. Hackshaw AK, Law MR, Wald NJ: The accumulated evidence on lung cancer and environmental tobacco smoke, *Br Med J* 315:980–988, 1997.

152. Reif JS, Dunn K, Ogilvie GK, et al.: Passive smoking and canine lung cancer risk, *Am J Epidemiol* 135:234–239, 1992.

153. Zierenberg-Ripoll A, Pollard RE, Stewart SL, et al.: Association between environmental factors including second-hand smoke and primary lung cancer in dogs, *J Small Anim Pract* 59:343–349, 2018.

154. Reif JS, Bruns C, Lower KS: Cancer of the nasal cavity and paranasal sinuses and exposure to environmental tobacco smoke in pet dogs, *Am J Epidemiol* 147:488–492, 1998.

155. Herrinton LJ, Friedman GD:Cigarette smoking and risk of non-Hodgkin's lymphoma subtypes, *Cancer Epidemiol Biomarkers* 7:25–28, Prev1998.

156. Linet MS, McLaughlin JK, Hsing AW, et al.: Is cigarette smoking a risk factor for non-Hodgkin's lymphoma or multiple myeloma? Results from the Lutheran brotherhood cohort study, *Leuk Res* 16:621–624, 1992.

157. Bertone ER, Snyder LA, Moore AS: Environmental tobacco smoke and risk of malignant lymphoma in pet cats, *Am J Epidemiol* 156:268–273, 2002.

158. Freedman DS, Tolbert PE, Coates R, et al.: Relation of cigarette smoking to non-Hodgkin's lymphoma among middle-aged men, *Am J Epidemiol* 148:833–841, 1998.

159. Marconato L, Leo C, Girelli R, et al.: Association between waste management and cancer in companion animals, *J Vet Intern Med* 23:564–569, 2009.

160. Bertone ER, Snyder LA, Moore AS: Environmental and lifestyle risk factors for oral squamous cell carcinoma in domestic cats, *J Vet Intern Med* 17:557–562, 2003.

161. Snyder LA, Bertone ER, Jakowski RM, et al.: p53 expression and environmental tobacco smoke exposure in feline oral squamous cell carcinoma, *Vet Pathol* 41:209–214, 2004.

162. Gibbons DL, Byers LA, Kurie JM: Smoking, p53 mutation, and lung cancer, *Mol Cancer Res* 12:3–13, 2014.

163. Hecht SS: Lung carcinogenesis by tobacco smoke, *Int J Cancer* 131:2724–2732, 2012.

164. Scesnaite A, Jarmalaite S, Mutanen P, et al.: Similar DNA methylation pattern in lung tumours from smokers and never-smokers with second-hand tobacco smoke exposure, *Mutagenesis* 27:423–429, 2012.

165. Hayes HM, Tarone RE, Cantor KP, et al.: Case-control study of canine malignant lymphoma: positive association with dog owner's use of 2,4-dichlorophenoxyacetic acid herbicides, *J Natl Cancer Inst* 83:1226–1231, 1991.

166. Carlo GL, Cole P, Miller AB, et al.: Review of a study reporting an association between 2,4-dichlorophenoxyacetic acid and canine malignant lymphoma: report of an expert panel, *Regul Toxicol Pharmacol* 16:245–252, 1992.

167. Hayes HM, Tarone RE, Cantor KP: On the association between canine malignant lymphoma and opportunity for exposure to 2,4-dichlorophenoxyacetic acid, *Environ Res* 70:119–125, 1995.

168. Kaneene JB, Miller R: Re-analysis of 2,4-D use and the occurrence of canine malignant lymphoma, *Vet Hum Toxicol* 41:164–170, 1999.

169. Reynolds PM, Reif JS, Ramsdell HS, et al.: Canine exposure to herbicide-treated lawns and urinary excretion of 2,4-dichlorophenoxyacetic acid, *Cancer Epidemiol Biomarkers Prev* 3:233–237, 1994.

170. Gavazza A, Presciuttini S, Barale R, et al.: Association between canine malignant lymphoma, living in industrial areas, and use of chemicals by dog owners, *J Vet Intern Med* 15:190–195, 2001.

171. Takashima-Uebelhoer BB, Barber LG, Zagarins SE, et al.: Household chemical exposures and the risk of canine malignant lymphoma, a model for human non-Hodgkin's lymphoma, *Environ Res* 112:171–176, 2012.

172. Knapp DW, Peer WA, Conteh A, et al.: Detection of herbicides in the urine of pet dogs following lawn chemical application, *Sci Total Environ* 456-457:34–41, 2013.
173. Glickman LT, Schofer FS, McKee LJ, et al.: Epidemiologic study of insecticide exposures, obesity, and risk of bladder cancer in household dogs, *J Toxicol Environ Health* 28:407–414, 1989.
174. Knapp DW, Glickman NW, Denicola DB, et al.: Naturally-occurring canine transitional cell carcinoma of the urinary bladder: a relevant model of human invasive bladder cancer, *Urol Oncol* 5:47–59, 2000.
175. Glickman LT, Raghavan M, Knapp DW, et al.: Herbicide exposure and the risk of transitional cell carcinoma of the urinary bladder in Scottish Terriers, *J Am Vet Med Assoc* 224:1290–1297, 2004.
176. Raghavan M, Knapp DW, Dawson MH, et al.: Topical flea and tick pesticides and the risk of transitional cell carcinoma of the urinary bladder in Scottish Terriers, *J Am Vet Med Assoc* 225:389–394, 2004.
177. Baker GL, Kahl LE, Zee BC, et al.: Malignancy following treatment of rheumatoid arthritis with cyclophosphamide. Long-term case-control follow-up study, *Am J Med* 83:1–9, 1987.
178. Weller RE, Wolf AM, Oyejide A: Transitional cell carcinomas of the bladder associated with cyclophosphamide therapy in a dog, *J Am Anim Hosp Assoc* 15:733–736, 1979.
179. Macy DW, Withrow SJ, Hoopes J: Transitional cell carcinoma of the bladder associated with cyclophosphamide administration, *J Am Anim Hosp Assoc* 19:965–969, 1983.
180. Cox PJ: Cyclophosphamide cystitis—identification of acrolein as the causative agent, *Biochem Pharmacol* 28:2045–2049, 1979.
181. Matz EL, Hsieh MH: Review of advances in uroprotective agents for cyclophosphamide- and ifosfamide-induced hemorrhagic cystitis, *Urology* 100:16–19, 2017.
182. Monach PA, Arnold LM, Merkel PA: Incidence and prevention of bladder toxicity from cyclophosphamide in the treatment of rheumatic diseases: a data-driven review, *Arthritis Rheum* 62:9–21, 2010.
183. Harper A, Blackwood L: Toxicity of metronomic cyclophosphamide chemotherapy in a UK population of cancer-bearing dogs: a retrospective study, *J Small Anim Pract* 58:227–230, 2017.
184. Matsuyama A, Schott CR, Wood GA, et al.: Evaluation of metronomic cyclophosphamide chemotherapy as maintenance treatment for dogs with appendicular osteosarcoma following limb amputation and carboplatin chemotherapy, *J Am Vet Med Assoc* 252:1377–1383, 2018.
185. Best MP, Fry DR: Incidence of sterile hemorrhagic cystitis in dogs receiving cyclophosphamide orally for three days without concurrent furosemide as part of a chemotherapeutic treatment for lymphoma: 57 cases (2007-2012), *J Am Vet Med Assoc* 243:1025–1029, 2013.
186. Charney SC, Bergman PJ, Hohenhaus AE, et al.: Risk factors for sterile hemorrhagic cystitis in dogs with lymphoma receiving cyclophosphamide with or without concurrent administration of furosemide: 216 cases (1990-1996), *J Am Vet Med Assoc* 222:1388–1393, 2003.
187. Mutsaers AJ, Widmer WR, Knapp DW: Canine transitional cell carcinoma, *J Vet Intern Med* 17:136–144, 2003.
188. Reif JS, Cohen D: The environmental distribution of canine respiratory tract neoplasms, *Arch Environ Health* 22:136–140, 1971.
189. Hayes HM, Hoover R, Tarone RE: Bladder cancer in pet dogs: a sentinel for environmental cancer? *Am J Epidemiol* 114:229–233, 1981.
190. Van Der Schalie WH, Gardner Jr HS, Bantle JA, et al.: Animals as sentinels of human health hazards of environmental chemicals, *Environ Health Perspect* 107:309–315, 1999.
191. Bukowski JA, Wartenberg D, Goldschmidt M: Environmental causes for sinonasal cancers in pet dogs, and their usefulness as sentinels of indoor cancer risk, *J Toxicol Environ Health Part A* 54:579–591, 1998.
192. Bukowski JA, Wartenberg D: An alternative approach for investigating the carcinogenicity of indoor air pollution: pets as sentinels of environmental cancer risk, *Environ Health Perspect* 105:1312–1319, 1997.
193. Hargis AM: A review of solar-induced lesions in domestic animals, *Comp Cont Edu* 3:287–294, 1981.
194. Dorn CR, Taylor DON, Schneider R, et al.: Survey of animal neoplasms in Alameda and Contra Costa Counties, California. II. Cancer morbidity in dogs and cats from Alameda County, *J Natl Cancer Inst* 40:307–318, 1968.
195. Schaffer PA, Wobeser B, Martin LE, et al.: Cutaneous neoplastic lesions of equids in the central United States and Canada: 3,351 biopsy specimens from 3,272 equids (2000-2010), *J Am Vet Med Assoc* 242:99–104, 2013.
196. Anderson DE, Badzioch M: Association between solar radiation and ocular squamous cell carcinoma in cattle, *Am J Vet Res* 52:784–788, 1991.
197. Madewell BR, Conroy JD, Hodgkins EM: Sunlight-skin cancer association in the dog: a report of three cases, *J Cutan Pathol* 8:434–443, 1981.
198. Saridomichelakis MN, Day MJ, Apostolidis KN, et al.: Basal cell carcinoma in a dog with chronic solar dermatitis, *J Small Anim Pract* 54:108–111, 2013.
199. Miller MA, Nelson SL, Turk JR, et al.: Cutaneous neoplasia in 340 cats, *Vet Pathol* 28:389–395, 1991.
200. Fu W, Cockerell CJ: The actinic (solar) keratosis: a 21st-century perspective, *Arch Dermatol* 139:66–70, 2003.
201. Khan SG, Bickers DR, Mukhtar H, et al.: Ras p21 farnesylation in ultraviolet B radiation - induced tumors in the skin of SKH-1 hairless mice, *J Invest Dermatol* 102:754–758, 1994.
202. Lowe NJ, Weingarten D, Wortzman M: Sunscreens and phototesting, *Clin Dermatol* 6:40–49, 1988.
203. Hanahan D, Weinberg RA: Hallmarks of cancer: the next generation, *Cell* 144:646–674, 2011.
204. Bernays ME, Flemming D, Peiffer Jr RL: Primary corneal papilloma and squamous cell carcinoma associated with pigmentary keratitis in four dogs, *J Am Vet Med Assoc* 214:215–217, 1999.
205. Hakanson N, Shively JN, Reed RE: Intraocular spindle cell sarcoma following ocular trauma in a cat: case report and literature review, *J Am Anim Hosp Assoc* 26:63–66, 1990.
206. Dickinson R, Bauer B, Gardhouse S, et al.: Intraocular sarcoma associated with a ruptured lens in a rabbit (*Oryctolagus cuniculus*), *Vet Ophthalmol* 16(Suppl 1):168–172, 2013.
207. Wertheimer N, Leeper E: Electrical wiring configurations and childhood cancer, *Am J Epidemiol* 109:273–284, 1979.
208. Reif JS, Lower KS, Ogilvie GK: Residential exposure to magnetic fields and risk of canine lymphoma, *Am J Epidemiol* 141:352–359, 1995.
209. National Research Council (US): *Committee on the Possible Effects of Electromagnetic Fields on Biologic Systems, Possible health effects of exposure to residential electric and magnetic fields*, Washington, DC, 1997, National Academies Press.
210. Thrall DE: Orthovoltage radiotherapy of acanthomatous epulides in 39 dogs, *J Am Vet Med Assoc* 184:826–829, 1984.
211. McEntee MC, Page RL, Théon A, et al.: Malignant tumor formation in dogs previously irradiated for acanthomatous epulis, *Vet Radiol Ultrasound* 45:357–361, 2004.
212. Kuttesch JF, Wexler LH, Marcus RB, et al.: Second malignancies after Ewing's sarcoma: radiation dose-dependency of secondary sarcomas, *J Clin Oncol* 14:2818–2825, 1996.
213. Hall EJ, Wuu CS: Radiation-induced second cancers: the impact of 3D-CRT and IMRT, *Int J Radiat Oncol Biol Phys* 56:83–88, 2003.
214. Suit H, Goldberg S, Niemierko A, et al.: Secondary carcinogenesis in patients treated with radiation: a review of data on radiation-induced cancers in human, non-human primate, canine and rodent subjects, *Radiat Res* 167:12–42, 2007.

215. White RA, Jefferies AR, Gorman NT: Sarcoma development following irradiation of acanthomatous epulis in two dogs, *Vet Rec* 118:668, 1986.
216. McChesney SL, Withrow SJ, Gillette EL, et al.: Radiotherapy of soft tissue sarcomas in dogs, *J Am Vet Med Assoc* 194:60–63, 1989.
217. Gillette SM, Gillette EL, Powers BE, et al.: Radiation-induced osteosarcoma in dogs after external beam or intraoperative radiation therapy, *Cancer Res* 50:54–57, 1990.
218. Patel TR, Chiang VL: Secondary neoplasms after stereotactic radiosurgery, *World Neurosurg* 81:594–599, 2014.
219. Lewis CG, Sunderman FW: Metal carcinogenesis in total joint arthroplasty: animal models, *Clin Orthop Relat Res* 329(Suppl):S264–S268, 1996.
220. Li XQ, Hom DL, Black J: Relationship between metallic implants and cancer: a case-control study in a canine population, *Vet Comp Orthop Traumatol* 6:70–74, 1993.
221. Selmic LE, Ryan SD, Boston SE, et al.: Osteosarcoma following tibial plateau leveling osteotomy in dogs: 29 cases (1997-2011), *J Am Vet Med Assoc* 244:1053–1059, 2014.
222. Arthur EG, Arthur GL, Keeler MR, et al.: Risk of osteosarcoma in dogs after open fracture fixation, *Vet Surg* 45:30–35, 2016.
223. Sartor AJ, Ryan SD, Sellmeyer T, et al.: Bi-institutional retrospective cohort study evaluating the incidence of osteosarcoma following tibial plateau levelling osteotomy (2000-2009), *Vet Comp Orthop Traumatol* 27:339–345, 2014.
224. Gilley RS, Hiebert E, Clapp K, et al.: Long-term formation of aggressive bony lesions in dogs with mid-diaphyseal fractures stabilized with metallic plates: incidence in a tertiary referral hospital population, *Front Vet Sci* 4:3, 2017.
225. Burton AG, Johnson EG, Vernau W, et al.: Implant-associated neoplasia in dogs: 16 cases (1983-2013), *J Am Vet Med Assoc* 247:778–785, 2015.
226. Rowland PH, Moise NS, Severson D: Myxoma at the site of a subcutaneous pacemaker in a dog, *J Am Anim Hosp Assoc* 27:649–651, 1991.
227. Pardo AD, Adams WH, McCracken MD, et al.: Primary jejunal osteosarcoma associated with a surgical sponge in a dog, *J Am Vet Med Assoc* 196:935–938, 1990.
228. Corbin EE, Cavanaugh RP, Fick JL, et al.: Foreign body reaction to a retained surgical sponge (gossypiboma) mimicking an implant associated sarcoma in a dog after a tibial plateau levelling osteotomy, *Vet Comp Orthop Traumatol* 26:147–153, 2013.
229. Rayner EL, Scudamore CL, Francis I, et al.: Abdominal fibrosarcoma associated with a retained surgical swab in a dog, *J Comp Pathol* 143:81–85, 2010.
230. Thieman Mankin KM, Dunbar MD, Toplon D, et al.: Rhabdomyosarcoma associated with the lead wire of a pacemaker generator implant, *Vet Clin Pathol* 43:276–280, 2014.
231. Orenstein MR, Schenker MB: Environmental asbestos exposure and mesothelioma, *Curr Opin Pulm Med* 6:371–377, 2000.
232. Glickman LT, Domanski LM, Maguire TG, et al.: Mesothelioma in pet dogs associated with exposure of their owners to asbestos, *Environ Res* 32:305–313, 1983.
233. Harbison ML, Godleski JJ: Malignant mesothelioma in urban dogs, *Vet Pathol* 20:531–540, 1983.
234. Machida N, Tanaka R, Takemura N, et al.: Development of pericardial mesothelioma in golden retrievers with a long-term history of idiopathic haemorrhagic pericardial effusion, *J Comp Pathol* 131:166–175, 2004.
235. Smith AN: The role of neutering in cancer development, *Vet Clin North Am Small Anim Pract* 44:965–975, 2014.
236. Moulton JE: Tumors of the mammary gland. In Moulton JE, editor: *Tumors in domestic animals*, ed 3, Berkley, CA, 1990, University of California Press, pp 518–552.
237. Schneider R, Dorn CR, Taylor DON: Factors influencing canine mammary cancer development and postsurgical survival, *J Natl Cancer Inst* 43:1249–1261, 1969.
238. Brodey RS, Goldschmidt MH, Roszel JR: Canine mammary gland neoplasms, *J Am Anim Hosp Assoc* 19:61–90, 1983.
239. Perez Alenza MD, Peña L, Del Castillo N, et al.: Factors influencing the incidence and prognosis of canine mammary tumours, *J Small Anim Pract* 41:287–291, 2000.
240. Beauvais W, Cardwell JM, Brodbelt DC: The effect of neutering on the risk of mammary tumours in dogs—a systematic review, *J Small Anim Pract* 53:314–322, 2012.
241. Kristiansen VM, Nodtvedt A, Breen AM, et al.: Effect of ovariohysterectomy at the time of tumor removal in dogs with benign mammary tumors and hyperplastic lesions: a randomized controlled clinical trial, *J Vet Intern Med* 27:935–942, 2013.
242. Kristiansen VM, Pena L, Diez Cordova L, et al.: Effect of ovariohysterectomy at the time of tumor removal in dogs with mammary carcinomas: a randomized controlled trial, *J Vet Intern Med* 30:230–241, 2016.
243. Panko WB, Patnaik AK, Harvey HJ, et al.: Estrogen receptors in canine mammary tumors, *Cancer Res* 42:2255–2259, 1982.
244. Mialot JP, Andre F, Martin PH, et al.: Etude de recepteurs des hormones steroides dans les tumeurs mammaires de la chienne. II. Correlations avec quelques caracteristques cliniques, *Rec Med Vet* 158:513–521, 1982.
245. Monson KR, Malbica JO, Hubben K: Determination of estrogen receptors in canine mammary tumors, *Am J Vet Res* 38:1937–1939, 1977.
246. Donnay I, Rauïs J, Devleeschouwer N, et al.: Comparison of estrogen and progesterone receptor expression in normal and tumor mammary tissues from dogs, *Am J Vet Res* 56:1188–1194, 1995.
247. Elling H, Ungemach FR: Simultaneous occurrence of receptors for estradiol, progesterone, and dihydrotestosterone in canine mammary tumors, *J Cancer Res Clin Oncol* 105:231–237, 1983.
248. Sartin EA, Barnes S, Kwapien RP, et al.: Estrogen and progesterone receptor status of mammary carcinomas and correlation with clinical outcome in dogs, *Am J Vet Res* 53:2196–2200, 1992.
249. Rutteman GR, Misdorp W, Misdorp W, et al.: OEstrogen (ER) and progestin receptors (PR) in mammary tissue of the female dog: different receptor profile in non-malignant and malignant states, *Br J Cancer* 58:594–599, 1988.
250. Rutteman GR: Hormones and mammary tumour disease in the female dog: an update, *In Vivo* 4:33–40, 1990.
251. Støvring M, Moe L, Glattre E: A population-based case-control study of canine mammary tumours and clinical use of medroxyprogesterone acetate, *APMIS* 105:590–596, 1997.
252. Zanninovic P, Simcic V: Epidemiology of mammary tumors in dogs, *Eur J Comp Anim Pract* 4:67–76, 1994.
253. Lantinga-van Leeuwen IS, Van Garderen E, Rutteman GR, et al.: Cloning and cellular localization of the canine progesterone receptor: co-localization with growth hormone in the mammary gland, *J Steroid Biochem Mol Biol* 75:219–228, 2000.
254. Mol JA, Lantinga-van Leeuwen I, Van Garderen E, et al.: Progestin-induced mammary growth hormone (GH) production, *Adv Exp Med Biol* 480:71–76, 2000.
255. Rijnberk A, Kooistra HS, Mol JA: Endocrine diseases in dogs and cats: Similarities and differences with endocrine diseases in humans, *Growth Horm IGF Res* 13:S158–S164, 2003.
256. Hayes HM, Milne KL, Mandell CP: Epidemiological features of feline mammary carcinoma, *Vet Rec* 108:476–479, 1981.
257. Misdorp W, Romijn A, Hart AAM: Feline mammary tumors: a case-control study of hormonal factors, *Anticancer Res* 11:1793–1797, 1991.
258. Overley B, Shofer FS, Goldschmidt MH, et al.: Association between ovarihysterectomy and feline mammary carcinoma, *J Vet Intern Med* 19:560–563, 2005.
259. National Cancer Institute: *Surveillance, epidemiology, and end results program public use data, (1973-2000)*, Bethesda, MD. 2003.

260. Villamil JA, Henry CJ, Hahn AW, et al.: Hormonal and sex impact on the epidemiology of canine lymphoma, *J Cancer Epidemiol*590753, 2009.

261. Torres de la Riva G, Hart BL, Farver TB, et al.: Neutering dogs: effects on joint disorders and cancers in golden retrievers, *PLoS One* 8:e55937, 2013.

262. Zink MC, Farhoody P, Elser SE, et al.: Evaluation of the risk and age of onset of cancer and behavioral disorders in gonadectomized Vizslas, *J Am Vet Med Assoc* 244:309–319, 2014.

263. Belanger JM, Bellumori TP, Bannasch DL, et al.: Correlation of neuter status and expression of heritable disorders, *Canine Genet Epidemiol* 4(6), 2017.

264. Ru G, Terracini B, Glickman LT: Host related risk factors for canine osteosarcoma, *Vet J* 156:31–39, 1998.

265. Cooley DM, Beranek BC, Schlittler DL, et al.: Endogenous gonadal hormone exposure and bone sarcoma risk, *Cancer Epidemiol Biomarkers Prev* 11:1434–1440, 2002.

266. Kent MS, Burton JH, Dank G, et al.: Association of cancer-related mortality, age and gonadectomy in golden retriever dogs at a veterinary academic center (1989-2016), *PLoS One* 13:e0192578, 2018.

267. White CR, Hohenhaus AE, Kelsey J, et al.: Cutaneous MCTs: associations with spay/neuter status, breed, body size, and phylogenetic cluster, *J Am Anim Hosp Assoc* 47:210–216, 2011.

268. Larsen AE, Grier RL: Evaluation of canine mast cell tumors for presence of estrogen receptors, *Am J Vet Res* 50:1779–1780, 1989.

269. Elling H, Ungemach FR: Sexual hormone receptors in canine mast cell tumour cytosol, *J Comp Pathol* 92:629–630, 1982.

270. Dow SW, Olson PN, Rosychuk RAW, et al.: Perianal adenomas and hypertestosteronemia in a spayed bitch with pituitary-dependent hyperadrenocorticism, *J Am Vet Med Assoc* 192:1439–1441, 1988.

271. Wilson GP, Hayes Jr HM: Castration for treatment of perianal gland neoplasms in the dog, *J Am Vet Med Assoc* 174:1301–1303, 1979.

272. Waters DJ, Sakr WA, Hayden DW, et al.: Workgroup 4: Spontaneous prostate carcinoma in dogs and nonhuman primates, *Prostate* 36:64–67, 1998.

273. Madewell BR, Gandour-Edwards R, DeVere White RW: Canine prostatic intraepithelial neoplasia: is the comparative model relevant? *Prostate* 58:314–317, 2004.

274. Teske E, Naan EC, Van Dijk EM, et al.: Canine prostate carcinoma: epidemiological evidence of an increased risk in castrated dogs, *Mol Cell Endocrinol* 197:251–255, 2002.

275. Sorenmo KU, Goldschmidt M, Shofer F, et al.: Immunohistochemical characterization of canine prostatic carcinoma and correlation with castration status and castration time, *Vet Comp Oncol* 1:48–56, 2003.

276. Bryan JN, Keeler MR, Henry CJ, et al.: A population study of neutering status as a risk factor for canine prostate cancer, *Prostate* 67:1174–1181, 2007.

277. Benchimol S, Minden MD: Viruses, oncogenes, and tumor suppressor genes. In Tannock IF, Hill RP, editors: *The basic science of oncology*, ed 3, New York, 1998, McGraw-Hill, pp 79–105.

278. Pfister HH: Biology and biochemistry of papillomaviruses, *Rev Physiol Biochem Pharmacol* 99:111–181, 1984.

279. Sundberg JP, Reszler AA, Williams ES, et al.: An oral papillomavirus that infected one coyote and three dogs, *Vet Pathol* 28:87–88, 1991.

280. Munday JS, Knight CG: Amplification of feline sarcoid-associated papillomaviruses DNA sequences from bovine skin, *Vet Dermatol* 21:341–344, 2010.

281. Belkin PV: Ocular lesions in canine oral papillomatosis, *Vet Med Small Anim Clin* 74:1520–1524, 1979.

282. Watrach AM, Small E, Case MT: Canine papilloma: progression of oral papilloma to carcinoma, *J Natl Cancer Inst* 45:915–920, 1970.

283. Nicholls PE, Starley MA: The immunology of animal papillomaviruses, *Vet Immunol Immunopathol* 73:101–127, 2000.

284. Tokita H, Konishi S: Studies on canine oral papillomatosis. II. Oncogenicity of canine oral papilloma virus to various tissues of dog with special reference to eye tumor, *Jpn J Vet Sci* 37:109–120, 1975.

285. Bregman CL, Hirth RS, Sundberg JP, et al.: Cutaneous neoplasms in dogs associated with canine oral papillomavirus, *Vet Pathol* 24:477–487, 1987.

286. Theilen GH, Madewell BR: Papillomatosis and fibromatosis. In Theilen GH, Madewell BR, editors: *Veterinary cancer medicine*, Philadelphia, 1987, Lea &Febinger, pp 267–281.

287. Calvert CA: Canine viral papillomatosis. In Greene GE, editor: *Infectious diseases of the dog and cat*, Philadelphia, 1991, WB Saunders, pp 288–290.

288. Callan MB, Preziosi D, Mauldin E: Multiple papillomavirus-associated epidermal hamartomas and squamous cell carcinomas in situ in a dog following treatment with prednisone and cyclosporine, *Vet Dermatol* 16:338–345, 2005.

289. Nagata M: Canine papillomatosis. In Bonagura JD, editor: *Kirk's current veterinary therapy XIII*, Philadelphia, 2000, WB Saunders, pp 569–571.

290. Bonney CH, Koch SA, Dice PF, et al.: Papillomatosis of conjunctiva and adnexa in dogs, *J Am Vet Med Assoc* 176:48–51, 1980.

291. Kuntsi-Vaattovaara H, Verstraete FJM, Newsome JT, et al.: Resolution of persistent oral papillomatosis in a dog after treatment with a recombinant canine oral papillomavirus vaccine, *Vet Comp Oncol* 1:57–63, 2003.

292. Bomholt A: Interferon therapy for laryngeal papillomatosis in adults, *Arch Otolaryngol* 109:550–552, 1983.

293. Sundberg JP, Smith EK, Herron AJ, et al.: Cutaneous verrucosis in a Chinese Sharpei dog, *Vet Pathol* 31:183–187, 1994.

294. Nagata M, Nanko H, Moriyana A, et al.: Pigmented plaques associated with papillomavirus infection in dogs: is this epidermodysplasia verruciformis? *Vet Dermatol* 6:179–186, 1995.

295. Bregman CL, Hinth RS, Sundberg JP, et al.: Cutaneous neoplasms in dogs associated with canine oral papillomavirus vaccine, *Vet Pathol* 24:477–487, 1987.

296. Meunier LD: Squamous cell carcinoma in beagles subsequent to canine oral papillomavirus vaccine, *Lab Anim Sci* 40:568, 1990 (Abstract).

297. Munday JS, Willis KA, Kiupel M, et al.: Amplification of three different papillomaviral DNA sequences from a cat with viral plaques, *Vet Dermatol* 19:400–404, 2008.

298. Schulman FY, Krafft AE, Janczewski T, et al.: Cutaneous fibropapilloma in a mountain lion *(Felis concolor)*, *J Zoo Wildl Med* 34:179–183, 2003.

299. Sundberg JP, Van Ranst M, Montali R, et al.: Feline papillomas and papillomaviruses, *Vet Pathol* 37:1–10, 2000.

300. Egberink HF, Horzinek MC: Feline viral papillomatosis. In Greene CE, editor: *Infectious diseases of the dog and cat*, 2nd ed Philadelphia, 1998, WB Saunders.

301. Lozano-Alarcon F, Lewis TP, Clark EG, et al.: Persistent papillomavirus infection in a cat, *J Am Anim Hosp Assoc* 32:392–396, 1996.

302. LeClerc SM, Clark EG, Haines DM: Papillomavirus infection in association with feline cutaneous squamous cell carcinoma *in situ*, *Proc Am Assoc Vet Derm/Am Coll Vet Derm* 13:125, 1997 (abstract).

303. Schulman FY, Krafft AE, Janczewski T: Feline cutaneous fibropapillomas: clinicopathologic findings and association with papillomavirus infection, *Vet Pathol* 38:291–296, 2001.

304. Teifke JP, Kidney BA, Lohr CV, et al.: Detection of papillomavirus DNA in mesenchymal tumour cells and not in the hyperplastic epithelium of feline sarcoids, *Vet Dermatol* 14:47–56, 2003.

305. Gill VL, Bergman PJ, Baer KE, et al.: Use of imiquimod cream (Aldara) in cats with multicentric squamous cell carcinoma in situ: 12 cases (2002-2005), *Vet Comp Oncol* 16:55–64, 2008.

306. Rojko JL, Hardy Jr WD: Feline leukemia virus and other retroviruses. In Sherding RG, editor: *The cat: diseases and clinical management*, 2nd ed? New York, 1994, Churchill Livingstone, pp 263–432.

307. Cotter SM: Feline viral neoplasia. In Greene CE, editor: *Infectious diseases of the dog and cat*, 2nd ed? Philadelphia, 1998, WB Saunders.

308. Hardy Jr WD, Hess PW, MacEwen EG, et al.: Biology of feline leukemia virus in the natural environment, *Cancer Res* 36:582–588, 1976.

309. Essex M: Feline leukemia and sarcoma viruses. In Klein G, editor: *Viral oncology*, New York, 1980, Raven Press.

310. Hardy Jr WD: The feline leukemia virus, *J Am Anim Hosp Assoc* 17:951, 1981.

311. Pedersen NC: Feline immunodeficiency virus. In Schellekens LT, Horzinek MC, editors: *Animal models in AIDS*, Amsterdam, 1990, Elsevier.

312. Hardy Jr WD: The feline sarcoma viruses, *J Am Anim Hosp Assoc* 17:981, 1981.

313. Benveniste RE, Sherr CJ, Todaro GJ: Evolution of type C viral genes: origin of feline leukemia virus, *Science* 190:886–888, 1975.

314. Daniels MJ, Golder MC, Jarrett O, et al.: Feline viruses in wildcats from Scotland, *J Wildl Dis* 35:121–124, 1999.

315. Marker L, Munson L, Basson PA, et al.: Multicentric T-cell lymphoma associated with feline leukemia virus infection in a captive Namibian cheetah *(Acinonyx jubatus)*, *J Wildl Dis* 39:690–695, 2003.

316. Schafer W, Bolognesi DP: Mammalian type C oncornaviruses: relationships between viral structure and cell surface antigens and their possible significance in immunological defense mechanisms, *Contemp Top Immunobiol* 6:127–167, 1977.

317. Bolognesi DP, Montelaro RC, Frank H, et al.: Assembly of type C oncornaviruses: a model, *Science* 199:183–186, 1978.

318. Hardy Jr WD: Immunology of oncornaviruses, *Vet Clin North Am* 4:133–146, 1974.

319. Sarma PS, Log T: Subgroup classification of feline leukemia and sarcoma viruses by viral interference and neutralization tests, *Virology* 54:160–169, 1973.

320. Sarma PS, Log T, Jain D, et al.: Differential host range of viruses of feline leukemia-sarcoma complex, *Virology* 64:438–446, 1975.

321. Hardy WD Jr, Hirshaut Y, Hess P: Detection of the feline leukemia virus and other mammalian oncornaviruses by immunofluorescence. In Dutcher RM, Chieco-Bianchi L, editors: *Unifying concepts of leukemia*, Basel: S Karger, 1973, pp 833–841.

322. Francis DP, Essex M, Gayzagian D: Feline leukemia virus: survival under home and laboratory conditions, *J Clin Microbiol* 9:154–156, 1979.

323. Dornsife RE, Gasper PW, Mullins JI: Induction of aplastic anemia by intrabone marrow inoculation of a molecularly cloned feline retrovirus, *Leuk Res* 13:745–755, 1989.

324. Hartmann K, Werner RM, Egberink H, et al.: Comparison of six in-house tests for the rapid diagnosis of feline immunodeficiency and feline leukaemia virus infections, *Vet Rec* 149:317–320, 2001.

325. Lauring AS, Anderson MM, Overbaugh J: Specificity in receptor usage by T-cell–tropic feline leukemia viruses: implications for the in vivo tropism of immunodeficiency-inducing variants, *J Virol* 75:8888–8898, 2001.

326. Lauring AS, Cheng HH, Eiden MV, et al.: Genetic and biochemical analyses of receptor and cofactor determinants for T-cell–tropic feline leukemia virus infection, *J Virol* 76:8069–8078, 2002.

327. Essex M, Cotter SM, Sliski AH, et al.: Horizontal transmission of feline leukaemia under natural conditions in a feline leukaemia cluster household, *Int J Cancer* 19:90–96, 1977.

328. Vail DM, Moore AS, Ogilvie GK, et al.: Feline lymphoma (145 cases): proliferation indices, CD3 immunoreactivity and their association with prognosis in 90 cats receiving therapy, *J Vet Intern Med* 12:349–354, 1998.

329. Louwerens M, London CA, Pedersen NC, et al.: Feline lymphoma in the post-feline leukemia virus era, *J Vet Intern Med* 19:329–335, 2005.

330. Jarrett O, Hardy Jr WD, Golder MC, et al.: The frequency of occurrence of feline leukaemia virus subgroups in cats, *Int J Cancer* 21:334–337, 1978.

331. Jarrett O, Russell PH: Differential growth and transmission in cats of feline leukaemia viruses of subgroups A and B, *Int J Cancer* 21:466–472, 1978.

332. Rosenberg Z, Pederson ZF, Haseltine WA: Comparative analysis of the genome of feline leukemia virus, *J Virol* 35:542–546, 1980.

333. Tzavaras T, Stewart M, McDougall A, et al.: Molecular cloning and characterization of a defective recombinant feline leukaemia virus associated with myeloid leukaemia, *J Gen Virol* 71:343–354, 1990.

334. Stewart MA, Warnock M, Wheeler A, et al.: Nucleotide sequences of a feline leukemia virus subgroup: a envelope gene and long terminal repeat and evidence for the recombinational origin of subgroup B viruses, *J Virol* 58:825–834, 1986.

335. Elder JM, Mullins JI: Nucleotide sequence of the envelope gene of Gardner-Arnstein feline leukemia virus B reveals unique sequence homologies with a murine mink cell focus-forming virus, *J Virol* 46:871–880, 1983.

336. Rigby MA, Rojko JL, Stewart MA, et al.: Partial dissociation of subgroup C phenotype and in vivo behaviour in feline leukaemia viruses with chimeric envelope genes, *J Gen Virol* 73:2839–2847, 1992.

337. Heding LD, Schaller JP, Blakeslee JR, et al.: Inactivation of tumor cell–associated feline oncornavirus for preparation of an infectious virus–free tumor cell immunogen, *Cancer Res* 36:1647–1652, 1976.

338. Essex M, Klein G, Snyder SP, et al.: Correlation between humoral antibody and regression of tumours induced by feline sarcoma virus, *Nature* 233:195–196, 1971.

339. Vedbrat S, Rasheed S, Lutz H, et al.: Feline oncornavirus–associated cell membrane antigen: a viral and not a cellularly coded transformation-specific antigen of cat lymphomas, *Virology* 124:445–461, 1983.

340. Snyder HW, Singhal MC, Zuckerman EE, et al.: The feline oncornavirus associated cell membrane antigen (FOCMA) is related to, but distinguishable from, FeLV-C gp70, *Virology* 131:315–327, 1983.

341. Macy DW: Vaccination against feline retroviruses. In August J, editor: *Consultations in feline internal medicine*, Philadelphia, 1994, WB Saunders, pp 33–39.

342. Dorn CR, Taylor DON, Schneider R, et al.: Survey of animal neoplasms in Alameda and Contra Costa counties, California. II. Cancer morbidity in dogs and cats from Alameda county, *J Natl Cancer Inst* 40:307–318, 1968.

343. Schneider R: Comparison and age- and sex-specific incidence rate patterns of the leukemia complex in the cat and the dog, *J Natl Cancer Inst* 70:971–977, 1983.

344. Goitsuka R, Tsuji M, Matsumoto Y, et al.: A case of feline large granular lymphoma, *Jpn J Vet Sci* 50:593–595, 1988.

345. Finn JP, Schwartz LW: A neoplasm of globule leukocytes in the intestine of a cat, *J Comp Pathol* 82:323–326, 1972.

346. Hardy Jr WD, McClelland AJ, Zuckerman EE, et al.: Development of virus non-producer lymphosarcomas in pet cats exposed to FeLV, *Nature* 288:90–92, 1980.

347. Hardy Jr WD, Zuckerman EE, McClelland AJ, et al.: The immunology and epidemiology of FeLV-nonproducer feline lymphosarcomas, *Cold Spring Harbor Conf Cell Prolif* 7:677, 1980.

348. Hardy Jr WD: Hematopoietic tumors of cats, *J Am Anim Hosp Assoc* 17:921–940, 1981.

349. Spodnick GJ, Berg J, Moore FM, et al.: Spinal lymphoma in cats: 21 cases (1976-1989), *J Am Vet Med Assoc* 200:373–376, 1992.

350. Hartmann K, Gerle K, Leutenegger C, et al.: *Feline leukemia virus: most important oncogene in cats? Abstracts from the Fourth International Feline Retrovirus Research Symposium*, 1998. Glasgow.

351. Teske E, van Straten G, van Noort R, et al.: Chemotherapy with cyclophosphamide, vincristine, and prednisolone (COP) in cats with malignant lymphoma: new results with an old protocol, *J Vet Intern Med* 16:179–186, 2002.

352. Shelton GH, Grant CK, Cotter SM, et al.: Feline immunodeficiency virus and feline leukemia virus infections and their relationships to lymphoid malignancies in cats: a retrospective study (1968-1988), *J Acquir Immune Defic Syndr* 3:623–630, 1990.

353. Hardy Jr WD, Zuckerman BE, MacEwen EG, et al.: A feline leukemia and sarcoma virus–induced tumor-specific antigen, *Nature* 270:249–251, 1977.

354. Hardy Jr WD, Zuckerman EE, Essex M, et al.: Feline oncornavirus–associated cell membrane antigen: anFeLV- and FeSV-induced tumor-specific antigen. In Clarkson B, Marks PA, Till JE, editors: *Differentiation of normal and neoplastic hematopoietic cells. Cold Spring Harbor*, New York, 1978, Cold Spring Harbor Laboratory Press.

355. Francis DP, Cotter SM, Hardy Jr WD, et al.: Comparison of virus-positive and virus-negative cases of feline leukemia and lymphoma, *Cancer Res* 39:3866–3870, 1979.

356. McClelland AJ, Hardy WD, Zuckerman EE: Prognosis of healthy feline leukemia virus infected cats. In Hardy WD, Essex M, McClelland AJ, editors: *Feline leukemia virus*, New York, 1980, Elsevier/North-Holland, pp 121–126.

357. Cotter SM: Feline leukemia virus: pathophysiology, prevention and treatment, *Cancer Invest* 10:173–181, 1992.

358. Cotter SM: Management of healthy feline leukemia virus–positive cats, *J Am Vet Med Assoc* 199:1470–1473, 1991.

359. August JR: Husbandry practices for cats infected with feline leukemia virus or feline immunodeficiency virus, *J Am Vet Med Assoc* 199:1474–1477, 1991.

360. Kociba GJ, Lange RD, Dunn CD, et al.: Serum erythropoietin changes in cats with feline leukemia virus–induced erythroid aplasia, *Vet Pathol* 20:548–552, 1983.

361. Snyder Jr HW, Singhal MC, Hardy Jr WD, et al.: Clearance of feline leukemia virus from persistently infected pet cats treated by extracorporeal immunoadsorption is correlated with an enhanced antibody response to FeLV gp70, *J Immunol* 132:1538–1543, 1984.

362. MacEwen EG: *Current immunotherapeutic approaches in small animals*, Columbus, OH, 1986, Proceedings of the KalKan Symposium on Oncology.

363. Kitchen LW, Mather FJ: Hematologic effects of short-term oral diethylcarbamazine treatment given to chronically feline leukemia virus infected cats, *Cancer Lett* 45:183–187, 1989.

364. Kitchen LW, Cotter SM: Effect of diethylcarbamazine on serum antibody to feline oncornavirus–associated cell membrane antigen in feline leukemia virus cats, *J Clin Lab Immunol* 25:101–103, 1988.

365. Barta O: Immunoadjuvant therapy. In Kirk RW, Bonagura JD, editors: *Kirk's current veterinary therapy XI: small animal practice*, Philadelphia, 1992, WB Saunders, pp 217–223.

366. Elmslie RE, Ogilvie GK, Dow SW, et al.: Evaluation of a biologic response modifier derived from *Serratia marcescens*: effects on feline macrophages and usefulness for the prevention and treatment of viremia in feline leukemia virus–infected cats, *Mol Biother* 3:231–238, 1991.

367. Gasper PW, Fulton R, Thrall MA: Bone marrow transplantation: update and current considerations. In Kirk RW, Bonagura JD, editors: *Kirk's current veterinary therapy XI: small animal practice*, Philadelphia, 1992, W.B. Saunders, pp 493–495.

368. Tompkins MB, Cummins JM: Response of feline leukemia virus–induced nonregenerative anemia to oral administration of an interferon-containing preparation, *Feline Pract* 12:6–15, 1982.

369. Tizard I: Use of immunomodulators as an aid to clinical management of feline leukemia virus–infected cats, *J Am Vet Med Assoc* 199:1482–1485, 1991.

370. Gingerich DA: Lymphocyte T-cell immunomodulator (LTCI): review of the immunopharmacology of a new veterinary biologic, *Intern J Applied Res Vet Med* 6:61–68, 2008.

371. Polas PV, Swenson CL, Sams R, et al.: In vitro and in vivo evidence that the antiviral activity of 2-3-dideoxycytidine is target cell–dependent in a feline retrovirus animal model, *Antimicrob Agents Chemother* 34:1414–1421, 1990.

372. Zeidner NS, Strobel JD, Perigo NA, et al.: Treatment of FeLV-induced immunodeficiency syndrome (FeLV-FAIDS) with controlled release capsular implantation of 2′,3′-dideoxycytidine, *Antiviral Res* 11:147–160, 1989.

373. DeClerq E, Sakuma T, Baba M, et al.: Antiviral activity of phosphonylmethoxyalkyl derivatives of purines and pyrimidines, *Antiviral Res* 8:261–272, 1987.

374. Hoover EA, Ebner JP, Zeidner NS, et al.: Early therapy of feline leukemia virus infection (FeLV-FAIDS) with 9-(2-phosphonylmethoxyethyl) adenine (PMEA), *Antiviral Res* 16:77–92, 1991.

375. Hoover EA, Zeidner NS, Mullins JI: Therapy of presymptomaticFeLV-induced immunodeficiency syndrome with AZT in combination with α-interferon, *Ann NY Acad Sci* 616:258–269, 1990.

376. Zeidner NS, Myles MH, Mathiason-DuBard CK, et al.: Alpha-Interferon (2b) in combination with zidovudine for the treatment of presymptomatic feline leukemia virus–induced immunodeficiency syndrome, *Antimicrob Agents Chemother* 34:1749–1756, 1990.

377. Zeidner NS, Mathiason-DuBard CK, Hoover EA: Reversal of feline leukemia virus infection by adoptive transfer of lectin/interleukin-2–activated lymphocytes, interferon-alpha and zidovudine, *J Immunother* 14:22–32, 1993.

378. Hardy Jr WD, McClelland AJ, Zuckerman EE, et al.: Prevention of the contagious spread of feline leukaemia virus and the development of leukaemia in pet cats, *Nature* 263:326–328, 1976.

379. Legendre AM, Hawks DM, Sebring R: Comparison of the efficacy of three commercial FeLV vaccines in a natural challenge, *J Am Vet Med Assoc* 199:1456–1462, 1991.

380. Hendrick MJ, Kass PH, McGill LD, et al.: Postvaccinal sarcomas in cats, *J Natl Cancer Inst* 86:341–343, 1994.

381. Macy DW: Unpublished data, 1994.

382. Varmus HE: Form and function of retroviral proviruses, *Science* 216:812–820, 1982.

383. Coffin JM: Structure, replication and recombination of retrovirus genomes: some unifying hypotheses, *J Gen Virol* 42:1–26, 1979.

384. Besmer P: Acute transforming feline retroviruses, *Contemp Top Microbiol Immunol* 107:1–27, 1993.

385. Essex M, Klein G, Synder SP, et al.: Antibody to feline oncornavirus–associated cell membrane antigen in neonatal cats, *Int J Cancer* 8:384–390, 1971.

386. Essex M, Cotter SM, Hardy Jr WD, et al.: Feline oncornavirus–associated cell membrane antigen. IV. Antibody titers in cats with naturally occurring leukemia, lymphoma, and other diseases, *J Natl Cancer Inst* 55:463–467, 1975.

387. Patnaik AK, Liu SK, Hurvitz AI, et al.: Nonhematopoietic neoplasms in cats, *J Natl Cancer Inst* 54:855–860, 1975.

388. Macy DW: Unpublished data, 1992.

389. Sieblink HJ, Chu I, Rimmelzwaan GF, et al.: *Isolation and partial characterization of infectious molecular clones of feline immunodeficiency virus directly obtained from bone marrow DNA of a naturally infected cat*, Davis, CA, 1990, Paper presented at the First International Conference of Feline Immunodeficiency Virus Researchers.

390. Hoise MJ, Jarrett O: Serological responses of cats to feline immunodeficiency virus, *AIDS* 4:215–220, 1990.

391. Yamamoto JK, Sparger E, Ho EW, et al.: Pathogenesis of experimentally-induced feline immunodeficiency virus infection in cats, *Am J Vet Res* 49:1246–1258, 1988.

392. Yamamoto JK, Hansen H, Ho EW, et al.: Epidemiologic and clinical aspects of feline immunodeficiency virus infection in cats from the continental United States and Canada and possible mode of transmission, *J Am Vet Med Assoc* 194:213–220, 1989.

393. North TW, North GLT, Pedersen NC: Feline immunodeficiency virus: a model for reverse transcriptase–targeted chemotherapy for acquired immune deficiency syndrome, *Antimicrob Agents Chemother* 33:915–919, 1989.

394. Fleming EJ, McCaw DL, Smith JA, et al.: Clinical hematologic and survival data from cats infected with feline immunodeficiency virus: 42 cases (1983-1988), *J Am Vet Med Assoc* 199:913–916, 1991.

395. Ishida T, Wahiza T, Toriyabe K, et al.: Feline immunodeficiency virus infection in cats of Japan, *J Am Vet Med Assoc* 194:221–225, 1989.
396. Sabine M, Michelsen J, Thomas F, et al.: Feline AIDS, *Aust Vet Pract* 18:105, 1988.
397. Pedersen NC, Ho EW, Brown ML, et al.: Isolation of a T-lymphotropic virus from domestic cats with an immunodeficiency-like syndrome, *Science* 235:790–793, 1987.
398. Swinney GR, Pauli JV, Jones BE, et al.: Feline T-lymphotrophic virus (FTLV) (feline immunodeficiency virus infection) in cats in New Zealand, *N Z Vet J* 37:41–43, 1989.
399. Hutson CA, Rideout BA, Pedersen NC: Neoplasia associated with feline immunodeficiency virus infection in cats of Southern California, *J Am Vet Med Assoc* 199:1357–1362, 1991.
400. Macy DW, Podolsiki CL, Collins J: *Prevalence of FeLV and FIV high risk cats in northeastern Colorado*, Auburn, AL, 1990, Paper presented at the Tenth Annual Conference of the Veterinary Cancer Society.
401. Pedersen WC, Barlough JE: Clinical overview of feline immunodeficiency virus, *J Am Vet Med Assoc* 199:1298–1305, 1991.
402. Neu H: FIV (FTLV)–Infektion der Katze: II Falle Beitragzur epidemiologic, klinischen Symptomatologie und zum Krankheitsverlauf, *Kleintierpraxis* 34:373, 1989.
403. Maclachlan NJ, Dubovi EJ: *Fenners Veterinary Virology*, 5th ed? Elsevier, 2017, pp 230–239.
404. Thomason NA, Dunowska M, Munday JS: The use of quantitative PCR to detect felis catus papillomavirus type 2 DNA from a high proportion of queens and their kittens, *Vet Microbiol* 174:211–217, 2015.
405. Munday JS, French A, Harvey CJ: Molecular and Immunohistochemical studies do not support a role for papillomaviruses in canine oral squamous cell carcinoma development, *Vet J* 204:223–225, 2015.
406. Hnilica KA: Viral, Rickettsial and Protozoal Skin Diseases. In Hnlicia KA, editor: *Small animal dermatology,y*, 3rd ed? St. Louis, 2001, Elsevier, pp 159–174.
407. Graf R, Gruntzig K, Boo G, et al.: Swiss Feline Cancer Registry 1965-2008: the influence of sex, breed and age on tumour types and tumour locations, *J Comp Pathol* 154:195–210, 2016.
408. Munday JS, Witham AL: Frequent detection of papillomavirus in clinically normal skin of cats infected and non infected with FIV, *Vet Dermatol* 21:307–310, 2010.
409. Sykes JE, Luff JA: Viral papillomatosis. In Sykes JE, editor: *Canine and feline infectious diseases*, New York, 2013, Elsevier, pp 261–268.
410. Hartman K: Feline leukemia virus Infection. In Greene CE, editor: *Infectious diseases of the dog and cat*, 4th ed? St. Louis, 2012, Elsevier, pp 132–148.

2
Tumor Biology and Metastasis

DAVID J. ARGYLE, CHAND KHANNA, AND NICOLE GIANCRISTOFARO

Cells of multicellular organisms form part of a specialized society that cooperate to promote survival of the organism. In this society, cell division, proliferation, and differentiation are strictly controlled, and a balance exists between normal cell birth and the natural cell death rate.[1] Derangement of these normal homeostatic mechanisms can lead to uncontrolled proliferation or loss of the ability to die, which may contribute to a normal cell taking on a malignant phenotype.

Cancer in animals is well documented throughout history but has taken on significance over the past hundred years for a number of reasons. Studies on chicken, feline, and bovine retroviruses have made significant contributions to our overall understanding of carcinogenesis through the discovery of oncogenes and tumor suppressor (TS) genes.[2] Further contributions to the understanding of viral oncogenesis have come from studies of the papillomaviruses in cattle and horses, complementing research into cervical cancer in women.[3-10] This complementary cancer research has paved the way for the development of programs of research in comparative medicine that has benefits for both humans and veterinary species. This chapter summarizes the current understanding of the molecular mechanisms of cancer development and metastasis.

Normal Cell Division

To understand the genesis of cancer, it is important to first understand the basic biology of normal cell division (i.e., normal cellular homeostasis). Within an animal all cells are subject to wear and tear, making cellular reproduction a necessity for maintenance of the individual. Reproduction of the gametes occurs by the process of meiosis, whereas reproduction of somatic cells involves two sequential phases known as *mitosis* and *cytokinesis*. Mitosis is nuclear division (karyokinesis), and cytokinesis involves the division of the cytoplasm, the two occurring in close succession. Nuclear division is preceded by a doubling of the genetic material of the cell during a period known as *interphase*. In addition to copying of the chromosomes, this period is characterized by marked cellular activity in terms of RNA, protein, and lipid synthesis. The alternation between mitosis and interphase in all tissues is often referred to as the *cell cycle*.

The Cell Cycle

The cell cycle comprises four phases (M phase, G1, S phase, and G2) (Fig. 2.1). Nonproliferating cells are usually arrested between the M (mitosis) and S (DNA synthesis) phases and are referred to as *G0 (quiescent) cells*. Most cells in normal tissues are in G0. Cells are stimulated to enter the cell cycle in response to external factors, including growth factors and cell adhesion. During the G1 phase of the cell cycle, cells are responsive to mitogenic signals. Once the cell cycle has traversed the restriction point (R) in the G1 phase, cell cycle transitions become autonomous.

Interphase (G1, S, and G2 phases) is the longest phase of the cell cycle. During interphase the chromatin is very long and slender; however, it shortens and thickens as interphase progresses. The M phase is further subdivided into four phases. The first phase is referred to as *prophase* and sees the first appearance of the chromosomes. As the phase progresses, the chromosomes appear as two identical sister chromatids joined at the *centromere*. As the nuclear membrane disappears, spindle fibers form and radiate from the two *centrioles,* each located at opposite poles of the cell. The spindle fibers serve to pull the chromosomes to opposite sides of the cell.

During *metaphase* the spindle fibers pull the centromeres of the chromosomes, which become aligned to the middle of the spindle, often referred to as the *equatorial plate*. During *anaphase* the centromeres split and the sister chromatids are pulled apart by the contraction of the spindle fibers. The final stage of cell division is *telophase,* characterized by the formation of a nuclear membrane around each group of chromosomes, followed by cytokinesis or separation of the cytoplasm to produce two identical diploid cells. Progression through the cell cycle lasts approximately 12 to 24 hours.

Control of the Cell Cycle

Progression through the cell cycle is mediated by the sequential activation and inactivation of a class of proteins called *cyclin-dependent kinases* (CDKs).[11-16] CDKs are enzymes that catalyze the addition of phosphate groups onto target substrates involved in the processes of DNA replication, protein synthesis, and cell division. CDKs act as "fine tuning" for cell cycle control and so must themselves be controlled in a strict and temporal fashion. CDK activity is controlled by regulatory subunits known as *cyclins*.[11,13] Although the levels of CDKs remain constant throughout the cell cycle, the concentration of cyclins varies in a phase-specific manner during the cell cycle. The periodic synthesis and destruction of cyclins provides the primary level of cell cycle control (see Fig. 2.1). The activity of cyclin/CDK complexes is also regulated by phosphorylation. Activation of CDK/cyclin complexes

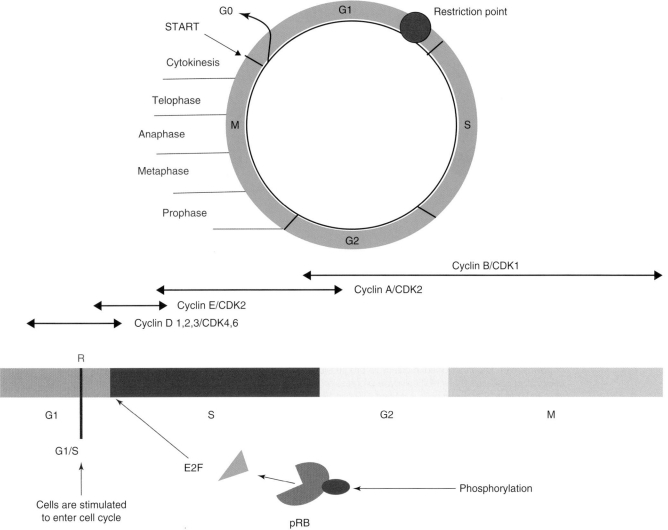

• **Fig. 2.1** The cell cycle and its control. The cell cycle is divided into four phases (G1, S, G2, and M) and G0, which represents cycle-arrested cells. Cells are stimulated to enter the cell cycle in response to external factors, including growth factors and cell adhesion molecules. During G1, cells are responsive to mitogenic signals. Once the cell cycle has traversed the restriction point (R) in the G1 phase, the cell cycle transitions become autonomous. Progression through the cell cycle is mediated by the sequential activation and inactivation of the cyclin-dependent kinases (CDKs). Control of CDK activity is through their interaction with specific cyclins (D, E, A, B) and with specific CDK inhibitors. G1-phase cyclin–CDK complexes commit the cell to cell cycle entry at the G1/S transition through phosphorylation of pRb, causing release of the E2F transcriptional factor and therefore an ability to overcome the Restriction point R and move into the S-phase. After completion of S phase, M-phase cyclin–CDK complex activity rises and drives the cell through the G2/M checkpoint by inducing chromosome condensation and creation of the mitotic spindle.

requires phosphorylation by *CDK-activating kinases* (CAKs); meanwhile, the phosphorylation at threonine and serine residues suppresses activity.[11–16] CDKs are also tightly regulated by a class of inhibitory proteins known as *CDK inhibitors* (CDKIs). CDKIs can block G1/S progression by binding CDKs/cyclin complexes and can be classified into two groups:

- INK4A family (p15[INK4b], p16[INK4a], p18[INK4c], and p19[INK4d]).[13] These act primarily on CDK4 and CDK6 complexes and prevent the association with cyclin D.
- CIP/KIP family (p21[Cip1], p27[Kip1], and p57[Kip2]).[13] These are less specific and can inactivate various cyclin/CDK complexes.

G1-phase cyclin–CDK complexes commit the cell to cell cycle entry at the G1/S transition through phosphorylation of Rb, causing release of the E2F transcriptional factor and therefore an ability to overcome the restriction point R and move into the S phase. After completion of S phase, M-phase cyclin–CDK complex activity rises and drives the cell through the G2/M checkpoint by inducing chromosome condensation and creation of the mitotic spindle. The corollary of all of these events is that loss of these control mechanisms can be a driving event in the development of cancer.[11–16]

Cellular Responses to DNA Damage

Cancer in animals and people is a common disease; however, considering the number of environmental stressors (that have the potential to cause DNA damage) to which cells are exposed on

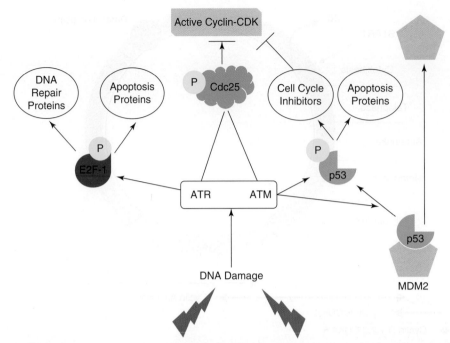

• **Fig. 2.2** ATM and ATR can be considered as "sensor" kinases that are responsive to DNA damage. If DNA is damaged during the cell cycle, there is activation of ATM and ATR and subsequent phosphorylation of downstream targets involved in cell cycle progression, repair, and cell death. These initiate a number of signaling pathways that inhibit cell cycle progression and stimulate the expression of genes involved in DNA repair (e.g., E2F-1 and p53). ATM and ATR can also target the Cdc25 family of phosphatases. These can block the cyclin-CDK activity and thus inhibit cell cycle progression.

a daily basis and the total number of cells in the body, the formation of cancer actually could be considered a very rare event. This is because the cell has a number of homeostatic mechanisms to protect it from accumulated damage. When normal cells are subjected to stress signals (e.g., radiation, DNA damage, oxygen depletion), most cells have the ability to undergo cell cycle arrest in G1, S, and G2, enter programmed cell death (apoptosis), or both. Within cells, numerous surveillance systems called *checkpoints* function to recognize and respond to DNA damage. Cell cycle checkpoints occur in the G1 phase in response to DNA damage, during S phase to monitor the quality of DNA replication and the occurrence of DNA damage, and during the G2/M phase to examine the status of the spindle. ATM and ATR are two key protein kinases that are involved in DNA damage responses.[17] They can be considered "sensor" kinases that are responsive to DNA damage. If DNA is damaged during the cell cycle, there is activation of ATM and ATR and subsequent phosphorylation of downstream targets involved in cell cycle progression, repair, and cell death. These initiate a number of signaling pathways that inhibit cell cycle progression and stimulate the expression of genes involved in DNA repair (e.g., E2F-1 and p53). ATM and ATR can also target the Cdc25 family of phosphatases. These can block cyclin-CDK activity (described previously) and thus inhibit cell cycle progression. Mutations in DNA damage–responsive elements, such as ATM, ATR, and p53, generally result in an increase in the accumulation of damaged DNA in cells, which leads to an increased risk of developing cancer (Fig. 2.2).

p53 Functions as a Genomic Guardian

p53 is a negative regulator of the cell cycle and is intimately involved is the cell's response to DNA damage or stress.[18] The p53

response to stress is largely mediated through the ATM kinase (see Fig. 2.2) and leads to the phosphorylation of the N terminus of p53. In normal cells p53 is short lived; however, phosphorylated p53 is stabilized and can then function as a transcriptional regulator binding to specific DNA regulatory sequences and transactivating a number of genes, including p21.[19,20] p21 has a high affinity for G1 CDK/cyclin complexes and acts as a CDKI inhibiting kinase activity, thereby arresting cells in G1.[21,22] Holding cells in G1 prevents the replication of damaged DNA, and the cell's own DNA repair machinery has the opportunity to repair damage before the cell reenters the active growth cycle (Fig. 2.3).

Cellular levels of p53 protein are regulated by the product of another gene called mouse double minute 2 oncogene (MDM2).[23] The principal role of MDM2 is to act as a negative regulator of p53 function. One mechanism for MDM2's effect on p53 is targeting p53 for degradation.[20,22] The p53 protein is maintained in normal cells as an unstable protein, and its interaction with MDM2 can target p53 for degradation via a ubiquitin proteosome pathway. MDM2 can also control p53 function by suppressing p53 transcriptional activity. MDM2 is a transcriptional target of p53, and expression is induced by the binding of p53 to an internal promoter within the *mdm2* gene. MDM2 can in turn bind to a domain within the amino terminus of p53, thereby inhibiting the transcriptional activity and G1 arrest function of p53 by masking access to the transcriptional machinery.[21,22,24] This pivotal role for MDM2 in the regulation of p53 checkpoint function has provided the rationale to therapeutically target MDM2 with a number of novel therapeutic inhibitors (i.e., Nutlin). The highly conserved structure of these targets across species and expected activity in many cancers provides a strong rationale for the development of these agents in veterinary patients. The recent discovery that elephants have multiple copies of p53 may explain why this species has a very low incidence of cancer.[25]

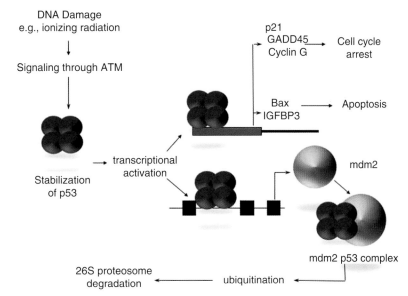

DNA Damage
e.g., ionizing radiation

Signaling through ATM

Stabilization
of p53

transcriptional
activation

p21
GADD45 ⟶ Cell cycle
Cyclin G   arrest

Bax ⟶ Apoptosis
IGFBP3

mdm2

mdm2 p53 complex

26S proteosome
degradation ⟵ ubiquitination ⟵

• **Fig. 2.3** The mediators of apoptosis. A wide variety of signals can initiate an apoptotic response, including Fas ligand (CD95 or FasL) and its interaction with the Fas receptor, tumor necrosis factor (TNF) and its receptor interaction, and certain oncogenes. The Fas and TNF receptors are members of the death receptor family. These are transmembrane proteins with cysteine-rich extracellular domains and intracellular regions that share a common structure termed the *death domain*. The proapoptotic ligands for these receptors are homotrimeric peptides that are either soluble or expressed at the surface of the adjacent cell. Ligand-induced receptor clustering promotes the binding of a soluble cytosolic adapter protein called *Fas-associated death domain* (FADD), which itself contains a death domain, in addition to a caspase binding site, to the clustered death domains of the receptors. This leads to activation of caspase 8 and downstream activation of effector caspases for apoptosis.

Cell Death

If DNA damage is extensive and the cell cannot repair itself, then the cell may be triggered to die by apoptosis. In contrast to necrosis, apoptosis is a distinct type of cell death most often characterized as the "programmed" self-destruction of cells that occurs in disease states and also as part of normal physiologic cell turnover. Whereas necrosis is characterized by swelling of the cell and lysis, apoptosis is marked by cellular and nuclear shrinkage followed by fragmentation and subsequent phagocytosis. These morphologic features of apoptosis result from a number of apoptosis effectors (i.e., caspases) and regulators (particularly the Bcl-2 protein family). The molecular mechanisms involved in apoptosis are shown in Fig. 2.4.[26] Apoptosis provides a controlled mechanism for eliminating cells that are irreversibly damaged; it involves an adenosine triphosphate (ATP)–dependent activation of cellular pathways, which move calcium from the endoplasmic reticulum to the cytoplasm and activation of endonucleases. As noted previously, some of these pathways are mediated through caspases. However, a wide variety of signals can initiate an apoptotic response, including Fas ligand (CD95 or FasL) and its interaction with the Fas receptor, tumor necrosis factor (TNF) and its receptor interaction, and certain oncogenes. The Fas and TNF receptors are members of the death receptor family. These transmembrane proteins with cysteine-rich extracellular domains and intracellular regions share a common structure termed the "death domain." The proapoptotic ligands for these receptors are homotrimeric peptides that are either soluble or expressed at the surface of the adjacent cell. Ligand-induced receptor clustering promotes the binding of a soluble cytosolic adapter protein called *Fas-associated death domain* (FADD), which itself contains a

death domain and a caspase binding site, to the clustered death domains of the receptors. This leads to activation of caspase 8 and downstream activation of effector caspases for apoptosis (Fig. 2.5).

If cells are damaged and unable to repair DNA, p53 expression can upregulate p21 and cause cell cycle arrest or can aid in directing the cell into programmed death or apoptosis through upregulation and expression of Bax (a proapoptotic Bcl-2 family protein) and also through priming of caspases. In this, the expression of p53 can also downregulate expression of the Bcl2 gene itself (a prosurvival, negative regulator of apoptosis).[22]

Key Points

- The cell cycle ensures a regulated process so that each cell can complete DNA replication before cell division occurs.
- The cell responds to growth and environmental signals through the cell cycle.
- Cancer is a common disease; however, the formation of cancer is actually a rare event, because of tightly regulated DNA repair mechanisms in the cell.
- Cellular responses to DNA damage are regulated through ATM and ATR, which act as "sensory kinases."
- The cellular response to DNA damage is either to inhibit cell cycle progression (allowing repair) or to facilitate entry into an apoptosis pathway. Failure to do this has the potential to promote the malignant phenotype.
- Components of the cell cycle that have a stimulatory effect include the cyclins and the CDKs. The negative influences come from a series of checkpoints that respond to external stimuli. These include tumor suppressor genes, such as p53 and Rb, and also genes involved in DNA repair.

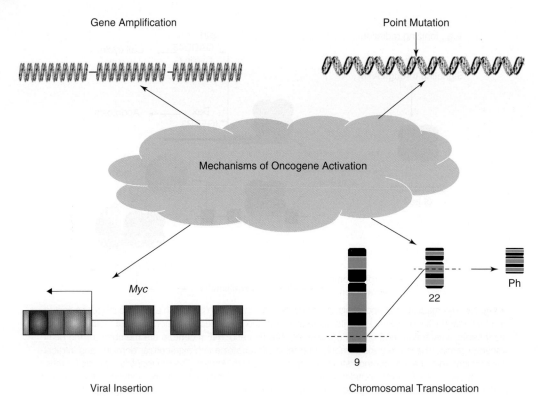

• **Fig. 2.4** Methods of oncogene activation. Oncogenes can be activated by chromosomal rearrangements (e.g., BCR/ABL–induced leukemia), gene amplification (e.g., amplification of mouse double minute 2 oncogene [MDM2] in some sarcomas), point mutations (e.g., changes in nucleotide sequence that alter protein production), or by viral insertions (e.g., the insertion of feline leukemia virus [FeLV] at the *myc* locus in FeLV-induced lymphomas).

• The process of DNA replication is also subject to the introduction of errors, and this is closely monitored by a class of enzymes called *DNA repair enzymes.* Consequently, a number of safeguards within the cell cycle ensure that normal cells are produced during division and that the DNA is replicated accurately. The next section describes how these systems are overcome to produce a malignant cancer cell.

From Normal Cell to Cancer Cell

It is difficult to define a cancer cell in absolute terms. Tumors are usually phenotypically recognized by the fact that their cells show abnormal growth patterns and are no longer under the control of normal homeostatic growth-controlling mechanisms, including apoptosis. Although the range of mechanisms involved in the development of tumors and the spectrum of tissues from which tumors are derived are diverse, they can be classified into three broad types:

• **Benign tumors:** Broadly speaking, these tumors arise in any of the tissues of the body and grow locally. Their clinical significance is the ability to cause local pressure, cause obstruction, or form a space-occupying lesion, such as a benign brain tumor. Benign tumors do not metastasize.
• **In situ tumors:** These are often small tumors that arise in the epithelium. Histologically, the lesion appears to contain cancer cells, but the tumor remains within the epithelial layer and does not invade the basement membrane or the supporting mesenchyme. A typical example of this is preinvasive squamous cell carcinoma (SCC) affecting the skin of cats, which is often referred to as *Bowen's disease.*

• **Cancer:** This often refers to a malignant tumor, characterized by unchecked cellular division and the capacity for both local invasion and distant metastasis.

Multistep Carcinogenesis

Cancer has been defined as the phenotypic end result of a whole series of changes that may have taken a long period of time to develop. Indeed, recent studies that have sequenced the genome of pancreatic and brain tumors have identified 63 and 60 genetic alterations on average in each cancer, respectively. From this large list of genetic alterations, a small number of commonly mutated genes are "drivers" of the cancer phenotype.[27,28]

The application of a cancer-producing agent (carcinogen) to tissues does not lead to the immediate production of a cancer cell. After an *initiation* step produced by the agent, a period of tumor *promotion* follows. This promotion may be caused by the same initiating agent or by other substances, such as normal growth promoters or hormones. The initiating step is a rapid event and affects the genetic material of the cell. If the cell does not repair this damage, then promoting factors may progress the cell toward a malignant phenotype. In contrast to initiation, progression (the stochastic accumulation of mutations that impose a survival advantage on the daughter cells) may be a very slow process and may not even manifest in the lifetime of the animal. Each stage of multistep carcinogenesis collectively results in an accumulation of genetic changes in the cell that ultimately provide a selection advantage that drives the progression toward a highly malignant cell. The age-dependent incidence of cancer suggests that between four and seven rate-limiting, stochastic events are required to produce the malignant phenotype.[29]

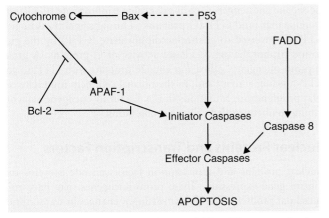

• **Fig. 2.5** p53 is involved in cell cycle control. The p53 response to stress may be mediated by DNA-dependent protein kinase (DNA-PK) or by the ATM kinase and leads to phosphorylation of the N terminus of p53. In normal cells, p53 is short lived; however, phosphorylated p53 is stabilized and can then function as a transcriptional regulator binding to sequences and transactivating a number of genes, including p21 and Bax. Consequently, the cell cycle is arrested or the cell undergoes programmed cell death (apoptosis). The cellular levels of the p53 protein are regulated by the product of another gene mouse double minute 2 oncogene (MDM2). The principal role of MDM2 is to act as a negative regulator of p53 function. One mechanism for MDM2 to downregulate p53 is to target p53 for degradation. The p53 protein is maintained in normal cells as an unstable protein, and its interaction with p53 can target p53 for degradation via a ubiquitin proteosome pathway. MDM2 can also control p53 function by suppressing p53 transcriptional activity. MDM2 is a transcriptional target of p53, and expression is induced by the binding of p53 to an internal promoter within the MDM2 gene. MDM2 can in turn bind to a domain within the amino terminus of p53, thereby inhibiting the transcriptional activity and G1 arrest function of p53 by masking access to the transcriptional machinery.

In 2011 a new phenomenon was described that challenges the slower, stepwise progression of cancer development; this phenomenon suggests that thousands of clustered chromosomal rearrangements could occur in a single event in localized and confined genomic regions in one or a few chromosomes. This event, known as *chromothrypsis,* occurs through one massive genomic rearrangement during a single catastrophic event in the cell's history.[30-32] Although chromothrypsis may occur as an early event in cancer cells, leading to more rapid transformation through loss of TS function or gain of oncogene function, the phenomenon has never been recapitulated in experimental models, but rather remains a cytogenomic observation in several pediatric cancers. Indeed, the lack of mechanistic understanding of chromothrypsis has limited its study in conventional animal models.[30-32]

Irrespective of speed of development, these events in tumor formation are a consequence of changes in genes or the regulation of gene expression. Over the past 30 years cancer research has generated a rich and complex body of information revealing that cancer is a disease involving dynamic changes in the genome. Seminal to our understanding of cancer biology has been the discovery of the so-called *cancer genes* or *oncogenes* and *TS genes.* Mutations that produce oncogenes with dominant gain of function and TS genes with recessive loss of function have been identified through their alterations in human and animal cancer cells and by their elicitation of cancer phenotypes in experimental models. A summary of the differences between oncogenes and TS genes is highlighted in Table 2.1.

TABLE 2.1	Key Differences Between Oncogenes and Tumor Suppressor Genes	
Oncogenes	**Tumor Suppressor Genes**	
Altered versions of proto-oncogenes that play a role in promoting cellular proliferation. Considered to be the cellular "gas pedal."	Genes involved in blocking cellular proliferation. Considered to be the cellular "brakes."	
Mutation at the cellular level causes a dominant gain of function.	Mutations are recessive and require loss of both alleles for a phenotypic change.	
Mutation causes a gain of function.	Mutation causes a loss of function.	
Mutations occur in somatic cells.	Mutations can occur in germ cells (inherited cancer predisposition) and/or can arise in somatic cells.	

Oncogenes

The RNA tumor viruses (retroviruses) provided the first evidence that genetic factors play a role in the development of cancer. The initial observation came in 1910, when Rous demonstrated that a filterable agent (later classified as a retrovirus and termed *avian leukosis virus*) was capable of producing lymphoid tumors in chickens.[33] Retroviruses have three core genes (*gag, pol,* and *env*) and an additional gene that gives the virus the ability to transform cells. Retroviral sequences responsible for transforming properties are called *viral oncogenes* (v-onc). The names of these genes are derived from the tumors in which they were first described (e.g., *v-ras* from rat sarcoma virus).

Viral oncogenes were subsequently shown to have cellular homologs called *cellular oncogenes* (c-onc). Later, the term *proto-oncogene* was used to describe cellular oncogenes that do not have transforming potential to form tumors in their native state but can be altered to lead to malignancy.[34] Most proto-oncogenes are key genes involved in the control of cell growth and proliferation, and their roles are complex. For simplicity, their sites and modes of action in the normal cell can be divided as follows (Table 2.2):
- Growth factors
- Growth factor receptors
- Protein kinases
- Signal transducers
- Nuclear proteins and transcription factors

Growth Factors

Growth factors (GFs) are molecules that act on the cell via cell surface receptors. Their contribution to carcinogenesis may be through excessive production of the GF or through ectopic expression in a cell type that does not normally express that GF.

Growth Factor Receptors

Several proto-oncogene–derived proteins form a part of cell surface receptors for GFs. The binding of GF ligand to receptor is the initial stage of the delivery of mitogenic signals to cells. Their role in carcinogenesis may be through structural alterations in these proteins, leading to enhanced or constitutive activation.

TABLE 2.2	Functional Classification of Tumor Oncogenes	
Oncogene	Name	Abbreviation
Growth factors	Platelet-derived growth factor	PDGF
	Epidermal growth factor	EGF
	Insulin-like growth factor-1	IGF-1
	Vascular endothelial growth factor	VEGF
	Transforming growth factor-β	TGF-β
	Interleukin-2	IL-2
Growth factor receptors	PDGF receptor	PDGFR
	EGF receptor	EGFR, erbB-1
	IGF-1 receptor	IGF-1R
	VEGF receptor	VEGFR
	IL-2 receptor	IL-2R
	Hepatocyte growth factor receptor	C-met
	Heregulin receptor	neu/erbB-2
	Stem cell factor receptor	C-Kit
Protein kinases	Tyrosine kinase	bcr-abl
	Tyrosine kinase	src
	Serine-threonine kinase	raf/mil
	Serine-threonine kinase	mos
G-protein signal transducers	GTPase	H-ras
	GTPase	K-ras
	GTPase	N-ras
Nuclear proteins	Transcription factor	ets
	Transcription factor	fos
	Transcription factor	jun
	Transcription factor	myb
	Transcription factor	myc
	Transcription factor	rel

GTPase, Guanosine triphosphatase.

Protein Kinases

Protein kinases are associated with the inner surface of the plasma membrane and are involved in signal transduction after ligand-receptor binding. Structural changes in these genes and proteins lead to increased kinase activity that can have profound effects on signal transduction pathways.

Signal Transduction

The binding of an extracellular GF to the membrane receptor leads to a series of events by which the mitogenic signal is transduced to the nucleus of the cell. Essential to this signaling is the successive phosphorylation of signaling intermediaries or the second messengers such as guanosine triphosphate (GTP) and proteins that bind GTP (G-proteins). During signal transduction GTP is converted to guanosine diphosphate (GDP) by the guanosine triphosphatase (GTPase) activity of G-proteins. A group of proto-oncogenes called *Ras* encode proteins with GTPase and GTP-binding activity and, in the normal cell, help modulate cellular proliferation. Mutations in the *Ras* proto-oncogene can contribute to uncontrolled cellular proliferation.

Nuclear Proteins and Transcription Factors

Nuclear proteins and transcription factors encode proteins that control gene expression. These proto-oncogenes may have roles in cellular proliferation. Not surprisingly, changes in transcription factor activity may contribute to the development of the malignant genotype.

Mechanisms by which Oncogenes Become Activated

The advent of recombinant DNA technology has allowed scientists to unravel a number of mechanisms by which the normal products of proto-oncogenes can be disrupted to produce uncontrolled cell division. The conversion of a proto-oncogene to an oncogene is a result of somatic events in the genetic material of the target tissue. The activated allele of the oncogene dominates the wild-type allele and results in a *dominant gain of function.* This means that only one allele needs to be affected to obtain phenotypic change; this is in contrast to TS genes, in which both alleles have to be lost for phenotypic change. The mechanisms of oncogene activation are outlined in this list and are shown in Fig. 2.4.[34–41]

- *Chromosomal translocation.* When proto-oncogenes are translocated within the genome (i.e., from one chromosome to another), their function can be greatly altered. The classic example in human medicine is the chromosomal breakpoint that produces the Philadelphia chromosome found in chronic myelogenous leukemia (CML). This involves translocation of the *c-abl* oncogene on chromosome 9 to a gene on chromosome 22 (*bcr*). The point where two genes come together is referred to as a *chromosomal breakpoint* (or *translocation breakpoint*).[42] The BCR/ABL hybrid gene produces a novel transcript whose protein product has elevated tyrosine kinase activity and can contribute to uncontrolled cellular proliferation. Transgenic mice for this chimeric gene develop lymphoblastic leukemia and lymphoma. Because this gene product is linked directly to CML formation, it is a logical target for tyrosine kinase inhibitors in the treatment of CML in humans.
- *Gene amplification.* Quantitation of gene copy number is possible by a number of molecular techniques, including comparative genomic hybridization, genotyping arrays, and Southern hybridization. Amplification of oncogenes can occur in a number of tumor types and has been demonstrated in childhood neuroblastoma, in which the *myc* proto-oncogene (nuclear transcription factor) is amplified up to 300 times.[43] Gene amplification is possibly the most common mechanism of proto-oncogene activation. A further example is the MDM2 proto-oncogene, which has been identified in dogs and horses, and recently was shown to be amplified in a proportion of canine soft tissue sarcomas.[44]
- *Point mutations.* These are single base changes in the DNA sequence of proto-oncogenes, leading to the production of abnormal proteins. Point mutations can arise through the actions of ionizing radiation, chemical carcinogens, or errors in DNA replication and repair. A mutation in a proto-oncogene

or the transcriptional machinery that controls its expression may disrupt homeostasis and result in sustained proliferation signals or failure to respond to negative feedback signals. A classic example is the *Ras* proto-oncogene, in which point mutations are a consistent finding in a number of human tumors. Point mutations have also been identified in a number of canine tumors, suggesting a model for human disease.[45–47]

- *Viral insertions.* The discovery of oncogenes was a direct result of studies on tumor-causing viruses. In some circumstances proto-oncogene function can be damaged by the insertion of viral elements.[48–50] Occasionally, novel retroviruses are isolated from leukemias or sarcomas in animals that have been viremic with a leukemia virus for some time. These viruses induce tumors very rapidly when inoculated into members of the species of origin and are referred to as *acutely transforming oncoviruses.* The prototype of the acutely transforming virus is the Rous sarcoma virus (RSV) isolated from a chicken in 1911.[51] Subsequently, many more have been isolated from animals infected with avian, feline, murine, or simian oncoviruses. These viruses are generated by a rare recombinant event between the leukemia virus, with which the animal was originally infected, and a cellular proto-oncogene. In this, part of the viral genome is deleted and replaced with the cellular oncogene. The virus then becomes acutely transforming because this oncogene is now under the transcriptional control of a very efficient viral promoter. This then allows infection of a cell and insertion of this continuously expressed oncogene into the cellular genome, leading to rapid progression and malignancy. Evidence suggests that these acutely transforming viruses are not transmitted naturally, but all events occur in the individual animal. Because the virus has itself lost some of its own genetic material, it is defective for replication; however, it is spread throughout an animal by the provision of help from the normal leukemia virus, which provides the missing proteins in co-infected cells. In addition to acutely transforming mechanisms, retroviruses can activate cellular oncogenes by integrating adjacent to them. A good example of this is the *myc* gene, which is frequently activated in feline T-cell lymphomas.[52] In one mode, the virus integrates adjacent to the oncogene, and transcription initiation in the viral long terminal repeat (LTR) proceeds into the adjacent oncogene, producing a hybrid mRNA. In a second form, the enhancer of the virus overrides the regulation of the c-*myc* transcription from its normal promoter.

Tumor Suppressor Genes

Changes in genes can lead either to stimulatory or inhibitory effects on cell growth and proliferation. The stimulatory effects are provided by the proto-oncogenes, as described earlier. Mutations or translocations of these genes produce positive signals leading to uncontrolled growth. In contrast, tumor formation can result from a loss of inhibitory functions associated with another class of cellular genes called the *TS genes.* The discovery of these genes began by observations of inherited cancer syndromes in children, in particular studies of retinoblastoma. In the early 1970s epidemiologic studies of both retinoblastoma and Wilms tumor led Knudson to propose his "two hit" theory of tumorigenesis.[53]

Retinoblastoma Provides the First Clues to the Existence of Tumor Suppressor Genes

Retinoblastoma occurs in two forms: a sporadic form and an inherited form (accounting for 40% of cases).[54] In the inherited form the mode of inheritance is autosomal dominant, and about half the children are affected by the condition. Knudson's model required the retinoblastoma tumor cells (in either sporadic or inherited forms) to acquire two separate genetic changes in the DNA before tumor development. The first or predisposing event could be inherited through the germ line (familial retinoblastoma) or it could arise de novo in somatic cells (sporadic form). The second event occurred in somatic cells. Thus in sporadic retinoblastoma both events arose in the retinal cells. However, in familial retinoblastoma, the individual had already inherited one mutant gene and required only a second hit in the remaining normal gene in somatic cells.

The mode of inheritance of retinoblastoma is dominant with incomplete penetrance. However, at the cellular level loss or inactivation of both alleles is required to change the cells' phenotype. The retinoblastoma gene codes for Rb, which was previously described as a normal cellular gene involved in control of the cell cycle (see earlier discussion). Rb is described as a TS and, in a cell with only one normal allele, that allele usually produces enough TS product to remain normal. Generically mutations in TS genes behave very differently from oncogene mutations. Whereas activating oncogene mutations are dominant to wild type (they emit their proliferating signals regardless of the wild-type gene product), suppressor mutations are recessive. Mutation in one gene copy usually has no effect, as long as a reasonable amount of wild-type protein remains. Consequently, some texts refer to TS genes as "recessive oncogenes."

More recently Knudson's hypothesis was confirmed when the Rb gene was cloned and characterized. The TS Rb is the principal member of a family of proteins that also encompass pRb2/p130 and p107. Rb plays a central role in regulating cell cycle progression in G1 to S phase (see Fig. 2.2). Indeed, disruption of Rb function has been found to be a common feature of many human cancers other than retinoblastoma. Rb function can be abrogated by point mutations, deletions, or complex formation with viral oncoproteins, such as SV40 large T antigen and adenoviral E1a protein.[55] The function of additional proteins associated with the Rb pathway is also subjected to deregulation in human cancers, including overexpression of D type cyclins, overexpression of CDK4, and downregulation of the CDKI cell cycle inhibitor p16.[56] Although loss of cell cycle control via the Rb pathway occurs commonly in many human tumors, little is known about the role of Rb, cyclin D, CDK4, and p16 in domesticated animal tumors.

The p53 Tumor Suppressor Gene

As described previously, p53 is a gene whose product is intimately involved as a negative regulator of the cell cycle control. Its discovery by Sir David Lane in 1979 marked a major milestone in cancer research and has allowed greater understanding of molecular mechanisms of cancer and identified potential targets for therapeutic intervention.[57]

The p53 protein has been described as the "guardian of the genome" by virtue of its ability to push cells into arrest or apoptosis, depending on the degree of DNA damage. Thus the p53 TS gene plays an important role in cell cycle progression, regulation of gene expression, and the cellular response mechanisms to DNA damage. Under normal physiologic conditions, wild-type p53 can bind specific DNA sequences and regulate transcription of a number of genes involved in cell cycle progression and apoptotic pathways, including *p21^{waf1/cip1}* and *Bax* (see Fig. 2.5). The p53-mediated mechanisms are responsible

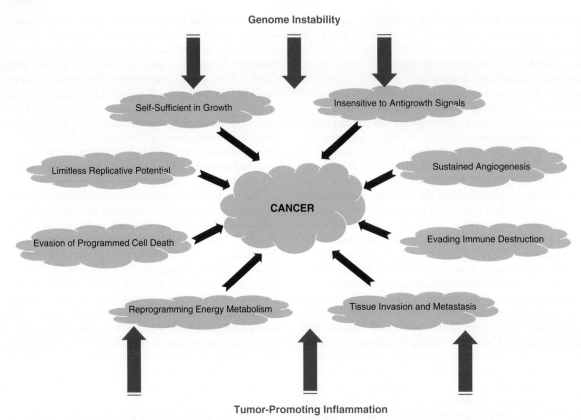

• **Fig. 2.6** The hallmarks of cancer. Cancer can be considered the end product of acquisition of eight fundamental characteristics. Underpinning these capabilities are the common denominator enabling characteristics of genome instability and tumor-promoting inflammation.

for tumor suppression and prevent accumulation of potentially oncogenic mutations and genomic instability. Failure of p53 to activate such cellular functions may ultimately result in abnormal uncontrolled cell growth, leading to tumorigenic transformation.[58–62]

p53 is the most frequently inactivated gene in human neoplasia, with functional loss commonly occurring through gene mutational events, including nonsense, missense and splice site mutations, allelic loss, rearrangements, and deletions. However, p53 function can also be abrogated by several nonmutational mechanisms, including nuclear exclusion, complex formation with a number of viral proteins, and through overexpression of the cellular oncogene MDM2.[63]

The homologs of p53 and MDM2 have both been identified in domestic animal species, and a number of studies indicate that this gene also has a central role in the progression of veterinary cancers.[64–68]

Key Points

Fig. 2.6; also see Table 2.1.
• Cancer is a genetic disease characterized by aberrant molecular changes in the genetic material of the cell.
• Cancer arises through mutations in DNA and/or changes in gene expression (epigenetic events).
• Cancer is a clonal disease resulting from the accumulation of mutations in oncogenes or tumor suppressor genes. Each successive change leads to a survival advantage for the cell, akin to darwinian natural selection.

• In this process of natural selection, the acquired characteristics that are advantageous to the cancer phenotype are often referred to as the *hallmarks of cancer.*
• Studies on viral carcinogenesis and/or monogenic cancer syndromes have facilitated the dissection of cancer biology and the identification of cancer-causing genes (oncogenes and tumor suppressor genes). However, most cancers encountered in clinical practice are sporadic (occurring as a result of changes in adult somatic cells) and not inherited.
• Proto-oncogenes are normal genes involved in growth and proliferation and can be "activated" to promote malignancy.
• Tumor suppressor genes are normal genes expressing proteins that inhibit growth and proliferation.
• If proto-oncogenes are the "accelerator pedal" in a cell, then tumor supressor genes are the "brakes."
• Gain of function in oncogenes and/or loss of function in tumor suppressor genes promotes the malignant phenotype.

Cancer Arises through Multiple Molecular Mechanisms

The advances in understanding of normal cell biology and the processes that lead to malignancy have increased dramatically over the past 30 years. The last decade has shown that transformation of a normal cell into a malignant cell requires very few molecular, biochemical, and cellular changes that can be considered as acquired capabilities.[42,43] Furthermore, despite the wide diversity of cancer types, these acquired capabilities appear to be common to all types of cancer. An optimistic view of increasing simplicity in cancer biology is further endorsed by the fact that all normal cells, irrespective of origin and phenotype, carry similar molecular machineries that regulate cell proliferation, differentiation, aging, and cell death.

Tumorigenesis is a multistep process, and these steps reflect genetic alterations that drive the progression of a normal cell into a highly malignant cancer cell. This is supported by the finding that genomes of tumor cells are invariably altered at multiple sites. The spectrum of changes ranges from subtle point mutations in growth regulatory genes to obvious changes in chromosomal complement.

Cancer cells have defects in regulatory circuits that govern cellular proliferation, homeostasis, and survival. A model has been proposed that suggests that the vast array of genetic abnormalities associated with cancer is a manifestation of eight alterations in cellular physiology that collectively contribute to malignant growth. First proposed in 2000 and updated in 2011, these "hallmarks" of cancer constitute an organizing principle for rationalizing the complexities of cancer and are underpinned by two overarching themes: *genome instability* and *chronic inflammation*.[69,70] The eight acquired characteristics can be summarized under these headings (see Fig. 2.6):

- Self-sufficient growth
- Insensitivity to antigrowth signals
- Evasion of programmed cell death (apoptosis)
- Limitless replicative potential
- Sustained angiogenesis
- Reprogramming energy metabolism
- Evading immune destruction
- Tissue invasion and metastasis

Cancer exhibits another dimension of complexity in that it contains an array of "normal" cells that contribute to the acquisition and maintenance of the cancer hallmarks by creating the tumor microenvironment (TME). The next section is an overview of these traits and the strategies by which they are acquired in cancer cells. The process of metastasis requires angiogenesis and invasion; therefore the traits of sustained angiogenesis and tissue invasion and metastasis are collectively reviewed under a final section on metastasis.

The Hallmarks of Cancer

In the preceding section we described the normal cell and the role of oncogenes and TS genes in cell cycle control and regulation. Directly or indirectly all components of the cancer phenotype (i.e., hallmarks of cancer) emerge from dysregulation of genes or the regulation of gene expression. Cancer-associated changes in the regulation of gene expression (epigenomics) have increasingly become the focus of cancer research. Amplifying this study of the regulation of gene expression has been a new understanding of therapeutic interventions that target various aspects of gene regulation (e.g., bromodomain inhibitors).[71]

Furthermore, understanding of the targets of the regulation of gene expression has expanded from the conventional view of epigenetic regulation of promoter activity to a new understanding of enhancer epigenomics and the description of "super enhancers." As suggested by the name, super enhancers may be considered to be have a broad control of a transcriptional signature. As such, the alteration in the activity of a single super enhancer may yield a change in many transcriptional components of the cancer phenotype.[72]

As described previously, cancer is a very common disease in animals and humans; however, the development of cancer is, in fact, a rare event. Despite the number of cells in the body, the proliferation and regulation of these cells, and the potential for malignant transformation, the development of a single cancer is rare. This is because of the cell's own natural defenses against progression toward the malignant phenotype. The ability of the cell to effect DNA repair or initiate cell death is a defense mechanism against malignant transformation and serves to maintain cellular homeostasis. Each of the acquired capabilities described previously represents a breach in a cell's homeostatic mechanisms. However, the biology of cancer cannot be understood by simply considering the phenotypic traits of the cancer cell. Rather, the cancer phenotype is defined by the interactions between the cancer cell, the TME, and the enabling effects of fundamental genomic instability and chronic inflammation.

Self-Sufficiency in Growth Signals

Normal cells require mitogenic stimuli for growth and proliferation. These signals are transmitted to the nucleus by the binding of signaling molecules to specific receptors, the diffusion of growth factors into the cell, extracellular matrix (ECM) components, or cell-to-cell adhesions or interactions.[73,74] As previously discussed, many oncogenes act by mimicking normal growth signals. Tumor cells are not dependent on external mitogenic stimuli for proliferation and sustained growth, but rather are self-sufficient. The liberation from dependency on exogenous signals severely disrupts normal cellular homeostasis. Arguably the most fundamental trait of cancer cells is their ability to sustain chronic proliferation. By deregulating these signals, cancer cells become masters of their own destinies, promoting signaling (typically through intracellular kinase domains) to promote progression through the cell cycle, increases in cell size, increases in cell survival, and changes in energy metabolism.

The cancer cell can acquire this capability in a number of ways:

- They may produce growth factor ligands themselves.
- They may induce stromal cells to produce such ligands.
- Receptor concentration on the cell surface may increase, leading to receptor homodimerization or heterodimerization, making the cell hyperresponsive to ligands.
- Structural alterations in the receptor may take place that cause ligand-independent "firing."
- Constitutive activation of the signaling pathway (downstream of the receptor) may occur. A good example of this is the constitutive activation of the PI3K-Akt pathway, through mutations in the catalytic subunit of the PI3 kinase.
- Disruptions in negative feedback mechanisms that attenuate proliferative signaling may occur; for example:
  - o Mutations in the *Ras* gene compromise the Ras GTPase activity, which acts as a negative feedback mechanism to ensure the effects of *Ras* are only transitory.
  - o *PTEN* is a tumor suppressor protein that counteracts PI3K signaling. *PTEN* loss has an effect similar to constitutive PI3K activation and promotes tumorigenesis.

Although the acquisition of growth signaling autonomy by cancer cells is conceptually satisfying, it is in fact too simplistic. One of the major problems of cancer research has been focusing on the cancer cell in isolation. It is now apparent that we must also consider the contribution of the TME to the survival of cancer cells. Within normal tissues paracrine and endocrine signals contribute greatly to growth and proliferation. Cell-to-cell growth signaling is also likely to operate in cancer cells and may be as important as some of the autonomous mechanisms of tumor growth. It recently was suggested that growth signals for the proliferation of carcinoma cells are derived from the tumor stromal elements (e.g., cancer- or carcinoma-associated fibroblasts [CAFs]). It is therefore possible that the survival of tumor cells not only relies on the acquisition of growth signal autonomy, but also may require the recruitment or modulation of stromal cells to provide these growth signals.

Insensitivity to Antigrowth Signals or Evading Growth Suppressors

Within the normal cell multiple antiproliferative signals operate to maintain cellular quiescence and homeostasis. These signals include soluble growth inhibitors that act via cell surface receptors and immobilized inhibitors that are embedded in the ECM and on the surface of nearby cells. The signals operate to push the cell either into G0 or into a postmitotic state (usually associated with the acquisition of specific differentiation–associated characteristics) and thus are intimately associated with cell cycle control mechanisms. Cells monitor their external environment during the progression through G1 and, on the basis of external stimuli, decide whether to proliferate, become quiescent, or enter into a postmitotic state.

Most cellular programs that negatively regulate cell growth and proliferation depend on the actions of TS genes. At the basic level most of the antiproliferative signals are funneled through the Rb protein and its close relatives. Disruption of Rb allows cell proliferation and renders the cell insensitive to antiproliferative signals, such as that provided by the well-characterized transforming growth factor-β (TGF-β).[54] The Rb protein integrates signals from diverse extracellular and intracellular sources and can control cell cycle progression. The other major TS is p53, which integrates intracellular signals and can promote either cell cycle arrest or apoptosis (depending on the degree of cellular stress or damage). However, the effects of p53 expression are highly context dependent. Loss of Rb or p53 is associated with the malignant phenotype through the cell's ability to evade antigrowth signals.

In addition to TS gene loss, cells can evade antigrowth signals by alternative cellular programs:

- Evasion of contact inhibition. Cell-to-cell contact in most normal cells results in an inhibitory signal against further cell proliferation. The role of this mechanism in vivo has been thought to be to maintain tissue homeostasis. In cell culture contact inhibition is abrogated in cancer cell monolayers, leading to their indefinite expansion. NF2 and LKB1 genes are considered tumor suppressor genes that are involved in this process, and loss of these genes in vivo may promote loss of contact inhibition that contributes to the progression of cancers.[75]
- Although TGF-β has antiproliferative effects in cancer, it is now appreciated that the TGF-β pathway can be corrupted in the later stages of malignancy and can contribute to cancer progression.[76]
- In this late effect TGF-β is found to activate a cellular program termed *epithelial-to-mesenchymal transition* (EMT) that promotes invasion and metastasis (see the following discussion).

Evading Cell Death: The Roles of Apoptosis, Autophagy, and Necrosis

The growth of any tumor depends not only on the rate of cell division, but also on the rate of cellular attrition (mainly provided by apoptotic mechanisms). Basic molecular and pathologic studies of tumors have confirmed that acquired resistance toward apoptosis and other types of death is a hallmark of all types of cancer.

Cancer cells, through a variety of strategies, can acquire resistance to cell death and apoptosis. One of the most common ways is through loss of function of the TS protein p53. Removal of normal p53 function leads to failure of the cells' sensor mechanism for DNA damage. When the cell suffers an insult, such as UV radiation, hypoxia, or exposure to DNA-damaging agents, signals are funneled through p53 to cause either cell cycle arrest or apoptosis. Failure of this mechanism can contribute to the progression of the cell toward malignancy and promote the accumulation of additional genetic defects that are not corrected at defined checkpoints in cell cycle progression.[59]

The mechanisms involved in apoptosis are now well established, as are the strategies by which cancer cells evade its actions. However, recently conceptual advances have been made involving other forms of "programmed cell death" as a barrier to cancer development. A notable example is the emerging role that autophagy plays in cancer development. *Autophagy* is a normal cellular response that operates at low basal levels in cells but can be induced in states of cellular stress, such as nutrient deficiency. In autophagy controlled breakdown of cellular organelles yields energy and cellular substrates that can be used for a variety of cellular functions. Recent evidence suggests that autophagy may be involved in both tumor cell survival and, paradoxically, tumor cell death, depending on the cellular state. The link between apoptosis and autophagy suggests that autophagy may represent another barrier for cells to overcome before they can attain malignancy. In contrast, it has also been shown that irradiation or cytotoxic drug treatment in late-stage tumors may promote autophagy, leading to cells attaining a state of reversible dormancy. The situation seems to suggest that autophagy is a barrier to tumor development in early disease, but in late-stage disease may allow cancer cells to survive severe cellular stress.[77,78]

In both autophagy and apoptosis the process does not lead to the release of any "proinflammatory" signals. In contrast, the process of necrosis, observed in larger tumors, causes release of signals that support an influx of inflammatory cells. For many years this has been considered a positive event, helping expose the immune system to tumor antigens and promote immune destruction. However, recent evidence suggests that some phenotypes of inflammatory macrophages can actually support tumor growth through fostering of angiogenesis, cancer cell proliferation, and invasion. Consequently, our understanding of macrophage phenotypes in cancer progression is an area of active research.[79,80]

Limitless Replicative Capacity

More than 30 years ago the pioneering observations of Hayflick established that when normal human or animal cells are grown in culture, they demonstrate a finite replicative life span.[81] That is, they are capable of a finite number of cell divisions, after which they undergo what has been termed *replicative senescence* and are incapable of any further cell division. The mechanism underlying the replicative clock that monitors this process has been the subject of intense research. This process has further evoked considerable interest because it is also one of the mechanisms that must be overcome to establish the "immortal" phenotype that is characteristic of the cancer cell.[69,70]

In mammalian cells DNA is organized into chromosomes within the nucleus, and these are capped by specialized

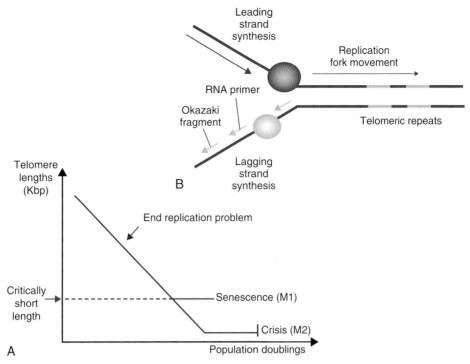

• **Fig. 2.7** A) Telomeric attrition in cultured cells. In mammalian cells the DNA is organized into chromosomes within the nucleus, and these are capped by specialized DNA-protein structures known as *telomeres*. The major function of these structures is protection, but they are progressively eroded at each cell division because of the inability of DNA to completely replicate itself. This is referred to as the "End Replication Problem", and arises because of the inability of chromosomes to completely replicate their extreme 5′ ends (B). The result is that there is progressive telomeric attrition as cell populations double. After an estimated 50 cell divisions, cells enter an irreversible (and prolonged) state of cellular senescence (sometimes referred to as *mortality stage 1* [M1]). This period is characterized by arrest of proliferation without loss of biochemical function or viability. At the end of this period, cells exhibit altered morphology and chromosomal instability, a state often referred to as *crisis* (mortality stage 2 [M2]).

DNA-protein structures known as *telomeres*.[81] The major function of these structures is protection, but they are progressively eroded at each cell division because of the inability of DNA to completely replicate itself. The result is progressive telomeric attrition as cell populations double. After an estimated 50 cell divisions, cells enter an irreversible (and prolonged) state of cellular senescence (sometimes referred to as *mortality stage 1* [M1]). This period is characterized by arrest of proliferation without loss of biochemical function or viability. At the end of this period cells exhibit altered morphology and chromosomal instability, a state often referred to as *crisis* (mortality stage 2 [M2]) (Fig. 2.7). Thus telomeric attrition is intimately involved with the aging of cells. Cancer cells must overcome replicative senescence and take on an immortal phenotype.

It has now been demonstrated in human tumors, and more recently in tumors of the dog, that telomere maintenance is a feature of virtually all cancer types.[82–89] Tumor cells succeed in telomere maintenance by the expression of the enzyme *telomerase*. From studies on cellular senescence, expression of the enzyme telomerase has emerged as a central unifying mechanism underlying the immortal phenotype of cancer cells and has thus become the most common marker of malignant cells. Telomerase is a ribonucleoprotein enzyme that maintains the protective structures at the ends of eukaryotic chromosomes, at the telomeres. In humans, telomerase expression is repressed in most somatic tissues, and telomeres shorten with each progressive cell division. In contrast, telomerase activity is a common finding in many human malignancies, resulting in stabilized telomere length. The telomerase complex consists of an RNA subunit that contains a domain complementary to the telomeric repeat sequence TTAGGG and a catalytic protein component. The catalytic protein component acts as a reverse transcriptase and can catalyze the addition of telomeric repeats onto the ends of chromosomes, using the RNA subunit as a template (see Fig. 2.7). It is now well documented that the level of telomerase in malignant tissue, compared with normal tissue, is much higher, and this differential is greater than that for classic enzymatic targets, such as thymidylate synthase, dihydrofolate reductase, or topoisomerase II.[90] Telomerase biology is complex, and the mechanisms by which telomerase becomes reactivated in tumor cells is the subject of intense research. However, this represents an exciting opportunity for further understanding the complex biology of cancer and also the identification of completely novel targets for therapy.

Sustained Angiogenesis

It is now well accepted that the development of new blood vessels from endothelial progenitors (vasculogenesis) or from existing blood vessels (angiogenesis) is required for cancer progression and metastasis.[91,92] Endothelial cells (EC) or endothelial progenitors are activated by tumor-derived growth factors and result in new capillaries at the tumor site.[93] In healthy tissue EC proliferation is controlled by a balance between protein factors that activate EC and those that antagonize activation. Malignant tumors provide signals that result in EC survival, motility, invasion, differentiation, and organization. These steps are required to create a supportive vasculature for the tumor. In many ways these required endothelial processes share parallel features with the processes required for the success of a metastatic cancer cell itself. The creation of new blood vessels requires the tumors to recruit circulating EC to their site, presumably through the release of growth factors, such as vascular endothelial growth factor (VEGF). Circulating EC must survive at their new site with the help of survival signals and form vascular tubes that then reorganize to sustain blood flow. The resulting vasculature of cancers is typically aberrant with often poorly organized and chaotic vascular structures that are leaky, with limited adventitial development and excessive branching.[94] Once developed, this angiogenic phenotype (the result of the angiogenic switch) is associated with a diverse pattern of ongoing angiogenesis and neovascularization. This ongoing process is likely complex and involves a wide variety of tumor and microenvironmental-derived growth factors and signaling molecules. Adding to this complexity, certain phases of cancer progression likely are associated with and require periods of antiangiogenesis. Indeed, these hypovascularized states may directly contribute to the progression of certain cancers.[95] Regulation of angiogenesis depends on the balance between proangiogenic and antiangiogenic factors. There is controversy as to the exact biologic function of thrombospondin-1 (TSP1) in angiogenesis. Although some studies suggest that TSP1 promotes neovascularization, TSP1 is commonly recognized as an endogenous angiogenesis inhibitor.[96]

Many lines of evidence support the importance of angiogenesis in the biology of metastasis. The vascularity of a primary tumor (measured by microvessel density) has been correlated with metastatic behavior for most human and many veterinary tumors. The expression of angiogenesis-associated growth or survival factors and their receptors (i.e., VEGFR) in serum and in tumors, respectively, has also been correlated with outcome; more recently functional imaging studies using magnetic resonance imaging (MRI) and other means has provided correlates of vascularity with poor outcome.[97,98] The strength of this biologic argument has supported the development of a number of novel therapeutic agents with antiangiogenic activities. These agents have moved through discovery and development and are now approved drugs for cancer. Additional information regarding angiogenesis and antiangiogenic therapy is provided in Chapter 15, Section C.

Reprogramming Energy Metabolism

The sustained growth and proliferation of a cancer requires a corresponding adjustment of energy metabolism to ensure this growth can be fueled. Under normal conditions, cells respire aerobically in that they metabolize glucose to pyruvate with a net gain in energy as ATP.[70] Cancer cells can undergo a "metabolic switch" so that glucose is metabolized to lactate, in the presence or absence of oxygen, causing a net energy deficit. A corresponding upregulation of glucose transporters (e.g., GLUT-1) occurs, which increases the uptake of glucose into the cytoplasm. This process is exploited in positron-emission tomography (PET) imaging because tumors preferentially uptake a radiolabeled analog of glucose (^{18}F-fluorodeoxyglucose [FDG]). This metabolic switch is sometimes referred to as the *Warburg effect* (Fig. 2.8).[99]

It is difficult to appreciate the survival advantage of this mechanism. One hypothesis is that the switch allows the diversion of glycolytic intermediates into other biosynthetic pathways that support the production of new cells. This is supported by the

observation that the Warburg effect also can be detected in growing cells in the embryo. An expansion of the theory of reprogramming of energy metabolism in cancer suggests that cancer cells have an advantage in a flexibility in their ability to derive ATP. This may come from a number of metabolic pathways that derive ATP from glucose metabolism under aerobic and anaerobic conditions, but it may also include efficiencies in metabolizing amino acids and lipids toward ATP and other biomolecule synthesis. Such metabolic flexibility may be necessary during primary tumor development, but even more so during metastatic progression (see next section).

Evading Immune Destruction

It is well defined that primary tumors and metastatic lesions can elicit both protective and suppressive immune responses.[79-80] B cells serve the host by the production of tumor-reactive antibodies. However, these antibodies may help define tumor-specific antigens (TSA) and aid in diagnosis, but they tend not to be protective for the host. Intense research has proven that the most protective forms of immunity against cancer are provided by the cell-mediated arm of the immune system, and immunocompromised animals are at increased risk of tumor development. (Tumor immunology is covered in detail in Chapter 14.)

The current and long-standing theory suggests that the cellular and tissue environment is constantly sampled and monitored by the immune system.[100] If a tumor is "altered self," then this should lead to eradication by a functioning immune system. Although there is a strong body of evidence to suggest that the immune system plays a major role in creating a barrier to tumor formation and progression, it is clear that when cancer arises, there is a failure of either surveillance or elimination mechanisms or both.[100] Epidemiologic evidence suggests that even the most immunogenic tumors have the ability to evolve mechanisms to subvert an apparently functioning immune system. This may arise through multiple mechanisms, but the best characterized of these include[101]:

- Inhibition of the effects of infiltrating cytotoxic T cells or natural killer (NK) cells
- Recruitment of immunosuppressive inflammatory cells (regulatory T cells [Treg] or myeloid-derived suppressor cells (MDSC) and tumor-promoting macrophages
- Defective antigen presentation; for example, by downregulation of the MHC class-1 machinery in cancer cells
- Failure of cancer cells to express co-stimulatory molecules, creating anergy or tolerance
- Expression of "immune checkpoint molecules," such as CTLA-4, or programmed-death-1 ligand/receptor (PD/PDL-1), which inhibit T-cell function

Tissue Invasion and Metastasis

The process of invasion and metastasis is covered in detail in subsequent sections of this chapter.

The Enabling Characteristics

As previously suggested, the hallmarks of cancer have been defined as functional capabilities that allow cancer cells to survive, proliferate, and disseminate. The fact that these critical hallmarks can be attained within a single cancer is explained by two key enabling characteristics of cancer – genome instability and tumor-promoting inflammation.

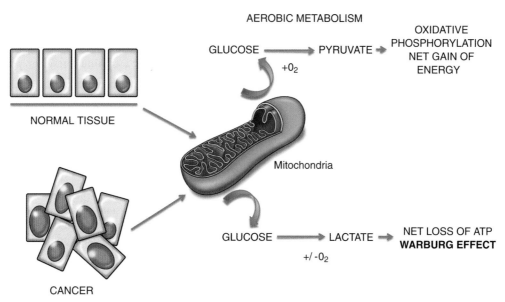

AEROBIC METABOLISM

• **Fig. 2.8** In normal tissues, cellular respiration in the presence of oxygen allows the production of a net gain in energy through metabolism of glucose to pyruvate. The *Warburg effect* in cancer cells refers to a metabolic switch that causes cancer cells to preferentially metabolize glucose to lactate irrespective of oxygen status, leading to a net loss of energy in the form of adenosine triphosphate (ATP).

Genome Instability

Most acquired hallmarks of cancer require changes in the genome through mutation, amplification, or chromosomal translocation. However, the process of random mutation is inefficient because of the complex and fastidious maintenance mechanisms of the normal cell that monitor DNA damage and regulate repair enzymes. As such, it is actually difficult to explain why cancers arise in animals at all, because the acquisition of all traits would seem an impossible task. To explain this, it may be argued that genomes must attain increased mutability or genome instability to overcome the redundant homeostatic mechanisms that ordinarily prevent the emergence of a cancer cell.[1,2]

A number of mechanisms have been suggested that may support the development of genomic instability.[70]

- Defects that affect various components of the DNA-maintenance machinery (caretakers of the genome), which may involve mutations in caretaker genes
- The loss of telomeric DNA, which may cause karyotypic instability and chromosomal changes (amplification/deletion)
- Inactivation of TS genes through genetic (mutation) or epigenetic (DNA methylation/histone modifications) mechanisms

Tumor-Promoting Inflammation

It has been recognized for decades that tumors contain inflammatory and immune cell infiltrates, which classically have been considered an attempt by the immune system to eradicate the tumor. However, recent evidence suggests that tumor-associated inflammation paradoxically may have a tumor-promoting effect. Inflammation can contribute to neoplastic progression through one of several mechanisms.[70, 80, 102,103]

- The supply of growth factors and growth signals to the TME that promote angiogenesis, cell proliferation, and invasion
- Induction signals that support the process of EMT
- Fostering of the progression of premalignant lesions to overt malignancy

- The production of reactive oxygen species that are mutagenic
Many of the cells that contribute to this are components of the innate immune system, particularly macrophages with a specific, cancer-promoting phenotype. Specifically, they form part of the TME that supports the maintenance of the cancer phenotype.

The Pathways to Cancer

The eight acquired capabilities of cancer cells and the two overarching enabling characteristics of genome instability and tumor inflammation have been outlined. It is important to stress that the pathways by which cells become malignant are highly variable. Mutations in certain oncogenes can occur early in the progression of some tumors and late in others. As a consequence, acquisition of the essential cancer characteristics may appear at different times in the progression of different cancers. Furthermore, in certain tumors a specific genetic event may, on its own, contribute only partially to the acquisition of a single capability, whereas in others it may contribute to the simultaneous acquisition of multiple capabilities. Regardless of the path taken, the hallmark capabilities of cancer remain common for multiple cancer types and help clarify mechanisms, prognosis, and the development of new treatments.

The highly complex signaling circuitry in cells is highly integrated and aligned with function. In the formation of a cancer cell, these circuits are "reprogrammed" to regulate the acquired capabilities of the cancer cell, or hallmarks of malignancy. The change is not simplistic, and considerable cross-talk occurs between circuits to support these hallmarks. This is in addition to a connection and signaling between the cancer cell and the TME

The Role of Tumor Microenvironment and Cancer Stem Cells

Over the past 10 years tumors have been increasingly considered as organ systems similar to the tissues from which they derive. This is in contrast to a reductionist view of cancer biology, which considers the tumor just a mass of tumor cells. In reality, the tumor is a complex system containing cancer cells and supporting cells, all of which contribute to the maintenance of the malignant population and support ultimate dissemination and metastasis. The major players in the cancer "organ system" are:

- Cancer cells and cancer stem cells (CSCs)
- Endothelial cells
- Pericytes
- Immune cells
- Tumor-associated fibroblasts

Cancer Cells and Cancer Stem Cells

The concept that a cancer can arise from any cell in the body, along with the stochastic model of tumorigenesis, has recently been challenged.[104–107] Although tumor heterogeneity is a well-established concept, a new dimension to heterogeneity has been established that suggests that a tumor may contain a hierarchical structure similar to many normal organ systems. Recent evidence suggests the existence of CSCs (sometimes termed *tumor-initiating cells*), which form the founder cell population for a tumor. It was first extensively documented for leukemia and multiple myeloma that only a small subset of cancer cells are capable of extensive proliferation. For example, when mouse myeloma cells were obtained from mouse ascites, separated from normal hematopoietic cells, and put in in vitro colony-forming assays, only 1 in 100 to 1 in 10,000 cancer cells were able to form colonies. Even when leukemic cells were transplanted in vivo, only 1% to 4% of cells could form spleen colonies.[106–114] Because the differences in clonogenicity among the leukemia cells mirrored the differences in clonogenicity among normal hematopoietic cells, the clonogenic leukemic cells were described as "leukemic stem cells."

It has also been shown for solid cancers that the cells are phenotypically heterogeneous and that only a small proportion of cells are clonogenic in culture and in vivo.[114–117] For example, only 1 in 1000 to 1 in 5000 lung cancer, ovarian cancer, or neuroblastoma cells were found to form colonies in soft agar. Just as in the context of leukemic stem cells, these observations led to the hypothesis that only a few cancer cells are actually tumorigenic and that these tumorigenic cells could be considered CSCs. Although the field and concept of CSCs is a controversial one, CSCs may prove to be a common constituent of many, if not all, cancer types. Features of the CSC model also fit well with a view of metastasis in which only a small number of cells within a tumor have the ability (and plasticity) to endure the stresses of metastatic progression, survive during a dormant period, and then progress, proliferate, and differentiate into the complex heterogenous metastatic lesion.

If tumor growth and metastasis are driven by a small population of CSCs, this might explain the failure to develop therapies that are consistently able to eradicate solid tumors.[104–107] Although currently available drugs can shrink tumors, these effects are usually transient and often do not appreciably extend the life of patients. One reason for the failure of these treatments is the acquisition of drug resistance by the cancer cells as they evolve; another possibility is that existing therapies fail to kill CSCs effectively.

Stem cell populations have been identified in human breast, bone, brain, colon, pancreas, liver, ovary, and skin cancers.[108–112] The actual origin of CSCs within solid tumors has not been clarified and may actually vary among tumor types. In some tumors the resident adult or somatic stem cell may serve as the

tumor-initiating cell, and in other tumors the initiating cell may be the resident progenitor or transit-amplifying cell. A characteristic of the CSCs is that they undergo asymmetric division and self-renew, providing a continual resident population of highly resistant cancer cells.

Existing cancer therapies have been largely developed against the bulk population of tumor cells because they are often identified by their ability to shrink tumors. Because most cells within a cancer have limited proliferative potential, an ability to shrink a tumor mainly reflects an ability to kill these cells. It seems that normal stem cells from various tissues tend to be more resistant to cytotoxic therapy than mature cell types from the same tissues. If the same is true of CSCs, then one would predict that these cells would be more resistant to cytotoxics than tumor cells with limited proliferative potential. Even therapies that cause complete regression of tumors might spare enough CSCs to allow regrowth of the tumors. Therapies that are more specifically directed against CSCs might result in much more durable responses and even cures of metastatic tumors. In veterinary oncology putative stem cell populations have been identified for breast, bone, brain, and liver tumors.[104–107,118–120] Interestingly, stem cell populations appear to have altered DNA repair pathways, which may explain their resistance to conventional drugs. Identification of these populations, coupled with the availability of microarray and microRNA array technology, is allowing the identification of potential therapeutic targets.

Recent research has linked the acquisition of CSC characteristics with the EMT program, described subsequently in the section on metastasis.[120] Cells that undergo EMT also take on characteristics reminiscent of the CSC phenotype. For example, they have the ability to self-renew and may support the ability of cells to colonize outside of the primary tumor. One may speculate that the signaling processes that support EMT may also serve to maintain the CSC population within a tumor and may also suggest plasticity in CSC populations.

Endothelial Cells

Much of the heterogeneity in tumors is found in the stromal compartment, and many of these cells are EC, which form the tumor-associated vasculature. VEGF and basic fibroblast growth factor are two prominent signaling molecules in the formation of these vessels. More modern sequencing techniques also have identified new pathways that may represent important signaling systems for neoangiogenesis and may represent therapeutic targets (e.g., Notch signaling).[121]

Pericytes

Pericytes are mesenchymal cells that wrap around the endothelial tubing of the blood vessels. Pericytes are considered a major cell type supporting the tumor vasculature.[122]

Immune Inflammatory Cells

As described previously, an environment of chronic inflammation is an important enabling characteristic that supports the acquisition of cancer-related traits. Cells of the innate immune system are particularly crucial for the maintenance of the tumor environment. In particular, tumor macrophages with a specific protumor phenotype can enhance cellular proliferation, invasion, and neoangiogenesis.[80]

Cancer-Associated Fibroblasts

Cancer-associated fibroblasts make up the supporting structure for many tumors but can also promote invasion, cell proliferation, and neoangiogenesis.[47] The importance of the various cell types that make up the TME cannot be overstated. Although a complex signaling network exists between and within cancer cells that maintains the cancer phenotype, superimposed on this are the complex signaling networks between stromal components and cancer cells. Although the potential evolution of cancer cells from early disease to late-stage disease has been discussed, it is quite possible that a similar evolution occurs in the supporting structures, dictated by the cancer itself. For example, incipient tumors may recruit stromal elements, which reciprocate by promoting cell proliferation and angiogenesis. Evolution of the cancer population may then feed back on the stromal population to further reprogram these cells to support the growing tumor. Of course, this could be extended to show the role of the stroma in promoting invasion and metastasis. These mechanisms underpin the complexity of understanding cancer pathogenesis, because the process is highly dynamic and context dependent.[123]

Key Points

- Cancer arises through multiple molecular mechanisms underpinned by changes at the genetic and/or epigenetic level.
- Cancer has been defined as the acquisition of eight fundamental characteristics shared across multiple cancer types. These hallmarks are enabled and supported by underlying genomic instability and tumor-associated inflammation.
- The normal circuitry in cells is reprogrammed to support these hallmarks and drive tumor progression.
- These circuits are interconnected and are also supported by cross-talk from cells making up the tumor microenvironment.
- Cancer stem cells may play a major role in maintaining the tumor in a way similar to the maintenance of normal organ systems by adult stem cells.

The Process of Tumor Metastasis

Metastasis is defined as the dissemination of neoplastic cells to discontinuous secondary (or higher order) sites, where they proliferate to form a macroscopic mass. Implicit in this process is the presence of a primary tumor. Metastases are not a direct extension of the primary tumor and are not dependent on the route of spread (i.e., hematogenous versus lymphatic versus peritoneal dissemination). The process of metastasis is believed to occur through the completion of a series of step-wise events. For this process to occur, a cancer cell must leave the site of the primary tumor, pass through the tumor basement membrane, and then through or between endothelial cells to enter the circulation (extravasation). While in the circulation, tumor cells must be able to resist anoikis (programmed cell death associated with loss of cellular contact), evade immune recognition and physical stress, and eventually arrest at distant organs. At that distant site the cell must leave the circulation and survive in the hostile microenvironment of the foreign tissue. These secondary sites are believed to be primed to receive metastatic cells through effects that are directed and mediated by the primary tumor itself (premetastatic niche). The distant site may be the eventual target organ for metastasis or may be a temporary (sanctuary) site. In either case, the cancer cell is thought to lie dormant for a variable and often protracted period before moving to its final location. After a break

in dormancy, cells receive signals to proliferate, create new blood vessels (angiogenesis) or co-opt existing blood vessels, and then successfully grow into a measurable metastatic lesion. Further progression likely is associated with the repetition of this process, resulting in the development of metastases from metastases. As such, the steps outlined here continue not only after the detection of the primary tumor, but also after the detection of metastases. From a therapeutic perspective, therefore it is never too late to target the biologic steps associated with metastatic progression as a means to improve outcomes for patients. The basic tenets of this model of metastasis have been intact for more than 40 years; however, a greater understanding of the biologic principles associated with each metastatic process is emerging.[124]

Metastasis-Associated Genes and Metastasis Suppressor Genes

Cancer cells are not unique in their ability to complete the individual steps required for metastasis (Fig. 2.9). For example, leukocytes and neuronal cells have the ability to invade tissue planes and cross vascular barriers. Several types of leukocytes demonstrate the phenotype of intermittent adherence to vascular endothelium and are able to resist anoikis. It is also true that stem cells of various phases of differentiation are able to perform many of these steps during development and in the adult.[125,126] Metastatic cells are unique in that each cell must be able to perform all the steps required for successful metastasis. An extension of this argument is that the genetic changes that permit the metastatic process are not unique to a metastatic cancer cell; however, the metastatic cell must have the appropriate set of genetic changes available to complete all the steps of the metastatic cascade.

Literally hundreds of genes and their resultant proteins have been suggested to contribute to the development of cancers and to their eventual ability to metastasize. A single genetic change in cancer can contribute many of the metastasis-associated processes (e.g., metastasis super enhancer), or several genes can work together toward a single metastasis-associated process. Metastatic cancers may achieve the metastatic phenotype through distinct constellations of genetic and epigenetic events that in their respective sums complete the list of necessary metastasis-associated processes needed for successful metastasis.[127]

Two classes of genes have been broadly defined as contributing to the metastatic phenotype. These include metastasis promoting genes[128,129] and metastasis suppressors.[129,130] These genes have functions in normal development and physiology (i.e., cell migration, tissue invasion, and angiogenesis, discussed earlier) that are subverted by the cancer cell in the acquisition of the metastatic phenotype.

The use of high throughput and genome-wide investigations has uncovered many putative metastasis-associated genes in cancer. It should be noted that many metastasis-associated genes have functions that also contribute to tumor formation and progression. Several of these metastasis-associated genes have been validated in canine and feline cancers.[131,132] For example, the metastasis-associated gene ezrin was identified using genomic approaches in murine and human studies of metastasis.[133] Ezrin is a membrane-cytoskeleton linker protein that functionally and physically connects the actin cytoskeleton to the cell membrane. The degree of ezrin expression in the primary tumor of dogs with osteosarcoma (OSA) was shown to predict a more aggressive course of disease, defined by metastasis to the lung. Furthermore, recent studies have confirmed the connection between ezrin and protein kinase C (PKC) signaling in murine, canine, and human OSA cells.[134,135]

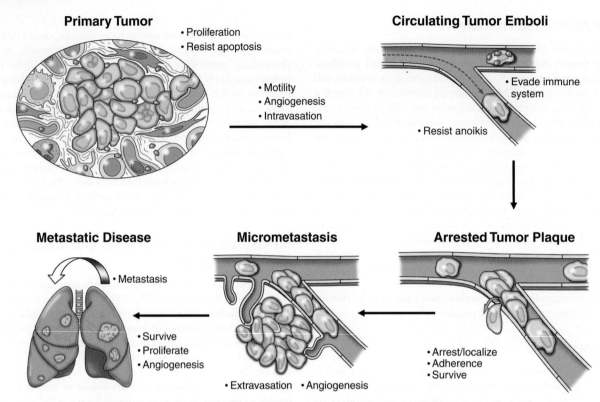

Primary Tumor
- Proliferation
- Resist apoptosis

- Motility
- Angiogenesis
- Intravasation

Circulating Tumor Emboli
- Evade immune system
- Resist anoikis

Metastatic Disease
- Metastasis
- Survive
- Proliferate
- Angiogenesis

Micrometastasis
- Extravasation   - Angiogenesis

Arrested Tumor Plaque
- Arrest/localize
- Adherence
- Survive

• **Fig. 2.9** The metastatic cascade. The metastatic cascade describes a set of discrete steps that cells must move through as a part of the process of metastasis. This complexity begins with the recognized complexity associated with primary tumor development, in which tumor cells must proliferate, resist apoptosis, and develop interactions with many host cells in the microenvironment. Subsequent steps allow metastatic cancer cells to enter and survive in the circulation. Cells then arrest at distant locations, extravasate, and survive in the microenvironment of the distant locations. Arrest of cells may be at the eventual secondary organ where metastasis becomes clinically evident, or cells may initially arrest at a "sanctuary site," where they may lie dormant before moving on to the eventual secondary site. The cellular programs that result in a break of dormancy are not well understood. Survival of cells at these sites of dormancy or the eventual secondary site is a significant hurdle for metastatic cells to overcome. Indeed, the majority of cells that arrive at distant locations are unable to survive in these distant locations. At secondary sites, tumor cells may proliferate and progress after the development of the angiogenic phenotype. It is likely that successful metastatic lesions at secondary sites are then the source of subsequent metastases within these secondary sites.

Metastasis suppressor genes have been identified in several human cancers. These genes also are thought to have normal functions in the regulation of motility, invasion, and angiogenesis. The loss of these genes is not thought to be associated with the formation of tumors; however, their loss is thought to contribute to specific steps in the metastatic cascade. The characterization, biology, and clinical effect of metastasis suppressor genes have been recently reviewed elsewhere.[136] The loss or reduced expression of metastasis suppressors has not been documented in canine or feline cancers to date.

The succeeding sections provide descriptions of the critical metastasis-associated processes (see Fig. 2.9). Examples of genetic changes or resulting protein changes that contribute to each process are highlighted in each section, with particular emphasis on those with demonstrated associations with veterinary malignancies.

Intravasation

After the successful growth of the primary tumor, intravasation of a cancer cell into the vascular or lymphatic circulation is the first necessary step in the metastatic cascade. The process of intravasation requires that a tumor cell be motile and able to digest, modulate, or escape the ECM.[137–139] The specific mechanisms used by cancer cells

to invade and intravasate include the classic model of enzymatic degradation of the ECM referred to as *mesenchymal invasion* (see later discussion on EMT). Unlike in mesenchymal invasion, tumor cells may also develop so-called *amoeboid invasion,* in which they individually slip between fibers of the ECM without evidence or a need for enzymatic degradation.[140] Finally, a distinct method, termed *collective invasion,* refers to the en masse regional extension of a tumor into surrounding tissues.[141] Such collective invasion is observed clinically in dogs with oral SCC and biologically high-grade/histologically low-grade fibrosarcoma. The low rate of distant metastasis associated with collective invasion suggests a lack of functional attributes necessary for true distant metastasis. It is likely that individual metastatic tumors may use distinct invasion programs at distinct points during metastatic progression. Not surprisingly, studies with intravital imaging (single cell imaging of cancer cells in animals) have demonstrated that only a minority of the cells in the primary tumor develop any of these forms of invasion.[142,143] Efforts are underway to define the genetic features of this minority population.[144,145]

In the classic mesenchymal form of invasion, matrix proteases and metalloproteases (MMPs) are believed to be necessary for the invasive phenotype. Expression of members of this enzyme family has been found in most human and several canine and feline malignancies, including canine OSA.[146–149] The activity of MMPs in OSA and mast cell tumors has been correlated with grade and metastatic propensity.[149,150] Similar correlative studies have been undertaken in human patients.[151] The importance of MMP activity during this early step in metastasis prompted the development of pharmacologic inhibitors of MMPs. Anticancer activity of these agents in preclinical animal models and in sporadic human patients was evident; however, in randomized trials, clinical benefit was not observed.[152,153] The failure of these clinical trials may be explained at many levels and does not refute the importance of invasion as a critical step for a metastatic cell. Rather, these results suggest potential redundancy in the types of invasion (mesenchymal versus amoeboid) that may exist within a given cancer.[154,155] Recent evidence also suggests that the expression of matrix-degrading enzymes and other growth factors may not be necessary in the tumor cells themselves but may be provided by inflammatory cells (i.e., macrophages) recruited by the growing tumor.[156]

Epithelial-Mesenchymal Transition

Observed primarily in the context of epithelial malignancies, the ability of tumor cells to engage in the early steps in the metastatic cascade has been linked to a transcriptional program referred to as EMT.[157] This transcriptional program has been largely ascribed to the effects of a family of transcription factors, including *twist, snail,* and *slug.*[158] Activation of these and other EMT transcription factors is not necessarily associated with a morphologic change in the cancer cell but may be associated with a loss of polarity (apicobasal) in epithelial cells, a greater proportion of cells losing cell-to-cell contacts similar to mesenchymal cells (observed in vitro), cell motility, and invasion. In the "mesenchymal" state, suggested by EMT, epithelial cancer cells (similar to cells involved in embryogenesis) develop the phenotypic ability to undergo invasion, migration, and intravasation.[159] Interestingly, cells that are able to take on these "mesenchymal" features share signaling programs and other phenotypes with tumor-initiating cell populations.[160]

Opponents of the EMT hypothesis are most critical of the use of the term *transition,* which suggests a switch in the phenotype of individual cells from an epithelial to a mesenchymal form. However, it is reasonable and generally agreed that the effects of EMT transcription factors contribute to the early phenotypes needed for metastatic progression. Limited data also suggests a need for mesenchymal cells to take on attributes of epithelial cells (likely later during metastatic progression) for successful metastasis, the so-called *mesenchymal-epithelial transition* (MET). For epithelial cancers MET is also understood to be a final step in EMT in which after the activation, development of an invasive phenotype, and colonization of a distant site, cells will revert to their original epithelial phenotypes.

The process of intravasation concludes when a cancer cell successfully enters the vascular or lymphatic circulation. Tumor cells may enter the circulation through established blood vessels, small arterioles, venules, or lymphatics, or through tumor-associated (or lined) blood vessels in a process referred to as *vasculogenic mimicry.*[161] For larger vascular structures the process of intravasation requires penetration of adventitial cells, including pericytes; digestion of the vascular basement membrane; and penetration between or through EC.[162] Penetration of the tumor-associated vasculature may be easier than invasion through normal vessels and may require only transit from the extracellular environment between EC into the circulation.

Survival in the Circulation (Resisting Anoikis)

Frisch and Francis reported the induction of apoptosis after disruption of the interaction between epithelial cells and the ECM.[163] This phenomenon was termed *anoikis,* from the Greek word for homelessness. In normal tissues, anoikis is a mechanism for maintaining tissue homeostasis and integrity.[164] For the metastatic cancer cell, survival during dissemination requires resistance to anoikis. In normal tissues, anoikis is prevented by two systems: cell-matrix anchorage and cell-cell interactions.[165] Anchorage of cells to the ECM is mediated primarily by transmembrane receptors referred to as *integrins.* The formation of active heterodimers triggers an intracellular cascade, resulting in activation of effectors of growth and survival.[166] Integrin family members have been identified in canine sarcomas and lymphomas.[167–172] Cell-cell anchorage in many epithelial tissues is mediated by cadherins, a family of calcium-binding glycoproteins. Intracellularly, cadherins form complexes with members of the catenin protein family that link them to the actin cytoskeleton, in addition to survival-promoting signal transduction cascades.[173] Loss of either cell-cell or cell-matrix interaction in normal cells triggers the activation of the caspase proteases, the hallmark of apoptotic cell death. Metastatic cancer must resist this contact-dependent death to be successful and must do so through two non–mutually exclusive mechanisms. The first is by maintaining cell-cell contacts with other tumor cells (homotypic interactions) or with host cells, such as platelets and inflammatory cells (heterotypic interactions), during metastatic progression. Both homotypic and heterotypic interactions generate intracellular signals that prevent the initiation of anoikis. Additionally, cancer cells may overexpress proteins that directly inhibit anoikis. For example, the integrin pair $\alpha_v\beta_3$ is frequently overexpressed in malignancy, including prostate cancer and melanoma.[174,175] This overexpression subverts the need for ligand binding and results in the generation of survival signals.[176] Proteins reported to be involved in resistance to anoikis include tropomyosin receptor kinase B (TrkB), focal adhesion kinase (FAK, the immediate effector of integrin signaling), galectin-3, and TGF-β, among others.[177] Several other molecular mediators of anoikis resistance have been identified and are reviewed elsewhere.[178] These molecules may be valuable novel antimetastasis targets.

Evasion of the Immune System

At all stages of metastatic progression, metastatic tumor cells must evade detection and destruction by the immune system. The ability of the host immune system to recognize and destroy tumor cells (immunosurveillance) was first proposed by Paul Ehrlich in 1909. Molecular support of the theory of immunosurveillance has come with studies of mice deficient in immunomodulatory and proinflammatory molecules, such as interferon-gamma (IFN-γ), interleukin-12 (IL-12), and perforin. Mice deficient in these molecules are known to develop tumors more readily than wild-type mice.[80] Clinical evidence for immunosurveillance against cancer was first reported by Coley more than 100 years ago. Through the administration of bacteria, Coley's toxin, Coley was able to induce fever and tumor regression in patients with cancer. Evidence in dogs with OSA further supports the potential value of cancer immunotherapy.[179] Indeed, survival times in dogs developing bacterial infection at the site of a limb salvage surgery are significantly longer than in dogs that do not develop infection. Interestingly, similar parallels may be seen in human OSA patients.[180] It is believed that in immunocompetent hosts, immunosurveillance removes a large number of cancer cells from the primary tumor, from the circulation, and at distant metastatic sites. Cancer cells use a wide variety of mechanisms to effect this evasion. The mechanisms for immunosurveillance and evasion of immunosurveillance by cancer are reviewed elsewhere and are summarized in Chapter 14.[181]

Modification of the immune system to treat cancer and prevent metastasis continues to be an attractive therapeutic strategy.[182] Clinical trials based on this concept have been reported throughout the veterinary literature in dogs with melanoma, soft tissue sarcoma, hemangiosarcoma, OSA, and others, using a variety of immune-based therapies.[185] This principle has been the basis for the development and approval of a therapeutic vaccine directed against a melanoma antigen in dogs with melanoma.[186]

Arrest in Target Tissues

The arrest of circulating tumor cells at distant sites is thought to occur by two distinct but potentially overlapping mechanisms. These include size-dependent "trapping" of tumor cells within the lumens of small vessels (capillaries and veins) in the target organ, and/or receptor-mediated interaction involving the tumor cell and the host vasculature.[187] Data supporting the trapping phenomenon comes from single-cell imaging studies in which metastatic cancer cells were observed to arrest primarily at distant vascular beds as a result of size-dependent restrictions of large tumor cells in small blood vessels.[188,189] This work was conducted primarily for metastasis to the liver and more recently for metastasis to the brain.[190] This trapping phenomenon suggests that the site for metastasis from a primary tumor is guided largely by the location of the first (small vessel) vascular bed encountered by a tumor cell. Alternatively, several groups have suggested the role of specific adhesion molecules as being necessary for initial tumor arrest in the microenvironment of the secondary metastatic sites.[191–193] Both of these mechanisms likely play a role in the initial seeding of distant metastatic target organs. The dominant mechanism of arrest may be primarily defined by tumor type or target organ.

Early Survival at Distant Sites

Once the cancer cell or cancer embolus has arrested at its distant sites, it may immediately move out of the circulation into the target organ or may stay within the circulation.[194] In either location the cancer cell must survive in a new microenvironment. Early survival of metastatic cells at secondary sites is a significant hurdle for the cancer cell. Several studies have shown the ability of cancer cells to arrest at multiple organs in the body. Within hours the number of remaining cells is reduced dramatically, and within days the number of viable cells may be as low as 0.1% of the original number of cells, even for the most aggressive cancer models.[195] To a large extent organ selectivity for cancers is defined by the organs in which a cancer cell can survive after initial arrest. The "seed and soil" hypothesis first articulated by Paget and then more recently by Fidler et al[193,213] suggests that the success of a cancer, or metastasis, is defined by interactions between the seed (tumor cell) and the soil (the tumor microenvironment).[196]

Arrest of tumor cells in target organs may or may not be receptor mediated (discussed earlier); however, adhesion requires receptor-ligand interactions. Contributors to these steps include the cell adhesion molecules (CAMs). Multiple CAMs have been identified and are named based on their cell specificity (e.g., N-CAM for neural and L-CAM for liver). CD44 is a specific adhesion molecule (H-CAM for homing) initially identified as the receptor for the matrix component hyaluronic acid on hematopoietic cells. Expression of splice variants of CD44 on tumor cells has been demonstrated to correlate with a poor prognosis in a wide variety of human tumors, from acute myelogenous leukemia (AML) and Hodgkin's disease to breast and colon cancer and OSA.[197] Chemokines are a class of chemotactic cytokines that function in leukocyte trafficking and function. In metastasis chemokines may also contribute to the metastatic process through enhanced metastatic cell survival.[198] Chemokines may be active in the recruitment of a leukocytic infiltrate to intravasated, circulating tumor cells, therein creating an embolus that can better resist shearing stress associated with circulation or through the generation of matrix-degrading proteins at the distant metastatic site.

The Premetastatic Niche and Modulation of the Microenvironment

It is increasingly clear that the sites (microenvironments) of successful secondary metastasis are modulated by the presence of a primary tumor and then by the arrival of metastatic cells at the secondary site. The concept of the premetastatic niche suggests that a primary tumor modulates the microenvironment of a secondary site before the arrival of most metastatic cells.[199] The modulation of the premetastatic niche appears to be accomplished by primary tumor–induced mobilization and recruitment of specific, primarily bone marrow–derived cells (bone marrow niche) to the secondary microenvironment.[200] These bone marrow–derived cells are myeloid in origin and express VEGFR. Interestingly, the sites of metastatic tumor arrest appear preferentially to include sites in which these myeloid-derived cells were first recruited. Furthermore, targeting these VEGFR-positive cells using pharmacologic and genetic tools has effectively prevented metastatic development in murine models.[201] Ongoing studies likely will uncover greater complexity of the populations of cells recruited to the premetastatic niche and potentially therapeutic targets for antimetastatic therapy.

After survival at the distant site, the tumor cell must proliferate and modulate its new environment. In most cases cancer cells are believed to extravasate from the circulation and then proliferate in the new organ. However, proliferation also may occur within blood vessels, in a process referred to as *intravascular metastases,* and then expand into the local tissue before further proliferation occurs.[201] In both situations modulation of the new environment is necessary for appropriate growth and progression of the metastatic lesions. We now recognize that part of this modulation is based on tumor-induced changes in the stroma.[202,203] These stromal changes may result in the production of growth factors or signals that are used by the tumor for further growth. These stromal cell–derived growth factors provide important signals for tumor cell proliferation and progression, including angiogenesis. The importance of tumor-stromal interaction suggests that the "induced" tumor-stroma may be a credible target for novel cancer therapeutics.[204]

Metastasis from Metastases

For most solid tumors the appearance of a single metastatic nodule is followed shortly by the development of additional metastases within the same target organ and tertiary sites. All these metastatic sites are unlikely to emerge from distinct and unique clones within the primary tumor and nearly simultaneously progress through the metastatic cascade to yield synchronous metastases at the distant site. It is reasonable, and perhaps more likely, that metastases develop from other metastatic sites. In this hypothesis a small number of successful clones colonize distant sites. As these clones move through progression to become successful metastases, the process of metastasis continues, resulting in metastasis from metastases. Although data supporting this hypothesis is limited, the implication for the treatment and management of cancer patients is substantial. If true, the process of metastasis from metastases would suggest that all steps in the metastatic cascade occur continuously, both before and after detection of metastases in patients. As such, all of the steps in the metastatic cascade may be targets for future therapeutic intervention.[205–211]

Ongoing Controversies and Areas of Research in the Field of Metastasis

Does the Metastatic Propensity for Tumors Emerge Early or Late in the Biology of Cancer?

The development of the metastatic phenotype traditionally has been believed to be a process that happens late in carcinogenesis. In this model, referred to as the *progression model,* the genetic changes responsible for primary tumor development in most cases are distinct and precede the steps that result in the metastatic phenotype.[212–213] The progression model argues that the metastatic phenotype is acquired within a small fraction of cells within the heterogeneous primary tumor. Support for the progression model came from work by Fidler and others, who demonstrated the ability to select for rodent cancers with greater metastatic potential, through the serial passage of metastatic tumor nodules back to naïve mice. This selection phenomenon suggested that a minority of tumor cell clones within a primary tumor were endowed with the metastatic phenotype and that this small proportion were enriched in the metastases compared with the primary tumor. Application of the progression model would suggest that a period exists between primary tumor development and acquisition of the full metastatic phenotype. This model was thought to be the basis of the improved outcome associated with early detection of cancers and the belief that effective and definitive therapy was most likely if a diagnosis was made early. Work from Ramaswamy et al provided data to support an alternative model, "the early oncogenic model" for metastasis.[214–217] This alternative suggests that the genetic events that contribute to initial primary tumor development are the same or emerge at the same time as the events that contribute to the metastatic phenotype. As such, the early oncogenic model suggests, the biology of a cancer is defined early and may not be something that can be reduced through early identification of a cancer. This is not to say that early detection of a cancer is not helpful for a patient, but rather that bad cancers may be "born" bad. This model may explain the phenomenon of "metastatic carcinoma of unknown primary site," in which metastatic disease is detected without an apparent primary tumor.

To add complexity to the question of the emergence of the metastatic phenotype, increasing evidence indicates that host (genomic) differences can influence the metastatic behavior of cancers without necessarily influencing primary tumor growth.[214,215] Using a genetically engineered mouse model of mammary cancer, Hunter et al have been able to identify specific host genes that influence metastatic behavior of tumors.[214–217] These findings have several important implications. First, they suggest that individuals might be predisposed to aggressive metastatic progression before the development of a tumor. In addition they suggest that some families in the population may be at high risk, not necessarily for tumor development, but for an aggressive metastatic course once a tumor develops. Most important, if a significant part of a patient's metastatic risk is encoded within the patient's constitutional genome rather than within the mutated tumor genome, it may be feasible to identify individuals at high risk for metastatic disease at the time of diagnosis of the primary tumor, or potentially before. This finding may be particularly relevant in the field of veterinary oncology, in which breed-associated genomic

differences may explain the more aggressive course of disease seen in some dog breeds compared with others. Taken together, the risk for metastatic progression is partly defined by the genetics of the patient, genetic changes that develop early in the process of tumor development, and the subsequent and incremental emergence of aggressive metastatic cells.

Where Is the Inefficiency in "Metastatic Inefficiency"?

As devastating as the metastatic process is, it is equally inefficient. Estimates of this inefficiency in animal models suggest that less than 1% of cancer cells that successfully enter the circulation are able to survive at distant sites.[218] The true metastatic efficiency of human cancers is likely to be much lower. In most studies to date it does not seem that entry of cancer cells into the circulation is the major barrier for successful metastases. Recent studies have identified high numbers of circulating tumor cells in cancer patients who are free of metastatic disease. The clinical importance of high numbers of circulating tumor cells is not clear[219]; however, for some cancers high numbers of circulating cancer cells apparently do not necessarily correlate with the risk for metastasis. Butler and Gullino estimated that 1 to 4×10^6 cells/g of tumor enter the systemic circulation each day in human cancers.[220] This data suggests that, although intravasation is necessary for metastasis, it is not sufficient nor is it process limiting. After removal of the primary tumor, these circulating cell counts drop, and in many cases no gross metastases develop. Although arrest at target organs may be a limitation for some cancers, early survival of cancer cells at distant sites appears to be a major hurdle for successful metastases and therefore is a significant contributor to metastatic inefficiency. Metastatic cancer cells appear to be highly vulnerable to death early after their arrival at a secondary site. The microenvironment of the secondary site is distinct from that of the primary tumor site and the initial tissues of origin of the cancer cell. These differences include changes in oxygen tension, pH, growth factor availability, and cellular binding partners. Collectively, these changes represent unique stressors to metastatic cancer cells.[221]

Metastatic cells must recognize, adapt, and endure these stresses to survive. Furthermore, appropriate modulation of the secondary microenvironment before the cancer cells arrive (premetastatic niche) and as a result of early and effective interaction with stromal and inflammatory cells within the new environment allow select populations of cells to survive and proliferate. The duration of this initial vulnerable state during metastatic progression may extend for the entire period of dormancy (see later). Also, metastatic cells likely must pass successfully through additional vulnerable states later during metastatic progression. Targeting metastatic cancer cells during these vulnerable states may be an effective treatment strategy for cancer metastasis.[222]

What is Dormancy and Where Do Dormant Cells Reside?

In spite of effective control of the primary tumor and aggressive multiagent and multimodality adjuvant therapy, the risk for metastases to distant sites remains high for several cancer histologies. Because most patients are free of gross metastases at the time of diagnosis, the development of metastases is presumed to emerge from microscopic cells that are not identifiable at the time of initial patient presentation.[223] The location, size, angiogenic state, and proliferative/apoptotic state of these microscopic cells are largely unknown. Indeed, these dormant cells may exist as single cancer cells or microscopic clusters; they may exist in a quiescent (outside the cell cycle) or balanced state of proliferation and apoptosis; they may lie dormant in the eventual secondary metastatic tissue site (e.g., the lung); or they may persist in sanctuary sites (e.g., the bone marrow). Recent insights gleaned from the CSC model may provide further support for the hypothesis that metastatic cells are capable of residence in transient sites such as the bone marrow, where they may rest in a dormant state before being recruited into the metastatic cascade. The signals that induce these presumed small populations of cells to break dormancy and emerge into gross metastases likely also involve TME interaction.[224,225]

Metastasis Biology: New Perspectives

Metastasis is a nearly universally grave development for cancer patients, irrespective of specific cancer histology. An emerging hypothesis proposes the existence of unique settings during the metastatic cascade when metastatic cells are vulnerable and stressed. Cellular adaptation to stress in these vulnerable cells is the most defining feature of metastatic proclivity and could be a target for new cancer drug development. Conversely, proliferation, apoptosis, invasion, and migration are neither sufficient nor necessary for metastatic success and therefore do not necessarily represent ideal targets for metastatic therapy.

Consistent with the *vulnerable cell hypothesis* is the concept of primary tumor reseeding. Some studies suggest that metastatic cells that leave the primary tumor likely distribute to all tissues in the body by hematogenous spread; however, survival of rare single metastatic cells at distant sites predicts the future development of gross metastases. Included in this list of metastatic sites is the microenvironment of the primary tumor, suggesting that local recurrence is also a product of distant metastasis. This *tumor reseeding hypothesis* also suggests a rationale to study the value of increased "surgical dose" in patients with nonlocalized tumors as a means to improve long-term outcomes. Conversely, the fact that the vast majority of metastatic cells in an organ will never survive or become a clinical problem should have us asking about the definitions of a metastatic site and the value of surgical resection of tissues that have microscopic evidence of metastasis but no clinically appreciated disease (i.e., a firm, fixed, and effaced lymph node).

Summary and Future Directions

This chapter has sought to simplify as far as possible the mechanisms of carcinogenesis and metastasis. Clearly, genomic instability and an environment of chronic inflammation support and provide a basis for the acquisition of the eight fundamental cancer characteristics. The identification of these pathways is providing excellent clues to the underlying mechanisms in cancer and the identification of potential therapeutic targets. However, despite the ability to make small molecules or antibodies, which aim at key targets in cancer survival, we are still a long way from a cure. The reasons for this are many but include inherent tumor heterogeneity (in part supplied by the existence of tumor stem cells), continual tumor evolution, and the immense and underestimated contribution of the tumor microenvironment. Unquestionably, multiple approaches will be required to maximize any possibility of therapeutic benefit.

References

1. McCance KL, Roberts LK: Cellular biology. In McCance KL, Huether SE, editors: *Pathophysiology: the biologic basis of disease in adults and children*, ed 3, St. Louis, 1997, Mosby.
2. Wyke J: Viruses and cancer. In Franks LM, Teich NM, editors: *The molecular and cellular biology of cancer*, ed 3, Oxford, 1997, Oxford University Press.
3. Vousden KH: Cell transformation by human papillomaviruses. In Minsen AC, Neil JC, McCrae MA, editors: *Viruses and cancer*, Cambridge, 1994, Cambridge University Press.
4. Campo MS, O'Neil BW, Barron RJ, et al.: Experimental reproduction of the papilloma-carcinoma complex of the alimentary canal in cattle, *Carcinogenesis* 15:1597–1601, 1994.
5. Campo MS, Jarrett WF, Barron R, et al.: Association of bovine papillomavirus type 2 and bracken fern with bladder cancer in cattle, *Cancer Res* 52:6898–6904, 1992.
6. Donner P, Greiser-Wilkie I, Moelling K: Nuclear localization and DNA binding of the transforming gene product of avian myelocytomatosis virus, *Nature* 296:262–266, 1982.
7. Reid SW, Smith KT, Jarrett WF: Detection, cloning and characterisation of papillomaviral DNA present in sarcoid tumours of *Equus asinus*, *Vet Rec* 135:430–432, 1994.
8. Gaukroger JM, Bradley A, Chandrachud L, et al.: Interaction between bovine papillomavirus type 4 and cocarcinogens in the production of malignant tumours, *J Gen Virol* 74(Pt 10):2275–2280, 1993.
9. Jarrett WF: Bovine papilloma viruses, *Clin Dermatol* 3:8–19, 1985.
10. Lancaster WD, Olson C, Meinke W: Bovine papillomavirus: presence of virus-specific DNA sequences in naturally occurring equine tumours, *Proc Nat Acad Sci U S A* 74:524–528, 1977.
11. Bertoli C, Skotheim JM, de Bruin RAM: Control of cell cycle transcription during G1 and S phases, *Nat Rev Mol Cell Biol* 14:518–528, 2013.
12. Casem ML: Cell Cycle. In Casem ML, editor: *Case studies in cell biology*, ed 1, Cambridge, 2016, MA: Academic Press, pp 299–326.
13. Romanel A, Jensen LJ, Cardelli L, et al.: Transcriptional regulation is a major controller of cell cycle transition dynamics, *PLOS One* 7:e29716, 2012.
14. Otto T, Sicinski P: Cell cycle proteins as promising targets in cancer therapy, *Nat Rev Cancer* 17:93–115, 2017.
15. Golias CH, Charalabopoulos A, Charalabopoulos: Cell proliferation and cell cycle control: a mini review, *Int J Clin Prac* 58:1134–1141, 2004.
16. Kong N, Fotouhi N, Wovkulich PM, et al.: Cell cycle inhibitors for the treatment of cancer, *Drugs Future* 28:881–896, 2003.
17. Maréchal A, Zou L: DNA Damage Sensing by the ATM and ATR kinases, *Cold Spring Harb Perspect Biol* 5:a012716, 2013.
18. Kastenhuber ER, Lowe SW: Putting p53 in context, *CELL* 170:1062–1078, 2017.
19. Lane DP: P53: guardian of the genome, *Nature* 358:15–16, 1992.
20. Brady CA, Attardi LD: p53 at a glance, *J Cell Sci* 123:2527–2532, 2010.
21. Levine AJ: P53, the cellular gatekeeper for growth and division, *Cell* 88:323–331, 1997.
22. Joerger AC, Fersht AR: The p53 pathway: origins, inactivation in cancer, and emerging therapeutic approaches, *Annu Rev Biochem* 85:375–404, 2016.
23. Wu X, Bayle JH, Olson D, et al.: The p53-mdm2 autoregulatory loop, *Genes Dev* 7:1126–1132, 1993.
24. Haupt Y, Maya R, Kazaz A, et al.: Mdm2 promotes the rapid degradation of p53, *Nature* 387:296–299, 1997.
25. Abegglen LM, Caulin AF, Chan A, et al.: Potential mechanisms for cancer resistance in elephants and comparative cellular response to DNA damage in humans, *J Am Med Assoc* 314:1850–1860, 2015.
26. Strasser A, Cory S, Adams JM: Deciphering the rules of programmed cell death to improve therapy of cancer and other diseases, *EMBO J* 30:3667–3683, 2011.
27. Jones S, Zhang X, Parsons DW, et al.: Core signaling pathways in human pancreatic cancers revealed by global genomic analyses, *Science* 321:1801–1806, 2008.
28. Parsons DW, Jones S, Zhang X, et al.: An integrated genomic analysis of human glioblastoma multiforme, *Science* 321:1807–1812, 2008.
29. McCance KL, Roberts LK: The biology of cancer. In McCance KL, Huether SE, editors: *Pathophysiology: the biological basis of disease in adults and children*, ed 3, St. Louis, 1997, Mosby.

30. Maher CA, Wilson RK: Chromothripsis and human disease: piecing together the shattering process, *Cell* 148:29–32, 2012.

31. Stephens PJ, Greenman CD, Fu B, et al.: Massive genomic rearrangement acquired in a single catastrophic event during cancer development, *Cell* 144:27–40, 2011.

32. Forment JV, Kaidi A, Jackson SP: Chromothripsis and cancer: causes and consequences of chromosome shattering, *Nat Rev Cancer* 12:663–670, 2012.

33. Jarrett O, Onions D: Leukaemogenic viruses. In Whittaker JA, editor: *Leukaemia*, ed 2, Oxford, 1992, Blackwell.

34. Balmain A, Brown K: Oncogene activation in chemical carcinogenesis, *Adv Cancer Res* 51:147–182, 1988.

35. Adams GE, Cox R: Radiation carcinogenesis. In Franks LM, Teich NM, editors: *The molecular and cellular biology of cancer*, ed 3, New York, 1997, Oxford University Press.

36. Neil JC, Hughs D, McFarlane R, et al.: Transduction and rearrangement of the myc gene by feline leukemia virus in naturally occurring T cell leukemias, *Nature* 308:814–820, 1984.

37. Onions DE, Lees G, Forrest D, et al.: Recombinant feline viruses containing the myc gene rapidly produce clonal tumours expressing T-cell antigen receptor gene transcripts, *Int J Cancer* 40:40–45, 1987.

38. Teich NM: Oncogenes and cancer. In Franks LM, Teich NM, editors: *The molecular and cellular biology of cancer*, ed 3, New York, 1997, Oxford University Press.

39. Tennent R, Wigley C, Balmain A: Chemical carcinogenesis. In Franks LM, Teich NM, editors: *The molecular and cellular biology of cancer*, ed 3, New York, 1997, Oxford University Press.

40. Huret JL, Senon S, Bernheim A, et al.: An atlas on genes and chromosomes in oncology and haematology, *Cell Mol Biol* 50:805–807, 2004.

41. Soto AM, Sonnenschein C: The somatic mutation theory of cancer: growing problems with the paradigm? *Bioessays* 26:1097–1107, 2004.

42. Ren R: Mechanisms of BCR–ABL in the pathogenesis of chronic myelogenous leukaemia? *Nat Rev Cancer* 5:172–183, 2005.

43. Huang M, Weiss WA: Neuroblastoma and MYCN, *Cold Spring Harb Perspect Med* 3:a014415, 2013.

44. Nasir L, Rutteman GR, Reid SWJ, et al.: Analysis of p53 mutational events and MDM2 amplification in canine soft-tissue sarcomas, *Cancer Lett* 174:83–89, 2001.

45. Mochizuki H, Breen M: Sequence analysis of RAS and RAF mutation hot spots in canine carcinoma, *Vet Comp Oncol* 15:1598–1605, 2017.

46. Crozier C, Wood GA, Foster RA, et al.: KRAS mutations in canine and feline pancreatic acinar cell carcinoma, *J Comp Pathol* 155:24–28, 2016.

47. Terragni R, Casadei Gardini A, Sabattini S, et al.: EGFR, HER-2 and KRAS in canine gastric epithelial tumors: a potential human model? *PLoS One* 9:e85388, 2014.

48. Smith AJ, Smith LA: Viral carcinogenesis, *Prog Mol Biol Transl Sci* 144:121–168, 2016.

49. Chen Y, Williams V, Filippova M, et al.: Viral carcinogenesis: factors inducing DNA damage and virus integration, *Cancers (Basel)* 6:2155–2186, 2014.

50. Smith AJ, Smith LA: Viral carcinogenesis. In Pruitt K, editor: *Progress in molecular biology and translational science*, Cambridge, 2016, MA: Academic Press, pp 121–168.

51. Weiss RA, Vogt PK: 100 years of Rous sarcoma virus, *J Exp Med* 208:2351–2355, 2011.

52. Mullins JI, Brody DS, Binari Jr RC, et al.: Viral transduction of c-myc gene in naturally occurring feline leukaemias, *Nature* 308:856–858, 1984.

53. Hino O, Kobayashi T, Mourning Dr, Alfred G: Knudson: the two–hit hypothesis, tumor suppressor genes, and the tuberous sclerosis complex, *Cancer Sci* 10:5–11, 2017.

54. Weinberg RA: The retinoblastoma protein and cell cycle control, *Cell* 81:323–330, 1995.

55. Du W, Searle JS: The Rb pathway and cancer therapeutics, *Curr Drug Targets* 10:581–589, 2009.

56. Sherr CJ, McCormick F: The RB and p53 pathways in cancer, *Cancer Cell* 2:103–112, 2002.

57. Soussi T: The history of p53: a perfect example of the drawbacks of scientific paradigms, *EMBO Rep* 11:822–826, 2010.

58. Oliner JD, Kinzler KW, Meltzer PS, et al.: Amplification of a gene encoding a p53 associated protein in human sarcomas, *Nature* 358:80–83, 1992.

59. Niazi S, Purohit M, Niazi JH: Role of p53 circuitry in tumorigenesis: a brief review, *Eur J Med Chem* 158:7–24, 2018.

60. Vogelstein B, Kinzler KW: P53 function and dysfunction, *Cell* 70:525–526, 1992.

61. Sluss HK, Jones SN: Analysing p53 tumour suppressor functions in mice, *Expert Opin Ther Targets* 7:89–99, 2003.

62. Harris CC: P53 tumor suppressor gene: from the basic research laboratory to the clinic—an abridged historical perspective, *Carcinogenesis* 17:1187–1198, 1996.

63. Joerger AC, Fersht AR: The p53 pathway: origins, inactivation in cancer, and emerging therapeutic approaches, *Annu Rev Biochem* 85:375–404, 2016.

64. Nasir L, Rutteman GR, Reid SW, et al.: Analysis of p53 mutational events and MDM2 amplification in canine soft-tissue sarcomas, *Cancer Lett* 174:83–89, 2001.

65. Nasir L, Burr P, Mcfarlane S, et al.: Cloning, sequence analysis and expression of the cDNAs encoding the canine and equine homologues of the mouse double minute 2 (mdm2) proto-oncogene, *Cancer Lett* 152:9–13, 2000.

66. Nasir L, Krasner H, Argyle DJ, et al.: A study of p53 tumour suppressor gene immunoreactivity in feline neoplasia, *Cancer Lett* 155:1–7, 2000.

67. Nasir L, Argyle DJ: Mutational analysis of p53 in two cases of Bull Mastiff lymphosarcoma, *Vet Rec* 145:23–24, 1999.

68. Nasir L, Argyle DJ, McFarlane ST, et al.: Nucleotide sequence of a highly conserved region of the canine p53 tumour suppressor gene, *DNA Sequence* 8:83–86, 1998.

69. Hanahan D, Weinberg RA: The hallmarks of cancer, *Cell* 100:57–70, 2000.

70. Hanahan D, Weinberg RA: Hallmarks of cancer: the next generation, *Cell* 144:646–674, 2011.

71. Bennett RL, Licht JD: Targeting epigenetics in cancer, *Annu Rev Pharmacol Toxicol* 58:187–207, 2018.

72. Morrow JJ, Bayles I, Funnell APW, et al.: Positively selected enhancer elements endow osteosarcoma cells with metastatic competence, *Nat Med* 24:176–185, 2018.

73. Self-sufficiency in growth signals. In Schwab M, editor: *Encyclopedia of cancer*, Berlin, 2011, Springer.

74. Pennati M, Cimino-Reale G, Gatti L, et al.: Strategies to strike survival networks in cancer, *Crit Rev Oncol* 21:269–308, 2016.

75. López-Lago MA, Okada T, Murillo MM, et al.: Loss of the tumor suppressor gene *NF2*, encoding merlin, constitutively activates integrin-dependent mTORC1 signaling, *Mol Cell Biol* 29:4235–4249, 2009.

76. Huang JJ, Blobe GC: Dichotomous roles of TGF-β in human cancer, *Biochem Soc Trans* 44:1441–1454, 2016.

77. Dikic I, Elazar Z: Mechanism and medical implications of mammalian autophagy, *Nat Rev Mol Cell Biol* 19:349–364, 2018.

78. Kimmelman AC: The dynamic nature of autophagy in cancer, *Genes Dev* 25:1999–2010, 2011.

79. Argyle D, Kitamura T: Targeting macrophage-recruiting chemokines as a novel therapeutic strategy to prevent the progression of solid tumors, *Front Immunol* 9:2629, 2018.

80. Raposo TP, Beirão BC, Pang LY, et al: Inflammation and cancer: till death tears them apart, *Vet J* 205:161–174, 2015.

81. Hayflick L: Mortality and immortality at the cellular level. A review, *Biochemistry* 62:1180–1190, 1997.

82. Blasco MA, Funk W, Villeponteau B, et al.: Functional characterization and developmental regulation of mouse telomerase RNA, *Science* 269:1267–1270, 1995.

83. Blasco MA, Lee H-W, Hande MP, et al.: Telomere shortening and tumour formation by mouse cells lacking telomerase RNA, *Cell* 91:25–34, 1997.

84. Biller BJ, Kitchel B, Casey D, et al.: Evaluation of an assay for detecting telomerase activity in neoplastic tissues of dogs, *Am J Vet Res* 59:1526–1528, 1998.

85. McKenzie K, Umbricht CB, Sukumar S: Applications of telomerase research in the fight against cancer, *Mol Med Today* 5:114–122.

86. Nasir L, Devlin P, Mckevitt T, et al.: Telomere lengths and telomerase activity in dog tissues: a potential model system to study human telomere and telomerase biology, *Neoplasia* 3:351–359, 2001.

87. Shay JW, Wright WE: Telomerase activity in human cancer, *Curr Opin Oncol* 8:66–71, 1996.

88. Yazawa M, Okuda M, Setoguchi A, et al.: Measurement of telomerase activity in dog tumours, *J Vet Med Sci* 61:1125–1129, 1999.

89. Zhu J, Wang H, Bishop JM, et al.: Telomerase extends the life-span of virus-transformed human cells without net telomere lengthening, *Proc Natl Acad Sci U S A* 96:3723–3728, 1999.

90. Akincilar SC, Unal B, Tergaonkar V: Reactivation of telomerase in cancer, *Cell Mol Life Sci* 73:1659–1670, 2016.

91. Folkman J: Tumor angiogenesis and tissue factor, *Nat Med* 2:167–168, 1996.

92. Folkman J: Angiogenesis: an organizing principle for drug discovery? *Nat Rev Drug Discov* 6:273–286, 2007.

93. Kerbel RS: Tumor angiogenesis: past, present and the near future, *Carcinogenesis* 21:505–515, 2000.

94. Nagy JA, Chang SH, Shih DC, et al.: Heterogeneity of the tumor vasculature, *Semin Thromb Hemost* 36:321–331, 2010.

95. Olive KP, Jacobetz MA, Davidson CJ, et al.: Inhibition of Hedgehog signaling enhances delivery of chemotherapy in a mouse model of pancreatic cancer, *Science* 324:1457–1461, 2009.

96. Huang T, Sun L, Yuan X, et al.: Thrombospondin-1 is a multifaceted player in tumor progression, *Oncotarget* 8:84546–84558, 2017.

97. Pircher A, Hilbe W, Heidegger I, et al.: Biomarkers in tumor angiogenesis and anti-angiogenic therapy, *Int J Mol Sci* 12:7077–7099, 2011.

98. Boss KM, Muradyan N, Thrall DE: DCE-MRI: a review and applications in veterinary oncology, *Vet Comp Oncol* 11:87–100, 2013.

99. Shanmugam M, McBrayer SK, Rosen ST: Targeting the Warburg effect in hematological malignancies: from PET to therapy, *Curr Opin Oncol* 21:531–536, 2009.

100. Sukari A, Nagasaka M, Al-Hadidi A, et al.: Cancer immunology and immunotherapy, *Anticancer Res* 36:5593–5606, 2016.

101. Vinay DS, Ryan EP, Pawelec G, et al.: Immune evasion in cancer: mechanistic basis and therapeutic strategies, *Semin Cancer Biol* 35(Suppl):S185–S198, 2015.

102. Sica A, Allavena P, Mantovani A: Cancer related inflammation: the macrophage connection, *Cancer Lett* 267:204–215, 2008.

103. Ben-Neriah Y, Karin M: Inflammation meets cancer, with NF-kappa B as the matchmaker, *Nat Immunol* 12:715–723, 2011.

104. Argyle DJ, Blacking T: From viruses to cancer stem cells: dissecting the pathways to malignancy, *Vet J* 177:311–323, 2008.

105. Blacking TM, Wilson H, Argyle DJ: Is cancer a stem cell disease? Theory, evidence and implications, *Vet Comp Oncol* 5:76–89, 2007.

106. Capodanno Y, Buishand FO, Pang LY, et al.: Notch pathway inhibition targets chemoresistant insulinoma cancer stem cells, *Endocr Relat Cancer* 25:131–144, 2018.

107. Pang LY, Saunders L, Argyle DJ: Epidermal growth factor receptor activity is elevated in glioma cancer stem cells and is required to maintain chemotherapy and radiation resistance, *Oncotarget* 8:72494–72512, 2017.

108. Park CH, Bergsage DE, McCulloc EA: Mouse myeloma tumour stem cells: primary cell culture assay, *J Natl Cancer Inst* 46:411, 1971.

109. Huntly BJ, Gilliland DG: Leukaemia stem cells and the evolution of cancer-stem-cell research, *Nat Rev Cancer* 5:311–321, 2005.

110. Kamel-Reid S, Letarte M, Sirard C, et al.: A model of human acute lymphoblastic leukemia in immune-deficient SCID mice, *Science* 246:1597–1600, 1989.

111. Lapidot T, Sirard C, Vormoor J, et al.: A cell initiating human acute myeloid leukaemia after transplantation into SCID mice, *Nature* 367:645–648, 1994.

112. Sirard C, Lapidot T, Vormoor J, et al.: Normal and leukemic SCID-repopulating cells (SRC) coexist in the bone marrow and peripheral blood from CML patients in chronic phase, whereas leukemic SRC are detected in blast crisis, *Blood* 87:1539–1548, 1996.

113. Bonnet D, Dick JE: Human acute myeloid leukemia is organized as a hierarchy that originates from a primitive hematopoietic cell, *Nat Med* 3:730–737, 1997.

114. Fidler IJ, Kripke ML: Metastasis results from preexisting variant cells within a malignant tumor, *Science* 197:893–895, 1977.

115. Heppner GH: Tumor heterogeneity, *Cancer Res* 44:2259–2265, 1984.

116. Nowell PC: Mechanisms of tumor progression, *Cancer Res* 46:2203–2207, 1986.

117. Southam CM, Brunschwig A: Quantitative studies of autotransplantation of human cancer, *Cancer* 14:971–978, 1961.

118. Pang LY, Argyle DJ: Using naturally occurring tumours in dogs and cats to study telomerase and cancer stem cell biology, *Biochim Biophys Acta* 1792380–391, 2009.

119. Pang LY, Argyle D: Cancer stem cells and telomerase as potential biomarkers in veterinary oncology, *Vet J* 185:15–22, 2010.

120. Pang LY, Cervantes-Arias A, Else RW, et al.: Canine mammary cancer stem cells are radio- and chemo-resistant and exhibit an epithelial-mesenchymal transition phenotype, *Cancer* 3:1744–1762, 2011.

121. Hida K, Maishi N, Annan DA, et al.: Contribution of tumor endothelial cells in cancer progression, *Int J Mol Sci* 19:E1272, 2018.

122. Meng MB, Zaorsky NG, Deng L, et al.: Pericytes: a double-edged sword in cancer therapy, *Future Oncol* 11:169–179, 2015.

123. Tao L, Huang G, Song H, et al.: Cancer associated fibroblasts: an essential role in the tumor microenvironment, *Oncol Lett* 14:2611–2620, 2017.

124. Mendoza M, Khanna C: Revisiting the seed and soil in cancer metastasis, *Int J Biochem Cell Biol* 41:1452–1462, 2009.

125. Sell S: Stem cell origin of cancer and differentiation therapy, *Crit Rev Oncol Hematol* 51:1–28, 2004.

126. Ramaswamy S, Ross KN, Lander ES, et al.: A molecular signature of metastasis in primary solid tumors, *Nat Genet* 33:49–54, 2003.

127. Patel SA, Vanharanta S: Epigenetic determinants of metastasis, *Mol Oncol* 11:79–96, 2017.

128. Clark EA, Golub TR, Lander ES, et al.: Genomic analysis of metastasis reveals an essential role for RhoC, *Nature* 406:532–535, 2000.

129. Shevde LA, Welch DR: Metastasis suppressor pathways–an evolving paradigm, *Cancer Lett* 198:1–20, 2003.

130. Steeg PS: Perspectives on classic article: metastasis suppressor genes, *J Natl Cancer Inst* 96:E4, 2004.

131. Paoloni M, Davis S, Lana S, et al.: Canine tumor cross-species genomics uncovers targets linked to osteosarcoma progression, *BMC Genom* 10:625, 2009.

132. Mayr B, Brem G, Reifinger M: Absence of S100A4 (mts1) gene mutations in various canine and feline tumours. Detection of a polymorphism in feline S100A4 (mts1), *J Vet Med A Physiol Pathol Clin Med* 47:123–128, 2000.

133. Khanna C, Wan X, Bose S, et al.: The membrane-cytoskeleton linker ezrin is necessary for osteosarcoma metastasis, *Nat Med* 10:182–186, 2004.

134. Ren L, Hong SH, Chen QR, et al.: Dysregulation of ezrin phosphorylation prevents metastasis and alters cellular metabolism in osteosarcoma, *Cancer Res* 72:1001–1012, 2012.

135. Hong SH, Osborne T, Ren L, et al.: Protein kinase C regulates ezrin-radixin-moesin phosphorylation in canine osteosarcoma cells, *Vet Comp Oncol* 9:207–218, 2011.

136. Shoushtari AN, Szmulewitz RZ, Rinker-Schaeffer CW: Metastasis-suppressor genes in clinical practice: lost in translation? *Nat Rev Clin Oncol* 8:333–342, 2011.

137. Liotta LA, Kohn EC: The microenvironment of the tumour-host interface, *Nature* 411:375–379, 2001.

138. Friedl P, Wolf K, Lammerding J: Nuclear mechanics during cell migration, *Curr Opin Cell Biol* 23:55–64, 2011.

139. Friedl P, Wolf K: Plasticity of cell migration: a multiscale tuning model, *J Cell Biol* 188 11–19, 2010.

140. Sabeh F, Shimizu-Hirota R, Weiss SJ: Protease-dependent versus -independent cancer cell invasion programs: three-dimensional amoeboid movement revisited, *J Cell Biol* 185:11–19, 2009.

141. Scott RW, Crighton D, Olson MF: Modeling and imaging 3-dimensional collective cell invasion, *J Vis Exp* 58:3525, 2011.

142. Condeelis J, Segall JE: Intravital imaging of cell movement in tumours, *Nat Rev Cancer* 3:921–930, 2003.

143. Condeelis J, Singer RH, Segall JE: The great escape: when cancer cells hijack the genes for chemotaxis and motility, *Annu Rev Cell Dev Biol* 21:695–718, 2005.

144. Wang W, Wyckoff JB, Frohlich VC, et al.: Single cell behavior in metastatic primary mammary tumors correlated with gene expression patterns revealed by molecular profiling, *Cancer Res* 62:6278–6288, 2002.

145. Wyckoff JB, Segall JE, Condeelis JS: The collection of the motile population of cells from a living tumor, *Cancer Res* 60:5401–5404, 2000.

146. Jankowski MK, Ogilvie GK, Lana SE, et al.: Matrix metalloproteinase activity in tumor, stromal tissue, and serum from cats with malignancies, *J Vet Intern Med* 16:105–108, 2002.

147. Loukopoulos P, O'Brien T, Ghoddusi M, et al.: Characterisation of three novel canine osteosarcoma cell lines producing high levels of matrix metalloproteinases, *Res Vet Sci* 77:131–141, 2004.

148. Hirayama K, Yakota H, Onai R, et al.: Detection of matrix metalloproteinases in canine mammary tumours: analysis by immunohistochemistry and zymography, *J Comp Pathol* 127:249–256, 2002.

149. Lana SE, Ogilvie GK, Hansen RA, et al.: Identification of matrix metalloproteinases in canine neoplastic tissue, *Am J Vet Res* 61:111–114, 2000.

150. Leibman NF, Lana SE, Hansen RA, et al.: Identification of matrix metalloproteinases in canine cutaneous mast cell tumors, *J Vet Intern Med* 14:583–586, 2000.

151. Coussens LM, Fingleton B, Matrisian LM: Matrix metalloproteinase inhibitors and cancer: trials and tribulations, *Science* 295:2387–2392, 2002.

152. Coussens LM, Fingleton B, Matrisian LM: Matrix metalloproteinase inhibitors and cancer: trials and tribulations, *Science* 295:2387–2392, 2002.

153. Moore AS, Dernell WS, Ogilvie GK, et al.: Doxorubicin and BAY 12–9566 for the treatment of osteosarcoma in dogs: a randomized, double-blind, placebo-controlled study, *J Vet Intern Med* 21:783–790, 2007.

154. Ramnath N, Creaven PJ: Matrix metalloproteinase inhibitors, *Curr Oncol Rep* 6:96–102, 2004.

155. Rucci N, Sanita P, Angelucci A: Roles of metalloproteases in metastatic niche, *Curr Mol Med* 11:609–622, 2011.

156. Qian BZ, Pollard JW: Macrophage diversity enhances tumor progression and metastasis, *Cell* 141:39–51, 2010.

157. Foroni C, Broggini M, Generali D, et al.: Epithelial-mesenchymal transition and breast cancer: role, molecular mechanisms and clinical impact, *Cancer Treat Rev* 38:389–397, 2012.

158. Peinado H, Olmeda D, Cano A: Snail, Zeb and bHLH factors in tumour progression: an alliance against the epithelial phenotype? *Nat Rev Cancer* 7:415–428, 2007.

159. Moreno-Bueno G, Peinado H, Molina P, et al.: The morphological and molecular features of the epithelial-to-mesenchymal transition, *Nat Protoc* 4:1591–1613, 2009.

160. Floor S, van Staveren WC, Larsimont D, et al.: Cancer cells in epithelial-to-mesenchymal transition and tumor-propagating-cancer stem cells: distinct, overlapping or same populations, *Oncogene* 30:4609–4621, 2011.

161. Hendrix MJ, Seftor EA, Hess AR, et al.: Vasculogenic mimicry and tumour-cell plasticity: lessons from melanoma, *Nat Rev Cancer* 3:411–421, 2003.

162. Kalluri R: Basement membranes: structure, assembly and role in tumour angiogenesis, *Nat Rev Cancer* 3:422–433, 2003.

163. Frisch SM, Francis H: Disruption of epithelial cell-matrix interactions induces apoptosis, *J Cell Biol* 124:619–626, 1994.

164. Taddei ML, Giannoni E, Fiaschi T, et al.: Anoikis: an emerging hallmark in health and diseases, *J Pathol* 226:380–393, 2012.

165. Grossmann J: Molecular mechanisms of "detachment-induced apoptosis–Anoikis", *Apoptosis* 7:247–260, 2002.

166. Guo W, Giancotti FG: Integrin signalling during tumour progression, *Nat Rev Mol Cell Biol* 5:816–826, 2004.

167. Fosmire SP, Dickerson EB, Scott AM, et al.: Canine malignant hemangiosarcoma as a model of primitive angiogenic endothelium, *Lab Invest* 84:562–572, 2004.

168. Akhtari M, Mansuri J, Newman KA, et al.: Biology of breast cancer bone metastasis, *Cancer Biol Ther* 7:3–9, 2008.

169. Restucci B, De Vico G, Maiolino P: Expression of beta 1 integrin in normal, dysplastic and neoplastic canine mammary gland, *J Comp Pathol* 113:165–173, 1995.

170. Olivry T, Moore PF, Naydan DK, et al.: Investigation of epidermotropism in canine mycosis fungoides: expression of intercellular adhesion molecule-1 (ICAM-1) and beta-2 integrins, *Arch Dermatol Res* 287:186–192, 1995.

171. Moore PF, Rossitto PV, Danilenko DM: Canine leukocyte integrins: characterization of a CD18 homologue, *Tissue Antigens* 36:211–220, 1990.

172. Selvarajah GT, Kirpensteijn J, van Wolferen ME, et al.: Gene expression profiling of canine osteosarcoma reveals genes associated with short and long survival times, *Mol Cancer* 8:72, 2009.

173. Fukata M, Kaibuchi K: Rho-family GTPases in cadherin-mediated cell-cell adhesion, *Nat Rev Mol Cell Biol* 2:887–897, 2001.

174. Seftor RE, Seftor EA, Gehlsen KR, et al.: Role of the alpha v beta 3 integrin in human melanoma cell invasion, *Proc Natl Acad Sci U S A* 89:1557–1561, 1992.

175. Zheng DQ, woodard AS, Fornaro M, et al.: Prostatic carcinoma cell migration via alpha(v)beta3 integrin is modulated by a focal adhesion kinase pathway, *Cancer Res* 59:1655–1664, 1999.

176. Ruoslahti E, Reed JC: Anchorage dependence, integrins, and apoptosis, *Cell* 77:477–478, 1994.

177. Paoli P, Giannoni E, Chiarugi P: Anoikis molecular pathways and its role in cancer progression, *Biochim Biophys Acta* 1833:3481–3498, 2013.

178. Nagaprashantha LD, Vatsyayan R, Lalsani PC, et al.: The sensors and regulators of cell-matrix surveillance in anoikis resistance of tumors, *Int J Cancer* 128:743–752, 2011.

179. Lascelles BD, Dernell WS, Correa MT, et al.: Improved survival associated with postoperative wound infection in dogs treated with limb-salvage surgery for osteosarcoma, *Ann Surg Oncol* 12:1073–1083, 2005.

180. Yu C, Xu S-F, Xu M, et al.: Postoperative infection and survival in osteosarcoma patients: reconsideration of immunotherapy for osteosarcoma, *Mol Clin Oncol* 3:495–500, 2015.

181. Smyth MJ, Hayakawa Y, Takeda K, et al.: New aspects of natural-killer-cell surveillance and therapy of cancer, *Nat Rev Cancer* 2:850–861, 2002.

182. Mocellin S, Rossi CR, Lisa M, et al.: Colorectal cancer vaccines: principles, results, and perspectives, *Gastroenterology* 127:1821–1837, 2004.

183. Mocellin S, Rossi CR, Nitti D: Cancer vaccine development: on the way to break immune tolerance to malignant cells, *Exp Cell Res* 299:267–278, 2004.

184. Rao B, Han M, Wang L, et al.: Clinical outcomes of active specific immunotherapy in advanced colorectal cancer and suspected minimal residual colorectal cancer: a meta-analysis and system review, *J Transl Med* 9:17, 2011.

185. Bergman PJ: Cancer immunotherapy, *Vet Clin N Am Small Anim Pract* 40:507–518, 2010.

186. Grosenbaugh DA, Leard AT, Bergman P, et al.: Safety and efficacy of a xenogeneic DNA vaccine encoding for human tyrosinase as

adjunctive treatment for oral malignant melanoma in dogs following surgical excision of the primary tumor, *Am J Vet Res* 72:1631–1638, 2011.

187. Bagge U, Skolnik G, Ericson LE: The arrest of circulating tumor cells in the liver microcirculation. A vital fluorescence microscopic, electron microscopic and isotope study in the rat, *J Cancer Res Clin Oncol* 105:134–140, 1983.

188. Chambers AF, MacDonald IC, Schmidt EE, et al.: Steps in tumor metastasis: new concepts from intravital videomicroscopy, *Cancer Metastasis Rev* 14:279–301, 1995.

189. Chambers AF, Naumov GN, Varghese HJ, et al.: Critical steps in hematogenous metastasis: an overview, *Surg Oncol Clin N Am* 10:243–255, 2001.

190. Kienast Y, von Baumgarten L, Fuhrmann M, et al.: Real-time imaging reveals the single steps of brain metastasis formation, *Nat Med* 16:116–122, 2010.

191. Li DM, Feng YM: Signaling mechanism of cell adhesion molecules in breast cancer metastasis: potential therapeutic targets, *Breast Cancer Res Treat* 128:7–21, 2011.

192. Zigler M, Kamiya T, Brantley EC, et al.: PAR-1 and thrombin: the ties that bind the microenvironment to melanoma metastasis, *Cancer Res* 71:6561–6566, 2011.

193. Villares GJ, Zigler M, Bar-Eli M: The emerging role of the thrombin receptor (PAR-1) in melanoma metastasis–a possible therapeutic target, *Oncotarget* 2:8–17, 2011.

194. Groom AC, MacDonald IC, Schmidt EE, et al.: Tumour metastasis to the liver, and the roles of proteinases and adhesion molecules: new concepts from in vivo videomicroscopy, *Can J Gastroenterol* 13:733–743, 1999.

195. Chambers AF: The metastatic process: basic research and clinical implications, *Oncol Res* 11:161–168, 1999.

196. Liu Q, Zhang H, Jiang X, et al.: Factors involved in cancer metastasis: a better understanding to "seed and soil" hypothesis, *Mol Cancer* 16:176, 2017.

197. Martin TA, Harrison G, Mansel RE, et al.: The role of the CD44/ezrin complex in cancer metastasis, *Crit Rev Oncol Hematol* 46:165–186, 2003.

198. Balkwill F: Chemokine biology in cancer, *Semin Immunol* 15:49–55, 2003.

199. Kaplan RN, Rafii S, Lyden D: Preparing the "soil": the premetastatic niche, *Cancer Res* 66:11089–11093, 2006.

200. Kaplan RN, Riba RD, Zacharoulis S, et al.: VEGFR1-positive haematopoietic bone marrow progenitors initiate the pre-metastatic niche, *Nature* 438:820–827, 2005.

201. Al-Mehdi AB, Tozawa K, Fisher AB, et al.: Intravascular origin of metastasis from the proliferation of endothelium-attached tumor cells: a new model for metastasis, *Nat Med* 6:100–102, 2000.

202. Cooper CR, Chay CH, Gendermalik JD, et al.: Stromal factors involved in prostate carcinoma metastasis to bone, *Cancer* 97 (Suppl 3):739–747, 2003.

203. De Wever O, Mareel M: Role of tissue stroma in cancer cell invasion, *J Pathol* 200:429–447, 2003.

204. Engels B, Rowley DA, Schreiber H: Targeting stroma to treat cancers, *Semin Cancer Biol* 22:41–49, 2011.

205. Folkman J: Tumor angiogenesis and tissue factor, *Nat Med* 2:167–168, 1996.

206. Folkman J: Angiogenesis: an organizing principle for drug discovery? *Nat Rev Drug Discov* 6:273–286, 2007.

207. Kerbel RS: Tumor angiogenesis: past, present and the near future, *Carcinogenesis* 21:505–515, 2000.

208. Nagy JA, Chang SH, Shih SC, et al.: Heterogeneity of the tumor vasculature, *Semin Thromb Hemost* 36:321–331, 2010.

209. Olive KP, Jacobetz MA, Davidson CJ, et al.: Inhibition of Hedgehog signaling enhances delivery of chemotherapy in a mouse model of pancreatic cancer, *Science* 324:1457–1461, 2009.

210. Pircher A, Hilbe W, Heidegger I, et al.: Biomarkers in tumor angiogenesis and anti-angiogenic therapy, *Int J Mol Sci* 12:7077–7099, 2011.

211. Boss KM, Muradyan N, Thrall DE: DCE-MRI: a review and applications in veterinary oncology, *Vet Comp Oncol* 11:87–100, 2013.

212. Fidler IJ, Kripke ML: Metastasis results from preexisting variant cells within a malignant tumor, *Science* 197:893–895, 1977.

213. Fidler IJ: The pathogenesis of cancer metastasis: the 'seed and soil' hypothesis revisited, *Nat Rev Cancer* 3:453–458, 2003.

214. Hunter K, Welch DR, Liu ET: Genetic background is an important determinant of metastatic potential, *Nat Genet* 34:23–24, 2003.

215. Hunter KW: Allelic diversity in the host genetic background may be an important determinant in tumor metastatic dissemination, *Cancer Lett* 200:97–105, 2003.

216. Hunter KW: Host genetics and tumour metastasis, *Br J Cancer* 90:752–755, 2004.

217. Khanna C, Hunter K: Modeling metastasis in vivo, *Carcinogenesis* 26:513–523, 2005.

218. Luzzi KJ, MacDonald IC, Schmiedt EE, et al.: Multistep nature of metastatic inefficiency: dormancy of solitary cells after successful extravasation and limited survival of early micrometastases, *Am J Pathol* 153:865–873, 1998.

219. Loberg RD, Fridman Y, Pienta BA, et al.: Detection and isolation of circulating tumor cells in urologic cancers: a review, *Neoplasia* 6:302–309, 2004.

220. Butler TP, Gullino PM: Quantitation of cell shedding into efferent blood of mammary adenocarcinoma, *Cancer Res* 35:512–516, 1975.

221. Psaila B, Lyden D: The metastatic niche: adapting the foreign soil, *Nat Rev Cancer* 9:285–293, 2009.

222. Chambers AF, Naumov GN, Vantyghem SA, et al.: Molecular biology of breast cancer metastasis. Clinical implications of experimental studies on metastatic inefficiency, *Breast Cancer Res* 2:400–407, 2000.

223. Paez D, Labonte MJ, Bohanes P, et al.: Cancer dormancy: a model of early dissemination and late cancer recurrence, *Clin Cancer Res* 18:645–653, 2012.

224. Barkan D, Kleinman H, Simmons JL, et al.: Inhibition of metastatic outgrowth from single dormant tumor cells by targeting the cytoskeleton, *Cancer Res* 68:6241–6250, 2008.

225. Barkan D, El Touny LH, Michalowski AM, et al.: Metastatic growth from dormant cells induced by a col-I-enriched fibrotic environment, *Cancer Res* 70:5706–5716, 2010.

3

The Pathology of Neoplasia

DEBRA A. KAMSTOCK, DUNCAN S. RUSSELL, AND BARBARA E. POWERS

Veterinary pathologists play a critical role in the management of companion animal neoplasia by providing diagnostic information that ultimately affects the prognosis and therapeutic decisions. The clinician should have an understanding of how these diagnoses are generated and communicated, while also having an awareness of the limitations of routine histopathologic assessment. A functional interdisciplinary working relationship between the pathologist and the clinician is essential to determine the optimal treatment for the cancer patient, especially as the diagnosis and treatment of neoplasia in veterinary medicine continues to become more complex. The cell of origin (histogenesis), which indicates the tumor type, needs to be identified as accurately as possible, and tumor subtypes should be identified, where applicable, especially when prognostically significant. Histologic grading of tumors is increasingly important, because for a number of tumor types, this has been shown to be a strong prognosticator of biologic behavior. Evaluation of surgical margins to assess excisional completeness also is often a critical component that may significantly affect the prognosis and therapeutic direction. Ancillary diagnostics, such as immunohistochemistry (IHC), immunocytochemistry (ICC), transmission electron microscopy (TEM), flow cytometry, or polymerase chain reaction (PCR) may be necessary to identify the tumor type or subtype correctly, to better estimate the prognosis, or to predict the response to therapy. As research and discovery continue in the field of veterinary neoplasia, prognostic and predictive markers, in addition to tumor classification, for practical application will continue to evolve.

Sample Handling

Multiple steps are involved in sample handling, from tissue procurement to the completed slide for the pathologist's review. Each step can affect the specimen's quality and the final microscopic interpretation. At the onset, the biopsy sample should be visually inspected by the clinician to confirm that the appropriate tissue has been obtained. If the biopsy is a needle-core or incisional specimen, the sample should be of sufficient size and consistency that it remains intact in formalin and is not lost in processing. Samples less than 1 mm^3 are usually inadequate, although a needle-core sample 1 mm wide but at least 5 mm long can be sufficient. If the biopsy samples are needle-core samples, more than one core of tissue should be obtained, if possible. Samples composed of extensive blood, mucus, fat, or necrotic debris are typically nondiagnostic and repeat biopsy should be considered.

Very small samples can be easily lost during shipping or in processing because of sample shrinkage during fixation and processing. Given these considerations, some techniques can be used to minimize tissue loss and maximize the likelihood of diagnosis. Samples less than 3 mm in size can be placed on paper (e.g., surgical glove paper) before fixation. These samples will be tacky and adhere to the paper. Very small or pale samples can be circled with pencil to draw attention to the samples at the laboratory. The paper can be folded around the sample, and the entire package can be placed in formalin for fixation and shipping. Alternatively, commercially available screened tissue cassettes can be used to house the sample during fixation and shipment. The sample is placed in the screened cassette at the time of surgery, and the cassette with the sample is placed directly into formalin for fixation. Extremely small samples can also be dyed with India ink or other commercially available dyes to assist in the identification of the sample.

If the specimen is an excisional biopsy, the entire sample should be submitted, if feasible, and margins of concern should be identified with suture or ink.[1] If the entire mass cannot be submitted, it is best to submit five or six sections, in the event some are nondiagnostic. When representative samples are taken, regardless of the tumor site, sections from the tumor/nontumor interface should be included. This allows evaluation of the interaction of the tumor with the surrounding normal tissue (e.g., invasiveness). If the clinician wishes to select sections that also contain surgical margins of interest, this should be explicitly stated on the submission form, and the physical tissue margins should be definitively marked (e.g., surgical ink). For large splenic tumors, multiple representative sections of solid or heterogenous tumor tissue, in addition to regions at the tumor/nontumor interface, should be collected if the entire spleen cannot be submitted; necrotic and hemorrhagic areas that are friable and collapse easily on manipulation should be avoided. Ultimately, caution should be used in handling all specimens; compression or crushing during the biopsy procedure or before fixation and excessive use of electrocautery, cryosurgery, or laser surgery all can cause specimen artifacts, which can reduce the sample's quality and impede diagnosis, particularly in small specimens.[2,3,4]

Biopsy samples for routine histopathology need to be preserved in a fixative. The most widely used fixative is 10% neutral buffered formalin, which is readily available and frequently supplied in individual specimen containers by many laboratories. During excessively cold weather, samples can freeze during shipment, which causes significant destructive tissue artifact. The addition of

20% ethylene glycol or ethanol to the formalin can prevent freezing and maintain tissue integrity. Before immersion in fixative, larger samples may need to be partially sectioned (bread-loafed) to facilitate appropriate fixation, which is critical to preserve microscopic tissue architecture; one side, such as the deep edge, should be left intact to retain tissue orientation.[1] Slices less than 1 cm thick should be avoided because the fixed tissue may curl and distort. The volume of tissue to fixative should approximate 1:10. If this is not feasible because of large tumor size, multiple representative sections can be submitted. The remaining biopsy sample should be retained in formalin, if possible, in case preliminary sections are nondiagnostic. When large samples are mailed, smaller volumes of fixative may be adequate if the specimen has been in the recommended initial volume for at least 12 hours, or the sample can be shipped chilled (without fixative) if previously in fixative for 48 to 72 hours.[1]

Submissions must include the biopsy sample and all necessary paperwork. Sample *containers* (not just the lid), must be properly labeled because samples can inadvertently become separated from submitted paperwork. A critical determinant of accurate biopsy results is the *information provided by the clinician,* typically on the submission form.[1] This information should include, but is not limited to, signalment, relevant clinical history, clinical findings, disease progression, imaging results, treatments (prior treatments can affect tissue/cellular features microscopically), clinical impression, and primary clinical differentials. The pathologist uses this information to generate and validate the microscopic diagnosis (or differential diagnoses). Without this, the diagnosis and/or prognostic interpretation may be inaccurate, culminating in improper patient management.[2,5] Clear communication of the anatomic location, which may include a photograph or drawing, is also important, especially in the consideration of specific tumor types (e.g., periarticular neoplasia), the prognosis (e.g., melanoma of the nail bed versus other cutaneous sites), and margin determination. If margins or areas of special clinical interest are marked on the sample, a clear description of these markings should be included on the submission form.

Once at the laboratory specimens are accessioned, visually examined, trimmed into processing cassettes, processed into paraffin blocks, sectioned, and stained. In most laboratories completed slides are ready for examination by the pathologist 24 to 48 hours after receipt. Samples such as bone require decalcification before trimming and sectioning and therefore take longer to process. Larger samples that are incompletely fixed, extremely bloody samples (e.g., spleen), or samples with abundant fatty tissue (e.g., mammary gland) may also require additional time for fixation. Once the specimen has been trimmed, most laboratories hold the remaining "wet" (fixed) tissues for a specified period in the event further evaluation is needed. Many laboratories file formalin-fixed paraffin-embedded (FFPE) tissue blocks and/or glass slides for prolonged periods, which allows for case review, additional diagnostics, or retrospective case studies.

Although the technique is infrequently used, frozen sections can provide the surgeon with a more rapid diagnosis. Samples are quick-frozen, sectioned on a cryostat, fixed, stained, and examined within 20 to 35 minutes. This technique is typically performed during surgery to assist with intraoperative decisions; essential requirements are appropriate equipment on site and a pathologist with expertise in interpreting frozen sections. Frozen sections may be helpful in establishing the identity of the tissue, completeness of excision, or adequacy of the tissue for more routine processing. Sometimes a provisional diagnosis can be made, or at least a distinction between benign and malignant processes can be determined. Frozen-section diagnoses are always confirmed by routine histopathology, often using the same tissue sample.[5]

Molecular-based tests, such as IHC and PCR, have become commonplace in veterinary medicine and can be performed on FFPE tissue. These samples often are viable indefinitely for these tests, although the time before fixation, time in fixation, fixative used, and storage time can negatively affect test performance. Exposure to sunlight or extreme temperatures during storage should also be avoided. Such factors should be considered in the interpretation of results. Individual laboratory guidelines for the samples required and shipping methods used should be followed to ensure optimal results. IHC requires unstained FFPE tissue sections on positively charged slides. PCR typically requires thick sections (10–20 μm FFPE curls) containing ample nonnecrotic tumor tissue to assure adequate DNA or RNA amounts. These can be sent to the testing laboratory at room temperature in an airtight container.

Terminology

The word *tumor* is derived from the Latin word for swelling (tumere: to swell), which initially was recognized as a hallmark of inflammation in the 1st century. In modern usage the term *tumor* typically refers to a neoplasm, which may be benign or malignant. *Neoplasia* is the formation of a new, abnormal growth of a tissue that is not responsive to normal physiologic control mechanisms and may be benign or malignant. The growth of this mass is not affected when the inciting stimulus is removed. *Cancer* specifically refers to a malignant neoplasm.[6] *Benign* tumors can be space occupying and can cause tissue distortion; however, they do not metastasize or have a high mortality. In contrast, *malignant* tumors (cancer) are more locally destructive, have the potential to metastasize, and may lead to death if left untreated.

All neoplasms arise in normal tissue and thus are composed of parenchymal and stromal cells; some may also be associated with inflammation. Tumor histogenesis and differentiation can be assessed with histopathology; they are based on the appearance of the tumor cells, their organization, and their association with the supporting stroma. Differentiation is controlled at the molecular level by gene expression. The potentially reversible process of *hyperplasia* (a nonneoplastic increase in the number of cells present) is also composed of parenchymal cells and stroma. Retention of near-normal architecture, similar to well-differentiated neoplasms, can make distinguishing between hyperplasia and benign neoplasia difficult. Neoplasia can also be defined as *clonal expansion* (uncontrolled proliferation of a clonal population of cells) that is no longer responsive to homeostatic mechanisms. Molecular techniques to determine clonality, such as PCR for antigen receptor rearrangement, can help differentiate these conditions. These tests are best recognized for use in canine and feline lymphomas.[7]

Metaplasia is the transformation of normal differentiated tissue of one kind into differentiated tissue of another and is not neoplastic. Metaplasia can reverse with cessation of the chronic inciting stimulus. An example is squamous metaplasia of the columnar epithelium of the prostate gland under the influence of estrogen. If stimuli persist and promotional events occur, metaplastic cells can become targets for carcinogenesis (e.g., bronchial squamous metaplasia in human smokers). In such cases metaplastic cells often acquire dysplastic changes. *Dysplasia* refers to abnormal epithelial growth and differentiation and can be a feature of neoplasia, but it is not necessarily a neoplastic condition. Dysplasia, such as in squamous epithelium exposed to ultraviolet radiation, can be a preneoplastic condition. *Anaplasia* is a loss of differentiation or atypical differentiation and is a feature of many, but not all, malignancies.

Tumor nomenclature often denotes the histogenesis and expected biologic behavior (benign or malignant) (Table 3.1). Benign tumors of both epithelial and mesenchymal origin typically are associated with the suffix *–oma* (e.g., papilloma, adenoma, osteoma, fibroma). Exceptions exist, such as melanoma – which, when considered malignant based on histopathologic features, should be classified specifically as *malignant* melanoma (it may be referred to as *melanocytoma* when benign). Mesothelioma and lymphoma are other examples that have no benign counterparts. *Leukemia,* a malignancy of blood cells in circulation (occasionally referred to as "liquid tumors"), also has no benign counterpart, although a leukemoid reaction is a nonmalignant condition that mimics leukemia.[2,5,8] Malignant tumors of epithelial origin are typically carcinomas (e.g., squamous cell carcinoma [SCC], transitional cell carcinoma [TCC]), whereas those of mesenchymal origin typically are associated with the suffix *–sarcoma* (e.g., osteosarcoma [OSA], fibrosarcoma [FSA], leiomyosarcoma). Some tumor classifications do not inherently denote biologic behavior (e.g., mast cell tumor [MCT], plasma cell tumor), and determination of such often depends on assessment of specific reported histopathologic features and/or published clinical studies.

Therefore a knowledge of the terminology used to describe tumor-associated histopathologic features is critical to a true understanding of the pathology report. Pathologic descriptions serve to communicate tumor histogenesis and histomorphologic evidence of malignant potential (Table 3.2). A low magnification assessment of the tumor periphery often provides insight into whether a tumor might be benign (e.g., well demarcated, compressive) or malignant (e.g., infiltrative). The tumor architecture may inform histogenesis—cords, rows, nests, rafts, and acini generally indicate epithelial origin; streams and bundles suggest mesenchymal origin; and solid sheets often indicate hematopoietic (round cell) origin. In addition to the overall appearance of a mass, detailed cellular features in the pathology report may also confer malignant potential (see Table 3.2). Cellular shape is significant because it indicates the cell of origin (histogenesis) and weighs heavily on the diagnosis. Shape may be reported as round, polygonal, spindle, or other. The degree of cellular *differentiation* is typically noted, which refers to the phenotypical maturation and subsequent recognition of a cell; marked *atypia* and *anaplasia* tend to reflect poor differentiation and often preclude cellular identification. *Monomorphic* and *pleomorphic* describe the overall cell population and refer to uniformity or variability, respectively, of the cell sizes and shapes and/or their respective nuclei. *Anisocytosis* and *anisokaryosis* refer specifically to cellular and nuclear size, respectively, and more specifically reflect the variability or range of size throughout the neoplastic cell population. *Karyomegalic* cells refer to those with extremely large nuclei.[9] Additional nuclear features reported may include binucleated or multinucleated cells, bizarre nuclei, and/or prominent or multiple nucleoli, in addition to mitotic figures. A *scirrhous* (also *desmoplastic*) response reflects fibroblastic proliferation with collagen deposition, observed in some malignant neoplasms, typically carcinomas.[10,11] *In situ* refers to a malignancy, usually limited to lesions of epithelial origin, that has not yet invaded beyond the natural confines of the basement membrane.[2,5]

Neoplasia can arise from any cell type, resulting in a significant number of different tumor types and classifications. As research continues to identify tumor-associated and cell-specific molecular alterations, tumor classifications and subclassifications are likely to change accordingly. Molecular techniques (e.g., IHC, PCR, flow cytometry) ideally will keep pace with new findings to support diagnostic application of newly discovered molecular characteristics and biomarkers. Broad encompassing techniques for large genomic, proteomic, and metabolomic fingerprinting of tumors are used as discovery tools to scan for alterations that define subclasses of tumor types previously unidentified by more traditional methods. The identification of specific genetic mutations, varied cell surface receptor expression, altered signaling pathways, or altered cellular metabolic responses to these genetic modifications may identify unique fingerprints for a tumor; these, when combined with traditional histologic methods, could allow more accurate subclassification, prognostication, and personalized treatment (see Chapter 8).

Histopathologic Features of Neoplasia

Despite advances in molecular techniques and other ancillary diagnostics, light microscopy remains the standard technique for tumor diagnosis. Neoplasia has certain histologic features that distinguish it from hyperplasia or inflammation, and some features differentiate benign from malignant neoplasia. In some cases these features can be difficult to observe. Definitive diagnosis of malignant versus benign, or even neoplasia versus inflammation or hyperplasia, may not always be possible. In these cases repeat biopsy or additional ancillary tests may be necessary to facilitate a definitive diagnosis.

When inflammation is present, reactive fibroblasts and endothelial cells (ECs) can display features similar to neoplasia[2] however, in reactive tissue with inflammation, the fibroblasts and ECs are oriented perpendicular to one another (reactive granulation tissue) and the lesion is associated with substantial cellular inflammation. Epithelioid macrophages in granulomatous inflammation can be mistaken for tumor cells, but the pattern of tissue involvement and the presence of other inflammatory cells (mixed inflammation) help rule out neoplasia. In some tumors, especially those with surface ulceration or intratumoral necrosis, an extensive amount of inflammation can obscure neoplasia. Other tumors, however, may be associated with inflammation as a defining histopathologic feature that influences tumorigenesis (e.g., feline injection-site sarcomas [ISSs], posttraumatic ocular sarcomas). In still other tumors, inflammatory infiltrates may be a recognized tumor-associated immune response (e.g., lymphocytic infiltrate in histiocytomas).[12]

Benign tumors may be most difficult to distinguish from hyperplasia (see Table 3.2) because both have a proliferation of well-differentiated cells that resembles normal tissue. Distortion or loss of normal tissue architecture occurs in benign neoplasia, and usually the tumor grows in an expansive manner, causing compression of adjacent tissue. These tumors typically are well demarcated and may have a fibrous tumor capsule. Hyperplasia tends to retain normal tissue orientation, does not compress adjacent tissue, and lacks a fibrous capsule. In general, if allowed to grow, benign neoplasia attains a larger size than a hyperplastic lesion. In some instances, such as sebaceous gland adenoma versus sebaceous gland hyperplasia or feline benign thyrofollicular proliferations (thyroid adenoma versus adenomatous hyperplasia), the distinction between adenoma and hyperplasia may be clinically irrelevant.[13]

TABLE 3.1   Nomenclature of Common Tumor Types in Veterinary Medicine

Tissue or Cell of Origin	Benign	Malignant
Epithelial		
Squamous	Squamous papilloma	Squamous cell carcinoma
Transitional	Papilloma	Transitional cell carcinoma
Glandular	Adenoma, cystadenoma	Adenocarcinoma, cystadenocarcinoma
Mesenchymal		
Fibrous tissue	Fibroma	Fibrosarcoma
Adipose tissue	Lipoma, infiltrative lipoma[a]	Liposarcoma
Cartilage	Chondroma	Chondrosarcoma
Bone	Osteoma	Osteosarcoma, multilobular osteochondrosarcoma
Muscle (smooth)	Leiomyoma	Leiomyosarcoma
Muscle (striated/skeletal)	Rhabdomyoma	Rhabdomyosarcoma
Endothelial cells, blood vasculature	Hemangioma	Hemangiosarcoma
Endothelial cells, lymphatic vasculature	Lymphangioma	Lymphangiosarcoma
Synovium	Villonodular hyperplasia (nonneoplastic)	Synovial cell sarcoma
Mesothelium	—	Mesothelioma
Melanocytes	Benign melanoma (melanocytoma)	Malignant melanoma, Melanosarcoma
Peripheral nerve	—	Malignant schwannoma, neurofibrosarcoma, peripheral nerve sheath tumor
Perivascular wall	—	Perivascular wall tumor (PVWT) (previously hemangiopericytoma)
Uncertain origin[b]	—	Malignant fibrous histiocytoma (MFH)
Hematopoietic and Lymphoreticular		
Lymphocytes	—	Lymphoma (tissue involvement) with subclassifications and leukemic (in circulation) forms
Plasma cells	Cutaneous plasmacytoma	Multiple myeloma, plasmacytoid or plasmablastic lymphoma
Granulocytes	—	Myeloid leukemia
Red blood cells	—	Erythroid leukemia
Platelets	—	Megakaryocytic or megakaryoblastic leukemia
Histiocytes (macrophages or dendritic cells)	Histiocytoma	Histiocytic sarcoma, malignant histiocytosis
Mast cells	—	Mast cell tumor[c]
Thymus[d]	Thymoma, noninvasive	Malignant thymoma (invasive), thymic carcinoma
Neural		
Glial cells	Astrocytoma, oligodendroglioma	Astrocytoma, glioblastoma multiforme, oligodendroglioma
Meninges	Meningioma	Malignant meningioma
Gonadal		
Germ cells[e]	Seminoma, dysgerminoma	Seminoma, Dysgerminoma
Supportive cells[e]	Sertoli cell tumor, granulosa cell tumor	Sertoli cell tumor, granulosa cell tumor
Interstitial cells[e]	Interstitial (Leydig) cell tumor, thecoma, luteoma	Interstitial (Leydig) cell tumor

[a]Infiltrative lipomas can be locally aggressive but do not metastasize.

[b]Histogenesis remains controversial; myofibroblasts, peripheral nerve sheath, or perivascular wall origin are considered. May be diagnosed by some as pleomorphic or anaplastic sarcoma.

[c]Theoretically, all mast cell tumors are potentially malignant, but grade I or low-grade mast cell tumors are often clinically benign.

[d]Thymic lymphoma can be classified as a hematopoietic neoplasm; however, thymoma and malignant thymoma (thymic carcinoma) are epithelial in origin.

[e]The terminology of these tumors does not distinguish between benign and malignant forms.

TABLE 3.2 Histologic Features of Hyperplasia and Benign and Malignant Neoplasia

Histologic Feature	Hyperplasia	Benign Neoplasia	Malignant Neoplasia
Tissue demarcation	Blends with normal tissue	Expansive and/or compressive, possibly encapsulated, well demarcated	Invasive, infiltrative, unencapsulated, poorly demarcated
Organization/architecture of cell population	Retention of normal tissue architecture	Fairly uniform, typically some retention of normal architecture	Moderately to markedly haphazard, loss of normal architecture
Cellular differentiation	Normal	Well differentiated	Moderately to poorly differentiated or undifferentiated
Cell and nuclear pleomorphism	None	Minimal	Moderate to marked
Cellular and nuclear atypia	None	Minimal to none	Moderate to marked; binucleated, multinucleated, karyomegalic, or bizarre nuclei may be observed
Anisocytosis/anisokaryosis	None	Minimal to none	Moderate to marked
Nucleoli	Normal, indiscernible	Normal, typically indiscernible	Prominent, large and/or multiple
Mitotic figures	Typically low	Typically low[a]	Typically high[a]
Necrosis	None	Minimal to none	Moderate to marked
Stromal reaction	None	None	Scirrhous or desmoplastic response[b]
Vascular invasion (blood or lymphatic vasculature)	Not present	Not present	Potential to exist

[a]Exceptions exist; see Table 3.3.
[b]Especially as can be seen with squamous cell and transitional cell carcinoma.

Histopathologic features that distinguish benign from malignant neoplasia were introduced in the earlier section Terminology and in Table 3.2. Ultimately, malignancies typically are characterized by invasive growth with effacement of normal tissue and poor organization of the tumor tissue itself. Cellular features of malignancy include increased cellular and nuclear pleomorphism; increased anisocytosis and anisokaryosis; increased and variable nuclear:cytoplasmic ratio; presence of binucleated, multinucleated, and/or karyomegalic cells or bizarre nuclei; abnormal nuclear chromatin; increased number of mitotic figures; bizarre mitotic figures; and abnormal, large, prominent and/or multiple nucleoli. Increased necrosis also is recognized as a feature of malignancy. Unequivocal intravascular (hematogenous or lymphogenous) invasion, histologic evidence of lymph node (LN) involvement, or widespread metastasis (confirmed by submission of multiple lesions at various sites) conclusively establish malignancy, regardless of other histopathologic features.[2,5,14]

In some tumors the histopathologic features do not correlate with expected biologic behavior. Examples include canine cutaneous histiocytoma, benign plasmacytoma, and pleomorphic feline cutaneous MCT.[15–17] These typically display some histologic features of malignancy but clinically are benign. Histologically low-grade yet biologically high-grade FSAs of the canine oral cavity have benign histologic features but are clinically malignant.[18] Similarly, bronchial carcinomas in cats retain organized epithelial structures composed of well-differentiated, ciliated, pseudostratified columnar epithelium even at distant metastatic sites, including the digit, eye, heart, and kidneys.[19] In these instances knowledge of the clinical history and tumor behavior is essential to distinguish benign from malignant neoplasia.

Challenges may also be encountered during evaluation for possible recurrence after therapy (surgery, radiation therapy [RT],

chemotherapy, or a combination thereof) because histopathologic features of treatment-associated tissue responses can be difficult to distinguish from overt neoplasia. This may be especially true after RT, which can induce the formation of bizarre reactive cells, including fibroblasts (*radiation atypical fibroblasts*), that display many features of malignancy, although these cells are not neoplastic.[20] Inflammation, fibrovascular proliferation, and EC and/or epithelial hyperplasia are other possible treatment-associated tissue responses that may preclude or obscure an appropriate assessment of neoplasia. If tumor cells are identified, the clinician may wish to know if these cells are viable, dead, or rendered viable but sterilized (reproductively dead) by RT or chemotherapy. Although the latter is not possible with routine microscopy, the presence of mitotic figures in the tumor cell population would indicate replicative potential.

Mitotic Figures

Mitotic figures (MFs) are observable, quantifiable tumor-associated histopathologic features that have been proven to be a reliable prognostic indictor for some tumors. The terminology, methodology of acquisition, and reporting of MFs, however, has varied over the years and thus is addressed here to provide the clinician with some insight and guidance when interpreting the MF information provided in the pathology report.

A MF provides visual confirmation of an actively dividing cell, specifically in mitosis. Mitosis occurs during the M-phase when replicated chromosomes of the cell are separated into two separate nuclei and, ultimately, cytokinesis gives rise to two separate cells. Mitotic stages are divided into prophase, prometaphase, metaphase, anaphase, and telophase, any of which may be visualized on routine microscopic evaluation, and all are considered

TABLE 3.3	Tumors That Tend to Defy the Typical Paradigm of Mitotic Figures and Expected Biologic Aggressiveness
High Mitotic Figures but Typically Benign	Low Mitotic Figures but Typically Malignant
Histiocytoma, trichoblastoma	Acanthomatous ameloblastoma, Adrenocortical carcinoma, Chondrosarcoma, Hepatocellular carcinoma, High/low fibrosarcoma of the canine oral cavity, Islet cell (β-cell) carcinoma, Malignant melanoma, Thyroid follicular cell carcinoma

MFs. MFs represent cell division and thus provide information about the growth fraction (GF) of a neoplastic mass. Through numerous studies, the presence of MFs in neoplastic tissue has proven to be a prognostic indicator of biologic behavior, either as an independent variable or as one factor in a grading scheme considered with other phenotypically observable histopathologic features (e.g., cell differentiation, nuclear features, necrosis).[9,21–30] In general, a higher number of MFs typically reflects a higher GF and increased potential for biologic aggressiveness; however, multiple exceptions exist (Table 3.3). Additionally, when the relevance of MFs for a specific tumor type has not been proven scientifically, caution is advised in simply extrapolating an interpretation of biologic behavior based on "high" or "low" "numbers of MFs.

The terminology used in histopathology reports and published veterinary studies to quantitatively report MFs (e.g., MFs, mitotic index, mitotic rate, mitotic activity, number of mitoses, mitotic count) has lacked standardization, as has the method of acquisition. This can create confusion as to how to interpret the pathology report and can complicate accurate comparison of data across studies. Additionally, even if the methodology is similar, microscopes can have variable lenses and magnifying components that affect the field of view (FOV) such that the area of tissue visualized at 400× magnification of one microscope may differ from that of another. Moreover, the advent and ever-increasing presence of digital pathology has introduced yet another variable with which to consider the FOV and total area of tissue evaluated, especially as it relates to previous studies and data acquired via traditional microscopic evaluation.

An effort to standardize terminology and the FOV, regardless of the instrument or technology used, recently has been introduced.[31] It has been proposed that the profession use the term "mitotic count" and that a standardized area of 2.37 mm^2 be the total area evaluated (this is most commonly acquired by evaluating 10 fields with a 40× objective, 22 field number ocular, and no tube lens); the number of fields viewed may vary, depending on equipment. The region of the tissue examined is yet another variable in need of standardization. Examples of various region approaches in the literature are consecutive regions, regions of highest mitotic activity, regions at the invasive edge, and random fields.[21,24,32,33] The authors believe that daily diagnostic application by pathologists should replicate the study-specific methods when a published grading scheme or published MF value as an independent variable is applied. The clinician should be familiar with the study-specific methodologies from which MFs and associated prognostic conclusions were drawn and should be aware of how the number of MFs reported on the pathology report were obtained. Standardization

of regions to be evaluated should be considered moving forward. Regions with the highest mitotic activity, whether at the invasive edge or elsewhere, may be the most representative of the GF.

Although efforts to improve standardization in methods for evaluating and reporting MFs certainly will be beneficial, the authors highlight that (1) applying such terminology or techniques to previously published studies may cause confusion and perhaps more inaccuracy; and (2) reporting of MFs is an estimate of biologic activity and is only one parameter of cell proliferation (reflective only of M-phase), as other evaluable proliferation indices (e.g., Ki67, PCNA, AgNORs) exist. The broader histopathologic picture still should be considered, as should all tumor-associated clinical parameters, including stage of disease, in the management of the cancer patient.

Lymph Node Metastasis

Histopathologic evidence of LN metastasis is a feature of malignancy, a negative prognostic indicator, and has a profound effect on the therapeutic plan. When LN "metastasis" is reported on a biopsy report, it is important the clinician recognize that this is the pathologist's *interpretation* based on histopathologic features observed. To that end, no firmly established nor standardized histologic criteria for LN metastasis in veterinary medicine exists, although recent attempts to establish a foundation have been made.[34] Ultimately, if a neoplastic cell population has colonized a tissue distant from its primary site, is forming a new mass lesion at that site, and is effacing and replacing the normal tissue architecture, these are irrefutable histopathologic features of overt metastasis. Similar findings in LN tissue are unequivocally supportive of metastasis. However, alternative findings may consist solely of individualized/isolated tumor cells (ITCs) or small aggregates of tumor cells in sinusoids and/or parenchyma, and these may be sparsely or frequently present.[34] Without standardized histologic criteria for metastasis, these types of histologic findings can result in interpathologist variability in interpretation and reporting of metastasis.

For this reason (1) the clinician should be cognizant of the histopathologic description of the LN on the pathology report, especially if the diagnosis itself states LN metastasis; and (2) outside of overt histopathologic evidence of metastasis as described previously, the pathologist should try to reserve an interpretive diagnosis (e.g., LN metastasis, no evidence of metastasis) and instead work to provide a descriptive diagnosis (e.g., rare isolated tumor cells are noted in the subcapsular sinus). Clinicians may find this frustrating and may not know how to interpret these descriptive findings, but until further research is pursued, the significance of these findings or the expected biologic behavior of the tumor simply remains unknown. In human medicine, evaluation for LN metastasis typically is reported as negative, ITCs, micrometastases, or macrometastases; however, the clinical and prognostic significance of ITCs and micrometastases is still under investigation.[35–39]

To improve the sensitivity of identification of nodal metastasis, perioperative or intraoperative evaluation for the sentinel LN (SLN) is becoming more commonplace in veterinary medicine (Chapter 9).[40] The pathologist also can improve sensitivity by using IHC (e.g., cytokeratin for carcinomas) or histochemical stains (e.g., toluidine blue for metachromatic granules in MCTs). This can aid in the identification of aberrant nodal cells and/or improve the efficiency by which these cells are detected visually.[34,41] Serial sectioning or multilevel sectioning can also improve detection sensitivity of metastasis by increasing the overall amount of tissue area evaluated.[41,42] The clinician should remember that the designation "clean" or "negative" node is based only on the tissue section (4–5 μm thick) or sections evaluated; on a routine basis, this is often less than 1% of the total tissue area. One study of 20 retrospectively evaluated LNs found that 25% of previously "negative" LNs could be reclassified after more comprehensive sectioning and staining.[41] Gross examination of the tissue by a pathologist or trained histotechnologist may assist with trimming in more suspicious areas based on color and/or texture, but an understanding of the total tissue area evaluated microscopically relative to the total area of the tissue submitted remains important.

Histologic Grading and Clinical Staging of Neoplasia

In certain tumors, histologic grading, which is based on microscopic evaluation of defined histopathologic criteria (many of which have been presented previously) is predictive of biologic behavior.[2,5,14] Grading can be a powerful estimate of expected clinical progression or clinical outcome, such as metastatic potential, disease-free interval, or overall survival. For some tumors, such as human and canine soft tissue sarcoma (STS), the histologic grade is more important than the tumor type.[2,22,32] Grade frequently affects clinical decisions, such as recommendations for adjuvant therapy. Although this grade can be a valuable component of the clinical picture, no grading scheme accurately predicts behavior in 100% of patients.[43] This introduces the critical difference between histologic grading and clinical staging; grading is based almost exclusively on histomorphologic characteristics of the primary tumor and does not typically incorporate clinical staging components, such as the presence of metastases or LN involvement.

Histomorphologic features used to determine grade may include cellular differentiation, number of MFs, invasiveness, necrosis, cellular or nuclear pleomorphism or atypia, nucleolar size and number, stromal reaction, and overall cellularity. For many routinely applied grading schemes, histologic features are described categorically (i.e., range of MFs, invasion pattern, percentage necrosis, degree of differentiation) and assigned a score. These grading schemes are time efficient, cost-effective, involve no new technology, and easily can be applied to routine diagnostic specimens. To ensure valid clinical application, grading must use the same methods and criteria as described in the relevant publication; clinicians should be familiar with these studies and ensure that accurate methods were applied by the pathologist in reporting grade.

Because of the nature of grading criteria, there is potential for subjectivity, and reproducibility between pathologists can be variable.[14,43,44] Despite this limitation, one human study of 440,000 cases found that interobserver variation did not alter the relationship between grade and outcome.[14] A recent international study that applied the World Health Organization (WHO) system of lymphoma classification to canine lymphomas demonstrated an overall accuracy of 83% among 17 pathologists.[45] With preparative training and careful application to well-described criteria, reasonable accuracy can be achieved. If the criteria are more loosely defined, pathologist concordance likely will be reduced.[44]

Some degree of grading variation is inevitable because of known biologic variation that defines tumor types and even individual tumors. Tumors often have considerable morphologic heterogeneity – this might directly reflect the expansion of differing clonal subpopulations and genetic instability that characterize many advanced tumors.[46] If heterogeneity is present, the most malignant-appearing areas (usually defined by cellularity, degree of differentiation, and mitotic activity) should be assessed for grading purposes. Grading of specific tumor subpopulations, such as those at the "invasive front," might also help to better prognosticate behavior.[47] Human biases have the potential to amplify natural biologic variation in tumors. In small biopsy samples, the sampling procedure can affect the representation of different components in a heterogeneous tumor. Some studies have demonstrated that pretreatment incisional biopsies are a reasonably accurate estimation of grade in the excisional sample; however, results might vary between tumor types.[48,49] If necrosis is considered directly in the grade, clinicians and/or pathologists might avoid these areas for diagnostic sampling. Therefore incisional biopsies could have a tendency to underestimate tumor grade.[48,49]

Guidelines for evaluating the prognostic utility of grading schemes have been described.[43,50] An awareness of study design, assessment of clinical outcomes and endpoints, statistical analysis, methods of marker evaluation, and specific study conclusions should all influence decisions to assign clinical relevance to specific histopathologic features and/or grade. Table 3.4 lists tumors for which strong data suggest that grade and/or specific histologic features are prognostic in dogs. Other canine tumors in which histomorphology has been linked to the prognosis include appendicular OSA[51,52]; multilobular osteochondrosarcoma (MLO)[53,54]; mandibular OSA[55]; chondrosarcoma[56]; hemangiosarcoma (HSA)[57]; urothelial carcinoma[10]; SCC of the tongue[58]; splenic sarcoma (nonangiomatous/nonlymphomatous)[59]; primary lung tumors[60]; ocular melanoma[61]; splenic liposarcoma[62]; and lingual HSA.[63] In cats, histologic features may be relevant in cutaneous MCTs[64,65]; primary lung tumors[66]; mammary carcinoma[67,68]; and uveal melanoma.[30,69] Independent validation of many veterinary grading schemes is limited, and some have been questioned in the recent literature.[43,70,71] In canine malignant mammary tumors, the histologic subtype may be more relevant than conventional grading.[72] As with MFs, grade is ultimately an estimate of biologic activity to be taken into account with other parameters and the overall clinical picture.

For tumors where grading systems are not well established, the pathologist may still estimate presumed biologic behavior based on the overall degree of tumor differentiation. This might be convenient for those tumors where there are insufficient data to directly associate histomorphology and prognosis. In these cases, the terms *well differentiated, moderately differentiated,* or *poorly differentiated* may infer a low-grade, medium-grade, and high-grade malignancy, respectively.[73] Pathologists who advocate for evidence-based medicine may chose not to include this in the final diagnosis unless clearly defined criteria and clinically validated data justify its prognostic utility; however, the degree of differentiation, should be reported in the histopathologic description.[74]

Many histomorphologic grading criteria are likely proxies for underlying molecular mechanisms that define most malignant tumors (Table 3.5). In human breast cancer morphologic phenotypes and grading criteria are associated with molecular signatures.[75] Tumoral necrosis, measured in multiple different grading schemes, might be related partly to inadequate perfusion, hypoxic injury, and vascularization. Tumoral neoangiogenesis is a hallmark of most malignant neoplasms and can be estimated by microvessel density. Important mediators in this process include the vascular endothelial growth factor (VEGF), thrombospondin-1, and hypoxia-inducible factor-1α. Underlying molecular mechanisms

TABLE 3.4	Canine Neoplasms with Grades or Histologic Features with Prognostic Significance		
Tumor Type	**Grades Given**	**Features of Importance**	**References**
Mast cell tumor, cutaneous	I, II, III	Cellularity, nuclear: cytoplasmic ratio, cell morphology, mitotic figures,[a] depth, necrosis, granularity	21
	2-tier: High, low	Mitotic figures (≥7 in 10 hpf) karyomegaly (nuclear diameter in ≥ 10% cells varying by at least twofold), multinucleation (3 or more nuclei), bizarre nuclei (≥3 in 10 hpf)	9
	I/Low, II/Low, II/High, III/High	Combination of the two previous grading schemes	9, 21 OPWG 2017 Consensus (http://vetcancersociety.org/vcs-members/vcs-groups/oncology-pathology-working-group/)
	Subcutaneous	Mitotic index ≤4, >4; growth pattern; multinucleation (two or more nuclei)	111
Soft tissue sarcoma	1, 2, 3	Differentiation, mitotic figures, necrosis	22,29
Lymphoma	Low, intermediate, high; I, II, III	Mitotic figures: low (0–5 mitoses in one 400× field), intermediate (6–10 mitoses), high (>10 mitoses)	32,45,147–149
		Nuclear size: small (<1.5× a RBC), intermediate (1.5–2× a RBC) and large (>2× a RBC)	
		Nuclear morphology: centroblastic, immunoblastic, centrocytes to centroblasts	
		Architecture and immunophenotype: diffuse large B-cell (DLBC), peripheral T cell not otherwise specified (PTC-NOS), T-cell lymphoblastic lymphoma (T-LBL), indolent nodular lymphoma (T-zone, marginal zone [mantle cell, and follicular])[b]	
Oral, lip, cutaneous and digital melanoma	Poor prognostic features	Mitoses: ≥4/10 hpf (oral/lip) or ≥3/10 hpf (cutaneous/digit); pigmentation: in <50% cells (oral/lip) or no to slight pigmentation (cutaneous/digit); atypical nuclei: in ≥30% (oral/lip) or in ≥20% cells (cutaneous/digit); Ki67 Index: >19.5 (oral/lip) or >15% (cutaneous/digit)	33,83,150,151
Mammary gland carcinoma	Prognostic significance by histologic subtype (per 2011 classification system)	Prolonged survival: carcinoma arising in benign mixed tumors, complex carcinoma, simple tubular carcinoma; Decreased survival: tubulopapillary carcinoma, intraductal papillary carcinoma, malignant myoepithelioma, adenosquamous carcinoma, comedocarcinoma, solid carcinoma, anaplastic carcinoma, carcinosarcoma	72,152,94
	System 1: Well, moderately, and poorly differentiated	Invasion, nuclear differentiation, lymphoid response	153–155
	System 2: Grades I (low), II (intermediate), III (high)	Tubule formation, nuclear pleomorphism, mitotic index	
Periarticular tumors	Tumor type/histogenesis dependent prognosis; (histiocytic sarcoma, synovial myxoma, synovial cell sarcoma)	Molecular markers (CD18, vimentins, cytokeratin, smooth muscle actin) and tumor constituents, (myxomatous matrix) that may assist in determining histogenesis.	156–159
Multilobular osteochondrosarcoma[c]	1, 2, 3	Borders, lobule size, organization, mitotic index, nuclear pleomorphism, necrosis	53,54
Pulmonary carcinoma[c]	1, 2, 3	Overall differentiation, nuclear pleomorphism, mitotic index, necrosis, nucleolar size, fibrosis, invasion	60

[a]Terminology regarding mitotic figures throughout the table reflects the terminology used in the respective study.

[b]The most common canine lymphoma subtypes, which have also been shown to carry prognostic relevance (the revised REAL/WHO Classification describes > 30 subcategories of lymphoma; prognostic significance is not validated for all subtypes). In general, the indolent subtypes have less aggressive biologic behavior. Mantle cell and follicular cell lymphomas are uncommon but are listed here for completeness. Of note, late stage indolent lymphomas may take on an aggressive phenotype.

[c]These studies do not meet the robust criteria recently described; however, because they remain the foundation of grading for these tumor types, they are included here with the caveat that clinicians should be cognizant of the limitations of study design.[50]

TABLE 3.5	Molecular Features Underlying Grading Criteria
Grading Criteria	**Underlying Molecular Mechanisms**
Mitotic activity	Cyclins, cyclin-dependent kinases (CDKs), proliferating cell nuclear antigen (PCNA), Ki67, bromodeoxyuridine (BrdUrd), labeling index (LI)/ growth fraction (GF)
Percent necrosis	Inflammatory mediators, including eicosanoids (prostaglandins), cytokines; microvessel density (MVD), including vascular endothelial growth factor (VEGF), thrombospondin-1 (TSP-1), and hypoxia-inducible factor 1-α
Invasiveness	Matrix metalloproteinases (MMPs), plasminogen activators (PA), integrin expression, cell adhesion molecules (E-cadherin, N-cadherin)
Stromal reaction	Transforming growth factor beta (TGF-β), platelet-derived growth factor (PDGF), basic fibroblast growth factor (bFGF), VEGF, MVD mediators
Nucleolar size	RNA transcriptional activity, silver staining nucleolar organizing regions (AgNORs)
Overall cellularity	Growth fraction, apoptosis factors (i.e., FasL, caspases), tumor doubling time

typically co-occur and, similarly, morphologic grading criteria are likely interconnected (e.g., tumoral necrosis, inflammation, stromal response, and invasive growth).[46]

As digital technologies become more readily available, grading schemes may change. Digitization has the potential to transform previously categorical morphologic criteria into more objective and repeatable continuous variables; it also will help assess the value of individual morphologic criteria used to estimate the prognosis.[76–78] Automated computerized morphologic examination is not routinely available in veterinary diagnostic pathology, but it might soon overcome the current limitations.

Grading may be supplemented by ancillary diagnostics to provide a more accurate prognostic estimate. For example, internal tandem duplications in exon 11 of the *c-kit* proto-oncogene have been linked to tumor grade, survival, and response to tyrosine kinase inhibitor therapies.[79–82] Measures of tumor growth fraction (e.g., Ki67 index) have been successfully applied to canine oral melanocytic tumors, particularly when routine morphologic interpretation offers an ambiguous assessment of the biologic course.[83] Recognition of cancer stem cells and an enhanced knowledge of tumor heterogeneity may continue to influence approaches to tumor grading.

The pathologist may assist in staging by assessing tumor size, depth of invasion, LN involvement, or confirmation of the neoplastic process at distant sites. This information is needed to stage tumors into WHO's TNM system (i.e., *t*umor size and/or invasion; *n*odal involvement; and distant *m*etastasis).[14] Categories for tumor size and depth of invasion vary according to tumor type. In human melanoma the Clark and Breslow scales are used to determine tumor size and depth of skin involvement. In human bladder cancer, tumor staging is largely based on the depth of tumor invasion into the bladder wall.[3,5] Similar concepts might be applicable for veterinary patients with tumors such as canine urothelial carcinoma and feline gastrointestinal lymphoma.[10,84] Cytologic assessment (i.e., fine-needle aspirate) of draining LNs

has been shown to be a sensitive alternative to histopathology for LN metastasis needed for staging.[85,86] However, if the cytologic assessment is negative, histologic evaluation still should be considered. In both processes of tumor grading or tumor staging, these procedures are useful only if they have been shown to correlate with clinical behavior.

Assessment of Tumor Margins

Margin assessment is an essential component of oncologic specimen review, especially when the surgical goal is curative-intent.[1,87] Although several important limitations are associated with this practice, routine histopathology is the most widely available method of determining excisional completeness. Histologic margins are a predictive marker of surgical treatment; however, margin status does not predict recurrence with absolute certainty.[1,87,88] Additionally, margin status at a primary site does not address the potential for metastases or the likelihood of a disease-free state.

The *surgical edge* refers to the surgically incised edge/excisional edge of the biopsy specimen. The *gross surgical margin* refers to the region between the surgical edge and the physically palpable and/or visual mass; typically determined before the surgical procedure and presumed to be tumor free. Microscopically the *histologic surgical margin* (histologic tumor-free margin [HTFM]) is the quantifiable tumor-free tissue between the neoplastic process and the surgically incised edge. Microscopic margin assessment should be performed for both benign and malignant lesions, although detailed characterization of the HTFM (e.g., objective measurement, tissue constituents and viability) may be limited to malignancies because recurrence of benign tumors is uncommon. Crucial determinants for obtaining accurate surgical margin information on the pathology report are (1) specimen handling and information submitted by the clinician; (2) the method of tissue trimming performed at the laboratory; and (3) observations reported by the pathologist.[1]

Histologic surgical margins should be interpreted with a knowledge of the intrinsic limitations of histopathology and factors that influence the pathologist's interpretation. The clinician is responsible for communicating the surgical goals as they relate to excisional outcomes (i.e., debulking versus curative-intent) and which tissue edges require microscopic scrutiny. In some cases annotated sketches or images might assist with trimming (regions selected from the gross specimen at the laboratory for processing and microscopic evaluation). Inking is the preferred method of identifying a surgical edge because it can be visualized at both the gross and microscopic levels.[5,89] Grossly the surgical ink affects regions of the specimen that are selected during trimming for microscopic examination. Importantly, ink allows the pathologist to identify a true surgical edge appropriately under the microscope (as opposed to artifact) and report the margin as it relates to a specific gross anatomic region. Surgical ink should be placed only on regions of the specimen that are true surgically incised edges or areas of specific clinical concern. Ink should also be allowed to dry according to the manufacturer's instructions (approximately 15 minutes) before fixative immersion. Even under ideal conditions, inking can be associated with a number of artifacts that may influence the histologic interpretation.[90] Continuous suturing of postexcisional specimens might mitigate artifacts associated with tissue alignment and cohesion.[91]

Histologic surgical margin outcomes are influenced by the method used to trim specimens at the laboratory.[1,92,93] One study of low-grade canine MCTs found that 23% of margin outcomes changed according to the sectioning technique.[94] The most common method of trimming for routine specimens is the *cross-sectioning* or *radial method.* The mass is bisected along its short axis, after which each remaining half is bisected along its long axis, creating quarter sections. This method is perpendicular sectioning and facilitates numeric quantification of the deep and four circumferential (lateral) margins. The overall amount of margin tissue evaluated is minimal, and this method may be particularly problematic for tumors with irregular geometry or discontinuous growth patterns (i.e., microsatellites). Additional techniques that can increase the overall percentage of margin tissue evaluated include *parallel, modified* (a combination of parallel and cross-sectioning), and *tangential* sectioning.[1] Tangential sectioning (sections taken parallel to the surgical edge) captures a greater percentage of the margin but can generate only a dichotomous margin outcome (i.e., tumor cells present versus not present). Shaved margins taken from the tumor bed might bypass some limitations associated with examination of the excised specimen.[87] Shavings from the tumor bed may be submitted in addition to the excised mass but should be submitted in a separate, appropriately labeled container. Möhs surgical technique is the most comprehensive histologic margin evaluation, but it is not widely available in a veterinary surgical setting.[95]

Reporting of the histologic surgical margins should be clear, concise, and thorough, furnishing the clinician with essential information needed to make informed decisions and recommendations for further management. Reporting should include (1) a description of the neoplastic cells closest to the surgical edge (e.g., individual cells, nests of cells, cells at the periphery of the mass itself); (2) an objective measurement of the HTFM (precluded for tangentially trimmed sections); and (3) a description of the tissue constituents (e.g., adipose tissue, dense connective tissue, muscle) and the quality of these constituents (e.g., normal, necrotic, inflamed), because different tissue types provide variable barriers against invasion and infiltration of neoplastic cells.[1,96,97] Vague terminology, such as clean, dirty, close, or narrow, should be avoided because these are subjective terms that introduce interpretative variability. Even though a pathologist might use *complete excision* to communicate a HTFM greater than 0 mm, this terminology introduces ambiguity by virtue of the fact that minimally adequate margins are poorly defined for most veterinary oncologic specimens.[87]

Of note, a quantified histologic surgical margin may be significantly less than a gross surgical margin. Margin measurements are influenced by architectural changes that begin at excision (inherent postexcisional tissue retraction) and end with sectioning and mounting of paraffin-embedded tissue onto the slide. Cadaveric canine skin undergoes a notable physical tissue length reduction ("shrinkage") immediately after excision, approximately 14% for circumferential measurements.[98] Myofibril contraction and tissue elasticity account for much of this effect.[98] This same process may result in increased tissue thickness, which can be influenced by tissue composition.[99] Tissue shrinkage also is affected by formalin fixation, and the degree of shrinkage varies relative to the tissue type.[99–101] For cutaneous biopsy specimens, shrinkage can be up to 30%.[99,100] Specimens may also undergo considerable tissue distortion during fixation, and this distortion may affect the observed HTFM.[87,98] In one study the reduction between the in vivo grossly normal surgical margin and the HTFM, once microscopic tumor infiltration had been taken into account, was reported to be as much as 30 mm and 24 mm in canine MCTs and STSs, respectively.[102]

Many tumor-specific studies have been performed with the goal of correlating surgical margins to clinical outcome. For canine MCTs a number of studies have reported positive associations between histologically complete margins and improved clinical outcomes.[88,103,104] Complete excision of canine STSs also has proven beneficial; dogs with incomplete margins have been reported as 10.5 times more likely to experience local recurrence.[22,26] Incomplete margins also have been linked to local recurrence of canine SCCs of the digit,[105] nasal planum,[106] and oral cavity[107,108]; MLOs[53]; and malignant canine mammary tumors.[72] Excisional status has been linked to survival time in canine noncutaneous HSA.[57]

Although the histologic margin status is an important clinical consideration, incompletely excised malignancies do not always recur, even after protracted follow-up periods. This is illustrated in canine low-grade STSs,[22,109] canine cutaneous MCTs, and subcutaneous MCTs.[110,111] Conversely, some neoplasms with highly invasive and/or metastatic phenotypes have a recurrence potential that is not necessarily related to complete histologic margin status. Recurrence is especially well recognized in feline ISSs, likely because of the tumor's infiltrative nature and pattern; one study of 13 recurrent tumors had only one that was histologically incomplete.[112] For canine oral malignant melanoma, the survival implications of excisional status are also ambiguous.[113] High-grade canine MCTs have a significant risk of local recurrence that is not associated with margin width.[114] Biologic factors that contribute to the potential for recurrence may include molecular signatures, field cancerization, tumor heterogeneity, and overall changes in the tumoral and peritumoral microenvironment.[87,115,116]

Histologic margin interpretation fundamentally centers on a morphologic, light microscopic interpretation by a trained anatomic pathologist. By definition this requires accurate identification of cells at the "leading front" of the neoplasm and recognition of the surgical edge (ideally identified by the presence of ink). Some degree of variation in margin measurement is expected. One study of canine MCTs found a median standard deviation of almost 2 mm in circumferential MCT measurements.[90] Although this difference may not be relevant in wide excisions, marginal excisions are especially prone to interpretive differences, particularly if the margins are classified as dichotomous variable (i.e., complete or incomplete).[90] Sometimes differentiating between inflammatory or reactive and neoplastic cells can be challenging, as with the edges of canine MCTs, granulation tissue in STSs, and carcinoma cells undergoing epithelial-mesenchymal transition.[87] The pathologist's approach to margin evaluation, and subsequent clinical interpretation, might also take into account growth patterns at the invasive front, which differ between tumor types.[78] In one study of low-grade canine MCTs and low/intermediate-grade canine STSs, circumferential and deep infiltration was 4 mm or 2 mm, respectively, from the subgross tumor edge.[78] Asymmetric invasion has been associated with a greater likelihood of incomplete excisions in canine MCTs.[78]

Collective data suggest that the adequacy of excision, and subsequent indications for possible adjuvant therapy, should not rest solely on the histologic margin status. Assessment of the likelihood of recurrence should be interpreted in parallel with a number of other variables, including tumor lineage, histologic grade where applicable, frequency of MFs, growth pattern, trimming technique, and margin composition.

Ancillary Diagnostics

Most oncologic cases in human medicine can be diagnosed by light microscopy using hematoxylin and eosin (H&E) stains.[5]

This likely reflects the situation in veterinary medicine. In a subset of cases, and for clinicians seeking further prognostic and/or predictive information, ancillary tests, such as histochemical stains, IHC, TEM, PCR, and flow cytometry, may be necessary (see Chapter 8). As molecular and genomic research in veterinary oncology continue to evolve, new ancillary tests also will likely emerge, resulting in greater sophistication in tumor diagnoses, prognostication, and theranostics, including more frequent identification of novel therapeutic targets.[117]

Special Histochemical Stains

Histochemical stains consist of chemical substances that, when applied to tissue sections, result in a direct chemical reaction with the tissue's constituents. For all intents and purposes, routine H&E is a histochemical stain in which hematoxylin reacts with nucleic acid and eosin with cytoplasmic protein. Some common histochemical stains that can be used in veterinary oncologic pathology to assist in the diagnosis of certain poorly differentiated tumors are listed in Table 3.6. Stains that identify extracellular matrices that may indirectly support tumor histogenesis include Masson trichrome (collagen; fibrocytic tumors), Alcian blue (proteoglycans; myxoma, myxosarcoma), and Congo red (amyloid; plasma cell tumors, amyloid producing odontogenic tumors). Although histochemical stains often are used for poorly differentiated tumors, the stains themselves do not differentiate between benign and malignant. With the advancement of IHC, many histochemical stains have lost popularity; however, they are still available and can be useful in the appropriate setting. Silver staining of nucleolar organizer regions (AgNOR) is an additional

histochemical staining technique that has demonstrated prognostic relevance in canine lymphoma,[118] MCTs,[119] and mammary tumors.[120]

Immunohistochemistry

IHC can aid the classification of several tumors in veterinary medicine and is a widely used diagnostic technique. IHC is a staining procedure that uses commercial antibodies to identify specific cellular and extracellular molecules ex vivo, such as cytoplasmic intermediate filaments, cell surface markers, or even secretory substances; all "molecules" or "markers" are tissue proteins, also referred to as *tissue antigens*. IHC can be performed on frozen sections or specimens routinely fixed in formalin and processed into paraffin blocks. Tissue sections are incubated with primary antibodies to specific cell proteins (antigens). Sections with bound primary antibody are then exposed to secondary antibodies directed against the primary antibody. The secondary antibodies are linked to peroxidase or avidin-biotin peroxidase complexes. The peroxidase catalyzes a reaction in the presence of dye that precipitates at the site of the complex and is visible with light microscopy.[121,122] As an alternative, alkaline phosphatase enzyme systems also are available. A list of common diagnostic IHC markers used in veterinary oncology, and the respective tumor types for which their use is indicated, is provided in Table 3.7. ICC uses similar technical aspects; however, it is performed on cytologic samples obtained from an aspirate or impression smear; this technique has been increasing in popularity over recent years.[123]

IHC also may be prognostically useful; for example, it can assist in evaluating proliferation or the tumor growth fraction through detection of markers such as Ki67 (MIB-1) and PCNA.[124] Prognosis also has been linked to markers of multidrug resistance (e.g., P-glycoprotein)[125] and altered proto-oncogenes or tumor suppressor genes (e.g., *p53, c-kit/CD117, p21, Rb,* and *PTEN*).[81,82,126–128] Other immunohistochemically detectable markers linked to the prognosis include VEGF and its receptors,[129] cyclooxygenase-2,[68,130–132] and platelet-derived growth factor receptor.[133] Many other potential prognostic markers in a variety of veterinary tumor types detectable by IHC have been and continue to be studied, (e.g., epidermal growth factor receptor, human epidermal growth factor receptor-2, urokinase plasminogen activator, heat shock proteins).[134–136] As the realm of IHC in veterinary medicine continues to expand, so, too, will the discovery of tumor-specific diagnostic markers and markers for prognostic (biologic aggressiveness) and predictive (therapeutic responsiveness) utility.

Although IHC can be a valuable tool, some complicating factors exist. A negative stain does not exclude a certain cell type. Technical components or tumor cell dedifferentiation, with loss of antigen expression, may result in a negative result. One of the more common technical problems that can cause negative staining is prolonged formalin fixation that results in excessive cross-linking of the antigenic components or loss of soluble proteins into the fixative. Antibody-specific antigens (epitopes) that have been masked by protein cross-linking often can be "unmasked" by pretreating sections with trypsin or pepsin or by using heat-induced epitope retrieval techniques.[121,122] Decalcification of tissue may also result in alteration of target proteins so that they are no longer recognized by the respective antibody. The type and duration of decalcifying solution, however, may mitigate these deleterious effects.[136,137] Areas of tissue necrosis, autolysis, hemorrhage, section drying, and sometimes collagenous matrix components can

TABLE 3.6	Special Histochemical Stains to Support Tumor Histogenesis	
Tumor Type (Reactive Constituent)	Histochemical Stain	Reference
Granular cell tumor (cytoplasmic lysosomes)	Periodic acid-Schiff (PAS)	160,161
Liposarcoma and lipid-rich neoplasms (lipid)	Oil Red-O, Sudan stains (black, III, IV)[a]	162–165
Mast cell tumor (cytoplasmic granules)	Toluidine blue, Giemsa, PAS[b]	17,34
Melanoma (melanin)	Fontana-Masson[c]	166,167
Neuroendocrine tumor (cytoplasmic granules)	Silver stains (Pascual's, Grimelius, Sevier-Munger), Churukian-Schenk	168,169
Plasma cell tumor (amyloid), APOT (amyloid)	Congo red	170–172
Rhabdomyosarcoma (myocyte cross striations)	Phosphotungstic acid-hematoxylin (PTAH)	173

[a]These stains must be performed on nonprocessed tissue because exposure to xylene during processing dissolves lipid components.

[b]May be used in feline and ferret mast cell tumors because the granules in these species are often better visualized with PAS.

[c]Reacts with melanin, which is also visible on routine light microscopy and therefore may be beneficial when trying to confirm melanin versus an alternative cellular pigment (e.g., hemosiderin, lipofuscin). Melanin bleach may provide similar information.

TABLE 3.7   Common Diagnostic Immunohistochemical Markers/Panels and Respective Tumor Types in Cats and Dogs

Tumor Type	Molecular Marker(s)	Localization/Expression	Comments	References
Carcinoma	Cytokeratin+a Vimentin−	Cytokeratin, Vimentin = Cyto	Coexpression can occur in mesothelioma and may reflect EMT in carcinomas.	47,174–176
Gastrointestinal stromal tumor (GIST) (interstitial cell of Cajal [ICC] origin)	KIT/ CD117+/− SMA+/− Desmin− S-100− Dog-1+	KIT = PM & Cyto SMA, Desmin = Cyto S-100 = N & Cyto Dog-1 = PM & Cyto	DOG1/TMEM16A. Mature ICCs do not express SMA but SMA positivity has been reported; suggested because of the close association of ICCs and intestinal smooth muscle or as ICCs and smooth muscle cells may arise from the same primitive stem cell.	177–179
Hemangiosarcoma/ Lymphangiosarcoma	Factor VIII-RAg/vWF+ CD31/PECAM-1+	Factor VIII-RAg/vWF = Cyto CD31/PECAM-1 = PM & Cyto	Factor VIII-RAg and CD31 do not differentiate between blood and lymphatic endothelial cell origin. Lymphatic endothelial-specific markers such as LYVE-1 and Prox-1 have been suggested as diagnostic markers. CD31/PECAM is also expressed, in lower levels, by monocytes, granulocytes, and subsets of T-cells.	180–184
Histiocytic sarcoma (HS)	CD18+, CD3−, CD79a−, Pax5−, Iba1+b Lysozyme+/−	CD18, CD3, CD79a = PM Pax5 = N Iba1, Lysozyme = Cyto	CD18 is expressed on all leukocytes. Its expression is typically highest on, yet not specific for, histiocytic cells. Iba1 expression shown in monocyte/macrophage lineage, dendritic cells and associated tumors. Additional, yet not commonly used, markers for subsets/ subclassification of histiocytic tumors: CD11d+ Hemophagocytic histiocytic sarcoma; CD90/Thy-1+ Cutaneous and systemic histiocytosis–canine dermal dendritic cell origin.	185–187
Leiomyoma, leiomyosarcoma	KIT/CD117− SMA+ Desmin+/− S-100− Dog-1−	KIT = PM & Cyto SMA, Desmin = Cyto S-100 = N & Cyto Dog-1 = PM & Cyto	Desmin confirms myogenic origin but does not differentiate between smooth, striated, or cardiac muscle.	177–179
Lymphoma, B cell	CD18+/−, CD3−, CD79a+, Pax5+ CD20+	CD18, CD3, CD79a = PM Pax5 = N CD20 = PM	CD18 expression is generally weak or absent. Pax5 (BSAP), a member of the highly conserved paired box (PAX) domain family of transcription factors. Expressed from early pro B to plasma cell where it is downregulated. CD20 = expressed in increasing concentrations from late pro-B to activated B cell (not plasma cells).	188–192
Lymphoma, T cell	CD18+/−, CD3+, CD79a−, Pax5−	CD18, CD3, CD79a = PM Pax5 = N	As for Lymphoma, B cell	189–191
Lymphoma, null cell	CD18−, CD3−, CD79a−, Pax5− (and exclusion of other round cell tumors)	CD18, CD3, CD79a = PM Pax5 = N	As for Lymphoma, B cell	188
Mast cell tumor	Tryptase+ KIT/ CD117+c	Tryptase = Cyto KIT/CD117 = PM and/ or cytoplasmic (Type I, II or III expression pattern)	*Histochemical* stains toluidine blue and Giemsa may be used to confirm mast cell origin. Tryptase IHC is fairly uncommon but is available if other diagnostic parameters are unrewarding. KIT/CD117 is not specific for mast cells (see table legend).	126,193
Melanocytic neoplasms (melanotic and amelanotic)	Melan-A+/− d PNL2+/− Tyrosinase+/− TRP-1+/− TRP-2+/− Vimentin+ S-100+	Melan-A = Cyto PNL2 = Cyto Tyrosinase = Cyto TRP-1&2 = Cyto Vim = Cyto S-100 = N & Cyto	Melan-A/MART-1. PNL2 is melanocyte-specific save for myeloid cells, especially neutrophils. Use of an immunohistochemical "cocktail" containing PNL2, Melan-A, TRP-1 and TRP-2 is reported to have excellent specificity and sensitivity. Both vimentin and S-100 have good sensitivity but poor specificity.	194–198
Mesothelioma	Cytokeratin+/− Vimentin+/−	As above	Coexpression expected for many mesotheliomas. TEM may demonstrate microvilli.	137,199
Neural astrocytic tumors (astrocytoma, glioblastoma, oligodendroglioma)	GFAP+ S-100+/− Olig2+/−	GFAP = Cyto S-100 = N & Cyto Olig2 = N	Astrocytomas are glial tumors, as are oligodendrogliomas; however, oligodendrogliomas are negative for GFAP. Olig-2 may also be expressed in some astrocytic tumors.	200–202

| TABLE 3.7 | Common Diagnostic Immunohistochemical Markers/Panels and Respective Tumor Types in Cats and Dogs—cont'd |

Tumor Type	Molecular Marker(s)	Localization/Expression	Comments	References
Neuroendocrine tumors	Chromogranin A$^{+/-}$ Synaptophysin$^{+/-}$ NSE$^+$ [Hormone-specific antibodies (e.g., antiglucagon, insulin, thyroglobulin and calcitonin (see Thyroid Tumor, later), may help determine specific histogenesis].	Chromogranin = Cyto Synaptophysin = Cyto NSE = Cyto	All are generic markers of NE origin. Recommended to run in concert because NE tumors are often variably immunoreactive. NSE is found in a number of cell types and therefore NE specificity, but it is useful in combination with other NE markers.	138,174,203
Plasma cell tumor	MUM-1/IRF4$^+$ CD18$^{+/-}$ CD3$^-$ CD79a$^{+/-}$ (Pax5$^-$)	MUM-1 = N CD18, CD3, CD79a = PM Pax5 = N	In humans, plasma cell neoplasms, multiple myeloma, and plasmablastic lymphomas are typically negative for Pax5. Pax5 expression via IHC in similar canine tumors, has not been reported.	204
Rhabdomyoma, rhabdomyosarcoma	Vimentin$^+$ Desmin$^+$ Myoglobin$^{+/-}$ SMA$^-$ (MyoD1$^{+/-}$ Myogenin$^{+/-}$; see comments)	Vimentin, Desmin, Myoglobin = Cyto MyoD1 and myogenin = N	Desmin (see Leiomyoma, leiomyosarcoma). Myoglobin is typically a late-stage marker; may be negative in poorly differentiated rhabdomyosarcomas. Myo-D1 and myogenin can be useful in undifferentiated tumors. (MyoD-1 and myogenin are not routinely available). PTAH is a histochemical stain that may highlight cross striations of skeletal muscle.	206–208
Sarcoma	Vimentin$^{+\ e}$ Cytokeratin$^-$	Cyto		174–176
Synovial cell sarcoma	Vimentin$^+$ Cytokeratin$^{+/-}$ CD18$^-$	Vimentin, cytokeratin = Cyto CD18 = PM	Histogenesis is controversial. Relevance of cytokeratin expression has been questioned. May recruit large numbers of CD18+ histiocytes, making distinction from articular/periarticular histiocytic sarcoma challenging.	209,210
Thyroid tumor: follicular epithelial origin (follicular carcinoma; follicular, solid, or mixed subtypes)	Thyroglobulin$^+$ TTF-1$^+$ Calcitonin$^-$ Chromogranin A$^-$ Synaptophysin$^-$ NSE$^-$	Thyroglobulin = Cyto TTF-1 = N Calcitonin = Cyto	Thyroglobulin = provides iodination sites for the production of thyroid hormones, TTF-1 = nuclear transcription factor specific to thyroid tissue save for pulmonary epithelium, calcitonin = polypeptide secreted by thyroid C-cells; counteracts effects of PTH by reducing blood Ca^{2+}	205,211–213
Thyroid tumor: C-cell /parafollicular cell origin (medullary C-cell carcinoma)	Thyroglobulin$^-$ TTF-1$^+$ Calcitonin$^+$ Chromogranin A$^+$ Synaptophysin$^+$ NSE$^+$	As above	As for Thyroid tumor: follicular epithelial origin	211–213

This table provides common diagnostic immunohistochemical markers used in veterinary oncologic pathology on formalin-fixed, paraffin-embedded tissue sections. Immunohistochemical stains should always be interpreted in conjunction with routine (hematoxylin & eosin) histopathologic evaluation and in the presence of appropriately stained positive and negative control tissues. *Positive immunoreactivity* supports histogenesis; however, *negative immunoreactivity* does not definitively rule out histogenesis because of the potential dedifferentiation of neoplastic cells with loss of antigen expression, in addition to the potential for technical error (false negative).

Ab, antibody; *BSAP*, B-cell–specific activator protein; *Cyto*, cytoplasmic; *DOG1*, discovered on gastrointestinal tumor 1; *EC*, endothelial cell; *EMT*, epithelial-mesenchymal transition; *Factor VIII-RAg/vWF*, factor VIII–related antigen/von Willebrand factor; *GFAP*, glial fibrillary acidic protein; *Gp*, glycoprotein; *IFP*, intermediate filament protein; *IHC*, immunohistochemistry; *MKs*, megakaryocytes; *MUM-1/IRF4*, multiple myeloma 1/interferon regulatory factor 4; *N*, nuclear; *NE*, neuroendocrine; *NSE*, neuron-specific enolase; *PECAM*, platelet endothelial cell adhesion molecule; *PM*, plasma membrane; *PTH*, parathyroid hormone; *PTAH*, phosphotungstic acid-hematoxylin; *RTK*, tyrosine kinase receptor; *SMA*, smooth muscle actin; *TEM*, Transmission electron microscopy; *TRP*, tyrosinase-related protein; *TTF-1*, thyroid transcription factor-1; *Vim*, vimentin.

aGeneric marker for tumors of epithelial origin.

bIba1 may be helpful in differentiating histiocytic tumors from other round cell tumors.[187]

cKIT/CD117 is supportive of but should *not be* considered diagnostic for mast cell tumor because it is not mast-cell specific; it has been shown to carry prognostic relevance in canine cutaneous mast cell tumor based on its cellular localization/expression pattern determined by means of IHC.[116]

dRare positivity in amelanotic melanomas.

eGeneric marker for tumors of mesenchymal cell origin.

result in excessive nonspecific background staining. A skilled pathologist who is familiar with the IHC stain should be asked to differentiate background stain from tumor-specific stain and to navigate technical difficulties. As with histochemical stains, IHC does not distinguish between neoplastic and nonneoplastic tissue. For example, normal bladder mucosal epithelium (urothelium), urothelial hyperplasia, and urothelial carcinoma (TCC) would all be immunopositive for cytokeratin. The distinction between neoplastic and nonneoplastic is made on routine H&E light microscopy based on hallmark features of neoplasia.

Evaluation and interpretation of IHC results should be performed with the knowledge of antibody sensitivity and specificity. For example, both vimentin and cytokeratin are highly sensitive for sarcomas and carcinomas, respectively, but lack specificity. S-100 can be used to support melanomas with good sensitivity, but it lacks specificity because it is expressed in a broad variety of cells, especially neural crest derivatives (e.g., Schwann cell, nerve, cartilage, bone, smooth muscle, adipose). Because most tumor markers have limitations, the best and most reliable results may be obtained using a panel of IHC stains, for which both marker-specific immunopositive and immunonegative results may be anticipated (e.g., rhabdomyosarcoma should be immunopositive for vimentin and desmin, but immunonegative for smooth muscle actin), rather than relying on a single stain. Additionally, IHC stains can be appropriately interpreted *only* in conjunction with appropriate species-specific controls. To support the diagnosis or determine the immunophenotype of feline intestinal lymphoma, appropriate positive control tissue, such as feline LN, spleen, or tonsil, must be run simultaneously. It must be of feline origin and contain normal lymphoid tissue if the pathologist is to confirm that the IHC stain was performed successfully and to interpret appropriately the immunoreaction of the test tissue. Similarly, a negative control, which consists of the test tissue treated either with nonspecific antibody or omission of the primary antibody, must also be run to assist in ruling out background/nonspecific staining. Laboratories that offer IHC should ensure all tests have been optimized and validated relative to each species for which the test is offered.

IHC can be a powerful tool for providing information that could not be otherwise determined on routine microscopy alone (e.g., confirmation of a tumor's histogenesis based on molecular markers). However, an IHC stain should never be interpreted in and of itself; rather, it always should be evaluated in conjunction with routine light microscopic findings and the relevant clinical information.

Transmission Electron Microscopy

As other ancillary diagnostic procedures have become more widely used, TEM is performed less frequently on tumor biopsy specimens, but it is still a notable ancillary resource. TEM requires specific technical support and equipment and is available only at a few diagnostic laboratories. Specimen preparation involves preserving very small representative tumor samples (1 × 1 mm) in special fixatives (e.g., glutaraldehyde), processing tissue into epoxy-based plastic blocks, and sectioning at 1 μm for thick sections to determine the adequacy of the sample and inclusion of appropriate tumor cells. Subsequently, sectioning is done at about 600 Å; the samples are stained with heavy metal–based stains and then examined with the aid of an electron microscope. Samples fixed in formalin can be used, although the quality of the subsequent sections is suboptimal.

TEM can help identify specific cellular features, such as intercellular junctions or basal lamina in epithelial cells, melanosomes in melanocytic cells, granules in mast cells, neurosecretory granules in neuroendocrine cells, mucin droplets in certain epithelial cells, and villous projections of mesothelial cells.[17,137,138] These features may be useful in distinguishing carcinoma from lymphoma and identifying melanoma, MCT, neuroendocrine tumor, and mesothelioma. TEM ultimately provides a level of magnification to visualize specific and detailed cellular components that cannot be appreciated with routine light microscopy.

Flow Cytometry and Polymerase Chain Reaction

Both flow cytometry and PCR have become fairly routine procedures in veterinary oncology and often are combined with histopathology, cytopathology, IHC, and/or ICC. These techniques can be useful for tumor classification and/or confirmation (especially hematopoietic tumors), particularly when H&E and/or IHC interpretation is ambiguous.[139–141] These techniques are discussed in detail in Chapter 8.

Clinical-Pathological Correlation and Second Opinions

Establishing a definitive histopathologic diagnosis can be precluded by the absence of relevant and necessary clinical information.[2,5] This may be especially true regarding primary bone tumors versus secondary tumors involving bone. Diagnosis of a surface or juxtacortical OSA depends both on imaging results and histopathologic features. Similarly, an osteoma may be difficult to distinguish from reactive bone without a corroborative radiograph. Periarticular neoplasia may be difficult to distinguish from other sarcomas, or even inflammatory or immune-mediated joint disease, unless radiographic or gross evidence of joint involvement and bone invasion is seen. Acanthomatous ameloblastoma may be difficult to distinguish from benign periodontal ligament tumors unless bone invasion is identified. Confirming bone involvement depends on deep biopsy samples that capture underlying bone or on clinical information that indicates bone involvement. The importance of communicating clinical data might be best illustrated by histologically low-grade yet biologically high-grade FSAs of the canine oral cavity.[18] Histologically these tumors may be mistaken for benign fibrous tissue, but the clinical presentation is a rapidly growing, invasive and destructive mass that often recurs after conservative surgery.[18] These examples demonstrate the need to furnish the pathologist with an accurate and thorough clinical history, all relevant clinical findings, and the results of all other diagnostic tests. Ultimately, providing any previous imaging scans (or other) results and reports themselves may be the easiest and most accurate means of relaying this information.

When extensive treatment may be pursued or *if a pathology diagnosis is not consistent with the clinical impression,* a second opinion should be considered.[142,143] In human medicine a review of mandatory second opinion surgical pathology at major hospitals revealed 1.4% to 5.8% major changes in the diagnosis that resulted in a change of therapy or prognosis. It was concluded that despite the extra cost, mandatory second opinions should be obtained whenever a major therapeutic endeavor is considered or if treatment decisions are based primarily on the pathologic diagnosis.[144–146] In veterinary medicine, diagnostic disagreement between first and second opinion pathology has been reported to be as high as 19%, including differences in histogenesis (tumor type) and benign versus malignant status, and up to 37% for differences that would affect the prognosis or treatment choices.[142,143]

The two major categories of errors that may occur at the pathology laboratory are technical errors (e.g., improper labeling, trimming, other) and errors in interpretation of the tissue.[2] If tissue is processed improperly because of equipment malfunction or because it is poorly sectioned, artifacts can occur that make the tissue specimen impossible to interpret. Errors in the pathologist's interpretation may occur in the absence of relevant (or receipt of erroneous) clinical information, or simply because the case is a challenging one. If a pathology service is staffed by medical rather than veterinary pathologists, certain tumors may be misdiagnosed (e.g., histiocytoma, MCT, transmissible venereal tumor, or perianal gland adenoma) because these do not have human counterparts. Many pathologists informally seek opinions from other pathologists when confronted with challenging cases. However, the clinician, should *never hesitate to ask for an official second opinion, nor should the original pathologist be offended by such a request.* A second or even a third pathologist can offer a different perspective on a difficult case and may suggest an alternative diagnosis, confirm the diagnosis of the primary pathologist, or confirm that an accurate diagnosis is not possible and suggest additional ancillary tests for diagnostic clarification. Because patient management is affected significantly by the histopathologic diagnosis, it is not at all unreasonable for the clinician to request a second opinion. A misdiagnosis can result in costly, ineffective, and ultimately unnecessary treatments (e.g., surgery, chemotherapy, RT, other) that can cause morbidity for patients and unwarranted stresses and costs for the client. Misdiagnoses may also result in insufficient treatment, resulting in cancer progression and, perhaps of greatest concern, unwarranted euthanasia. Considering these possible scenarios, second opinions are not only prudent but highly recommended.

For optimal management of the veterinary cancer patient, it is critical for the clinician to have a firm understanding of the procedures and processes involved in generating a diagnosis from a biopsy sample—from the time of tissue acquisition to the generation and interpretation of the final report. An awareness of the limitations of histopathologic assessment and an understanding of potentially beneficial ancillary tissue-based diagnostics also are paramount. However, biopsy assessment is only one aspect of a case; other components (e.g., history, clinical presentation, imaging or other diagnostic results, comorbidities) all should be considered collectively. Important factors are the willingness and ability of the clinician and pathologist to work collaboratively, with mutually open and receptive communication, to establish the most accurate diagnosis and optimal care for the veterinary cancer patient.

References

1. Kamstock DA, Ehrhart EJ, Getzy DM, et al.: Recommended guidelines for submission, trimming, margin evaluation, and reporting of tumor biopsy specimens in veterinary surgical pathology, *Vet Pathol* 48:19–31, 2011.
2. Spitalnik PF, di Saint-Agnese PA: The Pathology of Cancer. In Rubin BP, editor: *Clinical oncology, a multi-disciplinary approach,* ed 8th, Philadelphia W.B, 2001, Saunders Company, pp 47–61.
3. Clarke B, McCluggage WG: Iatrogenic lesions and artefacts in gynaecological pathology, *J Clin Pathol* 62:104–112, 2009.
4. Llamas-Velasco M, Paredes BE: Basic concepts in skin biopsy, Part I, *Actas Dermosifiliogr* 103:12–20, 2012.
5. Pfeifer J, Wick M: The pathologic evaluation of neoplastic diseases. In Murphy GLW, Lenhard R, editors: *Clinical oncology,* Washington DC, 1995, Pan American Health Organization, pp 75–95.
6. *Mosby Inc:Mosby's Medical Dictionary,* ed 8th, St Louis, 2009, MO Mosby.
7. Burnett RC, Vernau W, Modiano JF, et al.: Diagnosis of canine lymphoid neoplasia using clonal rearrangements of antigen receptor genes, *Vet Pathol* 40:32–41, 2003.
8. Jacobs RM, Messick H, Valli V: Tumors of the hemolymphatic system. In Meuten D, editor: *Tumors in domestic animals,* ed 4, Ames Iowa, 2002, Iowa State Press, pp 119–198.
9. Kiupel M, Webster JD, Bailey KL, et al.: Proposal of a 2-tier histologic grading system for canine cutaneous mast cell tumors to more accurately predict biological behavior, *Vet Pathol* 48:147–155, 2011.
10. Valli VE, Norris A, Jacobs RM, et al.: Pathology of canine bladder and urethral cancer and correlation with tumour progression and survival, *J Comp Pathol* 113:113–130, 1995.
11. Klobukowska HJ, Munday JS: High numbers of stromal cancer-associated fibroblasts are associated with a shorter survival time in cats with oral squamous cell carcinoma, *Vet Pathol* 53:1124–1130, 2016.
12. Moore PF, Schrenzel MD, Affolter VK, et al.: Canine cutaneous histiocytoma is an epidermotropic langerhans cell histiocytosis that expresses CD1 and specific beta(2)-integrin molecules, *Am J Pathol* 148:1699–1708, 1996.
13. Derwahl M, Studer H: Hyperplasia versus adenoma in endocrine tissues: are they different? *Trends Endocrin Met* 13:23–28, 2002.
14. Cullen JM, Breen M: An overview of molecular cancer pathogenesis, prognosis, and diagnosis. In Meuten D, editor: *Tumors in domestic animals,* ed 5, Ames Iowa, 2017, John Wiley & Sons Inc, pp 1–26.
15. Taylor DO, Dorn CR, Luis OH: Morphologic and biologic characteristics of canine cutaneous histiocytoma, *Cancer Res* 29:83–92, 1969.
16. Cangul IT, Wijnen M, van Garderen E, et al.: Clinico-pathological aspects of canine cutaneous and mucocutaneous plasmacytomas, *J Vet Med A* 49:307–312, 2002.
17. Johnson TO, Schulman FY, Lipscomb TP, et al.: Histopathology and biologic behavior of pleomorphic cutaneous mast cell tumors in fifteen cats, *Vet Pathol* 39:452–457, 2002.
18. Ciekot PA, Powers BE, Withrow SJ, et al.: Histologically low-grade, yet biologically high-grade, fibrosarcomas of the mandible and maxilla in dogs - 25 cases (1982-1991), *J Am Vet Med Assoc* 204:610–615, 1994.
19. Gottfried SD, Popovitch CA, Goldschmidt MH, et al.: Metastatic digital carcinoma in the cat: a retrospective study of 36 cats (1992-1998), *J Am Anim Hosp Assoc* 36:501–509, 2000.
20. Fajardo LF, Berthrong M, Anderson RE: Differential diagnosis of atypical cells in irradiated tissues. In Fajardo LF, Berthrong M, Anderson RE, editors: *Radiation pathology New York,* Oxford University Press, 2001, pp 421–430.
21. Patnaik AK, Ehler WJ, Macewen EG: Canine cutaneous mast-cell tumor - morphologic grading and survival-time in 83 dogs, *Vet Pathol* 21:469–474, 1984.
22. Kuntz CA, Dernell WS, Powers BE, et al.: Prognostic factors for surgical treatment of soft-tissue sarcomas in dogs:75 cases (1986-1996), *J Am Vet Med Assoc* 211:1147–1151, 1997.
23. Coindre JM: Grading of soft tissue sarcomas - review and update, *Arch Pathol Lab Med* 130:1448–1453, 2006.
24. Romansik EM, Reilly CM, Kass PH, et al.: Mitotic index is predictive for survival for canine cutaneous mast cell tumors, *Vet Pathol* 44:335–341, 2007.
25. Elston LB, Sueiro FA, Cavalcanti JN, et al.: The importance of the mitotic index as a prognostic factor for survival of canine cutaneous mast cell tumors: a validation study, *Vet Pathol* 46:362–364, 2009.

26. McSporran KD: Histologic grade predicts recurrence for marginally excised canine subcutaneous soft tissue sarcomas, *Vet Pathol* 46:928–933, 2009.

27. Berlato D, Murphy S, Monti P, et al.: Comparison of mitotic index and Ki67 index in the prognostication of canine cutaneous mast cell tumours, *Vet Comp Oncol* 13:143–150, 2015.

28. van Lelyveld S, Warland J, Miller R, et al.: Comparison between Ki-67 index and mitotic index for predicting outcome in canine mast cell tumours, *J Small Anim Pract* 56:312–319, 2015.

29. Dennis MM, McSporran KD, Bacon NJ, et al.: Prognostic factors for cutaneous and subcutaneous soft tissue sarcomas in dogs, *Vet Pathol* 48:73–84, 2011.

30. Edmondson EF, Hess AM, Powers BE: Prognostic significance of histologic features in canine renal cell carcinomas. 70 nephrectomies, *Vet Pathol* 52:260–268, 2015.

31. Meuten DJ, Moore FM, George JW: Mitotic count and the field of view area. time to standardize, *Vet Pathol* 53:7–9, 2016.

32. Valli VE, Kass PH, San Myint M, et al.: Canine lymphomas. association of classification type, disease stage, tumor subtype, mitotic rate, and treatment with survival, *Vet Pathol* 50:738–748, 2013.

33. Laprie C, Abadie J, Amardeilh MF, et al.: MIB-1 immunoreactivity correlates with biologic behaviour in canine cutaneous melanoma, *Vet Dermatol* 12:139–147, 2001.

34. Weishaar KM, Thamm DH, Worley DR, et al.: Correlation of nodal mast cells with clinical outcome in dogs with mast cell tumour and a proposed classification system for the evaluation of node metastasis, *J Comp Pathol* 151:329–338, 2014.

35. Gloyeske NC, Goreal W, O'Neil M, et al.: Outcomes of breast cancer patients with micrometastasis and isolated tumor cells in sentinel lymph nodes, *Mod Pathol* 24:40a–41a, 2011.

36. van der Heiden-van der Loo M, Schaapveld M, Ho VKY, et al.: Outcomes of a population-based series of early breast cancer patients with micrometastases and isolated tumour cells in axillary lymph nodes, *Ann Oncol* 24:2794–2801, 2013.

37. Ahmed SS, Thike AA, Iqbal J, et al.: Sentinel lymph nodes with isolated tumour cells and micrometastases in breast cancer: clinical relevance and prognostic significance, *J Clin Pathol* 67:243–250, 2014.

38. Sloothaak DAM, van der Linden RLA, van De Velde CJH, et al.: Prognostic implications of occult nodal tumour cells in stage I and II colon cancer. The correlation between micrometastasis and disease recurrence, *Eur J Surg Oncol* 43:1456–1462, 2017.

39. Sloothaak DA, Sahami S, van der Zaag-Loonen HJ, et al.: The prognostic value of micrometastases and isolated tumour cells in histologically negative lymph nodes of patients with colorectal cancer: a systematic review and meta-analysis, *Eur J Surg Oncol* 40:263–269, 2014.

40. Beer P, Pozzi A, Rohrer Bley C, et al.: The role of sentinel lymph node mapping in small animal veterinary medicine:a comparison with current approaches in human medicine, *Vet Comp Oncol* 16:178–187, 2018.

41. Casey KM, Steffey MA, Affolter VK: Identification of occult micrometastases and isolated tumour cells within regional lymph nodes of previously diagnosed non-metastatic (stage 0) canine carcinomas, *Vet Comp Oncol* 15:785–792, 2017.

42. Wong YP, Shah SA, Shaari N, et al.: Comparative analysis between multilevel sectioning with conventional haematoxylin and eosin staining and immunohistochemistry for detecting nodal micrometastases with stage I and II colorectal cancers, *Asian Pac J Cancer Prev* 15:1725–1730, 2014.

43. Meuten D, Munday JS, Hauck M: Time to standardize? Time to validate? *Vet Pathol* 55:195–199, 2018.

44. Northrup NC, Harmon BG, Gleger TL, et al.: Variation among pathologists in histologic grading of canine cutaneous mast cell tumors, *J Vet Diagn Invest* 17:245–248, 2005.

45. Valli VE, San Myint M, Barthel A, et al.: Classification of canine malignant lymphomas according to the world health organization criteria, *Vet Pathol* 48:198–211, 2011.

46. Hanahan D, Weinberg RA: Hallmarks of cancer: the next generation, *Cell* 144:646–674, 2011.

47. Nagamine E, Hirayama K, Matsuda K, et al.: Invasive front grading and epithelial-mesenchymal transition in canine oral and cutaneous squamous cell carcinomas, *Vet Pathol* 54:783–791, 2017.

48. Perry JA, Culp WT, Dailey DD, et al.: Diagnostic accuracy of pretreatment biopsy for grading soft tissue sarcomas in dogs, *Vet Comp Oncol* 12:106–113, 2014.

49. Shaw T, Kudnig ST, Firestone SM: Diagnostic accuracy of pretreatment biopsy for grading cutaneous mast cell tumours in dogs, *Vet Comp Oncol* 16:214–219, 2018.

50. Webster JD, Dennis MM, Dervisis N, et al.: Recommended guidelines for the conduct and evaluation of prognostic studies in veterinary oncology, *Vet Pathol* 48:7–18, 2011.

51. Kirpensteijn J, Kik M, Rutteman GR, et al.: Prognostic significance of a new histologic grading system for canine osteosarcoma, *Vet Pathol* 39:240–246, 2002.

52. Loukopoulos P, Robinson WE: Clinicopathological relevance of tumour grading in canine osteosarcoma, *J Comp Pathol* 136:65–73, 2007.

53. Dernell WS, Straw RC, Cooper MF, et al.: Multilobular osteochondrosarcoma in 39 dogs: 1979-1993, *J Am Anim Hosp Assoc* 34:11–18, 1998.

54. Straw RC, LeCouteur RA, Powers BE, et al.: Multilobular osteochondrosarcoma of the canine skull: 16 cases (1978-1988), *J Am Vet Med Assoc* 195:1764–1769, 1989.

55. Straw RC, Powers BE, Klausner J, et al.: Canine mandibular osteosarcoma: 51 cases (1980-1992), *J Am Anim Hosp Assoc* 32:257–262, 1996.

56. Farese JP, Kirpensteijn J, Kik M, et al.: Biologic behavior and clinical outcome of 25 dogs with canine appendicular chondrosarcoma treated by amputation: a Veterinary Society of Surgical Oncology retrospective study, *Vet Surg* 38:914–919, 2009.

57. Ogilvie GK, Powers BE, Mallinckrodt CH, et al.: Surgery and doxorubicin in dogs with hemangiosarcoma, *J Vet Intern Med* 10:379–384, 1996.

58. Carpenter LG, Withrow SJ, Powers BE, et al.: Squamous-cell carcinoma of the tongue in 10 dogs, *J Am Anim Hosp Assoc* 29:17–24, 1993.

59. Spangler WL, Culbertson MR, Kass PH: Primary mesenchymal (nonangiomatous/nonlymphomatous) neoplasms occurring in the canine spleen: anatomic classification, immunohistochemistry, and mitotic activity correlated with patient survival, *Vet Pathol* 31:37–47, 1994.

60. McNiel EA, Ogilvie GK, Powers BE, et al.: Evaluation of prognostic factors for dogs with primary lung tumors: 67 cases (1985-1992), *J Am Vet Med Assoc* 211:1422–1427, 1997.

61. Wilcock BP, Peiffer RL: Morphology and behavior of primary ocular melanomas in 91 dogs, *Vet Pathol* 23:418–424, 1986.

62. Gower KL, Liptak JM, Culp WT, et al.: Splenic liposarcoma in dogs: 13 cases (2002-2012), *J Am Vet Med Assoc* 247:1404–1407, 2015.

63. Burton JH, Powers BE, Biller BJ: Clinical outcome in 20 cases of lingual hemangiosarcoma in dogs: 1996-2011, *Vet Comp Oncol* 12:198–204, 2014.

64. Molander-McCrary H, Henry CJ, Potter K, et al.: Cutaneous mast cell tumors in cats: 32 cases (1991-1994), *J Am Anim Hosp Assoc* 34:281–284, 1998.

65. Wilcock BP, Yager JA, Zink MC: The morphology and behavior of feline cutaneous mastocytomas, *Vet Pathol* 23:320–324, 1986.

66. Hahn KA, McEntee MF: Prognosis factors for survival in cats after removal of a primary lung tumor: 21 cases (1979-1994), *Vet Surg* 27:307–311, 1998.

67. Weijer K, Head KW, Misdorp W, et al.: Feline malignant mammary tumors. I. Morphology and biology: some comparisons with human and canine mammary carcinomas, *J Natl Cancer Inst* 49:1697–1704, 1972.

68. De Campos CB, Damasceno KA, Gamba CO, et al.: Evaluation of prognostic factors and survival rates in malignant feline mammary gland neoplasms, *J Feline Med Surg* 18:1003–1012, 2016.
69. Kalishman JB, Chappell R, Flood LA, et al.: A matched observational study of survival in cats with enucleation due to diffuse iris melanoma, *Vet Ophthalmol* 1:25–29, 1998.
70. Schott CR, Tatiersky LJ, Foster RA, et al.: Histologic grade does not predict outcome in dogs with appendicular osteosarcoma receiving the standard of care, *Vet Pathol* 55:202–211, 2018.
71. Nemec A, Murphy B, Kass PH, et al.: Histological subtypes of oral non-tonsillar squamous cell carcinoma in dogs, *J Comp Pathol* 147:111–120, 2012.
72. Rasotto R, Berlato D, Goldschmidt MH, et al.: Prognostic significance of canine mammary tumor histologic subtypes: an observational cohort study of 229 cases, *Vet Pathol* 54:571–578, 2017.
73. Bonfiglio T, Rogers T: The pathology of cancer. In Rubin P, editor: *Clinical oncology*, ed 6th, American Cancer Society, 1983, pp 20–29.
74. Holmes MA: Philosophical foundations of evidence-based medicine for veterinary clinicians, *J Am Vet Med Assoc* 235:1035–1039, 2009.
75. Heng YJ, Lester SC, Tse GMK, et al.: The molecular basis of breast cancer pathological phenotypes, *J Pathol* 241:375–391, 2017.
76. Maiolino P, Cataldi M, Paciello O, et al.: Nucleomorphometric analysis of canine cutaneous mast cell tumours, *J Comp Pathol* 133:209–211, 2005.
77. Strefezzi RD, Xavier JG, Catao-Dias TL: Morphometry of canine cutaneous mast cell tumors, *Vet Pathol* 40:268–275, 2003.
78. Russell DS, Townsend KL, Gorman E, et al.: Characterizing microscopical invasion patterns in canine mast cell tumours and soft tissue sarcomas, *J Comp Pathol* 157:231–240, 2017.
79. Downing S, Chien MB, Kass PH, et al.: Prevalence and importance of internal tandem duplications in exons 11 and 12 of c-kit in mast cell tumors of dogs, *Am J Vet Res* 63:1718–1723, 2002.
80. London CA, Hannah AL, Zadovoskaya R, et al.: Phase I dose-escalating study of SU11654, a small molecule receptor tyrosine kinase inhibitor, in dogs with spontaneous malignancies, *Clin Cancer Res* 9:2755–2768, 2003.
81. Webster JD, Yuzbasiyan-Gurkan V, Kaneene JB, et al.: The role of c-KIT in tumorigenesis: evaluation in canine cutaneous mast cell tumors, *Neoplasia* 8:104–111, 2006.
82. London CA, Malpas PB, Wood-Follis SL, et al.: Multi-center, placebo-controlled, double-blind, randomized study of oral toceranib phosphate (SU11654), a receptor tyrosine kinase inhibitor, for the treatment of dogs with recurrent (either local or distant) mast cell tumor following surgical excision, *Clin Cancer Res* 15:3856–3865, 2009.
83. Bergin IL, Smedley RC, Esplin DG, et al.: Prognostic evaluation of Ki67 threshold value in canine oral melanoma, *Vet Pathol* 48:41–53, 2011.
84. Moore PF, Rodriguez-Bertos A, Kass PH: Feline gastrointestinal lymphoma: mucosal architecture, immunophenotype, and molecular clonality, *Vet Pathol* 49:658–668, 2012.
85. Langenbach A, McManus PM, Hendrick MJ, et al.: Sensitivity and specificity of methods of assessing the regional lymph nodes for evidence of metastasis in dogs and cats with solid tumors, *J Am Vet Med Assoc* 218:1424–1428, 2001.
86. Krick EL, Billings AP, Shofer FS, et al.: Cytological lymph node evaluation in dogs with mast cell tumours: association with grade and survival, *Vet Comp Oncol* 7:130–138, 2009.
87. Milovancev M, Russell DS: Surgical margins in the veterinary cancer patient, *Vet Comp Oncol* 15:1136–1157, 2017.
88. Scarpa F, Sabattini S, Marconato L, et al.: Use of histologic margin evaluation to predict recurrence of cutaneous malignant tumors in dogs and cats after surgical excision, *J Am Vet Med Assoc* 240:1181–1187, 2012.
89. Rochat MC, Mann FA, Pace LW, et al.: Identification of surgical biopsy borders by use of india ink, *J Am Vet Med Assoc* 201:873–878, 1992.
90. Kiser PK, Lohr CV, Meritet D, et al.: Histologic processing artifacts and inter-pathologist variation in measurement of inked margins of canine mast cell tumors, *J Vet Diagn Invest* 30:377–385, 2018.
91. Risselada M, Mathews KG, Griffith E: The effect of specimen preparation on post-excision and post-fixation dimensions, translation, and distortion of canine cadaver skin-muscle-fascia specimens, *Vet Surg* 45:563–570, 2016.
92. Kimyai-Asadi A, Goldberg LH, Jih MH: Accuracy of serial transverse cross-sections in detecting residual basal cell carcinoma at the surgical margins of an elliptical excision specimen, *J Am Acad Dermatol* 53:469–474, 2005.
93. Cates JM, Stricker TP: Surgical resection margins in desmoid-type fibromatosis: a critical reassessment, *Am J Pathol* 38:1707–1714, 2014.
94. Dores CB, Milovancev M, Russell DS: Comparison of histologic margin status in low-grade cutaneous and subcutaneous canine mast cell tumours examined by radial and tangential sections, *Vet Comp Oncol* 16:125–130, 2018.
95. Bernstein JA, Storey ES, Bauer RW: Moh's micrographic surgery for the management of a periocular mast cell tumor in a dog, *Vet Ophthalmol* 16:234–239, 2013.
96. Bray JP: Soft tissue sarcoma in the dog - part 2: surgical margins, controversies and a comparative review, *J Small Anim Pract* 58:63–72, 2017.
97. Enneking WF, Spanier SS, Goodman MA: A system for the surgical staging of musculoskeletal sarcoma, *Clin Orthop Relat Res* 106–120, 1980.
98. Upchurch DA, Malenfant RC, Wignall JR, et al.: Effects of sample site and size, skin tension lines, surgeon, and formalin fixation on shrinkage of skin samples excised from canine cadavers, *Am J Vet Res* 75:1004–1009, 2014.
99. Reimer SB, Seguin B, DeCock HE, et al.: Evaluation of the effect of routine histologic processing on the size of skin samples obtained from dogs, *Am J Vet Res* 66:500–505, 2005.
100. Kerns MJ, Darst MA, Olsen TG, et al.: Shrinkage of cutaneous specimens: formalin or other factors involved? *J Cutan Pathol* 35:1093–1096, 2008.
101. Johnson RE, Sigman JD, Funk GF, et al.: Quantification of surgical margin shrinkage in the oral cavity, *Head Neck* 19:281–286, 1997.
102. Milovancev M, Townsend KL, Bracha S, et al.: Reductions in margin length after excision of grade II mast cell tumors and grade I and II soft tissue sarcomas in dogs, *Vet Surg* 47:36–43, 2018.
103. Murphy S, Sparkes AH, Smith KC, et al.: Relationships between the histological grade of cutaneous mast cell tumours in dogs, their survival and the efficacy of surgical resection, *Vet Rec* 154:743–746, 2004.
104. Simpson AM, Ludwig LL, Newman SJ, et al.: Evaluation of surgical margins required for complete excision of cutaneous mast cell tumors in dogs, *J Am Vet Med Assoc* 224:236–240, 2004.
105. Marino DJ, Matthiesen DT, Stefanacci JD, et al.: Evaluation of dogs with digit masses: 117 cases (1981-1991), *J Am Vet Med Assoc* 207:726–728, 1995.
106. Lascelles BD, Parry AT, Stidworthy MF, et al.: Squamous cell carcinoma of the nasal planum in 17 dogs, *Vet Rec* 147:473–476, 2000.
107. Schwarz PD, Withrow SJ, Curtis CR, et al.: Mandibular resection as a treatment for oral-cancer in 81 dogs, *J Am Anim Hosp Assoc* 27:601–610, 1991.
108. Schwarz PD, Withrow SJ, Curtis CR, et al.: Partial maxillary resection as a treatment for oral-cancer in 61 dogs, *J Am Anim Hosp Assoc* 27:617–624, 1991.

109. Stefanello D, Morello E, Roccabianca P, et al.: Marginal excision of low-grade spindle cell sarcoma of canine extremities: 35 dogs (1996-2006), *Vet Surg* 37:461–465, 2008.

110. Seguin B, Besancon MF, McCallan JL, et al.: Recurrence rate, clinical outcome, and cellular proliferation indices as prognostic indicators after incomplete surgical excision of cutaneous grade 11 mast cell tumors: 28 dogs (1994-2002), *J Vet Intern Med* 20:933–940, 2006.

111. Thompson JJ, Pearl DL, Yager JA, et al.: Canine subcutaneous mast cell tumor: characterization and prognostic indices, *Vet Pathol* 48:156–168, 2011.

112. Phelps HA, Kuntz CA, Milner RJ, et al.: Radical excision with five-centimeter margins for treatment of feline injection-site sarcomas: 91 cases (1998-2002), *J Am Vet Med Assoc* 239:97–106, 2011.

113. Tuohy JL, Selmic LE, Worley DR, et al.: Outcome following curative-intent surgery for oral melanoma in dogs: 70 cases (1998-2011), *J Am Vet Med Assoc* 245:1266–1273, 2014.

114. Donnelly L, Mullin C, Balko J, et al.: Evaluation of histological grade and histologically tumour-free margins as predictors of local recurrence in completely excised canine mast cell tumours, *Vet Comp Oncol* 13:70–76, 2015.

115. Aparna MSP, Chatra L, Veena KM, et al.: Field cancerization: a review, *Arch Med Health Sci* 136–139, 2013.

116. Slaughter DP, Southwick HW, Smejkal W: Field cancerization in oral stratified squamous epithelium; clinical implications of multicentric origin, *Cancer* 6:963–968, 1953.

117. Davis B, Schwartz M, Duchemin D, et al.: Validation of a multiplexed gene signature assay for diagnosis of canine cancers from formalin-fixed paraffin-embedded tissues, *J Vet Intern Med* 31:854–863, 2017.

118. Kiupel M, Teske E, Bostock D: Prognostic factors for treated canine malignant lymphoma, *Vet Pathol* 36:292–300, 1999.

119. Kravis LD, Vail DM, Kisseberth WC, et al.: Frequency of argyrophilic nucleolar organizer regions in fine-needle aspirates and biopsy specimens from mast cell tumors in dogs, *J Am Vet Med Assoc* 209:1418–1420, 1996.

120. Bundgaard-Andersen K, Flagstad A, Jensen AL, et al.: Correlation between the histopathological diagnosis by AgNOR count and AgNOR area in canine mammary tumors, *J Vet Intern Med* 22:1174–1180, 2008.

121. Ramos-Vara JA: Principles and methods of immunohistochemistry, *Methods Mol Biol* 1641:115–128, 2017.

122. Ramos-Vara JA, Miller MA: When tissue antigens and antibodies get along: revisiting the technical aspects of immunohistochemistry—the red, brown, and blue technique, *Vet Pathol* 51:42–87, 2014.

123. Priest HL, Hume KR, Killick D, et al.: The use, publication and future directions of immunocytochemistry in veterinary medicine: a consensus of the Oncology-Pathology Working Group, *Vet Comp Oncol* 15:868–880, 2017.

124. Madewell BR: Cellular proliferation in tumors: a review of methods, interpretation, and clinical applications, *J Vet Intern Med* 15:334–340, 2001.

125. Bergman PJ, Ogilvie GK, Powers BE: Monoclonal antibody C219 immunohistochemistry against P-glycoprotein: sequential analysis and predictive ability in dogs with lymphoma, *J Vet Intern Med* 10:354–359, 1996.

126. Kiupel M, Webster JD, Kaneene JB, et al.: The use of KIT and tryptase expression patterns as prognostic tools for canine cutaneous mast cell tumors, *Vet Pathol* 41:371–377, 2004.

127. Sagartz JE, Bodley WL, Gamblin RM, et al.: p53 tumor suppressor protein overexpression in osteogenic tumors of dogs, *Vet Pathol* 33:213–221, 1996.

128. Koenig A, Bianco SR, Fosmire S, et al.: Expression and significance of p53, Rb, p21/waf-1, p16/ink-4a, and PTEN tumor suppressors in canine melanoma, *Vet Pathol* 39:458–472, 2002.

129. Santos A, Lopes C, Gartner F, et al.: VEGFR-2 expression in malignant tumours of the canine mammary gland: a prospective survival study, *Vet Comp Oncol* 14:e83–e92, 2016.

130. Gregorio H, Raposo T, Queiroga FL, et al.: High COX-2 expression in canine mast cell tumours is associated with proliferation, angiogenesis and decreased overall survival, *Vet Comp Oncol* 15:1382–1392, 2017.

131. Lavalle GE, Bertagnolli AC, Tavares WL, et al.: Cox-2 expression in canine mammary carcinomas: correlation with angiogenesis and overall survival, *Vet Pathol* 46:1275–1280, 2009.

132. Millanta F, Citi S, Della Santa D, et al.: COX-2 expression in canine and feline invasive mammary carcinomas: correlation with clinicopathological features and prognostic molecular markers, *Breast Cancer Res Treat* 98:115–120, 2006.

133. Iussich S, Maniscalco L, Di Sciuva A, et al.: PDGFRs expression in dogs affected by malignant oral melanomas: correlation with prognosis, *Vet Comp Oncol* 15:462–469, 2017.

134. Araujo MR, Campos LC, Damasceno KA, et al.: HER-2, EGFR, Cox-2 and Ki67 expression in lymph node metastasis of canine mammary carcinomas: association with clinical-pathological parameters and overall survival, *Res Vet Sci* 106:121–130, 2016.

135. Santos AA, Lopes CC, Ribeiro JR, et al.: Identification of prognostic factors in canine mammary malignant tumours: a multivariable survival study, *BMC Vet Res* 9:1, 2013.

136. Sunil Kumar BV, Bhardwaj R, Mahajan K, et al.: The overexpression of Hsp90B1 is associated with tumorigenesis of canine mammary glands, *Mol Cell Biochem* 440:23–31, 2018.

137. Warhol MJ, Hickey WF, Corson JM: Malignant mesothelioma: ultrastructural distinction from adenocarcinoma, *Am J Surg Pathol* 6:307–314, 1982.

138. Nakahira R, Michishita M, Yoshimura H, et al.: Neuroendocrine carcinoma of the mammary gland in a dog, *J Comp Pathol* 152:188–191, 2015.

139. Burkhard MJ, Bienzle D: Making sense of lymphoma diagnostics in small animal patients, *Vet Clin North Am Small Anim Pract* 43:1331–1347, 2013.

140. Kiupel M, Smedley RC, Pfent C, et al.: Diagnostic algorithm to differentiate lymphoma from inflammation in feline small intestinal biopsy samples, *Vet Pathol* 48:212–222, 2011.

141. Warren A, Center S, McDonough S, et al.: Histopathologic features, immunophenotyping, clonality, and eubacterial fluorescence in situ hybridization in cats with lymphocytic cholangitis/cholangiohepatitis, *Vet Pathol* 48:627–641, 2011.

142. Regan RC, Rassnick KM, Balkman CE, et al.: Comparison of first-opinion and second-opinion histopathology from dogs and cats with cancer: 430 cases (2001-2008), *Vet Comp Oncol* 8:1–10, 2010.

143. Regan RC, Rassnick KM, Malone EK, et al.: A prospective evaluation of the impact of second-opinion histopathology on diagnostic testing, cost and treatment in dogs and cats with cancer, *Vet Comp Oncol* 13:106–116, 2015.

144. Abt AB, Abt LG, Olt GJ: The effect of interinstitution anatomic pathology consultation on patient-care, *Arch Pathol Lab Med* 119:514–517, 1995.

145. Kronz JD, Westra WH: The role of second opinion pathology in the management of lesions of the head and neck, *Curr Opin Otolaryngol Head Neck Surg* 13:81–84, 2005.

146. Kronz JD, Westra WH, Epstein JI: Mandatory second opinion surgical pathology at a large referral hospital, *Cancer* 86:2426–2435, 1999.

147. Aresu L, Martini V, Rossi F, et al.: Canine indolent and aggressive lymphoma: clinical spectrum with histologic correlation, *Vet Comp Oncol* 13:348–362, 2015.

148. Comazzi S, Aresu L, Marconato L: Transformation of canine lymphoma/leukemia to more aggressive diseases: anecdotes or reality? *Front Vet Sci* 2:42, 2015.

149. Valli VE, Bienzel D, Meuten DJ: Tumors of the hemolymphatic system. In Meuten DJ, editor: *Tumors in domestic animals*, ed 5, Ames, Iowa, 2017, John Wiley & Sons, Inc, pp 203–273.

150. Smedley RC, Spangler WL, Esplin DG, et al.: Prognostic markers for canine melanocytic neoplasms: a comparative review of the literature and goals for future investigation, *Vet Pathol* 48:54–72, 2011.

151. Esplin DG: Survival of dogs following surgical excision of histologically well-differentiated melanocytic neoplasms of the mucous membranes of the lips and oral cavity, *Vet Pathol* 45:889–896, 2008.

152. Goldschmidt M, Pena L, Rasotto R, et al.: Classification and grading of canine mammary tumors, *Vet Pathol* 48:117–131, 2011.

153. Karayannopoulou M, Kaldrymidou E, Constantinidis TC, et al.: Histological grading and prognosis in dogs with mammary carcinomas: application of a human grading method, *J Comp Pathol* 133:246–252, 2005.

154. Goldschmidt MH, Pena L, Zappulli V: Tumors of the mammary gland. In Meuten DJ, editor: *Tumors in domestic animals*, ed 5th, Ames, Iowa, 2017, John Wiley & Sons, Inc, pp 733–757.

155. Pena L, De Andres PJ, Clemente M, et al.: Prognostic value of histological grading in noninflammatory canine mammary carcinomas in a prospective study with two-year follow-up: relationship with clinical and histological characteristics, *Vet Pathol* 50:94–105, 2013.

156. Vail DM, Powers BE, Getzy DM, et al.: Evaluation of prognostic factors for dogs with synovial sarcoma: 36 cases (1986-1991), *J Am Vet Med Assoc* 205:1300–1307, 1994.

157. Craig LE, Julian ME, Ferracone JD: The diagnosis and prognosis of synovial tumors in dogs: 35 cases, *Vet Pathol* 39:66–73, 2002.

158. Craig LE, Krimer PM, Cooley AJ: Canine synovial myxoma: 39 cases, *Vet Pathol* 47:931–936, 2010.

159. Klahn SL, Kitchell BE, Dervisis NG: Evaluation and comparison of outcomes in dogs with periarticular and nonperiarticular histiocytic sarcoma, *J Am Vet Med Assoc* 239:90–96, 2011.

160. Lu JE, Dubielzig R: Canine eyelid granular cell tumor: a report of eight cases, *Vet Ophthalmol* 15:406–410, 2012.

161. Liu CH, Liu CI, Liang SL, et al.: Intracranial granular cell tumor in a dog, *J Vet Med Sci* 66:77–79, 2004.

162. Kamstock DA, Fredrickson R, Ehrhart EJ: Lipid-rich carcinoma of the mammary gland in a cat, *Vet Pathol* 42:360–362, 2005.

163. Kwon HJ, Park MS, Kim DY, et al.: Round cell variant of myxoid liposarcoma in a Japanese Macaque (Macaca fuscata), *Vet Pathol* 44:229–232, 2007.

164. Avakian A, Alroy J, Rozanski E, et al.: Lipid-rich pleural mesothelioma in a dog, *J Vet Diagn Invest* 20:665–667, 2008.

165. Avallone G, Pellegrino V, Muscatello LV, et al.: Spindle cell lipoma in dogs, *Vet Pathol* 54:792–794, 2017.

166. Rannou B, Helie P, Bedard C: Rectal plasmacytoma with intracellular hemosiderin in a dog, *Vet Pathol* 46:1181–1184, 2009.

167. Rasheed S: Characterization of a differentiated cat melanoma cell line, *Cancer Res* 43:3379–3384, 1983.

168. Kuwata K, Shibutani M, Kemmochi Y, et al.: A neuroendocrine carcinoma of undetermined origin in a dog, *J Toxicol Pathol* 23:151–155, 2010.

169. Rizzo SA, Newman SJ, Hecht S, et al.: Malignant mediastinal extra-adrenal paraganglioma with spinal cord invasion in a dog, *J Vet Diagn Invest* 20:372–375, 2008.

170. Rowland PH, Valentine BA, Stebbins KE, et al.: Cutaneous plasmacytomas with amyloid in six dogs, *Vet Pathol* 28:125–130, 1991.

171. Kuwamura M, Kanehara T, Yamate J, et al.: Amyloid-producing odontogenic tumor in a Shih-Tzu dog, *J Vet Med Sci* 62:655–657, 2000.

172. Hirayama K, Endoh C, Kagawa Y, et al.: Amyloid-producing odontogenic tumors of the facial skin in three cats, *Vet Pathol* 54:218–221, 2017.

173. Yamate J, Murai F, Izawa T, et al.: A rhabdomyosarcoma arising in the larynx of a dog, *J Toxicol Pathol* 24:179–182, 2011.

174. Dabbs DJ: *Diagnostic immunohistochemistry theranostic and genomic applications*, ed 3, Philadelphia, 2010, Saunders.

175. Moore AS, Madewell BR, Lund JK: Immunohistochemical evaluation of intermediate filament expression in canine and feline neoplasms, *Am J Vet Res* 50:88–92, 1989.

176. Desnoyers MM, Haines DM, Searcy GP: Immunohistochemical detection of intermediate filament proteins in formalin fixed normal and neoplastic canine tissues, *Can J Vet Res* 54:360–365, 1990.

177. Frost D, Lasota J, Miettinen M: Gastrointestinal stromal tumors and leiomyomas in the dog: a histopathologic, immunohistochemical, and molecular genetic study of 50 cases, *Vet Pathol* 40:42–54, 2003.

178. Russell KN, Mehler SJ, Skorupski KA, et al.: Clinical and immunohistochemical differentiation of gastrointestinal stromal tumors from leiomyosarcomas in dogs: 42 cases (1990-2003), *J Am Vet Med Assoc* 230:1329–1333, 2007.

179. Dailey DD, Ehrhart EJ, Duval DL, et al.: DOG1 is a sensitive and specific immunohistochemical marker for diagnosis of canine gastrointestinal stromal tumors, *J Vet Diagn Invest* 27:268–277, 2015.

180. von Beust BR, Suter MM, Summers BA: Factor VIII-related antigen in canine endothelial neoplasms: an immunohistochemical study, *Vet Pathol* 25:251–255, 1988.

181. Giuffrida MA, Bacon NJ, Kamstock DA: Use of routine histopathology and factor VIII-related antigen/von Willebrand factor immunohistochemistry to differentiate primary hemangiosarcoma of bone from telangiectatic osteosarcoma in 54 dogs, *Vet Comp Oncol* 15:1232–1239, 2017.

182. Wilting J, Papoutsi M, Christ B, et al.: The transcription factor Prox1 is a marker for lymphatic endothelial cells in normal and diseased human tissues, *FASEB J* 16:1271–1273, 2002.

183. Galeotti F, Barzagli F, Vercelli A, et al.: Feline lymphangiosarcoma—definitive identification using a lymphatic vascular marker, *Vet Dermatol* 15:13–18, 2004.

184. Halsey CH, Worley DR, Curran K, et al.: The use of novel lymphatic endothelial cell-specific immunohistochemical markers to differentiate cutaneous angiosarcomas in dogs, *Vet Comp Oncol* 14:236–244, 2016.

185. Fulmer AK, Mauldin GE: Canine histiocytic neoplasia: an overview, *Can Vet J* 48:1041–1043, 2007.

186. Moore PF: A review of histiocytic diseases of dogs and cats, *Vet Pathol* 51:167–184, 2014.

187. Pierezan F, Mansell J, Ambrus A, et al.: Immunohistochemical expression of ionized calcium binding adapter molecule 1 in cutaneous histiocytic proliferative, neoplastic and inflammatory disorders of dogs and cats, *J Comp Pathol* 151:347–351, 2014.

188. Willmann M, Mullauer L, Guija de Arespacochaga A, et al.: Pax5 immunostaining in paraffin-embedded sections of canine non-Hodgkin lymphoma: a novel canine pan pre-B- and B-cell marker, *Vet Immunol Immunopathol* 128:359–365, 2009.

189. Ferrer L, Fondevila D, Rabanal R, et al.: Immunohistochemical detection of CD3 antigen (pan T marker) in canine lymphomas, *J Vet Diagn Invest* 5:616–620, 1993.

190. Milner RJ, Pearson J, Nesbit JW, et al.: Immunophenotypic classification of canine malignant lymphoma on formalin-mixed paraffin wax-embedded tissue by means of CD3 and CD79a cell markers, *Onderstepoort J Vet Res* 63:309–313, 1996.

191. Caniatti M, Roccabianca P, Scanziani E, et al.: Canine lymphoma: immunocytochemical analysis of fine-needle aspiration biopsy, *Vet Pathol* 33:204–212, 1996.

192. Felisberto R, Matos J, Alves M, et al.: Evaluation of Pax5 expression and comparison with BLA.36 and CD79alphacy in feline non-Hodgkin lymphoma, *Vet Comp Oncol* 15:1257–1268, 2017.

193. Walls AF, Jones DB, Williams JH, et al.: Immunohistochemical identification of mast cells in formaldehyde-fixed tissue using monoclonal antibodies specific for tryptase, *J Pathol* 162:119–126, 1990.

194. Smedley RC, Lamoureux J, Sledge DG, et al.: Immunohistochemical diagnosis of canine oral amelanotic melanocytic neoplasms, *Vet Pathol* 48:32–40, 2011.

195. Koenig A, Wojcieszyn J, Weeks BR, et al.: Expression of S100a, vimentin, NSE, and melan A/MART-1 in seven canine melanoma cells lines and twenty-nine retrospective cases of canine melanoma, *Vet Pathol* 38:427–435, 2001.

196. Giudice C, Ceciliani F, Rondena M, et al.: Immunohistochemical investigation of PNL2 reactivity of canine melanocytic neoplasms and comparison with Melan A, *J Vet Diagn Invest* 22:389–394, 2010.

197. Ramos-Vara JA, Miller MA: Immunohistochemical identification of canine melanocytic neoplasms with antibodies to melanocytic antigen PNL2 and tyrosinase: comparison with Melan A, *Vet Pathol* 48:443–450, 2011.

198. Ramos-Vara JA, Miller MA, Johnson GC, et al.: Melan A and S100 protein immunohistochemistry in feline melanomas: 48 cases, *Vet Pathol* 39:127–132, 2002.

199. McDonough SP, MacLachlan NJ, Tobias AH: Canine pericardial mesothelioma, *Vet Pathol* 29:256–260, 1992.

200. Lipsitz D, Higgins RJ, Kortz GD, et al.: Glioblastoma multiforme: clinical findings, magnetic resonance imaging, and pathology in five dogs, *Vet Pathol* 40:659–669, 2003.

201. Stoica G, Kim HT, Hall DG, et al.: Morphology, immunohistochemistry, and genetic alterations in dog astrocytomas, *Vet Pathol* 41:10–19, 2004.

202. Kovi RC, Wunschmann A, Armien AG, et al.: Spinal meningeal oligodendrogliomatosis in two boxer dogs, *Vet Pathol* 50:761–764, 2013.

203. Ferreira-Neves P, Lezmi S, Lejeune T, et al.: Immunohistochemical characterization of a hepatic neuroendocrine carcinoma in a cat, *J Vet Diagn Invest* 20:110–114, 2008.

204. Ramos-Vara JA, Miller MA, Valli VE: Immunohistochemical detection of multiple myeloma 1/interferon regulatory factor 4 (MUM1/IRF-4) in canine plasmacytoma: comparison with CD79a and CD20, *Vet Pathol* 44:875–884, 2007.

205. Beck J, Miller MA, Frank C, et al.: Surfactant protein A and napsin A in the immunohistochemical characterization of canine pulmonary carcinomas: comparison with thyroid transcription factor-1, *Vet Pathol* 54:767–774, 2017.

206. Andreasen CB, White MR, Swayne DE, et al.: Desmin as a marker for canine botryoid rhabdomyosarcomas, *J Comp Pathol* 98:23–29, 1988.

207. Murakami M, Sakai H, Iwatani N, et al.: Cytologic, histologic, and immunohistochemical features of maxillofacial alveolar rhabdomyosarcoma in a juvenile dog, *Vet Clin Pathol* 39:113–118, 2010.

208. Caserto BG: A comparative review of canine and human rhabdomyosarcoma with emphasis on classification and pathogenesis, *Vet Pathol* 50:806–826, 2013.

209. Fairley R: Synovial tumors in dogs, *Vet Pathol* 39:413–414, 2002.

210. Criag LE, Thompson KG: Tumors of the joint. In Meuten D, editor: *Tumors in domestic animals*, ed 5, Ames, Iowa, 2017, John Wiley & Sons, Inc, pp 337–345.

211. Liptak JM, Kamstock DA, Dernell WS, et al.: Cranial mediastinal carcinomas in nine dogs, *Vet Comp Oncol* 6:19–30, 2008.

212. Ramos-Vara JA, Miller MA, Johnson GC, et al.: Immunohistochemical detection of thyroid transcription factor-1, thyroglobulin, and calcitonin in canine normal, hyperplastic, and neoplastic thyroid gland, *Vet Pathol* 39:480–487, 2002.

213. Ramos-Vara JA, Miller MA, Johnson GC: Usefulness of thyroid transcription factor-1 immunohistochemical staining in the differential diagnosis of primary pulmonary tumors of dogs, *Vet Pathol* 42:315–320, 2005.

4

Epidemiology and the Evidence-Based Medicine Approach

AUDREY RUPLE, BRENDA N. BONNETT, AND RODNEY L. PAGE

Epidemiology is defined as the study of the distribution and determinants of disease in populations. Historically epidemiologic methods were used primarily in veterinary populations for the investigation of outbreaks and/or epidemics of infectious disease, yet the philosophies, attitudes, methodologies, and application of epidemiology are in fact more broadly applicable to research and clinical practice, regardless of species, disease, or discipline. In fact, epidemiologic principles form the foundation of evidence-based medicine (EBM), an approach to the practice of health care that is now well accepted in the human and veterinary medicine fields. For a clinician, using the EBM approach involves a commitment to base all decisions on the best available evidence and to be explicit about the level and quality of evidence on which decisions are based. An extensive literature is available on EBM and evidence-based practice in the human medicine field (e.g., The Cochrane Collaboration [http://www.cochrane.org/]) and in the veterinary field (e.g., Evidence-Based Veterinary Medicine Association [https://ebvma.org/]). The EBM approach can and should be applied to all interventions, including diagnosis and prognosis, choice of preventive and clinical therapies applied to individuals, and decisions about health policy or control programs for populations.

Pathophysiology forms the basis of our understanding of health and disease, but this knowledge, even combined with clinical acumen and experience, is not sufficient grounds for decision making across the spectrum of activities of health professionals. To have confidence that our interventions will be beneficial, we need to understand that personal and expert opinion are only anecdotal evidence, unless they are based on a valid appraisal of available evidence from the literature. In addition to embracing the philosophy of EBM, all clinicians must develop the knowledge and skills, such as information management, critical appraisal, and causal reasoning, that are needed to assess evidence to determine that their chosen interventions are both efficacious and effective (see glossary of terms in Table 4.1). Unfortunately, especially in veterinary medicine, there are many gaps in our evidence base, in terms of both validity and relevance of published studies.

In veterinary medicine, in general and in certain specialties including oncology, the trend has been toward a heightened sophistication of practice, including the use of advanced technologies in diagnostic testing (e.g., state-of-the-art imaging techniques and molecular characterization of tumors), therapeutic interventions (e.g., interventional surgery and targeted, small-molecule chemotherapy), and the expanding field of genomics in cancer research. This is attributable in part to the presumption that most clients want care for their pets at a level similar to that they themselves receive. Therefore many approaches and interventions have been adopted from human medicine and applied to animals despite considerable gaps in evidence as to their efficacy and/or effectiveness in the veterinary clinical situation. In addition, even where a sufficient quantity of studies is present, the quality and consistency of reporting is frequently inadequate to allow systematic review or adequate comparison between studies.[1] This issue is not unique to oncology and has spawned efforts to improve the reporting of veterinary studies, with a longer term goal of improving the quality of work.[1–7] To approach a level of care in veterinary oncology truly similar to that in humans, there will need to be an increased focus on EBM. Further information and articles pertinent to challenges of applying EBM in practice can be found on the website of the Evidence-Based Veterinary Medicine Association (https://ebvma.org) and the Centre for Evidence-Based Veterinary Medicine (http://www.nottingham.ac.uk/cevm/).

In this chapter, we focus on quantifying the occurrence of cancer (incidence, prevalence) and risk factors for cancer (causal reasoning, associations). An evidence-based approach to diagnosis, prognosis, and selection of therapeutic interventions will be proposed, although other authors in this text will present specific details of diagnosis, prognosis, and therapy for specific cancers. Rather than presenting an exhaustive or systematic review of the literature in this chapter, we will highlight the relevant literature. Our aim is to provide a guide for the application of epidemiologic principles to oncology, in general and for clinical practice.

Measures of Disease Occurrence

Complete and accurate cancer surveillance data are the foundation needed to make appropriate conclusions about the burden of disease, to make recommendations for cancer prevention and control, and for the design of analytic studies to identify causal associations between exposures and cancer risk. Here we cover the measures used to quantify cancer occurrence such as incidence, prevalence, and proportional measures and the types of data used to calculate them.

TABLE 4.1   Glossary of Terms

Term	Definition	Comments
Efficacy	How well a treatment works in those who receive it (e.g., correct formulation, dose).	May be proved in laboratory studies or clinical trials.
Effectiveness	How well a treatment works in those to whom it is offered.	Studies must occur in the environment and under conditions and with patients typical of those to whom it will be offered in practice.
Compliance	How closely a treatment protocol is followed.	Influenced by clinician, client, patient, formulation, duration, and so forth.
Coherence	How well findings reflect our understanding of biologic relationships/pathophysiology.	Limited by our current understanding.
Consistency	The extent to which new findings agree with previously published findings.	Limited by the current literature, traditional approaches, funding, and so forth.
Experimental studies	Traditional research approach done in a laboratory or highly controlled environment.	Potential for high validity, generally lower relevance to the clinical situation.
External validity	The extent to which a study's findings can be extrapolated to a wider population. Similar terms include relevance and generalizability.	A function of the study population, methods, data collection, treatments, and so forth.
Incidence rate	The rate at which new events occur in a population: (Number of new events in a specified period) $\div$ (Number of individuals at risk during this period) $\times 10^n$	Cancer incidence rates are available from population-based data (e.g., cancer registry data) or prospective (cohort or longitudinal) studies.
Internal validity	The extent to which a study's findings are likely correct for that study population.	Likelihood that systematic bias is responsible for the study findings reduces its validity (e.g., because of bias in selecting study participants, measuring the exposure, and confounding).
Observational studies	Epidemiologic studies that use existing comparisons in the species of interest in its "natural" environment (often client-owned animals, perhaps in veterinary practice settings).	Examples: (1) Case-control study: Researcher observes/describes exposures in individuals selected based on presence/absence of the outcome; (2) Cohort study: Individuals with different exposures are followed and incidence of outcome(s) is observed.
Randomized controlled trial (RCT)	*Randomized* refers to the random allocation of exposure. *Controlled* refers to appropriate comparison groups (e.g., placebo or standard treatment). *Trial* is generally conducted in a clinical setting.	Researcher exerts control over which individuals receive which treatments or exposures and observes outcomes.
Prevalence	The number of events in a given population at a designated time: Number of events at a designated time $\div$ Number of individuals at risk at the designated time.	Taking the number of canine cancers that are observed in a clinic or several clinics during a designated period of time and dividing by the total number of patients seen during the same period is a proportional measure, *not* prevalence.
Proportional morbidity or mortality	The number of events (e.g., disease, death) in a limited population (e.g., animals presenting to the clinic, total deaths) at a designated time.	Proportional measures are used when the underlying population at risk is not known.

Incidence

Incidence, or the number of newly diagnosed cancer cases divided by the total population at risk over a specified period of time, is the most useful disease occurrence statistic for comparison between populations over time. Incidence data are especially valid when they are generated from a large population-based cancer registry with histologically confirmed cases and complete ascertainment of the population at risk within a defined geographic area or theoretically from large prospective, longitudinal, or cohort studies. True incidence data are rarely obtainable in veterinary populations because of the scarcity of animal cancer registries and lack of information about the total animal population (census data) at risk.

Cancer incidence data has been provided from several population-based cancer registries (Table 4.2). Estimates of canine cancer incidence range from 99.3 to 804 per 100,000 dog-years.[8-17] Variation in estimates may be due in part to differences in actual cancer risks and/or variation in the base population. These registries included information from all cancer cases identified within a specified geographic region from a well-defined and enumerated population. One of the earliest, well-known cancer registries for

TABLE 4.2	Characteristics of Population-Based Companion Animal Cancer Registries and Cancer Incidence		
Registry	Period	Cases/Population at Risk	Incidence/Prevalence
California Animal Neoplasm Registry (CANR)[8,9]	1963–1966	1624/80,006 dogs 448/54,786 cats	381.2/100,000 dogs over 3-year period. 155.8/100,000 cats over the 3-year period.
Tulsa Registry of Canine and Feline Neoplasms[10] (Tulsa, Oklahoma)	1972–1973	899 cases/63,504 dogs; 59 cases/11,909 cats	1126 cases per 100,000 dogs; 470 cases per 100,000 cats
Norwegian Canine Cancer Registry[11,12] (Oslo, Norway)	1990–1998	14,401 tumors/census of dogs in Norway in 1992–93[13]	Boxers: 28 and 14/1000 dogs per year for total and malignant tumors, respectively. Bernese mountain dogs: 10 and 4/1000 dogs/year for total and malignant tumors, respectively.
Genoa Registry of Animal Tumors[13] (Genoa, Italy)	1985–2002	3303/107,981; 1,943,725 dog-years	Males: 99.3/100,000 dog-years Females: 272.1/100,000 dog-years, for total tumors (malignant and benign).
Animal Tumor Registry[14] (Venice, Italy)	2005	2509 dogs; 494 cats/296,318 dogs; 214,683 cats	282, 143 and 140/100,000 dogs for total, malignant and benign tumors, respectively; 77, 63, 14/100,000 cats for total, malignant and benign tumors, respectively.
Swiss Cancer Registry[15]	1955–2008	Registered Swiss dog population	13/100,000 dogs in 1955 to 695/100,000 dogs in 2008.
Danish Veterinary Cancer Registry (DVCR)[16]	2005–2008	1523 dogs/dogs registered in the Danish Dog Registry as of August 2006	Breeds with standardized morbidity ratios ≥2: Boxer, Bernese mountain dog, and West Highland white terrier. Measures for all dogs were not provided.
Piedmont Canine Cancer Registry[17]	2001–2008	1175 tumors/dogs recorded in registration system in Piedmont, Italy	804/100,000 dogs for malignant tumors; 897/100,000 dogs for benign tumors

companion animals was the California Animal Neoplasm Registry.[8,17] This comprehensive effort began in 1963 with the goal of identifying all neoplasms diagnosed over a 3-year period among animals living in the San Francisco Bay Area Counties of Alameda and Contra Costa. The denominator was estimated by conducting a survey in a probability sample of households in Alameda County to derive the age, sex, and breed distribution of pets and to determine whether the household had used veterinary services. Additional information on former and existing cancer registries for companion animals has been comprehensively reviewed.[18,19]

Prevalence

Cancer prevalence information from population-based registries is also useful for surveillance and comparison between populations. Prevalence is the number of total cancer cases divided by the number of dogs in the population at risk at one point in time. For example, the prevalence of canine cancer in April 2005 was 143 per 100,000 dogs in an Italian population (Table 4.2).[8,9]

Feline cancer prevalence has been reported from a population-based registry in Italy as 63 per 100,000 cats[14] (see Table 4.2). These data were based on a telephone survey conducted among 214,683

residents of two provinces in northern Italy over a 3-year period starting in 2005. Earlier prevalence data for feline cancers have ranged from 51.9/100,000 cat-years from the California Animal Neoplasm Registry[8,18] to 470.2/100,000 cat-years from the Tulsa Registry.[10]

In addition to population-based cancer registries, cancer occurrence data are abundantly available from veterinary teaching hospital databases and insurance databases. A caution to be noted when interpreting cancer occurrence information from hospital-based registries is that data may be inconsistently recorded or inaccurate and the size and characteristics of the underlying population at risk are not known[20,21]; thus neither true incidence nor prevalence measures can be calculated. Instead, the proportional morbidity ratio (PMR) is used to quantify cancer occurrence. For example, the PMR for a particular tumor type among a single breed is calculated as follows:

(Number of tumor type in breed ÷ number of total tumors in breed) ÷ (Number of tumor type in all other breeds ÷ number of total tumors in all other breeds).

Proportional measures are *not* to be interpreted as prevalence or incidence of cancer occurrence. As an example, Craig et al presents proportional statistics from a necropsy database and concludes that golden retrievers have an increased "risk" of tumors similar to that for Boxers.[22] However, only the proportion of dead dogs that had cancer are available in that study, and these data cannot be used to estimate risk. Although proportional measures, such as those presented in an article by Fleming et al,[23] have some usefulness for describing patterns within a breed, they are very risky to use for comparison across breeds in which population-based measures are unavailable and the degree of referral bias is unknown. In addition, in those data, 40% of deaths could not be classified pathologically and the unclassified proportion showed extreme variation across breed (e.g., 16%–60%). Fig. 4.1 shows a comparison between proportional mortality ratios and true mortality rate using a subset of data from Bonnett et al, a study with information on the population at risk and data from the Veterinary Medical Database (VMDB) study.[23,24] For golden retrievers, 30% of deaths (before 10 years of age in the Swedish insurance population) were a result of cancer.[24] For Leonbergers and Boxers, the proportional mortality was 28% and 37%, respectively.[24] Proportional values for these three breeds may be similar, but, in fact, Leonbergers and Boxers have a risk for death resulting from cancer (before 10 years of age) that is almost four times as high as that for golden retrievers (approximately 200 deaths per 10,000 years-at-risk versus 55 [$p > 0.05$]).[24] Irish wolfhounds and Bernese mountain dogs (BMDs) have an equal risk (approximately 300 deaths resulting from tumors per 10,000 dog-years at risk [DYAR]), but tumors account for more than 40% of deaths in BMDs and only 22% in Irish wolfhounds.[24] Note that these are deaths before 10 years of age. Comparing the proportional mortality values between the two studies, values for BMDs are very similar (42%, 45%), perhaps because almost all dogs of this breed would die before 10 years of age, whereas the values for golden retrievers are somewhat different (30%, 50%). Of course, there may be true differences between the two study populations, and/or the differences may be influenced by referral bias and the high proportion of unclassifiable deaths in the VMDB study.

To further illustrate this example, using just the breeds in Fig. 4.1 and data from the Swedish insurance database, if one ranked the breeds based on actual numbers of dogs that died because of tumors (e.g., perhaps how an oncology clinician would perceive the "risk" based on dogs that present to a specialty clinic), golden retrievers would be number one because they are among the more numerous breeds in this population. Likewise, if one ranked the breeds by the proportion of dead dogs that had tumors (e.g., similar to what would be reported in analysis of postmortem data), the top three would be BMDs, Boxers, and golden retrievers. So, in these examples, as has been frequently reported in the United States, based on proportional statistics, golden retrievers would be labeled as one of the highest risk breeds. However, in looking at the true incidence based on these Swedish data, they do not have an increased risk (before 10 years of age) compared with all breeds. There is likely considerable misunderstanding of the occurrence of cancer in dogs in the United States because of the lack of accurate incidence data and confusion about the interpretation of proportional statistics. Of course, where a breed is very common, such as the golden retriever, and given that a considerable proportion of them die of cancer, that will represent an important population burden of disease, even if they are not truly the "highest risk" breed. This is why golden retrievers were selected for the largest prospective cohort study conducted in a dog population, the Golden Retriever Lifetime Study (GRLS), to investigate the

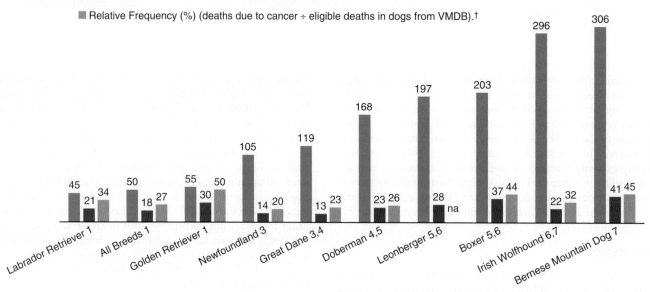

• **Fig. 4.1** Comparison of true mortality rate (blue column) and proportional mortality (red column) for selected dog breeds. True mortality is reported as the total number of deaths resulting from cancer per 10,000 dog-years-at-risk (e.g., the cancer mortality in Labrador retrievers was 45 deaths per 10,000 dogs per year). The proportional mortality is reported as the percentage of deaths resulting from cancer compared with all deaths reported in that breed (e.g., 21% of deaths in Labrador retrievers were caused by cancer). The 95% confidence intervals for mortality rates overlap for breeds with the same number (e.g., mortality risk in Labrador retrievers and golden retrievers was not different from that for all breeds combined, but was different from the other breeds listed in the table).[24,25]

risk factors for occurrence of cancer.[25] In addition, the Swedish data only include dogs up to 10 years of age; it is unknown how the statistics would look if dogs of all ages were included. As the authors of this study discuss, for cancer (or any cause of death) that occurs at older ages, a dog must live long enough to experience it (i.e., not die at a younger age because of any other cause), and deaths before 10 years of age are relevant to focus on for cancer prevention.[24]

Sources of Information on Cancer Occurrence

One of the largest clinic-based databases is the VMDB.[26] This database was started in 1964 by the National Cancer Institute, includes patient data from 26 university teaching hospitals in the United States and Canada, and contains more than 7 million records from all species covering the full range of diagnoses, including cancer. The VMDB is a widely used source of cancer surveillance information for companion animals; however, as discussed previously (and presented in Fig. 4.1), there is no information on the base population in these studies and only proportional measures can be calculated. Given that the data sources are teaching hospitals, the patients and disease diagnoses represented are likely to be influenced by referral bias, resulting in estimates of disease frequency that may not be typical of those seen in the general dog and cat population. In an analysis using VMDB medical records it was concluded that substantial referral bias may indeed exist in the data set, and the authors suggested the accuracy of prevalence estimates measured from the VMDB could be improved by statistical adjustment on the basis of geographic proximity of the patient's residence to the nearest university teaching hospital.[27]

The use of primary care data for investigations regarding the occurrence of cancer in companion animals is less affected by referral bias, but may be influenced by misclassification bias.[28] To date, primary care data have been an underused resource for determining cancer incidence, but advances in large-scale data collection and management suggest primary care data may become increasingly accessible for this purpose. For instance, the Veterinary Companion Animal Surveillance System (VetCompass), which began collecting clinical data from primary practices in the United Kingdom in 2009, now holds data on nearly 6 million animals collected from more than 500 veterinary practices across the United Kingdom (as of August 2017).[29] VetCompass began collecting clinical data in Australia in 2016[30] and pilot projects are underway in Spain, Germany, and New Zealand.[31] Projects related to cancer outcomes in companion animals are already underway,[29] and these data will likely become an increasingly important source of information for research concerning cancer occurrence.

Two well-established insurance databases are from the United Kingdom[32] and from Sweden.[24,32,33] A notable limitation of these databases is that not all cases are histologically confirmed. The benefits and limitations of these data have been discussed extensively in the literature.[34] From the UK database, using data from 1997 through 1998, cancer incidence among 130,684 dogs at risk was 747.9 per 100,000 dog-years.[35] From the Swedish data, the overall mortality rate for cancer was 50 per 10,000 dog-years-at-risk (which equates to 500 per 100,000).[24] Osteosarcoma (OSA) incidence rates were 6.1 and 5.0 dogs per 10,000 dog-years for males and females, respectively,[36] and among females, breast cancer incidence was 111 dogs per 10,000 dog-years.[37] The limitations of the Swedish data are that deaths are mainly in dogs 10 years of age or younger and it is unknown whether the diagnosis has been validated by histology,[20] but comparison across breeds

within the Swedish data is quite informative given that the limitations occur equally across breeds. Crudely comparing overall mortality rates for cancer, BMDs were approximately six times more likely to die of cancer compared with all dogs combined (306 versus 50 per 10,000 DYAR, respectively).[24] Where it was possible to do more sophisticated analyses, BMDs were shown to be 17 times more likely to die of cancer, compared with baseline, and adjusting for age, gender, and breed.[33] Even if specifics of the population may not be the same as other populations, data such as these are important for identifying high-risk breeds. Comparison across populations and over time is needed, with due consideration of data issues.

Studies on Swedish insurance data have also presented statistics on morbidity and mortality in cats.[38,39] As with dogs, the diagnoses are made by veterinarians, but further details are unavailable. The overall age-standardized mortality rate for death resulting from cancer in insured Swedish cats (generally <12 years of age) was 37 per 10,000 cat-years at risk. The most common types of cancer in the Swedish data were mammary, stomach/intestinal, and lymphoma. Siamese breeds were at increased risk of death caused by neoplasia; mammary cancer was the most common type,[40] in agreement with an earlier study.[41] Differences between populations and data are no doubt affected by differences in various factors (e.g., spay/neuter rates and age structure of the populations). Further study of neoplasia in cats is needed.

Notwithstanding the previous discussion on the relative paucity of population-based, histologically confirmed data on the incidence of cancer, there is no doubt that certain breeds are at high risk for cancer (e.g., the BMD, flat-coated retrievers, Boxers, and Scottish terriers). In the section that follows, we will present an overview of known and suspected risk factors for specific cancers, including breed-specific risks, which is not strictly limited by the level of evidence or quality of studies or data but that reflects the current state of knowledge. An important concern for the future, however, is that without true incidence data we are limited in our ability to track changes in occurrence over time, as proportional measures are influenced by changes both in the numerator and denominator. In other words, an increase in the popularity of a breed may lead to its apparent overrepresentation in proportional cancer measures; a change in the distribution of breeds may affect cancer prevalence, without any actual change in breed risk. Without incidence measures, it would be impossible to accurately evaluate the effectiveness of programs aimed at preventing or controlling disease.

Factors Associated with Cancer Risk

Observational studies are the tools of epidemiology used to identify and characterize the determinants of cancer risk. Information from descriptive studies such as case series may help generate hypotheses but is not adequate as a basis for evidence-based cancer prevention strategies. Results from case series are also no longer accepted for publication in at least one major veterinary medical journal.[6] Analytic observational studies such as case-control and cohort designs, on the other hand, are used to test research hypotheses, and when well designed, can provide valuable information for cancer prevention strategies.

The case-control study design is the most commonly used observational study design in veterinary epidemiology research and in cancer epidemiology research in general. This is the most efficient study design, in terms of cost and time, when evaluating associations with relatively rare outcomes, such as specific cancers. Unfortunately, as data collection is often retrospective, many potential sources of bias must be considered. The features of an ideally conducted study (e.g., with the least opportunity for systematic bias) include the complete ascertainment of all newly diagnosed cases with histopathologic confirmation of primary tumors and a random (or matched) selection of controls from the same base population as the cases. In a population-based case-control study design,[42,43] we can assume that if a control subject had been diagnosed with the tumor of interest, that control would have been a case in the study (i.e., the controls are from the same base population as the cases). The goal of the control group is to represent the exposure experience of the base population. For this reason, we are not interested in selecting the "healthiest" subjects as our comparison group.

In a hospital-based case-control study, both cases and controls are selected from the same hospital(s). The limitation with this design is that we cannot generalize the study results to a clearly defined base population. However, this design is valid and can still provide meaningful results. When using hospital-based case-control study design, it is preferable to randomly or systematically sample from the noncase population and to not include animals that have been diagnosed with other cancers.[44,45]

In a prospective cohort study, a group of animals is defined on the basis of exposure and followed over time to compare the incidence of disease (or other specified outcome) among the exposed and unexposed groups. The results obtained from a prospective cohort study are advantageous compared to results obtained from a case-control study for many reasons. One primary advantage is that we can assume temporality, or that the exposure came before the disease, when associations are observed from prospectively collected data. Systematic errors resulting from selection bias (e.g., referral bias) and differential recall bias (e.g., misclassification of exposure by disease status) are also not major concerns when interpreting results from a well-performed prospective cohort study. There is a need for more longitudinal (as opposed to retrospective), preferably population-based studies to strengthen the quality of evidence in the field of veterinary oncology.

Regardless of the observational study design used, nondifferential exposure misclassification will be a major concern, and the possibility and extent of misclassification should be considered when interpreting observational study results. Methods by which exposure misclassification can be reduced include using a precise and accurate questionnaire that has been properly validated or incorporating the use of biomarkers of exposure that can be quantified into the study design.

To estimate the magnitude of an association between an exposure and a cancer type, the relative risk, or risk ratio (RR), and odds ratio (OR) are calculated from data collected from cohort studies or cross-sectional and case-control studies, respectively. The RR is calculated as follows:

$$RR = \text{Incidence among exposed subjects} \div \\ \text{Incidence among unexposed subjects}$$

where incidence is the number of events divided by total animal-time of follow-up. The OR can be used to estimate the RR when incidence data are not available. The OR is calculated as follows:

$$OR = (\text{Number of exposed cases} \div \text{number of unexposed cases}) \div \\ (\text{Number of exposed controls} \div \text{number of unexposed controls})$$

TABLE 4.3	Guidelines for Interpreting Clinical Relevance from Odds Ratios or Relative Risk Measures	
Inverse Association ≈ Decreased Risk	Clinical Relevance	Positive Association ≈ Increased Risk
1.0	Not evident	1.0
0.7 to <1.0	Weak	>1.0–1.5
0.5 to <0.7	Moderate	>1.5–2.0
0.3 to <0.5	Strong	>2.0–3.5
<0.3	Very strong	>3.5

The RR and OR are similarly interpreted. A value greater than 1.0 indicates that the exposure is positively associated with disease (increases risk), whereas a value less than 1.0 indicates that the exposure is inversely associated with disease (decreases risk). A value of 1.0 indicates there is no association between exposure and disease. The 95% confidence interval (CI) indicates the precision of the RR or OR, and if the 95% CI includes 1.0, we interpret the RR or OR to be statistically nonsignificant. It must be remembered, however, that statistical significance does not necessarily equate with clinical importance. For the latter, the magnitude of the effect is also important to consider. Table 4.3 shows suggested guidelines for interpretation of risk estimates. When considering whether to implement preventive measures or health interventions at the population level, the following, in addition to the risk estimate, are also relevant: prevalence of the factor (i.e., likelihood of exposure) and the prevalence of the disease. These values are used to estimate the attributable risk or risk-reduction measures.

Findings from all observational studies are influenced by systematic error to some degree because there is inherent bias in the methods used to select the study population, measure exposures, and identify the outcome. The opportunity for any one study to report an association that is due in part to chance is a real concern, even with the use of valid study design methods and statistical analyses. Confidence in the evidence for a particular association is strengthened when it is observed repeatedly in multiple populations and with the use of more and more rigorous study design methods. Meta-analysis is a technique whereby results from multiple, similar studies can be combined to increase the power of findings. Several examples are available from the human literature relating to nutritional risk factors associated with pancreatic, breast, and colon cancer.[46–48] Unfortunately, in small animal oncology, studies have neither been performed nor reported consistently enough nor are there an adequate number of studies conducted to support meta-analyses being conducted regularly at this time. Notwithstanding these limitations, Table 4.4 presents risk factors, including breed risks, for some of the more common cancers in dogs and cats for which there are at least reasonable estimations of association.

The identification of modifiable risk factors for canine cancers is the first step in eventually reducing incidence. Table 4.5 presents analytic studies used to test hypotheses that selected factors were either associated with an increased or decreased risk of canine and feline cancers. Characteristics of the study design and analytic methods are highlighted as strengths

TABLE 4.4 Commonly Diagnosed Cancers and Suspected Risk Factors

Cancers	Suspected Risk Factors
Common Canine Cancers	
Mammary carcinoma	Obesity, increasing age, high dietary fat intake, late age at spay, and some breeds (e.g., English Springer spaniel, pointer, poodle, Boston terrier, Dachshund, German shepherd, Chihuahua)
Osteosarcoma	High weight, high height, increasing age, early castration/spay, some breeds (e.g., Irish wolfhound, Saint Bernard, Great Dane, Rottweiler, Irish setter, Doberman Pinscher, golden retriever, Labrador retriever, Leonberger)
Transitional cell carcinoma of the urinary bladder	Being neutered, exposure to phenoxy-acid containing herbicides, frequent flea dipping, increasing age, some breeds (e.g., Scottish terrier, Beagle, Shetland sheepdog, Wirehaired fox terrier, West Highland white terrier)
Mast cell tumors	Some breeds (e.g., Boxer, Rhodesian ridgeback, Vizsla, Boston terrier, Weimaraner, Chinese Shar-Pei, Bullmastiff, Dutch pug, Labrador retriever, American Staffordshire terrier, golden retriever, English setter, English pointer), increasing age
Lymphoma	ETS, exposure to chemicals containing 2,4-dichlorophenoxyacetic acid, increasing age, some breeds (e.g., Bullmastiff, Boxer, Scottish terrier, Gordon setter, Irish wolfhound, Basset hound, golden retriever)
Common Feline Cancers	
Lymphoma	FeLV, FIV, ETS increasing age
Sarcoma	Vaccine injection
Cutaneous squamous cell carcinoma	Solar irradiation

ETS, Environmental tobacco smoke; *FeLV*, feline leukemia virus; *FIV*, feline immunodeficiency virus.

TABLE 4.5 Selected Observational Studies of Canine and Feline Cancers by Type of Exposure

Exposure	Main Findings	Strengths/Limitations
ETS		
Reif, 1998[54]	Positive trend for number of packs smoked by owner and increased risk of canine nasal cancer among long-nosed (dolichocephalic) dogs.	Strengths: Evaluation of nose size as an effect modifier with biologic plausibility; collected information on potential confounders. Limitations: Use of controls with cancer.
Reif, 1992[55]	Statistically nonsignificant positive association for living with ≥1 versus no smokers and canine lung cancer risk. Association was stronger among short-nosed dogs (brachycephalic or mesocephalic).	Strengths: High participation rates among cases and controls. Limitations: Use of controls with cancer; limited statistical power.
Marconato, 2009[43]	Any ETS exposure was positively associated with canine lymphoma, compared with no exposure.	Strengths: Population-based study design. Limitations: Use of controls with cancer; limited ETS exposure information was collected.
Bertone, 2002[56]	Strong, statistically significant association for any household ETS exposure and malignant lymphoma in cats. Statistically significant trend reported for a stronger association with increasing years of ETS exposure.	Strengths: Statistical power to evaluate trends; cases confirmed by biopsy; respectable response rate among the cases and controls (>65%); use of a detailed questionnaire to assess ETS and other environmental exposures. Limitations: No clear biologic mechanism for the observed association.
Bertone, 2003[57]	Clinic-based case-control study had ETS exposure positively associated with feline oral SCC. Overall, results do not support a causal relationship between ETS exposure and feline SCC.	Strengths: Cases confirmed by biopsy; good response rates; use of a detailed questionnaire (see previous entry). Limitations: Prevalence of ETS exposure was low; limiting the statistical power to evaluate more than two levels of exposure.

Continued

TABLE 4.5	Selected Observational Studies of Canine and Feline Cancers by Type of Exposure—cont'd	
Exposure	Main Findings	Strengths/Limitations
Pesticides		
Hayes, 1991[63]	Any use of chemicals containing 2,4-dichlorophenoxyacetic acid (2,4-D) positively associated with canine malignant lymphoma, compared with no use. Lymphoma risk increased with greater number of applications of 2,4-D–containing chemicals.	Strengths: Complete ascertainment of newly diagnosed cases; high participation rates among cases and controls; collected extensive information on chemical use on lawns/yards (self-applied and commercially applied). Limitations: One control group composed of dogs with other cancers. NOTE: This and other limitations were addressed in subsequent analyses.
Glickman, 1989[65]	Residence location within one mile of a marsh (where chemicals were used for mosquito control) positively associated with canine TCC of the urinary bladder. Receiving flea dips more than two times/year versus no use was positively associated with TCC.	Strengths: Collected information on numerous sources of chemical exposure, including residential location to industries, pesticide use, flee/tick treatments. Limitations: 45% of control dogs had malignant neoplasia; information was not collected on individual dog exposure to the marsh or on specific chemicals used around the house/yard.
Glickman, 2004[44]	Access versus no access to phenoxy herbicide–treated lawns/yards positively associated with TCC of the urinary bladder among Scottish terriers. No association was observed for lawns/yards not treated with phenoxy herbicides.	Strengths: Collected information on brand name and active ingredients for household, lawn, and garden chemicals; results were specific for phenoxy herbicide exposure. Limitations: Limited statistical power to conduct subgroup analyses.
Raghavan, 2004[111]	Use of topical flea/tick products (e.g., shampoos, dips, powders, sprays, and collars) not associated with TCC of the urinary bladder among Scottish terriers.	Strengths: Collected detailed information on use of flea/tick products (e.g., type, brand, pattern of use) Limitation: 24% of control dogs had cancer; numbers for cases and controls were not presented by exposure level.
Environmental Pollutants		
Bettini, 2010[112]	Pulmonary anthracosis (high versus none) positively associated with canine lung cancer risk.	Strengths: Histologic confirmation of primary diagnosis of lung cancer; exposure assessment determined by histologic scoring of anthracosis; strong biologic mechanism supporting the a priori hypothesis. Limitations: Small number of cases limited the statistical analyses.
Marconato, 2009[43]	Living in geographic areas exposed to toxic waste positively associated with canine cancer risk (all tumors and lymphoma), compared with living in an unexposed area. No associations observed for canine mast cell tumors, canine mammary cancer, or feline cancers.	Strengths: Population-based study design, histologic confirmation of cases; odds ratios were adjusted for age, sex, and breed. Limitations: Same eligibility criterion (i.e., living at same address for 2 years before enrollment) was not applied to controls.
Gavazza, 2001[66]	Living in an industrial neighborhood was positively associated with canine lymphoma risk, compared with living in any other neighborhood. Use or storage of paints and solvents was positively associated with lymphoma risk, compared with no use of chemicals.	Strengths: Histopathologic or cytologic confirmation of cases; information was collected on potential confounders. Limitations: Very low prevalence of exposed cases and controls; only univariate analyses were conducted.
Bukowski, 1998[113]	Cumulative kerosene or coal heat exposure was positively associated with sinonasal cancer risk.	Strengths: High participation rate; covariate information was compared between respondents and nonrespondents; histopathologic confirmation of cases. Limitations: Use of controls with cancer.

TABLE 4.5	Selected Observational Studies of Canine and Feline Cancers by Type of Exposure—cont'd	
Exposure	**Main Findings**	**Strengths/Limitations**
Endogenous/Exogenous Sex Hormones		
Sonnenschein, 1991[75]	Earlier age at spaying was inversely associated with canine mammary cancer. Trend of decreasing risk was observed for younger age at spaying.	Strengths: Cases were limited to mammary carcinoma or adenocarcinoma. Limitations: Controls may not be representative of the base population.
Ru, 1998[76]	Neutered dogs, regardless of gender, had a greater risk of osteosarcoma, compared with intact dogs.	Strengths: Histologic or radiologic confirmation; large study size; collected information on potential confounders. Limitations: Medical conditions of the controls were not clearly described.
Glickman, 2004[44]	Neutered status versus intact was a risk factor for TCC of the urinary bladder among Scottish terriers.	Strengths: Cases were histologically confirmed. Limitations: Small study size did not permit for analyses by age at neutering.
Dias Pereira, 2008[114]	No overall association was observed for COMT genotype and canine mammary cancer risk. Older age at mammary cancer diagnosis was observed by COMT genotype.	Strengths: Strong biologic rationale for research hypothesis; cases were histologically confirmed. Limitations: Very small numbers in subgroup analyses; selection methods were not provided; information was not collected on potential confounders (e.g., hormone-related exposures).
Cooley, 2002[72]	Neutering before 1 year of age increased risk of canine osteosarcoma among Rottweilers, regardless of gender. Incidence rates decreased with later age at neutering. Reproductive factors (number of litters, number of live births, age at first pregnancy) were not associated with osteosarcoma among female dogs.	Strengths: Radiographic or histologic confirmation of cases; retrospective cohort study design. Limitations: Low participation rate.
Stovring, 1997[42]	MPA use was positively associated with canine mammary cancer.	Strengths: Population-based study design; histologic confirmation of cases. Limitations: Information was not collected on details of MPA use (e.g., frequency, dose, age at first use).
Teske, 2002[77]	Castration was positively associated with canine prostate cancer risk, compared with intact status.	Strengths: Strong biologic plausibility. Limitations: Only cytology was used to make cancer diagnosis.
Bryan, 2007[78]	Neutered versus intact status was a risk factor for the following canine cancers: TCC of the urinary bladder, prostate carcinoma, prostate adenocarcinoma, and TCC of the prostate.	Strengths: Histopathologic confirmation of cases; included analyses by histologic subtype. Limitations: Statistically nonsignificant measures were not presented.
Misdorp, 1991[115]	Ovariectomy was inversely associated with feline mammary cancer risk. Regular administration of progestogens increased risk. No association was observed for irregular progestogen administration or for parity.	Strengths: Histologic confirmation of cases; collection of detailed exogenous progestogens (frequency, brand, type); large study size. Limitations: Cases and controls were selected over different time periods.
Overley, 2005[116]	Intact versus neutered status was a risk factor for feline mammary cancer. Cats spayed before 1 year of age were at lower risk of mammary cancer than those spayed after 6 months of age. There was no risk benefit in cats spayed after 2 years of age.	Strengths: Histologic confirmation of cases; large study size. Limitations: Univariate analyses were performed, although detailed information was collected on exogenous hormone use, parity, and number of litters; large amount of missing data because of veterinarian nonresponse.
Torres de la Riva, 2013[79]	Male golden retrievers were more likely to develop lymphoma when neutered <1 year of age compared with intact dogs; Female golden retrievers were more likely to develop hemangiosarcoma when neutered at >1 year of age	Strengths: Large study size. Limitations: Cases were not histologically confirmed, only one breed of dog included.

Continued

TABLE 4.5	Selected Observational Studies of Canine and Feline Cancers by Type of Exposure—cont'd	
Exposure	**Main Findings**	**Strengths/Limitations**
Zink, 2014[80]	Neutering increased risk of developing mast cell tumors, hemangiosarcoma, lymphoma, and all other cancers in Vizslas compared with intact dogs. Neutering at <6 months of age was not associated with increased risk of developing cancer compared with neutering at older ages.	Strengths: Large study size, multivariable analyses were performed. Limitations: Cases were not histologically confirmed, only one breed of dog included.
Hart, 2014[81]	Neutering male golden retrievers and male and female Labrador retrievers or at any age had no significant effect on cancer occurrence compared with intact dogs; Neutering female golden retrievers at any point beyond 6 months of age was associated with increased risk of developing any cancer with the exception of lymphoma which was associated with an increased risk if neutering occurred before 6 months of age.	Strengths: Large study size, Cox proportional hazard models were used. Limitations: Population limited to dogs visiting a single Veterinary Teaching Hospital, only two breeds of dogs included, age categories at time of neutering were not consistent among analyses.
Hart, 2016[117]	Cancer occurrences in this population of German shepherd dogs were rare and there were no associations reported between neutering at any age and cancer outcomes.	Strengths: Large study size, Cox proportional hazard models were used. Limitations: Population limited to dogs visiting a single veterinary teaching hospital, only one breed of dog included, potential data quality issues.
Diet		
Perez Alenza, 1998[118]	Higher intake of red meat (as percentage of total calories) was positively associated with canine mammary carcinoma risk. No differences were observed for intake of fruits and vegetables, or biomarker levels of selenium, retinol, or individual fatty acids.	Strength: Used biomarkers of exposure; multivariable analyses included covariates for body conformation. Limitations: Use of a retrospective study design is not recommended for evaluating biomarkers of exposure and cancer risk because of possible disease and/or treatment effects on the biomarker measurement.
Sonnenschein, 1991[75]	Higher intake of fat and table food (as percentage of total calories) was inversely associated with canine mammary carcinoma. No associations were observed with protein or carbohydrates intake.	Strengths: Cases and controls were matched by age, spay status, and breed size, thus reducing the opportunity for confounding by these factors; the dietary assessment tool was validated using a 7-day food record, Limitations: Study size was too small to evaluate diet-cancer associations in subgroups.
Raghavan, 2005[119]	Vegetable intake (≥3 versus 0 times/week) was inversely associated with TCC of the urinary bladder in Scottish terriers. A trend was observed with greater servings of vegetables per week and decreased risk of TCC. No association was observed for weekly vitamin supplement intake, compared with no intake.	Strengths: Histopathology and/or cytology confirmation; use of a comprehensive dietary questionnaire; multivariable analyses. Limitations: Used a volunteer population; 61% of the cases were deceased at the start of the study; 24% of control dogs had neoplastic diseases.
Body Size		
Perez Alenza, 1998[118]	Obese body condition at 1 year of age and at 1 year before diagnosis was positively associated with canine mammary cancer, compared with normal or underweight body condition at the same time points.	Strengths: Objective measurements of weight and height were collected at presentation; body conformation was determined by a clinician at presentation. Limitations: Height, weight, and body conformation at 1 year of age and 1 year before diagnosis were based on owners' reports.
Sonnenschein, 1991[75]	Spayed dogs that were thin at 9–12 months of age had a lower risk of mammary cancer. Intact dogs that were not overweight in adulthood had a lower risk of mammary cancer.	Strengths: Cases were limited to mammary carcinoma or adenocarcinoma; designed to assess a timely hypothesis that early life factors are related to mammary cancer risk. Limitations: Controls may not be representative of the base population; subgroup analyses did not have ample statistical power to calculate precise measures.
Weeth, 2007[45]	BCSs ≥6 were inversely associated with canine cancer risk (all cancers, sarcomas, and carcinomas), compared with BCSs of 4–6. BCSs <3 were inversely associated with canine sarcoma risk, compared with scores of 4–6.	Strengths: Very large study size; 9-point BCS determined by physical examination; analyses were conducted by cancer type (sarcoma, carcinoma, round cell tumors) Limitations: Selection of cases and controls depended on availability of BCS in medical records; the inverse associations with higher BCS may be a result of reverse causation.

TABLE 4.5	Selected Observational Studies of Canine and Feline Cancers by Type of Exposure—cont'd	
Exposure	Main Findings	Strengths/Limitations
Ru, 1998[76]	Height (>61 versus <35.5 cm) and weight (>45 versus <23 kg) were positively associated with canine osteosarcoma risk, after adjusting for age and standard weight and height, respectively. Longer length of hind limbs and front limbs was positively associated with canine osteosarcoma risk, compared with shortest length.	Strengths: Histologic or radiologic confirmation; large study size; collected information on potential confounders. Limitations: Medical conditions of the controls were not clearly described; a proxy measure for height was used; there was a large percentage (22.5%) with missing weight information.
Glickman, 2004[44]	Greater weight was positively associated with TCC urinary bladder risk in Scottish terriers, comparing third versus first tertile. Greater weight-to-height ratio was also a risk factor for TCC.	Strengths: Cases were histologically confirmed. Limitations: Weight and height information was based on owners' reports.
Vaccines/Injection Site		
Kass, 2003[91]	Cats with sarcomas at a vaccine injection site (n = 662) were compared with cats with basal cell tumors or noninjection site sarcomas (n = 473). Univariate analyses showed no difference in the vaccine type (FVRCP, rabies, FeLV) between cases and controls. There were no differences between time at vaccination and tumor diagnosis between the two groups.	Strengths: Histologic confirmation of cases and controls; collected extensive vaccine information (date of injection, manufacturer, type, brand, site of injection). Limitations: Cases were identified on a volunteer basis from participating clinics; heterogeneous sarcoma case group.
Kass, 1993[90]	In 345 cats diagnosed with fibrosarcoma, 53.6% had tumors at the vaccine injection site. The time from FeLV vaccination to tumor diagnosis was significantly shorter among cats that had tumors at the cervical/interscapular region than cats that had tumors at noninjection sites.	Strengths: Biopsy-confirmed diagnoses; vaccination history was validated by veterinarian; collected vaccination details allowing for analyses by type of vaccine, time since vaccination and location of injection site. Limitations: Differential missing data by exposure status.
FeLV/FIV		
Hutson, 1991[120]	Among 1160 cats identified from an oncology referral and a general practice clinic, 2.5% were FIV positive. Of the FIV-positive cats, 62% were diagnosed with neoplasia (myeloproliferative disease, lymphoma, and SCC).	Strengths: Descriptive information of neoplasia among FIV-positive cats. Limitations: No evident population base; only count data were presented.
Gabor, 2001[121]	Among 101 cats with lymphosarcoma, 50% were FIV positive. These cats were more likely to be male domestic crossbreeds.	Strengths: Histopathologic confirmation of cases; FIV antibodies were determined using Western blot. Limitations: Convenience study population was used.
Shelton, 1990[96]	Coinfection with FIV and FeLV was present in 14.4% of 353 cats collected in several US cities. FIV and FeLV infection were strongly associated with risk of leukemia or lymphoma. A very imprecise positive association was also reported for coinfection and leukemia/lymphoma risk.	Strengths: FIV antibodies were determined using ELISA and Western blot. Limitations: Base population and subject recruitment methods were not well defined; low prevalence of coinfection among controls limited statistical power.
Solar Irradiation		
Dorn, 1971[122]	Among white cats, the observed incidence of SCC of the skin was greater than the expected incidence (p < 0.001). For SCC of the mouth–pharynx, white cats had no difference between observed and expected incidence.	Strengths: Population-based study population. Limitations: Amount of sun exposure was not quantified; the number of cats with SCC of the mouth–pharynx was small (n = 29).

BCS, Body condition score; COMT, catechol-O-methyltransferase; ELISA, enzyme-linked immunosorbent assay; ETS, environmental tobacco smoke; FeLV, feline leukemia virus; FIV, feline immunodeficiency virus; FVRCP, feline viral rhinotracheitis-calicivirus-panleukopenia; MPA, medroxyprogesterone acetate; SCC, squamous cell carcinoma; TCC, transitional cell carcinoma.

and weaknesses. Studies with the strongest level of evidence included several characteristics related to study design (e.g., hypothesis-driven, population-based, large study size, validated exposure assessment) and results (e.g., a precise measure of association, a modest-to-strong magnitude of association, statistically significant measure of association, statistically significant trend between exposure level and magnitude of association).

Highlighted Findings from Observational Studies

In this section, we discuss risk factors for which there is relatively strong evidence, those that relate to key issues in animal or human oncology, and those for which important controversies need to be addressed by further research. These categories coincide with those shown in Table 4.5.

Environmental Exposures

The identification of environmental exposures that are related to canine cancer risk have a broad public health interest, given the shared environments of companion animals and their owners, and they have similar etiology of some cancers.[49] In a comprehensive review, a historic perspective is provided on how studies in pet populations have informed human health with respect to the specific exposures of air pollution, environmental tobacco smoke (ETS), and pesticides.[50] The shared etiologic characteristics of cancers such as lymphoma, OSA, and mammary cancer also support the utility of looking to both pet and human populations to investigate environmental–cancer associations.[51]

There is experimental evidence for an underlying biologic mechanism for the compounds of cigarette smoke to have a causal relationship with canine carcinogenesis.[52,53] There are few observational studies that were designed to specifically evaluate associations between ETS exposure and canine cancer risk.[54,55] There is support for a positive association (3.4-fold increased risk) between ETS and lymphoma[43] and sinonasal cancers,[54] but not for lung cancer.[55] In a clinic-based case-control study, household ETS exposure was strongly associated with feline lymphoma.[56] The OR for any exposure, compared with no exposure, was 2.4, and statistically significant trends were reported for more years of ETS exposure, more smokers in the household, and number of cigarettes smoked per day in the household. In contrast, there is only weak observational evidence for ETS as a risk factor for oral squamous cell carcinoma in cats.[57] In summary, avoiding ETS exposure may reduce the risk of lymphoma in cats and dogs and the risk of sinonasal cancers in dogs.

Pesticides are a heterogeneous group of chemicals, some of which are known human and canine carcinogens.[58–60] Dogs may be exposed to pesticides in the home, in the yard/garden, and on application of flea and tick treatments. The most consistent observational evidence for pesticide exposure as a cancer risk factor is for phenoxy acid–containing herbicides and lymphoma risk, both in humans and dogs.[61] These data, however, have not been deemed strong enough to establish causality.[62] In a large case-control study (n = 491 cases and n = 945 controls), any use of pesticides that contained dichlorophenoxyacetic acid (2,4-D) was associated with a 30% increased risk of lymphoma compared with no use.[63,64] Although modest, the positive association also demonstrated a dose-dependent effect in which more frequent use of 2,4-D pesticides resulted in a stronger positive association with lymphoma risk (p for trend <0.02). Additional support for 2,4-D and canine bladder cancer risk is from the result of a small case-control study in Scottish terriers.[42]

Residential proximity to environmental hazard–containing sites has been used to estimate chemical exposure and canine cancer risk in several observational studies.[43,65,66] A 2.4-fold increase in risk of lymphoma was observed among dogs living in the cities containing illegal waste sites compared with dogs living in other cities.[43] No association was observed with mast cell tumors (MCTs) or breast cancer. Mortality caused by cancer is also higher among human populations living near the same waste sites compared with the general population.[67] Chemical mixtures that have been identified at hazard waste landfills include organic solvents, polychlorinated biphenyls, and heavy metals. These can reach human and pet populations through contaminated air, water, and/or soil,[68] and have been causally related to adverse human health effects, including childhood lymphoma.[69] The biologic plausibility and the observational findings from Marconato et al[43] both help strengthen the evidence that living near the waste sites increases risk of canine lymphoma.

Exposure misclassification is a primary limitation of using geographic proximity as a marker of exposure to an industrial or waste site because it may or may not be a good proxy for individual-level exposure. For example, a validation study would need to be conducted that provides information on whether dogs that live close to an industrial site are necessarily exposed at higher levels to environmental hazards compared with dogs that live further from the site. Misclassification of exposure that does not differ by disease status (e.g., nondifferential misclassification) typically results in an underestimate of the exposure–cancer association, although there are situations when the observed association results in an overestimate of the true association.[70,71]

Hormones and Neuter Status

Hormones may act as either growth factors or inhibitors, depending on the sex of the dog and the tissue type.[72–74] For some cancers, such as breast cancer, less exposure to sex hormones is protective; whereas for others, such as OSA, lymphoma, and prostate cancer, less exposure has been reported to increase risk.[72,75–82] Neuter/spay status and age at neuter/spay are the most commonly used measures of endogenous hormone exposure. In spite of some newer studies, there is limited evidence that the age of the dog at the time of neuter/spay can have an effect on the risk of developing cancer in certain breeds of dogs.[79,81] Given the widespread recommendation for early spay/neuter, especially in North America, this is a topic in need of further study.

In a mammary cancer case-control study, there was clear evidence that spayed dogs were at lower risk of mammary cancer.[75] In particular, the earlier age at which dogs were spayed the lower their mammary cancer risk compared with dogs that were not spayed. This finding has been supported by other observational studies of spay status and mammary cancer risk.[83]

Contrary to human epidemiologic and experimental evidence,[84,85] exposure to sex hormones such as androgens may be protective for canine prostate cancer.[82] From two case-control studies using large veterinary teaching hospital databases, neutered dogs had a 2.8- and 3.4-fold increased risk of prostate cancer compared with intact dogs.[77,78] The apparent opposite associations between hormone exposure and prostate cancer risk in men and dogs are likely a result of the higher rate of androgen-independent tumors in dogs than in men.[86,87]

Neuter status is also a risk factor for OSA and transitional cell carcinoma of the urinary bladder,[44,72,76,78] regardless of sex.[72,76] Cooley et al conducted a retrospective cohort study in 1999 among 683 Rottweilers and used a self-administered questionnaire to test the hypothesis that neuter/spay status was related to the development of OSA.[72] The owners were identified through eight national Rottweiler breed specialty clubs and had a purebred Rottweiler that was alive on January 1, 1995. The participation rate ([number of participants] ÷ [total number of invited owners] × 100) was 49%. This low participation rate suggests that selection bias may have influenced the results of this study. In other words, the participants of the study are likely to have systematic differences compared with those who did not participate. However, a strength of this study is the ability to calculate incidence because the total number of dog-months of observation were estimated retrospectively among dogs that were neutered/spayed and those that were not. During a total of 71,004 dog-months of observation, there were 86 cases of OSA. Collectively, the findings of a positive association between neuter/spay status and OSA from both case-control and cohort studies, and the biologic plausibility of the association, provide strong evidence that neutering/spaying dogs, regardless of sex, increases risk of OSA.

A number of reports have linked the age of dogs at the time of neuter/spay to increased risk of developing hemangiosarcoma, lymphoma, and MCTs in select breeds of dogs.[79–81] Using a retrospective analysis of medical records including dogs younger than 8 years of age from the Veterinary Medical Teaching Hospital at the University of California, Davis, an increased risk of developing hemangiosarcoma and MCTs was identified in female golden retrievers neutered at 12 months of age or older compared with intact female golden retrievers.[79] The same analysis revealed an increased risk of developing lymphoma in male golden retrievers neutered before 12 months of age compared with intact male golden retrievers.[79] A subsequent report that used a larger data set from the same location reported similar risks in golden retrievers, but showed there was no difference in risk of cancer occurrence in Labrador retrievers associated with neuter status.[81] Research from the same institution that examined cancer-related mortality in golden retrievers found that increasing age increased the odds of cancer-related mortality regardless of neuter status.[88] Neutered female golden retrievers were found to live statistically significantly longer than intact females and it was this increase in longevity that affected the rate of cancer occurrence rather than the hormonal differences caused by neutering. This conflicting result may be because of the fact that dogs of any age were included in this study whereas the previous reports limited results to dogs aged 8 years or younger.[79,81,88] Results of a survey of Vizsla owners indicate that neutering at any age was associated with increased risk of developing lymphoma and MCTs regardless of sex.[80] Increased risk associated with development of hemangiosarcoma was also indicated in both sexes regardless of the timing of neutering with the exception of males neutered at less than 12 months of age, which had no difference in risk compared with intact males.[80] Prospective research conducted to examine associations between age at neutering and cancer outcomes is needed in a wider variety of dog breeds before current recommendations regarding spay/neuter can be modified.

Risk Factors in Cats

In cats, the epidemiology of injection-site sarcomas has been well studied. A review from 2011 provides information on the current epidemiology, etiology, and clinical knowledge of feline injection-site sarcomas (FISSs).[89] Kass et al conducted one of the first epidemiologic studies investigating the hypothesis that vaccinations were related to feline fibrosarcoma risk in the early 1990s.[90] A main finding of this study was the shorter time interval from vaccination to FISS compared with the interval from vaccination to non-FISSs. This finding was not supported by a second, larger case-control study.[91] Although there is no doubt that the phenomenon of FISS exists, the administration of an injection itself is not sufficient to cause development of an FISS. The component causes (e.g., the nature of vaccines and adjuvants in the injected material and the role of the resulting inflammatory reaction), in addition to the physical injection that leads to the development of an FISS, are not well characterized. Further epidemiologic research designed with due consideration of the challenging methodological issues is needed to identify the various factors associated with FISSs.[92]

Cats infected with the feline immunodeficiency virus (FIV), the feline analog to the human immunodeficiency virus (HIV), are at increased risk of certain cancers.[93] FIV is a lentivirus typically transmitted by biting.[94] Lymphomas, particularly those of B-cell origin, are the most commonly diagnosed neoplasia among FIV-infected cats. Persistent feline leukemia virus (FeLV) infection is also known to have a strong role in feline neoplasia development,[95] and coinfection with FIV and FeLV may have synergistic effects on feline neoplasia risk.[96]

Diagnosis and Screening

As mentioned previously, numerous reporting guidelines have been produced for the human medical literature (e.g., http://methods.cochrane.org/mecir). One of these describes an approach to complete and accurate reporting of studies of diagnostic accuracy (Standards for Reporting of Diagnostic Accuracy [STARD]).[97,98] The application of this and another instrument in the veterinary field has been discussed.[99] Unfortunately, relatively few diagnostic interventions in veterinary medicine have been examined or evaluated as fully, in terms of reliability, accuracy, efficacy, and effectiveness, as is needed to support EBM practices. Guidelines for prognostic studies in veterinary oncology have also been reported.[100]

It may also be appropriate to use clinical trial methodology to evaluate the outcomes of diagnostic tests, for example, whether the animal is better off for having had the test performed.[101] In addition, recommendations about diagnostic tests and screening programs may have both positive and negative effects beyond any individual, on populations of animals and owners. Although new, sophisticated diagnostic tests used in humans are being evaluated for use in companion animals, it is important to remember that beyond the benefit in a specific case, efficacy and effectiveness of tests should consider the broadest aspects of cost–benefit. In human oncology, there has been much discussion about the problems inherent in certain widely applied screening processes and the consequences of false positives and negatives (e.g., prostate-specific antigen test for prostate cancer[102]). Owing to space constraints, we cannot expand on this crucially important area of cancer epidemiology.

Therapeutic Interventions

A review published in the *Journal of Veterinary Internal Medicine* highlighted that the quality of reporting of oncology studies in dogs and cats has not improved appreciably over time and that quality of reporting is highly correlated with the rate of positive outcomes (i.e., well-described studies are more likely to report positive effects of a treatment).[103] This may also be exacerbated by the fact that the profession increasingly depends on corporate contracts for funding of research, and, in addition to this having a major effects on which treatments are investigated, there may also be underreporting of studies in which either beneficial effects were not seen or where there were deleterious side effects. As mentioned previously, efforts are underway to produce reporting guidelines for companion animal intervention studies. However, guidelines for appropriate study design for clinical trials have been widely available for many decades, and the need for appropriate trials in oncology has been specifically advocated (see Chapter 18).[104] Longer-term analyses of survival after diagnosis and treatment, including both outcome and cost–benefit analysis, are needed to provide the information that owners and veterinarians need to choose the best options, with due consideration of quality-of-life issues.

Although there are good examples of randomized, controlled, blinded trials in veterinary oncology,[105,106] essentially all studies have some limitations in terms of either quality (validity) or relevance (extrapolation to other situations). For example, because many trials are performed on clients at specialty practices or veterinary teaching hospitals, animals have passed through numerous filters to be available for the study (e.g., referral, have a willing and capable owner, live long enough to have a confirmed diagnosis). Although this may improve the validity of the study (e.g., by increasing compliance and reducing loss to follow-up), it reduces the relevance to, for example, primary practice. Therefore clinicians must be able to apply the rules of evidence to determine both the quality and relevance of information for their specific situation and patients. Other authors in this text will present current information on treatments for cancer, and a further review of the literature is beyond the scope of this chapter. Hopefully, the quality of the veterinary literature will continue to improve over time, and the application of appropriate reporting guidelines and production of evidence-based reviews will assist clinicians to interpret and apply published information.

Knowledge Gaps and Future Directions

Even though systematic reviews and meta-analyses may not be currently possible, evidence-based reviews of the existing oncology literature in dogs and cats are needed to further elucidate what we know about breed risks, other risk factors, appropriate use of diagnostic and screening aids, therapies, prognoses, and so forth, and to identify the most crucial gaps in our knowledge. Appropriate assessment of existing oncology prevention and treatment strategies is also needed.

With increasingly available genomic information, our understanding of breeds and breed risk may change.[107,108] It is especially important to recognize the value of studying populations from different areas or countries. There are important differences and similarities in genetics (across and within breeds), environments, diets, and activities that will inform cancer etiology and management. Such complex relationships will be fully understood only by a multidisciplinary approach using various methodologies and study designs. These should include more population-based, longitudinal observational studies and outcomes-based approaches.[56,57,109] Although these may not yield results for many years, relying solely on traditional approaches (case-control studies and clinical trials of invasive or risky treatments) is not an effective strategy to reduce the population burden of cancer. In addition and beyond the scope of this chapter, there are important complex issues of human–animal interactions, in general and specifically related to the field of oncology. Thus there is a need for an increased understanding of the social and emotional factors underpinning many aspects of this diverse field.[110]

References

1. Sargeant JM, Thompson A, Valcour R, et al.: Quality of reporting of clinical trials of dogs and cats and associations with treatment effects, *J Vet Intern Med* 24:44–50, 2010.
2. Sargeant JM, O'Connor AM, Gardner IA, et al.: The REFLECT statement: reporting guidelines for randomized controlled trials in livestock and food safety, *J Food Prot* 73:579–603, 2010.
3. O'Connor AM, Sargeant JM, Gardner IA, et al.: The REFLECT statement: methods and processes of creating reporting guidelines for randomized controlled trials for livestock and food safety, *J Food Prot* 73:132–139, 2010.
4. Rishniw M, Pion PD, Herndon WE, et al.: Improving reporting of clinical trials in veterinary medicine, *J Vet Intern Med* 24:799–800, 2010.
5. O'Connor AM, Sargeant JM, Gardner IA, et al.: The REFLECT statement: methods and processes of creating reporting guidelines for randomized controlled trials for livestock and food safety, *J Food Prot* 73:132–139, 2010.
6. Hinchcliff KW, DiBartola SP: Quality matters: publishing in the era of CONSORT, REFLECT, and EBM, *J Vet Intern Med* 24(8–9), 2010.
7. Sargeant JM, O'Connor AM, Dohoo IR, et al.: Methods and processes of developing the strengthening the reporting of observational studies in epidemiology – veterinary (STROBE-Vet) statement, *J Vet Intern Med* 30:1887–1895, 2016.
8. Dorn CR, Taylor DO, Frye FL, et al.: Survey of animal neoplasms in Alameda and Contra Costa Counties, California. I. Methodology and description of cases, *J Natl Cancer Inst* 40:295–305, 1968.
9. Dorn CR, Taylor DO, Schneider R, et al.: Survey of animal neoplasms in Alameda and Contra Costa Counties, California. II. Cancer morbidity in dogs and cats from Alameda County, *J Natl Cancer Inst* 40:307–318, 1968.
10. MacVean DW, Monlux AW, Anderson Jr PS, et al.: Frequency of canine and feline tumors in a defined population, *Vet Pathol* 15:700–715, 1978.
11. Moe L, Gamlem H, Dahl K, et al.: Canine neoplasia–population-based incidence of vascular tumours, *APMIS Suppl* 125:63–68, 2008.
12. Nodtvedt A, Gamlem H, Gunnes G, et al.: Breed differences in the proportional morbidity of testicular tumours and distribution of histopathologic types in a population-based canine cancer registry, *Vet Comp Oncol* 9:45–54, 2011.
13. Merlo DF, Rossi L, Pellegrino C, et al.: Cancer incidence in pet dogs: findings of the Animal Tumor Registry of Genoa, Italy, *J Vet Intern Med* 22:976–984, 2008.
14. Vascellari M, Baioni E, Ru G, et al.: Animal tumour registry of two provinces in northern Italy: incidence of spontaneous tumours in dogs and cats, *BMC Vet Res* 5(39), 2009.
15. Grüntzig K, Graf R, Hässig M, et al.: The Swiss canine cancer registry: a retrospective study on the occurrence of tumours in dogs in Switzerland from 1955 to 2008, *J Comp Path* 152:161–171, 2015.
16. Bronden LB, Nielsen SS, Toft N, et al.: Data from the Danish veterinary cancer registry on the occurrence and distribution of neoplasms in dogs in Denmark, *Vet Rec* 166:586–590, 2010.
17. Baioni E, Scanziani E, Vincenti MC, et al.: Estimating canine cancer incidence: findings from a population-based tumour registry in northwestern Italy, *BMC Vet Res* 13:203, 2017.
18. Moe L, Bredal WP, Glattre E: Census of dogs in Norway, Oslo, 2001, Norwegian School of Veterinary Science.
19. Priester WA, McKay FW: The occurrence of tumors in domestic animals, *Natl Cancer Inst Monogr* 54:1–210, 1980.
20. Bronden LB, Flagstad A, Kristensen AT: Veterinary cancer registries in companion animal cancer: a review, *Vet Comp Oncol* 5:133–144, 2007.
21. Nødtvedt A, Berke O, Bonnett BN, et al.: Current status of canine cancer registration: report from an international workshop, *Vet Comp Oncol* 10:95–101, 2011.
22. Craig LE: Cause of death in dogs according to breed: a necropsy survey of five breeds, *J Am Anim Hosp Assoc* 37:438–443, 2001.
23. Fleming JM, Creevy KE, Promislow DE: Mortality in North American dogs from 1984 to 2004: an investigation into age-, size-, and breed-related causes of death, *J Vet Intern Med* 25:187–198, 2011.
24. Bonnett BN, Egenvall A, Hedhammar A, et al.: Mortality in over 350,000 insured Swedish dogs from 1995-2000: I. breed-, gender-, age- and cause-specific rates, *Acta Vet Scand* 46:105–120, 2005.
25. Guy MK, Page RL, Jensen WA, et al.: The golden retriever lifetime study: establishing an observational cohort study with translational relevance for human health, *Philos Trans R Soc Lond B Biol Sci* 370:20140230, 2015.
26. Veterinary Medical Database (VMDB) www.vmdb.org. accessed: 08/08/2017.
27. Bartlett PC, Van Buren JW, Neterer M, et al.: Disease surveillance and referral bias in the veterinary medical database, *Prev Vet Med* 94:264–271, 2010.

28. BSAVA: SAVSNET The next stage, *BSAVA Companion* 4–5, 2013.
29. Veterinary Companion Animal Surveillance System (VetCompass) www.rvc.ac.uk/vetcompass. accessed; 08/13/2017.
30. Latter M: VetCompass Australia – a leap forward for companion animals, *Aust Vet J* 94:N14, 2016.
31. O'Neill DG, Church DB, McGreevy PD, et al.: Approaches to canine health surveillance, *Canine Genet Epidemiol* 1:1–13, 2014.
32. Egenvall A, Hedhammar A, Bonnett BN, et al.: Survey of the Swedish dog population: age, gender, breed, location and enrollment in animal insurance, *Acta Vet Scand* 40:231–240, 1999.
33. Egenvall A, Bonnett BN, Hedhammar A, et al.: Mortality in over 350,000 insured Swedish dogs from 1995-2000: II. breed-specific age and survival patterns and relative risk for causes of death, *Acta Vet Scand* 46:121–136, 2005.
34. Egenvall A, Nodtvedt A, Penell J, et al.: Insurance data for research in companion animals: benefits and limitations, *Acta Vet Scand* 51:42, 2009.
35. Dobson JM, Samuel S, Milstein H, et al.: Canine neoplasia in the UK: estimates of incidence rates from a population of insured dogs, *J Small Anim Pract* 43:240–246, 2002.
36. Egenvall A, Nodtvedt A, von Euler H: Bone tumors in a population of 400 000 insured Swedish dogs up to 10 y of age: incidence and survival, *Can J Vet Res* 71:292–299, 2007.
37. Egenvall A, Bonnett BN, Ohagen P, et al.: Incidence of and survival after mammary tumors in a population of over 80,000 insured female dogs in Sweden from 1995 to 2002, *Prev Vet Med* 69:109–127, 2005.
38. Egenvall A, Nodtvedt A, Haggstrom J, et al.: Mortality of life-insured Swedish cats during 1999-2006: age, breed, sex, and diagnosis, *J Vet Intern Med* 23:1175–1183, 2009.
39. Egenvall A, Bonnett BN, Haggstrom J, et al.: Morbidity of insured Swedish cats during 1999-2006 by age, breed, sex, and diagnosis, *J Feline Med Surg* 12:948–959, 2010.
40. Rissetto K, Villamil JA, Selting KA, et al.: Recent trends in feline intestinal neoplasia: an epidemiologic study of 1,129 cases in the veterinary medical database from 1964 to 2004, *J Am Anim Hosp Assoc* 47:28–36, 2011.
41. Hayes HM, Milne KL, Mandell CP: Epidemiological features of feline mammary carcinoma, *Vet Rec* 108:476–479, 1981.
42. Stovring M, Moe L, Glattre E: A population-based case-control study of canine mammary tumours and clinical use of medroxyprogesterone acetate, *APMIS* 105:590–596, 1997.
43. Marconato L, Leo C, Girelli R, et al.: Association between waste management and cancer in companion animals, *J Vet Intern Med* 23:564–569, 2009.
44. Glickman LT, Raghavan M, Knapp DW, et al.: Herbicide exposure and the risk of transitional cell carcinoma of the urinary bladder in Scottish Terriers, *J Am Vet Med Assoc* 224:1290–1297, 2004.
45. Weeth LP, Fascetti AJ, Kass PH, et al.: Prevalence of obese dogs in a population of dogs with cancer, *Am J Vet Res* 68:389–398, 2007.
46. Paluszkiewicz P, Smolinska K, Debinska I, et al.: Main dietary compounds and pancreatic cancer risk. The quantitative analysis of case-control and cohort studies, *Cancer Epidemiol* 36:60–67, 2012.
47. Sun CL, Yuan JM, Koh WP, et al.: Green tea, black tea and breast cancer risk: a meta-analysis of epidemiological studies, *Carcinogenesis* 27:1310–1315, 2006.
48. Aune D, Chan DS, Lau R, et al.: Dietary fibre, whole grains, and risk of colorectal cancer: systematic review and dose-response meta-analysis of prospective studies, *BMJ* 343, 2011.
49. Backer LC, Grindem CB, Corbett WT, et al.: Pet dogs as sentinels for environmental contamination, *Sci Total Environ* 274:161–169, 2001.
50. Reif JS: Animal sentinels for environmental and public health, *Public Health Rep* 126:50–57, 2011.
51. Kelsey JL, Moore AS, Glickman LT: Epidemiologic studies of risk factors for cancer in pet dogs, *Epidemiol Rev* 20:204–217, 1998.
52. Hernandez JA, Anderson AE, Holmes WL, et al.: Pulmonary parenchymal defects in dogs following prolonged cigarette smoke exposure, *Am Rev Respir Dis* 93:78–83, 1966.
53. Cross FT, Palmer RF, Filipy RE, et al.: Carcinogenic effects of radon daughters, uranium ore dust and cigarette smoke in beagle dogs, *Health Phys* 42:33–52, 1982.
54. Reif JS, Bruns C, Lower KS: Cancer of the nasal cavity and paranasal sinuses and exposure to environmental tobacco smoke in pet dogs, *Am J Epidemiol* 147:488–492, 1998.
55. Reif JS, Dunn K, Ogilvie GK, et al.: Passive smoking and canine lung cancer risk, *Am J Epidemiol* 135:234–239, 1992.
56. Bertone ER, Snyder LA, Moore AS: Environmental tobacco smoke and risk of malignant lymphoma in pet cats, *Am J Epidemiol* 156:268–273, 2002.
57. Bertone ER, Snyder LA, Moore AS: Environmental and lifestyle risk factors for oral squamous cell carcinoma in domestic cats, *J Vet Intern Med* 17:557–562, 2003.
58. Dich J, Zahm SH, Hanberg A, et al.: Pesticides and cancer, *Cancer Causes Control* 8:420–443, 1997.
59. Hardell L: Pesticides, soft-tissue sarcoma and non-Hodgkin lymphoma—historical aspects on the precautionary principle in cancer prevention, *Acta Oncol* 47:347–354, 2008.
60. Andrade FH, Figueiroa FC, Bersano PR, et al.: Malignant mammary tumor in female dogs: environmental contaminants, *Diagn Pathol* 5(45), 2010.
61. Zahm SH, Blair A: Pesticides and non-Hodgkin's lymphoma, *Cancer Res* 52:5485s–5488s, 1992.
62. Garabrant DH, Philbert MA: Review of 2,4-dichlorophenoxyacetic acid (2,4-D) epidemiology and toxicology, *Crit Rev Toxicol* 32:233–257, 2002.
63. Hayes HM, Tarone RE, Cantor KP, et al.: Case-control study of canine malignant lymphoma: positive association with dog owner's use of 2,4-dichlorophenoxyacetic acid herbicides, *J Natl Cancer Inst* 83:1226–1231, 1991.
64. Hayes HM, Tarone RE, Cantor KP: On the association between canine malignant lymphoma and opportunity for exposure to 2,4-dichlorophenoxyacetic acid, *Environ Res* 70:119–125, 1995.
65. Glickman LT, Schofer FS, McKee LJ, et al.: Epidemiologic study of insecticide exposures, obesity, and risk of bladder cancer in household dogs, *J Toxicol Environ Health* 28:407–414, 1989.
66. Gavazza A, Presciuttini S, Barale R, et al.: Association between canine malignant lymphoma, living in industrial areas, and use of chemicals by dog owners, *J Vet Intern Med* 15:190–195, 2001.
67. Comba P, Bianchi F, Fazzo L, et al.: Cancer mortality in an area of Campania (Italy) characterized by multiple toxic dumping sites, *Ann N Y Acad Sci* 1076:449–461, 2006.
68. Upton AC, Kneip T, Toniolo P: Public health aspects of toxic chemical disposal sites, *Annu Rev Public Health* 10:1–25, 1989.
69. Vrijheid M: Health effects of residence near hazardous waste landfill sites: a review of epidemiologic literature, *Environ Health Perspect* 108:101–112, 2000.
70. Dosemeci M, Wacholder S, Lubin JH: Does nondifferential misclassification of exposure always bias a true effect toward the null value? *Am J Epidemiol* 132:746–748, 1990.
71. Wacholder S, Hartge P, Lubin JH, et al.: Non-differential misclassification and bias towards the null: a clarification, *Occup Environ Med* 52:557–558, 1995.
72. Cooley DM, Beranek BC, Schlittler DL, et al.: Endogenous gonadal hormone exposure and bone sarcoma risk, *Cancer Epidemiol Biomarkers Prev* 11:1434–1440, 2002.
73. Millanta F, Calandrella M, Bari G, et al.: Comparison of steroid receptor expression in normal, dysplastic, and neoplastic canine and feline mammary tissues, *Res Vet Sci* 79:225–232, 2005.
74. Rhodes L, Ding VD, Kemp RK, et al.: Estradiol causes a dose-dependent stimulation of prostate growth in castrated beagle dogs, *Prostate* 44:8–18, 2000.

75. Sonnenschein EG, Glickman LT, Goldschmidt MH, et al.: Body conformation, diet, and risk of breast cancer in pet dogs: a case-control study, *Am J Epidemiol* 133:694–703, 1991.

76. Ru G, Terracini B, Glickman LT: Host related risk factors for canine OSA, *Vet J* 156:31–39, 1998.

77. Teske E, Naan EC, van Dijk EM, et al.: Canine prostate carcinoma: epidemiological evidence of an increased risk in castrated dogs, *Mol Cell Endocrinol* 197:251–255, 2002.

78. Bryan JN, Keeler MR, Henry CJ, et al.: A population study of neutering status as a risk factor for canine prostate cancer, *Prostate* 67:1174–1181, 2007.

79. Torres de la Riva G, Hart BL, Farver TB, et al.: Neutering dogs: effects on joint disorders and cancers in Golden Retrievers, *PLoS One* 8:e55937, 2013.

80. Zink MC, Farhoody P, Elser SE, et al.: Evaluation of the risk and age of onset of cancer and behavioral disorders in gonadectomized Vizslas, *J Am Vet Med Assoc* 244:309–319, 2014.

81. Hart BL, Hart LA, Thigpen AP, et al.: Long-term health effects of neutering dogs: comparison of Labrador Retrievers with Golden Retrievers, *PLoS One* 9:e102241, 2014.

82. Johnston SD, Kamolpatana K, Root-Kustritz MV, et al.: Prostatic disorders in the dog, *Anim Reprod Sci*, 2000. 60-61:405–415.

83. Perez Alenza MD, Pena L, del Castillo N, et al.: Factors influencing the incidence and prognosis of canine mammary tumours, *J Small Anim Pract* 41:287–291, 2000.

84. Heinlein CA, Chang C: Androgen receptor in prostate cancer, *Endocr Rev* 25:276–308, 2004.

85. Gann PH, Hennekens CH, Ma J, et al.: Prospective study of sex hormone levels and risk of prostate cancer, *J Natl Cancer Inst* 88:1118–1126, 1996.

86. Sorenmo KU, Goldschmidt M, Shofer F, et al.: Immunohisto-chemical characterization of canine prostatic carcinoma and correlation with castration status and castration time, *Vet Comp Oncol* 1:48–56, 2003.

87. Navarro D, Luzardo OP, Fernandez L, et al.: Transition to androgen-independence in prostate cancer, *J Steroid Biochem Mol Biol* 81:191–201, 2002.

88. Kent MS, Burton JH, Dank G, et al.: Association of cancer-related mortality, age and gonadectomy in golden retriever dogs at a veterinary academic center (1989-2016), *PLoS One* 13:e0192578, 2018.

89. Martano M, Morello E, Buracco P: Feline injection-site sarcoma: past, present and future perspectives, *Vet J* 188:136–141, 2011.

90. Kass PH, Barnes WG, Spangler WL, et al.: Epidemiologic evidence for a causal relation between vaccination and fibrosarcoma tumorigenesis in cats, *J Am Vet Med Assoc* 203:396–405, 1993.

91. Kass PH, Spangler WL, Hendrick MJ, et al.: Multicenter case-control study of risk factors associated with development of vaccine-associated sarcomas in cats, *J Am Vet Med Assoc* 223:1283–1292, 2003.

92. Kass PH: Methodological issues in the design and analysis of epidemiological studies of feline vaccine-associated sarcomas, *Anim Health Res Rev* 5:291–293, 2004.

93. Magden E, Quackenbush SL, Vandewoude S: FIV associated neoplasms-A mini-review, *Vet Immunol Immunopathol* 143:227–234, 2011.

94. Yamamoto JK, Hansen H, Ho EW, et al.: Epidemiologic and clinical aspects of feline immunodeficiency virus infection in cats from the continental United States and Canada and possible mode of transmission, *J Am Vet Med Assoc* 194:213–220, 1989.

95. Rezanka LJ, Rojko JL, Neil JC: Feline leukemia virus: pathogenesis of neoplastic disease, *Cancer Invest* 10:371–389, 1992.

96. Shelton GH, Grant CK, Cotter SM, et al.: Feline immunodeficiency virus and feline leukemia virus infections and their relationships to lymphoid malignancies in cats: a retrospective study (1968-1988), *J Acquir Immune Defic Syndr* 3:623–630, 1990.

97. Bossuyt PM, Reitsma JB: The STARD initiative, *Lancet* 361:71, 2003.

98. Bossuyt PM, Reitsma JB, Bruns DE, et al.: Towards complete and accurate reporting of studies of diagnostic accuracy: the STARD initiative. Standards for reporting of diagnostic accuracy, *Clin Chem* 49:1–6, 2003.

99. Gardner IA: Quality standards are needed for reporting of test accuracy studies for animal diseases, *Prev Vet Med* 97:136–143, 2010.

100. Webster JD, Dennis MM, Dervisis N, et al.: Recommended guidelines for the conduct and evaluation of prognostic studies in veterinary oncology, *Vet Pathol* 48:7–18, 2011.

101. Lawrence J, Rohren E, Provenzale J: PET/CT today and tomorrow in veterinary cancer diagnosis and monitoring: fundamentals, early results and future perspectives, *Vet Comp Oncol* 8:163–187, 2010.

102. Chou R, Croswell JM, Dana T, et al.: Screening for prostate cancer: a review of the evidence for the U.S. Preventive Services Task Force, *Ann Intern Med* 155:762–771, 2011.

103. Sargeant JM, Thompson A, Valcour J, et al.: Quality of reporting of clinical trials of dogs and cats and associations with treatment effects, *J Vet Intern Med* 24:44–50, 2010.

104. Vail DM: Cancer clinical trials: development and implementation, *Vet Clin North Am Small Anim Pract* 37:1033–1057, 2007.

105. London CA, Malpas PB, Wood-Follis SL, et al.: Multi-center, placebo-controlled, double-blind, randomized study of oral toceranib phosphate (SU11654), a receptor tyrosine kinase inhibitor, for the treatment of dogs with recurrent (either local or distant) mast cell tumor following surgical excision, *Clin Cancer Res* 15:3856–3865, 2009.

106. Rau SE, Barber LG, Burgess KE: Efficacy of maropitant in the prevention of delayed vomiting associated with administration of doxorubicin to dogs, *J Vet Intern Med* 4:1452–1457, 2010.

107. Scott MC, Sarver AL, Gavin KJ, et al.: Molecular subtypes of osteosarcoma identified by reducing tumor heterogeneity through an interspecies comparative approach, *Bone* 49:356–367, 2011.

108. Modiano JF, Breen M, Burnett RC, et al.: Distinct B-cell and T-cell lymphoproliferative disease prevalence among dog breeds indicates heritable risk, *Cancer Res* 65:5654–5661, 2005.

109. Akesson A, Julin B, Wolk A: Long-term dietary cadmium intake and postmenopausal endometrial cancer incidence: a population-based prospective cohort study, *Cancer Res* 68:6435–6441, 2008.

110. Shaw J: Relationship-centered approach to cancer communication. In Withrow SJ, MacEwen EG, Page RL, editors: *Small animal clinical oncology*, ed 5, St. Louis, 2012, Elsevier, pp 272–279.

111. Raghavan M, Knapp DW, Dawson MH, et al.: Topical flea and tick pesticides and the risk of transitional cell carcinoma of the urinary bladder in Scottish Terriers, *J Am Vet Med Assoc* 225:389–394, 2004.

112. Bettini G, Morini M, Marconato L, et al.: Association between environmental dust exposure and lung cancer in dogs, *Vet J* 186:364–369, 2010.

113. Bukowski JA, Wartenberg D, Goldschmidt M: Environmental causes for sinonasal cancers in pet dogs, and their usefulness as sentinels of indoor cancer risk, *J Toxicol Environ Health A* 54:579–591, 1998.

114. Dias Pereira P, Lopes CC, Matos AJ, et al.: Influence of catechol-O-methyltransferase (COMT) genotypes on the prognosis of canine mammary tumors, *Vet Pathol* 46:1270–1274, 2009.

115. Misdorp W, Romijn A, Hart AA: Feline mammary tumors: a case-control study of hormonal factors, *Anticancer Res* 11:1793–1797, 1991.

116. Overley B, Shofer FS, Goldschmidt MH, et al.: Association between ovarihysterectomy and feline mammary carcinoma, *J Vet Intern Med* 19:560–563, 2005.

117. Hart BL, Hart LA, Thigpen AP, et al.: Neutering of German Shepherd dogs: associated joint disorders, cancers and urinary incontinence, *Vet Med and Sci* 2:191–199, 2016.

118. Perez Alenza D, Rutteman GR, Pena L, et al.: Relation between habitual diet and canine mammary tumors in a case-control study, *J Vet Intern Med* 12:132–139, 1998.

119. Raghavan M, Knapp DW, Bonney PL, et al.: Evaluation of the effect of dietary vegetable consumption on reducing risk of transitional cell carcinoma of the urinary bladder in Scottish Terriers, *J Am Vet Med Assoc* 227:94–100, 2005.
120. Hutson CA, Rideout BA, Pedersen NC: Neoplasia associated with feline immunodeficiency virus infection in cats of southern California, *J Am Vet Med Assoc* 199:1357–1362, 1991.
121. Gabor LJ, Love DN, Malik R, Canfield PJ: Feline immunodeficiency virus status of Australian cats with lymphosarcoma, *Aust Vet J* 79:540–545, 2001.
122. Dorn CR, Taylor DO, Schneider R: Sunlight exposure and risk of developing cutaneous and oral squamous cell carcinomas in white cats, *J Natl Cancer Inst* 46:1073–1078, 1971.

5

Paraneoplastic Syndromes

DENNIS B. BAILEY

Paraneoplastic syndromes (PNSs) are cancer-associated alterations in bodily structure and/or function that are not directly related to the physical effects of the primary or metastatic tumor. PNSs are most commonly caused by tumor production of small molecules (e.g., hormones, cytokines, or peptides) that are released into circulation, tumor depletion of normal small molecules, or host responses to the tumor (often immune mediated).[1]

Many PNSs parallel the underlying malignancy, and successful treatment of the tumor leads to disappearance of the PNS. Conversely, recurrence of the PNS after successful treatment can signal tumor recurrence and might even precede clinically detectable tumor. Some PNSs do not consistently resolve with treatment of the underlying malignancy, especially cancer cachexia and those of an immune or neurologic etiology.[1]

A PNS might be the first sign of malignancy, and a specific PNS often is associated with a relatively small group of tumor types. Therefore an understanding of PNSs is paramount for early cancer detection and appropriate therapy. In addition, a PNS may result in greater morbidity than that associated with the actual tumor. Therapy directed at the PNS might be warranted, especially when there is substantial morbidity and/or the underlying cancer cannot be effectively treated. Box 5.1 summarizes the most common PNSs of dogs and cats and the tumors associated with them.

Gastrointestinal Manifestations of Cancer

Cancer Anorexia and Cachexia

Several mechanisms contribute to weight loss in cancer patients. Hyporexia or anorexia is common in veterinary patients with advanced cancers, often a result of an enhanced inflammatory state and cytokines such as interleukin-1 (IL-1) and IL-6 interfering with the normal balance of anorexigenic and orexigenic signals.[2] Cancer cachexia is a profound destructive process characterized by skeletal muscle wasting, with or without loss of fat mass, and harmful abnormalities in fat and carbohydrate metabolism in spite of adequate nutrient intake.[2,3] Tumor necrosis factor-alpha (TNF-α), IL-1, and IL-6 play primary roles in cancer cachexia by inducing anorexia, increasing energy metabolism, and accelerating loss of lean body mass.[2] This results in large part from activation of nuclear factor kappa-B (NF-κB), which in turn activates the ubiquitin proteasome pathway. TNF-α, via NF-κB signaling, also upregulates myostatin, a member of the transforming growth factor-beta (TGF-β) superfamily that negatively regulates muscle mass.[2] TNF-α also interferes with the anabolic effects of growth hormone (GH) and insulin-like growth factor-1 (IGF-1).[2]

The exact diagnostic criteria for cancer cachexia continue to be debated, but moderate to severe weight loss is reported in 30% to 70% of people with various cancers.[4,5] Having said this, 40% to 60% of people are overweight or obese at the time of cancer diagnosis, and fewer than 10% have obvious malnutrition.[4] Therefore evidence of cachexia and sarcopenia was prevalent across all body mass index (BMI) categories.[4] Similarly, when body condition score (BCS) and weight loss were evaluated in dogs with various malignancies, 29% were classified as markedly overweight (BCS ≥7), and only 4% were classified as emaciated (BCS ≤3).[6] However, muscle wasting was identified in 35% of these dogs, and over the 12 months before cancer diagnosis, 14% of these dogs had lost 5% to 10% of body weight and 23% had lost >10% of body weight.[6] When BCS and muscle wasting were evaluated in cats presenting with various cancers, 44% had a BCS <5, although it is worth noting that a high percentage of these cats were diagnosed with gastrointestinal lymphoma or oral squamous cell carcinoma (SCC), tumor types in which difficulty with food intake or absorption may have been the primary causes for weight loss.[7] Muscle wasting was identified in 93% of cats, including 72% of cats with a BCS ≥5.[7] Across tumor types, low body weight and low BCS were negative prognostic factors for survival.[7]

For a detailed discussion regarding the metabolic alterations associated with cancer and nutritional support for veterinary cancer patients, the reader is directed to Chapter 16, Section B.

Gastrointestinal Ulceration

Mast cell tumors (MCTs) are the most common cause of PNS-associated gastrointestinal (GI) ulceration. Hyperhistaminemia is regarded as a main factor contributing to GI ulceration and perforation.[8,9] Histamine binds to gastric parietal cell H_2 receptors, stimulating gastric acid secretion. In addition, histamine exerts direct effects on the gastric mucosa, causing increased vascular permeability, localized protein exudation, and increased mucosal blood flow.[8] Histamine release can be spontaneous, or it can be triggered by tumor manipulation, chemotherapy, or radiation therapy (RT). Plasma histamine concentrations are elevated in dogs with macroscopic MCTs, although concentrations are not predictive of clinical signs of GI ulceration.[8,9] Symptomatic therapies such as histamine H_2 blockers, proton-pump inhibitors, misoprostol, sucralfate, and rehydration are warranted in dogs and cats with clinical signs of GI ulceration or prophylactically in patients with advanced-stage tumors. MCTs are covered in greater detail in Chapter 21.

• BOX 5.1 Paraneoplastic Syndromes and Associated Tumors

Cancer Cachexia
Multiple tumor types

Gastrointestinal Ulceration
MAST CELL TUMOR
Gastrinoma

Hypercalcemia
Dog
LYMPHOMA
ANAL SAC APOCRINE GLAND ADENOCARCINOMA
Multiple myeloma
Parathyroid tumors
Thymoma
Melanoma
Mammary tumors
Multiple others
Cat
LYMPHOMA
SQUAMOUS CELL CARCINOMA
MULTIPLE MYELOMA
Multiple others

Hypoglycemia
INSULINOMA
HEPATOCELLULAR ADENOMA/ADENOCARCINOMA
LEIOMYOMA/ LEIOMYOSARCOMA
Hemangiosarcoma
Lymphoma
Lymphocytic leukemia
Mammary carcinoma
Melanoma
Plasma cell tumor
Renal adenocarcinoma
Salivary adenocarcinoma

Hyperestrogenism
SERTOLI CELL TUMOR
Seminoma
Interstitial cell tumor
Granulosa cell tumor

Acromegaly
PITUITARY ADENOMA (CAT)

Ectopic ACTH
PRIMARY LUNG TUMOR

Hyperglobulinemia
MULTIPLE MYELOMA
Other myeloma-related disorders

Anemia
LYMPHOMA
LEUKEMIAS
HEMANGIOSARCOMA
Multiple others

Erythrocytosis
RENAL TUMORS

Nasal fibrosarcoma
Leiomyosarcoma
Schwannoma

Neutrophilic Leukocytosis
LUNG TUMORS
LYMPHOMA
Multiple others

Thrombocytopenia
LYMPHOMA
LEUKEMIAS
HEMANGIOSARCOMA
Multiple others

Disseminated Intravascular Coagulation
HEMANGIOSARCOMA
MAMMARY CARCINOMA (ESPECIALLY INFLAMMATORY)
PULMONARY ADENOCARCINOMA
Multiple others

Nodular Dermatofibrosis
RENAL CYSTADENOMA/CYSTADENOCARCIOMA (DOG)

Superficial Necrolytic Dermatitis
GLUCAGONOMA (PANCREAS, LIVER)

Feline Paraneoplastic Alopecia
PANCREATIC CARCINOMA (CAT)
BILIARY CARCINOMA (CAT)

Exfoliative Dermatitis
THYMOMA (CAT)

Glomerulonephritis
Primary erythrocytosis
Lymphocytic leukemia
Others

Myasthenia Gravis
THYMOMA
Osteosarcoma
Biliary carcinoma
Lymphoma
Oral sarcoma

Peripheral Neuropathy
INSULINOMA
LUNG TUMORS
MAMMARY TUMORS
Multiple others

Hypertrophic Osteopathy
PULMONARY METASTASIS (ESPECIALLY OSTEOSARCOMA)
PRIMARY LUNG TUMOR
Urinary tract tumors
Esophageal tumors
Other tumors and non-neoplastic etiologies

Fever
Multiple tumor types

An additional cause of PNS-associated gastroduodenal ulceration is gastrinoma, a gastrin-secreting pancreatic tumor, likely arising from the islet D-cells. Although these tumors are relatively rare, they have been reported in both dogs and cats.[10–13] Zollinger–Ellison syndrome refers to the triad of hypergastrinemia, a non–beta cell neuroendocrine tumor in the pancreas, and GI ulceration. Gastrinomas are covered in greater detail in Chapter 26.

Endocrinologic Manifestations of Cancer

Hypercalcemia

Cancer is diagnosed in 60% of dogs and 30% of cats with hypercalcemia.[14–16] In dogs, hypercalcemia of malignancy (HM) is associated most commonly with T-cell lymphoma (35%–55% of dogs with T-cell lymphoma develop HM) and anal sac apocrine gland adenocarcinoma (25% of dogs affected dogs develop HM).[15,17–22] Other reported cancers in dogs associated with HM include acute lymphoblastic leukemia, adrenal carcinoma, ameloblastoma, chronic lymphocytic leukemia, clitoral adenocarcinoma, hepatocellular carcinoma, nasal carcinoma, penile adenocarcinoma, pulmonary carcinoma, thymoma, osteosarcoma, mammary carcinoma, melanoma, multiple myeloma, pheochromocytoma, renal angiomyxoma, renal cell carcinoma, thymoma, and thyroid carcinoma.[17,23–32] In cats, HM is most commonly associated with lymphoma, SCC, and multiple myeloma.[16,33,34] Other reported HM-associated cancers in cats include fibrosarcoma, acute leukemia (including erythroleukemia), osteosarcoma, pulmonary carcinoma, renal carcinoma, thyroid carcinoma, and undifferentiated sarcoma.[16,35–37] Primary hyperparathyroidism, which usually is caused by a functional benign parathyroid adenoma or adenomatous hyperplasia, can also occur dogs and cats.[14–16]

HM is most commonly caused by soluble mediators released by the tumor cells into circulation that can then act on bone and kidneys through endocrine and paracrine pathways, which is referred to as humoral hypercalcemia of malignancy. Parathyroid hormone-related protein (PTHrP) is involved most commonly. PTHrP normally is released by fetal parathyroid glands and the placenta, where it is thought to play an important role in calcium transport across the placenta into the developing fetus, and by mammary glands, where it acts in a paracrine fashion to assist with mammary gland development and lactation.[38] PTHrP also is expressed in a wide variety of normal canine tissues: skin, anal sac, thyroid gland, mammary gland, tongue, esophagus, stomach, kidney, bladder, and lung.[39] Its function in many of these tissues is not well understood. There is 70% sequence homology of the first 13 N-terminal amino acids of PTHrP compared with PTH, which permits PTHrP to bind and activate PTH receptors on osteoblasts and renal tubular cells when released into circulation by tumor cells.[17,18,40,41]

Various other cytokines can also contribute to the pathogenesis of humoral HM, including IL-1, IL-6, TNF, and calcitriol.[17,18,40,41] HM can also be caused by osteolysis when tumors invade or metastasize to bone. Paracrine release of factors including IL-1, IL-6, TNF, receptor activator of nuclear factor kappa-B ligand (RANKL), TGF-α and -β, and prostaglandins (especially PGE_2) can increase local osteoclast number and activity.[17,18,37]

In dogs, hypercalcemia is commonly associated with polyuria/polydipsia (PU/PD), anorexia, vomiting, and occasionally muscle weakness or twitching. In cats, hypercalcemia is most commonly associated with anorexia and vomiting; PU/PD is much

less common.[16,37] PU/PD initially develops as a result of impaired action of antidiuretic hormone (ADH) on the tubular cells of the collecting duct. Dehydration is common. Renal damage can then result from renal vasoconstriction; mineralization of renal tubules, basement membranes, or interstitium; tubular degeneration or necrosis; and/or interstitial fibrosis.[37] Azotemia might or might not be reversible depending on the contributing underlying etiologies.

Measurement of ionized calcium is more accurate than total calcium, and equations that correct total calcium are not recommended.[42] However, in both dogs and cats, serum total calcium levels associated with HM tend to be higher compared with other etiologies.[15,16] In dogs and cats with humoral HM that are euhydrated and not azotemic, serum phosphate should be low to low-normal. When HM is suspected based on history, clinical signs, and baseline blood work, initial diagnostic evaluation should include a physical examination including careful palpation of peripheral lymph nodes and digital rectal examination (dogs), CBC, chemistry profile, urinalysis, thoracic radiographs, and abdominal ultrasound. If an underlying malignancy is not yet identified then cervical ultrasound; measurement of serum PTH, PTHrP, and calcitriol levels; survey bone radiographs; and/or bone marrow aspiration should be considered. Serum PTH should be low. Serum PTHrP usually is elevated, but it can be normal (not detectable). Serum calcitriol typically is normal, but it can be increased or decreased.[17,37,43]

The most effective treatment for HM is removal of the underlying cause: surgically removing the tumor or inducing a remission with chemotherapy or RT. Concurrent supportive care directed specifically at the hypercalcemia (Box 5.2) should be considered in patients that have a serum calcium concentration >16 mg/dL, patients with a calcium (mg/dL) times phosphate (mg/dL) product >60, patients that are clinically ill or azotemic, and patients with cancers that cannot be surgically removed and are unlikely to respond to chemotherapy or other therapies.[37,43] Intravenous fluid therapy with 0.9% sodium chloride (NaCl) is recommended first to correct existing dehydration and then to slightly volume expand to increase glomerular filtration rate and the filtered load of calcium. The high sodium content from 0.9% NaCl competes with calcium for renal tubular absorption, further enhancing

---

• BOX 5.2 Treatment for Hypercalcemia of Malignancy

Elimination of the inciting tumor is the primary goal for all categories of hypercalcemia.

Mild Hypercalcemia and Minimal Clinical Signs
Fluid therapy with 0.9% NaCl—rehydrated with subcutaneous or intravenous treatment

Moderate to Severe Hypercalcemia and Clinical Signs
Fluid therapy with 0.9% NaCl—correct dehydration over 4 to 6 hours, then continue at 100 to 125 mL/kg/day (1½–2 times maintenance rate)
Furosemide (2–4 mg/kg every 8–12 hours IV, SC, or PO)
Note: Only use after patient is fully rehydrated.
Prednisone (1–2 mg/kg q12–24 h PO)
Note: Only use after diagnosis obtained (see text).
Pamidronate (1.0–2.0 mg/kg diluted in 250 mL of NaCl IV over 2 hours every 2–4 weeks)
Zoledronate (0.1–0.25 mg/kg diluted in 60 mL of NaCl IV over 15 minutes every 2–4 weeks)

calciuresis. Once rehydrated, the loop diuretic furosemide can be used with continued saline diuresis to further promote urinary calcium loss. More refractory cases can be treated with bisphosphonates, which inhibit osteoclast-mediated bone resorption.[44] Pamidronate (1.0–2.0 mg/kg IV) is effective for treating HM in dogs induced by various cancers, and it also has been shown to be an effective treatment in both dogs and cats with hypercalcemia secondary to nonneoplastic conditions.[45] In humans, zoledronate is more effective at inducing normocalcemia and maintains normocalcemia for a longer duration.[46] It also is less nephrotoxic than pamidronate.[44,47] Zoledronate has not been evaluated for HM in veterinary patients, but it has been used safely in dogs with malignant osteolysis (dose 0.1–0.25 mg/kg IV).[47] In those rare situations in which marked hypercalcemia with life-threatening consequences (e.g., coma) require immediate correction, the use of salmon calcitonin (4-8 IU/kg, S.C., q8–12 hours) will more rapidly lower blood calcium than bisphosphonates; however, its use is limited by expense, availability, and the propensity for tachyphylaxis (rapid resistance to effects) to occur within days.[37]

Glucocorticoid steroids can quickly induce a rapid reduction in serum calcium level. However, *it is essential that a definitive cause for hypercalcemia be identified before any steroid therapy is initiated.* If lymphoma or another hematopoietic tumor is the underlying cause of HM, the premature use of steroids can interfere with the ability to confirm a diagnosis, necessitating additional diagnostics and/or discontinuation of the steroids and waiting for the cancer to become clinically evident again. In addition, steroids can induce resistance to other chemotherapy agents, decreasing the ability to attain a complete remission and shortening the length of survival.[48]

Hypoglycemia

The most common cause of paraneoplastic hypoglycemia in the dog is insulinoma (pancreatic beta-cell tumor).[49,50] Functional pancreatic beta-cell tumors typically produce excess amounts of insulin, but rarely they can also release IGF-1 or IGF-2.[51,52] The reader is directed to Chapter 26 for a discussion of insulinomas.

The non–islet cell tumors most commonly associated with paraneoplastic hypoglycemia are primary liver tumors (hepatocellular adenocarcinoma and adenoma) and smooth muscle tumors (leiomyosarcoma and leiomyoma, with tumors arising from liver, stomach, duodenum, and jejunum).[53–57] Case reports also exist for paraneoplastic hypoglycemia associated with a variety of other tumors, including hemangiosarcoma (HSA), lymphoma, lymphocytic leukemia, mammary carcinoma, melanoma, plasma cell tumor, renal adenocarcinoma, and salivary adenocarcinoma.[53,58–60] Tumor cell production of IGF-2 is the most common mechanism for paraneoplastic hypoglycemia in non–islet cell tumors.[1,53,54,61] Other mechanisms include production of IGF-1 or somatomedins, hypermetabolism of glucose, production of substances stimulating insulin release, production of hepatic glucose inhibitor, insulin binding by a monoclonal immunoglobulin (plasma cell tumors), insulin receptor proliferation, or rarely, ectopic insulin production.[1]

Insulinomas usually are small, and visualization on abdominal ultrasound is inconsistent.[49,50] The diagnosis is most often made by documenting hypoglycemia along with an inappropriately elevated serum insulin level. In contrast, most intraabdominal non–islet cell tumors causing hypoglycemia are large and readily identifiable on abdominal palpation or ultrasound.[53–56] The reader is directed to Chapter 26 for an extensive discussion of the

clinical consequences, diagnosis, and therapy of tumor-induced hypoglycemia.

Hyperestrogenism

The tumor most commonly associated with hyperestrogenism is the Sertoli cell tumor. Overall, 25% to 50% of dogs with Sertoli cell tumors will display clinical signs of hyperestrogenism.[62–64] Approximately half of canine Sertoli cell tumors develop in cryptorchid testes, and clinical hyperestrogenism occurs more commonly when Sertoli cell tumors develop in cryptorchid testes.[63–65] Therefore a Sertoli cell tumor must remain a differential diagnosis when a dog presents with clinical signs of hyperestrogenism, even if a testicular mass is not palpated on physical examination. Ultrasound is then indicated to screen for an inguinal or intraabdominal tumor. Paraneoplastic hyperestrogenism also can occur rarely in dogs with seminomas, interstitial cell tumors, and ovarian granulosa cell tumors.[66–68] This PNS has not been reported in cats.

Dogs with Sertoli cell tumors have significantly higher plasma estradiol-17β levels compared with healthy controls.[69] Sertoli cell tumors also have lower expression of 5α-reductase type 1 than normal testes, and plasma testosterone levels were lower in affected dogs.[69,70] Clinical signs of feminization secondary to Sertoli cell tumors correlated best with reductions in the testosterone/estradiol ratio rather than absolute increases in estradiol-17β.[69]

Clinical signs of hyperestrogenism include bilaterally symmetric alopecia, cutaneous hyperpigmentation, epidermal thinning, gynecomastia, galactorrhea, pendulous prepuce, penile atrophy, atrophy of the contralateral testicle, either prostatic atrophy or prostatomegaly (the latter secondary to squamous metaplasia), and attraction of other males.[62,63] Estrogen also can have myelotoxic effects. Bone marrow toxicosis is characterized initially by a transient increase in granulocytopoiesis and neutrophilic leukocytosis, followed by progressive bone marrow hypoplasia or aplasia leading to aplastic anemia (nonregenerative anemia, thrombocytopenia, and leukopenia).[63] Severely pancytopenic dogs can present with additional clinical signs associated with anemia (weakness, lethargy, pale mucous membranes, tachycardia), thrombocytopenia (petechia, ecchymoses, epistaxis, GI bleeding) and/or leukopenia (infection, sepsis). The clinical signs of hyperestrogenism will resolve with surgical removal of the Sertoli cell tumor, but this can take several months. Consequently, the mortality rate for dogs with severe myelotoxicosis and pancytopenia is high.[62,63]

Acromegaly (Hypersomatropism)

In cats, acromegaly is caused by hypersomatropism—excessive GH secretion by a functional pituitary adenoma arising from somatotroph cells.[71–73] In contrast, canine acromegaly most commonly results from progestin-induced GH secretion by mammary ductal epithelium. However, there are case reports of two GH-producing mammary tumors and one GH-producing pituitary tumor in dogs.[74,75]

GH antagonizes insulin by reducing insulin receptors and interfering with a wide range of postreceptor processes.[71–73] The vast majority of cats initially present with diabetes mellitus, and insulin resistance is common. Over time, the chronic exposure to excess GH results in overgrowth of connective tissue, bone, and viscera. Cats can develop broad facial features, prognathica inferior, diffuse thickening of the oropharyngeal tissues, hepatomegaly, renomegaly, adrenomegaly, hypertrophic cardiomyopathy, clubbing of the paws and distal extremities, and degenerative arthropathy.[71–73] Many effects of GH are mediated by IGF-1, and because GH assays are not readily available, measurement of serum IGF-1 remains the most practical way to confirm feline hypersomatotropism.[73] The reader is directed to Chapter 26 for a more detailed discussion regarding feline acromegaly.

Ectopic Adrenocorticotropic Hormone Syndrome

The ectopic production of adrenocorticotropic hormone (ACTH) or ACTH-like substances is a common PNS in humans.[1] About 3% to 5% of people with small cell lung cancer develop hyperadrenocorticism. This PNS also is reported in people with other carcinomas, including pancreatic carcinoma, thymic carcinoma, and carcinoids. This PNS results from expression of the proopiomelanocortin gene, which contains not only ACTH, but also melanocyte-stimulating hormone, lipotropin, endorphins, and enkephalins.[1] As a result, patients present with clinical signs typical of hyperadrenocorticism (Cushing's disease), but occasionally will also have other clinical signs such as hyperpigmentation. The diagnosis is made based on documentation of increased urine cortisol, a dexamethasone suppression test where serum cortisol is consistently suppressed, and elevated plasma levels of ACTH or ACTH precursors.[1] This PNS is very rare in veterinary oncology, with single case reports in dogs with a primary lung tumor, a metastatic neuroendocrine tumor arising in the pancreas, and a hepatic carcinoid.[76–78] When clinical signs cannot be controlled with surgery, trilostane is an effective alternative.[77]

Hematologic Manifestations of Cancer

Hyperglobulinemia and Bence Jones Proteinuria

Hyperglobulinemia, or more specifically monoclonal gammopathy or paraproteinemia, is seen most commonly with multiple myeloma, but also has been reported with all other myeloma-related disorders (MRD) including solitary plasma cell tumor of bone, extramedullary plasmacytoma (cutaneous and noncutaneous), IgM (Waldenström's) macroglobulinemia, plasma cell leukemia, Ig-secreting lymphoma, and Ig-secreting chronic lymphocytic leukemia.[79–82] MRD tumor cells typically produce an overabundance of a single type or component of immunoglobulin, which is referred to as the M component. On serum electrophoresis, a narrow-based spike typically is identified in the gamma region (i.e., monoclonal gammopathy), although on rare occasion it can extend into the beta region.[83] Biclonal spikes also have been reported in both dogs and cats.[80,84,85] M components can interfere with coagulation primarily by coating platelets, inhibiting platelet aggregation to damaged endothelial surfaces and release of platelet factor 3.[79,83] M components also can lead to hyperviscosity syndrome (see later).

Intact Ig molecules usually are released by plasma cells, but occasionally there is an imbalance in heavy and light chain production. If there is an excess of free light chain, they will be excreted in the urine—Bence Jones proteinuria. Bence Jones proteinuria is diagnosed on urine electrophoresis; it is not detected on routine urine dipstick.[86,87] Bence Jones proteins can cause light-chain renal tubular casts, leading to interstitial nephritis and possibly renal failure.[79,83]

Hyperviscosity Syndrome

Hyperviscosity syndrome refers to a constellation of clinical signs caused by an increase in blood viscosity. It can occur in patients with MRD (see Hyperglobulinemia, earlier), polycythemia vera (see Chapter 33, Section C), or paraneoplastic erythrocytosis (see Erythrocytosis, later).[79,88–91] In patients with MRD, hyperviscosity syndrome occurs most frequently in patients with IgM macroglobulinemia because IgM typically forms a high molecular weight pentamer.[79,91] When it occurs in patients with multiple myeloma, the M-component is more commonly IgA than IgG, as the former exists as a dimer and occasionally will polymerize, and the latter is a monomer.[79]

The clinical signs of hyperviscosity syndrome result from sludging of blood in small vessels, ineffective delivery of oxygen and nutrients, and coagulation abnormalities. Reported neurologic signs include stuporous mentation, ataxia, and seizures.[79,88,89] Ocular abnormalities include enlarged and tortuous retinal vessels, retinal hemorrhages, and retinal detachment, often resulting in acute-onset blindness.[79,88,92] Bleeding diathesis, hypertrophic cardiomyopathy, and congestive heart failure can also occur.[79,83,88,93]

In severe cases of hyperviscosity syndrome, emergency treatment is warranted. Plasmapheresis is indicated when hyperviscosity is caused by serum proteins.[93,94] Phlebotomy and intravenous fluids are indicated when hyperviscosity is caused by erythrocytosis.[90]

Anemia

The true prevalence of anemia in veterinary cancer patients is unknown, but it is likely one of the most common PNS observed. Anemia is reported in 30% to 43% of dogs and 43% to 58% of cats with lymphoma, and it is a negative prognostic factor in both species.[83,95–97] It also is commonly reported in dogs and cats with leukemias and HSA, and dogs with disseminated MCT and histiocytic sarcoma (HS).[83] The pathogenic mechanisms common to all anemias—blood loss, increased red blood cell (RBC) destruction (hemolysis), and decreased RBC production—can each play a role in cancer-related anemia, and multiple mechanisms can simultaneously contribute to the anemia observed in a given patient.

Anemia secondary to hemorrhage classically is regenerative, although it can take 2 to 3 days after the onset of bleeding for reticulocytosis to be present, and is accompanied by hypoproteinemia.[98] Acute, severe hemorrhage is most commonly associated with splenic HSA, but it also can occur in dogs with other benign and malignant splenic tumors, adrenal medullary and cortical carcinomas, hepatocellular carcinoma, and thyroid carcinoma.[98–101] Chronic, low-grade hemorrhage can occur with tumors involving the GI tract, nasal cavity, urinary bladder, and with tumors causing paraneoplastic GI ulceration (see earlier).[83] With chronic external hemorrhage iron deficiency can result, characterized by microcytosis, hypochromasia, low serum iron, and low saturation of transferrin.[102]

Hemolytic anemias can be immune mediated or non–immune mediated. Immune-mediated hemolytic anemia (IMHA) is characterized by severe anemia that is usually but not always adequately regenerative, along with spherocytes, autoagglutination, and/or a positive direct agglutination test (Coombs test).[103] Hemoglobinemia and/or hyperbilirubinemia are also commonly seen. IMHA is most commonly idiopathic in dogs and secondary to feline leukemia virus (FeLV) infection in cats, but it can be secondary to neoplasia in both species.[83,103] Lymphoma and leukemias are the cancers most frequently associated with IMHA in both small animals and humans.[83,103]

Non–immune mediated hemolytic anemia can arise secondary to microangiopathy, tumor cell erythrophagocytosis, or oxidative damage to erythrocytes. Microangiopathic hemolytic anemia (MAHA) is caused by endothelial cell injury and fibrin deposition, most commonly seen in patients with disseminated intravascular coagulation (DIC), and by inherent abnormalities in tumor vasculature, most notably with HSA.[83,104,105] These pathologic alterations cause shearing and destruction of erythrocytes, resulting in increased numbers of schistocytes in peripheral blood. Clinically significant tumor cell erythrophagocytosis is seen most commonly with HS, particularly the hemophagocytic variant.[106–108] In addition to a markedly regenerative anemia, common clinicopathologic abnormalities include a negative direct agglutination test, thrombocytopenia, hypoalbuminemia, and hypocholesterolemia. Erythrophagocytosis, with or without secondary anemia, has also been documented in dogs with lymphoma, plasma cell tumors, and acute megakaryoblastic leukemia, and in cats with lymphoma and mast cell tumor (MCT).[83] Oxidative injury to erythrocytes is characterized by Heinz bodies and/or eccentrocytes. In retrospective studies, 15% of dogs with eccentrocytosis, and 11% of cats with Heinz body anemia had underlying malignancies.[109,110] Lymphoma was the most common cancer for both species.

Nonregenerative anemias result from cancers directly or indirectly affecting erythropoiesis. Cancer cells can infiltrate the marrow and replace normal hematopoietic tissue, a condition called myelophthisis. This is seen most commonly with hematopoietic cancers, such as acute leukemias, lymphoma, multiple myeloma, mast cell neoplasia, and disseminated HS.[83,104,108,111–114] Aplastic anemia can result from paraneoplastic hyperestrogenism (see earlier). Decreased serum folate and cobalamin (vitamin B_{12}) concentrations have been reported in cats with GI lymphoma.[115] One of the most common causes of anemia in cancer patients is anemia of inflammatory disease (AID, also called anemia of chronic disease). This is characterized by a mild to moderate nonregenerative, normocytic, normochromic anemia. Inflammatory cytokines such as TNF-α, interferon-gamma (IFN-γ), IL-1, IL-6, and IL-10 reduce the production of endogenous erythropoietin in the face of hypoxemia, and suppress the erythroid progenitor response to erythropoietin.[102] IL-6 increases production of hepcidin by the liver. Hepcidin is an acute phase protein that causes increased cellular internalization and degradation of ferroportin, a membrane bound protein that exports iron from macrophages, hepatocytes, and duodenal enterocytes into the peripheral blood.[83,102] The net effect is the sequestration of iron, resulting in hypoferremia and decreased availability of iron for erythropoiesis.

Erythrocytosis (Polycythemia)

Paraneoplastic erythrocytosis has been reported in dogs with a variety or renal tumors (carcinoma; adenocarcinoma; fibrosarcoma; and lymphoma, with or without other organ involvement), nasal fibrosarcoma, cecal leiomyosarcoma, and spinal cord schwannoma.[60,116–124] It also has been reported in cats with renal adenocarcinoma.[125] Paraneoplastic erythrocytosis is associated with increased serum erythropoietin levels. The erythropoietin is most often produced by the tumor cells.[117,118,121,123] However, it also has been hypothesized that elevated erythropoietin levels might result from impaired renal blood flow causing local tissue hypoxia.[90,121] In people, paraneoplastic erythrocytosis can also result from tumor cells producing androgenic hormones and prostaglandins that enhance the effects of erythropoietin.[1]

It is important to rule out other causes for erythrocytosis. Relative erythrocytosis results from dehydration. Absolute erythrocytosis can be primary (polycythemia vera) or secondary to chronic respiratory disease, heart disease causing right-to-left shunting, or nonneoplastic renal disease.[90] Classically, dogs and cats with paraneoplastic erythrocytosis will have elevated serum erythropoietin levels, but there is considerable overlap with dogs and cats that are normal and even those with polycythemia vera.[90,126]

Paraneoplastic erythrocytosis typically resolves with removal of the primary tumor. However, patients presenting with hyperviscosity syndrome might require emergency treatment before surgery or chemotherapy induction (see Hyperviscosity Syndrome, earlier).[90,125]

Leukocytosis

Mild to moderate neutrophilic leukocytosis is common in dogs and cats with cancer, and is usually attributable to inflammation or tissue necrosis associated with the cancer; however, extreme neutrophilic leukocytosis (≥70,000 cells/μL), often with a left shift, monocytosis, and eosinophilia, has been reported in dogs with pulmonary carcinoma, renal tumors, intestinal T-cell lymphoma, metastatic fibrosarcoma, and adenomatous rectal polyps, and in cats with pulmonary SCC and dermal tubular adenocarcinoma.[83,127–133] This is thought to arise because of tumor production of granulocyte colony-stimulating factor (G-CSF) and/or granulocyte-macrophage colony-stimulating factor (GM-CSF).[83,131,132] Extreme neutrophilic leukocytosis, also referred to as a leukemoid response, can be difficult to distinguish from chronic myelogenous leukemia (CML), as the prevalence of the characteristic cytogenetic abnormalities identified in people with CML, although identified in dogs, has not been determined.[134,134b] This PNS is generally thought to have minimal clinical significance, although a retrospective study evaluating dogs with severe leukocytosis (≥50,000 white blood cells [WBC]/μL, with >50% neutrophils) resulting from a variety or neoplastic and nonneoplastic etiologies identified a high mortality rate.[135]

Eosinophilia is an uncommon PNS in veterinary cancer patients, but is seen most frequently in dogs and cats with MCT and lymphoma, particularly T-cell lymphoma.[136–140] Mast cells produce the eosinophilic cytokine IL-5 and other eosinophil chemotactic factors, and in people T-cell lymphomas have been documented to produce IL-5.[136,139] Eosinophilia also has been reported in dogs with oral fibrosarcoma, mammary carcinoma, and leiomyosarcoma, and in cats with oral SCC and bladder transitional cell carcinoma.[83,141–144] Eosinophilia is also frequently seen as part of a leukemoid response.

Thrombocytopenia

Thirteen percent to 36% of dogs with cancer present with thrombocytopenia before any treatment,[145,146] and 39% of thrombocytopenic cats are diagnosed with underlying neoplasia.[147] In both species, thrombocytopenia is especially common with hematopoietic and vascular cancers.[145–147] General mechanisms for thrombocytopenia include decreased platelet production, increased platelet destruction, increased platelet sequestration, and increased platelet consumption. However, in a series of 214 thrombocytopenic dogs with cancer, 61% had no identifiable explanation for their thrombocytopenia, although not all dogs had exhaustive diagnostic evaluations.[146]

As with anemia, decreased platelet production can result from myelophthisis and hyperestrogenism (see earlier). Cancer-associated immune-mediated thrombocytopenia is most commonly associated with lymphoma, multiple myeloma, and HS, but also has been reported with mammary adenocarcinoma, MCT, HSA, nasal adenocarcinoma, and fibrosarcoma.[148–151] Non–immune-mediated platelet destruction in cancer patients most commonly occurs secondary to microangiopathy. The spleen normally stores about one third of the body's platelets, and tumors causing diffuse splenomegaly can increase platelet sequestration. This occurs most commonly with splenic lymphoma and feline splenic MCT, but also can occur with highly vascularized tumors such as hemangioma and HSA.[83,151] Increased consumption can occur secondary to hemorrhage. Severe, acute hemorrhage frequently causes thrombocytopenia.[98] Chronic low-grade hemorrhage is more likely to cause thrombocytosis; thrombocytopenia results only when the regenerative capacity of the bone marrow has been exhausted.[151] More importantly, increased platelet consumption can result from the hypercoagulable state that is common in cancer patients (see later).[83,151] Platelet counts and kinetics were evaluated in 52 tumor-bearing and 24 normal dogs.[152] Tumor-bearing dogs had significantly lower platelet counts and shorter mean survival time of circulating platelets. In addition, mean platelet survival time was the shortest for dogs with metastatic cancers.

Coagulopathies and Disseminated Intravascular Coagulation

Hypocoagulability can result from thrombocytopenia and alterations in platelet function secondary to paraproteinemia (see earlier). Hemorrhagic diathesis also can result from blood hyperviscosity (see earlier). The most common clotting factor dysfunction seen in veterinary cancer patients results from the release of heparin by MCT, which acts as a cofactor for antithrombin III to inactivate clotting factors XII, XI, X, and IX.[139]

Hypercoagulability is much more common in cancer patients. In human cancer patients, thromboembolic disease can manifest as deep venous thrombosis, pulmonary thromboembolism (PE), migratory superficial thrombophlebitis (Trousseau's syndrome), nonbacterial thrombotic endocarditis, and DIC.[83] In dogs with various untreated cancers, platelet aggregation in response to agonists (collagen, adenosine diphosphonate, or platelet-activating factor) was significantly greater compared with healthy control dogs.[153,154] Thromboelastography documented hypercoagulability in 56% of dogs with lymphoma and 50% of dogs with various other cancers.[83,155] Although many of these patients did not necessarily have clinical manifestations of hypercoagulability, underlying cancer was identified in 27% of dogs with portal vein thrombosis, 30% with PE, and 54% with splenic vein thrombosis.[156–158]

DIC is a syndrome of systemic activation of coagulation, leading to widespread microthrombosis. Consumption of platelets and clotting factors can then lead to uncontrollable hemorrhage. Cancer is one of the most common causes of DIC. One study estimated 10% of dogs with cancer to have DIC.[159] Tumors with the highest incidences include HSA (with up to 50% of dogs affected at initial evaluation), mammary adenocarcinoma (particularly inflammatory mammary carcinoma), and pulmonary adenocarcinoma.[105,159,160] It is worth noting, though, that these studies focused primarily on acute phase DIC, characterized by obvious laboratory abnormalities and

clinical signs of organ dysfunction caused by microthrombosis and/or hemorrhage. The compensated chronic phase, where time exists for replenishment of coagulation factors, anticoagulation proteins, and platelets, is more difficult to diagnose and likely even more prevalent.[83]

The pathogenesis of thromboembolic disease in cancer patients is complex and multifactorial. One of the major causes for hemodynamic derangement is the inherent abnormalities of tumor microvasculature, including absent or incomplete endothelial coverage, vessel tortuosity, variations in vascular caliber, and blood flow turbulence.[83,105] Hyperviscosity or tumor invasion into blood vessels can further contribute.[83] There also is considerable "cross talk" between the inflammatory and coagulation pathways. Tissue factor, expressed on monocytes and endothelial cells during inflammation and on some cancer cells, complexes with factor VIIa to activate the extrinsic clotting cascade.[161] This is the major stimulus for thrombin production in DIC. In addition, TNF-α, IL-1, and IL-6 can directly activate certain clotting factors and downregulate protein C-thrombomodulin expression on endothelial cells.[83,161]

Thrombosis initially was thought to be merely a consequence of cancer, but more recent evidence supports that it might be a necessary intrinsic step in cancer progression. Fibrin deposition around neoplastic foci forms a provisional extracellular matrix for angiogenesis.[83,162] In addition, the formation of fibrin–platelet–tumor cell complexes increases adhesion to endothelium and enhances metastatic efficiency.[83,162]

Cutaneous Manifestations of Cancer

Nodular Dermatofibrosis

Nodular dermatofibrosis (ND) is a well-recognized PNS characterized by multiple slowly growing cutaneous collagenous nodules in association with bilateral renal cystadenocarcinomas or cystadenomas.[163–168] Almost all reported cases have been in German shepherd dogs, and pedigree analysis strongly indicates autosomal dominant inheritance.[168] The ND-associated mutation was mapped to the *BHD* gene on chromosome 5.[169] This is the causative gene for the human renal cancer syndrome Birt–Hogg–Dubé syndrome, which bears some similarities to renal cystadenocarcinoma/nodular dermatofibrosis. The function of folliculin, the protein encoded by the *BHD* gene, is unknown.

Most dogs present with multiple firm cutaneous nodules ranging in size from 2 mm to 5 cm that are not painful or pruritic (Fig. 5.1). Lesions are found predominantly on the limbs, although the head and trunk may be affected in advanced cases. Histologically, the nodules consist of irregular bundles of dense, well-differentiated collagen fibers in the dermis or subcutis.[165,166] ND almost always precedes systemic signs of illness related to tumor-induced renal failure or metastasis by months to years, although microscopically detectable renal changes can occur at a young age. Affected females almost always have concurrent uterine leiomyomas that carry little clinical significance.[163,164]

Currently, there is no effective therapy for the underlying cancer. Affected dogs develop multiple tumors bilaterally, precluding surgery, and chemotherapy has not been evaluated. Palliative surgical removal of cutaneous nodules can be considered when they are ulcerated or interfering with function. Mean time from first observation of ND until death is about 2.5 years.[163,168]

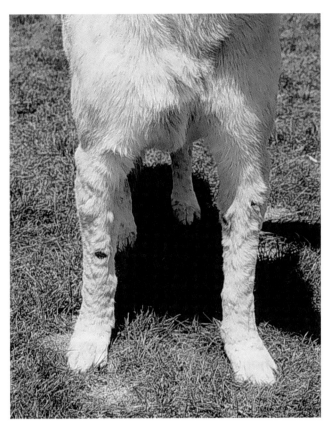

• **Fig. 5.1** Diffuse nodular dermatofibrosis (ND) in a German shepherd dog. The nodules are composed of extremely dense but well-differentiated collagen tissue (collagenous nevi) and are found predominately on the limbs, although the head and trunk may be affected in advanced cases.

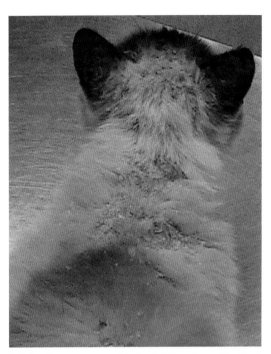

• **Fig. 5.2** Feline thymoma-associated exfoliative dermatitis. Regional alopecia involves the head, neck, and dorsal thorax with extensive scaling and focal crusts.

Superficial Necrolytic Dermatitis

Superficial necrolytic dermatitis (SND) is seen most commonly in dogs with hepatic disease (i.e., hepatocutaneous syndrome),[170–173] but it also reported as a paraneoplastic syndrome in dogs and cats with glucagon-secreting tumors in the pancreas and liver.[163,171–178] Necrolytic migratory erythema (NME) refers to the human analog of paraneoplastic SND.

The major dermatologic findings of SND are erosions and ulcerations, with alopecia, exudation, and adherent crusts on the feet, pressure points (such as the elbow or hock), flank, perineal area, muzzle, facial mucocutaneous junctions, and/or oral cavity. Hyperkeratosis and fissuring of foot pads occurs in all affected animals. Lesions may be painful and pruritic. Hypoaminoacidemia is a common feature in both paraneoplastic SND and hepatocutaneous syndrome.[163,171–174] It has been hypothesized that the elevated glucagon levels sustain gluconeogenesis and amino acid catabolism, resulting in hypoaminoacidemia that then leads to epidermal protein depletion and subsequent keratinocyte necrolysis.

Resolution of SND was reported in one dog with a solitary pancreatic glucagon secreting tumor that underwent surgery.[175] However, most dogs present with metastatic disease. Another dog was successfully treated with the somatostatin analog octeotride.[176] Amino acid infusions have been used in people with NME and dogs with hepatocutaneous syndrome.[163,171,172]

Feline Paraneoplastic Alopecia

Feline paraneoplastic alopecia has been reported in cats with pancreatic carcinoma and biliary carcinoma.[163,179–183] It is a nonpruritic, symmetric, progressive alopecia affecting primarily the ventrum and medial aspect of the limbs. Hair is easily epilated, and skin is shiny, inelastic, and thin, but not fragile. Foot pad involvement also is common. Affected pads are painful and can be dry, crusted, and fissured, or moist and erythematous. One study showed that *Malassezia* spp. dermatitis is rare in cats, and 7 of 15 affected cats had skin biopsy changes consistent with feline paraneoplastic alopecia, and pancreatic carcinoma was confirmed in 4 of these cats.[184] Given the aggressive biologic behaviors of pancreatic and biliary carcinomas, most cats presented with metastatic disease and were euthanized soon after diagnosis. However, in one cat with a solitary pancreatic tumor, skin changes resolved after surgery.[180]

Feline Thymoma-Associated Exfoliative Dermatitis

Paraneoplastic exfoliative dermatitis has been reported in cats with thymoma.[163,185–187] It begins as nonpruritic scaling and mild erythema on the head and pinnae, and then progressively involves the neck, trunk, and limbs (Fig. 5.2). With time, the scaling intensifies and alopecia develops. Keratosebaceous debris accumulates between the digits, in the nail beds, and in the ear canals. Crusts and ulcers may develop. One reported cat also had a secondary concurrent *Malassezia* spp. infection.[186] The underlying mechanism is unknown, but the presence of an interface dermatitis and lymphoid cellular infiltrate on histopathology suggests a tumor-induced immune-mediated process.[185] Most cats reported in the literature did not undergo treatment for their thymoma, but one that did undergo surgical removal had complete resolution of skin lesions.[186]

Renal Manifestations of Cancer

Glomerular Disorders

A variety of paraneoplastic glomerular disorders have been reported in people. Membranous nephropathy is reported most commonly and is associated with a variety of solid tumors.[1,188] It is hypothesized that tumor antigens are deposited in the glomeruli, and antibodies then bind to form immune complexes that activate complement.[1] Paraneoplastic glomerular disorders likely are underreported in veterinary cancer patients with only two case reports, one in a dog with primary erythrocytosis and one in a dog with lymphocytic leukemia.[189,190]

Miscellaneous Syndromes

Paraneoplastic nephrogenic diabetes insipidus was reported in a dog with intestinal leiomyosarcoma.[191] In addition, PU and PD and renal damage are commonly reported in dogs with paraneoplastic hypercalcemia, and occasionally in cats (see earlier). PU and PD also were reported in the rare cases of ectopic adrenocortoctropic hormone syndrome identified in dogs (see earlier).

Neurologic Manifestations of Cancer

Myasthenia Gravis

Paraneoplastic myasthenia gravis (MG) is reported most commonly in dogs and cats with thymoma,[192–200] but it also has been reported in dogs with osteosarcoma, cholangiocellular carcinoma, oral sarcoma, and nonepitheliotropic cutaneous lymphoma.[201–204] As with all forms of acquired MG, this is an immune-mediated disease where antibodies are formed against nicotinic acetylcholine (ACh) receptors on the postsynaptic sarcolemmal surface within the neuromuscular junction. Interestingly, patients with thymomas have been diagnosed with a variety of other immune-mediated diseases as well: exfoliative dermatitis and pemphigus vulgaris in cats;[185,200] polyarthritis, masticatory muscle myositis, perianal fistula, immune-mediated thrombocytopenia, and hypothyroidism in dogs.[192]

Generalized MG is associated with appendicular muscle weakness that is often but not always exercise induced. Concurrent weakness involving the muscles of the esophagus (megaesophagus), face, pharynx, and/or larynx can be present as well. Focal myasthenia gravis most commonly involves these latter muscle groups. The definitive diagnosis for acquired MG usually is made by demonstrating circulating antibodies against ACh receptors, although a small percentage of patients are seronegative. A positive edrophonium chloride challenge test is also helpful in dogs with generalized MG.

Surgical removal of the thymoma and/or RT is recommended to help reduce anti-ACh receptor antibody levels and improve clinical signs of MG, but response is inconsistent.[195–198] In recent studies, neither MG nor megaesophagus affected prognosis in dogs or cats with thymoma.[192,198,199] However, patients with megaesophagus have a high risk of aspiration pneumonia, and this is a common cause of perioperative morbidity and mortality.[192,193,198] Therefore, whenever possible, it is recommended that clinical signs of MG be controlled before anesthesia and surgery. Consultation with a neurologist regarding anticholinesterase therapy (pyridostigmine bromide) and immunosuppressive therapy is recommended.

Peripheral Neuropathy

Paraneoplastic peripheral nerve lesions are relatively common. When peroneal and ulnar nerve fibers were analyzed from dogs with a wide variety of cancers, paranodal/segmental demyelination and remyelination were seen most commonly, followed by axonal degeneration manifested by myelin ovoids and myelin globules.[205,206] These lesions are also reported in normal dogs with increasing age, but 16 of 21 dogs had a significantly greater number of lesions compared with age-matched controls.[205] Tumors associated with the highest percentages of abnormalities were bronchogenic carcinoma, mammary adenocarcinoma, melanoma, insulinoma, and osteosarcoma. Interestingly, though, none of the dogs in that study showed clinical signs consistent with a diffuse or localized neuropathy. Clinical paraneoplastic polyneuropathies, usually characterized by diffuse lower motor neuron signs, are much less common. They have been reported in dogs with insulinoma, multiple myeloma, lymphoma, fibrosarcoma, leiomyosarcoma, anaplastic sarcoma, pancreatic adenocarcinoma, prostatic adenocarcinoma, combined mixed mammary gland adenoma and pulmonary adenoma, and combined pulmonary carcinoma and metastatic HSA, and in a cat with renal lymphoma.[207–213]

Miscellaneous Manifestations of Cancer

Hypertrophic Osteopathy

Hypertrophic osteopathy (HO) is a generalized osteoproductive disorder of the periosteum that affects the long bones of the extremities, typically beginning on the digits and then progressing proximally. Lesions typically are bilaterally symmetric and involve all four limbs.[214] Paraneoplastic HO is most commonly associated with primary lung tumors or tumors that have metastasized to the lungs. Two studies both reported that the majority of dogs with paraneoplastic HO presented with pulmonary metastasis, and the most common tumor type was osteosarcoma.[214,215] Paraneoplastic HO without evidence of pulmonary involvement has been reported in dogs with renal transitional cell carcinoma and nephroblastoma, urinary bladder botryoid rhabdomyosarcoma, hepatocellular carcinoma, esophageal adenocarcinoma, prostatic carcinoma, and malignant schwannoma derived from the vagus nerve,[132,216–221] and in cats with adrenocortical carcinoma and renal adenoma.[222,223] Nonneoplastic diseases associated with HO include infectious/inflammatory lung disease, *Dirofilaria immitis* infection, bacterial endocarditis, patent ductus arteriosus with right-to-left shunting, *Spirocera lupi* esophageal granulomas, esophageal foreign body, and congenital megaesophagus.[214] Idiopathic HO has been reported in cats.[224,225] Cats with primary lung tumors can also develop digital metastasis, which can have a similar clinical presentation to HO.[226]

Affected patients most commonly present with swelling and/or edema of the distal limbs and lameness or difficulty ambulating. Limbs are often painful on palpation and/or warm to the touch.[214,215] One study also reported a high incidence of concurrent bilateral serous to mucopurulent ocular discharge and episcleral injection.[214] Fewer than half of affected patients have respiratory signs at the time of initial presentation.[214] When radiographs are taken of the distal extremities, symmetric periosteal new bone formation appears nodular or speculated, classically radiating 90 degrees from the long axis of the affected bones (Fig. 5.3). There also is often evidence of adjacent soft tissue swelling and edema.

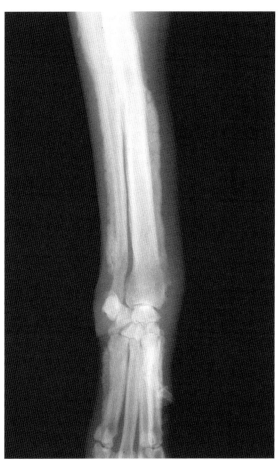

• **Fig. 5.3** Hypertrophic osteopathy (HO), seen radiographically in the distal forelimb of a dog with a primary lung tumor. Note the spiculated periosteal new bone formation radiating 90 degrees from the long axis of the radius, ulna, and metacarpal bones.

The pathogenesis of HO is not well understood. The classic pathophysiologic changes are increased peripheral blood flow, proliferation of vascular connective tissue, and ultimately bone spicule formation.[214] A neural reflex that originates in the thorax and is carried by afferent vagal fibers has been proposed,[132,214,220,221,227] and regression of HO has been reported in dogs after undergoing vagotomy.[221,227] More recently, humoral mechanisms have been hypothesized. People with lung cancer and HO have higher levels of serum growth hormone, growth hormone–releasing hormone, vascular endothelial growth factor (VEGF), and platelet-derived growth factor (PDGF).[228] Elevated levels of these and other hormones might result from tissue hypoxia, along with decreased pulmonary clearance because of pathologic shunting.[214,228] It also has been shown that circulating megakaryocytes and platelet clumps that normally become trapped in pulmonary capillary beds can bypass these capillaries, again due to pathologic shunting, and they subsequently can become lodged in the distal extremities and release PDGF.[229]

Whenever possible, the treatment for HO is removal of the underlying cancer. However, dogs more commonly present with pulmonary metastasis rather than a solitary lung mass. Pulmonary metastatectomy can be considered when there are only a few metastatic lesions.[230] Chemotherapy can be used for sensitive cancers as well.[231] In people, pamidronate and zoledronate are effective palliative treatments to control pain.[232] They have not been evaluated in veterinary patients with HO, but they have been used successfully to manage pain associated with primary bone tumors (see Chapter 25) and are thus a rational choice.

Fever

Paraneoplastic fever can result as part of an innate immune response against tumor antigens or areas of tumor necrosis. Fever is mediated primarily by TNF-α, IL-1, and IL-6 on the hypothalamus. These cytokines activate the arachidonic acid cascade, producing prostaglandin E_2, which acts on the thermoregulatory center of the hypothalamus.[233] The exact incidence of paraneoplastic fever is unknown, but in retrospective studies of fever of unknown origin, fewer than 10% of dogs were ultimately diagnosed with cancer.[234–236] Hematopoietic cancers were identified most frequently.

When an animal with cancer presents with fever, it is important to rule out concurrent infection. Tumors can become secondarily infected, especially if they are ulcerated or have large areas of necrosis. Gastrointestinal tumors can perforate the GI tract, resulting in septic peritonitis Sepsis secondary to myelophthisic leukopenia can also occur. Infections also can develop as a complication of cancer treatment: postoperative healing complications, severe neutropenia secondary to chemotherapy and sepsis, vomiting secondary to chemotherapy and subsequent aspiration pneumonia. A diagnosis of paraneoplastic fever is often made by ruling out other causes for fever. Paraneoplastic fever is most effectively treated by eliminating the inciting cancer. When this is not possible, if the fever is affecting quality of life then symptomatic treatment with and NSAID or antiinflammatory dose of steroids should be considered.

References

1. Boyiadzis M, Lieberman FS, Geskin LJ, et al.: Paraneoplastic syndromes. In DeVita VT, Hellman S, Rosenberg SA, editors: *Cancer: principles & practice of oncology*, ed 8, Philadelphia, 1997, Lippincott Williams & Wilkins, pp 2343–2362.
2. Freeman LM: Cachexia and sarcopenia: emerging syndromes of importance in dogs and cats, *J Vet Intern Med* 26:3–17, 2012.
3. Loviano A, Meguid RA, Meguid MM: Supportive care and quality of life: nutrition support. In DeVita VT, Hellman S, Rosenberg SA, editors: *Cancer: principles & practice of oncology*, ed 8, Philadelphia, 1997, Lippincott Williams & Wilkins, pp 2791–2804.
4. Ryan AM, Power DG, Daly L, et al.: Cancer-associated malnutrition, cachexia and sarcopenia: the skeleton in the closet 40 years later, *Proc Nutr Soc* 7(5):199–211, 2016.
5. Dewys WD, Begg C, Lavin PT, et al.: Prognostic effect of weight loss prior to chemotherapy in cancer patients. Eastern cooperative oncology group, *Am J Med* 69:491–497, 1980.
6. Michel KE, Sorenmo K, Shofer FS: Evaluation of body condition and weight loss in dogs presented to a veterinary oncology service, *J Vet Intern Med* 18:692–695, 2004.
7. Baez JL, Michel KE, Sorenmo K, et al.: A prospective investigation of the prevalence and prognostic significance of weight loss and changes in body condition in feline cancer patients, *J Feline Med Surg* 9:411–417, 2007.
8. Fox LE, Rosenthal RC, Twedt DC, et al.: Plasma histamine and gastrin concentrations in 17 dogs with mast cell tumors, *J Vet Intern Med* 4:242–246, 1990.
9. Ishiguro T, Kadosawa T, Takagi S, et al.: Relationship of disease progression and plasma histamine concentrations in 11 dogs with mast cell tumors, *J Vet Intern Med* 17:194–198, 2003.
10. Simpson KW, Dykes NL: Diagnosis and treatment of gastrinoma, *Semin Vet Med Surg (Small Anim)* 12:274–281, 1997.
11. Green RA, Gartrell CL: Gastrinoma. A retrospective study of four cases (1985–1995), *J Am Anim Hosp Assoc* 33:524–527, 1997.
12. English RV, Breitschwerdt EB, Grindem CB, et al.: Zollinger-Ellison syndrome and myelofibrosis in a dog, *J Am Vet Med Assoc* 192:1430–1434, 1988.

13. Middleton DJ: Duodenal ulceration associated with gastrin-secreting pancreatic tumor in a cat, *J Am Vet Med Assoc* 183: 461–462, 1983.

14. Elliott J, Dobson JM, Dunn JK, et al.: Hypercalcemia in the dog: a study of 40 cases, *J Small Anim Pract* 32: 564–567, 1991.

15. Messinger JS, Windham WR, Ward CR: Ionized hypercalcemia in dogs: a retrospective study of 109 cases (1998–2003), *J Vet Intern Med* 23:514–519, 2009.

16. Savary KC, Price GS, Vaden SL: Hypercalcemia in cats: a retrospective study of 71 cases (1991–1997), *J Vet Intern Med* 14: 184–189, 2000.

17. Lucas P, Lacoste H, deLorimier L-P, et al.: Treating paraneoplastic hypercalcemia in dogs and cats, *Vet Med* 314–330, 2007.

18. Vasilopulos RJ, Mackin A: Humoral hypercalcemia of malignancy: pathophysiology and clinical signs, *Compend Cont Educ Sm Anim Pract* 25:122–128, 2003.

19. Rebhun RB, Kent MS, Vorrofka SAEB, et al.: CHOP chemotherapy for the treatment of canine multicentric T-cell lymphoma, *Vet Comp Oncol* 9:38–44, 2010.

20. Brodsky EM, Mauldin GN, Lachowicz JL, et al.: Asparaginase and MOPP treatment of dogs with lymphoma, *J Vet Intern Med* 23:578–584, 2009.

21. Williams LE, Gliatto JM, Dodge RK, et al.: Carcinoma of the apocrine glands of the anal sac in dogs: 113 cases (1985–1995), *J Am Vet Med Assoc* 223:825–831, 2003.

22. Ross JT, Scavelli TD, Matthieson DT, et al.: Adenocarcinoma of the apocrine glands of the anal sac in dogs: a review of 32 cases, *J Am Anim Hosp Assoc* 27:349–355, 1991.

23. Pressler BM, Rotstein DS, Law JM, et al.: Hypercalcemia and high parathyroid hormone-related protein concentration associated with malignant melanoma in a dog, *J Am Vet Med Assoc* 221: 263–265, 2002.

24. Kleiter M, Hirt R, Kirtz G, et al.: Hypercalcaemia associated with chronic lymphocytic leukaemia in a Giant Schnauzer, *Aust Vet J* 79:335–338, 2001.

25. Furtado AR, Parrinello L, Merlo M, et al.: Primary penile adenocarcinoma with concurrent hypercalcemia of malignancy in a dog, *J Small Anim Pract* 56:289–292, 2015.

26. Robat CS, Cesario L, Gaeta R, et al.: Clinical features, treatment options, and outcome in dogs with thymoma: 116 cases (1999–2010), *J Am Vet Med Assoc* 243:1448–1454, 2013.

27. Merrick CH, Schleis SE, Smith AN, et al.: Hypercalemia of malignancy associated with renal cell carcinoma in a dog, *J Am Anim Hosp Assoc* 49:385–388, 2013.

28. Gajanayake I, Priestnall SL, Benigni L, et al.: Paraneoplastic hypercalcemia in a dog with benign renal angiomyxoma, *J Vet Diagn Invest* 22:775–780, 2010.

29. Neihaus SA, Winter JE, Goring RL, et al.: Primary clitoral adenocarcinoma with secondary hypercalcemia of malignancy in a dog, *J Am Anim Hosp Assoc* 46:193–196, 2010.

30. Henry CJ, Lanevschi A, Marks SL, et al.: Acute lymphoblastic leukemia, hypercalcemia, and pseudohyperkalemia in a dog, *J Am Vet Med Assoc* 208:237–239, 1996.

31. Dhaliwal RS, Tank KN: Parathyroid hormone-related peptide and hypercalcemia in a dog with functional keratinizing ameloblastoma, *Vet Comp Oncol* 3:90–100, 2005.

32. Anderson GM, Lane I, Fischer J, et al.: Hypercalcemia and parathyroid hormone-related protein in a dog with undifferentiated nasal carcinoma, *Can Vet J* 40, 1999. 341–341.

33. Klausner JS, Bell FW, Hayden DW, et al.: Hypercalcemia in two cats with squamous cell carcinoma, *J Am Vet Med Assoc* 196:103–105, 1990.

34. Sheafor SE, Gamblin RM, Couto CG: Hypercalcemia in two cats with multiple myeloma, *J Am Anim Hosp Assoc* 32: 503–508, 1996.

35. Anderson TE, Legendre AM, McEntee MM: Probable hypercalcemia of malignancy in a cat with bronchogenic adenocarcinoma, *J Am Anim Hosp Assoc* 36:52–55, 2000.

36. Bolliger AP, Graham PA, Richard V, et al.: Detection of parathyroid hormone-related protein in cats with humoral hypercalcemia of malignancy, *Vet Clin Pathol* 31:3–8, 2002.

37. Schenck PA, Chew DJ, Nagoda LA, et al.: Disorders of calcium: hypercalcemia and hypocalcemia. In DiBartola SP, editor: *Fluid, electrolyte, and acid-base disorders in small animal practice*, ed 4, St. Louis, 2012, Elsevier, pp 20–194.

38. Epstein FH: The physiology of parathyroid hormone-related protein, *N Engl J Med* 342:177–186, 2000.

39. Gröne A, Werkmeister JR, Steinmayer CL, et al.: Parathyroid hormone-related protein in normal and neoplastic canine tissues: immunohistochemical localization and biochemical extraction, *Vet Pathol* 31:308–315, 1994.

40. Rosol TJ, Capen CC: Mechanisms of cancer-induced hypercalcemia, *Lab Invest* 67:680–702, 1992.

41. Rosol TJ, Nagode LA, Couto CG, et al.: Parathyroid hormone (PTH)-related protein, PTH, and 1,25-dihydroxyvitamin D in dogs with cancer-associated hypercalcemia, *Endocrinology* 131:1157–1164, 1992.

42. Schenck PA, Chew DJ: Prediction of serum ionized calcium concentration by use of serum total calcium concentration in dogs, *Am J Vet Res* 66:1330–1336, 2005.

43. Vasilopulos RJ, Mackin A: Humoral hypercalcemia of malignancy: diagnosis and treatment, *Compend Cont Ed Sm Anim Pract* 25:129–137, 2003.

44. Milner RJ, Farese J, Henry CJ, et al.: Bisphosphonates in cancer, *J Vet Intern Med* 18:597–604, 2004.

45. Hostutler RA, Chew DJ, Jaeger JQ, et al.: Uses and effectiveness of pamidronate disodium for treatment of dogs and cats with hypercalcemia, *J Vet Intern Med* 19:29–33, 2005.

46. Major P, Lortholary A, Hon J, et al.: Zoledronic acid is superior to pamidronate in the treatment of hypercalcemia of malignancy: a pooled analysis of two randomized, controlled clinical trials, *J Clin Oncol* 19:558–567, 2001.

47. Fan TM, deLorimier LP, Garrett LD, et al.: The bone biologic effects of zoledronate in healthy dogs and dogs with malignant osteolysis, *J Vet Intern Med* 22:380–387, 2008.

48. Price GS, Page RL, Fischer B, et al.: Efficacy and toxicity of doxorubicin/cyclophosphamide maintenance therapy in dogs with multicentric lymphosarcoma, *J Vet Intern Med* 5:259–262, 1991.

49. Goutal CM, Brugmann BL, Ryan KA: Insulinoma in dogs: a review, *J Am Anim Hosp Assoc* 48:151–163, 2012.

50. Tobin RL, Nelson RW, Lucroy MD, et al.: Outcome of surgical versus medical treatment of dogs with beta cell neoplasia: 39 cases (1990-1997), *J Am Vet Med Assoc* 215:226–230, 1999.

51. Buishand FO, van Erp MG, Groenveld HA, et al.: Expression of insulin-like growth factor-1 by canine insulinomas and their metastases, *Vet J* 191:334–340, 2012.

52. Finotello R, Ressel L, Arvigo M, et al.: Canine pancreatic islet cell tumours secreting insulin-like growth factor type 2: a rare entity, *Vet Comp Oncol* 14:170–180, 2016.

53. Leifer CE, Peterson ME, Matus RE, et al.: Hypoglycemia associated with nonislet cell tumor in 13 dogs, *J Am Vet Med Assoc* 186:53–55, 1985.

54. Zini E, Glaus TM, Minuto F, et al.: Paraneoplastic hypoglycemia due to an insulin-like growth factor type-II secreting hepatocellular carcinoma in a dog, *J Vet Intern Med* 21:193–195, 2007.

55. Beaudry D, Knapp DW, Montgomery T, et al.: Smooth muscle tumors associated with hypoglycemia in four dogs. Clinical presentation, treatment, and tumor immunohistochemical staining, *J Vet Intern Med* 9:415–418, 1995.

56. Bagley RS, Levy JK, Malarkey DE: Hypoglycemia associated with intra-abdominal leiomyoma and leiomyosarcoma in six dogs, *J Am Vet Med Assoc* 208:69–71, 1996.

57. Cohen M, Post GS, Wright JC: Gastrointestinal leiomyosarcoma in 14 dogs, *J Vet Intern Med* 17:107–110, 2003.

58. Rossi G, Errico G, Perez P, et al.: Paraneoplastic hypoglycemia in a diabetic dog with an insulin growth factor-2-producing mammary carcinoma, *Vet Clin Pathol* 39:480–484, 2010.

59. Battaglia L, Petterino C, Zappulli V, et al.: Hypoglycaemia as a paraneoplastic syndrome associated with renal adenocarcinoma in a dog, *Vet Res Commun* 29:671–675, 2005.

60. Snead EC: A case of bilateral renal lymphosarcoma with secondary polycythaemia and paraneoplastic syndromes of hypoglycaemia and uveitis in an English Springer Spaniel, *Vet Comp Oncol* 3:139–144, 2005.

61. Zapf J: Role of insulin-like growth factor (IGF) II and IGF binding proteins in extrapancreatic tumour hypoglycaemia, *J Intern Med* 234:543–552, 1993.

62. Sanpera N, Masot M, Janer C, et al.: Oestrogen-induced bone marrow aplasia in a dog with a Sertoli cell tumour, *J Small Anim Pract* 43:365–369, 2002.

63. Sherdig RG, Wildon GP, Kociba GK: Bone marrow hypoplasia in eight dogs with Sertoli cell tumor, *J Am Vet Med Assoc* 178:497–501, 1981.

64. Weaver AD: Survey with follow-up of 67 dogs with testicular Sertoli cell tumours, *Vet Rec* 113:105–107, 1983.

65. Reif JS, Brodey RS: The relationship between cryptorchidism and canine testicular neoplasia, *J Am Vet Med Assoc* 155:2005–2010, 1969.

66. Kim O, Kim KS: Seminoma with hyperestrogenemia in a Yorkshire terrier, *J Vet Med Sci* 67:121–123, 2005.

67. Suess RP, Barr SC, Sacre BJ, et al.: Bone marrow hypoplasia in a feminized dog with an interstitial cell tumor, *J Am Vet Med Assoc* 200:1346–1348, 1992.

68. McCandlish IA, Munro C, Breeze RG, et al.: Hormone producing ovarian tumours in the dog, *Vet Rec* 105:9–11, 1979.

69. Mischke R, Meurer D, Hoppen HO, et al.: Blood plasma concentrations of oestradiol-17β, testosterone, and testosterone/estradiol ratio in dogs with neoplastic and degenerative testicular diseases, *Res Vet Sci* 73:267–272, 2002.

70. Peters MA, Mol JA, van Wolferen ME, et al.: Expression of insulin-like growth factor (IGF) system and steroidogenic enzymes in canine testis tumors, *Reprod Biol Endocrinol* 1:22–29, 2003.

71. Hurty CA, Flatland B: Feline acromegaly, a review of the syndrome, *J Am Anim Hosp Assoc* 41:292–297, 2005.

72. Peterson ME, Taylor RS, Greco DS, et al.: Acromegaly in 14 cats, *J Vet Intern Med* 4:192–201, 1990.

73. Niessen SJ, Church DB, Forcada Y: Hypersomatropism, acromegaly, and hyperadrenocortcism and feline diabetes mellitus, *Vet Clin North Am Small Anim Pract* 43:221–231, 2013.

74. vanKeulen LJ, Wesdorp JL, Kooistra HS: Diabetes mellitus in a dog with a growth hormone-producing acidophilic adenoma of the adenohypophysis, *Vet Pathol* 33:451–453, 1996.

75. Murai A, Nishii N, Morita T, et al.: GH-producing mammary tumors in two dogs with acromegaly, *J Vet Med Sci* 74:771–774, 2012.

76. Ogilvie GK, Weigel RM, Haschek WM, et al.: Prognostic factors for tumor remission and survival in dogs after surgery for primary lung tumor: 76 cases (1975–1985), *J Am Vet Med Assoc* 195:109–112, 1989.

77. Galac S, Kooistra HS, Voorhout G, et al.: Hyperadrenocorticism in a dog due to ectopic secretion of adrenocorticotropic hormone, *Domest Anim Endocrinol* 28:338–348, 2005.

78. Churcher RK: Hepatic carcinoid, hypercortisolism, and hypokalaemia in a dog, *Aust Vet J* 77:641–645, 1999.

79. MacEwen GE, Hurvitz A: Diagnosis and management of monoclonal gammopathies, *Vet Clin North Am* 7:119–132, 1977.

80. Mellor PJ, Haugland S, Murphy S, et al.: Myeloma-related disorders in cats commonly present as extramedullary neoplasms in contrast to myeloma in human patient: 24 cases with clinical follow up, *J Vet Intern Med* 20:1376–1383, 2006.

81. Giraudel JM, Pagès JP, Fuilfi JF: Monoclonal gammopathies in the dog: a retrospective study of 18 cases (1986–1999) and literature review, *J Am Anim Hosp Assoc* 39:135–147, 2002.

82. Rout ED, Shank AM, Waite AH, et al.: Progression of cutaneous plasmacytoma to plasma cell leukemia in a dog, *Vet Clin Pathol* 46:77–84, 2017.

83. Childress MO: Hematologic abnormalities in the small animal cancer patient, *Vet Clin North Am Small Anim Pract* 42:123–155, 2012.

84. Peterson EN, Meininger AC: Immunoglobulin A and immunoglobulin G biclonal gammopathy in a dog with multiple myeloma, *J Am Anim Hosp Assoc* 33:45–47, 1997.

85. Ramaiah SK, Seguin MA, Carwile HF, et al.: Biclonal gammopathy associated with immunoglobulin A in a dog with multiple myeloma, *Vet Clin Pathol* 31:83–89, 2002.

86. Grauer GF: Proteinuria: measurement and interpretation, *Top Companion Anim Med* 26:121–127, 2011.

87. Cowgill ES, Neel JA, Ruslander D: Light-chain myeloma in a dog, *J Vet Intern Med* 18:119–121, 2004.

88. Hammer AS, Couto CG: Complications of multiple myeloma, *J Am Anim Hosp Assoc* 30:9–14, 1994.

89. Forrester SD, Greco DS, Relford RL: Serum hyperviscosity syndrome associated with multiple myeloma in two cats, *J Am Vet Med Assoc* 200:79–82, 1992.

90. Nitsche EK: Erythrocytosis in dogs and cats: diagnosis and management, *Compend Cont Ed Small Anim Pract* 26:104–118, 2004.

91. Gentilini F, Calzolari C, Buonacucina A, et al.: Different biologic behavior of waldenström macroglobulinemia in two dogs, *Vet Comp Oncol* 3:87–97, 2005.

92. Hendrix DV, Gelatt KN, Smith PJ, et al.: Ophthalmic disease as a presenting complaint in five dogs with multiple myeloma, *J Am Anim Hosp Assoc* 34:121–128, 1998.

93. Boyle TE, Holowaychuk MK, Adams AK, et al.: Treatment of three cats with hyperviscosity syndrome and congestive heart failure using plasmapheresis, *J Am Anim Hosp Assoc* 47:50–55, 2011.

94. Bartages JW: Therapeutic plasmapheresis, *Semin Vet Med Surg (Small Anim)* 12:170–177, 1997.

95. Abbo AH, Lucroy MD: Assessment of anemia as an independent predictor of response to chemotherapy and survival in dogs with lymphoma, *J Am Vet Med Assoc* 231:1836–1842, 2007.

96. Miller AG, Morley PS, Rao S, et al.: Anemia is associated with decreased survival time in dogs with lymphoma, *J Vet Intern Med* 23:116–122, 2009.

97. Haney SM, Beaver L, Turrel J, et al.: Survival analysis of 97 cats with nasal lymphoma: a multi-institutional retrospective study (1986–2006), *J Vet Intern Med* 23:287–294, 2009.

98. Pintar J, Breitschwerdt EB, Hardie EM, et al.: Acute nontraumatic hemoabdomen in the dog: a retrospective analysis of 39 cases (1987–2001), *J Am Anim Hosp Assoc* 39, 2003. 528–522.

99. Aronsohn MG, Dubiel B, Roberts B, et al.: Prognosis for acute nontraumatic hemoperitoneum in the dog: a retrospective analysis of 60 cases (2003–2006), *J Am Anim Hosp Assoc* 45:72–77, 2009.

100. Whittemore JC, Preston CA, Kyles AE, et al.: Nontraumatic rupture of an adrenal gland tumor causing intra-abdominal or retroperitoneal hemorrhage in four dogs, *J Am Vet Med Assoc* 219:329–333, 2001.

101. Slensky KA, Volk SW, Schwarz T, et al.: Acute severe hemorrhage secondary to arterial invasion in a dog with thyroid carcinoma, *J Am Vet Med Assoc* 223:649–653, 2003.

102. Hohenhaus AE, Winzelberg SE: Nonregenerative anemia. In Ettinger SJ, Feldman EC, Côté, editors: *Textbook of veterinary internal medicine*, ed 8, St. Louis, 2017, Elsevier, pp 829–837.

103. McCullough S: Immune-mediated hemolytic anemia: understanding the nemesis, *Vet Clin North Am Small Anim Pract* 33:1295–1315, 2003.

104. Madewell BR, Feldman BF: Characterization of anemias associated with neoplasia in small animals, *J Am Vet Med Assoc* 176:419–425, 1980.

105. Hammer AS, Couto CG, Swardson C, et al.: Hemostatic abnormalities in dogs with hemangiosarcoma, *J Vet Intern Med* 5:11–14, 1991.

106. Moore PF, Affolter VK, Vernau W: Canine hemophagocytic histiocytic sarcoma: a proliferative disorder of CD11+ macrophages, *Vet Pathol* 43:632–645, 2006.

107. Dobson J, Villiers E, Roulois A, et al.: Histiocytic sarcoma of the spleen in flat-coated retrievers with regenerative anaemia and hypoproteinaemia, *Vet Rec* 158:825–829, 2006.

108. Moore PF: A review of histiocytic diseases of dogs and cats, *Vet Pathol* 51:67–184, 2014.

109. Caldin M, Carli E, Furlanello T, et al.: A retrospective study of 60 cases of eccentrocytosis in the dog, *Vet Clin Pathol* 34:224–231, 2005.

110. Christopher MM: Relationship of endogenous Heinz bodies to disease and anemia in cats: 120 cases (1978–1987), *J Am Vet Med Assoc* 194:1089–1095, 1989.

111. Matus RE, Leifer CE, MacEwen EG: Acute lymphoblastic leukemia in the dog: a review of 30 cases, *J Am Vet Med Assoc* 183:859–862, 1983.

112. Harvey JW: Myeloproliferative disorders in dogs and cats, *Vet Clin North Am Small Anim Pract* 11:349–381, 1981.

113. Madewell BR: Hematological and bone marrow cytological abnormalities in 75 dogs with malignant lymphoma, *J Am Animal Hosp Assoc* 22:235–240, 1986.

114. Marconato L, Vettini G, Giacoboni C, et al.: Clinicopathologic features and outcomes for dogs with mast cell tumors and bone marrow involvement, *J Vet Intern Med* 22:1001–1007, 2008.

115. Kiselow MA, Rassnick KM, McDonough SP, et al.: Outcome of cats with low grade lymphocytic lymphoma: 41 cases (1995–2005), *J Am Vet Med Assoc* 232:405–410, 2008.

116. Peterson ME: Inappropriate erythropoietin production from a renal carcinoma in a dog with polycythemia, *J Am Vet Med Assoc* 179:995–996, 1981.

117. Crow SE, Allen DP, Murphy CJ, et al.: Concurrent renal adenocarcinoma and polycythemia in a dog, *J Am Animal Hosp Assoc* 31:29–33, 1995.

118. Scott RC, Patnaik AK: Renal carcinoma with secondary polycythemia in the dog, *J Am Anim Hosp Assoc* 8:275–283, 1972.

119. Nelson RW, Hager D: Renal lymphosarcoma with inappropriate erythropoietin production in a dog, *J Am Vet Med Assoc* 182:1396–1397, 1983.

120. Gorse MJ: Polycythemia associated with renal fibrosarcoma in a dog, *J Am Vet Med Assoc* 192:793–794, 1988.

121. Durno AS, Webb JA, Gauthier MJ, et al.: Polycythemia and inappropriate erythropoietin concentrations in two dogs with renal T-cell lymphoma, *J Am Anim Hosp Assoc* 47:122–128, 2011.

122. Couto CG, Boudrieau RJ, Zanjani ED: Tumor-associated erythrocytosis in a dog with a nasal fibrosarcoma, *J Vet Intern Med* 3:183–185, 1989.

123. Sato K, Hikasa Y, Morita T, et al.: Secondary erythrocytosis associated with high plasma erythropoietin concentrations in a dog with cecal leiomyosarcoma, *J Am Vet Med Assoc* 220:486–490, 2002.

124. Yamauchi A, Ohta T, Okada T, et al.: Secondary erythrocytosis associated with schwannoma in a dog, *J Vet Med Sci* 66:1605–1608, 2004.

125. Klainbart S, Segev G, Loeb E, et al.: Resolution of renal adenocarcinoma-induced secondary inappropriate polycythemia after nephrectomy in two cats, *J Feline Med Surg* 10:264–268, 2008.

126. Cook SM, Lothrop CD: Serum erythropoietin concentrations measured by radioimmunoassay in normal, polycythemic, and anemic dogs and cats, *J Vet Intern Med* 8:18–25, 1994.

127. Lappin MR, Lattimer KS: Hematuria and extreme neutrophilic leukocytosis in a dog with renal tubular carcinoma, *J Am Vet Med Assoc* 192:1289–1292, 1988.

128. Thompson JP, Christopher MM, Ellison GW, et al.: Paraneoplastic leukocytosis associated with a rectal adenomatous polyp in a dog, *J Am Vet Med Assoc* 201:737–738, 1992.

129. Chinn DR, Myers RK, Matthews JA: Neutrophilic leukocytosis associated with metastatic fibrosarcoma in a dog, *J Am Vet Med Assoc* 186:806–809, 1985.

130. Madewell BR, Wilson DW, Hornoff WJ, et al.: Leukemoid blood response and bone infarcts in a dog with renal tubular adenocarcinoma, *J Am Vet Med Assoc* 197:1623–1625, 1990.

131. Sharkey LC, Rosol TJ, Grone A, et al.: Production of granulocyte colony-stimulating factor and granulocyte-macrophage colony-stimulating factor by carcinomas in a dog and a cat with paraneoplastic leukocytosis, *J Vet Intern Med* 10:405–408, 1996.

132. Peeters D, Clercx C, Thiry A, et al.: Resolution of paraneoplastic leukocytosis and hypertrophic osteopathy after resection of a renal transitional cell carcinoma producing granulocyte-macrophage colony-stimulating factor in a young bull terrier, *J Vet Intern Med* 15:407–411, 2001.

133. Dole RS, MacPhail CM, Lappin MR: Paraneoplastic leukocytosis with mature neutrophilia in a cat with pulmonary squamous cell carcinoma, *J Feline Med Surg* 6:391–395, 2004.

134. Keramatina A, Ahadi A, Akbari ME, et al.: Genomic profiling and chronic myelogenous leukemia: basic and clinical approach, *J Cancer Prev* 22:74–81, 2017.

134b Figueiredo JF, Culver S, Behling-Kelly E, et al.: Acute myeloblastic leukemia with associated BCR-ABL translocation in a dog, *Vet Clin Pathol* 41:362–368, 2012.

135. Lucroy MD, Madewell BR: Clinical outcome and associated diseases in dogs with leukocytosis and neutrophilia: 118 cases (1996–1998), *J Am Vet Med Assoc* 214:805–807, 1999.

136. Barrs VR, Beatty JA, McCandlish IA, et al.: Hypereosinophilic paraneoplastic syndrome in a cat with intestinal T cell lymphosarcoma, *J Small Anim Pract* 43:401–405, 2002.

137. Cave TA, Gault EA, Argyle DJ: Feline epitheliotrophic T-cell lymphoma with paraneoplastic eosinophilia – immunochemotherapy with vinblastine and recombinant interferon alpha-2b, *Vet Comp Oncol* 2:91–97, 2004.

138. Marchetti V, Benetti C, Citi S, et al.: Paraneoplastic hypereosinophilia in a dog with intestinal T-cell lymphoma, *Vet Clin Pathol* 34:259–263, 2005.

139. London CA: Mast cell tumors in the dog, *Vet Clin North Am Small Anim Pract* 33:473–489, 2003.

140. Bortnowski HB, Rosenthal RC: Gastrointestinal mast cell tumors and eosinophilia in two cats, *J Am Anim Hosp Assoc* 28:271–275, 1992.

141. Couto CG: Tumor associated eosinophilia in a dog, *J Am Vet Med Assoc* 184:837–838, 1984.

142. Fews D, Scase TJ, Battersby IA: Leiomyosarcoma of the pericardium, with epicardial metastases and peripheral eosinophilia in a dog, *J Comp Pathol* 138:224–228, 2008.

143. Sellon RK, Rottman JB, Jordan HL, et al.: Hypereosinophilia associated with transitional cell carcinoma in a cat, *J Am Vet Med Assoc* 201:591–593, 1992.

144. Losco PE: Local and peripheral eosinophilia in a dog with anaplastic mammary carcinoma, *Vet Pathol* 23:536–538, 1986.

145. Madewell BR, Feldman BF, O'Neil S: Coagulation abnormalities in dogs with neoplastic disease, *Thromb Haemost* 44:35–38, 1980.

146. Grindem CB, Breitschwerdt EB, Corbett WT, et al.: Thrombocytopenia associated with neoplasia in dogs, *J Vet Intern Med* 8:400–405, 1994.

147. Jordan HL, Grindem CB, Breitschwerdt EB: Thrombocytopenia in cats: a retrospective study of 41 cases, *J Vet Intern Med* 7:261–265, 1993.

148. Jain NC, Switzer JW: Autoimmune thrombocytopenia in dogs and cats, *Vet Clin North Am Small Anim Pract* 11:421–434, 1981.

149. Dircks BH, Schuberth H, Mischke R: Underlying diseases and clinicopathologic variables of thrombocytopenic dogs with and without platelet-bound antibodies detected by use of a flow cytometric assay: 83 cases (2004–2006), *J Am Vet Med Assoc* 235:960–966, 2009.

150. Helfand SC, Couto CG, Madewell BR: Immune-mediated thrombocytopenia associated with solid tumors in dogs, *J Am Anim Hosp Assoc* 21:787–794, 1985.

151. Chisholm-Chait A: Mechanisms of thrombocytopenia in dogs with cancer, *Comped Contin Educ Pract Vet* 22:1006–1017, 2000.

152. O'Donnell MR, Slichter SJ, Weiden PL, et al.: Platelet and fibrinogen kinetics in canine tumors, *Cancer Res* 41:1379–1383, 1981.

153. Thomas JS, Rogers KS: Platelet aggregation and adenosine triphosphate secretion in dogs with untreated multicentric lymphoma, *J Vet Intern Med* 13:319–322, 1999.

154. McNiel EA, Ogilvie GK, Fettman MJ, et al.: Platelet hyperfunction in dogs with malignancies, *J Vet Intern Med* 11:178–182, 1997.

155. Kristensen AT, Wiinberg B, Jessen LR, et al.: Evaluation of human recombinant tissue factor-activated thromboelastography in 49 dogs with neoplasia, *J Vet Intern Med* 22:140–147, 2008.

156. VanWinkle TJ, Bruce E: Thrombosis of the portal vein in eleven dogs, *Vet Pathol* 30:28–35, 1993.

157. LaRue MJ, Murtaugh RJ: Pulmonary thromboembolism in dogs: 47 cases (1986–1987), *J Am Vet Med Assoc* 197:1368–1372, 1990.

158. Laurenson MP, Hopper K, Herrera MA, et al.: Concurrent diseases and conditions in dogs with splenic vein thrombosis, *J Vet Intern Med* 4(1298):1304, 2010.

159. Murayama H, Miura T, Sakai M, et al.: The incidence of disseminated intravascular coagulation in dogs with malignant neoplasia, *J Vet Med Sci* 66:573–575, 2004.

160. Marconato L, Romanelli G, Stefanello D, et al.: Prognostic factors for dogs with mammary inflammatory carcinoma: 43 cases (2003–2008), *J Am Vet Med Assoc* 235:967–972, 2009.

161. Rudloff E, Kirby R: Disseminated intravascular coagulation. In Bonagura JD, Twedt DC, editors: *Kirk's current veterinary therapy XV*, St. Louis, 2014, Elsevier, pp 292–296.

162. Francis JL, Biggerstaff J, Amirkhosravi A: Hemostasis and malignancy, *Semin Thromb Hemost* 24:93–109, 1998.

163. Turek M: Cutaneous paraneoplastic syndromes in dogs and cats: a review of the literature, *Vet Dermatol* 14:279–296, 2003.

164. Lium G, Moe E: Hereditary multifocal renal cystadenocarcinomas and nodular dermatofibrosis in the German shepherd dog: macroscopic and histopathologic changes, *Vet Pathol* 22:447–455, 1985.

165. Suter M, Lott-Stoltz G, Wild P: Generalized nodular dermatofibrosis in six Alsatians, *Vet Pathol* 20:632–634, 1983.

166. Gilbert PA, Griffin CE, Walder EJ: Nodular dermatofibrosis and renal cystadenoma in a German shepherd dog, *J Am Anim Hosp Assoc* 26:253–256, 1990.

167. Atlee BA, DeBoer DJ, Ihrke PJ, et al.: Nodular dermatofibrosis in German shepherd dogs as a marker for renal cystadenocarcinoma, *J Am Anim Hosp Assoc* 27:481–487, 1991.

168. Moe L, Lium B: Hereditary multifocal renal cystadenocarcinomas and nodular dermatofibrosis in 51 German shepherd dogs, *J Small Anim Pract* 38:498–505, 1997.

169. Lingaas F, Comstock KE, Kirkness EF, et al.: A mutation in the canine *BHD* gene is associated with hereditary multifocal renal cystadenocarcinoma and nodular dermatofibrosis in the German shepherd dog, *Hum Mol Genet* 12:3043–3053, 2003.

170. Gross TL, Song MD, Havel PJ, et al.: Superficial necrolytic dermatitis (necrolytic migratory erythema) in dogs, *Vet Pathol* 30:75–81, 1993.

171. Cellio LM, Dennis J: Canine superficial necrolytic dermatitis, *Compend Contin Ed Small Anim Pract* 27:820–825, 2005.

172. Byrne KP: Metabolic epidermal necrosis-hepatocutaneous syndrome, *Vet Clin North Am Small Anim Pract* 29:1337–1355, 1999.

173. Allenspach K, Arnold P, Glaus T, et al.: Glucagon-producing neuroendocrine tumour associated with hypoaminoacidaemia and skin lesions, *J Small Anim Pract* 41:402–406, 2000.

174. Cave TA, Evans H, Hargreaves J, et al.: Metabolic epidermal necrosis in a dog associated with pancreatic adenocarcinoma, hyperglucagonaemia, hyperinsulinaemia and hypoaminoacidaemia, *J Small Anim Pract* 48:522–526, 2007.

175. Torres SMF, Caywood DD, O'Brien TD, et al.: Resolution of superficial necrolytic dermatitis following excision of a glucagon-secreting pancreatic neoplasm in a dog, *J Am Anim Hosp Assoc* 33:313–319, 1997.

176. Oberkirchner U, Linder KE, Zadrozny L, et al.: Successful treatment of canine necrolytic migratory erythema (superficial necrolytic dermatitis) due to metastatic glucagonoma with octreotide, *Vet Dermatol* 21:510–516, 2010.

177. Patel A, Whitbread TJ, McNeil PE: A case of metabolic epidermal necrosis in a cat, *Vet Dermatol* 7:221–226, 1996.

178. Asakawa MG, Cullen JM, Linder KE: Necrolytic migratory erythema associated with a glucagon-producing primary hepatic neuroendocrine carcinoma in a cat, *Vet Dermatol* 24:466–469, 2013.

179. Brooks DG, Campbell KL, Dennis JS, et al.: Pancreatic paraneoplastic alopecia in three cats, *J Am Anim Hosp Assoc* 30:557–563, 1994.

180. Tasker S, Griffon DJ, Nuttall TJ, et al.: Resolution of paraneoplastic alopecia following surgical removal of a pancreatic carcinoma in a cat, *J Small Anim Pract* 40:16–19, 1999.

181. Pascal-Tenorio A, Olivry T, Gross TL, et al.: Paraneoplastic alopecia associated with internal malignancies in the cat, *Vet Dermatol* 8:47–51, 1997.

182. Godfrey DR: A case of feline paraneoplastic alopecia with secondary Malassezia-associated dermatitis, *J Small Anim Pract* 39:394–396, 1998.

183. Barrs VR, Martin P, France M, et al.: What is your diagnosis? Feline paraneoplastic alopecia associated with pancreatic and bile duct carcinomas, *J Small Anim Pract* 40(559):595–596, 1999.

184. Mauldin EA, Morris DO, Goldschmidt MH: Retrospective study: the presence of Malassezia in feline skin biopsies. A clinicopathological study, *Vet Dermatol* 13:7–13, 2002.

185. Scott DW, Yager JA: Exfoliative dermatitis in association with thymoma in three cats, *Fel Pract* 23:8–13, 1995.

186. Forster-Van Hijfte MA, Curtis SF, et al.: Resolution of exfoliative dermatitis and Malassezia pachydermatis overgrowth in a cat after surgical thymoma resection, *J Small Anim Pract* 38:451–454, 1997.

187. Carpenter JL, Holzworth J: Thymoma in 11 cats, *J Am Vet Med Assoc* 181:248–251, 1982.

188. Lien YHH, Lai LW: Pathogenesis, diagnosis, and management of paraneoplastic glomerulonephritis, *Nat Rev Nephrol* 7:85–92, 2011.

189. Page RL, Stiff ME, McEntee MC, et al.: Transient glomerulonephropathy associated with primary erythrocytosis in a dog, *J Am Vet Med Assoc* 196:620–622, 1990.

190. Willard MD, Krehbiel JD, Schmidt GM, et al.: Serum and urine protein abnormalities associated with lymphocytic leukemia and glomerulonephritis in a dog, *J Am Anim Hosp Assoc* 17:381–386, 1981.

191. Cohen M, Post GS: Nephrogenic diabetes insipidus in a dog with intestinal leiomyosarcoma, *J Am Vet Med Assoc* 215:1818–1820, 1999.

192. Robat CS, Cesario L, Gaeta R, et al.: Clinical features, treatment options, and outcome in dogs with thymoma: 116 cases (1999-2010), *J Vet Med Assoc* 243:1448–1454, 2013.

193. Atwater SW, Powers BE, Park RD, et al.: Thymoma in dogs: 23 cases (1980-1991), *J Am Vet Med Assoc* 205:1007–1013, 1994.

194. Zitz JC, Birchard SJ, Couto GC, et al.: Results of excision of thymoma in cats and dogs: 20 cases (1984–2005), *J Am Vet Med Assoc* 232:1186–1192, 2008.

195. Lainesse MFC, Taylor SM, Myers SL, et al.: Focal myasthenia gravis as a paraneoplastic syndrome of canine thymoma: improvement following thymectomy, *J Am Anim Hosp Assoc* 32:111–117, 1996.

196. Klebanow ER: Thymoma and acquired myasthenia gravis in the dog: a case report and review of 13 additional cases, *J Am Anim Hosp Assoc* 28:63–69, 1992.

197. Bellah JR, Stiff ME, Russell RG: Thymoma in the dog: two case reports and review of 20 additional cases, *J Am Vet Med Assoc* 183:306–311, 1983.

198. Gores BR, Berg J, Carpenter JL, et al.: Surgical treatment of thymoma in cats: 12 cases (1987–1992), *J Am Vet Med Assoc* 204:1782–1785, 1994.
199. Smith AN, Wright JC, LaRue SM, et al.: Radiation therapy in the treatment of canine and feline thymomas: a retrospective study (1985–1999), *J Am Anim Hosp Assoc* 37:489–496, 2001.
200. Hill PB, Brain P, Collins D, et al.: Putative paraneoplastic pemphigus and myasthenia gravis in a cat with lymphocytic thymoma, *Vet Dermatol* 24:646–649, 2013.
201. Moore AS, Madewell BR, Cardinet GH, et al.: Osteogenic sarcoma and myasthenia gravis in a dog, *J Am Vet Med Assoc* 197:226–227, 1990.
202. Krotje LJ, Fix AS, Potthoff AD: Acquired myasthenia gravis and cholangiocellular carcinoma in a dog, *J Am Vet Med Assoc* 197:488–490, 1990.
203. Stepaniuk K, Legendre L, Watson S: Acquired myasthenia gravis associated with oral sarcoma in a dog, *J Vet Dent* 28:242–249, 2011.
204. Ridyart AE, Rhing SM, French AT, et al.: Myasthenia gravis associated with cutaneous lymphoma in a dog, *J Small Anim Pract* 41:348–351, 2000.
205. Braund KG, McGuire JA, Amling KA, et al.: Peripheral neuropathy associated with malignant neoplasms in dogs, *Vet Pathol* 24:16–21, 1987.
206. Braund KG: Remote effects of cancer on the nervous system, *Semin Vet Med Surg (Sm Anim)* 5:262–270, 1990.
207. Moore AS, Nelson RW, Henry CJ, et al.: Streptozocin for treatment of pancreatic islet cell tumors in dogs: 17 cases (1989–1999), *J Am Vet Med Assoc* 221:811–818, 2002.
208. Villiers E, Dobson J: Multiple myeloma with associated polyneuropathy in a German shepherd dog, *J Small Anim Pract* 39:249–251, 1998.
209. Presthus J, Teige: Peripheral neuropathy associated with lymphosarcoma in a dog, *J Small Anim Pract* 27:463–469, 1986.
210. Griffiths IR, Duncan ID, Swallow JS: Peripheral polyneuropathy in dogs: a study of five cases, *J Small Anim Pract* 18:101–106, 1977.
211. Dyer KR, Duncan ID, Hammang JP, et al.: Peripheral neuropathy in two dogs: correlation between clinical, electrophysiological, and pathological findings, *J Small Anim Pract* 27:133–146, 1986.
212. Mariani CL, Shelton SB, Alsup JC: Paraneoplastic polyneuropathy and subsequent recovery following tumor removal in a dog, *J Am Anim Hosp Assoc* 35:302–305, 1999.
213. Cavana P, Sammartano F, Capucchio MT, et al.: Peripheral neuropathy in a cat with renal lymphoma, *J Feline Med Surg* 11:869–872, 2009.
214. Withers SS, Johnson EG, Culp WTN, et al.: Paraneoplastic hypertrophic osteopathy in 30 dogs, *Vet Comp Oncol* 13:157–165, 2015.
215. Brodey RS: Hypertrophic osteoarthropathy in the dog: a clinicopathologic surgery of 60 cases, *J Am Vet Med Assoc* 159:1242–1256, 1971.
216. Seaman RL, Patton CS: Treatment of renal nephroblastoma in an adult dog, *J Am Anim Hosp Assoc* 39:76–79, 2003.
217. Halliwell WH, Ackerman N: Botryoid rhabdomyosarcoma of the urinary bladder and hypertrophic osteoarthropathy in a young dog, *J Am Vet Med Assoc* 165:911–913, 1974.
218. Randolph JF, Center SA, Flanders JA, et al.: Hypertrophic osteopathy associated with adenocarcinoma of the esophageal glands in a dog, *J Am Vet Med Assoc* 184:98–99, 1984.
219. Rendano VT, Slauson DO: Hypertrophic osteopathy in a dog with prostatic adenocarcinoma and without thoracic metastasis, *J Am Anim Hosp Assoc* 18:905–909, 1982.
220. Randall VD, Souza C, Vanderhart D, et al.: Hypertrophic osteopathy associated with hepatocellular carcinoma in a dog, *Can Vet J* 56:741–747, 2015.
221. Hara Y, Tagawa M, Ejima H, et al.: Regression of hypertrophic osteopathy following removal of intrathoracic neoplasia derived from the vagus nerve in a dog, *J Vet Med Sci* 57:133–135, 1995.
222. Johnson RL, Lenz SD: Hypertrophic osteopathy associated with a renal adenoma in a cat, *J Vet Diagn Invest* 23:171–175, 2011.
223. Becker TJ, Perry RL, Watson GL: Regression of hypertrophic osteopathy in a cat after surgical excision of an adrenocortical carcinoma, *J Am Anim Hosp Assoc* 35:499–505, 1999.
224. Foster SF: Idiopathic hypertrophic osteopathy in a cat, *J Feline Med Surg* 9:172–173, 2007.
225. de Melo Oscarino N, Fukushima FB, de Matos Gomes A, et al.: Idiopathic hypertrophic osteopathy in a cat, *J Feline Med Surg* 8:345–348, 2006.
226. Goldfinch N, Argyle DJ: Feline lung-digit syndrome: unusual metastatic patterns of primary lung tumours in cats, *J Feline Med Surg* 14:202–208, 2012.
227. Watson AD, Porges WL: Regression of hypertrophic osteopathy in a dog following unilateral intrathoracic vagotomy, *Vet Rec* 93:240–243, 1973.
228. Qian X, Qin J: Hypertrophic pulmonary osteoarthropathy with primary lung cancer, *Oncol Lett* 7:2079–2082, 2014.
229. Dickinson CJ, Martin JF: Megakaryocytes and platelet clumps as the cause of finger clubbing, *Lancet* 2:1434–1435, 1987.
230. Liptak JM, Monnet E, Dernell WS, et al.: Pulmonary metastatectomy in the management of four dogs with hypertrophic osteopathy, *Vet Comp Oncol* 2:1–12, 2004.
231. Hahn KA, Richardson RC: Use of cisplatin for control of metastatic malignant mesenchymoma and hypertrophic osteopathy in a dog, *J Am Vet Med Assoc* 195:351–353, 1989.
232. Jayaker BA, Abelson AG, Yao Q: Treatment of hypertrophic osteoarthropathy with zoledronic acid: case report and review of the literature, *Semin Arth Rheum* 41:291–296, 2011.
233. Ramsey IK, Tasker S: Fever. In Ettinger SJ, Feldman EC, Côté, editors: *Textbook of veterinary internal medicine*, ed 8, St. Louis, 2017, Elsevier, pp 195–203.
234. Dunn KJ, Dunn JK: Diagnostic evaluation in 101 dogs with pyrexia of unknown origin, *J Small Anim Pract* 39:574–580, 1998.
235. Chervier C, Chabanne L, Godde M, et al.: Causes, diagnostic signs, and the utility of investigations of fever in dogs: 50 cases, *Can Vet J* 53:525–530, 2012.
236. Battersby IA, Murphy KF, Tasker S, et al.: Restrospective study of fever in dogs: laboratory testing, diagnoses, and influence of prior treatment, *J Small Anim Pract* 47:370–376, 2006.

6

Diagnostic Imaging in Oncology

STEPHANIE NYKAMP AND ELISSA RANDALL

Diagnostic imaging is essential in the diagnosis, clinical staging, and evaluation of response to therapy of cancer patients. Radiography, ultrasound, computed tomography (CT), magnetic resonance imaging (MRI), positron emission tomography (PET), and nuclear scintigraphy can all be used to evaluate the cancer patient. Advanced functional imaging (e.g., PET/CT, PET/MR) may also prove valuable in predicting response to therapy. The choice of modality is dependent on availability and desired outcome, with each modality having advantages and disadvantages in regard to cost, sensitivity, and specificity. When evaluating the primary tumor, accurate detection of tumor margins is paramount. When evaluating for metastasis, the ideal modality would be both highly sensitive and specific so that all lesions are detected accurately. If such a modality is not available, initial imaging should be done with a modality that is highly sensitive and followed with one that is more specific.

The use of advanced imaging and improved techniques for functional imaging are improving the accuracy and precision of cancer imaging.[1] It should be noted that this can also result in stage migration. The effect of this additional information is not fully understood for many and should be used with caution when predicting outcome.[2] This chapter outlines the principles of each modality and their utility in assessing the veterinary cancer patient.

Imaging Modalities

Radiography

Conventional radiography has historically been the primary modality for assessment of cancer patients because it is readily available at a low cost, but it is gradually being replaced with other modalities that are more sensitive, specific, and becoming more readily available.

With few exceptions, radiography is a screening test rather than providing a definitive diagnosis. The most common application for radiographs is screening for pulmonary metastasis. In dogs and cats, thoracic radiographs are obtained with the patient in a recumbent position, and this results in atelectasis of the dependent lung. Three views (left and right lateral and dorsoventral or ventrodorsal) are recommended because this position-dependent atelectasis can reduce lesion conspicuity. The diagnosis would change in 12% to 15% of patients when only two views are obtained, with left lateral and ventrodorsal views being less sensitive than right lateral and ventrodorsal views.[3–5] Although the sensitivity of radiographs is lower than that of CT for the detection of pulmonary metastasis, they will likely continue to remain the initial screening test because of the low cost and high availability (Fig. 6.1).[6–8]

Radiography is also the primary method for the diagnosis and monitoring of dogs and cats with tumors of the appendicular skeleton (Fig. 6.2).[9] Detection of an aggressive bone lesion on radiographs is not definitive for neoplasia, but signalment, history, clinical signs, and travel history can help differentiate neoplasia from infectious causes.[9] Although radiographs remain the primary diagnostic tool for appendicular bone tumors, CT and MRI are more accurate for determining tumor margins, which is necessary to optimize outcomes when using advanced treatment techniques such as limb-sparing surgery or stereotactic radiosurgery.[10]

Limitations of radiography include superimposition of overlying structures and the relatively limited contrast resolution.[8] Radiology software exists that can suppress overlying bony structures using advanced processing and pattern recognition algorithms, which significantly increase sensitivity for detection of lung nodules[11]; however, they are of limited availability in veterinary medicine, and other imaging modalities have been used to overcome this limitation. When the preferred imaging modality is not immediately available, radiographs can be useful in detecting masses in other body regions (e.g., abdomen) as well. Radiographs may provide evidence that a mass is present such that abdominal ultrasound, CT, or MRI can then be performed to detect the origin of the mass.

Ultrasonography

Ultrasound is widely available and relatively inexpensive, resulting in widespread usage as a first-line diagnostic modality for a variety of diseases, including cancer diagnosis and staging and for restaging or evaluating response to treatment. The ability to evaluate the internal structure of organs and to better evaluate body cavities in the presence of effusion has resulted in ultrasound replacing survey and contrast radiographs as the primary method of abdominal imaging.

Ultrasound is very good for identifying and localizing lesions, but the sonographic appearance may not be specific to the nature of the lesion.[12–21] The lack of specificity is more apparent when assessing multicentric diseases, such as lymphoma and mast cell tumor, where the sonographic appearances are variable and a

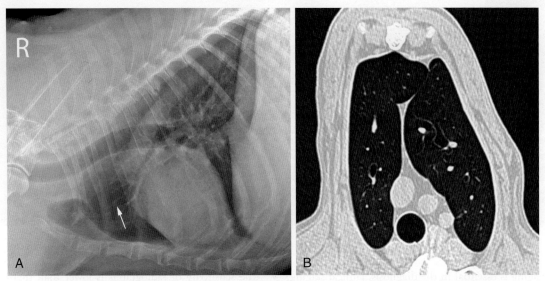

• **Fig. 6.1** A right lateral radiograph of the thorax (A) shows a pulmonary nodule in the ventral aspect of the second intercostal space *(arrow)*. Transverse CT image of the thorax at the same level (B) showed no evidence of the nodule, indicating this was a summation artifact on the radiograph resulting in a false-positive test for pulmonary metastasis.

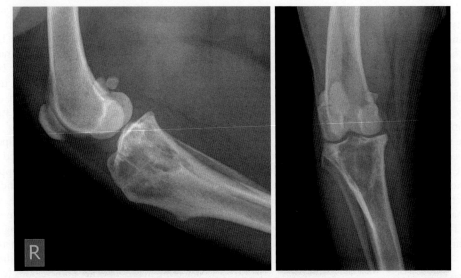

• **Fig. 6.2** Orthogonal radiographs of the stifle demonstrate an aggressive bone lesion in the proximal tibia that is characterized by moth-eaten bone lysis and cortical loss. The primary modality for the initial assessment of bone tumors remains radiography.

normal sonographic appearance does not necessarily exclude the presence of disease.[2,19] This limitation is overcome by the use of ultrasound-guided sampling techniques. Abdominal ultrasonography is also useful for the detection of comorbidities that may have an effect on treatment options for cancer patients.[2,19,20]

Although ultrasound findings are generally not specific, there are patterns that may be more indicative of neoplasia. Target lesions and focal nodules with a hyperechoic central region and hypoechoic rim have been associated with a higher predictive value for malignant neoplasia (Fig. 6.3). The positive-predictive value for malignancy is 74% when a single nodule is identified in either liver or spleen, and 81% when multiple target lesions are identified in one organ.[17] However, owing to the small sample size in this study, positive-predictive values may be overestimated. In dogs and cats with gastrointestinal disease, the loss of normal wall layering is strongly predicative of neoplasia compared with nonfungal inflammatory diseases.[15,22] Connecting peritoneal masses may be indicative of carcinomatosis in cats (Fig. 6.4).[23] Hypoechoic subcapsular thickening of the kidneys is associated with renal lymphoma in cats.[24] Ultrasound can also increase the suspicion of multiple organ involvement or detect intraabdominal metastases. This information will help guide sampling recommendations and may affect differential diagnoses and treatment decisions.

Color Doppler can be used to assess vascular invasion and the vascularity of masses (Fig. 6.5). Color Doppler displays the mean flow velocity and directional information using a color map, and this allows for visualization of smaller blood vessels and overall vascular pattern and distribution.[25] Spectral Doppler is required to determine maximum flow velocity, but this is more technically

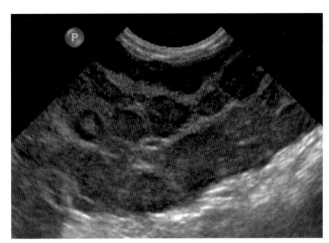

• **Fig. 6.3** A transverse ultrasound image of the liver demonstrates multifocal nodules, several of which have a target appearance with a central hyperechoic focus and a hypoechoic rim. Target lesions are associated with a higher positive-predicative value for malignant nodules than other sonographic patterns.

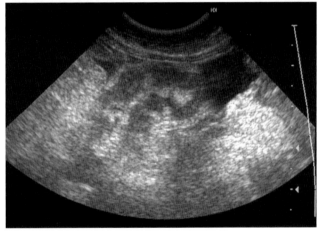

• **Fig. 6.4** A sagittal image of the midabdomen shows coalescing hypoechoic nodules within hyperechoic mesenteric fat and a moderate amount of echogenic abdominal fluid. These findings are strongly suggestive of carcinomatosis.

challenging. Vascular patterns may also be helpful in diagnosing malignant lesions. Owing to neovascularization of tumors, their blood supply tends to be more tortuous, with higher velocities than noted in normal tissue.[26–29] Ultrasound can also detect tumor invasion into local vasculature, which may influence the ranking of differential diagnoses and treatment decisions (e.g., adrenal mass invasion into the caudal vena cava) (Fig. 6.5).

Contrast-enhanced ultrasound improves detection of small blood vessels compared with power Doppler imaging because of reduced motion artifact and allows for evaluation of tissue perfusion.[30] First-generation contrast agents contained air within microbubbles, whereas second-generation agents contain perfluorocarbon or sulfur hexafluoride.[31] The microbubbles in second-generation ultrasound contrast agents are generally <2.5 μm, resulting in an intravascular agent that has a flow pattern similar to that of red blood cells and therefore can demonstrate the presence of blood vessels and can assess arterial, portal, and late phases in the liver.[31] There is some evidence that vascular tortuosity can

be used to predict malignancy, but this finding is not consistent.[32,33] In one study of liver masses, arterial hypervascularity was noted in the majority of hepatocellular carcinoma masses, but not other benign or malignant hepatic masses.[34] Multiphase evaluation of enhancement patterns with contrast-enhanced ultrasound can be used to differentiate between benign and malignant lesions. In both the liver and spleen, a nodule that remains hypoechoic in both the early vascular phase (5–10 seconds after injection) and late vascular phase (25–30 seconds after injection) is more commonly seen with malignant lesions whereas benign nodules most often become isoechoic to the surrounding parenchyma in both phases.[21,32,33,35,36] However, this distinction is less clear for renal lesions.[37] This differential contrast pattern has also been shown to increase the sensitivity for the diagnosis of liver metastasis.[31]

Elastography uses ultrasound to assess the relative hardness of tissues. This is an emerging technology in both human and veterinary medicine to increase the specificity of ultrasound for the diagnosis of various disease processes. In strain elastography, external pressure is applied with the transducer and the mechanical properties of the tissues are illustrated with a color map; hard tissues are typically displayed in yellow to red colors and soft tissues in green to blue colors.[38] Tissue stiffness tends to increase with disease.[39] Limitations include susceptibility to operator variability and the need to compare tissues with adjacent structures.[40] More research is required in this area to determine the utility of elastography in oncologic imaging.

Ultrasound-guided tissue sampling is fast and safe. Image guidance allows for direct needle placement in the lesion of interest, thus minimizing patient risk and increasing diagnostic accuracy.[41,42] Serious complications from image-guided biopsies are uncommon, but include needle-tract seeding of transitional cell carcinoma.[43] The most common complications of percutaneous lung biopsy are pulmonary hemorrhage and pneumothorax, but these are typically minor and self-limiting. The risk of these complications is higher when the needle passes through aerated lung before entering the lesion.[44,45] Hemorrhage associated with ultrasound guided sampling occurs in fewer than 6% of cases and is self-limiting in all but 1%.[46,47]

Ultrasound accuracy is dependent on the experience of the operator and quality of the images. CT and MRI provide advantages when evaluating abdominal disease because obtaining complete high-quality images is less user dependent and images can be reviewed by a radiologist more confidently. In addition, CT and MRI provide advantages in evaluating larger abdomens, complex or extensive masses, masses of undetermined origin, and areas difficult to assess with ultrasound, such as the cranial-dorsal abdomen, pelvic region, and retroperitoneal space.

Computed Tomography

In veterinary medicine, CT is still typically performed under general anesthesia, but with the increasing availability of faster multislice scanners more CT scans are being performed with sedation alone. This is particularly true for thoracic CTs to screen for pulmonary metastasis. This can also be facilitated with the use of Plexiglas tubes for restraint.[48] There are clear advantages in terms of speed and cost when anesthesia is not used, but pulmonary atelectasis can still occur, particularly if the patient was sedated, and this may have an effect on interpretation of thoracic CTs.[48]

The basic principles of CT will be discussed, but more detailed descriptions of CT protocols can be found elsewhere.[49] Slice thickness is an important consideration, as it affects both image

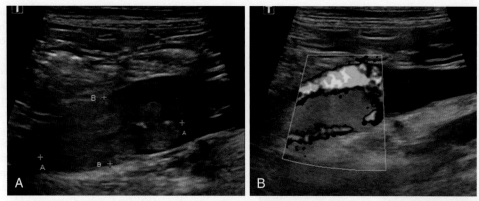

• **Fig. 6.5** Ultrasound images from a 10-year-old female spayed mixed breed dog. (A) A soft tissue mass is originating from the left adrenal gland (not visible) and invading into the caudal vena cava. (B) Color Doppler evaluation of the caudal vena cava with evidence of blood flow around the mass, but approximately 60% occlusion of the vessel by the mass and associated thrombus.

noise and partial volume averaging artifacts. Partial volume averaging can result in blurry margins, false attenuation measurements (Hounsfield units), and pseudolesions. Thin-slice images will have increased noise that can be offset by increasing mAs setting. This will improve image quality, but will also increase the radiation dose to the patient. Thin-slice imaging is more challenging on older scanners, as the heat load on the x-ray tube can slow the scan time, but newer generation CT scanners, particularly multislice helical scanners, have largely overcome the challenges, allowing large areas to be scanned quickly. The scan field of view (SFOV) is the area from which the image can be reconstructed. Because the reconstruction matrix size is constant, keeping the SFOV only as large as the anatomy to be imaged will improve spatial resolution. This is not critical for the majority of body parts, but a large SFOV used with whole-body CT can result in decreased resolution.

Although CT has decreased spatial resolution compared with radiographs, the reduced anatomic superimposition and superior contrast resolution result in CT being more sensitive to detect lesions throughout the body. For assessment of noncardiac thoracic disease, CT provides more information on the presence, location, and extent of disease in the majority of patients compared with survey radiographs.[6,50] Accuracy for detection of tracheobronchial lymphadenopathy is 93% for CT and 57% for radiographs, with a sensitivity of 83% and 0% respectively (using size, shape, and contrast enhancement on CT).[4] CT is also being used more frequently to evaluate the abdomen for primary and metastatic disease. The ability to image pelvic canal contents and visualize anatomy deep to gas-filled structures improves the sensitivity for detection of lesions.[51] For example, CT evaluation of insulinomas is superior to ultrasound, detection of sacral lymph node (LN) metastasis within the pelvic canal in dogs with apocrine gland anal sac adenocarcinomas is superior with CT compared with ultrasound, and the margins of soft tissue tumors, such as sarcomas and lipomas, are better delineated with contrast enhancement.[51–55] Tumors of the nasal cavity and head and neck have superior delineation on CT compared with radiographs or ultrasound.[53]

CT is also superior to palpation in determining tumor extent, as has been shown in cats with injection-site sarcomas,[54] and this is important implications in defining the aggressiveness of treatment with surgery and/or radiation therapy (RT). However, it is not possible to differentiate between peritumoral inflammation and local invasion, so more normal tissue may be included in

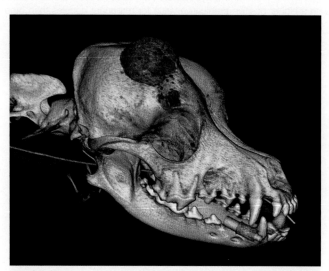

• **Fig. 6.6** A 3D reconstruction of a dog with a skull tumor can aid in assessment of tumor extension and surgical or radiation planning.

the treatment plan than necessary.[55,56] Detection of local tumor invasion is an important finding on CT and is evident by loss of adjacent fascial planes and vascular filling defects.[56] Large masses can cause compression of adjacent structures and, in these cases, it can be difficult to differentiate compression from invasion.[57] Although imaging characteristics are rarely pathognomonic for a specific tumor type, the CT appearance of fatty masses is highly predictive of lipoma, infiltrative lipoma, and liposarcoma.[58] Three-dimensional reconstructions are also very valuable for assessing skeletal structures and surgical planning (Fig. 6.6).

CT is more sensitive than radiographs in the detection of pulmonary metastasis and allows for detection of nodules as small as 1 mm in diameter compared with 7 to 9 mm for radiography.[7,8,50] In people, the high sensitivity of CT also results in detection of more benign lesions (up to 80%), with nodules <5 mm infrequently developing into metastasis.[59,60] The incidence of benign pulmonary nodules has not been fully investigated in veterinary medicine, but all nodules detected on CT developed into radiographically visible metastasis in one study of osteosarcoma in dogs.[50]

Ground-glass pulmonary lesions, also referred to as subsolid nodules, are characterized by an increased density that does not

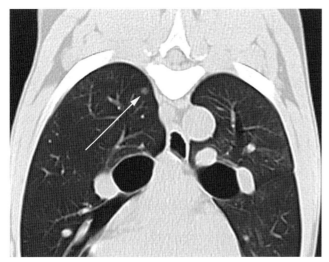

• **Fig. 6.7** Transverse computed tomography of the caudal thorax shows a focal ground-glass nodule *(arrow)* in the right caudal lung lobe. Ground-glass pulmonary lesions, also referred to as subsolid nodules, are characterized by an increased density that does not obscure the underlying pulmonary structures.

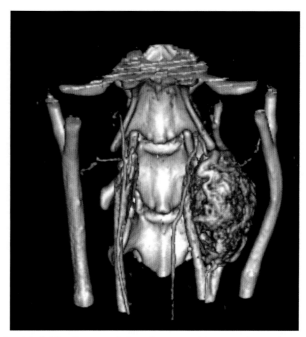

• **Fig. 6.8** A 3D volume rendering of computed tomography angiography of a thyroid mass shows the feeding blood vessels and highly vascular nature of the mass, consistent with a thyroid carcinoma.

obscure the underlying pulmonary structures (Fig. 6.7).[61] These nodules may be pure or mixed (containing some solid components). These lesions are frequently detected in people being staged for pulmonary metastasis, with up to 70% being caused by transient inflammation or hemorrhage.[62] Pure ground-glass lesions >8 mm have a high probability of malignancy, whereas those <4 mm are considered benign.[63] Lesions >22 mm, mixed lesions (partially ground-glass and partially solid), mixed lesions where the solid component grows to >2 mm in maximal diameter, and pure ground-glass lesions progressing to mixed lesions have a higher risk of being malignant.[61–63] Ground-glass lesions have not been fully investigated in veterinary medicine, but 75% of dogs with ground-glass lesions went on to develop radiographically visible metastasis in one pilot study.[50] To clearly discern the characteristics of pulmonary nodules, thin-slice techniques are required to avoid partial volume averaging, as this artifact can result in pure ground-glass nodules appearing to have a solid central component.[64]

Because CT has higher sensitivity to lesion detection than ultrasonography and radiography, there is increasing use of whole-body CT for cancer staging. In tumors with high metastatic potential, CT may detect muscular metastasis that may have been otherwise missed.[65] Whole-body CT for dogs with osteosarcoma has not been shown to be superior to radiography or nuclear scintigraphy for the detection bone metastasis, but concurrent neoplasia has been detected, and this may alter treatment options and prognosis.[50,66] Detection of metastatic and concurrent disease may be better with newer scanners and higher resolution reformatted images.

CT angiography (CTA) is being performed routinely to assess tumor vascularity, perfusion, and vascular invasion (Fig. 6.8). Multiphase CTA can improve detection of small tumors, such as insulinomas, and may be helpful in differentiating between benign and malignant lesions.[67,68] CTA is also advantageous in evaluating patients with pericardial effusion and thus enabling the detection of cardiac masses.[69] CTA may assist in predicting malignancy of hepatic and splenic masses and nodules, although more research is needed.[70] CTA also provides more accurate assessment of cranial

mediastinal and thyroid masses, which may assist in the determining the preferred treatment options for these patients.[71,72]

CT-guided biopsy is useful for the sampling of intracavitary lesions, such as pulmonary nodules, not readily identified with ultrasound. Manual CT-guided biopsy is performed using the internal laser of the scanner to orient to the transverse plane that includes the lesion of interest. Needle placement is assisted by radiopaque markers in bands in the sagittal or parasagittal plane. Barium can be used to create radiopaque bands, but commercially available opaque grids are also available that can be adhered to the skin (Fig. 6.9).[73]

Although MRI provides superior contrast resolution, CT is used for RT planning because it provides a map of electron density information that is used by most planning computers to calculate dose distribution.[74] Fusion of CT and MR images can aid in RT planning by maximizing both the spatial resolution of CT and the contrast resolution of MR. In human cancer therapy, CT combined with PET (PET/CT) is also used for RT planning, particularly with pulmonary lesions as PET/CT can differentiate between tumor and atelectic lung, which is not always possible with CT alone.[74]

Magnetic Resonance Imaging

MRI provides superior soft tissue resolution to CT and is highly sensitive to detection of pathology. MRI is generally considered superior to CT for neurologic and soft tissue imaging, but a study of feline injection-site sarcomas showed no difference in the evaluation of peritumoral lesions between CT and MRI.[75] MRI is also excellent for detecting infiltrative diseases of the musculoskeletal system, including accurate determination of the local extent of appendicular osteosarcoma lesions.[10,76]

With MRI, numerous imaging sequences are used to provide complementary information. T1-weighted images provide good spatial resolution to assess anatomy and are used with contrast

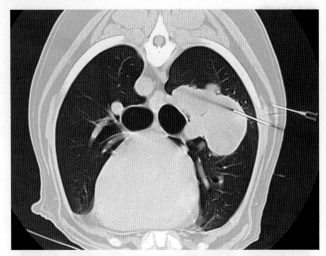

• **Fig. 6.9** Computed tomography (CT)-guided biopsy of the lung mass was facilitated by placement of a hypodermic needle into the body wall along the laser line that corresponded with the location of the mass. After placement of the marker needle, CT images were obtained to determine the best placement of the biopsy needle relative to the marker needle. This image shows the biopsy needle being placed ventral to the marker needle and perpendicular to the body wall. The tip of the needle is visible in the pulmonary mass.

to show vascular enhancement of tissues. T2-weighted images are water-weighted sequences that provide high-contrast images of water-dense pathology. On both T1- and T2-fast spin echo sequences, fat has a high signal intensity (bright) that can mask the margins of the pathology. The use of fat suppression techniques on T1 postcontrast and T2 images (e.g., Short-tau Inversion Recovery [STIR]) is important in cancer imaging to allow for clear assessment of the extent of pathology (Fig. 6.10). Diffusion-weighted imaging measures the random Brownian motion of water molecules in a voxel of tissue. Highly cellular tissues and swollen cells have restricted motion of water that can be detected with diffusion-weighted imaging.[77] Although this has been evaluated in humans, there is limited information on the effectiveness in veterinary medicine. Veterinary studies have found diffusion-weighted images and apparent diffusion coefficient maps helpful in diagnosing acute infarcts, which is hyperintense on diffusion-weighted images and hypointense on apparent diffusion coefficient maps.[78,79] However, in one study of 37 dogs, there was a wide range of apparent diffusion coefficient distribution within disease groups and significant overlap between groups when evaluating multiple tumor types, inflammatory disease, and infarcts.[80]

Because of the high contrast resolution, whole-body MRI has also been investigated in cancer patients. Whole-body diffusion-weighted MRI provides similar results to PET/CT in people with diffuse B-cell lymphoma.[81] In veterinary medicine, a protocol using large overlapping imaging fields and focused high-contrast sequences showed whole-body MRI can be performed in a reasonable time with sufficient quality to identify known lesions, but images were suboptimal for the skeletal system.[82] Further investigation to optimize protocols for veterinary patients is necessary.

Recently hepatocyte-specific MR contrast agents, such as gadoxetate disodium (Gd-EOB-DTPA), have been evaluated.[83,84] These agents accumulate in normal hepatocytes, potentially allowing for the differentiation between benign liver nodules and metastatic lesions, and aid in identification of primary liver tumors on delayed imaging.[84–86] These agents cause shortening of the T1 and T2 relaxation times, resulting in increased T1 signal intensity

compared with tissues that do not contain normal hepatocytes, allowing for the differentiation between hyperplastic and malignant nodules.[87]

Nuclear Scintigraphy

Nuclear medicine uses radiopharmaceuticals that accumulate in areas of interest based on physiologic processes. The low spatial resolution of these images precludes anatomic detail, but the functional information provided is advantageous in differentiating between occult and active disease processes. Scintigraphy lacks specificity, so it cannot differentiate between benign inflammatory lesions and malignant lesions. The two studies most commonly performed in cancer patents are thyroid and bone scintigraphy.

Bone scintigraphy provides physiologic information by detecting areas of increased bone activity (Fig. 6.11). Scintigraphy is highly sensitive for increased metabolic activity, but is not specific, and this can lead to false-positive diagnoses.[88,89] To reduce the risk of false-positive diagnoses, the use of supplementary imaging modalities, such as radiography, of suspected bone lesions is recommended.[50] Radiographs require at least a 30% to 50% change in mineral density to be detected, which means that early or small lesions may be missed on radiographs but detected with more sensitive CT scans.[50,90]

Thyroid scintigraphy is used to evaluate patients with ventral cervical masses. Thyroid scintigraphy can be used for the diagnosis of adenomatous hyperplasia in cats and can raise suspicion for thyroid carcinoma in cats and dogs. In cats, thyroid carcinoma typically has a large amount of hyperfunctional tissue, and ectopic hyperfunctional tissue may be present extending into the thorax (Fig. 6.12).[91] Thyroid carcinomas in dogs and cats are typically heterogeneous with irregular margins.[91,92] Imaging is typically performed with 99m-technetium pertechnetate ($^{99m}TcO_4^-$ There is a superscript negative sign beside the O and over the 4.) because of its availability and cost effectiveness.

Renal scintigraphy can be performed when nephrectomy is being considered for cats and dogs with a renal tumor or in cases in which adrenal tumors have invaded the renal vessels or compromised the adjacent kidney. A nuclear medicine glomerular filtration rate (GFR) study provides an assessment of global GFR, as well and right and left kidney GFR, so that the function of the single remaining kidney can be predicted.[93]

PET/CT or PET/MR is often preferred to scintigraphy to overcome some of the spatial limitations of nuclear scintigraphy.

Positron Emission Tomography/Computed Tomography (PET/CT) and MRI (PET/MR)

PET/CT and/or PET/MR combines the functional imaging of a nuclear medicine study and the high spatial resolution of CT and MR. The most commonly used radiopharmaceutical with PET imaging is the glucose analog 2-deoxy-2-^{18}F-fluorodeoxyglucose (FDG) bound to the positron emitter fluorine-18 (F-18). As a glucose analog, FDG is transported into hypermetabolic cells, where it becomes trapped after phosphorylation by hexokinase, as it is not a suitable substrate for glucose-6-phosphatase.[94] The F-18 portion of the radiopharmaceutical allows for it to be imaged, as the positrons emitted create two annihilation photons that travel 180 degrees from each other. These photons are detected by the PET detector ring.[94] Both tumors and inflammation result in increased glucose metabolism; therefore detection of a hypermetabolic lesion is not definitively indicative of neoplasia.

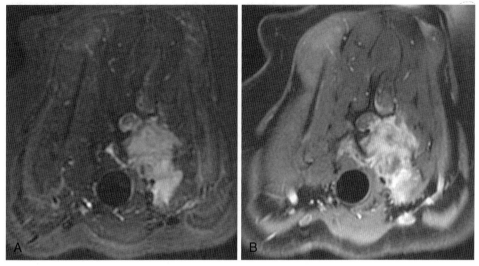

• **Fig. 6.10** A transverse Short-T1 Inversion Recovery (STIR) image (A) and T1 postcontrast image with fat suppression (B) shows the delineation of a peripheral nerve sheath tumor.

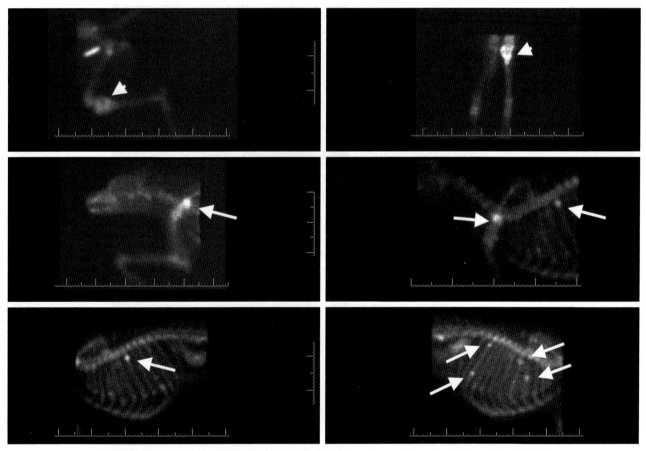

• **Fig. 6.11** Bone phase scintigraphy of the pelvic limbs *(top images)*, thoracic limbs and head *(middle images)*, and thorax *(bottom images)* show multifocal areas of increased radiopharmaceutical uptake *(hot spots)* in the ribs and scapula, consistent with bone metastasis *(arrows)*. The primary bone tumor is in the proximal tibia *(arrowhead)*.

However, F-18 FDG is the most commonly used PET radiopharmaceutical in human and veterinary medicine for detecting and staging cancer and evaluating response to treatment. Performing whole-body PET/CT provides additional information compared with traditional staging with thoracic radiographs and abdominal ultrasound; and, because of the metabolic component, can detect metastatic lesions before they would be detected with routine imaging, including CT alone (Fig. 6.13).

Other PET agents have been investigated in veterinary medicine. Labeling F-18 with sodium fluoride (NaF) results in a

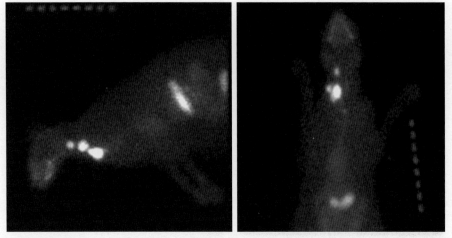

• **Fig. 6.12** Lateral (A) and ventral (B) thyroid scintigraphy images of the head, neck, and cranial thorax show multifocal areas of increased radiopharmaceutical uptake in the neck. This distribution of activity is consistent with a diagnosis of thyroid carcinoma.

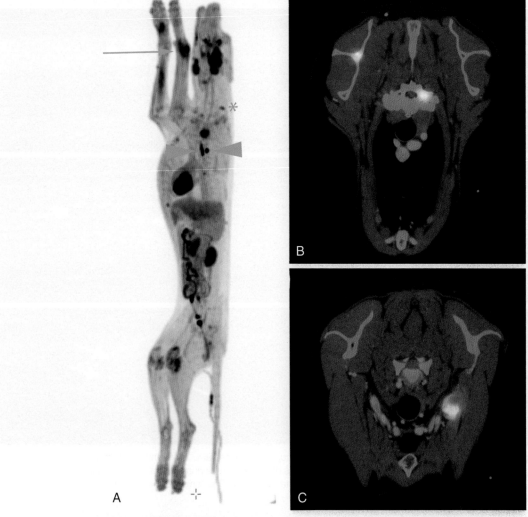

• **Fig. 6.13** F18-FDG PET/CT images from an 11-year-old mixed breed dog with osteosarcoma of the distal left radius. (A) Maximum intensity projection showing the primary tumor as hypermetabolic *(long arrow)* with areas of suspect metastatic disease in the lymph nodes *(*)* and bones (arrowhead, vertebra and scapula.) (B) Fused PET/CT image showing the hypermetabolic lesions in the right scapula and second thoracic vertebra, consistent with bone metastasis. (C) Fused PET/CT image showing an enlarged and hypermetabolic left axillary lymph node. *PET,* Positron emission tomography; *CT,* computed tomography.

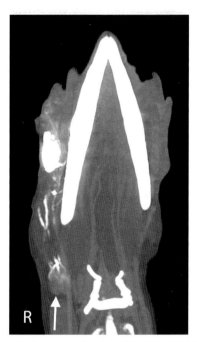

• **Fig. 6.14** A dorsal plane reconstruction of the head obtained 3 minutes after injection of a contrast medium around a rostral right mandibular mass demonstrates multiple lymphatic vessels draining into the right mandibular lymph node *(arrow)* identifying this as the sentinel lymph node. It is important to note that further cytologic or histopathologic assessment of the sentinel lymph node is required to determine whether there is evidence of metastasis within this lymph node.

bone-specific radiopharmaceutical that enables generation of highly detailed skeletal images that are superior for detection of bone metastasis compared with planar or single-photon emission computerized tomography (SPECT) imaging with Tc99m-methyl diphosphonate (Tc99m-MDP).[95] To date, the only reported use of NaF F-18 is in equine orthopedic disease and in four normal immature dogs.[96,97] Labeling F-18 with the thymidine analog FLT (3′-deoxy-3′[18F]fluorothymidine) allows the imaging of proliferating tissues, including neoplastic tissues. FLT reflects DNA synthesis and was successful in detecting initial disease, response to therapy, and predicting relapse in a small group of dogs with lymphoma.[98] PET/CT functional imaging of tumor hypoxia using dogs with spontaneously arising nasal tumors injected with copper(II)-diacetyl-bis(N^4-methylthiosemicarbazone) (Cu-ATSM) has also been performed and evaluated for radiation boost planning.[99]

The baseline metabolic rate of normal tissues must be known to accurately interpret PET images. The standardized uptake value (SUV) is a semiquantitative measure of FDG uptake that is directly proportional to the metabolic activity.[100] Increased SUV measurement correlates to subjective increased hypermetabolic activity visible on PET images. No specific cut-offs have been established for malignancy in veterinary medicine, whereas in human medicine an SUV_{max} >2.5 is predictive of malignancy in patients with solitary pulmonary nodules.[101] However, multiple studies have found that visual interpretation by an experienced reader is equivalent to or superior compared with SUV measurements.[102–104]

Multiple tumor types in dogs and cats have been shown to be hypermetabolic on PET or PET/CT, including but not limited to lymphoma, mast cell tumor, osteosarcoma, oral squamous cell carcinoma, mammary carcinoma, fibrosarcoma, and primary lung tumors.[98,105–111] F-18 FDG was shown to correlate with grade of

mast cell tumor in a small group of dogs.[112] Further specific uses of FDG and use of targeted agents will increase the usefulness of PET/CT in the future. The utility of PET/MRI in veterinary medicine is undergoing investigation.

Lymph Node Assessment

Assessing LNs for evidence of metastasis is an important part of staging cancer patients. B-mode ultrasound, CT, and MRI provide information on the size, shape, and echogenicity of LNs, providing a good initial assessment provided the LN is accessible. For example, only the medial iliac and cranial aspect of the internal iliac LNs are typically visible with abdominal ultrasound; as a result, ultrasonography is a less sensitive imaging modality than cross-sectional imaging techniques, such as CT and MRI, for the detection of nodal metastasis from perineal tumors where the sacral node is likely to be the draining node (e.g., apocrine gland anal sac adenocarcinomas).[52,113]

Using absolute LN size to determine malignancy can be problematic because of the substantial variation in dog breed sizes and the fact that metastatic LNs are not always enlarged. Many studies have looked at normalizing LN size to account for this variation, but with variable success.[114,115] CT assessment of sternal LNs suggest that a ratio of sternal LN height to the height of the second sternebra of >1 and a precontrast attenuation of 37.5 HU or greater is highly predictive of malignancy.[115] The presence of micrometastasis is also common and may not result in an absolute change in LN size.[4] A change in the shape of an LN from oval to round, as indicated by a short axis-to-long axis ratio of >0.7, and loss of definition of the LN hilus are seen more frequently with malignant than reactive LNs.[116,117] The signal characteristics of LNs should also be considered as, in combination with other parameters, this may be helpful in differentiating benign from malignant LNs. On ultrasound, both reactive and malignant LNs tend to be hypoechoic and may have a heterogeneous echogenicity, but there is no consistent pattern to differentiate these processes.[116,118] MRI perinodal contrast enhancement is seen more commonly in cats and dogs with reactive lymphadenitis.[119]

Metastatic disease to the LNs often alters the vascularity and these changes may be evident with Doppler ultrasonography. The blood supply to normal LNs is predominantly centered at the hilus, whereas malignant LNs trend to having a peripheral or mixed peripheral and hilar distribution with a greater number of vessels.[26,117,118] Displacement of the central hilar vessels, more than one central vessel, pericapsular vessels, and peripheral vessels that do not connect with the central vessel have all been associated with malignancy.[29] Vascular resistance may increase in malignant LNs as a result of vascular compression from tumor cells, and this can be detected by measuring resistive index and pulsatility index.[120] Increases in these parameters are suggestive of malignancy when seen in combination with other sonographic findings.[26,116] Fundamentally, however, there is no one sonographic measurement that is predictive of malignancy; using a combination of size, shape, and vascularity of the LN, in addition to fine-needle aspirate cytology of the LN, is recommended to increase the predictive value for detection of metastatic disease.[120]

Detection of the sentinel or draining LN is very important in the clinical staging and determining the treatment options and prognosis for animals and people with cancer (see Chapter 9). Assessment of LNs is based on size, shape, and contrast enhancement, but there is wide variation in accuracy using these parameters due in part to the subjectivity of evaluation.[4,118]

Micrometastasis may also be present, and this rarely alters the size or results in contrast enhancement of LNs, resulting in a false-negative diagnosis. In addition, contrast enhancement on CT may be a result of inflammation rather than metastatic disease, resulting in a false-positive diagnosis.[4] Considerable attention has been given to the evaluation of LNs with a variety of imaging modalities to determine whether there are characteristics that are specific to metastasis.[4,6]

Direct lymphangiography (injection of contrast medium into an LN or lymphatic vessel) and indirect lymphangiography (injection of contrast medium into the peritumoral tissues) can be used to image the lymphatic beds and identify the sentinel LN (Fig. 6.14).[121] Use of iodized oil contrast medium results in retention of the agent in the LN for up to 2 months after injection, which can aid in follow-up LN assessment, where contrast voids are consistent with new metastatic lesions, and make the LNs more conspicuous on radiation port films, which aids in RT planning.[121] Indirect lymphangiography is used to map the draining LNs from a superficial tumor.[122–125] A heterogeneous pattern of LN enhancement may also predict malignancy, because this pattern may be caused by loss of normal architecture secondary to tumor infiltration.[123] Sentinel LN mapping can also be performed with lymphoscintigraphy. Lymphatic drainage can be detected intraoperatively with the use of a gamma camera, hand-held gamma probe, and/or peritumoral injection of blue dyes.[126]

References

1. Wisner ER, Pollard RE: Trends in veterinary cancer imaging, *Vet Comp Oncol* 2:49–74, 2004.
2. Nerschbach V, Eberle N, Joetzke AE, et al.: Splenic and hepatic ultrasound and cytology in canine lymphoma: effects of findings on stage migration and assessment of prognosis, *Vet Comp Oncol Suppl* 1:82–94, 2016.
3. Ober CP, Ober CP, Barber D, et al.: Comparison of two- vs. three–view thoracic radiographic studies on conspicuity of structured interstitial patterns in dogs, *Vet Radiol Ultrasound* 47:542–545, 2006.
4. Paoloni MC, Adams WM, Dubielzig RR, et al.: Comparison of results of computed tomography and radiography with histopathologic findings in tracheobronchial lymph nodes in dogs with primary lung tumors: 14 cases (1999–2002), *J Am Vet Med Assoc* 228:1718–1722, 2006.
5. Lang J, Wortman JA, Glickmann LT, et al.: Sensitivity of radiographic detection of lung metastasis in the dog, *Vet Radiol Ultrasound* 27:74–78, 1986.
6. Prather AB, Berry CR, Thrall DE: Use of radiography in combination with computed tomography for the assessment of noncardiac thoracic disease in the dog and cat, *Vet Radiol Ultrasound* 46:114–121, 2005.
7. Eberle N, Fork M, Babo von V, et al.: Comparison of examination of thoracic radiographs and thoracic computed tomography in dogs with appendicular osteosarcoma, *Vet Comp Oncol* 9:131–140, 2010.
8. Nemanic S, London CA, Wisner ER: Comparison of thoracic radiographs and single breath-hold helical CT for detection of pulmonary nodules in dogs with metastatic neoplasia, *J Vet Intern Med* 20:508–515, 2006.
9. Schultz RM, Puchalski SM, Kent M, et al.: Skeletal lesions of histiocytic sarcoma in nineteen dogs, *Vet Radiol Ultrasound* 48:539–543, 2007.
10. Wallack ST, Wisner ER, Werner JA, et al.: Accuracy of magnetic resonance imaging for estimating intramedullary osteosarcoma extent in pre-operative planning of canine limb-salvage procedures, *Vet Radiol Ultrasound* 43:432–441, 2002.
11. Freedman MT, Lo S-CB, Seibel JC, et al.: Lung nodules: improved detection with software that suppresses the rib and clavicle on chest radiographs, *Radiology* 260:265–273, 2011.
12. Nyland TG, Mattoon JS: *Fundamentals of diagnostic ultrasound, Veterinary Diagnostic Ultrasound*, ed 3, St. Louis, 2015, Elsevier.
13. Besso JG, Penninck DG, Gliatto JM: Retrospective ultrasonographic evaluation of adrenal lesions in 26 dogs, *Vet Radiol Ultrasound* 38:448–455, 1997.
14. Hanson JA, Papageorges M, Girard E, et al.: Ultrasonographic appearance of splenic disease in 101 cats, *Vet Radiol Ultrasound* 42:441–445, 2001.
15. Penninck D, Smyers B, Webster CRL, et al.: Diagnostic value of ultrasonography in differentiating enteritis from intestinal neoplasia in dogs, *Vet Radiol Ultrasound* 44:570–575, 2003.
16. Cruz-Arambulo R, Wrigley R, Powers B: Sonographic features of histiocytic neoplasms in the canine abdomen, *Vet Radiol Ultrasound* 45:554–558, 2004.
17. Cuccovillo A, Lamb CR: Cellular features of sonographic target lesions of the liver and spleen in 21 dogs and a cat, *Vet Radiol Ultrasound* 43:275–278, 2002.
18. Ramirez S, Douglass JP, Robertson ID: Ultrasonographic features of canine abdominal malignant histiocytosis, *Vet Radiol Ultrasound* 43:167–170, 2005.
19. Sato AF, Solano M: Ultrasonographic findings in abdominal mast cell disease: a retrospective study of 19 patients, *Vet Radiol Ultrasound* 45:51–57, 2004.
20. Sacornrattana O, Dervisis NG, McNiel EA: Abdominal ultrasonographic findings at diagnosis of osteosarcoma in dogs and association with treatment outcome, *Vet Comp Oncol* 11:199–207, 2012.
21. O'Brien RT, Iani M, Matheson J, et al.: Contrast harmonic ultrasound of spontaneous liver noduels in 32 dogs, *Vet Radiol Ultrasound* 45:547–553, 2004.
22. Gaschen L: Ultrasonography of small intestinal inflammatory and neoplastic diseases in dogs and cats, *Vet Clin North Am Small Anim Pract* 41:329–344, 2011.
23. Monteiro CB, O'Brien RT: A retrospective study on the sonographic findings of abdominal carcinomatosis in 14 cats, *Vet Radiol Ultrasound* 45:559–564, 2004.
24. Valdés-Martínez A, Cianciolo R, Mai W: Association between renal hypoechoic subcapsular thickening and lymphosarcoma in cats, *Vet Radiol Ultrasound* 48:357–360, 2007.
25. Nyland TG, Mattoon JS: Fundamentals of diagnostic ultrasound. In Nyland TG, Mattoon JS, editors: *Veterinary diagnostic ultrasound*, ed 3, St. Louis, 2015, Elsevier, pp 1–49.
26. Prieto S, Gómez-Ochoa P, De Blas I, et al.: Pathologic correlation of resistive and pulsatility indicies in canine abdominal lymph nodes, *Vet Radiol Ultrasound* 50:525–529, 2009.
27. Santa della D, Gaschen L, Doherr MG, et al.: Spectral waveform analysis of intranodal arterial blood flow in abnormally large superficial lymph nodes in dogs, *Am J Vet Res* 69:478–485, 2008.
28. Nyman HT, Kristensen AT, Lee MH, et al.: Characterization of canine superficial tumors using gray-scale B mode, color flow mapping, and spectral Doppler ultrasonography - a multivariate study, *Vet Radiol Ultrasound* 47:192–198, 2006.
29. Salwei RM, O'Brien RT: Characterization of lymphomatous lymph nodes in dogs using contrast harmonic and power Doppler ultrasound, *Vet Radiol Ultrasound* 46:411–416, 2005.
30. Kim AY, Choi BI, Kim TK, et al.: Hepatocellular carcinoma: power Doppler US with a contrast agent—preliminary results, *Radiology* 209:135–140, 1998.
31. Nyman HT, Kristensen AT, Flagstad A: A review of the sonographic assessment of tumor metastases in liver and superficial lymph nodes, *Vet Radiol* 45:438–448, 2004.
32. Nakamura K, Sasaki N, Murakami M, et al.: Contrast-enhanced ultrasonography for characterization of focal splenic lesions in dogs, *J Vet Intern Med* 24:1290–1297, 2010.
33. Penninck D: Contrast enhanced sonographic assessment of feeding vessels as a discriminator between malignant vs. benign focal splenic lesions, *Vet Radiol Ultrasound* 52:457–461, 2011.

34. Kanemoto H, Ohno K, Nakashima K: Characterization of canine focal liver lesions wth contrast-enhanced ultrasound using a novel contrast agent – Sonazoid, *Vet Radiol* 50:188–194, 2009.

35. Dennis R, Kirberger RM, Barr F, et al.: Characterization of canine superficial tumors using gray-scale B mode, color flow mapping, and spectral Doppler ultrasonography – a multivariate study, *Vet Radiol Ultrasound* 47:192–198, 2016.

36. Ivančić M, Long F, Seiler GS: Contrast harmonic ultrasonography of splenic masses and associated liver nodules in dogs, *J Am Vet Med Assoc* 234:88–94, 2009.

37. Haers H, Vignoli M, Paes G, et al.: Contrast harmonic ultrasonographic appearance of focal space–occupying renal lesions, *Vet Radiol* 51:516–522, 2010.

38. Pollard R, Nyland TG, Berry CR, et al.: Advanced ultrasound techniques. In Nyland TG, Mattoon JS, editors: *Veterinary diagnostic ultrasound*, ed 3, St. Louis, 2015, Elsevier, pp 78–93.

39. Feliciano MAR, Maronezi MC, Pavan L, et al.: ARFI elastography as a complementary diagnostic method of mammary neoplasia in female dogs – preliminary results, *J Small Animal Practice* 55:504–508, 2014.

40. Holdsworth A, Bradley K, Birch S, et al.: Elastography of the normal canine liver, spleen and kidneys, *Vet Radiol Ultrasound* 55:620–627, 2014.

41. Wang KY, Panciera DL, Al-Rukibat RK, et al.: Accuracy of ultrasound-guided fine-needle aspiration of the liver and cytologic findings in dogs and cats: 97 cases (1990-2000), *J Am Vet Med Assoc* 224:75–78, 2004.

42. Penninck DG, Crystal MA, Matz ME, et al.: The technique of percutaneous ultrasound guided fine-needle aspiration biopsy and automated microcore biopsy in small animal gastrointestinal diseaes, *Vet Radiol Ultrasound* 34:433–436, 1993.

43. Nyland TG, Wallack ST, Wisner ER: Needle-tract implantation following US-guided fine-needle aspiration biopsy of transitional cell carcinoma of the bladder, urethra, and prostate, *Vet Radiol Ultrasound* 43:50–53, 2002.

44. Zekas LJ, Crawford JT, O'Brien RT: Computed tomography-guided fine-needle aspirate and tissue-core biopsy of intrathoracic lesions in thirty dogs and cats, *Vet Radiol Ultrasound* 46:200–204, 2005.

45. Wood EF, O'Brien RT, Young KM: Ultrasound-guided fine-needle aspiration of focal parenchymal lesions of the lung in dogs and cats, *J Vet Intern Med* 12:338–342, 1998.

46. Kerr LY: Ultrasound-guided biopsy, *Calif Vet* 42:9–10, 1988.

47. Léveillé R, Partington BP, Biller DS, et al.: Complications after ultrasound-guided biopsy of abdominal structures in dogs and cats: 246 cases (1984-1991), *J Am Vet Med Assoc* 203:413–415, 1993.

48. Oliveira CR, Ranallo FN, Pijanowski GJ: The Vetmousetrap™: a device for computed tomographic imaging of the thorax of awake cats, *Vet Radiol* 52:41–52, 2011.

49. Schwarz T, Saunders J: *Veterinary computed tomography*, ed 1, West Sussex, 2011, Wiley-Blackwell.

50. Oblak ML, Boston SE, Woods JP, et al.: Comparison of concurrent imaging modalities for staging of dogs with appendicular primary bone tumours, *Vet Comp Oncol* 13:28–39, 2013.

51. Robben JH, Pollak Y, Kirpensteijn J, et al.: Comparison of ultrasonography, computed tomography, and single-photon emission computed tomography for the detection and localization of canine insulinoma, *J Vet Intern Med* 19:15–22, 2005.

52. Pollard RE, Fuller MC, Steffey MA: Ultrasound and computed tomography of the iliosacral lymphatic centre in dogs with anal sac gland carcinoma, *Vet Comp Oncol* 15:299–306, 2017.

53. Codner EC, Lurus AG, Miller JB, et al.: Comparison of computed tomography with radiography as a noninvasive diagnostic technique for chronic nasal disease in dogs, *J Am Vet Med Assoc* 202:1106–1110, 1993.

54. Ferrari R, Di Giancamillo M, Stefanello D, et al.: Clinical and computed tomography tumour dimension assessments for planning wide excision of injection site sarcomas in cats: how strong is the agreement? *Vet Comp Oncol* 15:374–382, 2015.

55. Lederer K, Ludewig E, Hechinger H, et al.: Differentiation between inflammatory and neoplastic orbital conditions based on computed tomographic signs, *Vet Ophthalmol* 18:271–275, 2014.

56. Vliegen R, Dresen R, Beets G, et al.: The accuracy of multi-detector row CT for the assessment of tumor invasion of the mesorectal fascia in primary rectal cancer, *Abdominal Imaging* 33:604–610, 2008.

57. Yoon J, Feeney DA, Cronk DE, et al.: Computed tomographic evaluation of canine and feline mediastinal masses in 14 patients, *Vet Radiol Ultrasound* 45:542–546, 2004.

58. McEntee MC, Thrall DE: Computed tomographic imaging of infiltrative lipoma in 22 dogs, *Vet Radiol Ultrasound* 42:221–225, 2001.

59. Chalmers N, Best JJ: The significance of pulmonary nodules detected by CT but not by chest radiography in tumour staging, *Clin Radiol* 44:410–412, 1991.

60. MacMahon H, Austin JHM, Gamsu G, et al.: Guidelines for management of small pulmonary nodules detected on CT scans: a statement from the Fleischner Society, *Radiology* 237:395–400, 2005.

61. Pedersen JH, Saghir Z, Wille MMW, et al.: Ground-glass opacity lung nodules in the era of lung cancer CT screening: radiology, pathology, and clinical management, *Oncology* 30:266–274, 2016.

62. Lee SM, Park CM, Goo JM, et al.: Transient part-solid nodules detected at screening thin-section CT for lung cancer: comparison with persistent part-solid nodules, *Radiology* 255:242–251, 2010.

63. Park CM, Kim KG, Park E-A, et al.: Predictive CT findings of malignancy in ground-glass nodules on thin-section chest CT: the effects on radiologist performance, *Eur Radiol* 19:552–560, 2009.

64. Zhang Y, Shen Y, Qiang JW, et al.: HRCT features distinguishing pre-invasive from invasive pulmonary adenocarcinomas appearing as ground-glass nodules, *Eur Radiol* 26(1–8), 2016.

65. Terragni R, Ressel L: Whole body computed tomographic characteristics of skeletal and cardiac muscular metastatic neoplasia in dogs and cats, *Vet Radiol Ultrasound* 54:223–230, 2013.

66. Talbott JL, Boston SE, Milner RJ, et al.: Retrospective evaluation of whole body computed tomography for tumor staging in dogs with primary appendicular osteosarcoma, *Vet Surg* 46:75–80, 2017.

67. MAI W, Cáceres AV: Dual–phase computed tomographic angiography in three dogs with pancreatic insulinoma, *Vet Radiol Ultrasound* 49:141–148, 2008.

68. Griebie ER, David FH, Ober CP, et al.: Evaluation of canine hepatic masses by use of triphasic computed tomography and B-mode, color flow, power, and pulsed-wave Doppler ultrasonography and correlation with histopathologic classification, *Am J Vet Res* 78:1273–1283, 2017.

69. Scollan KF, Bottorff B, Stieger-Vanegas S, et al.: Use of multidetector computed tomography in the assessment of dogs with pericardial effusion, *J Vet Intern Med* 29:79–87, 2015.

70. Griebie ER, David FH, Ober CP, et al.: Evaluation of canine hepatic masses by use of triphasic computed tomography and B-mode, color flow, power, and pulsed-wave Doppler ultrasonography and correlation with histopathologic classification, *Am J Vet Res* 78:1273–1283, 2017.

71. Bertolini G, DRIGO M, Angeloni L, et al.: Incidental and nonincidental canine thyroid tumors assessed by multidetector row computed tomography: a single-centre cross sectional study in 4520 dogs, *Vet Radiol Ultrasound* 58:304–314, 2017.

72. Scherrer WE, Kyles AE, Samii VF, et al.: Computed tomographic assessment of vascular invasion and resectability of mediastinal masses in dogs and a cat, *N Z Vet J* 56:330–333, 2011.

73. Tidwell A: Computed tomography-guided percutaneous biopsy in the dog and cat: description of technique and preliminary evaluation in 14 patients, *Vet Radiol* 35:445–456, 1994.

74. Terezakis SA, Heron DE, Lavigne RF, et al.: What the diagnostic radiologist needs to know about radiation oncology, *Radiology* 261:30–44, 2011.

75. Nemanic S, Milovancev M, Terry JL, et al.: Microscopic evaluation of peritumoral lesions of feline injection site sarcomas identified by magnetic resonance imaging and computed tomography, *Vet Surg* 45:392–401, 2016.

76. Krimins RA, Fritz J, Gainsburg LA, et al.: Use of magnetic resonance imaging-guided biopsy of a vertebral body mass to diagnose osteosarcoma in a Rottweiler, *J Am Vet Med Assoc* 250:779–784, 2017.

77. Nagel KNA, Schouten MG, Hambrock T, et al.: Differentiation of prostatitis and prostate cancer by using diffusion-weighted MR imaging and MR-guided biopsy at 3 T, *Radiology* 267:164–172, 2013.

78. McConnell JF, Garosi L, Platt SR: Magnetic resonance imaging findings of presumed cerebellar cerebrovascular accident in twelve dogs, *Vet Radiol Ultrasound* 46:1–10, 2005.

79. Garosi L, McConnell JF, Platt SR, et al.: Clinical and topographic magnetic resonance characteristics of suspected brain infarction in 40 dogs, *J Vet Intern Med* 20:311–321, 2006.

80. Sutherland-Smith J, King R, Faissler D, et al.: Magnetic resonance imaging apparent diffusion coefficients for histologically confirmed intracranial lesions in dogs, *Vet Radiol Ultrasound* 52:142–148, 2011.

81. Lin C, Luciani A, Itti E, et al.: Whole-body diffusion-weighted magnetic resonance imaging with apparent diffusion coefficient mapping for staging patients with diffuse large B-cell lymphoma, *Eur Radiol* 20:2027–2038, 2010.

82. Kraft S, Randall E, Wilhelm M: Development of a whole body magnetic resonance imaging protocol in normal dogs and canine cancer patients, *Vet Radiol* 48:212–220, 2007.

83. Bratton AK, Nykamp SG, Gibson T: Evaluation of hepatic contrast enhancement with a hepatocyte-specific magnetic resonance imaging contrast agent (gadoxetic acid) in healthy dogs, *Am J Vet Res* 76:224–230, 2015.

84. Constant C, Hecht S, Craig LE, et al.: Gadoxetate disodium (GD-EOB-DTPA) contrast enhanced magnetic resonance imaging characteristics of hepatocellular carcinoma in dogs, *Vet Radiol Ultrasound* 57:594–600, 2016.

85. Louvet A, Duconseille AC: Feasibility for detecting liver metastases in dogs using gadobenate dimeglumine-enhanced magnetic resonance imaging, *Vet Radiol Ultrasound* 56:286–295, 2015.

86. Suh CH, Kim KW, Kim GY, et al.: The diagnostic value of Gd-EOB-DTPA-MRI for the diagnosis of focal nodular hyperplasia: a systematic review and meta-analysis, *Eur Radiol* 25:950–960, 2014.

87. Kanematsu M, Kondo H, Goshima S, et al.: Imaging liver metastases: review and update, *Eur J Radiol* 58:217–228, 2006.

88. Jankowski MK, Steyn PF, Lana SE, et al.: Nuclear scanning with 99mTc-HDP for the initial evaluation of osseous metastasis in canine osteosarcoma, *Vet Comp Oncol* 1:152–158, 2003.

89. Forrest LJ, Thrall DE: Bone scintigraphy for metastasis detection in canine osteosarcoma, *Vet Radiol Ultrasound* 35:124–130, 1994.

90. Rybak LD, Rosenthal DI: Radiological imaging for the diagnosis of bone metastases, *Q J Nucl Med* 45:53–64, 2001.

91. Peterson ME, Broome MR: Thyroid scintigraphy findings in 2096 cats with hyperthyroidism, *Vet Radiol Ultrasound* 56:84–95, 2014.

92. Berry CR, Daniel GB: *Textbook of veterinary nuclear medicine*, ed 2, Knoxville, 2006, American College of Veterinary Radiology.

93. Ragni RA, Moore AH: Kidney surgery, *Companion Anim* 18:16–24, 2013.

94. Workman RB, Coleman RE: *PET/CT Essentials for clinical practice*, New York, 2006, Springer-Verlag.

95. Grant FD, Fahey FH, Packard AB, et al.: Skeletal PET with 18F-fluoride: applying new technology to an old tracer, *J Nucl Med* 49:68–78, 2008.

96. Spriet M, Espinosa P, Kyme AZ, et al.: Positron emission tomography of the equine distal limb: exploratory study, *Vet Radiol Ultrasound* 57:630–638, 2016.

97. Valdés-Martínez A, Kraft SL, Brundage CM, et al.: Assessment of blood pool, soft tissue, and skeletal uptake of sodium fluoride F 18 with positron emission tomography-computed tomography in four clinically normal dogs, *Am J Vet Res* 73:1589–1595, 2012.

98. Lawrence J, Vanderhoek M, radiology DBV, et al.: Uses of 3′−deoxy−3′−[18F]fluorothymidine PET/CT for evaluating response to cytotoxic chemotherapy in dogs with non-Hodgkin's lymphoma, *Vet Radiol Ultrasound* 50:660–668, 2009.

99. Bradshaw TJ, Bowen SR, Deveau MA, et al.: Molecular imaging biomarkers of resistance to radiation therapy for spontaneous nasal tumors in canines, *Radiat Oncol Biol* 91:787–795, 2015.

100. Randall EK: PET-computed tomography in veterinary medicine, *Vet Clin North Am Small Anim Pract* 46:515–533, 2016.

101. Lowe VJ, Fletcher JW, Gobar L, et al.: Prospective investigation of positron emission tomography in lung nodules, *J Clin Oncol* 16:1075–1084, 1998.

102. Gould MK, Maclean CC, Kuschner WG, et al.: Accuracy of positron emission tomography for diagnosis of pulmonary nodules and mass lesions: a meta-analysis, *J Am Med Aassoc* 285:914–924, 2001.

103. Schöder H, Yeung HWD: Positron emission imaging of head and neck cancer, including thyroid carcinoma, *Semin Nucl Med* 34:180–197, 2004.

104. Lapela M, Eigtved A, Jyrkkiö S, et al.: Experience in qualitative and quantitative FDG PET in follow-up of patients with suspected recurrence from head and neck cancer, *Eur J Cancer* 36:858–867, 2000.

105. Seiler SMF, Baumgartner C, Hirschberger J, et al.: Comparative oncology: evaluation of 2-deoxy-2-[18F]fluoro-D-glucose (FDG) positron emission tomography/computed tomography (PET/CT) for the staging of dogs with malignant tumorsl, *PLoS ONE* 10: e0127800, 2015.

106. Randall EK, Kraft SL, Yoshikawa H, et al.: Evaluation of 18F-FDG PET/CT as a diagnostic imaging and staging tool for feline oral squamous cell carcinoma, *Vet Comp Oncol* 14:28–38, 2016.

107. Hansen AE, McEvoy F, Engelholm SA, et al.: FDG PET/CT imaging in canine cancer patients, *Vet Radiol Ultrasound* 52:201–206, 2011.

108. Leblanc AK, Jakoby BW, Daniel GB: 18FDG–PET Imaging in canine lymphoma and cutaneous mast cell tumor, *Vet Radiol Ultrasound* 50:215–223, 2009.

109. Leblanc AK, Miller AN, Galyon GD, et al.: Preliminary evaluation of serial 18FDG-PET/CT to assess response to toceranib phosphate therapy in canine cancer, *Vet Radiol Ultrasound* 53:348–357, 2012.

110. Kim J, Kwon SY, Cena R, et al.: CT and PET-CT of a dog with multiple pulmonary adenocarcinoma, *J Vet Med Sci* 76:615–620, 2014.

111. Ballegeer EA, Forrest LJ, Jeraj R, et al.: PET/CT following intensity-modulated radiation therapy for primary lung tumor in a dog, *Vet Radiol Ultrasound* 47:228–233, 2006.

112. LeBlanc AK, Jakoby BW, Townsend DW, et al.: 18FDG-PET imaging in canine lymphoma and cutaneous mast cell tumor, *Vet Radiol Ultrasound* 50:215–223, 2009.

113. Anderson CL, MacKay CS, Roberts GD, et al.: Comparison of abdominal ultrasound and magnetic resonance imaging for detection of abdominal lymphadenopathy in dogs with metastatic apocrine gland adenocarcinoma of the anal sac, *Vet Comp Oncol* 13:98–105, 2015.

114. Ballegeer EA, Adams WM, Dubielzig RR: Computed tomography characteristics of canine tracheobronchial lymph node metastasis, *Vet Radiol* 51:397–403, 2010.

115. Iwasaki R, Murakami M, Kawabe M, et al.: Metastatic diagnosis of canine sternal lymph nodes using computed tomography characteristics: a retrospective cross-sectional study, *Vet Comp Oncol* 68:536–538, 2017.

116. De Swarte M, Alexander K, Rannou B, et al.: Comparison of sonographic features of benign and neoplastic deep lymph nodes in dogs, *Vet Radiol Ultrasound* 52:451–456, 2011.

117. Nyman HT, Kristensen AT: Characterization of normal and abnormal canine superficial lymph nodes using gray-scale B-mode, color flow mapping, power, and spectral Doppler ultrasonography: a multivariate study, *Vet Radiol* 46:404–410, 2005.

118. Kinns J, MAI W: Association between malignancy and sonographic heterogeneity in canine and feline abdominal lymph nodes, *Vet Radiol Ultrasound* 48:565–569, 2007.

119. Johnson PJ, Elders R, Pey P, et al.: Clinical and magnetic resonance imaging features of inflammatory versus neoplastic lymph node mass lesions in dogs and cats, *Vet Radiol Ultrasound* 57:24–32, 2016.

120. Nyman HT, O Brien RT: The sonographic evaluation of lymph nodes, *Clin Tech Small Anim Pract* 22:128–137, 2007.

121. Mayer MN, Silver TI, Lowe CK, et al.: Radiographic lymphangiography in the dog using iodized oil, *Vet Comp Oncol* 11:151–161, 2012.

122. Majeski SA, Steffey MA, Fuller M, et al.: Indirect computed tomographic lymphography for iliosacral lymphatic mapping in a cohort of dogs with anal sac gland adenocarcinoma: technique description, *Vet Radiol Ultrasound* 58:295–303, 2017.

123. Soultani C, Patsikas MN, Karayannopoulou M, et al.: Assessment of sentinel lymph node metastasis in canine mammary gland tumors using computed tomographic indirect lymphography, *Vet Radiol Ultrasound* 58:186–196, 2016.

124. Grimes JA, Secrest SA, Northrup NC, et al.: Indirect computed tomography lymphangiography with aqueous contrast for evaluation of sentinel lymph nodes in dogs with tumors of the head, *Vet Radiol Ultrasound* 58:559–564, 2017.

125. Brissot HN, Edery EG: Use of direct lymphography to identify sentinel lymph node in dogs: a pilot study of 30 tumours, *Vet Comp Oncol* 15:740–753, 2017.

126. Worley DR: Incorporation of sentinel lymph node mapping in dogs with mast cell tumours: 20 consecutive procedures, *Vet Comp Oncol* 12:215–226, 2014.

7

Diagnostic Cytopathology in Clinical Oncology

KRISTEN R. FRIEDRICHS AND KAREN M. YOUNG

In veterinary oncology, cytologic evaluation plays several important roles that aid in clinical decision making, including making a preliminary or definitive diagnosis, planning diagnostic and treatment strategies, determining prognosis through staging, detecting recurrence, and monitoring response to therapy. An understanding of the advantages and limitations of cytologic evaluation is necessary to use this diagnostic modality effectively in clinical oncology.

Advantages of cytologic evaluation include the ability to evaluate the morphologic appearance of individual cells, the relatively low risk of procedures to the patient, the lower cost compared with surgical biopsy, and the speed with which results can be obtained. Cytologic evaluation also has several limitations. The amount of tissue sampled is small compared with that obtained from a surgical biopsy; therefore cytologic specimens may not be fully representative of the lesion. Sample quality may be poor because of factors intrinsic to the lesion or poor collection technique. Importantly, the inability to evaluate architectural relationships among cells in cytologic specimens may prevent distinction between reactive and neoplastic processes or between benign and malignant tumors. Examination of histologic samples, in which tissue architecture is preserved, may be required to make a definitive diagnosis of neoplasia, determine tumor type, and assess the extent of the lesion, including metastasis. Even then, ancillary tests such as immunohistochemical staining or tests for clonality may be required. Often, cytologic evaluation precedes a surgical biopsy and provides information that assists in formulating subsequent diagnostic and treatment procedures.

Some tumors, such as lymphoma, may often be definitively diagnosed and staged using cytologic evaluation exclusively, and treatment can be initiated without the need to collect histologic specimens. For other tumors, such as well-differentiated hepatocellular carcinoma, cytologic examination permits formulation of a list of differential diagnoses, and histologic evaluation must be performed for definitive diagnosis. At a minimum, categorization of a tumor as an epithelial, mesenchymal, or discrete round cell tumor often can be determined cytologically; this may be sufficient for initial discussions with the owner about diagnosis and prognosis. Staging the malignancy, monitoring therapy, and detecting recurrence using cytologic evaluation are more easily accomplished once a definitive diagnosis has been made and cytomorphologic

features of the tumor described. Staging procedures often include cytologic evaluation of regional lymph nodes (LNs). Importantly, LNs containing metastatic disease are not always enlarged, and thus normal-sized LNs should be sampled. For detection of solid tumor metastasis to regional LNs, fine-needle aspiration (FNA) is highly sensitive and specific[1]; however, metastatic disease may be present even if tumor cells are not identified in a sample collected from an LN; in this case, histologic evaluation may be required.

Sample Collection

Proper collection and preparation techniques are prerequisites to obtaining diagnostic samples of high quality. Supplies necessary for collecting cytologic samples from a variety of tissues, body cavities, and mucosal surfaces are available in most clinics. These include hypodermic needles and syringes, scalpel blades and handles, propylene urinary catheters, bone marrow aspiration needles, cotton swabs, clean glass slides, marking pencils, and collection vials and tubes (tubes with ethylenediaminetetraacetic acid [EDTA] and plain sterile tubes). For aspiration of internal lesions, obtained by guidance with ultrasonography or computed tomography (CT), longer spinal needles and extension sets (used to connect the spinal needle to the aspirating syringe) are useful. Cytologic specimens also can be made from tissues collected during surgical biopsy (see Chapter 9). All supplies should be assembled in one location for ready access. Although life-threatening situations are rarely encountered when collecting cytologic specimens, supplies and medications should be available to control bleeding and to treat anaphylaxis. The latter can occur rarely when aspirating mast cell tumors (MCTs) because of release of histamine.

For external or easily accessible lesions, such as cutaneous and subcutaneous masses or enlarged LNs, aspiration simply requires stabilization of the mass and consideration of underlying structures, such as large vessels and nerves. Some large abdominal masses can be aspirated blindly if they can be stabilized and if they are unlikely to be highly vascular or an abscess, aspiration of which may result in hemorrhage or dissemination of infection, respectively. Aspiration of intrathoracic and intraabdominal lesions is typically accomplished with guidance by imaging, either by ultrasonography or by CT, to aid in targeting the lesion and avoiding large vessels and other sensitive areas. Defects in cortical bone also can be identified with imaging, which can facilitate needle placement for aspiration of bone lesions. Cavity effusions are collected easily without imaging if fluid volume is significant; however, imaging can target smaller accumulations of fluid and provide a measure of safety. If there is particular concern for hemorrhage after aspiration, imaging can be repeated to look for evidence of bleeding at the aspiration site. Collection of cytologic specimens from the eye, brain, and lung requires special consideration and expertise.

Collection Techniques

Fine-needle aspiration (FNA) is by far the most common method for collecting cytologic specimens. Small-gauge needles (22–25 g) are sufficient for smaller lesions and result in less hemorrhage. Large-gauge needles (18–20 g) may be required to collect sufficient material from masses containing abundant matrix (i.e., firm masses and sarcomas), but specimens may contain more blood. Medium-sized syringes (12–15 cc) yield more vacuum for aspiration than smaller syringes (3–6 cc). The intent of aspiration is to draw cells into the needle shaft, not to fill the syringe with material unless the lesion is fluid-filled. After the needle is inserted into the lesion, vacuum is maintained in the syringe while the needle is redirected into the tissue several times to collect a broad representation of cells. This is especially important when aspirating LNs to evaluate for metastasis. After aspiration, vacuum is released before removing the needle from the tissue, the needle is removed from the tissue and then from the syringe, the syringe is filled with air and reattached to the needle, and the cells are expelled onto a glass slide. An alternative technique, often referred to as "fenestration," is to obtain cells without aspiration by holding the needle by the hub between the thumb and middle finger while covering the hub opening with the forefinger (to prevent blood or other fluids from escaping) and rapidly and repeatedly inserting the needle into the lesion with redirection until cells are packed into the needle shaft.[2] This method often yields as much cellular material as the aspiration technique and produces less hemorrhage and patient discomfort. Similar to the aspiration technique, a syringe is used to expel the material in the needle onto a glass slide. Alternatively, a syringe, preloaded with air, can be attached to the needle used for the fenestration technique before needle insertion into the tissue of interest, which allows easy expression of fenestrated material onto slides on exit from the tissue. A second clean slide is then placed on top of the sample and the two slides are pulled apart in parallel, taking care not to exert pressure on the sample. The aim is to obtain a monolayer of intact cells. Failure to spread the specimen immediately leads to a sample that is too thick to interpret; conversely, aggressive pressure on the sample may rupture many if not all cells, also leading to a nondiagnostic specimen.

Cytologic material may be collected from mucosal surfaces such as the respiratory, gastrointestinal, and genital tracts by saline washes or with a brush or biopsy forceps inserted through an endoscope. Cytologic materials collected using an endoscopic brush are gently rolled onto a glass slide and often result in highly cellular smears. In contrast, rolling a cotton swab over the surface of a lesion is only moderately successful at collecting sufficient material for cytologic evaluation of tumors. Traumatic catheterization is the preferred method for collecting cytologic material from bladder masses because of the potential risk of seeding tumor cells when transitional cell carcinomas (TCCs) are aspirated transabdominally.[3] Traumatic catheterization is accomplished with an open-ended polypropylene urinary catheter attached to a large syringe (50–60 cc). The catheter is inserted into the urethra and bounced off the bladder wall in the region of the lesion (typically using ultrasonographic guidance), taking care not to perforate the bladder wall. Saline can be flushed into the bladder to facilitate collection of cells and cellular particles, some of which may be large enough to process for histologic evaluation.

Imprinting and scraping are excellent means of preparing cytologic specimens from tissues obtained by surgical biopsy. When making imprints, a fresh surface should be exposed on the piece of tissue using a scalpel blade and then gently blotted on absorbent paper until little blood or tissue fluid appears on the paper. The tissue is held with forceps, and the fresh surface is gently pressed repeatedly onto the glass slide, using slightly different pressure with each imprint. The final specimen will contain a row of imprints of varying thickness, one or more of which should be suitable for evaluation. Common mistakes when preparing imprints include insufficient blotting and application of too much pressure, resulting in excessive blood or cellular disruption, respectively. Sometimes mucosal or connective tissue is obtained instead of tumor cells if the incorrect surface is imprinted onto the slide. When tumors such as sarcomas contain abundant matrix, imprinting will often not yield sufficient numbers of cells for evaluation. The surface of these lesions should be cross-hatched with a scalpel blade and imprinted without blotting; this may liberate cells embedded in matrix. Alternatively, the surface of firm lesions can be scraped several times in one direction with a scalpel blade held at 45 degrees to the tissue. The material on the edge of the blade is then gently spread on a glass slide. When using samples obtained by surgical biopsy to prepare cytologic specimens, care must be taken not to disrupt surfaces or margins important for histologic evaluation, especially for excisional biopsies in which assessment of tumor margins is fundamental to the evaluation.

Tissue particles or mucus collected by saline washes or by traumatic catheterization can be retrieved with a pipette and gently pressed between two glass slides. If washes or cavity fluids are cell-poor, cells in the fluid must be concentrated to prepare slides of sufficient cellularity. Collected fluid can be centrifuged, the supernatant decanted, and the cell pellet or sediment resuspended in a small amount of remaining fluid and then spread onto a glass slide. Similar to preparation of blood smears, the feathered edge of the fluid should be included on the slide because nucleated cells will accumulate there and may be best evaluated at the edge. Alternatively, when spreading the suspended cell pellet fluid on a glass slide, the spreader slide can be abruptly lifted off the slide, leaving a line of fluid—and concentrated cells—on the slide instead of a feathered edge. The best method to concentrate cells in cell-poor fluid samples is to use a cytocentrifuge, but most veterinary practices lack this equipment.

Cytologic Stains

A variety of quick stains are available for immediate examination of cytologic specimens and include quick Romanowsky stains, such as Diff-Quik. A specific set of staining jars should be kept exclusively for cytologic specimens and not used concurrently for dermatologic specimens. The jars containing the stain components should be capped between uses to prevent evaporation and contamination of the fixative and stains. Maintenance, including scheduled replacement of stain components, is important to avoid artifacts such as stain precipitate and contamination with organisms or debris that might be misinterpreted. Slides should be completely air-dried before fixation in the methanol fixative. Stains must thoroughly penetrate the smear, and in well-stained smears nuclei should be purple (Fig. 7.1A). A thick sample requires more contact time with the stains; understained slides (Fig. 7.1B) can be restained for a longer period of time, and overstained slides can be destained with methanol and restained for a shorter period of time. If the slides will be sent to an outside diagnostic laboratory, clinicians are encouraged to stain a slide to ensure that sufficient material was collected and that cells are intact before submitting additional unstained slides for evaluation. Additional specimens should be collected if only noncellular material is present or if all the cells are ruptured. For some lesions, the first slide prepared may be the only slide that contains cellular material. It is best to send this slide unstained to the diagnostic laboratory, but, if it is stained, be sure to include it with the other slides.

Quick Romanowsky stains provide good nuclear detail and usually sufficient cytoplasmic detail for cytologic interpretation. Mast cell granules occasionally fail to stain with aqueous quick stains (Fig. 7.2A). Wright–Giemsa and modified Wright stains provide a broader palette of colors and excellent staining of

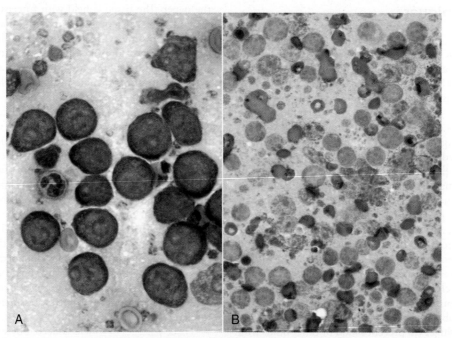

• **Fig. 7.1** Fine-needle aspirate of a lymph node from a dog with lymphoma. (A) Well-stained specimen. Lymphocytes are three times the diameter of an erythrocyte and larger than a neutrophil and have multiple prominent nucleoli. Cytoplasmic fragments are visible in the background. Part of a swollen magenta nucleus with a prominent nucleolus is present at the lower right edge. (B) Poorly stained specimen. Cytoplasmic fragments are visible, but cellular detail is poor.

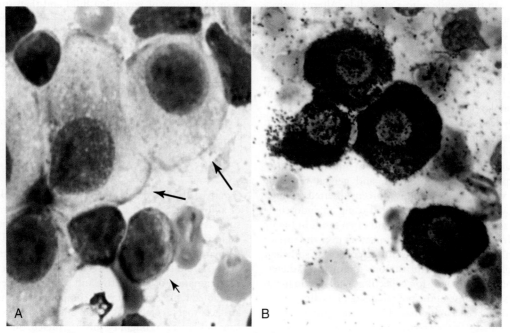

• **Fig. 7.2** Fine-needle aspirate of a mast cell tumor. (A) Granules in mast cells *(large arrows)* fail to stain when the specimen is stained with an aqueous quick stain. Small lymphocytes *(small arrow)* are also present. (B) Granules are prominent in a Wright-stained specimen from the same tumor.

cytoplasmic granules (Fig. 7.2B), but require more steps and longer staining times or the use of an automated stainer. Fixation of wet smears is required for Papanicolaou staining, which is not frequently used in veterinary cytology. Heat fixation is not required or recommended for cytologic specimens.

Cytochemical and immunocytochemical staining may be necessary to determine the specific tumor type. A complete list of available special stains and antibodies is beyond the scope of this chapter; consultation with a veterinary cytopathologist is recommended when considering the necessity and use of these stains. Cytochemical stains identify specific chemical compounds or structures within the cytoplasm or nucleus and include stains such as Prussian blue for iron; periodic acid–Schiff (PAS) for carbohydrates; alkaline phosphatase for identifying osteoblasts[4]; and a wide variety of leukocyte markers, including Sudan black B, peroxidase, chloracetate esterase, and nonspecific esterases. Immunocytochemical staining procedures use antibodies to identify specific proteins or peptides within or on the surface of the cells. Common antibodies used in veterinary oncology include those directed against CD3 (T cells), CD79a and CD20 (B cells), cytokeratin (epithelial cells), vimentin (mesenchymal cells), and Melan A (melanocytes). Use of a single stain or antibody is discouraged, as cell lineage is rarely identified, a single marker is often expressed by a variety of lineages, and aberrant expression by neoplastic cells can occur; a panel of stains or antibodies usually is necessary for complete identification.

Examination and Description of Cytologic Specimens

A good microscope, ideally equipped with a digital camera to document cytologic findings for the medical record or for consultation, should be used for examining cytologic specimens. The 4×, 10×, and 20× objectives are useful for scanning the slide and assessing cellular arrangements and general cell shape, whereas the 40× ("high dry") and 50× or 100× (oil-immersion) objectives are required for examining cellular detail. To improve clarity, the 40× objective requires an additional optical interface, which can be provided by applying a drop of immersion oil or permanent mounting medium to the slide followed by a coverslip. As a note of warning, the 40× objective lens is easily coated with oil applied to the slide for viewing the specimen with oil-immersion objectives; if this occurs, the lens should be cleaned immediately with glass cleaner and lens paper to prevent accumulation of oil inside the objective lens. Proper use, including correct placement of the condenser for viewing stained and unstained specimens, and maintenance of the microscope are essential to adequate examination of cytologic specimens.

Consider the following when examining the slide preparation: (1) Is the specimen of sufficient quality to permit a clinically useful interpretation? Clinical decisions should not be made from specimens that are poorly cellular or have too many ruptured cells. (2) Based on the tissue sampled, do the cells represent the expected population, an abnormal population, or both? It is important to become familiar with the cytologic appearance of "normal" cells in frequently aspirated tissues, such as lymph node and liver. (3) Does the abnormal population represent inflammation, hyperplasia, or a neoplasm? Whenever inflammation is found in a lesion suspected to be a tumor, caution is advised in making a definitive diagnosis of neoplasia. Although some tumors are accompanied by neutrophilic inflammation, experienced

cytopathologists recognize that primary inflammatory lesions can convincingly mimic neoplastic lesions. (4) If neoplasia is likely, what is the tissue of origin and is the tumor benign or malignant? These questions can sometimes be answered by cytologic evaluation of the lesion but often require confirmation with histologic examination.

Specimens of Diagnostic Quality

What constitutes adequate cellularity depends on the type of tumor. Aspirates of mesenchymal tumors, which often contain extracellular matrix, tend to be less cellular than those of epithelial and discrete round cell tumors. The degree of cellularity also has an effect on the level of confidence expressed in the interpretation, and diagnostic opinions are often qualified with "possible" or "probable" for poorly cellular specimens compared with "diagnostic for" or "consistent with" for highly cellular specimens. All cytologic specimens contain some ruptured cells, but to render a meaningful interpretation the majority of cells should be intact. Material from ruptured cells is recognized as stringy strands of chromatin or swollen magenta nuclei, often with obvious nucleoli, and free cytoplasmic fragments (see Fig. 7.1A). Large lymphocytes and cells from endocrine tumors are highly susceptible to rupture, and extra care should be taken not to exert pressure on the cells when preparing cytologic specimens from these lesions.

Nonneoplastic Cells and Noncellular Material Found in Cytologic Specimens

The submandibular salivary gland occasionally is aspirated instead of the mandibular LNs and is recognized by clusters of foamy cells in a background of mucin and blood. When tissue containing a metastatic tumor is aspirated, the specimen may contain only neoplastic cells or may contain normal cells from the tissue (e.g., lymphoid populations in an LN), which helps confirm location of the tumor. Necrosis can be found in tumors that have outgrown their blood supply. Necrotic cells lack detail and consist of gray-pink, indistinct cytoplasm and amorphous nuclei (Fig. 7.3); they

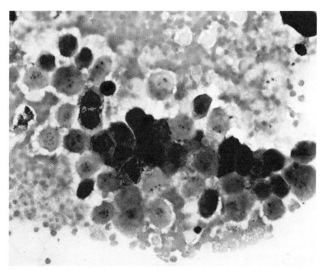

• **Fig. 7.3** Cells from a mass in the bladder obtained by traumatic catheterization. The cells are gray and have indistinct morphologic features, typical of necrotic cells.

should not be confused with apoptotic or pyknotic cells, which retain distinct cytoplasmic borders that surround condensed nuclear fragments.

Aspiration usually results in some degree of sampling hemorrhage leading to the presence of few or many erythrocytes admixed with nucleated cells. Aspiration of splenic lesions and thyroid and vascular tumors may result in pronounced hemorrhage and abundant blood in the cytologic specimen. Preexisting intralesional hemorrhage is indicated by the presence of macrophages containing erythrocytes or hemosiderin. Small numbers of peripheral leukocytes, primarily neutrophils, will accompany hemorrhage, but the presence of neutrophils in numbers greater than their proportion in blood is supportive of inflammation. Neutrophilic inflammation may accompany tumors, most notably squamous cell carcinoma and large tumors with necrotic centers; however, inflammation can induce criteria of malignancy in nonneoplastic populations, especially fibroblasts and squamous cells, and surgical biopsy may be required to confirm suspected neoplasia when inflammation is prominent. Some tumors are associated with infiltration of specific inflammatory cells (e.g., eosinophils in MCTs).

For tumors that produce ground substance(s), such as sarcomas, or that elicit a scirrhous response, such as some carcinomas, extracellular matrix may be observed in cytologic specimens. Collagen and osteoid consist of collections of smooth or fibrillar magenta material, whereas chondroid matrix typically forms larger lakes of bright pink-to-purple material. Mucinous material may be secreted by a variety of tumors, including salivary, biliary, and intestinal carcinomas and myxomatous sarcomas. Mucin or myxoid matrix is pale blue to pink, and cells surrounded by mucin are often aligned in rows. Ultrasound gel may be a contaminant on slides prepared from ultrasound-guided aspirates if the needle is not cleaned before expelling cells onto the slide. Ultrasound gel appears as bright magenta, granular material when stained with cytologic stains and, if abundant, may impair cytologic examination.

Description of Neoplastic Populations

Determination of the number of cells exfoliated and the shape and arrangement of cells early in the cytologic evaluation aids in formulating an initial list of differential diagnoses, permitting placement of tumors in three broad categories: epithelial, mesenchymal, and discrete round cell tumors. Briefly, cells from epithelial tumors exfoliate well and are round, cuboidal, columnar, or polygonal cells arranged in cohesive sheets or clusters; cells from mesenchymal tumors exfoliate poorly and are spindle, stellate, or oval cells arranged individually or in noncohesive aggregates; and cells from discrete round cell tumors exfoliate well and are individualized round cells that are arranged in a monolayer. Cellular arrangements observed in cytologic specimens and their associated histologic correlates and tissue types have been described.[5]

Proper terminology should be used to succinctly describe cell populations and convey important information. The terms *homogeneous* and *heterogeneous* describe cell populations (Figs. 7.4 and 7.5). Homogeneous denotes a population of one cell (excluding erythrocytes and associated leukocytes), which is typical of most tumors. Heterogeneous refers to mixed populations of cells, which are commonly found in aspirates of inflammatory lesions; however, some neoplasms will contain heterogeneous populations of cells (e.g., MCTs accompanied by eosinophils and fibroblasts [see Fig. 7.5] and squamous cell carcinomas with associated neutrophilic inflammation [see later]). The terms *monomorphic* and *pleomorphic* describe the morphologic appearance of cells within a single population. Monomorphic describes cells of a single lineage in which the cells have a uniform morphologic appearance (see Fig. 7.4A). Monomorphic features typically are associated with benign tumors, but a number of malignant tumors are cytologically monomorphic. In contrast, pleomorphic is used to describe cells of a single lineage that have variable morphologic features (see Fig. 7.4B). Pleomorphic features comprise a set of criteria

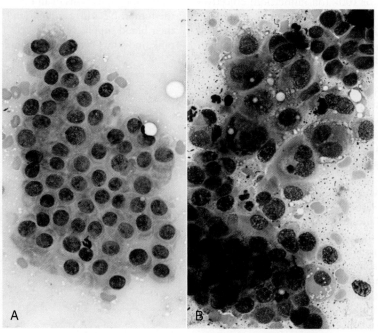

• **Fig. 7.4** Cells from a pulmonary carcinoma (A) and a transitional cell carcinoma (TCC) (B). Note that in both specimens, cells comprise a homogeneous population of epithelial cells; however, cells from the pulmonary carcinoma are monomorphic, whereas those from the TCC are pleomorphic.

of malignancy and suggest malignant behavior, but these features may be observed in nonneoplastic cells found in primary inflammatory lesions.

Criteria of malignancy are cellular features within a single population that suggest malignant behavior, with greater emphasis placed on nuclear criteria. The more criteria observed, the more likely the tumor is malignant. Cellular and cytoplasmic criteria of malignancy include variation in cell size (*anisocytosis*), abnormal cellular arrangement (3-dimensional [3D] clusters instead of a monolayer), cells that are smaller or larger than their normal counterpart, variable nuclear-to-cytoplasmic (N:C) ratios or N:C ratios that differ from what is expected for the cell type, intensely basophilic cytoplasm (*hyperchromasia*), abnormal vacuolation or granulation, and aberrant phagocytic activity. The nucleus is the most important component of the cell when determining the biologic behavior of a neoplasm. Nuclear criteria of malignancy include variation in nuclear size (*anisokaryosis*), unusual nuclear shape, multinuclearity, variation in nuclear size within the same multinucleated cell, nuclear fragments, multiple nucleoli that vary in size and shape within the same nucleus or among cells, increased mitoses, and nonsymmetric mitoses (Fig. 7.6). When Papanicolaou stain is used, additional nuclear features such as irregular thickening of the nuclear membrane can be evaluated. Cellular gigantism (cell >10 times the diameter of an erythrocyte) and the presence of macronuclei (>5 times the diameter of an erythrocyte) or macronucleoli (larger than an erythrocyte) are particularly disturbing criteria of malignancy. In nonneoplastic cells, the chromatin pattern is finely stippled in replicating or metabolically active cells and condensed in mature quiescent cells. Finely stippled chromatin is also common in rapidly proliferating neoplastic cells, and chromatin that is irregularly clumped or ropy is unusual and suggestive of a neoplastic process. Some nonneoplastic cells, including mesothelial cells, fibroblasts, and squamous epithelial cells, may have criteria of malignancy when they are highly proliferative in the presence of inflammation. Conversely, some malignant tumors such as apocrine gland tumors of the anal sac have few criteria of malignancy.

Sending Cytologic Samples to a Diagnostic Laboratory

When using a referral diagnostic laboratory, two to four unstained smears should be sent. If a highly cellular smear has been stained and examined by the oncologist for confirmation of sample quality and the cellularity of the remaining unstained smears is in question, send the stained smear in addition to the unstained smears. All slides should be packed in rigid slide containers to prevent breakage during shipment. For shipment by commercial mail services, slide holders are placed in a cardboard box with sufficient padding; padded envelopes are not recommended because these may not provide sufficient protection. Slides should not be refrigerated before or during shipment. Exposure to formalin or formalin fumes should be avoided during the preparation and shipment of cytologic specimens because this will permanently alter staining characteristics and render the sample nondiagnostic; surgical biopsy specimens preserved in formalin should be sent separately from cytologic specimens, or each type of sample should be sealed in separate plastic bags. If cavity fluids or mucosal washes are submitted, include two freshly made unstained smears along with the fluid (in EDTA) or wash (sealed container). Plain tubes (red top) or sterile vials are required for specimens that may be cultured. For all submitted glass slides, indicate how the slides were prepared and whether a concentration method was used for cavity effusions.

Interpretation of Cytologic Specimens

The final interpretation of a cytologic specimen should be based not only on the cytologic findings but also on signalment, history, clinicopathologic findings, and imaging results. This information should be provided in a concise but complete summary to the individual evaluating the sample. When submitting samples to a cytopathologist, the exact location of the lesion should be clearly described because "thoracic mass" could indicate a mass located in the skin, subcutis, body wall, mediastinum, thoracic cavity, or pulmonary parenchyma; the differential diagnoses will be different for different locations. For clinicians who perform an initial evaluation of the cytologic specimen, observational and interpretative skills can be developed by comparing their findings with

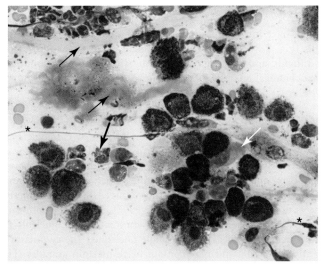

• **Fig. 7.5** Fine-needle aspirate of a mast cell tumor. Note the heterogeneous populations of cells, including mast cells, eosinophils *(thick arrow)*, fibroblasts *(white arrow)*, and lymphocytes. Extracellular matrix *(thin arrows)*, likely collagen, is also present and stringy chromatin *(asterisks)* from broken nuclei is noted.

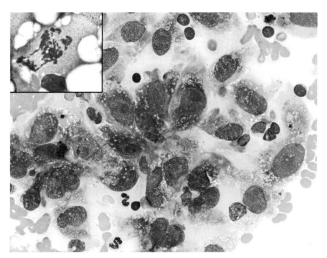

• **Fig. 7.6** Fine-needle aspirate of a hemangiosarcoma with multiple criteria of malignancy. *Inset:* An atypical mitotic figure from a liposarcoma.

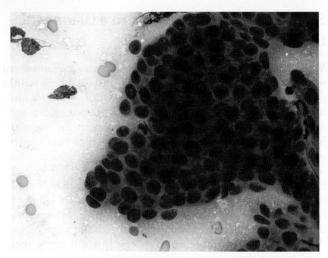

• **Fig. 7.7** Fine-needle aspirate of a basal cell tumor (trichoblastoma). Note the monomorphic population of cohesive cells aligned in rows.

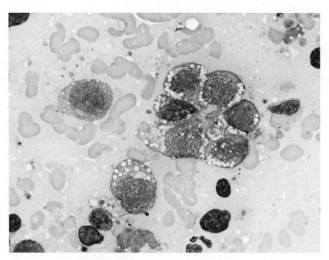

• **Fig. 7.8** Fine-needle aspirate of an anaplastic colonic carcinoma. The tumor cells have high N:C ratios and are sometimes individualized.

those described in the cytopathologist's complete report and by considering the information obtained from other diagnostic tests.

Confidence in cytologic interpretation is based on the quality of the specimen, the completeness of the clinical information provided, and the experience of the cytopathologist. Terms that express the degree of certainty, such as "consistent with," "diagnostic for," "cannot rule out," "probable," and "possible," may be used and interpreted differently by cytopathologists and clinicians.[6] If the certainty of an interpretation or diagnosis is unclear, the clinician should consult the cytopathologist. Correlations between cytologic and histologic interpretations or diagnoses are highly variable, depending on tissue types, disease processes, and methods of collection and preparation.

Epithelial, Mesenchymal, and Discrete Round Cell Tumors

The ability to identify specific tumor types by cytologic evaluation can aid in treatment planning and prognostication. Even if a specific diagnosis cannot be made, classification of the tumor as an epithelial, mesenchymal, or discrete round cell neoplasm can provide sufficient information to formulate a differential diagnosis and plan additional diagnostic procedures.

Tumors of Epithelial Tissues

Tumors derived from epithelial tissue comprise the largest category of neoplasms and include tumors of epithelial surfaces, such as the skin and respiratory, gastrointestinal, and urogenital tracts, and tumors of glands and organs. Given their diverse origin, the cytomorphologic appearance of these neoplasms can be highly variable; however, some features are shared by most epithelial tumors. Epithelial cells have intercellular junctions that connect the cells to each other and do not elaborate extracellular matrix. Therefore cells exfoliate well, resulting in highly cellular specimens, and are arranged in cohesive sheets or clusters in cytologic smears (Fig. 7.7). The cytoplasmic borders of individual cells typically are distinct, but this can vary in certain types of tumors. Poorly differentiated epithelial tumors have few or no identifying features and tend to be round cells with moderate-to-high N:C ratios and basophilic cytoplasm. In some cases, the cells no

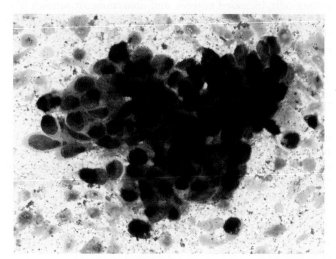

• **Fig. 7.9** Fine-needle aspirate of a basal cell tumor (trichoblastoma) in which the cells are heavily pigmented.

longer have intercellular junctions and appear as discrete round cells (Fig. 7.8). Determining the tissue of origin in these cases is difficult, and histologic evaluation, with or without immunohistochemical analysis, is necessary to define the specific tumor type.

Tumors of Adnexa in Skin with Basilar or Sebaceous Cells

Differentiating among adnexal tumors of skin by cytologic evaluation may be difficult when identifying features are absent or when multiple cell types are present. Some of these tumors have a large component of basilar cells that are small cuboidal or round cells with high N:C ratios and are arranged in tightly cohesive sheets or in palisading rows (see Fig. 7.7). Nuclei are uniformly round with condensed to reticular chromatin, and nucleoli are indistinct or appear as a small single nucleolus. The cytoplasm is lightly basophilic and may contain black melanin granules (Fig. 7.9). Tumors that originate from the hair follicle and matrical cysts often have a central cystic space filled with mature squamous cells, keratin flakes, or keratin debris, and this material may be aspirated when the mass is sampled. Tumors with sebaceous differentiation contain clusters of large round cells filled with oily

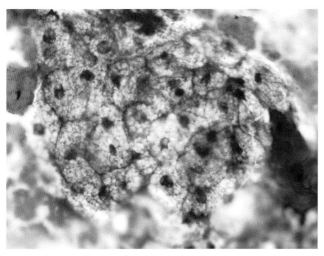

• **Fig. 7.10** Fine-needle aspirate of a sebaceous adenoma.

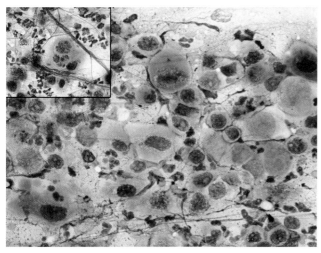

• **Fig. 7.11** Fine-needle aspirate of a squamous cell carcinoma (SCC). Note the marked anisocytosis and anisokaryosis, variable N:C ratios, perinuclear vacuolation, and angular cytoplasmic borders in some cells. *Inset*: A neutrophilic infiltrate often accompanies SCC.

appearing vacuoles that partially obscure the small central nucleus (Fig. 7.10). Necrotic cellular debris may be found in both benign and malignant forms of these tumors. Cutaneous basilar epithelial neoplasms include trichoblastoma, trichoepithelioma, pilomatricoma, feline basal cell tumors, sebaceous epithelioma, apocrine ductal adenoma, and others; histologic examination is usually required to identify the specific type. Fortunately, the majority of adnexal tumors are benign. Malignant types are infrequent; some resemble their benign counterparts but have frequent mitoses, whereas others have pleomorphic features that predict their biologic behavior.

Tumors of the Epidermis

Squamous cell carcinoma (SCC) is the most common malignancy of the epidermis; the tumor has varying degrees of differentiation, even within a single tumor, and the cytologic specimen may consist primarily of basilar cells, more mature keratinized cells, or both (Fig. 7.11). Pleomorphism can be marked, including moderate-to-marked anisocytosis and anisokaryosis, hyperchromasia, and marked nuclear atypia. Keratin does not stain with Romanowsky

stains, and cytologic features suggestive of keratinization include individualization of cells, sharp angular cytoplasmic margins, and smooth and glassy turquoise cytoplasm. Cells that appear keratinized may have small condensed nuclei or absent nuclei, representing a normal maturational process, but may have a large intact nucleus with fine-to-reticular chromatin and multiple visible nucleoli. An immature nucleus concurrent with mature cytoplasm signifies "asynchronous maturation." Perinuclear vacuolation or magenta cytoplasmic inclusions (keratohyaline granules) may be observed in the more mature squamous cells. Keratinization within a tumor typically is accompanied by neutrophilic inflammation (Fig. 7.11, inset). Differentiating between SCC and a primary inflammatory lesion with dysplastic squamous epithelium can be a cytologic dilemma: in both cases, the cells may have criteria of malignancy and asynchronous maturation. Location, appearance of the lesion, and ultimately histologic examination aid in differentiating inflammatory and neoplastic lesions.

Tumors of Glands

Salivary Gland Tumors

Salivary gland tumors may be composed of ductular cells, secretory cells, or both. Salivary ductular cells or poorly differentiated secretory cells resemble basilar epithelial cells with minimal pleomorphism even when these tumors are malignant; mild-to-moderate anisokaryosis may be present and nucleoli may be prominent. Tumors with a predominance of secretory cells include well-differentiated forms (acinic carcinoma) and more pleomorphic forms. The neoplastic cells are arranged in 3D clusters, sometimes resembling acini seen histologically, and have moderate and variable N:C ratios. The cytoplasm contains few-to-many secretory vacuoles of varying sizes. Cells with a single large vacuole that displaces the nucleus to an eccentric location may be noted and are referred to as *signet-ring cells*. In pleomorphic salivary adenocarcinomas, anisokaryosis and the presence of visible nucleoli of varying number, shape, and size are typical. Some tumors may produce mucin, which appears as pale pink or blue material that aligns surrounding erythrocytes into streaming rows.

Mammary Gland Tumors

Mammary gland tumors are classified histologically into benign and malignant tumors based on the type, arrangement, and invasiveness of neoplastic epithelium and on the presence or absence of neoplastic and nonneoplastic mesenchymal components. This classification system cannot be applied to cytologic specimens, nor can biologic behavior reliably be ascertained by cytology. Cytologic specimens from mammary masses may contain ductular cells, secretory cells, mesenchymal cells, or a combination of these. Cells from ductular or tubular mammary tumors resemble basilar epithelial cells with low-to-moderate N:C ratios and occasionally contain basophilic granular cytoplasmic inclusions. Pleomorphic features are mild-to-moderate, even when these tumors are malignant. Tumors of secretory origin have few-to-many criteria of malignancy, including moderate-to-marked anisocytosis and anisokaryosis, variably sized secretory vacuoles within the cytoplasm with some signet-ring formation, and nuclear criteria of malignancy (Fig. 7.12). If present, the mesenchymal component may consist of mildly to moderately pleomorphic spindle cells with or without fibrillar magenta extracellular matrix. The spindle cells represent myoepithelial cells or fibroblasts and may be neoplastic or nonneoplastic. The background of many mammary tumors contains lakes of blue secretory material, vacuolated macrophages containing similar material, and low numbers of neutrophils. Although biologic behavior is difficult to determine cytologically, the greater the number of malignant criteria present within any of the cell types, the more likely the tumor is malignant; however, even tumors with mild pleomorphism may be malignant. Features that define inflammatory mammary carcinomas histologically, such as the presence of tumor emboli in lymphatic vessels, cannot be appreciated cytologically, and this diagnosis is suspected when epithelial cells have cytologic criteria of malignancy and when typical clinical signs such as erythema, swelling, and warmth are identified. Mammary hyperplasia cannot be differentiated cytologically from neoplastic proliferation of tubular cells in the absence of pleomorphic features, and knowing the stage of the reproductive cycle in intact females can be helpful.

Perianal Gland Tumors

Perianal gland tumors, also called *circumanal* or *hepatoid tumors,* have a characteristic appearance and with experience can be differentiated from tumors of the apocrine gland of the anal sac. Cells are arranged in cohesive clusters and resemble hepatocytes, having uniformly low N:C ratios and abundant amphophilic granular cytoplasm with distinct margins (Fig. 7.13). Nuclei are uniformly round

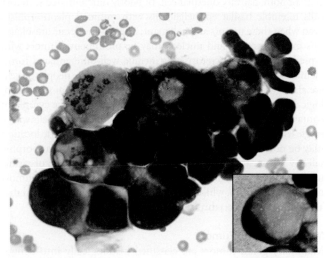

• **Fig. 7.12** Fine-needle aspirate of a mammary adenocarcinoma. *Inset:* Signet-ring cell.

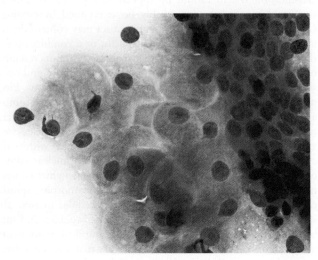

• **Fig. 7.13** Fine-needle aspirate of a perianal adenoma with characteristic hepatoid cells *(left)* and reserve cells *(right).*

and centrally located, with reticular chromatin and a single nucleolus. A population of reserve cells with high N:C ratios may be found at the periphery of the clusters. Occasionally, a perianal gland tumor may consist exclusively of reserve cells and is termed a *perianal gland epithelioma.* Although the majority of these tumors are benign, pleomorphic features are not prominent even in the malignant tumors.

Tumors of the Apocrine Gland of the Anal Sac

Tumors of the apocrine gland of the anal sac and perianal gland tumors are the most common tumors in the perianal region and with experience can be reliably differentiated cytologically. Although not of neuroendocrine origin, apocrine adenocarcinomas resemble other tumors with a neuroendocrine appearance (see later). Even though pleomorphism is minimal, these tumors are malignant and frequently metastasize to the medial iliac LNs and eventually beyond. Pleomorphism is usually limited to mild to moderate anisokaryosis with occasional macronuclei.

Tumors of the Prostate Gland

Tumors of the prostate gland have features similar to other glandular tumors. Sometimes the cells contain circular granular eosinophilic inclusions (see Transitional Cell Carcinomas [TCCs]). Primary prostatic carcinomas cannot be easily differentiated cytologically from TCCs that arise within the prostate.

Tumors of the Urogenital System

Transitional Cell Carcinomas

TCCs may be located in the bladder, urethra, ureter, prostate, or vagina. Needle aspiration of tumor tissue is avoided to prevent potential seeding of tumor cells along the needle tract.[3] Traumatic catheterization of the bladder and prostatic washes are the preferred means of obtaining cytologic specimens. Cells from a TCC are individualized round cells with some cells forming cohesive sheets and clusters. Criteria of malignancy typically are prominent and include marked anisocytosis and anisokaryosis; variation in N:C ratios; marked basophilia; coarse chromatin patterns; and variation in nucleolar size, shape, and number (see Fig. 7.4B). Multinuclearity is common. Large circular eosinophilic or magenta granular inclusions, representing accumulations of glycosaminoglycans, occasionally are found in the cytoplasm, but this feature is not pathognomonic for TCCs (Fig. 7.14). Moderately

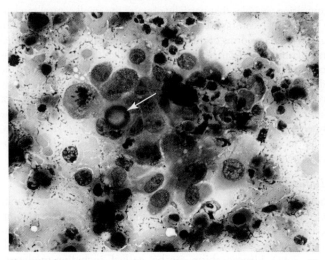

• **Fig. 7.14** Cells from a transitional cell carcinoma of the prostate. The *arrow* indicates a cytoplasmic eosinophilic inclusion that represents an accumulation of glycosaminoglycans.

pleomorphic TCCs must be differentiated from hyperplastic transitional epithelium that occurs secondary to inflammatory processes in the bladder; this can be challenging because inflammation sometimes accompanies TCCs. Transitional cell polyps are sampled infrequently and typically consist of sheets of epithelial cells with a uniform or mildly pleomorphic appearance.

Tumors of Organs

Hepatocellular Tumors

In the liver, primary tumors may arise from hepatocytes or from biliary epithelium. Hepatic carcinoids may be considered as primarily hepatic in origin (see Neuroendocrine Tumors). Hepatocellular tumors include benign adenomas, or hepatomas, and carcinomas. Unfortunately, hepatic nodules and masses, whether areas of hyperplasia, regeneration, benign tumors, or malignant tumors, may be indistinguishable cytologically because all these entities may consist of well-differentiated hepatocytes with some atypia. Histologic examination is recommended for a definitive diagnosis. Features of hepatocellular atypia that should raise concern for a neoplastic process include anisocytosis and anisokaryosis, variations in N:C ratios, decreased volume and increased basophilia of the cytoplasm, and the presence of more than two nuclei per cell and multiple visible nucleoli. In addition, the cells may appear disorganized and form 3D clusters rather than appearing in a uniform monolayer. The presence of capillaries coursing through the hepatocellular sheets is suggestive of hepatocellular carcinoma.[7] In our experience, the absence of cytoplasmic lipofuscin granules suggests formation of new cells and thus a benign or malignant neoplasm. However, all these features may be observed in hyperplastic or regenerative hepatic nodules. Undifferentiated hepatocellular carcinomas may have few cytologic features that identify them as hepatocellular in origin and may resemble other undifferentiated carcinomas that have metastasized to the liver.

Biliary Tumors

Biliary tumors include both benign biliary cystadenomas and carcinomas. Biliary cystic tumors consist of cystic spaces lined by attenuated biliary epithelium that is indistinguishable from normal biliary epithelium. Cytologic specimens consist of small-to-large sheets of monomorphic cuboidal epithelial cells, arranged in a monolayer, with moderately high N:C ratios, basophilic cytoplasm, and uniform central round nuclei. The cytoplasm may contain secretory vacuoles. Biliary carcinomas also may have a monomorphic appearance or may be pleomorphic with polygonal cells arranged in sheets and 3D clusters; in this case, the cells may have variable N:C ratios, deeply basophilic cytoplasm, and central-to-eccentric oval nuclei. Secretory vacuoles may be numerous, single, or absent. Nuclear and nucleolar pleomorphism is prominent.

Tumors of the Exocrine Pancreas

Tumors of the exocrine pancreas may arise from ductular or acinar epithelium. Cells from ductular carcinomas resemble biliary carcinomas and consist of monomorphic sheets of cuboidal cells with high N:C ratios, basophilic cytoplasm, and central round nuclei. Nuclear pleomorphism is typically mild, but criteria of malignancy may be present. Exocrine pancreatic adenocarcinoma typically has markedly pleomorphic features. The distinctive cytoplasm of exocrine pancreas, consisting of intensely basophilic cytoplasm with numerous small eosinophilic globules, may be observed in a proportion of cells supporting pancreatic origin.

Renal Carcinomas

Renal carcinomas have few defining cytologic characteristics. Variably pleomorphic cuboidal epithelial cells may be arranged in loose sheets, clusters, tubules, and acini. The cells have moderate-to-high N:C ratios and may contain a few discrete cytoplasmic vacuoles. Nuclei are generally round and centrally or basally located, with variably distinct nucleoli. Cytologically, renal carcinomas may be mistaken for neuroendocrine tumors.

Pulmonary Carcinomas or Adenocarcinomas

Pulmonary carcinomas or adenocarcinomas may occur in animals with respiratory signs or may be found incidentally when thoracic radiographs are taken for another reason. Cats with primary pulmonary tumors may be presented for lameness resulting from metastasis to the digits. Primary lung tumors are often minimally pleomorphic (see Fig. 7.4A), although moderately to markedly pleomorphic features may be observed. Cells are cuboidal to polygonal, are arranged in cohesive sheets and clusters, and have moderate-to-high N:C ratios. Within a single tumor, some cells may contain many discrete vacuoles (Fig. 7.15). Apical cilia typically are lacking. If the tumor is large and has outgrown its blood supply, there may be large amounts of necrotic cellular debris accompanied by neutrophilic inflammation. Aspirates from the center of necrotic lesions may not contain intact epithelial cells, and repeat aspiration from the periphery of the lesion is recommended. When numerous large sheets and clusters of epithelial cells are aspirated from a pulmonary mass, a diagnosis of neoplasia is straightforward; however, when only a few small sheets of deeply basophilic epithelium are found, it is difficult to differentiate a pulmonary neoplasm from consolidated hyperplastic respiratory epithelium resulting from a primary inflammatory process.

Thymoma and Thymic Carcinoma

Thymoma and thymic carcinoma result from neoplastic transformation of the supporting epithelium in the thymus. However, neoplastic epithelial cells often comprise only a small proportion of cells aspirated from a thymoma. The majority of cells are small lymphocytes, and in dogs well-differentiated mast cells often are present (Fig. 7.16). Epithelial cells, when observed, are polyhedral cells with abundant cytoplasm and central oval nuclei and are

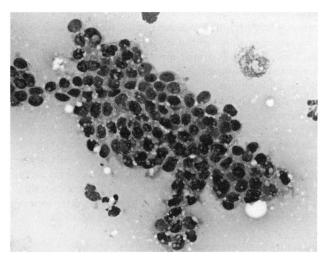

• **Fig. 7.15** Fine-needle aspirate of a pulmonary carcinoma. Note the monomorphic population with numerous small cytoplasmic vacuoles.

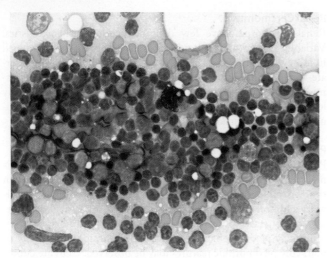

• **Fig. 7.16** Fine-needle aspirate of a thymoma in a dog. The majority of cells are small lymphocytes. A mast cell and an eosinophil also are present.

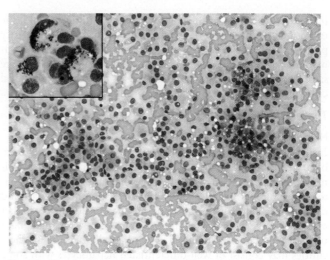

• **Fig. 7.17** Fine-needle aspirate of a thyroid carcinoma in a dog. Note the loosely cohesive sheets of cells in a background of free nuclei and abundant blood. *Inset*: Some of the tumor cells contain blue-black granules thought to be tyrosine granules.

arranged individually or in small sheets. Criteria of malignancy among the epithelial cells are minimal in thymomas. Histologic examination or molecular diagnostic tests (e.g., flow cytometry) are often necessary to confirm a thymoma diagnosis (see Chapter 34, Section B). In thymic carcinomas, the epithelial component is much more prominent as are criteria of malignancy.

Nasal Carcinomas and Adenocarcinomas

Nasal carcinomas and adenocarcinomas, like primary lung tumors, typically are only mildly to moderately pleomorphic. Cytoplasmic vacuolation also may vary, with the majority of cells having few-to-no secretory vacuoles. Apical cilia are typically lacking. Small numbers of highly pleomorphic epithelial cells arranged in sheets or clusters accompanied by marked neutrophilic inflammation likely represent hyperplastic respiratory epithelium and not a tumor. Surgical biopsy is often required to make a diagnosis of neoplasia, especially when cytoplasmic features are not definitive and when concurrent inflammation is present.

Gastrointestinal Tumors

Epithelial gastrointestinal tumors include adenocarcinomas of the stomach, small intestine, and large intestine, and these tumors have similar cytologic features. Aspirates of these tumors typically consist of highly pleomorphic epithelial cells arranged in sheets and clusters. The cells typically contain few-to-many secretory vacuoles. The background may contain abundant mucus produced by the tumor cells or pink fibrillar collagen representing a scirrhous response secondary to the tumor. Anaplastic carcinomas of the gastrointestinal tract may resemble discrete round cell tumors (Fig. 7.8). Polyps may occur anywhere in the gastrointestinal tract and typically have a benign cytologic appearance with uniform, hyperchromatic cuboidal to columnar epithelial cells arranged in dense sheets. Occasional goblet cells with a large pale blue cytoplasmic inclusion may be observed. Histologic examination of a full thickness surgical biopsy is required to definitively differentiate invasive carcinomas and carcinoma in situ from noninvasive polyps.

Endocrine and Neuroendocrine Tumors

Endocrine and neuroendocrine tumors comprise a diverse collection of tumor types. If the primary location of the tumor is

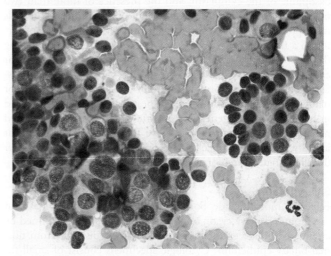

• **Fig. 7.18** Fine-needle aspirate of anal sac apocrine adenocarcinoma. Note the rosette of tumor cells *(right)*. Mild anisokaryosis and a macronucleus are seen *(left)*, although this tumor is typically monomorphic.

not known, a specific tumor type may be impossible to determine owing to the cytologic similarity among these tumors. In general, aspirates of endocrine and neuroendocrine tumors are highly cellular and consist of loosely cohesive sheets and clusters of epithelial cells with ill-defined intercellular junctions and cytoplasmic margins (Fig. 7.17). The cells are fragile, and numerous free nuclei from ruptured cells are scattered in the background. Nuclei of intact cells may be arranged in a rosette (Fig. 7.18), suggestive of acinar formation. Within intact cells, nuclei are round and centrally located with reticular chromatin. Nucleoli are often indistinct, but one to two nucleoli may be observed. The cytoplasm may contain a few clear, distinct vacuoles. There are usually few criteria of malignancy, even in carcinomas, and anisocytosis and anisokaryosis are mild to moderate, with large nuclei observed occasionally. Mitotic figures may be present. Some tumors of endocrine origin are biologically active, and tumor type may be identified based on clinical presentation and laboratory findings.

Thyroid Carcinomas

Thyroid carcinomas in dogs are highly vascularized, and aspirates may yield abundant blood as well as some hemosiderophages. In addition to displaying general features of endocrine tissue, cells from thyroid tumors may contain blue-black cytoplasmic granules (see Fig. 7.17, inset), believed to represent tyrosine granules, and amorphous pink material that may represent colloid. In the absence of these features, thyroid tumors cannot be differentiated cytologically from C-cell tumors and parathyroid tumors that occur in the same location. Most thyroid tumors in dogs are nonfunctional carcinomas, whereas in cats thyroidal masses or nodules are functional adenomas or adenomatous hyperplasia. Ectopic thyroid tissue may undergo transformation and be found in unexpected locations, such as the thoracic inlet and mediastinum.

Parathyroid Tumors

Parathyroid tumors are typically adenomas but are often functional and result in hypercalcemia through the systemic actions of parathyroid hormone. Parathyroid tumors have the typical features of endocrine tissue. Occasionally, eosinophilic spiculate inclusions are found in the cytoplasm.[8]

Chemodectomas or Paragangliomas

Chemodectomas or paragangliomas are neuroendocrine tumors of chemoreceptor cells found in the carotid or aortic bodies located in the submandibular region and at the base of the heart, respectively. In some tumors, the cells have numerous small pink granules. Otherwise, they do not have cytologic features that distinguish them from other endocrine tumors, such as ectopic thyroid tumors.

Adrenal Cortical and Medullary Tumors

Adrenal cortical and medullary tumors are cytologically similar and have a typical neuroendocrine appearance. Adrenal cortical tumors of the zona glomerulosa and fasciculata often contain few-to-many discrete clear vacuoles. Pleomorphism is minimal and differentiation between adrenal adenoma and adenocarcinoma is not always possible cytologically. Pheochromocytomas of the adrenal medulla lack distinct cytoplasmic vacuoles but may contain pink granules and will stain positively with silver stains and express synaptophysin and chromogranin A.[9]

Insulinomas

Insulinomas, or beta-cell tumors, have typical neuroendocrine features without additional defining characteristics except for the clinical presentation of hypoglycemia. Insulinomas may metastasize to liver, regional lymph nodes, mesentery, and omentum, and these metastatic sites may be the first place the tumor is recognized.

Carcinoids of Lung, Liver, Intestine, and Colon

Carcinoids of lung, liver, intestine, and colon are rare neuroendocrine tumors. They must be distinguished from other neuroendocrine tumors that have metastasized based on history, clinical presentation, presence of other primary tumors, and histologic examination.

Tumors of Mesenchymal Tissues

Tumors derived from mesenchymal or connective tissues can be diverse in their cytologic appearances, but they have some common features. Cells are often embedded in extracellular matrix produced by tumor cells and exfoliate poorly. Thus cytologic samples tend to have low cellularity, although exceptions occur. Cells do not have intercellular junctions and are arranged individually

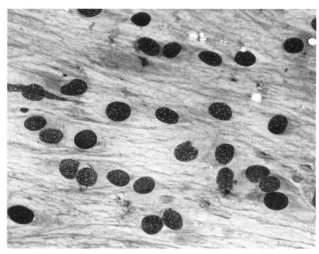

• **Fig. 7.19** Fine-needle aspirate of a myxosarcoma in a dog. Note the individualized spindle cells.

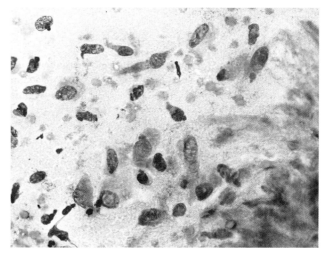

• **Fig. 7.20** Imprint of granulation tissue composed of pleomorphic fibroblasts.

(Fig. 7.19); however, in cases in which cellularity is high or when scraping and imprint methods are used to prepare slides, cells may be found in dense noncohesive aggregates that are disorganized. Cell shape is typically oval, spindle, or stellate, and the tumors are often grouped according to the most common shape. Cytoplasmic margins are characteristically indistinct, and nuclei are generally round, oval, or elongate. Some mesenchymal tumors lack further distinguishing features, and knowledge of the location and other clinical information is necessary to formulate a list of differential diagnoses in anticipation of the definitive diagnosis based on histologic and immunohistochemical staining. Even then, some of these tumors may be reported as soft tissue sarcomas without identifying the specific lineage of origin.

Reactive or hyperplastic mesenchymal cells that accompany inflammatory and neoplastic lesions present a diagnostic dilemma because these cells may have criteria of malignancy (Fig. 7.20). When a mass is composed of heterogeneous cell populations, caution is advised in making a definitive cytologic diagnosis of a mesenchymal tumor; this is especially true when concurrent neutrophilic inflammation is present. Additional diagnostic measures should be taken to confirm the presence of a neoplasm before making major treatment decisions.

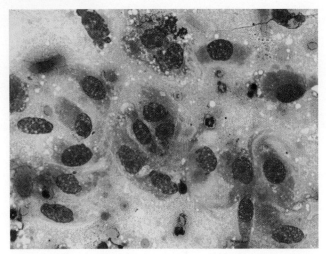

• **Fig. 7.21** Fine-needle aspirate of a fibrosarcoma in a dog. Note the cellular pleomorphism and pink background, possibly glycosaminoglycans.

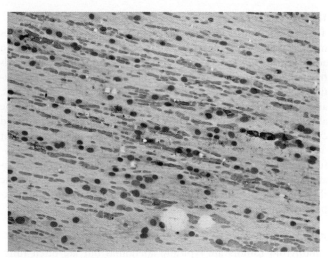

• **Fig. 7.22** Fine-needle aspirate of a myxosarcoma (same tumor as Fig. 7.19). Note the myxomatous background in which tumor cells and erythrocytes are aligned in rows.

Mesenchymal Tumors Composed of Spindle and Stellate Cells

Tumors of Fibroblasts

Tumors of fibroblasts may have morphologic features of well-differentiated fibroblasts, including monomorphic elongate spindle or fusiform cells with moderate N:C ratios, basophilic cytoplasm, and central oval nuclei with one to several small nucleoli; however, a population of well-differentiated fibroblasts may represent reactive fibroplasia, as is found in scars or granulation tissue (see Fig. 7.20), a fibroma, or a well-differentiated fibrosarcoma. Unfortunately, there are no clear cytomorphologic characteristics that can reliably differentiate among these entities. The presence of accompanying inflammation warrants an interpretation of reactive fibroblasts even when pleomorphic features are present. Epithelioid macrophages found in pyogranulomatous lesions are frequently mistaken for neoplastic fibroblasts by inexperienced clinicians. High cellularity, marked pleomorphism, especially with respect to the nucleus, and absence of inflammation along with a supportive clinical picture lend credible evidence for a cytologic diagnosis of fibrosarcoma. Malignant fibroblasts may vary in shape and N:C ratio and may have numerous nuclear criteria of malignancy. Anisocytosis and anisokaryosis may be moderate to marked (Fig. 7.21). Neoplastic fibroblasts may contain pink cytoplasmic granules. Accompanying collagen, consisting of fibrillar bands of pink extracellular material, may support the origin of the cells as fibroblasts; however, similar matrix can be seen with a variety of other mesenchymal neoplasms. Cells from myxosarcoma resemble cells of fibrosarcoma, but are embedded in a lightly eosinophilic matrix that aligns the cells in streaming rows (Fig. 7.22; see Fig. 7.19). Feline injection site sarcomas (ISSs) are highly pleomorphic mesenchymal tumors, primarily of fibroblastic origin, that occur at sites of previous injections, most often of vaccines containing adjuvant. In addition to containing pleomorphic mesenchymal cells, aspirates of feline ISSs may contain large multinucleated tumor cells (Fig. 7.23) and moderate numbers of small lymphocytes.

Tumors of the Perivascular Wall or Nerve Sheath

Tumors of the perivascular wall or nerve sheath, such as hemangiopericytoma, peripheral nerve sheath tumor (PNST), and schwannoma, often exfoliate well; samples are highly cellular with cells

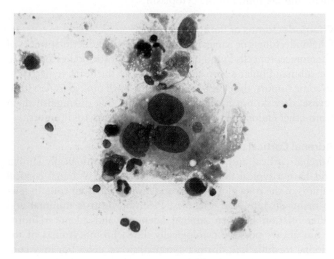

• **Fig. 7.23** Fine-needle aspirate of a vaccine-associated fibrosarcoma in a cat. Note the extreme atypia in the multinucleated tumor cell.

arranged both individually and in dense aggregates (Fig. 7.24). Cells are usually spindle and plump with wispy veil-like cytoplasmic extensions; oval-to-stellate forms also are found. The lightly basophilic cytoplasm frequently contains a few small clear round vacuoles. Nuclei are oval and centrally located with finely stippled chromatin and often one to three small nucleoli. Binuclearity is observed in a small proportion of cells, and multinucleate cells with peripheralized nuclei, so-called "crown cells," may be noted. Anisocytosis and anisokaryosis are mild to moderate. Linear capillaries may be embedded within aggregates of tumor cells in aspirates of perivascular wall tumors.

Tumors of Vascular and Lymphatic Endothelium

Tumors of vascular and lymphatic endothelium include hemangioma/hemangiosarcoma (HSA) and lymphangioma/lymphangiosarcoma, respectively. Tumors of vascular endothelium are more common than those of lymphatic endothelium. Aspirates of hemangioma may contain a uniform population of long thin spindle cells in a background of abundant blood; however, cellularity is rarely sufficient for a definitive diagnosis of this benign

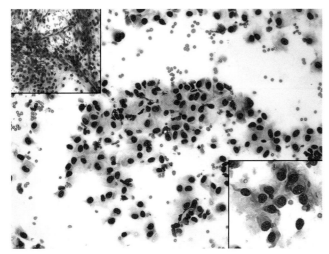

• **Fig. 7.24** Fine-needle aspirate of a perivascular wall tumor (hemangio-pericytoma). Note how well the cells exfoliated. *Upper left inset*: Vessels are often associated with the tumor cells. *Lower right inset*: Cells are spindle, stellate, or oval.

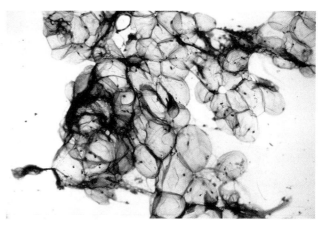

• **Fig. 7.25** Fine-needle aspirate of well-differentiated adipocytes from a lipoma.

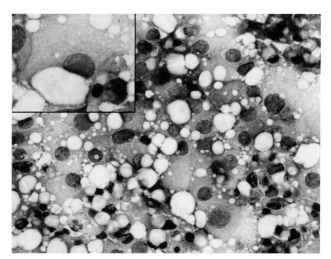

• **Fig. 7.26** Fine-needle aspirate of a liposarcoma in a dog. Note that the polygonal cells contain lipid vacuoles. *Inset*: A large lipid vacuole in a tumor cell.

vascular tumor. Aspiration of suspected HSA is approached cautiously because of the potential consequence of hemorrhage, but cellular yields may be sufficient to reach a tentative diagnosis. The neoplastic cells are often markedly pleomorphic and consist of spindle, stellate, and oval cells that have deeply basophilic cytoplasm containing punctate vacuoles (see Fig. 7.6); some neoplastic cells may contain mature red blood cells.[10] Large, irregular, or indented oval nuclei typically have coarse chromatin and multiple prominent nucleoli that vary in shape and size. Multinucleated cells are found occasionally. Anisocytosis and anisokaryosis are often marked. A small amount of pink extracellular matrix may be associated with the neoplastic cells. Erythroid precursors and macrophages containing erythrocytes or hemosiderin may accompany HSA, especially within the spleen. Important markers of vascular differentiation are CD31 and von Willebrand factor. HSAs occur primarily in the spleen and right atrium with metastasis to liver and lung, but also occur in the dermis and subcutis and rarely arise from bone. Tumor cells are typically not found in hemorrhagic effusions that result from rupture of the tumor.

Tumors of Adipose Tissue

Tumors of adipose tissue comprise lipomas and liposarcomas. Lipomas are common tumors of dogs, and although the gross appearance and texture of these tumors is characteristic, they often are aspirated to rule out other types of tumors that require more immediate attention. Aspirates of lipomas consist of abundant lipid that often dissolves during fixation in methanol-based fixatives, leaving an acellular smear. Adipose tissue that adheres throughout the staining procedure consists of clusters of large round cells with a small nucleus peripheralized by a single clear lipid vacuole (Fig. 7.25). Supporting stromal strands and capillary vessels are sometimes visible within the cluster of adipocytes, and free fat may be present. Normal subcutaneous adipose tissue cannot be differentiated from a lipoma or infiltrating lipoma cytologically; therefore caution is recommended when making a conclusive cytologic diagnosis of lipoma if the gross appearance or texture of the mass is not typical. Liposarcomas are uncommon and can adopt a variety of cytologic appearances. Cells may be spindle, stellate, or round with variable N:C ratios. Clear lipid vacuoles of varying sizes are present within a basophilic or amphophilic cytoplasm (Fig. 7.26).

Nuclei are round to oval and often display criteria of malignancy. Confirming the presence of lipid using Oil Red O stain is best accomplished on unfixed smears. With inflammation of adipose tissue (panniculitis or steatitis), the sample often contains moderately pleomorphic fibroblasts and histiocytes that contain lipid or lipid-like vacuoles; these cells are easily mistaken for a neoplastic population. The presence of even low numbers of neutrophils within these lesions favors a conservative interpretation, and surgical biopsy should be pursued for definitive diagnosis.

Mesenchymal Tumors Composed of Thin Elongate Cells

Tumors of Smooth Muscle and Stroma

Tumors of smooth muscle and stroma, such as leiomyoma, leiomyosarcoma, and gastrointestinal stromal tumor (GIST), have a similar cytologic appearance. Aspirates of these tumors, whether benign or malignant, often are highly cellular and consist of long thin mesenchymal cells arranged in aggregates and linear bundles. Nuclei are often elongate or "cigar-shaped" (Fig. 7.27). Pleomorphism is typically mild. The most common sites for these tumors are the gastrointestinal tract and female reproductive tract, especially the uterus and vagina. Immunohistochemical detection of smooth muscle actin or KIT (CD117) expression in smooth muscle tumors and GIST, respectively, is required to distinguish these tumors.

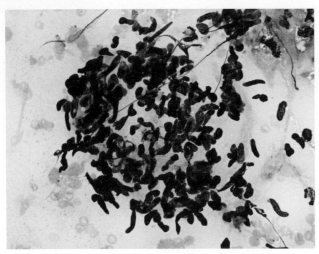

• **Fig. 7.27** Fine-needle aspirate of a gastrointestinal stromal tumor (GIST). Many cells are disrupted, but elongated (cigar-shaped) nuclei are visible.

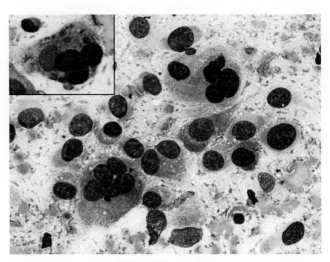

• **Fig. 7.28** Fine-needle aspirate of a proliferative and lytic lesion in bone. The diagnosis was osteosarcoma. The pleomorphic cells tend to be round or oval with eccentric nuclei and sometimes paranuclear clear zones. *Inset*: A multinucleated tumor cell contains prominent pink granules.

Tumors of Striated Muscle

Tumors of striated muscle, rhabdomyoma and rhabdomyosarcoma, are uncommon and can have a variety of cytomorphologic appearances. Rhabdomyomas occurring in the tongue and pharynx may present cytologically as a "granular cell tumor" composed of individual round or polygonal cells containing numerous fine pink cytoplasmic granules and a central round nucleus. Electron microscopic examination reveals the pink granules to be numerous mitochondria. Rhabdomyosarcomas typically comprise individualized pleomorphic spindle cells with low numbers of elongate strap cells that may or may not demonstrate cross-striations within the cytoplasm. Strap cells characteristically have several round-to-oval nuclei arranged in a linear row. Normal muscle fibers are bright blue, with prominent cross-striations when viewed at high magnification, and have randomly distributed pale oval nuclei.

Mesenchymal Tumors Composed of Round or Oval Cells

Tumors of Bone Origin

Tumors of bone origin include osteosarcoma, osteoma, multilobular tumor of bone, and giant cell tumor of bone. Osteosarcoma (OSA) is the most common tumor of bone in dogs and results in a mixed osteolytic and osteoproliferative lesion radiographically. Aspirates of OSA may be highly or poorly cellular, depending on the collection technique and the nature of the lesion. Cytologic features that support osteoblasts as the cells of origin include oval cells with basophilic cytoplasm containing paranuclear clearing, and eccentric nuclei with criteria of malignancy (Fig. 7.28). The cytoplasm occasionally contains fine-to-coarse magenta granules or few small clear vacuoles. N:C ratios are moderate to high, and anisocytosis is moderate to occasionally marked. Alkaline phosphatase staining of cytologic samples has been shown to differentiate tumors of osteoblast origin (osteosarcoma and multilobular tumor of bone) from other vimentin-positive tumors of bone. Often, bright magenta extracellular matrix or osteoid is found. Large multinucleated osteoclasts are typically scattered among the neoplastic osteoblasts. Multilobular tumor of bone and giant cell tumor of bone are composed predominantly of osteoblasts and osteoclasts, respectively. In giant cell tumor of bone (or osteoclastoma), spindle cells are found; it is possible these cells, rather than the osteoclasts, may be the neoplastic cells. Both tumors have characteristic locations or radiographic appearances. The cytologic appearance of plasma cell tumor and OSA may overlap because both contain cells

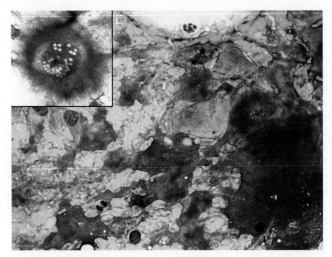

• **Fig. 7.29** Fine-needle aspirate of a chondrosarcoma with pleomorphic tumor cells and abundant magenta matrix that sometimes surrounds the tumor cells *(inset)*.

with eccentric nuclei and paranuclear clearing; for inexperienced clinicians, this may constitute a diagnostic dilemma in dogs, and less frequently in cats, that have osteolytic lesions. Clinical presentation and laboratory abnormalities may be useful in distinguishing these malignancies. Caution is recommended when making a cytologic diagnosis of OSA at the site of a pathologic fracture as hyperplastic and reactive osteoblasts may have a degree of pleomorphism that can be mistaken for a well-differentiated neoplasm.

Tumors of Chondrocytes

Tumors of chondrocytes are less common than osteosarcoma and may arise in any location where cartilage occurs, including epiphyseal bone, nasal cavity, and large airways. Although the amount of matrix present in any given tumor can vary, the most characteristic cytologic finding in aspirates of chondrosarcoma is the large amount of purple extracellular matrix that envelops and often obscures the neoplastic chondroblasts (Fig. 7.29). Neoplastic chondroblasts are round with moderate-to-high N:C ratios but may be spindle or stellate. A few cytoplasmic vacuoles or magenta

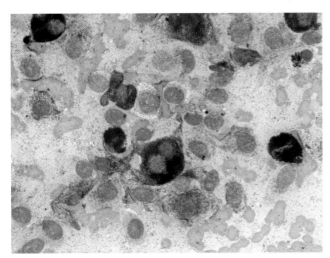

• **Fig. 7.30** Fine-needle aspirate of a melanoma in a dog. Note the fine melanin granules in the tumor cells and in the background.

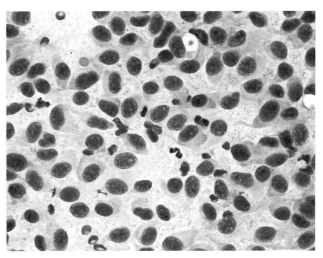

• **Fig. 7.31** Fine-needle aspirate of a melanoma in which melanin granules are not visible (amelanotic melanoma).

granules are common, and nuclei are round with finely stippled chromatin and variably prominent nucleoli.

Periarticular Tumors

Periarticular tumors are predominantly histiocytic sarcomas (HSs) with other sarcomas (synovial myxoma, pleomorphic sarcoma, fibrosarcoma, and undifferentiated sarcoma) diagnosed less frequently.[11] Descriptions of synovial cell sarcoma histologically as monophasic (spindle) or biphasic (epithelioid and spindle) may encompass these different tumor types or a periarticular tumor of undefined cell lineage.[12,13] Cytomorphologic appearances of periarticular tumors correspond to the specific tumor type described elsewhere under mesenchymal tumors with round or spindle cells or under tumors with frequent multinucleated cells.

Tumors of Melanocytes

In malignant melanoma, the cells can adopt the appearance of epithelial (sheets of cohesive cells), mesenchymal (individualized oval or spindle cells), or discrete round cell tumors, and all three cytologic appearance may be evident in the same tumor. Individual melanoblasts are round, oval, or spindle cells with moderately high N:C ratios, lightly basophilic cytoplasm, and round or oval nuclei with fine chromatin and distinct nucleoli. Criteria of malignancy consist primarily of anisokaryosis and nucleolar pleomorphism. Highly pigmented tumors do not present a diagnostic challenge, and fine black melanin granules may be so numerous that they obscure all cellular detail. Cells with varying degrees of pigmentation are typically found within the same tumor, and melanin granules may be sparse in some cells (Fig. 7.30). Amelanotic tumors present a greater diagnostic challenge. Usually, a faint scattering of fine gray-black melanin granules is found in a few cells to support a diagnosis, but cells may be completely devoid of pigmentation (Fig. 7.31). In these circumstances, moderately pleomorphic tumor cells aspirated from masses on the digits or in the oral cavity should alert the clinician to the possibility of this highly malignant tumor. Because melanocytes are of neuroectodermal origin, the cells may express certain neural markers, such as S-100 and neuron-specific enolase, in addition to vimentin and often Melan A.

An additional cytologic challenge is the identification of metastatic lesions within lymph nodes. Most lymph nodes draining pigmented melanomas contain melanophages, which are macrophages containing abundant melanin; in the authors' experience, this is especially true after surgical removal or biopsy of the primary mass. These melanophages may be mistaken for metastatic cells, but they differ from neoplastic melanoblasts as melanophages typically contain coarse collections of melanin within phagolysosomes rather than the fine granulation typically found within melanoblasts.

Most dermal tumors of melanocytic origin are benign and are termed *melanocytomas*. They consist of polygonal or spindle cells containing black cytoplasmic granules. Several of the adnexal tumors may contain melanin pigment and must be differentiated from melanocytomas. These typically are of epithelial origin and should be distinguished by their cellular arrangement in cohesive sheets (see Fig. 7.9).

Mesenchymal Tumors Composed of Cells Arranged in Dense Aggregates

Cells aspirated from some mesenchymal tumors, including rhabdomyosarcoma, perivascular wall tumor, PNST, amelanotic melanoma, and the epithelioid form of HSA, form dense aggregates and clusters that are more characteristic of epithelial cells. Careful examination typically reveals some spindle cells with indistinct margins and spaces between the closely packed cells indicating the lack of intercellular junctions. Slide preparation by imprinting and scraping also may yield clusters and sheets of mesenchymal cells that mimic epithelial populations.

Mesenchymal Tumors with Frequent Multinucleated Cells

Although any neoplasm can have a few multinucleated cells, multinuclearity is especially common in certain sarcomas. These include HSs, feline ISSs, pleomorphic sarcoma (also called malignant fibrous histiocytosis or anaplastic sarcoma with giant cells), rhabdomyosarcoma, and some plasmacytomas in which the multinucleated cells are part of the tumor population. In OSA, multinucleated osteoclasts are often present and are not part of the neoplastic population of cells.

Discrete Round Cell Tumors

The majority of discrete round cell tumors are of hematopoietic origin, including neoplasms of mast cells, plasma cells, lymphocytes, and histiocytes. Transmissible venereal tumors (TVTs) are also included in this category, and there are a variety of epithelial and mesenchymal tumors that sometimes appear as round cell tumors. These tumors share certain cytomorphologic features. Cells exfoliate easily leading to highly cellular specimens in which the cells are individualized in noncohesive monolayers. As the moniker indicates, the cells are round and have distinct cytoplasmic margins and round nuclei, although nuclear shape may vary in pleomorphic forms of these tumors.

Mast Cell Tumors

MCTs consist of cells with numerous purple cytoplasmic granules that fill the cytoplasm and often obscure the nucleus (see Figs. 7.2 and 7.5). In cats, granules are finer than they are in canine mast cells. Even in poorly granulated MCTs, there often are enough granules in some cells to suggest that they are mast cells. One notable exception is when the granules fail to take up stain when one of the aqueous quick stains is used, so clinicians using these stains should be alert to this artifact (see Fig. 7.2). The nucleus is generally centrally located but may be eccentric. Criteria of malignancy are observed infrequently and may include anisocytosis, anisokaryosis, binuclearity, multinuclearity, nuclear pleomorphism, and the presence of mitotic figures. Marked pleomorphism is uncommon and when present suggests a higher-grade tumor; however, at present grading is based on histologic findings. Markedly pleomorphic MCT cells may have sparse or absent granulation, marked variation in cell and nuclear size, and lobulated or ameboid nuclei. In dogs, aspirates of MCTs often contain numerous eosinophils along with a small proportion of reactive fibroblasts and thick bands of collagen (see Fig. 7.5). Proposed cytologic grading systems for mast tumors in dogs have not been validated yet; these systems suggest that marked pleomorphism, poor granulation, and the presence of mitotic figures may predict a more aggressive behavior. A novel cytologic grading scheme adapted from two-tier histologic grading criteria was predictive of a poorer outcome and had high sensitivity and specificity compared with histologic grading.[14]

Determining the presence of metastasis in tissues, including LNs, liver, and spleen, that have resident mast cells, may be difficult. Features that support metastatic disease include the presence of large numbers of mast cells suggestive of tissue effacement, mast cells with pleomorphic features, and mast cells arranged in groups instead of singly. If cytologic evaluation cannot distinguish between resident mast cells and metastasis, a surgical biopsy should be evaluated.

Other neoplasms in which the cells contain cytoplasmic granules may be mistaken for mast cell tumors and include granulated T-cell lymphoma, natural killer (NK) cell lymphoma, and granular cell tumors. When cells from MCTs are agranular or when the granules fail to stain with aqueous stains, the tumor may be mistaken for plasmacytoma, histiocytoma, atypical lymphoma, or squamous cell carcinoma. Reactive nonneoplastic mast cells may be found in increased numbers at sites of fibrosis because of the role mast cells play in wound healing.

Plasma Cell Tumors

Plasma cell tumors composed of well-differentiated plasma cells are easily recognized owing to the characteristic features of plasma cells—abundant royal blue cytoplasm, paranuclear clear zone (Golgi apparatus), eccentric round nucleus, and clumped

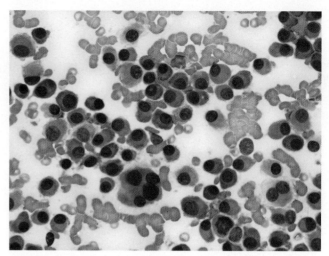

• **Fig. 7.32** Fine-needle aspirate of a plasmacytoma. Many cells have the characteristic appearance of plasma cells. Multinuclearity is a common feature of this tumor.

chromatin. Multinuclearity is common in plasmacytomas, and in more pleomorphic forms of this tumor the nuclei may be multilobulated (Fig. 7.32). Neoplastic plasma cells may appear immature and resemble large lymphocytes with higher N:C ratios and finer chromatin. Sometimes the cells contain Russell bodies, collections of immunoglobulin within the endoplasmic reticulum, and are termed *Mott cells*. Plasma cell tumors may occur in the skin, oral mucosa, bone marrow, liver, and spleen, and the specific diagnostic criteria for plasma cell myeloma, extramedullary plasma cell myeloma, and plasmacytoma are presented in Chapter 33, Section D. Reactive plasma cell proliferations consist of a mixture of inflammatory cells and are rarely mistaken for a neoplastic process in a cutaneous mass; however, when plasmacytosis is identified in bone marrow, reactive and neoplastic conditions must be distinguished.

Lymphoma

Lymphoma comprises many variants, and entire chapters are written on their cytologic features. Definitive diagnosis of lymphoma based on examination of cytologic specimens is often possible; however, some types of lymphoma or lymphoma in certain tissues may be difficult to diagnose cytologically. As with many discrete round cell neoplasms, it is the homogeneity of the population, rather than the morphologic features, that suggest a neoplastic process. In lymphoid organs or other tissues in which there is a reactive or polyclonal infiltrate of lymphocytes, small lymphocytes should predominate and comprise more than 50% of the lymphoid cells, even as the proportion of large and intermediate lymphocytes increases. Plasma cells and other inflammatory cells also may be found in these reactive lesions. As the proportion of intermediate and large lymphocytes approaches or exceeds 50%, it becomes more difficult to differentiate between a reactive and neoplastic process; this is especially true for the spleen and certain LNs, such as mandibular and mesenteric nodes, that are continuously exposed to antigen. Because of this, sampling of other LNs or tissues is preferred. In addition, cats can mount strong lymphocytic responses that can cytologically resemble lymphoma. In contrast, there are certain types of lymphoma, such as T-cell-rich B-cell lymphoma and Hodgkin's-like lymphoma, that contain a mixture of clonal (neoplastic) and

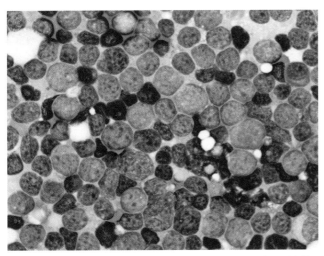

• **Fig. 7.33** Fine-needle aspirate of a lymph node from a dog with T-cell lymphoma. Note that most of the cells are about two times the diameter of an erythrocyte and that nucleoli are indistinct in many cells.

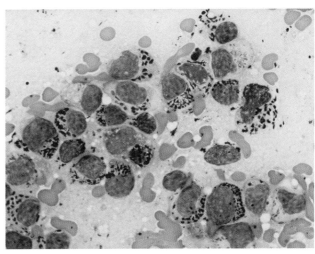

• **Fig. 7.34** Fine-needle aspirate of a mesenteric lymph node from a cat with large granular lymphoma. Note the prominent coarse eosinophilic granules in the tumor cells.

polyclonal (nonneoplastic) populations of lymphocytes. When a diagnosis of lymphoma is not obvious from the cytologic specimen, additional procedures should be performed, including surgical biopsy with histologic evaluation, immunophenotyping, assessment of clonality, or a combination of these (see Chapter 33, Sections A and B).

Lymphoma can be diagnosed cytologically when large or intermediate lymphocytes comprise the majority of the nodal population. Large and intermediate lymphocytes are defined as those larger than or the same size as a neutrophil, respectively, or that are greater than two times or one and a half to two times the diameter of an erythrocyte, respectively. Cytologic types include immunoblastic or centroblastic types, composed of large cells with visible nucleoli and deeply basophilic cytoplasm (see Fig. 7.1A), and lymphoblastic types composed of medium-sized cells often having indistinct nucleoli (Fig. 7.33). Mitotic figures and tingible-body macrophages, which are macrophages containing nuclear debris from tumor cells, may be increased, but this is not a defining characteristic. Cytologic diagnosis of small-cell lymphoma is more challenging, especially in tissues such as lymph node and spleen with a resident population of small lymphocytes or in tissues such as liver and small intestine in which lymphocytic inflammation is common. In these cases, additional diagnostic testing is required for confirmation and may include one or more of the following: histologic examination, preferably of a whole node or full-thickness piece of intestine; immunophenotyping by immunocytochemical/histochemical staining or flow cytometry; and polymerase chain reaction for antigen receptor rearrangement (PARR) to detect clonality (see Chapter 8). Because lymphocytes are fragile, free nuclei and cytoplasmic fragments frequently are observed in aspirates of lymphoma (see Fig. 7.1A); however, these features can be found in samples from reactive lymphocytic populations and are not criteria for neoplasia.

Infrequently, neoplastic lymphocytes are highly pleomorphic and exhibit moderate to marked anisocytosis, indented or deeply clefted nuclei, ameboid nuclei, multinuclearity, cytoplasmic vacuoles, and aberrant phagocytic behavior. When present, a few, some, or most of the neoplastic lymphocytes in a given tumor may have these features and may be mistaken for neoplastic histiocytes.[15] Sometimes neoplastic lymphocytes contain fine or coarse pink cytoplasmic granules, suggestive of a T- or NK-cell

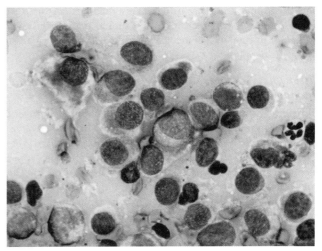

• **Fig. 7.35** Fine-needle aspirate of a histiocytoma. Note the discrete round cells with a variable appearance. A few small lymphocytes also are present.

phenotype. In large granular lymphoma, the lymphocytes contain large, coarse, pink granules and are thought to be cytotoxic T or NK cells (Fig. 7.34).

Tumors of Histiocytic Origin

Cutaneous Histiocytoma

Cutaneous histiocytoma originates from epidermal dendritic or Langerhans cells and is typically found on the head or limbs of young dogs. The cells are round and have pale blue to colorless cytoplasm and a round, sometimes indented, central nucleus with fine to reticular chromatin and indistinct nucleoli (Fig. 7.35). Occasionally, the cytoplasm is more basophilic, and the nucleus more eccentrically located; in these cases, the cells may be mistaken for immature plasma cells and the mass called a plasmacytoma. Finding a few mitotic figures is common, but binuclearity is infrequent. Often the tumor cells are highlighted by a pale purple proteinaceous background. In mature lesions, there may be an infiltrate of small lymphocytes representing the

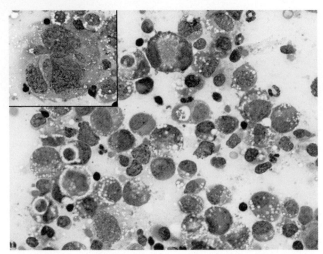

• **Fig. 7.36** Fine-needle aspirate of a histiocytic sarcoma. Note extreme pleomorphism, phagocytosis, and bizarre multinucleated cell *(inset)*.

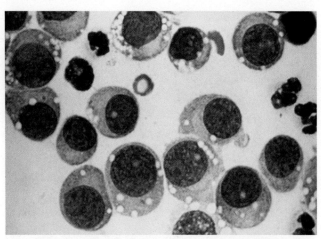

• **Fig. 7.37** Fine-needle aspirate of a transmissible venereal tumor (TVT). Note the coarse chromatin and small discrete vacuoles in the cytoplasm that are often referred to as a "string of pearls." (Courtesy Dr. Robert Hall.)

T-cell–mediated immune response that likely leads to the spontaneous resolution of these tumors. Presumed histiocytomas that do not resolve or that increase in size should undergo histologic evaluation to rule out cutaneous lymphoma or a more aggressive histiocytic neoplasm.

Histiocytic Sarcomas of Dendritic and Macrophage Lineage

Histiocytic sarcomas of dendritic and macrophage lineage are malignant tumors and are variably called HS, *malignant histiocytosis* (MH), and *hemophagocytic histiocytic sarcoma* (HHS), depending on clinical presentation, cytomorphologic appearance, and specific cell lineage (see Chapter 34, Section F). These tumors have at least three cytologic appearances. First, the tumor may be composed of a highly pleomorphic population of discrete round cells with extreme variations in N:C ratios, cell size, and nuclear size (Fig. 7.36).[16] The cytoplasm is basophilic and may contain numerous vacuoles, thought to be lysosomes, or phagocytosed erythrocytes, leukocytes, other tumor cells, or cellular debris. Nuclei are typically round but may vary in shape and have indented or irregular margins. Chromatin is coarse to clumped, and nucleoli are prominent and vary in number, size, and shape. Multinuclearity and bizarre mitotic figures are common. Many of these tumors are infiltrated by low numbers of small lymphocytes, plasma cells, and neutrophils. The second form comprises round, oval, and spindle cells with a more sarcoma-like appearance. Pleomorphism is less striking, but criteria of malignancy are present and warrant a cytologic interpretation of malignancy. Cytoplasmic vacuolation and phagocytic behavior also are less frequent. Nuclear shape is typically round to oval or elongate. These two forms are consistent with a tumor of dendritic cell origin.

The third form is HHS, in which neoplastic macrophages constitute a "wolf in sheep's clothing" because the cells resemble phagocytic macrophages found in inflammatory lesions and seldom exhibit criteria of malignancy.[17] The cells have moderate N:C ratios; vacuolated cytoplasm that frequently contains hemosiderin or phagocytosed erythrocytes, neutrophils, or platelets; and round central nuclei with reticular chromatin and one to two variably prominent nucleoli. More prominent pleomorphic features may be seen in a few cells. The neoplastic macrophages may form dense sheets in spleen, liver, or bone marrow, which may be

the sole warning of their malignant nature. Rarely is a definitive diagnosis of HHS made cytologically and histologic examination is required; a clinical presentation of hemolytic anemia nonresponsive to immunosuppressive therapy, with or without other peripheral blood cytopenias, warrants consideration of HHS. In the absence of defined masses, a histologic diagnosis may also be difficult.

Differential diagnoses for these tumors depend on cytologic appearance. Few tumors are as pleomorphic as the round cell variant of HS; however, differential diagnoses may include anaplastic carcinoma and pleomorphic lymphoma. Differential diagnoses for the spindle-cell variant include a variety of other sarcomas. Differentials for HHS are not tumors at all, but include reactive macrophage proliferations secondary to other tumors or other inflammatory processes (hemophagocytic syndrome).

Transmissible Venereal Tumor

Transmissible venereal tumor (TVT) is a unique transmissible tumor thought to be of histiocytic origin. Its morphologic appearance is distinctive, and cytologic evaluation can provide a definitive diagnosis, especially when the tumor is located in typical locations, such as mucous membranes of external genitalia and nasal cavity. The N:C ratio is moderate to high. The nucleus is centrally or eccentrically located and has coarse chromatin and one or more prominent nucleoli (Fig. 7.37). The cytoplasm is lightly basophilic and contains characteristic clear vacuoles, often giving a "string of pearls" appearance. Mitotic figures are frequent. Mature lesions may contain infiltrating small lymphocytes. When found in atypical locations, such as the torso, limbs, and lymph nodes, TVT may be mistaken for lymphoma, HS, or amelanotic melanoma.

Mesenchymal and Epithelial Tumors That May Appear as Discrete Round Cell Tumors

Mesenchymal and epithelial tumors that may appear as discrete round cell tumors include amelanotic melanoma, granular cell tumor, anaplastic carcinoma, OSA, chondrosarcoma, rhabdomyosarcoma, and liposarcoma. Histologic examination of the tumor and immunohistochemical evaluation may be required to ascertain the lineage of these round cell imposters.

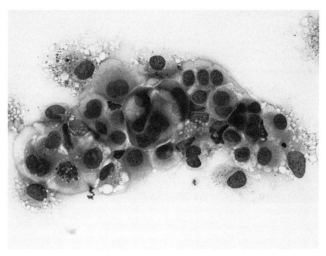

• **Fig. 7.38** Reactive mesothelial cells in pleural fluid from a cat with chylothorax. These cells may be highly pleomorphic and have criteria of malignancy, but they represented hyperplastic mesothelium in this cat.

Tumor Metastases and Tumors Exfoliating into Cavity Effusions

Specific tumor types preferentially metastasize to certain organs or sites, depending on location of the primary tumor, vascular or lymphatic dissemination, and many other factors. Regional lymph nodes, lung, liver, and spleen are common metastatic sites, but any tissue or organ can be involved, including skin, bone, bone marrow, and the central nervous system. Cytologic identification of tumor metastases begins with recognizing an abnormal population of cells in the metastatic site followed by determining the tissue of origin, if possible, based on cytomorphologic features.

Both primary and metastatic tumors may exfoliate into cavities, including the thoracic, abdominal, and pericardial cavities, or into cerebrospinal or synovial fluid. Although neoplastic cells in these abnormal locations may be categorized as epithelial, mesenchymal, or discrete round cell tumors, the specific origin of the primary tumor is only rarely determined by examining cells in the effusion. A major cytologic challenge when examining cells in cavity effusions is distinguishing reactive mesothelium, mesothelioma, and carcinoma (i.e., carcinomatosis). Mesothelium undergoes hyperplasia and exfoliation whenever an effusion forms in the thoracic, abdominal, or pericardial cavities, and reactive mesothelial cells can adopt all the criteria of malignancy described for tumor cells, including marked anisocytosis and anisokaryosis, macrocytosis and macrokaryosis, multinuclearity, variation of nuclear size within the same cell, nucleolar pleomorphism, and abnormal mitotic figures (Fig. 7.38). Identification of a mass and histologic examination often are required for a definitive diagnosis.

References

1. Langenbach A, McManus PM, Hendrick MJ, et al.: Sensitivity and specificity of methods for assessing the regional lymph nodes for evidence of metastasis in dogs and cats with solid tumors, *J Am Vet Med Assoc* 218:1424–1428, 2001.
2. Akhtar M, Ali MA, Huq M, et al.: Fine-needle biopsy: comparison of cellular yield with and without aspiration, *Diagn Cytopathol* 5:162–165, 1989.
3. Nyland TG, Wallack ST, Wisner ER: Needle-tract implantation following US-guided fine-needle aspiration biopsy of transitional cell carcinoma of the bladder, urethra, and prostate, *Vet Rad Ultrasound* 43:50–53, 2002.
4. Barger A, Graca R, Bailey K, et al.: Use of alkaline phosphatase staining to differentiate canine osteosarcoma from other vimentin-positive tumors, *Vet Pathol* 42:161–165, 2005.
5. Masserdotti C: Architectural patterns in cytology: correlation with histology, *Vet Clin Pathol* 35:388–396, 2006.
6. Christopher MM, Hotz CS, Shelly SM, et al.: Interpretation by clinicians of probability expressions in cytology reports and effect on clinical decision-making, *J Vet Intern Med* 24:496–503, 2010.
7. Masserdotti C, Drigo M: Retrospective study of cytologic features of canine well-differentiated hepatocellular carcinoma, *Vet Clin Pathol* 41:382–390, 2012.
8. Alleman AR, Choi US: Endocrine system. In Raskin RE, Meyer DJ, editors: *Canine and feline cytology: a color atlas and interpretation guide*, ed 2, St. Louis, 2010, Saunders.
9. Barthez PY, Marks SL, Woo J, et al.: Pheochromocytoma in dogs: 61 cases (1984–1995), *J Vet Intern Med* 11:272–278, 1997.
10. Bertazzolo W, Dell'Orco M, Bonfanti U, et al.: Canine angiosarcoma: cytologic, histologic, and immunohistochemical correlations, *Vet Clin Pathol* 34:28–34, 2005.
11. Craig LE, Julian ME, Ferracone JD: The diagnosis and prognosis of synovial tumors in dogs: 35 cases, *Vet Pathol* 39:66–73, 2002.
12. Vail DM, Powers BE, Getzy DM, et al.: Evaluation of prognostic factors for dogs with synovial sarcoma: 36 cases (1986-1991), *J Am Vet Med Assoc* 205:1300–1307, 1994.
13. Monti P, Barnes D, Adrian AM, et al.: Synovial cell sarcoma in a dog: a misnomer-Cytologic and histologic findings and review of the literature, *Vet Clin Pathol* 47:181–185, 2018.
14. Camus MS, Priest HL, Koehler JW, et al.: Cytologic criteria for mast cell tumor grading in dogs with evaluation of clinical outcome, *Vet Pathol* 53:1117–1123, 2016.
15. Flatland B, Fry MM, Newman SJ, et al.: Large anaplastic spinal B-cell lymphoma in a cat, *Vet Clin Pathol* 37:389–396, 2008.
16. Affolter VK, Moore PF: Localized and disseminated histiocytic sarcoma of dendritic cell origin in dogs, *Vet Pathol* 39:74–83, 2002.
17. Moore PF, Affolter VK, Vernau W: Canine hemophagocytic histiocytic sarcoma: a proliferative disorder of CD11d⁺ macrophages, *Vet Pathol* 43:632–645, 2006.

8

Molecular Diagnostics

ANNE C. AVERY, KARA MAGEE, MELISSA C. PAOLONI, AND CHAND KHANNA

Goals of Molecular Diagnostic Testing in Oncology

Molecular diagnostic testing in oncology is performed to achieve one of several goals: (1) to determine whether a patient has cancer, typically in circumstances in which visual examination of tissue by cytology or histology cannot distinguish a reactive from a neoplastic process; (2) to establish a prognosis; and (3) to guide treatment. Some of these goals currently are realized in veterinary oncology; the polymerase chain reaction for antigen receptor rearrangement (PARR) assay is used to confirm hematopoietic malignancy in both canine and feline patients, and the presence of *c-kit* gene mutations can inform the prognosis in canine mast cell disease. Increasingly, global analysis of oncogenes and gene expression is being used in human oncology, and advances in technology and ongoing veterinary research will make such testing available, affordable, and informative in veterinary medicine within the next few years.

The presence of a particular mutation or chromosomal abnormality can help subclassify a tumor. For example, in people, leukemia/small cell lymphoma (CLL/SCL) and mantle cell lymphoma (MCL) are both neoplasms of mature B cells, with a similar (but not identical) immunophenotype. However, MCL almost always has a rearrangement between the immunoglobulin heavy chain locus (IgH) and the *CCND1* gene (encoding cyclinD1), whereas this rearrangement is very rare in CLL/SCL.[1] The prognosis for and treatment of these two diseases are quite different, so the distinction is important to make.

Molecular diagnostic testing also can help guide therapy. This may be best illustrated by the development of tyrosine kinase inhibitors (TKIs). These drugs inhibit signaling through tyrosine kinase receptors, such as KIT, platelet-derived growth factor receptor (PDGFR), and epidermal growth factor receptor (EGFR). Tumors with mutations in these receptors that result in their constitutive activation may respond well to TKIs, whereas those without such mutations may require different kinds of therapy. Thus testing for mutations in these genes has become commonplace in human medicine (e.g., *EGFR* in small cell lung carcinoma, stem cell factor [SCF] receptor *[c-kit]* in gastrointestinal stromal cell tumors). Similarly, mast cell tumors in dogs that harbor a *c-kit* mutation may respond better to TKIs than those without the mutation.[2]

Oncogenes and chromosomal translocations uniquely distinguish neoplastic from normal tissue. As such, sensitive detection of mutations can be used to quantify residual disease in patients that have been treated. The best example of this is detection of the *bcr-abl* fusion gene, which can allow oncologists to detect as few as $1:10^3$ neoplastic cells in the peripheral blood of people with chronic myelogenous leukemia.[4] Tumor-specific primers that recognize the unique immunoglobulin genes found in both canine and human B-cell lymphomas have been used to quantify tumor burden and monitor disease in both dogs and people with lymphoma.[1,4,5]

The previous examples describe testing for single genetic alterations that are known to be shared by most tumors of the same type. Increasingly, the field of oncology is moving toward personalized, or precision, medicine (PMED). The goal of PMED is to identify genetic mutations and activated signaling pathways that are found in an individual's cancer, even when such changes have not yet been described in a particular cancer type. (PMED is discussed at the end of this chapter.)

For the purposes of this chapter, molecular diagnostics refers to the analysis of genes and gene expression. The goal of this chapter is to review several molecular techniques useful in the diagnosis and classification of cancer. Advanced molecular methodologies and diagnostics likely will continue to improve, become increasingly inexpensive, simpler to use, and more broadly available to veterinarians over the next few years.

Genomic Dysregulation in Cancer

Most molecular diagnostics target genomic dysregulation that may exist in cancer cells. Such dysregulation may occur at the level of the copy number of a gene; a point mutation in that gene that changes its function; epigenetic modification of deoxyribonucleic acid (DNA) that changes the level of expression; or large-scale changes to chromosomes that remove genes from their normal regulatory environment. Different methods are required for identifying each of these types of changes.

Methods for Analyzing Genes

DNA represents the genetic code of all species. This code consists of a series of continuous nucleic acid sugar strands linked through hydrogen bonds. This series of nucleic acids takes on a tertiary folded structure through modification by binding proteins called *histones*. The folded and wrapped DNA strand is packaged within the chromosomes of the cell. The earliest techniques used to assess the genetic changes of cancer defined gains, losses, or structural changes in chromosomes, referred to as *cytogenetics*. Subsequently, polymerase chain reaction (PCR)-based methods and high-throughput sequencing have allowed us to detect smaller discrete mutations in DNA that do not involve changes in large portions of the chromosome. Small deletions and insertions in genes, in addition to single-nucleotide changes, are now routinely detected.

Detection of Chromosomal Abnormalities

Historically these techniques involved the examination of metaphase preparations made from chromosomes. The metaphase preparations were then stained (banded) to help in the identification of distinct chromosome morphologies. These techniques allowed detection of gross abnormalities in the chromosome number (ploidy) and the presence of chromosomal translocations; they also led to the identification of genes associated with tumor development and progression. Cytogenetic analysis has been most useful in the clinical assessment of leukemias, for which metaphase preparations are relatively easy to develop from whole blood samples.[6] For most human leukemias, cytogenetic descriptors are used to define distinct subgroups into prognostic groups and to guide treatment decisions.

The use of cytogenetic approaches in the management of companion animals has been limited because of the difficulty involved in using conventional chromosomal banding to identify canine chromosomes. The development of chromosome-specific "paints" that allow the identification of specific canine chromosomes has improved the opportunity to apply cytogenetic descriptors to canine cancers. Using these techniques, Breen et al have identified a chromosomal translocation in canine chronic myelogenous leukemia and chronic monocytic leukemia that is the equivalent of the *bcr-abl* Philadelphia chromosome found in human chronic myelogenous leukemia.[3,7]

For the most part traditional cytogenetic techniques, including the use of chromosome-specific paints, are labor intensive and have been replaced by alternative modalities. Comparative genomic hybridization (CGH) arrays can define gains and losses in chromosome number in tumor specimens rapidly and with highly reproducible results. In CGH analysis the investigator labels genomic DNA from a normal individual and from a patient's tumor cells with two different-colored fluorescent probes. The labeled DNA then is hybridized to an array of DNA probes that span most of the genome. These probes are printed onto a chip or slide, such that the location of each individual probe is identified. The degree of hybridization to each probe is determined by the level of fluorescence detected by laser excitation. Equal hybridization of the DNA from both sources to an individual probe indicates a normal copy number, whereas increased binding by the tumor DNA indicates the presence of chromosomal duplication in the area of the genome covered by that probe (Fig. 8.1). Similarly, higher binding by the DNA from the normal individual indicates chromosomal loss in the area.

CGH arrays are useful for localizing chromosomal regions where investigators should focus their search for genes important to that cancer. Studies of a number of cancers have shown widespread gains and losses of genomic regions. Breen et al have shown that a subset of T-cell lymphomas (histologically defined as peripheral T-cell lymphoma, unspecified) exhibits copy number gain in regions common to most examples of this histologic type, but not present in other T-cell lymphoma subtypes.[8] This finding will help identify genes within the duplicated areas that might be useful for diagnostics and therapy and for understanding the genesis of the neoplasm. A similar study in canine malignant

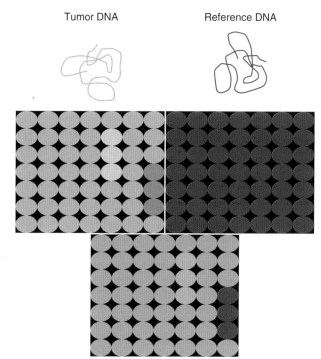

Tumor DNA   **Reference DNA**

• **Fig. 8.1** The principle of array analysis. A chip or slide is printed such that each position on the chip (there are thousands) has a single probe, which can range in size, depending on the type of array. DNA from a tumor tested is labeled with one dye *(green)*, and DNA from the reference sample with another *(red)*. Both samples are hybridized to the same chip. The separate red and green panels indicate that the tumor DNA exhibits both chromosomal gain (increased green fluorescence) and loss (decreased green fluorescence). When the two DNA preparations are cohybridized, a yellow signal indicates equal degrees of red and green fluorescence. When a gain in copy number occurs in a region of DNA, the signal is green. When a loss in copy number occurs, the signal is red. This is one of several ways microarrays can be performed.

histiocytosis (MH) demonstrated that MH frequently exhibits loss of chromosomal regions that contain tumor suppressor genes,[9] and transitional cell carcinomas (TCCs) were found to commonly exhibit complete gain of a chromosome.[10] The latter discovery led to the development of a diagnostic test for detection of canine TCC by enumerating chromosomal copy numbers.[11] Thus such genetic characterization offers opportunities to develop specific diagnostics, therapies, and management strategies.

Whole genome sequencing (WGS, discussed later in the chapter) can also detect chromosomal rearrangements. Because this technology rapidly is becoming less expensive and very efficient, WGS likely will replace CGH arrays within the next decade.

PCR-Based Techniques—Detection of Mutations and Novel Genes and Assessment of Clonality

PCR is the process of amplifying a small specific segment of DNA for the purpose of further analysis. Two small segments of DNA (commonly about 20 bases long) that are complementary to the DNA sequence surrounding the area to be amplified are synthesized. These primers are then used to amplify the DNA that lies between them (typically less than 1000 bases). This amplified

DNA product can be analyzed in a number of ways for mutations and to quantify the product for measurement of gene expression; or, in the case of lymphoid malignancy, the DNA can be separated by size to look for clonal populations of B and T cells. The same methods can be applied to the analysis of ribonucleic acid (RNA) once the RNA has been transcribed into DNA (reverse transcriptase PCR [RT-PCR]).

For primer synthesis the sequence of the target gene typically must be known. The publication of good quality canine[12] and feline[13] genomes has been invaluable in this regard—it is now possible simply to use the known sequences, rather than hope for sequence similarities with mice and humans.

Detection of Genetic Insertions and Deletions

PCR-based assays commonly are used in human oncology to detect insertions or deletions in genes relevant to the prognosis or treatment of a neoplasm. In veterinary medicine detection of internal tandem duplications in the *c-kit* gene in canine mast cell tumors is now a routine part of the diagnosis for the purpose of obtaining prognostic information. The primary mutations described are internal tandem duplications (ITDs) in two different exons, exon 8 and exon 11.[14] The mutations involve the duplication of a small segment of DNA so that it is repeated, resulting in a larger gene (Fig. 8.2). Approximately 14% to 20% of canine mast cell tumors have a duplication in either exon 8 or exon 11.[14] Dogs with tumors that carry the ITDs consistently have been shown to have a worse outcome than dogs with a wild-type *c-kit* gene.[15,16]

Detection of this type is fairly simple, because the presence of a larger (or smaller, in the case of deletions) PCR product is determined by size separation. As more genes are identified as targets of therapy, such assays likely will become more frequent. Suter et al identified an internal duplication in the *flt3* gene using the same methods[17] and provided preliminary evidence that the response to a small molecule inhibitor is predicted by the presence of this mutation in cell lines. Thus we are likely to see routine use of mutation detection in the near future.

Detection of Single-Base Mutations

Some cancers will have predictable, single-base mutations that can be detected by standard sequencing. However, sequencing can be insensitive; therefore a variety of PCR-based assays have been developed for mutation analysis. The best example of this type of assay currently in use is detection of a single nucleotide change found in the *BRAF* gene in 80% of cases of canine TCC.[18] The mutation found in the canine gene is equivalent to a *BRAF* mutation common in a variety of human cancers (V600E), and it causes constitutive activation of the BRAF protein. BRAF is a serine/threonine kinase, which activates a series of downstream signaling pathways to drive cellular metabolism and proliferation.[19]

Breen et al developed a PCR-based assay to detect this mutation (in dogs the mutation is called V595E).[20] The purpose of the assay is to diagnose TCC in urine samples with suspicious cells, which can often be difficult by cytology alone. The method used for detection is a technique called *droplet digital PCR* (ddPCR). ddPCR can detect the V595E mutation when it is present in as little as .01% of the DNA.[20] This method was considerably more sensitive than standard sequencing, which could not detect the mutation when it was present in less than 10% of the DNA. ddPCR probably will be used more commonly in the future, because it provides a way of quantifying mutations and DNA copy number changes with high precision.

Detection of Fusion Gene Products by PCR

One mechanism by which chromosomal translocation causes malignant transformation of cells is to create novel proteins with altered function. The best studied of these fusion genes, the Philadelphia chromosome, is the *bcr-abl* fusion gene found in greater than 90% of all human chronic myelogenous leukemias (CMLs) and occasionally acute lymphoblastic leukemia (ALL) and acute myelogenous leukemia (AML).[21] ABL is a tyrosine kinase that has myriad activities in cell growth and differentiation. It is encoded on human chromosome 9, and in CML is translocated to chromosome 22. The site of the translocation varies within the *bcr* (breakpoint cluster region) gene, so that a new fusion gene, *bcr-abl*, is formed. The new fusion protein allows for the constitutive activation of the ABL tyrosine kinase, which in turn promotes the development of CML. This novel protein is the product of a novel RNA transcript, which can be readily detected by RT-PCR. This assay can detect as few as 1:10³ tumor cells[4] and therefore can be used both for diagnosis of CML and for quantifying residual disease after treatment.

Assays for a large number of translocations in human cancers have been developed over the past 10 years.[22] These assays are now routinely available for characterization of human tumors, particularly leukemia and sarcoma. The finding that canine leukemia and lymphoma can exhibit the same translocations as their human counterparts[7,23] suggests that detection of novel fusion genes will provide inexpensive and sensitive diagnostic testing both for detecting cancer and for monitoring disease in the near future.

Assessment of Clonality in Lymphoma and Leukemia

A clonality assay demonstrates that a group of cells is derived from a single clone. The term usually is used to refer to detection of the unique genes found in each individual B or T cell—immunoglobulin genes in B cells and T-cell receptor (TCR) genes in T cells. The portion of these genes that encodes the antigen binding region is the portion that varies between cells, both in size and sequence. Once a B or T cell is mature and divides in response to antigenic stimulation, the immunoglobulin and T-cell receptor genes are passed on to the daughter cells.[24,25]

In the course of a normal immune response to a pathogen, B and T cells are activated, expand, and eventually die, leaving behind a small number of residual memory cells. On the other hand, when a cell becomes neoplastic, it no longer responds to growth controls and undergoes unlimited expansion. Therefore if it can be established that most of the cells in a particular collection of lymphocytes have the same immunoglobulin or T-cell receptor gene, these cells most likely are neoplastic rather than reactive.[26]

When immunoglobulin and T-cell receptor genes rearrange during the course of B-cell and T-cell development, respectively, the length and sequence of the resultant gene differs from cell to cell. This happens for many reasons; for example, nucleotides are added between V, D, and J segments as they rearrange into a contiguous formation. The clonality assay takes advantage of this development. A sample consisting of many different lymphocytes, as in a reactive process (e.g., the lymph nodes of a dog with chronic pyoderma or poor dental hygiene), will have multiple, different-sized, T-cell receptor and immunoglobulin genes. On the other hand, in a sample consisting of neoplastic lymphocytes, the immunoglobulin gene or the T-cell receptor gene (depending on whether it is a B-cell or a T-cell lymphoma) will be a single size (Fig. 8.3). (All methods used in veterinary medicine to detect clonally rearranged T-cell receptor genes target the TCR gamma gene.)

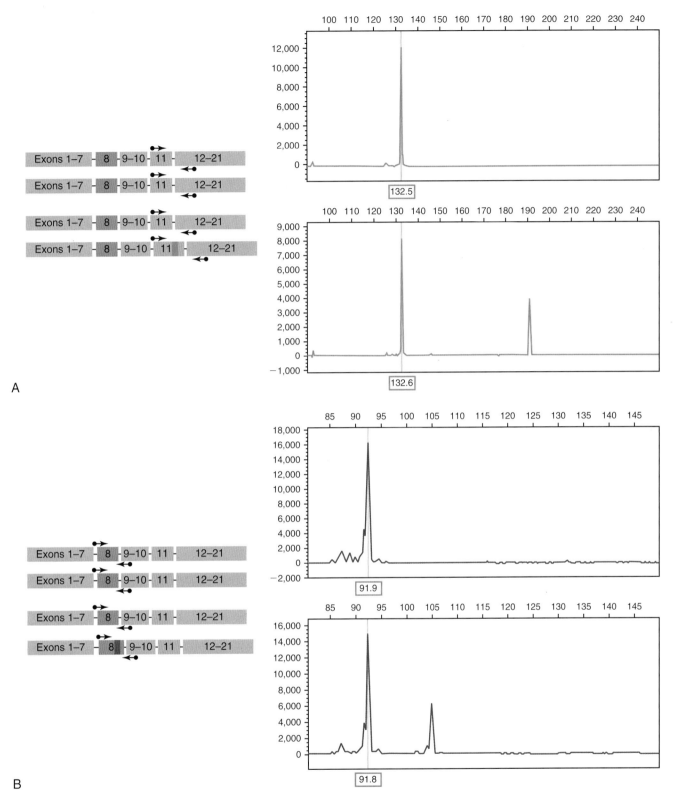

A

B

• **Fig. 8.2** Detection of *c-kit* mutations by polymerase chain reaction (PCR). (A) Two different tumor types are depicted: one has two copies of a wild-type *c-kit* gene, and the other has one copy of a *c-kit* gene containing an internal tandem duplication in exon 11. On the right are shown the PCR products detected after amplification with primers surrounding the duplication *(arrows)* for each tumor. (B) Same as in (A), but in this case the second tumor has an internal duplication in exon 8, and the PCR products are amplified with primers flanking the region of the duplication.

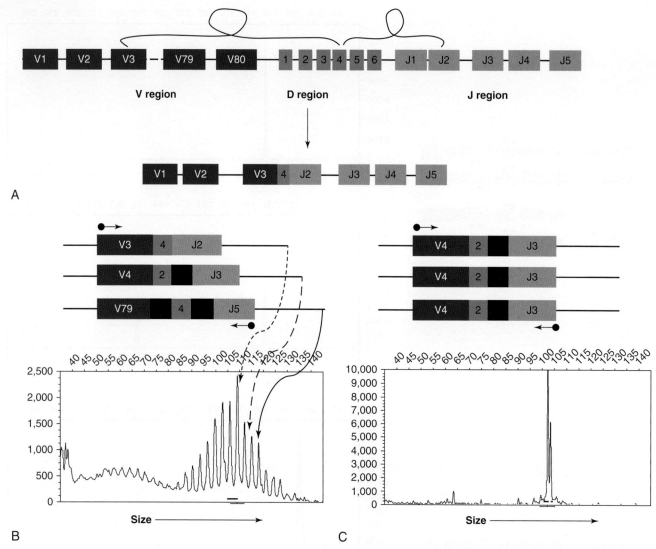

• **Fig. 8.3** Rearrangement of immunoglobulin genes. (A) There are approximately 80 V region genes, 6 D region genes, and 5 J region genes. Single V, D, and J genes are brought together at random to create a single VDJ gene segment, which encodes the antigen-binding portion of an antibody, and the intervening sequence is removed. (B) In the process of bringing together V, D and J genes, a variable number of nucleotides *(black)* are added between V and D, and D and J. As a result, each individual B cell will have a VDJ gene segment with a unique length. When DNA from a heterogeneous population of B cells is isolated and amplified with primers bracketing the VDJ gene segment *(small arrows)*, the polymerase chain reaction (PCR) products will be different lengths. The lower panel shows the PCR products separated by size by capillary gel electrophoresis; it illustrates multiple different-sized PCR products. (C) When a population of B cells comprises cells derived from a single clone, all the VDJ gene segments will be identically sized. PCR amplification of the VDJ gene segment will yield a single-sized product *(see lower panel)*. All the principles illustrated here apply to T-cell receptor (TCR) genes. For the clonality assay, the T-cell receptor γ-chain is amplified, although in theory the TCR β-chain could also be used.

Clonality assays are accomplished by isolating DNA from cells suspected to be neoplastic. PCR primers directed at the conserved regions of T-cell receptor or immunoglobulin genes are used to amplify the variable regions, and the PCR products are separated by size using a variety of methods. The presence of a single-sized PCR product indicates clonality, whereas the presence of multiple PCR products supports a reactive process.[27] This assay has been reported by a number of laboratories for both dogs and cats[27]; it is termed the *PCR for antigen receptor rearrangements* (PARR) assay to distinguish it from other types of clonality assays.[28] It should be noted, however, that the term "PARR" is not used in the human literature, where the assay instead is referred to as a *clonality assay*.

The PARR assay can detect approximately 1:100 neoplastic cells. The sensitivity and specificity of the assay differ between laboratories; however, because the results are significantly affected by the conditions under which the assay is run and the technique used to separate the PCR products, clinicians must consult the laboratory providing the testing about the sensitivity and specificity of the assay as performed under their conditions.

The main application of the PARR assay is to establish clonality in a sample that is cytologically or histologically ambiguous. Another application is to compare two neoplasms arising at different times to determine whether they have the same clonal origin.[29] The PARR assay increasingly is used to distinguish inflammatory bowel disease from gastrointestinal (GI) lymphoma in dogs[30,31] and cats[32,33] and to aid in the diagnosis of nodular splenic lymphoma, which can be difficult to distinguish from nodular hyperplasia.[34]

Clonality assays sometimes can be useful for establishing the lineage (B cell vs. T cell) in cytologically unambiguous lymphomas if additional case material is not obtainable from the patient. However, flow cytometry or immunohistochemistry generally is preferable for this purpose, for several reasons: first, aberrant rearrangements occasionally can be seen in nonlymphoid tumors, such as myelogenous leukemias.[35] Second, simply knowing whether a neoplasm is derived from a B cell or a T cell may not be clinically useful. Both lineages can give rise to markedly different tumor types with significantly different outcomes. For example, the two most common forms of T-cell lymphoma (peripheral T-cell lymphoma and T-zone lymphoma) both have clonally rearranged T-cell receptor genes. Peripheral T-cell lymphoma, however, has a median survival time of 150 days,[36] whereas T-zone lymphoma is indolent and may not require treatment at all.[37]

The principle of the clonality assay also can be used to quantify tumor cells in blood, bone marrow, or node and to monitor minimum residual disease. For this type of analysis PCR primers specific for the immunoglobulin or T-cell receptor gene carried by the tumor are used instead of the broadly reactive primers used to screen samples. In this way the investigator is certain that only tumor DNA is amplified, and not nonneoplastic lymphocytes. The specificity of this reaction permits determination of the number of tumor cells in a sample of blood, even when those cells are as rare as $1:10^4$ cells. Yamazaki et al demonstrated that with current chemotherapy protocols, all seven dogs they examined had at least $1:10^4$ cells in their peripheral blood, even though the dogs achieved clinical remission.[5] Although this kind of analysis may not be practical for routine diagnostics, it is a powerful research tool to compare the efficacy of novel chemotherapy regimens, and it also can be used to refine current protocols. Indeed, this method subsequently was used by Sato et al to evaluate the responsiveness of B-cell lymphoma to individual components of the cyclophosphamide, hydroxydaunorubicin, Oncovin and prednisone or prednisolone (CHOP) chemotherapy protocol.[38]

Assessment of Clonality in Nonlymphoid Neoplasms

Nonlymphoid cells do not have unique DNA sequences that differ from cell to cell, so other methods must be used for clonality assessment. The question of whether a collection of cells is neoplastic arises in a variety of circumstances—eosinophilia in the cat, for example, or pleural effusion in a dog, which is dominated by cells that could be either reactive or neoplastic mesothelium. One way to determine whether the cells in these cases are derived from the same clone is to examine the pattern of X chromosome inactivation. One copy of the X chromosome in the cells of female animals is inactivated by DNA methylation. The purpose of the inactivation is to ensure that both male and female animals have the same "dosage" of genes found on the X chromosome. Inactivation is thought to be random, so in a nonneoplastic collection of cells, any given cell would have an equal chance of either the maternal or paternal X chromosome being inactivated. If the cells are all derived from the same clone, however, the same X chromosome would be inactivated in each cell.

In female animals, X chromosome inactivation can be measured using the androgen receptor gene. This gene contains repeated DNA elements (CAG repeats), the number of which varies. If an animal is heterozygous for the number of repeats, it is possible to determine whether the same X chromosome is

inactivated in all the cells in a particular sample. Because not all animals will be heterozygous, the assay is useful only in a subset of female animals—68% of cats[39] and 50% of dogs.[40] The assay has been used for canine patients with possible chronic myelogenous leukemia[40] and for cats with possible myelodysplastic syndrome.[39] In dogs this assay has been named the *canine androgen receptor assay* (CANARA assay).[41]

Whole Genome and Whole Exome Sequencing—Next Generation Sequencing

Next generation sequencing (also known as *massively parallel sequencing*) is a technology that allows investigators to sequence the entire genome of an individual (or an individual's tumor). Sequencing an entire genome was considered an enormous and expensive endeavor not many years ago, but it is now a routine part of investigating the biology of cancer. Thousands of human cancers have been fully sequenced, and the cost and efficiency of this process means that individual tumors can be sequenced to aid clinical decision making. The main types of information that can be obtained from whole genome sequencing of a tumor include (1) mutations in potential oncogenes or tumor suppressor genes, including single nucleotide variants (SNVs) and insertions and deletions (indels); (2) structural changes in chromosomes, including fusion genes and copy number variations (CNVs), in which whole genetic regions may be duplicated; and (3) the mutational load of a particular tumor, which may predict responsiveness to checkpoint inhibitor therapy and also identify potential neoantigens that may be targeted in immunotherapy strategies. The principles of next generation sequencing are described in the next section.

Quantifying Genes and Gene Expression

The complete genetic code, or DNA sequence, is present within every cell in the body. The effective genetic information that uniquely defines each cell type within the body is defined by the genes expressed (transcribed) as messenger RNA (mRNA). The complete profile of mRNA expression is more responsible for the phenotype of a cancer than the individual genes, although mutations in a gene often are individual drivers of a cancer phenotype. To assess the level of expression of one or a few genes, three methods could be used: (1) real-time quantitative PCR (RT-qPCR), which has been used for many years; (2) ddPCR, which is a more recent development that has many advantages over RT-qPCR and which probably will replace RT-qPCR for most applications; and (3) non-PCR–based gene counting methods, such as Nanostring.

If the goal is to measure expression of all the genes in a tumor, microarrays and, more recently, RNA sequencing (RNA seq) methods have been used. Assessment of the global level of gene expression is called *gene expression profiling*.

Real-Time PCR and Droplet Digital PCR

RT-qPCR refers to the quantitative (Q) measurement of DNA—either genes or, more commonly, RNA that has be reversed transcribed to cDNA.[42] The principle of RT-qPCR is that DNA is amplified using primers, just as in a routine PCR reaction, but at each round of amplification, the amount of PCR product is quantified. Unlike endpoint PCR, in which the reaction runs to completion and the product is separated by size, real-time PCR is quantitative and relies on the change in the amount of PCR product, as measured by fluorescence, as the reaction progresses.

Real-time PCR typically uses fluorescently labeled DNA probes. These are short segments of DNA complementary to the target sequence between the two primer sites. A fluorescent molecule attached to the probe is quenched (no fluorescence detectable) until the 5′ to 3′ exonuclease activity of the Taq polymerase releases the fluorescent molecule. As the amount of PCR product increases proportional to the starting material, the amount of fluorescence increases (Fig. 8.4A). The expression level of a gene of interest is normalized to housekeeping genes and can be compared between samples.

ddPCR rapidly is replacing RT-qPCR because it has a number of distinct advantages.[43] In this method, RNA is reverse transcribed into cDNA and then the cDNA is dispersed into thousands of oil droplets, in such a proportion that the oil droplet will have either one copy of the gene of interest or no copies (see Fig. 8.4B). Also in the oil droplet is the other material for a PCR reaction (primers, fluorescent probes as described previously, and polymerase). An endpoint PCR reaction is performed in each droplet (all droplets are amplified simultaneously), and the number of fluorescent droplets is counted. This is called "digital" PCR because the level of gene expression is correlated with the count of positive droplets. By contrast, RT-qPCR measures the level of gene by the cumulative fluorescence of all the cDNA in the sample.

The reason ddPCR is an improvement on RT-qPCR is that for the latter, scrupulous attention must be paid to primer efficiency, and the range of gene expression over which it is useful is limited.

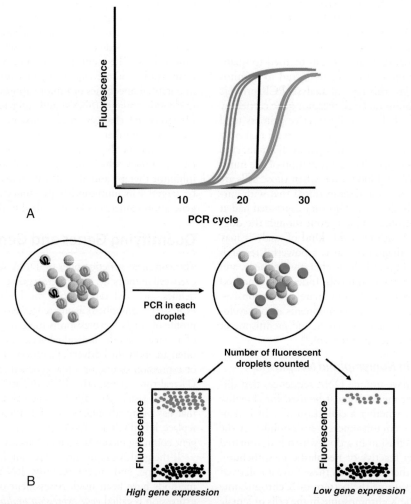

• **Fig. 8.4** Comparison of a real-time quantitative polymerase chain reaction (RT-qPCR) assay and a droplet digital PCR (ddPCR) assay. (A) An RT-qPCR assay shows different levels of expression of a gene in two different tumors. The green lines are from a tumor (performed in triplicate) that expresses high levels of the gene being measured; the blue lines are from a tumor that expresses lower levels of the gene being measured. At the end of the reaction (cycle 40 in this example), the two samples have almost the same level of fluorescence. In RT-qPCR, gene expression is assessed by measuring the difference in fluorescence in the early cycles. The difference in fluorescence at cycle 22 is significant. The same curves are generated for a housekeeping gene (not shown) to normalize the amount of input complementary DNA (cDNA) for both samples. (B) In ddPCR, RNA is reverse transcribed into cDNA, and the cDNA (which includes all genes) then is partitioned into thousands of oil droplets, using special instrumentation, together with the other materials for a PCR reaction (primers, polymerase, fluorescent probes). Many droplets will be empty; some will have cDNA but not the gene of interest *(black)*; and some will have the gene of interest. The PCR reaction is performed to endpoint (e.g., 30 cycles). The amount of RNA of the gene of interest is reflected by the number of fluorescent droplets. As with RT-qPCR, a similar reaction using a housekeeping gene is performed to normalize input cDNA levels.

With ddPCR, as long as the PCR reaction produces a fluorescent signal, the efficiency with which the reaction achieves that signal is not as relevant to the results. The technology is also less limited by the amount of sample available.

Gene Expression Profiling

Gene expression profiling refers to the quantification of thousands of mRNAs simultaneously, to create a picture of global gene expression in the cell population. The pattern of gene expression is called a *gene expression profile.* In most cases gene expression profiling is comparative. Investigators can compare expression profiles of tumor cells to the normal cellular counterpart, to similar tumors with different clinical outcomes, to tumor cells from the same patient before and after therapy, or between primary and metastatic lesions, to determine how different pathways have changed. Such information has proven invaluable in a variety of settings. For example, in a study of cervical cancer in people, investigators analyzed gene expression profiles of tumors that responded to chemotherapy and radiation and compared those with tumors that did not. Their study revealed that activation of the PI3K/Akt signaling pathway was associated with a poor response, suggesting one potential therapeutic target.[44] It is important to note that the collective signature of an expression profile can be an informative predictor of disease biology or response to therapy; however, alterations in the expression of a single gene are rarely informative and require extensive post hoc validation.

Another example of how gene expression profiling has advanced oncology is the studies of B-cell lymphoma by Staudt and colleagues. Noting that diffuse large B-cell lymphoma (DLBCL) has a heterogeneous outcome in people, this group compared the gene expression profiles of 96 DLBCLs with B cells derived from different stages of normal B-cell development.[45] They found that the gene expression profile of DLBCL could be categorized either as similar to germinal center B cells or similar to activated B cells. Importantly, these two categories had prognostic significance; germinal center–like DLBCL patients have a better prognosis. The distinction between germinal center DLBCL and activated B-cell DLBCL is now well established as a prognostic indicator in people. Studies of canine lymphoma have offered conflicting data with regard to subclassification of canine DLBCL into germinal center and activated B-cell subtypes based on gene expression profiling, so additional study is necessary.[46,47] Staudt et al made another important discovery about human B-cell lymphoma, using gene expression profiling, that provided insights into immunity to cancer. Expression profiles of lymph nodes from patients with follicular B-cell lymphoma demonstrated that the type of immune response signature was prognostic in this disease. Patients whose lymph node gene expression patterns exhibited evidence of T-cell activation had a better overall survival than patients whose gene expression patterns resembled activated macrophages.[48] The expression profile of the tumor cells themselves was not predictive. This finding suggests that the immune response contributes to survival in patients with follicular B-cell lymphoma, a result corroborated in other types of B-cell lymphoma.[49,50]

Microarrays

Microarrays are solid chips on which DNA probes that are complementary to thousands of different genes are imprinted.[51] Such platforms expand the study of expression of single genes to a larger scale needed for an expression signature to be defined. RNA from a tumor is transcribed into cDNA and labeled with a fluorescent molecule. The labeled cDNA is then hybridized with the probes on the chip, and the level of fluorescence is proportional to the number of copies of RNA molecules in the sample (Fig. 8.5). A microarray experiment can be performed in a large variety of ways, but ultimately the goal is to measure expression of all the genes in the sample.

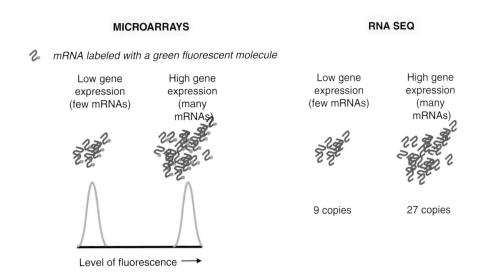

• **Fig. 8.5** Comparison of the measurement of gene expression using microarrays and RNA seq. Microarrays are carried out by labeling all the messenger RNAs *(mRNAs)* (reverse transcribed into cDNAs) in a sample with a fluorescent molecule, and then allowing that molecule to anneal to a chip coated with thousands of DNA probes complementary to each cDNA. The level of fluorescence at each position on the chip (corresponding to an individual gene) reflects the total number of mRNA molecules in the sample, but the number of mRNA molecules is not counted. RNA seq, on the other hand, uses technology that allows every single expressed gene to be sequenced. Because the sequence of every gene is known, the absolute number of mRNAs for each gene in the sample can be counted.

RNA seq

As does a microarray, RNA seq measures global gene expression.[52] In microarrays the amount of mRNA from an individual gene is measured by the cumulative fluorescence contributed by all copies of the mRNA transcribed from a given gene (see Fig. 8.5). RNA seq, however, uses massively parallel sequencing, also known as Next Gen sequencing, to sequence every mRNA in a sample. The sequence allows for identification of the gene from which it was derived. Because all mRNAs are sequenced, this methodology allows the investigator to count the number of individual mRNAs. Genes that are highly expressed will have high numbers of mRNAs.

Although RNA seq experiments involve a great deal more bioinformatic complexity, they also can provide information not obtainable using microarrays. This includes the ability to identify potential mutations in coding regions because sequence information is being obtained, and the ability to identify some fusion genes that create fusion transcripts.

Personalized Medicine in Cancer

Foundations of Precision Medicine: the Genetic Basis of Cancer

Cancer is a genetic disease that arises as a consequence of the stepwise accumulation of disruptive mutations in genes that regulate cell life and death. Clonal expansion of cell populations bearing cancer gene mutations fuels the formation of malignant tumors. This genetic model of cancer emerged in the latter 20th century as a product of advances in genetics, evolution, and cancer medicine. Through this mutational process, cancers acquire specific key properties, including self-sufficient growth signaling, resistance to growth inhibitory signaling, invasion and metastasis, unlimited replication potential, angiogenic signaling, immune modulation, DNA instability, metabolic dysregulation, and immune evasion.[53]

The genetic model and its downstream phenotypes have since been validated in many cancer types and provide a framework for our growing genomic understanding of cancer. The concept of personalized or precision medicine stems from the previously described genomic underpinning of cancer and its nascent and emerging complexity. Indeed, truly personalized and genomic medicine now seeks to define the genomic drivers of a particular patient's cancer and match these alterations to specific therapeutics. PMED is ushering in a new era in cancer therapy in which clinical and translational value are applied to advances in the genomic analysis of cancer. The discoveries and tools described previously have provided new opportunities to tailor cancer therapy to the individual molecular characteristics of a specific cancer, in a specific patient, to guide diagnosis, prognosis, and treatment selection. In many cases these genetic alterations can be matched to specific therapeutic agents as a means to uniquely improve outcomes for patients. Tumor samples and matched germline samples (from peripheral blood or cheek swabs) may be collected, preserved, and then analyzed for genetic alterations in a core set of cancer genes, which ultimately are matched to an individualized therapeutic prescription.

How Precision Medicine Differs from the Current Practice of Oncology

The use of patient-specific information as a means to deliver PMED is not new to the treatment of cancer patients. Through the history of cancer medicine, treatments have been administered in a patient-specific and personalized manner. Even in the modern era, the use of molecular data to guide the therapy of specific individuals with cancer is not entirely novel. The use of specific immunohistochemical or cytogenetic markers to guide the diagnosis and prognosis has been a critical and routine practice in pathology laboratories for many decades. Furthermore, in some cancers molecular markers have been used to guide treatment selection. For example, in human breast cancer a long-standing practice has been to define the expression of hormone receptors as a means to deliver specific therapeutics that alter downstream signaling pathways.[54] *C-kit* mutation status has been used in veterinary medicine to direct therapy for mast cell tumors,[2,55] but conflicting data in the literature raise questions about this approach, and more investigation is needed.[16]

Although genomic data is expected to affect patient outcomes dramatically, genomic data has been slow to enter the clinic. One of the first pilot studies incorporating molecular profiling to guide therapy in advanced cancers was published in 2010.[56] This study faced considerable challenges, but the researchers found that 27% of 68 patients treated according to molecular profiling recommendations (i.e., PMED) experienced a longer progression-free survival than during the most recent treatment on which they had progressed. Although it is perhaps intuitively beneficial to incorporate precise target identification into patient treatment, this approach still faces significant hurdles, and it remains to be proven through prospective trials that treatment based on PMED outperforms a physician's choice of treatment. Now, multiple clinical trials incorporating genomics-guided therapy selection are underway to test this very hypothesis. In one such trial, the Stand Up To Cancer and Melanoma Research Alliance Dream Team Clinical Trial, molecularly guided therapy in non-V600E mutant BRAF metastatic melanoma is being assessed. This is now an ongoing randomized clinical trial.

Returning clinically relevant and actionable information based on genomic analysis within a window that enables effective treatment selection is a substantial challenge. Notable hurdles include those associated with tumor biopsy; sample preservation and transport; nucleic acid extraction and quality control; genomic sequencing infrastructure and platform; data analysis and integration; generation of digestible genomic reports for physicians, veterinarians, and scientists alike; and performance of tumor board reviews to provide a treatment recommendation. Additional hurdles involve the implementation of precision medicine in the clinic.

In the broadest sense, the clinician seeking a PMED approach for a patient must first ask what data would be most helpful.

"I need new treatment options." In the setting of a rare tumor or a patient with unusual tumor biology, new ideas for therapy may be needed. In this setting an optimal PMED platform will identify specific drivers of this patient's cancer biology and propose new treatments. For such a clinical question, an optimal PMED platform likely will include an analysis of mutations in cancer-associated genes, with drug matching to target the presumed aberrant mutational targets of the individual cancer. The validation of the value of this approach has been difficult using conventional clinical trial designs and may demand novel perspectives on evidence for clinical validation. Because many solid tumors are clinical problems as a result of metastatic progression (e.g., canine osteosarcoma), the optimal PMED platform will derive a list of "shed" mutational targets from circulating biofluids (i.e., so-called liquid biopsy) alone or in combination with tumor analysis.

"I have some idea on treatments but want to prioritize the best therapy." It is not uncommon that the selection of the best treatment for a cancer histology is unclear and often defaults to the clinician's preference (e.g., selection of a specific cytotoxic chemotherapy for canine bladder carcinoma). A distinct PMED approach may provide assistance in known drug selection. The theoretical value of selecting the best drug, based on intrinsic resistance and sensitivity signatures, may be effectively provided through transcriptomic, proteomic, and cell-based PMED platforms. The validation of these drug selection strategies will require prospective validation in specific cancers in which cohorts of individuals may receive a PMED-described medication compared with clinician's best choice. Such transcriptomic, proteomic, and cell-based PMED platforms are less likely to identify specific drivers of cancer biology and generate new options for therapy.

An ever-growing array of tests designed to inform diagnostic and treatment decisions in the human clinic is available from more than 100 academic and 50 commercial laboratories. These tests range in scope from single genes to gene panels, exomes, and even whole genomes. Indeed, the multiomic analysis of cancer (multiple modalities used in a single cancer) is now common and has reulted in a need to display and share such multiomic data. In everyday clinical practice the cost is still prohibitive, and the expertise and infrastructure required to bring them to bear on patient care are also largely lacking. Finally, more comprehensive data showing improvements in genomics-correlated clinical outcomes is needed to support the use of these tests.

The Path to PMED for Veterinary Cancer Patients

Although much work remains to be done to chart the genomic landscapes of companion animal cancers, the PMED approach nonetheless is poised to have a dramatic effect on the care of canine cancer patients. Indeed, we have published on the clinical feasibility of this approach in dogs.[57] PMED now represents a cutting edge opportunity in veterinary cancer care and is the subject of ongoing prospective clinical trials. In fact, not only would this approach make great headway in the care of canine cancer patients, but also, given the unique aspects of naturally occurring cancer in pet dogs and the forward-thinking perspectives of the veterinary profession on the whole, veterinary oncology may be able to provide key data validating this model and refining its implementation for human medicine. As a means to change the biology of an important canine cancer problem, we have initiated a research agenda that will deliver personalized medicine for the canine cancer hemangiosarcoma through clinical trials that have recently launched.

Using Molecular Diagnostics as a Clinician

It has been historically acceptable for one laboratory to describe the performance of a specific assay in their hands and for clinicians to expect similar if not identical results from the same analysis performed by a distinct laboratory. Indeed, based on this expected consistency of analysis among laboratories, there was little need for distinct laboratories performing the same assay to publish their own independent results and experiences. Standardization has yet to come to the field of molecular diagnostics, and clinicians should expect the publication of a laboratory experience with a given assay and should not expect the performance of the assay to be the same across laboratories. Further complicating the issue of assay performance, characterized by sensitivity, specificity, and positive and negative predictive values, is the need to understand carefully the relevance of the patient populations used in manuscripts that describe assay performance. Assay performance is closely regulated in the human molecular diagnostics field (e.g., Clinical Laboratory Improvement Amendments [CLIA] laboratory certification), but such regulation is absent in the veterinary reference laboratory diagnostic model. Therefore rigor and the requirement of transparency appropriately become the responsibility of the diagnostic scientist and must be demanded and understood by the attending clinician.

Summary

Molecular diagnostics is becoming more integrated into veterinary medicine and at the same time becoming more affordable. One important feature of such advanced diagnostics is that many of these techniques save money for owners and eliminate the need for invasive procedures for their pets. For example, sensitive methods for detecting lymphoma through a combination of cytology, flow cytometry, and PARR assays can mean that a diagnosis of splenic lymphoma can be made without splenectomy. Detection of the *c-kit* mutation can guide therapy so that the most efficacious (and therefore cost-effective) drugs are used. More expensive exploratory techniques, such as whole genome sequencing and proteomic analysis of tumors, will almost certainly lead to discovery of new testing that can further simplify diagnoses. Veterinarians are encouraged to participate in these developmental studies when they can, by providing biologic materials and clinical data to researchers, because ultimately patients and their owners will derive great benefit from current research.

References

1. Jevremovic D, Viswanatha DS: Molecular diagnosis of hematopoietic and lymphoid neoplasms, *Hematol Oncol Clin North Am* 23:903–933, 2009.
2. London CA, Malpas PB, Wood-Follis SL, et al.: Multi-center, placebo-controlled, double-blind, randomized study of oral toceranib phosphate (SU11654), a receptor tyrosine kinase inhibitor, for the treatment of dogs with recurrent (either local or distant) mast cell tumor following surgical excision, *Clin Cancer Res* 15:3856–3865, 2009.
3. Cruz Cardona JA, Milner R, Alleman AR, et al.: BCR-ABL translocation in a dog with chronic monocytic leukemia, *Vet Clin Pathol* 40:40–47, 2011.
4. Morley A: Quantifying leukemia, *N Engl J Med* 339:627–629, 1998.
5. Yamazaki J, Baba K, Goto-Koshino Y, et al.: Quantitative assessment of minimal residual disease (MRD) in canine lymphoma by using real-time polymerase chain reaction, *Vet Immunol Immunopathol* 126:321–331, 2008.
6. Knuutila S: Cytogenetics and molecular pathology in cancer diagnostics, *Ann Med* 36:162–171, 2004.
7. Breen M, Modiano JF: Evolutionarily conserved cytogenetic changes in hematological malignancies of dogs and humans—man and his best friend share more than companionship, *Chromosome Res* 16:145–154, 2008.
8. Thomas R, Seiser EL, Motsinger-Reif A, et al.: Refining tumor-associated aneuploidy through 'genomic recoding' of recurrent DNA copy number aberrations in 150 canine non-Hodgkin lymphomas, *Leuk Lymphoma* 52:1321–1335, 2011.
9. Hedan B, Thomas R, Motsinger-Reif A, et al.: Molecular cytogenetic characterization of canine histiocytic sarcoma: a spontaneous model for human histiocytic cancer identifies deletion of tumor suppressor genes and highlights influence of genetic background on tumor behavior, *BMC Cancer* 11:201–215, 2011.

10. Shapiro SG, Raghunath S, Williams C, et al.: Canine urothelial carcinoma: genomically aberrant and comparatively relevant, *Chromosome Res* 23:311–331, 2015.

11. Mochizuki H, Shapiro SG, Breen M: Detection of copy number imbalance in canine urothelial carcinoma with droplet digital polymerase chain reaction, *Vet Pathol* 53:764–772, 2016.

12. Hoeppner MP, Lundquist A, Pirun M, et al.: An improved canine genome and a comprehensive catalogue of coding genes and non-coding transcripts, *PLoS One* 9:e91172, 2014.

13. Montague MJ, Li G, Gandolfi B, et al.: Comparative analysis of the domestic cat genome reveals genetic signatures underlying feline biology and domestication, *Proc Natl Acad Sci U S A* 111:17230–17235, 2014.

14. Letard S, Yang Y, Hanssens K, et al.: Gain-of-function mutations in the extracellular domain of KIT are common in canine mast cell tumors, *Mol Cancer Res* 6:1137–1145, 2008.

15. Takeuchi Y, Fujino Y, Watanabe M, et al.: Validation of the prognostic value of histopathological grading or c-kit mutation in canine cutaneous mast cell tumours: a retrospective cohort study, *Vet J* 196:492–498, 2013.

16. Weishaar KM, Ehrhart EJ, Avery AC, et al.: c-Kit mutation and localization status as response predictors in mast cell tumors in dogs treated with prednisone and toceranib or vinblastine, *J Vet Intern Med* 32:394–405, 2018.

17. Suter SE, Small GW, Seiser EL, et al.: FLT3 mutations in canine acute lymphocytic leukemia, *BMC Cancer* 11:38, 2011.

18. Decker B, Parker HG, Dhawan D, et al.: Homologous mutation to human BRAF V600E is common in naturally occurring canine bladder cancer - evidence for a relevant model system and urine-based diagnostic test, *Mol Cancer Res* 13:993–1002, 2015.

19. Holderfield M, Deuker MM, McCormick F, et al.: Targeting RAF kinases for cancer therapy: BRAF-mutated melanoma and beyond, *Nat Rev Cancer* 14:455–467, 2014.

20. Mochizuki H, Shapiro SG, Breen M: Detection of BRAF mutation in uring DNA as a molecular diagnostic for canine urothelial and prostatic carcinoma, *PLoS One* 10:e0144170, 2015.

21. Wong S, Witte ON: The BCR-ABL story: bench to bedside and back, *Annu Rev Immunol* 22:247–306, 2004.

22. Osumi K, Fukui T, Kiyoi H, et al.: Rapid screening of leukemia fusion transcripts in acute leukemia by real-time PCR, *Leuk Lymphoma* 43:2291–2299, 2002.

23. Ulve R, Rault M, Bahin M, et al.: Discovery of human-similar gene fusions in canine cancers, *Cancer Res* 77:5721–5727, 2017.

24. Blom B, Spits H: Development of human lymphoid cells, *Annu Rev Immunol* 24:287–320, 2006.

25. Delves PJ, Roitt IM: The immune system. First of two parts, *N Engl J Med* 343:37–49, 2000.

26. Swerdlow SH: Genetic and molecular genetic studies in the diagnosis of atypical lymphoid hyperplasias versus lymphoma, *Hum Pathol* 34:346–351, 2003.

27. Keller SM, Vernau W, Moore PF: Clonality testing in veterinary medicine: a review with diagnostic guidelines, *Vet Pathol* 53:711–725, 2016.

28. Burnett RC, Vernau W, Modiano JF, et al.: Diagnosis of canine lymphoid neoplasia using clonal rearrangements of antigen receptor genes, *Vet Pathol* 40:32–41, 2003.

29. Burnett RC, Blake MK, Thompson LJ, et al.: Evolution of a B-cell lymphoma to multiple myeloma after chemotherapy, *J Vet Intern Med* 18:768–771, 2004.

30. Lane J, Price J, Moore A, et al.: Low-grade gastrointestinal lymphoma in dogs: 20 cases (2010 to 2016), *J Small Anim Pract* 59:147–153, 2018.

31. Ohmura S, Leipig M, Schopper I, et al.: Detection of monoclonality in intestinal lymphoma with polymerase chain reaction for antigen receptor gene rearrangement analysis to differentiate from enteritis in dogs, *Vet Comp Oncol* 15:194–207, 2017.

32. Gress V, Wolfesberger B, Fuchs-Baumgartinger A, et al.: Characterization of the T-cell receptor gamma chain gene rearrangements as an adjunct tool in the diagnosis of T-cell lymphomas in the gastrointestinal tract of cats, *Res Vet Sci* 107:261–266, 2016.

33. Moore PF, Rodriguez-Bertos A, Kass PH: Feline gastrointestinal lymphoma: mucosal architecture, immunophenotype, and molecular clonality, *Vet Pathol* 49:658–668, 2012.

34. Sabattini S, Lopparelli RM, Rigillo A, et al.: Canine splenic nodular lymphoid lesions: immunophenotyping, proliferative activity and clonality assessment, *Vet Pathol* 55:645–653, 2018.

35. Stokol T, Nickerson GA, Shuman M, et al.: Dogs with acute myeloid leukemia have clonal rearrangements in T and B cell receptors, *Front Vet Sci* 4:76, 2017.

36. Avery PR, Burton J, Bromberek JL, et al.: Flow cytometric characterization and clinical outcome of CD4+ T-cell lymphoma in dogs: 67 cases, *J Vet Intern Med* 28:538–546, 2014.

37. Flood-Knapik KE, Durham AC, Gregor TP, et al.: Clinical, histopathological and immunohistochemical characterization of canine indolent lymphoma, *Vet Comp Oncol* 11:272–286, 2013.

38. Sato M, Yamazaki J, Goto-Koshino Y, et al.: Evaluation of cytoreductive efficacy of vincristine, cyclophosphamide, and doxorubicin in dogs with lymphoma by measuring the number of neoplastic lymphoid cells with real-time polymerase chain reaction, *J Vet Intern Med* 25:285–291, 2011.

39. Mochizuki H, Goto-Koshino Y, Takahashi M, et al.: X-chromosome inactivation pattern analysis for the assessment of cell clonality in cats, *Vet Pathol* 49:963–970, 2012.

40. Mochizuki H, Goto-Koshino Y, Takahashi M, et al.: Demonstration of the cell clonality in canine hematopoietic tumors by X-chromosome inactivation pattern analysis, *Vet Pathol* 52:61–69, 2015.

41. Delcour NM, Klopfleisch R, Gruber AD, et al.: Canine cutaneous histiocytomas are clonal lesions as defined by X-linked clonality testing, *J Comp Pathol* 149:192–198, 2013.

42. Wong ML, Medrano JF: Real-time PCR for mRNA quantitation, *Biotechniques* 39:75–85, 2005.

43. Quan PL, Sauzade M, Brouzes E: dPCR: a technology review, *Sensors (Basel)* 18:E1271, 2018.

44. Schwarz JK, Payton JE, Rashmi R, et al.: Pathway-specific analysis of gene expression data identifies the PI3K/Akt pathway as a novel therapeutic target in cervical cancer, *Clin Cancer Res* 18:1464–1471, 2012.

45. Alizadeh AA, Eisen MB, Davis RE, et al.: Distinct types of diffuse large B-cell lymphoma identified by gene expression profiling, *Nature* 403:503–511, 2000.

46. Aresu L, Ferraresso S, Marconato L, et al.: New molecular and therapeutic insights into canine diffuse large B cell lymphoma elucidates the role of the dog as a model for human disease, *Haematologica*, 2018; epub ahead of print. https://doi.org/10.3324/haematol.2018.207027.

47. Richards KL, Motsinger-Reif AA, Chen HW, et al.: Gene profiling of canine B-cell lymphoma reveals germinal center and postgerminal center subtypes with different survival times, modeling human DLBCL, *Cancer Res* 73:5029–5039, 2013.

48. Dave SS, Wright G, Tan B, et al.: Prediction of survival in follicular lymphoma based on molecular features of tumor-infiltrating immune cells, *N Engl J Med* 351:2159–2169, 2004.

49. Lenz G, Wright G, Dave SS, et al.: Stromal gene signatures in large-B-cell lymphomas, *N Engl J Med* 359:2313–2323, 2008.

50. Rimsza LM, Roberts RA, Miller TP, et al.: Loss of MHC class II gene and protein expression in diffuse large B-cell lymphoma is related to decreased tumor immunosurveillance and poor patient survival regardless of other prognostic factors: a follow-up study from the Leukemia and Lymphoma Molecular Profiling Project, *Blood* 103:4251–4258, 2004.

51. Bumgarner R: Overview of DNA microarrays: types, applications, and their future, *Curr Protoc Mol Biol Chapter* 22, 2013. Unit 22 21.

52. Wang Z, Gerstein M, Snyder M: RNA-Seq: a revolutionary tool for transcriptomics, *Nat Rev Genet* 10:57–63, 2009.

53. Hanahan D, Weinberg RA: Hallmarks of cancer: the next generation, *Cell* 144:646–674, 2011.

54. Zhang MH, Man HT, Zhao XD, et al.: Estrogen receptor-positive breast cancer molecular signatures and therapeutic potentials (Review), *Biomed Rep* 2:41–52, 2014.

55. London CA, AL Hannah, Zadovoskaya R, et al.: Phase I dose-escalating study of SU11654, a small molecule receptor tyrosine kinase inhibitor, in dogs with spontaneous malignancies, *Clin Cancer Res* 9:2755–2768, 2003.

56. Von Hoff DD, Stephenson Jr JJ, Rosen P, et al.: Pilot study using molecular profiling of patients' tumors to find potential targets and select treatments for their refractory cancers, *J Clin Oncol* 28:4877–4883, 2010.

57. Paoloni M, Webb C, Mazcko C, et al.: Prospective molecular profiling of canine cancers provides a clinically relevant comparative model for evaluating personalized medicine (PMed) trials, *PLoS One* 9:e90028, 2014.

9

Biopsy and Sentinel Lymph Node Mapping Principles

NICOLE P. EHRHART

A biopsy refers to a procedure that involves obtaining a tissue specimen for microscopic (i.e., histopathologic) analysis to establish a precise diagnosis. Histopathologic interpretation of tissue removed from a tumor is not foolproof and is highly dependent on the quality of the biopsy sample submitted. Therefore it is important to understand basic principles of biopsy procurement and submission to obtain an accurate diagnosis. If the tissue diagnosis is incorrect, every subsequent step in the treatment of the patient may also be incorrect.

Fine-needle aspiration cytology (FNAC) is a simple and rapid way to obtain information about a tumor and is often the first step in the diagnostic workup. Results of FNAC help guide the diagnostic tests for staging. Studies have shown that FNAC is a reliable and useful method to guide further workup when neoplasia is suspected or to rule out neoplasia.[1,2] Nonetheless, FNAC gives limited information and may be nondiagnostic or equivocal. Inflammation, necrosis, and hemorrhage may result in cytopathologic changes that do not accurately represent the underlying disease process. Histologic confirmation may be necessary for definitive diagnosis of neoplasia.

There are many available techniques for obtaining tissue specimens, ranging from needle-core techniques to complete surgical excision. The choice of technique depends on the anatomic location of the tumor, the overall health of the patient, suspected tumor type, and clinician preference. Biopsy techniques can be grouped under one of two major categories: pretreatment biopsy (e.g., needle-core biopsy, punch biopsy, wedge biopsy, etc.) or excisional biopsy. Pretreatment biopsy is performed to obtain additional information about the tumor before definitive treatment. Posttreatment (i.e., excisional) biopsy refers to the process of obtaining histopathologic information after surgical removal of the tumor. Excisional biopsy is best used to obtain a more complete picture of the disease process (e.g., histologic grade, histologic subtype, degree of invasion into regional vasculature and lymphatics, etc.) and provides an opportunity to evaluate completeness of excision. It is rarely ever the best first step in obtaining a tissue diagnosis. Although excisional biopsy is attractive to many clinicians because it allows for definitive treatment and diagnosis in one step, it is often used inappropriately in the management of a cancer patient, resulting in incomplete surgical margins. Incomplete surgical margins can result in local tumor recurrence and the need for radiation therapy or a wider, more extensive surgery. All of these sequelae compromise the optimum treatment pathway for the patient and will involve more morbidity and expense than a properly performed first excision. The issue to be determined before surgery then is: how aggressive should the surgery to remove the tumor be? It is intuitive that wide, ablative surgery (e.g., body wall resection) would be inappropriate for a simple lipoma. It also follows that marginal excision (shell out) is inappropriate for definitive treatment of an aggressive infiltrative tumor such as a soft tissue sarcoma. Thus thorough knowledge of the tumor type is imperative before attempting surgical excision. The best way to obtain this information is often via biopsy.

Specific indications for pretreatment biopsy are as follows:
1. When FNAC is nondiagnostic or equivocal
2. When the type of recommended treatment (radiation, chemotherapy, surgery) would be altered by knowledge of the tumor type or grade
3. When the extent of recommended treatment (ablative surgery, wide excision, marginal excision) would be altered by knowledge of the tumor type or grade
4. When the tumor is in a difficult area to reconstruct (maxillectomy, locations requiring extensive flaps, head and neck, etc.) and planning is needed to prepare the patient and client appropriately
5. When knowledge of the tumor type or histologic grade would change the willingness of the client to proceed with curative-intent treatment

If any one of the listed criteria is met, a pretreatment biopsy should be pursued.

There are occasions when pretreatment biopsy would be contraindicated. These include cases when the type of treatment or extent of surgery would not be changed by knowing the tumor type (e.g., testicular mass, solitary splenic mass) or when the surgical procedure to obtain the biopsy is as risky as definitive removal (e.g., spinal cord biopsy). In these cases, the patient would best be served by excisional biopsy of the tumor if staging results support this choice.

Biopsy Methods

The more commonly used methods of tissue procurement are needle-core biopsy, punch biopsy, incisional (wedge) biopsy, and excisional biopsy.

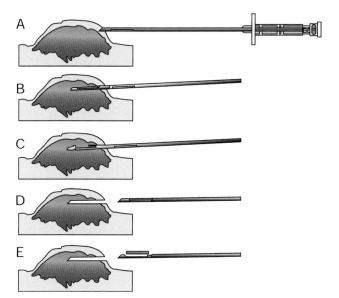

• **Fig. 9.1** Mechanism of action of needle-core biopsy for typical solid tumor. (A) A small stab incision is made with a scalpel blade to allow for insertion of the instrument. With the instrument closed, the needle is advanced into the tumor, taking care to ensure the capsule is penetrated. (B) The outer canula is fixed in place while the inner canula with the specimen notch is advanced into the mass. This allows the tumor tissue to protrude into the specimen notch. (C) The inner canula is held steady while the outer canula is advanced. This traps the tumor specimen in the notch. (D) The instrument is removed. (E) The inner canula is advanced again to allow access to the tissue within the specimen notch.

Needle-Core Biopsy

Needle-core biopsy utilizes various types of needle core instruments (Tru-Cut, etc.) to obtain soft tissue (Fig. 9.1). Most of these needles use spring or pneumatically powered needles, although manually operated devices are still available as well. Specialized core instruments are used for bone biopsies and will be covered in Chapter 25. These instruments are generally 14-gauge in diameter and procure a piece of tissue that is about 1 mm wide and 1.0 to 1.5 cm long. In spite of this small sample size, the structural relationship of the tissue and tumor cells can usually be visualized by the pathologist. Virtually any accessible mass can be sampled by this method. It may be used for externally located lesions or for deeply seated lesions (kidney, liver, prostate, etc.) with image-guidance via closed methods or at the time of open surgery.

The most common use of the needle-core biopsy is for externally palpable masses. Except for highly inflamed and necrotic cancers (especially in the oral cavity), where incisional biopsy is preferred, needle-core biopsies can be done on an outpatient basis with local anesthesia and sedation. The area to be biopsied is clipped and cleaned. The skin or overlying tissue is aseptically prepared as for minor surgery. If the overlying tissue (usually skin and muscle) is intact, it is blocked with local anesthetic in the region that the biopsy needle will penetrate. Tumor tissue itself is very poorly innervated and generally does not require local anesthesia. The mass is then fixed in place with one hand or by an assistant. A small 1- to 2-mm stab incision is made in the overlying skin with a scalpel blade to allow insertion of the biopsy instrument. The stab incision is necessary to prevent dulling of the needle tip and allow better penetration into the underlying tissue. Through the same skin incision, several needle cores are removed from different sites to get a "cross section" of tissue types within the mass.

The stab incision can be sutured with a single interrupted suture. The tissue is gently removed from the instrument with a scalpel blade or hypodermic needle and placed in formalin and/or alternative media (e.g., culture media) or snap frozen as necessary. For smaller-gauge needle-core biopsy instruments, the tissue may be flushed off the needle with saline. Samples may be gently rolled on a glass slide for cytologic preparations before fixation. With experience, the operator can generally tell from the appearance of the core sample whether diagnostic material has been attained. Small, discontinuous segments of tissue and fluid within the trough will only rarely be diagnostic and usually imply the need for incisional biopsy. Soft tissue sarcomas in particular may not yield good tissue cores because of necrosis and fibrous septa that often permeate the mass. Cystic masses are also problematic.

Needle biopsy tracts are probably a minimal risk for local tumor seeding but should be removed en bloc with the tumor at subsequent resection. Therefore it is important to plan where the stab incision and needle biopsy tract should be placed to make subsequent excision simpler. Avoid excessive tunneling through uninvolved tissues by choosing the most direct path from the skin to the tumor to obtain a representative sample.

Many of these needles are "disposable" with plastic casings and therefore cannot be steam sterilized. It is not uncommon, however, for veterinary practices to resterilize these instruments (using ethylene oxide or hydrogen peroxide gas) and use them repeatedly until they become dull.

Needle-core biopsy instruments are inexpensive, easy to use, and needle-core biopsy procedures can be performed as outpatient procedures. They are generally more accurate than cytology but likely have lower accuracy than incisional or excisional biopsies, especially when a tumor is heterogeneous, inflamed, cystic, or contains a large amount of necrosis. It is important to understand that for a 5-cm diameter mass, one needle-core biopsy sample represents less than 1% of the tumor tissue. The smaller the biopsy specimen, the less representative it may be for the entire tumor.

Needle-core biopsy can be performed with the aid of image-guidance. Utilization of image-guidance for needle-core biopsy is very helpful for obtaining tissue from deeply seated lesions. Ultrasound-, fluoroscopic-, and computed tomographic-assistance may be used to obtain samples from tumors located in areas where percutaneous biopsy would be risky or unlikely to yield a representative sample. In situations in which the lesion is located within a body cavity, the risk of tumor seeding from uncontrolled hemorrhage or fluid leakage as a result of image-guided biopsy must be taken into account before deciding if image-guided needle-core biopsy techniques will hold an advantage over more direct access in a given patient.

Punch Biopsy

Punch biopsy tools were originally designed for biopsy of the skin (Fig. 9.2). They deliver a shorter and wider (2–8 mm) biopsy than does a needle core. They can be used on any external tumor (skin, oral, perianal) or tumors where there is direct access (e.g., liver biopsy during laparotomy). They do not work as well for tumors located under intact skin unless the skin is incised first. Preparation of the site is the same as for needle-core biopsy. If the lesion is cutaneous, the punch biopsy instrument is placed on the surface of the area of interest and rotated back and forth using pressure to penetrate the involved tissue. If the skin is intact over the tumor, the skin is first incised using a scalpel. The punch is then introduced through the skin incision to the surface of the tumor. Once

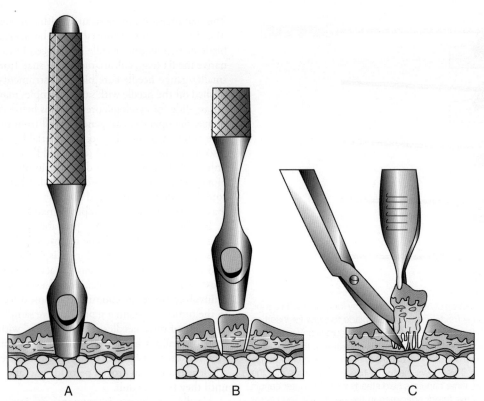

• **Fig. 9.2** Mechanism of action of punch biopsy. (A) The instrument is applied with pressure and back and forth rotation to allow the instrument to penetrate the mass. (B) The punch is removed or angled across the base to sever the deep attachment. (C) If needed, the specimen can be gently grasped with forceps and cut at the base with metzenbaum scissors.

the punch has cut into the tumor, the core is gently lifted, and the base of the core is cut off with scissors. One or two sutures may be placed to close the incision and tamponade bleeding.

Incisional Biopsy

Incisional biopsy is utilized when neither cytology nor needle-core biopsy has yielded diagnostic material (Fig. 9.3). Incisional biopsy is also preferred for ulcerated and necrotic lesions because larger samples can be obtained, making it more likely for the surgeon to sample representative areas. Most tumors are very poorly innervated and may be biopsied without the need for local anesthesia or sedation as long as the overlying normal skin and tissue has been anesthetized. Preparation involves clipping the hair over the incision site. After an aseptic preparation is made, surgical drapes are used to protect the field from the surrounding environment. Under aseptic conditions, the skin, if intact over the tumor, is incised and a wedge of tumor tissue is removed from the mass. It is not necessary to remove a wedge of intact skin overlying the tumor if it appears to be normal and not fixed to the underlying tumor. It is important for the surgeon to confirm at the time of the biopsy that he or she has not simply removed a small section of the reactive tissue surrounding the tumor. This can be difficult in some cases; however, most tumors have coloration and texture that is distinct from that of the surrounding normal and reactive tissue. If needed, cytologic assessment of touch impressions can be made using the resected tissue to confirm that neoplastic cells are present in the removed tissue.

Many authors have recommended that the surgeon acquire a composite biopsy of normal and abnormal tissue to assure accuracy in diagnosis on histopathologic examination. Although this may be helpful to the pathologist in benign skin disease and subtle lesions, it is not recommended in cases in which neoplasia is suspected, as this may result in extending the biopsy incision into previously uninvolved tissues. This can compromise the surgical margins needed to remove the mass entirely at the time of definitive surgery and exposes previously uninvolved tissues to freshly incised tumor. Instead, a representative sample of the tumor itself should be submitted. This may require obtaining multiple samples via the same incision to ensure that a representative sample has been achieved. Care must be taken to ensure that any biopsy tract (incisional or other) will not compromise subsequent curative-intent resection, contaminate uninvolved tissue needed for reconstruction, or compromise subsequent radiation therapy. The surgeon should avoid widely opening uninvolved tissue planes that could become contaminated with released tumor cells. Small incisions, even through expendable muscle bellies, are preferred to contaminating an entire intramuscular compartment. The incisional biopsy tract is always removed in continuity with the tumor at the time of curative-intent resection.

Specialized Biopsy Techniques

Specialized biopsy techniques will generally be covered under specific individual tumors. However, some general comments follow.

Endoscopic Biopsies

These techniques use flexible or occasionally rigid scopes that allow visualized or blind biopsy of hollow lumens, especially gastrointestinal, respiratory, and urogenital systems. Although these

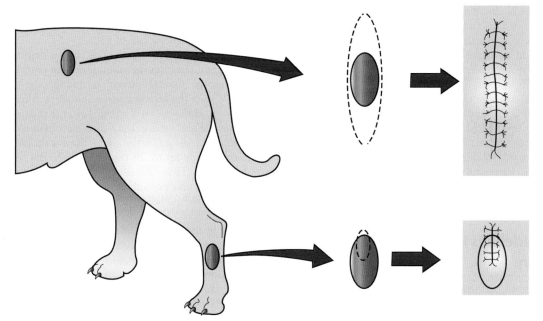

• **Fig. 9.3** Excisional *(top)* contrasted with incisional *(bottom)* biopsy. The top tumor should be small enough that excisional biopsy will not negatively influence other possible treatments. The bottom tumor, however, requires knowledge of the tumor type before excision to ensure appropriate surgical "dose" is used at the time of definitive removal. Note that the biopsy incision is oriented in such a way to make it easiest to include during wide excision and minimize difficulty with closure.

techniques are convenient, cost effective, and generally safe, they may suffer from inadequate visualization and limited biopsy sample size compared with other techniques. For example, an endoscopic biopsy result of ulcerative gastritis in a dog with a firm, infiltrative mass of the lesser curvature of the stomach does not rule out gastric adenocarcinoma.

Laparoscopy and Thoracoscopy

Evaluation of the abdomen and thorax via minimally invasive techniques, when performed by an experienced operator, can yield important information regarding stage of disease and can procure tissue for biopsy. In addition, laparoscopic- and thoracoscopic-assisted removal results in smaller incisions and more rapid recovery times compared with open procedures. The option to convert to an open procedure should be available if problems are encountered that cannot be adequately addressed using minimally invasive methods. As specialists become more proficient at these techniques, more and more options are becoming available for tumor removal.

Image-Guided Biopsy

Diagnostic imaging has greatly expanded the ability to stage various neoplasias. The use of positron emission tomography–computed tomography (PET–CT) in veterinary medicine has also led to significant advances in sentinel node mapping, novel staging methods, and the ability to assess response to treatment. In addition, the use of radiographic-, fluoroscopic-, ultrasonographic-, CT-, and magnetic resonance imaging (MRI)-guided needle aspirates or core biopsies can prevent the need for more invasive diagnostic procedures. Commonly biopsied tissue includes lung, kidney, liver, spleen, prostate, and, more recently, brain.

Excisional Biopsy

This method is utilized when the treatment would not be altered by knowledge of tumor type (e.g., "benign" skin tumors, solitary splenic mass, testicular tumor, etc.). It is more frequently performed than indicated but when used on properly selected cases, it can be both diagnostic and therapeutic as well as cost effective.

Sentinel Lymph Node Mapping and Biopsy

In veterinary medicine, assessment of nodal metastasis has been largely predicated on palpation or imaging of nodal size and architecture with cytologic sampling when abnormal. Sentinel lymph node (SLN) mapping and subsequent biopsy are performed to identify the first lymph node (LN) to which a cancer is likely to spread from a primary tumor and to sample that LN for evidence of metastasis. If the SLN is free of metastasis, subsequent LNs in the drainage pattern are also likely to be negative. This method was initially studied in human cutaneous melanoma to detect lymphatic drainage patterns before surgery. It is now a widely utilized staging procedure in many human cancers, but the evidence for its usefulness in staging has been primarily from the application of this technique in human breast cancer patients. The SLN has been classically defined as the first node detectable after peritumoral injection of a radioactive marker and subsequent scintigraphy. Visual identification in surgery is typically aided by the use of vital dye injection (e.g., methylene blue) in conjunction with use of a portable gamma probe in the operating room to detect the LN with the greatest radioactivity. In one study of 19 dogs with cutaneous mast cell tumors,[3] the SLN was different from the regional anatomic LN in eight (42%) of these dogs. SLN mapping and biopsy identified LN metastasis in these eight dogs and clients were offered adjunctive therapy that otherwise would not have been considered.[3]

Indirect lymphography is an alternative to scintigraphic SLN mapping. This procedure involves injection of a contrast agent in the periphery of the tumor and serial or real-time imaging to follow contrast uptake in the draining lymphatic basin. This method uses contrast enhancement of nearby LNs and lymphatic channels to identify the SLN. In this technique, the contrast medium is injected in four quadrants around or within the tumor. The first contrasting node(s) is identified via imaging providing a surgical target (as opposed to extensive dissection within the lymphatic basin to find a lymph node with vital dye). A vital dye, such as methylene blue, is injected intraoperatively in the same locations as the contrast agent. The use of the vital dye provides the surgeon with visual confirmation of the SLN. Some authors have advocated using lipid-based contrast medium because it slows clearance and therefore may permit imaging for longer periods compared with water-soluble contrast agents. In a recent study, this method was successful at identifying the sentinel lymph node in 96.6% of veterinary patients with solid tumors of various histologies.[4]

General Guidelines for Tissue Procurement and Fixation

1. When properly performed, a pretreatment biopsy will *not* negatively influence survival. The metastatic cascade involves a series of complex events that are not dependent on the number of neoplastic cells in circulation (see Chapter 2). On the other hand, neoplastic cells contaminate the *local* tissues surrounding the mass and, in some cases, successfully attach and grow within these normal tissues. Careful hemostasis, obliteration of dead space, and avoidance of seromas or hematomas will minimize local contamination of the incisional biopsy site. Definitive surgery to remove the tumor along with the associated biopsy tract should take place as soon as possible after the biopsy procedure. Surgical drains should not be placed in biopsy sites, if possible, because the drain tract can become contaminated with tumor cells and seed tumor cells through uninvolved tissue planes. In particular, care should be taken during biopsy not to "spill" cancer cells within the thoracic or abdominal cavities, where they may seed pleural or peritoneal surfaces.

2. When biopsies are performed on the limbs or the tail, the incision should be made along the long axis of the limb or tail rather than transversely. Transverse incisions are much more difficult to resect completely. If a biopsy is near the midline, the incision should be oriented parallel to the midline.

3. Avoid taking the junction of normal and abnormal tissue for pretreatment biopsy. Care should be taken not to incise normal tissue that cannot be resected or would be used in reconstructing the surgical defect. Avoid biopsies that contain only ulcerated or inflamed tissues.

4. The larger the sample, the more likely it is to be diagnostic. Tumors are not homogeneous and usually contain areas of necrosis, inflammation, and reactive tissue. Several samples from one mass are more likely to yield an accurate diagnosis than a single sample.

5. Biopsies should not be obtained with electrocautery or laser, as it can deform (autolysis or polarization) the cellular architecture of the tissue sample. Electrocautery is better utilized for hemostasis after blade removal of a diagnostic specimen.

6. Care should be taken not to unduly deform the specimen with forceps, suction, or other handling methods before fixation.

7. Intraoperative diagnosis of disease by frozen sections, although not routinely available in veterinary medicine, is used widely in human hospitals. Special equipment and training are required for this technique to be fully utilized. One study in veterinary medicine revealed an accurate and specific diagnosis rate of 83%.[5]

8. If evaluation of margins of excision is desired, it is best if the surgeon indicates the surgical margin on the specimen using tissue ink. Several commercial inking systems are available for this use. The resected tissue should be blotted with a paper towel, as the dyes will adhere better to the tissue when the tissue is slightly tacky. The tissue ink is "painted" on the surgical margins using a cotton swab. The dye should then be allowed to dry for up to 20 minutes before the tissue is placed in formalin. Tissue already fixed in formalin can be marked, but the dyes may not adhere as well and drying time is extended. When the pathologist reads the slides and sees tumor cells at the inked edge, you can be certain tumor cells have been left in the patient. Different colored ink can also be used to denote different sites on the tumor, such as proximal margin or deep margin. Even with inking, proper fixation, and processing, the clinician must realize the entire margin will not be examined by the pathologist. Rather, representative sections will be obtained from the inked margin. Therefore any guidance that the clinician can give to the pathologist as to the most important sections to assess for tumor cells will help the pathologist pay particular attention to such areas. It is essential that both the pathologist and the clinician communicate if the pathology report is confusing or does not match the clinical picture. Of course, margin evaluation is necessary only for excisional biopsy or after curative-intent surgery and does not apply to needle-core or incisional biopsies, which by definition will have inadequate margins.

9. Stainless steel vascular clips or staples in the resected specimen will damage the microtomes used by the pathology laboratory. Remove them before the tissue is submitted.

10. Proper fixation is essential. Tissue is generally fixed in 10% buffered neutral formalin with 1 part tissue to 10 parts fixative. If more than one lesion has been biopsied, they should each be placed in a separate well identified container. Certain tissues such as eye, nerve, and muscle may require special fixation techniques. The clinician may want to call and consult with the pathologist on how to submit tissue for special circumstances.

11. Tissue should not be thicker than 1 cm or it will not fix properly. Masses greater than 1 cm in diameter can be sliced like a loaf of bread, leaving the deep inked margin intact, to allow fixation. Extremely large masses can be incompletely sliced as described earlier, fixed in a large bucket of formalin for 2 to 3 days, and then shipped in a container with 1 part tissue to 1 part formalin. A less ideal but alternative approach is to have the surgeon take representative smaller samples from the mass (e.g., soft and hard pieces, red and pale pieces, deep and superficial pieces, etc.) and the lateral and deep margins in the hope that they are representative. The rest of the mass can be saved in the clinic in formalin in case more tissue needs to be evaluated. This extra tissue should never be frozen. Freezing causes severe artifact in the tissue.

12. A *detailed* history should accompany all biopsy requests. Interpretation of surgical biopsies is a combination of art and science. Without all of the essential diagnostic information (e.g., signalment, history of recurrences, invasion into bone, rate of growth, etc.), the pathologist will be significantly compromised in his or her ability to deliver accurate and clinically useful information.

13. A veterinary-trained pathologist is preferred over a pathologist trained in human diseases. Although many cancers are histologically similar across species lines, enough differences exist to result in interpretive errors.

In 2011 the American College of Veterinary Pathologists, along with several medical and surgical oncologists, published a comprehensive set of recommendations and guidelines for submission, trimming, margin evaluation, and reporting of tumor biopsy specimens.[6] This landmark paper was the first collaborative attempt to standardize pathology reporting in veterinary oncology and has been endorsed by a large international group of veterinary pathologists and oncology specialists. It is recommended that clinicians utilize diagnostic laboratories that adhere to these guidelines so that results are standardized and easier to interpret.

Interpretation of Results

The job of the pathologist is to determine (1) tumor versus no tumor, (2) benign versus malignant, (3) histologic type, (4) histologic grade (if available clinically), and to (5) assess surgical margins (if excisional biopsy). Making an accurate diagnosis is not as simple as putting a piece of tissue in formalin and waiting for results. Many pitfalls can occur to render the end result inaccurate. Potential errors can take place at any level of diagnosis and it is up to the clinician in charge of the case to interpret the full meaning of the biopsy result. In cases in which the biopsy result does not correlate with the clinical behavior of the tumor, a second opinion should be requested. A study published in 2009 reviewed first- and second-opinion histopathology reports.[7] There was diagnostic agreement between first and second opinions in 70% of cases. In 20% of cases, there was partial agreement, where the diagnosis did not change but information such as grade or presence of lymphatic or vascular invasion was disparate. In 10% of cases, there was complete diagnostic disagreement. Of these, 7% were a disagreement between malignant versus nonmalignant disease and 3% were disagreements about the cell of origin of the tumor. If the biopsy result does not correlate with the biologic behavior of the tumor, several options are possible:

1. Call the pathologist and express your concern over the biopsy result. This exchange of information should be helpful for both parties and not looked upon as an affront to the pathologist's authority or expertise. It may lead to
   a. Resectioning of available tissue or paraffin blocks
   b. Special stains for certain possible tumor types (e.g., toluidine blue for mast cells)
   c. A second opinion by another pathologist

2. If the tumor is still present in the patient, and particularly if widely varied options exist for therapy, a second (or third) biopsy should be performed.

A carefully performed, submitted, and interpreted biopsy is the most important step in management and subsequent prognosis of the patient with cancer. The biopsy report is key in decision making regarding therapeutic options, prognosis, and overall case management. All too often tumors are not submitted for histologic evaluation after removal because "the owner didn't want to pay for it." Histopathology interpretation should not be an elective decision. Instead, it should be as automatic as closing the skin after surgery. The charge for submission and interpretation of the biopsy should be included in the surgery fee, but histopathology interpretation is not optional. Because of increasing medicolegal concerns, it is not medical curiosity alone that mandates knowledge of tumor type. Understanding how and when to perform a biopsy, how to submit a biopsy specimen for histopathologic interpretation, and how to interpret the report are of paramount importance in the treatment of veterinary cancer patients.

References

1. Ghisleni G, Roccabianca P, Ceruti R, et al.: Correlation between fine-needle aspiration cytology and histopathology in the evaluation of cutaneous and subcutaneous masses from dogs and cats, *Vet Clin Pathol* 35:24–30, 2006.
2. Sharkey LC, Wellman ML: Diagnostic cytology in veterinary medicine: a comparative and evidence-based approach, *Clinics Lab Med* 31:1–19, 2011.
3. Worley DR: Incorporation of sentinel lymph node mapping in dogs with mast cell tumours: 20 consecutive procedures, *Vet Comp Oncol* 12:215–226, 2014.
4. Brissot HN, Edery EG: Use of indirect lymphography to identify sentinel lymph node in dogs: a pilot study in 30 tumours, *Vet Comp Oncol* 15:740–753, 2017.
5. Whitehair JG, Griffey SM, Olander HJ, et al.: The accuracy of intraoperative diagnoses based on examination of frozen sections. A prospective comparison with paraffin-embedded sections, *Vet Surg* 22:255–259, 1993.
6. Kamstock DA, Ehrhart EJ, Getzy DM, et al.: Recommended guidelines for submission, trimming, margin evaluation, and reporting of tumor biopsy specimens in veterinary surgical pathology, *Vet Pathol* 48:19–31, 2011.
7. Regan RC, Rassnick KM, Balkman CE, Bailey DB, McDonough SP: Comparison of first-opinion and second-opinion histopathology from dogs and cats with cancer: 430 cases (2001-2008), *Vet Comp Oncol* 8:1–10, 2010.

10

Surgical Oncology

JAMES P. FARESE, JULIUS M. LIPTAK, AND STEPHEN J. WITHROW

Complete surgical removal of localized cancer cures more cancer patients than any other form of treatment,[1] in part because this modality is generally applied as the sole treatment for local disease, early stage disease, and tumors with limited potential to metastasize. In humans, 60% of patients who are cured of cancer are cured by surgery alone.[2] Before this hope for cure can be realized in veterinary medicine, surgeons must have a thorough understanding of anatomy, physiology, resection, and reconstruction options for all organs; expected tumor behavior; and the various alternatives or adjuvants to surgery. Surgical oncologists should not only be good technical surgeons, but also dedicated tumor biologists. Surgery will likely play a role at one point or another in the management of most cancer patients.

Surgical procedures may include any of the following: diagnosis (biopsy), resection for cure, resection for palliation of symptoms, and a wide variety of ancillary procedures to enhance and complement other forms of treatment.

Surgical resection of cancer was introduced in the 16th century BC and remained relatively underutilized until the development of general anesthesia (1840s), antisepsis (1860s), and effective analgesia, which made aggressive resection safer and more tolerable for the patient. Dr. William Halstead developed the basic principles of surgical oncology in the 1890s. In the 21st century, radical resection has increasingly been customized to meet the needs of the patient. Further refinements in surgery have been made possible with newer equipment, advanced imaging, modifications in analgesic drugs and techniques, use of blood products, and advancements in critical care medicine.

Most dogs and cats with cancerous conditions are geriatric; however, with normal major organ function, dogs and cats at an advanced age can still be good candidates for surgery, and age has not been shown to affect the tumor-related prognosis for tumor types. In fact, dogs with osteosarcoma that are younger than 2 years of age have a worse prognosis than dogs that are older than 2 years of age after amputation alone.[3] In most instances older animals will tolerate aggressive surgical intervention as well as younger patients do. Screening for comorbidities (e.g., thoracic radiographs and abdominal ultrasound) is recommended before major surgical procedures, especially in older dogs and cats.

Surgery for Diagnosis

Although biopsy principles are covered in Chapter 9, it is worth emphasizing that properly timed, performed, and interpreted biopsies are one of the most crucial steps in the management of the cancer patient. Not only does the surgeon need to procure adequate and representative tissue to establish a diagnosis, but also the biopsy must not compromise subsequent curative surgical resection or radiation field planning.

Levels of Tumor Excision

The aggressiveness of surgical resection, or surgical dose, is categorized as intralesional (or debulking), marginal, wide, and radical (Fig. 10.1). These categories were first proposed for musculoskeletal tumors by Dr. William Enneking, but they have since gained wide acceptance for all solid tumors.[4] The most common mistake in surgical oncology is to use too low a surgical dose, particularly because of the fear of being unable to close the resultant defect. In human medicine, two surgical teams are sometimes involved in the excision of tumors, one team for surgical resection and another team for subsequent reconstruction, to avoid this situation. Because this is unrealistic in veterinary medicine, the use of sterile surgical markers to delineate margins before incision assists in orientating the surgeon and overcoming the subconscious concerns of wound closure.

Surgery for Cure

Before a surgeon can provide the optimal operation for the patient with cancer, the following questions need to be considered:
1. What is the histologic type, histologic grade, and clinical stage of the cancer to be treated?
2. What are the expected local and systemic effects of this tumor?
3. Is a cure possible and at what price in terms of function and cosmetics?
4. Is an operation indicated at all?
5. Are there alternative options to surgery, or does surgery need to be combined with other modalities?

A recurring theme in surgical management of cancer is that the first surgery has the best chance of cure. Several reasons for this improvement in survival have been proposed. Untreated tumors often have had less chronologic time to metastasize and acquire more biologically aggressive phenotypes than recurrent cancers. Untreated tumors and adjacent normal tissues have near normal anatomy, which facilitates surgical dissection and resection. Recurrent tumors may contaminate previously uninvolved tissue planes, thereby requiring wider resection than otherwise would have been needed on the initial tumor excision.

If one thinks about a given cancer as resembling a crab, incomplete surgery removes the body of the crab but leaves the legs behind. The "body" of most tumors is often quiescent and hypoxic, whereas the leading edge of the tumor (legs) is the most invasive and well vascularized. Thus subtotal removal may selectively leave behind the most aggressive components of the tumor.

Patients with recurrent cancer often have less normal tissue for closure. Furthermore, changes in vascularity and local immune responses may accompany local tumor recurrence.

Curative-intent surgery is best performed at the first surgery, and the surgeon should have all the necessary diagnostic information to develop an appropriate treatment plan. Radiographs and

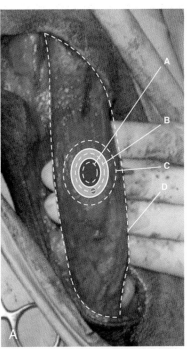

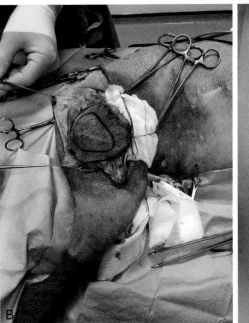

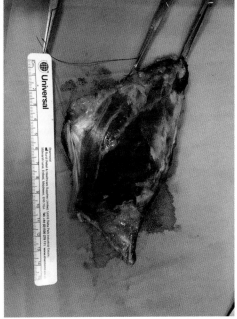

• **Fig. 10.1** (A) The four levels of tumor excision proposed by Dr. William Enneking for resection of human musculoskeletal tumors. A tumor is seen within the semitendinosus muscle belly *(blue)*, and the tumor pseudocapsule is surrounded by a reactive zone *(yellow)*. Note the satellite tumor in the reactive zone *(green)*, and the levels of surgical excision: intracapsular *(A)*, marginal *(B)*, wide *(C)*, and radical *(D) (dotted lines)*. (B) *1*, Intraoperative image of a radical excision of a biceps muscle sarcoma completely contained within the muscle fascia. The biopsy tract is excised en bloc with the tumor. With this plan the entire tissue compartment (i.e., the entire biceps femoris muscle belly) is removed to ensure complete removal. *2*, The excised specimen as seen from the medial aspect.

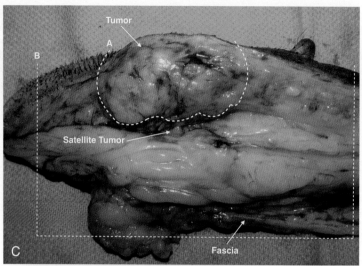

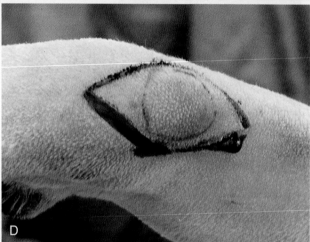

• **Fig. 10.1, cont'd** (C) Wide resection of tumor involves adequate lateral and deep margins. The width of lateral margins is determined by the tumor type and ranges from 1 cm for benign tumors and carcinomas to 3 cm for soft tissue sarcomas and up to 5 cm for vaccine-associated sarcomas. Malignant tumors may have satellite tumor cells outside the tumor pseudocapsule *(arrow)*. Deep margins are not determined by depth but, rather, by tumor-resistant fascial layers. A minimum of one fascial layer should be included in the resection. The deep margin is the most common site of failure. Dotted lines show the dissection planes for marginal *(A)* and wide *(B)* excisions. Note how a marginal dissection in this example leads to residual tumor cells in the surgical field. (D) Planned marginal resection of a soft tissue sarcoma on the distal limb of a dog. Marginal resection results in removal of the measurable tumor burden, but microscopic tumor cells may remain in the surgical wound. (**A** Photo courtesy of Dr. Paolo Buracco, University of Torino. **D** from Johnston SA, Tobias KM: *Veterinary surgery: small animal,* ed 2, St Louis, 2018, Elsevier.)

ultrasonography have been used routinely for many years, and the increased availability of computed tomography (CT) and magnetic resonance imaging (MRI) has added greatly to our ability to determine the extent of a solid tumor and optimize the surgical approach. CT is now readily available at most specialty hospitals and allows good visualization of neoplastic tissue (particularly when it enhances well with an intravenously administered contrast agent), adjacent muscle bellies and fascial planes, intraabdominal and intrathoracic organs, regional lymph nodes (LNs), and bone (Fig. 10.2). CT is commonly used for imaging thoracic wall tumors to determine which ribs need to be resected, oral tumors to assess the degree of bone involvement, adrenal tumors to assess caudal vena caval or renal involvement, and cutaneous or subcutaneous masses to better assess local tumor invasion and extent of disease. Reconstructed CT images allow the surgeon to choose the orientation in which to visualize a mass in relation to

adjacent tissues, and multiplanar views and three-dimensional (3D) reconstructions can be manipulated at a computer workstation to help the surgeon envision a surgical plan before the time of surgery with complicated cases (e.g., large skull tumors). Furthermore, for more complex surgeries, CT images can be used to print 3D models to further assist the surgeon in preoperative planning and intraoperative decision making.[5] MRI is preferred for tumors of the central and peripheral nervous system and perhaps tumors of the intraabdominal organs and cutaneous and subcutaneous tissues. MRI is useful for determining the proximity of tumors to important neurovascular structures and for assessing soft tissue components and intramedullary involvement of canine osteosarcoma before limb-sparing surgery is performed.

Advanced imaging has greatly enhanced the surgeon's ability to assess the anatomic location and extent of various cancers; however, imaging needs to be interpreted in conjunction with

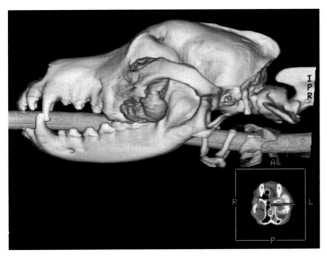

• **Fig. 10.2** Computed tomography of a dog with suspected multilobular osteochondrosarcoma of the inferior orbit is used to provide three-dimensional reconstructed images. This enables the surgeon to determine the size and extent of the tumor and to plan the surgical margins and approach accurately. Computed tomography is preferred for imaging of bone and intrathoracic masses. (From Johnston SA, Tobias KM: *Veterinary surgery: small animal,* ed 2, St Louis, 2018, Elsevier.)

TABLE 10.1	Classification and Resection of Wound Margins	
Type	**Plane of Dissection**	**Result**
Intracapsular	Tumor removed piecemeal or curetted, "debulking"	Residual macroscopic disease
Marginal	Tumor removed on or adjacent to the tumor pseudocapsule, "shelled out"	Usually leaves microscopic disease
Wide	Tumor removed with margins of normal tissue lateral and deep to the tumor; tumor capsule is not compromised	Possible skip lesions
Radical	Tumor removed with an entire compartment or structure (e.g., amputation)	No local residual cancer

clinical palpation, assessment of mobility, and expected biologic behavior. Some cancers deemed inoperable by imaging are in fact mobile and operable. Leading edges of some cancers are compressed against adjacent tissue and can appear more invasive. Before declaring a mass inoperable, surgeons should always take the opportunity to palpate the local tumor with the patient under heavy sedation or anesthesia before or after imaging, explore the history of the tumor's growth pattern and, in many cases, obtain a tissue sample. Positive prognostic factors typically include a slow growth rate, mobility within adjacent tissues, no previous surgery, discrete tumor borders, small tumor size, and a low-grade nature. Conversely, surgery may be less effective for the same tumor type and grade if the mass is ill defined, recurrent, or has a recent history of rapid growth.

The surgical oncologist must be able to assimilate all of the information and make an informed decision. We must also remind ourselves and our clients that there is much we do not know (e.g., incomplete margins do not necessarily ensure local tumor recurrence[6]) and that surgical judgment regarding expected local behavior and likely resection is often qualitative and is an imperfect "science."

The actual surgical technique will vary with the site, size, and stage of the tumor, in addition to the skill and experience of the surgeon. The same tumor type in dogs and cats may vary with regard to the required surgical approach and technique and the prognosis. The following are some general statements that need to be emphasized with surgical oncology.

1. All incisional biopsy tracts should be excised en bloc with the primary tumor because tumor cells are capable of growth within the biopsy incisions. Fine-needle aspiration (FNA) cytology tracts are of minor, but not zero, concern, whereas punch biopsy tracts are of intermediate concern.[7] With this in mind, the surgeon should keep all biopsy incisions to a minimal length and should position and orient them such that they can be easily removed with the definitive resection.

2. Early vascular ligation (especially venous) should be attempted to diminish release of large tumor emboli into the systemic circulation. This is probably only clinically meaningful for tumors with a well-defined venous supply, such as splenic and lung tumors. Small numbers of cancer cells are constantly being released into the venous (and lymphatic) circulation by most tumors. Larger, macroscopic cell aggregates may be a greater concern, however, and these may be prevented from vascular escape with early venous ligation.

3. Local control of malignant cancer requires that a margin of normal tissue be removed around the tumor. Resection of the "bad from the good" can and should be classified in more detail than radical versus conservative (Table 10.1; also, see Fig. 10.1).[8] Tumors with a high probability of local recurrence (e.g., high-grade soft tissue sarcoma, high-grade mast cell tumors, feline injection-site sarcomas, feline mammary carcinoma) should have 2 to 3 cm margins laterally and at least one uninvolved fascial layer for deep margins. Tumors are not flat, and wide removal in one plane does not ensure complete excision. Fixation of cancer to adjacent structures mandates removal of the adherent area en bloc with the tumor. Invasive cancer should not be "shelled out" if a cure is expected. Many cancers are surrounded by a pseudocapsule. This pseudocapsule is almost invariably composed of compressed and viable tumor cells, not healthy, reactive host cells. If a malignant tumor is entered at the time of resection or if the margins are incomplete, that procedure is often no better therapeutically than a large incisional biopsy. When possible, resection of the previous scar and the entire wound bed with "new" margins (never entering the previous surgical field) is indicated, including a minimum of one tissue plane away from or deep to the mass. For example, invasion of cancer into the medullary cavity of a bone requires subtotal or total bone resection, not curettage. The width of surgical margins necessary for complete excision of a given tumor type is an ongoing debate, and our current practices are based on minimal objective data. As a community we have answered most of the questions about how much tissue we can safely remove, but it will serve our patients well to determine how little extra tissue is necessary to excise and consistently achieve the same success. We must challenge recommendations that are reported in the literature if they are based solely on a surgeon's personal experience or opinion, in the absence of objective findings.

4. Tumors should be handled gently to avoid the risk of seeding tumor cells into the surgical wound.[9] Copious lavage of all cancer wound beds helps mechanically remove small numbers of exfoliated tumor cells; however, it should not replace gentle tissue handling and the careful technique required to avoid entering the tumor bed.

5. If more than one malignant mass is being removed, separate surgical packs should be used for each site to avoid iatrogenic tumor cell implantation from one site to a second site. In addition, gloves and instruments should be changed before closure to minimize the possibility of seeding of tumor cells in the incision.

The aggressiveness of resection should be tempered only rarely by fears of wound closure. It is better to leave a wound partially or even in some cases completely open with no cancer cells than to close it and have residual cancer. Numerous innovative reconstructive techniques are available for closure of cancer wounds, and the surgeon is limited only by his or her ingenuity and willingness to try new reconstructive techniques.[10] Practice on a cadaveric specimen is recommended before unfamiliar reconstructive surgical techniques are performed. Reliable microvascular-free composite transfers of muscle and skin are hampered because of the unique canine skin and muscle anatomy, but they are being developed.[11]

Marginal Excision

Aggressive surgical excision may not be recommended in some cases because of the tumor's type, size, and location; the patient's age (i.e., recurrence with a less aggressive surgery may not be expected to occur within the expected life span of the patient); and other factors. In such cases marginal excision may be performed (see Fig. 10.1D). The surgeon should tailor the level of excision to the needs of the patient and client, and the expectations and goals of the procedure must be clearly established and explained to the client before surgery.

Lymph Node Removal

Controversy surrounds the surgical management of regional LNs draining the primary tumor site.[12,13] As a general rule, epithelial cancers are more likely to metastasize to LNs than are mesenchymal cancers. However, any enlarged LN requires investigation for complete staging. Lymphadenomegaly may develop secondary to metastasis (firm, irregular, and sometimes fixed to surrounding tissue) or hyperplasia, or to reactivity to various tumor factors, infection, or inflammation. Metastasis is often a poor prognostic sign, and a reactive LN may represent a beneficial host response. Enlarged LNs as a result of cancer metastasis and invasion are generally effaced by tumor cells; although these can often be diagnosed with FNA cytology, histopathology is superior to cytology for the diagnosis of LN metastasis.[14] LN extirpation should be considered under a number of circumstances:

1. If the LN is positive for cancer and not fixed to surrounding normal tissues, it may be possible to remove it with some therapeutic intent. Frequently, however, multiple LNs drain a primary tumor site (e.g., mandibular, medial retropharyngeal, and parotid LNs for oral tumors), and lymphadenectomy is incomplete. LN metastasis at the time of initial diagnosis is often a poor prognostic sign; however, patients that develop metastasis after local tumor control may benefit from lymphadenectomy. Although it usually is not practical, removal of the primary tumor, intervening lymphatic ducts, and draining LN has been

recommended (en bloc resection). Limb amputation for excision of a malignant digit tumor with metastasis to the popliteal LN and mastectomy procedures that include the regional LN are examples of en bloc resections. Few other anatomic sites are amenable to this approach. Lymphadenectomy can have a beneficial effect on survival with specific tumor types, such as dogs with apocrine gland anal sac adenocarcinomas (AGASACs) metastatic to the sacral or sublumbar LNs,[15] dogs with cutaneous mast cell tumors and LN metastasis,[16] and cats with mammary carcinoma and LN metastasis.[17] Lymphadenectomy may also provide a palliative benefit for dogs with metastatic AGASAC LNs causing tenesmus.

2. Normal-sized LNs can be metastatic.[18] Normal-sized LNs that are known to drain a primary tumor site may be randomly sampled (biopsy or cytology) to gain further staging information. This is particularly important if adjuvant therapy decisions (radiation therapy [RT] or chemotherapy) would be predicated on confirmation of residual or metastatic cancer. Intrathoracic or intraabdominal LNs are perhaps most crucial because they are not readily or safely accessible for histologic or cytologic examination (e.g., sublumbar LNs at the aortic trifurcation), even under ultrasound guidance. In such cases the surgeon must educate the owner about the situation and either remove the primary tumor without further knowledge of LN involvement or recommend removal of the normal-sized LNs concurrently, for staging and possibly therapeutic purposes.

3. LNs identified as sentinel LNs using various mapping procedures (see Chapter 9 for more details).

LN removal is generally *not* performed under the following circumstances:

1. LNs in critical areas (e.g., some mesenteric LNs) or in cases in which the tumor cells have eroded through the capsule and become adherent (fixed) to surrounding tissues. In this scenario, LNs may not be resectable without leaving residual disease in the wound bed (necessitating adjuvant therapy to achieve local tumor control), or an attempt at removal may cause serious harm to the patient by injuring important adjacent structures. In such instances the prudent course usually is to aspirate or biopsy the LN for diagnostic purposes and leave it in situ, or to treat the LN with other modalities, such as RT.

2. Prophylactic removal of normal LNs or chains of LNs is not beneficial and may be harmful.[12] Regional LNs may in fact be the initiator of favorable local and systemic immune responses, and elective removal has been associated with poor survival in certain human cancers.[12,19,20]

Surgery for Distant Disease

Metastasectomy for pulmonary metastasis has been described in dogs.[21] Resection of liver metastasis for carcinomas (especially gastrointestinal cancers) increasingly is being performed in human oncology. As more effective adjuvant therapies evolve and minimally invasive techniques are further developed, the need for cytoreductive metastasectomy will likely increase.

Palliative Surgery

Palliative surgery is an attempt to improve the quality of the patient's life (pain relief or improved function), but not necessarily survival time.[22] This type of surgery requires careful consideration of the expected morbidity of the procedure versus the expected gain for the patient and owner. In essence it comes down to a decision of when to discontinue therapy. One of the most difficult decisions in surgical oncology is the decision not to operate. Treatment of any kind should never be worse than no treatment.

However, in many situations palliative surgery may be beneficial. Examples include mastectomy for infected, metastatic mammary tumors; anal sacculectomy for dogs with a large local AGASAC causing tenesmus and distant metastasis; and splenectomy for a dog with a ruptured splenic tumor.

Cytoreductive Surgery

Incomplete removal of a tumor (planned or unplanned), in which gross tumor is left behind, is referred to as *intralesional, debulking,* or *cytoreductive surgery*. It is commonly performed but rarely indicated.[23] A theoretical indication is to enhance the efficacy of other treatment modalities; for example, debulking an infiltrative lipoma in a swollen limb before RT. Debulking is a practical consideration before cryosurgery to reduce the amount of tissue to freeze and the duration of the cryotherapy. Cytoreduction may also help with treatment planning and dosimetry for certain types of RT. However, the improved tumor control achieved is more a result of geometric and dosimetry considerations than intentional and incomplete removal of tumor cells. Removing 99.9% of a 1 cm tumor (1×10^9, or 1 billion cells) still leaves a million residual cancer cells. Immunotherapy and chemotherapy theoretically could be helped by reducing tumor volume (e.g., LN removal for oral melanoma with the use of a melanoma vaccine),[24,25] but to date few well-controlled clinical trials have shown a benefit in veterinary medicine. If tumors are debulked with the anticipation of postoperative RT, the margins of debulked tumor should be marked with radiopaque metal clips to allow proper treatment planning based on radiographs or CT of the surgical site. The orientation of the incision should be considered carefully if RT is possible postoperatively.

Nonsurgical Locally Ablative Procedures

Ablative techniques to eradicate local (or metastatic) disease have a place in oncology, but they are based only rarely on evidence of outcomes.[26] Indications for the use of local ablative therapy vary, but they generally are limited to small, discrete lesions <2 cm. A limitation of all these techniques is that completeness of cell kill and margin analysis cannot be determined after treatment. If the operator picked the correct tumor, site, and dose delivery, then local control may be achieved; however, monitoring for regrowth is the only way to ensure that treatment has been adequate. As a general rule, recurrent disease tends to be more invasive and difficult to control than primary disease, so the first ablative procedure should be well planned and executed. All of the local ablative treatments require special equipment and training to be performed properly. Selective tumor cell kill that spares adjacent normal tissue is often claimed for these techniques, but it is unlikely to be consistently true.

Radiofrequency Ablation

The most common nonsurgical locally ablative procedures in human medicine include radiofrequency (RF) ablation, microwave ablation, and cryoablation. RF ablation involves delivery of a high-frequency (300–500 KHz) alternating current via a needle-like probe. The procedure typically is performed with either ultrasound or CT guidance and is commonly used to treat primary and secondary hepatic tumors. The minimally invasive nature of this technique makes it ideal for the treatment of metastatic liver lesions. For the treatment of metastatic colorectal cancer to the liver, RF has 5-year survival rates similar to those for surgery. Microwave ablation is similar to RF, but higher frequency currents (900–2459 MHz) are delivered. Microwave ablation is a newer technology with less evidence supporting its use, but it is often used for the same indications as RF ablation. RF and microwave ablation have been reported in dogs as experimental models.[27,28]

Cryoablation

Cryosurgery, or cryoablation, is a much older form of local therapy that has local anticancer effects by means of direct cell kill and vascular collapse. It has been used extensively in veterinary medicine, most commonly for skin, nasal planum, eyelid, perianal, and oral cavity tumors.[29–31] Cryotherapy continues to be an attractive treatment option for owners not interested in invasive procedures and for palliation of advanced (i.e., nonresectable or metastatic) oral tumors. Cryotherapy can be used as an adjunct to cytoreductive surgery. There is one report of image-guided cryoablation of a nasal mass in a dog that recurred after intensity-modulated RT (IMRT).[32] In humans laparoscopic and percutaneous cryoablation of select neoplasms (e.g., breast and renal tumors) has become an attractive, minimally invasive treatment option.[33,34]

Hyperthermia

Hyperthermia is the elevation of tissue temperature above normal physiologic levels. The term *hyperthermia* encompasses a wide range of temperatures and modalities. A variety of methods and devices are used clinically to induce hyperthermia in tissues. Noninvasive methods using RF currents, microwaves, or ultrasound are the most common. Heating of solid tumors typically is nonuniform because of the heating devices available, nonuniform distribution of blood flow in the tumor, and heat-dissipating activity of adjacent normal tissue. A number of studies demonstrated an improved outcome when hyperthermia was combined with RT for the treatment of solid tumors in dogs.[35–38] The ideal strategy for clinical hyperthermia treatment, including thermal dose, fractionation, and time and temperature goals, has yet to be identified.

Photodynamic Therapy

The practice of using sunlight to treat disease is ancient, but modern refinements have allowed the interactions between light and drugs to evolve into a highly effective cancer treatment called *photodynamic therapy* (PDT). PDT relies on light of an appropriate activating wavelength, oxygen, and a photosensitizer (PS) that accumulates within a tumor. The excited PS interacts with molecular oxygen, creating reactive oxygen species that are responsible for causing vascular stasis and necrosis, membrane damage, and apoptosis, and for initiating a signaling cascade resulting in an influx of inflammatory cells. Although initially studied as a single modality, PDT may also be useful when combined with other cancer treatments. Early studies show that a combination of PDT and low-dose cisplatin increased efficacy in both *in vitro* and murine models, and similar synergy has been observed when doxorubicin is combined with PDT.[39,40] In veterinary medicine PDT most commonly has been used in the treatment of feline squamous cell carcinoma (SCC). Most SCCs are superficial, localized, and rarely metastasize, making them well suited for treatment with PDT. An early description of chloro-aluminum sulfonated phthalocyanine–based PDT in 10 cats with superficial SCC or carcinoma in situ reported a 70% complete response rate, demonstrating the potential for PDT as a skin cancer treatment.[41] With a number of recent technologic improvements, PDT has the potential to become integrated into the mainstream of cancer treatment.[42]

Electrochemotherapy

Electrochemotherapy (ECT) is the use of chemotherapeutic drugs, most typically bleomycin or cisplatin, in combination with electric pulses that cause reversible permeabilization of the cell membrane, enabling the entry of drugs into the cells (or electroporation).[43,44] The antitumor effects of ECT are multiple[45] and include immunogenic cell death, resulting in eradication of clonogenic tumor cells. More recently ECT has been combined with different immunotherapies, especially gene electrotransfer of interleukin-12, to enhance the systemic antitumor effects of ECT.[46–49] Treatment-related adverse effects are usually mild and include wound dehiscence.

ECT is indicated primarily for the treatment of incompletely excised cutaneous and subcutaneous tumors, but also for the sole treatment of small primary tumors. Most published studies are uncontrolled and retrospective in design; however, ECT has shown some efficacy in the treatment of canine mast cell tumors (MCTs),[48–53] canine perianal adenomas and adenocarcinomas,[54,55] canine nasal tumors,[56] canine and feline localized lymphoma,[57] and canine and feline spontaneous soft tissue sarcomas.[58,59]

In one study 37 dogs with incompletely excised cutaneous MCTs were treated with cisplatin ECT; the local recurrence rate was 16%, with a median time to local recurrence of 1200 days.[52] In another study 28 dogs with incompletely excised cutaneous MCTs were treated with bleomycin ECT; the local recurrence rate was 18%, with a median time to local recurrence of 52.8 days.[50] In a retrospective comparative study 51 dogs with cutaneous MCTs were divided into four groups: ECT only, ECT applied intraoperatively, ECT applied postoperatively, and ECT applied for recurrent MCTs.[53] Objective responses were reported in all dogs with complete responses (CRs) recorded in 93%, 90%, 80%, and 64% of dogs treated with ECT postoperatively, intraoperatively, alone, and for recurrent disease, respectively.

In one study, of 21 dogs with primary nasal tumors, 11 dogs were treated with minimally invasive ECT and 10 dogs were treated with cytoreductive surgery and chemotherapy.[56] Partial and CRs were reported in 64% and 27% of dogs treated with ECT, respectively. Dogs treated with ECT had significantly better 12- and 32-month survival rates (60% and 30%, respectively) than dogs treated with surgery and chemotherapy (10% and 0%, respectively).

Surgery and Chemotherapy

The combined use of chemotherapy and surgery is becoming more commonplace in veterinary oncology, and the knowledge an oncologic surgeon must possess to master the use of combination therapy is ever expanding.[60,61] Many chemotherapeutic agents impede wound healing to some extent. In spite of this risk, few clinically relevant problems occur when surgery is performed on a patient receiving chemotherapy.[62,63] General recommendations are to wait 7 to 10 days after surgery to begin chemotherapy, especially for high-risk procedures such as intestinal anastomosis.[64]

The use of intraoperative[65] or perioperative chemotherapy[66,67] is receiving increased attention and could have greater implications for wound healing. Neoadjuvant chemotherapy is also becoming more popular and in some instances may greatly facilitate excision of a solid tumor.[68]

Surgery and Radiation Therapy

Theoretically both preoperative and postoperative RT have advantages.[61,69] Regardless, RT results in some impairment of wound healing potential, and the timing of surgery and RT must be considered.[70] Radiation damage to normal tissues (stem cells, blood vessels, lymphatics) may be progressive and potentially permanent as the total radiation dose, dose per fraction, and field size increase; therefore close collaboration between the radiation oncologist and the surgeon is critical in designing the most effective regimen. If RT is given preoperatively, surgery can be performed after any acute radiation effects have resolved (generally 3–4 weeks). Postoperative RT is recommended 7 to 14 days after surgery to allow adequate wound healing. In spite of the theoretical problems, surgery can often be safely performed on irradiated tissues and complications are not prohibitive.

The benefit of surgery and RT is clear for some tumor types; however, in some instances the improvement in outcome over single-modality therapy is controversial. Canine nasal tumors are one example of this controversy.[71,72] Early reports showed no benefit of surgery and postoperative RT over RT alone; however, a recent study demonstrated that preoperative RT was beneficial when exenteration of the nasal cavity was performed 6 to 10 weeks after completion of RT.[72] With the advent of stereotactic radiation therapy (SRT) and IMRT (see Chapter 13), such approaches are even more attractive because the overlying skin or underlying mucosa can be spared the full effects of radiation, thereby diminishing concerns about incisional healing after RT. In the past surgeons were reluctant to operate in a radiation field; these more focused forms of RT hopefully will allow the surgeon to operate with fewer wound healing complications and to create novel treatment plans that combine RT and surgery for select tumors. Radiation side effects are greatly diminished with a more conformal approach, and this in turn makes owners more willing to have their pets undergo RT.

Access to more sophisticated radiation techniques, such as SRT and IMRT, is rapidly increasing, and with these developments a new paradigm is emerging in veterinary radiation oncology. For example, bone sarcomas in locations not amenable to limb-sparing surgery now can be treated with curative-intent therapy,[73] and treatment protocols for large solid tumors previously deemed nonresectable are being investigated. Combinations of SRT and surgery also are being explored.

Although these new treatment options represent great advances, familiar challenges remain. In the case of dogs with appendicular osteosarcoma, fracture may occur after SRT. In addition, although some of these cases are amenable to surgical stabilization, postoperative infection rates are very high with the presence of orthopedic implants, and healing of the fracture does not occur because of the effects of RT on bone healing. Thus the role of the surgeon continues to evolve in the management of cases treated with RT.

Prevention of Cancer

Certain common cancers in dogs and cats can be prevented. The recent elucidation of the canine genome as it relates to genetic susceptibility to certain cancers likely will increase the surgical indications for prevention. It is well known that early (<1 year) oophorectomy reduces the risk of mammary cancer in the dog by 200-fold compared with intact dogs (and to a lesser degree in cats). Castration of the male dog helps prevent perianal adenomas and, obviously, testicular cancer. Removal of in situ SCC (precancerous) from the skin of white cats or removal of in situ adenomatous polyps from the rectum of dogs may also prevent malignant transformation of these tumors. Elective removal of cryptorchid testes, which are at high risk for tumor development, is another example of preventive surgery.

Miscellaneous Oncologic Surgery

Veterinary surgeons are being called on increasingly to facilitate the medical management of cancer patients. The placement of long-term vascular access catheters for delivery of fluids, chemotherapy, or anesthetic and analgesic agents has become commonplace, and ports are routinely placed to aid in the evacuation of malignant thoracic effusions (e.g., mesothelioma). Operative placement of various enteral and parenteral feeding tubes also is common.

Surgeons and radiation oncologists may work together to treat large cancers or tumor beds after excision with intraoperative RT. Surgical intervention for oncologic emergencies is not infrequent; such emergencies include intractable pain, bleeding, pathologic fracture, infection, and bowel perforation or obstruction.

The comprehensive veterinary oncology team also now includes the discipline of interventional radiology to help manage or palliate certain malignancies. Examples include the use of self-expanding nitinol stents to treat dogs with malignant urethral obstruction[74] and double pigtail stents for the treatment of malignant ureteral obstructions resulting from trigonal transitional cell carcinoma of the urinary bladder.[75]

Equipment advances also are facilitating tumor excisions (e.g., harmonic scalpel[76] and LigaSure), and laparoscopic and thoracoscopic evaluation of body cavities for clinical staging purposes increasingly is performed. Minimally invasive approaches for excision of cancers within body cavities are becoming more commonplace, and given the potential for reduced morbidity, veterinary surgeons may feel more comfortable performing surgery in the face of advanced disease for certain solid cancers (e.g., thoracoscopic partial lung lobectomy of a solitary metastatic lung nodule at the time of amputation for an appendicular osteosarcoma). A few other examples of minimally invasive surgery performed in companion animals for cancerous diseases include thoracoscopic pericardiectomy for heart-based tumors[77,78]; thoracoscopic right atrial mass resection[78]; thoracoscopic and thoracoscopic-assisted lung lobectomy[79,80]; laparoscopic-assisted intestinal surgery[81]; laparoscopic liver, pancreatic, and prostatic biopsy[82]; laparoscopic and laparoscopic-assisted splenectomy[83–85]; and laparoscopic adrenalectomy.[86,87]

Discussion

Surgery is the principal treatment for local or regionally confined cancer; however, just because a surgical procedure is possible does not mean that surgery is justified. Surgical resection of the external genitalia used to be routine treatment for dogs with transmissible venereal tumors, but now chemotherapy alone is curative in more than 90% of dogs. Radical mastectomy does not affect survival in most dogs with mammary gland tumors, but more aggressive

surgery is beneficial in cats with mammary carcinomas.[17,88–90] More surgery is not always better surgery. Long-term follow-up of well-staged and graded tumors with defined surgical technique and margins is necessary to demonstrate the true value of any operation. A great deal of progress in surgical technique and surgical thinking needs to take place before the use of surgery can be optimized.

A better understanding of expected tumor biology and more precise staging methods (e.g., molecular diagnostics, angiograms, ultrasound, CT, MRI, positron emission tomography/CT) will facilitate more precise surgical operations. Surgical techniques will continue to improve and undergo refinement,[75,91–93] but until surgeons become biologists, the big breakthroughs will be slow in coming. Surgeons should be investigating the influence of anesthesia, infection, immune function, blood transfusions, growth factors, oncogenes, and cytokines, to name a few factors, on the outcome of our patients.[94–100]

In spite of these anticipated advances in technology and biology, the most difficult aspect to learn is surgical judgment. As Cady has said, "Biology is king; selection of cases is queen; and the technical details of surgical procedures are the princes and princesses of the realm, who frequently try to overthrow the powerful forces of the king or queen, usually to no long-term avail, although with some temporary apparent victories."[101]

References

1. Chabner BA, Curt GA, Hubbard SM: Surgical oncology research development: the perspective of the National Cancer Institute, *Cancer Treat Rep* 68:825–829, 1984.
2. Poston GJ: Is there a surgical oncology? In Poston GJ, Beauchamp RD, Ruers TJM, editors: *Textbook of surgical oncology*, ed 1, London, 2007, Informa Healthcare, pp 1–4.
3. Spodnick GJ, Berg J, Rand WM, et al.: Prognosis for dogs with appendicular osteosarcoma treated by amputation alone: 162 cases (1978-1988), *J Am Vet Med Assoc* 200:995–999, 1992.
4. Dernell WS, Withrow SJ: Preoperative patient planning and margin evaluation, *Clin Tech Small Anim Pract* 13:17–21, 1998.
5. Winer JN, Verstraete FJM, Cissell DD, et al.: The applicatiomn of 3-dimensional printing for preoperative planning in oral and maxillofacial surgery in dogs and cats, *Vet Surg* 46:942–951, 2017.
6. Bacon NJ, Dernell WS, Ehrhart N, et al.: Evaluation of primary re-excision after recent inadequate resection of soft tissue sarcomas in dogs: 41 cases (1999-2004), *J Am Vet Med Assoc* 230:548–554, 2007.
7. Withrow SJ: Risk associated with biopsies for cancer. In Bonagura J, editor: *Kirk's current veterinary therapy XII: small animal practice*, ed 12, Philadelphia, 1995, Saunders, pp 24–26.
8. Enneking WF: *Musculoskeletal tumor surgery*, ed 1, New York, 1983, Churchill-Livingstone.
9. Gilson SK, Stone EA: Surgically induced tumor seeding in eight dogs and two cats, *J Am Vet Med Assoc* 196:1811–1815, 1990.
10. Pavletic MM: *Atlas of small animal wound management and reconstructive surgery*, ed 4, Ames, 2018, Wiley-Blackwell.
11. Dundas JM, Fowler JD, Schmon CL: Modification of the superficial cervical axial pattern skin flap for oral reconstruction, *Vet Surg* 34:206–213, 2005.
12. Cady B: Lymph node metastases: indicators, but not governors of survival, *Arch Surg* 119:1067–1072, 1984.
13. Gilson SD: Clinical management of the regional lymph node, *Vet Clin North Am Small Anim Pract* 25:149–167, 1995.
14. Grimes JA, Matz BM, Christopherson PW, et al.: Agreement between cytology and histopathology for regional lymph node metastasis in dogs with melanocytic neoplasms, *Vet Pathol* 54:579–587, 2017.

15. Williams LE, Gliatto JM, Dodge RK, et al.: Carcinoma of the apocrine glands of the anal sac in dogs: 113 cases (1985-1995), *J Am Vet Med Assoc* 223:825–831, 2003.

16. Hume CT, Kiupel M, Rigatti L, et al.: Outcomes of dogs with grade 3 mast cell tumors: 43 cases (1997-2007), *J Am Anim Hosp Assoc* 47:37–44, 2011.

17. Novosad CA, Bergman PJ, O'Brien MG, et al.: Retrospective evaluation of adjunctive doxorubicin for the treatment of feline mammary gland adenocarcinoma: 67 cases, *J Am Anim Hosp Assoc* 42:110–120, 2006.

18. Williams LE, Packer RA: Association between lymph node size and metastasis in dogs with oral malignant melanoma: 100 cases (1987-2011), *J Am Vet Med Assoc* 222:1234–1236, 2003.

19. Olson RM, Woods JE, Soule EH: Regional lymph node management and outcome in 100 patients with head and neck melanoma, *Am J Surg* 142:470–473, 1981.

20. Veronesi U, Adamus J, Bandiera DC, et al.: Delayed regional lymph node dissection in stage I melanoma of the skin of the lower extremities, *Cancer* 49:2420–2430, 1982.

21. O'Brien MG, Straw RC, Withrow SJ, et al.: Resection of pulmonary metastases in canine osteosarcoma: 36 cases (1983-1992), *Vet Surg* 22:105–109, 1993.

22. Milch RA: Surgical palliative care, *Semin Oncol* 32:165–168, 2005.

23. Moore GE: Debunking debulking, *Surg Gyn Obstet* 150:395–396, 1980.

24. Morton DL: Changing concepts of cancer surgery: surgery as immunotherapy, *Am J Surg* 135:367–371, 1978.

25. Broomfield S, Currie A, van der Most RG, et al.: Partial, but not complete, tumor-debulking surgery promotes protective antitumor memory when combined with chemotherapy and adjuvant immunotherapy, *Cancer Res* 65:7580–7584, 2005.

26. Withrow SJ, Poulson JM, Lucroy MD: Miscellaneous treatments for solid tumors. In Withrow SJ, Vail DM, editors: *Withrow and MacEwen's small animal clinical oncology*, ed 4, St. Louis, 2007, Saunders, pp 785–823.

27. Huang J, Li T, Liu N, et al.: Safety and reliability of hepatic radiofrequency ablation near the inferior vena cava: an experimental study, *Int J Hyperthermia* 27:116–123, 2011.

28. Qiu-Jie S, Zhi-Yu H, Xiao-Xia N: Feasible temperature of percutaneous microwave ablation of dog liver abutting the bowel, *Int J Hyperthermia* 27:124–131, 2011.

29. Harvey HJ: Cryosurgery of oral tumors in dogs and cats, *Vet Clin North Am Small Anim Pract* 10:821–830, 1980.

30. Holmberg DL: Cryosurgical treatment of canine eyelid tumors, *Vet Clin North Am Small Anim Pract* 10:831–836, 1980.

31. Fernandez De Queiroz G, Matera JM, Dagli M: Clinical study of cryosurgery efficacy in the treatment of skin and subcutaneous tumors in dogs and cats, *Vet Surg* 37:438–443, 2008.

32. Murphy SM, Lawrence JA, Schmiedt CW, et al.: Image-guided transnasal cryoablation of a recurrent nasal adenocarcinoma in a dog, *J Small Anim Pract* 52:329–333, 2011.

33. Manenti G, Perretta T, Gaspari E, et al.: Percutaneous local ablation of unifocal subclinical breast cancer: clinical experience and preliminary results of cryotherapy, *Eur Radiol* 21:2344–2353, 2011.

34. Klatte T, Grubmüller B, Waldert M, et al.: Laparoscopic cryoablation versus partial nephrectomy for the treatment of small renal masses: systematic review and cumulative analysis of observational studies, *Eur Urol* 60:435–443, 2011.

35. Dewhirst MW, Sim DA, Sapareto S, et al.: Importance of minimum tumor temperature in determining early and long-term responses of spontaneous canine and feline tumors to heat and radiation, *Cancer Res* 44:43–50, 1984.

36. Thrall DE, LaRue SM, Yu D, et al.: Thermal dose is related to duration of local control in canine sarcomas treated with thermoradiotherapy, *Clin Cancer Res* 11:5206–5214, 2005.

37. Gillette EL, McChesney SL, Dewhirst MW, et al.: Response of canine oral carcinomas to heat and radiation, *Int J Radiat Oncol Biol Phys* 13:1861–1867, 1987.

38. Gillette SM, Dewhirst MW, Gillette EL, et al.: Response of canine soft tissue sarcomas to radiation or radiation plus hyperthermia: a randomized phase II study, *Int J Hyperthermia* 8:309–320, 1992.

39. Casas A, Fukuda H, Riley P, et al.: Enhancement of aminolevulinic acid based photodynamic by Adriamycin, *Cancer Lett* 121:105–113, 1997.

40. Lanks KW, Gao JP, Sharma T: Photodynamic enhancement of doxorubicin cytotoxicity, *Cancer Chemother Pharmacol* 35:17–20, 1994.

41. Roberts WG, Klein MK, Loomis M, et al.: Photodynamic therapy of spontaneous cancers in felines, canines, and snakes with chloro-aluminum sulfonated phthalocyanine, *J Natl Cancer Inst* 83:18–23, 1991.

42. Agostinis P, Berg K, Cengel KA, et al.: Photodynamic therapy of cancer: an update, *CA Cancer J Clin* 61:250–281, 2011.

43. Cemazar M, Tamzali Y, Sersa G, et al.: Electrochemotherapy in veterinary oncology, *J Vet Intern Med* 22:826–831, 2008.

44. Tozon N, Tratar UL, Znidar K, et al.: Operating procedures of the electrochemotherapy for treatment of tumor in dogs and cats, *J Vis Exp* 116:e54760, 2016.

45. Spugnini EP, Baldi F, Mellone P, et al.: Patterns of tumor response in canine and feline cancer patients treated with electrochemotherapy: preclinical data for the standardization of this treatment in pets and humans, *J Translat Med* 5:48, 2007.

46. Chuang TF, Lee SC, Liao KW, et al.: Electroporation-mediate IL-12 gene therapy in a transplanatable canine model, *Int J Cancer* 125:698–707, 2009.

47. Calvet CY, Mir LM: The promising alliance of anti-cancer electrochemotherapy with immunotherapy, *Cancer Metastasis Rev* 35:165–177, 2016.

48. Cemazar M, Avgustin JA, Pavlin D, et al.: Efficacy and safety of electrochemotherapy combined with peritumoral IL-12 gene electrotransfer of canine mast cell tumours, *Vet Comp Oncol* 15:641–654, 2016.

49. Salvadori C, Svara T, Rocchigiani G, et al.: Effects of electrochemotherapy with cisplatin and peritumoral IL-12 gene electrotransfer on canine mast cell tumors: a histopathologic and immunohistochemical study, *Radiol Oncol* 51:286–294, 2017.

50. Spugnini EP, Vincenzi B, Baldi F, et al.: Adjuvant electrochemotherapy for the treatment of incompletely resected canine mast cell tumors, *Anticancer Res* 26:4585–4590, 2006.

51. Kodre V, Cemazar M, Pecar J, et al.: Electrochemotherapy compared to surgery for treatment of canine mast cell tumours, *In Vivo* 23:55–62, 2009.

52. Spugnini EP, Vincenzi B, Citro G, et al.: Evaluation of cisplatin as an electrochemotherapy agent for the treatment of incompletely excised mast cell tumors in dogs, *J Vet Intern Med* 25:407–411, 2011.

53. Lowe R, Gavazza A, Impellizeri JA, et al.: The treatment of canine mast cell tumours with electrochemotherapy with or without surgical excision, *Vet Comp Oncol* 15:775–784, 2016.

54. Tozon N, Kodre V, Sersa G, et al.: Effective treatment of perianal tumors in dogs with electrochemotherapy, *Anticancer Res* 25:839–846, 2005.

55. Spugnini EP, Dotsinsky I, Mudrov N, et al.: Biphasic pulses enhance bleomycin efficacy in a spontaneous canine perianal tumors model, *J Exp Clin Cancer Res* 26:483–487, 2007.

56. Maglietti F, Tellado M, Olaiz N, et al.: Minimally invasive electrochemotherapy procedure for treating nasal duct tumors in dogs using a single needle electrode, *Radiol Oncol* 51:422–430, 2017.

57. Spugnini EP, Citro G, Mellone P, et al.: Electrochemotherapy for localized lymphoma: a preliminary study in companion animals, *J Exp Clin Cancer Res* 26:515–518, 2007.

58. Orlowski S, Mir LM: Treatment of spontaneous soft tissue sarcomas in cat, *Methods Mol Med* 37:305–311, 2000.

59. Spugnini EP, Vincenzi B, Citro G, et al.: Adjuvant electrochemotherapy for the treatment of incompletely excised spontaneous canine sarcomas, *In Vivo* 21:819–822, 2007.

60. Cornell K, Waters DJ: Impaired wound healing in the cancer patient: effects of cytotoxic therapy and pharmacologic modulation by growth factors, *Vet Clin North Am Small Anim Pract* 25:111–131, 1995.

61. McEntee MC: Principles of adjunct radiotherapy and chemotherapy, *Vet Clin North Am Small Anim Pract* 25:133–148, 1995.

62. Ferguson MK: The effect of antineoplastic agents on wound healing, *Surg Gyn Obstet* 154:421–429, 1982.

63. Graves G, Cunningham P, Raaf JH: Effect of chemotherapy on the healing of surgical wounds, *Clin Bull* 10:144–149, 1980.

64. Laing EJ: The effects of antineoplastic agents on wound healing: guidelines for combined use of surgery and chemotherapy, *Compend Contin Educ Pract Vet* 11:136–143, 1989.

65. Dernell WS, Withrow SJ, Straw RC, et al.: Intracavitary treatment of soft tissue sarcomas in dogs using cisplatin in a biodegradable polymer, *Anticancer Res* 17:4499–4506, 1997.

66. Fisher B, Gunduz N, Saffer EA: Influence of the interval between primary tumor removal and chemotherapy on kinetics and growth of metastases, *Cancer Res* 43:1488–1492, 1983.

67. Fisher B: Cancer surgery: a commentary, *Cancer Treat Rep* 68:31–41, 1984.

68. Bray J, Polton G: Neoadjuvant and adjuvant chemotherapy combined with anatomical resection of feline injection-site sarcoma: results in 21 cats, *Vet Comp Oncol* 14:147–160, 2016.

69. Tepper J, Million RR: Radiation therapy and surgery, *Am J Clin Oncol* 11:381–385, 1988.

70. Sequin B, McDonald DE, Kent MS, et al.: Tolerance of cutaneous or mucosal flaps placed into a radiation therapy field of dogs, *Vet Surg* 34:214–222, 2005.

71. MacEwen EG, Withrow SJ, Patnaik AK: Nasal tumors in the dog: retrospective evaluation of diagnosis, prognosis, and treatment, *J Am Vet Med Assoc* 170:45–48, 1977.

72. Adams WM, Bjorling DE, McAnulty JF, et al.: Outcome of accelerated radiotherapy alone or accelerated radiotherapy followed by exenteration of the nasal cavity in dogs with intranasal neoplasia: 53 cases (1990–2002), *J Am Vet Med Assoc* 227:936–941, 2005.

73. Farese JP, Milner R, Thompson MS, et al.: Stereotactic radiosurgery for the treatment of lower extremity osteosarcoma in dogs, *J Am Vet Med Assoc* 225:1567–1572, 2004.

74. Weisse C, Berent A, Todd K, et al.: Evaluation of palliative stenting for management of malignant urethral obstructions in dogs, *J Am Vet Med Assoc* 229:226–234, 2006.

75. Berent AC, Weisse C, Beal MW, et al.: Use of indwelling, double-pigtail stents for treatment of malignant ureteral obstruction in dogs: 12 cases (2006–2009), *J Am Vet Med Assoc* 238:1017–1025, 2011.

76. Royals SR, Ellison GW, Adin CA: Use of an ultrasonically activated scalpel for splenectomy in 10 dogs with naturally occurring splenic disease, *Vet Surg* 34:174–178, 2005.

77. Jackson J, Richter KP, Launer DP: Thoracoscopic partial pericardectomy in 13 dogs, *J Vet Intern Med* 13:529–533, 1999.

78. Crumbaker DM, Rooney MB, Case JB: Thoracoscopic subtotal pericardiectomy and right atrial mass resection in a dog, *J Am Vet Med Assoc* 237:551–554, 2010.

79. Wormser C, Singhal S, Holt DE, et al.: Thoracoscopic-assisted pulmonary surgery for partial and complete lung lobectomy in dogs and cats: 11 cases (2008-2013), *J Am Vet Med Assoc* 245:1036–1041, 2014.

80. Bleakley S, Duncan CG, Monnet E: Thoracoscopic lung lobectomy for primary lung tumors in 13 dogs, *Vet Surg* 44:1029–1035, 2015.

81. Barry KS, Case JB, Winter MD, et al.: Diagnostic usefulness of laparoscopy versus exploratory laparotomy for dogs with suspected gastrointestinal obstruction, *J Am Vet Med Assoc* 251:307–314, 2017.

82. Holak P, Adamiak Z, Jałyński M, et al.: Laparoscopy-guided prostate biopsy in dogs–a study of 13 cases, *Pol J Vet Sci* 13:765–766, 2010.

83. Shaver SL, Mayhew PD, Steffey MA, et al.: Short-term outcome of multiple port laparoscopic splenectomy in 10 dogs, *Vet Surg* 44(Suppl 1):71–75, 2015.

84. Wright T, Singh A, Mayhew PD, et al.: Laparoscopic-assisted splenectomy in dogs: 18 cases (2012-2014), *J Am Vet Med Assoc* 248:916–922, 2016.

85. Mayhew PD, Sutton JS, Singh A, et al.: Complications and short-term outcomes associated with single-port laparoscopic splenectomy in dogs, *Vet Surg* 47:O67–O74, 2018.

86. Jiménez Peláez M, Bouvy BM, Dupré GP: Laparoscopic adrenalectomy for treatment of unilateral adrenocortical carcinomas: technique, complications, and results in seven dogs, *Vet Surg* 37:444–453, 2008.

87. Pitt KA, Mayhew PD, Steffey MA, et al.: Laparoscopic adrenalectomy for removal of unilateral noninvasive pheochromocytomas in 10 dogs, *Vet Surg* 45:O70–O76, 2016.

88. MacEwen EG, Hayes AA, Harvey HJ, et al.: Prognostic factors for feline mammary tumors, *J Am Vet Med Assoc* 185:201–204, 1984.

89. Golinger RC: Breast cancer controversies: surgical decisions, *Semin Oncol* 7:444–459, 1980.

90. Gemignani F, Mayhew PD, Giuffrida MA, et al.: Association of surgical approach with complication rate, progression-free survival time, and disease-specific survival time in cats with mammary adenocarcinoma: 107 cases (1991-2014), *J Am Vet Med Assoc* 252:1393–1402, 2018.

91. Bartels KE: Lasers in veterinary medicine: where have we been, and where are we going? *Vet Clin North Am Small Anim Pract* 32:495–515, 2002.

92. Gillams AR: Mini-review: the use of radiofrequency in cancer, *Br J Cancer* 92:1825–1829, 2005.

93. Kennedy JE: High-intensity focused ultrasound in the treatment of solid tumours, *Nature Rev* 5:321–327, 2005.

94. Kodama M, Kodama T, Nishi Y, et al.: Does surgical stress cause tumor metastasis? *Anticancer Res* 12:1603–1616, 1992.

95. Blumberg N, Heal JM: Perioperative blood transfusion and solid tumor recurrence: a review, *Cancer Invest* 5:615–625, 1987.

96. Pollock RE, Lotzová E, Stanford SD: Surgical stress impairs natural killer cell programming of tumor for lysis in patients with sarcomas and other solid tumors, *Cancer* 70:2192–2202, 1992.

97. Medleau L, Crowe DT, Dawe DL: Effect of surgery on the in vitro response of canine peripheral blood lymphocytes to phytohemagglutinin, *Am J Vet Res* 44:859–860, 1983.

98. Murthy SM, Goldschmidt RA, Rao LN, et al.: The influence of surgical trauma on experimental metastasis, *Cancer* 64:2035–2044, 1989.

99. Navarro M, Lozano R, Román A, et al.: Anesthesia and immunosuppression in an experimental model, *Eur Surg Res* 22:317–322, 1990.

100. Meakins JL: Surgeons, surgery, and immunomodulation, *Arch Surg* 126:494–498, 1991.

101. Cady B: Basic principles in surgical oncology, *Arch Surg* 132:338–346, 1997.

11

Interventional Oncology

WILLIAM T.N. CULP

The field of interventional radiology has grown dramatically over the past decade and has expanded the available diagnostic and treatment options for veterinary patients. Similarly, the field of interventional oncology (IO), with a focus on image-guided therapies for neoplasia, has quickly joined surgery, chemotherapy, and radiation therapy as a 4th pillar of treatment options for oncologic disease in companion animals. IO combines the use of minimally invasive techniques, advanced instrumentation, image guidance, and creative thinking to allow clinicians to offer treatments that can improve pain control, increase quality of life, and potentially alter prognosis favorably. Although this discipline is expanding rapidly, the available scientific evidence is limited. However, significant work into the evaluation of these procedures is underway.

Principles of Interventional Oncology

Imaging

Image guidance allows those individuals performing IO procedures to do so in a minimally invasive fashion. It is required for clinicians performing IO procedures to have a strong understanding of anatomy and anatomic assessment with various imaging modalities. Although there are numerous anatomic descriptions of normal anatomy in dogs and cats, very limited data are available for the description of anatomic changes associated with pathologic conditions that may commonly be treated with IO techniques. However, some basic imaging concepts are applicable in most situations, as the goals of many IO techniques are to either close down a lumen that is naturally open (e.g., embolization) or open a lumen that is obstructed by a malignancy (e.g., stenting).

The most commonly used imaging modality in veterinary medicine for the performance of IO techniques is fluoroscopy. Fluoroscopy provides a real-time assessment of anatomic structures and allows clinicians performing these procedures to use radiopaque instrumentation and contrast medium. Basic fluoroscopic equipment and techniques can be used for most stenting procedures, but advanced capabilities such as digital subtraction angiography and road-mapping are recommended when performing assessments of tumoral blood supply or vascular obstructions. It is important to be cognizant of the potential for increased exposure to radiation when performing these procedures, and appropriate training in management of radiation exposure should be a priority for those performing IO procedures.

As stated previously, fluoroscopic vascular guides for performing IO procedures are limited. The fluoroscopic abdominal anatomy has recently been described and can be used to assist with intravascular locoregional therapies in the abdomen.[1] In this study, the branching patterns of the major abdominal arteries and associated anatomic landmarks (generally vertebral bodies) were described to assist with vascular access and instrument positioning during abdominal IO procedures. Consistency in the location of many of the major abdominal arteries was noted, which will hopefully decrease anesthesia time and improve understanding of the normal anatomy, so that abnormal or altered anatomy can be appreciated when it is encountered.[1]

Recently ultrasound has been used more commonly during veterinary IO procedures. The main indications for ultrasound usage are to guide access to fluid-filled organs for implant placement or drainage or to access tumors for ablation. Ultrasound is an excellent imaging modality for these procedures, as it allows for rapid manipulation of images and real-time assessment of implant positioning. In veterinary patients, percutaneous access to the renal pelvis during antegrade ureteral stent placement is a common indication for the use of ultrasound guidance. In human IO procedures, ultrasound is commonly used to obtain vascular access as well.

Computed tomography (CT) is a crucial component of the preprocedural assessment of many cases undergoing an IO procedure. At the author's clinic, in veterinary IO cases being treated with an intravascular technique a contrast-enhanced CT is generally performed before the IO procedure to allow for assessment both of the vascular supply to a tumor and the extent of the tumor. CT is also being utilized more commonly as a tool for the assessment of tumor response. This modality is excellent for assessing tumor size and generating tumor volumes both pre- and postprocedure.

Instrumentation

Although IO incorporates certain equipment commonly used in veterinary practices, much of the instrumentation and devices used are specific to this discipline. To facilitate the minimally invasive nature that is desired to perform IO techniques, access to organs is obtained and maintained through the use of access needles and catheters and the placement of sheaths. Needles and catheters are often similar to what is regularly used in veterinary practices, but variations in diameter, length, and shape are available for different indications.

Sheaths can be used multifunctionally and are also available in different variations. Some of the more popular sheaths used during veterinary IO procedures include those equipped with a hemostatic valve and sidearm to allow for contrast injection. These sheaths are often placed intravascularly to allow for serial insertion of instrumentation into a blood vessel without concern for losing access. Sheaths can also be created with a "peel-away" design. This type of sheath allows for instrumentation that may have a sizeable external attachment piece to be introduced into a lumen or cavity.

One of the main workhorses of most IO procedures is the guide wire. The guide wire demonstrates much of its utility as a means of getting into a location in the least invasive way possible and in a relatively safe fashion. The guide wire also acts as means of placement of specialized catheters, sheaths, stents, and balloons, as these devices very commonly are designed with an inner cannula that allows them to slide over a guide wire into position. Guide wires are available in a variety of lengths, diameters, shapes, and stiffness; these variations are particularly important to consider when attempting to gain access through a severely obstructed lumen.

Specialized catheters are generally used to gain or maintain access in a luminal structure (including blood vessel) or for establishing a coaxial system, by which a smaller catheter or other device can also be placed. Specialized catheters are often used to generate contrast studies when planning ballooning and stenting procedures. In companion animals, the catheters used for contrast studies and vascular procedures are generally 4 to 5 French in diameter, although larger catheters may be used to allow for easier drainage of an obstructed organ. In addition, much smaller catheters (microcatheters) can be used to access smaller caliber vessels during intraarterial chemotherapy delivery or embolization; as an example, the author commonly uses microcatheters that are 1.7 to 2.4 French in diameter for prostatic embolization procedures.

Stents are devices placed into a luminal structure or passage to counteract a disease-induced stricture. The use of stents is commonplace in medicine, and the disease processes treated by stenting are constantly expanding. There are descriptions of stents used to treat malignant obstructions in the urethra, ureter, trachea, esophagus, colon, and blood vessels in companion animals.[2-10] In addition, stents have been used to treat malignant obstructions of the biliary tract and nasopharynx in the author's clinic.

Stents can be simple catheters or other tube-like devices that are placed to simply allow for a lumen to be open, or specially designed with varying metals in a variety of configurations and sizes. Stents that contain interstices can be covered or uncovered, and can be delivered with a balloon (balloon-expandable stents) or be self-expanding. If stents are covered, they can be impregnated with antineoplastic substances such as chemotherapy or radiation beads.

An embolic agent is a substance placed into a blood vessel to cause temporary or permanent occlusion of blood flow. This alteration of blood flow could be a partial or total occlusion of the blood supply depending on the eventual goal. Many different embolic agents have been described, and advances in these products are continuing on a regular basis. Currently, major embolic agents commonly used during the treatment of neoplasia include particles and liquid embolics such as cyanoacrylate or ethylene–vinyl alcohol copolymer, although many other agents may be considered.

Interventional Oncology Treatment Categories

Stenting of Malignant Strictures

The use of stents in the treatment of companion animals has become commonplace over the past decade. Increased availability of specialized equipment and imaging modalities has improved

the ability of veterinarians to be able to offer advanced procedures such as stenting. Although stenting procedures are now considered an important component of oncologic therapy, research is still limited.

Most of the available literature describing stenting in companion animals is focused on the description of the procedure and initial outcomes in a small cohort of animals; however, experience is growing, and our assessment of these procedures should expand with that growth. Stenting should be evaluated both from a procedural and clinical outcome standpoint. In many human trials, the technical success of a stenting procedure is determined and generally focuses on whether an obstruction could be bypassed and whether a stent could be successfully placed. Clinical success is often defined as stent patency at a defined period of time after the procedure.

Intraluminal stent placement for the treatment of malignant urethral obstruction is likely the most commonly performed veterinary IO technique. Urethral stent placement is generally considered an attractive option for the relief of malignant obstruction, as the procedure can be performed with minimal invasion and often rapidly relieves obstruction. In dogs, female cats, and male cats that have had a perineal urethrostomy, urethral stents can be placed via the distal urethra without need for an incision.

Several studies have described outcomes in dogs and cats undergoing urethral stenting. In four canine urethral stent studies, 95 dogs undergoing stent placement to treat malignant urethral obstructions have been reported.[2-4] In the first study, both self-expanding and balloon-expandable stents were utilized to relieve obstruction, and stent placement was found to be rapid, safe, and effective at restoring luminal patency.[4] Stent placement was successful in relieving urinary obstruction in 97% of cases in the four published studies.[2-4,11] Reported major complications of urethral stenting have included incontinence (26%–37%), reobstruction (16%), and stent migration (11%)[2,3]; in addition, stranguria poststent placement is also a common finding.[2,4] Of 19 owners surveyed in one study, 16 were satisfied with the outcome and felt that they would recommend urethral stent placement to other owners.[3] When treatment with nonsteroidal antiinflammatory drugs (NSAIDs) before or chemotherapy after stent placement was pursued, median survival times were significantly increased versus when medical therapy was not pursued.[2] Urethral stent placement has been shown to be successful in relieving malignant obstructions in cats as well.[12,13]

Ureteral stenting to relieve a malignant obstruction is generally required when a lower urinary tract carcinoma grows from the bladder, urethra, and/or prostate to obstruct the ureteral orifice in the bladder. This procedure can be performed with minimal invasion using ultrasound and fluoroscopic guidance (Fig. 11.1). As the ureteral orifice is generally obscured by the tumor, it is usually recommended to percutaneously gain access into the renal pelvis and place a guide wire across the obstruction in an antegrade fashion. Dilation of a tract through the tumor then occurs from retrograde placement of a sheath and dilator. The ureteral stent is also passed retrograde through the stent and positioned with its pigtails in the renal pelvis and bladder. In one study evaluating 12 dogs undergoing ureteral stent placement via percutaneous access, stents were successfully placed in all dogs.[5] In dogs with azotemia before stent placement, improvements in blood urea nitrogen (BUN) and serum creatinine concentrations were noted in all dogs.[8] In addition, all dogs with follow-up ultrasonography demonstrated improved hydronephrosis and hydroureter.[5]

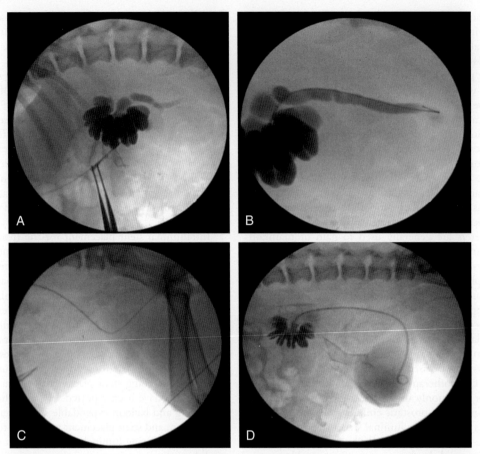

• **Fig. 11.1** Fluoroscopic images during a percutaneous ureteral stenting procedure in a 5-year-old male castrated pit bull terrier. (A) An over-the-needle catheter has been placed in the renal pelvis and a contrast nephroureterogram has been performed. (B) A guide wire is being passed down the ureter to the point of the ureteral obstruction. (C) The guide wire can be seen extending through the ureter, through the bladder and out the urethra in this male dog. (D) Final placement of the ureteral stent with a pigtail in the renal pelvis and a pigtail in the bladder.

Whenever possible, surgical resection of gastrointestinal tumors should be pursued. However, tumors occasionally grow undetected in companion animals for extended periods of time, resulting in large and/or invasive tumors that may be considered poor surgical candidates. Stenting of malignant obstructions in the gastrointestinal tract has been described for the esophagus and colon in companion animals.[7,9,10] These procedures can be performed using a natural orifice; the author prefers to use a combination of endoscopic and fluoroscopic guidance during the procedure to improve precision of stent placement. In a case report of a dog with an esophageal squamous cell carcinoma, stent placement resulted in an improvement in clinical signs for 12 weeks until euthanasia for unrelated reasons.[9] Colonic stenting has been reported in two cats and one dog.[7,10] All cases demonstrated clinical improvement after stenting.

Stents have also been used to treat malignant obstruction of the trachea and extraluminal compression of blood vessels.[6,8] A cat with a tracheal carcinoma was evaluated for respiratory distress and noted to have near complete obstruction of the tracheal lumen. Intraluminal tracheal stenting relieved the clinical signs and no complications were noted.[8] Endovascular stenting was used to relieve Budd–Chiari syndrome in three dogs with confirmed or suspected neoplastic obstructions. All three dogs demonstrated resolution of clinical sings and extended survival times ranging from 7 to 20 months.[6]

Intraarterial Chemotherapy

The use of intraarterial (IA) delivery of chemotherapy has long been considered in oncology.[14] The proposed theoretical advantages of IA drug delivery are that local drug concentration is increased (i.e., at the level of the tumoral blood supply), tumor toxicity is not cell cycle specific because of high drug concentrations, and the decrease in systemic exposure to drugs leads to a decrease in potential systemic side effects.[14,15] Several studies have demonstrated that IA infusion of drugs increases the concentration of drug in the target organ.[16,17] In one study, IA drug delivery resulted in greater target organ concentrations of drugs compared with intravenous (IV) administration.[16] Studies have further shown that drug concentration was influenced by blood flow rate, i.e., vessels with a low arterial blood flow will have a higher local concentration of drug[16,18]; however, many questions still remain about the magnitude of these proposed advantages (i.e., if these advantages do exist, do they exist at a level that makes IA delivery a reasonable alternative to IV delivery?) and the pharmacologic activity of a drug in a higher concentration in the tumor.

The IA delivery of drugs comes with certain challenges, many of which are magnified in a veterinary patient. Obtaining vascular access in an artery requires a small incision or ultrasound-guided intravascular access. When the artery used for access is not ligated but instead repaired, the access site needs to be monitored closely postprocedure for bleeding. In addition, as opposed to humans, dogs and cats require anesthesia during IA procedures. IA delivery also exposes the treating clinician and patient to radiation during the fluoroscopic procedure. Lastly, because of anesthesia and equipment costs, IA procedures are more expensive than traditional drug delivery via an IV route.

IA chemotherapy can be used as a sole therapy, but in humans this technique is often employed in a neoadjuvant setting as a means of margin sterilization or downstaging, or in combination with radiation therapy as a radiation sensitizer.[19–24] Cisplatin is well established as a radiosensitizing agent, although the exact mechanisms of this are still being elucidated.[22,25] Several human studies have demonstrated improvements in both local tumor control rates and survival times when IA chemotherapy is combined with radiation therapy.[21,23,25] In a study evaluating the combination of IA cisplatin with radiation therapy for the treatment of canine bladder cancer, two dogs demonstrated an objective reduction in tumor size.[26] Side effects and toxicity were minimal in these two dogs.[26]

IA chemotherapy has been described in the treatment regimen of canine appendicular osteosarcoma in a few studies.[27–29] In one study,[27] dogs with extremity osteosarcoma were divided into six groups: untreated, radiation alone, IA cisplatin alone, IV cisplatin alone, radiation therapy plus IA cisplatin, and radiation therapy plus IV cisplatin. After treatment, the tumors were resected and evaluated. In all radiation therapy groups, radiation was delivered in different doses. There was a direct relationship between the number of radiation doses (whether given with or without cisplatin) on percent necrosis of the tumor. The radiation doses predicted to result in 80% or 90% tumor necrosis when radiation therapy was the sole treatment were approximately 42 and 50 Gy, respectively. The radiation doses decreased to approximately 28 and 36 Gy, respectively, when combined with IA cisplatin.[27]

In a second osteosarcoma study,[28] IA cisplatin was administered in two doses on days 1 and 21. Dogs in this study were randomized to receive IA cisplatin alone or IA cisplatin plus radiation therapy. Three weeks after treatment, a limb-sparing surgery was performed. This study demonstrated the when IA cisplatin is administered with moderate doses of radiation, a high percent tumor necrosis was achieved. Dogs with less than 75% necrosis had a significantly greater local tumor recurrence rate at 1 year, of approximately 65%, compared with a 15% local tumor recurrence rate in dogs with greater than 75% necrosis.[28]

More recently, the early tumor response of IA chemotherapy was described in the treatment of lower urinary tract neoplasia in dogs.[30] In this study, two treatment groups were established: (1) NSAID and IA carboplatin and (2) NSAID and IV carboplatin. Arterial access was obtained through either the carotid or femoral artery. Complications in the IA chemotherapy group were minor, and adverse events such as anemia, lethargy, and anorexia were significantly less likely in the group receiving IA chemotherapy compared with that receiving IV chemotherapy. The dogs in the IA chemotherapy group had a significantly greater decrease in tumor length, length percentage, width percentage, longest unidimensional measurement, and longest unidimensional measurement percentage after treatment compared with the IV chemotherapy group.[30] It is important to note that this study evaluated only short-term outcome, and larger scale studies are needed to further evaluate the use of IA chemotherapy for lower urinary tract neoplasia.[30]

Embolization and Chemoembolization

Embolization was first described in the early 1970s when autologous blood clot was used as an embolic agent.[31] Currently, embolic agents are generally categorized into permanent and temporary, with temporary agents such as gelatin sponge, collagen, and thrombin rarely used to treat neoplastic disease. More commonly, permanent embolic agents such as particles (e.g., polyvinyl alcohol beads) and liquid agents (e.g., cyanoacrylate, alcohol, and ethylene vinyl alcohol copolymer) are used, although there are also indications for the use of other permanent agents such as coils, plugs, and balloons.

Embolization is focused on the principle of directly targeting the specific blood supply of the tumor with the purpose of slowing or eliminating blood flow to that tumor. Pursuing embolization often stems from the desire to achieve one of two goals: (1) treating a tumor primarily by diminishing the blood supply so that tumor death occurs, or (2) preoperatively treating a tumor to decrease blood loss during a major surgical resection. In veterinary patients, the second reason is rarely used; however, further consideration for this option should be given, especially in tumors that are at particular risk for experiencing blood loss such as liver, nasal, and thyroid tumors. The main reason for embolization currently in companion animals is as a primary treatment in cases that are deemed to be nonresectable or patients considered to be poor surgical candidates.

The concept of embolization has been most evaluated in the treatment of liver neoplasia in humans, with the publication of hundreds of scientific articles. The liver has a unique dual blood supply, as it receives a large portion of normal blood flow from the portal vein as opposed to the hepatic artery.[32] Interestingly, much of hepatic tumoral blood supply is arterial in origin, thus allowing the hepatic arterial branches and their subsequent downstream branches to be catheterized and treated. The outcomes associated with transarterial embolization of liver masses in humans have been favorable, with randomized clinical trials demonstrating a survival benefit.[33]

Many other organs can also be considered for targeting with embolization despite not having a dual blood supply like the liver. In humans, embolization has been described in many different organs, and the literature evaluating embolization in other locations is growing. The concept for treatment in many of these organs is to specifically select the blood supply to the tumor while avoiding normal blood supply to the remainder of the organ. Tumors often stimulate neovascularization, and these abnormal new blood vessels can be targeted by superselective catheterization. In addition, some organs may not be needed (e.g., prostate), allowing these tumors to be targeted with embolization without major concern for loss of function.

Chemoembolization differs from embolization in that chemotherapy is simultaneously delivered to a tumor at the time of embolization. This provides the theoretical advantages of IA chemotherapy, as described earlier, with the additional aspect that chemotherapy elimination from the target organ/tumor is altered as a result of diminished blood flow.[34,35] After embolization, hypoxia within tumor cells increases vessel permeability, and these factors alter cell membrane function and cause chemotherapy to be sequestered in higher concentrations within tumor cells.[34] This likely plays a major role in reduction of systemic drug exposure and a reported decrease in side effects and toxicity.[34]

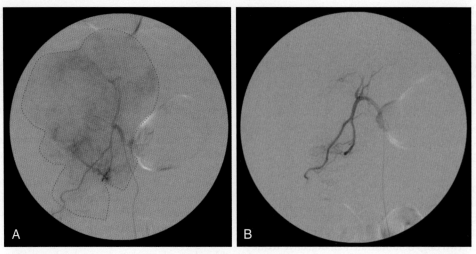

• **Fig. 11.2** Fluoroscopic images preembolization (A) and postembolization (B) of a liver tumor in an 11-year-old male castrated mixed breed dog. Note the outline of the tumor marked by the dashes (A), and the lack of tumor opacification postembolization (B).

Traditional chemoembolization involves the administration of a slurry containing a contrast medium, embolic agent, and a chemotherapy agent. Many chemotherapy agents have been described in humans including doxorubicin, epirubicin, cisplatin, and mitomycin C.[33,36] Much research is being invested into the evaluation of other means of delivering chemotherapy to tumors in combination with embolization. Drug-eluting beads (DEBs) have now been evaluated in several human studies and have demonstrated some promise.[33,37] These beads are generally made of a biocompatible polymer that can bind chemotherapeutic agents.[35,37] The drug can be released in the tumoral blood supply in a controlled and sustained manner; consequently, the chance of systemic side effects from the chemotherapy may be decreased.[35] Further evaluation of the efficacy of DEBs compared with traditional transarterial chemoembolization needs to be performed to determine whether there is a benefit of one delivery agent over the other.[33]

An additional agent, called lipiodol, is also often used during chemoembolization. Lipiodol is an iodinated poppy seed lipid–based medium that has several proposed benefits: (1) it is radiopaque and can be used in the slurry to replace contrast medium, (2) it acts as an embolic agent on its own, and (3) it preferentially concentrates in tumor tissue longer than in nontumor tissue.[35,38] Most descriptions of liver chemoembolization include lipiodol in the injected embolic slurry.

The superiority of embolization and chemoembolization to each other remains controversial.[34,35] Embolization (also called bland embolization) has an established antitumor effect, with the rationale being that embolization results in ischemic tumor cell death.[35] Proponents of embolization also highlight the prevention of chemotherapy toxicity. However, investigators who prefer chemoembolization cite the added benefit of chemotherapy-induced cytotoxicity.[35]

Liver embolization (Fig. 11.2) has been described in a few case series in dogs, and is currently the most evaluated embolization technique in companion animals.[39,40] Recently, in an experimental model, temporary hepatic arterial embolization was performed using gelatin sponge particles in five dogs with normal livers and no complications were encountered.[41] In one study describing embolization in dogs with large hepatic masses, one dog was treated with bland embolization and one dog was treated with chemoembolization.[40] Clinical improvement was noted in the dog treated with bland embolization, but the dog died at home approximately 4 months posttreatment.[40] Doxorubicin was administered with polyvinyl alcohol particles and lipiodol in the dog treated with chemoembolization; however, the dog died approximately 3 weeks after treatment as a consequence of an unrelated traumatic event.[40] In another study, superselective catheterization of the hepatic arterial branch was not achieved in two dogs.[39] Both dogs underwent transarterial chemotherapy and lipiodol administration, and one dog also received an additional embolic agent. When hepatic tumor size was evaluated after treatment, both dogs demonstrated stable disease at 1 month, but progressive disease at 3 months after treatment.[39] A hepatocellular carcinoma in a cat treated with bland embolization has also been reported.[42] In this cat, CT revealed a decrease in tumor size at 71 days posttreatment. Surgical resection was pursued 231 days after embolization and no recurrence was noted at 481 days after tumor removal.[42]

Prostatic artery embolization (PAE) is a growing field in both human and veterinary medicine. In humans, PAE has been used mostly as a treatment for benign prostatic hyperplasia (BPH) or to treat prostate-induced hematuria.[43] Experimentally, dogs have undergone PAE in a model of BPH.[44] In this study, four of seven dogs with induced BPH had reduction of prostate size after embolization.[44] The use of PAE to treat prostatic neoplasia has also recently been reported in dogs.[45] Ten dogs with confirmed prostatic carcinoma underwent PAE via a vascular approach in the left carotid artery. Tumor size was evaluated preembolization and approximately 1 month postembolization. In all dogs, prostatic tumor size decreased after embolization, and an improvement in clinical signs was noted based on an owner questionnaire.[45]

Other reported cases of embolization include a metastatic bone lesion treated with bland arterial embolization[40] and a cystic nasal adenocarcinoma in a cat. In the nasal adenocarcinoma case, chemoembolization using a combination of carboplatin, polyvinyl alcohol beads, and contrast was performed.[46] Nasal embolization is regularly performed in the author's practice as a primary treatment for nasal tumors. A femoral vascular approach is used,

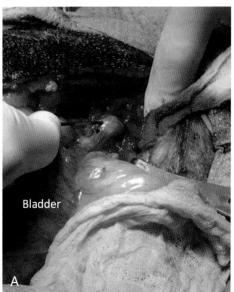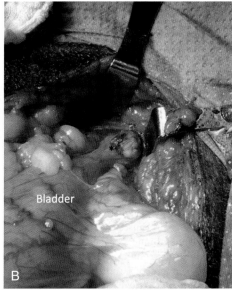

• **Fig. 11.3** Intraprocedural images during radiofrequency ablation (RFA) of a prostatic carcinoma in 15-year-old male castrated mixed breed dog. (A) The RFA electrode has been introduced into the prostate (*) and ultrasound will be used to determine location and depth. (B) After RFA, the ablation zone can be visually seen by the alteration in color of the prostate.

because this allows for selection of both carotid arteries and subsequent bilateral treatment. A coaxial catheterization system is used to allow for superselection of the nasal blood supply.

Ablation

Ablation is a mainstay of IO treatments in humans, and the applications in veterinary patients are expanding. General categories of ablation are chemical and thermal ablation. Chemical ablation usually focuses on the intralesional injection of liquid agents, with ethanol being the most common. Thermal ablation is often subdivided into hyperthermic and hypothermic therapies. The hyperthermic ablative techniques include radiofrequency ablation (RFA), microwave ablation (MWA), high-intensity focused ultrasound (HIFU), and laser ablation, whereas cryoablation is the major hypothermic ablation technique.

Most ablation procedures are performed percutaneously with image guidance, although these procedures can also be performed with minimally invasive or open surgical approaches. For chemical ablation, a needle is usually placed intralesionally and a liquid ablation agent (most commonly ethanol) is injected to cause tissue destruction. Thermal ablation techniques such as RFA, MWA, and cryoablation are performed after the introduction of a probe into the tumor.

After introduction of an RFA electrode into a tumor, the electrode is connected to a generator that produces an electrical current that is transmitted through the electrode into the tumor; the circuit is completed through grounding pads attached to the patient. The electrical current causes ionic agitation of the tissue, which generates heat resulting in coagulation and cellular necrosis.[47] Electrode tips come in a variety of lengths and may be just a single tip or an array of expandable tines. The goal of RFA is to treat a margin of grossly normal tissue beyond the tumor to limit the potential for local recurrence.[48]

RFA is the most studied thermal ablation technique in humans and has been shown to be an excellent treatment option in several studies.[48,49] Most of the work with RFA in veterinary patients has

been in the treatment of parathyroid masses in an effort to control hypercalcemia.[50–52] Recently, the treatment of a prostatic carcinoma in a dog using RFA was described (Fig. 11.3); as the dog was undergoing surgery for removal of metastatic lymph nodes, the RFA procedure was performed via a celiotomy.[53] At surgery, the electrode was placed into the prostatic tumor using ultrasound-guidance and RFA was successfully performed. No signs of residual disease were noted at 8 months post-RFA.

MWA uses electromagnetic energy to cause friction and heat, also resulting in coagulative necrosis.[48] MWA is a more recently described option for tumor ablation and there is significant promise with this modality, especially for veterinary patients. Higher intratumoral temperatures and faster ablations with less char and less pain are often achievable with MWA compared with RFA.[54,55] In addition, this modality does not require grounding pads on the patient, which is beneficial in smaller animals or animals in which grounding pad placement is difficult and may lead to burn injury.

The use of MWA has recently been evaluated in a few veterinary clinical cases.[53,56,57] To date, MWA has been reported to treat liver neoplasia in five dogs, a metastatic pulmonary lesion in one dog, and renal carcinoma in one dog.[53,56,57] In the dogs with liver tumors,[57] a ventral celiotomy was performed and MWA was used to treat hepatic lesions directly. No procedural complications were encountered. A dog with suspected radiation-induced scapular and humeral osteosarcoma was diagnosed with hypertrophic osteopathy after developing a pulmonary metastatic lesion. The metastatic nodule was treated with thoracoscopically guided MWA. Post-MWA evaluation demonstrated resolution of the clinical signs associated with hypertrophic osteopathy.[56] Lastly, a dog with a solitary left renal carcinoma was treated with percutaneous MWA via ultrasound guidance.[53] No complications were reported and the dog is currently 32 months post-MWA with no evidence of disease.[53]

Cryoablation causes cell death by forming ice crystals within cells, through the use of alternating freeze–thaw cycles.[47] Tumors of the head have received the most attention in companion animals when considering cryoablation. Long-term control of a nasal adenocarcinoma was achieved in one dog,[58] and a combination of transarterial embolization, systemic chemotherapy, and cryoablation resulted in partial tumor remission in a dog with a maxillary fibrosarcoma.[59]

Other thermal ablation techniques demonstrating promise and being used more regularly in human patients include HIFU and laser ablation.[60] The use of HIFU for the treatment of a hepatocellular adenoma has been reported in one dog,[61] and investigation into other options is currently ongoing. Laser ablation performed with ultrasound guidance has been described for the palliative treatment of lower urinary tract transitional cell carcinoma in dogs.[62] In a series of dogs undergoing this procedure, the median survival time was 380 days.[62]

Irreversible electroporation (IRE) is another promising ablation technique. For this technique, high-frequency electrical energy is applied to tumor tissue and causes electroporation with increased permeability of cell membranes.[63] The damage results in cellular apoptosis. Although this technique has not been used in companion animals with spontaneous tumors, the potential is tremendous, as the nonthermal electrical characteristic of IRE prevents damage to adjacent structures, such as vessels and nerves, and a higher specificity in tumor targeting.[63]

Drainage

IO techniques provide minimally invasive options for establishing drainage secondary to malignant obstructive disease. The drainage can occur from organs that should normally be able to drain independently (e.g., gallbladder, renal pelvis, and bladder) and body cavities containing malignant effusions. Access to these organs is often possible with ultrasound guidance.

Drainage catheters are generally designed with several features that assist in catheter placement and enhance maintenance of the catheter when in position, including a stiffening cannula, insertion needle, and pigtail (often with a lock). A modified Seldinger technique can often be used for placement of a drainage catheter. Using ultrasound guidance, an over-the-needle catheter is introduced into the organ or cavity in which the drainage catheter will be placed; alternatively, the insertion needle within the drainage catheter can just be directly inserted. If an over-the-needle catheter is used, a guide wire can be inserted through the catheter into the organ or cavity. The over-the-needle catheter is then removed, and the drainage catheter (with stiffening cannula) is passed over the guide wire into the drainage site. Once appropriately positioned, the stiffening cannula can be removed and the drainage catheter advanced over the guide wire, if required. Once the drainage catheter is properly positioned, the guide wire can be removed, and the pigtail loop can be locked.

Veterinary IO has a promising future. Currently, IO techniques are offered in many specialty practices. As knowledge of the options and exposure to the instrumentation increases, so will the experience with these cases and critical evaluation in the veterinary literature. It is likely that advances in IO diagnostics and treatments will mirror what is seen in human medicine and the translational potential is outstanding.

References

1. Culp WT, Mayhew PD, Pascoe PJ, et al.: Angiographic anatomy of the major abdominal arterial blood supply in the dog, *Vet Radiol Ultrasound* 56:474–485, 2015.
2. Blackburn AL, Berent AC, Weisse CW, et al.: Evaluation of outcome following urethral stent placement for the treatment of obstructive carcinoma of the urethra in dogs: 42 cases (2004–2008), *J Am Vet Med Assoc* 242:59–68, 2013.
3. McMillan SK, Knapp DW, Ramos-Vara JA, et al.: Outcome of urethral stent placement for management of urethral obstruction secondary to transitional cell carcinoma in dogs: 19 cases (2007–2010), *J Am Vet Med Assoc* 241:1627–1632, 2012.
4. Weisse C, Berent A, Todd K, et al.: Evaluation of palliative stenting for management of malignant urethral obstructions in dogs, *J Am Vet Med Assoc* 229:226–234, 2006.
5. Berent AC, Weisse C, Beal MW, et al.: Use of indwelling, double-pigtail stents for treatment of malignant ureteral obstruction in dogs: 12 cases (2006–2009), *J Am Vet Med Assoc* 238:1017–1025, 2011.
6. Schlicksup MD, Weisse CW, Berent AC, et al.: Use of endovascular stents in three dogs with Budd-Chiari syndrome, *J Am Vet Med Assoc* 235:544–550, 2009.
7. Culp WT, Macphail CM, Perry JA, et al.: Use of a nitinol stent to palliate a colorectal neoplastic obstruction in a dog, *J Am Vet Med Assoc* 239:222–227, 2011.
8. Culp WT, Weisse C, Cole SG, et al.: Intraluminal tracheal stenting for treatment of tracheal narrowing in three cats, *Vet Surg* 36:107–113, 2007.
9. Hansen KS, Weisse C, Berent AC, et al.: Use of a self-expanding metallic stent to palliate esophageal neoplastic obstruction in a dog, *J Am Vet Med Assoc* 240:1202–1207, 2012.
10. Hume DZ, Solomon JA, Weisse CW: Palliative use of a stent for colonic obstruction caused by adenocarcinoma in two cats, *J Am Vet Med Assoc* 228:392–396, 2006.
11. Radhakrishnan A: Urethral stenting for obstructive uropathy utilizing digital radiography for guidance: feasibility and clinical outcome in 26 dogs, *J Vet Intern Med* 31:427–433, 2017.
12. Christensen NI, Culvenor J, Langova V: Fluoroscopic stent placement for the relief of malignant urethral obstruction in a cat, *Aust Vet J* 88:478–482, 2010.
13. Brace MA, Weisse C, Berent A: Preliminary experience with stenting for management of non-urolith urethral obstruction in eight cats, *Vet Surg* 43:199–208, 2014.
14. Eckman WW, Patlak CS, Fenstermacher JD: A critical evaluation of the principles governing the advantages of intra-arterial infusions, *J Pharmacokinet Biopharm* 2:257–285, 1974.
15. Aigner KR: Intra-arterial infusion: overview and novel approaches, *Semin Surg Oncol* 14:248–253, 1998.
16. Chen HS, Gross JF: Intra-arterial infusion of anticancer drugs: theoretic aspects of drug delivery and review of responses, *Cancer Treat Rep* 64:31–40, 1980.
17. Bertino JR, Boston B, Capizzi RL: The role of chemotherapy in the management of cancer of the head and neck: a review, *Cancer* 36:752–758, 1975.
18. von Scheel J, Golde G: Pharmacokinetics of intra-arterial tumour therapy. An experimental study, *Arch Otorhinolaryngol* 239:153–161, 1984.
19. Stephens FO: Clinical experience in the use of intra-arterial infusion chemotherapy in the treatment of cancers in the head and neck, the extremities, the breast and the stomach, *Recent Results Cancer Res* 86:122–127, 1983.
20. Sakata K, Aoki Y, Karasawa K, et al.: Analysis of the results of combined therapy for maxillary carcinoma, *Cancer* 71:2715–2722, 1993.
21. Robbins KT, Kumar P, Regine WF, et al.: Efficacy of targeted supradose cisplatin and concomitant radiation therapy for advanced head and neck cancer: the Memphis experience, *Int J Radiat Oncol Biol Phys* 38:263–271, 1997.
22. Boeckman HJ, Trego KS, Turchi JJ: Cisplatin sensitizes cancer cells to ionizing radiation via inhibition of nonhomologous end joining, *Mol Cancer Res* 3:277–285, 2005.
23. Rabbani A, Hinerman RW, Schmalfuss IM, et al.: Radiotherapy and concomitant intraarterial cisplatin (RADPLAT) for advanced squamous cell carcinomas of the head and neck, *Am J Clin Oncol* 30:283–286, 2007.

24. Mendenhall WM, Riggs CE, Vaysberg M, et al.: Altered fractionation and adjuvant chemotherapy for head and neck squamous cell carcinoma, *Head Neck* 32:939–945, 2010.

25. Myint WK, Ng C, Raaphorst GP: Examining the non-homologous repair process following cisplatin and radiation treatments, *Int J Radiat Biol* 78:417–424, 2002.

26. McCaw DL: Radiation and cisplatin for treatment of canine urinary bladder carcinoma, *Veterinary Radiology* 29:264–268, 1988.

27. Powers BE, Withrow SJ, Thrall DE, et al.: Percent tumor necrosis as a predictor of treatment response in canine osteosarcoma, *Cancer* 67:126–134, 1991.

28. Withrow SJ, Thrall DE, Straw RC, et al.: Intra-arterial cisplatin with or without radiation in limb-sparing for canine osteosarcoma, *Cancer* 71:2484–2490, 1993.

29. Heidner GL, Page RL, McEntee MC, et al.: Treatment of canine appendicular osteosarcoma using cobalt 60 radiation and intraarterial cisplatin, *J Vet Intern Med* 5:313–316, 1991.

30. Culp WT, Weisse C, Berent AC, et al.: Early tumor response to intraarterial or intravenous administration of carboplatin to treat naturally occurring lower urinary tract carcinoma in dogs, *J Vet Intern Med* 29:900–907, 2015.

31. Lubarsky M, Ray CE, Funaki B: Embolization agents-which one should be used when? Part 1: large-vessel embolization, *Semin Intervent Radiol* 26:352–357, 2009.

32. Breedis C, Young G: The blood supply of neoplasms in the liver, *Am J Pathol* 30:969–977, 1954.

33. Molvar C, Lewandowski RJ: Intra-arterial therapies for liver masses: data distilled, *Radiol Clin North Am* 53:973–984, 2015.

34. Gbolahan OB, Schacht MA, Beckley EW, et al.: Locoregional and systemic therapy for hepatocellular carcinoma, *J Gastrointest Oncol* 8:215–228, 2017.

35. Pesapane F, Nezami N, Patella F, et al.: New concepts in embolotherapy of HCC, *Med Oncol* 34:58, 2017.

36. De Maio E, Fiore F, Daniele B, et al.: Transcatheter arterial procedures in the treatment of patients with hepatocellular carcinoma: a review of literature, *Crit Rev Oncol Hematol* 46:285–295, 2003.

37. Carter S, Martin Ii RC: Drug-eluting bead therapy in primary and metastatic disease of the liver, *HPB (Oxford)* 11:541–550, 2009.

38. Nakakuma K, Tashiro S, Hiraoka T, et al.: Studies on anticancer treatment with an oily anticancer drug injected into the ligated feeding hepatic artery for liver cancer, *Cancer* 52:2193–2200, 1983.

39. Cave TA, Johnson V, Beths T, et al.: Treatment of unresectable hepatocellular adenoma in dogs with transarterial iodized oil and chemotherapy with and without an embolic agent: a report of two cases, *Vet Comp Oncol* 1:191–199, 2003.

40. Weisse C, Clifford CA, Holt D, et al.: Percutaneous arterial embolization and chemoembolization for treatment of benign and malignant tumors in three dogs and a goat, *J Am Vet Med Assoc* 221:1430–1436, 2002.

41. Oishi Y, Tani K, Ozono K, et al.: Transcatheter arterial embolization in normal canine liver, *Vet Surg* 46:797–802, 2017.

42. Iwai S, Okano S, Chikazawa S, et al.: Transcatheter arterial embolization for treatment of hepatocellular carcinoma in a cat, *J Am Vet Med Assoc* 247:1299–1302, 2015.

43. Golzarian J, Antunes AA, Bilhim T, et al.: Prostatic artery embolization to treat lower urinary tract symptoms related to benign prostatic hyperplasia and bleeding in patients with prostate cancer: proceedings from a multidisciplinary research consensus panel, *J Vasc Interv Radiol* 25:665–674, 2014.

44. Sun F, Sanchez FM, Crisostomo V, et al.: Transarterial prostatic embolization: initial experience in a canine model, *AJR Am J Roentgenol* 197:495–501, 2011.

45. Culp WTN, Johnson EG, Palm CA, et al.: Prostatic artery embolization: early results of a novel treatment for prostatic neoplasia in canine patients. In: *Proceedings*, Veterinary Society of Surgical Oncology Meeting. Napa, CA, 2016.

46. Marioni-Henry K, Schwarz T, Weisse C, et al.: Cystic nasal adenocarcinoma in a cat treated with piroxicam and chemoembolization, *J Am Anim Hosp Assoc* 43:347–351, 2007.

47. Gillams AR: Image guided tumour ablation, *Cancer Imaging* 5:103–109, 2005.

48. Facciorusso A, Serviddio G, Muscatiello N: Local ablative treatments for hepatocellular carcinoma: an updated review, *World J Gastrointest Pharmacol Ther* 7:477–489, 2016.

49. Rombouts SJ, Vogel JA, van Santvoort HC, et al.: Systematic review of innovative ablative therapies for the treatment of locally advanced pancreatic cancer, *Br J Surg* 102:182–193, 2015.

50. Rasor L, Pollard R, Feldman EC: Retrospective evaluation of three treatment methods for primary hyperparathyroidism in dogs, *J Am Anim Hosp Assoc* 43:70–77, 2007.

51. Pollard RE, Long CD, Nelson RW, et al.: Percutaneous ultrasonographically guided radiofrequency heat ablation for treatment of primary hyperparathyroidism in dogs, *J Am Vet Med Assoc* 218:1106–1110, 2001.

52. Bucy D, Pollard R, Nelson R: Analysis of factors affecting outcome of ultrasound-guided radiofrequency heat ablation for treatment of primary hyperparathyroidism in dogs, *Vet Radiol Ultrasound* 58:83–89, 2017.

53. Culp WTN, Johnson EG, Palm CA, et al.: Use of thermal ablation techniques in the treatment of canine urogenital neoplasia. In Proceedings. Veterinary Interventional Radiology and Interventional Endoscopy Society Meeting, Cabo San Lucas, Mexico, 2017.

54. Simon CJ, Dupuy DE: Image-guided ablative techniques in pelvic malignancies: radiofrequency ablation, cryoablation, microwave ablation, *Surg Oncol Clin N Am* 14:419–431, 2005.

55. Vogl TJ, Naguib NN, Lehnert T, et al.: Radiofrequency, microwave and laser ablation of pulmonary neoplasms: clinical studies and technical considerations—review article, *Eur J Radiol* 77:346–357, 2011.

56. Mazzaccari K, Boston SE, Toskich BB, et al.: Video-assisted microwave ablation for the treatment of a metastatic lung lesion in a dog with appendicular osteosarcoma and hypertrophic osteopathy, *Vet Surg* 46:1161–1165, 2017.

57. Yang T, Case JB, Boston S, et al.: Microwave ablation for treatment of hepatic neoplasia in five dogs, *J Am Vet Med Assoc* 250:79–85, 2017.

58. Murphy SM, Lawrence JA, Schmiedt CW, et al.: Image-guided transnasal cryoablation of a recurrent nasal adenocarcinoma in a dog, *J Small Anim Pract* 52:329–333, 2011.

59. Weisse C, Berent A, Solomon S: Combined transarterial embolization, systemic cyclophosphamide, and cryotherapy ablation for "Hi-Lo" maxillary fibrosarcoma in a dog, In: *Proceedings*. 8th Annual Meeting, Veterinary Endoscopy Society, 22.

60. Brace C: Thermal tumor ablation in clinical use, *IEEE Pulse* 2:28–38, 2011.

61. Kopelman D, Inbar Y, Hanan?el A, et al.: Magnetic resonance-guided focused ultrasound surgery (MRgFUS). Four ablation treatments of a single canine hepatocellular adenoma, *HPB (Oxford)* 8:292–298, 2006.

62. Cerf DJ, Lindquist EC: Palliative ultrasound-guided endoscopic diode laser ablation of transitional cell carcinomas of the lower urinary tract in dogs, *J Am Vet Med Assoc* 240:51–60, 2012.

63. Lyu T, Wang X, Su Z, et al.: Irreversible electroporation in primary and metastatic hepatic malignancies: a review, *Medicine (Baltimore)* 96:e6386, 2017.

12

Cancer Chemotherapy

DANIEL L. GUSTAFSON AND DENNIS B. BAILEY

General Principles of Cancer Chemotherapy

Mechanism of Cancer Therapy

The use of chemical elixirs for the treatment of cancer can be traced through the medicinal customs and practices of multiple cultures. The modern use of pharmacologic agents to treat cancer began in the mid-1940s when Alfred Gilman and Louis Goodman showed the efficacy of nitrogen mustard in tumor-bearing mice, and these results were quickly translated and verified in human patients. These results and the efforts of others such as Sydney Farber with antifolates and George Hitchings and Gertrude Elion with purine analogs rapidly advanced the growing interest of treating cancer with drugs. The beginning of a systematic screening program for anticancer drugs at the National Cancer Institute (NCI) in 1955 set the framework for cancer chemotherapy development in both the public and private sectors and led to the characterization of many of the agents still in clinical use today.[1,2]

The basis of anticancer drug activity is the targeting of dividing cells through interference with processes involved in progression through the cell cycle. As shown in Fig. 12.1, the major classes of drugs used to treat cancer work at various steps in the processes of DNA replication (S phase) and subsequent cell division (M phase). Another set of therapeutic agents, the signal transduction inhibitors, work by interfering with the signaling processes that trigger entry into the cell cycle and continuing cellular proliferation. This newer class of agents is discussed in Chapter 15, Section B. DNA synthesis is a complicated process involving anabolic processes to create the purine and pyrimidine nucleotide triphosphates required for replication, unwinding of the template DNA to provide access to the replication machinery, and the high-fidelity process of creating complementary strands. Anticancer drugs may work at any of these steps, including the antimetabolites that inhibit anabolic processes required for providing the nucleotide building blocks, topoisomerase inhibitors that interfere with the enzymatic process of DNA unwinding, and alkylating/DNA binding agents that can either act in a bifunctional manner to cross-link DNA through either interstrand or intrastrand interactions blocking strand separation and template processing, or in a monofunctional manner interfering with the replication machinery through multiple mechanisms of altered binding and base recognition. The resulting effects of interacting at these levels of DNA replication can include the generation of DNA strand breaks, incomplete replication, and triggering of apoptotic signaling such that cell death is the ultimate result.

Processes in cell division not involving DNA replication are also targets for anticancer agents. The most prominent of these targets is tubulin, with several classes of drugs having antitubulin activity. The mechanism of action of these agents involves either inhibiting the polymerization of tubulin or stabilizing the polymerized form so that depolymerization is blocked. The result of blocking either of these processes is the inhibition of microtubule function in the dividing cell. Microtubule function is critical to progression through mitosis via spindle fiber formation and the separation of chromosome pairs into daughter cells. Blockade of this process by antitubulin agents has proved to be an effective strategy because cells blocked in this part of the cell cycle (M phase) can undergo apoptosis, other mechanisms of cell death and loss of viability.

Terminology and Concepts

Terms that are related to the efficacy and toxicity of cancer chemotherapy are important concepts for understanding their pharmacologic activity. The *therapeutic index* for a given chemotherapeutic agent is the ratio between the toxic dose and the therapeutic dose for that drug. For most cytotoxic drugs used to treat cancer, the therapeutic index is an abstract parameter because the administered dose is based on the *maximum tolerated dose* (MTD) rather than dose response. The MTD is an empirically derived value that represents the highest dose of a given drug that can be administered with few patients experiencing unacceptable or irreversible adverse effects (AEs). MTD is initially derived from a limited population sample and then refined with additional clinical experience. This is an important concept in cancer drug administration in that drug doses are generally based on this value rather than assessments of efficacy. A newer concept for drugs used to treat cancer is the *biologically effective dose* (BED), based on a measured response at a putative target or surrogate that is related to the mechanism of action of the agent. Determination of the BED is currently more related to the use of signal transduction inhibitors and molecularly targeted agents; however, the concept is not exclusive to these agents and this approach may be useful when applied to cytotoxic chemotherapy using dosing protocols not based on the MTD. *Dose intensity* (DI) is a measure of dose per unit of time and thus allows comparisons between protracted and compacted dosing schedules. Comparisons of DI between, for example, every 3 weeks and every week dosing allows for determining whether the total dose of the drug or the DI relates to toxicity or therapeutic outcome and the effect that altering dosing

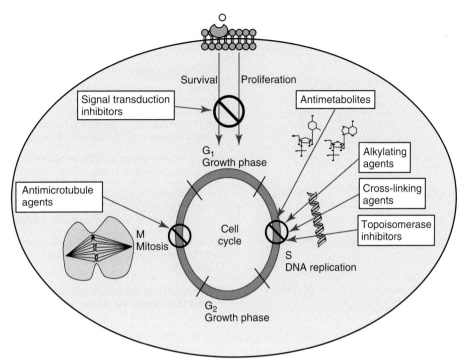

• **Fig. 12.1** Cell cycle specificity of the major classes of drugs used in cancer chemotherapy. Although agents may have effects throughout the cell cycle, the phase where the major effect is realized is highlighted.

schedules can have on outcome. *Therapeutic gain* is often evaluated when combining two drugs or a drug with radiation therapy, and quantitatively describes any improved tumor response relative to increased normal tissue toxicity when agents are used in a planned schedule. The basis for a positive therapeutic gain is the additive or synergistic tumor effects that exceed any summative toxicity patterns in normal tissues accomplished with combination therapy.

Indications and Goals of Therapy

The therapeutic intent and goals of a given chemotherapeutic regimen are important contributors to how a given drug is selected or assessed. *Primary induction chemotherapy* refers to drug therapy administered as the first treatment for patients with hematopoietic cancers and advanced cancers for which no alternative treatment exists. *Primary neoadjuvant chemotherapy* is the utilization of chemotherapeutic drugs before treatment with other modalities, primarily surgical removal of the primary tumor, with the intent of decreasing tumor size and/or clinical stage (*downstaging*) for improved control and preventing possible postoperative growth of micrometastasis. *Adjuvant chemotherapy* is the treatment with chemotherapeutic drugs after the surgical removal or radiation control of the primary tumor. The purpose is to treat occult disease, residual tumor cells after incomplete excision of the primary tumor, and/or micrometastases. In general, chemotherapy is most effective in the adjuvant setting potentially owing to factors associated with the smaller size of residual disease and developing metastases, leading to enhanced drug delivery and more favorable growth kinetics associated with a larger dividing fraction of cells. *Consolidation therapy*, used most commonly with hematopoietic cancers, is the reintensification of therapy after remission is attained to further reduce the likelihood of relapse. *Maintenance therapy* is also used after remission is attained but involves low-intensity therapy given over a protracted period of time. *Rescue*

or *salvage therapy* is the use of chemotherapy after a tumor fails to respond to a previous therapy or after tumor recurrence. *Palliative chemotherapy* is delivered to decrease clinical signs in the case of unresectable or disseminated disease that is associated with functional disturbances or pain. The outcome of this therapy is based more on quality of life issues as opposed to other metrics of tumor response. The more subjective nature of assessing the effect of palliative chemotherapy, especially in terms of pain control, makes systematic testing of protocols difficult and treatment recommendations more at the discretion of the clinician and client. In cases in which organ function is affected by tumor growth, more objective endpoints may exist in terms of functional improvements after treatment. Doses and scheduling of palliative intent therapies may also differ, as strict adherence to schedules originating from trials where objective responses were measured may not be relevant and more patient-based endpoints may be employed. *Radiosensitization* is the enhancement of cytotoxicity when irradiation and chemotherapeutic agents are combined such that a therapeutic gain is obtained. The basis for chemotherapeutic exposure leading to enhanced radiosensitivity can be multifaceted and involve (1) the enrichment of the tumor cell population in a more sensitive phase of the cell cycle, (2) increased tumor oxygenation through cytoreduction or alterations in tumor vascularization, and (3) selective killing of inherently radioresistant hypoxic cell fractions.

As a preliminary metric, the clinical measurements of the tumor response to cancer chemotherapy are useful for predicting the effect of treatment on the extent of disease or time interval of tumor control. Table 12.1 describes conventional measures of treatment response.

Tumor Susceptibility and Resistance

Tumor Cell Sensitivity

Individual cell sensitivity to anticancer agents has been addressed empirically through the screening of tumor cell panels associated

TABLE 12.1	Measures of Response in Cancer Therapy and Treatment	
Response Term	Abbreviation	Description
Complete remission/response	CR	Complete disappearance of tumor(s) and symptoms of disease.
Partial remission/response	PR	Decrease in tumor volume of ≥50% or decrease in tumor maximum diameter of >30%.
Stable disease	SD	Neither an increase nor a decrease in tumor size (e.g., <30% reduction or <20% increase in tumor maximum diameter).
Progressive disease	PD	Increase in tumor volume of >25% or increase of tumor maximum diameter of >20%; appearance of new lesions.
Median response duration/median survival time	MRD/MST	The median value for a group of individuals treated with a given therapy in terms of the length of time they achieved a complete or partial remission (MRD) or length of survival after implementation of therapy (MST).
Progression-free interval/progression-free survival	PFI/PFS	The amount of time elapsed without evidence of progressive tumor growth (PFI) or survival without progressive growth of the tumor from treatment start (PFS).
Disease-free interval/disease-free survival	DFI/DFS	The amount of time that elapses without disease recurrence (DFI) or survival (DFS) of the patient after therapy.

with a given histotype. Human cancer cell line databases that include both genomic and drug response data are publicly available and include the NCI60 (https://dtp.cancer.gov), Cancer Cell Line Encyclopedia (CCLE) (https://portals.broadinstitute.org/ccle), and Genomics of Drug Sensitivity in Cancer (CCSG) (https://www.cancerrxgene.org). The rich gene expression and other features of these cell lines allow for drug sensitivity and genotypic characteristics to be explored.[3] The use of canine tumor cell line panels to screen drug sensitivity is becoming established as a viable way to identify potential drug combinations for further testing as well.[4]

Chemosensitivity depends on a number of factors, including drug uptake into the cell, interaction with a cellular target, generation of lethal damage to important cellular macromolecules, repair of potentially lethal damage, and the cell's response to generated damage as depicted in Fig. 12.2. Uptake of some cancer chemotherapeutic agents occurs via passive diffusion because of their lipid-soluble properties, whereas other compounds are actively transported into tumor cells. Melphalan is actively transported into cells by two amino acid transporters,[5] and blocking transport with amino acid substrates or analogs can significantly affect cytotoxicity.[6] Other examples include nucleoside transporters used by Ara-C [7] and gemcitabine[8] and the reduced folate carrier system involved in methotrexate uptake.[9] The intracellular target(s) for specific chemotherapeutic agents can play a role in determining sensitivity based on their levels and the nature of the interaction. For example, topoisomerase IIα levels can play a role in the sensitivity of tumor cells to doxorubicin (DOX),[10,11] as altered levels via decreased gene copy or transcriptional downregulation leads to a decrease in sensitivity (resistance). The opposite is true for thymidylate synthetase levels and 5-fluorouracil (5-FU) toxicity, where increased levels of enzyme correlate with a decrease in sensitivity to 5-FU.[12] Although the nature of the interaction with the target is different for DOX and 5-FU, the fact that altered target levels can modulate response show how quantitative interactions with the target can alter drug sensitivity.

The extent of cellular damage, potential repair of that damage, and the cellular response occur in a tightly knit continuum that

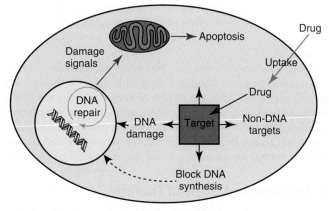

• **Fig. 12.2** Processes involved in the pharmacologic activity and associated chemosensitivity of chemotherapeutic agents in tumor cells. Associated processes include drug uptake, interaction with drug target, effect on DNA and associated DNA repair, and the cellular response to these effects.

determines cellular fate. The generation of cellular damage is a consequence of interaction with a cellular target and can be either a primary or a secondary event. In general, for DNA-damaging agents, the resulting DNA lesions are a result of the interplay of DNA binding and DNA repair. For example, DNA strand breaks that result from O^6-methyl guanine lesions are because of aberrant mismatch repair processes and subsequent replication.[13] DNA damage also triggers response pathways that can result in cell cycle arrest to allow for repair and subsequent survival, or the triggering of apoptotic machinery that ultimately results in cell death. The definition of cellular response, be it mitotic catastrophe, apoptosis, necrosis, autophagy, or cellular stasis, is dependent on an intricate interplay of survival and death signaling and is often specific to the agent, the dose at the critical target, and the cell lineage.[14] Alterations in pro- and antiapoptotic signaling clearly play a role in tumorigenesis and response to therapy,[15] and the effect of antiapoptotic signaling in lymphoma by the mediators bcl-2 and survivin seem the most clear both in regard to chemosensitivity[16–18] and response to therapy in humans and dogs[19–21]; however, a clear understanding of the role of damage response and active cell death pathways in chemosensitivity and response in solid tumors is still lacking.

Tumor Cell Resistance

Acquired resistance, or selection of resistant cells, during the treatment process is thought to be one of the major mechanisms of therapeutic failure during cancer drug therapy. Resistance of tumor cells to chemotherapeutic agents can be drug and mechanism dependent or can occur through a multidrug mechanism. In general, acquired resistance to a specific agent can develop via a variety of mechanisms associated with drug uptake, drug metabolism/detoxification, target modification, damage repair, or damage recognition and response. Changes in intracellular drug concentrations can come about either because of a decrease in drug uptake or through increased efflux. Decreased expression of transporters known to play a role in drug uptake has been observed in resistance to treatment with melphalan in human breast cancer cells,[22] and acquired resistance to methotrexate in KB carcinoma cells.[23] The induction of drug efflux pumps in response to drug treatment is a primary mechanism for multidrug resistance and will be discussed later in this section.

Alterations in metabolic or detoxification pathways within tumor cells are another mechanism by which acquired resistance may be acquired. As many chemotherapeutic agents are electrophilic based on their DNA-binding properties, enhancement of conjugation reactions with nucleophiles such as glutathione is a plausible mechanism of resistance.[24] Induction of glutathione-S-transferases has been shown to be a mechanism by which tumor cells can acquire resistance to nitrogen mustards.[25,26] Although tumor cells themselves generally have limited drug metabolism capabilities, some metabolic pathways can play a role in the resistance phenotype. For example, the sensitivity of tumor cells to 5-FU is inversely correlated with the expression of dihydropyrimidine dehydrogenase,[27–29] the enzyme predominantly responsible for the metabolism of 5-FU to the inactive 5-FUH$_2$ metabolite.[30] For the prodrug gemcitabine, which must be phosphorylated to the di- and triphosphate forms before eliciting an inhibitory effect on DNA synthesis,[31,32] the enzyme responsible for this metabolic activation, deoxycytidine kinase,[33,34] is decreased in pancreatic tumor cells made resistant to this drug.[35] This interplay between metabolic detoxification and activation, predominantly with nucleotide analogs, leads to complex scenarios involving upregulation of catabolic processes and the downregulation of anabolic processes influencing the cellular pharmacology of these agents.

Modifications in the cellular target of a given drug usually pertain to mutations in the target protein leading to a decrease in affinity or absence of drug interaction. These modifications can include a decrease in the levels of a specific target responsible for the generation of a toxic product, increases in target levels to ameliorate the effect of target inhibition, or target mutations such that the drug can no longer interact in a manner detrimental to the tumor cell. Decreased topoisomerase II gene expression and activity has been observed in human lung and colon cells with acquired resistance to the epipodophyllotoxins etoposide and teniposide,[36] whose antitumor activity involves topoisomerase II–dependent DNA strand break formation.[37] Target amplification as a mechanism of acquired resistance has been observed in methotrexate resistance, where gene amplification and increased dihydrofolate reductase (DHFR) levels allow for cells to overcome DHFR inhibition.[38] Mutations in targets such as β-tubulin in the case of

paclitaxel[39] and topoisomerase I for camptothecin[40] affect binding of drug and interaction with the target, thus conferring resistance.

Damage repair in cancer cells treated with chemotherapy commonly refers to DNA repair processes, as a majority of chemotherapy agents work at the level of the DNA. Resistance conferred through alteration in DNA repair includes not only the induction of specific processes to repair discrete lesions but also more global DNA repair processes such as postreplication and mismatch repair.[41] Multiple studies have shown that enhanced removal of platinum adducts from tumor cell DNA correlates with acquired resistance to cisplatin,[42–44] although the exact mechanism(s) and protein(s) responsible for repair of these lesions are unknown. The bulky DNA adducts generated by many cancer chemotherapeutic agents can cause replicative gaps in DNA that require postreplication surveillance and repair. The ability of cells to bypass these bulky lesions and interstrand cross-links during DNA replication is important in tolerance to agents causing these types of DNA damage (cisplatin, mitomycin C, melphalan), and multiple DNA repair pathways can account for this release from the DNA replication block.[45] The fact that DNA repair pathways and processes are redundant and nondiscrete and that both lesion-specific and global processes seem to play a role in determining drug resistance highlights the problems associated with attributing specific resistance phenotypes to specific proteins or pathways. This problem may be addressed with unbiased genomic or proteomic approaches that profile multiple factors.

Tumor cell drug resistance associated with alterations in cellular damage recognition and response is generally associated with defects in apoptosis.[15] Generally, these alterations in apoptosis signaling are not a response to therapy but rather are preexisting and play a role in initial sensitivity. This is exemplified in a study showing that although survivin expression was shown to be predictive for response to CHOP (Cyclophosphamide, Hydroxydaunorubicin, Oncovin [vincristine], and Prednisone) therapy in canine lymphoma, survivin expression in patient-matched samples pretreatment and at relapse showed no significant difference.[21] This suggests that the role of antiapoptotic, prosurvival signaling diminishes the initial response to drug therapy as opposed to facilitating survival of initially drug-sensitive clones through an acquired mechanism.

Some mechanisms of acquired resistance result in a phenotype in which the tumor is resistant to multiple chemotherapeutic agents, or multidrug resistant (MDR). Some of the mechanisms discussed earlier, including DNA repair, enhanced metabolism or detoxification, and resistance to apoptosis can result in resistance to multiple agents; however, the "MDR phenotype" generally refers to tumor cells expressing individual or multiple members of the ATP-binding cassette (ABC) transporter family, which plays a primary role in active efflux of drugs from cells. Forty-eight ABC genes have been identified in the human genome,[46] and currently 15 members of the ABC transporter family have been recognized that include a cancer drug as a substrate for transport.[47] These include the well-studied and well-characterized PGP/MDR1 (ABCB1), MXR/BCRP (ABCG2), MRP1 (ABCC1), and MRP2 (ABCC2). The basic function of the ABC transporters is conserved across the family and involves the ATP-dependent transport of xenobiotics and endogenous substrates from the inside of the cell to the extracellular space. The role of ABC transporters in multidrug resistance of canine and feline cancers is poorly explored; however, ABCB1 is expressed in canine lymphoma,[48] mammary tumors,[49] and canine and feline primary pulmonary carcinomas.[50] ABCC1, ABCC2, ABCC5, ABCC10, and ABCG2 are expressed in canine mammary tumors as well.[49,51] The normal tissue distribution of the ABC transporters is also beginning to be investigated in dogs, with initial studies showing relatively similar tissue distributions and presumed function.[52,53] Feline ABCG2 has specific amino acid changes that lead to transporter dysfunction with regard to a number of substrates, suggesting that cats may have altered pharmacokinetic disposition for drugs that are ABCG2 substrates.[54]

Combination Therapies

The success of combination chemotherapy compared with single-agent treatment is attributed to providing maximal cell kill within the range of tolerable host toxicity, providing a broader range of interactions between the drugs and the heterogeneous tumor cell population, and slowing the development of cellular drug resistance. However, certain guidelines should be followed when designing a combination protocol.[55] Only drugs with known efficacy as single agents against the cancer of interest should be included, with preference for drugs that can induce a complete remission in at least some patients. Whenever possible, drugs with nonoverlapping toxicities should be used. This potentially will result in a wider range of AEs, but a lower risk of a severe or life-threatening episode. Lastly, drugs should be used at their optimal dose and schedule, and drug combinations should be given at consistent intervals.

The success of combination therapies as opposed to single-agent therapy is best illustrated in veterinary oncology by treatment protocols for canine lymphoma. DOX is the most active single-agent therapy tested, and the addition of DOX to other active protocols (i.e., cyclophosphamide [CP], vincristine, and prednisone) empirically increases median remission duration and median survival time compared with either DOX alone or combinations without DOX (see Chapter 33, Table 33.4).[56–72] In contrast, in dogs with appendicular osteosarcoma (OSA), adjuvant treatment with combinations of platinum and DOX empirically does not show any improvement in disease-free interval or survival over those treated with single-agent DOX or platinum protocols (see Chapter 25, Table 25.2).[73]

The concept of summation dose-intensity (SDI) can be used to compare different combination chemotherapy protocols.[74,75] The contribution of each drug is based on its fractional dose-intensity (DI) (relative to maximum DI when the drug is used as a single agent) and its relative antitumor potency compared with the other drugs included in the protocol. The individual contributions of each drug are then added together. SDI > 1 implies a benefit over monotherapy using the single-most active drug at its MTD and optimum dosing schedule. SDI = 1 implies equality, and SDI < 1 implies diminished efficacy.

Toxicities Associated with Drug Therapy of Cancer

Chemotherapy may fail to produce a positive clinical benefit for the reasons described earlier but may also fail because of unacceptable toxicity. Anticipating and managing AEs requires a thorough understanding of drug activity profiles and clinical experience modifying chemotherapeutic administration. The first step in the process of successfully managing cancer in companion animals is always a clear and frank discussion with the owner regarding the potential for benefit, toxicity, cost, and time commitment. A common understanding about the goals of therapy, and committing to

a continuing dialog as needs may change throughout treatment, cannot be underestimated.

Dosing conventions have been developed from formal phase I studies for an increasing number of agents investigated specifically in companion animals. Nonetheless, suggested starting doses represent an estimate of the MTD from a small population of animals, and safe individual patient dosing may vary substantially. There are numerous reasons for pharmacokinetic variability in cancer drugs among a population of patients.[76] Concurrent illness or organ dysfunction, extreme tumor burden, specific breed sensitivities (e.g., Collies with ABCB1 *mut/mut*), or idiosyncratic considerations (anticipated drug–drug interactions or drug allergies) will mandate modifications of the protocol and dosing. Concurrent illness and organ dysfunction can have profound effects on selection of anticancer agents and dosing. In general, predictable dose adjustments for pets with renal or hepatic disease have not been developed and treatment should be approached conservatively. Interestingly, in cats, the glomerular filtration rate (GFR) can be used to define an individual dose for carboplatin that will permit some patients with renal disease to be safely dosed that would not have been safe if dosed by conventional methods.[77] Chemotherapeutic dosing in obese patients often raises questions about drug partitioning in lipid storage sites around the body. Distribution of many pharmaceutical agents may be affected in obese patients; however, there is no accepted scale for empiric dose adjustments in humans. Individual factors such as the specific drug, degree of obesity, and other comorbidities may convince a clinician to dose reduce or cap the dose of a chemotherapeutic agent.[78] Some reviews suggest that dose reductions based on body mass may ultimately be detrimental to outcomes in obese patients.[79] It is the initial chemotherapeutic intervention that is expected to result in the greatest opportunity to benefit the patient and, therefore, thoroughly assessing the patient's specific medical limitations and then proceeding with thoughtfully designing, administering, and completing a therapeutically robust protocol is highly desirable.

As individual patient tolerance and response to each compound in a multiagent protocol is observed, future modifications may be anticipated more accurately. The greatest benefit achievable with anticancer cytotoxic therapy requires a commitment to dose intensity. Optimal dose intensity demands therapeutic monitoring to either reduce *or* increase the dose based on the patient's capacity to maintain an acceptable quality of life during effective therapy. The decision to increase the dose of an agent is conceptually challenging but important. To make a recommendation to increase dosing of a cytotoxic compound, owner understanding and monitoring of the patient's hematologic values and clinical events during the first treatment cycle are critical. A dose of a cytotoxic agent that does not result in any change in the target normal tissue (e.g., blood neutrophil count) is likely ineffective and could potentially be increased at the next infusion with continued follow-up to determine adequacy of dose adjustments (Fig. 12.3). Dose reductions are deleterious to the optimum delivery of chemotherapy but are to be anticipated. Specific guidelines for dose adjustments of antineoplastic agents are not standardized and are done empirically with a 10% to 25% reduction in dose generally considered for patients experiencing severe or unacceptable hematologic or gastrointestinal AEs. Close monitoring and preemptive management of signs may permit successful management of any potential future clinical signs, and clinical management is based on the extent and severity of the resulting signs as described in Table 12.2.

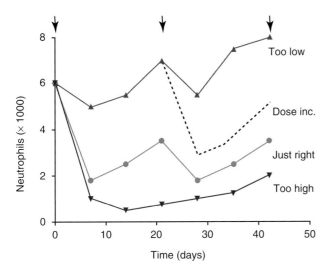

• **Fig. 12.3** Blood neutrophil patterns after chemotherapy treatments *(arrows)*. The appropriate dose *(circles)* results in noticeable nadirs with return to normal before the next dose. Doses that are too high or too low should prompt dose adjustments, including potential dose increases *(dashed line)*.

The AEs for anticancer agents may be categorized into acute toxicities (at the time or within 24–48 hours after treatment), acute delayed effects (2–14 days), or cumulative/chronic toxicity (weeks, months, or years). Acute toxicity may include infusion hypersensitivities because of histamine release associated with allergic (L-asparaginase) or allergic-like (DOX) reactions, or vehicle-induced mast cell degranulation (e.g., paclitaxel, etoposide). Routine management of these events with antihistamines and corticosteroids may significantly mitigate this problem. Acute nausea and vomiting may occur with specific agents (e.g., cisplatin, dacarbazine, streptozotocin) or when the infusion is too rapid (e.g., DOX). Preemptive antiemetic management often manages these AEs. Drugs with vesicant properties can cause moderate or severe tissue necrosis if not administered safely through a suitable catheter. Vinca alkaloid, DOX, mechlorethamine, and actinomycin D extravasations can be very severe situations that should be avoided, even if sedation is required or rescheduling is required for safe catheter placement. Owners need to be informed about this possibility before treatment and a management plan for this situation should be developed. Management recommendations for extravasations are included in the individual drug descriptions in the text that follows.

TABLE 12.2   Guidelines for Common Chemotherapy-Induced Toxicity

	Prophylaxis	Grade 2/Mild Toxicity	Grade 3/Moderate Toxicity	Grade 4/Severe Toxicity
Neutropenia		1000–1500/ μL	500–999/μL	<500/μL, with or without fever
Broad-spectrum antibiotics	Not recommended	No	Oral.[a] If fever, then hospitalize and IV.[b] CBC in 2–5 days.	Oral.[a] If fever, then hospitalize and IV.[b] CBC in 24 hours.
Parenteral fluids (SQ or IV) and supportive care	No	No	Not routine unless febrile.	Not routine unless febrile.
Nausea/vomiting		<3 vomiting episodes	3–5 episodes/day for 2–4 days	>5 episodes/24 hours or >4 days
Antiemetics[c]	Oral, if prior experience warrants.	Oral or IV as indicated.	IV	IV
H₂ blocker,[d] proton pump inhibitor[e]	Oral, if prior experience warrants.	Oral or IV as indicated.	IV	IV
Parenteral fluids (SQ or IV) and supportive care	No	As indicated.	Yes	Yes, hospitalize.
Diarrhea		2 stools/day over baseline	3–6 stools/day over baseline	>6 stools/day
Diet adjustment	Yes	Yes	Yes	Yes
Antidiarrheals[f]	Yes	Yes	Yes	Yes
Parenteral fluids (SQ or IV) and supportive care	No	No	Yes	Yes, hospitalize.

CBC, Complete blood count; *IV,* intravenous; *SQ,* subcutaneous.

[a]Enrofloxacin (dog: 10 mg/kg PO q24h, cat: 2.5–5 mg/kg PO q24h) or Clavamox (13.75 mg/kg PO q12h).

[b]Ampicillin (20 mg/kg IV q8h) or ampicillin/sulbactam (30 mg/kg IV q8h) and enrofloxacin (dog: 10 mg/kg IV q24h, cat: 2.5–5 mg/kg IV q24h).

[c]Maropitant (dogs: 1 mg/kg IV or SC, 2 mg/kg PO, once daily, cats: 1 mg/kg PO, SC, or IV). Ondansetron (0.5–1.0 mg/kg IV or PO, q12–24h).

[d]Famotidine (0.5–1.0 mg/kg PO, SQ, or IV).

[e]Pantoprazole (1 mg/kg IV or SQ as needed).

[f]Loperamide (0.08 mg/kg PO q8h); tylosin (10 mg/kg PO q12h); metronidazole 15 to 25 mg/kg PO q12h).

Delayed acute effects from chemotherapy often include bone marrow suppression and nausea, vomiting, and diarrhea. In the majority of instances these effects are self-limiting, and the incidence of hospitalization is low. Table 12.2 reviews the general therapeutic strategies for management of the most common types of AEs experienced in companion animals after chemotherapy.[80]

Examples of potential cumulative and/or chronic toxicity include hepatic dysfunction after multiple doses of lomustine (CCNU), cardiac abnormalities after exceeding a safe cumulative dose of DOX (dogs), and renal disease after cisplatin (dogs) or DOX (cats) use. Screening recommendations and strategies to reduce the risks of such chronic effects have been developed and are incorporated into standard protocol procedures. It is critical to the success of treatment that owners be thoroughly informed about monitoring guidelines for the signs of chemotherapy-induced toxicity. Owner online educational resources are readily available at www.csuanimalcancercenter.org. It is advisable to instruct the owner regarding monitoring and early responses when his or her pet experiences nausea and vomiting, diarrhea, or hematuria and it is important to inform the owner about how to obtain an accurate body temperature. These "at home" aids will allow the clinician to assess the management options should a concern arise.

Safety Concerns of Cancer Drug Therapy

Handling cytotoxic chemotherapy drugs is classified as an occupational health hazard by the National Institute for Occupational Safety and Health (www.cdc.gov/niosh/topics/hazdrug/). Cytotoxic chemotherapy drugs are mutagenic, carcinogenic, teratogenic, abortifacient, and increase the risk of stillbirth.[81–84] Veterinary hospitals that handle chemotherapy drugs must be aware of and comply with evolving federal and state guidelines, and only trained personnel should be involved with handling these drugs or the patients that receive them. Clients must also be informed about potential hazards, particularly for women who are pregnant or breastfeeding, and for young children.

Chemotherapy should be stored, prepared, and used in designated areas that are clearly labeled. Ideally, these areas should be dedicated solely for these tasks, with access restricted for unauthorized personnel. Eating, drinking, smoking, chewing gum, using tobacco, applying cosmetics, or storing food or drinks must be prohibited in these areas. Chemotherapy ideally should be prepared in a class II, type B2 biologic safety cabinet (BSC). This type of BSC provides inward airflow, downward HEPA-filtered laminal airflow, and HEPA-filtered exhausted air that is 100% ventilated outside. The use of a closed-system transfer device (CSTD) such as PhaSeal, Equashield, Chemoclave, or Onguard is recommended as well. A CSTD mechanically prevents the escape of drug or vapor out of the system into the environment and reduces the risk of accidental needle puncture.[85] These precautions reduce environmental contamination, but do not obviate the need for personal protective equipment (PPE). Double-gloving is recommended using powder-free latex or nitrile gloves that are chemotherapy rated by ASTM International standards. Gowns should be disposable, impermeable, closed-front style, and long-sleeved with elastic or knit cuffs. Eye and face protection should be used when there is a high risk for splashes or aerosols, such as with intralesional chemotherapy injections. Respiratory protection using a fitted respirator with an N95 rating is required when engineering mechanisms cannot control exposure of an aerosolized drug (e.g., a drug spill). Guidelines for limiting exposure to hazardous drugs

in the workplace has been addressed through the United States Department of Labor.[86]

Chemotherapy must be administered in a quiet location without distraction. Oral chemotherapy drugs should be intact; tablets should never be split or crushed, and capsules should never be opened. Oral liquid preparations are not recommended because of a risk of inaccurate dosing and environmental contamination if some of the medication is spit out. For intravenous (IV) chemotherapy, the smallest gauge and shortest length of catheter to accommodate therapy should be used, and it must be placed via a "clean stick." Only nonheparinized saline flushes should be used. IV pumps should be avoided, except for multihour infusions (e.g., cytosine arabinoside, dacarbazine). Chemical restraint should be considered as-needed to ensure the safety of the patient and treating personnel.

When dealing with chemotherapy spills, there is no universal cleaning agent; however, use of a sodium hypochlorite (bleach) solution, a strong detergent, and water will deactivate and remove most hazardous drug residues.[86] Alcohol will not deactivate chemotherapy drugs and can spread contamination. Chemotherapy drugs and their metabolites can be excreted in urine, feces, saliva, and vomitus. Urinary levels of some active drugs may remain high for days after treatment,[87] and fecal excretion may also be expected. Contaminated excreta should be handled like a chemotherapy spill.

Pharmacologic Principles in Cancer Therapy

Pharmacokinetics

Pharmacokinetic (PK) considerations in cancer drug therapy are important because of the relationship between drug exposure and pharmacodynamic (PD) response, be it efficacy or toxicity, that is more exact than the relationship between drug dose and PD response.[88] PK considerations are also important with regard to interactions with other drugs,[89] herbal products,[90,91] and genetic differences among breeds and individuals that can cause changes in drug exposure at a given dose.[92] Cytotoxic chemotherapy is usually dosed on an MTD-based schedule reflecting only acceptable toxicity and thus limits any informative role of drug half-life and effective therapeutic concentrations from initial dosing considerations. The most important PK parameters are those that have a relationship with either a response to therapy (efficacy) or toxicity, which is most often either the area under the plasma/serum concentration versus time curve (AUC) or the maximum drug concentration achieved (C_{max}), illustrated in Fig. 12.4. The relationships of AUC and C_{max} in the clinical pharmacology of DOX illustrate the complex associations with PK considerations. The C_{max} during DOX infusion in humans is related to the incidence of cardiotoxicity both in adult[93] and pediatric[94] patients, but is also associated with longer remissions in leukemia patients.[95] A relationship between AUC values and decreased white blood cells has also been established with DOX[96]; however, no clear relationships between AUC and efficacy exist.[97] These data have allowed for adjustments in DOX dosing protocols such that intermediate infusion times (10–30 minutes) are utilized to decrease the C_{max} and thus cardiotoxicity, while still maintaining peak levels associated with effective therapy.

PK studies that relate drug exposure to responses are an important first step in establishing relationships that may be exploited for dose modification based on patient characteristics or therapeutic drug monitoring. These data are generally lacking for the drugs

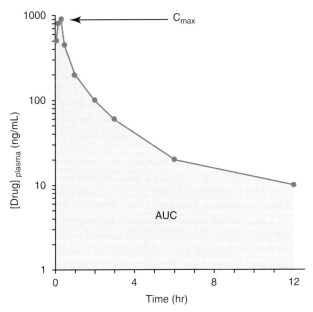

• **Fig. 12.4** Illustration of pharmacokinetic parameters C_{max} and area under the curve *(AUC)* in a theoretical drug plasma concentration versus time plot.

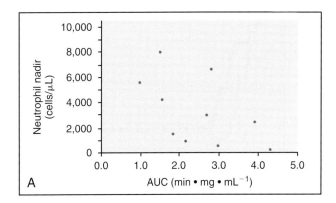

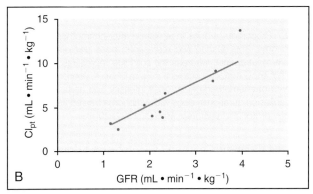

• **Fig. 12.5** Relationship between (A) neutrophil nadir and carboplatin exposure and (B) platinum clearance and glomerular filtration rate *(GFR)* in cats being treated for cancer. *AUC*; Area under the curve. (From Bailey DB, Rassnick KM, Erb HN, et al: Effect of glomerular filtration rate on clearance and myelotoxicity of carboplatin in cats with tumors, *Am J Vet Res* 65:1502, 2004.)

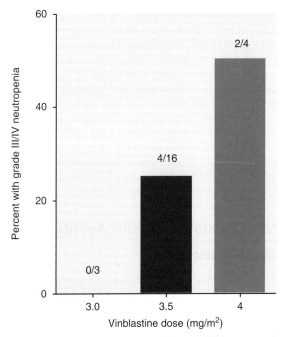

• **Fig. 12.6** Relationship of prevalence of grade III/IV neutropenia with vinblastine dose in dogs being treated for cancer. (Data from Bailey DB, Rassnick KM, Kristal O, et al: Phase I dose escalation of single-agent vinblastine in dogs, *J Vet Intern Med* 22:1397, 2008.)

used to treat cancer in companion animals, with a few exceptions. Studies on the PK and myelotoxicity of carboplatin in cats have shown a clear relationship between drug exposure and the neutrophil nadir and also drug clearance and GFR (Fig. 12.5). The fact that PK parameters can be correlated both with a toxic endpoint and a physiologic function allows for the calculation of a dosing metric relating the GFR of an individual cat to a dose that produces a drug exposure (AUC) that results in acceptable toxicity.[77] It remains to be determined whether such individualized dosing results in improved outcome in a heterogeneous population. The current drug-dosing convention for cancer drugs is the use of body surface area (BSA) for dose normalization (mg/m²). Exceptions to this paradigm are the use of body weight (mg/kg) for dogs that weigh less than 15 kg and for cats with DOX dosing, based on empiric evidence showing a better toxicity profile for smaller animals when mg/kg dosing is used.[98] The approximate calculation for BSA in dogs and cats based on weight is as follows:

$$m^2 = \frac{A \times (\text{weight in grams})^{\frac{2}{3}}}{10,000}$$

where *A* is equal to 10.1 for dogs and 10.0 for cats.

Pharmacodynamics

Pharmacodynamic (PD) considerations for cytotoxic chemotherapy are generally related to standard measures of response (i.e., CR, PR, SD, etc.) and AEs.[99] A majority of the literature in veterinary oncology relates PD responses to specific drugs or combinations, doses, or schedules. Fig. 12.6 shows the relationships between vinblastine dose and the incidence of grade III or IV neutropenia observed in a Phase I cohort of dogs.[100] These results relate a dose to a PD response with the absence of exposure PK data. PD endpoints can also be used as indicators of efficacy and potentially as targets of therapy. The proportion of dogs in remission after treatment for lymphoma is increased in the group that experienced grade III or IV neutropenia compared with the group that did not (Fig. 12.7).[101] In this example, outcome was related to overall drug effects on normal

tissues as indicated by the degree of neutropenia (PD response), whereas dose intensity did not have a significant effect. Again, these data did not include exposure (PK) assessment and in this case only

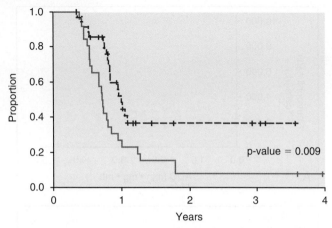

• **Fig. 12.7** Proportion of dogs in remission after chemotherapy treatment for lymphoma. The *dashed line* represents those animals experiencing grade III/IV neutropenia, whereas the *solid line* represents those animals that did not show that level of toxicity. (From Ghan A, Johnson JL, Williams LE: Impact of chemotherapeutic dose intensity and hematologic toxicity on first remission duration in dogs with lymphoma treated with a chemoradiotherapy protocol, *J Vet Intern Med* 21:1332, 2007.)

relates the therapeutic outcome to an observed drug response. A lack of complete PK/PD data relationships in veterinary medicine reduces the opportunities for therapeutic drug monitoring and the potential for optimizing efficacy.

Pharmaceutics

Pharmaceutics is the science associated with dosage form design with regard to formulation and optimizing drug delivery via a specific route. For example, improved formulations of clinical agents such as paclitaxel have made these compounds available for use in veterinary patients. The excipient (drug carrier) used in the original clinical formulation of paclitaxel (Taxol®) was cremaphor-EL, which causes hypersensitivity reactions when used in dogs.[102,103] A new water-soluble micellar formulation of paclitaxel (Paccal® Vet) appears effective without associated hypersensitivity reactions in dogs with mast cell tumors (MCTs).[103,104] (This preparation was not commercially available at the time this chapter was written.) The ability of new formulations and delivery methods to alter the efficacy and toxicity profile of agents is a rapidly expanding field. It is expected that new technologies in drug formulation and targeting will be incorporated into veterinary medicine to alter drug delivery and distribution in a more favorable manner.

Specific Chemotherapeutic Agents

Alkylating Agents

The alkylating agents comprise antitumor drugs whose mechanism of action involves the covalent binding of alkyl groups to cellular macromolecules. The cellular target of these agents is DNA, where they form monofunctional or bifunctional adducts that generate inter- or intrastrand cross-links.

Nitrogen Mustards

Mechlorethamine (Mustargen)

Basic Pharmacology. Mechlorethamine is frequently referred to as "nitrogen mustard" and was the first cytotoxic agent to show

antineoplastic activity.[105–107] Mechlorethamine undergoes spontaneous hydrolysis to 2-hydroxyethyl-2-chloroethylmethylamine and bis-2-hydroxyethylmethylamine, yielding nucleophilic reactive centers capable of forming DNA cross-links.[108]

Clinical Pharmacology. Mechlorethamine rapidly disappears from the plasma after administration, primarily through spontaneous degradation, although some percentage of the drug is enzymatically metabolized.[109] Mechlorethamine uptake into cells seems to be carrier mediated, with decreased uptake as a mechanism for resistance.[110]

Experience with mechlorethamine as a single agent is not reported, although gastrointestinal (GI) and bone marrow toxicities are dose-limiting toxicities (DLTs) of conventional mechlorethamine-containing protocols. This drug is a strong vesicant and can cause severe tissue necrosis if extravasated. In case of extravasation, sodium thiosulfate (0.17 mmol/L, or 2.5%) should be administered through the catheter before it is removed, or it can be injected directly into the affected site after the catheter has been removed. The volume injected should be equal to that of the intended mechlorethamine dose.

Clinical Use. Mechlorethamine is used predominantly in multiagent protocols for lymphoma in dogs and cats.[111–113,114] Dosing of mechlorethamine in these protocols is reported as 3 mg/m² IV on days 0 and 7 of a 21- or 28-day cycle.

Melphalan

Basic Pharmacology. Melphalan (L-phenylalanine mustard) is a nitrogen mustard containing DNA cross-linking agent with a similar structure and pharmacology to chlorambucil. The major difference is that melphalan is actively transported into tumor cells by amino acid transporters,[5] and its uptake can be blocked by the amino acid leucine. Melphalan has direct alkylating activity and does not require metabolic activation.

Clinical Pharmacology. Melphalan can be given orally, with an oral bioavailability of approximately 30%. A relatively high percentage of melphalan (20%–35%) is excreted unchanged in the urine, with a majority of the remainder of the dose undergoing spontaneous chemical decomposition to inert products.[115] The primary toxicity is myelosuppression—neutropenia and thrombocytopenia.

Clinical Use. The primary indication for melphalan in companion animals is for management of multiple myeloma. The initial dose of 0.1 mg/kg daily for 10 to 14 days should be reduced to 0.05 mg/kg daily based on control of the paraproteinemia and hematologic screening for both dogs and cats. Alternate dosing regimens have also been used for dogs: 7 mg/m² daily for 5 days every 3 weeks or 2 mg/m² daily for 10 days with a 10-day off cycle and repeated as needed.[116]

Cyclophosphamide

Basic Pharmacology. CP is a nitrogen mustard–containing prodrug that is inactive in the absence of metabolic activation, which occurs via microsomal mixed function oxidases predominantly in the liver.[117] The activation of CP involves ring oxidation to 4-hydroxycyclophosphamide (4-OHCP), spontaneous and reversible ring opening to the amino aldehyde aldophosphamide, and the subsequent irreversible breakdown of aldophosphamide to phosphoramide mustard and acrolein. Phosphoramide mustard is considered the most active CP metabolite and is capable of bifunctional alkylation and cross-linking.[118]

Clinical Pharmacology. In dogs and cats, PO and IV administration are equally effective, and this has been verified by PK studies showing similar exposure to the active 4-OHCP metabolite.[119,120] The major DLT of CP is neutropenia. GI toxicity (nausea and vomiting) is not common but has been observed.[121] In dogs, sterile hemorrhagic cystitis (SHC) can result from the metabolite acrolein.[122] It is uncommon with conventional IV dosing, but there are reports after even just a single IV administration.[123,124] The incidence is higher with chronic oral dosing, and a cumulative dose is a risk factor.[125,126] Concurrent treatment with furosemide (1–2 mg/kg PO or IV) significantly reduces the risk of SHC.[123,125] CP should be discontinued permanently in patients that develop SHC. Chlorambucil is often a suitable replacement. Treatment for SHC is largely symptomatic with nonsteroidal antiinflammatory drugs (NSAIDs), oxybutynin (0.2–0.3 mg/kg PO q8–12 h), and/or pentosan polysulfate sodium (20 mg/kg PO twice weekly for 5 weeks, then once weekly for 12 weeks). In extreme cases, intravesicular dimethyl sulfoxide (DMSO) or dilute formalin, or surgery can be considered.[127,128]

Clinical Use. CP is commonly included in multiagent protocols for lymphoma in both dogs and cats. Standard bolus dosages are 200 to 250 mg/m^2 in both dogs and cats. Bone marrow ablation protocols in dogs have used doses in the range of 500 to 750 mg/m^2 before hematopoietic cell transplantation.[129–131] CP has also been dosed using a fractionated schedule (50–75 mg/m^2 PO for 3–4 consecutive days) in both dogs and cats in combination protocols for sarcomas and mammary carcinoma.[132–136] The use of CP in low-dose continuous (metronomic) chemotherapy protocols is discussed in detail in Chapter 15, Section C of this text.

Ifosfamide

Basic Pharmacology. Ifosfamide is a nitrogen mustard–containing prodrug that, like CP, requires metabolic activation by microsomal mixed function oxidases before generating the isofosforamide mustard metabolite capable of bifunctional alkylation.[137]

Clinical Pharmacology. The major difference between the clinical use of ifosfamide and CP is a result of differences in the relative metabolism of the parent drugs, with dechloroethylation accounting for up to 25% of the metabolism of ifosfamide,[138] whereas this number is much smaller for CP. This difference in metabolism accounts for an increase in the formation of the neurotoxic metabolite chloracetaldehyde after ifosfamide dosing and potentially for the less favorable metabolism profile observed with ifosfamide after oral dosing.[139] The primary DLT associated with ifosfamide treatment is a dose-related myelosuppression, but nephrotoxicity and damage to the bladder epithelium are not uncommon. Vigorous hydration is required with ifosfamide administration, and mesna, a urinary epithelial protectant, must be administered to avoid severe cystitis.

Clinical Use. Ifosfamide has been evaluated in dogs and cats with cancer and is recommended primarily for management of sarcomas. The recommended dose for dogs is 375 mg/m^2 IV and for cats is 900 mg/m^2 IV, both as slow infusions and saline diuresis, every 3 weeks.[140,141] The basis for such discrepancies in the MTD between species is not understood but reflects profound and interesting differences in metabolism pathways and most likely reduced generation of bioactive metabolites. A phase II study in feline injection site sarcomas (ISSs) reported moderate objective response rates.[142]

Chlorambucil

Basic Pharmacology. Chlorambucil (*p*-bis[chloro-2-ethyl] aminophenyl-4-butanoic acid) is a nitrogen mustard derivative that enters cells via passive diffusion[143] and has direct bifunctional alkylating ability responsible for the cytotoxic activity.[144]

Clinical Pharmacology. Chlorambucil is orally bioavailable with rapid absorption. Hepatic metabolism is extensive, with the pharmacologically active phenylacetic acid being the primary metabolite and presumably responsible for much of the clinical activity.[145,146] The major DLT is myelosuppression, including granulocytopenia and thrombocytopenia.

Clinical Use. Chlorambucil is used primarily for chronic lymphocytic leukemia, Waldenström's macroglobulinemia and feline low-grade (small cell) GI lymphoma. It also is used as part of metronomic therapy for a variety of cancers, including bladder transitional cell carcinoma (TCC) (see Chapter 15, Section C).[147] Chronic oral dosing typically begins at 3 to 6 mg/m^2 once daily. Doses as high as 4 mg/m^2/d are well tolerated long term in dogs, but often the dose can be lowered based on control of cancer.[148] In cats, to maintain dose intensity without splitting tablets, a dosage of 2 mg every-other-day or Monday–Wednesday–Friday is commonly used. An oral bolus dose of 20 mg/m^2 every 2 weeks also has been reported with excellent response in feline low-grade GI lymphoma.[149]

Nitrosoureas

Lomustine (Cyclohexylchloroethylnitrosurea)

Basic Pharmacology. Cyclohexylchloroethylnitrosurea (CCNU, CeeNU) is a nitrosourea-based agent that is highly lipid soluble and enters cells by passive diffusion.[150] Under aqueous conditions and at physiologic pH, CCNU will spontaneously decompose to a reactive center capable of DNA alkylation[151,152] and DNA–DNA and DNA–protein cross-links.[153]

Clinical Pharmacology. The highly lipophilic properties of CCNU allows for rapid crossing of biologic membranes including the blood–brain barrier. CCNU undergoes extensive hepatic metabolism,[154] predominantly by hydroxylation of the cyclohexyl ring, to metabolites with at least equivalent alkylating activity that presumably play an important role in the cytotoxic activity.[155] This extensive hepatic metabolism is presumably responsible for the lack of oral bioavailability of the parent compound but rapid appearance of metabolites after oral dosing.[156] The major DLT is myelosuppression with acute neutropenia followed by cumulative and potentially irreversible thrombocytopenia.[157] In cats, the neutrophil nadir can occur anywhere from 1 to 4 weeks post-treatment.[158] In dogs, and much less commonly in cats, chronic administration may result in hepatic enzyme elevations and possible hepatic dysfunction requiring discontinuation of the drug temporarily (i.e., drug holiday) or permanently.[159–161] The most consistent and dramatic hematologic abnormality is a marked elevation in alanine aminotransferase (ALT). Concurrent administration with Denamarin™, a product that increases glutathione levels and provides antioxidant properties, reduces the risk of ALT elevation, and decreases the magnitude of elevations in ALT, aspartate aminotransferase (AST), alkaline phosphatase (ALKP), and bilirubin.[162] Pulmonary fibrosis has been reported rarely in cats.[163]

Clinical Use. CCNU (70–90 mg/m^2 PO every 3 weeks) is most often used alone or in multiagent protocols for canine lymphoma, MCTs, and histiocytic sarcoma. In cats, CCNU (40–60 mg/m^2 PO or 10 mg per cat every 4–6 weeks) is used primarily for MCTs and lymphoproliferative disorders.

Streptozotocin

Basic Pharmacology. Streptozotocin is a naturally occurring nitrosourea capable of DNA alkylation and inhibition of DNA synthesis in both bacteria and mammalian cells.[164,165] Cellular uptake of streptozotocin is dependent on the GLUT2 transporter and expression of this transporter determines sensitivity of both insulinoma[166] and pancreatic beta cells.[167]

Clinical Pharmacology. Streptozotocin is rapidly cleared from the blood after IV administration with a reported half-life of 15 to 40 minutes in humans.[168] Streptozotocin has unique activities, including inducing diabetes in animals[169,170] and lack of significant bone marrow toxicity.[171,172]

Clinical Use. Streptozotocin is used to manage insulinoma. Limited reports of efficacy have appeared in the literature, although transient normoglycemia occurred in the experience of the authors.[173] The drug is dosed at 500 mg/m^2 as an IV infusion every 2 weeks with saline diuresis to avoid renal toxicity.

Other Alkylating Agents
Dacarbazine
Basic Pharmacology. Dacarbazine (DTIC) is a prodrug that requires metabolic activation by the hepatic cytochrome P450 system[174,175] to the resulting 5-aminoimidazole carboxamide and the active methylating intermediate methyldiazonium ion.[176] Resulting DNA methylation products are 3-methyl adenine, 7-methyl guanine, and O^6-methyl guanine,[177] which are presumably responsible for the cytotoxic activity.

Clinical Pharmacology. DTIC has poor oral bioavailability and is administered intravenously. Use in cats is not recommended because of a lack of information regarding their ability to convert the parent drug to the active form. DTIC is extensively metabolized in the liver and excreted in the urine. The major DLT is GI toxicity, although occasional severe myelosuppression can be observed.

Clinical Use. In dogs, DTIC is used as a single agent, or in combination with DOX or CCNU, for lymphoproliferative diseases in a relapse setting.[178–181] It also has been used in combination with DOX, with or without vincristine, for hemangiosarcoma.[182,183] As a single agent, an IV infusion dose of 800 to 1000 mg/m^2 every 3 weeks has been used.[178] When combined with other cytotoxics, the dose must be reduced (600–800 mg/m^2 IV)[179,181,183] or spread out over several days (200 mg/m^2/d IV for 5 days).[180,182]

Procarbazine
Basic Pharmacology. Procarbazine (PCB), like DTIC, is a prodrug requiring chemical or metabolic alteration for the generation of active metabolites.[184,185] The mechanism of action of PCB could involve multiple interactions, including inhibition of DNA and RNA synthesis, but a predominant role for DNA methylation to form O^6-methyl guanine seems likely.[186]

Clinical Pharmacology. PCB is rapidly and completely absorbed after oral administration followed by rapid disappearance of the parent compound and subsequent appearance of metabolites.[187] PCB and/or metabolites equilibrate rapidly between the blood and cerebrospinal fluid.[188] IV delivery has been tested in humans with the appearance of neurotoxicity not seen with oral delivery, suggesting that first-pass metabolism associated with oral dosing significantly alters the spectrum of exposure to parent drug versus metabolites.[189]

Clinical Use. PCB most frequently is used in combination with mechlorethamine or CCNU, vincristine, and prednisone for lymphoma.[111–113,190,191] It is dosed at 50 mg/m^2/d PO for 14 days of a 21- or 28-day cycle. Every other day dosing or use of reformulated capsules is required for smaller dogs and cats owing to the limitations of available capsule sizes.

Antitumor Antibiotics

The antitumor antibiotics consist of natural products from microbial fermentation including the anthracyclines, mitomycins, and actinomycins that have yielded clinically useful compounds with diverse mechanisms of action. Included in the discussion here are the anthracycline DOX, the anthracenedione (synthetic analog) mitoxantrone (MTO), and actinomycin D.

Doxorubicin
Basic Pharmacology. The cellular pharmacology of DOX is dominated by its ability to react with a number of cellular components and a multimodal mechanism of cellular toxicity. Its activities include DNA intercalation and inhibition of RNA and DNA polymerases[192] and topoisomerase II,[193] alkylation of DNA,[194] reactive oxygen species (ROS) generation,[195,196] perturbation of cellular Ca^{2+} homeostasis,[197,198] inhibition of thioredoxin reductase,[199] and interaction with plasma membrane components.[200] These processes are involved in both the antitumor effects and AEs of DOX, with their relative contributions still open to some debate.

Clinical Pharmacology. After intravenous dosing, DOX is extensively distributed to tissues, with binding to cellular DNA[201] and anionic lipids[202,203] determining the magnitude of tissue uptake.[204] Elimination occurs through renal and biliary elimination of parent drug and metabolism to doxorubicinol and the 7-hydroxy aglycone. Metabolism to doxorubicinol is via side chain reduction mediated by aldo-keto reductases[205] and 7-hydroxy aglycone by reductive cleavage of the sugar moiety both by the liver and extrahepatic tissues.[206]

Rapid administration of DOX can cause an anaphylactoid-like reaction associated with increased plasma histamine levels.[207] Routine pretreatment with diphenhydramine typically is not needed as long as DOX is administered over 15 to 30 minutes. DOX is a vesicant and in the event of an extravasation, cold compresses should be applied. Dexrazoxane (Zinecard, 10 mg per 1 mg DOX IV) has been shown to substantially reduce the extent of tissue damage and should be given IV (different vein from site of extravasation) immediately after extravasation, and ideally again 24 and 48 hours later.[208]

The acute DLTs associated with DOX are myelosuppression and GI toxicity. In dogs, cardiotoxicity is well established.[209,210] Acute cardiotoxicity manifests as transient arrhythmias associated with transient increases in circulating histamine and catecholamines and is usually of little clinical significance. Cumulative cardiotoxicity manifests as a decrease in myocardial contractility and/or arrhythmias, which often leads to congestive heart failure. The damage is irreversible and carries a grave prognosis. The mechanism of cumulative cardiotoxicity by DOX is complicated,[211] and may involve ROS generation,[212] altered calcium homeostasis,[213] topoisomerase-IIβ–mediated DNA double-strand breaks,[214] or upregulation of death receptors on cardiomyocytes.[215] It is controversial whether or not every dog should have cardiac evaluation with echocardiogram and electrocardiography before receiving DOX, but evaluation should be considered in dogs with known heart disease and breeds predisposed to dilated cardiomyopathy (e.g., Boxer, Doberman Pinscher). Dogs with normal baseline myocardial function should be able to safely receive a cumulative DOX dose of 150 to 240 mg/m^2. For dogs with impaired systolic function or dogs in which the cumulative dose has reached this maximum, dexrazoxane can be administered immediately before DOX to help prevent cardiotoxicity.[216] In cats, DOX can cause cumulative nephrotoxicity[217] and should be used cautiously in cats with underlying renal disease, with close monitoring of renal function parameters.

Clinical Use. DOX is the most active single agent available for a wide variety of cancers in companion animals. The drug may be used alone or in combination protocols for a variety of cancers including lymphoma, HSA, OSA, histiocytic sarcoma, feline ISS, mammary carcinoma, thyroid carcinoma, and colonic adenocarcinoma. Conventional dosing regimens are 30 mg/m^2 via IV infusion (15–30 minutes) every 3 weeks in dogs larger than 15 kg, and either 25 mg/m^2 or 1 mg/kg for dogs smaller than 15 kg and all cats.

Mitoxantrone

Basic Pharmacology. Mitoxantrone (MTO) is a synthetic DOX analog and maintains similar activity as DOX in terms of DNA intercalation and the inhibition of RNA and DNA polymerases and topoisomerase II.[218,219] However, MTO does not cause oxidative damage to cells[220] and has a reduced potential to undergo one-electron reduction and generate ROS.[221]

Clinical Pharmacology. After IV administration, MTO is extensively distributed to tissues, with residual levels being long lasting. MTO is not extensively metabolized and a fraction of the drug (<30%) is excreted unchanged in the urine and feces.[222–224] The DLT is myelosuppression. Cardiotoxicity has not been reported in dogs and only rarely in humans.

Clinical Use. MTO is administered at a dose of 5.0 to 5.5 mg/m^2 in dogs and 6 mg/m^2 in cats as a slow IV bolus every 3 weeks. It is considered a front-line drug for treating canine TCC and anal sac adenocarcinoma.[225,226] MTO has been used as a cardiac-sparing alternative to DOX in dogs with underlying myocardial dysfunction or that have reached their maximum cumulative dose of DOX with the potential for similar outcomes,[227] and as a rescue agent in relapsed canine lymphoma with mixed results.[228]

Actinomycin D (Dactinomycin)

Basic Pharmacology. Actinomycin D, or dactinomycin (DACT), consists of two symmetric polypeptide chains attached to a central phenoxazone ring. DACT has been shown to interact with double-stranded DNA in multiple ways in a sequence-dependent manner,[229–231] and also bind to single-stranded DNA.[232] The resulting interactions of DACT with both double- and single-stranded DNA results in a potent inhibition of transcription, thus inhibiting RNA and protein synthesis.[233,234] DACT is taken up into cells by passive diffusion,[235] and the sensitivity of cells may depend on uptake and retention,[236] with ABCB1 playing a role in DACT efflux.[237]

Clinical Pharmacology. After IV administration, DACT is rapidly distributed to tissues and then slowly eliminated from tissues. Metabolism is minimal, with 20% of DACT excreted unchanged in the urine and 14% in the feces.[238] The major DLTs of DACT are myelosuppression and GI toxicity.[238] It is a vesicant and can cause severe tissue damage if extravasated.

Clinical Use. DACT is used in multiagent protocols for dogs with lymphoproliferative diseases in the relapse setting or as a DOX substitute in dogs with cardiac abnormalities. It is administered IV at 0.5–0.75 mg/m^2 every 1–3 weeks.

Antimetabolites

The antimetabolites comprise agents that inhibit the use of cellular metabolites in the course of cell growth and division. Therefore these agents are generally analogs of compounds used in the normal course of metabolism and in the case of cancer chemotherapeutics, specifically anabolic processes associated with DNA replication.

Cytosine Arabinoside

Basic Pharmacology. Cytosine arabinoside (cytarabine, Ara-C) acts as an analog to deoxycitidine and is phosphorylated in cells to generate arabinosylcytosine triphosphate (ara-CTP), which acts as a competitive inhibitor of DNA polymerase α.[239] Ara-CTP is also incorporated into DNA, which correlates with cytotoxicity,[240] and thus presumably is the primary mechanism of action. Incorporation into DNA cannot be excised[241] and inhibits both the function of the DNA template and subsequent synthesis.[242] Ara-C has also been reported to have a differentiating function in leukemic cells through decreased c-*myc* expression.[243] Ara-C is actively transported into tumor cells via nucleoside transporters [244] and phosphorylated sequentially by deoxycytidine kinase, dCMP kinase, and nucleoside diphosphate kinase.[245]

Clinical Pharmacology. Ara-C is water-soluble and dosed by intravenous infusion. It distributes rapidly in total body water and crosses into the central nervous system (CNS) with cerebrospinal fluid concentrations reaching approximately 60% of plasma levels at steady-state.[246] The primary mode of metabolism is deamination by the liver and extrahepatic tissues. Observed DLTs are myelosuppression and occasionally GI signs.

Clinical Use. Ara-C is administered at a dose of 600 mg/m^2, ideally as a CRI over a 2- to 5-day duration. However, a more convenient method of administration in dogs and cats is to divide that dose into 4 SC injections given twice daily for 2 consecutive days. Ara-C was not effective as a single agent at inducing remission in naïve canine lymphoma,[247] but is a component of the rescue protocol DMAC (dexamethasone, melphalan, actinomycin-D, Ara-C).[248] However, results of a recent small study suggest improved responses in dogs with naïve, stage V multicentric lymphoma when Ara-C (150 mg/m^2/day as a continuous rate infusion) was infused over 5 days after the first and second cycle of a conventional CHOP-based protocol compared with the CHOP protocol alone.[249] Bone marrow support with human granulocyte colony stimulating factor and erythropoietin were coadministered with Ara-C and patients in this treatment group did not experience increased AEs. Low-dose subcutaneous Ara-C (50 mg/m^2 BID for 2 days or 100 mg/m^2 as a constant rate infusion for 1 day) has been reported to improve clinical signs in dogs with meningoencephalitis of unknown origin when combined with prednisone.[250,251]

Methotrexate

Basic Pharmacology. Methotrexate (MTX) is a folate analog that inhibits the enzyme dihydrofolate reductase, thus depleting reduced folate pools required for purine and thymidylate biosynthesis.[252] MTX is also converted to polyglutamates that act as direct inhibitors of folate-dependent enzymes that play a role in de novo purine and thymidylate synthesis.[253,254] MTX enters cells via active transport through the reduced folate carrier.[9]

Clinical Pharmacology. The oral bioavailability of MTX is high at lower doses but becomes variable as doses increase,[255] and thus is usually dosed orally at lower doses and intravenously at higher doses. The PK of MTX is well understood across species[256] and is dominated by enterohepatic recycling that accounts for the observed GI side effects at doses that do not cause hematopoietic toxicities. At higher doses, both GI toxicity and myelosuppression are observed. MTX does not undergo substantial hepatic metabolism except when administered at high doses and is primarily excreted unchanged in the urine.[256]

Clinical Use. MTX was used in original multiagent protocols for treatment of lymphoproliferative disorders in dogs and cats. With the development of other less toxic and more potent agents, MTX has been eliminated from conventional treatment regimens and is rarely used in veterinary oncology.

Gemcitabine

Basic Pharmacology. Gemcitabine (GCB), or 2,2-difluo-rodeoxy–cytidine (dFdC), is actively transported into cells by nucleoside transporters[257] and metabolized by phosphorylation to mono- (dFdCMP), di- (dFdCDP), and triphosphorylated (dFdCTP) species.[245] The effect of dFdC treatment on cells is the inhibition of DNA synthesis through dFdCTP inhibition of DNA polymerase,[258] dFdCDP inhibition of ribonucleotide reductase and subsequent depletion of deoxyribonucleotide pools,[31] and dFdCTP incorporation into DNA leading to strand termination.[32] The dFdCTP incorporated into newly synthesized DNA appears resistant to normal DNA repair[259] and its presence is critical for triggering apoptosis by this agent.[260] Recent studies suggest that the primary deamination metabolite of dFdC, dFdU, may also play a role in cytotoxicity.[261]

Clinical Pharmacology. GCB is dosed intravenously because oral dosing leads to low systemic exposure,[262] presumably because of extensive first-pass metabolism in the liver through deamination to the dFdU metabolite.[263] Infusion length also seems to be a potentially important variable as longer, constant rate infusions have been shown to lead to increased intracellular dFdCTP levels and enhanced response as opposed to shorter infusions.[264] The DLT of GCB is hematologic in both humans and dogs.[245,265]

Clinical Use. The role of GCB in veterinary oncology is still being defined. A preliminary study indicated efficacy when GCB (800 mg/m^2 IV over 30–60 minutes, once a week) was used in combination with piroxicam for canine TCC[266]; however, no benefit has been demonstrated for canine lymphoma, OSA, mammary carcinoma, or hepatocellular carcinoma.[265,267–269] Single-agent doses have ranged from 400 to 800 mg/m^2 IV over 30 to 60 minutes, once a week, but standardized dosing regimens need to be established before clinically relevant phase II efficacy studies can be done. Low-dose GCB has been shown to be tolerated well in combination with carboplatin in dogs and cats.[270–272] GCB was not well tolerated as a radiosensitizer for head and neck carcinomas in dogs and cats owing to unacceptable hematologic and local tissue toxicity.[273]

5-Fluorouracil

Basic Pharmacology. 5-Fluorouracil (5-FU) is a halogenated analog of uracil that enters cells using a facilitated-transport system shared by adenine, uracil, and hypoxanthine.[274] 5-FU is converted to active nucleotide forms intracellularly by a series of phosphorylase and kinase reactions to yield mono-, di-, and triphosphate forms of both fluorouridine and fluorodeoxyuridine,[275,276] which are incorporated into RNA and DNA interfering with synthesis and function.[277–279] The 5-FU metabolite FdUMP is an inhibitor of thymidylate synthetase, leading to depletion of thymidine 5′-monophosphate and thymidine 5′-triphosphate.[280] The alterations in thymidine and deoxyuridine phosphate pools caused by thymidylate synthetase inhibition, effects on DNA synthesis and integrity, and effects on RNA synthesis and processing are all thought to play a role in cytotoxicity induced by 5-FU.

Clinical Pharmacology. 5-FU is dosed IV and is extensively metabolized in many tissues by dihydropyrimidine dehydrogenase to dihydrofluorouracil, which is further catabolized to α-fluoro-β-alanine, ammonia and CO_2.[281,282] Approximately 90% of an administered dose is metabolized, and both 5-FU and its catabolites undergo biliary excretion with <5% of the parent drug renally excreted. 5-FU causes a dose-dependent myelosuppression, GI toxicity, and neurotoxicity in dogs. Inadvertent ingestion of a topical 5-FU cream is toxic and/or fatal.[283] 5-FU is **contraindicated** in cats because of severe CNS toxicity.

Clinical Use. 5-FU is infrequently used for management of organ epithelial tumors (hepatic, pancreatic, renal, mammary). The reported dose is 150 mg/m^2 IV weekly. It also may be administered topically and intralesionally to dogs, although convincing reports of efficacy are not available.

Rabacfosadine (Tanovea)

Basic Pharmacology. Rabacfosadine (RFD) is a multiactivation-step prodrug that results in the intracellular generation of the nucleotide analog 9-(2-phosphonylmethoxyethyl)guanine (PMEG).[284] The metabolic sequelae of RFD involve cellular uptake of the parent compound and subsequent hydrolysis by cathepsin A to cPrPMEDAP and deamination by N^6-methyl-AMP aminohydrolase to generate intracellular PMEG.[285–287] PMEG is then phosphorylated to the diphosphate form (PMEGpp) that competes with dGTP as a substrate for DNA polymerases with resulting incorporation into DNA resulting in chain termination.[288,289] Distribution studies of RFD have shown preferential uptake into PBMCs and lymphoid tissue and selective metabolism of cPrPMEDAP in liver and kidney via dealkylation to the less toxic PMEDAP metabolite, presumably leading to selective toxicity in target as opposed to normal tissue.[285]

Clinical Pharmacology. The most common AEs observed with RFD are GI. Neutropenia, thrombocytopenia, elevated liver enzymes, and proteinuria are also reported. RFD can cause dermatologic toxicity, characterized by otitis externa or focal pruritic, alopecic, and erythematous lesions adjacent to the pinna, on the dorsum, or in the inguinal areas. The underlying mechanism is unknown, but it has been proposed that it is secondary to drug distribution to the skin. Anecdotally, concurrent treatment with antiinflammatory doses of prednisone may reduce the frequency of dermatologic changes. Although uncommon, the most severe and irreversible toxicity associated with RFD is idiosyncratic pulmonary fibrosis.[285,290–294]

Clinical Use. The standard dose of RFD in dogs is 1 mg/kg IV every 21 days as a single agent[294] or every 42 days when alternated with DOX.[292] RFD has been evaluated as a single agent in dogs for cutaneous T-cell lymphoma,[290] multiple myeloma,[291] relapsed B-cell lymphoma,[294] and in naïve canine multicentric lymphoma in combination with DOX.[292] The established efficacy of RFD in relapsed lymphoma makes it a reasonable choice in the salvage setting.[294] Efficacy of RFD in combination with DOX in the treatment of naïve lymphoma also establishes this protocol as an option for first-line therapy.[292] As of the time this chapter was written, RFD has conditional licensure by the FDA and can be used only for canine lymphoma.

Antimicrotubule Agents

The antimicrotubule agents currently used in veterinary medicine are structurally complex agents belonging to the taxane or vinca alkaloid class of compounds. These agents have a mechanism of action involving interference with the polymerization or depolymerization of the microtubules that play critical roles in cell function and division.

Taxanes (Paclitaxel and Docetaxel)

Basic Pharmacology. The clinically used taxanes (paclitaxel [PTX] and docetaxel [DTX]) both act by stabilizing microtubules against depolymerization and thus inhibit reorganization dynamics required for carrying out cellular functions.[295-297] This alteration in microtubule function causes an abnormal organization of spindle microtubules involved in chromosome segregation during mitosis, leading to mitotic arrest.[298] PTX and DTX share identical mechanisms with the increased potency of DTX [299] attributable to an approximately 2-fold higher affinity for tubulin binding compared with PTX.[300]

Clinical Pharmacology. The clinical use of the taxanes is complicated by their poor solubility and the use of excipients including cremophor EL (PTX) and polysorbate 80 (DTX) to allow for intravenous administration. Both PTX and DTX are rapidly distributed throughout the body and eliminated slowly, primarily by hepatic metabolism and biliary excretion. Renal elimination is 10% or less for both compounds. Toxicities associated with taxanes include hypersensitivity reactions that are attributable to the cremophor EL and polysorbate 80 utilized in formulation. Diarrhea and neutropenia are the major dose-limiting taxane-specific toxicities observed.

Clinical Use. The use of PTX has not been frequently described in either dogs or cats. This is likely because of the requirement for significant pretreatment with antihistamines and corticosteroids followed by a prolonged infusion that must be monitored for acute hypersensitivity. One report evaluated dogs treated with PTX at a dose of 165 mg/m² slow IV infusion every 3 weeks.[103] Although a few measurable responses were identified for various tumor types, hypersensitivity was frequent (64%) despite pretreatment, and significant bone marrow toxicity was observed, leading to the conclusion that the recommended dose for further evaluation is 132 mg/m² as a slow IV infusion every 3 weeks. As discussed earlier in the section on pharmaceutics, a water-soluble micellar preparation is effective for nonresectable MCT, but at the time this chapter was written it was no longer commercially available.[301] PTX in cats has been used at 80 mg/m² slow IV infusion every 3 weeks with similar need for pretreatment.[302]

Hypersensitivity is more manageable with DTX as opposed to PTX. In a small group of dogs with mammary carcinoma, DTX was administered at a dosage of 30 mg/m² IV over 30 minutes with routine pretreatment (steroids, diphenhydramine).[303] Low-grade cutaneous hypersensitivities were reported but easily managed. Similarly, cats were successfully treated at a dosage of 2.25 mg/kg IV over 1 hour with pretreatment.[304] To overcome hypersensitivity reactions a strategy was developed to administer DTX orally with cyclosporine as an absorption aid. This strategy was investigated in phase I studies in dogs and cats with cancer where the MTD of DTX was 1.63 mg/kg and 1.75 mg/kg PO (by gavage) every 2 to 3 weeks, respectively, when combined with cyclosporine (5 mg/kg PO).[305,306] Although no hypersensitivity reactions were reported, diarrhea was the DLT. Subsequent phase II evaluation of this dosing strategy in dogs demonstrated modest activity against oral squamous cell carcinoma (SCC).[307]

Vinca Alkaloids (Vinblastine, Vincristine, Vindesine, Vinorelbine)

The vinca alkaloids as a class of antitumor agents consist of the naturally occurring vincristine (VCR) and vinblastine (VBL) and a semisynthetic derivative and metabolite of VBL, vindesine, and the semisynthetic derivative of VBL, vinorelbine. These agents all share a similar mechanism of action and focus will be on VCR and VBL in this section because of their use in veterinary medicine.

Basic Pharmacology. The vinca alkaloids bind to a distinct site on tubulin[308] and inhibit microtubule assembly.[309] This inhibition of microtubule function leads to a disruption in the mitotic spindle apparatus resulting in metaphase arrest and cytotoxicity.[310,311] The vinca alkaloids enter cells by a simple diffusion process. Exposure time and concentration seem to be important variables in determining cytotoxicity.

Clinical Pharmacology. The vinca alkaloids are administered by IV infusion, rapidly distribute to tissues, and are slowly eliminated primarily by hepatic metabolism and biliary excretion of parent drug and metabolites. Urinary excretion of parent drug and metabolites is relatively low: 10% to 20%. One of the metabolites of VBL is desacetylvinblastine (vindesine), which is active and has been identified in dogs.[312] VBL and VCR differ in their respective toxicities, with VCR being less myelosuppressive than VBL but causing more peripheral neurotoxic and GI effects, including significant ileus. All vinca alkaloids are vesicants. If extravasated, 5 to 10 mL saline can be infused around the affected area. The addition of hyaluronidase (150 U/1 mL extravasated drug) to the saline has been reported but is not widely available. Warm compresses should be applied as well. A solution of DMSO and flucinolone acetonide (Synotic) mixed with 10 mg of flunixin meglumine should be applied topically after each heat application.

Clinical Use. VCR is used predominantly as a component in multiagent protocols for dogs and cats with lymphoma. It is also used as a single agent for dogs with transmissible venereal tumor. The dose for VCR is 0.5 to 0.75 mg/m² IV bolus weekly in both dogs and cats, or as defined in the protocol.

VBL is most often used to manage canine MCT either as a single agent or in combination with other agents. It also is used to treat canine bladder TCC,[313] as a rescue for lymphoma,[314] and in place of VCR in multiagent protocols to help minimize adverse GI AEs.[315] Several dose-schedule variations exist in dogs. When given weekly, starting dosages of 2.0 to 2.67 mg/m² IV are used most commonly, but dosage escalations up to 3.0 mg/m² have been reported.[316,317] Doses as high as 3.0 to 3.5 mg/m² IV are well tolerated when the dose interval is extended to q2 weeks.[100,313] In cats, VBL has been administered at a dosage of 1.5 mg/m² IV as part of a COP-based protocol.[315]

Vinorelbine is administered at a starting dosage of 15 mg/m² IV over 5 minutes once weekly in dogs, and 11.5 mg/m² in cats.[318-321] There is preliminary evidence to support activity against primary lung tumors, histiocytic sarcoma, and MCTs, but insufficient numbers of patients have been evaluated to accurately quantify tumor response at this time.

Topoisomerase Inhibitors

The topoisomerase inhibitors represent classes of drugs that inhibit either the type I or type II topoisomerase enzymes that are involved in the unlinking and unwinding of the DNA strand for replication and transcription. The major classes of topoisomerase II inhibitors used in veterinary oncology are the anthracyclines, which have already been discussed, and the epipodophyllotoxins of which etoposide and teniposide are the clinically relevant members. The major class of topoisomerase I inhibitors used in human oncology are the camptothecins, which have found little use so far in veterinary medicine and will not be discussed here.

Epipodophyllotoxins (Etoposide and Teniposide)

Basic Pharmacology. Etoposide (VP-16) and teniposide (VM-26) both inhibit the catalytic activity of topoisomerase II[322] by stabilizing a protein–DNA cleavage complex[323] that ultimately results in the generation of single- and double-strand DNA breaks.[324] These compounds enter tumor cells by simple diffusion across the cell membrane, and increased levels of topoisomerase II in proliferating tumor cells increases selectivity.[325]

Clinical Pharmacology. Etoposide has been evaluated in dogs both IV and orally. Etoposide administered IV is associated with severe histamine release in dogs associated with the polysorbate 80 vehicle as described earlier with the use of IV DTX. Oral dosing has shown low and highly variable bioavailability in dogs, making this route of delivery difficult to use.[326] Etoposide is eliminated after dosing by hepatic metabolism, and renal elimination of both parent drug (30%–40% of the dose) and glucoronide metabolites. The major DLT of IV etoposide in the dog is hypersensitivity.[327]

Clinical Use. Based on the hypersensitivity reactions experienced in dogs after IV etoposide and the low bioavailability of orally administered etoposide, it is not recommended for use. Strategies to overcome the vehicle induced hypersensitivity by reformulation or to improve bioavailability are required to continue evaluating etoposide. No studies have been reported in cats.

Corticosteroids

Prednisone

Basic Pharmacology. Prednisone and prednisolone are corticosteroids that presumably induce killing of hematopoietic cancer cells through interaction with the glucocorticoid receptor[328] and the induction of apoptosis.[329] Mechanisms of apoptosis induction by corticosteroids in hematologic cancers is still not completely understood and multiple mechanisms exist whereby tumor cells of hematopoietic origin resist steroid-induced killing.[330]

Clinical Pharmacology. Prednisone is generally well tolerated in dogs over short time periods (weeks) when administered as a tapering schedule to a tolerable baseline dose dependent on the response of the patient and the cancer. The adrenal–pituitary axis can become suppressed with, signs of iatrogenic hyperadrenocorticism causing severe disease in dogs if prednisone is continued at immunosuppressive doses. Cats tolerate exogenous steroids well for prolonged periods.

Clinical Use. Prednisone is widely used for management of lymphoid malignancies, MCTs, insulinoma, and brain tumors in dogs and cats. It is also useful for the management of paraneoplastic hypercalcemia. Dogs are often dosed at 2 mg/kg (or 40 mg/m²) PO daily at the beginning of multiagent protocols for lymphoma and are weaned off the drug over 3 to 4 weeks. Cats are tolerant of prednisone or prednisolone and are maintained at 5 mg PO q24h or BID as needed. Prednisone is also used to manage signs and side effects of chemotherapy-induced toxicity such as hypersensitivities or hemorrhagic cystitis. Antiinflammatory doses are used in dogs (0.5–1.0 mg/kg) PO once daily and reduced as indicated by signs.

Others

Platinum (Carboplatin and Cisplatin)

Basic Pharmacology. The activity of platinum containing antitumor agents is through covalent binding to DNA through displacement reactions resulting in bifunctional lesions and interior intrastrand cross-links.[331] Intrastrand adducts, in particular N^7-d(GpG) and N^7-d(ApG) account for the majority of platinum-DNA damage and are highly correlated with drug-induced cell killing.[332] Reactions with water are an important component of the pharmacology of cisplatin (CDDP) owing to some of the aquated species potentially crossing cell membranes more rapidly.[333]

Clinical Pharmacology. Both CDDP and carboplatin are administered intravenously. Metabolism of both CDDP and carboplatin occurs primarily through reactions with water and elimination by binding to plasma and tissue proteins. Urinary elimination of unbound and bound forms accounts for nearly 50% of the cisplatin dose 5 days after administration. Carboplatin is predominantly excreted in the urine with approximately 65% of the dose recovered in the urine 24 hours after administration.[333] Strong correlations exist between carboplatin exposure and renal function such that simple formulas have been derived in both humans[334] and cats[335] for dosing calculations based on renal function. The DLTs associated with CDDP are GI (nausea and vomiting) and renal. Pretreatment with antiemetics, and vigorous saline diuresis is required. CDDP is **contraindicated** in cats because of fatal pulmonary vasculitis and edema.[336] In contrast, the DLT associated with carboplatin is myelosuppression. GI AEs are less common and less severe, the drug is not nephrotoxic, and it can be safely administered to cats.

Clinical Use. CDDP (50–70 mg/m² IV infusion administered with saline diuresis and antiemetics every 3 weeks) is indicated primarily for canine OSA. It also has activity against bladder TCC, mesothelioma, carcinomatosis, and germinal cell tumors.[337,338] A variety of other tumor types have been reported to be marginally sensitive to CDDP.

In dogs, carboplatin (300 mg/m² or 10 mg/kg IV as a slow bolus every 3 weeks) often is preferred to CDDP because of its more favorable toxicity profile and ease of delivery. Although no formal comparisons exist, carboplatin appears to have similar efficacy to CDDP for canine OSA but is inferior for TCC.[73,339] Carboplatin also is used for anal sac adenocarcinoma, SCC, intestinal carcinoma, prostatic carcinoma, mesothelioma, and carcinomatosis.[271,340–342]

The traditional dose of carboplatin in cats is 200 to 240 mg/m² IV as a slow bolus every 3 weeks.[343] A significant proportion of cats require every 4 week regimens owing to prolonged neutropenia. As in humans, an individualized dose of carboplatin may be calculated based on GFR and a targeted area under the concentration versus time curve (AUC_{Target}).[77,344] When GFR is measured using serum iohexol clearance (commercially available through Michigan State University), the dosing equation is:

$$\text{Carboplatin dose} = AUC_{Target} \times [(1.3 \times GFR) + 1.4] \times \text{Body weight(kg)}$$

Based on a phase I study, the maximum tolerated AUC_{Target} is 2.75 min × mg/mL.[345] Limited efficacy information is available with either dosing strategy, but clinical responses have been reported in cats with injection site sarcoma, HSA, colonic adenocarcinoma, and oral SCC.[77,343,346]

Hydroxyurea

Basic Pharmacology. Hydroxyurea (HU) enters cells via passive diffusion[347] and is an inhibitor of ribonucleotide reductase,[348] resulting in depletion of deoxyribonucleotide pools.[349]

This interaction with ribonucleotide reductase can also lead to the allosteric inhibition of other enzymes in the DNA precursor synthesis pathway that make up the replitase complex.[350] The magnitude of decrease in cellular deoxyribonucleotide pools induced by hydroxyurea treatment correlates with inhibition of DNA synthesis observed.[351]

Clinical Pharmacology. HU is dosed orally and distributes rapidly to all tissues. Elimination is through hepatic metabolism and urinary elimination of the parent compound. AEs associated with HU treatment include GI effects, myelosuppression (including anemia), and rarely pulmonary fibrosis, with cats being more susceptible to myelosuppressive effects and potentially methemoglobinemia at higher doses. In dogs, a painful detachment of the claw (nail) from the quick (onycholysis) is often observed after chronic HU treatment.

Clinical Use. HU is used primarily for management of bone marrow disorders such as polycythemia vera and granulocytic leukemias. It also has been used to treat canine MCT.[352] HU is safe to use at 50 to 60 mg/kg orally once daily initially for 2 weeks followed by 30 mg/kg/d to lessen myelosuppressive and onycholytic effects.

L-Asparaginase

Basic Pharmacology. The enzymatic function of L-asparaginase is the hydrolysis of L-asparagine to L-aspartic acid. This depletion of circulating L-asparagine leads to inhibition of protein synthesis in tumor cells lacking L-asparagine synthetase, causing induction of apoptosis.[353]

Clinical Pharmacology. L-Asparaginase can be dosed subcutaneously, intramuscularly, or intraperitoneally and blood levels of the protein remain for weeks. Hypersensitivity reactions can lead to a shorter half-life through enhanced clearance. The AEs associated with L-asparaginase treatment are a result of either hypersensitivity reactions, which may be accentuated after repeated exposures, or to decreased protein synthesis from depleted L-asparagine pools.[354] Furthermore, neutralizing antibodies may be produced to this foreign protein that can result in limited effectiveness after repeated dosing. Hypersensitivity may be managed using pretreatment antihistamines and occasionally dexamethasone if allergic reactions are severe enough to warrant its use. Patients receiving multiple doses should remain under observation for at least 30 minutes after treatment before being discharged, and owners should be advised to observe their pet for 1 to 4 hours after treatment for signs of hypersensitivity.

Clinical Use. L-Asparaginase (400 IU/kg IM or SQ or 10,000 IU/m² IM or SQ) is used exclusively for lymphoproliferative disorders. To avoid development of resistance to L-asparginase, it is often used only in patients at the time of initial induction (especially if clinically ill) or at the time or relapse. A polyethylene glycol (PEG)ylated form of L-asparaginase is available to mitigate neutralizing antibody production; however, its use in veterinary medicine is limited because of cost.

Targeted Agents

Tyrosine Kinase Inhibitors

Tyrosine kinase inhibitors (TKIs) are small-molecule inhibitors that block, with varying specificity, receptor tyrosine kinases (RTKs) expressed on the cell surface by acting as competitive inhibitors of adenosine triphosphate (ATP) binding. ATP binding is required for RTK autophosphorylation and subsequent downstream signaling.

Toceranib (TOC) phosphate (Palladia), masitinib (MAS, Kinavet, Masivet), and imatinib mesylate (Gleevec) have been used most commonly in veterinary oncology. At the time of writing, MAS no longer has Food and Drug Administration (FDA) approval in the United States, but it remains available in Europe.

Basic Pharmacology. The TKIs used in veterinary oncology inhibit RTKs in the split kinase family. The primary targets of TOC are KIT (stem cell factor receptor, CD117), vascular endothelial growth factor receptor 2 (VEGFR2), platelet-derived growth factor receptor β (PDGFRβ), and FMS-like tyrosine kinase-3 (Flt-3).[355–357] However, TOC is structurally very similar to the human TKI sunitinib, which has been shown to in addition block VEGFR3, PDGFRα, RET, and colony-stimulating factor receptor (CSF1R).[358] MAS targets KIT, PDGFR, and Lyn (an intracellular kinase in the Src family).[359] Imatinib targets KIT, Abl, and PDGFR.[360]

TOC has a reported oral bioavailability of approximately 80% in dogs and feeding does not affect absorption characteristics.[361] TOC is highly protein bound in the plasma (>90%) and undergoes hepatic metabolism to a single alicyclic N-oxide metabolite.[362] The half-life of TOC ranges between 13 and 17 hours, and it is estimated that approximately 90% of TOC and its metabolite are excreted in feces and 10% in urine.[361,362]

Clinical Pharmacology. TKIs can target tumor cells directly by inhibiting normal or mutated RTKs expressed on their surface that promote cell division and survival. They also can have an antiangiogenic effect through inhibition of VEGFR and PDGFR on endothelial cells and pericytes, respectively.[355,356]

AEs likely result from chronic inhibition of RTKs on normal cells that require these pathways for cell survival and proliferation. As to be expected, TKIs that target multiple RTKs often have more toxic effects. In both dogs and cats, the most common AEs associated with TOC and MAS are diarrhea, vomiting, hyporexia, and less commonly, GI bleeding.[357,363–366] Neutropenia has been reported with both drugs, but it is relatively uncommon and usually mild. Hemolytic anemia has been reported in dogs receiving MAS.[363] Protein-losing nephropathies have been reported in dogs receiving TOC or MAS, and in cats receiving MAS.[363,366,367] TOC has also been associated with hypertension in dogs; this AE is generally controllable with standard hypertension medications. TOC can cause muscle cramping, which usually resolves with NSAIDs and/or a short drug holiday.[356,357] Imatinib has been observed to cause idiosyncratic hepatotoxicity in dogs.[356]

Clinical Use. The label dose for TOC in dogs is 3.25 mg/kg PO q48h. However, subsequent use has shown doses of 2.5 to 2.75 mg/kg either every-other-day or Monday–Wednesday–Friday to be effective and better tolerated.[356,368,369] TOC is approved for canine MCT. It also has activity against anal sac adenocarcinoma, gastrointestinal stromal tumor, thyroid carcinoma, and nasal adenocarcinoma.[368,370] In dogs with OSA, the addition of TOC-based maintenance protocols after amputation and conventional chemotherapy did not improve DFI or survival, although a small percentage of dogs with gross metastatic OSA do experience short-term benefit.[371,372] TOC has been used in cats with a recommended starting dosage of 2.7 mg/kg Monday, Wednesday, and Friday, with biologic responses being reported in cats with mast cell disease.[364,365]

The recommended dosage for MAS in dogs is 12.5 mg/kg PO q24h, with a standard dosage reduction to 9.0 mg/kg q24h in the event of unacceptable toxicity.[363] It is indicated primarily for nonresectable or recurrent MCT. In healthy cats, MAS was well tolerated at a dosage of 50 mg (10.9–14.8 mg/kg) PO q48h,[366] but data supporting efficacy are lacking. The recommended dosage for imatinib in dogs and cats is 10 mg/kg PO q24h, but caution should be used because this is based on small numbers of patients, with most treated for less than 1 month,[356,373,374] with the primary indication being mast cell neoplasia.

Future Directions in Drug Therapies for Cancer

Individualized Dosing

Population Pharmacokinetics

The convention for drug dosing is to normalize the dose to the weight or surface area of the patient. This is done even though there are often no data to support a relationship between a given drug's exposure in the patient and either of these parameters. These conventions are based on the idea that body weight or BSA is related to drug distribution and/or elimination in a manner that allows for consistent drug exposure in treated individuals. Dosing in mg/kg or mg/m^2 is a crude attempt at individualized dosing, and for some drugs, substantial variability is expected. Studies specifically aimed at determining what demographic characteristics in the patient population determine variability in drug exposure are termed *population pharmacokinetic studies.*

Molecular Profiling

Tumor Sensitivity

Tumors have traditionally been classified by descriptive characteristics such as organ of origin, histology, aggressiveness, and extent of spread. That empiric rubric is being challenged, as molecular classifications made possible by microarrays and other profiling technologies become increasingly common and persuasive.[375,376] The reductionist program would suggest that, eventually, all differences among traditional tumor types will be reduced to statements about molecules in the tumors and about the interactions among those molecules; hence it might then be possible to study physiologic processes in one type of cancer and extrapolate the results in a predictive manner to another type through commonalities in their molecular constitutions. But what if we want to do the same thing at the pharmacologic level-to extrapolate and predict drug sensitivity based on molecular characteristics of the tumor? These types of decisions are already being used in human medicine at a discrete level for the use of antiestrogens in estrogen receptor–positive breast cancers,[377] and the use of select molecularly targeted agents based on the mutation/expression status of target molecules[378,379]; however, responses to traditional chemotherapy agents, which still make up the backbone of available therapies both in human and veterinary medicine, are more complex and do not generally sort as responders and nonresponders based on single, or even a few, molecular characteristics. Examples do exist in which this is the case, such as overexpression of ABCB1 and the multidrug resistance phenotype,[380] but generally a multitude of genes involved in drug activation, detoxification, DNA repair, stress responses, and a myriad of other known and unknown pathways play a role in determining tumor cell chemosensitivity. Therefore a mechanism that can evaluate multiple factors in a tumor indiscriminately and determine whether it is sensitive or insensitive to a given chemotherapeutic agent would be an invaluable adjunct in determining which drugs to use for which individual tumor.

Predictive Evaluations

Current clinical practice in both human and veterinary oncology bases the choice of cytotoxic chemotherapy on descriptive histopathology characteristics. For example, a diagnosis of OSA in a veterinary patient would lead to the use of adjuvant DOX and/or a platinum-based drug (carboplatin or CDDP) after surgical resection of the tumor. Why are these drugs used? The easy answer is that studies have shown that dogs receiving either of these drugs after surgery live significantly longer than dogs receiving surgery alone.[381] Studies in human patients have shown in a variety of tumor types that in vitro chemosensitivity testing of tumor biopsies and tailoring therapy can lead to increases in antitumor response.[382–385] Therefore basing therapy on an empirical assessment of drug sensitivity rather than on tumor type alone is a strategy that could lead to preferred outcomes. Issues with the use of chemosensitivity assessment in clinical practice are the technical difficulties associated with tissue procurement and culturing and measures of drug response. Another approach to predicting the chemosensitivity of tumors has evolved around gene expression profiling and an informatics approach.[386,387] Although much attention has been focused on recent evidence of research impropriety and improper validation of predictors used for clinical trials in human lung and breast cancer,[388,389] and this has dampened some enthusiasm for using genomic predictors in chemosensitivity profiling, it should be noted that extensive review of these data by statisticians[390] and NCI review panels has found that the errors made were in data handling and consistency in analysis. Thus these unfortunate events should not be an indictment of "omics" approaches in making clinical decisions but rather a stark reminder that correct and careful research approaches and data analysis must be adhered to.

Novel Combinations

The approval of the first targeted agent for veterinary applications in the United States (TOC) has provided access to a multitargeted TKI. Biologic agents, including species-specific cytokines, peptides, monoclonal antibodies, chimeric molecules, and targeted toxins will also invariably become more prevalent as experimental therapies in veterinary medicine. The use of these novel agents in combination with traditional cytotoxic chemotherapy will likely follow the development pathway seen in human oncology, which includes adding these agents to standard protocols in a disease-specific manner. Thus changes to current standards of practice and care should be expected as these newer agents are incorporated and tested.

References

1. Chabner BA, Roberts TG: Timeline: chemotherapy and the war on cancer, *Nat Rev Cancer* 5:65–72, 2005.
2. DeVita VT, Chu E: A history of cancer chemotherapy, *Cancer Res* 68:8643–8653, 2008.
3. Sharma SV, Haber DA, Settleman J: Cell line-based platforms to evaluate the therapeutic efficacy of candidate anticancer agents, *Nat Rev Cancer* 10:241–253, 2010.
4. Fowles JS, Dailey DD, Gustafson DL, et al.: The Flint Animal Cancer Center (FACC) canine tumour cell line panel: a resource for veterinary drug discovery, comparative oncology and translational medicine, *Vet Comp Oncol* 15:481–492, 2017.
5. Begleiter A, Lam H-YP, Grover J, et al.: Evidence for active transport of melphalan by two amino acid carriers in l5178y lymphoblasts in vitro, *Cancer Res* 39:353–359, 1979.

6. Vistica D: Cytotoxicity as an indicator for transport mechanism: evidence that murine bone marrow progenitor cells lack a high-affinity leucine carrier that transports melphalan in murine 11210 leukemia cells, *Blood* 56:427–429, 1980.

7. Wiley JS, Jones SP, Sawyer WH, et al.: Cytosine arabinoside influx and nucleoside transport sites in acute leukemia, *J Clin Invest* 69:479–489, 1982.

8. Mackey JR, Mani RS, Selner M, et al.: Functional nucleoside transporters are required for gemcitabine influx and manifestation of toxicity in cancer cell lines, *Cancer Res* 58:4349–4357, 1998.

9. Goldman ID, Lichtenstein NS, Oliverio VT: Carrier-mediated transport of the folic acid analogue, methotrexate, in the l1210 leukemia cell, *J Biol Chem* 243:5007–5017, 1968.

10. Withoff S, Keith WN, Knol AJ, et al.: Selection of a subpopulation with fewer DNA topoisomerase II alpha gene copies in a doxorubicin-resistant cell line panel, *Br J Cancer* 74:502–507, 1996.

11. Wang H, Jiang Z, Wong YW, et al.: Decreased cp-1 (nf-y) activity results in transcriptional down-regulation of topoisomerase iialpha in a doxorubicin-resistant variant of human multiple myeloma rpmi 8226, *Biochem Biophys Res Commun* 237:217–224, 1997.

12. Moran RG, Spears CP, Heidelberger C: Biochemical determinants of tumor sensitivity to 5-fluorouracil: ultrasensitive methods for the determination of 5-fluoro-2′-deoxyuridylate, 2′-deoxyuridylate, and thymidylate synthetase, *Proc Natl Acad Sci USA* 76:1456–1460, 1979.

13. Karran P, Bignami M: DNA damage tolerance, mismatch repair and genome instability, *BioEssays* 16:833–839, 1994.

14. Brown JM, Attardi LD: The role of apoptosis in cancer development and treatment response, *Nat Rev Cancer* 5:231–237, 2005.

15. Igney FH, Krammer PH: Death and anti-death: tumour resistance to apoptosis, *Nat Rev Cancer* 2:277–288, 2002.

16. Reed JC, Kitada S, Takayama S, et al.: Regulation of chemoresistance by the bcl-2 oncoprotein in non-Hodgkin's lymphoma and lymphocytic leukemia cell lines, *Ann Oncol* 5(Suppl 1):61–65, 1994.

17. Schmitt CA, Rosenthal CT, Lowe SW: Genetic analysis of chemoresistance in primary murine lymphomas, *Nat Med* 6:1029–1035, 2000.

18. Ambrosini G, Adida C, Altieri DC: A novel anti-apoptosis gene, survivin, expressed in cancer and lymphoma, *Nat Med* 3:917–921, 1997.

19. Kramer M, Hermans J, Parker J, et al.: Clinical significance of bcl2 and p53 protein expression in diffuse large b-cell lymphoma: a population-based study, *J Clin Oncol* 14:2131–2138, 1996.

20. Sohn SK, Jung JT, Kim DH, et al.: Prognostic significance of bcl-2, bax, and p53 expression in diffuse large B-cell lymphoma, *Am J Hematol* 73:101–107, 2003.

21. Rebhun RB, Lana SE, Ehrhart EJ, et al.: Comparative analysis of survivin expression in untreated and relapsed canine lymphoma, *J Vet Intern Med* 22:989–995, 2008.

22. Moscow JA, Swanson CA, Cowan KH: Decreased melphalan accumulation in a human breast cancer cell line selected for resistance to melphalan, *Br J Cancer* 68:732–737, 1993.

23. Saikawa Y, Knight CB, Saikawa T, et al.: Decreased expression of the human folate receptor mediates transport-defective methotrexate resistance in KB cells, *J Biol Chem* 268:5293–5301, 1993.

24. Tew KD: Glutathione-associated enzymes in anticancer drug resistance, *Cancer Res* 54:4313–4320, 1994.

25. Wang AL, Tew KD: Increased glutathione-*S*-transferase activity in a cell line with acquired resistance to nitrogen mustards, *Cancer Treat Rep* 69:677–682, 1985.

26. Lewis AD, Hickson ID, Robson CN, et al.: Amplification and increased expression of alpha class glutathione *S*-transferase-encoding genes associated with resistance to nitrogen mustards, *Proc Natl Acad Sci USA* 85:8511–8515, 1988.

27. Beck A, Etienne MC, Cheradame S, et al.: A role for dihydropyrimidine dehydrogenase and thymidylate synthase in tumour sensitivity to fluorouracil, *Eur J Cancer* 30A:1517–1522, 1994.

28. Ishikawa Y, Kubota T, Otani Y, et al.: Dihydropyrimidine dehydrogenase activity and messenger rna level may be related to the antitumor effect of 5-fluorouracil on human tumor xenografts in nude mice, *Clin Cancer Res* 5:883–889, 1999.

29. Scherf U, Ross DT, Waltham M, et al.: A gene expression database for the molecular pharmacology of cancer, *Nat Genet* 24:236–244, 2000.

30. Heggie GD, Sommadossi JP, Cross DS, et al.: Clinical pharmacokinetics of 5-fluorouracil and its metabolites in plasma, urine, and bile, *Cancer Res* 47:2203–2206, 1987.

31. Heinemann V, Xu YZ, Chubb S, et al.: Inhibition of ribonucleotide reduction in ccrf-cem cells by 2′,2′-difluorodeoxycytidine, *Mol Pharmacol* 38:567–572, 1990.

32. Huang P, Chubb S, Hertel LW, et al.: Action of 2′,2′-difluorodeoxycytidine on DNA synthesis, *Cancer Res* 51:6110–6117, 1991.

33. Heinemann V, Hertel LW, Grindey GB, et al.: Comparison of the cellular pharmacokinetics and toxicity of 2′,2′-difluorodeoxycytidine and 1-beta-d-arabinofuranosylcytosine, *Cancer Res* 48:4024–4031, 1988.

34. Bouffard DY, Laliberte J, Momparler RL: Kinetic studies on 2′,2′-difluorodeoxycytidine (gemcitabine) with purified human deoxycytidine kinase and cytidine deaminase, *Biochem Pharmacol* 45:1857–1861, 1993.

35. Nakano Y, Tanno S, Koizumi K, et al.: Gemcitabine chemoresistance and molecular markers associated with gemcitabine transport and metabolism in human pancreatic cancer cells, *Br J Cancer* 96:457–463, 2007.

36. Long BH, Wang L, Lorico A, et al.: Mechanisms of resistance to etoposide and teniposide in acquired resistant human colon and lung carcinoma cell lines, *Cancer Res* 51:5275–5283, 1991.

37. Chen GL, Yang L, Rowe TC, et al.: Nonintercalative antitumor drugs interfere with the breakage-reunion reaction of mammalian DNA topoisomerase II, *J Biol Chem* 259:13560–13566, 1984.

38. Alt FW, Kellems RE, Bertino JR, et al.: Selective multiplication of dihydrofolate reductase genes in methotrexate-resistant variants of cultured murine cells, *J Biol Chem* 253:1357–1370, 1978.

39. Giannakakou P, Sackett DL, Kang Y-K, et al.: Paclitaxel-resistant human ovarian cancer cells have mutant β-tubulins that exhibit impaired paclitaxel-driven polymerization, *J Biol Chem* 272:17118–17125, 1997.

40. Andoh T, Ishii K, Suzuki Y, et al.: Characterization of a mammalian mutant with a camptothecin-resistant DNA topoisomerase I, *Proc Natl Acad Sci USA* 84:5565–5569, 1987.

41. Chaney SG, Sancar A: DNA repair: enzymatic mechanisms and relevance to drug response, *J Natl Cancer Inst* 88:1346–1360, 1996.

42. Behrens BC, Hamilton TC, Masuda H, et al.: Characterization of a cis-diamminedichloroplatinum(II)-resistant human ovarian cancer cell line and its use in evaluation of platinum analogues, *Cancer Res* 47:414–418, 1987.

43. Masuda H, Tanaka T, Matsuda H, et al.: Increased removal of DNA-bound platinum in a human ovarian cancer cell line resistant to cis-diamminedichloroplatinum(II), *Cancer Res* 50:1863–1866, 1990.

44. Parker RJ, Eastman A, Bostick-Bruton F, et al.: Acquired cisplatin resistance in human ovarian cancer cells is associated with enhanced repair of cisplatin-DNA lesions and reduced drug accumulation, *J Clin Invest* 87:772–777, 1991.

45. Nojima K, Hochegger H, Saberi A, et al.: Multiple repair pathways mediate tolerance to chemotherapeutic cross-linking agents in vertebrate cells, *Cancer Res* 65:11704–11711, 2005.

46. Borst P, Elferink RO: Mammalian abc transporters in health and disease, *Annu Rev Biochem* 71:537–592, 2002.

47. Fletcher JI, Haber M, Henderson MJ, et al.: ABC transporters in cancer: more than just drug efflux pumps, *Nat Rev Cancer* 10:147–156, 2010.

48. Lee JJ, Hughes CS, Fine RL, et al.: P-glycoprotein expression in canine lymphoma: a relevant, intermediate model of multidrug resistance, *Cancer* 77:1892–1898, 1996.

49. Honscha KU, Schirmer A, Reischauer A, et al.: Expression of ABC-transport proteins in canine mammary cancer: consequences for chemotherapy, *Reprod Domest Anim* 44(Suppl 2):218–223, 2009.

50. Hifumi T, Miyoshi N, Kawaguchi H, et al.: Immunohistochemical detection of proteins associated with multidrug resistance to anti-cancer drugs in canine and feline primary pulmonary carcinoma, *J Vet Med Sci* 72:665–668, 2010.

51. Nowak M, Madej JA, Dziegiel P: Expression of breast cancer resis-tance protein (bcrp-1) in canine mammary adenocarcinomas and adenomas, *In Vivo* 23:705–709, 2009.

52. Conrad S, Viertelhaus A, Orzechowski A, et al.: Sequencing and tissue distribution of the canine *mrp2* gene compared with *mrp1* and *mdr1*, *Toxicology* 156:81–91, 2001.

53. Yabuuchi H, Tanaka K, Maeda M, et al.: Cloning of the dog bile salt export pump (bsep; abcb11) and functional comparison with the human and rat proteins, *Biopharm Drug Dispos* 29:441–448, 2008.

54. Ramirez CJ, Minch JD, Gay JM, et al.: Molecular genetic basis for fluoroquinolone-induced retinal degeneration in cats, *Pharma-cogenet Genomics* 21:66–75, 2011.

55. Devita VT, Chu E: Principles of medical oncology. In Devita VT, Hellman S, Rosenberg SA, editors: *Cancer: Principles & Practice of Oncology*, ed 8, Philadelphia, 1997, Lippincott Williams and Wilkins, pp 337–342.

56. Page RL, Macy DW, Ogilvie GK, et al.: Phase III evaluation of doxorubicin and whole-body hyperthermia in dogs with lym-phoma, *Int J Hyperthermia* 8:187–197, 1992.

57. Carter RF, Harris CK, Withrow SJ, et al.: Chemotherapy of canine lymphoma with histopathological correlation- doxorubicin alone compared to cop as 1st treatment regimen, *J Am Anim Hosp Assoc* 23:587–598, 1987.

58. Postorino NC, Susaneck SJ, Withrow SJ, et al.: Single agent ther-apy with adriamycin for canine lymphosarcoma, *J Am Anim Hosp Assoc* 25:221–225, 1989.

59. Valerius KD, Ogilvie GK, Mallinckrodt CH, et al.: Doxorubicin alone or in combination with asparaginase, followed by cyclophos-phamide, vincristine, and prednisone for treatment of multicentric lymphoma in dogs: 121 cases (1987–1995), *J Am Vet Med Assoc* 210:512–516, 1997.

60. Mutsaers AJ, Glickman NW, DeNicola DB, et al.: Evaluation of treatment with doxorubicin and piroxicam or doxorubicin alone for multicentric lymphoma in dogs, *J Am Vet Med Assoc* 220:1813–1817, 2002.

61. Cotter SM: Treatment of lymphoma and leukemia with cyclophos-phamide, vincristine, and prednisone.1. Treatment of dogs, *J Am Anim Hosp Assoc* 19:159–165, 1983.

62. MacEwen EG, Brown NO, Patnaik AK, et al.: Cyclic combina-tion chemotherapy of canine lymphosarcoma, *J Am Vet Med Assoc* 178:1178–1181, 1981.

63. MacEwen EG, Hayes AA, Matus RE, et al.: Evaluation of some prognostic factors for advanced multicentric lymphosarcoma in the dog: 147 cases (1978–1981), *J Am Vet Med Assoc* 190:564–568, 1987.

64. Khanna C, Lund EM, Redic KA, et al.: Randomized controlled trial of doxorubicin versus dactinomycin in a multiagent protocol for treatment of dogs with malignant lymphoma, *J Am Vet Med Assoc* 213:985, 1998.

65. Greenlee PG, Filippa DA, Quimby FW, et al.: Lymphomas in dogs: a morphologic, immunologic, and clinical study, *Cancer* 66:480–490, 1990.

66. Stone MS, Goldstein MA, Cotter SM: Comparison of 2 protocols for induction of remission in dogs with lymphoma, *J Am Anim Hosp Assoc* 27:315–321, 1991.

67. Myers NC, Moore AS, Rand WM, et al.: Evaluation of a multidrug chemotherapy protocol (acopa II) in dogs with lymphoma, *J Vet Intern Med* 11:333–339, 1997.

68. Boyce KL, Kitchell BE: Treatment of canine lymphoma with COPLA/LVP, *J Am Anim Hosp Assoc* 36:395–403, 2000.

69. Morrison-Collister KE, Rassnick KM, Northrup NC, et al.: A combination chemotherapy protocol with mopp and ccnu consoli-dation (tufts velcap-sc) for the treatment of canine lymphoma, *Vet Comp Oncol* 1:180–190, 2003.

70. Zemann BI, Moore AS, Rand WM, et al.: A combination chemo-therapy protocol (velcap-l) for dogs with lymphoma, *J Vet Intern Med* 12:465–470, 1998.

71. Keller ET, MacEwen EG, Rosenthal RC, et al.: Evaluation of prognostic factors and sequential combination chemotherapy with doxorubicin for canine lymphoma, *J Vet Intern Med* 7:289–295, 1993.

72. Garrett LD, Thamm DH, Chun R, et al.: Evaluation of a 6-month chemotherapy protocol with no maintenance therapy for dogs with lymphoma, *J Vet Intern Med* 16:704–709, 2002.

73. Selmic LE, Burton JH, Thamm DH, et al.: Comparison of carbo-platin and doxorubicin-based chemotherapy protocols in 470 dogs after amputation for treatment of appendicular osteosarcoma, *J Vet Intern Med* 28:554–563, 2014.

74. Frei E, Elias A, Wheeler C, et al.: The relationship between high-dose treatment and combination chemotherapy: the concept of summation dose intensity, *Clin Cancer Res* 4:2027, 1998.

75. Simon R, Korn EL: Selecting drug combinations based on total equivalent dose (dose intensity), *J Natl Cancer Inst* 82:1469–1476, 1990.

76. Undevia SD, Gomez-Abuin G, Ratain MJ: Pharmacokinetic vari-ability of anticancer agents, *Nat Rev Cancer* 5:447–458, 2005.

77. Bailey DB, Rassnick KM, Erb HN, et al.: Effect of glomerular fil-tration rate on clearance and myelotoxicity of carboplatin in cats with tumors, *Am J Vet Res* 65:1502–1507, 2004.

78. Thompson LA, Lawson AP, Sutphin SD, et al.: Description of cur-rent practices of empiric chemotherapy dose adjustment in obese adult patients, *J Oncol Pract* 6:141–145, 2010.

79. Hunter RJ, Navo MA, Thaker PH, et al.: Dosing chemotherapy in obese patients: actual versus assigned body surface area (BSA), *Cancer Treat Rev* 35:69–78, 2009.

80. Vail DM: Supporting the veterinary cancer patient on chemo-therapy: neutropenia and gastrointestinal toxicity, *Top Companion Anim Med* 24:122–129, 2009.

81. Valanis B, Vollmer WM, Steele P: Occupational exposure to anti-neoplastic agents: self-reported miscarriages and stillbirths among nurses and pharmacists, *J Occup Environ Med* 41:632–638, 1999.

82. Sessink PJ, Kroese ED, van Kranen HJ, et al.: Cancer risk assess-ment for health care workers occupationally exposed to cyclophos-phamide, *Int Arch Occup Environ Health* 67:317–323, 1995.

83. Ebert U, Loffler H, Kirch W: Cytotoxic therapy and pregnancy, *Pharmacol Ther* 74:207–220, 1997.

84. Autio K, Rassnick KM, Bedford-Guaus SJ: Chemotherapy dur-ing pregnancy: a review of the literature, *Vet Comp Oncol* 5:61–75, 2007.

85. Kicenuik K, Northrup N, Dawson A, et al.: Treatment time, ease of use and cost associated with use of equashield, Phaseal*, or no closed system transfer device for administration of cancer chemo-therapy to a dog model, *Vet Comp Oncol* 15:163–173, 2017.

86. Pharmacists ASoH- S: Ashp guidelines on handling hazardous drugs, *Am J Health Syst Pharm* 63:1172, 2006.

87. Knobloch A, Mohring SA, Eberle N, et al.: Cytotoxic drug residues in urine of dogs receiving anticancer chemotherapy, *J Vet Intern Med* 24:384–390, 2010.

88. Evans WE, Relling MV: Clinical pharmacokinetics-pharmacodynamics of anticancer drugs, *Clin Pharmacokinet* 16:327–336, 1989.

89. Eckhoff GA: Mechanisms of adverse drug-reactions and interac-tions in veterinary-medicine, *J Am Vet Med Assoc* 176:1131–1133, 1980.

90. He SM, Yang AK, Li XT, et al.: Effects of herbal products on the metabolism and transport of anticancer agents, *Expert Opin Drug Metab Toxicol* 6:1195–1213, 2010.

91. Tarirai C, Viljoen AM, Hamman JH: Herb-drug pharmacokinetic interactions reviewed, *Expert Opin Drug Metab Toxicol* 6:1515–1538, 2010.

92. Mealey KL: Therapeutic implications of the *mdr-1* gene, *J Vet Pharmacol Ther* 27:257–264, 2004.

93. Legha SS, Benjamin RS, Mackay B, et al.: Reduction of doxorubicin cardiotoxicity by prolonged continuous intravenous infusion, *Ann Intern Med* 96:133–139, 1982.

94. Berrak SG, Ewer MS, Jaffe N, et al.: Doxorubicin cardiotoxicity in children: reduced incidence of cardiac dysfunction associated with continuous-infusion schedules, *Oncol Rep* 8:611–614, 2001.

95. Preisler HD, Gessner T, Azarnia N, et al.: Relationship between plasma adriamycin levels and the outcome of remission induction therapy for acute nonlymphocytic leukemia, *Cancer Chemother Pharmacol* 12:125–130, 1984.

96. Piscitelli SC, Rodvold KA, Rushing DA, et al.: Pharmacokinetics and pharmacodynamics of doxorubicin in patients with small cell lung cancer, *Clin Pharmacol Ther* 53:555–561, 1993.

97. Danesi R, Fogli S, Gennari A, et al.: Pharmacokinetic-pharmacodynamic relationships of the anthracycline anticancer drugs, *Clin Pharmacokinet* 41:431–444, 2002.

98. Arrington KA, Legendre AM, Tabeling GS, et al.: Comparison of body surface area-based and weight-based dosage protocols for doxorubicin administration in dogs, *Am J Vet Res* 55:1587–1592, 1994.

99. Veterinary co-operative oncology group – common terminology criteria for adverse events (VCOG-CTCAE) following chemotherapy or biological antineoplastic therapy in dogs and cats v1.0, *Vet Comp Oncol* 2:195–213, 2004.

100. Bailey DB, Rassnick KM, Kristal O, et al.: Phase I dose escalation of single-agent vinblastine in dogs, *J Vet Intern Med* 22:1397–1402, 2008.

101. Vaughan A, Johnson JL, Williams LE: Impact of chemotherapeutic dose intensity and hematologic toxicity on first remission duration in dogs with lymphoma treated with a chemoradiotherapy protocol, *J Vet Intern Med* 21:1332–1339, 2007.

102. Eschalier A, Lavarenne J, Burtin C, et al.: Study of histamine release induced by acute administration of antitumor agents in dogs, *Cancer Chemother Pharmacol* 21:246–250, 1988.

103. Poirier VJ, Hershey AE, Burgess KE, et al.: Efficacy and toxicity of paclitaxel (taxol) for the treatment of canine malignant tumors, *J Vet Intern Med* 18:219–222, 2004.

104. von Euler H, Akerlund-Denneberg N, Rivera P, et al.: Efficacy and safety in an open label single arm multi center phase III trial of a new formulation of paclitaxel (Paccal® vet) in dogs with mast cell tumours grade II and III, *ESVONC Annual Congress*, 2009.

105. Goodman LS, Wintrobe MM, et al.: Nitrogen mustard therapy; use of methyl-bis (beta-chloroethyl) amine hydrochloride and tris (beta-chloroethyl) amine hydrochloride for Hodgkin's disease, lymphosarcoma, leukemia and certain allied and miscellaneous disorders, *J Am Med Assoc* 132:126–132, 1946.

106. Jacobson LO, Spurr CL, et al.: Studies on the effect of methyl bis (beta-chloroethyl) amine hydrochloride on diseases of the hemopoietic system, *J Clin Invest* 25:909, 1946.

107. Rhoads CP: Nitrogen mustards in the treatment of neoplastic disease; official statement, *J Am Med Assoc* 131:656–658, 1946.

108. Kohn KW, Spears CL, Doty P: Inter-strand crosslinking of DNA by nitrogen mustard, *J Mol Biol* 19:266–288, 1966.

109. Skipper HE, Bennett LL, Langham WH: Over-all tracer studies with C[14] labeled nitrogen mustard in normal and leukemic mice, *Cancer* 4:1025–1027, 1951.

110. Goldenberg GJ, Vanstone CL, Israels LG, et al.: Evidence for a transport carrier of nitrogen mustard in nitrogen mustard-sensitive and -resistant l5178y lymphoblasts, *Cancer Res* 30:2285–2291, 1970.

111. Rassnick KM, Mauldin GE, Al-Sarraf R, et al.: MOPP chemotherapy for treatment of resistant lymphoma in dogs: a retrospective study of 117 cases (1989–2000), *J Vet Intern Med* 16:576–580, 2002.

112. Rassnick KM, Bailey DB, Malone EK, et al.: Comparison between l-CHOP and an l-CHOP protocol with interposed treatments of CCNU and MOPP (l-CHOP-CCNU-MOPP) for lymphoma in dogs, *Vet Comp Oncol* 8:243–253, 2010.

113. Brodsky EM, Maudlin GN, Lachowicz JL, et al.: Asparaginase and MOPP treatment of dogs with lymphoma, *J Vet Intern Med* 23:578–584, 2009.

114. Martin OA, Price J: Mechlorethamine, vincristine, melphalan and prednisolone rescue chemotherapy protocol for resistant feline lymphoma, *J Feline Med Surg1098612X17735989*, 2017.

115. Tew KD, Colvin OM, Chabner BA: Alkylating agents. In Chabner BA, Longo DL, editors: *Cancer chemotherapy & biotherapy: Principles and practice*, Philadelphia, 2001, Lippincott Williams & Wilkins, pp 373–414.

116. Fernandez R, Chon E: Comparison of two melphalan protocols and evaluation of outcome and prognostic factors in multiple myeloma in dogs, *J Vet Intern Med* 32:1060–1069, 2018.

117. Cohen JL, Jao JY: Enzymatic basis of cyclophosphamide activation by hepatic microsomes of the rat, *J Pharmacol Exp Ther* 174:206–210, 1970.

118. Colvin M, Brundrett RB, Kan MN, et al.: Alkylating properties of phosphoramide mustard, *Cancer Res* 36:1121–1126, 1976.

119. Warry E, Hansen RJ, Gustafson DL, et al.: Pharmacokinetics of cyclophosphamide after oral and intravenous administration to dogs with lymphoma, *J Vet Intern Med* 25:903–908, 2011.

120. Stroda KA, Murphy JD, Hansen RJ, et al.: Pharmacokinetics of cyclophosphamide and 4-hydroxycyclophosphamide in cats after oral, intravenous, and intraperitoneal administration of cyclophosphamide, *Am J Vet Res* 78:862–866, 2017.

121. Fetting JH, McCarthy LE, Borison HL, et al.: Vomiting induced by cyclophosphamide and phosphoramide mustard in cats, *Cancer Treat Rep* 66:1625–1629, 1982.

122. Cox PJ: Cyclophosphamide cystitis—identification of acrolein as the causative agent, *Biochem Pharmacol* 28:2045–2049, 1979.

123. Charney SC, Bergman PJ, Hohenhaus AE, et al.: Risk factors for sterile hemorrhagic cystitis in dogs with lymphoma receiving cyclophosphamide with or without concurrent administration of furosemide: 216 cases (1990–1996), *J Am Vet Med Assoc* 222:1388–1393, 2003.

124. Peterson JL, Couto CG, Hammer AS, et al.: Acute sterile hemorrhagic cystitis after a single intravenous administration of cyclophosphamide in three dogs, *J Am Vet Med Assoc* 201:1572–1574, 1992.

125. Chan CM, Frimberger AE, Moore AS: Incidence of sterile hemorrhagic cystitis in tumor-bearing dogs concurrently treated with oral metronomic cyclophosphamide chemotherapy and furosemide: 55 cases (2009–2015), *J Am Vet Med Assoc* 249:1408–1414, 2016.

126. Matsuyama A, Woods JP, Mutsaers AJ: Evaluation of toxicity of a chronic alternate day metronomic cyclophosphamide chemotherapy protocol in dogs with naturally occurring cancer, *Can Vet J* 58:51–55, 2017.

127. Laing EJ, Miller CW, Cochrane SM: Treatment of cyclophosphamide-induced hemorrhagic cystitis in five dogs, *J Am Vet Med Assoc* 193:233–236, 1988.

128. Weller RE: Intravesical instillation of dilute formalin for treatment of cyclophosphamide-induced hemorrhagic cystitis in two dogs, *J Am Vet Med Assoc* 172:1206–1209, 1978.

129. Frimberger AE, Moore AS, Rassnick KM, et al.: A combination chemotherapy protocol with dose intensification and autologous bone marrow transplant (VELCAP-HDC) for canine lymphoma, *J Vet Intern Med* 20:355–364, 2006.

130. Warry EE, Willcox JL, Suter SE: Autologous peripheral blood hematopoietic cell transplantation in dogs with T-cell lymphoma, *J Vet Intern Med* 28:529–537, 2014.

131. Willcox JL, Pruitt A, Suter SE: Autologous peripheral blood hematopoietic cell transplantation in dogs with B-cell lymphoma, *J Vet Intern Med* 26:1155–1163, 2012.

132. Sorenmo KU, Jeglum KA, Helfand SC: Chemotherapy of canine hemangiosarcoma with doxorubicin and cyclophosphamide, *J Vet Intern Med* 7:370–376, 1993.

133. Sorenmo K: Canine mammary gland tumors, *Vet Clin North Am Small Anim Pract* 33:573–596, 2003.

134. Jeglum KA, deGuzman E, Young KM: Chemotherapy of advanced mammary adenocarcinoma in 14 cats, *J Am Vet Med Assoc* 187:157–160, 1985.

135. Mauldin GN, Matus RE, Patnaik AK, et al.: Efficacy and toxicity of doxorubicin and cyclophosphamide used in the treatment of selected malignant tumors in 23 cats, *J Vet Intern Med* 2:60–65, 1988.

136. Barber LG, Sorenmo KU, Cronin KL, et al.: Combined doxorubicin and cyclophosphamide chemotherapy for nonresectable feline fibrosarcoma, *J Am Anim Hosp Assoc* 36:416–421, 2000.

137. Creaven PJ, Allen LM, Alford DA, et al.: Clinical pharmacology of isophosphamide, *Clin Pharmacol Ther* 16:77–86, 1974.

138. Norpoth K: Studies on the metabolism of isopnosphamide (NSC-109724) in man, *Cancer Treat Rep* 60:437–443, 1976.

139. Lind MJ, Roberts HL, Thatcher N, et al.: The effect of route of administration and fractionation of dose on the metabolism of ifosfamide, *Cancer Chemother Pharmacol* 26:105–111, 1990.

140. Rassnick KM, Frimberger AE, Wood CA, et al.: Evaluation of ifosfamide for treatment of various canine neoplasms, *J Vet Intern Med* 14:271–276, 2000.

141. Rassnick KM, Moore AS, Northrup NC, et al.: Phase I trial and pharmacokinetic analysis of ifosfamide in cats with sarcomas, *Am J Vet Res* 67:510–516, 2006.

142. Rassnick KM, Rodriguez CO, Khanna C, et al.: Results of a phase II clinical trial on the use of ifosfamide for treatment of cats with vaccine-associated sarcomas, *Am J Vet Res* 67:517–523, 2006.

143. Begleiter A, Goldenberg GJ: Uptake and decomposition of chlorambucil by l5178y lymphoblasts in vitro, *Biochem Pharmacol* 32:535–539, 1983.

144. Jiang BZ, Bank BB, Hsiang YH, et al.: Lack of drug-induced DNA cross-links in chlorambucil-resistant chinese hamster ovary cells, *Cancer Res* 49:5514–5517, 1989.

145. Mitoma C, Onodera T, Takegoshi T, et al.: Metabolic disposition of chlorambucil in rats, *Xenobiotica* 7:205–220, 1977.

146. Goodman GE, McLean A, Alberts DS, et al.: Inhibition of human tumour clonogenicity by chlorambucil and its metabolites, *Br J Cancer* 45:621–623, 1982.

147. Schrempp DR, Childress MO, Stewart JC, et al.: Metronomic administration of chlorambucil for treatment of dogs with urinary bladder transitional cell carcinoma, *J Am Vet Med Assoc* 242:1534–1538, 2013.

148. Custead MR, Weng HY, Childress MO: Retrospective comparison of three doses of metronomic chlorambucil for tolerability and efficacy in dogs with spontaneous cancer, *Vet Comp Oncol* 15:808–819, 2017.

149. Stein TJ, Pellin M, Steinberg H, et al.: Treatment of feline gastrointestinal small-cell lymphoma with chlorambucil and glucocorticoids, *J Am Anim Hosp Assoc* 46:413–417, 2010.

150. Begleiter A, Lam HP, Goldenberg GJ: Mechanism of uptake of nitrosoureas by l5178y lymphoblasts in vitro, *Cancer Res* 37:1022–1027, 1977.

151. Montgomery JA, James R, McCaleb GS, et al.: The modes of decomposition of 1,3-bis(2-chloroethyl)-1-nitrosourea and related compounds, *J Med Chem* 10:668–674, 1967.

152. Colvin M, Brundrett RB, Cowens W, et al.: A chemical basis for the antitumor activity of chloroethylnitrosoureas, *Biochem Pharmacol* 25:695–699, 1976.

153. Kohn KW: Interstrand cross-linking of DNA by 1,3-bis(2-chloroethyl)-1-nitrosourea and other 1-(2-haloethyl)-1-nitrosoureas, *Cancer Res* 37:1450–1454, 1977.

154. Hill DL, Kirk MC, Struck RF: Microsomal metabolism of nitrosoureas, *Cancer Res* 35:296–301, 1975.

155. Wheeler GP, Johnston TP, Bowdon BJ, et al.: Comparison of the properties of metabolites of ccnu, *Biochem Pharmacol* 26:2331–2336, 1977.

156. Lee FY, Workman P, Roberts JT, et al.: Clinical pharmacokinetics of oral ccnu (lomustine), *Cancer Chemother Pharmacol* 14:125–131, 1985.

157. Heading KL, Brockley LK, Bennett PF: Ccnu (lomustine) toxicity in dogs: a retrospective study (2002-07), *Aust Vet J* 89:109–116, 2011.

158. Rassnick KM, Gieger TL, Williams LE, et al.: Phase I evaluation of CCNU (lomustine) in tumor-bearing cats, *J Vet Intern Med* 15:196–199, 2001.

159. Hosoya K, Lord LK, Lara-Garcia A, et al.: Prevalence of elevated alanine transaminase activity in dogs treated with CCNU (lomustine), *Vet Comp Oncol* 7:244–255, 2009.

160. Kristal O, Rassnick KM, Gliatto JM, et al.: Hepatotoxicity associated with CCNU (lomustine) chemotherapy in dogs, *J Vet Intern Med* 18:75–80, 2004.

161. Musser ML, Quinn HT, Chretin JD: Low apparent risk of CCNU (lomustine)-associated clinical hepatotoxicity in cats, *J Feline Med Surg* 14:871–875, 2012.

162. Skorupski KA, Hammond GM, Irish AM, et al.: Prospective randomized clinical trial assessing the efficacy of denamarin for prevention of CCNU-induced hepatopathy in tumor-bearing dogs, *J Vet Intern Med* 25:838–845, 2011.

163. Skorupski KA, Durham AC, Duda L, et al.: Pulmonary fibrosis after high cumulative dose nitrosurea chemotherapy in a cat, *Vet Comp Oncol* 6:120–125, 2008.

164. Reusser F: Mode of action of streptozotocin, *J Bacteriol* 105:580–588, 1971.

165. Bhuyan BK: The action of streptozotocin on mammalian cells, *Cancer Res* 30:2017–2023, 1970.

166. Schnedl WJ, Ferber S, Johnson JH, et al.: Stz transport and cytotoxicity: specific enhancement in glut2-expressing cells, *Diabetes* 43:1326–1333, 1994.

167. Hosokawa M, Dolci W, Thorens B: Differential sensitivity of glut1- and glut2-expressing beta cells to streptozotocin, *Biochem Biophys Res Commun* 289:1114–1117, 2001.

168. Adolphe AB, Glasofer ED, Troetel WM, et al.: Preliminary pharmacokinetics of streptozotocin, an antineoplastic antibiotic, *J Clin Pharmacol* 17:379–388, 1977.

169. Schein PS, Cooney DA, Vernon ML: The use of nicotinamide to modify the toxicity of streptozotocin diabetes without loss of antitumor activity, *Cancer Res* 27:2324–2332, 1967.

170. Schein PS, Rakieten N, Cooney DA, et al.: Streptozotocin diabetes in monkeys and dogs, and its prevention by nicotinamide, *Proc Soc Exp Biol Med* 143:514–518, 1973.

171. Schein PS: 1-Methyl-1-nitrosourea and dialkylnitrosamine depression of nicotinamide adenine dinucleotide, *Cancer Res* 29:1226–1232, 1969.

172. Panasci LC, Fox PA, Schein PS: Structure-activity studies of methylnitrosourea antitumor agents with reduced murine bone marrow toxicity, *Cancer Res* 37:3321–3328, 1977.

173. Moore AS, Nelson RW, Henry CJ, et al.: Streptozocin for treatment of pancreatic islet cell tumors in dogs: 17 cases (1989–1999), *J Am Vet Med Assoc* 221:811–818, 2002.

174. Audette RC, Connors TA, Mandel HG, et al.: Studies on the mechanism of action of the tumour inhibitory triazenes, *Biochem Pharmacol* 22:1855–1864, 1973.

175. Reid JM, Kuffel MJ, Miller JK, et al.: Metabolic activation of dacarbazine by human cytochromes p450: the role of cyp1a1, cyp1a2, and cyp2e1, *Clin Cancer Res* 5:2192–2197, 1999.

176. Nagasawa HT, Shirota FN, Mizuno NS: The mechanism of alkylation of DNA by 5-(3-methyl-1-triazeno)imidazole-4-carboxamide (mic), a metabolite of dic (NSC-45388): non-involvement of diazomethane, *Chem Biol Interact* 8:403–413, 1974.

177. Kleihues P, Kolar GF, Margison GP: Interaction of the carcinogen 3,3-dimethyl-1-phenyltriazene with nucleic acids of various rat tissues and the effect of a protein-free diet, *Cancer Res* 36:2189–2193, 1976.
178. Griessmayr PC, Payne SE, Winter JE, et al.: Dacarbazine as single-agent therapy for relapsed lymphoma in dogs, *J Vet Intern Med* 23:1227–1231, 2009.
179. Flory AB, Rassnick KM, Al-Sarraf R, et al.: Combination of CCNU and DTIC chemotherapy for treatment of resistant lymphoma in dogs, *J Vet Intern Med* 22:164–171, 2008.
180. Van Vechten M, Helfand SC, Jeglum KA: Treatment of relapsed canine lymphoma with doxorubicin and dacarbazine, *J Vet Intern Med* 4:187–191, 1990.
181. Dervisis NG, Dominguez PA, Sarbu L, et al.: Efficacy of temozolomide or dacarbazine in combination with an anthracycline for rescue chemotherapy in dogs with lymphoma, *J Am Vet Med Assoc* 231:563–569, 2007.
182. Finotello R, Stefanello D, Zini E, et al.: Comparison of doxorubicin-cyclophosphamide with doxorubicin-dacarbazine for the adjuvant treatment of canine hemangiosarcoma, *Vet Comp Oncol* 15:25–35, 2017.
183. Dervisis NG, Dominguez PA, Newman RG, et al.: Treatment with dav for advanced-stage hemangiosarcoma in dogs, *J Am Anim Hosp Assoc* 47:170–178, 2011.
184. Gale GR, Simpson JG, Smith AB: Studies of the mode of action of N-isopropyl-alpha-(2-methylhydrazino)-p-toluamide, *Cancer Res* 27:1186–1191, 1967.
185. Moloney SJ, Wiebkin P, Cummings SW, et al.: Metabolic activation of the terminal N-methyl group of N-isopropyl-alpha-(2-methylhydrazino)-p-toluamide hydrochloride (procarbazine), *Carcinogenesis* 6:397–401, 1985.
186. Schold SC, Brent TP, von Hofe E, et al.: O^6-alkylguanine-DNA alkyltransferase and sensitivity to procarbazine in human brain-tumor xenografts, *J Neurosurg* 70:573–577, 1989.
187. Shiba DA, Weinkam RJ: Quantitative analysis of procarbazine, procarbazine metabolites and chemical degradation products with application to pharmacokinetic studies, *J Chromatogr B Biomed Sci Appl* 229:397–407, 1982.
188. Oliverio VT, Denham C, Devita VT, et al.: Some pharmacologic properties of a new antitumor agent, N-isopropyl-alpha-(2-methylhydrazino)-p-toluamide, hydrochloride (NSC-77213), *Cancer Chemother Rep* 42:1–7, 1964.
189. Chabner BA, Sponzo R, Hubbard S, et al.: High-dose intermittent intravenous infusion of procarbazine (NSC-77213), *Cancer Chemother Rep* 57:361–363, 1973.
190. Northrup NC, Gieger TL, Kosarek CE, et al.: Mechlorethamine, procarbazine and prednisone for the treatment of resistant lymphoma in dogs, *Vet Comp Oncol* 7:38–44, 2009.
191. Brown PM, Tzannes S, Nguyen S, et al.: Lopp chemotherapy as a first-line treatment for dogs with T-cell lymphoma, *Vet Comp Oncol* 16:108–113, 2018.
192. Zunino F, Gambetta R, Di Marco A: The inhibition in vitro of DNA polymerase and rna polymerase by daunomycin and adriamycin, *Biochem Pharmacol* 24:309–311, 1975.
193. Tewey KM, Chen GI, Nelson EM, et al.: Intercalative anti-tumor drugs interfere with the breakage-reunion reaction of mammalian DNA topoisomerase, *J Biol Chem* 259:9182–9187, 1984.
194. Taatjes DJ, Gaudiano G, Resing K, et al.: Alkylation of DNA by the anthracycline, antitumor drugs adriamycin and daunomycin, *J Med Chem* 39:4135–4138, 1996.
195. Doroshow JH: Role of hydrogen peroxide and hydroxyl radical in the killing of ehrlich tumor cells by anticancer quinones, *Proc Natl Acad Sci USA* 83:4514–4518, 1985.
196. Bachur NR, Gordon SL, Gee MV: A general mechanism for microsomal activation of quinone anticancer agents to free radicals, *Cancer Res* 38:1745–1750, 1978.
197. Pessah IN, Durie EL, Schiedt MJ, et al.: Anthraquinone-sensitized Ca^{++} release channel from rat cardiac sarcoplasmic reticulum:

198. Oakes SG, Schlager JJ, Santone KS, et al.: Doxorubicin blocks the increase in intracellular Ca^{++}, part of a second messenger system in n1e-115 murine neuroblastoma cells, *J Pharmacol Exp Ther* 252:979–983, 1990.
199. Mau BL, Powis G: Inhibition of cellular thioredoxin reductase by diaziquone and doxorubicin: relationship to the inhibition of cell proliferation and decreased ribonucleotide reductase activity, *Biochem Pharmacol* 43:1621–1626, 1992.
200. Morre DJ, Kim C, Paulik M, et al.: Is the drug-responsive nadh oxidase of the cancer cell plasma membrane a molecular target for adriamycin? *J Bioenerg Biomembr* 29:269–280, 1997.
201. Terasaki T, Iga T, Sugiyama Y, et al.: Experimental evidence of characteristic tissue distribution of adriamycin: tissue DNA concentration as a determinant, *J Pharm Pharmacol* 34:597–600, 1982.
202. Nicolay K, Timmers RJM, Spoelstra E, et al.: The interaction of adriamycin with cardiolipin in model and rat liver mitochondrial membranes, *Biochim Biophys Acta* 778:359–371, 1984.
203. Goormaghtigh E, Chatelain P, Caspers J, et al.: Evidence of a specific complex between adriamycin and negatively-charged phospholipids, *Biochim Biophys Acta* 597:1–14, 1980.
204. Gustafson DL, Rastatter JC, Colombo T, et al.: Doxorubicin pharmacokinetics: macromolecule binding, metabolism and elimination in the context of a physiological model, *J Pharm Sci* 91:1488–1501, 2002.
205. Ahmed NK, Felsted RL, Bachur NR: Daunorubicin reduction mediated by aldehyde and ketone reductases, *Xenobiotica* 11:131–136, 1981.
206. Pan SS, Bachur NR: Xanthine oxidase catalyzed reductive cleavage of anthracycline antibiotics and free radical formation, *Mol Pharmacol* 17:95–99, 1980.
207. Eschalier A, Lavarenne J, Burtin C, et al.: Study of histamine release induced by acute administration of antitumor agents in dogs, *Cancer Chemother Pharmacol* 21:246–250, 1988.
208. Thamm DH, Vail DM: Aftershocks of cancer chemotherapy: managing adverse effects, *J Am Anim Hosp Assoc* 43:1–7, 2007.
209. Billingham ME, Mason JW, Bristow MR, et al.: Anthracycline cardiomyopathy monitored by morphologic changes, *Cancer Treat Rep* 62:865–872, 1978.
210. Alves de Souza RC, Camacho AA: Neurohormonal, hemodynamic, and electrocardiographic evaluations of healthy dogs receiving long-term administration of doxorubicin, *Am J Vet Res* 67:1319–1325, 2006.
211. Ghigo A, Li M, Hirsch E: New signal transduction paradigms in anthracycline-induced cardiotoxicity, *Biochim Biophys Acta* 1863:1916–1925, 2016.
212. Chatterjee K, Zhang J, Honbo N, et al.: Doxorubicin cardiomyopathy, *Cardiology* 115:155–162, 2010.
213. Pessah IN, Durie EL, Schiedt MJ, et al.: Anthraquinone-sensitized Ca^{2+} release channel from rat cardiac sarcoplasmic reticulum: possible receptor-mediated mechanism of doxorubicin cardiomyopathy, *Mol Pharmacol* 37:503–514, 1990.
214. Zhang S, Liu X, Bawa-Khalfe T, et al.: Identification of the molecular basis of doxorubicin-induced cardiotoxicity, *Nat Med* 18:1639–1642, 2012.
215. Zhao L, Zhang B: Doxorubicin induces cardiotoxicity through upregulation of death receptors mediated apoptosis in cardiomyocytes, *Sci Rep* 7:44735, 2017.
216. FitzPatrick WM, Dervisis NG, Kitchell BE: Safety of concurrent administration of dexrazoxane and doxorubicin in the canine cancer patient, *Vet Comp Oncol* 8:273–282, 2010.
217. O'Keefe DA, Sisson DD, Gelberg HB, et al.: Systemic toxicity associated with doxorubicin administration in cats, *J Vet Intern Med* 7:309–317, 1993.
218. Foye WO, Vajragupta O, Sengupta SK: DNA-binding specificity and rna polymerase inhibitory activity of bis(aminoalkyl)anthraquinones and bis(methylthio)vinylquinolinium iodides, *J Pharm Sci* 71:253–257, 1982.

219. Crespi MD, Ivanier SE, Genovese J, et al.: Mitoxantrone affects topoisomerase activities in human breast cancer cells, *Biochem Biophys Res Commun* 136:521–528, 1986.
220. Patterson LH, Gandecha BM, Brown JR: 1,4-bis(2-[(2-hydroxyethyl)amino]ethylamino)-9,10-anthracenedione, an anthraquinone antitumour agent that does not cause lipid peroxidation in vivo; comparison with daunorubicin, *Biochem Biophys Res Commun* 110:399–405, 1983.
221. Nguyen B, Gutierrez PL: Mechanism(s) for the metabolism of mitoxantrone: electron spin resonance and electrochemical studies, *Chem Biol Interact* 74:139–162, 1990.
222. Alberts DS, Peng YM, Leigh S, et al.: Disposition of mitoxantrone in cancer patients, *Cancer Res* 45:1879–1884, 1985.
223. Lu K, Savaraj N, Loo TL: Pharmacological disposition of 1,4-dihydroxy-5-8-bis[[2 [(2-hydroxyethyl)amino]ethyl]amino]-9,10-anthracenedione dihydrochloride in the dog, *Cancer Chemother Pharmacol* 13:63–66, 1984.
224. Chiccarelli FS, Morrison JA, Cosulich DB, et al.: Identification of human urinary mitoxantrone metabolites, *Cancer Res* 46:4858–4861, 1986.
225. Henry CJ, McCaw DL, Turnquist SE, et al.: Clinical evaluation of mitoxantrone and piroxicam in a canine model of human invasive urinary bladder carcinoma, *Clin Cancer Res* 9:906–911, 2003.
226. Turek MM, Forrest LJ, Adams WM, et al.: Postoperative radiotherapy and mitoxantrone for anal sac adenocarcinoma in the dog: 15 cases (1991–2001), *Vet Comp Oncol* 1:94–104, 2003.
227. Wang SL, Lee JJ, Liao AT: Comparison of efficacy and toxicity of doxorubicin and mitoxantrone in combination chemotherapy for canine lymphoma, *Can Vet J* 57:271–276, 2016.
228. Lucroy MD, Phillips BS, Kraegel SA, et al.: Evaluation of single-agent mitoxantrone as chemotherapy for relapsing canine lymphoma, *J Vet Intern Med* 12:325–329, 1998.
229. Takusagawa F, Dabrow M, Neidle S, et al.: The structure of a pseudo intercalated complex between actinomycin and the DNA binding sequence d(GpC), *Nature* 296:466–469, 1982.
230. Takusagawa F, Goldstein BM, Youngster S, et al.: Crystallization and preliminary x-ray study of a complex between d(ATGCAT) and actinomycin D, *J Biol Chem* 259:4714–4715, 1984.
231. Brown SC, Mullis K, Levenson C, et al.: Aqueous solution structure of an intercalated actinomycin D-dATGCAT complex by two-dimensional and one-dimensional proton nmr, *Biochemistry* 23:403–408, 1984.
232. Wadkins RM, Jovin TM: Actinomycin D and 7-aminoactinomycin D binding to single-stranded DNA, *Biochemistry* 30:9469–9478, 1991.
233. Goldberg IH, Rabinowitz M, Reich E: Basis of actinomycin action. I. DNA binding and inhibition of RNA-polymerase synthetic reactions by actinomycin, *Proc Natl Acad Sci USA* 48:2094–2101, 1962.
234. Reich E, Franklin RM, Shatkin AJ, et al.: Action of actinomycin D on animal cells and viruses, *Proc Natl Acad Sci USA* 48:1238–1245, 1962.
235. Kessel D, Wodinsky I: Uptake in vivo and in vitro of actinomycin D by mouse leukemias as factors in survival, *Biochem Pharmacol* 17:161–164, 1968.
236. Inaba M, Johnson RK: Decreased retention of actinomycin D as the basis for cross-resistance in anthracycline-resistant sublines of p388 leukemia, *Cancer Res* 37:4629–4634, 1977.
237. Diddens H, Gekeler V, Neumann M, et al.: Characterization of actinomycin-D-resistant cho cell lines exhibiting a multidrug-resistance phenotype and amplified DNA sequences, *Int J Cancer* 40:635–642, 1987.
238. Galbraith WM, Mellett LB: Tissue disposition of 3h-actinomycin D (NSC-3053) in the rat, monkey, and dog, *Cancer Chemother Rep* 59:1601–1609, 1975.
239. Furth JJ, Cohen SS: Inhibition of mammalian DNA polymerase by the 5′-triphosphate of 1-beta-d-arabinofuranosylcytosine and the 5′-triphosphate of 9-beta-d-arabinofuranoxyladenine, *Cancer Res* 28:2061–2067, 1968.
240. Kufe DW, Major PP, Egan EM, et al.: Correlation of cytotoxicity with incorporation of ara-C into DNA, *J Biol Chem* 255, 1980. 8997–8900.
241. Major PP, Egan EM, Herrick DJ, et al.: Effect of ara-C incorporation on deoxyribonucleic acid synthesis in cells, *Biochem Pharmacol* 31:2937–2940, 1982.
242. Mikita T, Beardsley GP: Functional consequences of the arabinosylcytosine structural lesion in DNA, *Biochemistry* 27:4698–4705, 1988.
243. Bianchi Scarra GL, Romani M, Coviello DA, et al.: Terminal erythroid differentiation in the k-562 cell line by 1-beta-d-arabinofuranosylcytosine: accompaniment by c-myc messenger RNA decrease, *Cancer Res* 46:6327–6332, 1986.
244. Plagemann PG, Marz R, Wohlhueter RM: Transport and metabolism of deoxycytidine and 1-beta-d-arabinofuranosylcytosine into cultured novikoff rat hepatoma cells, relationship to phosphorylation, and regulation of triphosphate synthesis, *Cancer Res* 38:978–989, 1978.
245. Garcia-Carbonero R, Ryan DP, Chabner BA: Cytidine analogs. In Chabner BA, Longo DL, editors: *Cancer chemotherapy & biotherapy: principles and practice*, Philadelphia, 2001, Lippincott Williams & Wilkins, pp 265–294.
246. Scott-Moncrieff JC, Chan TC, Samuels ML, et al.: Plasma and cerebrospinal fluid pharmacokinetics of cytosine arabinoside in dogs, *Cancer Chemother Pharmacol* 29:13–18, 1991.
247. Ruslander D, Moore AS, Gliatto JM, et al.: Cytosine arabinoside as a single agent for the induction of remission in canine lymphoma, *J Vet Intern Med* 8:299–301, 1994.
248. Alvarez FJ, Kisseberth WC, Gallant SL, et al.: Dexamethasone, melphalan, actinomycin D, cytosine arabinoside (DMAC) protocol for dogs with relapsed lymphoma, *J Vet Intern Med* 20:1178–1183, 2006.
249. Marconato L, Bonfanti U, Stefanello D, et al.: Cytosine arabinoside in addition to VCAA-based protocols for the treatment of canine lymphoma with bone marrow involvement: does it make the difference? *Vet Comp Oncol* 6:80–89, 2008.
250. Menaut P, Landart J, Behr S, et al.: Treatment of 11 dogs with meningoencephalomyelitis of unknown origin with a combination of prednisolone and cytosine arabinoside, *Vet Rec* 162:241–245, 2008.
251. Smith PM, Stalin CE, Shaw D, et al.: Comparison of two regimens for the treatment of meningoencephalomyelitis of unknown etiology, *J Vet Intern Med* 23:520–526, 2009.
252. Allegra CJ, Fine RL, Drake JC, et al.: The effect of methotrexate on intracellular folate pools in human mcf-7 breast cancer cells: evidence for direct inhibition of purine synthesis, *J Biol Chem* 261:6478–6485, 1986.
253. Allegra CJ, Chabner BA, Drake JC, et al.: Enhanced inhibition of thymidylate synthase by methotrexate polyglutamates, *J Biol Chem* 260:9720–9726, 1985.
254. Fabre I, Fabre G, Goldman ID: Polyglutamylation, an important element in methotrexate cytotoxicity and selectivity in tumor versus murine granulocytic progenitor cells in vitro, *Cancer Res* 44:3190–3195, 1984.
255. Wan SH, Huffman DH, Azarnoff DL, et al.: Effect of route of administration and effusions on methotrexate pharmacokinetics, *Cancer Res* 34:3487–3491, 1974.
256. Bischoff KB, Dedrick RL, Zaharko DS, et al.: Methotrexate pharmacokinetics, *J Pharm Sci* 60:1128–1133, 1971.
257. Mackey JR, Mani RS, Selner M, et al.: Functional nucleoside transporters are required for gemcitabine influx and manifestation of toxicity in cancer cell lines, *Cancer Res* 58:4349–4357, 1998.
258. Gandhi V, Plunkett W: Modulatory activity of 2′,2′-difluorodeoxycytidine on the phosphorylation and cytotoxicity of arabinosyl nucleosides, *Cancer Res* 50:3675–3680, 1990.
259. Gandhi V, Legha J, Chen F, et al.: Excision of 2′,2′-difluorodeoxycytidine (gemcitabine) monophosphate residues from DNA, *Cancer Res* 56:4453–4459, 1996.

260. Huang P, Plunkett W: Fludarabine- and gemcitabine-induced apoptosis: incorporation of analogs into DNA is a critical event, *Cancer Chemother Pharmacol* 36:181–188, 1995.

261. Veltkamp SA, Pluim D, van Eijndhoven MA, et al.: New insights into the pharmacology and cytotoxicity of gemcitabine and 2′,2′-difluorodeoxyuridine, *Mol Cancer Ther* 7:2415–2425, 2008.

262. Veltkamp SA, Jansen RS, Callies S, et al.: Oral administration of gemcitabine in patients with refractory tumors: a clinical and pharmacologic study, *Clin Cancer Res* 14:3477–3486, 2008.

263. Veltkamp SA, Pluim D, van Tellingen O, et al.: Extensive metabolism and hepatic accumulation of gemcitabine after multiple oral and intravenous administration in mice, *Drug Metab Dispos* 36:1606–1615, 2008.

264. Tempero M, Plunkett W, Ruiz Van Haperen V, et al.: Randomized phase II comparison of dose-intense gemcitabine: thirty-minute infusion and fixed dose rate infusion in patients with pancreatic adenocarcinoma, *J Clin Oncol* 21:3402–3408, 2003.

265. Turner AI, Hahn KA, Rusk A, et al.: Single agent gemcitabine chemotherapy in dogs with spontaneously occurring lymphoma, *J Vet Intern Med* 20:1384–1388, 2006.

266. Marconato L, Zini E, Lindner D, et al.: Toxic effects and antitumor response of gemcitabine in combination with piroxicam treatment in dogs with transitional cell carcinoma of the urinary bladder, *J Am Vet Med Assoc* 238:1004–1010, 2011.

267. McMahon M, Mathie T, Stingle N, et al.: Adjuvant carboplatin and gemcitabine combination chemotherapy postamputation in canine appendicular osteosarcoma, *J Vet Intern Med* 25:511–517, 2011.

268. Marconato L, Lorenzo RM, Abramo F, et al.: Adjuvant gemcitabine after surgical removal of aggressive malignant mammary tumours in dogs, *Vet Comp Oncol* 6:90–101, 2008.

269. Elpiner AK, Brodsky EM, Hazzah TN, et al.: Single-agent gemcitabine chemotherapy in dogs with hepatocellular carcinomas, *Vet Comp Oncol* 9:260–268, 2011.

270. McMahon M, Mathie T, Stingle N, et al.: Adjuvant carboplatin and gemcitabine combination chemotherapy postamputation in canine appendicular osteosarcoma, *J Vet Intern Med* 25:511–517, 2011.

271. Dominguez PA, Dervisis NG, Cadile CD, et al.: Combined gemcitabine and carboplatin therapy for carcinomas in dogs, *J Vet Intern Med* 23:130–137, 2009.

272. Martinez-Ruzafa I, Dominguez PA, Dervisis NG, et al.: Tolerability of gemcitabine and carboplatin doublet therapy in cats with carcinomas, *J Vet Intern Med* 23:570–577, 2009.

273. LeBlanc AK, LaDue TA, Turrel JM, et al.: Unexpected toxicity following use of gemcitabine as a radiosensitizer in head and neck carcinomas: a veterinary radiation therapy oncology group pilot study, *Vet Radiol Ultrasound* 45:466–470, 2004.

274. Wohlhueter RM, McIvor RS, Plagemann PG: Facilitated transport of uracil and 5-fluorouracil, and permeation of orotic acid into cultured mammalian cells, *J Cell Physiol* 104:309–319, 1980.

275. Reyes P: The synthesis of 5-fluorouridine 5′-phosphate by a pyrimidine phosphoribosyltransferase of mammalian origin. I. Some properties of the enzyme from p1534j mouse leukemic cells, *Biochemistry* 8:2057–2062, 1969.

276. Houghton JA, Houghton PJ: Elucidation of pathways of 5-fluorouracil metabolism in xenografts of human colorectal adenocarcinoma, *Eur J Cancer Clin Oncol* 19:807–815, 1983.

277. Kufe DW, Major PP: 5-Fluorouracil incorporation into human breast carcinoma rna correlates with cytotoxicity, *J Biol Chem* 256:9802–9805, 1981.

278. Kufe DW, Major PP, Egan EM, et al.: 5-Fluoro-2′-deoxyuridine incorporation in l1210 DNA, *J Biol Chem* 256:8885–8888, 1981.

279. Tanaka M, Yoshida S, Saneyoshi M, et al.: Utilization of 5-fluoro-2′-deoxyuridine triphosphate and 5-fluoro-2′-deoxycytidine triphosphate in DNA synthesis by DNA polymerases alpha and beta from calf thymus, *Cancer Res* 41:4132–4135, 1981.

280. Santi DV, McHenry CS, Sommer H: Mechanism of interaction of thymidylate synthetase with 5-fluorodeoxyuridylate, *Biochemistry* 13:471–481, 1974.

281. Naguib FN, el Kouni MH, Cha S: Enzymes of uracil catabolism in normal and neoplastic human tissues, *Cancer Res* 45:5405–5412, 1985.

282. Grem JL: 5-Fluoropyrimidines. In Chabner BA, Longo DL, editors: *Cancer chemotherapy & biotherapy: principles and practice*, ed 3, Philadelphia, 2001, Lippincott Williams & Wilkins, pp 185–264.

283. Snavely NR, Snavely DA, Wilson BB: Toxic effects of fluorouracil cream ingestion on dogs and cats, *Arch Dermatol* 146:1195–1196, 2010.

284. Rose WC, Crosswell AR, Bronson JJ, et al.: In vivo antitumor activity of 9-[(2-phosphonylmethoxy)ethyl]-guanine and related phosphonate nucleotide analogues, *J Natl Cancer Inst* 82:510–512, 1990.

285. Reiser H, Wang J, Chong L, et al.: Gs-9219—a novel acyclic nucleotide analogue with potent antineoplastic activity in dogs with spontaneous non-Hodgkin's lymphoma, *Clin Cancer Res* 14:2824–2832, 2008.

286. Compton ML, Toole JJ, Paborsky LR: 9-(2-Phosphonylmethoxyethyl)-N^6-cyclopropyl-2,6-diaminopurine (CPR-PMEDAP) as a prodrug of 9-(2-phosphonylmethoxyethyl)guanine (PMEG), *Biochem Pharmacol* 58:709–714, 1999.

287. Naesens L, Hatse S, Segers C, et al.: 9-(2-Phosphonylmethoxyethyl)-N^6-cyclopropyl-2,6-diaminopurine: a novel prodrug of 9-(2-phosphonylmethoxyethyl)guanine with improved antitumor efficacy and selectivity in choriocarcinoma-bearing rats, *Oncol Res* 11:195–203, 1999.

288. Ho HT, Woods KL, Konrad SA, et al.: Cellular metabolism and enzymatic phosphorylation of 9-(2-phosphonylmethoxyethyl) guanine (PMEG), a potent antiviral agent, *Adv Exp Med Biol* 312:159–166, 1992.

289. Kramata P, Votruba I, Otova B, et al.: Different inhibitory potencies of acyclic phosphonomethoxyalkyl nucleotide analogs toward DNA polymerases alpha, delta and epsilon, *Mol Pharmacol* 49:1005–1011, 1996.

290. Morges MA, Burton JH, Saba CF, et al.: Phase II evaluation of VDC-1101 in canine cutaneous T-cell lymphoma, *J Vet Intern Med* 28:1569–1574, 2014.

291. Thamm DH, Vail DM, Kurzman ID, et al.: GS-9219/VDC-1101—a prodrug of the acyclic nucleotide PMEG has antitumor activity in spontaneous canine multiple myeloma, *BMC Vet Res* 10:30, 2014.

292. Thamm DH, Vail DM, Post GS, et al.: Alternating rabacfosadine/doxorubicin: efficacy and tolerability in naive canine multicentric lymphoma, *J Vet Intern Med* 31:872–878, 2017.

293. Vail DM, Thamm DH, Reiser H, et al.: Assessment of GS-9219 in a pet dog model of non-Hodgkin's lymphoma, *Clin Cancer Res* 15:3503–3510, 2009.

294. Saba CF, Vickery KR, Clifford CA, et al.: Rabacfosadine for relapsed canine B-cell lymphoma: efficacy and adverse event profiles of 2 different doses, *Vet Comp Oncol* 16:E76–E82, 2018.

295. Schiff PB, Fant J, Horwitz SB: Promotion of microtubule assembly in vitro by taxol, *Nature* 277:665–667, 1979.

296. Schiff PB, Horwitz SB: Taxol stabilizes microtubules in mouse fibroblast cells, *Proc Natl Acad Sci USA* 77:1561–1565, 1980.

297. Ringel I, Horwitz SB: Studies with RP 56976 (taxotere): a semisynthetic analogue of taxol, *J Natl Cancer Inst* 83:288–291, 1991.

298. Jordan MA, Toso RJ, Thrower D, et al.: Mechanism of mitotic block and inhibition of cell proliferation by taxol at low concentrations, *Proc Natl Acad Sci USA* 90:9552–9556, 1993.

299. Bissery MC, Guenard D, Gueritte-Voegelein F, et al.: Experimental antitumor activity of taxotere (RP 56976, NSC 628503), a taxol analogue, *Cancer Res* 51:4845–4852, 1991.

300. Diaz JF, Andreu JM: Assembly of purified gdp-tubulin into microtubules induced by taxol and taxotere: reversibility, ligand stoichiometry, and competition, *Biochemistry* 32:2747–2755, 1993.

301. Vail DM, von Euler H, Rusk AW, et al.: A randomized trial investigating the efficacy and safety of water soluble micellar paclitaxel (Paccal Vet) for treatment of nonresectable grade 2 or 3 mast cell tumors in dogs, *J Vet Intern Med* 26:598–607, 2012.

302. Kim J, Doerr M, Kitchell BE: Exploration of paclitaxel (taxol) as a treatment for malignant tumors in cats: a descriptive case series, *J Feline Med Surg* 17:186–190, 2015.

303. Simon D, Schoenrock D, Baumgartner W, et al.: Postoperative adjuvant treatment of invasive malignant mammary gland tumors in dogs with doxorubicin and docetaxel, *J Vet Intern Med* 20:1184–1190, 2006.

304. Shiu KB, McCartan L, Kubicek L, et al.: Intravenous administration of docetaxel to cats with cancer, *J Vet Intern Med* 25:916–919, 2011.

305. McEntee MC, Rassnick KM, Bailey DB, et al.: Phase I and pharmacokinetic evaluation of the combination of orally administered docetaxel and cyclosporin a in tumor-bearing cats, *J Vet Intern Med* 20:1370–1375, 2006.

306. McEntee MC, Rassnick KM, Lewis LD, et al.: Phase I and pharmacokinetic evaluation of the combination of orally administered docetaxel and cyclosporin a in tumor-bearing dogs, *Am J Vet Res* 67:1057–1062, 2006.

307. Waite A, Balkman C, Bailey D, et al.: Phase II study of oral docetaxel and cyclosporine in canine epithelial cancer, *Vet Comp Oncol* 12:160–168, 2014.

308. Correia JJ: Effects of antimitotic agents on tubulin-nucleotide interactions, *Pharmacol Ther* 52:127–147, 1991.

309. Wilson L, Jordan MA, Morse A, et al.: Interaction of vinblastine with steady-state microtubules in vitro, *J Mol Biol* 159:125–149, 1982.

310. Bruchovsky N, Owen AA, Becker AJ, et al.: Effects of vinblastine on the proliferative capacity of l cells and their progress through the division cycle, *Cancer Res* 25:1232–1237, 1965.

311. Tucker RW, Owellen RJ, Harris SB: Correlation of cytotoxicity and mitotic spindle dissolution by vinblastine in mammalian cells, *Cancer Res* 37:4346–4351, 1977.

312. Creasey WA, Marsh JC: Metabolism of vinblastine (VBL) in the dog, *Proc Am Assoc Cancer Res* 14:57, 1973 (abstract).

313. Arnold EJ, Childress MO, Fourez LM, et al.: Clinical trial of vinblastine in dogs with transitional cell carcinoma of the urinary bladder, *J Vet Intern Med* 25:1385–1390, 2011.

314. Lenz JA, Robat CS, Stein TJ: Vinblastine as a second rescue for the treatment of canine multicentric lymphoma in 39 cases (2005 to 2014), *J Small Anim Pract* 57:429–434, 2016.

315. Krick EL, Cohen RB, Gregor TP, et al.: Prospective clinical trial to compare vincristine and vinblastine in a cop-based protocol for lymphoma in cats, *J Vet Intern Med* 27:134–140, 2013.

316. Vickery KR, Wilson H, Vail DM, et al.: Dose-escalating vinblastine for the treatment of canine mast cell tumour, *Vet Comp Oncol* 6:111–119, 2008.

317. Serra Varela JC, Pecceu E, Handel I, et al.: Tolerability of a rapid-escalation vinblastine-prednisolone protocol in dogs with mast cell tumours, *Vet Med Sci* 2:266–280, 2016.

318. Grant IA, Rodriguez CO, Kent MS, et al.: A phase II clinical trial of vinorelbine in dogs with cutaneous mast cell tumors, *J Vet Intern Med* 22:388–393, 2008.

319. Poirier VJ, Burgess KE, Adams WM, et al.: Toxicity, dosage, and efficacy of vinorelbine (navelbine) in dogs with spontaneous neoplasia, *J Vet Intern Med* 18:536–539, 2004.

320. Wouda RM, Miller ME, Chon E, et al.: Clinical effects of vinorelbine administration in the management of various malignant tumor types in dogs: 58 cases (1997–2012), *J Am Vet Med Assoc* 246:1230–1237, 2015.

321. Pierro JA, Mallett CL, Saba CF: Phase I clinical trial of vinorelbine in tumor-bearing cats, *J Vet Intern Med* 27:943–948, 2013.

322. Minocha A, Long BH: Inhibition of the DNA catenation activity of type II topoisomerase by VP16-213 and VM26, *Biochem Biophys Res Commun* 122:165–170, 1984.

323. Chen GL, Yang L, Rowe TC, et al.: Nonintercalative antitumor drugs interfere with the breakage-reunion reaction of mammalian DNA topoisomerase II, *J Biol Chem* 259:13560–13566, 1984.

324. Long BH, Musial ST, Brattain MG: Single- and double-strand DNA breakage and repair in human lung adenocarcinoma cells exposed to etoposide and teniposide, *Cancer Res* 45:3106–3112, 1985.

325. Sullivan DM, Latham MD, Ross WE: Proliferation-dependent topoisomerase II content as a determinant of antineoplastic drug action in human, mouse, and chinese hamster ovary cells, *Cancer Res* 47:3973–3979, 1987.

326. Flory AB, Rassnick KM, Balkman CE, et al.: Oral bioavailability of etoposide after administration of a single dose to tumor-bearing dogs, *Am J Vet Res* 69:1316–1322, 2008.

327. Pommier YG, Goldwasser F, Strumberg D: Topoisomerase II inhibitors: epipodophyllotoxins, acridines, ellipticines, and bis-dioxopiperazines. In Chabner BA, Longo DL, editors: *cancer chemotherapy & biotherapy: principles and practice*, ed 3, Philadelphia, 2001, Lippincott Williams & Wilkins, pp 538–578.

328. Baxter JD, Harris AW, Tomkins GM, et al.: Glucocorticoid receptors in lymphoma cells in culture: relationship to glucocorticoid killing activity, *Science* 171:189–191, 1971.

329. Greenstein S, Ghias K, Krett NL, et al.: Mechanisms of glucocorticoid-mediated apoptosis in hematological malignancies, *Clin Cancer Res* 8:1681–1694, 2002.

330. Moalli PA, Rosen ST: Glucocorticoid receptors and resistance to glucocorticoids in hematologic malignancies, *Leuk Lymphoma* 15:363–374, 1994.

331. Fichtinger-Schepman AM, van der Veer JL, den Hartog JH, et al.: Adducts of the antitumor drug cis-diamminedichloroplatinum(II) with DNA: formation, identification, and quantitation, *Biochemistry* 24:707–713, 1985.

332. Zwelling LA, Anderson T, Kohn KW: DNA-protein and DNA interstrand cross-linking by cis- and trans-platinum(II) diamminedichloride in l1210 mouse leukemia cells and relation to cytotoxicity, *Cancer Res* 39:365–369, 1979.

333. Reed E, Kohn KW, Chabner BA, et al.: *Platinum analogues. Cancer chemotherapy: principles and practice*, Philadelphia, 1990, JB Lippincott Co., pp 465–490.

334. Calvert AH, Newell DR, Gumbrell LA, et al.: Carboplatin dosage: prospective evaluation of a simple formula based on renal function, *J Clin Oncol* 7:1748–1756, 1989.

335. Bailey DB, Rassnick KM, Erb HN, et al.: Effect of glomerular filtration rate on clearance and myelotoxicity of carboplatin in cats with tumors, *Am J Vet Res* 65:1502–1507, 2004.

336. Knapp DW, Richardson RC, DeNicola DB, et al.: Cisplatin toxicity in cats, *J Vet Intern Med* 1:29–35, 1987.

337. Knapp DW, Henry CJ, Widmer WR, et al.: Randomized trial of cisplatin versus firocoxib versus cisplatin/firocoxib in dogs with transitional cell carcinoma of the urinary bladder, *J Vet Intern Med* 27:126–133, 2013.

338. Barabas K, Milner R, Lurie D, et al.: Cisplatin: a review of toxicities and therapeutic applications, *Vet Comp Oncol* 6:1–18, 2008.

339. Allstadt SD, Rodriguez CO, Boostrom B, et al.: Randomized phase III trial of piroxicam in combination with mitoxantrone or carboplatin for first-line treatment of urogenital tract transitional cell carcinoma in dogs, *J Vet Intern Med* 29:261–267, 2015.

340. Wouda RM, Borrego J, Keuler NS, et al.: Evaluation of adjuvant carboplatin chemotherapy in the management of surgically excised anal sac apocrine gland adenocarcinoma in dogs, *Vet Comp Oncol* 14:67–80, 2016.

341. Murphy S, Hayes A, Adams V, et al.: Role of carboplatin in multi-modality treatment of canine tonsillar squamous cell carcinoma—a case series of five dogs, *J Small Anim Pract* 47:216–220, 2006.

342. Charney SC, Bergman PJ, McKnight JA, et al.: Evaluation of intracavitary mitoxantrone and carboplatin for treatment of carcinomatosis, sarcomatosis and mesothelioma, with or without malignant effusions: a retrospective analysis of 12 cases (1997–2002), *Vet Comp Oncol* 3:171–181, 2005.

343. Kisseberth WC, Vail DM, Yaissle J, et al.: Phase I clinical evaluation of carboplatin in tumor-bearing cats: a veterinary cooperative oncology group study, *J Vet Intern Med* 22:83–88, 2008.

344. Bailey DB, Rassnick KM, Prey JD, et al.: Evaluation of serum iohexol clearance for use in predicting carboplatin clearance in cats, *Am J Vet Res* 70:1135–1140, 2009.

345. Bailey DB, Rassnick KM, Dykes NL, et al.: Phase I evaluation of carboplatin by use of a dosing strategy based on a targeted area under the platinum concentration-versus-time curve and individual glomerular filtration rate in cats with tumors, *Am J Vet Res* 70:770–776, 2009.

346. Arteaga TA, McKnight J, Bergman PJ: A review of 18 cases of feline colonic adenocarcinoma treated with subtotal colectomies and adjuvant carboplatin, *J Am Anim Hosp Assoc* 48:399–404, 2012.

347. Morgan JS, Creasey DC, Wright JA: Evidence that the antitumor agent hydroxyurea enters mammalian cells by a diffusion mechanism, *Biochem Biophys Res Commun* 134:1254–1259, 1986.

348. Turner MK, Abrams R, Lieberman I: Meso-alpha, beta-diphenylsuccinate and hydroxyurea as inhibitors of deoxycytidylate synthesis in extracts of ehrlich ascites and l cells, *J Biol Chem* 241:5777–5780, 1966.

349. Skoog L, Nordenskjold B: Effects of hydroxyurea and 1-beta-d-arabinofuranosyl-cytosine on deoxyribonucleotide pools in mouse embryo cells, *Eur J Biochem* 19:81–89, 1971.

350. veer Reddy GP, Pardee AB: Inhibitor evidence for allosteric interaction in the replitase multienzyme complex, *Nature* 304:86–88, 1983.

351. Bianchi V, Pontis E, Reichard P: Changes of deoxyribonucleoside triphosphate pools induced by hydroxyurea and their relation to DNA synthesis, *J Biol Chem* 261:16037–16042, 1986.

352. Rassnick KM, Al-Sarraf R, Bailey DB, et al.: Phase II open-label study of single-agent hydroxyurea for treatment of mast cell tumours in dogs, *Vet Comp Oncol* 8:103–111, 2010.

353. Story MD, Voehringer DW, Stephens LC, et al.: l-Asparaginase kills lymphoma cells by apoptosis, *Cancer Chemother Pharmacol* 32:129–133, 1993.

354. Chabner BA, Sallan SE: Enzyme therapy: l-asparaginase. In Chabner BA, Longo DL, editors: *Cancer chemotherapy & biotherapy: principles and practice*, ed 3, Philadelphia, 2001, Lippincott Williams & Wilkins, pp 647–656.

355. London CA, Hannah AL, Zadovoskaya R, et al.: Phase I dose-escalating study of SU11654, a small molecule receptor tyrosine kinase inhibitor, in dogs with spontaneous malignancies, *Clin Cancer Res* 9:2755–2768, 2003.

356. London CA: Tyrosine kinase inhibitors in veterinary medicine, *Top Companion Anim Med* 24:106–112, 2009.

357. London CA, Malpas PB, Wood-Follis SL, et al.: Multi-center, placebo-controlled, double-blind, randomized study of oral toceranib phosphate (SU11654), a receptor tyrosine kinase inhibitor, for the treatment of dogs with recurrent (either local or distant) mast cell tumor following surgical excision, *Clin Cancer Res* 15:3856–3865, 2009.

358. Papaetis GS, Syrigos KN: Sunitinib: a multitargeted receptor tyrosine kinase inhibitor in the era of molecular cancer therapies, *BioDrugs* 23:377–389, 2009.

359. Dubreuil P, Letard S, Ciufolini M, et al.: Masitinib (AB1010), a potent and selective tyrosine kinase inhibitor targeting kit, *PLoS One* 4:e7258, 2009.

360. Fabian MA, Biggs WH, Treiber DK, et al.: A small molecule-kinase interaction map for clinical kinase inhibitors, *Nat Biotechnol* 23:329–336, 2005.

361. Yancey MF, Merritt DA, Lesman SP, et al.: Pharmacokinetic properties of toceranib phosphate (Palladia, SU11654), a novel tyrosine kinase inhibitor, in laboratory dogs and dogs with mast cell tumors, *J Vet Pharmacol Ther* 33:162–171, 2010.

362. Yancey MF, Merritt DA, White JA, et al.: Distribution, metabolism, and excretion of toceranib phosphate (Palladia, SU11654), a novel tyrosine kinase inhibitor, in dogs, *J Vet Pharmacol Ther* 33:154–161, 2010.

363. Hahn KA, Ogilvie G, Rusk T, et al.: Masitinib is safe and effective for the treatment of canine mast cell tumors, *J Vet Intern Med* 22:1301–1309, 2008.

364. Merrick CH, Pierro J, Schleis SE, et al.: Retrospective evaluation of toceranib phosphate (Palladia*) toxicity in cats, *Vet Comp Oncol* 15:710–717, 2017.

365. Harper A, Blackwood L: Toxicity and response in cats with neoplasia treated with toceranib phosphate, *J Feline Med Surg* 19:619–623, 2017.

366. Daly M, Sheppard S, Cohen N, et al.: Safety of masitinib mesylate in healthy cats, *J Vet Intern Med* 25:297–302, 2011.

367. Tjostheim SS, Stepien RL, Markovic LE, et al.: Effects of toceranib phosphate on systolic blood pressure and proteinuria in dogs, *J Vet Intern Med* 30:951–957, 2016.

368. London C, Mathie T, Stingle N, et al.: Preliminary evidence for biologic activity of toceranib phosphate (Palladia*) in solid tumours, *Vet Comp Oncol* 10:194–205, 2012.

369. Weishaar KM, Ehrhart EJ, Avery AC, et al.: C-kit mutation and localization status as response predictors in mast cell tumors in dogs treated with prednisone and toceranib or vinblastine, *J Vet Intern Med* 32:394–405, 2018.

370. Elliott JW, Swinbourne F, Parry A, et al.: Successful treatment of a metastatic, gastrointestinal stromal tumour in a dog with toceranib phosphate (Palladia), *J Small Anim Pract* 58:416–418, 2017.

371. London CA, Gardner HL, Mathie T, et al.: Impact of toceranib/piroxicam/cyclophosphamide maintenance therapy on outcome of dogs with appendicular osteosarcoma following amputation and carboplatin chemotherapy: a multi-institutional study, *PLoS One* 10:e0124889, 2015.

372. Kim C, Matsuyama A, Mutsaers AJ, et al.: Retrospective evaluation of toceranib (Palladia) treatment for canine metastatic appendicular osteosarcoma, *Can Vet J* 58:1059–1064, 2017.

373. Isotani M, Ishida N, Tominaga M, et al.: Effect of tyrosine kinase inhibition by imatinib mesylate on mast cell tumors in dogs, *J Vet Intern Med* 22:985–988, 2008.

374. Lachowicz JL, Post GS, Brodsky E: A phase I clinical trial evaluating imatinib mesylate (Gleevec) in tumor-bearing cats, *J Vet Intern Med* 19:860–864, 2005.

375. Su AI, Welsh JB, Sapinoso LM, et al.: Molecular classification of human carcinomas by use of gene expression signatures, *Cancer Res* 61:7388–7393, 2001.

376. Golub TR, Slonim DK, Tamayo P, et al.: Molecular classification of cancer: class discovery and class prediction by gene expression monitoring, *Science* 286:531–537, 1999.

377. Moseson DL, Sasaki GH, Kraybill WG, et al.: The use of antiestrogens tamoxifen and nafoxidine in the treatment of human breast cancer in correlation with estrogen receptor values: a phase II study, *Cancer* 41:797–802, 1978.

378. Flaherty KT, Puzanov I, Kim KB, et al.: Inhibition of mutated, activated BRAF in metastatic melanoma, *N Engl J Med* 363:809–819, 2010.

379. Paez JG, Janne PA, Lee JC, et al.: Egfr mutations in lung cancer: correlation with clinical response to gefitinib therapy, *Science* 304:1497–1500, 2004.

380. Ueda K, Cornwell MM, Gottesman MM, et al.: The *mdr1* gene, responsible for multidrug-resistance, codes for p-glycoprotein, *Biochem Biophys Res Commun* 141:956–962, 1986.

381. Mauldin G, Matus R, Patnaik A, et al.: Efficacy and toxicity of doxorubicin and cyclophosphamide used in the treatment of selected malignant tumors in 23 cats, *J Vet Intern Med* 2:60–65, 1988.

382. Herzog TJ, Krivak TC, Fader AN, et al.: Chemosensitivity testing with chemofx and overall survival in primary ovarian cancer, *Am J Obstet Gynecol* 203:68 e61–66, 2010.

383. Wakatsuki T, Irisawa A, Imamura H, et al.: Complete response of anaplastic pancreatic carcinoma to paclitaxel treatment selected by chemosensitivity testing, *Int J Clin Oncol* 15:310–313, 2010.

384. Ugurel S, Schadendorf D, Pfohler C, et al.: In vitro drug sensitivity predicts response and survival after individualized sensitivity-directed chemotherapy in metastatic melanoma: a multicenter phase II trial of the dermatologic cooperative oncology group, *Clin Cancer Res* 12:5454–5463, 2006.

385. Staib P, Staltmeier E, Neurohr K, et al.: Prediction of individual response to chemotherapy in patients with acute myeloid leukaemia using the chemosensitivity index CI, *Br J Haematol* 128:783–791, 2005.

386. Lee JK, Havaleshko DM, Cho H, et al.: A strategy for predicting the chemosensitivity of human cancers and its application to drug discovery, *Proc Natl Acad Sci USA* 104:13086–13091, 2007.

387. Staunton JE, Slonim DK, Coller HA, et al.: Chemosensitivity prediction by transcriptional profiling, *Proc Natl Acad Sci USA* 98:10787–10792, 2001.

388. Potti A, Dressman HK, Bild A, et al.: Retraction: genomic signatures to guide the use of chemotherapeutics, *Nat Med* 17:135, 2011.

389. Bonnefoi H, Potti A, Delorenzi M, et al.: Retraction—validation of gene signatures that predict the response of breast cancer to neoadjuvant chemotherapy: a substudy of the EORTC 10994/big 00-01 clinical trial, *Lancet Oncol* 12:116, 2011.

390. Baggerly KA, Coombes KR: Deriving chemosensitivity from cell lines: forensic bioinformatics and reproducible research in high-throughput biology, *Ann Appl Stat* 3:1309–1334, 2009.

13

Radiation Oncology

SUSAN M. LARUE AND IRA K. GORDON

Radiation therapy (RT) has been used to treat cancers in both veterinary and human medicine since shortly after the discovery of x-rays by Roentgen in 1895, and the fields have followed similar paths. Dr. Henri Coutard, a radiation oncologist at the Curie Institute in Paris, carefully evaluated the effect of dose per fraction, total dose, overall treatment time, field size, and tumor size on tumor control and adverse radiation effects.[1] Alois Pommer, an Austrian veterinarian, published extensively starting in the 1930s on fractionated irradiation of benign and malignant diseases and established an RT protocol widely used for many years.[2] It was not until the 1970s and 1980s that scientists acquired a broader understanding of radiation biology, rationally explaining the benefit of dividing dose into smaller fractions.[3] Close to 60% of human patients with serious cancers undergo RT at some point during treatment.[4] Over the past 20 years, major technological advances have improved tumor control and reduced adverse effects from irradiation. RT has also proven to be an effective treatment modality for solid tumors in animal cancer patients; however, early use of the newer modalities was limited due to the paucity of veterinary treatment centers. The past decade has been marked by the opening of numerous veterinary RT centers and the commissioning of more advanced RT technologies. Modalities, such as stereotactic RT (SRT), image-guided RT, and intensity-modulated RT (IMRT) have allowed more targeted treatment, decreasing adverse radiation effects and providing improved radiation options for tumors in a variety of locations.[5] More than 70 facilities in North America are actively treating animals with RT and 27 of those reporting SRT capabilities.[6] The American College of Veterinary Radiology (specialty in radiation oncology) has residency training programs at 13 treatment centers.[7] International expansion has included Europe, Asia, Australia, and South America.[6]

The management of cancer patients is complex, and determining the best treatment modality or combination of modalities can be challenging. In most instances, when local control of a solid tumor cannot be obtained surgically without excessively compromising function, appearance, or quality of life, consultation with a radiation oncologist is advised. Surgery followed or preceded by fractionated RT may allow a more conservative surgery and yield comparable or better tumor control and/or functional outcome than either surgery or RT alone. RT alone is indicated in areas where surgical options are limited, such as nasal tumors, heart-based tumors, and some brain tumors.[8–10] SRT has provided treatment alternatives in patients where surgery is not an option and in locations that were not previously amenable to unmodulated RT, such as abdominal tumors.[11] In addition to treating serious cancers with what is referred to as "curative intent," RT also plays an important role in the palliative management of advanced cancers, the treatment of endocrinopathies associated with endocrine adenomas, as an adjuvant treatment for lymphoma, and for certain benign conditions.[12–19] New technology and treatment approaches have led to an unwieldy collection of acronyms, the most common of which are listed in Table 13.1.

Principles of Radiation Biology

Radiation dose is described by the amount of energy absorbed by the tissue. The unit of absorbed dose is the Gray (Gy); 1 Gy equals one joule absorbed per kilogram of tissue. Ionizing radiation kills cells by damaging critical molecules in the cell, primarily deoxyribonucleic acid (DNA), which eventually leads to cell death.[20] Megavoltage photons, the predominant form of radiation used in veterinary medicine, interact with tissue primarily by the Compton effect, producing high energy electrons that cause ionization events either to critical molecules (direct action) or from water molecules located within nanometers of critical molecules (indirect action).[21–25] These events produce highly reactive free radicals that result in biologic damage that may kill the cell or render it incapable of reproducing.[20,25] This type of cell death, referred to as mitotic catastrophe, is due to chromosomal aberrations, primarily from double strand breaks.[20,26] Although mitotic death is still the primary mode of radiation-associated cell death, other mechanisms have been recognized, including apoptosis, radiation bystander effect, radiation abscopal effect, autophagy, and senescence.

Repair of Radiation-Induced DNA Damage

A critical determinant of a cell population's sensitivity to radiation is the ability of cells to repair DNA damage caused by radiation. 1 Gy of radiation from photons causes approximately 2500 base damages, 1000 single strand breaks, and 40 double strand breaks in DNA in each cell.[20] Mammals have developed highly conserved pathways to sense and repair single and double strand breaks as well as other forms of DNA damage.[27,28] The double strand breaks are the most lethal as they may lead to severe chromosomal aberrations.[20,28] Most of this damage is repaired by cells within 6 to 24 hours.[29,30] Genes involved in control of intrinsic radiosensitivity are primarily genes involved in cell-cycle progression and DNA repair.[31,32] A given dose of radiation is preferentially cytotoxic to proliferating cells, including tumor cells and renewing cell

TABLE 13.1	Acronyms Commonly Used in Radiation Oncology	
GTV	Gross tumor volume	The extent of gross disease as determined by palpation, direct visualization, or indirectly through imaging techniques. (GTV cannot be defined after a tumor has been surgically excised.)
CTV	Clinical target volume	The region of suspected subclinical tumor involvement, including normal tissue with presumed microscopic extension. Additional volumes such as lymph nodes may be included in the CTV.
PTV	Planning target volume	The volume including the CTV and an additional margin to account for variations in size, shape, and position of the CTV during therapy. The PTV margin also accounts for setup and physical uncertainties.
SIB	Simultaneous integrated boost	A portion of the tumor, generally central, that is prescribed a higher dose than the rest of the tumor. Allows for high-dose delivery to the central core of the tumor and a dose fall-off toward the periphery.
OAR	Organ at risk	Normal organs/tissues in proximity to a target structure that may influence prescribed dose or treatment plan parameters.
MLC	Multileaf collimator	A beam-shaping device made up of individual independently moving "leaves" of shielding material (usually tungsten).
OBI	On-board imaging	An imaging system and tool on a radiation delivery device used to confirm the match of treatment setup to the planned setup.
PRT	Palliative radiation therapy	A radiation treatment course delivered with the intent to minimize tumor-related symptoms and improve quality of life with few short-term side effects.
DRT	Definitive radiation therapy	A radiation treatment course delivered with the intent of achieving long-term tumor control or durable tumor response.
3DCRT	Three-dimensional conformal radiation therapy	Radiation planning technique utilizing cross-sectional imaging (i.e., computed tomography scan) and treatment-planning software to optimize radiation beam angles, blocks, and beam-shaping devices (i.e., wedges) with the goal of maximizing doses to targets and minimizing doses to organs at risk. Typically involves static blocks and gantry angles.
IMRT	Intensity modulated radiation therapy	Radiation planning technique and delivery technique by modulating fluence within each of multiple radiation fields. Requires "inverse" treatment planning.
SRT	Stereotactic radiation therapy	Radiation-planning technique involving minimal margins applied to the target and maximizing dose fall-off outside of target and near OARs. Most commonly used in high dose-per-fraction protocols.
SRS	Stereotactic radiosurgery	Generally implies a single fraction, high-dose radiation treatment course involving minimal margins applied to the target and maximizing dose fall-off outside of target and near OARs.
VMAT	Volumetric modulated arc therapy	A radiation delivery technique involving the radiation gantry rotating about the patient while delivering IMRT.
QA	Quality assurance	Processes that insure all aspects of radiation treatment quality and safety. These processes frequently involve independent measurements that verify radiation dose delivered for comparison to expected values or values calculated by a treatment planning system.

populations (e.g., epithelial stem cells), although slowly dividing and nondividing cells (e.g., bone and cells of the nervous system) are also affected by radiation and often limit the dose deliverable during RT.[3,33] Tumor cells are also capable of DNA repair, although DNA mutations may alter repair capabilities.[23]

Cell Cycle Effects

The period of the cell cycle in which DNA undergoes synthesis is known as S-phase. Before and after S-phase are periods without overt activity by the DNA; these periods are called the G1 phase and the G2 phase. The G2 phase is followed by mitosis (M phase). Cells are distributed throughout the cell cycle in a tumor or tissue at a given time. Individual cell sensitivity to irradiation varies depending on the phase of the cell cycle at the time of irradiation. Cells in late S-phase are most resistant to irradiation, and cells in late G2 or M phase are most sensitive.[29,30] Cells with a long G1 period may be resistant early in that phase.[34]

Oxygen Effects

Because of their rapid growth and abnormal vasculature, tumors often become hypoxic.[35,36] Oxygen is a critical factor in the response to irradiation, because reactive oxygen species generate much of the damage from radiation.[20] As a result, normoxic cells are up to three-fold more sensitive to radiation than hypoxic cells.[20] Additionally, tumor hypoxia is associated with the upregulation of hypoxia-inducible proteins that may prepare the tumor cells to handle stresses and can also affect tumor metabolism and metastatic potential.[36,37]

Relative Biologic Effectiveness

Although this chapter primarily discusses the effects of photons (x-rays and gamma rays) and electrons, other forms of radiation can be used for treatment, including protons, neutrons, and carbon particles. The relative biologic effectiveness (RBE) is not a physical measurelike the linear energy transfer (LET), which measures the amount of energy transferred per unit path length. LET is a factor in RBE, but RBE also considers factors such as biologic endpoint, fractionation, radiation dose rate, and dose. The RBE of 1 Gy of electrons and photons is the same, but 1 Gy of neutrons or heavy charged particles such as carbon causes substantially more damage.[38,39] RBE essentially compares the biologic difference between specific types of radiation relative to the effect of photons. Protons, which are commonly used in human radiation facilities, have a slightly higher RBE than photons and electrons.[40] Protons and heavy charged particles also share unique properties in dose distribution that can be beneficial in treatment planning.[41,42]

Alternative Methods of Radiation Cell Death

Radiation-induced apoptosis is the second most common form of cell death after irradiation, but it is highly cell-type dependent.[43] Lymphoid tissues are particularly prone to apoptosis, which may be the dominant form of cell death in these tissues.[43] Apoptosis can occur spontaneously in tumors, although the degree of occurrence can vary even within the same tumor type.[44] Radiation responsive tumors may undergo greater levels of radiation-induced apoptosis than more radioresistant tumors.[45] Apoptosis of endothelial cells may indirectly affect tumor cell kill by leading to vascular collapse. Vascular collapse has been recognized to play a role in the overall response to radiation therapy.[46] Apoptosis of endothelium primarily occurs when high-dose fractions are administered and may play a more important role when hypofractionated radiation is delivered.[47–49]

The bystander effect, defined as biologic effects observed in cells not traversed by radiation but in proximity, may affect some cells, but this has not been well quantified in vivo.[50] Autophagy, cell senescence, oxidative stress, and immune response may also play roles.[50,51] Abscopal effects refer to distant sites, such as when a tumor irradiated in one part of the body affects tumors in other locations.[50] Abscopal effects may be associated with an enhanced immune response.[50]

Tumor Stem Cells

As early as 1973, it was recognized that the number of injected tumor cells from a variety of spontaneous cell lines to induce tumor formation in 50% of recipients varied from 21 to 24,000 cells.[52,53] This tumor-forming ability in vivo appears to correlate in many cases with the percentage of cells within the tumor bulk possessing a stem-cell-like phenotype. Cancer stem cell markers, such as CD24 and CD44, have been identified, but the relationship between the markers and stem cell characteristics remains under investigation.[54,55] It is hypothesized that the number or percentage of tumor stem cells and their intrinsic radiation sensitivity predict radiocurability.[55] Tumor stem cells are being intensively investigated as a potential target for therapy.

Principles of Fractionated Radiation Therapy

Time, Dose, and Fraction Size

Early radiation oncologists found that higher total doses could be given if the doses were divided into smaller doses, known as fractions. Coutard, a radiation oncologist at the Curie Institute in Paris, observed that tumor response was improved and less injury of normal tissue occurred when radiation was fractionated.[1] Coutard's recommendations were 2 Gy fractions delivered Monday through Friday for 6 to 8 weeks with a total dose of 60 to 80 Gy. In veterinary medicine, standard fractionation denotes a regimen delivering 2.7 to 4.0 Gy per fraction, three to five times per week, to a total dose of 42 to 57 Gy. Hyperfractionation refers to schedules in which the dose per fraction is reduced and the total dose is increased. In human radiation oncology, this approach has been associated with improved outcome for a number of tumor types, including oropharyngeal carcinoma.[56] Accelerated RT describes a treatment regimen in which the overall time of treatment is reduced.[57] Hypofractionation describes the administration of higher doses per fraction given in a smaller number of fractions. Compared with most conventional human protocols, the protocols used in veterinary medicine would be considered hypofractionated and accelerated. The response of tumor and normal tissues to conventionally fractionated RT (regardless of human or veterinary oncologist prescribed) has been described by Withers as the "Four Rs" of RT: repair of DNA damage, redistribution of cells in the cell cycle, reoxygenation of tumor cells, and repopulation of tumor and normal tissues.[3]

Division of the total radiation dose into fractions is important for a number of reasons. The first reason is to exploit potential differences in repair capabilities between tumors and normal tissues. Slowly dividing cells are somewhat less sensitive to small doses of radiation than more rapidly dividing cells; however, they appear to become relatively more sensitive if radiation is delivered in larger doses per fraction. If smaller doses per fraction are used, normal tissues with slowly dividing cells can be spared relative to tumor tissues with rapidly dividing cells.[58]

Other events that occur between radiation fractions are cell cycle redistribution and reoxygenation. When a fraction of RT is administered, many of the cells in the sensitive portions of the cell cycle are killed. During the interval between fractions, cells from the late S-phase, which are more likely to be alive than other cells, progress to more sensitive parts of the cell cycle. This is known as redistribution.[29,30] Tumor hypoxia is a common feature occurring in many solid tumors due to decreased vascular density and malformed tumor vessels. Chronic hypoxia, also known as diffusion-limited hypoxia, is caused by limitation in oxygen diffusion to cells further away from tumor vessels.[36,37,59] Perfusion-limited related hypoxia is due to temporary closing or blockage of malformed blood vessels. The tumor microenvironment is constantly changing and is itself affected by radiation.[36] After a fraction of radiation, oxygenated cells die, allowing hypoxic cells closer access to vessels. The location of acutely hypoxic cells varies based on the opening and closing of vessels and is transient. Tumor hypoxia cannot be predicted by tumor size or histologic type but is thought to contribute to treatment failure. In experimental models, the pattern for reoxygenation and the extent of the reoxygenation varies.[60,61]

The length of time over which RT is administered is important primarily because of tumor repopulation but also because of rapidly proliferating normal tissues, such as mucosa and skin. Tumor cells that have not been destroyed by irradiation continue to replicate during the course of therapy. This process is exacerbated by a phenomenon known as accelerated repopulation.[3,62,63] It is believed that after approximately 4 weeks of therapy, tumors repopulate more rapidly than initially.[3,63] The reason for this is not clear, but the phenomenon could be related to (1) a reduction in the cell cycle time, (2) an increase in the number of tumor cells that are actively dividing (growth fraction),

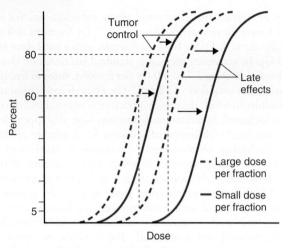

• **Fig. 13.1** Radiotherapy delivered in small fractions (*solid lines*) can produce a higher probability of tumor control with the small level of late effects as radiotherapy delivered in large fractions (*broken lines*).

(3) a reduction in the number of tumor cells that normally die (cell loss factor), or (4) an increase in the number of tumor stem cells. Regardless of the cause, when treatment lasts longer than 4 weeks, repopulation may affect the outcome unless total dose is increased to account for this phenomenon. Repopulation may have a greater adverse effect on rapidly dividing tumors than on slowly dividing tumors.

Repopulation of rapidly proliferating (also known as acutely responding) normal tissues is also affected by time. The same total dose of radiation administered over a short period results in somewhat more severe acute effects than if administered over a longer course.[3,64–66] Nonproliferating (late responding) normal tissues are not significantly affected by the length of time over which therapy is administered;[33,64–65] they are more affected by dose per fraction and total dose.[3,33] Additionally, fractions should be separated by at least 6 hours to allow repair of DNA damage to normal tissues.[66] Cells of the brain and spinal cord may require additional time for complete repair.[66]

The total dose administered to a patient should have a low probability for causing significant late normal tissue reactions in the region of therapy; however, the response of tissues also depends on the fraction size. For example, 48 Gy administered in 4 Gy fractions has a higher probability of causing late effects than 48 Gy administered in 3 Gy fractions (Fig. 13.1). The probability of tumor control is minimally affected because rapidly proliferating tissues, including tumors, are not as sensitive to the change in dose per fraction. The benefits of protocols that use small doses per fraction are clear: they allow a higher total dose to be administered without increasing the probability of damage to late-responding normal tissues. Conversely, extending overall treatment time may allow for greater accelerated repopulation.[3,62,67–68]

Radiation Effects to Normal Tissues

Reactions from RT are classified as acute, late, consequential, and early delayed. Acute effects occur during or shortly after RT. Acute effects involve rapidly proliferating tissues, such as the oral mucosa, intestinal epithelium, and epithelial structures of the eyes and skin. Concurrent chemotherapy can exacerbate acute radiation effects.[69] Although the severity of acute effects may vary between patients, these effects generally are self-limiting and recovery is rapid; however, acute effects can

be unpleasant for the patient and distressing to the owner, and in rare instances they can be life-threatening if proper care is not given. Acute effects will heal with modest pain management in the vast majority of cases over the course of weeks or occasionally months. In veterinary patients, the most important provision to allow healing during this time is prevention of self-trauma of the irradiated site. Pain management plays an important role and should be addressed. Pain management for cancer patients is discussed in Chapter 16A of this text and specific protocols have been published.[70] Additional treatment is based on common sense, supportive care, and the knowledge that the signs will resolve with time.

Early delayed radiation effects have been recognized only in neurologic tissues. Occurring between 2 weeks and 4 months after treatment, they may take several forms.[71] Somnolence may develop in patients receiving whole brain irradiation.[72] Early delayed effects may simulate tumor recurrence or may cause neurologic signs not previously associated with the tumor, and so careful imaging evaluation is necessary. Early delayed effects may be due to demyelination or from cerebral edema–associated cytokine release with tumor cell death. Early delayed effects will generally respond to corticosteroid administration and supportive care.[71]

Late effects are mechanistically more complex than acute effects and involve more slowly proliferating tissues, such as bone, lung, heart, kidneys, and nervous system. The dose of radiation administered to the patient is limited by the tolerance of these normal tissue structures in the field. Late reactions can be difficult to treat; it is the radiation oncologist's obligation to minimize the incidence of late effects with appropriate dose prescriptions and careful radiation planning and treatment. When late effects occur, they may be quite severe, resulting in fibrosis, necrosis, loss of function, and even death.[73] Late effects occur from the loss of normal tissue stem cells with concurrent radiation-induced vascular changes and inflammation. These changes are multifactorial, but the cytokine transforming growth factor beta (TGFβ) is believed to play a critical role in radiation fibrosis.[74] Strategies attempted in human radiation oncology to mitigate late radiation effects include the use of antioxidants and free radical scavengers (e.g., superoxide dismutase, vitamin E, thiol radioprotectors), vascular directed therapies (e.g., clopidogrel, statins, pentoxifylline), antiinflammatory agents (corticosteroids), inhibitors of the renin-angiotensin system (e.g., ACE inhibitors), and stem cell therapies.[73] Consequential late effects, the result of extensive damage to stem cells of acutely responding tissues such as colon, are indistinguishable clinically and histologically from late effects and should be managed in a similar fashion.[75]

An unusual late effect associated with RT is the occurrence of radiation-associated secondary tumors. Ionizing radiation is a complete carcinogen, capable of initiating, promoting, and progressing cellular changes that lead to cancer. Therefore it is possible to see radiation-induced neoplasia develop in an RT field. It appears that radiation with high LET such as neutrons result in carcinogenesis at a higher frequency than the megavoltage photons typically used in veterinary RT.[76] Age influences the risk of radiation carcinogenesis because younger patients have the potential to live longer after radiation, and information from nuclear accidents suggest that they are more likely to develop secondary tumors.[76,77] Certain tissues such as the thyroid gland are also more prone to development of radiation-induced tumors.[78] Secondary tumors have been reported in dogs in both clinical and research settings.[79,80]

For a tumor to be considered radiation induced, the following criteria must be met:

1. The malignancy must arise within the irradiated field.
2. Sufficient latency must have elapsed between the time of irradiation and development of the tumor (typically at least 1 year).
3. The original tumor and the new tumor must have different histologic diagnoses.
4. The tissue in which the new tumor forms must have been previously normal before radiation exposure.

The overall incidence of radiation-induced tumors in patients treated with RT is thought to be extremely low (up to 2% of patients treated).[78]

In veterinary patients, severe late reactions such as fibrosis and tissue necrosis should be managed under the guidance of an oncologic surgeon and/or radiation oncologist experienced in dealing with radiation injury.

Chemical Modifiers of Radiation

Although rarely used clinically in veterinary medicine, many drugs can modify the cellular and tissue response to radiation.[81] Radioprotectors (e.g., amifostine/WR-2721) are compounds that decrease the amount of radiation damage to targeted normal cells without providing similar protection to tumor cells.[82,83] Radiosensitizers are chemicals that achieve greater tumor inactivation than would be expected from the additive effect of treatment with either radiation or the chemical alone and have included common chemotherapeutic agents such as carboplatin and gemcitabine.[82] Mechanisms of action also include targeting hypoxic cells by increasing sensitivity, increasing oxygen delivery, decreasing oxygen consumption, and the use of hypoxia molecular target inhibitors.[84] Newer concepts include employing gold nanoparticles and targeted therapies, including immune checkpoint inhibitors.[85,86]

STEREOTACTIC RADIATION THERAPY: BIOLOGIC AND ONCOLOGIC PRINCIPLES

Although time, dose, and fraction size are still the underpinnings of SRT, some of the biologic mechanisms appear to be different from conventionally fractionated RT. It can be confusing, because the term "stereotactic RT technology" describes the physical equipment and software required to deliver focal treatment with location confirmation. Although generally associated with hypofractionated protocols, the technology can be used for administration of traditionally fractionated RT. For instance, the use of image-guided and intensity-modulated RT has been described for the treatment of urinary tract tumors in dogs.[87] For purposes of this chapter, the term SRT will refer to the use of high doses per fraction (hypofractionation) using SRT technology and techniques.

Unlike conventionally fractionated RT, which spares normal tissues by improved repair, SRT overcomes the radiobiologic limitations by stereotactically verified positioning and treatment delivery techniques that leave a minimal volume of normal tissue in the high dose area. SRT, by definition, requires: (1) a tumor for targeting (not microscopic disease); (2) treatment planning and administration that will provide a dramatic dose drop off between the tumor and the surrounding normal tissue structures; and (3) a method of stereotactically verifying patient positioning.[88,89] The result is that normal late-responding tissue structures are spared through dose avoidance rather than by administering small doses per fraction.

The normal tissue structures still receive the dose, and the dose per fraction is higher than for traditional RT; however, the total dose to normal tissue structures is lower than what is typical for fractionated RT because of the steep dose drop-off between tumor and critical normal tissue structures. Normal tissue tolerance data are just evolving for SRT, as are reports of long-term outcome, in both human and veterinary medicine. Estimates of tolerance have been based on limited clinical data, toxicity observation, and educated guessing.[90] It is inappropriate to extrapolate dose constraints from fractionated protocols. An additional clinical difference between SRT and fractionated RT is that with SRT, acutely responding normal tissues in the surrounding region, such as skin, esophagus, and colon, are susceptible to consequential late effects due to the short overall treatment time.[91,92] Dose constraints therefore must also be applied to these tissues. SRT is generally hypofractionated and delivered in one to five fractions over a period of 1 to 2 weeks, minimizing the effect of accelerated repopulation. Early stereotactic treatment using a gamma-knife necessitated delivery in a single fraction (referred to as stereotactic radiosurgery [SRS]). Current technology allowing precise repositioning makes limited fractionation feasible. Even this minimal fractionation should allow higher total doses to be administered safely to late-responding tissues in the region and presumably take advantage of tumor reoxygenation and redistribution. Biologic response after SRT has not been conclusively evaluated. Experimental data imply that direct tumor cell death cannot account for the efficacy of SRT and SRS. Tumor cell death will be discussed later, but based on cell culture and rodent experiments, which suggest that 10^{8-9} tumor cells must die to eradicate a 1-gram tumor, the doses used to obtain tumor control in human tumors treated with SRS or SRT are far lower.[93-97] High dose, hypofractionated RT has been shown to cause vascular damage in mouse tumor models, which leads to greater-than-expected tumor control, leading to the conclusion that tumor vascular injury leads to indirect tumor cell death.[46,49]

From a practical standpoint, SRT minimizes the number of anesthesia episodes required in older and sometimes debilitated patients and is also generally more convenient for the owner; however, these factors should not be the overarching rationale for prescribing SRT. Although acute effects are minimal and tumor-associated signs, such as discomfort or dysfunction, often improve rapidly, the ultimate decision should be based on choosing the modality that provides the best long-term tumor control and/or best quality of life. Long-term tumor control and late effects are still being quantified, but recent publications demonstrate comparable survival times (STs) in nasal and brain tumors and improved outcome in the treatment of feline acromegaly when compared with conventionally fractionated protocols.[8,9,98] SRT technology has also resulted in the improved treatment of tumor sites infrequently previously irradiated in veterinary medicine, including the adrenal gland, brachial plexus, and trigeminal nerve.[11,99,100]

No all-embracing RT protocol exists. With increased understanding of underlying biology, protocols continue to be manipulated to exploit tumor characteristics for improved control or to increase sparing of normal tissues. Regardless of whether using finely fractionated RT or SRT, the protocol should be chosen based on the specific normal tissues present in the irradiated field. For example, brain and spinal cord are less tolerant to the effects of irradiation than muscle or bone. Another factor that must be considered when selecting the appropriate dose is the volume of tissue in the field. Large volumes of normal tissues are more susceptible to damage from irradiation than smaller volumes. For many tumor locations, a 5% probability for late effects is tolerated, because without the treatment, patients may not live long enough to develop late effects; however, for structures such as the spinal cord, where a late effect such as paralysis is viewed as unacceptable, a 1% probability of effects is used. Conversely, for procedures like SRT limb-sparing for canine osteosarcoma (OSA), the risk of fracture is affected by the region and condition of lytic bone at the time of treatment. Owners may choose to accept a higher risk of fracture to maintain limb function, because a future amputation can be used as a salvage procedure.[101]

It is not within the scope of this chapter to prescribe specific radiation doses or fractionation schedules, because many factors must be considered. Rather, referring veterinarians must know what to expect when sending patients to a radiation oncology center and should be able to explain the fundamental principles to clients. The radiation oncologist should inform the referring veterinarian and owner of the probabilities of tumor control, acute effects, and late effects expected with a specific protocol. The goal of RT is to destroy the reproductive capacity of the tumor without excessive damage to surrounding normal tissues. The relationship of three parameters (overall treatment time, total dose, and fraction size) as well as other factors, such as chemotherapy, previous surgery, and underlying medical conditions such as diabetes, must be carefully considered in the development of an RT plan.

THE LINEAR QUADRATIC FORMALISM AND BIOLOGIC EFFECTIVE DOSE

Many mathematical models have been used to describe or predict the effect of radiation on cells and tissues. The linear quadratic formalism has been useful for evaluating the effect of radiation in fraction sizes commonly used in RT and has been a tool for modifying radiation protocols based on projected effect on late-responding tissues.[102–105] Mechanistically, this model corresponds radiation injury to chromosome aberrations.[106–108] After a tissue or population of cells is exposed to any dose of radiation, a fraction of the cells will be killed. The proportion of remaining cells is known as the surviving fraction (S). The sensitivity of a tumor or tissue to radiation can be shown as a graph of the radiation dose (D) versus the surviving fraction (Fig. 13.2).[109] The relationship between a dose of radiation and the surviving fraction of cells is commonly described by the linear quadratic equation: $S(D) = e^{-(\alpha D + \beta D^2)}$, where S is the surviving fraction at a dose (D).[103] Alpha (α) and beta (β) are constants that vary according to the tissue, with α corresponding to the cell death that increases linearly with dose, and β corresponding to the cell death that increases in proportion to the square of the dose (also known as the quadratic component). The α/β ratio is a useful number that is the dose in Gy when cell kill from the linear and quadratic components of the cell survival curve are equal. Cells with a higher α/β ratio have a more linear appearance when plotted on a log scale, and cells with a low α/β ratio have a parabolic shape. The α/β ratio is also an important description of the radiosensitivity of a cell. At low dose fractions, tissues or cells with low α/β ratio are relatively radiation resistant compared with tissues or cells with high α/β ratio. It has been suggested that tissues and cells with low α/β ratios have a greater capacity for repair of sublethal radiation damage.[110] Sublethal radiation damage is defined as damage that can become lethal if it interacts with additional damage.[29,30] Sublethal damage repair is the reason that cell survival increases when a radiation dose is split into two fractions separated by a time interval.[29,30]

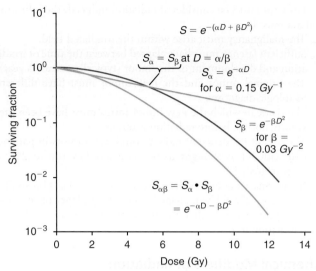

• **Fig. 13.2** Illustration of the alpha/beta model in which cell killing occurs by either a single-event process or a double-event process such that the overall killing by either process is the product of the two, and the alpha/beta ratio is the dose at which both processes contribute equally to the total killing. Note that the upper curve is survival for the alpha component only, the middle curve is for the beta component only, and the lower curve is for both components. (From Wilson PF, Bedford JS. Radiobiological principles. In: Hoppe RT, Phillips TL, Roach M, III, eds. *Leibel and Phillips Textbook of Radiation Oncology.* 3rd ed. St. Louis: Elsevier; 2010:3–30.)

Most early-responding tissues and tumors have a high α/β ratio, whereas late-responding tissues have a low α/β ratio.[103] Tumors that may have a low α/β ratio can influence the optimal radiation prescription in terms of total dose, time, and fraction size. Tumors that may have lower α/β ratios include melanoma, prostatic tumors, soft tissue sarcomas, transitional cell carcinomas, and OSA, but these are generalities and the α/β ratio may differ from tumor to tumor.[110–112]

The concept of biologic effective dose (BED) is used to predict how changes in dose prescription may preferentially affect different cells or tissues based on their α/β ratio in the linear quadratic model of survival. The formula for BED is as follows: BED = nd [1 + d/(α/β)], where n is the number of fractions and d is the dose per fraction. If the α/β ratio of a tissue is known or can be estimated, the BED can be calculated for any dose prescription. It is possible to use this formula to assess how dosimetry changes or errors alter the effective dose of a protocol. It is important to note that there are several limitations to the use of this equation, including that it does not account for differences in the overall length of time of the radiation protocol or accelerated repopulation. More complicated additions to the formula can be used to take overall treatment time into account.[105] Although experimental and clinical data provide confirmation of α/β ratios for most tissues, linear quadratic parameters for tumors are uncertain; therefore calculations made with this model for tumor control prediction may not be valid.[113] Nevertheless, this formula is a useful tool when considering hyperfractionating a standard radiation protocol to create a new protocol that increases normal tissue tolerance, which could allow increased total dose, or to adjust a protocol when there has been an extensive delay in treatment. The validity of BED for SRT is unclear. It has been useful for estimating late effects based on data from conventionally fractionated RT; however, BED-derived constraints for acutely responding tissues may overestimate tolerance of acutely responding tissues because of the shortened overall treatment time in SRT. Work is ongoing to establish SRT constraints for acutely responding tissues.[91,92]

PALLIATIVE RADIATION THERAPY

Palliative RT (PRT) is an important tool in cancer treatment, and its use in veterinary medicine for a wide variety of tumor types is increasing. PRT is not ideally intended to provide long-term or definitive tumor control; rather, it is intended to relieve pain or improve function or quality of life in patients in which other factors (e.g., advanced metastatic disease, comorbidities) are likely to lead to early demise. Because curing the patient is no longer the goal, the treatment should not negatively affect quality of life by causing acute radiation effects. Radiation protocols used for palliation are far less aggressive and more flexible than when treating with curative intent. PRT is most often hypofractionated compared with curative-intent protocols, often administered in 6 to 10 Gy per fraction, in one to six total fractions once or twice weekly. Conversely, PRT can be delivered in conventional or modestly hypofractionated schedules once or twice daily for a shorter treatment regimen. Most publications have focused on metastatic or primary bone tumors, principally canine OSA (see Chapter 25), but it is also reported for nasal tumors, hemangiosarcoma, soft tissue sarcoma, mast cell tumors, GI lymphomas, and oral tumors.[114-117] Palliative RT is more convenient and less expensive for the owner than fractionated RT or SRT with curative intent. It is, however, important to remember that palliative RT is not a substitute for curative-intent protocols despite the convenience. Some palliative RT protocols may have an increased probability of causing late radiation effects based on biologic effective dose calculations[102,103]; however, because they are prescribed to patients that have a poor long-term prognosis, these late effects generally do not have time to manifest. Curative-intent RT protocols require strict adherence to radiation biologic principles; palliative RT protocols, on the other hand, are far more flexible. As in human hospital settings, the protocols may vary dramatically between centers and, regardless of the protocol, most palliative RT patients receive some level of benefit. Because the duration of response after palliation is limited, some owners elect pursuing a second course.[118] PRT is not restricted to specific modalities of radiation administration. SRT is also an option for palliative treatment. It may provide quicker and more durable response for the primary or metastatic lesion being treated and ideally maintain quality of life until death from disseminated disease.

Radiation Therapy Equipment

Ionizing radiation can be administered by an external source (teletherapy) through placement of radioactive isotopes interstitially (brachytherapy) or by systemic or cavitary injection of radioisotopes, such as iodine-131 (^{131}I). Teletherapy, also referred to as external beam RT, is the most commonly used method of RT in veterinary medicine. External beam RT usually is classified as orthovoltage or megavoltage radiotherapy, based on the energy of the photon. Orthovoltage machines produce x-rays with an energy of 150 to 500 kVp; megavoltage radiation emits photons with an average energy greater than 1 million electron volts (1 MeV). Although some veterinary radiation oncology centers continue to treat with orthovoltage machines, megavoltage radiation is the most commonly used type of external beam RT. Megavoltage radiation for therapy can be obtained from cobalt machines or linear accelerators.[6] Because megavoltage radiation has excellent tissue-penetrating capabilities, RT can be performed on deeply seated tumors for which orthovoltage therapy would not be an option.

Orthovoltage x-rays, which have low energy, distribute maximum doses to the skin surface. Acute effects to the skin can be quite severe, causing discomfort to the patient, and late effects to the skin and subcutaneous tissues can be dose limiting. Megavoltage radiation has a higher energy than orthovoltage, and the photons must interact with tissues, allowing the dose to build up before the maximum dose can be achieved. The skin therefore can receive a significantly lower dose than the underlying tumor. This skin-sparing effect of megavoltage radiation allows the optimal dose to be administered to a more deeply seated tumor without causing severe reactions to the skin. When the tumor involves or is in close proximity to the skin, megavoltage radiation can be used successfully by placing a sheet of tissue-equivalent material, called a bolus, over the tumor. This allows the dose buildup to occur before reaching the skin so that the skin and associated tumor can receive the maximum dose of radiation.

The absorption of megavoltage radiation, unlike that of orthovoltage radiation, is minimally dependent on the composition of the tissue. This characteristic permits even distribution of the dose throughout the tissues in the field. Orthovoltage radiation is preferentially absorbed by bone.[119] If a tumor adjacent to or overlying bone is administered a meaningful dose of orthovoltage radiation, the probability that late effects to the bone (bone necrosis) will develop is quite high.[119,120] Treatment with orthovoltage should be limited to small, superficial tumors, such as nasal planum tumors, or to superficial tumor beds after surgical excision.

Interaction of megavoltage radiation with tissues is quite predictable; this has allowed the development of accurate computerized treatment planning systems. These planning systems allow treatment of the tumor with multiple beams administered from different angles. The goal of computerized treatment planning is to ensure a desired minimum tumor dose to a region specified by the radiation oncologist and to spare normal tissue structures when possible. Three-dimensional conformal RT uses CT or MRI images, which are imported or contoured using a tablet. The summation of multiple beams coming from different directions provides a higher dose to the tumor than surrounding tissues.

In addition to photons, radiation treatments in veterinary medicine also include electron-beam therapy. Various energies of electrons are commonly incorporated in the capabilities of modern linear accelerators. Electron beam therapy is most favorable for superficial targets, because electrons do not penetrate to nearly the depth of a photon beam, which can allow for sparing of deep structures.

Although not yet commonly utilized in veterinary medicine due to the technical demands and cost, proton beam radiation equipment is becoming widely available in human treatment facilities and offers dosimetric benefits that photons cannot. A machine called a cyclotron speeds up protons, imparting high energy that determines the travel depth of the proton. Unlike photon therapy, protons deposit radiation dose in the targeted range and minimal dose exits the tumor.[42]

Radiation Planning and Delivery Techniques

Advances in treatment planning and imaging over the past decade have led to the development of image-based, 3D conformal RT (3D-CRT), which permits better conformity between

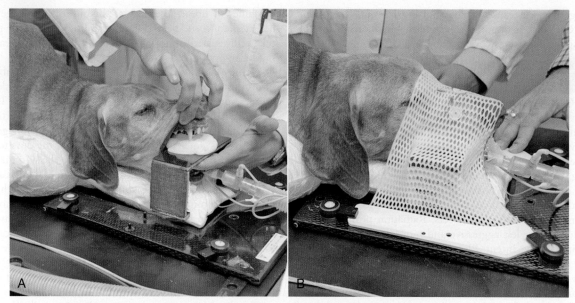

• **Fig. 13.3** (A) Teeth being placed in preformed acrylic bite block that is inserted into a carbon fiber indexed frame. Neck is resting on a vacuum-lock bag. (B) An acrylic face mask being placed.

the irradiated high-dose volume and the geometric shape of the tumor. 3D-CRT requires importation of CT images into a treatment planning system. The animal must be positioned for the imaging in a fashion that can be closely replicated on a day-to-day basis for treatment. Acrylic face masks and Vac-Lok Cushions are commonly used for positioning (Fig. 13.3). The radiation oncologist identifies important normal tissue structures known as organs at risk, gross tumor volume (GTV), clinical target volume (CTV), and planning target volume (PTV) on these images. By definition, the GTV only includes gross tumor whereas the CTV includes the GTV plus an expansion based on the known clinical behavior of the specific tumor to account for regional microscopic disease.[121] For example, the CTV expansions for a sarcoma are generally larger than for a carcinoma. If the patient has had cytoreductive surgery and only microscopic tumor remains, there is no GTV and the CTV is based on the scar, regions of surgical disruption, and an expansion for microscopic disease beyond the surgical site.[121] In addition to the GTV and CTV, the PTV includes expansion for an internal margin that accounts for variations in size and shape relative to anatomic landmarks (e.g., filling of bladder, respiratory movements) and set-up margin (SM). The SM accounts for uncertainties in patient positioning and alignment during planning imaging and subsequent treatments.[121] The better the immobilization device, the smaller the SM expansion can be. SM expansions will vary based on the location of the tumor because some sites, such as the head, are more amenable to rigid immobilization devices, such as bite blocks, which provide better replicability. Decreasing the PTV expansion by using good immobilization and available imaging affects the volume of normal tissue treated, is a key component to successful 3D-CRT, and is critical to other advanced treatment modalities. PTV expansions are both facility and region specific and ideally are determined with input by both the medical radiation physicist and the radiation oncologist. Somewhat more sophisticated beam shaping is performed by taking advantage of fixed multileaf collimators. The major advantage of 3D-CRT is that dose-volume histograms can be obtained for the tumor and normal tissue structures. This

provides a quantitative method of evaluating treatment plans and enhances quality assurance.

IMRT and related modalities, such as TomoTherapy, allow even greater sculpting of the radiation dose. IMRT requires a treatment planning system that uses inverse treatment planning. Inverse planning requires that the various tumor structures (GTV, CTV, and PTV) as well as critical normal tissue structures be identified and contoured into the planning system. Optimization objectives for each structure are entered, and a sophisticated algorithm attempts to meet all objectives. This is standard of care for the treatment of prostate tumors, head and neck cancers, vertebral cancers, some brain cancers, and pelvic cancers in humans. A major benefit associated with IMRT is that dose to adjacent normal tissue structures can be minimized, dramatically reducing acute effects. Patients are more comfortable and require less pain medication.[122] The tumor dose can be increased without exceeding normal tissue tolerance, presumably leading to improved tumor control. Fractionation schedules and other factors, such as immobilization, margins, and CTV expansions, are similar to 3D-CRT. TomoTherapy, a form of IMRT that uses a helical delivery system to sculpt the beam, and volumetric-modulated arc RT are also being used in veterinary medicine.[11,123] IMRT is proving useful for the treatment of tumors or tumor beds with complex geometry located near important normal tissues, such as nasal tumors, oral tumors, and urogenital tumors.[123,124]

SRT is a treatment technique made possible by highly conformal radiation treatment techniques, such as IMRT and proton therapy, in combination with precise positioning devices and localization methods, such as cone-beam computed tomography (CBCT). In SRT, the usual wide margins (CTV) to account for microscopic disease extension are not applied, and PTV expansion may be decreased to spare important adjacent normal tissues (Fig. 13.4). Highly conformal radiation is applied to a specific gross (tumor) target with rapid dose fall-off within a small margin. This technique minimizes the radiation dose reaching normal structures adjacent to the treated target. Table 13.2 shows a comparison of characteristics of traditionally fractionated RT compared with SRT.

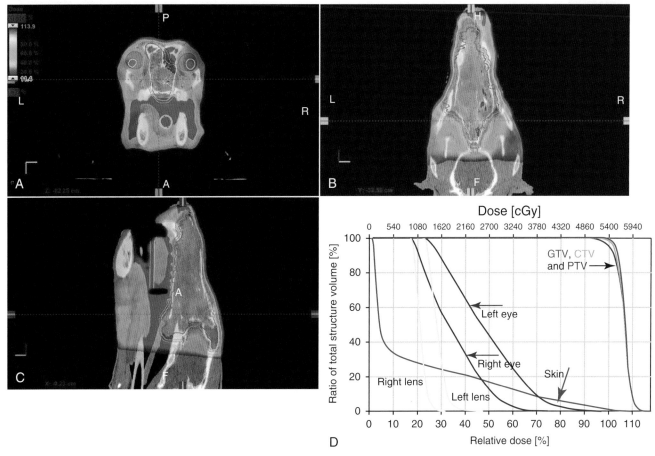

• **Fig. 13.4** A canine nasal tumor with axial (A), dorsal (B), and sagittal (C) sections through a canine nasal tumor. Dose is in color wash with the prescribed dose in orange. (D) The dose volume histogram. Note the high dose to the tumor compared with regional normal tissue structures.

TABLE 13.2	Characteristics of Traditionally (Finely) Fractionated Radiation Therapy vs. Stereotactic Radiation Therapy		
General Characteristics	3D/IMRT	SRT	
Dose/fraction	2.5–4.2 Gy	6–24 Gy	
Number of fractions	10–25	1–5	
Target definition	CTV/PTV gross disease and clinical extension Tumors may not have sharp boundaries	GTV/CTV/ITP/PTV Well-defined tumors: GTV = CTV	
Margins	cm	mm	
Primary imaging modalities for planning	CT	CT/MR/PET-CT	
Redundancy in geometric verification	No	Yes	
Maintenance of high spatial targeting accuracy for the entire treatment	Moderately enforced, moderate patient position control and monitoring	Strictly enforced (sufficient immobilization and high-frequency position monitoring through integrated image guidance)	
Need for respiratory motion management	Minimal, usually managed by increasing ITV	High particularly for tumors thorax and cranial abdomen	
Staff training	High	High, plus special SRT training	
Radiobiologic understanding	Well understood	Poorly understood	
Interaction with systemic therapies	Yes; principles well established	Yes; minimally understood	
Immobilization devices	Vac-Lok bags, pillows, and acrylic mesh	Vac-Lok bags, pillows, and acrylic mesh + bite blocks for head and neck tumors	
Purpose	Palliative/curative	Palliative/curative	

Modified from Benedict SH, Yenice KM, Followill D, et al. Stereotactic body radiation therapy: the report of AAPM Task Group 101. *Med Phys.* 2010;37:4078–4101. *CT,* Computed tomography; *CTV,* clinical target volume; *GTV,* gross tumor volume; *IMRT,* intensity modulated radiation therapy; *ITV,* internal target volume; *PTV,* planning target volume; *SRT,* stereotactic radiation therapy.

Immobilization and Localization Techniques

As radiation delivery techniques become more conformal and treatment margins are reduced, the importance of precise patient positioning and target localization/verification become increasingly important. A variety of techniques are used to achieve the requisite level of accuracy for any given patient and RT procedure. A port film is a radiograph taken, typically by the treatment beam, at the beginning of an RT and periodically throughout the treatment course to ensure proper radiation positioning and alignment of the treatment beam and patient for 3D-CRT. Commonly obtained as a double exposure from the treatment machine with an initial exposure of the treatment field followed by exposure of a wide field of the surrounding anatomy, it results in a radiographic image with a dark central area indicative of the treatment field with lighter exposure of the surrounding anatomy for reference. Digital radiography technology is now frequently implemented and may be integrated into a linear accelerator. An electronic portal imaging device (EPID) is a digital imaging plate mounted on a linear accelerator with a robotic arm for extending and retracting the plate in precise positions. EPIDs allow for more routine or daily treatment localization/verification, with rapid image acquisition, analysis, and storage of these images. An on-board imager (OBI) is a high-resolution digital imaging system (x-ray source and digital capture system) separate from the primary beam from the treatment machine itself. OBI systems are typically kilovoltage energy systems that provide superior contrast to images generated from a megavoltage linear accelerator beam. CBCT platforms are integrated into linear accelerators whereby a volumetric CT image can be generated by rotating the x-ray source and digital reading plate around the patient during an exposure. CBCT allows for improved localization, particularly for soft tissue structures that are difficult to immobilize relative to cutaneous or bony anatomic landmarks. Surface-guidance RT utilizes 3D camera technology or other means to accurately detect the patient surface, often in real-time during RT.

TUMORS COMMONLY TREATED WITH RADIATION

Oral Tumors

Many oral tumors, such as acanthomatous ameloblastomas (AAs) and rostral squamous cell carcinomas (SCCs), respond well to both complete surgical excision and RT. For less radiation responsive tumors such as fibrosarcomas, complete surgical excision is preferred; however, postoperative RT is recommended after incomplete histologic excision (see Chapter 23, Section A). For large oral tumors, aggressive surgery can lead to functional and/or cosmetic abnormalities. In these cases pretreatment planning for both surgery and RT may be indicated.[125] RT after surgery should start as soon as possible and can start immediately after surgery. However, in the face of excessive tension on the suture line or indication of delayed healing, RT should be postponed until healing has occurred. The therapeutic gain from following surgery with RT will be lost if the radiation is delayed for too long. The introduction of IMRT allows better sparing of important structures in the area and minimizes inadvertent dosing to salivary glands, tongue, lips, and skin, making patients more comfortable during treatment.[122]

Efficacy of Treatment

AAs are very radiation responsive. Tumor control with RT can be close to 90%.[126] A relationship has been demonstrated between tumor (T) stage and local control.[127] The reported 3-year progression-free survival time (PFS) for T1 tumors (less than 2 cm) and T2 tumors (2–4 cm) is 86%; it is only about 30% for T3 tumors (over 4 cm).[127] In a retrospective study of 57 dogs with AAs that were treated with RT reported that the overall median time to first event and median survival time (MST) were 1210 and 1441 days, respectively.[128] Dogs younger than 8.3 years old (the median age in the study) had a significantly longer MST (2322 days) than dogs older than 8.3 years (1106 days). Dogs that received doses higher than 40 Gy had significantly longer MST than dogs that received 40 Gy or less (2994 days vs. 143 days). It was previously suggested that RT could result in transformation of AAs into malignant epithelial tumors, but this possibility has since been refuted.[126,128]

Canine oral SCCs are responsive to radiation, although the prognosis is site dependent, with tumors located more rostrally having better probability of control.[129] Tumors at the base of the tongue or tonsil are highly metastatic and are likely to recur locally or regionally. In one study of oral SCC the reported PFS at 1 and 3 years is 72% and 40%, respectively, for all T stages.[130] Another study of fractionated RT (48–57 Gy in 3–4 Gy fractions) in 14 dogs with oral SCC, the median disease-free interval (DFI), and MST were 365 and 450 days, respectively.[131] In cats, oral SCC has a poor prognosis.[132] Although many cats show an initial response and may even show dramatic reductions in tumor size, tumor recurrence is common. Combining curative-intent RT with etanidazole or mitoxantrone therapy has resulted in MSTs of 116 to 170 days.[81,133] Seven cats with mandibular SCC were treated with hemimandibulectomy and mandibular node excision followed by RT; the MST was 420 days, but some cats do not adapt to bilateral mandibulectomies.[134] Nine cats with oral SCC received accelerated RT (14 fractions of 3.5 Gy in 9 days), which resulted in an MST of 86 days.[135] In a different approach, SRT (20 Gy) was delivered to 18 cats with oral SCC. Acute radiation effects were minimal and initially cats improved clinically, but MST was only 106 days.[136] Although RT is likely to play a role in the treatment of this disease, new approaches are indicated.

Oral fibrosarcomas (FSAs) are unlikely to metastasize but can be difficult to control locally. Oral FSAs are less radiosensitive than AAs and SCCs, although tumor control probabilities ranging from 33% to 67% at 1 year have been reported.[137,138] In one study of oral FSAs treated with RT, the PFS at 1 year and 3 years were 76% and 55%, respectively.[130] Surgical cytoreduction improves the probability of tumor control by RT.[137] This should be taken into consideration during surgical planning with a focus on removing gross disease and obtaining a tension-free closure. An MST of 540 days was reported in eight dogs with oral sarcomas treated with surgery followed by RT.[139] In tumors too large to be surgically resected to a subclinical level, RT alone is indicated; the probability of long-term tumor control is low with conventional RT, but new strategies using IMRT or SRT are currently being evaluated.

Malignant melanoma (MM) is the most common oral tumor in dogs and is associated with a high rate of regional and distant metastasis.[140] Higher doses of radiation per fraction (4 Gy and above) are believed to improve response rates for melanoma.[111] In one study, 38 dogs with nonmetastatic oral MM were treated with 48 Gy delivered in 4 Gy fractions on a Monday-Wednesday-Friday schedule.[130] The overall median PFS was 17.8 months, and the median PFS was 38.0 months, 11.7 months, and 12.0 months for dogs T1, T2, and T3 tumors, respectively. In a retrospective study of 140 dogs, most of which had regional or distant metastasis at presentation,[141] coarsely fractionated (9–10 Gy weekly fractions to a total dose of 30–36 Gy) and conventionally fractionated (2–4 Gy fractions to as high as 45 Gy or more) protocols were used with or without surgery or chemotherapy. The median times to first event and MST were 5 and 7 months, respectively. Tumor recurrence was the first event in only 27% of the dogs, whereas new metastases or death accounted for the remaining 63%. In a retrospective study of 39 dogs with incompletely resected oral MM treated with coarsely fractionated RT plus platinum-based chemotherapy, the MST was 363 days.[142] The dogs received six weekly fractions of 6 Gy, with cisplatin (10–30 mg/m²) or carboplatin (90 mg/m²) administered 1 hour before irradiation. The local recurrence rate was 15% and the median time to metastasis was 311 days.[142] Five cats with oral MM were treated with 8 Gy delivered on days 0, 7, and 21. All died from progressive disease and the MST was 146 days.[143]

Radiation Considerations

Reproducibility of treatment fields for oral tumors can be aided by positioning and immobilization devices. Depending on the size and location of the target, IMRT allows better sparing of surrounding normal structures such as the eyes and salivary glands. MM may have a low α/β ratio, making them more responsive to coarsely fractionated protocols.[144]

Treatment-Related Toxicities

Treatment toxicity depends on the time-dose-fraction size of the protocol and the specific normal structures in the treatment field. For oral tumors, this can include the skin, nasal cavity, and eyes. The major acute complications associated with RT of the oral cavity are mucositis and skin effects. Mucositis always occurs to some degree in patients that have received irradiation to the oral cavity, pharynx, and/or esophagus. Mucositis typically begins during the second week of therapy and reaches a maximum severity during or shortly after the last week of therapy. Clinical signs include thickened saliva and tenderness of the mouth. Patients may be reluctant to eat or drink and require supportive care. Low-salt foods are less irritating to the oral mucosa than regular commercial diets. Infrequently, placement of a gastrostomy or esophagostomy tube may be necessary to facilitate feeding. Oral mucositis should subside within 2 weeks after therapy. The extent of skin effects will vary based on the field size and location. Erythema, hair loss, dry and moist desquamation, and swelling of lips can occur. The effects may start late in the course of treatment or shortly after completion of treatment. Blotting the skin gently with moist towels can help keep the area clean. Never rub or scrub the area, and an E-collar may be useful to keep the patient from rubbing or pawing at the area. Pain management is important for both mucositis and skin effects.

Rarely, animals treated with chemotherapy subsequent to a course of RT can develop a return of radiation side effects such as mucositis or moist desquamation of the skin, a phenomenon known as radiation recall.[145] Radiation recall is a poorly understood phenomenon that can occur with many different antineoplastic drugs, although it is most commonly associated with doxorubicin, taxanes, and gemcitabine.[145] It is drug specific for individual patients and rechallenge does not necessarily induce the reaction.[145]

Late complications of radiation specific to the oral cavity include osteoradionecrosis, xerostomia, and oronasal fistula development. Xerostomia (dryness of the mouth due to salivary dysfunction) is a common complication in human patients undergoing RT of the head and neck region[146,147]; however, clinically significant xerostomia is not commonly recognized in animals. IMRT technology should provide improved sparing of salivary glands and in human patients has resulted in significantly lower proportion of patients with grade II or worse xerostomia.[147] Osteoradionecrosis, or development of nonvital bone susceptible to pathologic fracture after RT, is an uncommon complication that can occur in any bone in a radiation field, typically years after treatment. The mandible is the most susceptible bone to osteoradionecrosis but, as with most late effects, the risk can be minimized by administering radiation in lower doses per fraction.[148] The role of SRT for the treatment of oral tumors is unclear.[149] Human patients who have failed traditional RT regimens are sometimes treated with salvage SRT.[149]

Nasal Tumors

Nasal tumors (see Chapter 24, Section B) in dogs are difficult to control. Surgery, cryosurgery, or immunotherapy alone do not appear to improve survival over no treatment.[150–153] RT provides the best reported tumor control for canine nasal tumors and likely needs to be part of any curative-intent treatment regimen.

Efficacy of Treatment

RT has long been the standard of care for nasal and sinonasal tumors. The location is not generally amenable to complete surgical resection, and although early reports of orthovoltage radiation pulse surgery showed improved outcomes,[154,155] most reports combining RT and surgery have not demonstrated therapeutic gain compared with radiation alone.[156,157] Interestingly, over the past 20 years, advancements in treatment planning technology from point calculations to 2D, 2.5D, and 3D-CRT technologies have not been associated with improved tumor control or survival. Megavoltage RT alone planned with 3D-CRT has been reported to provide an MST of approximately 1 year.[158–160] Histologic subpopulations may be prognostically significant; however, most publications are hampered by inadequate patient numbers. Cribriform erosion has been associated with a poor prognosis with fractionated RT protocols.[161,162]

Two publications have evaluated outcome in dogs with nasal tumors treated with IMRT.[122,123] Thirty-one dogs treated with IMRT were compared with 36 historical controls treated with the same prescription using 2D treatment planning. The MSTs were 420 days and 410 days, respectively.[123] In another report, 12 dogs treated with IMRT to a dose commonly used for 2D or 3D-CRT planning had an MST of 446 days.[122] Patient numbers in both studies were low, and there was no stratification for prognostic factors. Although definitive conclusions cannot be made regarding tumor control, the decrease in acute effects to the region in both studies was profound with minimal grade II and III cutaneous and mucosal toxicity noted. Although the ipsilateral eye could not be spared, minimal side effects to the contralateral eye were noted.[123]

SRT has been investigated in 29 dogs with solid nasal tumors with three daily fractions of 10 Gy.[10] Clinical signs improved in all dogs. Acute effects were minimal; however, approximately 10% of dogs developed significant oronasal or nasocutaneous fistulas. The MST was 586 days with 69% and 22% alive 1 and 2 years post-SRT, respectively.[9] Developing patient selection criteria and modifying normal tissue radiation constraints should be a priority, so late tissue effects can be minimized.

Lymphoproliferative nasal tumors in cats respond well and durably to RT (these are addressed later in the chapter in the section on lymphoma; also see Chapter 33, Section B).[163] Carcinomas and sarcomas in cats respond comparably to nasal tumors in dogs: 48 Gy administered in 4 Gy fractions over 4 weeks resulted in a 1- and 2-year survival rates of 44.3% and 16.6%, respectively.[164] The histologic type and clinical stage of the tumor did not affect the prognosis.

Nine dogs with recurrent nasal tumors previously treated with 3D-CRT (median 50 Gy) were reirradiated.[165] The overall MST from initial treatment was 31 months with an increased incidence of late effects. Retreatment becomes a more viable option with new modalities, such as IMRT and SRT, that can better spare local normal tissues.

The response to feline nasal planum SCC is affected by the tumor stage.[166] Cats with T1 tumors had 1- and 5-year survival rates of 85% and 56%, respectively, and the mean ST was 53 months (the median was not reached). However, larger, more invasive tumors showed a less favorable response when treated with 40 Gy in 4 Gy fractions over 3.5 weeks.[166] Tumor control should be improved by reducing the dose per fraction and increasing the total dose. For small, superficial SCC lesions of the nasal planum in cats, strontium (Sr)-90 plesiotherapy is a viable option. Because Sr-90 emits a low-energy β-particle, very high doses can be administered to the surface of a lesion without unacceptable complications or damage to underlying tissue. In one study, 49 cats with SCC of the nasal planum were administered a median of 128 Gy in a single fraction with a complete response rate of 88% and median PFI of 1710 days.[167] Larger, invasive SCC lesions are usually not amenable to treatment with Sr-90.[167]

Radiation Considerations

Canine and feline sinonasal tumors are challenging to treat with radiation because they are anatomically complex with frequent involvement of the nasal sinuses, cribriform plate, and nasopharynx. The geometry of the nasal cavity is problematic, because the target is larger caudally than rostrally, making it difficult to achieve even dose distribution. The dose sculpting benefits of inverse treatment planning used for IMRT and SRT make these modalities the treatment of choice for nasal tumors. Regardless of radiation modality used, clients should be advised of the potential for persistent nasal symptoms and long-term radiation effects.

Treatment-Related Toxicities

After treatment with 3D-CRT, radiation toxicities of nasal tumors are similar to those described previously for the oral cavity, with mucositis affecting the oral cavity and tongue, and dry to moist desquamation of skin. Regardless of radiation modality used, the nasal cavity will never be completely normal after turbinate destruction from the tumor and from radiation damage. In dry environments, room humidifiers can make patients more comfortable, and intermittent antibiotics may be necessary to treat periodic bouts of rhinitis. Fungal infections after the treatment of nasal tumors has also been reported.[9] Long-term use of pentoxifylline and vitamin E are recommended to help mitigate radiation effects in patients treated with SRT.[168] Nasal discharge, sneezing, and epistaxis may indicate tumor recurrence and can be challenging to differentiate from posttreatment rhinitis. Deep nasal culture and sensitivity may help direct antibiotic treatment. If there is no durable clinical response from antibiotic treatment, then a CT is recommended to evaluate for recurrence.

Ocular radiation complications are extremely common when 3D-CRT planning is used because of the proximity of the nasal cavity and frontal sinus to the orbit.[169] Effects to the eyes are dose related and vary in severity.[170] Acute effects include blepharitis,

blepharospasm, conjunctivitis, and keratoconjunctivitis sicca (KCS).[169,170] KCS may be temporary or permanent, depending on the dose administered and the sensitivity of the patient.[169,171] KCS is treated with artificial tears and steroids to prevent corneal ulceration. If corneal ulceration is present, healing may be delayed as a result of radiation damage to the corneal stem cells.[172] Late effects include vascular changes, which may have subtle effects on vision but in most cases do not result in blindness. Radiation-induced cataracts may occur and the latent period is related to dose.[173] As with other cataracts, these can be removed with phacoemulsification. When treating nasal or facial tumors, it may be necessary for the eye to receive the full treatment dose. At doses above 40 Gy, degenerative angiopathy of retinal vessels can progress over 2 years and result in retinal degeneration.[172] Optic nerve axonal degeneration has been reported to occur secondary to the retinal changes.[172] IMRT and SRT allow greater sparing of ocular tissues, resulting in diminished acute and late toxicities.[9,123]

Tumors in the Cranial Vault

Brain tumors can be treated successfully with RT and/or surgery (see Chapter 31). In the treatment of brain tumors, surgery may be indicated to relieve life-threatening clinical signs. Although appropriate studies are still needed, reported STs after radiation for brain tumors in dogs with less severe neurologic signs are frequently comparable to surgery alone.[174] Adjuvant RT is indicated in patients with incomplete surgical resection; RT alone should be performed in dogs and cats with cancer at surgically inaccessible sites or in locations where surgical morbidity is high.

Efficacy of Treatment

Published STs of canine brain tumors treated with RT compare favorably to surgery, although directly comparable data is lacking and combinations of surgery and RT may be superior to either modality alone. There is little published information on irradiation of nonpituitary feline brain tumors, because most feline meningiomas are effectively treated surgically.[175] Nevertheless, radiation outcomes for cats appear comparable to canine brain tumors, and RT should be considered when the tumor location is not amenable to surgical resection. In one study, 46 dogs with brain tumors associated with neurologic disease were treated with RT alone[176]; the MST was 23.3 months with 1- and 2-year survival rates of 69% and 47%, respectively. No prognostic clinical factors were identified. The outcome in this study was superior to those from previous reports in which the MST was about 1 year.[177–179] Differences may be due to improved treatment planning capabilities, which was supported by a study of 31 dogs treated with 3D-CRT that had an MST of 19 months.[180] In another study also involving 31 dogs with meningioma, postoperative RT improved the MST from 7 months with surgery alone to 16.5 months with surgery followed by RT.[181]

Thirty dogs with image-based diagnoses of intracranial meningiomas were treated with SRT, with most receiving 24 Gy in three fractions. The overall MST for any cause of death was 561 days and treatment was well tolerated.[8] In another study, 39 dogs with image-based meningiomas were treated with stereotactic volume-modulated arc RT (VMAT) receiving 33 Gy in five fractions. The 2-year overall survival rate was 74.3% and treatment was well tolerated.[182]

Forty-two dogs with presumed gliomas were treated with VMAT alone or in combination with temozolomide. The MSTs for RT alone and RT and temozolomide were 383 days and 420 days, respectively; there was no significant difference between the groups. A control arm of 30 dogs with glial tumors was treated medically and their MST was 94 days.[183]

Pituitary tumors in dogs and cats generally are responsive to radiation, and surgical access is limited. Dogs with pituitary tumors treated with fractionated RT have MSTs varying between 1 and 2 years.[184,185] A study comparing 19 dogs with pituitary tumors receiving RT (48 Gy in 16 daily fractions of 3 Gy) to untreated dogs found 1-, 2-, and 3-year survival rates of 93%, 87%, and 55% in the RT group and 45%, 32%, and 25% in the unirradiated group, respectively.[186] Fractionated pituitary irradiation in dogs is more effective at delaying tumor growth than in controlling adrenocorticotropic hormone (ACTH) secretion.[186,187] Eucortisolism is seen in some patients after RT; however, pre-ACTH and post-ACTH cortisol levels should be monitored at regular intervals so that medications can be modified, if indicated.

Cats seem to have marked clinical improvement of associated endocrinopathies when treated with RT.[188] In one study, 53 cats with functional pituitary adenomas associated with feline acromegaly were treated with SRT.[98] Diagnosis was based on history, physical examination, laboratory results, and cross-sectional imaging of the pituitary region. The overall MST was 1072 days. Of the 41 cats where insulin information was available, 95% experienced a decrease in required insulin dose, with 32% achieving diabetic remission. Hypothyroidism developed in 14% of treated cats. Interestingly, three cats with no pituitary enlargement, but who met other criteria, were treated and responded.[98] Previous studies using fractionated RT showed durable response to neurologic disease but limited endocrine responses (Chapter 26).[188,189]

Two recent manuscripts explored the treatment of trigeminal nerve sheath tumors with SRT, with MSTs ranging from 441 to 745 days.[190,191] In both studies, all tumors had an intracranial component. Extension into the cranial nerve can involve one to three of the branches, and administering dose to involved branches could be important for tumor control.[191]

Radiation Considerations

The integration of 3-D imaging, patient positioning devices, and advanced treatment planning techniques have the potential to improve tumor targeting and sparing of normal brain tissue. For many brain tumors, IMRT will not provide an improved dose distribution compared with 3D-CRT; however, dose sculpting may be beneficial for cranial nerve tumors. An additional consideration in patients undergoing RT for a brain tumor is the anesthetic risk associated with increased intracranial pressure or brainstem disease; an appropriate anesthetic regimen should be selected to minimize the risk of complications. Specifically, patients should be ventilated while under anesthesia to decrease blood P_{CO_2}, and anesthetic agents that decrease (or at least do not increase) intracranial pressure should be selected. SRT limits the number of anesthetic episodes, which may be beneficial in unstable patients.

Treatment-Related Toxicities

For most brain tumors, acute effects to the skin can be avoided with megavoltage RT. Occasionally, ocular and otic side effects or mucositis to the caudal oral cavity may be seen if these structures are in or adjacent to the treatment field. The radiation tolerance is lower when the entire brain is treated; this limits prescription of a dose that is adequate for tumor control but still has an acceptable probability of late effects. The radiation tolerance of brain and spinal tissues is generally considered to be less than that of other commonly treated tissues, and volume may be an important factor for brain and spinal lesions. Early delayed effects can occur 1 to 3 months after treatment and may be due to transient demyelination or from edema associated with cytokine release from dying tumor cells. Animals with early delayed effects may have signs similar to or different from those at the initial presentation or they may be stuporous. Early delayed effects occur in up to 40% of humans undergoing brain RT; symptoms include headache, lethargy, and exacerbation of focal neurologic signs.[192] In animals, clinical signs often are transient, but response time can be slow. Early delayed effects are treated with the administration of systemic corticosteroids, and sometimes supportive care is required. MRI may show an apparent increase in tumor size and tumor enhancement during this time. Focal enhancement in a normal brain associated with edema and demyelination may also be present.[193] In a study of SRT for canine meningiomas, 37% of dogs showed mild-to-moderate exacerbation of neurologic signs 3 to 16 weeks after treatment.[8] Most dogs responded to systemic corticosteroids and supportive care, and dosimetric information relating to the toxicity helped establish dose constraints for the brain.[8]

Late effects probably occur in veterinary patients more often than identified. Late effects generally occur at least 6 months after treatment but can also occur years later. Brain necrosis is the most commonly identified effect. The probability of late brain effects depends on the total dose, fraction size, and the volume of brain irradiated. In a study of 83 dogs with brain masses treated with a hypofractionated protocol (38 Gy administered in five weekly fractions), brain necrosis was confirmed or suspected in 14% of dogs.[194] Signs are similar to those associated with early delayed effects, although the response to corticosteroids is limited. Clinically distinguishing between late effects and tumor recurrence can often be difficult. CT or MRI evaluation can be misleading. Not all brain tumors completely regress after treatment, therefore the presence of a mass does not always indicate a recurring tumor. A prudent course is to obtain a CT or MRI evaluation 6 months after treatment to serve as a reference if clinical signs develop in the future.

Superficial Tumors of the Trunk and Extremities

Many tumors involving the trunk or extremities are amenable to treatment by RT. Combining RT and surgery has the potential to enhance tumor control and improve the functional outcome over either modality alone. For many invasive tumors, conservative surgery with adjuvant RT can provide a viable alternative to radical surgery. For tumors in nonresectable locations, SRT alone may provide a good outcome depending on tumor type and volume. The surgeon and radiation oncologist should consult before therapeutic intervention is started to develop an overall treatment approach.

Soft tissue sarcomas (STSs) are common tumors arising in a wide range of locations, most commonly arising as subcutaneous masses. Hemangiopericytomas, FSAs, neurofibrosarcomas, myxosarcomas, and nerve sheath tumors are classified together as STSs because of their similar biologic behavior (see Chapter 22). Metastases are uncommon with grade I and grade II STSs; therefore local tumor control is the primary concern, whereas grade III tumors have more aggressive metastatic potential. STSs are locally invasive, and tumor cells may extend far beyond the bulk of the tumor. Surgery alone can result in long-term tumor control if the tumor can be excised completely.[195] When wide excision is not feasible, recurrence rates after narrow excision are reported to vary from <10% to >70% depending on histologic grade, completeness of excision, tumor size, tumor invasiveness, and tumor location. Accordingly, risk assessment for local recurrence and the potential recommendation for adjuvant therapy requires consideration of all of these factors. Based on these risks, combining RT and surgery may be beneficial in cases where complete excision may not be possible. RT can be administered first with the hope of converting an inoperable tumor into an operable one. This approach has the benefit of reducing the volume of normal tissues irradiated. More commonly, surgical excision is performed first as a cytoreductive procedure and then followed by RT to eliminate the residual subclinical disease. In one study, 48 dogs with STS were treated with surgical cytoreduction followed by RT; eight dogs (16%) developed tumor recurrence, and the 5-year survival rate was 78%.[196] In another study of 38 dogs with STS of the body and extremities, treatment with surgery followed by RT resulted in an MST of 2270 days.[139] Recent publications indicate that many low-grade STSs may not recur despite incomplete excision[197–199]; however, the level of surgical training can affect outcome.[200]

STS can be treated with RT alone; however, tumor control is not as durable as with a combination of RT and surgery.[137] RT alone is useful for tumors near the paw/pads, where surgical options are limited, and in tumors wrapping around the limbs. Pads in the radiation field initially may slough; however, if appropriate fractionation schemes are used, the pads regrow and can function normally.

Injection site sarcomas (ISSs) are a significant problem in cats (see Chapter 22). These tumors are challenging to control locally and seem unresponsive to aggressive RT or conservative surgery alone. In one study, 33 cats with histologically confirmed ISS were treated with RT followed by surgery.[201] The median DFI and MST were 398 and 600 days, respectively. In another study, 25 cats with subclinical disease after surgery were treated with RT alone (57 Gy delivered in 3 Gy fractions) and, in some cases, with adjuvant chemotherapy.[202] The overall MST was 701 days. Local recurrence was observed in 28.6% of cats. In cats with local recurrence, one tumor developed outside the treatment field, and the remaining tumors recurred in the radiation field. Similar findings were reported in 78 cats treated with surgical cytoreduction followed by RT.[203] In this study, cats that underwent only one surgery before RT had a lower recurrence rate than cats that had more than one surgery. The ST and DFI shortened as the time between surgery and the start of RT lengthened. In a study of 79 cats treated with either pre- or postoperative RT, PCV >25% was associated with better outcome (MST 760 days) than in cats with PCV <25% (MST 306 days).[204]

Cats with surgically nonresectable disease present a greater challenge. Escalation of the radiation dose by delivering the dose in smaller fractions is probably necessary for these patients. IMRT or SRT may be beneficial for obtaining adequate dose to the tumor, because appropriate sparing of the lungs, viscera, and spinal cord is critical in these patients. SRT was used to treat 11 cats with nonresectable ISSs. Acute radiation effects were minimal and cats tolerated the treatment well; however, this modality should be considered palliative as the overall MST was 301 days.[205]

Cutaneous mast cell tumors (MCTs) can be treated successfully with RT (see Chapter 21). The obvious advantage is that greater margins may be obtained with RT than with surgery. The probability of control may be improved if surgical cytoreduction is performed first. In a study of 37 dogs with grade II MCTs treated with cytoreduction and RT, tumor control at 1 and 2 years exceeded 90%.[206] In 56 dogs with incompletely resected MCTs,

the median DFI was 32.7 months.[207] Controversy exists regarding whether the addition of RT is necessary after incomplete excision of MCT due to moderate recurrence rates; however, a study of 64 dogs showed lower recurrence rates (8% vs. 38%) and significantly longer MSTs (2930 days vs. 710 days) in dogs receiving adjuvant RT compared with dogs not receiving RT.[208]

RT also is indicated for cutaneous MCT with regional LN metastasis. In one study, 19 dogs with MCT and regional node involvement were treated with surgical cytoreduction of the primary site, radiation to the primary tumor and regional node, and prednisone.[209] The median disease-free ST was 1240 days. In a study of 21 dogs with grade II, stage II MCTs treated with surgical resection and adjuvant chemotherapy, the addition of RT for locoregional control resulted in a longer MST (2056 days) than dogs not treated with adjuvant RT (1103 days).[210] Palliative RT is commonly used to treat symptomatic locoregional MCT in dogs when systemic spread has occurred.

Radiation Considerations

Many tumors of the limbs and trunk extend very close to the skin surface. Point calculations or 3D-CRT modalities are commonly and successfully used. Application of an appropriate thickness of a bolus material over the skin is frequently needed when treating with megavoltage photons to avoid underdosing the superficial region. When an extremity is in a radiation field, a 1- to 2-cm strip of tissue should be shielded to avoid the risk of lymphedema, which can present as painful swelling of the distal limb. For microscopic or macroscopic ISSs in cats, radiation planning is challenging with 3D-CRT. Inverse planning allows better sculpting around body curvatures and allows a higher dose to be delivered to the target structures.

Treatment-Related Toxicities

When treating superficial tumors, early effects to the skin are expected and are restricted to the radiation field. The severity of these effects are dose related. Depilation is common and in some cases may be permanent. The hair may not return for several months and varies in relation to the dose administered to the skin and the individual patient's sensitivity. Damage to the melanocytes may result in hypopigmentation or hyperpigmentation of the skin and/or alteration of the coat color when regrowth occurs, often resulting in whitish-gray fur (leukotrichia). Dry desquamation may accompany epilation; this generally does not cause any problem or discomfort for the patient and usually is not treated. Moist desquamation, which usually appears 3 to 5 weeks after the start of therapy, is associated with pruritus and pain, which can vary in severity. Self-mutilation exacerbates the problem and may lead to ulceration or necrosis. Pain management is an important part of the overall treatment plan. NSAIDs are usually the first line of therapy if there are no contraindications. Tramadol, amantadine, and gabapentin are often added to the regimen. Severe late effects to the skin are rare with fractionated RT but include fibrosis and necrosis.

Bone Tumors

Although OSAs are not considered highly radiation-responsive tumors, RT may be considered as part of a multimodality therapy when surgical excision is not an option (see Chapter 25). RT can be combined with chemotherapy and surgery for limb-sparing protocols.[211,212] SRT is currently being evaluated as a limb-sparing alternative. In one study, SRS was performed on 11 dogs with appendicular OSA[213]; although radiation dose varied and not all dogs received adjuvant chemotherapy, good limb function and tumor control were observed in some of the patients. A recent study of 46 dogs with OSA treated with SRT showed a median survival of 9.7 months, which is comparable to reports of amputation plus chemotherapy, but a high rate of pathologic fracture.[101]

Treatment of axial OSA has been particularly challenging because of the proximity to important normal tissue structures, particularly when treating vertebral tumors. In a retrospective study of multimodality therapy for axial OSAs, dogs that underwent curative-intent RT protocols had a longer duration of tumor control (265 days) than those treated with a palliative regimen (79 days).[214] SRT was delivered to nine dogs with primary or secondary vertebral OSA.[96] The protocols and doses varied based on proximity to spinal cord. Five of six dogs had improved pain control, but the overall MST was only 139 days.[191] As more information becomes available regarding dose constraints and optimal fractionation, RT may have value, but it should currently be considered a palliative procedure.

The mechanism of the amelioration of pain caused by bony neoplasia is not completely understood, but decreases in intratumoral pressure, local antiinflamatory effects, tumor cell apoptosis, and cytotoxicity to osteoclasts have been proposed.[215] Relief of pain may occur almost immediately or may be delayed, sometimes as long as 2 weeks after the start of RT. Human studies have indicated that a single large dose may be comparable or superior to multifraction protocols using more conventional doses per fraction.[216] In a recent study of 58 dogs, 8 Gy was administered on 2 consecutive days, providing onset of pain relief within 2 days in 91% of patients.[217] Commonly in veterinary medicine, 7 to 10 Gy fractions have been administered on days 0, 7, and 21.[218,219] In one study, 12 of 15 dogs with appendicular bone tumors treated with palliative RT had improved limb function, and the MST was 130 days.[219] In another study, dogs with appendicular OSA were given either three fractions of 10 Gy or two fractions of 8 Gy[118]; 74% of 95 dogs experienced pain relief for a median duration of 73 days. No difference in response was found between the two treatment groups. Sometimes localized pain recurs before metastatic disease becomes life limiting. Palliative RT can be readministered as long as the owners understand that continued administration of large doses per fraction eventually leads to late effects. Clearly, most palliative OSA RT protocols help relieve pain; the preference of the protocol chosen by the attending radiation oncologist will likely be based on the geographic location of the clients and the availability of staffing.

Radiation Considerations

RT is unlikely to have a substantial palliative effect if a displaced pathologic fracture from a bone tumor is already present. Additional monitoring during anesthesia recovery is recommended to prevent the patient from trying to stand prematurely. Nonslick flooring may be helpful in preventing injury to the affected limb while recovering from anesthesia.

Treatment-Related Toxicities

All dogs with bone tumors are at risk of developing pathologic fracture unless the affected limb is amputated. This risk may be increased with radiation therapy due to palliative benefit, resulting in increased weight-bearing load and other potential effects of radiation on bone maintenance. For limb sparing using SRT/SRS, patient selection is crucial. A study of 46 dogs treated with SRT for OSA had pathologic fracture rates of 27%, 56%, and 62% at

3, 6, and 9 months, respectively.[101] Area of bone involvement was prognostic for fracture as dogs with involvement of subchondral bone had a median time to fracture of 4.2 months versus 16.3 months in dogs without.[101] Occasional grade III acute and late skin toxicity was also seen in this study, particularly for tumors involving the radius.[101] Proximity of the tumor to the skin must be considered, particularly in locations such as the distal radius where minimal soft tissue exists between the bone and skin. Bisphosphonates at time of diagnosis or before SRT may be helpful for bone maintenance.[220,221] Prophylactic stabilization with a bone plate or interlocking nail has been investigated, but this was associated with high rates of severe complications.[222,223]

Lymphoma

RT can be important in the treatment of localized lymphoma, and it has an emerging role as an adjuvant therapy in the treatment of systemic lymphoma. Lymphocytes are exquisitely radiation sensitive[224] and may undergo apoptosis in addition to classic mitotic death after exposure to radiation.[225] Humans with non-Hodgkin lymphoma commonly receive combined modality treatment with RT and chemotherapy, primarily for stage I or stage II disease,[226] although this treatment may have a role in more advanced stages as well.[227] Combined modality treatment or RT alone is also beneficial in humans for primary lymphomas of bone, cutaneous B-cell lymphoma, and mycosis fungoides.[228–231]

In one study of 10 cats, extranodal lymphomas (nasal cavity, retrobulbar area, mediastinum, subcutaneous tissue, maxilla, and mandible) were treated with megavoltage RT with or without concurrent chemotherapy.[232] Complete responses were achieved in 80% of cats and partial responses in two cats. The median remission time for the cats that experienced complete responses was 114 weeks, and three cats were alive and disease free at 131 weeks. Three cats developed disease outside the radiation field, which suggests that adjuvant chemotherapy or extending the field for part of the treatment to include additional nodes may improve locoregional control.

RT has also been used to treat cutaneous lymphoma in dogs. RT of localized lymphoma has been reported to result in prolonged remission times.[233] Humans with cutaneous B-cell lymphoma are commonly treated with RT, which generally results in long-term control of disease. The extent of skin involvement and the presence of extracutaneous disease are prognostic.[231] Mycosis fungoides is sometimes treated with total skin electron irradiation in humans. As with cutaneous B-cell lymphoma, the stage of disease is prognostic, but human patients with disease confined to the skin may have prolonged remission times.

Half-body RT has been investigated as an adjuvant multicentric canine lymphoma. An 8 Gy dose to lymphoma cells reduces the surviving fraction to 0.005, which is much greater than the estimated cell kill from one cycle of chemotherapy.[224] In one study, RT was administered at the end of the chemotherapy protocol, whereas another sandwiched the RT after the first chemotherapy cycle.[234,235] Although the protocols were well tolerated, the additional expense was not justified by patient outcome.

Whole abdomen RT has also been used as a salvage technique for feline GI lymphoma.[117] In a study of 11 cats with relapsed or resistant alimentary lymphoma treated with 4 Gy fractions on 2 consecutive days, 10 cats had either partial or complete clinical remission. Acute effects associated with RT were minimal. The post-RT MST was 214 days.[117]

An emerging approach in the management of dogs with hematologic malignancies, such as lymphoma and leukemia, is total body irradiation (TBI) followed by either autologous or allogeneic transplantation of peripheral blood hematopoietic progenitor cells. After consolidation with a standard CHOP-based chemotherapy protocol, dogs are given a high-dose cyclophosphamide, followed 2 weeks later with progenitor cell mobilization using 5 days of recombinant human granulocyte colony-stimulating factor. Peripheral blood mononuclear cells are then harvested, and the CD34+ cells are enumerated, with the goal of obtaining >2 x 10^6/kg CD34+ cells. The next day, 10 to 12 Gy of TBI is administered over 2 days, and the harvested cells are immediately infused intravenously once RT is completed. In a toxicity study of 10 dogs, all dogs experienced grade IV neutropenia, lymphopenia, and thrombocytopenia.[236,237] Neutrophils recovered to at least 500/uL by day 12; however, thrombocytopenia often persisted for weeks. Using this treatment strategy, the median DFI and MST were 271 days and 463 days, respectively, for 24 dogs with high-grade B-cell lymphoma, with 33% of dogs living >2 years. When using the same protocol to treat 13 dogs with high-grade T-cell lymphoma in first remission, the median DFI and MST were 184 and 240 days, respectively, with 15% of dogs being long-term survivors.[237,238]

Other Tumors

RT is used for a variety of tumors in the thoracic and abdominal cavities. The principles of patient selection for RT with tumors in these regions are the same as for any other region. RT should be considered for any tumor that cannot be excised completely. In one study, dogs with thyroid carcinomas treated with 48 Gy delivered in 4 Gy fractions had PFS rates of 80% at 1 year and 72% at 3 years.[239] Thymomas are radiation responsive in human patients.[240] In a study of seven cats with thymoma treated with RT, the MST was close to 2 years (see Chapter 34, Section B).[241]

Eighteen dogs with primary disease of the urinary bladder (7), urethra (1), or prostate (10) were treated with IMRT assisted by image guidance to verify tumor position.[124] In all dogs, the radiation dose ranged from 54 to 58 Gy, delivered in 20 daily fractions. The majority of patients were treated with adjuvant chemotherapy and non-steroid antiinflammatory drugs (NSAIDs). Acute and late tissue toxicities were limited, and treatment was well tolerated. The overall MST was 654 days. Location of the primary tumor had no effect on either local tumor control or survival. A modified treatment protocol in a larger number of dogs resulted in increased radiation effects such as urinary incontinence (personal communication, B. Clerc-Renaud).

Perianal adenocarcinomas and apocrine gland anal sac adeno-carcinomas (AGASACA) (see Chapter 23, Section H) can be difficult to control locally with surgery alone and may metastasize to the regional sublumbar LNs. RT may be used in the adjuvant setting to treat residual microscopic or gross locoregional disease. A study of 28 dogs with locoregionally advanced (stage IIIb) AGASAC treated with either surgery or RT showed a significantly longer median PFS for dogs treated with IMRT (14.7 months) compared with dogs treated surgically (6.0 months).[242] Perianal gland carcinomas are generally slow to disseminate systemically, so full-course RT or SRT of involved regional LNs may be warranted. Mucositis also can occur whenever any portion of the alimentary system is included in the RT field. Colitis is a common acute effect during RT for colorectal tumors. Severe large bowel diarrhea may be seen. Anusitis from irradiation is worsened by the diarrhea, making the patient quite uncomfortable. High-bulk

diets and regional hygiene are recommended. Steroid enemas seem beneficial in some patients with colitis.[243] Late effects from RT to the pelvic region can occur, and these can be clinically significant.[75] This can be addressed by administering the radiation in smaller doses per fraction.[75]

Because of the rapid drop-off between tumor dose and regional tissues, SRT has introduced treatment to a much wider variety of tumors in the thorax and abdomen. Nine dogs with canine adrenocortical tumors with vascular invasion were treated with SRT (VMAT). The overall MST was 1030 days with minimal toxicity. The endocrine panels in two of three dogs with cortisol-secreting tumors normalized.[11] SRT has been used to treat extensive abdominal LN involvement in dogs with AGASACA, and this was well tolerated and provided durable palliation in three dogs (personal communication, Dr. Tiffany Martin). SRT was used to treat six dogs with heart base tumors.[244] The MST was not reached, and four dogs were progression free at 408, 451, 751, and 723 days posttreatment. Treatment-related complications included coughing, congestive heart failure, and tachyarrhythmias.[244] Palliative RT can be useful for tumors causing airway, bowel, or urinary tract obstruction or neurologic dysfunction. Mediastinal lymphoma often responds rapidly to irradiation. Relief from respiratory distress can be achieved within hours of a single dose of RT.

References

1. Coutard H: Roentgen therapy of epitheliomas of the tonsillar region, hypopharynx and larynx from 1920 to 1926, *Am J Roentgenol* 28:313–331, 1932.
2. Pommer A: X-ray therapy in veterinary medicine. In Brandly CA, Jungher EL, editors: *Advances in veterinary science*, Academic Press, 1958, pp 98–136.
3. Withers HR: The four R's of radiotherapy, *Adv Radiat Biol* 5:241–271, 1975.
4. DeVita Jr VT: Progress in cancer management, Keynote address, *Cancer* 51:2401–2409, 1983.
5. Farrelly J, McEntee MC: A survey of veterinary radiation facilities in 2010, *Vet Radiol Ultrasound* 55:638–643, 2014.
6. Gieger T: Veterinary radiation facilities. Available at: https://vetcancersociety.org/vcs-members/links-of-interest-2/radiation-facilities/.
7. Geiger T: ACVR website.approved veterinary radiation oncology residency programs. Available at: https://www.acvr.org/page/approved-radiation-oncology-residency-programs.
8. Griffin LR, Nolan MW, Selmic LE, et al.: Stereotactic radiation therapy for treatment of canine intracranial meningiomas, *Vet Comp Oncol* 14:e158–e170, 2016.
9. Gieger TL, Nolan MW: Linac-based stereotactic radiation therapy for canine nonlymphomatous nasal tumours: 29 cases (2013-2016), *Vet Comp Oncol* 16:E68–E75, 2018.
10. Nolan MW, Arkans MM, LaVine D, et al.: Pilot study to determine the feasibility of radiation therapy for dogs with right atrial masses and hemorrhagic pericardial effusion, *J Vet Cardiol* 19:132–143, 2017.
11. Dolera M, Malfassi L, Pavesi S, et al.: Volumetric-modulated arc stereotactic radiotherapy for canine adrenocortical tumours with vascular invasion, *J Small Anim Pract* 57:710–717, 2016.
12. Zhao P, Lu S, Yang Y, et al.: Three-dimensional conformal radiation therapy of spontaneous benign prostatic hyperplasia in canines, *Oncol Res* 19:225–235, 2011.
13. Beckmann K, Carrera I, Steffen F, et al.: A newly designed radiation therapy protocol in combination with prednisolone as treatment for meningoencephalitis of unknown origin in dogs: a prospective pilot study introducing magnetic resonance spectroscopy as monitor tool, *Acta Vet Scand* 57(4), 2015.

14. Poirier VJ, Mayer-Stankeova S, Buchholz J, et al.: Efficacy of radiation therapy for the treatment of sialocele in dogs, *J Vet Intern Med* 32:107–110, 2018.

15. Hubler M, Volkert M, Kaser-Hotz B, et al.: Palliative irradiation of Scottish Fold osteochondrodysplasia, *Vet Radiol Ultrasound* 45:582–585, 2004.

16. Kapatkin AS, Nordquist B, Garcia TC, et al.: Effect of single dose radiation therapy on weight-bearing lameness in dogs with elbow osteoarthritis, *Vet Comp Orthop Traumatol* 29:338–343, 2016.

17. Rossi F, Cancedda S, Leone VF, et al.: Megavoltage radiotherapy for the treatment of degenerative joint disease in dogs: results of a preliminary experience in an italian radiotherapy centre, *Front Vet Sci* 5:74, 2018.

18. Rivers B, Walter P, McKeever J: Treatment of canine acral lick dermatitis with radiation therapy: 17 cases (1979-1991), *J Am Anim Hosp Assoc* 29:541–544, 1993.

19. Owen L: Canine lick granulama treated with radiotherapy, *J Sm Anim Pract* 30:454–456, 1989.

20. Ward JF: DNA damage produced by ionizing radiation in mammalian cells: identities, mechanisms of formation, and reparability, *Prog Nucleic Acid Res Mol Biol* 35:95–125, 1988.

21. Compton AH: A Quantum theory of the scattering of X-rays by light elements, *Phys Rev* 21:483–502, 1923.

22. Hall EJ, Giacca A: Physics and chemistry of radiation absorption. In Hall EJ, Giacca A, editors: *Radiobiology for the radiologist*, ed 8, Philadelphia, 2019, Wolters Kluwer, pp 1–10.

23. Baskar R, Dai J, Wenlong N, et al.: Biological response of cancer cells to radiation treatment, *Front Mol Biosci* 1:24, 2014.

24. Lasnitzki I: A quantitative analysis of the direct and indirect action of X radiation on malignant cells, *Br J Radiol* 20:240–247, 1947.

25. Ward JF: Radiation-induced strand breakage in DNA, *Basic Life Sci* 5B:471–472, 1975.

26. Carrano AV: Chromosome aberrations and radiation-induced cell death. I. Transmission and survival parameters of aberrations, *Mutat Res* 17:341–353, 1973.

27. Willers H, Dahm-Daphi J, Powell SN: Repair of radiation damage to DNA, *Br J Cancer* 90:1297–1301, 2004.

28. Santivasi WL, Xia F: Ionizing radiation-induced DNA damage, response, and repair, *Antioxid Redox Signal* 21:251–259, 2014.

29. Elkind MM, Sutton H: X-ray damage and recovery in mammalian cells in culture, *Nature* 184:1293–1295, 1959.

30. Elkind MM, Sutton H: Radiation response of mammalian cells grown in culture. 1. Repair of X-ray damage in surviving Chinese hamster cells, *Radiat Res* 13:556–593, 1960.

31. Pawlik TM, Keyomarsi K: Role of cell cycle in mediating sensitivity to radiotherapy, *Int J Radiat Oncol Biol Phys* 59:928–942, 2004.

32. Lange SS, Takata K, Wood RD: DNA polymerases and cancer, *Nat Rev Cancer* 11:96–110, 2011.

33. Withers HR, Thames HD: Dose fractionation and volume effects in normal tissues and tumors, *Am J Clin Oncol* 11:313–329, 1988.

34. Terasima T, Tolmach LJ: Changes in x-ray sensitivity of HeLa cells during the division cycle, *Nature* 190:1210–1211, 1961.

35. Thomlinson RH, Gray LH: The histological structure of some human lung cancers and the possible implications for radiotherapy, *Br J Cancer* 9:539–549, 1955.

36. Vaupel P, Mayer A: Tumor hypoxia: causative mechanisms, microregional heterogeneities, and the role of tissue-based hypoxia markers, *Adv Exp Med Biol* 923:77–86, 2016.

37. Vaupel P: Tumor microenvironmental physiology and its implications for radiation oncology, *Semin Radiat Oncol* 14:198–206, 2004.

38. Hall EJ, Giacca AJ: Linear Energy transfer and relative biologica effectiveness. In Hall EJ, Giacca AJ, editors: *Radiobiology for the radiologist*, ed 8, Philadelphia, 2019, Wolters Kluwer, pp 101–110.

39. Anonymous: International Commison on Radiological Protection: Relative biological effectiveness (RBE), quality factor (Q), and radiation weighting factor (Wr). In *Anonymous. ICRP ed 60*, Oxford, 2004, Elsevier Science.

40. Paganetti H: Relative biological effectiveness (RBE) values for proton beam therapy. Variations as a function of biological endpoint, dose, and linear energy transfer, *Phys Med Biol* 59:R419–R472, 2014.

41. Tessonnier T, Mairani A, Brons S, et al.: Experimental dosimetric comparison of (1)H, (4)He, (12)C and (16)O scanned ion beams, *Phys Med Biol* 62:3958–3982, 2017.

42. Tommasino F: Durante M: Proton radiobiology, *Cancers (Basel)* 7:353–381, 2015.

43. Hendry JH: Survival of cells in mammalian tissues after low doses of irradiation: a short review, *Int J Radiat Biol Relat Stud Phys Chem Med* 53:89–94, 1988.

44. West CM, Hendry JH: Intrinsic radiosensitivity as a predictor of patient response to radiotherapy, *BJR Suppl* 24:146–152, 1992.

45. Hendry JH, West CM: Apoptosis and mitotic cell death: their relative contributions to normal-tissue and tumour radiation response, *Int J Radiat Biol* 71:709–719, 1997.

46. Song CW, Levitt SH: Vascular changes in Walker 256 carcinoma of rats following X irradiation, *Radiology* 100:397–407, 1971.

47. Song CW, Kim MS, Cho LC, et al.: Radiobiological basis of SBRT and SRS, *Int J Clin Oncol* 19:570–578, 2014.

48. Paris F, Fuks Z, Kang A, et al.: Endothelial apoptosis as the primary lesion initiating intestinal radiation damage in mice, *Science* 293:293–297, 2001.

49. Garcia-Barros M, Paris F, Cordon-Cardo C, et al.: Tumor response to radiotherapy regulated by endothelial cell apoptosis, *Science* 300:1155–1159, 2003.

50. Marin A, Martin M, Linan O, et al.: Bystander effects and radiotherapy, *Rep Pract Oncol Radiother* 20:12–21, 2015.

51. Verheij M: Clinical biomarkers and imaging for radiotherapy-induced cell death, *Cancer Metastasis Rev* 27:471–480, 2008.

52. Hewitt HB, Blake E, Proter EH: The effect of lethally irradiated cells on the transplantability of murine tumours, *Br J Cancer* 28:123–135, 1973.

53. Hill RP, Milas L: The proportion of stem cells in murine tumors, *Int J Radiat Oncol Biol Phys* 16:513–518, 1989.

54. Jaggupilli A, Elkord E: Significance of CD44 and CD24 as cancer stem cell markers: an enduring ambiguity, *Clin Dev Immunol* 2012:708036, 2012.

55. Gerweck LE, Wakimoto H: At the crossroads of cancer stem cells, radiation biology, and radiation oncology, *Cancer Res* 76:994–998, 2016.

56. Horiot JC, Le FR, N'Guyen T, et al.: Hyperfractionated compared with conventional radiotherapy in oropharyngeal carcinoma: an EORTC randomized trial, *Eur J Cancer* 26:779–780, 1990.

57. Horiot JC, Bontemps P, Van Den Bogaert W, et al.: Accelerated fractionation (AF) compared to conventional fractionation (CF) improves loco-regional control in the radiotherapy of advanced head and neck cancers: results of the EORTC 22851 randomized trial, *Radiother Oncol* 44:111–121, 1997.

58. Thames HD, Hendry JH: Response of tissues to fractionated irradiation: effect of repair. In *Anonymous. Fractionation in radiotherapy*, Philadelphia, 1987, Taylor and Francis, pp 53–99.

59. Vaupel P, Mayer A: Tumor oxygenation status: facts and fallacies, *Adv Exp Med Biol* 977:91–99, 2017.

60. Rockwell S, Moulder JE: Hypoxic fractions of human tumors xenografted into mice: a review, *Int J Radiat Oncol Biol Phys* 19:197–202, 1990.

61. Rockwell S, Moulder JE, Martin DF: Tumor-to-tumor variability in the hypoxic fractions of experimental rodent tumors, *Radiother Oncol* 2:57–64, 1984.

62. Withers HR, Taylor JM, Maciejewski B: The hazard of accelerated tumor clonogen repopulation during radiotherapy, *Acta Oncol* 27:131–146, 1988.

63. Barendsen GW, Roelse H, Hermens AF, et al.: Clonogenic capacity of proliferating and nonproliferating cells of a transplantable rat rhabdomyosarcoma in relation to its radiosensitivity, *J Natl Cancer Inst* 51:1521–1526, 1973.

64. Hall EJ, Giaccia AJ: Time, dose, and fractionation in radiotherapy. In Hall EJ, Giaccia AJ, editors: *Radiobiology for the radiologist*, ed 8, Philadelphia, 2019, Wolters Kluwer, pp 417–436.

65. Fowler JF: Fractionated radiation therapy after strandqvist, *Acta Radiol Oncol* 23:209–216, 1984.

66. Dische S, Saunders MI: The CHART regimen and morbidity, *Acta Oncol* 38:147–152, 1999.

67. Amdur RJ, Parsons JT, Fitzgerald LT, et al.: The effect of overall treatment time on local control in patients with adenocarcinoma of the prostate treated with radiation therapy, *Int J Radiat Oncol Biol Phys* 19:1377–1382, 1990.

68. Amdur RJ, Parsons JT, Mendenhall WM, et al.: Split-course versus continuous-course irradiation in the postoperative setting for squamous cell carcinoma of the head and neck, *Int J Radiat Oncol Biol Phys* 17:279–285, 1989.

69. Trotti A: Toxicity in head and neck cancer: a review of trends and issues, *Int J Radiat Oncol Biol Phys* 47:1–12, 2000.

70. Carsten RE, Hellyer PW, Bachand AM, et al.: Correlations between acute radiation scores and pain scores in canine radiation patients with cancer of the forelimb, *Vet Anaesth Analg* 35:355–362, 2008.

71. Keime-Guibert F, Napolitano M, Delattre JY: Neurological complications of radiotherapy and chemotherapy, *J Neurol* 245:695–708, 1998.

72. Freeman JE, Johnston PG, Voke JM: Somnolence after prophylactic cranial irradiation in children with acute lymphoblastic leukaemia, *Br Med J* 4:523–525, 1973.

73. Stewart FA, Dorr W: Milestones in normal tissue radiation biology over the past 50 years: from clonogenic cell survival to cytokine networks and back to stem cell recovery, *Int J Radiat Biol* 85:574–586, 2009.

74. Dancea HC, Shareef MM, Ahmed MM: Role of radiation-induced TGF-beta signaling in cancer therapy, *Mol Cell Pharmacol* 1:44–56, 2009.

75. Anderson CR, McNiel EA, Gillette EL, et al.: Late complications of pelvic irradiation in 16 dogs, *Vet Radiol Ultrasound* 43:187–192, 2002.

76. Hendee WR: Estimation of radiation risks. BEIR V and its significance for medicine, *JAMA* 268:620–624, 1992.

77. Kamran SC, Berrington de GA, Ng A, et al.: Therapeutic radiation and the potential risk of second malignancies, *Cancer* 122:1809–1821, 2016.

78. Hall EJ, Wuu CS: Radiation-induced second cancers: the impact of 3D-CRT and IMRT, *Int J Radiat Oncol Biol Phys* 56:83–88, 2003.

79. Hosoya K, Poulson JM, Azuma C: Osteoradionecrosis and radiation induced bone tumors following orthovoltage radiation therapy in dogs, *Vet Radiol Ultrasound* 49:189–195, 2008.

80. Gillette SM, Gillette EL, Powers BE, et al.: Radiation-induced osteosarcoma in dogs after external beam or intraoperative radiation therapy, *Cancer Res* 50:54–57, 1990.

81. Evans SM, LaCreta F, Helfand S, et al.: Technique, pharmacokinetics, toxicity, and efficacy of intratumoral etanidazole and radiotherapy for treatment of spontaneous feline oral squamous cell carcinoma, *Int J Radiat Oncol Biol Phys* 20:703–708, 1991.

82. Citrin DE, Mitchell JB: Altering the response to radiation: sensitizers and protectors, *Semin Oncol* 41:848–859, 2014.

83. Smith TA, Kirkpatrick DR, Smith S, et al.: Radioprotective agents to prevent cellular damage due to ionizing radiation, *J Transl Med* 15:232, 2017.

84. Salem A, Asselin MC, Reymen B, et al.: Targeting hypoxia to improve non-small cell lung cancer outcome, *J Natl Cancer Inst* 110:14–30, 2018.

85. Schuemann J, Berbeco R, Chithrani DB, et al.: Roadmap to clinical use of gold nanoparticles for radiation sensitization, *Int J Radiat Oncol Biol Phys* 94:189–205, 2016.

86. Reichert ZR, Wahl DR, Morgan MA: Translation of targeted radiation sensitizers into clinical trials, *Semin Radiat Oncol* 26:261–270, 2016.

87. Nolan MW, Kogan L, Griffin LR, et al.: Intensity-modulated and image-guided radiation therapy for treatment of genitourinary carcinomas in dogs, *J Vet Intern Med* 26:987–995, 2012.

88. Potters L, Kavanagh B, Galvin JM, et al.: American Society for Therapeutic Radiology and Oncology (ASTRO) and American College of Radiology (ACR) practice guideline for the performance of stereotactic body radiation therapy, *Int J Radiat Oncol Biol Phys* 76:326–332, 2010.

89. Timmerman R, Galvin J, Michalski J, et al.: Accreditation and quality assurance for Radiation Therapy Oncology Group: multicenter clinical trials using stereotactic body radiation therapy in lung cancer, *Acta Oncol* 45:779–786, 2006.

90. Benedict SH, Yenice KM, Followill D, et al.: Stereotactic body radiation therapy: the report of AAPM Task Group 101, *Med Phys* 37:4078–4101, 2010.

91. LaCouture TA, Xue J, Subedi G, et al.: Small bowel dose tolerance for stereotactic body radiation therapy, *Semin Radiat Oncol* 26:157–164, 2016.

92. Srivastava R, Asbell SO, LaCouture T, et al.: Low toxicity for lung tumors near the mediastinum treated with stereotactic body radiation therapy, *Pract Radiat Oncol* 3:130–137, 2013.

93. Jang WI, Kim MS, Bae SH, et al.: High-dose stereotactic body radiotherapy correlates increased local control and overall survival in patients with inoperable hepatocellular carcinoma, *Radiat Oncol* 8:250, 2013.

94. Nagata Y: Stereotactic body radiotherapy for early stage lung cancer, *Cancer Res Treat* 45:155–161, 2013.

95. Timmerman R, Paulus R, Galvin J, et al.: Stereotactic body radiation therapy for inoperable early stage lung cancer, *JAMA* 303:1070–1076, 2010.

96. Staehler M, Bader M, Schlenker B, et al.: Single fraction radiosurgery for the treatment of renal tumors, *J Urol* 193:771–775, 2015.

97. Kim YJ, Cho KH, Kim JY, et al.: Single-dose versus fractionated stereotactic radiotherapy for brain metastases, *Int J Radiat Oncol Biol Phys* 81:483–489, 2011.

98. Wormhoudt TL, Boss MK, Lunn K, et al.: Stereotactic radiation therapy for the treatment of functional pituitary adenomas associated with feline acromegaly, *J Vet Intern Med* 32:1383–1391, 2018.

99. Dolera M, Malfassi L, Bianchi C, et al.: Frameless stereotactic volumetric modulated arc radiotherapy of brachial plexus tumours in dogs: 10 cases, *Br J Radiol* 90:20160617, 2017.

100. Swift KE, McGrath S, Nolan MW, et al.: Clinical and imaging findings, treatments, and outcomes in 27 dogs with imaging diagnosed trigeminal nerve sheath tumors: a multi-center study, *Vet Radiol Ultrasound* 58:679–689, 2017.

101. Kubicek L, Vanderhart D, Wirth K, et al.: Association between computed tomographic characteristics and fractures following stereotactic radiosurgery in dogs with appendicular osteosarcoma, *Vet Radiol Ultrasound* 57:321–330, 2016.

102. Fowler JF: 21 years of biologically effective dose, *Br J Radiol* 83:554–568, 2010.

103. Fowler JF: The linear-quadratic formula and progress in fractionated radiotherapy, *Br J Radiol* 62:679–694, 1989.

104. Fowler JF: Short and long fractionated schedules in radiotherapy and a proposed improvement, *Br J Radiol* 60:777–779, 1987.

105. Fowler JF: Potential for increasing the differential response between tumors and normal tissues: can proliferation rate be used? *Int J Radiat Oncol Biol Phys* 12:641–645, 1986.

106. Bedford JS: Sublethal damage, potentially lethal damage, and chromosomal aberrations in mammalian cells exposed to ionizing radiations, *Int J Radiat Oncol Biol Phys* 21:1457–1469, 1991.

107. Bedford JS, Mitchell JB, Griggs HG, et al.: Radiation-induced cellular reproductive death and chromosome aberrations, *Radiat Res* 76:573–586, 1978.

108. Bedford JS, Cornforth MN: Relationship between the recovery from sublethal X-ray damage and the rejoining of chromosome breaks in normal human fibroblasts, *Radiat Res* 11:406–423, 1987.

109. Wilson PF, Bedford JS: Radiobiological principles. In Hoppe RT, Phillips TL, Roach III M, editors: *Leibel and Phillips textbook of radiation oncology*, ed 3, St. Louis, 2010, Elsevier, pp 3–30.

110. Fitzpatrick CL, Farese JP, Milner RJ, et al.: Intrinsic radiosensitivity and repair of sublethal radiation-induced damage in canine osteosarcoma cell lines, *Am J Vet Res* 69:1197–1202, 2008.

111. van den Aardweg GJMJ, Kilic E, de Klein N, et al.: Dose fractionation effects in primary and metastatic human uveal melanoma cell lines, *Invest Ophthalmol Vis Sci* 44:4660–4664, 2003.

112. Parfitt SL, Milner RJ, Salute ME, et al.: Radiosensitivity and capacity for radiation-induced sublethal damage repair of canine transitional cell carcinoma (TCC) cell lines, *Vet Comp Oncol* 9:232–240, 2011.

113. van Leeuwen CM, Oei AL, Crezee J, et al.: The alfa and beta of tumours: a review of parameters of the linear-quadratic model, derived from clinical radiotherapy studies, *Radiat Oncol* 13:96, 2018.

114. Buchholz J, Hagen R, Leo C, et al.: 3D conformal radiation therapy for palliative treatment of canine nasal tumors, *Vet Radiol Ultrasound* 50:679–683, 2009.

115. Bregazzi VS, LaRue SM, Powers BE, et al.: Response of feline oral squamous cell carcinoma to palliative radiation therapy, *Vet Radiol Ultrasound* 42:77–79, 2001.

116. Hillers KR, Lana SE, Fuller CR, et al.: Effects of palliative radiation therapy on nonsplenic hemangiosarcoma in dogs, *J Am Anim Hosp Assoc* 43:187–192, 2007.

117. Parshley DL, LaRue SM, Kitchell B, et al.: Abdominal irradiation as a rescue therapy for feline gastrointestinal lymphoma: a retrospective study of 11 cats (2001-2008), *J Feline Med Surg* 13:63–68, 2011.

118. Ramirez III O, Dodge RK, Page RL, et al.: Palliative radiotherapy of appendicular osteosarcoma in 95 dogs, *Vet Radiol Ultrasound* 40:517–522, 1999.

119. Einstein A: Concerning an heuristic point of view toward the emission and transformation of light, *Ann Phys* 17:132–148, 1905.

120. Barak F, Werner A, Walach N, et al.: Extensive late bone necrosis after postoperative orthovoltage irradiation of breast carcinoma. Report of a case, *Acta Radiol Oncol* 23:485–488, 1984.

121. Ling CC, Humm J, Larson S, et al.: Towards multidimensional radiotherapy (MD-CRT): biological imaging and biological conformality, *Int J Radiat Oncol Biol Phys* 47:551–560, 2000.

122. Hunley DW, Mauldin GN, Shiomitsu K, et al.: Clinical outcome in dogs with nasal tumors treated with intensity-modulated radiation therapy, *Can Vet J* 51:293–300, 2010.

123. Lawrence JA, Forrest LJ, Turek MM, et al.: Proof of principle of ocular sparing in dogs with sinonasal tumors treated with intensity-modulated radiation therapy, *Vet Radiol Ultrasound* 51:561–570, 2010.

124. Nolan MW, Custis JT, Harmon JF, et al.: Intensity-modulated radiation therapy for local control of canine urogenital carcinomas, *J Vet Intern Med* 26:987–995, 2012.

125. Mendenhall WM, Dagan R, Bryant CM, et al.: Radiation oncology for head and neck cancer: current standards and future changes, *Oral Maxillofac Surg Clin North Am* 31:31–38, 2019.

126. Thrall DE: Orthovoltage radiotherapy of acanthomatous epulides in 39 dogs, *J Am Vet Med Assoc* 184:826–829, 1984.

127. Theon AP, Rodriguez C, Griffey S, et al.: Analysis of prognostic factors and patterns of failure in dogs with periodontal tumors treated with megavoltage irradiation, *J Am Vet Med Assoc* 210:785–788, 1997.

128. McEntee MC, Page RL, Theon A, et al.: Malignant tumor formation in dogs previously irradiated for acanthomatous epulis, *Vet Radiol Ultrasound* 45:357–361, 2004.

129. Evans SM, Shofer F: Canine oral nontonsillar squamous cell carcinomas: prognostic factors for recurrence and survival following orthovoltage radiation therapy, *Vet Radiol* 29:133–137, 1988.

130. Theon AP, Rodriquez C, Madewell BR: Analysis of prognostic factors and patterns of failure in dogs with malignant oral tumors treated with megavoltage irradiation, *J Am Vet Med Assoc* 210:778–784, 1997.

131. LaDueMiller T, Price GS, Page RL, et al.: Radiotherapy of canine non-tonsillar squamous cell carcinoma, *Vet Radiol Ultrasound* 37:74–77, 1996.

132. Postorino-Reeves NC, Turrel JM, Withrow SJ: Oral squamous cell carcinoma in the cat, *J Am An Hosp Assoc* 29:1–4, 1993.

133. Ogilvie GK, Moore AS, Obradovich JE: Toxicoses and efficacy associated with administration of mitoxantrone to cats with malignant tumors, *J Am Vet Med Assoc* 202:1839–1844, 1993.

134. Hutson CA, Willauer CC, Walder EJ, et al.: Treatment of mandibular squamous cell carcinoma in cats by use of mandibulectomy and radiotherapy: seven cases (1987-1989), *J Am Vet Med Assoc* 201:777–781, 1992.

135. Fidel JL, Sellon RK, Houston RK, et al.: A nine-day accelerated radiation protocol for feline squamous cell carcinoma, *Vet Radiol Ultrasound* 48:482–485, 2007.

136. Yoshikawa H, Ehrhart EJ, Charles JB, et al.: Assessment of predictive molecular variables in feline oral squamous cell carcinoma treated with stereotactic radiation therapy, *Vet Comp Oncol* 14:39–57, 2016.

137. McChesney SL, Withrow SJ, Gillette EL, et al.: Radiotherapy of soft tissue sarcomas in dogs, *J Am Vet Med Assoc* 194:60–63, 1989.

138. Gillette SM, Dewhirst MW, Gillette EL, et al.: Response of canine soft tissue sarcomas to radiation or radiation plus hyperthermia: a randomized phase II study, *Int J Hyperthermia* 8:309–320, 1992.

139. Forrest LJ, Chun R, Adams WM, et al.: Postoperative radiotherapy for canine soft tissue sarcoma, *J Vet Intern Med* 14:578–582, 2000.

140. Todoroff RJ, Brodey RS: Oral and pharyngeal neoplasia in the dog: a retrospective survey of 361 cases, *J Am Vet Med Assoc* 175:567–571, 1979.

141. Proulx DR, Ruslander DM, Dodge RK, et al.: A retrospective analysis of 140 dogs with oral melanoma treated with external beam radiation, *Vet Radiol Ultrasound* 44:352–359, 2003.

142. Freeman KP, Hahn KA, Harris FD, et al.: Treatment of dogs with oral melanoma by hypofractionated radiation therapy and platinum-based chemotherapy (1987-1997), *J Vet Intern Med* 17:96–101, 2003.

143. Farrelly J, Denman DL, Hohenhaus AE, et al.: Hypofractionated radiation therapy of oral melanoma in five cats, *Vet Radiol Ultrasound* 45:91–93, 2004.

144. Bentzen SM, Overgaard J, Thames HD, et al.: Clinical radiobiology of malignant melanoma, *Radiother Oncol* 16:169–182, 1989.

145. Burris III HA, Hurtig J: Radiation recall with anticancer agents, *Oncologist* 15:1227–1237, 2010.

146. van der Veen J, Nuyts S: Can intensity-modulated-radiotherapy reduce toxicity in head and neck squamous cell carcinoma? *Cancers (Basel)* 9:E135, 2017.

147. Ghosh-Laskar S, Yathiraj PH, Dutta D, et al.: Prospective randomized controlled trial to compare 3-dimensional conformal radiotherapy to intensity-modulated radiotherapy in head and neck squamous cell carcinoma: Long-term results, *Head Neck* 38(Suppl 1):E1481–E1487, 2016.

148. Kuhnt T, Stang A, Wienke A, et al.: Potential risk factors for jaw osteoradionecrosis after radiotherapy for head and neck cancer, *Radiat Oncol* 11:101, 2016.

149. Siddiqui F, Patel M, Khan M, et al.: Stereotactic body radiation therapy for primary, recurrent, and metastatic tumors in the head-and-neck region, *Int J Radiat Oncol Biol Phys* 74:1047–1053, 2009.

150. Hahn KA, Knapp DW, Richardson RC, et al.: Clinical response of nasal adenocarcinoma to cisplatin chemotherapy in 11 dogs, *J Am Vet Med Assoc* 200:355–357, 1992.

151. Henry CJ, Brewer Jr WG, Tyler JW, et al.: Survival in dogs with nasal adenocarcinoma: 64 cases (1981-1995), *J Vet Intern Med* 12:436–439, 1998.

152. Holmberg DL, Fries C, Cockshutt J, et al.: Ventral rhinotomy in the dog and cat, *Vet Surg* 18:446–449, 1989.

153. Langova V, Mutsaers AJ, Phillips B, et al.: Treatment of eight dogs with nasal tumours with alternating doses of doxorubicin and carboplatin in conjunction with oral piroxicam, *Aust Vet J* 82:676–680, 2004.

154. Adams WM, Bjorling DE, McAnulty JE, et al.: Outcome of accelerated radiotherapy alone or accelerated radiotherapy followed by exenteration of the nasal cavity in dogs with intranasal neoplasia: 53 cases (1990-2002), *J Am Vet Med Assoc* 227:936–941, 2005.

155. Thrall DE, Harvey CE: Radiotherapy of malignant nasal tumors in 21 dogs, *J Am Vet Med Assoc* 183:663–666, 1983.

156. Yoon JH, Feeney DA, Jessen CR, et al.: External-beam Co-60 radiotherapy for canine nasal tumors: a comparison of survival by treatment protocol, *Res Vet Sci* 84:140–149, 2008.

157. Northrup NC, Etue SM, Ruslander DM, et al.: Retrospective study of orthovoltage radiation therapy for nasal tumors in 42 dogs, *J Vet Intern Med* 15:183–189, 2001.

158. McEntee MC, Page RL, Heidner GL, et al.: A retrospective study of 27 dogs with intranasal neoplasms treated with cobalt radiation, *Vet Radiol* 32:135–139, 1991.

159. Nadeau M, Kitchell BE, Rooks RL, et al.: Cobalt radiation with or without low-dose cisplatin for treatment of canine naso-sinus carcinomas, *Vet Radiol Ultrasound* 45:362–367, 2004.

160. Theon AP, Madewell BR, Harb MF, et al.: Megavoltage irradiation of neoplasms of the nasal and paranasal cavities in 77 dogs, *J Am Vet Med Assoc* 202:1469–1475, 1993.

161. Adams WM, Kleiter MM, Thrall DE, et al.: Prognostic significance of tumor histology and computed tomographic staging for radiation treatment response of canine nasal tumors, *Vet Radiol Ultrasound* 50:330–335, 2009.

162. Kondo Y, Matsunaga S, Mochizuki M, et al.: Prognosis of canine patients with nasal tumors according to modified clinical stages based on computed tomography: a retrospective study, *J Vet Med Sci* 70:207–212, 2008.

163. Straw RC, Withrow SJ, Gillette EL, et al.: Use of radiotherapy for the treatment of intranasal tumors in cats: six cases (1980-1985), *J Am Vet Med Assoc* 189:927–929, 1986.

164. Theon AP, Peaston AE, Madewell BR, et al.: Irradiation of nonlymphoproliferative neoplasms of the nasal cavity and paranasal sinuses in 16 cats, *J Am Vet Med Asoc* 204:78–83, 1994.

165. Bommarito DA, Kent MS, Selting KA, et al.: Reirradiation of recurrent canine nasal tumors, *Vet Radiol Ultrasound* 52:207–212, 2011.

166. Theon AP, Madewell BR, Shearn VI, et al.: Prognostic factors associated with radiotherapy of squamous cell carcinoma of the nasal plane in cats, *J Am Vet Med Assoc* 206:991–996, 1995.

167. Hammond GM, Gordon IK, Theon AP, et al.: Evaluation of strontium Sr 90 for the treatment of superficial squamous cell carcinoma of the nasal planum in cats: 49 cases (1990-2006), *J Am Vet Med Assoc* 231:736–741, 2007.

168. Delanian S, Lefaix JL: Current management for late normal tissue injury: radiation-induced fibrosis and necrosis, *Semin Radiat Oncol* 17:99–107, 2007.

169. Pinard CL, Mutsaers AJ, Mayer MN, et al.: Retrospective study and review of ocular radiation side effects following external-beam Cobalt-60 radiation therapy in 37 dogs and 12 cats, *Can Vet J* 53:1301–1307, 2012.

170. Roberts SM, Lavach JD, Severin GA, et al.: Ophthalmic complications following megavoltage irradiation of the nasal and paranasal cavities in dogs, *J Am Vet Med Assoc* 190:43–47, 1987.

171. Jeganathan VS, Wirth A, MacManus MP: Ocular risks from orbital and periorbital radiation therapy: a critical review, *Int J Radiat Oncol Biol Phys* 79:650–659, 2011.

172. Ching SV, Gillette SM, Powers BE, et al.: Radiation-induced ocular injury in the dog: a histological study, *Int J Radiat Oncol Biol Phys* 19:321–328, 1990.

173. Hall P, Granath F, Lundell M, et al.: Lenticular opacities in individuals exposed to ionizing radiation in infancy, *Radiat Res* 152:190–195, 1999.

174. Hu H, Barker A, Harcourt-Brown T, et al.: Systematic review of brain tumor treatment in dogs, *J Vet Intern Med* 29:1456–1463, 2015.

175. Gordon LE, Thacher C, Matthiesen DT, et al.: Results of craniotomy for the treatment of cerebral meningioma in 42 cats, *Vet Surg* 23:94–100, 1994.

176. Bley CR, Sumova A, Roos M, et al.: Irradiation of brain tumors in dogs with neurologic disease, *J Vet Intern Med* 6:849–854, 2005.

177. Turrel JM, Fike JR, LeCouteur RA, et al.: Radiotherapy of brain tumors in dogs, *J Am Vet Med Assoc* 184:82–86, 1984.

178. Evans SM, Dayrell-Hart B, Powlis W, et al.: Radiation therapy of canine brain masses, *J Vet Intern Med* 7:216–219, 1993.

179. Spugnini EP, Thrall DE, Price GS, et al.: Primary irradiation of canine intracranial masses, *Vet Radiol Ultrasound* 41:377–380, 2000.

180. Keyerleber MA, McEntee MC, Farrelly J, et al.: Three-dimensional conformal radiation therapy alone or in combination with surgery for treatment of canine intracranial meningiomas, *Vet Comp Oncol* 13:385–397, 2015.

181. Axlund TW, McGlasson ML, Smith AN: Surgery alone or in combination with radiation therapy for treatment of intracranial meningiomas in dogs: 31 cases (1989-2002), *J Am Vet Med Assoc* 221:1597–1600, 2002.

182. Dolera M, Malfassi L, Pavesi S, et al.: Stereotactic Volume modulated arc radiotherapy in canine meningiomas: imaging-based and clinical neurological posttreatment evaluation, *J Am Anim Hosp Assoc* 54:77–84, 2018.

183. Dolera M, Malfassi L, Bianchi C, et al.: Frameless stereotactic radiotherapy alone and combined with temozolomide for presumed canine gliomas, *Vet Comp Oncol* 16:90–101, 2018.

184. Dow SW, LeCouteur RA, Rosychuk RAW, et al.: Response of dogs with functional pituitary macroadenomas and macrocarcinomas to radiation, *J Sm Anim Pract* 31:287–294, 1990.

185. Theon AP, Feldman EC: Megavoltage irradiation of pituitary macrotumors in dogs with neurologic signs, *J Am Vet Med Assoc* 213:225–231, 1998.

186. Kent MS, Bommarito D, Feldman E, et al.: Survival, neurologic response, and prognostic factors in dogs with pituitary masses treated with radiation therapy and untreated dogs, *J Vet Intern Med* 21:1027–1033, 2007.

187. Sawada H, Mori A, Lee P, et al.: Pituitary size alteration and adverse effects of radiation therapy performed in 9 dogs with pituitary-dependent hypercortisolism, *Res Vet Sci* 118:19–26, 2018.

188. Mayer MN, Greco DS, LaRue SM: Outcomes of pituitary tumor irradiation in cats, *J Vet Intern Med* 20:1151–1154, 2006.

189. Sellon RK, Fidel J, Houston R, et al.: Linear-accelerator-based modified radiosurgical treatment of pituitary tumors in cats: 11 cases (1997-2008), *J Vet Intern Med* 23:1038–1044, 2009.

190. Hansen KS, Zwingenberger AL, Theon AP, et al.: Treatment of MRI-diagnosed trigeminal peripheral nerve sheath tumors by stereotactic radiotherapy in dogs, *J Vet Intern Med* 30:1112–1120, 2016.

191. Swift KE, LaRue SM: Outcome of 9 dogs treated with stereotactic radiation therapy for primary or metastatic vertebral osteosarcoma, *Vet Comp Oncol* 16:E152–E158, 2018.

192. Leibel SA, Sheline GE: Tolerance of the central and peripheral neverous system in therapeutic irradiation. In Lett JT, Altman KI, editors: *Advances in radiation biology*, New York, 1987, Academic Press, p 257.

193. Graeb DA, Steinbok P, Robertson WD: Transient early computed tomographic changes mimicking tumor progression after brain tumor irradiation, *Radiology* 144:813–817, 1982.

194. Brearley MJ: Hypofractionated radiation therapy of brain masses in dogs: a retrospective analyisi of survival in 83 cases (1991-1996), *J Vet Intern Med* 13:408–412, 1999.

195. Kuntz CA, Dernell WS, Powers BE, et al.: Prognostic factors for surgical treatment of soft-tissue sarcomas in dogs: 75 cases (1986-1996), *J Am Vet Med Assoc* 211:1147–1151, 1997.

196. McKnight JA, Mauldin GN, McEntee MC, et al.: Radiation treatment for incompletely resected soft-tissue sarcomas in dogs, *J Am Vet Med Assoc* 217:205–210, 2000.

197. Baker-Gabb M, Hunt GB, France MP: Soft tissue sarcomas and mast cell tumours in dogs; clinical behaviour and response to surgery, *Aust Vet J* 81:732–738, 2003.

198. McSporran KD: Histologic grade predicts recurrence for marginally excised canine subcutaneous soft tissue sarcomas, *Vet Pathol* 46:928–933, 2009.

199. Bray JP, Polton GA, McSporran KD, et al.: Canine soft tissue sarcoma managed in first opinion practice: outcome in 350 cases, *Vet Surg* 43:774–782, 2014.

200. Monteiro B, Boston S, Monteith G: Factors influencing complete tumor excision of mast cell tumors and soft tissue sarcomas: a retrospective study in 100 dogs, *Can Vet J* 52:1209–1214, 2011.

201. Cronin K, Page RL, Spodnick G, et al.: Radiation therapy and surgery for fibrosarcoma in 33 cats, *Vet Radiol Ultrasound* 39:51–56, 1998.

202. Bregazzi VS, LaRue SM, McNiel E, et al.: Treatment with a combination of doxorubicin, surgery, and radiation versus surgery and radiation alone for cats with vaccine-associated sarcomas: 25 cases (1995-2000), *J Am Vet Med Assoc* 218:547–550, 2001.

203. Cohen M, Wright JC, Brawner WR, et al.: Use of surgery and electron beam irradiation, with or without chemotherapy, for treatment of vaccine-associated sarcomas in cats: 78 cases (1996-2000), *J Am Vet Med Assoc* 219:1582–1589, 2001.

204. Mayer MN, Treuil PL, LaRue SM: Radiotherapy and surgery for feline soft tissue sarcoma, *Vet Radiol Ultrasound* 50:669–672, 2009.

205. Nolan MW, Griffin LR, Custis JT, et al.: Stereotactic body radiation therapy for treatment of injection-site sarcomas in cats: 11 cases (2008-2012), *J Am Vet Med Assoc* 243:526–531, 2013.

206. Frimberger AE, Moore AS, LaRue SM, et al.: Radiotherapy of incompletely resected, moderately differentiated mast cell tumors in the dog: 37 cases (1989-1993), *J Am Anim Hosp Assoc* 33:320–324, 1997.

207. LaDue T, Price GS, Dodge R, et al.: Radiation therapy for incompletely resected canine mast cell tumors, *J Am Anim Hosp Assoc* 39:57–62, 1998.

208. Kry KL, Boston SE: Additional local therapy with primary re-excision or radiation therapy improves survival and local control after incomplete or close surgical excision of mast cell tumors in dogs, *Vet Surg* 43:182–189, 2014.

209. Chaffin K, Thrall DE: Results of radiation therapy in 19 dogs with cutaneous mast cell tumor and regional lymph node metastasis, *Vet Radiol Ultrasound* 43:392–395, 2002.

210. Lejeune A, Skorupski K, Frazier S, et al.: Aggressive local therapy combined with systemic chemotherapy provides long-term control in grade II stage 2 canine mast cell tumour: 21 cases (1999-2012), *Vet Comp Oncol* 13:267–280, 2015.

211. LaRue SM, Withrow SJ, Powers BE, et al.: Limb-sparing treatment for osteosarcoma in dogs, *J Am Vet Med Assoc* 195:1734–1744, 1989.

212. Thrall DE, Dewhirst MW, Page RL, et al.: A comparison of temperatures in canine solid tumours during local and whole-body hyperthermia administered alone and simultaneously, *Int J Hyperthermia* 6:305–317, 1990.

213. Farese JP, Milner R, Thompson MS, et al.: Stereotactic radiosurgery for treatment of osteosarcomas involving the distal portions of the limbs in dogs, *J Am Vet Med Assoc* 225:1567–1572, 2004.

214. Dickerson ME, Page RL, LaDue TA, et al.: Retrospective analysis of axial skeleton osteosarcoma in 22 large-breed dogs, *J Vet Intern Med* 15:120–124, 2001.

215. Vakaet LA, Boterberg T: Pain control by ionizing radiation of bone metastasis, *Int J Dev Biol* 48:599–606, 2004.

216. Steenland E, Leer JW, van Houwelingen H, et al.: The effect of a single fraction compared to multiple fractions on painful bone metastases: a global analysis of the dutch bone metastasis study, *Radiother Oncol* 52:101–109, 1999.

217. Knapp-Hoch HM, Fidel JL, Sellon RK, et al.: An expedited palliative radiation protocol for lytic or proliferative lesions of appendicular bone in dogs, *J Am Anim Hosp Assoc* 45:24–32, 2009.

218. Dernell WS, Van Vechten BJ, Straw RC, et al.: Outcome following treatment of vertebral tumors in 20 dogs (1986-1995), *J Am An Hosp Assoc* 36:245–251, 2000.

219. McEntee MC, Page RL, Novotney CA, et al.: Palliative radiotherapy for canine appendicular osteosarcoma, *Vet Radiol Ultrasound* 34:367–370, 1993.

220. Wolfe TD, Pillai SP, Hildreth III BE, et al.: Effect of zoledronic acid and amputation on bone invasion and lung metastasis of canine osteosarcoma in nude mice, *Clin Exp Metastasis* 28:377–389, 2011.

221. Arrington SA, Damron TA, Mann KA, et al.: Concurrent administration of zoledronic acid and irradiation leads to improved bone density, biomechanical strength, and microarchitecture in a mouse model of tumor-induced osteolysis, *J Surg Oncol* 97:284–290, 2008.

222. Boston SE, Duerr F, Bacon N, et al.: Intraoperative radiation for limb sparing of the distal aspect of the radius without transcarpal plating in five dogs, *Vet Surg* 36:314–323, 2007.

223. Boston SE, Vinayak A, Lu X, et al.: Outcome and complications in dogs with appendicular primary bone tumors treated with stereotactic radiotherapy and concurrent surgical stabilization, *Vet Surg* 46:829–837, 2017.

224. Fertil B, Malaise E: Intrinsic radiosensitivity of human cell lines is correlated with radioresponsiveness of human tumors: analysis of 101 published survival curves, *Int J Radiol Oncol Biol Phys* 11:1699–1707, 1985.

225. Bump EA, Braunhut SJ, Palayoor ST, et al.: Novel concepts in modification of radiation sensitivity, *Int J Radiol Oncol Biol Phys* 29:249–253, 1994.

226. Vose JM: Current approaches to the management of non-Hodgkin's lymphoma, *Semin Oncol* 25:483–491, 1998.

227. Yahalom J: Radiation therapy in the treatment of lymphoma, *Curr Opin Oncol* 11:370–374, 1999.

228. Fidias P, Spiro I, Sobczak ML, et al.: Long-term results of combined modality therapy in primary bone lymphomas, *Int J Radiat Oncol Biol Phys* 45:1213–1218, 1999.

229. Giger U, Evans SM, Hendrick MJ, et al.: Orthovoltage radiotherapy of primary lymphoma of bone in a dog, *J Am Vet Med Assoc* 195:627–630, 1989.

230. Kirova YM, Piedbois Y, Haddad E, et al.: Radiotherapy in the management of mycosis fungoides: indications, results, prognosis. Twenty years experience, *Radiother Oncol* 51:147–151, 1999.

231. Kirova YM, Piedbois Y, Le Bourgeois JP: Radiotherapy in the management of cutaneous B-cell lymphoma. Our experience in 25 cases, *Radiother Oncol* 52:15–18, 1999.

232. Elmslie RE, Ogilvie GK, Gillette EL, et al.: Radiotherapy with and without chemotherapy for localized lymphoma in 10 cats, *Vet Radiol* 32:277–280, 1991.

233. Meleo KA: The role of radiotherapy in the treatment of lymphoma and thymoma, *Vet Clin North Am Sm Anim Pract* 27:115–129, 1997.

234. Gustafson NR, Lana SE, Mayer MN, et al.: A preliminary assessment of whole-body radiotherapy interposed within a chemotherapy protocol for canine lymphoma, *Vet Comp Oncol* 2:125–131, 2004.

235. Williams LE, Johnson JL, Hauck ML, et al.: Chemotherapy followed by half-body radiation therapy for canine lymphoma, *J Vet Intern Med* 18:703–709, 2004.

236. Escobar C, Grindem C, Neel JA, et al.: Hematologic changes after total body irradiation and autologous transplantation of hematopoietic peripheral blood progenitor cells in dogs with lymphoma, *Vet Pathol* 49:341–343, 2012.

237. Warry EE, Willcox JL, Suter SE: Autologous peripheral blood hematopoietic cell transplantation in dogs with T-cell lymphoma, *J Vet Intern Med* 28:529–537, 2014.

238. Willcox JL, Pruitt A, Suter SE: Autologous peripheral blood hematopoietic cell transplantation in dogs with B-cell lymphoma, *J Vet Intern Med* 26:1155–1163, 2012.

239. Pack L, Roberts RE, Dawson SD, et al.: Definitive radiation therapy for infiltrative thyroid carcinoma in dogs, *Vet Radiol Ultrasound* 42:471–474, 2001.

240. Ohara K, Tatsuzaki H, Fuji H, et al.: Radioresponse of thymomas verified with histologic response, *Acta Oncol* 37:471–474, 1998.

241. Smith AN, Wright JC, Brawner Jr WR, et al.: Radiation therapy in the treatment of canine and feline thymomas: a retrospective study (1985-1999), *J Am Anim Hosp Assoc* 37:489–496, 2001.

242. Meier V, Besserer J, Roos M, et al.: A complication probability study for a definitive-intent, moderately hypofractionated image-guided intensity-modulated radiotherapy protocol for anal sac adenocarcinoma in dogs, *Vet Comp Oncol* 218; epub ahead of print. DOI: 10.1111/vco.12441

243. Fuccio L, Guido A, Laterza L, et al.: Randomised clinical trial: preventive treatment with topical rectal beclomethasone dipropionate reduces post-radiation risk of bleeding in patients irradiated for prostate cancer, *Aliment Pharmacol Ther* 34:628–637, 2011.

244. Magestro LM, Gieger TL, Nolan MW: Stereotactic body radiation therapy for heart-base tumors in six dogs, *J Vet Cardiol* 20:186–197, 2018.

14

Cancer Immunotherapy

STEVEN DOW AND AMANDA GUTH

The main role of the immune system is recognition of "foreign" proteins. In the case of cancer, this role includes immune recognition of mutated or altered forms of self-proteins that arise during tumorigenesis (commonly referred to as "tumor antigens" [TAs]). However, it is now apparent that powerful regulatory cells and expression of certain molecules whose main functions are to prevent rampant, uncontrolled immune responses can also serve to block natural development of effective antitumor immune response. Therefore immunotherapy approaches in treatment of various cancers must take into account the ability to overcome these negative regulators of tumor immunity to be successful.

Under appropriate conditions, the immune system is capable of controlling cancer. For example, it is well established that the incidence of virally induced cancers is increased in immunosuppressed individuals. Further, cancer incidence increases in aged individuals and correlates with the progression of immunesenescence (aging and exhaustion of the immune response) that is thought to reduce immunosurveillance of cancer, a topic discussed in the text that follows. Moreover, in some cases, spontaneous remission of tumors is observed without any therapeutic intervention, most likely attributed to a successful immune response. Biologically, tumor-specific T cells are observed in the tumor tissue and tumor-draining lymph nodes, providing evidence that these cells have encountered and recognized the tumor cells as foreign. Finally, in some cases, paraneoplastic autoimmunity develops, suggesting that the antitumor immune response has somehow gone unchecked by regulatory cells.

Recently the field of immunotherapy took an exciting twist with the development in human medicine of therapeutic antibodies designed to target immune suppressive molecules (checkpoint molecules) and/or their ligands expressed on T cells and antigen-presenting cells, such as programmed death molecule-1 (PD-1) and cytotoxic T-lymphocyte antigen-4 (CTLA-4). By using antibodies to block negative signaling by certain checkpoint molecules such as PD-1 and CTLA-4, remarkable, and durable, antitumor responses have been observed in a significant, but minority, subset of patients with advanced tumors such as melanoma, renal cell carcinoma, and non–small cell lung cancer.[1–5] The development of checkpoint targeted immunotherapies has reignited the field of immunotherapy for cancer, and similar antibodies for treatment of cancer in dogs are under development by several different groups, including ours.

Improving knowledge of the immune system and how it is regulated will increase our ability to design better immunotherapies. In addition, immunotherapy has the potential to work in conjunction with chemotherapies, radiation therapy, and surgery. This chapter will first discuss the role of the immune system in regulating tumor development, then the various classes of immunotherapies both currently in use and those under investigation. The biological basis for the therapies, their use in human and companion animals, and their successes and limitations will be discussed.

Immune System Control of Tumor Development and Growth

Immune Surveillance of Cancer

Forty years ago, Thomas and Burnet, while studying how lymphocytes could respond to newly formed antigens on transformed cells, put forth the concept that the immune system could actively respond to and eliminate neoplastic cells, an idea known as immune surveillance.[6] In contrast, later studies showed that genetically manipulated immunodeficient (athymic) mice did not demonstrate an increased incidence of spontaneously or carcinogen-induced cancer.[7,8] Such observations led to the immune surveillance concept falling out of favor.

Since the development of more sensitive and sophisticated technologies, many of the ideas behind the concept of the immune surveillance hypothesis are now again accepted, and currently, this modification of the original hypothesis is referred to as the immunoediting hypothesis,[9] which consists of three phases: (1) "elimination"—removal of the immunogenic tumor cells by the immune system; however, less immunogenic cells can survive; (2) "equilibrium"—tumor growth and immune destruction are equal; and (3) "escape"—tumor growth ensues due to decreased immunogenicity, immune suppression, and rapid tumor cell growth.[9] However, despite recent data, a controversy still remains around the immune surveillance hypothesis, discussed in a review by Schreiber et al.[9]

Mechanisms of Immune Evasion by Tumors

Given the fact that cancer can develop in immunocompetent individuals, clearly tumor cells are able to avoid recognition by the immune system.[10] This is accomplished by various mechanisms discussed in the text that follows, which involve both changes in the tumor cells themselves and ways in which the tumor and the tumor stromal environment can manipulate the immune system and prevent antitumor immunity. These mechanisms of immune evasion pose a significant challenge to the development of effective immunotherapies. Fig. 14.1 demonstrates some of these key mechanisms.

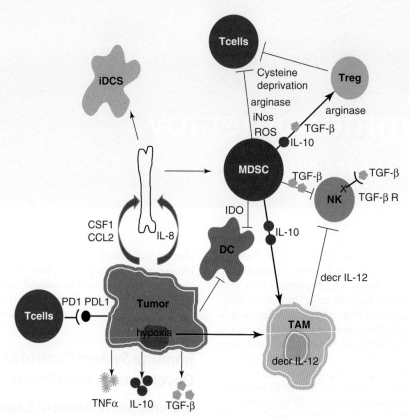

• **Fig. 14.1** Mechanisms of tumor cell evasion via hijacking the immune system. *DC,* Dendritic cell; *iDC,* immature dendritic cell; *MDSC,* myeloid-derived suppressor cell; *TAM,* tumor-associated macrophage; *Treg,* regulatory T-cell.

Failure of Tumor Cells to Activate the Immune System

One of the most exciting achievements in human cancer therapy and immunotherapy has been development of monoclonal antibodies (mAbs) that either block or activate signaling through so-called checkpoint molecules.[11–14] Checkpoint molecules are expressed primarily by T cells, and are divided into two classes, including those that negatively regulate T cells (coinhibitory checkpoint molecules) and those that stimulate T cells (costimulatory checkpoint molecules). At present, there are at least 16 identified checkpoint molecules, which include eight coinhibitory receptors (PD-1, CTLA-4, TIM-3, VISTA, BTLA, B7-H3, B7-H4, and LAG3) and eight costimulatory receptors (CD28, OX40, GITR, ICOS, CD137, CD27, CD40L, and CD122).[15] All of these molecules are potential targets for tumor immunotherapy using antibodies that either activate (costimulatory checkpoint molecules) or inhibit (coinhibitory molecules) signaling. These checkpoint molecules have been evaluated as targets for tumor immunotherapy in rodent models, and most have also been evaluated in human clinical trials.[1–5] At present, PD-1 (and its ligand PD-L1) and CTLA-4 antibodies have been approved for treatment of cancer in humans. Of the costimulatory checkpoint molecule targeted therapeutics, antibodies targeting OX40 and GITR are the most promising and furthest advanced in human trials.[16–18]

In particular, the PD-1/PD-L1 axis has been targeted to reverse immunosuppression in cancer.[11,12,19,20] PD-1 and CTLA-4 are expressed primarily on T cells and NK cells, whereas PD-L1 is expressed by myeloid cells (monocytes, macrophages, and dendritic cells) and by certain tumor cells.[21–23] We and others have reported recently that some tumors in dogs express PD-L1, and we have also shown that macrophages in dogs express PD-L1.[24]

We also demonstrated that PD-L1 is regulated by T cell cytokines in dogs.[24] Several new monoclonal antibody therapeutics targeting checkpoint molecules have been approved, including Yervoy (Ipilimumab) targeting CTLA-4 and Keytruda (pembrolizumab) and Opdivo (nivolumab) targeting PD-1, for treatment of four different cancers (melanoma, head and neck cancer, bladder cancer, and Hodgkin lymphoma). In addition, pembrolizumab has recently received expanded approval for treatment of any cancer with high levels of microsatellite instability, which is associated with generation of neoantigens recognized by tumor-infiltrating T cells. An antibody therapeutic targeting PD-L1 (Tecentriq, atezolizumab) was also recently approved in humans. Responses in patients with advanced, heavily pretreated tumors to checkpoint targeted therapies are reported in approximately 20% of patients, and many of these responses are durable and in some cases complete.[25]

Currently, similar therapies are not yet available for veterinary patients. Due to target–antigen specificity, the Food and Drug Administration (FDA)-approved antibodies do not cross-react with canine antigens and the constant domain portion of the antibodies is specific for humans (aka humanized antibodies). However, there is growing interest in developing similar antibodies in a canonized form for use in veterinary medicine. For example, we reported recently the target specificity and functional properties of canine specific PD-1 targeted antibodies.[26] In addition, a clinical trial evaluating a canine version of this antibody is currently in progress in dogs with cancer. Results of the first trial of a canine chimeric antibody targeting canine PD-L1 were also reported recently.[27] Development of checkpoint molecule targeted therapies for dogs is likely to continue rapidly and to eventually exert a tremendous effect on veterinary oncology.

Tumors also can express other immune suppressive molecules that work in modulating the tumor microenvironment. An example would be CD73, an ecto-5′-nucleotidase that catalyzes the breakdown of AMP to the adenosine. When expressed on tumors, this creates a local microenvironment rich in adenosine, which is immunosuppressive.[28] Indoleamine deoxygenase is another highly immune suppressive molecule expressed locally by tumors and tumor-infiltrating myeloid cells.[29,30]

Lastly, tumor cells are also capable of avoiding immune elimination by failing to be recognized by the immune system in the first place. For example, some tumor cells can down-modulate major histocompatibility complex (MHC) surface expression to escape recognition by T cells. MHC Class I expression can be lost on tumor cells due to changes in protein synthesis, structure, or allelic loss.[31,32] Moreover, defects in antigen processing and presentation can occur that can also lead to decreased MHC expression.[31,32] A decrease in MHC class II expression is also observed in certain human hematopoietic cancers, although it should be noted that most tumors are normally MHC class II negative.[33,34] Reduced expression of MHC class II has been recently correlated with poor outcome in dogs with B cell lymphoma.[35] Thus tumor cells themselves can actively and directly suppress antitumor T cell responses through such mechanisms as decreased expression of MHC molecules and increased expression of inhibitory molecules.

Active Immune Suppression by Myeloid-Derived Suppressor Cells

A population of cells in the tumor microenvironment that plays a major role in tumor immunosuppression is myeloid-derived suppressor cells (MDSCs). These cells consist of immature monocytes and granulocytes released from the bone marrow into the blood in response to sustained inflammation, including cancer.[36-44] Sometimes included in the functional description of this group of cells are tumor-associated macrophages (TAMs), which have the same ability, and use similar mechanisms as MDSCs, to induce potent tumor immunosuppression.[45,46] Numerous studies demonstrate increased numbers of MDSCs in humans with cancer[47-49] and in mouse cancer models.[40,50] Furthermore, it has been shown that the presence of these cells correlates with clinical disease stage and metastatic tumor burden in humans with solid tumors.[48] MDSCs are released from the bone marrow in response to cytokines released in inflammation, including granulocyte-macrophage colony stimulating factor (GM-CSF) and interleukin-3 (IL-3).[51] MDSCs can be recruited to the tumor microenvironment by multiple chemokines, many of which are produced by the tumor during times of hypoxia and are regulated by hypoxia-inducible factor 1α (HIF-1α) production.[45,52-60] Once within the tumor microenvironment (TME), MDSCs differentiate into macrophages or neutrophils and actively suppress the local antitumor immune responses and promote tumor invasion and metastasis via the production of matrix metalloproteinases (MMPs).[43,61] Moreover, TAMs stimulate tumor angiogenesis and promote metastasis.[45] Of note, there is still no clear consensus on how to identify MDSC in humans, mice, or dogs, thus making it more difficult to clearly define the role that MDSCs play in cancer.

The ability of MDSCs to suppress the antitumor response is the subject of many recent studies.[42,62,63] Numerous mechanisms of suppression have been reported and MDSCs have the ability to suppress not only T cells, but also natural killer (NK) cells and DCs. They are also able to potentiate T regulatory cells (Tregs, discussed in the text that follows) and differentiate into TAMs in the tumor (see Fig. 14.1). Current known mechanisms of immune

suppression by MDSCs include suppression of T cells through production of inducible nitric oxide species (iNOS), reactive oxygen species (ROS), arginase, and cysteine deprivation.[42] MDSCs can produce transforming growth factor-beta(TGF-β) and IL-10, which stimulate Tregs and TAMs, and MDSC can cause downregulation of the IL-12 production by TAMs, a cytokine involved in T-cell activation.[62] MDSCs cause NK cell anergy (lack of function) also by this decreased IL-12 production and through membrane-bound TGF-β.[62,63] Thus given the ability of these cells to use multiple pathways to induce tumor immunosuppression, the development of effective immunotherapies that can target these cells and either eliminate them or lead to their maturation, rather than ones that target specific pathways of suppression, is critical for that therapy's success.

Induction of Regulatory T Cells by Tumors

Numbers of regulatory T cells (Tregs) are expanded in cancer patients, in tumor tissues, tumor-draining lymph nodes, bone marrow, and blood.[64-66] These cells are phenotypically defined by surface expression of CD4 and CD25 but are most specifically identified by the intracellular transcription factor, forkhead box P3 (FoxP3).[67,68] Other surface markers used to identify Tregs include CTLA-4, GITR, Lag3, and folate receptor 4 (FR-4).[69-72] Tregs are capable of directly suppressing tumor-specific CD4+ and CD8+ T cells and NK cells and are enriched in the tumor microenvironment by conversion of CD4 T cells to Tregs by locally produced factors such as IL-6 and TGF-β.[73-76] Proliferation of tumor-specific Tregs occurs after antigen recognition, or recruitment of these cells via chemokine signaling (i.e., CCR5).[77] Recent work has also suggested a role for the chemokine CCL-1 in specifically converting T cells to Tregs and inducing their suppressive nature.[78]

Many studies demonstrate that increased numbers of Treg cells are correlated with a poor prognosis.[64,79-81] In addition, Tregs present in metastatic lymph nodes inhibit the ability of tumor-infiltrating lymphocytes to mount an effective antitumor response.[82] Work in the author's laboratory demonstrated that canine Treg cells can also be identified via the expression of CD4 and foxp3.[83] Moreover, they reported previously that cancer-bearing dogs had increased numbers of Tregs compared with healthy dogs and that this difference was greater in certain types of canine cancer.[65,83] Therefore current therapies aimed at depleting Treg cells in humans could be applied to veterinary medicine. In particular, many studies have shown that the use of cyclophosphamide or anti-Treg-specific antibodies decreases the numbers of Tregs present in tumors and in circulation of tumor-bearing patients.[84-88] In addition, it was shown that the tyrosine kinase inhibitor drug toceranib (Palladia) can deplete canine Tregs both in vitro and in vivo.[89]

Impaired Dendritic Cell Activation and Function

Another important mechanism of tumor suppression is through impairment of the potent antigen-presenting cells, dendritic cells (DCs). Numerous studies have denoted that overall numbers of DCs are decreased in various human cancers studied, including head and neck squamous cell carcinoma (HNSCC),[90] breast and prostate cancer, and malignant glioma.[91] A recent study showed that indoleamine 1 (IDO1), expression in the tumor microenvironment led to increased DC apoptosis.[28] The aforementioned tumor studies demonstrated fewer circulating myeloid DCs with a concurrent increase in immature DCs (iDCs) with reduced ability to present antigen and stimulate T cells; thus they induce

T-cell tolerance rather than activate T cells.[91–93] The DCs present in the tumor tend to be immature and dysfunctional. Studies of DCs in numerous human cancers demonstrate minimal activation, decreased ability to stimulate in an alloreactive fashion, and decreased expression of costimulatory molecules.[90,91,94–99] A similar study done in dogs with canine transmissible venereal tumors (CTVTs) showed that the tumor environment caused downregulation of DC surface markers of activation and MHC, and decreased endocytic capabilities and decreased allogenic mixed lymphocyte reaction (MLR) responses.[56] Possible mechanisms causing the DC dysfunction include the overexpression of the protein S100A9,[100] accumulation of triglycerides in the DCs which leads to decreased capacity to present antigen,[101] and downregulation of toll-like receptor (TLR)-9 expression.[102] Moreover, factors such as IL-10 and vascular endothelial growth factor (VEGF) can negatively affect DC function and maturation.[103,104] Lastly, some DCs in the tumor are considered to be regulatory based on low expression of surface markers MHC II, CD86, and CD11c with high expression of costimulatory molecules CD80, CD40, CD106, and CD11b. These cells secrete regulatory factors such as IL-10 and nitric oxide (NO) and inhibit proliferation of naïve CD4+ T cells to antigen presented by mature, functional DCs.[105] Overall, the microenvironment of the tumor leads to attraction of immature and regulatory DCs that, due to their decreased activation and function, can potently inhibit the development of antitumor T cell responses even when copious amounts of antigen are present.

Production of Immunosuppressive Cytokines

In addition to the suppressive milieu established by tumor-infiltrating cells, tumor cells themselves are capable of producing immunosuppressive cytokines.[106] A few key immunosuppressive cytokines produced by tumor cells are IL-10, VEGF, and TGF-β.[106,107] These cytokines act to suppress antitumor T cell responses and inhibit DC function. IL-10 promotes Treg production and function[108] and, in an autocrine and/or paracrine fashion, may potentially affect tumor cell proliferation and survival.[109] In human cancer patients, increased levels of serum IL-10 are observed in patients with either pancreatic carcinoma or non-Hodgkin lymphoma (NHL).[110,111] In addition, elevated levels of IL-10 in diffuse large B-cell lymphoma of humans correlate with a poor prognosis.[112] TGF-β acts similarly to IL-10 in that it is a potent immunosuppressive cytokine that can potentiate Treg proliferation and function.[74,113–115] It can also enhance tumor progression; carcinomas can produce excess TGF-β, which in turn increases the epithelial-to-mesenchymal transition, tumor invasion, and metastasis and inhibits tumor-specific CD8+ T cells.[115] Moreover, tumor-produced tumor necrosis factor-alpha (TNF-α) leads to promotion of tumor cell survival via induction of antiapoptotic proteins.[116] Finally, TNF-α has been shown to promote tumor angiogenesis and metastasis and hamper cytotoxic T-cell and macrophage responses.[117]

One study in veterinary medicine examined a lymph node of a dog with metastatic melanoma. This study revealed an overexpression of IL-10 and TGF-β concurrent with a lack of expression of IL-2, IL-4, or interferon-gamma (IFN-γ) cytokines typically associated with antitumor immunity, thus demonstrating that tumor immunosuppression occurs in veterinary patients as well.[118] For a review of cytokines relevant to tumor immunotherapy, see Table 14.1.

TABLE 14.1	Biological Activities of Key Cytokines Relevant to Tumor Immunotherapy
Cytokine	Major Activity
IL-2	Growth factor for T cells, including regulatory T cells; induces proliferation and differentiation of T cells to effector T cells; enhances CTL and NK cell cytotoxicity, production of LAK cells, induces B-cell proliferation. Approved for use clinically by the FDA.
IL-3	Multicolony-stimulating factor, promotes production/differentiation and proliferation of macrophages, monocytes, granulocytes, and dendritic cells; secreted by activated T cells and supports growth and differentiation of T cells.
IL-4	Key Th2 cytokine; induces differentiation of naïve CD4 T cells toward Th2 phenotype, inhibits macrophage activation, induces B cell growth and differentiation, stimulates isotype switching and IgG and IgE production. Up-regulates MHC Class II production.
IL-6	Supports B-cell proliferation and differentiation to plasma cells; proinflammatory, antiapoptotic cytokine that may contribute to tumor development associated with chronic inflammation. Causes upregulation of PD-1 on monocytes that are triggered to produce IL-10 after ligation of this receptor.
IL-8	Chemotactic/activation factor for neutrophils and T cells; induces matrix metalloproteinase-2 activity; plays a role in inflammation and tumor metastasis.
IL-10	Immunosuppressive cytokine produced by activated DCs, macrophages, and T cells; induces regulatory T cell function; also overexpressed by some tumors and tumor-associated leukocytes.
IL-11	Stimulates proliferation of hematopoietic stem cells; induces megakaryocyte maturation resulting in increased platelet production.
IL-12	Key Th1 cytokine produced by DCs, macrophages; stimulates synthesis of IFN-γ and TNF-α by T cells and NKs, thus decreasing angiogenesis, enhances cytotoxicity of CTLs and NK cells, stimulates differentiation of naïve CD4+ T cells to T cells with the Th1 phenotype.
IL-13	Th2 promoting cytokine, produced by NKT cells; inhibits inflammatory cytokine production by macrophages; possible inhibitory role in tumor immunosurveillance.
IL-15	T cell growth factor; supports survival of memory CD8+ T cells; promotes NK cell activation and survival and triggers cytotoxic activity.
IL-17	Induces proinflammatory response. Role in cancer is currently controversial—depending on context, may either promote or inhibit tumor growth.
IL-19	Promotes T-cell differentiation toward the Th2 phenotype.
IL-21	Member of IL-2 cytokine family; enhances cytotoxicity and proliferation of CTL and NK cells.

TABLE 14.1	Biological Activities of Key Cytokines Relevant to Tumor Immunotherapy—cont'd
Cytokine	**Major Activity**
IL-23	Member of IL-12 cytokine family; upregulates the production of MMP9 in tumors; increases angiogenesis while reducing CD8 TILs. Stimulates CD4+ T cells to become Th17 cells.
GM-CSF	Promotes growth and differentiation of pleuripotent progenitor cells; stimulates growth of cells of the granulocyte, macrophage, and eosinophil lineage.
CSF-1	Promotes differentiation of stem cells into monocytes and macrophages.
G-CSF	Stimulates bone marrow to produce granulocytes and stem cells. Stimulates neutrophil survival, function, and maturation.
IFN-α, β	Induce apoptosis of tumor cells; enhances CTL effector function, activates NK cells, modulates MHC Class I/II expression, inhibits tumor angiogenesis.
IFN-γ	Key Th1 cytokine produced by activated T cells and NK cells; promotes the differentiation of naïve CD4+ T cells to Th1 phenotype; activates macrophages, increases MHC Class I/II expression.
TNF-α	Produced by Th1 T cells, CTLs, activated DCs and macrophages; induces NO production by macrophages, induces tumor apoptosis; important proinflammatory cytokine.
TGF-β	Immunosuppressive cytokine; inhibits macrophage activation and B-cell growth; overexpressed by some tumors.

CSF-1, Colony-stimulating factor-1; *CTL,* cytotoxic T-lymphocyte; *DCs,* dendritic cells; *FDA,* Food and Drug Administration; *G-CSF,* granulocyte colony-stimulating factor; *GM-CSF,* granulocyte-macrophage colony stimulating factor; *IFN,* interferon; *IgE,* immunoglobulin E; *IgG,* immunoglobulin G; *IL,* interleukin; *LAK,* lymphokine-activated killer; *MHC,* major histocompatibility; *MMP,* matrix metalloproteinase; *NK,* natural killer; *NKT,* natural killer T-cell; *NO,* nitric oxide; *PD-1,* programmed death molecule-1; *TGF,* transforming growth factor; *Th1,* T-helper 1; *Th2,* T-helper 2; *TILs,* tumor-infiltrating lymphocytes; *TNF,* tumor necrosis factor.

TABLE 14.2	Ways to Manipulate MDSCs to Decrease Immunosuppression			
Depletion/Inhibit Proliferation	**Promote Maturation**	**Inhibit Recruitment**	**Block Interactions**	**Block Function**
Liposomal clodronate	Zoledronate[263]	cFMS kinase inhibitor (GW2580)[264]	Anti-CD40 Ab[265]	Nitroaspirin[266]
Gemcitabine[267]	ATRA[268]	NSAIDs[269]	Anti-PD-1/PD-L1 Ab[270]	Arginase 1 inhibitor (NOHA)[271]
5-FU[272]	Docetaxel[273]			Triterpenoid[274]
Sunitinib[275]	Sunitinib[275]			Sildenafil[276]
Docetaxel[273]	Decitabine[277]			
Cox 2 inhibitor (SC58236)[269]	Activated NKT cells[278]			
KIT-specific Ab[279]	VSSP vaccine[280]			
25-Hydroxyvitamin D3[281]				
CXCR2 antagonist (S-265610)[55]				
CXCR4 antagonist (AMD3100)[55]				
PROK2-specific Ab[282]				

Ab, Antibody; *ATRA,* all-*trans* retinoic acid; *5-FU,* 5-fluorouracil; *MDSCs,* myeloid-derived suppressor cells; *NKT,* natural killer T cells; *NSAIDs,* nonsteroidal antiinflammatory drugs; *PD-1,* programmed death molecule-1; *PD-L1,* ligand of PD-1; *VSSP,* very small size proteoliposome.

Strategies to Control Tumor Growth Through Immune Activation

Blocking Checkpoint Molecules

With the recent advancements in human immunotherapy, many companies are pursuing development of checkpoint inhibitor antibodies besides ones that block PD-1 and CTLA-4. Antibodies targeting PD-1, CTLA-4, and PD-L1 are now approved for treatment of a variety of different cancers in humans, including the broad category of all tumor cells with high levels of microsatellite instability. Currently, there are clinical trials looking at the use of antibodies targeting the other inhibitory checkpoint molecules Tim-3 and Lag-3, and studies evaluating costimulatory checkpoint molecules such as OX40, CD28, and ICOS. In addition, clinical trials evaluating PD-1 and PD-L1 antibodies in dogs with cancer are currently underway.[27]

Depletion of Immunosuppressive MDSCs

In light of many recent studies, it has become clear that an effective immunotherapy must be able to overcome or be combined with other treatments that can overcome the immunosuppression present in the tumor microenvironment. As mentioned earlier, both checkpoint molecules and myeloid-derived suppressor cells (MDSCs) are a key component of such immunosuppression. Although a few of the human antibodies that target checkpoint molecules were discussed earlier, Table 14.2 lists the various potential ways in which MDSCs may be manipulated to enhance the effectiveness of immunotherapy.

Nonspecific Immune Activation to Generate Antitumor Activity Using Biological Response Modifiers

In the 1900s, William Coley observed that cancer patients who developed bacterial infections survived longer than those who did not (reviewed[119]). Building on these observations, Coley developed "Coley's toxins" consisting of killed cultures of *Streptococcus pyogenes* and *Serratia marcescens* that he gave to patients with inoperable sarcomas. Although with this "vaccine" Coley saw cure rates of approximately 15%, his therapy was discontinued because of its significant failure rate and intolerable side effects. However, this seminal work laid the foundation for further studies aimed at nonspecific, pan immune activation to treat cancer through the use of biological response modifiers (BRMs).

Bacillus of Calmette and Guerin and *Corynebacterium parvum*

One of the most well-known and clinically used BRM is bacillus of Calmette and Guerin (BCG), a live, attenuated strain of *Mycobacterium bovis*. Currently, in human medicine, BCG is intravesically instilled into the bladder, where it is considered to be effective as a means to treat and prevent relapse of noninvasive transitional cell carcinoma.[120,121] One proposed mechanism for its antitumor effects relates to the recruitment of neutrophils and their ability to promote urothelial cell turnover.[122] This recruitment most likely relates to the ability of BCG to elicit Th1 inflammatory cytokines,[123,124] a cytokine profile associated with inducing cytolytic cells to kill the target tumor cells (compared with a Th2-cytokine response, which is typically associated with antiinflammatory immune responses).

BCG immunotherapy has been evaluated in dogs with cancer,[125] but its clinical use as an immunotherapy in dogs is limited. Although BCG can be safely instilled into canine bladders,[126] the rate of true superficial (as opposed to infiltrative) bladder cancers is extremely low in dogs compared with humans.[127] Recent uses of BCG in dogs includes treatment of CTVT in conjunction with vincristine,[128] or in combination with human chorionic gonadotropin (LDI-100), to treat dogs with mast cell tumors.[129] In this study, response rates for grade I and II MCTs were comparable to those for single-agent vinblastine, but without the myelosuppression.

Another BRM studied in human and veterinary medicine is *Corynebacterium parvum*. In human and dog melanoma studies, *C. parvum* displayed antitumor activity as an adjunct to surgery.[130,131] However, the efficacy of *C. parvum* as an immunotherapy in other canine cancers has been disappointing.[132]

Immunotherapy with Live Attenuated *Salmonella*

As a tumor grows, the core may become necrotic as the initial tumor cells are deprived of nutrients. Layered upon the necrotic core are tumor cells that exist in an area of hypoxia—they are out of reach of blood vessels that can supply them with oxygen. These cells remain viable and pose a challenge to most immunotherapies, chemotherapies, and even small-molecule drugs because of their restricted location. Recently researchers have begun to genetically modify facultative anaerobic bacteria that can penetrate and survive in these regions. In fact, it has been shown that several strains of *Salmonella*, including *S. typhimurium* and *S. choleraesuius,* target tumors after systemic administration. These bacteria penetrate the necrotic core and feed on the dead cells while also emitting natural toxins that will destroy surrounding, viable cells. Using a mouse melanoma model, treatment with VNP20009, an attenuated *Salmonella typhimurium*, was able to slow tumor growth and specifically target primary tumor and metastatic lesions.[133] Although this study showed that the effects were independent of B and T cells, possible indirect effects of the *Salmonella* include production of inflammatory cytokines, such as TNF-α.[134] Recently, another proposed mechanism involves the ability of *Salmonella* to induce melanoma cells to express gap junctions that can interact with DCs and cause bits of tumor cell proteins to be loaded and expressed on the surface of these DCs for presentation to T cells.[135] Unfortunately, in human trials, the bacteria failed to colonize some patients and did not provide any antitumor activity.[136]

Administration of VNP20009 in dogs resulted in a more positive outcome than in humans. In a Phase I clinical trial, VNP20009 was administered to dogs with a variety of malignant tumors.[137] In this study, 41 dogs received intravenous infusions of VNP20009 either weekly or biweekly at escalating doses. Fever and vomiting were reported as dose-limiting toxicities. Bacterial colonization was seen in approximately 40% of dogs and significant clinical responses observed in 15% of patients, with an overall rate of 37% of dogs experiencing either a transient response or stable disease. Thus the use of VNP20009 in specific dog tumors should be further investigated, perhaps in combination with modified *Salmonella* engineered to deliver tumor cytotoxic agents.

Liposome-Encapsulated Muramyl Tripeptide

Bacterial cell components, such as peptides derived from mycobacterial cell walls, were evaluated for potential immunogenicity. One such product is muramyl tripeptide-phosphatidylethanolamine (MTP-PE), an NOD2 receptor agonist, that when encapsulated in a liposome (L-MTP-PE) can efficiently activate monocytes and macrophages to produce proinflammatory cytokines, such as IL-1α and -β, IL-6, IL-7, IL-8, IL-12 and TNF-α.[138] L-MTP-PE has been assessed in Phase I and II trials of people with osteosarcoma (OSA), renal carcinoma, and metastatic melanoma.[138–140] Moreover, this drug has been approved for use in treating pediatric osteosarcoma in Europe under the name Mepact (mifamurtide).[141]

L-MTP-PE has been evaluated in veterinary medicine in a variety of studies.[142–146] The survival benefit of L-MTP-PE therapy has been most clearly demonstrated in dogs with appendicular OSA.[147] In this study, dogs receiving L-MTP-PE after limb amputation had a median survival time (MST) of 222 days whereas dogs that received placebo had a MST of 77 days. However, as most of the dogs in both groups developed metastatic disease, further studies evaluated the efficacy of L-MTP-PE in conjunction with chemotherapy.[142] In this study, dogs receiving L-MTP-PE after treatment with cisplatin had a MST of 14.4 months versus 9.8 months in dogs that received cisplatin only. Interestingly, only 73% of dogs receiving L-MTP-PE developed metastatic disease compared with 93% in the cisplatin-only group. However, in a second trial, these investigators saw no significant survival advantage in dogs with OSA that received L-MTP-PE concurrently with cisplatin. The authors postulated that cisplatin attenuated antimetastatic potential of L-MTP-PE because of impaired immune effectors. L-MTP-PE was also evaluated for efficacy in canine hemangiosarcoma (HSA).[144] Dogs that received L-MTP-PE with chemotherapy after splenectomy had a MST of 9 months versus 5.7 months seen with dogs receiving chemotherapy alone. In another study only dogs with stage I oral melanoma that received L-MTP-PE had an increased survival over placebo-treated dogs.[145] No differences were observed in dogs with more advanced disease.

Liposome–DNA Complexes

Bacterial DNA can also stimulate the innate immune system via its CpG oligonucleotides, particularly when complexed with cationic liposomes, in a form known as cationic lipid–DNA complexes (CLDCs).[148] Complexing bacterial plasmid DNA to liposomes allows for more efficient delivery of the CpG DNA to the endosomal compartment of antigen presenting cells, such as DCs, where it is released from the liposomes and binds to its receptor, TLR-9.[149,150] In mouse studies, CLDCs stimulate the immune system largely through induction of NK cell activity and release of IFN-γ.[148] Moreover, CLDCs were also shown to stimulate the production of type I IFN,[151] and thus are potent nonspecific immunostimulants.

The use of CLDCs in dogs has been evaluated in metastatic OSA and in dogs with soft tissue sarcoma (STS).[152,153] Intravenous administration of a modified CLDC that encodes for IL-2 was performed in dogs with stage IV OSA.[152] Dogs that received the CLDC developed fevers and showed changes in their leukogram profile indicative of immune stimulation. Moreover, NK cell activity was observed, as assessed by target cell lysis, and monocytes showed increased expression of B7.2 on their surface, indicating activation. Treatment was associated with a significant increase in survival times compared with historical controls. Another study examined the use of CLDC in canine STS.[153] Administration of CLDC, IV, once weekly for 6 weeks resulted in an objective response in 15% of the dogs and a decrease in tumor microvessel density in half of the dogs receiving the treatment. Thus CLDC has excellent potential to be used as a stand-alone immunotherapeutic in veterinary medicine for a variety of cancer types.

Oncolytic Viruses

Oncolytic viruses are defined as viruses capable of replicating in and lysing tumor cells, thus making them likely candidates for drug or gene delivery to tumors. This section focuses on oncolytic viruses as means of directly killing the cells, and a later section focuses on using viral vectors as a means of gene delivery. A beneficial side effect of these viruses is that they not only kill the tumor cells, but they also cause release of tumor antigens for processing by the immune system. With safety being the main concern, modern genetics has allowed for modifications of the virus to make them less pathogenic and also target tumor cells specifically. A recent review of the use of oncolytic virotherapy for canine cancer describes the biology behind this therapy and recent veterinary studies assessing these therapies.[154] Adenoviruses that have undergone genetic modification of their early genes, 1A (E1A) and 1B (E1B), preferentially target rapidly dividing tumor cells and have been used to target canine OSA cells.[155–157] Canine distemper virus (CDV) has also been investigated as a treatment for B and T cell lymphoma in dogs.[158] In vitro studies using fluorescently labeled, attenuated CDV and canine lymphoma cells demonstrated that CDV infected lymphoid cells via binding of the cell membrane protein CD150, which is overexpressed on malignant B cells, and induced cellular apoptosis.[158] More recently, many groups have begun looking at Pox viruses in oncolytic viral therapy, although this research has been done only in in vitro cultures or xenograft mice.[159–162] There is also a report on the use of an attenuated strain of Newcastle disease virus in in vitro cultures on both human and canine lymphoma cells and compared cell death with peripheral blood mononuclear cells (PBMCs).[163] They reported a 34% increase in cell death in canine lymphoma cells compared with normal PBMCs. Furthermore, this group injected one dog with a T-cell lymphoma and found

viral particles in kidney, salivary gland, lung, and stomach. Lastly, a clinical study of dogs with various cancer types were treated with a recombinant form vesicular stomatitis virus (VSV), that expresses IFN-β and the sodium iodide symporter (NIS).[164] This study was designed to assess for safety and efficacy. They determined that there was no viral shedding two of the five dogs (both with T-cell lymphoma) had a transient partial response during the 28-day observation posttreatment time period. Five of the 9 dogs demonstrated stable disease for the same 28-day time period and the remaining two dogs had progressive disease. One of the dogs with stable disease (anal adenocarcinoma) had resection of the tumor after completion of the study and evidence of an uncharacteristic T cell infiltration into the tumor tissue was observed, suggesting a possible immune effect of the VSV therapy.

Toll-Like Receptor and NOD-Like Receptor Agonists

TLRs are part of the innate immune system and are proteins expressed on the surfaces of macrophages and dendritic cells and serve the purpose of recognizing microbial pathogens. As discussed earlier, CLDC contains CpG DNA, which can bind to TLR-9. Lipopolysaccharide (LPS) is a known ligand for TLR-4. Recently the TLR-7 agonist imiquimod was studied as a topical therapy in combination with an autologous cellular vaccine in dogs with invasive meningioma,[165] and as a single therapy in cats with squamous cell carcinoma.[166] As noted earlier, MTP functions as an NOD2 receptor agonist, and can be preferentially targeted to activate macrophages by liposome encapsulation.[167]

Nonspecific Tumor Immunotherapy Using Recombinant Cytokine Therapy

Interleukin-2

IL-2 is a cytokine that is released by T cells after their activation via interactions of antigen-loaded MHC and costimulatory molecules expressed on the surface of antigen presenting cells. Its function is to induce clonal expansion of T cells in an antigen-specific fashion and activate DCs, macrophages, and B cells, which in turn release proinflammatory cytokines. Moreover, IL-2 stimulates NK cells, thus playing an important role in inducing both the innate and adaptive arms of the immune system.

The therapeutic use of IL-2 in humans is fraught with toxicity[168–170]; however, the use of IL-2 therapy in veterinary medicine holds some promise. Helfand et al demonstrated that intravenously injected recombinant human IL-2 (rhIL-2) activates canine lymphocytes, causing only mild gastrointestinal toxicity, even at high doses for 4 consecutive days.[171] Another study demonstrated the ability of rhIL-2 to induce canine lymphokine activated killer (LAK) cells and, incidentally, showed that LAK cells from tumor-bearing dogs did not kill tumor cells as efficiently compared with normal dogs.[172] Further evaluation of toxicity and efficacy of rhIL-2 was done using dogs with primary lung cancer and with lung metastases in an aerosol formulation.[173] In this study, complete regression was seen in two of the four dogs with pulmonary metastases and these dogs remained disease-free for at least 12 months after treatment. One of the two dogs with a primary lung tumor had stabilized disease for more than 8 months, whereas the other dog had progressive disease. Assessment of the lymphocytes obtained from bronchoalveolar lavage showed increased cytolytic activity after 15 days of IL-2 treatment. In addition, minimal toxicity was noted in this study. Finally, IL-2 gene therapy using viral vectors has been examined for treatment of feline fibrosarcomas and canine melanoma and was shown to be safe and effective.[174–176] Therefore given its comparatively low toxicity and promising effectiveness, rIL-2 therapy is a plausible treatment for canine cancer.

Interleukin 12

IL-12, produced by antigen-stimulated DCs, macrophages, and B cells, plays a role in stimulating the growth and function of T cells and enhances the cytolytic activity of both T cells and NK cells. Similar to IL-2, IL-12 therapy in humans lead to serious side effects, and is thus currently not used clinically. Current investigation into the use of IL-12 in veterinary medicine revolves around recombinant gene therapy for treatment of canine head and neck tumors,[177] with some in vitro work looking at its use in feline hyperthermia-induced gene therapy.[178] More recently, in an experimental model of CTVT, intratumoral delivery of the IL-12 gene resulted in decreased tumor growth and complete tumor remission.[179] Similar studies in dogs using IL-12 electrogene therapy resulted in reduced tumor volume of 9 out of 11 dogs with mast cell tumors[180] and increases in intratumoral IFN-γ and antiangiogenic effects in nine dogs with various cancers,[181] and in six dogs treated with concurrent metronomic chemotherapy.[182] However, no significant clinical responses were observed in these studies. Interestingly, both studies demonstrated increased levels of tumor-infiltrating lymphocytes, suggesting immune specificity of this therapy.

Interleukin-15

IL-15 is structurally similar to and uses similar signaling molecules as IL-2. IL-15 plays a role in stimulation of NK cells and in promoting proliferation of T cells. However, from an immunotherapy standpoint, IL-15 holds more promise than IL-2 in that (1) it does not cause activation-induced cell death of CD4+ T cells after prolonged periods of exposure, but rather sustains T-cell proliferation[183]; (2) it plays a critical role in CD8+ T cell memory formation and maintenance[184]; and (3) unlike IL-2, it does not appear to play a role in the development of Tregs.[185]

Clinical evaluation has been underway now in several trials in human cancer patients. An initial safety study in nonhuman primates was recently conducted.[186] Twelve daily doses of clinical grade human recombinant IL-15 revealed that neutropenia was the dose-limiting and documented an increase in circulating NK cells and memory CD8+ T cells.

In veterinary medicine, one study combined intralesional IL-15 and IL-6 plasmid DNA injections in beagles with CTVT.[187] With this treatment, investigators observed a threefold increase in the proportion of CD8+ T cells that infiltrated the tumors and an enhancement of IFN-γ-producing cells and increased cytolytic activity against the tumor. Lastly, in 2015, one group reported on the generation of recombinant canine IL-15.[188] They demonstrated that *in* vitro, recombinant IL-15 could expand canine NK cells and could cause expansion of lymphocytes in peripheral blood when administered to dogs intravenously. Thus IL-15 therapy shows promise as an effective immunotherapy in both human and veterinary medicine.

Interferons

Interferons (IFNs) are proteins produced by lymphocytes that play an important role in immune responses to pathogens and cancer. Broadly, they can influence cell proliferation, play a role in the induction of apoptosis, upregulate antigen presentation to T cells, and enhance the ability of the adaptive immune system to mount a cytolytic immune response. Moreover, IFNs have antiangiogenic properties. The IFNs are typically classified as either type I (IFN-α, -β, and -ω) or type II (IFN-γ).

Interferon-α, Interferon-β, and Interferon-ω

The type I IFNs can affect cellular proliferation through various mechanisms including interactions with cell cycle proteins (i.e., c-myc and retinoblastoma) and induction of apoptosis via Bcl-2/Bax and TNF/Fas interactions. Their antiangiogenic properties of downregulating VEGF and basic fibroblast growth factor (bFGF)[189] make them attractive as immunotherapies and they have been used successfully to treat pediatric hemangiomas.[190]

Clinical trials using the type I IFNs have met limited success because of the high occurrence of severe toxicity and overall limited response rates. Nonetheless, their effectiveness was assessed in melanoma, multiple myeloma, renal cell carcinoma, leukemia, other cancers, and in conjunction with chemotherapies. The best response, in terms of disease-free survival, was seen in renal cell carcinoma and melanoma when used as single agents.[191,192]

The use of type I IFNs in veterinary medicine is limited and they are used mostly for feline viral diseases.[193] One study showed that recombinant feline IFN-ω was safe and easy to use for treating feline fibrosarcomas. As this was a safety study, the therapeutic effects of this treatment were not evaluated. Another recently published study also used recombinant feline IFN-ω with or without chemotherapy to study its effects in treating mammary tumors in vitro.[194] This study reported that the antitumor cell effects of recombinant IFN-ω and chemotherapy were additive and suggested further investigation into its clinical use as an adjuvant therapy.

Interferon-γ

IFN-γ plays an important role in stimulating the immune system. It is secreted mostly by NK cells, DCs and antigen-activated T cells and counteracts the effects of many of the immunosuppressive cytokines. It is a physiologic activator of macrophages, leading to increased antigen presentation and increased lysosomal function and NO production by macrophages. NO production by macrophages is an efficient mechanism of tumor cytolysis. IFN-γ can also cause increased MHC Class I and II expression on a variety of cells, including tumors. Increased MHC expression has been confirmed to occur on in vitro IFN-γ treated canine tumor cells lines[195] and in vivo after treatment with IFN-γ.[196] Thus its role in antitumor immunity is characterized by increased tumor cell lysis and increased tumor antigen presentation to the adaptive immune response.

The use of IFN-γ in veterinary medicine is currently being investigated. A recently published study examined the use of IFN-γ in combination with a single injection of autologous, ex vivo activated DCs in dogs with various malignant or benign tumors.[197] In the seven dogs enrolled in the study, the investigators noted four complete responses and two partial responses against malignant tumors and saw moderate partial responses against fast-growing benign tumors. Another study looked at the use of adenoviral IFN-γ gene transfer as an adjuvant therapy to treat a dog with astrocytoma.[198] After therapy and surgery, the dog was tumor free for more than 450 days. Finally, a safety study was done in cats with fibrosarcomas using a triple gene therapy that included IFN-γ along with IL-2 and GM-CSF.[176] In this study, cats tolerated the therapy, although six of the eight cats developed local recurrence of disease within 1 year of treatment.

Specific Immunotherapy for Cancer: Tumor Vaccines

The development of a tumor vaccine that is safe, effective, and long-lasting is an ultimate goal of immunotherapy. Whereas the effects of traditional cancer treatments such as chemotherapy, surgery, and radiation therapy typically result in noticeable clinical responses within hours to days after treatment, cancer vaccine therapeutic responses typically take weeks to months to lead to an appreciable clinical response. This difference in response time, coupled with the lack of congruent and objective ways to measure efficacy, make it difficult to develop tumor vaccines.

Nonetheless, despite the challenges to tumor vaccine development, there are many different varieties of tumor vaccines currently in use either clinically or as part of Phase I, II, and III clinical trials. In fact, in April of 2010, the first FDA-approved therapeutic cancer vaccine for human prostate cancer was approved. In the following section, we will discuss only those showing success in human trials and those relevant to veterinary medicine.

Tumor Antigen Targets for Immunization

Tumor antigens (TAs) are proteins are other molecules that are either unique to cancer cells or significantly more abundant in cancer cells compared with normal cells. These proteins include the broad categories of oncogenes, oncofetal proteins, and cancer testes antigens. Although TAs offer potential targets for vaccine development, their downside is that some of them tend to be individual or certain tumor type specific. Nonetheless, much work has been accomplished characterizing TAs for various forms of cancer and a table of currently studied TAs can be found in a 2009 publication by a panel of experts organized by the National Cancer Institute (NCI).[199] Although numerous TAs exist, the use of these TAs in tumor vaccines is not trivial. As mentioned earlier, the tumor is highly capable of inducing a potent, immunosuppressive microenviroment by various mechanisms; thus standard vaccine procedures using TAs can be rendered useless in this powerful environment. In fact, there are little data available showing a clear correlation between in vitro TA responses and prognosis. The success of most tumor vaccines has been limited to animal models of induced disease.[200,201] However, through the use of better vaccine strategies and by combining therapies that can ultimately overcome tumor immunosuppression, more promising specific immunotherapies are being developed. In the text that follows we will discuss the various platforms used to develop tumor vaccines.

Tumor Vaccine Approaches

Whole Tumor Cell and Tumor Cell Lysate Vaccines

One of the more simple approaches to tumor vaccine development is through the use of whole tumor cell or tumor cell lysate vaccines. These can either be made directly from the patient in the form of an autologous vaccine or from cell lines of similar tumor types from the same species as an allogeneic vaccine. Whole cell preparations are most often produced made by lethally irradiating tumor cells and/or tissues. Tumor lysate vaccines, including membrane protein fraction vaccines, are made by mechanically disrupting the tumor cells and/or tissues. Both whole cell and tumor-lysate vaccines are typically administered with some form of adjuvant to enhance the immune response. These polyvalent vaccines may be superior to specific peptide or protein (subunit) vaccines in that they contain a heterogeneous population of TAs.

One study out of our laboratory assessed the use of an allogeneic HSA tumor lysate vaccine in combination with chemotherapy.[202] In this Phase I/II study, 28 dogs were evaluated and received eight immunizations of tumor lysate plus CLDC (see the section "Liposome–DNA Complexes") over a 22-week period while concurrently receiving doxorubicin. The vaccine was well tolerated; adverse effects were limited to moderate diarrhea and anorexia. Tumor-specific antibody responses were detected in four to five of the six dogs tested, depending on which HSA cell-line they were screened against. Moreover, overall survival times of dogs receiving the combination treatment were significantly better than chemotherapy-only treated historical controls.

Whole cell and tumor lysate vaccines can also be modified to enhance their immunogenicity. Aside from different adjuvant strategies, combination of these vaccines with modifiers such as immunostimulatory cytokines has been examined. One clinical trial of 16 dogs with STS or melanoma assessed the use of an autologous, whole cell vaccine transfected with human GM-CSF.[203] Three dogs in the study demonstrated objective tumor responses that included regression of primary and metastatic lesions. On histologic examination of tumor tissue in the dogs that received the vaccine, an impressive inflammatory response was noted. Another recent study using a similar human GM-CSF adjuvanted, autologous vaccine looked at its efficacy in treating dogs with B cell lymphoma.[204] Dogs in remission after a 19-week standard CHOP (Cyclophosphamide, Hydroxydaunorubicin, Oncovin [vincristine], and Prednisone) protocol were randomized into placebo or vaccine treatment groups. No improvement in median length to remission, nor overall survival, was seen. Another study investigated the use of an allogeneic melanoma vaccine in combination with a xenogeneic melanoma protein, human glycoprotein 100 (hpg100).[205] In this Phase II trial, the vaccine was well tolerated and the researchers observed an overall response rate of 17% and a tumor control rate (including complete and partial responses and stable disease greater than 6 weeks duration) of 35%. Lastly, some positive results have been seen with an autologous B cell lymphoma vaccine where the cells were transfected loaded with tumor RNA and activated through CD40, particularly in prolonging remission duration of salvage therapy.[206]

Immunization Against Defined Tumor Antigens Using Plasmid DNA

Vaccines that use specific gene sequences of TAs encoded in plasmid DNA have shown some clinical promise with their ability to invoke both cellular and humoral immunity. The ease of working with bacterial DNA and the ability to quickly produce large quantities of plasmid DNA make this an attractive vaccine platform. Moreover, the DNA sequences of a majority of TAs are known and can be easily inserted into the plasmid DNA and expressed under the control of a constitutively active bacterial promoter. Typically given intradermally or intramuscularly, the proteins expressed by transcription and translation of the plasmid are readily picked up by DCs, processed and presented in the context of MHC Class I and II, thus providing a more "natural" stimulation of the immune system. Moreover, the unmethylated dinucleotide-CpG residues, or CpG motifs, present in high frequency in the bacterial DNA provide additional stimulation of DCs, triggering them to induce a Th1-type immune response.[207]

No DNA vaccines have been licensed for human use yet. However, many DNA vaccines have been tested in clinical trials and results have thus far been disappointing for various reasons (see review[208]). Nonetheless, the first conditionally licensed veterinary cancer vaccine is based on the DNA plasmid technology.[209] The ONCEPT Vaccine (Merial, Inc.) for canine malignant melanoma (CMM) uses xenogeneic DNA plasmids that contain the gene encoding human tyrosinase (huTyr). Initial studies showed the development of an antibody-mediated immune response against the huTyr protein that cross-reacted to canine tyrosinase (also see Chapter 19 for more details).[210] Improved survival of dogs treated with this vaccine compared with historical control animals has been reported with no severe side effects noted.[209,211] Further studies of this plasmid DNA technology demonstrated that the vaccine could induce antigen-specific IFN-γ+ T cells in normal beagle dogs.[212] The same group that developed the CMM vaccine has reportedly completed Phase I trials of murine CD20 for treatment of canine B cell lymphoma and is initiating a Phase II trial soon.[213] Lastly, a recently developed vaccine against the dog telomerase reverse transcriptase protein, for use in canine lymphoma patients, has demonstrated positive results, significantly increasing survival in dogs with B-cell lymphoma when added to conventional chemotherapy.[214,215]

Tumor Vaccination Using Viral Vector Vaccines

As discussed earlier (section "Oncolytic Viruses"), viruses have been used to target tumor cells, in particular ones with innate oncolytic properties. However, viruses can also be used as vectors for expression of particular TAs. Typically, attenuated or replication-defective forms of the virus are used to allow for effective stimulation of the innate and adaptive immune responses without the risk of spreading and rapidly dividing within the host. The most commonly used viral platform for both human and veterinary studies is the Poxviridae family. The poxviruses are easy to work with, are amenable to large amounts of foreign DNA, and are highly immunogenic, allowing for strong immune responses against weak TAs, such as carcinoembryonic antigen (CEA).[216] In humans, one of the most commonly used viral vaccine platform is the canarypox virus ALVAC. Recent published human clinical trials using ALVAC include combining CEA-expressing ALVAC with chemotherapy for metastatic colorectal cancer,[217] ALVAC expressing huGM-CSF or IL-2 for treatment of melanoma or leiomyosarcoma,[218] and intranodal injection of ALVAC expressing gp100 in high-risk melanoma patients.[219] Interestingly, although all of these studies reported that the vaccine was safe to use and that immunologic responses were observed, the efficacy of these therapies is limited.[220]

Vaccination Against Tumor Antigens Using Dendritic Cells

DCs possess very potent antigen presenting abilities and are an attractive target for cancer vaccine strategies. Besides their role in vivo in processing and presenting TAs derived either naturally or from tumor vaccines, there are many clinical trials published that examine the use of ex vivo activated and expanded DCs injected back into the donor as a way of activating tumor-specific T cells in vivo. The drawback to this method is that the ex vivo processing of DCs typically is expensive, takes about 7 to 10 days, requires growth in a combination of cytokines, and can be used only autologously. Nonetheless, ex vivo prepared DCs have shown clinical efficacy, particularly in human patients with metastatic disease.[221,222] Recently, it has been determined that the potency of the DCs produced ex vivo depends on the combination of cytokines used.[223] DCs generated with GM-CSF and IFN-α or GM-CSF and IL-15 display potent priming of T-cell–mediated and CD8+ T-cell–mediated immune responses in vitro. Moreover, the use of mature DCs is better than use of immature DCs, as immature DCs actually induce immune tolerance via expansion of

IL-10–secreting T cells.[224] However, the methods of maturation matter as well, with studies showing DCs activated with a mixture of IFN-α, polyinosinic-polycytidylic acid, IL-1β, TNF, and IFN-γ elicit many fold more antimelanoma CTLs in vitro than the standard IL-1β, TNF, IL-6, prostaglandin E_2 (PGE_2) cocktail.[225] Finally, new methods of targeting antigens to DCs through anti-DC receptor (i.e., lectin receptors such as DEC-205, DC-SIGN, or DNGR-1) antibody–TA fusions, appropriate selection of adjuvants to deliver antigens to DCs, and combination therapies using chemotherapy and DC activation are being investigated.[221,223]

DC vaccination in veterinary medicine has been and is still currently being explored. An initial study of three dogs with oral melanoma showed that bone marrow derived DCs transduced with an adenovirus expressing human gp100 could safely be used. In this study, dogs received three subcutaneous vaccines over 4 months.[226] One of the dogs, which was disease-free 4 years later, developed a robust CTL response against the gp100. Another dog that relapsed after 22 months had no evidence of antigp100 CTLs. A similar study performed in normal dogs was done to assess the immune response of DCs pulsed with canine melanoma cell (CMM2) lysates, where a good delayed-type hypersensitivity (DTH) response was seen against CMM2 after vaccination.[227]

Another study described earlier (section "Interferon-γ") saw success using ex vivo activated DCs and IFN-γ for treating canine solid tumors. Finally, a very recent study looked at the safety of using a DC–mammary tumor cell fusion hybrid vaccine.[228] In this case normal dog PBMCs were used to generate DCs that were subsequently fused to canine mammary tumor cells. Injection of normal beagle dogs with this fusion plus CpG adjuvant resulted in a robust antibody response against the fusion partner tumor cell line and three unrelated canine mammary tumor cells. However, no CTL responses were noted. Hence, development of DC vaccines for use in veterinary medicine is currently being explored in various tumor models and using various strategies to optimize the induced antitumor immune response.

Antibody Therapy for Cancer

Monoclonal Antibodies

The use of mAb therapy for cancer has been studied for more than four decades after the development of hybridoma technology by Kohler and Milstein in 1975.[229] This technique consisted of antibody-producing cells fused with mouse myeloma cells, thus becoming immortalized and capable of continuously producing antibody that can be purified out of the culture media. Initially, the use of mAbs clinically was limited because of the responses mounted by the host against the foreign mouse proteins. However, recent technology allowed for "humanizing" these antibodies by genetically grafting the mouse hypervariable region of interest onto the human immunoglobulin, thus resulting in an antibody that is 95% human. Moreover, mice genetically rendered to express human immunoglobulins can successfully generate 100% human antibodies in response to various antigens.[230] Using humanized antibodies improves antibody-dependent cell-mediated cytotoxicity (ADCC), improves antibody stability, and decreases immunogenicity of the antibody itself. The use of mAbs in human medicine has increased over the years. Table 14.3 lists those approved by the FDA for use as human cancer treatments and some recent mAbs tested in human clinical trials.[231] As a general guide, mAb names ending in -omab are murine based, -ximab and -zumab are chimeric, and -umab are humanized versions of the antibodies.

TABLE 14.3 Approved Monoclonal Antibodies

Target	mAb	Indication	Year Approved by the FDA
EpCAM	Edrecolomab	Colorectal	1995
CD20	Rituximab	Non-Hodgkin lymphoma	1997
HER2	Trastuzumab	Breast cancer	1998
CD33	Gemtuzumab	Acute myelogenous leukemia	2000
CD52	Alemtuzumab	Chronic lymphocytic leukemia, T-cell lymphoma	2001
CD20	Ibritumomab[a] tiuxetan	Non-Hodgkin lymphoma	2002
VEGF	Bevacizumab	Colorectal	2004
VEGFR	Cetuximab	Colorectal	2004
EpCAM × CD3	Catumaxomab	Hepatocarcinoma	2005
EGFR	Panitumumab	Colorectal	2006
CD20	Ofatumumab	Chronic lymphocytic leukemia	2009
CTLA-4	Ipilimumab	Melanoma	2011
CD30	Brentuximab vedotin	Lymphoma	2011
HER2	Pertuzumab	Breast cancer	2012
	Ado-trastuzumab	Breast cancer	2013
CD20	Obinutuzumab	Chronic lymphocytic leukemia	2013
VEGFR	Ramucirumab	Gastric cancer	2014
PD-1	Pembrolizumab	Melanoma	2014
CD20	Tositumomab[b]	Acute lymphocytic leukemia	2014
PD-1	Nivolumab	Melanoma	2014
GD2	Dinutuximab	Neuroblastoma	2015
CD38	Daratumumab	Myeloma	2015
EGFR	Necitumumab	Lung cancer	2015
SLAMF7	Elotuzumab	Myeloma	2015
PD-L1	Atezolizumab	Urothelial cancer	2016
CD19/CD3	Blinatumomab	Acute lymphocytic leukemia	2017
PD-L1	Avelumab	Gastric cancer	2017
	Durvalumab	Urothelial cancer	2017

CD, cluster of determination; CTLA-4, Cytotoxic T-lymphocyte antigen-4; EGFR, epidermal growth factor receptor; EpCAM, epithelial cell adhesion molecule; GD2, glycolipid antigen disialoganglioside 2; HER-2, human epidermal growth factor receptor 2; PD-1, programmed death molecule-1; PD-L1, ligand of PD-1; SLAMF, signaling lymphocytic activation molecule family F; VEGF, vascular endothelial growth factor; VEGFR, vascular endothelial growth factor receptor.

[a]111In/90Y-labeled.
[b]131I-labeled.

With the current excitement surrounding immune checkpoint inhibitor therapy, it is anticipated that fully caninized antibodies may be available for cancer therapy in the near future. In fact, a chimerized anti-PD-L1 antibody was tested in a small clinical trial in Japan with some positive results.[27] There has already been USDA approval of the Cytopoint (Zoetis), a canonized antibody that targets canine IL-31, which is involved in allergic skin disease and pruritus in dogs.

Conjugated Monoclonal Antibodies

Another use of mAbs is linking them to potential toxins, immunocytokines, or radioisotopes. Initial studies involved linking chemical toxins to immunoglobulins to generate molecules called immunotoxins. Such chemicals tested were ricin and diphtheria toxins, but these conjugates were immunogenically and chemically unstable. Development of recombinant immunotoxins helped address this issue, although the current concern with immunotoxins is their ability to nonspecifically kill any cell expressing the antibody-specific receptor.

Recently Paoloni et al developed an "immunocytokine" that targets necrotic areas of the tumor and is linked to IL-12.[232] A dose escalation was performed with this drug, called NHS-IL12, and it was demonstrated that it could be safely administered to dogs with melanoma at the appropriate dose, and that IL-12 could be measured in dog serum postadministration and was correlated with an increase in systemic IL-10 levels. Interestingly, they observed increased IFN-γ levels that correlated with adverse reactions. In five of seven dogs, they observed an increased infiltration of CD8+ T cells. Some partial responses and stable disease were observed in the dogs in the study.

mAbs can also be linked to radionuclides. The concept behind these antibodies is that the antibody targets tumor tissue and the energy released by the radioisotope attached to the antibody can penetrate bulky solid tumors and can also kill surrounding tumor and stromal cells. Examples of radiolabeled mAbs in clinical use in humans are found in Table 14.3. The current use of radiolabeled mAbs in dogs is limited to imaging modalities rather than treatment of cancer.

Cancer Immunotherapy Using Adoptive Transfer of T Cells

Adoptive T-cell transfer (ACT) is a technique whereby cells are collected from a cancer patient, expanded, and activated in culture and then transferred back into the patient. Although this technique allows for the enhancement of tumor-specific T cells, it is labor intensive, expensive, and time-consuming; thus its use is limited in both human and veterinary patients. In the text that follows, we will discuss historical methods to generate these cells and new techniques currently being investigated to improve this form of immunotherapy. As mentioned at the beginning of this chapter, one limitation to most immunotherapies is the fact that tumors can orchestrate an immunosuppressive environment. Thus even if one instilled thousands of activated, tumor-specific T cells into a cancer patient, the majority of these cells will become inactivated on reaching the tumor, particularly when dealing with solid tumors.[233] It is currently being recognized that strategies to overcome immunosuppression must be implemented to enhance the efficiency of tumor-specific T cells in ACT studies. One technique to address this suppression is performing lymphodepletion before ACT.[234–236] Recent studies have also suggested the isolation of CD4+ T cells for ACT, rather than cytotoxic CD8+ T cells, as CD4+ T cells are capable of activating both innate immune cells and CD8+ T cells.[237,238] However, CD4+ T cells contain Treg cells; thus strategies to block the development of Treg cells during CD4+ T cell ACT have been investigated.[237] In addition, the availability of TAs appears to also play a role in the strength of CD4+ ACT therapy.[239] Similarly, the addition of cytokines and/or blocking antibodies against suppressor cells, along with ACTs, has been shown to enhance the effectiveness of this therapy.[237,240–242]

More recently, there has been interest in developing chimeric antigen receptor (CAR) T cells for canine immunotherapy. CAR-T cells are generated via transfection of antibody genes specific for a tumor target into a T cell.[243–247] This directs the engineered T cells specifically to the tumor tissue. Success with this technology has been seen in humans with chronic lymphocytic leukemia where the T cells target the CD19+ B cells.[244,245] In terms of veterinary use, initial in vitro studies were performed looking at autologous T cells transfected with the *HER2* gene to target canine osteosarcoma cells.[248] More recently, Panjwani et al transfected canine T cells with CD20-targeting RNA for dogs with B cell lymphoma.[249] This was the first study to show that these cells could be made, expanded, and safely administered to dogs.

Transfer of Lymphokine-Activated Killer Cells

Initial T-cell transfer studies involved the generation of lymphokine-activated killer (LAK) cells. This was done by culturing PBMCs in high concentrations of IL-2, thus selecting for a population of cells with potent tumor cell lysis ability. Clinical trials using this technique in humans were disappointing and unfeasible despite promising mouse studies.[250] The use of LAK cells in veterinary medicine is limited to studies of cats with FeLV or FIV.[251]

Transfer of Tumor-Infiltrating Lymphocytes

One source of potent antitumor T cells is in the tumor itself. These cells, called tumor-infiltrating lymphocytes (TILs), when expanded using IL-2, exhibit potent cytolytic activity that is many folds higher than LAK cells against tumors in both a specific and nonspecific way.[252] Although they are considered the best source of T cells for ACT,[253,254] their use in human medicine is limited because of a few variables such as time of isolation, the tumor they were isolated from, and the functional state of the cells when isolated.[250] Nonetheless, limited success has been observed in cases of treating human melanoma with TILs, particularly when combined with nonmyeloablative chemotherapy such as fludarabine and cyclophosphamide, which deplete lymphocytes but spare bone marrow stem cells.[255] In one study, 6 of 13 melanoma patients had significant tumor regression and four had a mixed response including regression of some lesions and growth of others.[255] In a follow-up study involving a larger number of patients (34 in total), tumor regression was seen in 51% of the patients that received chemotherapy before the TIL transfer and IL-2 treatment.[256] In addition to the use of nonmyeloablative treatments, recent studies have investigated the use of other forms of Th1 stimulation along with ACT. One group has investigated the use of adding CpG-ODNs to their TILs to increase their efficacy.[257] In a study using ex vivo isolated human TILs, instillation of the activated TILs with CpG-ODN into athymic nude, tumor-bearing mice, resulted in decreased tumor burden and prolonged survival. Regardless of the human clinical trials' results, the use of TILs in veterinary medicine is absent, perhaps owing to the lack of reliable efficacy across multiple tumor types.

Natural Killer Cell Immunotherapy

Lastly, there is a growing interest in using NK cells for immunotherapy. A recent canine immunotherapy review states that the author's institution is currently conducting a phase II canine clinical trial using autologouse NK cells that were activated ex vivo for treatment of appendicular OSA.[258]

The Future of Cancer Immunotherapy

The use of immunotherapy for the treatment of cancer is an exciting and ever-evolving field of research and application. With the advancement of techniques used to assess immune responses to tumors, better ways of predicting responses, including development of Response Evaluation Criteria in Solid Tumors (RECIST), and an understanding that tumor responses to immunotherapies may be delayed compared with conventional chemotherapy, radiation therapy and surgery, one can more reliably assess the clinical efficacy and safety of novel immunotherapies. Moreover, a better understanding of the disease pathology in our veterinary patients has led to a movement toward using spontaneous canine and feline cancers as models for human disease, thus allowing for testing of novel immunotherapies in our small animal patients that will benefit not only them, but human cancer patients as well.[259,260]

However, the development of a successful immunotherapy protocol is not without limitations. One of the main reasons for failure of many immunotherapies is due to the immunosuppressive microenvironment established by the tumor. Thus immunotherapies that are best able to overcome this suppression will prove the most successful.[261] In addition, the use of certain drugs and/or proteins that can deplete or inactivate the key players in immune suppression, i.e., MDSCs and Tregs, and therapies that target checkpoint molecules may be best used in concert with novel vaccines or other immunotherapies to optimize their effectiveness. Along those lines, the use of newer and more potent adjuvants, such as various preparations of CpG motifs, to stimulate the immune system will be a critical component of newer vaccines. It has now become clear that the most successful adjuvants are ones that not only stimulate a strong primary response against the tumor, but ones that also lead to the development of a robust central memory response.

One of the more successful categories of immunotherapies currently used in human medicine is mAbs. Advances in technology led to the development of humanized, nonimmunogenic forms of antibodies against key cellular receptors, either to activate key antitumor immune cells or lead to cytolytic activity against tumor cells. However, similar advances in treating dogs with mAbs are not currently available, although development of such reagents is underway by many investigators and companies.

It should be understood that many, if not all, immunotherapies developed should work in concert and synergize with current cancer treatment modalities. Given the ability of tumor cells to become resistant to chemotherapy and radiation therapy and their ability to suppress the immune system, one would be naïve to think that a single-modality treatment is the most effective means of tumor control. Although the immune system can be manipulated to mount an effective antitumor immune response, it is best used in cases of residual and metastatic disease, where radiation therapy, chemotherapy, and/or surgery are used to cytoreduce and down-stage large tumors. Moreover, it is becoming very clear that the immune system is a key player involved in the tumor responses to radiation and chemotherapy, thus finding ways to incorporate immunotherapy into current standard of care may actually enhance the effectiveness of these modalities. For example, we have observed that the use of liposomal clodronate therapy to eliminate MDSCs can enhance the tumor response to chemotherapy in dogs with malignant histiocytosis.[262] We hypothesize that the immunosuppressive cells present in the tumor microenvironment are capable of protecting tumor cells from the effects of chemotherapy, thus by removing these tumor cells, we can enhance the effectiveness of the chemotherapy. We predict that the use of immunotherapy as part of a protocol to treat canine and feline diseases should soon become routine. By understanding the role of the immune system in cancer in our small animal patients, we can develop better immunotherapies that will not only benefit these patients, but also ones that will be applicable to human medicine.

References

1. Perez-Gracia JL, Labiano S, Rodriguez-Ruiz ME, Sanmamed MF, Melero I: Orchestrating immune check-point blockade for cancer immunotherapy in combinations, *Curr Opin Immunol* 27:89–97, 2014.
2. Quezada SA, Peggs KS: Exploiting CTLA-4, PD-1 and PD-L1 to reactivate the host immune response against cancer, *Br J Cancer* 108(8):1560–1565, 2013.
3. Topalian SL, Drake CG, Pardoll DM: Immune checkpoint blockade: a common denominator approach to cancer therapy, *Cancer Cell* 27(4):450–461, 2015.
4. Wu YL, Liang J, Zhang W, Tanaka Y, Sugiyama H: Immunotherapies: the blockade of inhibitory signals, *Int J Biol Sci* 8(10):1420–1430, 2012.
5. Venur VA, Joshi M, Nepple KG, Zakharia Y: Spotlight on nivolumab in the treatment of renal cell carcinoma: design, development, and place in therapy, *Drug Des Devel Ther* 11:1175–1182, 2017.
6. Burnet M: Cancer; a biological approach. I. The processes of control, *Br Med J* 1(5022):779–786, 1957.
7. Stutman O: Tumor development after 3-methylcholanthrene in immunologically deficient athymic-nude mice, *Science* 183(124):534–536, 1974.
8. Rygaard J, Povlsen CO: The mouse mutant nude does not develop spontaneous tumours. An argument against immunological surveillance, *Acta Pathol Microbiol Scand B Microbiol Immunol* 82(1):99–106, 1974.
9. Schreiber TH, Podack ER: A critical analysis of the tumour immunosurveillance controversy for 3-MCA-induced sarcomas, *Br J Cancer* 101(3):381–386, 2009.
10. Rabinovich GA, Gabrilovich D, Sotomayor EM: Immunosuppressive strategies that are mediated by tumor cells, *Annu Rev Immunol* 25:267–296, 2007.
11. Dolan DE, Gupta S: PD-1 pathway inhibitors: changing the landscape of cancer immunotherapy, *Cancer Control* 21(3):231–237, 2014.
12. Jin HT, Ahmed R, Okazaki T: Role of PD-1 in regulating T-cell immunity, *Curr Top Microbiol Immunol* 350:17–37, 2011.
13. Lonberg N, Korman AJ: Masterful antibodies: checkpoint blockade, *Cancer Immunol Res* 5(4):275–281, 2017.
14. Robert C, Soria JC, Eggermont AM: Drug of the year: programmed death-1 receptor/programmed death-1 ligand-1 receptor monoclonal antibodies, *Eur J Cancer* 49(14):2968–2971, 2013.
15. Webb ES, Liu P, Baleeiro R, Lemoine NR, Yuan M, Wang YH: Immune checkpoint inhibitors in cancer therapy, *J Biomed Res ePub ahead of print*, 2017.
16. Linch SN, McNamara MJ, Redmond WL: OX40 Agonists and Combination Immunotherapy: putting the Pedal to the Metal, *Front Oncol* 5:34, 2015.
17. Aspeslagh S, Postel-Vinay S, Rusakiewicz S, Soria JC, Zitvogel L, Marabelle A: Rationale for anti-OX40 cancer immunotherapy, *Eur J Cancer* 52:50–66, 2016.
18. Knee DA, Hewes B, Brogdon JL: Rationale for anti-GITR cancer immunotherapy, *Eur J Cancer* 67:1–10, 2016.
19. Henick BS, Herbst RS, Goldberg SB: The PD-1 pathway as a therapeutic target to overcome immune escape mechanisms in cancer, *Expert Opin Ther Targets* 18(12):1407–1420, 2014.
20. McDermott DF, Atkins MB: PD-1 as a potential target in cancer therapy, *Cancer Med* 2(5):662–673, 2013.
21. Shi F, Shi M, Zeng Z, et al.: PD-1 and PD-L1 upregulation promotes CD8(+) T-cell apoptosis and postoperative recurrence in hepatocellular carcinoma patients, *Int J Cancer* 128(4):887–896, 2011.
22. Mu CY, Huang JA, Chen Y, et al.: High expression of PD-L1 in lung cancer may contribute to poor prognosis and tumor cells immune escape through suppressing tumor infiltrating dendritic cells maturation, *Med Oncol* 28(3):682–688, 2011.
23. Nomi T, Sho M, Akahori T, et al.: Clinical significance and therapeutic potential of the programmed death-1 ligand/programmed death-1 pathway in human pancreatic cancer, *Clin Cancer Res* 13(7):2151–2157, 2007.
24. Hartley G, Faulhaber E, Caldwell A, et al.: Immune regulation of canine tumour and macrophage PD-L1 expression, *Vet Comp Oncol* 15(2):534–549, 2017.
25. Brahmer JR, Tykodi SS, Chow LQ, et al.: Safety and activity of anti-PD-L1 antibody in patients with advanced cancer, *N Engl J Med* 366(26):2455–2465, 2012.
26. Coy J, Caldwell A, Chow L, et al.: PD-1 expression by canine T cells and functional effects of PD-1 blockade, *Vet Comp Oncol* 15(4):1487–1502, 2017.
27. Maekawa N, Konnai S, Takagi S, et al.: A canine chimeric monoclonal antibody targeting PD-L1 and its clinical efficacy in canine oral malignant melanoma or undifferentiated sarcoma, *Scientific reports* 7(1):8951, 2017.
28. Jin D, Fan J, Wang L, et al.: CD73 on tumor cells impairs antitumor T-cell responses: a novel mechanism of tumor-induced immune suppression, *Cancer Res* 70(6):2245–2255, 2010.
29. Holmgaard RB, Zamarin D, Munn DH, et al.: Indoleamine 2,3-dioxygenase is a critical resistance mechanism in antitumor T cell immunotherapy targeting CTLA-4, *J Exp Med* 210(7):1389–1402, 2013.
30. Platten M, von Knebel Doeberitz N, Oezen I, et al.: Cancer Immunotherapy by Targeting IDO1/TDO and Their Downstream Effectors, *Front Immunol* 5:673, 2014.
31. Reinis M. Immunotherapy of MHC class I-deficient tumors. *Future oncology* 6(10):1577–1589
32. Garrido F, Algarra I, Garcia-Lora AM: The escape of cancer from T lymphocytes: immunoselection of MHC class I loss variants harboring structural-irreversible "hard" lesions, *Cancer immunology, immunotherapy : CII* 59(10):1601–1606, 2010.
33. Rimsza LM, Farinha P, Fuchs DA, et al.: HLA-DR protein status predicts survival in patients with diffuse large B-cell lymphoma treated on the MACOP-B chemotherapy regimen, *Leuk Lymphoma* 48(3):542–546, 2007.
34. Rimsza LM, Roberts RA, Miller TP, et al.: Loss of MHC class II gene and protein expression in diffuse large B-cell lymphoma is related to decreased tumor immunosurveillance and poor patient survival regardless of other prognostic factors: a follow-up study from the Leukemia and Lymphoma Molecular Profiling Project, *Blood* 103(11):4251–4258, 2004.
35. Rao S, Lana S, Eickhoff J, et al.: Class II MHC expression predicts survival in canine B cell lymphoma, *J Vet Intern Med* 25(5):1097–1105, 2011.
36. Kusmartsev S, Gabrilovich DI: Immature myeloid cells and cancer-associated immune suppression, *Cancer Immunol Immunother* 51(6):293–298, 2002.
37. Yang L, DeBusk LM, Fukuda K, et al.: Expansion of myeloid immune suppressor Gr+CD11b+ cells in tumor-bearing host

directly promotes tumor angiogenesis, *Cancer Cell* 6(4):409–421, 2004.

38. Hiratsuka S, Watanabe A, Aburatani H, Maru Y: Tumour-mediated upregulation of chemoattractants and recruitment of myeloid cells predetermines lung metastasis, *Nat Cell Biol* 8(12):1369–1375, 2006.

39. Kusmartsev S, Gabrilovich DI: Role of immature myeloid cells in mechanisms of immune evasion in cancer, *Cancer Immunol Immunother* 55(3):237–245, 2006.

40. Bunt SK, Yang L, Sinha P, et al.: Reduced inflammation in the tumor microenvironment delays the accumulation of myeloid-derived suppressor cells and limits tumor progression, *Cancer Res* 67(20):10019–10026, 2007.

41. Gabrilovich DI, Nagaraj S: Myeloid-derived suppressor cells as regulators of the immune system, *Nat Rev Immunol* 9(3):162–174, 2009.

42. Ostrand-Rosenberg S, Sinha P: Myeloid-derived suppressor cells: linking inflammation and cancer, *J Immunol* 182(8):4499–4506, 2009.

43. Ye XZ, Yu SC, Bian XW: Contribution of myeloid-derived suppressor cells to tumor-induced immune suppression, angiogenesis, invasion and metastasis, *J Genet Genomics* 37(7):423–430, 2010.

44. Youn JI, Gabrilovich DI: The biology of myeloid-derived suppressor cells: the blessing and the curse of morphological and functional heterogeneity, *Eur J Immunol* 40(11):2969–2975, 2010.

45. Murdoch C, Muthana M, Coffelt SB, Lewis CE: The role of myeloid cells in the promotion of tumour angiogenesis, *Nat Rev Cancer* 8(8):618–631, 2008.

46. Qian BZ, Pollard JW: Macrophage diversity enhances tumor progression and metastasis, *Cell* 141(1):39–51, 2010.

47. Almand B, Clark JI, Nikitina E, et al.: Increased production of immature myeloid cells in cancer patients: a mechanism of immunosuppression in cancer, *J Immunol* 166(1):678–689, 2001.

48. Diaz-Montero CM, Salem ML, Nishimura MI, et al.: Increased circulating myeloid-derived suppressor cells correlate with clinical cancer stage, metastatic tumor burden, and doxorubicin-cyclophosphamide chemotherapy, *Cancer Immunol Immunother* 58(1):49–59, 2009.

49. Mandruzzato S, Solito S, Falisi E, et al.: IL4 Ralpha+ myeloid-derived suppressor cell expansion in cancer patients, *J Immunol* 182(10):6562–6568, 2009.

50. Melani C, Chiodoni C, Forni G, Colombo MP: Myeloid cell expansion elicited by the progression of spontaneous mammary carcinomas in c-erbB-2 transgenic BALB/c mice suppresses immune reactivity, *Blood* 102(6):2138–2145, 2003.

51. Casacuberta-Serra S, Pares M, Golbano A, et al.: Myeloid-derived suppressor cells can be efficiently generated from human hematopoietic progenitors and peripheral blood monocytes, *Immunol Cell Biol* 95(6):538–548, 2017.

52. Bosco MC, Puppo M, Blengio F, et al.: Monocytes and dendritic cells in a hypoxic environment: Spotlights on chemotaxis and migration, *Immunobiology* 213(9-10):733–749, 2008.

53. Du R, Lu KV, Petritsch C, et al.: HIF1alpha induces the recruitment of bone marrow-derived vascular modulatory cells to regulate tumor angiogenesis and invasion, *Cancer Cell* 13(3):206–220, 2008.

54. Sawanobori Y, Ueha S, Kurachi M, et al.: Chemokine-mediated rapid turnover of myeloid-derived suppressor cells in tumor-bearing mice, *Blood* 111(12):5457–5466, 2008.

55. Yang L, Huang J, Ren X, et al.: Abrogation of TGF beta signaling in mammary carcinomas recruits Gr-1+CD11b+ myeloid cells that promote metastasis, *Cancer Cell* 13(1):23–35, 2008.

56. Liu CC, Wang YS, Lin CY, et al.: Transient downregulation of monocyte-derived dendritic-cell differentiation, function, and survival during tumoral progression and regression in an in vivo canine model of transmissible venereal tumor, *Cancer Immunol Immunother* 57(4):479–491, 2008.

57. Zhao L, Lim SY, Gordon-Weeks AN, et al.: Recruitment of a myeloid cell subset (CD11b/Gr1 mid) via CCL2/CCR2 promotes the development of colorectal cancer liver metastasis, *Hepatology (Baltimore, Md)* 57(2):829–839, 2013.

58. Liu Y, Cao X: Characteristics and significance of the pre-metastatic niche, *Cancer Cell* 30(5):668–681, 2016.

59. Alfaro C, Teijeira A, Onate C, et al.: Tumor-produced interleukin-8 attracts human myeloid-derived suppressor cells and elicits extrusion of neutrophil extracellular traps (NETs), *Clin Cancer Res* 22(15):3924–3936, 2016.

60. Zhang H, Ye YL, Li MX, et al.: CXCL2/MIF-CXCR2 signaling promotes the recruitment of myeloid-derived suppressor cells and is correlated with prognosis in bladder cancer, *Oncogene* 36(15):2095–2104, 2017.

61. Joyce JA, Pollard JW: Microenvironmental regulation of metastasis, *Nat Rev Cancer* 9(4):239–252, 2009.

62. Sinha P, Clements VK, Bunt SK, Albelda SM, Ostrand-Rosenberg S: Cross-talk between myeloid-derived suppressor cells and macrophages subverts tumor immunity toward a type 2 response, *J Immunol* 179(2):977–983, 2007.

63. Li H, Han Y, Guo Q, Zhang M, Cao X: Cancer-expanded myeloid-derived suppressor cells induce anergy of NK cells through membrane-bound TGF-beta1, *J Immunol* 182(1):240–249, 2009.

64. Miller AM, Lundberg K, Ozenci V, et al.: CD4+CD25 high T cells are enriched in the tumor and peripheral blood of prostate cancer patients, *J Immunol* 177(10):7398–7405, 2006.

65. O'Neill K, Guth A, Biller B, Elmslie R, Dow S: Changes in regulatory T cells in dogs with cancer and associations with tumor type, *J Vet Intern Med* 23(4):875–881, 2009.

66. Biller BJ, Guth A, Burton JH, Dow SW: Decreased ratio of CD8+ T cells to regulatory T cells associated with decreased survival in dogs with osteosarcoma, *J Vet Intern Med* 24(5):1118–1123, 2010.

67. Nomura T, Sakaguchi S: Naturally arising CD25+CD4+ regulatory T cells in tumor immunity, *Curr Top Microbiol Immunol* 293:287–302, 2005.

68. Fontenot JD, Rudensky AY: A well adapted regulatory contrivance: regulatory T cell development and the forkhead family transcription factor Foxp3, *Nat Immunol* 6(4):331–337, 2005.

69. Camisaschi C, Casati C, Rini F, et al.: LAG-3 expression defines a subset of CD4(+)CD25(high)Foxp3(+) regulatory T cells that are expanded at tumor sites, *J Immunol* 184(11):6545–6551, 2010.

70. Shimizu J, Yamazaki S, Takahashi T, et al.: Stimulation of CD25(+) CD4(+) regulatory T cells through GITR breaks immunological self-tolerance, *Nat Immunol* 3(2):135–142, 2002.

71. Wing K, Onishi Y, Prieto-Martin P, et al.: CTLA-4 control over Foxp3+ regulatory T cell function, *Science* 322(5899):271–275, 2008.

72. Yamaguchi T, Hirota K, Nagahama K, et al.: Control of immune responses by antigen-specific regulatory T cells expressing the folate receptor, *Immunity* 27(1):145–159, 2007.

73. Qin FX: Dynamic behavior and function of Foxp3+ regulatory T cells in tumor bearing host, *Cell Mol Immunol* 6(1):3–13, 2009.

74. Chen W, Jin W, Hardegen N, et al.: Conversion of peripheral CD4+CD25- naive T cells to CD4+CD25+ regulatory T cells by TGF-beta induction of transcription factor Foxp3, *J Exp Med* 198(12):1875–1886, 2003.

75. Chen W, Wahl SM: TGF-beta: the missing link in CD4+CD25+ regulatory T cell-mediated immunosuppression, *Cytokine Growth Factor Rev* 14(2):85–89, 2003.

76. Hawiger D, Wan YY, Eynon EE, Flavell RA: The transcription cofactor Hopx is required for regulatory T cell function in dendritic cell-mediated peripheral T cell unresponsiveness, *Nat Immunol* 11(10):962–968, 2010.

77. Huehn J, Hamann A: Homing to suppress: address codes for Treg migration, *Trends Immunol* 26(12):632–636, 2005.

78. Hoelzinger DB, Smith SE, Mirza N, Dominguez AL, Manrique SZ, Lustgarten J: Blockade of CCL1 inhibits T regulatory cell suppressive function enhancing tumor immunity without affecting T effector responses, *J Immunol* 184(12):6833–6842, 2010.

79. Curiel TJ, Coukos G, Zou L, et al.: Specific recruitment of regulatory T cells in ovarian carcinoma fosters immune privilege and predicts reduced survival, *Nat Med* 10(9):942–949, 2004.

80. Sasada T, Kimura M, Yoshida Y, Kanai M, Takabayashi A: CD4+CD25+ regulatory T cells in patients with gastrointestinal malignancies: possible involvement of regulatory T cells in disease progression, *Cancer* 98(5):1089–1099, 2003.

81. Turk MJ, Guevara-Patino JA, Rizzuto GA, et al.: Concomitant tumor immunity to a poorly immunogenic melanoma is prevented by regulatory T cells, *J Exp Med* 200(6):771–782, 2004.

82. Viguier M, Lemaitre F, Verola O, et al.: Foxp3 expressing CD4+CD25(high) regulatory T cells are overrepresented in human metastatic melanoma lymph nodes and inhibit the function of infiltrating T cells, *J Immunol* 173(2):1444–1453, 2004.

83. Biller BJ, Elmslie RE, Burnett RC, et al.: Use of FoxP3 expression to identify regulatory T cells in healthy dogs and dogs with cancer, *Vet Immunol Immunopathol* 116(1-2):69–78, 2007.

84. Teng MW, Swann JB, von Scheidt B, et al.: Multiple antitumor mechanisms downstream of prophylactic regulatory T-cell depletion, *Cancer Res* 70(7):2665–2674, 2010.

85. Piconese S, Valzasina B, Colombo MP: OX40 triggering blocks suppression by regulatory T cells and facilitates tumor rejection, *J Exp Med* 205(4):825–839, 2008.

86. Berraondo P, Nouze C, Preville X, et al.: Eradication of large tumors in mice by a tritherapy targeting the innate, adaptive, and regulatory components of the immune system, *Cancer Res* 67(18):8847–8855, 2007.

87. Matar P, Rozados VR, Gonzalez AD, et al.: Mechanism of antimetastatic immunopotentiation by low-dose cyclophosphamide, *Eur J Cancer* 36(8):1060–1066, 2000.

88. Ghiringhelli F, Menard C, Puig PE, et al.: Metronomic cyclophosphamide regimen selectively depletes CD4+CD25+ regulatory T cells and restores T and NK effector functions in end stage cancer patients, *Cancer immunol immunother CII* 56(5):641–648, 2007.

89. Mitchell L, Thamm DH, Biller BJ: Clinical and immunomodulatory effects of toceranib combined with low-dose cyclophosphamide in dogs with cancer, *J Vet Intern Med* 26(2):355–362, 2012.

90. Hoffmann TK, Muller-Berghaus J, Ferris RL, et al.: Alterations in the frequency of dendritic cell subsets in the peripheral circulation of patients with squamous cell carcinomas of the head and neck, *Clin Cancer Res* 8(6):1787–1793, 2002.

91. Pinzon-Charry A, Ho CS, Laherty R, et al.: A population of HLA-DR+ immature cells accumulates in the blood dendritic cell compartment of patients with different types of cancer, *Neoplasia* 7(12):1112–1122, 2005.

92. Steinman RM, Hawiger D, Nussenzweig MC: Tolerogenic dendritic cells, *Annu Rev Immunol* 21:685–711, 2003.

93. Fuchs EJ, Matzinger P: Is cancer dangerous to the immune system? *Semin Immunol* 8(5):271–280, 1996.

94. Enk AH, Jonuleit H, Saloga J, Knop J: Dendritic cells as mediators of tumor-induced tolerance in metastatic melanoma, *Int J Cancer* 73(3):309–316, 1997.

95. Nestle FO, Burg G, Fah J, et al.: Human sunlight-induced basal-cell-carcinoma-associated dendritic cells are deficient in T cell costimulatory molecules and are impaired as antigen-presenting cells, *Am J Pathol* 150(2):641–651, 1997.

96. Chaux P, Favre N, Martin M, Martin F: Tumor-infiltrating dendritic cells are defective in their antigen-presenting function and inducible B7 expression in rats, *Int J Cancer* 72(4):619–624, 1997.

97. Ishida T, Oyama T, Carbone DP, Gabrilovich DI: Defective function of Langerhans cells in tumor-bearing animals is the result of defective maturation from hemopoietic progenitors, *J Immunol* 161(9):4842–4851, 1998.

98. Almand B, Resser JR, Lindman B, et al.: Clinical significance of defective dendritic cell differentiation in cancer, *Clin Cancer Res* 6(5):1755–1766, 2000.

99. Troy AJ, Summers KL, Davidson PJ, et al.: Minimal recruitment and activation of dendritic cells within renal cell carcinoma, *Clin Cancer Res* 4(3):585–593, 1998.

100. Cheng P, Corzo CA, Luetteke N, et al.: Inhibition of dendritic cell differentiation and accumulation of myeloid-derived suppressor cells in cancer is regulated by S100A9 protein, *J Exp Med* 205(10):2235–2249, 2008.

101. Herber DL, Cao W, Nefedova Y, et al.: Lipid accumulation and dendritic cell dysfunction in cancer, *Nat Med* 16(8):880–886, 2010.

102. Hartmann E, Wollenberg B, Rothenfusser S, et al.: Identification and functional analysis of tumor-infiltrating plasmacytoid dendritic cells in head and neck cancer, *Cancer Res* 63(19):6478–6487, 2003.

103. Gerlini G, Tun-Kyi A, Dudli C, et al.: Metastatic melanoma secreted IL-10 down-regulates CD1 molecules on dendritic cells in metastatic tumor lesions, *Am J Pathol* 165(6):1853–1863, 2004.

104. Gabrilovich DI, Chen HL, Girgis KR, et al.: Production of vascular endothelial growth factor by human tumors inhibits the functional maturation of dendritic cells, *Nat Med* 2(10):1096–1103, 1996.

105. Zhang M, Tang H, Guo Z, et al.: Splenic stroma drives mature dendritic cells to differentiate into regulatory dendritic cells, *Nat Immunol* 5(11):1124–1133, 2004.

106. Lin WW, Karin M: A cytokine-mediated link between innate immunity, inflammation, and cancer, *J Clin Invest* 117(5):1175–1183, 2007.

107. Ridge J, Terle DA, Dragunsky E, Levenbook I: Effects of gamma-IFN and NGF on subpopulations in a human neuroblastoma cell line: flow cytometric and morphologic analysis, *Vitro Cell Dev Biol Anim* 32(4):238–248, 1996.

108. Maloy KJ, Salaun L, Cahill R, et al.: CD4+CD25+ T(R) cells suppress innate immune pathology through cytokine-dependent mechanisms, *J Exp Med* 197(1):111–119, 2003.

109. Sredni B, Weil M, Khomenok G, et al.: Ammonium trichloro(dioxoethylene-o,o')tellurate (AS101) sensitizes tumors to chemotherapy by inhibiting the tumor interleukin 10 autocrine loop, *Cancer Res* 64(5):1843–1852, 2004.

110. Ebrahimi B, Tucker SL, Li D, et al.: Cytokines in pancreatic carcinoma: correlation with phenotypic characteristics and prognosis, *Cancer* 101(12):2727–2736, 2004.

111. Ozdemir F, Aydin F, Yilmaz M, et al.: The effects of IL-2, IL-6 and IL-10 levels on prognosis in patients with aggressive non-Hodgkin's lymphoma (NHL), *J Exp Clin Cancer Res* 23(3):485–488, 2004.

112. Lech-Maranda E, Bienvenu J, Michallet AS, et al.: Elevated IL-10 plasma levels correlate with poor prognosis in diffuse large B-cell lymphoma, *Eur Cytokine Netw* 17(1):60–66, 2006.

113. Becker C, Fantini MC, Neurath MF: TGF-beta as a T cell regulator in colitis and colon cancer, *Cytokine Growth Factor Rev* 17(1-2):97–106, 2006.

114. Ghiringhelli F, Puig PE, Roux S, et al.: Tumor cells convert immature myeloid dendritic cells into TGF-beta-secreting cells inducing CD4+CD25+ regulatory T cell proliferation, *J Exp Med* 202(7):919–929, 2005.

115. Derynck R, Akhurst RJ, Balmain A: TGF-beta signaling in tumor suppression and cancer progression, *Nat Genet* 29(2):117–129, 2001.

116. Luo JL, Maeda S, Hsu LC, et al.: Inhibition of NF-kappaB in cancer cells converts inflammation- induced tumor growth mediated by TNFalpha to TRAIL-mediated tumor regression, *Cancer Cell* 6(3):297–305, 2004.

117. Elgert KD, Alleva DG, Mullins DW: Tumor-induced immune dysfunction: the macrophage connection, *J Leukoc Biol* 64(3):275–290, 1998.

118. Catchpole B, Gould SM, Kellett-Gregory LM, Dobson JM: Immunosuppressive cytokines in the regional lymph node of a dog suffering from oral malignant melanoma, *J Small Anim Pract* 43(10):464–467, 2002.

119. Richardson MA, Ramirez T, Russell NC, Moye LA: Coley toxins immunotherapy: a retrospective review, *Altern Ther Health Med* 5(3):42–47, 1999.

120. Alexandroff AB, Jackson AM, O'Donnell MA, James K: BCG immunotherapy of bladder cancer: 20 years on, *Lancet* 353(9165):1689–1694, 1999.

121. van der Meijden AP: Non-specific immunotherapy with bacille Calmette-Guerin (BCG), *Clin Exp Immunol* 123(2):179–180, 2001.
122. Vita F, Siracusano S, Abbate R, et al.: BCG prophylaxis in bladder cancer produces activation of recruited neutrophils, *Can J Urol* 18(1):5517–5523, 2011.
123. Ludwig AT, Moore JM, Luo Y, et al.: Tumor necrosis factor-related apoptosis-inducing ligand: a novel mechanism for Bacillus Calmette-Guerin-induced antitumor activity, *Cancer Res* 64(10):3386–3390, 2004.
124. Herr HW, Morales A: History of bacillus Calmette-Guerin and bladder cancer: an immunotherapy success story, *J Urol* 179(1):53–56, 2008.
125. Klein WR, Rutten VP, Steerenberg PA, Ruitenberg EJ: The present status of BCG treatment in the veterinary practice, *Vivo* 5(6):605–608, 1991.
126. Debruyne FM, van der Meijden AP, Schreinemachers LM, et al.: Intravesical and intradermal BCG-RIVM application: a toxicity study, *Prog Clin Biol Res* 185B:151–159, 1985.
127. Knapp DW, Glickman NW, Denicola DB, Bonney PL, Lin TL, Glickman LT: Naturally-occurring canine transitional cell carcinoma of the urinary bladder: a relevant model of human invasive bladder cancer, *Urol Oncol* 5(2):47–59, 2000.
128. Mukaratirwa S, Chitanga S, Chimatira T, et al.: Combination therapy using intratumoral bacillus Calmette-Guerin (BCG) and vincristine in dogs with transmissible venereal tumours: therapeutic efficacy and histological changes, *J S Afr Vet Assoc* 80(2):92–96, 2009.
129. Henry CJ, Downing S, Rosenthal RC, et al.: Evaluation of a novel immunomodulator composed of human chorionic gonadotropin and bacillus Calmette-Guerin for treatment of canine mast cell tumors in clinically affected dogs, *Am J Vet Res* 68(11):1246–1251, 2007.
130. Lipton A, Harvey HA, Balch CM, et al.: *Corynebacterium parvum* versus bacille Calmette-Guerin adjuvant immunotherapy of stage II malignant melanoma, *J Clin Oncol* 9(7):1151–1156, 1991.
131. MacEwen EG, Patnaik AK, Harvey HJ, et al.: Canine oral melanoma: comparison of surgery versus surgery plus *Corynebacterium parvum*, *Cancer Invest* 4(5):397–402, 1986.
132. Misdorp W: Incomplete surgery, local immunostimulation, and recurrence of some tumour types in dogs and cats, *Vet Q* 9(3):279–286, 1987.
133. Luo X, Li Z, Lin S, et al.: Antitumor effect of VNP20009, an attenuated *Salmonella*, in murine tumor models, *Oncol Res* 12(11-12):501–508, 2001.
134. Leschner S, Westphal K, Dietrich N, et al.: Tumor invasion of *Salmonella enterica* serovar *typhimurium* is accompanied by strong hemorrhage promoted by TNF-alpha, *PLoS One* 4(8):e6692, 2009.
135. Saccheri F, Pozzi C, Avogadri F, et al.: Bacteria-induced gap junctions in tumors favor antigen cross-presentation and antitumor immunity, *Sci Transl Med* 2(44):44ra57, 2010.
136. Toso JF, Gill VJ, Hwu P, et al.: Phase I study of the intravenous administration of attenuated *Salmonella typhimurium* to patients with metastatic melanoma, *J Clin Oncol* 20(1):142–152, 2002.
137. Thamm DH, Kurzman ID, King I, et al.: Systemic administration of an attenuated, tumor-targeting *Salmonella typhimurium* to dogs with spontaneous neoplasia: phase I evaluation, *Clin Cancer Res* 11(13):4827–4834, 2005.
138. Kleinerman ES, Jia SF, Griffin J, et al.: Phase II study of liposomal muramyl tripeptide in osteosarcoma: the cytokine cascade and monocyte activation following administration, *J Clin Oncol* 10(8):1310–1316, 1992.
139. Asano T, Kleinerman ES: Liposome-encapsulated MTP-PE: a novel biologic agent for cancer therapy, *J Immunother Emphasis Tumor Immunol* 14(4):286–292, 1993.
140. Gianan MA, Kleinerman ES: Liposomal muramyl tripeptide (CGP 19835A lipid) therapy for resectable melanoma in patients who were at high risk for relapse: an update, *Cancer Biother Radiopharm* 13(5):363–368, 1998.
141. Anderson PM, Tomaras M, McConnell K: Mifamurtide in osteosarcoma—a practical review, *Drugs Today (Barc)* 46(5):327–337, 2010.
142. Kurzman ID, MacEwen EG, Rosenthal RC, et al.: Adjuvant therapy for osteosarcoma in dogs: results of randomized clinical trials using combined liposome-encapsulated muramyl tripeptide and cisplatin, *Clin Cancer Res* 1(12):1595–1601, 1995.
143. Fox LE, King RR, Shi F, et al.: Induction of serum tumor necrosis factor-alpha and interleukin-6 activity by liposome-encapsulated muramyl tripeptide-phosphatidylethanolamine (L-MTP-PE) in normal cats, *Cancer Biother* 9(4):329–340, 1994.
144. Vail DM, MacEwen EG, Kurzman ID, et al.: Liposome-encapsulated muramyl tripeptide phosphatidylethanolamine adjuvant immunotherapy for splenic hemangiosarcoma in the dog: a randomized multi-institutional clinical trial, *Clin Cancer Res* 1(10):1165–1170, 1995.
145. MacEwen EG, Kurzman ID, Vail DM, et al.: Adjuvant therapy for melanoma in dogs: results of randomized clinical trials using surgery, liposome-encapsulated muramyl tripeptide, and granulocyte macrophage colony-stimulating factor, *Clin Cancer Res* 5(12):4249–4258, 1999.
146. Teske E, Rutteman GR, vd Ingh TS, et al.: Liposome-encapsulated muramyl tripeptide phosphatidylethanolamine (L-MTP-PE): a randomized clinical trial in dogs with mammary carcinoma, *Anticancer Res* 18(2A):1015–1019, 1998.
147. MacEwen EG, Kurzman ID, Rosenthal RC, et al.: Therapy for osteosarcoma in dogs with intravenous injection of liposome-encapsulated muramyl tripeptide, *J Natl Cancer Inst* 81(12):935–938, 1989.
148. Dow SW, Fradkin LG, Liggitt DH, Willson AP, Heath TD, Potter TA: Lipid-DNA complexes induce potent activation of innate immune responses and antitumor activity when administered intravenously, *J Immunol* 163(3):1552–1561, 1999.
149. Zaks K, Jordan M, Guth A, et al.: Efficient immunization and cross-priming by vaccine adjuvants containing TLR3 or TLR9 agonists complexed to cationic liposomes, *J Immunol* 176(12), 2006. 7335–4735.
150. Hemmi H, Takeuchi O, Kawai T, et al.: A Toll-like receptor recognizes bacterial DNA, *Nature* 408(6813):740–745, 2000.
151. Sellins K, Fradkin L, Liggitt D, Dow S: Type I interferons potently suppress gene expression following gene delivery using liposome(-) DNA complexes, *Mol Ther* 12(3):451–459, 2005.
152. Dow S, Elmslie R, Kurzman I, et al.: Phase I study of liposome-DNA complexes encoding the interleukin-2 gene in dogs with osteosarcoma lung metastases, *Hum Gene Ther* 16(8):937–946, 2005.
153. Kamstock D, Guth A, Elmslie R, et al.: Liposome-DNA complexes infused intravenously inhibit tumor angiogenesis and elicit antitumor activity in dogs with soft tissue sarcoma, *Cancer Gene Ther* 13(3):306–317, 2006.
154. MacNeill AL: On the potential of oncolytic virotherapy for the treatment of canine cancers, *Oncolytic Virother* 4:95–107, 2015.
155. Smith BF, Curiel DT, Ternovoi VV, et al.: Administration of a conditionally replicative oncolytic canine adenovirus in normal dogs, *Cancer Biother Radiopharm* 21(6):601–606, 2006.
156. Le LP, Rivera AA, Glasgow JN, et al.: Infectivity enhancement for adenoviral transduction of canine osteosarcoma cells, *Gene Ther* 13(5):389–399, 2006.
157. Hemminki A, Kanerva A, Kremer EJ, et al.: A canine conditionally replicating adenovirus for evaluating oncolytic virotherapy in a syngeneic animal model, *Mol Ther* 7(2):163–173, 2003.
158. Suter SE, Chein MB, von Messling V, et al.: In vitro canine distemper virus infection of canine lymphoid cells: a prelude to oncolytic therapy for lymphoma, *Clin Cancer Res* 11(4):1579–1587, 2005.
159. Gentschev I, Ehrig K, Donat U, et al.: Significant growth inhibition of canine mammary carcinoma xenografts following treatment with oncolytic vaccinia virus GLV-1h68, *J Oncol* 736907, 2010.

160. Gentschev I, Adelfinger M, Josupeit R, et al.: Preclinical evaluation of oncolytic vaccinia virus for therapy of canine soft tissue sarcoma, *PLoS One* 7(5):e37239, 2012.

161. Patil SS, Gentschev I, Adelfinger M, et al.: Virotherapy of canine tumors with oncolytic vaccinia virus GLV-1h109 expressing an anti-VEGF single-chain antibody, *PLoS One* 7(10):e47472, 2012.

162. Adelfinger M, Bessler S, Frentzen A, et al.: Preclinical testing oncolytic vaccinia virus strain GLV-5b451 expressing an anti-VEGF single-chain antibody for canine cancer therapy, *Viruses* 7(7):4075–4092, 2015.

163. Sanchez D, Pelayo R, Medina LA, et al.: Newcastle disease virus: potential therapeutic application for human and canine lymphoma, *Viruses* 8(1), 2015.

164. Naik S, Galyon GD, Jenks NJ, et al.: Comparative oncology evaluation of intravenous recombinant oncolytic vesicular stomatitis virus therapy in spontaneous canine cancer, *Mol Cancer Ther* 17(1):316–326, 2018.

165. Andersen BM, Pluhar GE, Seiler CE, et al.: Vaccination for invasive canine meningioma induces in situ production of antibodies capable of antibody-dependent cell-mediated cytotoxicity, *Cancer Res* 73(10):2987–2997, 2013.

166. Gill VL, Bergman PJ, Baer KE, et al.: Use of imiquimod 5% cream (Aldara) in cats with multicentric squamous cell carcinoma in situ: 12 cases (2002-2005), *Vet Comp Oncol* 6(1):55–64, 2008.

167. Fogler WE, Fidler IJ: Comparative interaction of free and liposome-encapsulated nor-muramyl dipeptide or muramyl tripeptide phosphatidylethanolamine (^{3}H-labelled) with human blood monocytes, *Int J Immunopharmacol* 9(2):141–150, 1987.

168. Siegel JP, Puri RK: Interleukin-2 toxicity, *J Clin Oncol* 9(4):694–704, 1991.

169. Vial T, Descotes J: Clinical toxicity of interleukin-2, *Drug Saf* 7(6):417–433, 1992.

170. Margolin KA, Rayner AA, Hawkins MJ, et al.: Interleukin-2 and lymphokine-activated killer cell therapy of solid tumors: analysis of toxicity and management guidelines, *J Clin Oncol* 7(4):486–498, 1989.

171. Helfand SC, Soergel SA, MacWilliams PS, et al.: Clinical and immunological effects of human recombinant interleukin-2 given by repetitive weekly infusion to normal dogs, *Cancer Immunol Immunother* 39(2):84–92, 1994.

172. Funk J, Schmitz G, Failing K, Burkhardt E: Natural killer (NK) and lymphokine-activated killer (LAK) cell functions from healthy dogs and 29 dogs with a variety of spontaneous neoplasms, *Cancer Immunol Immunother* 54(1):87–92, 2005.

173. Khanna C, Anderson PM, Hasz DE, et al.: Interleukin-2 liposome inhalation therapy is safe and effective for dogs with spontaneous pulmonary metastases, *Cancer* 79(7):1409–1421, 1997.

174. Jourdier TM, Moste C, Bonnet MC, et al.: Local immunotherapy of spontaneous feline fibrosarcomas using recombinant poxviruses expressing interleukin 2 (IL2), *Gene Ther* 10(26):2126–2132, 2003.

175. Quintin-Colonna F, Devauchelle P, Fradelizi D, et al.: Gene therapy of spontaneous canine melanoma and feline fibrosarcoma by intratumoral administration of histoincompatible cells expressing human interleukin-2, *Gene Ther* 3(12):1104–1112

176. Jahnke A, Hirschberger J, Fischer C, et al.: Intra-tumoral gene delivery of feIL-2, feIFN-gamma and feGM-CSF using magnetofection as a neoadjuvant treatment option for feline fibrosarcomas: a phase-I study, *J Vet Med A Physiol Pathol Clin Med* 54(10):599–606, 2007.

177. Cutrera J, Torrero M, Shiomitsu K, et al.: Intratumoral bleomycin and IL-12 electrochemogenetherapy for treating head and neck tumors in dogs, *Methods Mol Biol* 423:319–325, 2008.

178. Siddiqui F, Li CY, Zhang X, et al.: Characterization of a recombinant adenovirus vector encoding heat-inducible feline interleukin-12 for use in hyperthermia-induced gene-therapy, *Int J Hyperthermia* 22(2):117–134, 2006.

179. Chuang TF, Lee SC, Liao KW, et al.: Electroporation-mediated IL-12 gene therapy in a transplantable canine cancer model, *Int J Cancer* 125(3):698–707, 2009.

180. Pavlin D, Cemazar M, Cor A, et al.: Electrogene therapy with interleukin-12 in canine mast cell tumors, *Radiol Oncol* 45(1):31–39, 2011.

181. Cicchelero L, Denies S, Haers H, et al.: Intratumoural interleukin 12 gene therapy stimulates the immune system and decreases angiogenesis in dogs with spontaneous cancer, *Vet Comp Oncol* 15(4):1187–1205, 2017.

182. Cicchelero L, Denies S, Vanderperren K, et al.: Immunological, anti-angiogenic and clinical effects of intratumoral interleukin 12 electrogene therapy combined with metronomic cyclophosphamide in dogs with spontaneous cancer: a pilot study, *Cancer Lett* 400:205–218, 2017.

183. Marks-Konczalik J, Dubois S, Losi JM, et al.: IL-2-induced activation-induced cell death is inhibited in IL-15 transgenic mice, *Proc Natl Acad Sci U S A* 97(21):11445–11450, 2000.

184. Zhang X, Sun S, Hwang I, et al.: Potent and selective stimulation of memory-phenotype CD8+ T cells in vivo by IL-15, *Immunity* 8(5):591–599, 1998.

185. Antony PA, Restifo NP: CD4+CD25+ T regulatory cells, immunotherapy of cancer, and interleukin-2, *J Immunother* 28(2):120–128, 2005.

186. Waldmann TA, Lugli E, Roederer M, et al.: Safety (toxicity), pharmacokinetics, immunogenicity, and impact on elements of the normal immune system of recombinant human IL-15 in rhesus macaques, *Blood* 117(18):4787–4795, 2011.

187. Chou PC, Chuang TF, Jan TR, et al.: Effects of immunotherapy of IL-6 and IL-15 plasmids on transmissible venereal tumor in beagles, *Vet Immunol Immunopathol* 130(1-2):25–34, 2009.

188. Lee SH, Shin DJ, Kim SK: Generation of recombinant canine interleukin-15 and evaluation of its effects on the proliferation and function of canine NK cells, *Vet Immunol Immunopathol* 165(1-2):1–13, 2015.

189. Streck CJ, Zhang Y, Miyamoto R, et al.: Restriction of neuroblastoma angiogenesis and growth by interferon-alpha/beta, *Surgery* 136(2):183–189, 2004.

190. Folkman J: Successful treatment of an angiogenic disease, *N Engl J Med* 320(18):1211–1212, 1989.

191. Coates A, Rallings M, Hersey P, Swanson C: Phase-II study of recombinant alpha 2-interferon in advanced malignant melanoma, *J Interferon Res* 6(1):1–4, 1986.

192. Rosenthal MA, Cox K, Raghavan D, et al.: Phase II clinical trial of recombinant alpha-2 interferon for biopsy-proven metastatic or recurrent renal carcinoma, *Br J Urol* 69(5):491–494, 1992.

193. Zeidner NS, Mathiason-DuBard CK, Hoover EA: Reversal of feline leukemia virus infection by adoptive transfer of activated T lymphocytes, interferon alpha, and zidovudine, *Semin Vet Med Surg (Small Anim)* 10(4):256–266, 1995.

194. Penzo C, Ross M, Muirhead R, et al.: Effect of recombinant feline interferon-omega alone and in combination with chemotherapeutic agents on putative tumour-initiating cells and daughter cells derived from canine and feline mammary tumours, *Vet Comp Oncol* 7(4):222–229, 2009.

195. Whitley EM, Bird AC, Zucker KE, Wolfe LG: Modulation by canine interferon-gamma of major histocompatibility complex and tumor-associated antigen expression in canine mammary tumor and melanoma cell lines, *Anticancer Res* 15(3):923–929, 1995.

196. Hsiao YW, Liao KW, Chung TF, et al.: Interactions of host IL-6 and IFN-gamma and cancer-derived TGF-beta1 on MHC molecule expression during tumor spontaneous regression, *Cancer Immunol Immunother* 57(7):1091–1104, 2008.

197. Mito K, Sugiura K, Ueda K, et al.: IFN{gamma} markedly cooperates with intratumoral dendritic cell vaccine in dog tumor models, *Cancer Res* 70(18):7093–7101, 2010.

198. Pluhar GE, Grogan PT, Seiler C, et al.: Anti-tumor immune response correlates with neurological symptoms in a dog with spontaneous astrocytoma treated by gene and vaccine therapy, *Vaccine* 28(19):3371–3378, 2010.

199. Cheever MA, Allison JP, Ferris AS, et al.: The prioritization of cancer antigens: a national cancer institute pilot project for the acceleration of translational research, *Clin Cancer Res* 15(17):5323–5337, 2009.

200. Smyth MJ, Dunn GP, Schreiber RD: Cancer immunosurveillance and immunoediting: the roles of immunity in suppressing tumor development and shaping tumor immunogenicity, *Adv Immunol* 90:1–50, 2006.

201. Whiteside TL: Immune responses to malignancies, *J Allergy Clin Immunol* 125(2 Suppl 2):S272–283, 2010.

202. U'Ren LW, Biller BJ, Elmslie RE, et al.: Evaluation of a novel tumor vaccine in dogs with hemangiosarcoma, *J Vet Intern Med* 21(1):113–120, 2007.

203. Hogge GS, Burkholder JK, Culp J, et al.: Preclinical development of human granulocyte-macrophage colony-stimulating factor-transfected melanoma cell vaccine using established canine cell lines and normal dogs, *Cancer Gene Ther* 6(1):26–36, 1999.

204. Turek MM, Thamm DH, Mitzey A, et al.: Human granulocyte-macrophage colony-stimulating factor DNA cationic-lipid complexed autologous tumour cell vaccination in the treatment of canine B-cell multicentric lymphoma, *Vet Comp Oncol* 5(4):219–231, 2007.

205. Alexander AN, Huelsmeyer MK, Mitzey A, et al.: Development of an allogeneic whole-cell tumor vaccine expressing xenogeneic gp100 and its implementation in a phase II clinical trial in canine patients with malignant melanoma, *Cancer Immunol Immunother* 55(4):433–442, 2006.

206. Sorenmo KU, Krick E, Coughlin CM, et al.: CD40-activated B cell cancer vaccine improves second clinical remission and survival in privately owned dogs with non-Hodgkin's lymphoma, *PLoS One* 6(8):e24167, 2011.

207. Mutwiri G, Pontarollo R, Babiuk S, et al.: Biological activity of immunostimulatory CpG DNA motifs in domestic animals, *Vet Immunol Immunopathol* 91(2):89–103, 2003.

208. Liu MA: DNA vaccines: an historical perspective and view to the future, *Immunol Rev* 239(1):62–84, 2011.

209. Bergman PJ, Camps-Palau MA, McKnight JA, et al.: Development of a xenogeneic DNA vaccine program for canine malignant melanoma at the Animal Medical Center, *Vaccine* 24(21):4582–4585, 2006.

210. Liao JC, Gregor P, Wolchok JD, et al.: Vaccination with human tyrosinase DNA induces antibody responses in dogs with advanced melanoma, *Cancer Immun* 6(8), 2006.

211. Bergman PJ, McKnight J, Novosad A, et al.: Long-term survival of dogs with advanced malignant melanoma after DNA vaccination with xenogeneic human tyrosinase: a phase I trial, *Clin Cancer Res* 9(4):1284–1290, 2003.

212. Goubier A, Fuhrmann L, Forest L, et al.: Superiority of needle-free transdermal plasmid delivery for the induction of antigen-specific IFNgamma T cell responses in the dog, *Vaccine* 26(18):2186–2190, 2008.

213. Bergman PJ: Cancer immunotherapy, *Vet Clin North Am Small Anim Pract* 40(3):507–518, 2010.

214. Gavazza A, Lubas G, Fridman A, et al.: Safety and efficacy of a genetic vaccine targeting telomerase plus chemotherapy for the therapy of canine B-cell lymphoma, *Hum Gene Ther* 24(8):728–738, 2013.

215. Peruzzi D, Gavazza A, Mesiti G, et al.: A vaccine targeting telomerase enhances survival of dogs affected by B-cell lymphoma, *Mol Ther* 18(8):1559–1567, 2010.

216. von Mehren M, Arlen P, Tsang KY, et al.: Pilot study of a dual gene recombinant avipox vaccine containing both carcinoembryonic antigen (CEA) and B7.1 transgenes in patients with recurrent CEA-expressing adenocarcinomas, *Clin Cancer Res* 6(6):2219–2228, 2000.

217. Kaufman HL, Lenz HJ, Marshall J, et al.: Combination chemotherapy and ALVAC-CEA/B7.1 vaccine in patients with metastatic colorectal cancer, *Clin Cancer Res* 14(15):4843–4849, 2008.

218. Hofbauer GF, Baur T, Bonnet MC, et al.: Clinical phase I intratumoral administration of two recombinant ALVAC canarypox viruses expressing human granulocyte-macrophage colony-stimulating factor or interleukin-2: the transgene determines the composition of the inflammatory infiltrate, *Melanoma Res* 18(2):104–111, 2008.

219. Spaner DE, Astsaturov I, Vogel T, et al.: Enhanced viral and tumor immunity with intranodal injection of canary pox viruses expressing the melanoma antigen, gp100, *Cancer* 106(4):890–899, 2006.

220. Lech PJ, Russell SJ: Use of attenuated paramyxoviruses for cancer therapy, *Expert Rev Vaccines* 9(11):1275–1302, 2010.

221. Melief CJ: Cancer immunotherapy by dendritic cells, *Immunity* 29(3):372–383, 2008.

222. Palucka K, Ueno H, Roberts L, et al.: Dendritic cells: are they clinically relevant? *Cancer J* 16(4):318–324, 2010.

223. Palucka K, Ueno H, Banchereau J: Recent developments in cancer vaccines, *J Immunol* 186(3):1325–1331, 2011.

224. Slingluff Jr CL, Petroni GR, Yamshchikov GV, et al.: Clinical and immunologic results of a randomized phase II trial of vaccination using four melanoma peptides either administered in granulocyte-macrophage colony-stimulating factor in adjuvant or pulsed on dendritic cells, *J Clin Oncol* 21(21):4016–4026, 2003.

225. Giermasz AS, Urban JA, Nakamura Y, et al.: Type-1 polarized dendritic cells primed for high IL-12 production show enhanced activity as cancer vaccines, *Cancer Immunol Immunother* 58(8):1329–1336, 2009.

226. Gyorffy S, Rodriguez-Lecompte JC, Woods JP, et al.: Bone marrow-derived dendritic cell vaccination of dogs with naturally occurring melanoma by using human gp100 antigen, *J Vet Intern Med* 19(1):56–63, 2005.

227. Tamura K, Yamada M, Isotani M, et al.: Induction of dendritic cell-mediated immune responses against canine malignant melanoma cells, *Vet J* 175(1):126–129, 2008.

228. Bird RC, Deinnocentes P, Church Bird AE, et al.: An autologous dendritic cell canine mammary tumor hybrid-cell fusion vaccine, *Cancer Immunol Immunother* 60(1):87–97, 2011.

229. Kohler G, Milstein C: Continuous cultures of fused cells secreting antibody of predefined specificity, *Nature* 256(5517):495–497, 1975.

230. Osbourn J, Jermutus L, Duncan A: Current methods for the generation of human antibodies for the treatment of autoimmune diseases, *Drug Discov Today* 8(18):845–851, 2003.

231. Abes R, Teillaud JL: Modulation of tumor immunity by therapeutic monoclonal antibodies, *Cancer Metastasis Rev* 30(1):111–124, 2011.

232. Paoloni M, Mazcko C, Selting K, et al.: Defining the pharmacodynamic profile and therapeutic index of NHS-IL12 immunocytokine in dogs with malignant melanoma, *PLoS One* 10(6):e0129954, 2015.

233. Rosenberg SA, Yang JC, Restifo NP: Cancer immunotherapy: moving beyond current vaccines, *Nat Med* 10(9):909–915, 2004.

234. Gattinoni L, Finkelstein SE, Klebanoff CA, et al.: Removal of homeostatic cytokine sinks by lymphodepletion enhances the efficacy of adoptively transferred tumor-specific CD8+ T cells, *J Exp Med* 202(7):907–912, 2005.

235. Paulos CM, Wrzesinski C, Kaiser A, et al.: Microbial translocation augments the function of adoptively transferred self/tumor-specific CD8+ T cells via TLR4 signaling, *J Clin Invest* 117(8):2197–2204, 2007.

236. Dudley ME, Yang JC, Sherry R, et al.: Adoptive cell therapy for patients with metastatic melanoma: evaluation of intensive myeloablative chemoradiation preparative regimens, *J Clin Oncol* 26(32):5233–5239, 2008.

237. Quezada SA, Simpson TR, Peggs KS, et al.: Tumor-reactive CD4(+) T cells develop cytotoxic activity and eradicate large

established melanoma after transfer into lymphopenic hosts, *J Exp Med* 207(3):637–650, 2010.

238. Xie Y, Akpinarli A, Maris C, et al.: Naive tumor-specific CD4(+) T cells differentiated in vivo eradicate established melanoma, *J Exp Med* 207(3):651–667, 2010.

239. Corthay A, Lorvik KB, Bogen B: Is secretion of tumour-specific antigen important for cancer eradication by CD4(+) T cells?—Implications for cancer immunotherapy by adoptive T cell transfer, *Scand J Immunol* 73(6):527–530, 2011.

240. Hanson HL, Donermeyer DL, Ikeda H, et al.: Eradication of established tumors by CD8+ T cell adoptive immunotherapy, *Immunity* 13(2):265–276, 2000.

241. Klebanoff CA, Finkelstein SE, Surman DR, et al.: IL-15 enhances the in vivo antitumor activity of tumor-reactive CD8+ T cells, *Proc Natl Acad Sci U S A* 101(7):1969–1974, 2004.

242. May KF, Chen L, Zheng P, Liu Y: Anti-4-1BB monoclonal antibody enhances rejection of large tumor burden by promoting survival but not clonal expansion of tumor-specific CD8+ T cells, *Cancer Res* 62(12):3459–3465, 2002.

243. Casucci M, Bondanza A, Falcone L, et al.: Genetic engineering of T cells for the immunotherapy of haematological malignancies, *Tissue Antigens* 79(1):4–14, 2012.

244. Cruz CR, Micklethwaite KP, Savoldo B, et al.: Infusion of donor-derived CD19-redirected virus-specific T cells for B-cell malignancies relapsed after allogeneic stem cell transplant: a phase 1 study, *Blood* 122(17):2965–2973, 2013.

245. Riches JC, Gribben JG: Advances in chimeric antigen receptor immunotherapy for chronic lymphocytic leukemia, *Discov Med* 16(90):295–302, 2013.

246. Cheadle EJ, Gornall H, Baldan V, et al.: CAR T cells: driving the road from the laboratory to the clinic, *Immunol Rev* 257(1):91–106, 2014.

247. Cieri N, Mastaglio S, Oliveira G, et al.: Adoptive immunotherapy with genetically modified lymphocytes in allogeneic stem cell transplantation, *Immunol Rev* 257(1):165–180, 2014.

248. Mata M, Vera JF, Gerken C, et al.: Toward immunotherapy with redirected T cells in a large animal model: ex vivo activation, expansion, and genetic modification of canine T cells, *J Immunother* 37(8):407–415, 2014.

249. Panjwani MK, Smith JB, Schutsky K, et al.: Feasibility and safety of RNA-transfected CD20-specific chimeric antigen receptor T cells in dogs with spontaneous B cell lymphoma, *Mol Ther* 24(9):1602–1614, 2016.

250. Yannelli JR, Wroblewski JM: On the road to a tumor cell vaccine: 20 years of cellular immunotherapy, *Vaccine* 23(1):97–113, 2004.

251. Blakeslee J, Noll G, Olsen R, Triozzi PL: Adoptive immunotherapy of feline leukemia virus infection using autologous lymph node lymphocytes, *J Acquir Immune Defic Syndr Hum Retrovirol* 18(1):1–6, 1998.

252. Yron I, Wood TA, Spiess PJ, Rosenberg SA: In vitro growth of murine T cells. V. The isolation and growth of lymphoid cells infiltrating syngeneic solid tumors, *J Immunol* 125(1):238–245, 1980.

253. Rosenberg SA, Restifo NP, Yang JC, et al.: Adoptive cell transfer: a clinical path to effective cancer immunotherapy, *Nat Rev Cancer* 8(4):299–308, 2008.

254. Dudley ME, Rosenberg SA: Adoptive-cell-transfer therapy for the treatment of patients with cancer, *Nat Rev Cancer* 3(9):666–675, 2003.

255. Dudley ME, Wunderlich JR, Yang JC, et al.: A phase I study of nonmyeloablative chemotherapy and adoptive transfer of autologous tumor antigen-specific T lymphocytes in patients with metastatic melanoma, *J Immunother* 25(3):243–251, 2002.

256. Rosenberg SA, Dudley ME: Cancer regression in patients with metastatic melanoma after the transfer of autologous antitumor lymphocytes, *Proc Natl Acad Sci U S A* 101(Suppl 2):14639–14645, 2004.

257. Xu L, Wang C, Wen Z, et al.: CpG oligodeoxynucleotides enhance the efficacy of adoptive cell transfer using tumor infiltrating lymphocytes by modifying the Th1 polarization and local infiltration of Th17 cells, *Clin Dev Immunol* 410893, 2010.

258. Park JS, Withers SS, Modiano JF, et al.: Canine cancer immunotherapy studies: linking mouse and human, *J Immunother Cancer* 4:97, 2016.

259. Khanna C, London C, Vail D, et al.: Guiding the optimal translation of new cancer treatments from canine to human cancer patients, *Clin Cancer Res* 15(18):5671–5677, 2009.

260. Withrow SJ, Khanna C: Bridging the gap between experimental animals and humans in osteosarcoma, *Cancer Treat Res* 152:439–446, 2009.

261. Stewart TJ, Smyth MJ: Improving cancer immunotherapy by targeting tumor-induced immune suppression, *Cancer Metastasis Rev* 30(1):125–140, 2011.

262. Hafeman SD, Varland D, Dow SW: Bisphosphonates significantly increase the activity of doxorubicin or vincristine against canine malignant histiocytosis, *Vet Comp Oncol* 10(1):44–56, 2012.

263. Melani C, Sangaletti S, Barazzetta FM, et al.: Amino-biphosphonate-mediated MMP-9 inhibition breaks the tumor-bone marrow axis responsible for myeloid-derived suppressor cell expansion and macrophage infiltration in tumor stroma, *Cancer Res* 67(23):11438–11446, 2007.

264. Priceman SJ, Sung JL, Shaposhnik Z, et al.: Targeting distinct tumor-infiltrating myeloid cells by inhibiting CSF-1 receptor: combating tumor evasion of antiangiogenic therapy, *Blood* 115(7):1461–1471, 2010.

265. Pan PY, Ma G, Weber KJ, et al.: Immune stimulatory receptor CD40 is required for T-cell suppression and T regulatory cell activation mediated by myeloid-derived suppressor cells in cancer, *Cancer Res* 70(1):99–108, 2010.

266. De Santo C, Serafini P, Marigo I, et al.: Nitroaspirin corrects immune dysfunction in tumor-bearing hosts and promotes tumor eradication by cancer vaccination, *Proc Natl Acad Sci U S A* 102(11):4185–4190, 2005.

267. Suzuki E, Kapoor V, Jassar AS, et al.: Gemcitabine selectively eliminates splenic Gr-1+/CD11b+ myeloid suppressor cells in tumor-bearing animals and enhances antitumor immune activity, *Clin Cancer Res* 11(18):6713–6721, 2005.

268. Mirza N, Fishman M, Fricke I, et al.: All-trans-retinoic acid improves differentiation of myeloid cells and immune response in cancer patients, *Cancer Res* 66(18):9299–9307, 2006.

269. Sinha P, Clements VK, Fulton AM, Ostrand-Rosenberg S: Prostaglandin E2 promotes tumor progression by inducing myeloid-derived suppressor cells, *Cancer Res* 67(9):4507–4513, 2007.

270. Curran MA, Montalvo W, Yagita H, Allison JP: PD-1 and CTLA-4 combination blockade expands infiltrating T cells and reduces regulatory T and myeloid cells within B16 melanoma tumors, *Proc Natl Acad Sci U S A* 107(9):4275–4280, 2010.

271. Serafini P, Mgebroff S, Noonan K, Borrello I: Myeloid-derived suppressor cells promote cross-tolerance in B-cell lymphoma by expanding regulatory T cells, *Cancer Res* 68(13):5439–5449, 2008.

272. Vincent J, Mignot G, Chalmin F, et al.: 5-Fluorouracil selectively kills tumor-associated myeloid-derived suppressor cells resulting in enhanced T cell-dependent antitumor immunity, *Cancer Res* 70(8):3052–3061, 2010.

273. Kodumudi KN, Woan K, Gilvary DL, et al.: A novel chemoimmunomodulating property of docetaxel: suppression of myeloid-derived suppressor cells in tumor bearers, *Clin Cancer Res* 16(18):4583–4594, 2010.

274. Nagaraj S, Youn JI, Weber H, et al.: Anti-inflammatory triterpenoid blocks immune suppressive function of MDSCs and improves immune response in cancer, *Clin Cancer Res* 16(6):1812–1823, 2010.

275. Ko JS, Zea AH, Rini BI, et al.: Sunitinib mediates reversal of myeloid-derived suppressor cell accumulation in renal cell carcinoma patients, *Clin Cancer Res* 15(6):2148–2157, 2009.

276. Serafini P, Meckel K, Kelso M, et al.: Phosphodiesterase-5 inhibition augments endogenous antitumor immunity by reducing myeloid-derived suppressor cell function, *J Exp Med* 203(12):2691–2702, 2006.

277. Daurkin I, Eruslanov E, Vieweg J, Kusmartsev S: Generation of antigen-presenting cells from tumor-infiltrated CD11b myeloid cells with DNA demethylating agent 5-aza-2'-deoxycytidine, *Cancer Immunol Immunother* 59(5):697–706, 2010.

278. Ko HJ, Lee JM, Kim YJ, et al.: Immunosuppressive myeloid-derived suppressor cells can be converted into immunogenic APCs with the help of activated NKT cells: an alternative cell-based antitumor vaccine, *J Immunol* 182(4):1818–1828, 2009.

279. Pan PY, Wang GX, Yin B, et al.: Reversion of immune tolerance in advanced malignancy: modulation of myeloid-derived suppressor cell development by blockade of stem-cell factor function, *Blood* 111(1):219–228, 2008.

280. Fernandez A, Mesa C, Marigo I, et al.: Inhibition of tumor-induced myeloid-derived suppressor cell function by a nanoparticulated adjuvant, *J Immunol* 186(1):264–274, 2011.

281. Lathers DM, Clark JI, Achille NJ, Young MR: Phase 1B study to improve immune responses in head and neck cancer patients using escalating doses of 25-hydroxyvitamin D3, *Cancer Immunol Immunother* 53(5):422–430, 2004.

282. Shojaei F, Singh M, Thompson JD, Ferrara N: Role of Bv8 in neutrophil-dependent angiogenesis in a transgenic model of cancer progression, *Proc Natl Acad Sci U S A* 105(7):2640–2645, 2008.

15
Molecular/Targeted Therapy of Cancer

SECTION A: GENE THERAPY FOR CANCER

DAVID J. ARGYLE

Since its development, recombinant DNA technology has been vigorously applied to the advancement of medicine. New molecular techniques have been used to study the role of specific genes and their products in disease, to improve diagnosis, and to produce novel therapeutics. Gene therapy, in its simplest definition, is the introduction of genes into cells in vivo to treat a disease,[1] and it has been applied to many chronic, intractable diseases such as single gene defects and cancer. This definition could probably now be extended to the delivery of all forms of nucleic acids for treatment. More than 2000 clinical gene therapy trials have been conducted worldwide, and as could be predicted with any developing technology, there have been a litany of disappointments interspersed with a few prominent successes, particularly in ocular and immunodeficiency diseases.[2] Cancer has proved to be an attractive target for gene therapy, with clinical studies that have included delivery of "killing genes," immune-modulating genes, and genes that can alter host tumor microenvironment (e.g., tumor vasculature).[1] Early human cancer trials, including those to deactivate oncogenes or restore tumor suppressor gene function, proved to have little clinical utility, but the past 20 years have seen a growing number of clinical successes in human medicine that have paralleled our increased understanding of and experience with the delivery technology.[2-5] Furthermore, the exponential growth of data around cancer genomes, biology, and immunology is allowing the exploitation of gene therapy technologies to improve patient outcomes and a drive toward precision medicine. The gene therapy field in veterinary oncology has proved to be much slower that in human medicine, hindered by the paucity of biology data, costs of development, and (in some cases), the regulatory environment. However, a number of studies are now emerging that suggest that this technology may prove to be a useful adjunct in veterinary oncology.

Delivery Vehicles for Cancer Gene Therapy

Effective gene therapy relies on our ability to introduce genes efficiently into target cells or tissues in vivo, or the ex vivo delivery of genes to autologous cells and subsequent adoptive transfer back to the patient. It is the efficient and safe transfer of genes that has proved to be the greatest hurdle to clinical development over the past 20 years, and a herculean effort has been placed into developing robust vector systems for clinical use. The major delivery vehicles that have been exploited fall into the two broad categories of viral vectors and nonviral (usually plasmid-based) vectors. Vector systems are summarized in Table 15.1 and Fig. 15.1.

The great advantage to viral vectors for gene delivery is their ability to infect cells and our ability to exploit their replicative machinery. The majority of systems use replication-defective viruses to overcome concerns that recombination within the host may lead to the production of wild-type virus with pathogenic potential. The common systems rely on oncogenic retroviruses (e.g., murine leukemia virus [MuLV]), adenoviruses (e.g., human adenovirus type 5 [AD5]), adeno-associated viruses (AAVs), or lentiviruses. Lentiviral vectors have a better safety profile than retroviral vectors and are more efficient at delivering genes to nondividing cells.[6-11] Among the various viral-based vector systems, the AAVs are proving to have the greatest utility in the treatment of human diseases. Alipogene tiparvovec (marketed as Glybera), an AAV-vector based treatment for lipoprotein lipase deficiency, was one of the first gene therapy products to be licensed by the European Medicines Agency in 2012 and was an important milestone in drug development[2]; however, the drug was withdrawn in 2017 by the parent company because of lack of demand and the 1 million euro price tag.

Most of the viral systems for cancer gene therapy involve the local delivery of virus to tumor deposits (e.g., by intratumoral injection), or ex vivo delivery of transgene to autologous cells. Systemic delivery of virus is hindered by rapid clearance of viruses from the body by the immune and complement systems. To overcome this, work has progressed to explore cellular delivery of viruses by the systemic route. In this delivery system, viral producer cells are delivered to the patient, and virus production is triggered when the cells reach the tumor. Endothelial cells, T cells, macrophages, dendritic cells, and mesenchymal stem cells (MSCs) are also being explored as potential cell delivery systems. The advantage of these systems is that virus could potentially be delivered to metastatic disease and primary tumors.[12-16]

Concerns relating to virus safety, an inability to produce high enough viral titers for clinical trials, and the cost of viral vectors have led to the development of nonviral delivery systems for gene therapy.[17-18] Such methodologies have included the use of cationic liposomes, "naked" (plasmid) DNA, synthetic viruses, transposons, and bacteria (summarized in Table 15.1). Cationic liposomes are microscopic vesicles that enter cells by endocytosis and have been used to safely and efficiently deliver genes to

TABLE 15.1	Gene Therapy Vector Systems
Viral Vectors	
Retroviruses (oncoviruses)	Originally the gold-standard vector. Gene is packaged into replication-defective viral particles using a packaging cell line. The therapeutic gene is integrated into the host cell genome when the virus is delivered to the target cell. Limited by their inability to infect postmitotic cells.
Retroviruses (lentivirus)	Many are based on HIV-1. These vectors have become safer in recent years and have many of the benefits of the oncoviruses and also will infect postmitotic cells. Construction of the vector takes place in a packaging cell line and the therapeutic gene is integrated into the host cell genome.
Adenoviruses	Have become the most popular viral delivery mechanism. Gene is packaged into a replication incompetent adenovirus (usually E1 deleted). Gene expression remains episomal when delivered to the host cell. Concerns have been raised about the safety of adenoviral vectors, in particular potential toxic side effects at high doses. Adenoviruses can infect a wide range of pre- and postmitotic cells. Conditionally replicating adenoviruses are being explored as oncolytic vectors.
Adeno-associated viruses (AAV)	Gaining popularity as a vector as they are potentially safer than adenoviruses. They infect a wide variety of mammalian cell types but are limited by the amount of DNA they can deliver. Gene expression in the host cell is episomal. However, in the natural host, integration is possible.
Nonviral Vectors	
Naked DNA	This is a simple form of gene delivery in which "naked" plasmid DNA is directly injected into the tumor. Vectors are derived from bacterial plasmids and are engineered to express the therapeutic gene under the control of a strong promoter. Naked DNA can be taken up by many tissues, but typically the efficiency for delivery is lower than that for viral gene delivery.
Particle bombardment (gene gun)	This is a more sophisticated approach to the delivery of naked DNA. In this system plasmid DNA is typically adsorbed onto gold particles. Helium is then used as a motive force to fire the gold particles into cells or tissues via a hand-held "gene gun."
Liposome/DNA conjugates	In this system naked DNA is coated with liposomes to improve uptake by endocytosis. This enhances the efficiency of gene delivery.
Ligand/DNA conjugates	Ligands are used to specifically target DNA to tumor tissue.

HIV-1, Human immunodeficiency virus-1.

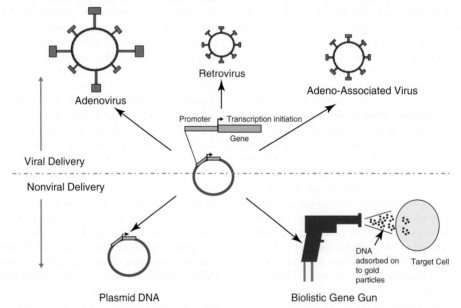

• **Fig. 15.1** Viral and nonviral gene delivery. Adenoviral vectors are produced in "producer cell lines." They enter the cell by transduction and their genetic material is transported to the nucleus. In contrast to retroviruses, the DNA is not integrated into the host genome, but gene expression is achieved episomally. Retroviral vectors are also produced is specialized producer cell lines. They enter the cell by transduction but their RNA genome is reverse transcribed into proviral DNA. This integrates into the host genome, where expression of the transgene takes place. DNA plasmid vectors contain a gene cassette that incorporates the therapeutic transgene under the control of a promoter. The plasmid can be delivered by direct injection as naked or liposome encapsulated DNA, by direct injection or systemically wrapped in nanomedicine particles, or by direct injection utilizing a helium-driven "biolistic" gene gun.

tumor cells through direct injection and systemic delivery.[15,16] They have a selectivity for endothelial cells, are considered efficient gene delivery systems, and are relatively safe. Naked DNA delivery (the delivery of plasmid DNA alone containing the gene of interest) results in uptake by tumor cells and antigen-presenting cells after simple direct injection.[17] A modification of this is particle-mediated gene delivery using a "gene gun." In this approach, DNA is adsorbed onto gold particles and fired into tissues under high pressure (using helium as the motive force).[17,18] However, the majority of these naked DNA approaches are still inefficient and are not able to be given systemically (see Table 15.1).[19–23]

Plasmid vectors for gene therapy have a number of limitations[19–23]:

- Plasmid DNA preparations contain several topological variants of the plasmid, including the unwanted open circular and linear forms of the molecule.
- Plasmids are inefficient at delivering genes compared with viruses, thus requiring vehicles, physical forces, or specialized modifications for uptake and nuclear localization. Some delivery methods lead to breakage of the plasmid DNA backbone, which increases the likelihood of genome integration and/or less efficient expression.
- Plasmids are nonreplicating episomes, so transgene expression is transient and is diluted by cell division.
- Bacterial sequences in plasmids, such as unmethylated cytosine-phosphate-guanine (CpG) dinucleotides, have the potential to be recognized by the mammalian immune system via toll-like receptor (TLR)-9, potentially precipitating not only transgene silencing but also immune response.
- Plasmids typically encode antibiotic resistance-encoding genes for selection of plasmid-harboring bacteria. The use of antibiotics and their resistance genes in the preparation of plasmid vectors, however, is discouraged by regulatory bodies such as the Food and Drug Administration (FDA) and the European Medicines Agency because of the risk of transfer and replication of resistance genes to bacteria in the human microbiome and possibly into the environment.
- Residual antibiotics that remain from vector production may trigger an immune reaction in patients.

In human gene therapy, these issues have led to the development of minimal plasmid vectors, with extensive deletions (minivectors).[17]

Targeting Cancer Gene Therapy

In terms of delivery, one of the major barriers is the ability to give vectors systemically, to target them to cancer tissues, and to ensure that therapeutic transgenes are not expressed in normal cells. Targeting also ensures that enough vector can reach the target of interest, without being dispersed to irrelevant sites. Numerous strategies have been attempted to provide levels of targeting and to spare normal tissue, and many have been explored in isolation or as combination strategies (e.g., dual and triple targeting).

1. **Transductional targeting.** This involves surface modification (usually of virus), to allow delivery and/or entry to cells via specific surface receptor. This approach has largely been applied to adenoviral vectors and has included modifications to the *cox*sackie and *a*denovirus *r*eceptor (CAR) (which gives adenovirus its normal cellular tropism), and/or the use of "adaptors." An adaptor molecule can ablate native CAR-based tropism and target the virus to an alternate cellular receptor molecule. For example, bispecific fusion proteins (e.g., diabodies, composed of two single-chain antibodies [scFv], with one scFv recognizing the fiber knob and the other a tumor-associated antigen [TAA]) can be used as an adaptor to target adenovirus to a specific tumor type[24,25] (Fig. 15.2).

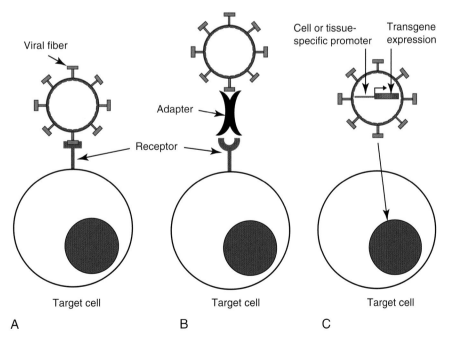

• **Fig. 15.2** Vector targeting. The specificity of viral vectors can be improved utilizing either transductional targeting (A), where the viral surface proteins are modified so they will only enter the cell of interest; transductional targeting, where the vector is modified using an "adapter" (B); or transcriptional targeting (C), where the expression of the therapeutic transgene is under the control of a tissue or cell-specific promoter. Transcriptional targeting can also be employed in nonviral vectors and directly delivered to the patient.

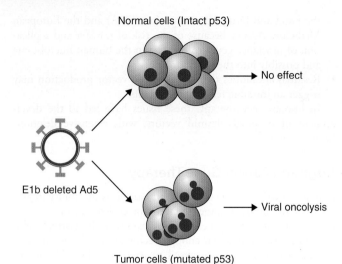

Normal cells (Intact p53)

No effect

E1b deleted Ad5

Viral oncolysis

Tumor cells (mutated p53)

• **Fig. 15.3** Conditionally replicating adenovirus. The ONYX-015 vector is an E1b-deleted Adenovirus that conditionally replicates in cells with a nonfunctional *p53* gene. p53 protein has the potential to shut down cell cycling when infected with wild-type adenovirus but is prevented from doing so through the actions of the product of viral E1b. E1b-deficient viruses cannot replicate in normal cells with p53 intact. However, in cells that have no functional p53 protein, viral replication can proceed and cause cell lysis.

2. **Transcriptional targeting.** This strategy exploits unique gene expression in specific cell types once the vector has entered the cell.[26–30] Although every gene is represented in every cell of the body, expression of any one gene requires specific transcription factors that may be unique to a particular cell or tissue type. Certain genes have been identified that are expressed in cancer cells but are not expressed in normal cells (e.g., telomerase) or are expressed only in a specific tissue type (e.g., prostate-specific antigen [PSA]). By using the promoter sequences for these genes to drive transgene expression, targeted expression in cancer cells only (e.g., using the promoter for telomerase) or to a specific tissue type (e.g., to the prostate using the promoter for PSA) can be achieved (see Fig. 15.2).

3. **Replication-competent oncolytic viruses.** Progress has been made in the development of viruses that conditionally replicate in cancer cells.[31,32] One of the first examples to be used in clinical trials was the ONYX-015 vector, an E1b-deleted adenovirus that conditionally replicates in cells with a nonfunctional *p53* gene. p53 protein has the potential to shut down cell cycling when infected with wild-type adenovirus but is prevented from doing so through the actions of the product of viral E1b. E1b-deficient viruses cannot replicate in normal cells with p53 intact; however, in cells that have no functional p53 protein, viral replication can proceed and cause cell lysis (Fig. 15.3). Many other conditionally replicating viruses are being developed that rely on specific cancer cell defects (e.g., reoviruses that conditionally replicate in cells with intact Ras signaling pathways) or are transcriptionally targeted. Replication-competent viruses are described in more detail in the text that follows.

Gene Therapy Strategies for Cancer

In the following sections, the broad approaches that can be applied to cancer treatments are outlined. In reality, experience tells us

that the optimal approach for patients will be a combination of approaches, including a combined approach with more conventional treatments.

Rescue of the Cancer Cell Through Gene Replacement or Repair Technologies

Early cancer gene therapy strategies focused on the ablation of oncogenes or the replacement of defective tumor suppressor genes.[1] One of the most studied genes in cancer development has been the tumor suppressor gene *p53,* acting as a genomic guardian for the cell and being "switched on" when a cell is exposed to DNA damaging agents. The *p53* gene product causes the cell to either stop dividing or undergo apoptosis, depending on the degree of damage. In many cancers (50% of human cancers), this gene is defective and the second allele is missing. Damaged cells fail to stop dividing and can accumulate further damaging events, which can allow selection for a malignant phenotype. A number of studies have addressed this by attempting to replace the defective *p53* gene with its normal counterpart[31]; however, problems associated with this approach include:

• The current technology is unable to efficiently deliver a normal *p53* gene to every cancer cell in a tumor mass.
• Cancer is a multigenetic abnormality, and the delivery of one correct gene to a tumor cell may still not have the desired phenotypic effect.

Gene replacement for cancer therapy proved to be disappointing clinically, but gene repair is possible, at least in the laboratory setting. Gene repair has been achieved using lentiviral-mediated zinc finger nucleases and exploiting endogenous repair mechanisms. In addition, newly developed gene editing approaches such as *T*ranscriptional *A*ctivator-*L*ike *N*ucleases (TALENS), and *C*lustered *R*egularly *I*nterspaced *S*hort *P*alindromic *R*epeats (CRISPR) provide novel ways to manipulate the genome.[33] At present, these technologies are laboratory based and are being used to develop newly engineered cancer models. Their utility in actual "gene repair" treatments is very far from clinical exploitation.

Gene Silencing in Cancer Cells

Gene silencing usually refers to the delivery and use of small interfering double-stranded RNA (siRNA) molecules to cancer cells to ablate the deleterious effects of activated oncogenes. In the cell, exogenously delivered siRNA is directed to the RNA-induced silencing complex (RISC). This complex is then directed to the target mRNA of the offending gene. By degradation of mRNA, expression of the target gene is suppressed, which is known as posttranscriptional gene silencing (PTGS).[34]

Proponents of RNA interference (RNAi)-based cancer therapy have argued a high efficiency and potential low cost compared with the other methods of gene therapy,[34,35] and high specificity compared with other modalities of cancer therapy such as chemotherapy. The major advantage of RNAi is the potential to target multiple genes of various cellular pathways involved in tumor progression.[36] Simultaneous inhibition of multiple genes is an effective approach to treat cancer and to reduce the possibility of multidrug resistance. RNAi suffers from some of the same issues as conventional gene delivery, in that its efficiency is dependent on an efficient delivery system. siRNA can be delivered directly to tumors but systemic delivery is vulnerable to

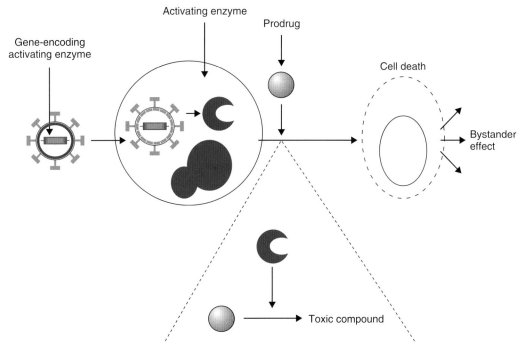

• **Fig. 15.4** Gene-directed enzyme prodrug therapy. In gene-directed enzyme prodrug therapy (GDEPT), an activating gene is delivered to the cancer cells. A relatively inactive prodrug is then given to the patient systemically. In cells processing the activating gene, the prodrug is converted to a highly toxic drug, which can kill the cancer cell. The advantage of this system is the evidence of bystander effect. In this, only a small proportion of cancer cells need to receive the activating gene, as toxic metabolites leak across gap junctions and kill surrounding cancer cells.

enzymatic inactivation and renal clearance. A number of delivery systems are in clinical trials, including nanoparticles for systemic use. At present, no clinical trials have been performed in veterinary species.

Gene-Directed Enzyme Prodrug Therapy

Gene-directed enzyme prodrug therapy (GDEPT) involves the delivery of a "suicide" gene (usually viral or bacterial enzyme) to cancer cells that has the ability to convert a relatively nontoxic prodrug to an active compound within the cancer cell (Fig. 15.4). At the clinical level, the gene would be delivered to the patient's tumor and the enzyme activity would be confined to the cancer cells.[37] These systems have been combined with transcriptionally targeted vectors (described previously) to improve the targeting and eventual therapeutic index.[32] Once the patient's cells have been transduced, they would then be given a prodrug systemically. In the cancer cells, this novel enzyme can convert the prodrug to a more active compound that has the ability to kill the cancer cell (see Fig. 15.4). A number of successful approaches have been developed in vitro, based on this system. For example, the *Escherchia. coli* nitroreductase gene has been used in preclinical models to cause reduction of an inactive prodrug (CB1954, a weak alkylating agent) to promote cell killing in cancer cells.[37] However, because of the low efficiency of existing vectors, the success of this therapy will largely depend on the extent of the bystander effect. In this, the activation of the prodrug in the cell causes cell death and also leakage of toxic metabolites to neighboring cells. Consequently, it is estimated that only a small fraction of the cells need receive the gene for there to be a dramatic effect on tumor volume. Furthermore, in

mouse models, a distant bystander effect on tumor metastases has been demonstrated that is mediated through the patient's immune system.[38] The in situ destruction of tumor cells is mediated through necrosis rather than apoptosis, creating an ideal inflammatory environment for the exposure and presentation of tumor antigens to the immune system. This allows the patient's immune system to recognize tumor metastases and has caused regression in a number of preclinical model systems. Owing to the presence of this phenomenon, complete tumor regression has been reported in model systems, even when only 10% of the tumor cells have been transduced with suicide genes. To date, five basic mechanisms have been proposed as mediators of the bystander effect[38]:
- Release of activated soluble toxic factors as cells die
- Passive diffusion of toxic factors from intact cells
- Transference of toxic compounds through gap junctions
- Phagocytosis of apoptotic bodies released from transduced cells
- Stimulation of host immune response in the tumor microenvironment

It is likely that a combination of these mechanisms operates to support bystander tumor cell killing.

In reality, the use of GDEPT in human clinical trials has been disappointing, with many of the preclinical successes not translated into large-scale clinical successes. Human clinical trials have included colon, liver, lung, prostate, breast, glioma, and ovarian cancers with variable results[38]; however, it should be noted that the apparent safety concerns related to suicide gene therapy have often limited trials to patients with highly aggressive tumors and poor clinical performance scores. This may have significantly limited any potential for clinical success.

Utilizing Stem Cells to Deliver "Suicide Genes"

The attractiveness of enzyme–prodrug cancer gene therapy has been described earlier, but it relies on the ability to specifically target prodrugs to tumors. Prodrug cancer gene therapy driven by MSCs has been suggested as a treatment modality that could achieve this.[39–42] Thanks to their immunosuppressive properties, allogeneic MSCs can substitute for autologous stem cells in delivering the therapeutic agent in targeted tumor therapy, and the tumor-homing ability of MSCs holds therapeutic advantages compared with vehicles such as proteins, antibodies, nanoparticles, and to some extent viruses.

Gene-Directed Immunotherapy

The search for an effective cancer vaccine over the past 150 years has led to extensive studies of the immune response of cancer patients. These studies have suggested that cell-mediated immune responses are important components of the antitumor immune response. Cytokines are small glycoprotein molecules that orchestrate the immune response, tissue repair, and hematopoiesis, and it has been demonstrated that the relative amounts of individual cytokines can direct the immune system toward either a mainly humoral or a mainly cell-mediated response. In particular, cytokines such as interleukin-2 (IL-2), interferon-gamma (IFN-γ), IL-12, and IL-18 have the ability to promote cell-mediated responses. Furthermore, evidence derived from animal models suggested that local production of cytokines around a tumor mass can lead to production of an antitumor immune response and a reversal of T-cell anergy (nonresponsiveness).[43,44] Thus there appears a rationale for using cytokine molecules in cancer patients to improve the antitumor immune response to tumors that present weakly antigenic epitopes or epitopes that evade immune recognition. In the 1980s and 1990s, a number of clinical studies were undertaken using recombinant cytokine proteins to improve the survival of human cancer patients. However, cytokines tend to be autocrine or paracrine in nature and the levels of protein required to demonstrate a biologic effect were often too toxic for the patient to withstand. However, a more promising approach has been to deliver the actual cytokine genes to cancer cells rather than delivery of the protein to the whole patient.[45–47] Many trials have now combined this approach with gene-directed immunotherapy. In this approach, cytokine genes, and the prodrug-activating gene, are delivered to cancer cells. The conversion of an inactive prodrug by the activating gene leads to destruction of the cancer cells by necrosis. The codelivery of cytokines that enhance cell-mediated immune responses such as IL-2, IFN-γ, IL-12, and IL-18 enhances the antitumor response and may potentially improve the distant bystander effect against micrometastatic disease.[1] This approach has also been adopted in a number of small-scale veterinary studies, including one on canine malignant melanoma, which used cells to deliver IL-2 to tumors.[48,49] These studies have had encouraging results and warrant further larger scale trials.

More recently, cancer immunotherapy based on the genetic modification of autologous T cells has gained a great deal of attention for successes in the treatment of leukemias and lymphomas resistant to standard therapies.[50,51] In this, autologous CD8+ T cells are engineered to recognize and kill tumor cells bearing specific surface antigens. This is achieved through cellular modification by the incorporation of a chimeric antigen receptor (CAR) to redirected T cells, and combines the specificity of a monoclonal antibody with the proliferative and cytotoxic ability of an activated CD8+ T cell.[50–52] A similar approach has been employed in dogs, creating CD20-directed CAR T-cells that demonstrated feasibility, if with only modest clinical responses.[53]

Gene Modification to Improve Chemotherapy and/or Radiation Therapy Outcomes

An alternative approach to gene therapy for cancer involves the delivery of genes to normal cells of the bone marrow to protect them against the cytotoxic effects of conventional chemotherapeutic drugs. In particular, the multidrug resistance (MDR) gene has been cloned and delivered to normal bone marrow cells. When patients are given high doses of chemotherapy, the normal cells with the MDR gene are able to export the toxic drugs across their membranes, reducing potential side effects.[54–56] However, this approach does not protect gastrointestinal cells, which limits its usefulness. Furthermore, there is also a danger that the MDR gene could transfer to malignant cells, rendering them insensitive to the effects of standard drugs.

An alternative approach is to enhance the sensitivity of cancer cells to either chemotherapy or radiation therapy (RT) to improve clinical outcomes. As an example, the transcription factor Slug has been identified as a potential mediator of radio-resistance and has been found to have an antiapoptotic effect. A recent study demonstrated that the modulation of Slug expression by siRNA affected oral squamous cell carcinoma sensitivity to RT through upregulating p53 upregulated modulator of apoptosis (PUMA).[57] Furthermore, inhibition of the Notch and epidermal growth factor receptor (EGFR) pathways in cancer have been shown to modulate chemotherapy and radiosensitivity, opening the possibility of gene modulation during treatment with standard conventional modalities.[58,59] The limitation, as with all other gene therapy approaches, is in the capacity for efficient gene delivery.

The Use of Replication-Competent Viral Vectors

Progress has been made in the development of replication-competent viruses that conditionally replicate in cancer cells.[60–63] As an example, the ONYX-015 vector (as described earlier) was one of the earliest vectors to enter into clinical trials. Since that time, oncolytic viruses (OVs) have been emerging as important therapeutics in cancer management, combining both tumor-specific cell killing, together with stimulation of host immunity.[64] OVs represent a diverse group of agents that cause lysis during their natural life cycle (e.g., vaccinia) or can be engineered to be lytic by toxic transgene expression. OVs can cause selective tumor cell killing by virtue of virus-specific receptors on the surface of the cancer cell and/or by the tumor cell replicative machinery. In addition, tumor lysis can lead to the promotion of antitumor immunity. There are some wild-type viruses that are in clinical use (e.g., reoviruses, vaccinia virus and Newcastle disease virus), but many are attenuated and/or engineered to improve selectivity or mode of action (e.g., E1b-deleted Ad5).[64,65]

The effectiveness of OVs has been demonstrated in preclinical models and has led to the FDA approval and conditional European Medicine Agency's approval of the first OV for use in human melanoma, the immunostimulatory herpesvirus, talimogene laherparepvec. In this, the Herpes simplex virus has been engineered such that both copies of the viral gene coding for ICP34.5 have been deleted and replaced with the gene coding for human granulocyte-macrophage colony-stimulating factor (GM-CSF), and the gene coding for ICP47 (ICP47 suppresses the immune response to the virus) has been removed. To date, increased survival or protection from metastasis has not been definitively demonstrated.[66]

In veterinary oncology, there have been a number of limited clinical studies. Recent pilot safety studies have been performed in dogs using systemically delivered recombinant oncolytic reovirus and vesicular stomatitis virus.[67,68] This demonstrated the feasibility and safety of this approach and opens the door to future studies to demonstrate efficacy in the clinical setting. A cautionary note, however, is that the majority of dogs in the United States and Europe are vaccinated against some viruses such as canine adenovirus and these types of vectors may not be able to overcome host immunity with long-term treatments.[1,69]

Safety Considerations in Gene Therapy

One of the major considerations in gene therapy revolves around issues of safety, in particular the safety of the vectors used for gene delivery. In 1999, gene therapy suffered a major setback with the death of a patient as a direct result of adenovirus gene therapy. Problems associated with vector delivery include inappropriate inflammatory responses caused by vector delivery (e.g., adenoviruses), the generation of replication-competent viruses (although this is unlikely with new generation vectors), and insertional mutagenesis caused by integrating viruses (e.g., retroviruses).[1]

Until recently, many gene therapy trials had utilized retroviral vectors for gene delivery. There are many advantages to using retroviruses as outlined in Table 15.1; however, retroviruses are also associated with serious diseases of domestic animals and the use of these in gene therapy poses a risk of insertional mutagenesis and/or the production of replication-competent viruses during the manufacturing process. Realistically, insertional mutagenesis leading to a malignant transformation is an unlikely event because cancer is a multistep process. In fact, there may be a greater risk of malignant transformation from external beam RT than from the use of retroviruses to treat cancer. The production of replication-competent retroviruses during the production process would also be unlikely because of the rigorous testing that is required before clinical application. Many of these issues are resolving with the development of new generation vectors.[1] As an example, in the use of retroviruses and to prevent insertional mutagenesis in normal tissues, one group recently described the use of zinc finger nucleases (engineered DNA-editing enzymes) that allows the insertion of DNA to a site of choice within the genome.[69] This adds a further level of safety in a high-risk procedure.

One might imagine that the delivery of naked DNA may offer a safer alternative. However, all of the potential safety issues using this technology are still not fully answered. These include potential risks of autoimmunity and also the actual fate of the DNA when it has been delivered to the patient; in the case of the former, however, there would appear to be no evidence of autoimmunity being a problem in preclinical models.

One of the most exciting developments in cancer gene therapy is the use of conditionally replicating OVs. However, the safety of these vector systems needs special consideration as many of them in their native form could pose a risk to both human and animal health. Despite this, published trial data have not demonstrated any significant safety issues. Local delivery has been associated in human medicine with mild flulike symptoms, which have resolved with symptomatic treatment with paracetamol/acetaminophen.[65] In addition, OVs do not reach a maximum tolerated dose (MTD), mainly because of a high tolerance for the virus. However, as OVs with greater potency are developed, or used in combination with other treatments, then safety should remain a concern. One of the major issues may be the development of resistance through immune clearance. Although immunosuppressive therapy has been suggested as part of the treatment with OVs, this should be considered with caution relating to both safety and ensuring that the optimal performance of the virus is not blocked.[65]

Conclusions

Gene therapy promises a completely new approach to the treatment of cancer and represents an emerging area of therapeutics. It has suffered over the past 20 years as clinical trials in human medicine have not delivered what they had originally promised. However, many of these studies were conducted in patients with high-grade or end-stage disease and many studies were conducted prematurely without refining the delivery technologies. Clearly, there are a number of technical issues such as safety surrounding the delivery and efficiency of the vectors that need to be resolved before gene therapy becomes established clinical practice. Despite gene therapy being very much in its infancy, the field is advancing at a rapid rate and resent successes have given the field a significant optimistic boost. A number of clinical trials have begun in companion animals, and products are in development for clinical application. However, although these treatments would appear to be powerful in preclinical models, it is likely that their greatest benefit will be in the management of patients with minimal disease states. Thus gene therapy will probably have its greatest advantage not as a stand-alone treatment but as an adjunct to more conventional therapies such as surgery, RT, or chemotherapy.

SECTION B: SIGNAL TRANSDUCTION AND CANCER

CHERYL A. LONDON

In normal cells, signals are generated that begin at the outside of the cell and are transmitted through the cytoplasm to the nucleus, regulating cell growth, differentiation, survival, and death. Several components of cellular signal transduction pathways are typically dysregulated in cancer cells, resulting in uncontrolled cell growth and thereby contributing to tumorigenesis. Because many tumors have similar alterations in signal transduction components, these have become promising targets for therapeutic intervention. This section focuses primarily on the role of a particular group of signal transducers called *protein kinases,* their role in normal cells, the mechanisms by which they contribute to tumorigenesis, and the use of agents designed to inhibit them when they become dysfunctional.

Protein Kinases and Normal Cells

Protein kinases play critical roles in normal cell signal transduction, acting to tightly regulate cellular processes such as growth and differentiation. These proteins work through phosphorylation; that is, they bind adenosine triphosphate (ATP) and use it to add phosphate groups to key residues on themselves (a process called *autophosphorylation*) and on other molecules, thereby stimulating a downstream signal inside the cell. This process typically occurs in response to external signals generated by growth factors

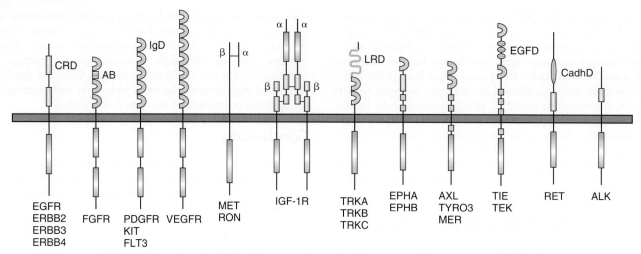

• **Fig. 15.5** Structure of receptor tyrosine kinases. The structures of receptor tyrosine kinase families implicated in a variety of malignancies are shown. *AB*, Acid box; *ALK*, anaplastic lymphoma kinase; *CadhD*, cadherin-like domain; *CRD*, cysteine-rich domain; *EGFD*, epidermal growth factor-like domain; *EGFR*, epidermal growth factor receptor; *Eph*, member of ephrin receptor family; *FGFR*, fibroblast growth factor receptor; *IgD*, immunoglobulin-like domain; *LRD*, leucine-rich domain; *IGF-1R*, insulin like growth factor receptor 1; *PDGFR*, platelet-derived growth factor receptor; *TIE*, tyrosine kinase receptor on endothelial cells; *TRK*, member of nerve growth factor receptor family; *VEGFR*, vascular endothelial growth factor receptor. The symbols α and β indicate specific RTK subunits. (Reprinted with permission from Blackwell Publishing, London CA, *Vet Comp Oncol* 2:177–193, 2004.)

(GFs) or other stimuli that initiate the cascade. Protein kinases are classified as tyrosine kinases (TKs) if they phosphorylate proteins on tyrosine residues or serine/threonine kinases if they phosphorylate proteins on serine and threonine residues. In some cases, the kinases perform both functions (i.e., dual-function kinases). Protein kinases can be expressed on the cell surface, in the cytoplasm, and in the nucleus. The human genome encodes more than 500 kinases, of which 90 are classified as TKs.[70]

TKs on the cell surface that are activated through binding of GFs are called receptor TKs (RTKs). Of the 90 identified TKs, approximately 60 are known to be RTKs. Each RTK contains an extracellular domain that binds the GF, a transmembrane domain, and a cytoplasmic kinase domain that positively and negatively regulates phosphorylation of the RTK (Fig. 15.5).[71–73] Most RTKs are monomers on the cell surface and are dimerized through the act of GF binding; this changes the three-dimensional structure of the receptor, permitting ATP to bind and autophosphorylation to occur, generating a downstream signal through subsequent binding of adaptor proteins and nonreceptor kinases.[71] Dysregulation of RTKs resulting in pathway activation/uncontrolled signaling is known to contribute to several human cancers, and work is ongoing to characterize such abnormalities in canine and feline cancers. Examples of RTKs known to play prominent roles in specific cancers include KIT, Met, EGFR, and ALK, all which can be activated by overexpression, mutation, and/or chromosomal translocation.[74–78]

Although RTK signaling is critical for regulating typical cell functions, it is also an important driver of angiogenesis, a process considered essential for continued tumor cell growth. The RTKs involved in angiogenesis include the vascluar endothelial growth factor receptors (VEGFRs), platelet-derived growth factor receptors (PDGFRs), fibroblast growth factor receptors (FGFRs), and Tie-1 and Tie-2 (receptors for angiopoietin).[79–82] VEGFRs are expressed on vascular endothelium and VEGFR signaling drives endothelial migration and proliferation.[79] PDGFR-alpha and

-beta are expressed in stroma and pericytes that are critical for the maintenance of newly formed blood vessels.[81,82] FGFR-1 and -2 are expressed on vascular endothelium and work with VEGFR to promote increased expression of VEGF.[81] Tie-1 and Tie-2 are expressed on blood vessels in tumors and are important in the recruitment of pericytes and smooth muscle cells to the newly forming vascular channels.[83]

Kinases in the cytoplasm act as bridges, conducting signals generated by RTKs to the nucleus through a series of intermediates that become phosphorylated.[84] The cytoplasmic kinases may be directly on the inside of the cell membrane or free in the cytoplasm. With respect to tumor cell biology, two particular cytoplasmic pathways are often dysregulated in cancer. The first includes members of the RAS-RAF-MEK-ERK/p38/JNK families (Fig. 15.6).[85,86] Most of these are serine/threonine kinases and their activation leads to ERK phosphorylation, translocation into the nucleus, and subsequent alteration of transcription factor and nuclear kinase activity important for controlling the cell cycle. Some examples of dysregulation in human cancers include RAS mutations in lung cancer, colon cancer, and several hematologic malignancies and BRAF mutations in cutaneous melanomas and papillary thyroid carcinomas.[87–89] Interestingly, BRAF mutations synonymous to those in human malignant melanomas are also found in canine transitional cell carcinomas, with more than 80% of tumors testing positive.[90]

The second cytoplasmic pathway includes phosphatidyl inositol-3 kinase (PI3K) and its associated downstream signal transducers AKT, nuclear factor κB (NFκB), and mTOR, among others (Fig. 15.7).[91,92] PI3K is activated by RTKs and in turn activates AKT, which alters several additional proteins involved in the regulation of cell survival, cycling, and growth.[93] AKT phosphorylates targets that promote apoptosis (BAD, procaspase-9, and Forkhead transcription factors) and activates NFκB, a transcription factor that has antiapoptotic activity.[91–93] AKT also phosphorylates other proteins such as mTOR, p21, p27, and GSK3. This leads

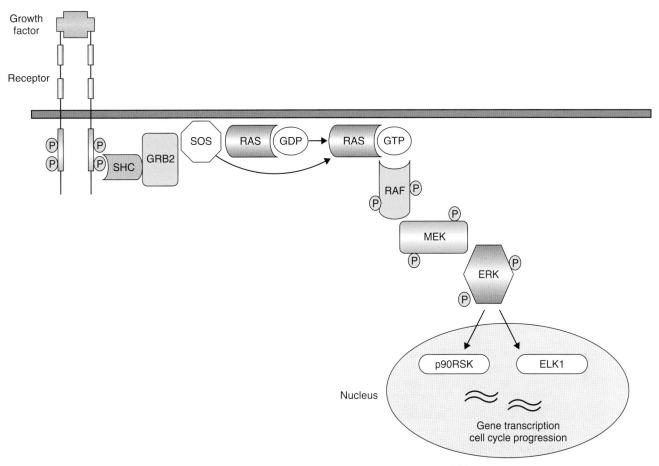

• **Fig. 15.6** Ras signal transduction. Activated receptor tyrosine kinases recruits SOS to the plasma membrane through binding of SHC and GRB2. SOS replaces bound GDP with GTP, thereby activating RAS. The downstream target RAF is then phosphorylated by RAS, leading to subsequent activation of MEK, then ERK. ERK has several substrates both in the nucleus and in the cytoplasm, including ETS transcription factors such as ELK1 and RSK, which regulate cell cycle progression. (Reprinted with permission from Blackwell Publishing, London CA, Vet Comp Oncol 2:177–193, 2004.)

to redistribution of these proteins either in or out of the nucleus, ultimately inhibiting apoptosis while promoting cell cycling.[91–93] Abnormalities of PI3K resulting in pathway activation are commonly found in human cancers including mutations (breast and colorectal cancers and glioblastoma) and gene amplifications (gastric, lung, ovarian cancers).[94] This pathway may also become dysregulated through loss of activity of phosphatase and tensin homolog (PTEN), a phosphatase that dephosphorylates AKT and terminates signaling.[91,95,96] PTEN mutations and/or decreased PTEN expression are present in several human cancers (e.g., glioblastoma and prostate cancer)[94,95] and have been documented in canine cancers (osteosarcoma, melanoma).[97–99]

RTK-induced signaling ultimately influences cellular events by affecting transcription and the proteins that control cell cycling. The cyclins and their kinase partners (cyclin-dependent kinases [CDKs]) act to regulate the progression of cells through various phases of the cell cycle (Fig. 15.8).[100–102] There are several cyclins (A–F); however, cyclins D and E play key roles in cell cycling through regulation of restriction point passage by the activation of their respective CDKs (CDK4 and CDK6 for cyclin D and CDK2 for cyclin E). Coordinated function of cyclins D and E is required for cells to progress from G1 into S phase (Fig. 15.8). In many cases, RTK-generated signals induce expression of cyclin D, which complexes with CDK4 and CDK6, resulting in phosphorylation

of the tumor suppressor Rb, partially repressing its function.[101,102] Functional cyclin D/CDK complexes induce transcription of cyclin E, and active cyclin E/CDK complexes further reduce Rb activity through phosphorylation. This in turn initiates the process of DNA replication necessary for cells to cycle. Dysregulation of the cylins and CDKs is common in human cancers; for example, overexpression of cyclins D and E is often present in breast, pancreatic, and head and neck carcinomas.[102] Consequently, CDK4/CDK6 have become relevant targets for therapeutic intervention, particularly in the setting of breast cancer.[103]

Protein Kinases and Cancer Cells

Dysfunction of protein kinases is a common event in tumors. Although this has been best characterized in human cancers, data indicate that dog and cat cancers experience similar dysregulation (Table 15.2). Kinases may be dysregulated through a variety of mechanisms, including mutation, overexpression, fusion proteins, or autocrine loops. In many cases, these alterations result in phosphorylation of the kinase in the absence of an appropriate signal. Mutations documented in kinases include a single amino acid change through a point mutation, deletion of amino acids, or insertion of amino acids, usually in the form of an internal tandem duplication (ITD). For example, a point mutation

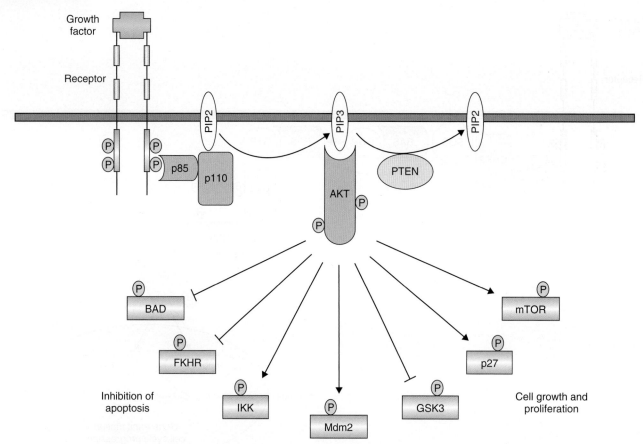

• **Fig. 15.7** PI3 kinase signal transduction. After receptor tyrosine kinase activation, PI3 kinase is recruited to the phosphorylated receptor through binding of the p85 adaptor subunit leading to activation of the catalytic subunit (p110). This activation results in the generation of the second messenger phosphatidylinositol-3,4,5-triphosphate (PIP3). PIP3 recruits AKT to the membrane and after its phosphorylation, several downstream targets are subsequently phosphorylated leading to either their activation or inhibition. The cumulative effect results in cell survival, growth, and proliferation. (Reprinted with permission from Blackwell Publishing, London CA, *Vet Comp Oncol* 2:177–193, 2004.)

occurs in the *BRAF* gene (V600E, exon 15) in approximately 60% of human cutaneous melanomas.[87,104,105] This amino acid change causes a conformation change in B-Raf, mimicking its activated form and thereby inducing constitutive downstream ERK signaling and abnormal promotion of cell growth and survival.[106,107] RAS is another kinase that is dysregulated through point mutation in several hematopoietic neoplasms (multiple myeloma, juvenile chronic myelogenous leukemia [CML], acute myelogenous leukemia [AML], and chronic myelomonocytic leukemia [CMML]) and in lung cancer, colon cancer, and several others.[86,108,109]

Another example of a mutation involves KIT, an RTK that normally is expressed on hematopoietic stem cells, melanocytes, in the central nervous system, and on mast cells.[110] In approximately 30% of canine grade 2 and grade 3 mast cell tumors (MCTs), mutations consisting of ITDs are found in the juxtamembrane domain of KIT, resulting in constitutive activation in the absence of ligand binding. These mutations are associated with a higher risk of local recurrence and metastasis.[111–113] Additional activating mutations in the extracelluar domain of KIT (specifically exons 8 and 9) have also been identified in canine MCTs.[114] Interestingly, KIT mutations consisting of deletions in the juxtamembrane domain are also found in approximately 50% of human patients with gastrointestinal stromal tumors (GISTs) and are also found

in canine GISTs.[115–118] There are other well-characterized mutations involving RTKs in human cancers including FLT3 ITDs in AML,[119–122] EGFR point mutations in lung carcinomas,[123,124] and PI3K-α mutations in several types of carcinomas.[94]

Overexpression of kinases usually involves the RTKs and may result in enhanced response of the cancer cells to normal levels of growth factor; or, if the levels are high enough, the kinase may become activated through spontaneous dimerization in the absence of signal/growth factor. In humans, the RTK HER2 (also known as ErbB2, a member of the EGFR family) is overexpressed in both breast and ovarian carcinomas and this often correlates with a more aggressive phenotype.[125,126,73] EGFR is also overexpressed in human lung, bladder, cervical, ovarian, renal, and pancreatic cancers, and some tumors have as many as 60 copies of the gene per cell.[76,127,128] As with HER2, such overexpression is linked to a worse outcome in affected patients.[76]

Fusion proteins are generated when a portion of the kinase becomes attached to another gene through chromosomal rearrangement and the normal mechanisms that control protein function are disrupted. One of the best characterized fusion proteins is BCR-ABL, which is found in 90% of patients with CML.[129–132] ABL is a cytoplasmic TK that, when fused to BCR, results in dysregulation of ABL, inappropriate activity of the protein, and

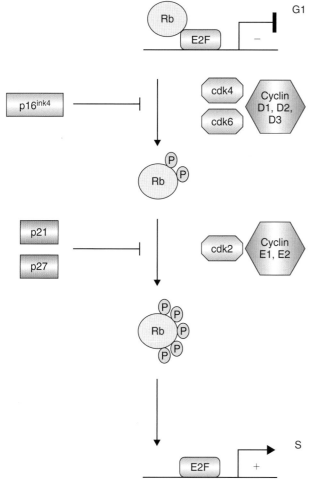

• **Fig. 15.8** Cyclin and CDK regulation of G1–S transition. CDK inhibitors such as p16ink4 and p21 restrict the activity of cyclin D– and cyclinE–dependent kinases. Progressive Rb phosphorylation by the cyclins results in liberation of E2F and the resultant transcription of S phase genes. (Reprinted with permission from Blackwell Publishing, London CA, *Vet Comp Oncol* 2:177–193, 2004.)

TABLE 15.2	Receptor Tyrosine Kinases Associated with Human Cancer
Tyrosine Kinase	**Cancer Association**
EGFR family	Breast, ovary, lung,[a] stomach, colon, glioblastoma
Insulin receptor family	Sarcomas, cervix, kidney
PDGFR family	Glioblastoma, ovary, CMML, GISTs
KIT	AML, GISTs,[a] seminoma, MCTs,[a,b] melanoma
FLT3	AML[a]
VEGFR family	Angiogenesis,[a,b] Kaposi's sarcoma, hemangiosarcoma/angiosarcoma,[a] melanoma
FGFR family	AML, lymphoma, breast, prostate, multiple myeloma, TCC
NGFR family	Thyroid cancer, neuroblastoma, fibrosarcoma, AML
Met/Ron	Thyroid cancer, osteosarcoma,[a] rhabdomyosarcoma, liver, kidney, colon
EPHR family	Melanoma, stomach, colon, breast, esophagus
AXL	AML
Tie family	Angiogenesis, stomach, hemangioblastoma
RET family	Thyroid cancer, multiple endocrine neoplasia
ALK	Non-Hodgkin's lymphoma, lung

[a]Also associated with canine cancer.

[b]Also associated with feline cancer.

ALK, Anaplastic lymphoma kinase; *AML,* acute myelogenous leukemia; *CMML,* chronic myelomonocytic leukemia; *EGFR,* epidermal growth factor receptor; *EPHR,* ephrin receptor; *FGFR,* fibroblast growth factor receptor; *GISTs,* gastrointestinal stromal tumors; *MCTs,* mast cell tumors; *NGFR,* nerve growth factor receptor; *PDGFR,* platelet-derived growth factor receptor; *TCC,* transitional cell carcinoma; *Tie,* tyrosine kinase receptor on endothelial cells; *VEGFR,* vascular endothelial growth factor receptor.

resultant malignant transformation. Other examples of fusion proteins include TEL-PDGFR-β in CMML, FIP1-PDGFR-α in hypereosinophilic syndrome with mastocytosis, and EML4-ALK in non-small-cell lung cancer (NSCLC).[133]

Autocrine loops of activation primarily occur when the tumor cell expresses both the RTK and the corresponding GF; in most cases, one or the other usually is also overexpressed, resulting in constitutive activation of the RTK. Examples include coexpression of transforming growth factor-alpha (TGF-) and EGFR in glioblastoma and squamous cell carcinoma, insulin-like growth factor-1 (IGF-α) and its ligand, IGF-1R, in breast and colorectal cancer, and VEGF and VEGFR in melanoma.[73,134–136] In canine cancers, possible autocrine loops have been documented in osteosarcoma (OSA) (coexpression of MET and its ligand, HGF) and hemangiosarcoma (HSA, coexpression of KIT and its ligand, SCF).[137–139]

Inhibition of Kinases

Given the detailed molecular characterization of signal transducer dysregulation in cancer cells, significant efforts have been directed at developing strategies to inhibit those transducers that participate in tumorigenesis through direct effects on cancer cells or through modulation of the local tumor microenvironment (stroma and neovasculature). The two most successful approaches to date have been monoclonal antibodies (mAbs) and small molecule inhibitors.

Several mAbs have been developed to target the extracellular domain of RTKs known to be important in a variety of tumors. These antibodies may prevent the growth factor from binding, promote internalization of the RTK and subsequent degradation, or may induce an immune response against the cancer cell. One of the most successful examples is a humanized mAb called trastuzumab (Herceptin). This antibody targets HER2, which as previously discussed is overexpressed in approximately 30% of human breast cancers.[140] Initial clinical trials of trastuzumab as single-agent treatment for HER2-positive breast cancer resulted in a response rate of approximately 25% in the setting of metastatic disease.[141] The response rate approached 50% when trastuzumab was combined with chemotherapy.[142] When used in the adjuvant setting, multiple studies have demonstrated that trastuzumab significantly improves survival rates of women with HER2-positive disease; consequently, it is now part of the routine standard of care for this type of cancer.[143,144] Other examples of mAbs that have significant activity in human cancers include rituximab (Rituxan), which targets CD20 expressed in a number of B-cell malignancies[145,146] and cetuximab (Erbitux), which targets ErbB1/HER1/EGFR known to be overexpressed in several carcinomas.[76,140,147]

Small molecule inhibitors work primarily by blocking the ATP binding site of kinases, essentially acting as either reversible or irreversible competitive inhibitors; a smaller number of these inhibitors work by preventing necessary protein–protein interactions (allosteric inhibition).[148] In the absence of ATP, the kinase is unable to phosphorylate itself or downstream signaling elements, thereby interrupting a survival/growth signal essential to the tumor cell, ultimately resulting in cell death. As the molecular characterization of tumors has improved, the development and application of small molecule inhibitors has rapidly expanded in human oncology, and their use is markedly altering how cancers are managed. Such inhibitors are often easy to synthesize in large quantities, frequently orally bioavailable, and can readily enter cells to bind the intended target.

The first small molecule inhibitor to be approved for human use was imatinib (Gleevec), an orally administered drug that binds the ATP pocket of ABL and the RTKs KIT and PDGFR-α.[149] As previously discussed, BCR-ABL fusion proteins are present in 90% of human patients with CML, making ABL a good target for therapeutic intervention. The application of imatinib to CML has been transformative, with significant biologic activity demonstrated in several clinical trials resulting in the approval of imatinib for first-line care of affected individuals.[150-155] In the chronic phase of the CML, imatinib induces a remission rate of close to 95%, and most patients remain in remission for longer than 1 year. Unfortunately, the remission rate is much lower for patients in blast crisis (20%–50%), often lasting less than 10 months. Resistance to imatinib has been well characterized and is primarily a result of the development of mutations in ABL that prevent drug binding, although gene amplification has also been documented.[156,157] Imatinib also has clinical activity against human GIST, in which 50% to 60% of the tumors have point mutations or deletions in the juxtamembrane domain of KIT resulting in constitutive activation.[158,159] Imatinib therapy for GIST patients results in response rates of 50% to 70%, far better than the 5% response rate observed with standard chemotherapy.[160,161] A small number of GISTs have activating mutations in PDGFR-α instead of KIT mutations; these patients also respond to imatinib.[162]

There are now more than 30 FDA-approved protein kinase inhibitors for the treatment of human cancers, ranging from those that target specific mutations in a single kinase to those that are multitargeted in nature, affecting both tumor cells and the microenvironment. For example, a subset of people with NSCLC have tumors with activating mutations in EGFR (in exons 19 or 21) that respond to erlotinib (Tarceva) or gefitinib (Iressa), small molecule inhibitors of EGFR.[163] Response rates in patients with EGFR mutations can be as high as 80% compared with less than 10% to 20% for those without, demonstrating that the efficacy of targeted therapies is often dependent on the presence of a known activated signaling element. Resistance to erlotinib/gefitinib is often mediated by a second mutation at codon 790 (T790M), and a protein kinase inhibitor osimertinib (Tagrisso), which targets this specific resistance mutation, has been approved.[164] A small number of patients with NSCLC also exhibit activation of the RTK ALK through its fusion to EML4.[165] A small molecule inhibitor of ALK, crizotinib (Xalkori) has demonstrated significant activity against lung cancer patients whose tumors express the EML4–ALK translocation. Objective response rates of greater than 50% to crizotinib

are typical in this subset of patients, with many more of patients experiencing long-term disease stabilization.[165,166]

Vemurafenib (Zelboraf) is a small molecule inhibitor of B-raf that has significant activity against cutaneous malignant melanomas that possess activating mutations in the *BRAF* gene. Response rates in the setting of *BRAF* mutant melanoma exceed 50%, compared with less than 5% for patients treated with dacarbazine.[167] Inhibition of mTOR has become of interest in several cancers, given the activation of the PI3K pathway and the critical role of mTOR in mediating its effects. Rapamycin (Rapamune), a drug used for many years as an immunosuppressive agent, is the prototypic mTOR inhibitor.[168,169] Temisorlimus (Torisel) and everolimus (Zortress), two rapamycin analogs, have been approved for use in patients with metastatic renal carcinoma, and other mTOR inhibitors are currently under investigation for their potential utility in treating soft tissue and bone sarcomas.[168,169]

Several new kinase inhibitors target signal transduction pathways in hematologic malignancies. Ibrutinib (Imbruvica) blocks signaling through the BTK cytoplasmic kinase that is critical for B cell receptor activity.[170] It is approved for use in several B-cell malignancies including CLL, follicular lymphoma, and Waldenström's macroglobulinemia; response rates in these diseases typically exceed 70% to 80% and are often durable in nature. With respect to T-cell malignancies, small molecule inhibitors of PI3Kγδ (tenalisib, duvelisib) have shown significant activity against peripheral and cutaneous T-cell lymphomas, with response rates ranging from 40% to 50%.[171]

Whereas the inhibitors discussed earlier tend to inhibit a restricted set of kinases, there are other inhibitors that exhibit more broadly targeted inhibition. Sunitinib (Sutent) is a small molecule inhibitor of several RTKs including VEGFR1/2, PDGFR-α/β, KIT, FLT3, CSFR1, and RET.[172] The multitargeted nature of this inhibitor may be responsible for its observed activity in several types of cancer including GIST, renal cell carcinoma, thyroid carcinoma, and insulinoma, among others.[172] Although such agents often have significant clinical activity, they are typically associated with a broader range of toxicities that may limit their use.

Kinase Inhibitors in Veterinary Medicine

There are now two small molecule inhibitors approved for use in dogs in veterinary oncology. Toceranib (TOC) phosphate (Palladia) is a multitargeted inhibitor closely related to sunitinib that exhibits a similar target profile including VEGFR, PDGFR, KIT, FLT3, and CSF1R. TOC has demonstrated activity against MCT and sarcomas and carcinomas. In the original phase I study, 28% of dogs experienced objective responses to treatment, with an additional 26% experiencing stable disease for an overall clinical benefit of 54%.[173] A pivotal study of TOC was subsequently conducted in dogs with recurrent or metastatic intermediate or high-grade MCTs, resulting in an objective response rate of 42.8% (21 complete responses (CR), 42 partial responses (PR)), with an additional 16 dogs experiencing stable disease for an overall clinical benefit of 60%.[174] Dogs whose MCT harbored activating mutations in KIT were roughly twice as likely to respond to TOC than those without mutations (69% vs 37%). After approval of TOC in 2009, it has been used to treat a number of different solid tumors.[175] Biologic activity has been reported in dogs with anal sac adenocarcinoma, thyroid carcinoma, head and neck carcinoma, and nasal carcinoma. Work is ongoing to more clearly define the role of TOC in the treatment of canine and feline cancer.

Mastinib (MAS, Kinavet, Masivet) is a small molecule inhibitor of KIT, PDGFR-α/β and Lyn that has been evaluated in both dogs and cats, although it is not currently approved by the US FDA. In dogs with MCTs, MAS significantly improved time to progression compared with placebo, and outcome was improved in dogs with MCT harboring KIT mutations.[176] Subsequent follow-up of patients treated with long-term MAS identified an increased number of patients with long-term disease control compared with those treated with placebo (40% vs 15% alive at 2 years).[177] Small studies have also evaluated the efficacy of imatinib for the treatment of canine and feline MCT.[178–180] Imatinib was well tolerated, and objective antitumor responses were observed in dogs with both mutant and wild-type KIT. Responses have also been observed in cats with MCT.[181,182]

Other small molecule inhibitors are currently under development for the treatment of canine cancer. RV1001 is an orally bioavailable PI3Kδ inhibitor that has demonstrated significant activity against naïve and relapsed T- and B-cell lymphomas in dogs. In phase I and II clinical trials, objective response rates ranged from 62% to 77% (respectively), with hepatotoxicity as the primary dose limiting event.[183] Verdinexor (KPT-335) is an orally bioavailable small molecule inhibitor of XPO-1, a nuclear export protein shuttle responsible for transporting several tumor suppressor proteins, thereby extinguishing their function. Blockade of XPO1 forces retention of these proteins, including such key cellular regulators as p53, p21, RB, FOXO, and NFκB. Verdinexor has been evaluated in both phase I and II studies in dogs with lymphoma; objective response rates in both studies were approximately 35%, with several dogs experiencing long-term stable disease, and hyporexia was determined to be the dose-limiting toxicity.[184,185]

Conclusion

With the advent of molecular techniques, the characterization of signal transduction pathways that are dysfunctional in cancer cells has become commonplace. Advances in computer modeling and small molecule engineering have led to the rapid development of inhibitors capable of blocking specific pathways critical for cancer cell proliferation and survival. The success of kinase inhibitors such as imatinib and crizotinib indicate that the application of this therapeutic strategy can markedly improve clinical outcomes. Perhaps the greatest challenges will be determining how these novel therapeutics can be effectively combined with standard treatment regimens such as surgery, chemotherapy, and radiation therapy to provide optimal anticancer efficacy without enhancing toxicity, and identifying strategies to use these therapeutics that are less likely to result in drug resistance.

SECTION C: ANTIANGIOGENIC AND METRONOMIC THERAPY

ANTHONY J. MUTSAERS AND BARBARA BILLER

Tumor Angiogenesis

For a solid tumor to grow beyond a few millimeters in size, it must recruit a blood supply to provide adequate nutrients and oxygen to the dividing cell mass and remove waste products.[186,187] Inducing angiogenesis is a hallmark of cancer progression,[188] yet angiogenesis is also a prominent aspect of normal physiology and transient pathology (e.g., in wound healing) and is tightly regulated. A large number of proangiogenic growth factors and signaling pathways promote the process of blood vessel growth.[186] Similarly, endogenous inhibitors of angiogenesis are temporally expressed to suppress vessel expansion and maintain angiogenic balance.[189] The net effect depends on this relative balance, which is tipped toward promoting angiogenesis during tumor growth. Therapeutic interventions aim to tip the scales back toward inhibiting angiogenesis.[190] Importantly, the vessels produced to support tumor growth are vastly different from normal vasculature. Tumor vessels are characterized by profound leakiness and sparse intermittent coverage of the endothelium by structural mural components, such as pericytes. These abnormalities inherent in tumor vessels contribute to the poor perfusion and high interstitial fluid pressure that are consistent features of the tumor microenvironment.

"Classical" angiogenesis occurs through the sprouting of new vessels from existing vasculature. The term vasculogenesis describes the de novo formation of new blood vessels from bone marrow–derived progenitor cell populations that respond to locally produced proangiogenic signals.[191,192] Numerous cell types that originate from bone marrow, including circulating endothelial progenitor cells (CEPs), may contribute to tumor angiogenesis by traveling to tumor sites and incorporating into existing vessel walls.[193–196] Finally, in certain circumstances, cancer cells may also access a blood supply through means other than sprouting new vessels. In certain highly vascular tissue environments, cancers may use *vessel co-option* to grow along existing blood vessels, which may ultimately lead to vessel collapse as the tumor grows.[197] In other contexts, cancer cells may produce microvascular channels that conduct fluid through a tumor cell–lined network in a process first described in uveal melanoma, known as *vasculogenic mimicry*.[197,198] The relative contributions of classical angiogenesis, CEP contribution, vessel co-option, and vasculogenic mimicry are likely cancer cell, organ/tissue environment, and stage dependent, potentially evolving as the tumor mass grows and becomes more heterogeneous and therapy resistant.

In addition to blood vessels, lymphatics are important components of the tumor microenvironment and a prominent feature of tissue homeostasis, immunosurveillance, and a gateway to metastatic spread.[199] Lymphatic vessel growth regulation is physiologically similar in principle to that of blood vessels,[200] and therefore targeting lymphangiogenesis may also represent an attractive treatment strategy in clinical oncology worthy of focused research.[201]

Antiangiogenic Therapy

Angiogenesis became a validated therapeutic target in oncology with the widespread approval of drugs that inhibit a potent signaling pathway for blood vessel growth, the vascular endothelial growth factor (VEGF) receptor tyrosine kinase pathway.[202–206] Drugs such as bevacizumab (Avastin), the humanized anti-VEGF monoclonal antibody, and small molecule receptor tyrosine kinase inhibitors (RTKIs) such as sunitinib (Sutent) in human oncology and TOC phosphate (Palladia) in veterinary medicine are considered to be efficacious, at least in part, because of the antiangiogenic effects of VEGFR signaling inhibition.[207,208]

Multiple mechanisms have been proposed to explain the antitumor effects of antiangiogenic therapies.[204] The first and most intuitive is *vascular collapse* resulting in impaired oxygen delivery to the tumor, leading to nutrient starvation, hypoxia, and death of cancer cells that cannot survive in this environment.[209] Conversely, a second perhaps paradoxical mechanism involves more efficient delivery of oxygen, nutrients, and indeed other drugs (such as chemotherapeutics) to tumor cells by the process of *vessel normalization*.[210,211] Normalization occurs when smaller, tortuous, inefficient, and leaky tumor vessels are selectively destroyed by the therapy, resulting in improved blood flow through more established vasculature, increasing perfusion to the tumor as a whole.[212] Vascular normalization has been demonstrated clinically using functional magnetic resonance imaging (fMRI) in patients treated with VEGF pathway inhibitors.[213,214] The most common clinical approach to targeting tumor angiogenesis has been either inhibition of overexpressed proangiogenic stimuli or supplementation of factors that inhibit angiogenesis, to tip the overall balance in favor of suppressing vessel growth.

Inhibition of Proangiogenic Factors

Currently, most RTKIs target numerous receptors to varying degrees.[208,215] TOC is an example of an RTKI that complements its direct effects on tumor cells (e.g., via mutated c-*kit* inhibition) with angiogenesis inhibition because it directly targets VEG-FRs.[216] In addition, drugs that inhibit PDGFRs, such as TOC, disrupt signaling pathways important for blood vessel support structures, such as the stromal pericyte component of larger vessels.[217,218] These drugs need not necessarily be purely antiangiogenic, as blood vessel receptors such as VEGFR and PDGFR may also be expressed by certain cancer cells, resulting in an autocrine growth factor loop within the tumor.[219,220] The end result is that, in specific instances, targeting angiogenic pathways may have concurrent direct antitumor cell and antiangiogenic effects.

Significant cross-influence exists between growth signaling pathways, and as a result there is strong interaction between tumor oncogene and suppressor gene expression and regulation of blood vessel expansion through growth factors such as VEGF. Therefore many drugs that target oncogenes have demonstrated antiangiogenic "off-target" effects as a byproduct of VEGF reduction.[221–223] For example, the anti-HER2 (*ErbB-2*) human MAb trastuzumab (Herceptin) and anti-EGFR antibodies such as cetuximab (Erbitux) are examples of drugs that indirectly suppress angiogenesis because neutralization of their oncogenic targets leads to a dramatic reduction in tumor cell VEGF production, which increases again at the time of targeted drug resistance.[224,225] Through reduction in VEGF or other growth factor expression, there is an antiangiogenic component to many forms of cancer treatment, including not only targeted inhibitors but also cytotoxic chemotherapy and RT. Therefore antiangiogenic effects are not necessarily restricted to treatment modalities that target known angiogenesis pathways directly.

Angiogenic Inhibitor Supplementation

Since the discovery of endogenous proteins and protein fragments that inhibit blood vessel growth, such as angiostatin, endostatin, and thrombospondins, there has been clinical interest in using angiogenesis inhibitors as cancer therapeutics.[189,226] In veterinary medicine, thrombospondin-1 mimetic peptides were evaluated in dogs with multiple tumor types. Treatment with the mimetic peptides ABT-526 and ABT-510 in a prospective clinical trial of 242 dogs with multiple tumor types showed an objective response or substantially stabilized disease in 42 dogs and a lack of dose-limiting toxicity.[227] Interestingly, most objective responses were recorded after 60 days of continuous drug treatment. Subsequently, an updated formulation, ABT-898, demonstrated a response rate of 32% in 28 dogs with soft tissue

sarcoma.[228] Results of a prospective randomized placebo-controlled clinical trial in dogs with multicentric lymphoma treated at first relapse revealed significantly improved time to tumor progression and remission duration, but not remission rate, when ABT-526 was used in combination with lomustine chemotherapy, compared with dogs treated with lomustine alone.[229] No ABT-526–specific toxicities were noted in this trial. In addition to thrombospondin-1, preliminary studies documenting detection of the endogenous inhibitors angiostatin and endostatin in normal and tumor-bearing dogs have been reported.[230,231] In a pilot study of endostatin as a therapeutic agent, 13 dogs with soft tissue sarcomas were treated with the canine endostatin gene delivered via liposome–DNA complexes.[232] Although endostatin gene expression was not detected in the tumors after treatment, objective responses were documented in two dogs, and eight dogs experienced stable disease, suggesting potential nonspecific antitumor activity.

Targeting Tumor Endothelial Cell Markers

Tumor endothelial cells (ECs) differ from normal endothelia in their gene and protein expression.[233] These differences may represent an opportunity for a favorable therapeutic index when drugs are designed to bind differentially expressed targets on tumor-specific endothelium. If not naturally destructive to these cells, drugs can be designed to carry a payload to induce local cytotoxicity, producing an antiangiogenic effect. A phage vector delivering tumor necrosis factor-alpha (RGD-A-TNF) to αV integrins on tumor endothelium is an example of this strategy that has undergone evaluation in dogs.[234] Through serial biopsy, this dose escalation trial demonstrated selective targeting of tumor endothelium via αV integrin-targeted expression of TNF, and treatment of a cohort of tumor-bearing dogs at the MTD resulted in partial remission in 2 of 14 and stable disease in 6 of 14 dogs.

Other Antiangiogenic Agents

A vast array of drugs not necessarily designed as anticancer therapeutics may derive at least a portion of their activity through inhibition of angiogenesis. Two examples investigated in a veterinary setting include inhibitors of matrix metalloproteinases (MMPs) and cyclooxygenases (COXs). The MMPs are a family of enzymes that degrade the extracellular matrix and basement membrane, thereby mediating tumor invasion, angiogenesis, and metastasis.[235] Unfortunately, clinical evaluation of compounds that inhibit these enzymes has to date been largely unrewarding,[236,237] including results from a large randomized trial of 303 dogs with OSA, in which treatment with the MMP inhibitor Bay12-9566 or placebo after doxorubicin (DOX) chemotherapy did not improve overall survival.[238] Inhibition of the proinflammatory COX enzymes has been reported in numerous tumor types in veterinary oncology.[239–241] The effects of COX inhibition on angiogenesis were evaluated with piroxicam treatment of canine transitional cell carcinoma (TCC). In a study of 18 dogs, piroxicam treatment was associated with reduced urinary concentrations of the proangiogenic growth factor basic fibroblast growth factor (bFGF) and induction of apoptosis.[242] In a subsequent study evaluating these parameters in 12 dogs treated with piroxicam in combination with cisplatin, reductions in urinary bFGF and VEGF were associated with response to the combination regimen.[243]

Another agent with demonstrated antiangiogenic effects, thalidomide, has been approved for treatment of human multiple myeloma.[244] Thalidomide has been evaluated in veterinary oncology for treatment of canine hemangiosarcoma (HSA) and other tumors as a single agent and in combination with chemotherapy, including metronomic chemotherapy protocols.[245,246] Targeting angiogenesis in combination with chemotherapy has been considered a useful strategy,[204] particularly as drug delivery may be enhanced through a "normalized" vasculature.[210] Many reported early clinical trials utilize a cocktail of multiple drugs, such as COX inhibitor, kinase inhibitor, thalidomide, and/or chemotherapy agent(s). Multiple drug trial design may increase the chances of documenting anticancer activity, but is challenging to decipher the relative contributions of a particular agent to the outcome of the treatment protocol.

Metronomic Chemotherapy

Ideal anticancer therapies would be highly efficacious, widely available at low cost, and associated with a low risk of causing adverse events. Keeping this in mind, along with the statement of Fidler and Ellis that "Cancer is a chronic disease and should be treated like other chronic diseases," one path taken toward the identification of optimal therapies has been the exploration of metronomic drug delivery.[247] Characterized by chronic administration of chemotherapeutic agents at low doses, metronomic chemotherapy (or low-dose continuous chemotherapy) is being used with increasing understanding and frequency in the treatment of humans and companion animals with cancer.

The term metronomic chemotherapy (MC) was originally introduced by Hanahan and colleagues in 2000 to describe the concept that the continuous administration of certain cytotoxic drugs targeted tumor ECs, impairing their ability to repair and recover as long as no extended drug-free gaps were allowed.[248] Although a number of cytotoxic chemotherapy agents achieve at least a portion of their therapeutic efficacy through inhibition of tumor angiogenesis, their delivery at the MTD in conventional chemotherapy protocols necessitates a break period to permit recovery of normal cell populations.[249,250] When many of the same drugs are instead delivered in a metronomic fashion, the therapeutic target shifts from the rapidly dividing tumor cell population to the more slowly proliferating tumor endothelium. Although this approach was initially designed to overcome the development of chemotherapeutic drug resistance via inhibition of tumor angiogenesis, additional mechanisms of action have since been uncovered. These include activation of antitumor immunity, induction of tumor dormancy, and inhibition of cancer stem cells. Compared with typical MTD treatment regimens, the low toxicity profile, ease of administration for orally delivered drugs, and decreased cost make MC protocols particularly appealing in veterinary oncology. However, mechanistic and clinical evaluation in veterinary patients is still at a relatively early stage.

Mechanisms of Action

Tumor Angiogenesis

When different types of cells in culture were exposed to continuous ultralow doses of chemotherapy, proliferating EC populations displayed an exquisite sensitivity compared with other cell types, including tumor cells in many instances.[251,252] Although the reasons for EC selectivity are not entirely clear, the explanation likely goes beyond mere targeting of rapidly dividing cells. Experimental evidence has suggested that upregulation of thrombospondin-1

occurs during treatment with metronomic cyclophosphamide and possibly other chemotherapy agents.[253,254] The resulting angiogenic suppression may be complemented by decreased tumor cell production of proangiogenic growth factors such as VEGF, through reduced tumor cell mass.

Other components of angiogenesis may also be targeted by metronomic delivery of chemotherapy. Mechanistically, tumor angiogenesis involves recruitment of CEPs.[195] These CEP cells may be most influential in rebuilding tumor vessels during the break period after the acute damage of MTD chemotherapy exposure.[255] Preclinical models have demonstrated that CEPs acutely decrease with MTD treatment, only to rapidly rebound during the break period (similar to other bone marrow-derived cells), when they may contribute to EC repopulation.[256] In contrast, metronomic chemotherapy delivery does not appear to be associated with a CEP surge, leading instead to a sustained antiangiogenic effect.[256–258]

Immunomodulatory Effects

The ability of tumors to grow undetected by the host immune system is a well-recognized feature of malignancy. Through the dynamic process of immunoediting the phenotype of neoplastic cells evolves to escape immune detection. Two major immune cells, regulatory T lymphocytes (Treg), and myeloid-derived suppressor cells (MDSCs), are key players in this process. Although they limit pathologic inflammation under normal conditions, Treg and MDSC efficiently suppress antitumor immune responses in cancer patients.[259–261] Treg are particularly adept at inhibiting effector (cytotoxic) T cells through direct cell-to-cell contact and secretion of immunosuppressive cytokines such as TGF-β and IL-10. MDSC and other immune cells such as poorly functional dendritic cells and inhibitory macrophages also help establish tumor tolerance and an immunosuppressive tumor microenvironment.

Although it may seem counterintuitive, a number of chemotherapeutic agents display both immunostimulatory and immunosuppressive effects, a difference that sometimes depends only on the dose and schedule of drug administration. One of the best examples of this concept is illustrated by the alkylating agent cyclophosphamide (CYC). Whereas high doses have long been used as a myeloablative preconditioning therapy for procedures such as bone marrow transplantation, metronomic delivery of CYC is associated with multiple immunostimulatory effects including decreases in the number and function of Treg, dendritic cell activation, and stimulation of tumor-specific cytotoxic T cells.[262]

The clinical effect of metronomic CYC chemotherapy on the host immune system was first demonstrated in a key study by Ghiringhelli in which human patients with advanced cancer experienced a selective decrease in circulating Treg numbers with marked restoration of T effector cell proliferation and NK cell function.[263] Numerous additional studies have since uncovered direct and specific inhibitory effects of low-dose CYC on Treg function, often with corresponding increases in effector T-cell function and decreased expression of immunosuppressive cytokines.[262,264] Worth noting, however, are results of studies in mouse tumor models and in human cancer patients documenting stimulation of MDSC recruitment and rebounding tumor growth during administration of metronomic CYC.[265–267]

Immunomodulatory effects of CYC have also been reported in dogs with spontaneous cancer. Metronomic administration of CYC, for example, appears to be immunostimulatory based on two small studies in which circulating Treg were significantly decreased when CYC was given alone or in combination with TOC.[268,269] Interestingly, dogs receiving the two drugs concurrently had significant increases in serum concentrations of IFN-γ that were inversely correlated with Treg numbers after 6 weeks of treatment.[269]

Administration of low, noncytotoxic concentrations of other chemotherapeutic agents such as paclitaxel, DOX, methotrexate and gemcitabine have also been shown to improve antitumor immunity. Mechanisms for this vary but include dendritic cell activation, improvement of cytotoxic T-cell function and reduction of MDSC activity.[270–272] For example, administration of low doses of paclitaxel to mice with metastatic lung tumors led to a selective decrease in Treg number and function without interfering with tumor-specific cytotoxic T cell function.[273] The nucleoside analog gemcitabine appears to decrease MDSC accumulation within tumor tissues, likely in part through the differentiation of MDSC into functionally active immunostimulatory DCs.[265,266]

Similar to CYC, the alkylating agent temozolomide (TMZ) has also been shown to reduce circulating Treg numbers in human cancer patients.[274] Denies and colleagues recently investigated daily low dose TMZ therapy in 30 tumor-bearing dogs, administered either alone or in combination with daily low-dose CYC.[275] In these dogs the primary study endpoints were circulating Treg numbers and plasma concentrations of TSP-1 and VEGF. The investigators found that dogs receiving CYC (12.5 mg/m^2/day) or the combination of CYC and TMZ (6.6 mg/m^2/day) had significantly lower percentages of Treg after 2 weeks of therapy whereas dogs receiving TMZ alone did not. Neither drug nor the combination was found to influence pre- and posttreatment plasma concentrations of TSP-1 or VEGF. As TMZ has been well tolerated in dogs at higher doses in conventional chemotherapy protocols, additional pharmacodynamic studies may lead to identification of a biologically effective dose when used in the metronomic setting.[276,277]

Other Targets of Metronomic Chemotherapy

Dormancy is a stage of tumor development in which viable neoplastic cells are present but inactive as a result of dynamic equilibrium between apoptosis and proliferation. Dormancy may arise in the early phases of tumor progression before conditions are in place to adequately support tumor cell proliferation and again in the posttreatment remission period. Not surprisingly, reactivation of dormant tumor cells represents one reason for the development of progressive disease after completion of conventional MTD chemotherapy protocols.[278] Similar to dormant tumor cells, cancer stem cells (CSCs) may also be present both before and after conventional anticancer therapy. Also known as tumor initiating cells, CSCs display a unique and formidable phenotype within the tumor cell population, characterized by their capabilities for self-renewal and DNA repair. Accumulating experimental data suggest MC may be able to target CSCs and dormant tumor cells because of the tendency of both cell populations to reside in close proximity to tumor vasculature.[279] For instance, in mice with glioma and hepatocellular carcinoma, antiangiogenic therapy was found to disrupt this close association, leading to apoptosis of CSC and bystander damage to dormant tumor cells immediately adjacent tumor vasculature.[280,281] Whether this mechanism of action of MC will translate into a therapeutic benefit for human or veterinary patients awaits further investigation.

Clinical Trial Evaluation

Summary of Human Clinical Trials

Nearly 20 years ago, the results of a pivotal clinical trial were reported in which women with metastatic breast cancer received daily low dose CYC and twice weekly methotrexate. This study found a disease control rate (defined as a complete or partial response or durable stable disease) of 32% and a low incidence (13%) of mild to moderate leukopenia.[282] As most of the women had already failed MTD chemotherapy protocols containing CYC, these results stimulated significant interest in further investigation of MC for the treatment of advanced cancers.

Since that time, numerous phase I and II studies have described the clinical benefits of MC, many reporting encouraging tumor control rates and very low toxicity rates. The majority of these studies have paired a conventional chemotherapy drug with a noncytotoxic drug that also targets angiogenesis. Noncytotoxic drugs typically include those with indirect effects on angiogenesis such as COX inhibitors, tetracyclines, and thalidomide or those with more direct effects such as bevacizumab.

In a meta-analysis of 80 published human clinical trials, the most frequently used cytotoxic drugs were CYC (43%) followed by capecitabine, etoposide, and vinorelbine.[283] In this systematic literature review, most studies (80%) were reports from single-arm trials, often relying on historical controls. In 72% of the trials, the patient sample size was 50 or less. Of the few trials with multiple arms (n = 16), only seven were randomized. Recent clinical data compiled from larger MC clinical trials for cancer patients living in India have found that methotrexate and celecoxib are used most often, likely owing to the wide availability and low cost of these agents.[284]

To date there has been only one double-blinded, placebo-controlled randomized clinical trial reported in human cancer patients.[285] This study compared a four-drug metronomic regimen of daily celecoxib and thalidomide with alternating periods of etoposide and CYC to placebo in 108 pediatric patients with solid tumors (mostly OSA or primitive neuroectodermal tumors). The primary study end point was the progression-free rate (PFR) as defined by the proportion of patients without disease progression at 6 months after starting MC. Unfortunately, there was no difference in PFR between the two groups as more than 96% of patients developed progressive disease within 3 months. Interestingly, patients receiving MC for a tumor type other than a bone sarcoma demonstrated significantly longer overall progression-free survival (PFS) time compared with those receiving placebo. The authors concluded that MC may not display efficacy across all classes of pediatric solid tumors, underscoring the importance of tumor histology in predicting treatment response.

Summary of Veterinary Clinical Trials

Similar to human clinical studies, veterinary clinical trials evaluating MC have been mostly small, phase I and II and/or retrospective. Metronomic administration of CYC, given alone or in combination with a nonsteroidal antiinflammatory drug (NSAID), has been the approach most often tested; however, the treatment protocol, disease setting and outcomes assessed have all varied considerably. The majority of trials have investigated dogs with various malignancies and advanced disease, using the disease control rate as the main indicator of tumor response. A handful of studies have also examined pharmacodynamic measures of response including biomarkers of angiogenesis or immunomodulation.[268,269,277]

Veterinary Trials with Alkylating Agents

Thus far there have been roughly 20 published reports of clinical trials investigating metronomic delivery of an alkylating agent in dogs with cancer; only two have included cats. Of these about 80% have utilized CYC with the remainder employing other alkylators. An early trial by Lana et al tested the administration of oral CYC (12.5–25 mg/m²/day) alternating with etoposide (50 mg/m² PO, daily) and combined with daily piroxicam for the adjuvant treatment of dogs with splenic HSA.[286] These investigators found that the approach had similar efficacy and less toxicity compared with control dogs receiving conventional DOX chemotherapy. The metronomic protocol was well tolerated over a 6-month period although two of nine dogs developed a transient sterile hemorrhagic cystitis (SHC). A more recent investigation by Wendelburg and colleagues found a similar result when comparing metronomic CYC chemotherapy versus conventional DOX chemotherapy for dogs with splenic HSA.[287] In this study, however, the median overall survival time (OST) was strikingly short (3.4 months) for dogs receiving either adjuvant metronomic or conventional chemotherapy and not significantly different from dogs treated with splenectomy alone.

Metronomic delivery of CYC has also been investigated in the maintenance setting after completion of adjuvant MTD chemotherapy in dogs with HSA or OSA. For dogs with HSA treated with splenectomy and six doses of DOX, daily or every other day CYC plus an NSAID had no effect on PFS or OST.[288] In dogs with OSA, the addition of daily CYC with an NSAID after limb amputation and four doses of carboplatin yielded similar PFS and OST as dogs treated with amputation and carboplatin alone.[289] In a larger multicenter study, dogs with OSA were randomized to receive piroxicam and CYC with or without TOC after limb amputation and four doses of adjuvant carboplatin.[290] Compared with historical control dogs treated with amputation and four doses of carboplatin, there was no improvement in the median PFS or OST in dogs of either treatment arm.

Other alkylating agents including chlorambucil, lomustine, and TMZ have also been evaluated in veterinary treatment protocols. In most of these trials the primary study endpoint has been toxicity, with tumor response evaluation a secondary goal.[275,291–293] When administration of lomustine at a daily oral dose of 2.84 mg/m² was tested in 81 dogs with a various malignancies, an unexpectedly high incidence of adverse events occurred and led to the discontinuation of the therapy in nearly 30%.[293] Oral chlorambucil is typically well tolerated when given at 4 mg/m²/day in metronomic protocols. But when given at higher daily doses of 6 or 8 mg/m², a retrospective study found significantly increased gastrointestinal and bone marrow toxicities with no improvement in tumor response.[292] Chlorambucil at 4 mg/m²/day combined with monthly doses of lomustine was also well tolerated based on investigation of eight dogs with glioma. In this study, three of the dogs developed grade I or II thrombocytopenia after 8 to 16 months of chronic therapy but there was no neutropenia attributable to chlorambucil and no grade III, IV, or V bone marrow toxicity.[291]

Combination of Metronomic Chemotherapy with Other Treatment Modalities

The question of whether concurrent MC and conventional MTD chemotherapy can be safely administered has been the focus of several recent clinical trials. In dogs with various malignancies, the combination of MTD DOX with concurrent metronomic CYC was found to be well tolerated in a recent phase I study.[294] DOX (30 mg/m² intravenous [IV]) was given once every 3 weeks for four treatments with concurrent daily oral CYC. Dose escalation for CYC was performed according to a standard 3 + 3 cohort schema starting at 10 mg/m²/day and extending to 15 mg/m² by 2.5 mg/m² increments. There were no significant toxicities in dogs of any cohort but the duration of the treatment period was potentially too short to determine the incidence of SHC or DOX-induced cardiomyopathy. Unfortunately, administration of DOX was associated with nonselective depletion of circulating lymphocytes such that any potential benefits of Treg depletion by low-dose CYC would have been lost.

RT combined with MC is another area under active investigation in both people and companion animals. In one study, Cancedda et al treated 50 dogs with macroscopic soft tissue sarcoma using a 5 × 6 Gray hypofractionated RT protocol. Twenty of these dogs then received daily oral piroxicam and thalidomide plus every other day oral CYC. The addition of this MC protocol had no effect on PFS but treated dogs displayed a significantly longer OST compared with dogs treated with RT alone (757 vs 286 days, respectively).[295] RT has also been combined with metronomic dosing of lomustine in the treatment of dogs with OSA.[296] When combined with palliative RT, the lomustine was well tolerated but did not extend the OST compared with dogs receiving RT alone.

As in the human oncology field, there is significant interest in combining MC with immunotherapy for dogs and cats with cancer; however, published reports are few. Cicchelero et al investigated the immunologic and antiangiogenic effects of intratumoral electrogene therapy with IL-12 in six dogs that also received daily oral CYC at 12.5 mg/m².[297] Although study design did not permit determination of the contribution of each treatment separately, there was a significant decrease in circulating Treg numbers from pretreatment values and decreased intratumoral blood volume in five of the six dogs. The intratumoral concentration of the angiogenic inhibitor TSP-1 was significantly increased compared with baseline for the duration of the 35-day study period.

Adverse Events

Despite the therapeutic index achieved by treating activated versus dormant vasculature, there is still potential risk that drug effects on vessels have unwanted consequences. For bevacizumab, potential side effects of a vascular etiology include hypertension, edema, hemorrhage, thromboembolism, proteinuria, intestinal perforation, and impaired wound healing.[298] Similarly, in veterinary oncology, side effects for TOC may include hypertension, proteinuria, dose-dependent gastrointestinal upset, bleeding, myelosuppression, azotemia, anemia, lethargy, lameness, or disruption of the hypothalamic–pituitary–thyroid axis.[299–302]

CYC is a commonly employed drug for metronomic scheduling but is associated with the potential for SHC.[303] The incidence of SHC may be more frequent in metronomic protocols. Recent reports document that cystitis may occur in up to 34% of cases, and SHC risk increases with longer treatment duration, which is common with metronomic therapy.[304,288,289] These toxicity results echo the finding that cumulative dose is a risk factor for SHC in dogs with lymphoma treated with MTD CYC.[305] Close urinary monitoring is strongly recommended for patients receiving MC, and recent studies demonstrate reduced SHC with concurrent use of furosemide as a preventative therapy.[306,307] Chlorambucil has also been used as an alternative to CYC that negates the risk of SHC. With these drugs and any type of therapy intended to be administered continuously for long periods of time, adverse events associated with cumulative dosing must be investigated, as these side effects may not be observed in more commonly reported short-term clinical trials.

Although not initially expected, acquired resistance to antiangiogenic therapy has become evident from clinical trial results. Given the genetically stable nature of the blood vessel/EC target compared with the mutation-prone cancer cell population, antiangiogenic treatment was originally postulated to be less likely to demonstrate drug resistance.[308] Proposed mechanisms of resistance to antiangiogenic therapies involve both tumor and host-mediated pathways that can be intrinsic or induced by treatment.[309] One alarming consequence of antiangiogenic treatment that emerged from preclinical studies with certain antiangiogenic RTKIs is the potential to alter the host microenvironment (e.g., in the lungs), leading to metastatic conditioning.[310,311] This phenomenon of increased invasion and metastasis as a result of antiangiogenic drug treatment was observed with sunitinib, an RTKI with a similar target spectrum to TOC.[311] However, a randomized clinical trial of TOC used in the adjuvant setting for canine OSA revealed no difference in the disease-free interval.[290]

Biomarkers

The incorporation of biomarkers into clinical decision making is increasingly important in the era of targeted therapeutics.[312] The aims of validated biomarkers include (1) predicting patients who will or will not respond to treatment, (2) monitoring response to therapy, or (3) determining the therapeutic dose for agents that often possess optimal biologic activity at doses well below the traditionally defined MTD. The use of validated biomarkers to guide the application of antiangiogenic agents is relevant in all three of these areas.

Tumor tissue expression and/or blood-based circulating growth factor levels have been the most popular approaches to predicting response to antiangiogenic treatment, with VEGF being the most studied molecule.[313–315] For example, in a pilot study of MC and celecoxib therapy in 15 dogs with various cancers, low baseline plasma VEGF was predictive of response.[316] The temporal comparison of pretreatment with posttreatment levels may provide the most useful information for certain surrogate biomarkers, as was demonstrated with urinary bFGF and VEGF with piroxicam treatment of canine TCC.[242,243] Biomarkers that are particularly valuable for antiangiogenic therapy may be those that define tumor response because inhibiting angiogenesis does not necessarily result in reduced tumor volume in the short term. A static tumor response sharply contrasts that observed with successful MTD chemotherapy approaches that result in overt measurable tumor shrinkage. Imaging modalities that can provide information about vascular function are potentially valuable tools for monitoring tumor angiogenesis and the effects of antiangiogenic therapy.[317] Dynamic contrast-enhanced MRI (DCE-MRI) has been studied for its ability to quantitatively assess vascular parameters.[318] A study by MacLeod and colleagues demonstrated blood volume and permeability measurements in canine intracranial masses using this modality.[319]

The area of dose optimization also represents an unmet need for biomarkers in antiangiogenic and metronomic chemotherapy. In the absence of dose limiting toxicities, the choice of drug dose may be highly empirical without information on target modulation. The assessment of Treg may provide insight as a dose optimization biomarker. A study that utilized serial sampling in canine soft tissue sarcoma demonstrated dose-dependent reduction in Treg with MC treatment. Reduced Treg were observed at 15 mg/m² but not 12.5 mg/m² doses, leading to the conclusion that 15 mg/m² may be a more appropriate dose for future clinical trials.[268] In addition to Treg levels, temporal evaluation of other markers has been studied. Assessment of CECs and/or CEPs has been applied for biomarker analysis of dosing antiangiogenic and metronomic therapy.[320–322] For example, in the study by Rusk and colleagues, decreasing CEC levels in dogs treated with the thrombospondin-1 mimetic peptide ABT-526 may have indicated adequate exposure to the antiangiogenic drug, which in this study was utilized at a single dose.[227] However, total CEC levels were not associated with soft tissue sarcoma response to TSP peptides in another trial.[228]

Finally, in dogs with solid tumors, temporal increases in plasma VEGF over 30 days of TOC treatment occurred at doses considerably lower than the FDA-approved MTD.[323] These results suggested that biologic activity of TOC through VEGF pathway inhibition occurs within an optimal dose range that has an improved adverse event profile compared with the MTD. Blood pressure changes may also reflect the biologic activity of this class of drugs and measuring hypertension has also been suggested as a surrogate biomarker for VEGF pathway inhibitors, including TOC.[324,300]

Conclusion

Numerous forms of conventional and targeted cancer therapies produce antiangiogenic effects that may contribute to their overall efficacy, and the field of tumor angiogenesis has come of age with the successful application of drugs that inhibit the VEGF receptor and other relevant pathways. The metronomic application of chemotherapy has antiangiogenic effects and demonstrates significant immunomodulatory activity that warrants further study, particularly in combination with other targeted approaches. However, well-powered prospective clinical trials to evaluate efficacy are currently lacking. Optimization of drug choices, combinations, and tumor applications remain as significant challenges, as does the emergence of drug resistance. Biomarker research may provide insight into patients that are more likely to benefit, optimal dosing for agents with activity below the MTD, and predict clinical benefit that may often manifest as sustained stable disease.

SECTION D: NOVEL AND EMERGING THERAPEUTIC AGENTS

DOUGLAS H. THAMM AND DAVID J. ARGYLE

The recent explosion in available tumor bioinformatic information, rational and combinatorial drug design, and high-throughput drug screening have resulted in a massive increase in potential therapeutic targets and anticancer treatment strategies. An exhaustive survey of all potential novel targets for cancer therapy would be impossible, and thus this review is designed to present a brief overview of some of the more promising and well developed, "druggable" targets that have been discovered recently, with an emphasis on those for which in vitro or in vivo data in veterinary species are available.

DNA Methylation

In addition to the information encoded within the genome sequence, epigenetic changes are of great importance in the modification and maintenance of gene expression. These changes take place through a number of mechanisms, including polymerase enzyme modulation, microRNAs, chromatin condensation, and DNA methylation. Mammalian DNA is methylated at cytosines within CpG dinucleotide sequences. During tissue differentiation, methylation pattern is one governor of tissue-specific gene expression and thus phenotype.[325–327]

Two different methylation-related phenomena have been identified in cancer. Tumor DNA in dogs and other mammals is globally hypomethylated,[328,329] specifically in pericentromeric satellite sequences. This may lead to decreased genome stability and an increase in the incidence of oncogenic chromosome defects. Indeed, the purposeful induction of genomic hypomethylation by reduction in germline DNA methyltransferase-1 (DNMT1) levels in genetically engineered mice is associated with a high incidence of T-cell lymphomas displaying trisomy 15.[330] Cancer cells also acquire sequence-specific promoter hypermethylation and transcriptional repression in normally unmethylated regions, several of which have been shown to be associated with known tumor suppressor genes, including Rb, p16, p73, and the von Hippel–Lindau protein (VHL),[325,326,331–334] or other important tumor-associated genes, such as E-cadherin, estrogen, retinoic acid receptors, and P-glycoprotein.[335,336] In addition, downregulation of expression of cytokines, tumor antigens, and/or antigen presentation machinery has been demonstrated to be regulated by promoter methylation in some cancers, which could contribute to tumor immune avoidance.[337–339]

The methylation of DNA is controlled by four known DNMTs, of which DNMT1 may be the most important in cancer.[325–327] A variety of agents can inhibit DNMT function. The two best studied are 5-azacytidine (Vidaza, Celgene) and 5-aza-deoxycitidine (decitabine, Dacogen, Otsuka), nucleoside analogs that incorporate into DNA and inhibit DNMT activity, but allow replication to proceed. A large number of single-agent human clinical trials with these agents have been reported, and significant activity has been demonstrated in hematopoietic neoplasia, leading to the US FDA approval of 5-azacytidine and decitabline for the treatment of myelodysplastic syndrome.[340,341] Encouraging response rates to the nucleoside analog decitabine have also been seen in patients with imatinib-refractory chronic myelogenous leukemia.[342,343] Results in advanced solid tumors have been generally disappointing[344–346]; however, studies in combination with standard antineoplastic therapy and other targeted agents are ongoing.[347] Interestingly, the commonly used cardiac medications procainamide and hydralazine also possess demethylating activity,[335,348] and clinical trials have demonstrated alterations in promoter methylation and reactivation of silenced genes after administration of well-tolerated doses of hydralazine to human cervical cancer patients.[349] Hydralazine–valproic acid (VPA) combinations have demonstrated activity in myelodysplastic syndrome and cutaneous T-cell lymphoma in early human trials.[350,351] Procainamide and hydralazine have long track records of use in veterinary medicine, and as such could serve as inexpensive and available drugs for the evaluation of methylation inhibition in veterinary cancer patients.

Recent genome-wide studies have demonstrated significant changes in patterns of specific gene methylation in canine lymphomas, some of which appear capable of providing prognostic information.[352,353] Multiple in vitro studies have demonstrated selective growth inhibition and/or induction of apoptosis in canine and feline tumor cells treated with demethylating agents.[354–358] Importantly, a phase I clinical trial of the demethylating agent 5-azacitidine has been performed in dogs with urothelial carcinomas. Objective responses were reported, but there was no correlation between gene methylation changes after treatment and clinical outcome.[359]

Two potential problems exist regarding the wide clinical implementation of DNMT inhibitors for cancer treatment. As discussed earlier, induction of long-term genome-wide hypomethylation could decrease chromosome stability leading to potentially tumorigenic chromosome rearrangements.[327] Demethylation could also trigger the reactivation of genes promoting a more aggressive or metastatic phenotype.[327] In support of this theory, treatment of nonmetastatic breast cancer cells with 5-azacytidine was shown to upregulate expression of urokinase-like plasminogen activator, an enzyme important in tumor invasion and metastasis, leading to enhanced metastatic potential.[360]

Histone Deacetylase

Another critical determinant of gene expression is the condensation of chromatin in the form of heterochromatin, which results in transcriptional silencing. This is accomplished by a number of pathways, one of which is the acetylation and deacetylation of histones, controlled by histone acetyltransferases and histone deacetylases (HDACs). The HDACs specifically maintain chromatin in a condensed form, and can associate with specific transcription factors resulting in transcription repression. Histone acetylation reduces electrostatic charge interactions between histones leading to chromatin decondensation. Histone acetylation may be key in regulating the expression of genes associated with cellular proliferation, differentiation and survival, both in development and carcinogenesis.[361,362] Induction of HDAC expression, leading to transcriptional repression, is a common feature in human cancers such as colon cancer,[363] and negatively regulates the expression of multiple tumor suppressor genes, including *p53* and *VHL*.[364] Certain HDAC isoforms are capable of acetylating nonhistone proteins, such as DNMT1, tubulin, and p53, which can alter protein stability, intracellular trafficking, and protein–protein or protein–DNA interactions.[365–367] Differential expression of certain HDAC isoforms has been associated with outcome in a variety of human tumors, with HDACs 2 and 6 studied most completely.[368]

Pharmacologic inhibition of HDAC can affect multiple facets of the malignant phenotype. HDAC inhibition inhibits colon carcinogenesis in the APC mouse model.[363] Angiogenesis can be inhibited through upregulation of VHL and subsequent inhibition of hypoxia-inducible factor-1alpha (Hif-1α) function and vascular endothelial growth factor production[364,369,370]; decreased expression of other proangiogenic factors, such as basic fibroblast growth factor, angiopoietin-2, and Tie-2[369,370]; inhibition of endothelial nitric oxide synthase and endothelial cell proliferation and tube formation[371,372]; and inhibition of the commitment of endothelial progenitor cells to the endothelial lineage.[373] Inhibition of HDACs can enhance apoptosis in tumor and endothelial cells,[370,374–376] and directly inhibit tumor cell proliferation.[375,377–379] Consistent with its role as a transcriptional repressor, inhibition of HDACs has been shown to induce differentiation in thyroid and prostate cancer, neuroblastoma, and the leukemias.[380–384] HDAC inhibition enhances the in vitro and in vivo efficacy of multiple standard cytotoxic therapies, antibodies and small molecules.[367,370,376,385–393]

Two HDAC inhibitors, vorinostat (SAHA, Zolinza, Merck) and romidepsin (FK228, Istodax, Celgene), have been approved by the FDA for the treatment of cutaneous T-cell lymphoma,[394–396] and a large number of additional agents are in intermediate- to late-stage clinical trials. A number of studies are being conducted evaluating HDAC inhibitors for various other hematologic and solid tumors, and early studies combining these drugs with other targeted and cytotoxic therapies have been reported.[397–400]

Recent in vitro studies have demonstrated potent induction of histone acetylation, growth inhibition, and induction of apoptosis in a variety of canine tumor cell lines treated with either vorinostat or the novel HDAC inhibtior OSU-HDAC42 (AR-42)[401,402]; and inhibition of canine prostate cancer metastasis to bone was observed after AR-42 treatment in a murine xenograft model.[403] Synergy between vorinostat and the DNMT inhibitor zebularine has been observed in canine OSA cell lines.[358] The commercially available anticonvulsant drug VPA can function as an HDAC inhibitor, and is capable of inhibiting tumor cell invasion, P-glycoprotein expression, proliferation and angiogenesis, and enhancing chemosensitivity.[404,367,381] VPA was recently shown to enhance the efficacy of DOX in canine OSA cell lines in vitro, and to synergize with DOX in a canine OSA xenograft.[391] A recent study demonstrated that VPA could be administered before a standard dose of DOX in tumor-bearing dogs, at dosages sufficient to enhance histone acetylation in tumor and peripheral blood mononuclear cells, but not associated with toxicity or apparent potentiation of DOX's adverse effects.[392]

The Proteasome

The abundance of cellular proteins is tightly controlled at the levels of both production and destruction. Protein production can be modified at the transcriptional and posttranscriptional level, and therapies based on these approaches are relatively abundant. Until relatively recently, little attention had been paid to the manipulation of protein degradation as a therapeutic modality. The ubiquitin–proteasome pathway (UPP) is responsible for the degradation of the majority of intracellular proteins, and is responsible for the regulation of many proteins with key roles in cancer.

The 26S proteasome is a large multiprotein complex containing ubiquitin recognition domains, which bind ubiquitinated proteins tagged for degradation, and proteolytic domains with trypsin-like, chymotrypsin-like, and caspase-like activity, which degrade proteins into short polypeptide sequences.[405] It is responsible for the degradation of a variety of proteins responsible for cell-cycle regulation, angiogenesis, apoptosis, and chemotherapy and radiation sensitivity (Table 15.3).[405–407]

Tumor cells are generally more sensitive to the effects of proteasome inhibition than are normal cells. Various studies have demonstrated a 3- to 40-fold increase in susceptibility to proteasome inhibitor-associated apoptosis when comparing tumor cells with corresponding normal tissues.[407–411] The mechanisms for this differential sensitivity are unclear, but proliferating cells generally appear more sensitive than do quiescent cells.[405,407] In

TABLE 15.3	Molecular Targets and Consequences of Proteasome Inhibition	
Process	Proteins Degraded by Proteasome	Cellular Consequences
NFκB activation	IκB	Accumulation of IκB inhibits nuclear translocation and activity of NFκB, leading to decreased proliferation, survival, invasion, angiogenesis.
Apoptosis	p53, Bax, tBid, Smac, JNK, Noxa	Accumulation of these proteins directly or indirectly promotes apoptosis through various pathways.
Cell cycle regulation	p21, p27, other CDK inhibitors, cyclins, p53	Accumulation of CDK inhibitors can cause cell-cycle arrest and apoptosis. The increased expression of multiple cyclins can send contradictory signals to the cell resulting in apoptosis.
Signal transduction	MKP-1 phosphatase	Accumulation dephosphorylates p44/42 MAP kinase, leading to decreased MAPK pathway signaling, proliferation, survival, +/– angiogenesis.
Oncogenic transformation	c-Fos, c-jun, c-myc, N-myc	Unclear how overabundance of these proteins exerts an antitumor effect.
Unfolded protein response	Various damaged/ misfolded proteins	Accumulation of damaged proteins leads to endoplasmic reticulum stress and apoptosis.
Chemo / radiation sensitivity	IκB, P-glycoprotein, topoisomerase IIα, DNA damage repair enzyme downregulation	NFκB is induced in response to DNA damage; normal proteasome function is required for correct folding of P-GP; downregulation of topoisomerase IIα may reduce sensitivity to doxorubicin.

NFκB, Nuclear factor κB.

Adapted from Adams J: The development of proteasome inhibitors as anticancer drugs, *Cancer Cell* 5:417–421, 2004; Rajkumar SV, Richardson PG, Hideshima T, et al: Proteasome inhibition as a novel therapeutic target in human cancer, *J Clin Oncol* 23:630–639, 2005; Voorhees PM, Dees EC, O'Neil B, et al: The proteasome as a target for cancer therapy, *Clin Cancer Res* 9:6316–6325, 2003.

addition, dysregulation of UPP function appears to occur in many types of cancer, thus potentially rendering them more sensitive to inhibition.[407,412]

Although a number of chemicals appear capable of proteasome inhibition in vitro, only the boronic acid derivatives appear suitable for clinical use and only two drugs, bortezomib (Velcade, Takeda) and carfilzomib (Kyprolis, Amgen), have received FDA approval, for the treatment of human multiple myeloma and mantle cell lymphoma.[413–417] Several additional proteasome inhibitors are in clinical development. Meaningful antitumor activity has been observed in patients with other hematopoietic neoplasms,[418–420] but less activity has been seen in solid tumors to date.[421–424]

Bortezomib and the investigational proteasome inhibitor ONX0912 have demonstrated in vitro and/or in vivo (xenograft) antiproliferative effects in canine melanoma and OSA cells,[393,425,426] and drugs targeting valosin-containing protein, another regulator of cellular proteostasis, have shown in vitro activity against canine lymphoma cells.[427,428]

Toxicology studies with bortezomib have been performed in dogs,[429] and a biologically effective and tolerable dose has been established in golden retrievers with golden retriever muscular dystrophy.[430] There are no published reports of proteasome inhibitor use in veterinary clinical oncology.

Heat Shock Protein 90

Given the complex nature of cancer and the multiple pathways that can be subjugated to contribute to the malignant phenotype, an optimal cancer drug might target a variety of oncogenic pathways simultaneously. One molecular target that has the potential to interrupt a wide variety of pathways important in cancer is heat shock protein 90 (HSP90), a molecular chaperone responsible for the conformational maturation of many proteins involved in diverse oncogenic activities such as cell adhesion/migration/invasion, signal transduction, cell cycle progression, angiogenesis, and survival (Table 15.4). HSP90 and other chaperones are responsible for ensuring the correct folding and prevention of aggregation of their client proteins.[431] Misfolding and aggregation of proteins lead to ubiquitination and proteasomal destruction, resulting in proteins with diminished function and greatly shortened half-lives.[432] Although several classes of compound are capable of inhibiting HSP90 chaperone function,[433–435] the best studied are ansamycin antibiotics of the geldanamycin class.

Many HSP90 inhibitors appear to demonstrate significant preferential activity against malignant cells versus normal cells. The HSP90 derived from most tumor cells has a binding affinity for the HSP90 inhibitor 17-allylaminogeldanamycin (17-AAG) approximately 100-fold higher than HSP90 derived from normal cells.[436] This may occur as a result of the overaccumulation of mutated, misfolded, and overexpressed signaling proteins in tumor cells leading to increased HSP90 chaperone activity and a greater proportion of the molecule in the bound, active, and 17-AAG sensitive state.[436]

Tumor cells display considerable variation in sensitivities to HSP90 inhibition. Although the mechanisms underlying this differential sensitivity are incompletely characterized, some important characteristics include reliance on certain kinase cascades, expression of apoptotic and cell-cycle regulators, and P-glycoprotein expression.[437]

Many receptor tyrosine kinases targeted by the geldanamycins may have important roles in canine and feline tumors. For example, geldanamycins are capable of inhibiting the function of mutant and wild-type KIT,[438] which is important in canine MCT[439]; MET,[440] which is expressed in multiple canine tumor types[441,442]; PDGF receptor,[443] which is expressed in feline injection-site sarcoma and OSA[444,445]; and IGF-1 receptor,[438] which is expressed and functional in canine OSA and melanoma.[446–448] The geldanamycins are likewise able to attenuate the function of the Hif-1 protein, a key transcription factor responsible for sensing and responding to hypoxia and activating the angiogenic switch.[433,449,450] They are also able to deplete key antiapoptotic proteins such as mutant p53 and survivin,[451–454] contributing to enhanced in vitro sensitivity to standard cytotoxic therapies such as RT and chemotherapy when used in combination.[455–460]

Under certain circumstances, HSP90 inhibitors could have negative effects on cancer outcomes. For example, 17-AAG has been shown to protect colon carcinoma cells from cisplatin-mediated toxicity,[461] whereas it has additive or synergistic activity when combined with cisplatin against human neuroblastoma and OSA cells.[455] In addition, although 17-AAG inhibited primary tumor formation, it potentiated bone-specific mammary carcinoma metastasis by enhancing osteoclastogenesis in one murine model.[462]

The impressive preclinical data generated with compounds such as HSP90 inhibitors has led to published phase I human clinical trials of multiple agents,[463–469] including some early combinatorial studies,[465–467,470,471] although none are yet approved.

TABLE 15.4	Molecules and Processes Targeted by HSP90 Inhibition	
Process	**Targets**	**References**
Invasion and migration	Urokinase-like plasminogen activator,[a] FAK phosphorylation	507–509
Cell cycle progression	Cyclin D3, cdk4	510
Signal transduction	Akt, Kit, Raf-1, EGFR, HER2, Jun, Lyn, Src, IGF-1R, PDGFR, Met, Bcr-Abl, ILK, androgen receptor, progesterone receptor, glucocorticoid receptor	437,438,440,455–458,460,461,510–514
Hypoxic response / angiogenesis	Hif-1, VEGF, Glut-1, nitric oxide synthase	433,434,437,449,450,456,515
Antiapoptosis	Wild-type and mutant p53, survivin	435,451–454,512,516
Cell senescence	Telomerase	517,518

[a]Urokinase-like plasminogen activator activity appears to be inhibited by geldanamycin class drugs through a mechanism other than HSP90 inhibition. *EGFR*, Epidermal growth factor receptor; *HIF-1*, hypoxia-inducible factor-1; *IGF-1R*, insulin-like growth factor receptor 1; *ILK*, integrin-linked kinase; *PDGFR*, platelet-derived growth factor receptor; *VEGF*, vascular endothelial growth factor.

Evidence of biologic effect in the form of upregulation of HSP70 chaperone expression in peripheral blood mononuclear cells (PBMCs) has been observed.

There is in vitro evidence of antitumor activity of HSP90 inhibitors in canine OSA, pulmonary carcinoma, and MCT cell lines.[472–476] The HSP90 inhibitor STA-1474 has been evaluated in a phase I clinical trial in dogs with spontaneous cancer. Upregulation of HSP70 after drug administration was observed in both tumor cells and PBMCs, and clinical responses were observed in dogs with MCT, OSA, melanoma, and thyroid carcinoma.[477]

Poly ADP-Ribose Polymerase and Poly ADP-Ribose Glycohydrolase

Poly ADP-ribose polymerase (PARP) is a "nick-sensor" that signals the presence of DNA damage and facilitates DNA repair.[478] The first PARP enzyme was discovered by Chambon et al and is now recognized as a superfamily of 18 members,[479] although only PARP-1 and PARP-2 are known to act in DNA damage.[480] The PARP family are also involved in the regulation of several transcription factors, such as NFκB in modulating the expression of chemokines, adhesion molecules, inflammatory cytokines, and mediators.[478] Poly ADP-ribose glycohydrolase (PARG) is the main enzyme in catabolizing PAR to ADP-ribose. To date, only one single PARG gene has been detected in mammals, encoding for three RNAs, which generate three isoforms.[478]

PARP has multiple intracellular functions, including signaling DNA damage and recognizing and binding to DNA strand breaks generated by DNA-damaging agents (cytotoxic drugs and ionizing radiation).[481] Activation of PARP is one of the earliest DNA damage responses. PARP is also a modulator of DNA base excision repair, which constitutes a major mechanism for genomic stability. There is increasing evidence demonstrating that both PARP and PARG repair DNA.[479] When PARP binds to DNA strand breaks, it activates an enzyme causing shuttling of PARP and, subsequently, opening of the chromatin. PARG enters the nucleus, moves to the PARP substrate, and DNA strand breaks are repaired. Because of excessive PARG, PAR decreases and thus chromatin returns to its original structure.

PARP inhibition has been suggested as an important approach in sensitizing cancer cells to conventional cancer therapy, leading to early clinical trials with PARP inhibitors as single agents and in combination.[481–483] PARP inhibitors have been shown to be lethal in BRCA-deficient cells because of persistence of DNA lesions that would normally be repaired in a BRCA-dependent fashion,[484] suggesting that PARP inhibitors might be an effective monotherapy in these cancers. Indeed, single-agent antitumor activity is observed in *BRCA*-mutant breast and ovarian cancer patients,[485–487] which has led to the FDA approval of olaparib (Lynparza, AstraZeneca), rucaparib (Rubraca, Clovis Oncology), and niraparib (Zejula, Tesaro) for the treatment of BRCA-mutant ovarian cancer; however, one might expect that their major benefit would be to enhance conventional cytotoxic drug treatment or RT, and studies have demonstrated that PARP inhibition potentiates the cytotoxicity of anticancer drugs and ionizing radiation through inhibition of DNA repair in cancer cells.

Inhibition of PARG could also be one of the pathways selected for cancer management because of its effects on increased sensitivity to both radiation and chemotherapy. Although PARG inhibitors have lagged behind PARP inhibitors, a number of molecules

have been developed that target these pathways, with varying degrees of specificity. In experimental mouse models these have shown promise in breast, colon, lung, brain tumors, and melanoma, either as monotherapy or combined with conventional drugs or RT.[488–492]

Recent studies suggest that polymorphisms in BRCA1 and BRCA2 may predispose certain dog breeds to mammary tumors[493]; however, evidence of a similar functional deficit in DNA repair to those observed in BRCA-mutant humans, which might confer sensitivity to PARP inhibitors, is lacking, as is any information regarding in vitro or in vivo efficacy of this class of drug in canine or feline cancer.

Nuclear Export

The transport of proteins between the nucleus and cytoplasm is a tightly regulated process. Export of proteins from the nucleus to the cytoplasm is governed by a series of proteins called the exportins. Exportin 1 (XPO1, CRM1) is a member of this series that is responsible for the nuclear export of a broad variety of target proteins, including a large number of known tumor suppressor proteins, including p53, survivin, Rb, p21, and IkB.[494] XPO1 is upregulated in many cancers versus normal tissues, and increased expression can be associated with higher tumor grade and inferior treatment outcomes.[495–497]

Multiple small molecule inhibitors of XPO1 have been developed and evaluated preclinically. Small molecule elective inhibitors of nuclear export (SINE) inactivate XPO1 and have shown considerable selective antiproliferative and proapoptotic activity in multiple solid and hematopoietic human tumor types,[498–501] and early-phase human clinical trials have been conducted with the SINE selinexor with evidence of objective antitumor activity.[502–504]

The SINE KPT-335 has in vitro antiproliferative activity in canine tumor cell lines derived from melanoma, lymphoma, MCT, and OSA, and nuclear exclusion of target proteins such as P21 and p53 after KPT-335 treatment has been demonstrated.[505,506] Oral KPT-335 was evaluated in a phase I clinical trial in tumor-bearing dogs: hepatotoxicity, hyporexia, and weight loss were dose limiting, and clinical responses were observed in several dogs with lymphoma.[506] KPT-335 is being developed as a veterinary cancer therapeutic, but at the time of writing it does not have FDA approval.

References

1. Argyle DJ: Gene therapy in veterinary medicine, *Vet Rec* 144:369–376, 1999.
2. Kumar SR, Markusic DM, Biswas M, et al.: Clinical development of gene therapy: results and lessons from recent successes, *Mol Ther Methods Clin Dev* 3:16034, 2016.
3. Naldini L: Medicine: A comeback for gene therapy, *Science* 326:805–806, 2009.
4. Herzog RW, Cao O, Srivastava A: Two decades of clinical gene therapy–success is finally mounting, *Discov Med* 9:105–111, 2010.
5. Couzin-Frankel J: Breakthrough of the year 2013. Cancer immunotherapy, *Science* 342:1432–1433, 2013.
6. Bartosch B, Cosset FL: Strategies for retargeted gene delivery using vectors derived from lentiviruses, *Curr Gene Ther* 4:427–443, 2004.
7. Tomanin R, Scarpa M: Why do we need new gene therapy viral vectors? Characteristics, limitations and future perspectives of viral vector transduction, *Curr Gene Ther* 4:357–372, 2004.

8. Lachmann RH: Herpes simplex virus-based vectors, *Int J Exp Pathol* 85:177–190, 2004.
9. Buning H, Braun-Falco M, Hallek M: Progress in the use of adeno-associated viral vectors for gene therapy, *Cells Tissues Organs* 177:139–150, 2004.
10. Mah C, Byrne BJ, Flotte TR: Virus-based gene delivery systems, *Clin Pharmacokinet* 41:901–911, 2002.
11. Dornburg R: The history and principles of retroviral vectors, *Front Biosci* 8:D818–D835, 2003.
12. Culver KW, Ram Z, Wallbridge S, et al.: In vivo gene transfer with retroviral vector-producer cells for treatment of experimental brain tumors, *Science* 256:1550–1552, 1992.
13. Hu YL, Fu YH, Tabata Y, et al.: Mesenchymal stem cells: a promising targeted-delivery vehicle in cancer gene therapy, *J Control Release* 147:154–162, 2010.
14. Basel MT, Shrestha TB, Bossmann SH, et al.: Cells as delivery vehicles for cancer therapeutics, *Ther Deliv* 5:555–567, 2014.
15. Muta M, Matsumoto G, Hiruma K, et al.: Study of cancer gene therapy using IL-12-secreting endothelial progenitor cells in a rat solid tumor model, *Oncol Rep* 10, 2003. 1765–176.
16. Pereboeva L, Komarova S, Mikheeva G, et al.: Approaches to utilize mesenchymal progenitor cells as cellular vehicles, *Stem Cells* 21:389–404, 2003.
17. Ramamoorth M, Narvekar A: Non-viral vectors in gene therapy- an overview, *J Clin Diagn Res* 9:GE01–GE06, 2015.
18. Hardee CL, Arévalo-Soliz LR, Hornstein BD, et al.: Advances in non-viral DNA vectors for gene therapy, *Genes (Basel)* 8: E65, 2017.
19. Shim G, Kim D, Le QV, et al.: Nonviral delivery systems for cancer gene therapy: strategies and challenges, *Curr Gene Ther* 18: 3–20, 2018.
20. Tranchant I, Thompson B, Nicolazzi C, et al.: Physicochemical optimisation of plasmid delivery by cationic lipids, *J Gene Med* 6:S24–S35, 2004.
21. Hirko A, Tang FX, Hughes JA: Cationic lipid vectors for plasmid DNA delivery, *Curr Med Chem* 10:1185–1193, 2003.
22. Yang N, Sun WH: Gene and non-viral approaches to cancer gene therapy, *Nat Med* 1:481–483, 1995.
23. Keller ET, Burkholder JK, Shi F, et al.: In-vivo particle mediated cytokine gene transfer into canine oral mucosa and epidermis, *Cancer Gene Ther* 3:186–191, 1996.
24. Dachs GU, Dougherty GJ, Stratford IJ, et al.: Targeting gene therapy to cancer, *Oncol Res* 9:313–325, 1997.
25. Glasgow JN, Everts M, Curiel DT: Transductional targeting of adenovirus vectors for gene therapy, *Cancer Gene Ther* 13: 830–844, 2006.
26. Blackwood L, Onions DE, Argyle DJ: The feline thyroglobulin promoter: towards targeted gene therapy of hyperthyroidism, *Domest Anim Endocrinol* 185–201, 2001.
27. Vile RG, Hart IR: In-vitro and in-vivo targeting of gene expression to melanoma cells, *Cancer Res* 53:962–967, 1993.
28. Pang LY, Argyle DJ: Cancer stem cells and telomerase as potential biomarkers in veterinary oncology, *Vet J* 185:15–22, 2010.
29. Pang L, Argyle DJ: Using naturally occurring tumours in dogs and cats to study telomerase and cancer stem cell biology, *Biochim Biophys Acta* 1792:380–391, 2009.
30. Fullerton NE, Boyd M, Mairs RJ, et al.: Combining a targeted radiotherapy and gene therapy approach for adenocarcinoma of prostate, *Prostate Cancer Prostatic Dis* 7:355–363, 2004.
31. Edelman J, Edelman J, Nemunaitis J: Adenoviral p53 gene therapy in squamous cell cancer of the head and neck region, *Curr Opin Mol Ther* 5:611–617, 2003.
32. Bortolanza S, Hernandez-Alcoceba R, Kramer G, et al.: Evaluation of the tumor specificity of a conditionally replicative adenovirus controlled by a modified human core telomerase promoter, *Mol Ther* 9:S375, 2004.
33. Cox DBT, Platt RJ, Zhang F: Therapeutic genome editing: prospects and challenges, *Nat Med* 21:121–131, 2015.
34. Fire AZ: Gene silencing by double-stranded RNA, *Cell Death Differentiation* 14:1998–2012, 2007.
35. Bora RS, Gupta D, Mukkur TK, et al.: RNA interference therapeutics for cancer: challenges and opportunities, *Mol Med Rep* 6: 9–15, 2012.
36. Tabernero J, Shapiro GI, LoRusso PM, et al.: First-in-humans trial of an RNA interference therapeutic targeting VEGF and KSP in cancer patients with liver involvement, *Cancer Discov* 3: 406–417, 2013.
37. Blackwood L, O'Shaughnessy PJ, Reid SJ, et al.: E. coli nitroreductase/CB1954: in vitro studies into a potential system for feline cancer gene therapy? *Vet J* 161:269–279, 2001.
38. Gholami A: Suicide gene therapy: a special focus on progress and concerns about cancer treatment, *Trends Pharmaceut Sci* 3:221–236, 2017.
39. Cihova M, Altanerova V, Altaner C: Stem cell based cancer gene therapy, *Mol Pharma* 8:1480–1487, 2011.
40. Le Blanc K: Immunomodulatory effects of fetal and adult mesenchymal stem cells, *Cytotherapy* 5:485–489, 2003.
41. Koppula PR, Chelluri LK, Polisetti N, et al.: Histocompatibility testing of cultivated human bone marrow stromal cells—a promising step towards pre-clinical screening for allogeneic stem cell therapy, *Cell Immunol* 259:61–66, 2009.
42. Griffin MD, Ritter T, Mahon BP: Immunological aspects of allogeneic mesenchymal stem cell therapies, *Hum Gene Ther* 21:1641–1655, 2010.
43. Lasek W, Basak G, Switaj T, et al.: Complete tumour regressions induced by vaccination with IL-12 gene-transduced tumour cells in combination with IL-15 in a melanoma model in mice, *Cancer Immunol Immunother* 53:363–372, 2004.
44. Yamazaki M, Straus FH, Messina M, et al.: Adenovirus-mediated tumor-specific combined gene therapy using herpes simplex virus thymidine/ganciclovir system and murine interleukin-12 induces effective antitumor activity against medullary thyroid carcinoma, *Cancer Gene Ther* 11:8–15, 2004.
45. Nagayama Y, Nakao K, Mizuguchi H, et al.: Enhanced antitumor effect of combined replicative adenovirus and nonreplicative adenovirus expressing interleukin-12 in an immunocompetent mouse model, *Gene Ther* 10:1400–1403, 2003.
46. Liu YQ, Huang H, Saxena A, et al.: Intratumoral co-injection of two adenoviral vectors expressing functional interleukin-18 and inducible protein-10, respectively, synergizes to facilitate regression of established tumors, *Cancer Gene Ther* 9:533–542, 2002.
47. Goto H, Osaki T, Nishino K, et al.: Construction and analysis of new vector systems with improved interleukin-18 secretion in a xenogeneic human tumor model, *J Immunother* 25: S35–S41, 2002.
48. Quintin-Colonna F, Devauchelle P, Fradelizi D, et al.: Gene therapy of spontaneous canine melanoma and feline fibrosarcoma by intratumoral administration of histoincompatible cells expressing human interleukin-2, *Gene Ther* 3:1104–1112, 1996.
49. Glikin GC, Finocchiaro LM: Clinical trials of immunogene therapy for spontaneous tumors in companion animals, *Sci World J* 2014:718520, 2014.
50. Davila ML, Riviere I, Wang X, et al.: Efficacy and toxicity management of 19-28z CAR T cell therapy in B cell acute lymphoblastic leukemia, *Sci Transl Med* 6(224ra25), 2014.
51. Maude SL, Frey N, Shaw PA, et al.: Chimeric antigen receptor T cells for sustained remissions in leukemia, *N Engl J Med* 371:1507–1517, 2014.
52. Lee DW, Kochenderfer JN, Stetter-Stevenson M, et al.: T cells expressing CD19 chimeric antigen receptors for acute lymphoblastic leukaemia in children and young adults: a phase 1 dose-escalation trial, *Lancet* 385:517–528, 2015.
53. Panjwan MK, Smith JB, Schutsky K, et al.: Feasibility and safety of RNA-transfected CD20-specific chimeric antigen receptor T cells in dogs with spontaneous B cell lymphoma, *Mol Ther* 24:1602–1614, 2016.

54. Carpinteiro A, Peinert S, Ostertag W, et al.: Genetic protection of repopulating hematopoietic cells with an improved MDR1-retrovirus allows administration of intensified chemotherapy following stem cell transplantation in mice, *Int J Cancer* 98:785–792, 2002.

55. Schiedlmeier B, Schilz AJ, Kuhlcke K, et al: Multidrug resistance 1 gene transfer can confer chemoprotection to human peripheral blood progenitor cells engrafted in immunodeficient mice, *Hum Gene Ther* 13:233–242, 2002.

56. Fairbairn LJ, Rafferty JA, Lashford LS: Engineering drug resistance in human cells, *Bone Marrow Transplant* 25:S110–S113, 2000.

57. Jiang F, Zhou L, Wei C, et al.: Slug inhibition increases radiosensitivity of oral squamous cell carcinoma cells by upregulating PUMA, *Int J Oncol* 49:709–719, 2016.

58. Capodanno Y, Buishand FO, Pang LY, et al.: Notch pathway inhibition targets chemoresistant insulinoma cancer stem cells, *Endocr Relat Cancer* 25:131–144, 2018.

59. Pang LY, Saunders L, Argyle DJ: Epidermal growth factor receptor activity is elevated in glioma cancer stem cells and is required to maintain chemotherapy and radiation resistance, *Oncotarget* 8:72494–72512, 2017.

60. Chiocca EA, Abbed KM, Tatter S, et al.: A phase I open-label, dose-escalation, multi-institutional trial of injection with an E1B-attenuated adenovirus, ONYX-015, into the peritumoral region of recurrent malignant gliomas, in the adjuvant setting, *Mol Ther* 10:958–966, 2004.

61. Post DE, Fulci G, Chiocca EA, et al.: Replicative oncolytic herpes simplex viruses in combination cancer therapies, *Curr Gene Ther* 4:41–51, 2004.

62. Shah AC, Benos D, Gillespie GY, et al.: Oncolytic viruses: clinical applications as vectors for the treatment of malignant gliomas, *J Neurooncol* 65:203–226, 2003.

63. Dirven CMF, van Beusechem VW, Lamfers MLM, et al.: Oncolytic adenoviruses for treatment of brain tumours, *Exp Opin Biol Ther* 2:943–952, 2002.

64. Russell SJ, Peng K-W: Oncolytic virotherapy: a contest between apples and oranges, *Mol Ther* 25:1107–1116, 2017.

65. Lawler SE, Speranza M-C, Cho C-F, et al.: Oncolytic viruses and cancer treatment: a review, *JAMA Oncol* 3:841–849, 2017.

66. Conry RM, Westbrook B, McKee S, et al.: Talimogene laherparepvec: first in class oncolytic virotherapy, *Hum Vaccin Immunother* 14:839–846, 2018.

67. Hwang CC, Igase M, Sakurai M, et al.: Oncolytic reovirus therapy: pilot study in dogs with spontaneously occurring tumours, *Vet Comp Oncol* 16:229–238, 2018.

68. Naik S, Galyon GD, Jenks NJ, et al.: Comparative oncology evaluation of intravenous recombinant oncolytic vesicular stomatitis virus therapy in spontaneous canine cancer, *Mol Cancer Ther* 17:316–326, 2018.

69. Hemminki A, Kanerva A, Kremer EJ, et al.: A canine conditionally replicating adenovirus for evaluating oncolytic virotherapy in a syngeneic animal model, *Mol Ther* 7:163–173, 2003.

70. Manning G, Whyte DB, Martinez R, et al.: The protein kinase complement of the human genome, *Science* 298:1912–1934, 2002.

71. Lemmon MA, Schlessinger J: Cell signaling by receptor tyrosine kinases, *Cell* 141:1117–1134, 2010.

72. Madhusudan S, Ganesan TS: Tyrosine kinase inhibitors in cancer therapy, *Clin Biochem* 37:618–635, 2004.

73. Zwick E, Bange J, Ullrich A: Receptor tyrosine kinases as targets for anticancer drugs, *Trends Mol Med* 8:17–23, 2002.

74. Barreca A, Lasorsa E, Riera L, et al.: Anaplastic lymphoma kinase in human cancer, *J Mol Endocrinol* 47:R11–R23, 2011.

75. Fletcher JA: Role of KIT and platelet-derived growth factor receptors as oncoproteins, *Semin Oncol* 31:4–11, 2004.

76. Laskin JJ, Sandler AB: Epidermal growth factor receptor: a promising target in solid tumours, *Cancer Treat Rev* 30:1–17, 2004.

77. Ma PC, Jagadeeswaran R, Jagadeesh S, et al.: Functional expression and mutations of c-Met and its therapeutic inhibition with SU11274 and small interfering RNA in non-small cell lung cancer, *Cancer Res* 65:1479–1488, 2005.

78. Ma PC, Maulik G, Christensen J, et al.: c-Met: structure, functions and potential for therapeutic inhibition, *Cancer Metastasis Rev* 22:309–325, 2003.

79. Thurston G, Gale NW: Vascular endothelial growth factor and other signaling pathways in developmental and pathologic angiogenesis, *Int J Hematol* 80:7–20, 2004.

80. Eskens FA: Angiogenesis inhibitors in clinical development; where are we now and where are we going? *Br J Cancer* 90:1–7, 2004.

81. Cherrington JM, Strawn LM, Shawver LK: New paradigms for the treatment of cancer: the role of anti- angiogenesis agents, *Adv Cancer Res* 79:1–38, 2000.

82. McCarty MF, Liu W, Fan F, et al.: Promises and pitfalls of anti-angiogenic therapy in clinical trials, *Trends Mol Med* 9:53–58, 2003.

83. Thurston G: Role of Angiopoietins and Tie receptor tyrosine kinases in angiogenesis and lymphangiogenesis, *Cell Tissue Res* 314:61–68, 2003.

84. Blume-Jensen P, Hunter T: Oncogenic kinase signalling, *Nature* 411:355–365, 2001.

85. Johnson GL, Lapadat R: Mitogen-activated protein kinase pathways mediated by ERK, JNK, and p38 protein kinases, *Science* 298:1911–1912, 2002.

86. Downward J: Targeting RAS signalling pathways in cancer therapy, *Nat Rev Cancer* 3:11–22, 2003.

87. Davies H, Bignell GR, Cox C, et al.: Mutations of the *BRAF* gene in human cancer, *Nature* 417:949–954, 2002.

88. Kumar R, Angelini S, Snellman E, et al.: BRAF mutations are common somatic events in melanocytic nevi, *J Invest Dermatol* 122:342–348, 2004.

89. Mercer KE, Pritchard CA: Raf proteins and cancer: B-Raf is identified as a mutational target, *Biochim Biophys Acta* 1653:25–40, 2003.

90. Decker B, Parker HG, Dhawan D, et al.: Homologous mutation to human BRAF V600E is common in naturally occurring canine bladder cancer—evidence for a relevant model system and urine-based diagnostic test, *Mol Cancer Res* 13:993–1002, 2015.

91. Fresno Vara JA, Casado E, de Castro J, et al.: PI3K/Akt signalling pathway and cancer, *Cancer Treat Rev* 30:193–204, 2004.

92. Franke TF, Hornik CP, Segev L, et al.: PI3K/Akt and apoptosis: size matters, *Oncogene* 22:8983–8998, 2003.

93. Mitsiades CS, Mitsiades N, Koutsilieris M: The Akt pathway: molecular targets for anti-cancer drug development, *Curr Cancer Drug Targets* 4:235–256, 2004.

94. Markman B, Atzori F, Perez-Garcia J, et al.: Status of PI3K inhibition and biomarker development in cancer therapeutics, *Ann Oncol* 21:683–691, 2010.

95. Simpson L, Parsons R: PTEN: life as a tumor suppressor, *Exp Cell Res* 264:29–41, 2001.

96. Weng LP, Smith WM, Dahia PL, et al.: PTEN suppresses breast cancer cell growth by phosphatase activity-dependent G1 arrest followed by cell death, *Cancer Res* 59:5808–5814, 1999.

97. Kanae Y, Endoh D, Yokota H, et al.: Expression of the PTEN tumor suppressor gene in malignant mammary gland tumors of dogs, *Am J Vet Res* 67:127–133, 2006.

98. Koenig A, Bianco SR, Fosmire S, et al.: Expression and significance of p53, Rb, p21/waf-1, p16/ink-4a, and PTEN tumor suppressors in canine melanoma, *Vet Pathol* 39:458–472, 2002.

99. Levine RA, Forest T, Smith C: Tumor suppressor PTEN is mutated in canine osteosarcoma cell lines and tumors, *Vet Pathol* 39:372–378, 2002.

100. Swanton C: Cell-cycle targeted therapies, *Lancet Oncol* 5:27–36, 2004.

101. Ortega S, Malumbres M, Barbacid M: Cyclin D-dependent kinases, INK4 inhibitors and cancer, *Biochim Biophys Acta* 1602:73–87, 2002.

102. Malumbres M, Barbacid M: To cycle or not to cycle: a critical decision in cancer, *Nat Rev Cancer* 1:222–231, 2001.

103. Iwata H. Clinical development of CDK4/6 inhibitor for breast cancer, *Breast Cancer* 2018.

104. Wellbrock C, Ogilvie L, Hedley D, et al.: V599EB-RAF is an oncogene in melanocytes, *Cancer Res* 64:2338–2342, 2004.

105. Pollock PM, Meltzer PS: A genome-based strategy uncovers frequent BRAF mutations in melanoma, *Cancer Cell* 2: 5–7, 2002.

106. Wan PT, Garnett MJ, Roe SM, et al.: Mechanism of activation of the RAF-ERK signaling pathway by oncogenic mutations of B-RAF, *Cell* 116:855–867, 2004.

107. Dhillon AS, Kolch W: Oncogenic B-Raf mutations: crystal clear at last, *Cancer Cell* 5:303–304, 2004.

108. Brose MS, Volpe P, Feldman M, et al.: BRAF and RAS mutations in human lung cancer and melanoma, *Cancer Res* 62: 6997–7000, 2002.

109. Malumbres M, Barbacid M: RAS oncogenes: the first 30 years, *Nat Rev Cancer* 3:459–465, 2003.

110. Galli SJ, Zsebo KM, Geissler EN: The kit ligand, stem cell factor, *Adv Immunol* 55:1–95, 1994.

111. Downing S, Chien MB, Kass PH, et al.: Prevalence and importance of internal tandem duplications in exons 11 and 12 of c-kit in mast cell tumors of dogs, *Am J Vet Res* 63:1718–1723, 2002.

112. London CA, Galli SJ, Yuuki T, et al.: Spontaneous canine mast cell tumors express tandem duplications in the proto-oncogene c-kit, *Exp Hematol* 27:689–697, 1999.

113. Zemke D, Yamini B, Yuzbasiyan-Gurkan V: Mutations in the juxtamembrane domain of c-KIT are associated with higher grade mast cell tumors in dogs, *Vet Pathol* 39:529–535, 2002.

114. Letard S, Yang Y, Hanssens K, et al.: Gain-of-function mutations in the extracellular domain of KIT are common in canine mast cell tumors, *Mol Cancer Res* 6:1137–1145, 2008.

115. Demetri GD: Targeting the molecular pathophysiology of gastrointestinal stromal tumors with imatinib. Mechanisms, successes, and challenges to rational drug development, *Hematol Oncol Clin North Am* 16:1115–1124, 2002.

116. Demetri GD: Differential properties of current tyrosine kinase inhibitors in gastrointestinal stromal tumors, *Semin Oncol* 38(Suppl 1):S10–S19, 2011.

117. Frost D, Lasota J, Miettinen M: Gastrointestinal stromal tumors and leiomyomas in the dog: a histopathologic, immunohistochemical, and molecular genetic study of 50 cases, *Vet Pathol* 40:42–54, 2003.

118. Gregory-Bryson E, Bartlett E, Kiupel M, et al.: Canine and human gastrointestinal stromal tumors display similar mutations in c-KIT exon 11, *BMC Cancer* 10:559, 2010.

119. Kondo M, Horibe K, Takahashi Y, et al.: Prognostic value of internal tandem duplication of the FLT3 gene in childhood acute myelogenous leukemia, *Med Pediatr Oncol* 33: 525–529, 1999.

120. Nakoa M, Yokota S, Iwai T, et al.: Internal tandem duplication of the flt3 gene found in acute myeloid leukemia, *Leukemia* 10:1911–1918, 1996.

121. Yokota S, Kiyoi H, Nakao M, et al.: Internal tandem duplication of the FLT3 gene is preferentially seen in acute myeloid leukemia and myelodysplastic syndrome among various hematological malignancies. A study on a large series of patients and cell lines, *Leukemia* 11:1605–1609, 1997.

122. Iwai T, Yokota S, Nakao M, et al.: Internal tandem duplication of the FLT3 gene and clinical evaluation in childhood acute myeloid leukemia, The Children's Cancer and Leukemia Study Group, Japan, *Leukemia* 13:38–43, 1999.

123. Pao W, Chmielecki J: Rational, biologically based treatment of EGFR-mutant non-small-cell lung cancer, *Nat Rev Cancer* 10:760–774, 2010.

124. Wen J, Fu J, Zhang W, et al.: Genetic and epigenetic changes in lung carcinoma and their clinical implications, *Mod Pathol* 24:932–943, 2011.

125. Paik S, Hazan R, Fisher ER, et al.: Pathologic findings from the National Surgical Adjuvant Breast and Bowel Project: prognostic significance of erbB-2 protein overexpression in primary breast cancer, *J Clin Oncol* 8:103–112, 1990.

126. Slamon DJ, Clark GM, Wong SG, et al.: Human breast cancer: correlation of relapse and survival with amplification of the HER-2/neu oncogene, *Science* 235:177–182, 1987.

127. Libermann TA, Nusbaum HR, Razon N, et al.: Amplification, enhanced expression and possible rearrangement of EGF receptor gene in primary human brain tumours of glial origin, *Nature* 313:144–147, 1985.

128. Libermann TA, Nusbaum HR, Razon N, et al.: Amplification and overexpression of the EGF receptor gene in primary human glioblastomas, *J Cell Sci Suppl* 3:161–172, 1985.

129. Golub TR, Barker GF, Lovett M, et al.: Fusion of PDGF receptor beta to a novel ets-like gene, tel, in chronic myelomonocytic leukemia with t(5;12) chromosomal translocation, *Cell* 77:307–316, 1994.

130. Gotlib J, Cools J, Malone 3rd JM, et al.: The FIP1L1-PDGFRalpha fusion tyrosine kinase in hypereosinophilic syndrome and chronic eosinophilic leukemia: implications for diagnosis, classification, and management, *Blood* 103:2879–2891, 2004.

131. Melo JV, Hughes TP, Apperley JF: Chronic myeloid leukemia, *Hematology (Am Soc Hematol Educ Program)*132–152, 2003.

132. Van Etten RA: Mechanisms of transformation by the BCR-ABL oncogene: new perspectives in the post-imatinib era, *Leuk Res* 28(Suppl 1):S21–S28, 2004.

133. Medves S, Demoulin JB: Tyrosine kinase gene fusions in cancer: translating mechanisms into targeted therapies, *J Cell Mol Med*, 2011.

134. Sciacca L, Costantino A, Pandini G, et al.: Insulin receptor activation by IGF-II in breast cancers: evidence for a new autocrine/paracrine mechanism, *Oncogene* 18:2471–2479, 1999.

135. Ekstrand AJ, James CD, Cavenee WK, et al.: Genes for epidermal growth factor receptor, transforming growth factor alpha, and epidermal growth factor and their expression in human gliomas in vivo, *Cancer Res* 51:2164–2172, 1991.

136. Graeven U, Fiedler W, Karpinski S, et al.: Melanoma-associated expression of vascular endothelial growth factor and its receptors FLT-1 and KDR, *J Cancer Res Clin Oncol* 125:621–629, 1999.

137. Fosmire SP, Dickerson EB, Scott AM, et al.: Canine malignant hemangiosarcoma as a model of primitive angiogenic endothelium, *Lab Invest* 84:562–572, 2004.

138. MacEwen EG, Kutzke J, Carew J, et al.: c-Met tyrosine kinase receptor expression and function in human and canine osteosarcoma cells, *Clin Exp Metastasis* 20:421–430, 2003.

139. Ferracini R, Angelini P, Cagliero E, et al.: MET oncogene aberrant expression in canine osteosarcoma, *J Orthop Res* 18:253–256, 2000.

140. Harris M: Monoclonal antibodies as therapeutic agents for cancer, *Lancet Oncol* 5:292–302, 2004.

141. Vogel CL, Cobleigh MA, Tripathy D, et al.: First-line Herceptin monotherapy in metastatic breast cancer, *Oncology* 61(Suppl 2):37–42, 2001.

142. Slamon DJ, Leyland-Jones B, Shak S, et al.: Use of chemotherapy plus a monoclonal antibody against HER2 for metastatic breast cancer that overexpresses HER2, *N Engl J Med* 344:783–792, 2001.

143. Arteaga CL, Sliwkowski MX, Osborne CK, et al.: Treatment of HER2-positive breast cancer: current status and future perspectives, *Nat Rev Clin Oncol*, 2011.

144. Mukai H: Treatment strategy for HER2-positive breast cancer, *Int J Clin Oncol* 15:335–340, 2010.

145. Cabanillas F: Front-line management of diffuse large B cell lymphoma, *Curr Opin Oncol* 22:642–645, 2010.

146. Vidal L, Gafter-Gvili A, Salles G, et al.: Rituximab maintenance for the treatment of patients with follicular lymphoma: an updated systematic review and meta-analysis of randomized trials, *J Natl Cancer Inst* 103:1799–1806, 2011.

147. Brand TM, Iida M, Wheeler DL: Molecular mechanisms of resistance to the EGFR monoclonal antibody cetuximab, *Cancer Biol Ther* 11:777–792, 2011.

148. Zhang J, Yang PL, Gray NS: Targeting cancer with small molecule kinase inhibitors, *Nat Rev Cancer* 9:28–39, 2009.

149. de Kogel CE, Schellens JH: Imatinib, *Oncologist* 12:1390–1394, 2007.

150. Mauro MJ, Druker BJ: STI571: targeting BCR-ABL as therapy for CML, *Oncologist* 6:233–238, 2001.

151. Kantarjian H, Sawyers C, Hochhaus A, et al.: Hematologic and cytogenetic responses to imatinib mesylate in chronic myelogenous leukemia, *N Engl J Med* 346:645–652, 2002.

152. Beham-Schmid C, Apfelbeck U, Sill H, et al.: Treatment of chronic myelogenous leukemia with the tyrosine kinase inhibitor STI571 results in marked regression of bone marrow fibrosis, *Blood* 99:381–383, 2002.

153. Druker BJ, Talpaz M, Resta DJ, et al.: Efficacy and safety of a specific inhibitor of the BCR-ABL tyrosine kinase in chronic myeloid leukemia, *N Engl J Med* 344:1031–1037, 2001.

154. Druker BJ, Sawyers CL, Kantarjian H, et al.: Activity of a specific inhibitor of the BCR-ABL tyrosine kinase in the blast crisis of chronic myeloid leukemia and acute lymphoblastic leukemia with the Philadelphia chromosome, *N Engl J Med* 344:1038–1042, 2001.

155. Sawyers CL: Rational therapeutic intervention in cancer: kinases as drug targets, *Curr Opin Genet Dev* 12:111–115, 2002.

156. Weisberg E, Griffin JD: Resistance to imatinib (Glivec): update on clinical mechanisms, *Drug Resist Updat* 6:231–238, 2003.

157. Nardi V, Azam M, Daley GQ: Mechanisms and implications of imatinib resistance mutations in BCR-ABL, *Curr Opin Hematol* 11:35–43, 2004.

158. Duffaud F, Blay JY: Gastrointestinal stromal tumors: biology and treatment, *Oncology* 65:187–197, 2003.

159. Heinrich MC, Rubin BP, Longley BJ, et al.: Biology and genetic aspects of gastrointestinal stromal tumors: KIT activation and cytogenetic alterations, *Hum Pathol* 33:484–495, 2002.

160. Miettinen M, Sarlomo-Rikala M, Lasota J: Gastrointestinal stromal tumors: recent advances in understanding of their biology, *Hum Pathol* 30:1213–1220, 1999.

161. Miettinen M, Sarlomo-Rikala M, Lasota J: Gastrointestinal stromal tumours, *Ann Chir Gynaecol* 87:278–281, 1998.

162. Heinrich MC, Corless CL, Duensing A, et al.: PDGFRA activating mutations in gastrointestinal stromal tumors, *Science* 299:708–710, 2003.

163. Peled N, Yoshida K, Wynes MW, et al.: Predictive and prognostic markers for epidermal growth factor receptor inhibitor therapy in non-small cell lung cancer, *Ther Adv Med Oncol* 1:137–144, 2009.

164. Singh M, Jadhav HR: Targeting non-small cell lung cancer with small-molecule EGFR tyrosine kinase inhibitors, *Drug Discov Today* 23:745–753, 2018.

165. Bang YJ: The potential for crizotinib in non-small cell lung cancer: a perspective review, *Ther Adv Med Oncol* 3:279–291, 2011.

166. Shaw AT, Yeap BY, Solomon BJ, et al.: Effect of crizotinib on overall survival in patients with advanced non-small-cell lung cancer harbouring ALK gene rearrangement: a retrospective analysis, *Lancet Oncol* 12:1004–1012, 2011.

167. Chapman PB, Hauschild A, Robert C, et al.: Improved survival with vemurafenib in melanoma with BRAF V600E mutation, *N Engl J Med* 364:2507–2516, 2011.

168. Markman B, Dienstmann R, Tabernero J: Targeting the PI3K/Akt/mTOR pathway—beyond rapalogs, *Oncotarget* 1:530–543, 2010.

169. Vilar E, Perez-Garcia J, Tabernero J: Pushing the envelope in the mTOR pathway: the second generation of inhibitors, *Mol Cancer Ther* 10:395–403, 2011.

170. Pal Singh S, Dammeijer F, Hendriks RW: Role of Bruton's tyrosine kinase in B cells and malignancies, *Mol Cancer* 17:57, 2018.

171. Horwitz SM, Koch R, Porcu P, et al.: Activity of the PI3K-delta,gamma inhibitor duvelisib in a phase 1 trial and preclinical models of T-cell lymphoma, *Blood* 131:888–898, 2018.

172. Papaetis GS, Syrigos KN: Sunitinib: a multitargeted receptor tyrosine kinase inhibitor in the era of molecular cancer therapies, *BioDrugs* 23:377–389, 2009.

173. London CA, Hannah AL, Zadovoskaya R, et al.: Phase I dose-escalating study of SU11654, a small molecule receptor tyrosine kinase inhibitor, in dogs with spontaneous malignancies, *Clin Cancer Res* 9:2755–2768, 2003.

174. London CA, Malpas PB, Wood-Follis SL, et al.: Multi-center, placebo-controlled, double-blind, randomized study of oral toceranib phosphate (SU11654), a receptor tyrosine kinase inhibitor, for the treatment of dogs with recurrent (either local or distant) mast cell tumor following surgical excision, *Clin Cancer Res* 15:3856–3865, 2009.

175. London C, Mathie T, Stingle N, et al.: Preliminary evidence for biologic activity of toceranib phosphate (Palladia) in solid tumours, *Vet Comp Oncol* 10:194–205, 2012.

176. Hahn KA, Ogilvie G, Rusk T, et al.: Masitinib is safe and effective for the treatment of canine mast cell tumors, *J Vet Intern Med* 22:1301–1309, 2008.

177. Hahn KA, Legendre AM, Shaw NG, et al.: Evaluation of 12- and 24-month survival rates after treatment with masitinib in dogs with nonresectable mast cell tumors, *Am J Vet Res* 71:1354–1361, 2010.

178. Isotani M, Ishida N, Tominaga M, et al.: Effect of tyrosine kinase inhibition by imatinib mesylate on mast cell tumors in dogs, *J Vet Intern Med* 22:985–988, 2008.

179. Marconato L, Bettini G, Giacoboni C, et al.: Clinico-pathological features and outcome for dogs with mast cell tumors and bone marrow involvement, *J Vet Intern Med* 22:1001–1007, 2008.

180. Yamada O, Kobayashi M, Sugisaki O, et al.: Imatinib elicited a favorable response in a dog with a mast cell tumor carrying a c-kit c.1523A>T mutation via suppression of constitutive KIT activation, *Vet Immunol Immunopathol* 142:101–106, 2011.

181. Isotani M, Tamura K, Yagihara H, et al.: Identification of a c-kit exon 8 internal tandem duplication in a feline mast cell tumor case and its favorable response to the tyrosine kinase inhibitor imatinib mesylate, *Vet Immunol Immunopathol* 114:168–172, 2006.

182. Isotani M, Yamada O, Lachowicz JL, et al.: Mutations in the fifth immunoglobulin-like domain of kit are common and potentially sensitive to imatinib mesylate in feline mast cell tumours, *Br J Haematol* 148:144–153, 2009.

183. Gardner HL, Rippy SB, Bear MD, et al.: Phase I/II evaluation of RV1001, a novel PI3Kδ inhibitor, in spontaneous canine lymphoma, *PLoS One* 13:e0195357, 2018.

184. London CA, Bernabe LF, Barnard S, et al.: Preclinical evaluation of the novel, orally bioavailable Selective Inhibitor of Nuclear Export (SINE) KPT-335 in spontaneous canine cancer: results of a phase I study, *PLoS One* 9:e87585, 2014.

185. Sadowski AR, Gardner HL, Borgatti A, et al.: Phase II study of the oral selective inhibitor of nuclear export (SINE) KPT-335 (verdinexor) in dogs with lymphoma, *BMC Vet Res* 14:250, 2018.

186. Folkman J: Angiogenesis in cancer, vascular, rheumatoid and other disease, *Nat Med* 1:27–31, 1995.

187. Folkman J: Tumor angiogenesis: therapeutic implications, *N Engl J Med* 285:1182–1186, 1971.

188. Hanahan D, Weinberg RA: Hallmarks of cancer: the next generation, *Cell* 144:646–674, 2011.

189. Folkman J: Endogenous angiogenesis inhibitors, *APMIS* 112:496–507, 2004.

190. Ferrara N, Kerbel RS: Angiogenesis as a therapeutic target, *Nature* 438:967–974, 2005.

191. Patel-Hett S, D'Amore PA: Signal transduction in vasculogenesis and developmental angiogenesis, *Int J Dev Biol* 55:353–363, 2011.

192. Stewart KS, Kleinerman ES: Tumor vessel development and expansion in Ewing's sarcoma: a review of the vasculogenesis process and clinical trials with vascular-targeting agents, *Sarcoma* 165837, 2011.

193. Asahara T, Murohara T, Sullivan A, et al.: Isolation of putative progenitor endothelial cells for angiogenesis, *Science* 275:964–967, 1997.

194. Purhonen S, Palm J, Rossi D, et al.: Bone marrow-derived circulating endothelial precursors do not contribute to vascular endothelium and are not needed for tumor growth, *Proc Natl Acad Sci U S A* 105:6620–6625, 2008.

195. Shaked Y, Ciarrocchi A, Franco M, et al.: Therapy-induced acute recruitment of circulating endothelial progenitor cells to tumors, *Science* 313:1785–1787, 2006.

196. Kerbel RS, Benezra R, Lyden DC, et al.: Endothelial progenitor cells are cellular hubs essential for neoangiogenesis of certain aggressive adenocarcinomas and metastatic transition but not adenomas, *Proc Natl Acad Sci USA* 105:E54, 2008.

197. Dome B, Hendrix MJ, Paku S, et al.: Alternative vascularization mechanisms in cancer: pathology and therapeutic implications, *Am J Pathol* 170:1–15, 2007.

198. Hendrix MJ, Seftor EA, Hess AR, et al.: Vasculogenic mimicry and tumour-cell plasticity: lessons from melanoma, *Nat Rev Cancer* 3:411–421, 2003.

199. Tammela T, Alitalo K: Lymphangiogenesis: molecular mechanisms and future promise, *Cell* 140:460–476, 2010.

200. Adams RH, Alitalo K: Molecular regulation of angiogenesis and lymphangiogenesis, *Nat Rev Mol Cell Biol* 8:464–478, 2007.

201. Holopainen T, Bry M, Alitalo K, et al.: Perspectives on lymphangiogenesis and angiogenesis in cancer, *J Surg Oncol* 103:484–488, 2011.

202. Potente M, Gerhardt H, Carmeliet P: Basic and therapeutic aspects of angiogenesis, *Cell* 146:873–887, 2011.

203. Kerbel RS: Tumor angiogenesis, *N Engl J Med* 358:2039–2049, 2008.

204. Kerbel RS: Antiangiogenic therapy: a universal chemosensitization strategy for cancer? *Science* 312:1171–1175, 2006.

205. Khosravi SP, Fernandez PI: Tumoral angiogenesis: review of the literature, *Cancer Invest* 26:104–108, 2008.

206. Carmeliet P, Jain RK: Molecular mechanisms and clinical applications of angiogenesis, *Nature* 473:298–307, 2011.

207. Motzer RJ, Hoosen S, Bello CL, et al.: Sunitinib malate for the treatment of solid tumours: a review of current clinical data, *Expert Opin Investig Drugs* 15:553–561, 2006.

208. Ivy SP, Wick JY, Kaufman BM: An overview of small-molecule inhibitors of VEGFR signaling, *Nat Rev Clin Oncol* 6:569–579, 2009.

209. Franco M, Man S, Chen L, et al.: Targeted anti-vascular endothelial growth factor receptor-2 therapy leads to short-term and long-term impairment of vascular function and increase in tumor hypoxia, *Cancer Res* 66:3639–3648, 2006.

210. Jain RK: Normalization of tumor vasculature: an emerging concept in antiangiogenic therapy, *Science* 307:58–62, 2005.

211. Carmeliet P, Jain RK: Principles and mechanisms of vessel normalization for cancer and other angiogenic diseases, *Nat Rev Drug Discov* 10:417–427, 2011.

212. Goel S, Duda DG, Xu L, et al.: Normalization of the vasculature for treatment of cancer and other diseases, *Physiol Rev* 91:1071–1121, 2011.

213. Sorensen AG, Emblem KE, Polaskova P, et al.: Increased survival of glioblastoma patients who respond to antiangiogenic therapy with elevated blood perfusion, *Cancer Res* 72:402–407, 2012.

214. Batchelor TT, Sorensen AG, di TE, et al.: AZD2171, a pan-VEGF receptor tyrosine kinase inhibitor, normalizes tumor vasculature and alleviates edema in glioblastoma patients, *Cancer Cell* 11:83–95, 2007.

215. Fabian MA, Biggs III WH, Treiber DK, et al.: A small molecule-kinase interaction map for clinical kinase inhibitors, *Nat Biotechnol* 23:329–336, 2005.

216. London CA, Malpas PB, Wood-Follis SL, et al.: Multi-center, placebo-controlled, double-blind, randomized study of oral toceranib phosphate (SU11654), a receptor tyrosine kinase inhibitor, for the treatment of dogs with recurrent (either local or distant) mast cell tumor following surgical excision, *Clin Cancer Res* 15:3856–3865, 2009.

217. Hahn KA, Ogilvie G, Rusk T, et al.: Masitinib is safe and effective for the treatment of canine mast cell tumors, *J Vet Intern Med* 22:1301–1309, 2008.

218. Pietras K, Hanahan D: A multitargeted, metronomic, and maximum-tolerated dose "chemo-switch" regimen is antiangiogenic, producing objective responses and survival benefit in a mouse model of cancer, *J Clin Oncol* 23:939–952, 2005.

219. Mentlein R, Forstreuter F, Mehdorn HM, et al.: Functional significance of vascular endothelial growth factor receptor expression on human glioma cells, *J Neurooncol* 67:9–18, 2004.

220. Jackson MW, Roberts JS, Heckford SE, et al.: A potential autocrine role for vascular endothelial growth factor in prostate cancer, *Cancer Res* 62:854–859, 2002.

221. Kerbel RS, Viloria-Petit A, Klement G, et al.: "'Accidental' antiangiogenic drugs: anti-oncogene directed signal transduction inhibitors and conventional chemotherapeutic agents as examples, *Eur J Cancer* 36:1248–1257, 2000.

222. Lopez-Ocejo O, Viloria-Petit A, Bequet-Romero M, et al.: Oncogenes and tumor angiogenesis: the HPV-16 E6 oncoprotein activates the vascular endothelial growth factor (VEGF) gene promoter in a p53 independent manner, *Oncogene* 19:4611–4620, 2000.

223. Ebos JM, Tran J, Master Z, et al.: Imatinib mesylate (STI-571) reduces Bcr-Abl-mediated vascular endothelial growth factor secretion in chronic myelogenous leukemia, *Mol Cancer Res* 1:89–95, 2002.

224. du Manoir JM, Francia G, Man S, et al.: Strategies for delaying or treating in vivo acquired resistance to trastuzumab in human breast cancer xenografts, *Clin Cancer Res* 12:904–916, 2006.

225. Viloria-Petit A, Crombet T, Jothy S, et al.: Acquired resistance to the antitumor effect of epidermal growth factor receptor-blocking antibodies in vivo: a role for altered tumor angiogenesis, *Cancer Res* 61:5090–5101, 2001.

226. O'Reilly MS, Boehm T, Shing Y, et al.: Endostatin: an endogenous inhibitor of angiogenesis and tumor growth, *Cell* 88:277–285, 1997.

227. Rusk A, McKeegan E, Haviv F, et al.: Preclinical evaluation of antiangiogenic thrombospondin-1 peptide mimetics, ABT-526 and ABT-510, in companion dogs with naturally occurring cancers, *Clin Cancer Res* 12:7444–7455, 2006.

228. Sahora A, Rusk A, Henkin J, et al.: Prospective study of thrombospondin-1 mimetic peptides, ABT-510 and ABT-898, in dogs with soft tissue sarcoma, *J Vet Intern Med* 26:1169–1176, 2012.

229. Rusk A, Cozzi E, Stebbins M, et al.: Cooperative activity of cytotoxic chemotherapy with antiangiogenic thrombospondin-I peptides, ABT-526 in pet dogs with relapsed lymphoma, *Clin Cancer Res* 12:7456–7464, 2006.

230. Pirie-Shepherd SR, Coffman KT, Resnick D, et al.: The role of angiostatin in the spontaneous bone and prostate cancers of pet dogs, *Biochem Biophys Res Commun* 292:886–891, 2002.

231. Troy GC, Huckle WR, Rossmeisl JH, et al.: Endostatin and vascular endothelial growth factor concentrations in healthy dogs, dogs with selected neoplasia, and dogs with nonneoplastic diseases, *J Vet Intern Med* 20:144–150, 2006.

232. Kamstock D, Guth A, Elmslie R, et al.: Liposome-DNA complexes infused intravenously inhibit tumor angiogenesis and elicit antitumor activity in dogs with soft tissue sarcoma, *Cancer Gene Ther* 13:306–317, 2006.

233. St Croix B, Rago C, Velculescu V, et al.: Genes expressed in human tumor endothelium, *Science* 289:1197–1202, 2000.

234. Paoloni MC, Tandle A, Mazcko C, et al.: Launching a novel preclinical infrastructure: comparative oncology trials consortium directed therapeutic targeting of TNFalpha to cancer vasculature, *PLoS One* 4:e4972, 2009.

235. Hua H, Li M, Luo T, et al.: Matrix metalloproteinases in tumorigenesis: an evolving paradigm, *Cell Mol Life Sci* 68:3853–3868, 2011.

236. Hirte H, Vergote IB, Jeffrey JR, et al.: A phase III randomized trial of BAY 12-9566 (tanomastat) as maintenance therapy in patients with advanced ovarian cancer responsive to primary surgery and paclitaxel/platinum containing chemotherapy: a National Cancer Institute of Canada Clinical Trials Group Study, *Gynecol Oncol* 102:300–308, 2006.

237. Moore MJ, Hamm J, Dancey J, et al.: Comparison of gemcitabine versus the matrix metalloproteinase inhibitor BAY 12-9566 in patients with advanced or metastatic adenocarcinoma of the pancreas: a phase III trial of the National Cancer Institute of Canada Clinical Trials Group, *J Clin Oncol* 21:3296–3302, 2003.

238. Moore AS, Dernell WS, Ogilvie GK, et al.: Doxorubicin and BAY 12-9566 for the treatment of osteosarcoma in dogs: a randomized, double-blind, placebo-controlled study, *J Vet Intern Med* 21:783–790, 2007.

239. Mohammed SI, Khan KN, Sellers RS, et al.: Expression of cyclooxygenase-1 and 2 in naturally-occurring canine cancer, *Prostaglandins Leukot Essent Fatty Acids* 70:479–483, 2004.

240. Knapp DW, Richardson RC, Chan TC, et al.: Piroxicam therapy in 34 dogs with transitional cell carcinoma of the urinary bladder, *J Vet Intern Med* 8:273–278, 1994.

241. Knapp DW, Richardson RC, Bottoms GD, et al.: Phase I trial of piroxicam in 62 dogs bearing naturally occurring tumors, *Cancer Chemother Pharmacol* 29:214–218, 1992.

242. Mohammed SI, Bennett PF, Craig BA, et al.: Effects of the cyclooxygenase inhibitor, piroxicam, on tumor response, apoptosis, and angiogenesis in a canine model of human invasive urinary bladder cancer, *Cancer Res* 62:356–358, 2002.

243. Mohammed SI, Craig BA, Mutsaers AJ, et al.: Effects of the cyclooxygenase inhibitor, piroxicam, in combination with chemotherapy on tumor response, apoptosis, and angiogenesis in a canine model of human invasive urinary bladder cancer, *Mol Cancer Ther* 2:183–188, 2003.

244. Suvannasankha A, Fausel C, Juliar BE, et al.: Final report of toxicity and efficacy of a phase II study of oral cyclophosphamide, thalidomide, and prednisone for patients with relapsed or refractory multiple myeloma: a Hoosier Oncology Group Trial, HEM01-21, *Oncologist* 12:99–106, 2007.

245. Bray JP, Orbell G, Cave N, et al.: Does thalidomide prolong survival in dogs with splenic haemangiosarcoma? *J Small Anim Pract* 59:85–91, 2018.

246. Finotello R, Henriques J, Sabattini S, et al.: A retrospective analysis of chemotherapy switch suggests improved outcome in surgically removed, biologically aggressive canine haemangiosarcoma, *Vet Comp Oncol* 15:493–503, 2017.

247. Fidler IJ, Ellis LM: Chemotherapeutic drugs—more really is not better, *Nat Med* 6:500–502, 2000.

248. Hanahan D, Bergers G, Bergsland E: Less is more, regularly: metronomic dosing of cytotoxic drugs can target tumor angiogenesis in mice, *J Clin Invest* 105:1045–1047, 2000.

249. Kerbel RS, Kamen BA: The anti-angiogenic basis of metronomic chemotherapy, *Nat Rev Cancer* 4:423–436, 2004.

250. Pasquier E, Kavallaris M, Andre N: Metronomic chemotherapy: new rationale for new directions, *Nat Rev Clin Oncol* 7:455–465, 2010.

251. Drevs J, Fakler J, Eisele S, et al.: Antiangiogenic potency of various chemotherapeutic drugs for metronomic chemotherapy, *Anticancer Res* 24:1759–1763, 2004.

252. Bocci G, Nicolaou KC, Kerbel RS: Protracted low-dose effects on human endothelial cell proliferation and survival in vitro reveal a selective antiangiogenic window for various chemotherapeutic drugs, *Cancer Res* 62:6938–6943, 2002.

253. Bocci G, Francia G, Man S, et al.: Thrombospondin 1, a mediator of the antiangiogenic effects of low-dose metronomic chemotherapy, *Proc Natl Acad Sci USA* 100:12917–12922, 2003.

254. Hamano Y, Sugimoto H, Soubasakos MA, et al.: Thrombospondin-1 associated with tumor microenvironment contributes to low-dose cyclophosphamide-mediated endothelial cell apoptosis and tumor growth suppression, *Cancer Res* 64:1570–1574, 2004.

255. Shaked Y, Kerbel RS: Antiangiogenic strategies on defense: on the possibility of blocking rebounds by the tumor vasculature after chemotherapy, *Cancer Res* 67:7055–7058, 2007.

256. Bertolini F, Paul S, Mancuso P, et al.: Maximum tolerable dose and low-dose metronomic chemotherapy have opposite effects on the mobilization and viability of circulating endothelial progenitor cells, *Cancer Res* 63:4342–4346, 2003.

257. Daenen LG, Shaked Y, Man S, et al.: Low-dose metronomic cyclophosphamide combined with vascular disrupting therapy induces potent antitumor activity in preclinical human tumor xenograft models, *Mol Cancer Ther* 8:2872–2881, 2009.

258. Shaked Y, Emmenegger U, Man S, et al.: Optimal biologic dose of metronomic chemotherapy regimens is associated with maximum antiangiogenic activity, *Blood* 106:3058–3061, 2005.

259. Toh B, Abastado JP: Myeloid cells: prime drivers of tumor progression, *Oncoimmunology* 1:1360–1367, 2012.

260. Umansky V, Sevko A: Tumor microenvironment and myeloid-derived suppressor cells, *Cancer Microenviron* 6:169–177, 2013.

261. Finn OJ: Immuno-oncology: understanding the function and dysfunction of the immune system in cancer, *Ann Oncol* 23(Suppl 8):viii6–9, 2012.

262. Penel N, Adenis A, Bocci G: Cyclophosphamide-based metronomic chemotherapy: after 10 years of experience, where do we stand and where are we going? *Crit Rev Oncol Hematol* 82:40–50, 2012.

263. Ghiringhelli F, Menard C, Puig PE, et al.: Metronomic cyclophosphamide regimen selectively depletes CD4+CD25+ regulatory T cells and restores T and NK effector functions in end stage cancer patients, *Cancer Immunol Immunother* 56:641–648, 2007.

264. Kerbel RS, Shaked Y: The potential clinical promise of 'multimodality' metronomic chemotherapy revealed by preclinical studies of metastatic disease, *Cancer Lett* 400:293–304, 2017.

265. Salem ML, Al-Khami AA, El-Nagaar SA, et al.: Kinetics of rebounding of lymphoid and myeloid cells in mouse peripheral blood, spleen and bone marrow after treatment with cyclophosphamide, *Cell Immunol* 276:67–74, 2012.

266. Angulo I, de las Heras FG, Garcia-Bustos JF, et al.: Nitric oxide-producing CD11b(+)Ly-6G(Gr-1)(+)CD31(ER-MP12)(+) cells in the spleen of cyclophosphamide-treated mice: implications for T-cell responses in immunosuppressed mice, *Blood* 95:212–220, 2000.

267. Noguchi M, Moriya F, Koga N, et al.: A randomized phase II clinical trial of personalized peptide vaccination with metronomic low-dose cyclophosphamide in patients with metastatic castration-resistant prostate cancer, *Cancer Immunol Immunother* 65:151–160, 2016.

268. Burton JH, Mitchell L, Thamm DH, et al.: Low-dose cyclophosphamide selectively decreases regulatory T cells and inhibits angiogenesis in dogs with soft tissue sarcoma, *J Vet Intern Med* 25:920–926, 2011.

269. Mitchell L, Thamm DH, Biller BJ: Clinical and immunomodulatory effects of toceranib combined with low-dose cyclophosphamide in dogs with cancer, *J Vet Intern Med* 26:355–362, 2012.

270. Nars MS, Kaneno R: Immunomodulatory effects of low dose chemotherapy and perspectives of its combination with immunotherapy, *Int J Cancer* 132:2471–2478, 2013.

271. Shurin GV, Tourkova IL, Kaneno R, et al.: Chemotherapeutic agents in noncytotoxic concentrations increase antigen presentation by dendritic cells via an IL-12-dependent mechanism, *J Immunol* 183:137–144, 2009.

272. Suzuki E, Kapoor V, Jassar AS, et al.: Gemcitabine selectively eliminates splenic Gr-1+/CD11b+ myeloid suppressor cells in tumor-bearing animals and enhances antitumor immune activity, *Clin Cancer Res* 11:6713–6721, 2005.

273. Zhu Y, Liu N, Xiong SD, et al.: CD4+Foxp3+ regulatory T-cell impairment by paclitaxel is independent of toll-like receptor 4, *Scand J Immunol* 73:301–308, 2011.

274. Ridolfi L, Petrini M, Granato AM, et al.: Low-dose temozolomide before dendritic-cell vaccination reduces (specifically)
CD4+CD25++Foxp3+ regulatory T-cells in advanced melanoma
patients, *J Transl Med* 11:135, 2013.
275. Denies S, Cicchelero L, de Rooster H, et al.: Immunological and
angiogenic markers during metronomic temozolomide and cyclophosphamide in canine cancer patients, *Vet Comp Oncol* 15:594–
605, 2017.
276. Cancedda S, Rohrer Bley C, Aresu L, et al.: Efficacy and
side effects of radiation therapy in comparison with radiation therapy and temozolomide in the treatment of measurable canine malignant melanoma, *Vet Comp Oncol* 14:
e146–e157, 2016.
277. Treggiari E, Elliott JW, Baines SJ, et al.: Temozolomide alone
or in combination with doxorubicin as a rescue agent in 37
cases of canine multicentric lymphoma, *Vet Comp Oncol* 16:
194–201, 2018.
278. Aguirre-Ghiso JA: Models, mechanisms and clinical evidence for
cancer dormancy, *Nat Rev Cancer* 7:834–846, 2007.
279. Calabrese C, Poppleton H, Kocak M, et al.: A perivascular niche for
brain tumor stem cells, *Cancer Cell* 11:69–82, 2007.
280. Folkins C, Man S, Xu P, et al.: Anticancer therapies combining
antiangiogenic and tumor cell cytotoxic effects reduce the tumor
stem-like cell fraction in glioma xenograft tumors, *Cancer Res*
67:3560–3564, 2007.
281. Martin-Padura I, Marighetti P, Agliano A, et al.: Residual dormant
cancer stem-cell foci are responsible for tumor relapse after antiangiogenic metronomic therapy in hepatocellular carcinoma xenografts, *Lab Invest* 92:952–966, 2012.
282. Colleoni M, Rocca A, Sandri MT, et al.: Low-dose oral methotrexate and cyclophosphamide in metastatic breast cancer: antitumor
activity and correlation with vascular endothelial growth factor levels, *Ann Oncol* 13:73–80, 2002.
283. Lien K, Georgsdottir S, Sivanathan L, et al.: Low-dose metronomic chemotherapy: a systematic literature analysis, *Eur J Cancer*
49:3387–3395, 2013.
284. Parikh PM, Hingmire SS, Deshmukh CD: Selected current data
on metronomic therapy (and its promise) from India, *South Asian J
Cancer* 5:37–47, 2016.
285. Pramanik R, Agarwala S, Gupta YK, et al.: Metronomic chemotherapy vs best supportive care in progressive pediatric solid
malignant tumors: a randomized clinical trial, *JAMA Oncol* 3:
1222–1227, 2017.
286. Lana S, U'Ren L, Plaza S, et al.: Continuous low-dose oral chemotherapy for adjuvant therapy of splenic hemangiosarcoma in dogs,
J Vet Intern Med 21:764–769, 2007.
287. Wendelburg KM, Price LL, Burgess KE, et al.: Survival time of
dogs with splenic hemangiosarcoma treated by splenectomy with
or without adjuvant chemotherapy: 208 cases (2001-2012), *J Am
Vet Med Assoc* 247:393–403, 2015.
288. Matsuyama A, Poirier VJ, Mantovani F, et al.: Adjuvant doxorubicin with or without metronomic cyclophosphamide for
canine splenic hemangiosarcoma, *J Am Anim Hosp Assoc* 53:
304–312, 2017.
289. Matsuyama A, Schott CR, Wood GA, et al.: Evaluation of metronomic cyclophosphamide chemotherapy as maintenance treatment
for dogs with appendicular osteosarcoma following limb amputation and carboplatin chemotherapy, *J Am Vet Med Assoc* 252:1377–
1383, 2018.
290. London CA, Gardner HL, Mathie T, et al.: Impact of toceranib/
piroxicam/cyclophosphamide maintenance therapy on outcome of
dogs with appendicular osteosarcoma following amputation and
carboplatin chemotherapy: a multi-institutional study, *PLoS One*
10:e0124889, 2015.
291. Bentley RT, Thomovsky SA, Miller MA, et al.: Canine
(pet dog) tumor microsurgery and intratumoral concentration and safety of metronomic chlorambucil for spontaneous glioma: a phase I clinical trial, *World Neurosurg* 116:
E534–E542, 2018.
292. Custead MR, Weng HY, Childress MO: Retrospective comparison of three doses of metronomic chlorambucil for tolerability and
efficacy in dogs with spontaneous cancer, *Vet Comp Oncol* 15:808–
819, 2017.
293. Tripp CD, Fidel J, Anderson CL, et al.: Tolerability of metronomic
administration of lomustine in dogs with cancer, *J Vet Intern Med*
25:278–284, 2011.
294. Rasmussen RM, Kurzman ID, Biller BJ, et al.: Phase I lead-in and
subsequent randomized trial assessing safety and modulation of
regulatory T cell numbers following a maximally tolerated dose
doxorubicin and metronomic dose cyclophosphamide combination chemotherapy protocol in tumour-bearing dogs, *Vet Comp
Oncol* 15:421–430, 2017.
295. Cancedda S, Marconato L, Meier V, et al.: Hypofractionated
radiotherapy for macroscopic canine soft tissue sarcoma: a retrospective study of 50 cases treated with a 5 x 6 Gy protocol with
or without metronomic chemotherapy, *Vet Radiol Ultrasound* 57:
75–83, 2016.
296. Duffy ME, Anderson CL, Choy K, et al.: Metronomic administration of lomustine following palliative radiation therapy for appendicular osteosarcoma in dogs, *Can Vet J* 59:136–142, 2018.
297. Cicchelero L, Denies S, Vanderperren K, et al.: Immunological,
anti-angiogenic and clinical effects of intratumoral interleukin 12
electrogene therapy combined with metronomic cyclophosphamide in dogs with spontaneous cancer: a pilot study, *Cancer Lett*
400:205–218, 2017.
298. Shih T, Lindley C: Bevacizumab: an angiogenesis inhibitor for the
treatment of solid malignancies, *Clin Ther* 28:1779–1802, 2006.
299. London CA: Tyrosine kinase inhibitors in veterinary medicine, *Top
Companion Anim Med* 24:106–112, 2009.
300. Tjostheim SS, Stepien RL, Markovic LE, et al.: Effects of toceranib
phosphate on systolic blood pressure and proteinuria in dogs, *J Vet
Intern Med* 30:951–957, 2016.
301. Piscoya SL, Hume KR, Balkman CE: A retrospective study of proteinuria in dogs receiving toceranib phosphate, *Can Vet J* 59:611–
616, 2018.
302. Hume KR, Rizzo VL, Cawley JR, et al.: Effects of toceranib phosphate on the hypothalamic-pituitary-thyroid axis in tumor-bearing
dogs, *J Vet Intern Med* 32:377–383, 2018.
303. Charney SC, Bergman PJ, Hohenhaus AE, et al.: Risk factors
for sterile hemorrhagic cystitis in dogs with lymphoma receiving
cyclophosphamide with or without concurrent administration
of furosemide: 216 cases (1990-1996), *J Am Vet Med Assoc* 222:
1388–1393, 2003.
304. Matsuyama A, Woods JP, Mutsaers AJ: Evaluation of toxicity of
a chronic alternate day metronomic cyclophosphamide chemotherapy protocol in dogs with naturally occurring cancer, *Can Vet J*
58:51–55, 2017.
305. Gaeta R, Brown D, Cohen R, et al.: Risk factors for development
of sterile haemorrhagic cystitis in canine lymphoma patients receiving oral cyclophosphamide: a case-control study, *Vet Comp Oncol*
12:277–286, 2014.
306. Setyo L, Ma M, Bunn T, et al.: Furosemide for prevention of
cyclophosphamide-associated sterile haemorrhagic cystitis in dogs
receiving metronomic low-dose oral cyclophosphamide, *Vet Comp
Oncol* 15:1468–1478, 2017.
307. Chan CM, Frimberger AE, Moore AS: Incidence of sterile hemorrhagic cystitis in tumor-bearing dogs concurrently treated with oral
metronomic cyclophosphamide chemotherapy and furosemide: 55
cases (2009-2015), *J Am Vet Med Assoc* 249:1408–1414, 2016.
308. Kerbel RS: A cancer therapy resistant to resistance, *Nature*
390:335–336, 1997.
309. Ebos JM, Lee CR, Kerbel RS: Tumor and host-mediated pathways
of resistance and disease progression in response to antiangiogenic
therapy, *Clin Cancer Res* 15:5020–5025, 2009.
310. Paez-Ribes M, Allen E, Hudock J, et al.: Antiangiogenic
therapy elicits malignant progression of tumors to increased
local invasion and distant metastasis, *Cancer Cell* 15:
220–231, 2009.

311. Ebos JM, Lee CR, Cruz-Munoz W, et al.: Accelerated metastasis after short-term treatment with a potent inhibitor of tumor angiogenesis, *Cancer Cell* 15:232–239, 2009.

312. Park JW, Kerbel RS, Kelloff GJ, et al.: Rationale for biomarkers and surrogate end points in mechanism-driven oncology drug development, *Clin Cancer Res* 10:3885–3896, 2004.

313. Drevs J, Schneider V: The use of vascular biomarkers and imaging studies in the early clinical development of anti-tumour agents targeting angiogenesis, *J Intern Med* 260:517–529, 2006.

314. Sandri MT, Johansson HA, Zorzino L, et al.: Serum EGFR and serum HER-2/neu are useful predictive and prognostic markers in metastatic breast cancer patients treated with metronomic chemotherapy, *Cancer* 110:509–517, 2007.

315. Lindauer A, Di GP, Kanefendt F, et al.: Pharmacokinetic/pharmacodynamic modeling of biomarker response to sunitinib in healthy volunteers, *Clin Pharmacol Ther* 87:601–608, 2010.

316. Marchetti V, Giorgi M, Fioravanti A, et al.: First-line metronomic chemotherapy in a metastatic model of spontaneous canine tumours: a pilot study, *Invest New Drugs* 30:1725–1730, 2011.

317. Drevs J, Schneider V: The use of vascular biomarkers and imaging studies in the early clinical development of anti-tumour agents targeting angiogenesis, *J Intern Med* 260:517–529, 2006.

318. Morgan B, Thomas AL, Drevs J, et al.: Dynamic contrast-enhanced magnetic resonance imaging as a biomarker for the pharmacological response of PTK787/ZK 222584, an inhibitor of the vascular endothelial growth factor receptor tyrosine kinases, in patients with advanced colorectal cancer and liver metastases: results from two phase I studies, *J Clin Oncol* 21:3955–3964, 2003.

319. MacLeod AG, Dickinson PJ, LeCouteur RA, et al.: Quantitative assessment of blood volume and permeability in cerebral mass lesions using dynamic contrast-enhanced computed tomography in the dog, *Acad Radiol* 16:1187–1195, 2009.

320. Shaked Y, Emmenegger U, Man S, et al.: Optimal biologic dose of metronomic chemotherapy regimens is associated with maximum antiangiogenic activity, *Blood* 106:3058–3061, 2005.

321. Twardowski PW, Smith-Powell L, Carroll M, et al.: Biologic markers of angiogenesis: circulating endothelial cells in patients with advanced malignancies treated on phase I protocol with metronomic chemotherapy and celecoxib, *Cancer Invest* 26:53–59, 2008.

322. Bertolini F, Mancuso P, Shaked Y, et al.: Molecular and cellular biomarkers for angiogenesis in clinical oncology, *Drug Discov Today* 12:806–812, 2007.

323. Bernabe LF, Portela R, Nguyen S, et al.: Evaluation of the adverse event profile and pharmacodynamics of toceranib phosphate administered to dogs with solid tumors at doses below the maximum tolerated dose, *BMC Vet Res* 9:190, 2013.

324. Robinson ES, Khankin EV, Karumanchi SA, et al.: Hypertension induced by VEGF signaling pathway inhibition: mechanisms and potential use as a biomarker, *Semin Nephrol* 30:591–601, 2010.

325. Brueckner B, Lyko F: DNA methyltransferase inhibitors: old and new drugs for an epigenetic cancer therapy, *Trends Pharmacol Sci* 25:551–554, 2004.

326. Herman JG, Baylin SB: Gene silencing in cancer in association with promoter hypermethylation, *N Engl J Med* 349:2042–2054, 2003.

327. Szyf M: DNA methylation and cancer therapy, *Drug Resist Updat* 6:341–353, 2003.

328. Pelham JT, Irwin PJ, Kay PH: Genomic hypomethylation in neoplastic cells from dogs with malignant lymphoproliferative disorders, *Res Vet Sci* 74:101–104, 2003.

329. Ehrlich M: DNA methylation in cancer: too much, but also too little, *Oncogene* 21:5400–5413, 2002.

330. Gaudet F, Hodgson JG, Eden A, et al.: Induction of tumors in mice by genomic hypomethylation, *Science* 300:489–492, 2003.

331. Catto JW, Azzouzi AR, Rehman I, et al.: Promoter hypermethylation is associated with tumor location, stage, and subsequent progression in transitional cell carcinoma, *J Clin Oncol* 23:2903–2910, 2005.

332. Baylin SB, Herman JG: DNA hypermethylation in tumorigenesis: epigenetics joins genetics, *Trends Genet* 16:168-174.

333. van Doorn R, Zoutman WH, Dijkman R, et al.: Epigenetic profiling of cutaneous T-cell lymphoma: promoter hypermethylation of multiple tumor suppressor genes including BCL7a, PTPRG, and p73, *J Clin Oncol* 23:3886–3896, 2005.

334. Fujiwara-Igarashi A, Goto-Koshino Y, Mochizuki H, et al.: Inhibition of p16 tumor suppressor gene expression via promoter hypermethylation in canine lymphoid tumor cells, *Res Vet Sci* 97:60–63, 2014.

335. Segura-Pacheco B, Trejo-Becerril C, Perez-Cardenas E, et al.: Reactivation of tumor suppressor genes by the cardiovascular drugs hydralazine and procainamide and their potential use in cancer therapy, *Clin Cancer Res* 9:1596–1603, 2003.

336. Tomiyasu H, Goto-Koshino Y, Fujino Y, et al.: Epigenetic regulation of the ABCB1 gene in drug-sensitive and drug-resistant lymphoid tumour cell lines obtained from canine patients, *Vet J* 199:103–109, 2014.

337. Saleh MH, Wang L, Goldberg MS: Improving cancer immunotherapy with DNA methyltransferase inhibitors, *Cancer Immunol Immunother* 65:787–796, 2016.

338. Sigalotti L, Fratta E, Coral S, et al.: Epigenetic drugs as immunomodulators for combination therapies in solid tumors, *Pharmacol Ther* 142:339–350, 2014.

339. Peng D, Kryczek I, Nagarsheth N, et al.: Epigenetic silencing of TH1–type chemokines shapes tumour immunity and immunotherapy, *Nature* 527:249–253, 2015.

340. Silverman LR, Demakos EP, Peterson BL, et al.: Randomized controlled trial of azacitidine in patients with the myelodysplastic syndrome: a study of the cancer and leukemia group B, *J Clin Oncol* 20:2429–2440, 2002.

341. Kantarjian H, Issa JP, Rosenfeld CS, et al.: Decitabine improves patient outcomes in myelodysplastic syndromes: results of a phase III randomized study, *Cancer* 106:1794–1803, 2006.

342. Issa JP, Gharibyan V, Cortes J, et al.: Phase II study of low-dose decitabine in patients with chronic myelogenous leukemia resistant to imatinib mesylate, *J Clin Oncol* 23:3948–3956, 2005.

343. Cashen AF, Schiller GJ, O'Donnell MR, et al.: Multicenter, phase II study of decitabine for the first-line treatment of older patients with acute myeloid leukemia, *J Clin Oncol* 28:556–561, 2010.

344. Aparicio A, Eads CA, Leong LA, et al.: Phase I trial of continuous infusion 5-aza-2'-deoxycytidine, *Cancer Chemother Pharmacol* 51:231–239, 2003.

345. Momparler RL, Bouffard DY, Momparler LF, et al.: Pilot phase I-II study on 5-aza-2'-deoxycytidine (Decitabine) in patients with metastatic lung cancer, *Anticancer Drugs* 8:358–368, 1997.

346. Linnekamp JF, Butter R, Spijker R, et al.: Clinical and biological effects of demethylating agents on solid tumours - a systematic review, *Cancer Treat Rev* 54:10–23, 2017.

347. Pohlmann P, DiLeone LP, Cancella AI, et al.: Phase II trial of cisplatin plus decitabine, a new DNA hypomethylating agent, in patients with advanced squamous cell carcinoma of the cervix, *Am J Clin Oncol* 25:496–501, 2002.

348. Villar-Garea A, Fraga MF, Espada J, et al.: Procaine is a DNA-demethylating agent with growth-inhibitory effects in human cancer cells, *Cancer Res* 63:4984–4989, 2003.

349. Zambrano P, Segura-Pacheco B, Perez-Cardenas E, et al.: A phase I study of hydralazine to demethylate and reactivate the expression of tumor suppressor genes, *BMC Cancer* 5:44, 2005.

350. Candelaria M, Herrera A, Labardini J, et al.: Hydralazine and magnesium valproate as epigenetic treatment for myelodysplastic syndrome. Preliminary results of a phase-II trial, *Ann Hematol* 90:379–387, 2011.

351. Espinoza-Zamora JR, Labardini-Mendez J, Sosa-Espinoza A, et al.: Efficacy of hydralazine and valproate in cutaneous T-cell lymphoma, a phase II study, *Expert Opin Investig Drugs* 26:481–487.

352. Yamazaki J, Jelinek J, Hisamoto S, et al.: Dynamic changes in DNA methylation patterns in canine lymphoma cell lines demonstrated by genome-wide quantitative DNA methylation analysis, *Vet J* 231:48–54, 2018.

353. Ferraresso S, Arico A, Sanavia T, et al.: DNA methylation profiling reveals common signatures of tumorigenesis and defines epigenetic prognostic subtypes of canine diffuse large B-cell lymphoma, *Sci Rep* 7:11591, 2017.

354. Fujita M, Kaneda M: DNA methylation inhibitor causes cell growth retardation and gene expression changes in feline lymphoma cells, *J Vet Med Sci* 79:1352–1358, 2017.

355. Harman RM, Curtis TM, Argyle DJ, et al.: A comparative study on the in vitro effects of the DNA methyltransferase inhibitor 5-azacytidine (5-AzaC) in breast/mammary cancer of different mammalian species, *J Mammary Gland Biol Neoplasia* 21:51–66, 2016.

356. Noguchi S, Mori T, Igase M, et al.: A novel apoptosis-inducing mechanism of 5-aza-2'-deoxycitidine in melanoma cells: demethylation of TNF-alpha and activation of FOXO1, *Cancer Lett* 369:344–353, 2015.

357. Flesner BK, Kumar SR, Bryan JN: 6-thioguanine and zebularine down-regulate DNMT1 and globally demethylate canine malignant lymphoid cells, *BMC Vet Res* 10:290, 2014.

358. Thayanithy V, Park C, Sarver AL, et al.: Combinatorial treatment of DNA and chromatin-modifying drugs cause cell death in human and canine osteosarcoma cell lines, *PLoS One* 7:e43720, 2012.

359. Hahn NM, Bonney PL, Dhawan D, et al.: Subcutaneous 5-azacitidine treatment of naturally occurring canine urothelial carcinoma: a novel epigenetic approach to human urothelial carcinoma drug development, *J Urol* 187:302–309, 2012.

360. Guo Y, Pakneshan P, Gladu J, et al.: Regulation of DNA methylation in human breast cancer. Effect on the urokinase-type plasminogen activator gene production and tumor invasion, *J Biol Chem* 277:41571–41579, 2002.

361. Berger SL: Histone modifications in transcriptional regulation, *Curr Opin Genet Dev* 12:142–148, 2002.

362. Jenuwein T, Allis CD: Translating the histone code, *Science* 293:1074–1080, 2001.

363. Zhu P, Martin E, Mengwasser J, et al.: Induction of HDAC2 expression upon loss of APC in colorectal tumorigenesis, *Cancer Cell* 5:455–463, 2004.

364. Kim MS, Kwon HJ, Lee YM, et al.: Histone deacetylases induce angiogenesis by negative regulation of tumor suppressor genes, *Nat Med* 7:437–443, 2001.

365. Glozak MA, Sengupta N, Zhang X, et al.: Acetylation and deacetylation of non-histone proteins, *Gene* 363:15–23, 2005.

366. Sadoul K, Boyault C, Pabion M, et al.: Regulation of protein turnover by acetyltransferases and deacetylases, *Biochimie* 90:306–312, 2008.

367. Marchion DC, Bicaku E, Daud AI, et al.: Valproic acid alters chromatin structure by regulation of chromatin modulation proteins, *Cancer Res* 65:3815–3822, 2005.

368. Weichert W: HDAC expression and clinical prognosis in human malignancies, *Cancer Lett* 280:168–176, 2009.

369. Zgouras D, Becker U, Loitsch S, et al.: Modulation of angiogenesis-related protein synthesis by valproic acid, *Biochem Biophys Res Commun* 316:693–697, 2004.

370. Qian DZ, Wang X, Kachhap SK, et al.: The histone deacetylase inhibitor NVP-LAQ824 inhibits angiogenesis and has a greater antitumor effect in combination with the vascular endothelial growth factor receptor tyrosine kinase inhibitor PTK787/ZK222584, *Cancer Res* 64:6626–6634, 2004.

371. Michaelis M, Michaelis UR, Fleming I, et al.: Valproic acid inhibits angiogenesis in vitro and in vivo, *Mol Pharmacol* 65:520–527, 2004.

372. Rossig L, Li H, Fisslthaler B, et al.: Inhibitors of histone deacetylation downregulate the expression of endothelial nitric oxide synthase and compromise endothelial cell function in vasorelaxation and angiogenesis, *Circ Res* 91:837–844, 2002.

373. Rossig L, Urbich C, Bruhl T, et al.: Histone deacetylase activity is essential for the expression of HoxA9 and for endothelial commitment of progenitor cells, *J Exp Med*, 2005.

374. Phillips A, Bullock T, Plant N: Sodium valproate induces apoptosis in the rat hepatoma cell line, FaO, *Toxicology* 192:219–227, 2003.

375. Tang R, Faussat AM, Majdak P, et al.: Valproic acid inhibits proliferation and induces apoptosis in acute myeloid leukemia cells expressing P-gp and MRP1, *Leukemia* 18:1246–1251, 2004.

376. Roh MS, Kim CW, Park BS, et al.: Mechanism of histone deacetylase inhibitor Trichostatin A induced apoptosis in human osteosarcoma cells, *Apoptosis* 9:583–589, 2004.

377. Maeda T, Nagaoka Y, Kawai Y, et al.: Inhibitory effects of cancer cell proliferation by novel histone deacetylase inhibitors involve p21/WAF1 induction and G2/M arrest, *Biol Pharm Bull* 28:849–853, 2005.

378. Takai N, Desmond JC, Kumagai T, et al.: Histone deacetylase inhibitors have a profound antigrowth activity in endometrial cancer cells, *Clin Cancer Res* 10:1141–1149, 2004.

379. Olsen CM, Meussen-Elholm ET, Roste LS, et al.: Antiepileptic drugs inhibit cell growth in the human breast cancer cell line MCF7, *Mol Cell Endocrinol* 213:173–179, 2004.

380. Fortunati N, Catalano MG, Arena K, et al.: Valproic acid induces the expression of the Na+/I- symporter and iodine uptake in poorly differentiated thyroid cancer cells, *J Clin Endocrinol Metab* 89:1006–1009, 2004.

381. Gottlicher M: Valproic acid: an old drug newly discovered as inhibitor of histone deacetylases, *Ann Hematol* 83(Suppl 1):S91–S92, 2004.

382. Gottlicher M, Minucci S, Zhu P, et al.: Valproic acid defines a novel class of HDAC inhibitors inducing differentiation of transformed cells, *EMBO J* 20:6969–6978, 2001.

383. Stockhausen MT, Sjolund J, Manetopoulos C, et al.: Effects of the histone deacetylase inhibitor valproic acid on Notch signalling in human neuroblastoma cells, *Br J Cancer* 92:751–759, 2005.

384. Thelen P, Schweyer S, Hemmerlein B, et al.: Expressional changes after histone deacetylase inhibition by valproic acid in LNCaP human prostate cancer cells, *Int J Oncol* 24:25–31, 2004.

385. Chobanian NH, Greenberg VL, Gass JM, et al.: Histone deacetylase inhibitors enhance paclitaxel-induced cell death in ovarian cancer cell lines independent of p53 status, *Anticancer Res* 24:539–545, 2004.

386. Fuino L, Bali P, Wittmann S, et al.: Histone deacetylase inhibitor LAQ824 down-regulates Her-2 and sensitizes human breast cancer cells to trastuzumab, taxotere, gemcitabine, and epothilone B, *Mol Cancer Ther* 2:971–984, 2003.

387. Kim MS, Blake M, Baek JH, et al.: Inhibition of histone deacetylase increases cytotoxicity to anticancer drugs targeting DNA, *Cancer Res* 63:7291–7300, 2003.

388. Maggio SC, Rosato RR, Kramer LB, et al.: The histone deacetylase inhibitor MS-275 interacts synergistically with fludarabine to induce apoptosis in human leukemia cells, *Cancer Res* 64:2590–2600, 2004.

389. Watanabe K, Okamoto K, Yonehara S: Sensitization of osteosarcoma cells to death receptor-mediated apoptosis by HDAC inhibitors through downregulation of cellular FLIP, *Cell Death Differ* 12:10–18, 2005.

390. Chinnaiyan P, Vallabhaneni G, Armstrong E, et al.: Modulation of radiation response by histone deacetylase inhibition, *Int J Radiat Oncol Biol Phys* 62:223–229, 2005.

391. Wittenburg LA, Bisson L, Rose BJ, et al.: The histone deacetylase inhibitor valproic acid sensitizes human and canine osteosarcoma to doxorubicin, *Cancer Chemother Pharmacol* 67:83–92, 2011.

392. Wittenburg LA, Gustafson DL, Thamm DH: Phase I pharmacokinetic and pharmacodynamic evaluation of combined valproic acid/doxorubicin treatment in dogs with spontaneous cancer, *Clin Cancer Res* 16:4832–4842, 2010.

393. Wittenburg LA, Ptitsyn AA, Thamm DH: A systems biology approach to identify molecular pathways altered by HDAC inhibition in osteosarcoma, *J Cell Biochem* 113:773–783, 2012.

394. Whittaker SJ, Demierre MF, Kim EJ, et al.: Final results from a multicenter, international, pivotal study of romidepsin in refractory cutaneous T-cell lymphoma, *J Clin Oncol* 28:4485–4491, 2010.

395. Duvic M, Talpur R, Ni X, et al.: Phase 2 trial of oral vorinostat (suberoylanilide hydroxamic acid, SAHA) for refractory cutaneous T-cell lymphoma (CTCL), *Blood* 109:31–39, 2007.

396. Olsen EA, Kim YH, Kuzel TM, et al.: Phase IIb multicenter trial of vorinostat in patients with persistent, progressive, or treatment refractory cutaneous T-cell lymphoma, *J Clin Oncol* 25:3109–3115, 2007.

397. Munster PN, Thurn KT, Thomas S, et al.: A phase II study of the histone deacetylase inhibitor vorinostat combined with tamoxifen for the treatment of patients with hormone therapy-resistant breast cancer, *Br J Cancer* 104:1828–1835, 2011.

398. Kirschbaum M, Frankel P, Popplewell L, et al.: Phase II study of vorinostat for treatment of relapsed or refractory indolent non-Hodgkin's lymphoma and mantle cell lymphoma, *J Clin Oncol* 29:1198–1203, 2011.

399. Otterson GA, Hodgson L, Pang H, et al.: Phase II study of the histone deacetylase inhibitor Romidepsin in relapsed small cell lung cancer (Cancer and Leukemia Group B 30304), *J Thorac Oncol* 5:1644–1648, 2010.

400. Stathis A, Hotte SJ, Chen EX, et al.: Phase I study of decitabine in combination with vorinostat in patients with advanced solid tumors and non-Hodgkin's lymphomas, *Clin Cancer Res* 17:1582–1590, 2011.

401. Kisseberth WC, Murahari S, London CA, et al.: Evaluation of the effects of histone deacetylase inhibitors on cells from canine cancer cell lines, *Am J Vet Res* 69:938–945, 2008.

402. Murahari S, Jalkanen AL, Kulp SK, et al.: Sensitivity of osteosarcoma cells to HDAC inhibitor AR-42 mediated apoptosis, *BMC Cancer* 17:67, 2017.

403. Elshafae SM, Kohart NA, Altstadt LA, et al.: The effect of a histone deacetylase inhibitor (AR-42) on canine prostate cancer growth and metastasis, *Prostate* 77:776–793, 2017.

404. Blaheta RA, Michaelis M, Driever PH, et al.: Evolving anticancer drug valproic acid: insights into the mechanism and clinical studies, *Med Res Rev* 25:383–397, 2005.

405. Adams J: The development of proteasome inhibitors as anticancer drugs, *Cancer Cell* 5:417–421, 2004.

406. Rajkumar SV, Richardson PG, Hideshima T, et al.: Proteasome inhibition as a novel therapeutic target in human cancer, *J Clin Oncol* 23:630–639, 2005.

407. Voorhees PM, Dees EC, O'Neil B, et al.: The proteasome as a target for cancer therapy, *Clin Cancer Res* 9:6316–6325, 2003.

408. Hideshima T, Richardson P, Chauhan D, et al.: The proteasome inhibitor PS-341 inhibits growth, induces apoptosis, and overcomes drug resistance in human multiple myeloma cells, *Cancer Res* 61:3071–3076, 2001.

409. Masdehors P, Omura S, Merle-Beral H, et al.: Increased sensitivity of CLL-derived lymphocytes to apoptotic death activation by the proteasome-specific inhibitor lactacystin, *Br J Haematol* 105:752–757, 1999.

410. Orlowski RZ, Eswara JR, Lafond-Walker A, et al.: Tumor growth inhibition induced in a murine model of human Burkitt's lymphoma by a proteasome inhibitor, *Cancer Res* 58:4342–4348, 1998.

411. Soligo D, Servida F, Delia D, et al.: The apoptogenic response of human myeloid leukaemia cell lines and of normal and malignant haematopoietic progenitor cells to the proteasome inhibitor PSI, *Br J Haematol* 113:126–135, 2001.

412. Masdehors P, Merle-Beral H, Maloum K, et al.: Deregulation of the ubiquitin system and p53 proteolysis modify the apoptotic response in B-CLL lymphocytes, *Blood* 96:269–274, 2000.

413. Jagannath S, Barlogie B, Berenson J, et al.: A phase 2 study of two doses of bortezomib in relapsed or refractory myeloma, *Br J Haematol* 127:165–172, 2004.

414. Jagannath S, Durie BG, Wolf J, et al.: Bortezomib therapy alone and in combination with dexamethasone for previously untreated symptomatic multiple myeloma, *Br J Haematol* 129:776–783, 2005.

415. Richardson PG, Sonneveld P, Schuster MW, et al.: Bortezomib or high-dose dexamethasone for relapsed multiple myeloma, *N Engl J Med* 352:2487–2498, 2005.

416. Richardson PG, Barlogie B, Berenson J, et al.: A phase 2 study of bortezomib in relapsed, refractory myeloma, *N Engl J Med* 348:2609–2617, 2003.

417. Robak T, Huang H, Jin J, et al.: Bortezomib-based therapy for newly diagnosed mantle-cell lymphoma, *N Engl J Med* 372:944–953, 2015.

418. O'Connor OA, Wright J, Moskowitz C, et al.: Phase II clinical experience with the novel proteasome inhibitor bortezomib in patients with indolent non-Hodgkin's lymphoma and mantle cell lymphoma, *J Clin Oncol* 23:676–684, 2005.

419. Goy A, Younes A, McLaughlin P, et al.: Phase II study of proteasome inhibitor bortezomib in relapsed or refractory B-cell non-Hodgkin's lymphoma, *J Clin Oncol* 23:667–675, 2005.

420. Cortes J, Thomas D, Koller C, et al.: Phase I study of bortezomib in refractory or relapsed acute leukemias, *Clin Cancer Res* 10:3371–3376, 2004.

421. Davis NB, Taber DA, Ansari RH, et al.: Phase II trial of PS-341 in patients with renal cell cancer: a University of Chicago phase II consortium study, *J Clin Oncol* 22:115–119, 2004.

422. Maki RG, Kraft AS, Scheu K, et al.: A multicenter Phase II study of bortezomib in recurrent or metastatic sarcomas, *Cancer* 103:1431–1438, 2005.

423. Markovic SN, Geyer SM, Dawkins F, et al.: A phase II study of bortezomib in the treatment of metastatic malignant melanoma, *Cancer* 103:2584–2589, 2005.

424. Shah MH, Young D, Kindler HL, et al.: Phase II study of the proteasome inhibitor bortezomib (PS-341) in patients with metastatic neuroendocrine tumors, *Clin Cancer Res* 10:6111–6118, 2004.

425. Rossi UA, Finocchiaro LME, Glikin GC: Bortezomib enhances the antitumor effects of interferon-beta gene transfer on melanoma cells, *Anticancer Agents Med Chem* 17:754–761, 2017.

426. Ito K, Kobayashi M, Kuroki S, et al.: The proteasome inhibitor bortezomib inhibits the growth of canine malignant melanoma cells in vitro and in vivo, *Vet J* 198:577–582, 2013.

427. Gareau A, Rico C, Boerboom D, et al.: In vitro efficacy of a first-generation valosin-containing protein inhibitor (CB-5083) against canine lymphoma, *Vet Comp Oncol*, 2018; epub ahead of print.

428. Nadeau ME, Rico C, Tsoi M, et al.: Pharmacological targeting of valosin containing protein (VCP) induces DNA damage and selectively kills canine lymphoma cells, *BMC Cancer* 15:479, 2015.

429. Bouchard PR, Juedes MJ, Nix D, et al.: Nonclinical discovery and development of bortezomib (PS-341, VELCADE), a proteasome inhibitor for the treatment of cancer, Proc 55th Annual Meeting, *Am Coll Vet Pathol*, 2004.

430. Araujo KP, Bonuccelli G, Duarte CN, et al.: Bortezomib (PS-341) treatment decreases inflammation and partially rescues the expression of the dystrophin-glycoprotein complex in GRMD dogs, *PLoS One* 8:e61367, 2013.

431. Neckers L: Hsp90 inhibitors as novel cancer chemotherapeutic agents, *Trends Mol Med* 8:S55–61, 2002.

432. Isaacs JS, Xu W, Neckers L: Heat shock protein 90 as a molecular target for cancer therapeutics, *Cancer Cell* 3:213–217, 2003.

433. Kurebayashi J, Otsuki T, Kurosumi M, et al.: A radicicol derivative, KF58333, inhibits expression of hypoxia-inducible factor-1alpha and vascular endothelial growth factor, angiogenesis and growth of human breast cancer xenografts, *Jpn J Cancer Res* 92:1342–1351, 2001.

434. Osada M, Imaoka S, Funae Y: Apigenin suppresses the expression of VEGF, an important factor for angiogenesis, in endothelial cells via degradation of HIF-1alpha protein, *FEBS Lett* 575:59–63, 2004.

435. Plescia J, Salz W, Xia F, et al.: Rational design of shepherdin, a novel anticancer agent, *Cancer Cell* 7:457–468, 2005.

436. Kamal A, Thao L, Sensintaffar J, et al.: A high-affinity conformation of Hsp90 confers tumour selectivity on Hsp90 inhibitors, *Nature* 425:407–410, 2003.

437. Maloney A, Clarke PA, Workman P: Genes and proteins governing the cellular sensitivity to HSP90 inhibitors: a mechanistic perspective, *Curr Cancer Drug Targets* 3:331–341, 2003.

438. Fumo G, Akin C, Metcalfe DD, et al.: 17–Allylamino-17–demethoxygeldanamycin (17–AAG) is effective in down-regulating mutated, constitutively activated KIT protein in human mast cells, *Blood* 103:1078–1084, 2004.

439. Downing S, Chien MB, Kass PH, et al.: Prevalence and importance of internal tandem duplications in exons 11 and 12 of c-kit in mast cell tumors of dogs, *Am J Vet Res* 63:1718–1723, 2002.

440. Maulik G, Kijima T, Ma PC, et al.: Modulation of the c-Met/hepatocyte growth factor pathway in small cell lung cancer, *Clin Cancer Res* 8:620–627, 2002.

441. Liao AT, McMahon M, London CA: Characterization, expression and function of c-Met in canine spontaneous cancers, *Vet Comp Oncol* 3:61–72, 2005.

442. MacEwen EG, Kutzke J, Carew J, et al.: c-Met tyrosine kinase receptor expression and function in human and canine osteosarcoma cells, *Clin Exp Metastasis* 20:421–430, 2003.

443. Sakagami M, Morrison P, Welch WJ: Benzoquinoid ansamycins (herbimycin A and geldanamycin) interfere with the maturation of growth factor receptor tyrosine kinases, *Cell Stress Chaperones* 4:19–28, 1999.

444. Katayama R, Huelsmeyer MK, Marr AK, et al.: Imatinib mesylate inhibits platelet-derived growth factor activity and increases chemosensitivity in feline vaccine-associated sarcoma, *Cancer Chemother Pharmacol* 54:25–33, 2004.

445. Levine RA: Overexpression of the sis oncogene in a canine osteosarcoma cell line, *Vet Pathol* 39:411–412, 2002.

446. MacEwen EG, Pastor J, Kutzke J, et al.: IGF-1 receptor contributes to the malignant phenotype in human and canine osteosarcoma, *J Cell Biochem* 92:77–91, 2004.

447. Serra M, Pastor J, Domenzain C, et al.: Effect of transforming growth factor-beta1, insulin-like growth factor-I, and hepatocyte growth factor on proteoglycan production and regulation in canine melanoma cell lines, *Am J Vet Res* 63:1151–1158, 2002.

448. Thamm DH, Huelsmeyer MK, Mitzey AM, et al.: RT-PCR-based tyrosine kinase display profiling of canine melanoma: IGF-1 receptor as a potential therapeutic target, *Melanoma Res* 20:35–42, 2010.

449. Mabjeesh NJ, Post DE, Willard MT, et al.: Geldanamycin induces degradation of hypoxia-inducible factor 1alpha protein via the proteosome pathway in prostate cancer cells, *Cancer Res* 62:2478–2482, 2002.

450. Isaacs JS, Jung YJ, Mimnaugh EG, et al.: Hsp90 regulates a von Hippel Lindau-independent hypoxia-inducible factor-1 alpha-degradative pathway, *J Biol Chem* 277:29936–29944, 2002.

451. Muller L, Schaupp A, Walerych D, et al.: Hsp90 regulates the activity of wild type p53 under physiological and elevated temperatures, *J Biol Chem* 279:48846–48854, 2004.

452. Muller P, Ceskova P, Vojtesek B: Hsp90 is essential for restoring cellular functions of temperature-sensitive p53 mutant protein but not for stabilization and activation of wild-type p53: implications for cancer therapy, *J Biol Chem* 280:6682–6691, 2005.

453. Walerych D, Kudla G, Gutkowska M, et al.: Hsp90 chaperones wild-type p53 tumor suppressor protein, *J Biol Chem* 279:48836–48845, 2004.

454. Fortugno P, Beltrami E, Plescia J, et al.: Regulation of survivin function by Hsp90, *Proc Natl Acad Sci U S A* 100:13791–13796, 2003.

455. Bagatell R, Beliakoff J, David CL, et al.: Hsp90 inhibitors deplete key anti-apoptotic proteins in pediatric solid tumor cells and demonstrate synergistic anticancer activity with cisplatin, *Int J Cancer* 113:179–188, 2005.

456. Bisht KS, Bradbury CM, Mattson D, et al.: Geldanamycin and 17-allylamino-17-demethoxygeldanamycin potentiate the in vitro and in vivo radiation response of cervical tumor cells via the heat shock protein 90-mediated intracellular signaling and cytotoxicity, *Cancer Res* 63:8984–8995, 2003.

457. Jones DT, Addison E, North JM, et al.: Geldanamycin and herbimycin A induce apoptotic killing of B chronic lymphocytic leukemia cells and augment the cells' sensitivity to cytotoxic drugs, *Blood* 103:1855–1861, 2004.

458. Machida H, Matsumoto Y, Shirai M, et al.: Geldanamycin, an inhibitor of Hsp90, sensitizes human tumour cells to radiation, *Int J Radiat Biol* 79:973–980, 2003.

459. Munster PN, Basso A, Solit D, et al.: Modulation of Hsp90 function by ansamycins sensitizes breast cancer cells to chemotherapy-induced apoptosis in an RB- and schedule-dependent manner, *Clin Cancer Res* 7:2228–2236, 2001.

460. Solit DB, Basso AD, Olshen AB, et al.: Inhibition of heat shock protein 90 function down-regulates Akt kinase and sensitizes tumors to Taxol, *Cancer Res* 63:2139–2144, 2003.

461. Vasilevskaya IA, Rakitina TV, O'Dwyer PJ: Geldanamycin and its 17–allylamino-17–demethoxy analogue antagonize the action of cisplatin in human colon adenocarcinoma cells: differential caspase activation as a basis for interaction, *Cancer Res* 63:3241–3246, 2003.

462. Price JT, Quinn JMW, Sims NA, et al.: The heat shock protein 90 inhibitor, 17–allylamino-17-demethoxygeldanamycin, enhances osteoclast formation and potentiates bone metastasis of a human breast cancer cell line, *Cancer Res* 65:4929–4938, 2005.

463. Goetz MP, Toft D, Reid J, et al.: Phase I trial of 17–allylamino-17-demethoxygeldanamycin in patients with advanced cancer, *J Clin Oncol* 23:1078–1087, 2005.

464. Grem JL, Morrison G, Guo XD, et al.: Phase I and pharmacologic study of 17–(allylamino)-17-demethoxygeldanamycin in adult patients with solid tumors, *J Clin Oncol* 23:1885–1893, 2005.

465. Pacey S, Wilson RH, Walton M, et al.: A phase I study of the heat shock protein 90 inhibitor alvespimycin (17-DMAG) given intravenously to patients with advanced solid tumors, *Clin Cancer Res* 17:1561–1570, 2011.

466. Richardson PG, Chanan-Khan AA, Alsina M, et al.: Tanespimycin monotherapy in relapsed multiple myeloma: results of a phase 1 dose-escalation study, *Br J Hematol* 150:438–445, 2010.

467. Ramanathan RK, Egorin MJ, Erlichman C, et al.: Phase I pharmacokinetic and pharmacodynamic study of 17-dimethylaminoethylamino-17-demethoxygeldanamycin, an inhibitor of heat-shock protein 90, in patients with advanced solid tumors, *J Clin Oncol* 28:1520–1526, 2010.

468. Cercek A, Shia J, Gollub M, et al.: Ganetespib, a novel Hsp90 inhibitor in patients with KRAS mutated and wild type, refractory metastatic colorectal cancer, *Clin Colorectal Cancer* 13:207–212, 2014.

469. Oki Y, Younes A, Knickerbocker J, et al.: Experience with HSP90 inhibitor AUY922 in patients with relapsed or refractory non-Hodgkin lymphoma, *Haematologica* 100:e272–e274, 2015.

470. Johnson ML, Yu HA, Hart EM, et al.: Phase I/II study of HSP90 inhibitor AUY922 and erlotinib for EGFR-mutant lung cancer with acquired resistance to epidermal growth factor receptor tyrosine kinase inhibitors, *J Clin Oncol* 33:1666–1673, 2015.

471. Bendell JC, Jones SF, Hart L, et al.: A phase I study of the Hsp90 inhibitor AUY922 plus capecitabine for the treatment of patients with advanced solid tumors, *Cancer Invest* 33:477–482, 2015.

472. Lin TY, Bear M, Du Z, et al.: The novel HSP90 inhibitor STA-9090 exhibits activity against Kit-dependent and -independent malignant mast cell tumors, *Exp Hematol* 36:1266–1277, 2008.

473. McCleese JK, Bear MD, Fossey SL, et al.: The novel HSP90 inhibitor STA-1474 exhibits biologic activity against osteosarcoma cell lines, *Int J Cancer* 125:2792–2801, 2009.

474. Massimini M, Palmieri C, De Maria R, et al.: 17-AAG and apoptosis, autophagy, and mitophagy in canine osteosarcoma cell lines, *Vet Pathol* 54:405–412, 2017.

475. Graner AN, Hellwinkel JE, Lencioni AM, et al.: HSP90 inhibitors in the context of heat shock and the unfolded protein response: effects on a primary canine pulmonary adenocarcinoma cell line, *Int J Hyperthermia*1–15, 2016.

476. Clemente-Vicario F, Alvarez CE, Rowell JL, et al.: Human genetic relevance and potent antitumor activity of heat shock protein 90 inhibition in canine lung adenocarcinoma cell lines, *PLoS One* 10:e0142007, 2015.

477. London CA, Bear MD, McCleese J, et al.: Phase I evaluation of STA-1474, a prodrug of the novel HSP90 inhibitor ganetespib, in dogs with spontaneous cancer, *PLoS One* 6:e27018, 2011.

478. Fauzee NJ, Pan J, Wang YL: PARP and PARG inhibitors—new therapeutic targets in cancer treatment, *Pathol Oncol Res* 16:469–478, 2010.

479. D'Amours D, Desnoyers S, D'Silva I, et al.: Poly(ADP-ribosyl)ation reactions in the regulation of nuclear functions, *Biochem J* 342(Pt 2):249–268, 1999.

480. Hochegger H, Dejsuphong D, Fukushima T, et al.: Parp-1 protects homologous recombination from interference by Ku and Ligase IV in vertebrate cells, *EMBO J* 25:1305–1314, 2006.

481. Plummer R, Jones C, Middleton M, et al.: Phase I study of the poly(ADP-ribose) polymerase inhibitor, AG014699, in combination with temozolomide in patients with advanced solid tumors, *Clin Cancer Res* 14:7917–7923, 2008.

482. Plummer R, Stephens P, Aissat-Daudigny L, et al.: Phase 1 dose-escalation study of the PARP inhibitor CEP-9722 as monotherapy or in combination with temozolomide in patients with solid tumors, *Cancer Chemother Pharmacol* 74:257–265, 2014.

483. Dent RA, Lindeman GJ, Clemons M, et al.: Phase I trial of the oral PARP inhibitor olaparib in combination with paclitaxel for first- or second-line treatment of patients with metastatic triple-negative breast cancer, *Breast Cancer Res* 15:R88, 2013.

484. De Soto JA, Wang X, Tominaga Y, et al.: The inhibition and treatment of breast cancer with poly (ADP-ribose) polymerase (PARP-1) inhibitors, *Int J Biol Sci* 2:179–185, 2006.

485. Sandhu SK, Schelman WR, Wilding G, et al.: The poly(ADP-ribose) polymerase inhibitor niraparib (MK4827) in BRCA mutation carriers and patients with sporadic cancer: a phase 1 dose-escalation trial, *Lancet Oncol* 14:882–892, 2013.

486. Coleman RL, Sill MW, Bell-McGuinn K, et al.: A phase II evaluation of the potent, highly selective PARP inhibitor veliparib in the treatment of persistent or recurrent epithelial ovarian, fallopian tube, or primary peritoneal cancer in patients who carry a germline BRCA1 or BRCA2 mutation - An NRG Oncology/Gynecologic Oncology Group study, *Gynecol Oncol* 137:386–391, 2015.

487. Drew Y, Ledermann J, Hall G, et al.: Phase 2 multicentre trial investigating intermittent and continuous dosing schedules of the poly(ADP-ribose) polymerase inhibitor rucaparib in germline BRCA mutation carriers with advanced ovarian and breast cancer, *Br J Cancer* 114:723–730, 2016.

488. Albert JM, Cao C, Kim KW, et al.: Inhibition of poly(ADP-ribose) polymerase enhances cell death and improves tumor growth delay in irradiated lung cancer models, *Clin Cancer Res* 13:3033–3042, 2007.

489. Donawho CK, Luo Y, Penning TD, et al.: ABT-888, an orally active poly(ADP-ribose) polymerase inhibitor that potentiates DNA-damaging agents in preclinical tumor models, *Clin Cancer Res* 13:2728–2737, 2007.

490. Li M, Threadgill MD, Wang Y, et al.: Poly(ADP-ribose) polymerase inhibition down-regulates expression of metastasis-related genes in CT26 colon carcinoma cells, *Pathobiology* 76:108–116, 2009g.

491. Tentori L, Leonetti C, Scarsella M, et al.: Systemic administration of GPI 15427, a novel poly(ADP-ribose) polymerase-1 inhibitor, increases the antitumor activity of temozolomide against intracranial melanoma, glioma, lymphoma, *Clin Cancer Res* 9:5370–5379, 2003.

492. Dungey FA, Caldecott KW, Chalmers AJ: Enhanced radiosensitization of human glioma cells by combining inhibition of poly(ADP-ribose) polymerase with inhibition of heat shock protein 90, *Mol Cancer Ther* 8:2243–2254, 2009.

493. Rivera P, Melin M, Biagi T, et al.: Mammary tumor development in dogs is associated with BRCA1 and BRCA2, *Cancer Res* 69:8770–8774, 2009.

494. Xu D, Grishin NV, Chook YM: NESdb: a database of NES-containing CRM1 cargoes, *Mol Biol Cell* 23:3673–3676, 2012.

495. Shen A, Wang Y, Zhao Y, et al.: Expression of CRM1 in human gliomas and its significance in p27 expression and clinical prognosis, *Neurosurgery* 65:153–159, 2009.

496. Kojima K, Kornblau SM, Ruvolo V, et al.: Prognostic impact and targeting of CRM1 in acute myeloid leukemia, *Blood* 121:4166–4174, 2013.

497. Yao Y, Dong Y, Lin F, et al.: The expression of CRM1 is associated with prognosis in human osteosarcoma, *Oncol Rep* 21:229–235, 2009.

498. Azmi AS, Aboukameel A, Bao B, et al.: Selective inhibitors of nuclear export block pancreatic cancer cell proliferation and reduce tumor growth in mice, *Gastroenterology* 144:447–456, 2013.

499. Lapalombella R, Sun Q, Williams K, et al.: Selective inhibitors of nuclear export show that CRM1/XPO1 is a target in chronic lymphocytic leukemia, *Blood* 120:4621–4634, 2012.

500. Tai YT, Landesman Y, Acharya C, et al.: CRM1 inhibition induces tumor cell cytotoxicity and impairs osteoclastogenesis in multiple myeloma: molecular mechanisms and therapeutic implications, *Leukemia* 28:155–165, 2014.

501. Gravina GL, Mancini A, Sanita P, et al.: KPT-330, a potent and selective exportin-1 (XPO-1) inhibitor, shows antitumor effects modulating the expression of cyclin D1 and survivin in prostate cancer models, *BMC Cancer* 15:941, 2015.

502. Alexander TB, Lacayo NJ, Choi JK, et al.: Phase I study of selinexor, a selective inhibitor of nuclear export, in combination with fludarabine and cytarabine, in pediatric relapsed or refractory acute leukemia, *J Clin Oncol* 34:4094–4101, 2016.

503. Abdul Razak AR, Mau-Soerensen M, Gabrail NY, et al.: First-in-class, first-in-human phase I study of selinexor, a selective inhibitor of nuclear export, in patients with advanced solid tumors, *J Clin Oncol* 34:4142–4150, 2016.

504. Kuruvilla J, Savona M, Baz R, et al.: Selective inhibition of nuclear export with selinexor in patients with non-Hodgkin lymphoma, *Blood* 129:3175–3183, 2017.

505. Breit MN, Kisseberth WC, Bear MD, et al.: Biologic activity of the novel orally bioavailable selective inhibitor of nuclear export (SINE) KPT-335 against canine melanoma cell lines, *BMC Vet Res* 10:160, 2014.

506. London CA, Bernabe LF, Barnard S, et al.: Preclinical evaluation of the novel, orally bioavailable Selective Inhibitor of Nuclear Export (SINE) KPT-335 in spontaneous canine cancer: results of a phase I study, *PLoS One* 9:e87585, 2014.

507. Xie Q, Gao CF, Shinomiya N, et al.: Geldanamycins exquisitely inhibit HGF/SF-mediated tumor cell invasion, *Oncogene* 24:3697–3707, 2005.

508. Zagzag D, Nomura M, Friedlander DR, et al.: Geldanamycin inhibits migration of glioma cells in vitro: a potential role for hypoxia-inducible factor (HIF-1alpha) in glioma cell invasion, *J Cell Physiol* 196:394–402, 2003.

509. Masson-Gadais B, Houle F, Laferriere J, et al.: Integrin alphavbeta3, requirement for VEGFR2–mediated activation of SAPK2/p38 and for Hsp90–dependent phosphorylation of focal adhesion kinase in endothelial cells activated by VEGF, *Cell Stress Chaperones* 8:37–52, 2003.

510. Smith V, Sausville EA, Camalier RF, et al.: Comparison of 17–dimethylaminoethylamino-17–demethoxy-geldanamycin (17DMAG) and 17–allylamino-17–demethoxygeldanamycin (17AAG) in vitro: effects on Hsp90 and client proteins in melanoma models, *Cancer Chemother Pharmacol* 56:126–137, 2005.

511. Burger AM, Fiebig HH, Stinson SF, et al.: 17-(Allylamino)-17-demethoxygeldanamycin activity in human melanoma models, *Anticancer Drugs* 15:377–387, 2004.

512. Park JW, Yeh MW, Wong MG, et al.: The heat shock protein 90–binding geldanamycin inhibits cancer cell proliferation, down-regulates oncoproteins, and inhibits epidermal growth factor-induced invasion in thyroid cancer cell lines, *J Clin Endocrinol Metab* 88:3346–3353, 2003.

513. Blagosklonny MV: Hsp-90-associated oncoproteins: multiple targets of geldanamycin and its analogs, *Leukemia* 16:455–462, 2002.

514. Aoyagi Y, Fujita N, Tsuruo T: Stabilization of integrin-linked kinase by binding to Hsp90, *Biochem Biophys Res Commun* 331:1061–1068, 2005.

515. Kaur G, Belotti D, Burger AM, et al.: Antiangiogenic properties of 17–(dimethylaminoethylamino)-17-demethoxygeldanamycin: an orally bioavailable heat shock protein 90 modulator, *Clin Cancer Res* 10:4813–4821, 2004.

516. Hawkins LM, Jayanthan AA, Narendran A: Effects of 17-allyl-amino-17-demethoxygeldanamycin (17-AAG) on pediatric acute lymphoblastic leukemia (ALL) with respect to Bcr-Abl status and imatinib mesylate sensitivity, *Pediatr Res* 57:430–437, 2005.

517. Villa R, Folini M, Porta CD, et al.: Inhibition of telomerase activity by geldanamycin and 17-allylamino, 17-demethoxygeldanamycin in human melanoma cells, *Carcinogenesis* 24:851–859, 2003.

518. Haendeler J, Hoffmann J, Rahman S, et al.: Regulation of telomerase activity and anti-apoptotic function by protein-protein interaction and phosphorylation, *FEBS Lett* 536:180–186, 2003.

16

Supportive Care for the Cancer Patient

SECTION A: MANAGEMENT OF CHRONIC CANCER PAIN

MICHAEL W. NOLAN, CONSTANZA MENESES, TIMOTHY M. FAN, AND B. DUNCAN X. LASCELLES

This chapter explains the underlying mechanisms of cancer-induced pain. It also provides a guide for assessment and treatment of pain in canine and feline cancer patients. Finally, the future of analgesic therapies is discussed. Given the modicum of clinical studies in dogs and cats, the information in this chapter cannot be based solely on peer-reviewed investigations. Rather, it is a combination of the authors' experiences and the experiences of others who collectively are contributing to the treatment of cancer patients. It also is based on considered extrapolations from physician-based medicine and from veterinary research on other chronically painful conditions, such as osteoarthritis (OA).

Mechanisms of Cancer-Induced Pain

In veterinary medicine several types of tumors have been associated with painful symptoms (Table 16.1). However, the presence and manifestation of pain in cancer patients are not predictable, and its prevalence and severity depend on numerous factors commonly linked to the characteristics of the patient, the cancer type, the anatomic location, and associated therapeutic interventions.

The generation of noxious (painful) signals generally starts in the peripheral nervous system (PNS), triggered by tissue compromise, invasion, and injury generated by the tumor itself. Pronociceptive mediators (e.g., cytokines, interleukins, chemokines, prostanoids, endothelins, and growth factors) can be released by both cancer cells and the immune cells that infiltrate the tumor microenvironment.[1–7] The release of these factors sets off an inflammatory signaling cascade, which modifies the intracellular homeostasis of the surrounding sensory neurons' primary afferent fibers and cell bodies located at the level of the dorsal root ganglia (DRG). This powerfully modulates excitatory synaptic transmission in the central nervous system (CNS), sensitizing spinal cord neurons and enhancing nociceptive transmission within supraspinal circuits.[4,8,9]

Central neuronal plasticity and hyperexcitability can originate either from increased and sustained peripheral inputs or from primary or metastatic CNS tumors, or both. Significant overlap is seen between mechanisms underlying peripheral and central

plasticity. Cancer models of pain in rodents have shown that persistent noxious signals can lead to genetic alterations that modify the synaptic ultrastructure of spinal neurons (e.g., recruitment of wide dynamic range neurons in the superficial spinal cord) and induce dysregulation of the neuron–glia–immune system and the descending inhibitory/facilitatory system.[10–16] It has been hypothesized that these events could preserve the nociceptive transmission without the need for algesic mediators.[8] Currently, the exact intracellular signaling pathways that explain the interconnected mechanisms among all these elements remains unclear. However, new research has identified the potential role of various therapeutic targets for cancer pain management (see the section Future Analgesic Therapies later in the chapter). The failure of clinical studies regarding this signaling pathway might be representative of the current limitation of translating data from the commonly used animal models to humans, as has been discussed in several reviews of translational pain research.[17–20]

Pain as a Consequence of Cancer Therapy

Clinical interventions represent an important and often underappreciated source of discomfort in patients. Invasive diagnostic interventions, such as tumor biopsy and bone marrow aspiration, are obvious examples, but other potential sources for at least transient iatrogenic pain include positioning for radiographic studies (which could exacerbate or upset orthopedic diseases such as OA) and physical examination (e.g., digital rectal examination, tumor palpation).

Surgery is perhaps the most obvious cause for treatment-related pain in cancer patients. Surgery is the most common treatment for canine and feline tumors, and it causes a visible wound. The control of acute perioperative pain in cancer patients is very important, and readers are referred to appropriate texts for information on perioperative pain control.[21] Though phantom limb pain is commonly discussed with regard to amputation of tumor-bearing limbs, little is known about the epidemiology of pain in animals related to chronic tumor surgery.

Radiation therapy (RT) can also cause painful side effects. Late radiation-induced neuropathies and tissue fibrosis can cause significant disability. Fortunately, although those late effects are both chronic and progressive, they are also uncommon, affecting about 5% of patients 2 to 3 years after finishing a typical definitive course of RT. Uncomfortable acute radiation side effects, such as dermatitis and oral mucositis, are far more common. The incidence and severity of these side effects depend on a variety of factors, including the radiation prescription, the planning technique and treatment delivery modality, and the anatomic site and species. In veterinary medicine radiation-induced pain is more

TABLE 16.1	Tumor Types Most Likely to Be Associated with Pain[a]
Category	**Notes**
Tumors involving bone	Primary bone tumors (both of the appendicular and axial skeleton) and metastasis to bone are painful. Just as in humans, sometimes metastasis to bone can be relatively nonpainful; however, this should be considered the exception.
Central nervous system tumors	Extradural tumors that expand and put pressure on neural tissue are often associated with pain. Tumors originating from within the neural tissue are often not associated with pain until later in the course of the disease. In humans with primary brain tumors or metastases to the brain, up to 90% suffer from headaches; it should be presumed that animals also suffer such headaches.
Gastrointestinal tumors	Pain from gastrointestinal tumors may be very difficult to localize and may manifest as vague signs and behavioral changes. Colonic and rectal pain is often manifested as perineal discomfort.
Inflammatory mammary carcinoma	Inflammatory carcinomas can be particularly painful, manifested as reluctance to move and perform activities.
Genitourinary tract tumors	Stretching of the renal capsule appears to produce significant pain. Bladder tumors appear to be predictably associated with pain. Tumors of the distal genitourinary tract are often manifested as perineal pain or pain that appears to be located in the lumbar region.
Prostate tumors	Pain may be manifested as lower back or abdominal pain.
Oral and pharyngeal tumors	Soft tissue tumors that project from the surface appear to be relatively nonpainful. Tumors involving bone or that are growing within the tissues of the maxilla or mandible appear to be significantly more painful. Soft tissue tumors of the pharynx and caudal oral cavity are particularly painful.
Intranasal tumors	Pain caused by intranasal tumors usually manifests as a diminished willingness to engage in normal behaviors.
Invasive soft tissue sarcomas	In the authors' experience, injection-site sarcomas in cats can be particularly painful, and the size of the lesion does not necessarily correlate with the degree of pain. Other invasive sarcomas in both species are painful. In the authors' experience, one form of soft tissue sarcoma, the peripheral nerve sheath tumor, is often associated with pain, both spontaneous and associated with palpation.
Invasive cutaneous tumors	Especially those that are ulcerative.
Liver and biliary tumors	Especially those that are expansile, stretching the liver capsule.
Disseminated intrathoracic and intraabdominal tumors (e.g., mesothelioma, malignant histiocytosis)	The signs associated with such tumors are particularly vague; however, intracavitary analgesia (e.g., an intraabdominal local anesthetic) often can markedly improve the animal's demeanor.
Lung tumors	Although significant pain is reported in humans with lung cancer, animals often appear to show few signs of pain. However, even in those animals, provision of an analgesic can often improve demeanor.
Pain after surgical removal of a tumor	Chronic postoperative pain has not been documented in animals, but it is a common problem after oncologic surgery in humans. Phantom pain (e.g., phantom limb pain), a form of neuropathic pain, does appear to exist in animals.

[a]Very often it is difficult for the veterinarian to appreciate that pain may be present. However, the administration of an analgesic to animals suffering from these conditions is reported by owners to result in an improvement in demeanor. In the face of lack of evidence to the contrary, it is suggested that this improvement is due to the alleviation of pain.

commonly observed in dogs than cats, and the most evident pain signs include decreased interaction with the surroundings, lameness, or increased interest in the affected site (e.g., licking, chewing).[22] Acute radiation-associated pain (RAP) is poorly responsive to standard antiinflammatory and analgesic therapies and thus can be quite difficult to treat. Although acute side effects are transient and self-limiting, the discomfort they cause can have significant implications for long-term oncologic outcomes, because the discomfort can result in early termination of treatment regimens, with a consequent decrease in radiotherapeutic efficacy. Development of more effective RAP therapies is hindered because little is known about the etiology of RAP. Indeed, the first model of RAP was described only recently.[23] Until the underlying pathophysiology is better understood, treatment of RAP will remain empiric.

In humans, pain results from a wide range of chemotherapy-associated complications. Extravasation reactions are perhaps the best recognized potential source of chemotherapy-associated pain in dogs, and they have been reported with both conventional cytotoxic agents (e.g., doxorubicin) and drugs that are generally regarded as "safer" (e.g., bisphosphonates).[24,25] Chemotherapy also represents a significant cause of chronic neuropathic pain in human cancer patients.[26] The risk of chemotherapy-induced peripheral neuropathy (CIPN) varies from patient to patient, depending on the drug agent, treatment protocol, and coexisting neuropathic disorders.[27] In general terms the pathophysiology involves (1) recruitment and activation of immune and glial cells, which leads to the production and release of pronociceptive mediators in the DRG and spinal cord[28–31]; (2) oxidative stress, with increased production of reactive oxygen species (associated with mitochondrial dysfunction)[32,33]; and (3) increased activity of both voltage-gated and ligand-gated ion channels (including voltage-activated sodium, calcium, and transient receptor potential [TRP] channels).[34-36] The resulting inflammatory response and neuronal injury lead to the increased nocifensive behaviors observed in patients undergoing chemotherapy. In these patients, pain usually has an insidious development, but acute or subacute onset can be observed. Clinically, reported signs include paresthesia, abdominal pain, painful muscle cramps, burning-like sensations, numbness, and a specific paclitaxel-associated acute pain syndrome.[37] Cisplatin, oxaliplatin, gemcitabine, vincristine, and others drugs can induce both peripheral and central modifications. To date, only two reports have confirmed CIPN in veterinary medicine.[38,39] This low rate of reporting may reflect a truly low incidence of CIPN in dog and cats or, alternatively, it may reflect the inability to diagnose accurately what may be a higher incidence of low-grade subclinical CIPN. Currently no systematic studies in veterinary medicine have annotated the prevalence of cancer pain caused by chemotherapy. Given the difficulty in assessing pain, especially chronic conditions resulting from prolonged courses of chemotherapy, only subjective states of chemotherapy-induced pain have been evaluated, from the pet owner's perspectives.[40-42]

Assessment of Cancer Pain

The prevalence of cancer-related pain in humans ranges from 33% in patients after curative treatment to 64% in the setting of metastatic disease.[43] Despite the fact that pharmacologic strategies have improved in the past 10 years, a significant fraction of surviving cancer patients still endure pain that is ineffectively managed[44]; this makes chronic pain one of the key elements underlying deterioration in the quality of life of these patients. In small animal practices cancer is one of the leading causes of morbidity and mortality.[45] Even though currently no documentation exists of the actual prevalence of cancer pain in dogs and cats, it is reasonable to deduce that a significant population of companion animals experiences cancer-related pain during their disease progression, in a manner similar to humans.

Assessment of pain in animals, although often difficult, is extremely important. It is likely that the tolerance of pain by an individual animal varies greatly and is further complicated by the innate ability of dogs and cats to mask significant disease and pain. It is important to remember that cancer pain significantly differs from other types of chronic painful conditions, and differences in clinical and behavioral manifestations among individuals and breeds can be influenced by the type of cancer, tumor location, disease progression, and general state of the patient. In general, if a tumor is considered to be painful in humans, it is appropriate to give an animal with a similar condition the benefit of the doubt and treat it for pain.

The approach of the author (BDXL) to the assessment of cancer pain is to evaluate these aspects (Fig. 16.1):
- Physical examination findings
- Owner observations using clinical metrology instruments (CMIs)
- Activity
- Quantitative sensory testing

Physical Examination

Physiologic variables, such as heart rate, respiratory rate, temperature, and pupil size, are not reliable measures of acute perioperative pain in dogs and are unlikely to be useful in chronic pain states. However, physiologic parameters and the use of complementary clinical techniques (i.e., imaging and laboratory studies)

allow for a broader and more comprehensive view of the patient's general state and disease progression when establishing an analgesic regimen. Additionally, the examination of every patient must include palpation of the tumor area. One of the most useful ways of determining if a tumor is painful is to palpate the area and evaluate the animal's response. This may not correlate precisely with the amount of pain the animal spontaneously experiences, but if a tumor is painful on manipulation or palpation, it is highly likely that spontaneous pain is associated with it. As veterinarians we struggle to measure spontaneous pain. It is perhaps reassuring that the way to measure spontaneous pain in rodent models is the subject of considerable debate among researchers.

Clinical Metrology Instruments

In humans the importance of patient-reported outcomes (PROs) is widely recognized.[46] PROs may refer to a large variety of different health data reported by patients, such as symptoms, functional status, quality of life (QOL), and health-related quality of life (HRQOL).[46] QOL is a complex, abstract, multidimensional concept that defines an individual's satisfaction with life in domains he or she considers important. The designation HRQOL reflects an attempt to restrict this complex concept to aspects of life that are specifically related to the individual's health and that potentially could be modified by health care.[47] In veterinary medicine assessing the effect of cancer in a companion animal's life has become a fundamental practice to ensure an animal's welfare. Assessment of the QOL has become a worldwide outcome measure in cancer patients, and it is an extremely useful tool when making decisions about treatment and continuity of life.

A pragmatic approach to the recognition of cancer-related pain has been adopted in veterinary oncology and pain research, and the establishment of CMIs in clinical and research practice is essential to reduce the inherent variability in pain assessment in animals.[48] CMIs use a proxy to provide information about the effect of both disease and interventions in pets. The use of validated questionnaires has made pet owners an important component in the assessment of animals with painful diseases. Table 16.2 presents a list of pain behaviors associated with cancer and/or cancer therapy in cats and dogs. Owners have the advantage of being able to detect behavioral changes in their pets in nonstressful circumstances. However, to evaluate properly behaviors affected by pain, in addition to the animal's QOL, pet owners need to be educated by veterinary practitioners on what signs and behaviors may indicate pain.

Owner-completed questionnaires have been designed to measure the severity of pain in dogs and cats. Several features are evaluated to determine pain severity and subsequent analgesic efficacy. The best developed and validated of these were created to measure chronic musculoskeletal pain; in dogs they are the Liverpool Osteoarthritis in Dogs[49,50]; the Canine Brief Pain Inventory[51,52]; and the Helsinki Chronic Pain Index[53]; and in cats it is the Feline Musculoskeletal Pain Index.[54-57] Some work has focused on developing cancer-specific owner questionnaires in dogs and cats undergoing either chemotherapy or RT.[40-42,58-65] In general, questionnaires include questions about the owner's perceptions of the pet's physical state (appetite, sleep patterns, gastrointestinal problems), interaction with the owner (anxiety, depression, happiness), activity levels (mobility, play activity), and perceived pain level, in addition to the owner's level of worry about the pet's health issues.[42,60,64,65] Several QOL scoring systems have been created to evaluate cancer patients; however, the use of nonvalidated instruments currently represents a source of bias in the measurement

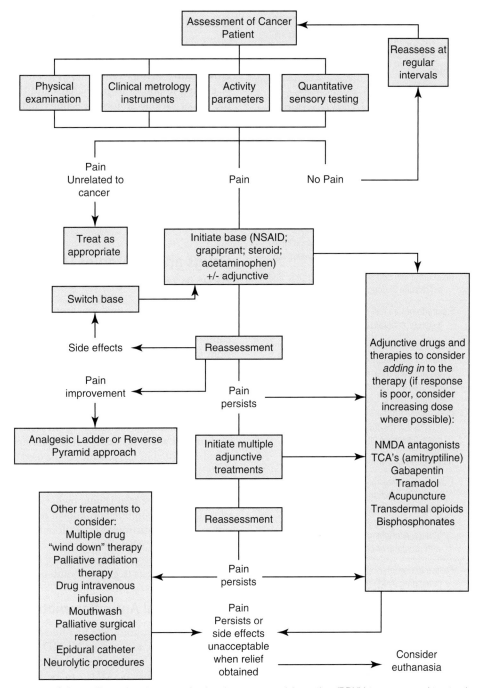

• **Fig. 16.1** Scheme illustrating the strategic planning process of the author (BDXL) to assess and treat pain in cancer patients. *NSAID,* nonsteroidal anti-imflammatory; *NMDA,* N-methyl ᴅ-aspartate; *TCA's.*

of the effects of various cancer treatments.[42] Recent publications have advocated rigorous assessment of the validity and reliability of these metrology instruments.[42,65] Table 16.3 shows QOL instruments and validation criteria that have been developed for use in veterinary cancer patients.

Activity

Reduced mobility is a common symptom in pain conditions. In the mid-2000s, accelerometers were validated as surrogate measures of distance moved in dogs[66] and cats,[67] and since then accelerometry

has been shown to detect increased activity in response to nonsteroidal antiinflammatory drugs (NSAIDs)[50,68,69] and an anti-nerve growth factor (NGF) antibody[70] in dogs with OA. Objective measurements of mobility or activity may be a particularly good outcome measure in cats, whose activity is spontaneous and not influenced by owners taking them on walks; improvements in this spontaneous activity in the home environment have been detected in cats with OA that were fed a diet rich in omega-3 fatty acids,[71] NSAIDs,[56,57,72] and anti-NGF neutralizing antibody.[73] Activity monitors may allow for disruption of sleep-wake cycles associated with pain, although recent initial work in this area by the authors

TABLE 16.2	Behaviors That May Be Seen with Cancer and Cancer Therapy–Associated Pain in Cats and Dogs
Behavior	**Notes**
Activity	Decreased activity and diminished engagement in the activities of daily living (playing); altered gait or lameness can be associated with generalized pain but is more often associated with limb or joint pain; quality of sleep may be adversely affected, manifesting as increased restlessness or altered sleep-wake cycles.
Appetite	Often diminished with chronic cancer pain.
Attitude	Any change in behavior can be associated with cancer pain—aggressiveness, dullness, shyness, 'clinging,' increased dependence.
Facial expression	Head hung low and squinted eyes in cats. Sad expression in dogs, head carried low.
Grooming	Failure to groom can result from a painful oral lesion or generalized pain.
Response to palpation	(One of the best ways to diagnose and monitor pain.) Pain can be elicited by palpation of the affected area, or manipulation of the affected area, which exacerbates the pain present. This is manifested as an aversion response from the animal (i.e., the animal attempts to escape the procedure, or yowls, cries, hisses, or bites).
Respiration	May be elevated with severe cancer pain.
Self-traumatization	Licking at an area (bone with primary bone cancer, the abdomen with intraabdominal cancer) can indicate pain. Scratching can indicate pain (e.g., scratching at cutaneous tumors, scratching and biting at the flank with prostatic or colonic neoplasia).
Urinary and bowel elimination	Failure to use litter box (cats); urinating and defecating inside (dogs).
Vocalization	Vocalization is rare in response to cancer pain in dogs and cats; however, owners of dogs often report frequent odd noises (whining, grunting) associated with cancer pain. Occasionally cats will hiss, utter spontaneous plaintive meows, or purr in association with cancer pain.

did not uncover any effects of osteoarthritis pain. Recent work has extended our understanding of factors affecting accelerometer output in dogs.[74] Accelerometry is performed in client-owned animals, in their home environments, with the accelerometers mounted on collars. Human chronic cancer patients with pain are more likely to present with sedentary behavioral patterns and fatigue.[75] Similar studies have not been performed in small animals with cancer, but accelerometry and activity measures hold promise as a tool to assess pain and cancer-related changes in activity. Approximately 10 activity monitors are marketed specifically for small animals, although current understanding of what the output of each activity monitor actually relates to is limited.

Quantitative Sensory Testing

Objective methods to measure central sensitization secondary to chronic pain recently have been developed in veterinary medicine. Quantitative sensory testing (QST) consists of the measurement of evoked responses to mechanical and thermal stimuli through the use of various devices. Feasibility and repeatability studies of these modalities have being performed in normal and osteoarthritic dogs.[76,77] Currently, published QST studies in dogs or cats with cancer pain exist, although the authors (MN, BDXL) have used QST to assess sensitivity associated with RT. The use of QST and related testing modalities has significant potential to help us understand the pathophysiology of cancer pain and potentially in the "cage-side" diagnosis of cancer pain–related abnormalities in sensory processing.

Drugs and Strategies Used for Management of Pain in Cancer Patients

The drugs that can be used for chronic cancer pain management are listed in Tables 16.4 and 16.5. The following discussions are not a comprehensive appraisal of each class of drug, but rather are suggestions for their use for cancer pain. Fig. 16.1 presents an assessment and treatment scheme to help the reader easily devise a strategic plan to manage pain in cancer patients. If pain scores improve after the initial base treatment, an analgesic ladder or a reverse pyramid approach can be applied (i.e., the number and dosages of drugs administered can be reduced). If pain persist, a more aggressive and multimodal analgesic strategy must be implemented. The adjunctive drugs listed in this scheme can be used on their own, or potentially two "base" analgesics could be combined (e.g., an NSAID and acetaminophen). However, the way this influences the side effects likely to be seen is unknown, except in the case of NSAIDs plus steroids, a combination known to increase the risk of serious adverse events (gastrointestinal ulceration). Euthanasia should be considered only when pain persists and significantly affects the patient's QOL or when the necessary analgesic relief caused unacceptable side effects (e.g., moribund, unresponsive, comatose).

Nonsteroidal Antiinflammatory Drugs

NSAIDs are commonly the first line of treatment in cancer pain. Several excellent reviews on NSAID use in small animals have been published, and the reader is referred to these.[72,78–82] The choice of available NSAIDs can be bewildering, but a few key points should be kept in mind.
- On a population basis, all NSAIDs are probably equally efficacious in relieving pain; however, for a given patient, one drug often is more effective than another.
- Gastrointestinal side effects associated with NSAID use appear to be more common with drugs that preferentially block COX-1 over COX-2.
- No difference in renal toxicity is seen between COX-1 selective drugs and COX-2 selective drugs.
- Liver toxicity can occur with any NSAID.
- No NSAID is completely safe, but the approved NSAIDs are significantly safer than the older, nonapproved NSAIDs.
- Longer term or continuous NSAID use appears to be more effective than short-term or reactive use[80]; however, when the disease is relatively stable, gradual dose reduction may be possible while maintaining efficacy.[69]

TABLE 16.3 Summary of Validated Quality of Life Instruments in Veterinary Cancer Pain Models

Study	Cancer Treatment	Species	Study Design	Face Validity	Internal Consistency	Factor Analysis	Reliability	Discriminatory Validity	Responsiveness	Criterion Validity
"Development and psychometric testing of the Canine Owner-Reported Quality of Life questionnaire, an instrument designed to measure quality of life in dogs with cancer"[58]	Chemotherapy Surgery Radiation therapy Palliative stents Medication for palliative or supportive care	Canine	Key-informant interviews, questionnaire development, and field trial	+	+	+ (4-factor)	+		(+)	
"Psychometric properties of the Canine Symptom Assessment Scale, a multidimensional owner-reported questionnaire instrument for assessment of physical symptoms in dogs with solid tumors"[42]	Medical Radiation therapy Palliative	Canine	Owner survey	+	+	+ (3-factor)				+ (against subscales of the CBPI)
"Quality of life survey for use in a canine cancer chemotherapy setting"[64]	Chemotherapy	Canine	Owner and clinician survey	+						
"Health-related quality of life in canine and feline cancer patients"[40]	Chemotherapy Surgery Radiation therapy	Canine Feline	Owner and clinician survey	+				+		
"Health-related quality of life scale for dogs with pain secondary to cancer"[60]	Without treatment	Canine	Owner survey							

Canine brief pain inventory.

TABLE 16.4   Suggested Dosages of Analgesics to Alleviate Chronic Cancer Pain in Dogs[a]

Drug	Dosage	Comments
Amantadine	4–5 mg/kg given orally (PO) every 24 hours (q24hrs)	Loose stools and excess GI gas can be seen at higher doses for a few days. Should not be combined with drugs such as selegiline or sertraline until more is known about drug interactions. Should not be used in seizure patients, and caution should be exercised in patients in heart failure.
Amitriptyline	0.5–2 mg/kg PO q24hrs	Has not been evaluated for clinical toxicity in the dog. Should be used cautiously in combination with tramadol.
Fentanyl, transdermal	2–5 mcg/kg/hrs	Can be very useful in short-term control of cancer pain. Long-term use is limited by need to change patch every 4–7 days. Clinicians should be aware of the abuse potential and danger to children of fentanyl patches.
Gabapentin	3–10 mg/kg PO q6–12hrs	Has not been evaluated in dogs as an analgesic. Most likely side effect is sedation.
Grapiprant	2 mg/kg PO q24hrs	Mild GI disturbances can be observed but generally are infrequent. Other EP_4 receptor antagonists (piprant NSAIDs) are being evaluated as anticancer agents for humans, but no studies of grapiprant in veterinary cancer patients have been performed.
Pamidronate	1–1.5 mg/kg diluted in 4 mL/kg normal saline (NaCl), given intravenously (IV) slowly over 2 hrs. Repeat every 4–6 wks.	Inhibits osteoclast activity and thus provides analgesia only in patients suffering from a primary or metastatic bone tumor that is causing osteolysis. Nephrotoxicity may be a concern.
Paracetamol (acetaminophen) + codeine (30 or 60 mg)	10–15 mg/kg of acetaminophen PO q12hrs	Sedation can be seen as a side effect with doses at or above 2 mg/kg codeine.
Paracetamol (acetaminophen)	10–15 mg/kg PO q12hrs	Associated with fewer GI side effects than regular NSAIDs; has not been noted to be associated with renal toxicity. However, toxicity has not been evaluated clinically in dogs. Can be combined with regular NSAIDs for severe cancer pain, but combination has not been evaluated for toxicity.
Prednisolone	0.25–1 mg/kg PO q12–24hrs; taper to q48hrs if possible after 14 days	Do NOT use concurrently with NSAIDs. Can be particularly useful in providing analgesia when a significant inflammatory component is associated with the tumor, and for CNS or nerve tumors.
Prednisone	0.25–1 mg/kg PO q12–24hrs; taper to q48hrs if possible after 14 days	Do NOT use concurrently with NSAIDs. Can be particularly useful in providing analgesia when a significant inflammatory component is associated with the tumor and for CNS or nerve tumors. In animals with diminished liver function, prednisolone may be more appropriate.
Tramadol	4–5 mg/kg PO q6–12hrs	Has not been evaluated for efficacy or toxicity in dogs. On balance, tramadol does not appear to be effective for osteoarthritis pain.
Zoledronate	0.1–0.2 mg/kg in 50–100 mL 0.9% NaCl, given IV over 15 min Maximum of 4 mg per dog; can be repeated q21–28days	This drug inhibits osteoclast activity and can provide analgesia in cases suffering from a primary or metastatic bone tumor that is causing osteolysis. Nephrotoxicity may be a concern.

CNS, Central nervous system; *GI*, gastrointestinal; *NSAIDs*, nonsteroidal antiinflammatory drugs; *PO*, oral.

Empty cells denote that the aspect of validity has not been determined.

[a]None of these drugs have been evaluated for efficacy in the treatment of cancer pain. **None of these drugs are approved or licensed for use in chronic cancer pain**. Nonsteroidal antiinflammatory drugs (NSAIDs) have not been included in this table. NSAIDs should be used as a first line of pain relief if it is clinically appropriate to use them and should be used at their approved dosage. The dosages given are based on the authors' experience and the experience of others working in the area of clinical cancer pain control.

TABLE 16.5	Suggested Dosages of Analgesics to Alleviate Chronic Cancer Pain in Cats[a]	
Drug	**Dosage (mg/kg)**	**Notes**
Paracetamol (acetaminophen)	Contraindicated	Contraindicated – small doses rapidly cause death in cats.
Amantadine	3–5 mg/kg PO q24hrs	This drug has not been evaluated for toxicity but is well tolerated in dogs and humans, with occasional side effects of agitation and GI irritation. May be a useful addition to NSAIDs in the treatment of chronic cancer pain conditions. Amantadine powder can be purchased and formulated into appropriately sized capsules. The kinetics have recently been evaluated in cats.
Amitriptyline	0.5–2 mg/kg PO q24hrs	This drug appears to be well tolerated for up to 12 months of daily administration. May be a useful addition to NSAIDs for treatment of chronic pain conditions.
Aspirin	10 mg/kg PO q48hrs	Can cause significant gastrointestinal ulceration.
Buprenorphine	0.01–0.02 mg/kg sublingual q8–12hrs	The sublingual route is not resented by cats and may be a good way to provide postoperative analgesia at home. Feedback from owners indicates that after 2–3 days dosing at this dosage, anorexia develops. Smaller doses (5–10 mcg/kg) may be more appropriate for long-term administration, especially in combination with other drugs.
Butorphanol	0.2–1 mg/kg PO q6hrs	One study suggests that using oral butorphanol after surgery may be beneficial. Generally considered to be a poor analgesic in cats except for visceral pain, but the author has found it to be useful as part of a multimodal approach to cancer pain therapy.
Carprofen	Not enough data to enable recommendations for long-term administration	—
Etodolac	Not recommended	—
Firocoxib	—	Use has not been reported in clinical cases; however, firocoxib has a half-life of 8–12 hours in the cat, and at 3 mg/kg provided antipyretic effects in a pyrexia model.
Flunixin meglumine	1 mg/kg PO daily for 7 days	Daily dosing for 7 days results in an increased rate of metabolism of the drug; however, a rise in liver enzymes suggests that liver toxicity may be a problem with prolonged dosing.
Gabapentin	10 mg/kg q12hrs	Appears to be particularly effective in chronic pain in cats when an increase in sensitivity has occurred or when the pain appears to be excessive compared to the lesion present.
Ketoprofen	1 mg/kg PO q24hrs	Probably well tolerated as pulse therapy for chronic pain, with approximately 5 days of "rest" between treatments. Has also been used by some long term at a dosage of 1 mg/kg every 3 days. Another approach has been to use 0.5 mg/kg daily for 5 days (weekdays), and then no drug over the weekend, with this regimen repeated.
Meloxicam	0.1 mg/kg PO on day 1; then 0.05 mg/kg PO daily for 4 days; then 0.05 mg/kg every other day thereafter (approved in the EU at 0.05 mg/kg daily indefinitely for musculoskeletal pain)	The liquid formulation makes it very easy to gradually and accurately reduce the dosage. However, a decreasing regimen (as suggested here) has not been evaluated for efficacy in cats, although it has been found to be successful in dogs. The lowest dosage that has been demonstrated to be effective (in osteoarthritis pain) is 0.035 mg/kg/day. Meloxicam should be dosed accurately using syringes.
Piroxicam	1 mg/cat PO daily for a maximum of 7 days. If longer term medication is considered, suggest every other day dosing	Daily dosing for 7 days results in a slight increase in the half-life.
Prednisolone	0.5–1 mg/kg PO q24hrs	Can be very effective. **NOT to be combined with concurrent NSAID administration.**
Prednisone	0.5–1 mg/kg PO q24hrs	Can be very effective. **NOT to be combined with concurrent NSAID administration.** In animals with diminished liver function, prednisolone may be more appropriate.

Continued

TABLE 16.5	Suggested Dosages of Analgesics to Alleviate Chronic Cancer Pain in Cats[a]—cont'd	
Drug	Dosage (mg/kg)	Notes
PSGAGs (polysulphated glycosaminoglycans) (Adequan)	5 mg/kg subcutaneously twice weekly for 4 weeks; then once weekly for 4 weeks; then once monthly (other suggested regimens call for once weekly injections for 4 weeks, then once monthly)	There is no clinical evidence that it provides any effect; however, anecdotal information suggests improvement can be seen after a few injections.
Robenacoxib	1–2 mg/kg q24hrs	Recently gained approval in the EU and other countries for long-term administration to cats for chronic musculoskeletal disorder pain. It is the first NSAID that is a coxib, has a short half-life, and demonstrates tissue selectivity.
Tolfenamic acid	4 mg/kg PO q24hrs for 3 days maximum	Has not been evaluated for chronic pain, but recent objective measurements demonstrated analgesia in the cat when administered perioperatively.
Tramadol	1–2 mg/kg once to twice daily	Recent evidence suggests it may be effective for chronic pain in the cat. Tablets are very bitter and aversive to cats.
Transdermal fentanyl patch	2–5 µg/kg/hrs	The patch may provide 5–7 days of analgesia in some cases and should be left on for longer than 3 days. After removal, the decay in plasma levels is slow.
Vedaprofen	0.5 mg/kg q24hrs for 3 days	Has not been evaluated for chronic pain but was evaluated for controlling pyrexia in upper respiratory infection and for controlling postoperative pain after ovariohysterectomy.

[a]None of these drugs have been evaluated for efficacy in the treatment of cancer pain. **None of these drugs are approved or licensed for use in chronic cancer pain**. Some drugs are approved for inflammatory or painful conditions in the cat in certain countries, and dosages for the control of cancer pain are extrapolated from these. The dosages given come from the authors' experience, and the experience of others working in the area of clinical cancer pain control.

GI, Gastrointestinal; *NSAIDs*, nonsteroidal antiinflammatory drugs; *PO*, oral.

The choice of NSAID predominantly depends on the patient's response (closely evaluated both by the veterinarian and by the owner). Currently, limited evidence is available in small animal medicine on the incidence of adverse events in patients prescribed NSAID therapy,[83,84] and most of what we know is related to administration to dogs with OA. Veterinary professionals (including veterinary surgeons and nurses) more commonly associate side effects with postoperative use of NSAIDs rather than chronic administration in dogs.[82]

Unfortunately, pain treatment in cats has not evolved to an equivalent maturity in scientific and clinical analysis, and a consequent suboptimal analgesic efficiency currently exists in the management of felines.[85,86] Emesis, anorexia, lethargy, renal insufficiency, dehydration, and death have been observed after the use of oral NSAID formulations in cats.[87] Moreover, no NSAIDs have been licensed in North America for long-term administration in cats, and two NSAIDs, meloxicam and robenacoxib, have been approved in the European Union only for long-term treatment of musculoskeletal pain. However, a number of these compounds probably can be used safely (see Table 16.5). The key to safe chronic administration of an NSAID in cats is to use the smallest effective dosage and avoid using it (or use a reduced dosage) in cats with renal insufficiency. Another factor the author (BDXL) considers important is to select drugs with a short half-life to minimize the likelihood of adverse toxicities.

The patient on NSAIDs must be monitored for toxicity. The owner should be informed of the potential for toxicity and the signs to watch for (lethargy, depression, vomiting, melena, increased water consumption). Blood work (and urinalysis) should be performed regularly to monitor renal and liver function. Baseline health panels (complete blood count and serum chemistry) should be obtained when therapy is started, and these parameters should be monitored on a regular basis thereafter. The author

(BDXL) repeats evaluations after 2 to 4 weeks and then at 1- to 4-month intervals as dictated by the individual patient and client.

If pain relief with NSAIDs is inadequate, a comprehensive multimodal therapeutic plan can be established. A common first additional option among veterinarians seems to be tramadol[82]; however, the recognized analgesic effect of tramadol has been questioned in clinical efficacy studies of chronic pain in dogs, with conflicting results.[88] Acetaminophen or acetaminophen/codeine combinations often can be used in conjunction with NSAIDs, but the influence of this combination on adverse events is unknown. Other agents that are used to treat chronic pain include amantadine, an *N*-methyl D-aspartate (NMDA) antagonist; anticonvulsants (e.g., gabapentin); and tricyclic antidepressants (e.g., as amitriptyline). These can all be combined with NSAIDs, although we do not know the full extent of side effects. Readers are cautioned that they should not assume that combinations of different adjunctive drugs are without side effects; quite the contrary, there is much to be learned about potential adverse interactions, especially in cancer patients that may be on other therapies.

Piprant NSAIDs

Grapiprant is a highly selective EP_4 prostaglandin PGE_2 receptor antagonist, a member of the piprant class of NSAIDs. In experimental settings, this drug has shown antiinflammatory function in models of acute and chronic inflammation in rodents.[89,90] Recently grapiprant was approved by the US Food and Drug Administration (FDA) as a veterinary drug for chronic OA pain in dogs. The recommended clinical dosage for canine OA pain is 2 mg/kg given orally (PO). The advantage of this drug may be the wide safety margin (see Table 16.4).[91,92] In cats, no adverse events have been associated with oral administration of grapiprant in toxicokinetic analyses (15 mg/kg, PO, once daily for 28 days),[93] but no studies have been performed to evaluate the efficacy of grapiprant for the treatment of cats with chronic painful diseases. Interestingly, the EP$_4$ receptor has been implicated in cancer metastasis in murine models. EP$_4$ activity on tumor and host cells promotes breast cancer progression via tumor cell migration, invasion, angiogenesis, and lymphangiogenesis.[94–98] Therefore EP$_4$ pharmacologic blockade may not only mitigate pain, but also attenuate multiple protumorigenic properties. This potential benefit has yet to be studied in the setting of clinical veterinary oncology.

Acetaminophen

Acetaminophen is a nonacidic NSAID. Many authorities do not consider it an NSAID because it probably acts by somewhat different mechanisms.[99] Some evidence indicates an antiinflammatory effect in dogs.[100] The exact mechanism of action remains controversial,[101] and the antiinflammatory features of this drug are associated mainly with the inhibition of central prostaglandin synthesis.[102] Other potential antinociceptive mechanisms include the serotonergic descending inhibitory pathway,[103] the endocannabinoid system,[104] and possibly brain TRPV-1 and TRPA1 receptors.[105,106] Although highly toxic in the cat, it can be effectively used in dogs for pain control in the acute setting.[100,107] No studies of toxicity in dogs have been done, but if toxicity is encountered, it probably will affect the liver. In common with all NSAIDs and opioids, acetaminophen should be used cautiously in dogs with liver dysfunction. The author (BDXL) often uses acetaminophen as the first line of analgesic therapy in dogs with renal compromise, in which NSAIDs should be avoided, and in dogs that appear to be otherwise intolerant to NSAIDs (e.g., vomiting or gastrointestinal ulceration).

Opioids

Opioids are considered an effective part of the management of cancer pain in humans, particularly when they are used as part of a multimodal approach (i.e., including NSAIDs or adjunctive analgesics). The use of opioids in cancer patients is recommended in moderate to severe cases of pain. Moreover, a recommended measure is to combine the use of opioid and nonopioid drugs both to relieve pain and to reduce the opioid dosage and consequent adverse events.

Oral morphine, transdermal fentanyl, oral butorphanol, sublingual buprenorphine (cats only), and oral codeine have been tested for the alleviation of chronic cancer pain. However, none of these drugs has been fully evaluated for clinical toxicity when administered long term or for efficacy against chronic cancer pain. Furthermore, recent evidence has indicated that oral opioids may not reach effective plasma concentrations in dogs when dosed at the currently recommended levels due to a high first-pass effect in dogs.[108–111] Given this fact, and the ongoing opioid crisis in the human population, we do not recommend using or dispensing oral opioids in companion animals. Also of concern is the dispensing of fentanyl patches, although data does support efficacy in dogs and cats.[112,113]

Currently no information is available on the long-term use of oral opioids for chronic pain in the cat. Buprenorphine, a partial µ-agonist, appears to produce predictable analgesia when given sublingually[114] and is well accepted by most cats. The small volume required (maximum 0.066 mL/kg [20 µg/kg]) makes administration simple. Based on clinical feedback from owners, this is an acceptable technique for home use. Inappetence can occur after several days of treatment, but lower doses (5–10 µg/kg) may be able to overcome this problem. When buprenorphine is administered concurrently with other drugs, less frequent dosing of buprenorphine often is required.[114]

Tramadol

Tramadol, a synthetic derivative of codeine, is classified as an opioidergic/monoaminergic drug.[115,116] The pharmacodynamic effects of tramadol result from complex interactions between opiate, adrenergic, and serotonin receptor systems. However, tramadol undergoes extensive metabolism. Thus the analgesic efficacy of tramadol may vary between species because of differences in the metabolic profiles of this drug. Tramadol is considered efficacious in a variety of human conditions, including cancer pain.[117] The benefits arise in part from opioid receptor–mediated activity of the active metabolite, *O*-desmethyltramadol (M1), which arises from hepatic demethylation of tramadol. Several studies have reported lower circulating concentrations of tramadol M1 metabolite in dogs compared with humans and cats,[108,118–123] and clinical benefits have not been observed after oral administration in dogs with chronic pain associated with OA.[88] It is important to highlight that little is known about the side effects of tramadol in dogs, and almost nothing is known about the side effects when tramadol is combined with other drugs in human or canine medicine.

In contrast to dogs, oral administration of tramadol induces antinociceptive behaviors in cats in a dose-dependent manner. The analgesic effects of tramadol in cats are supported by pharmacokinetic data that cats do produce the active metabolite M1.[124,125] Recently, prospective studies in a research colony of cats with naturally occurring OA demonstrated that oral tramadol at 3 mg/kg every 12 hours for 19 days resulted in measurable pain relief without clinically important adverse effects. The most common adverse events were mydriasis, sedation, and euphoria.[126] Tramadol is difficult to administer to cats because of its highly aversive taste. Even custom flavoring of compounded liquid formulations has been largely ineffective at improving palatability. Nonetheless, the drug can be of significant value in cats that will tolerate oral administration and in cats with feeding tubes (e.g., esophagostomy and gastrostomy).

Serotonin syndrome, which is manifested as altered mental status and neuromuscular and autonomic dysfunction, can follow co-administration of two or more drugs that affect serotonin signaling. Thus caution is advised when prescribing tramadol in patients also receiving drugs such as trazodone or mirtazapine, which are commonly used in veterinary cancer patients.

The dosages given in Tables 16.4 and 16.5 are for the regular form of tramadol, but not for the prolonged release form, which has not yet been thoroughly evaluated for toxicity in the dog or cat.

N-Methyl D-Aspartate Antagonists

The NMDA receptor appears to be central to the induction and maintenance of central sensitization,[127,128] and the use of NMDA receptor antagonists is beneficial when central sensitization has become established (i.e., especially chronic pain). Ketamine, tiletamine, dextromethorphan, and amantadine have NMDA antagonist properties, among other actions.

Ketamine is not obviously useful for the management of chronic pain because of the formulation available and the tendency for dysphoric side effects even at low doses. Furthermore, oral ketamine has not been evaluated in dogs or cats for long-term administration. Intraoperative "microdose" ketamine, administered intravenously (IV), appears to provide beneficial effects for a variety of oncologic surgical procedures, including limb amputations,[129] and this may reduce the incidence of chronic pain later. Other reports suggest a benefit to using ketamine perioperatively in low doses,[130] and the authors recommend its use in cancer surgery to help control pain later postoperatively.

Amantadine has been used for the treatment of neuropathic pain in humans,[131] and one study suggests a benefit to adding amantadine to an NSAID treatment in dogs that do not get complete relief from the NSAID alone.[132] The toxic side effects have been evaluated in dogs but not cats, and the dosages suggested are considered safe.[133] Amantadine should be avoided in patients with congestive heart failure, a history of seizures, or those on selegiline, sertraline, or tricyclic antidepressants.

The active metabolite of dextromethorphan may not be produced in dogs, probably negating its use in that species for chronic pain.[134]

Anticonvulsant Drugs

Many anticonvulsants (e.g., carbamazepine, phenytoin, baclofen, and more recently, gabapentin) have been used to treat chronic pain, including neuropathic pain, in humans, in addition to chemotherapy-induced peripheral neuropathies. Gabapentin and pregabalin are among the most effective drugs available for neuropathic pain in humans. Although the exact mechanism of action of these drugs is unclear, one potential mode by which they exert their analgesic effect is by binding to the α_2-δ protein subunit of voltage-gated calcium channels, thereby reducing excitatory neurotransmitter release through channel modulation or channel trafficking. Although considerable information is available on gabapentin disposition in dogs and cats,[135–138] and some information has been reported on its use as an anticonvulsant in dogs,[139] no information has been produced about its use for the control of chronic or long-term pain.

A potential analgesic value can be attributed to gabapentin (and theoretically to pregabalin). Although the indications for gabapentin and pregabalin presently are unclear in veterinary patients, these drugs do appear to be useful for cancer pain in some patients and are probably particularly effective in cancers that have some neurogenic or nerve destruction component. However, further clinical trials are required to assess the efficacy of these drugs in domestic animals.

Tricyclic Antidepressants

Tricyclic antidepressants have been used for many years for the treatment of chronic pain syndromes in people and are becoming widely used for the modulation of behavioral disorders in animals. Within the CNS are descending inhibitory serotonergic and noradrenergic pathways that reduce pain transmission in the spinal cord. Tricyclic antidepressants (e.g., amitriptyline, clomipramine, fluoxetine, imipramine, maprotiline, and paroxetine) primarily inhibit the reuptake of various monoamines (serotonin for clomipramine, fluoxetine, and paroxetine; noradrenaline for imipramine, amitriptyline, and maprotiline). Tricyclic antidepressants can also interact directly with 5-hydroxytryptamine and peripheral noradrenergic receptors and may also contribute other actions, such as voltage-gated sodium channel blockade and reduction in peripheral prostaglandin E_2-like activity or tumor necrosis factor production. However, human medicine has a relative lack of controlled, clinical trials specifically evaluating the efficacy of antidepressants in treating cancer pain,[140] with the exception of two studies demonstrating a lack of efficacy in the treatment of chemotherapy-induced peripheral neuropathy.[141,142]

The tricyclic antidepressant amitriptyline appears to be effective in cats for pain alleviation in interstitial cystitis,[143] and many practitioners are reporting efficacy in other chronically painful conditions in the cat, including OA. Amitriptyline has been used daily for periods up to 1 year for interstitial cystitis, and few side effects are reported. The authors have also used amitriptyline in cats for cancer pain, with some encouraging results. Only two case reports have been documented on the use of oral amitriptyline for neuropathic pain in dogs (dosages of 1.1 mg/kg and 1.3 mg/kg PO were used); the reports described improvement in the patients' clinical signs after long-term administration (longer than 3 months).[144] In dogs, pharmacokinetic analyses have shown that oral administration of amitriptyline at a dosage of 4 mg/kg produces low amitriptyline plasma concentrations, suggesting that this dosage is an inappropriate therapeutic option for dogs.[145] More experimental and clinical comparative analyses are needed to validate amitriptyline as a safe and clinically relevant therapeutic option in veterinary medicine. Amitriptyline probably should not be used concurrently with other drugs that modify the serotonergic system (e.g., amantadine, tramadol) until more is known about drug interactions.

Sodium Channel Blockade

Alterations in the level of expression, cellular localization, and distribution of sodium channels are seen in many pain states. These aberrantly expressed sodium channels result in hyperexcitability and ectopic activity in peripheral and central nerves that encode nociceptive information. Low doses of lidocaine and other sodium channel blockers readily block these aberrantly expressed sodium channels, producing pain relief. Low-dose IV lidocaine has proven as effective as other commonly used medications for the treatment of neuropathic pain in humans,[146] and the author (BDXL) uses such an approach to downregulate central sensitization in veterinary cancer patients. The use of transdermal lidocaine patches for the treatment of cancer pain is attracting increasing interest.[147] Much of this interest revolves around using the patch to administer a low systemic level of lidocaine that blocks the aberrantly expressed sodium channels. Studies have been performed evaluating the kinetics of lidocaine absorbed from patches applied to dogs and cats.[148–150] Peak plasma concentrations of lidocaine were obtained between 10 and 24 hours after application in dogs and at 65 hours after application in cats. The results of these studies indicate that, similar to what is seen in humans, systemic absorption of lidocaine from the patch is minimal. Potential systemic toxicity associated with lidocaine administration, including bradycardia, hypotension, cardiac arrest, muscle or facial twitching, tremors, seizures, nausea, and vomiting, was not noted in any study. Dosing guidelines have been suggested,[151] although to date no reports have been published evaluating the analgesic efficacy of topical lidocaine (whether in patches or cream) in veterinary cancer patients; however, the technique holds promise.

Steroids

Glucocorticoids provide an effective strategy for counteracting inflammatory pain. The mechanism of actions of steroids involves inhibition of collagenase and proinflammatory cytokines.

Moreover, they are able to trigger lipocortin synthesis and thus block the production of eicosanoids, such as prostaglandins.[152–155] This pharmacologic targeting can exert an effect both on the PNS and on the CNS because free steroids can cross the blood-brain barrier.[155,156] Currently, in human patients, the evidence is conflicting on the usefulness of steroids for preventing painful conditions such as acute or recurrent migraines.[157–159] Studies in neuropathic pain models in rodents have demonstrated that steroids could inhibit or attenuate this pain, but the underlying mechanism remains unknown.[160,161] Steroid use has been shown to provide analgesia in certain human cancer patient subpopulations, including those with bone cancer, spinal cord compression, or brain tumors.[162–166] Likewise, corticosteroids may provide benefit to veterinary cancer patients, including those with ulcerated or inflamed cutaneous mast cell tumors or with cerebral edema secondary to intracranial neoplasia. However, the analgesic utility of drugs such as prednisone and dexamethasone have not been systematically evaluated in dogs and cats with cancer, and nuisance side effects (polyuria/polydipsia, panting, behavioral changes, anxiety) have the potential to diminish QOL in a substantial fraction of treated patients. Additionally, exogenous steroids should not be used concurrently with NSAIDs because this dramatically increases the risk of side effects, especially gastrointestinal ones.

Bisphosphonates

Malignant bone disease creates a unique pain state with a neurobiologic signature distinct from that of inflammatory and neuropathic pain.[167–169] Bone cancer–related pain is thought to be initiated and perpetuated by dysregulated osteoclast activity and activation of nociceptors by prostaglandins, cytokines, and hydrogen ions released within resorptive pits. Therapies that block osteoclast activity not only have the potential to markedly reduce bone pain, but may also mitigate other skeletal complications associated with neoplastic conditions, including pathologic fractures, neuronal compression, and hypercalcemia of malignancy.

Bisphosphonates are synthetic analogs of pyrophosphate, and their primary effect is to inhibit osteoclast activity through inhibition of the mevalonate pathway. Bisphosphonates accumulate in metabolically active bone by virtue of their chemical structure, and after osteoclast-mediated bone resorption, they are released and disrupt cellular functions, resulting in osteoclast death. The antiresorptive activities of bisphosphonates has been demonstrated in normal and cancer-bearing dogs by means of a reduction in urine N-telopeptide excretion and enhanced bone mineral density.[170] This activity contributes to the risk of osteonecrosis, which is most frequently reported in the mandible.[171,172] Mandibular osteonecrosis is uncommonly reported in tumor-bearing dogs that are being treated with bisphosphonates,[173] and it is this activity which is also the mechanism likely responsible for significant analgesia that may last for several months in approximately 30% of dogs treated with injectable bisphosphonate drugs.[170,174]

Oral absorption of bisphosphonates tends to be poor, and IV dosing is the preferred route of administration in dogs and cats. In human cancer patients potential acute adverse effects include nephrotoxicity, electrolyte abnormalities, and acute-phase reactions[175,176]; however, it is the experience of the author (TF) that these notable toxicities are not observed in companion animals receiving IV bisphosphonate therapies. For many years pamidronate was the drug of choice for dogs with malignant bone pain. It may be administered at a dosage of 1 to 2 mg/kg over 2 hours as a constant rate infusion ([CRI] diluted in saline) every 3 to 4 weeks.

Zoledronate is now preferred because of its 100-fold greater antiresorptive potency relative to pamidronate and more rapid infusion rate. It is dosed at 0.1 mg/kg, diluted in physiologic saline, and administered as a CRI over 15 minutes. Many practitioners give a maximum dose of 4 mg per dog. The infusion time is important; longer or shorter treatment times may increase the risk of nephrotoxicity.[177]

At odds with the fact that clinically apparent analgesic benefit is often in excess of a month, many veterinary oncologists currently recommend that bisphosphonate injections be repeated at 3- to 5-week intervals. Although this dosing regimen is not substantiated by investigations of how bisphosphonate therapy modifies the biomechanical integrity of bone having undergone malignant osteolysis or by clinical data reflecting the effect of such therapy on the risk of pathologic fracture, one hope for such frequent administration is that modulation of bone turnover will reduce the risk of pathologic fracture. In addition to the inhibitory effects of bisphosphonates on osteoclasts, in vitro reports suggest that they may also exert directly beneficial effects on cancer cells, including canine osteosarcoma (OSA) and fibrosarcoma lines.[178,179] Hence, the intent to maximize potential antineoplastic effects also has been proffered as a rationale for ongoing monthly administration of bisphosphonates. However, caution must be exercised, because the preclinical data is inconclusive and conflicting. For example, one recent publication describing experiments performed in a canine OSA xenograft model suggests that zoledronate therapy may actually increase the incidence of pulmonary metastasis.[180] To better define the ideal treatment protocol, clinical trials are underway investigating the effect of monthly zoledronate administration on metastatic propensity in canine OSA. Such comparative oncologic studies of zoledronate's potential influence in canine OSA metastatic progression might help explain the absence of benefit exerted by adjuvant zoledronate in the upfront setting of pediatric OSA.[181]

Palliative-Intent Radiation Therapy

RT often is administered with the goal of controlling cancer. Because higher doses of radiation typically are associated with a higher probability of favorable tumor control, definitive-intent RT protocols are intensive and typically involve delivery of large total doses of radiation to the tumor. In this situation the goal is to maximize the antineoplastic efficacy of RT. By contrast, some patients are irradiated with the primary goal of reducing cancer-associated symptoms, including cancer pain. Palliative-intent RT can be given using a variety of administration techniques. For example, samarium is a radioisotope that has been evaluated for use in dogs.[182] Although the use of samarium Sm153 lexidronam in veterinary medicine is still limited, the results of a noncontrolled clinical study with subjective assessments reported improvement in lameness scores in 63% of dogs, suggesting that this therapy may be useful in the palliation of pain in dogs with bone tumors in which curative-intent treatment is not pursued.[183] External beam RT is most commonly applied. Regardless of the delivery system, the dose-response relationships for radiation-induced reductions in cancer pain have not been well studied, but they are not necessarily the same as the dose-response relationships for tumor control. In fact, they are likely quite different. This is exemplified by the fact that malignant bone pain in humans often can be effectively treated with low total dose, hypofractionated radiation protocols. For example, high-quality data shows that the pain relief associated with a single 8 Gy fraction is equivalent to that achieved with 30 Gy in 10 fractions in patients with painful bone metastases.[184]

In veterinary medicine the use of RT for palliation of patients with malignant osteolytic bone pain has been reported in several diseases, including feline oral squamous cell carcinoma[185–187] and canine oral melanoma.[188–193] The best studied use of RT for pain control is palliation of canine appendicular OSA. Interestingly, Weinstein and collaborators[194] demonstrated that a single fraction of 8 Gy failed to measurably reduce lameness in dogs with appendicular OSA. However, a subset of those dogs did have improved limb function and, in a separate study, 91% of dogs experienced clinically appreciable analgesia after delivery of 16 Gy in two consecutive daily fractions of 8 Gy.[195] Higher doses of radiation have been investigated in other studies. Although dissimilar methodology precludes direct comparison, results are similar with response rates up to 92%, median time to onset of pain relief ranging from 2 to 14 days, and median duration of pain relief ranging from 67 to 95 days.[195,196] Unfortunately, the lack of both proper controls, and failure to use validated objective measures of cancer pain make complete and reliable interpretation of these studies challenging.

Analgesia for Radiation Side Effects

Whereas palliative-intent RT can be used to relieve cancer pain, definitive-intent RT can itself result in painful side effects. RAP can result from acute or late radiation side effects. Although late side effects can be quite severe, they are also relatively uncommon. Thus the most commonly encountered forms of RAP occur during and shortly after a course of RT.

As mentioned previously, painful RT side effects are common in dogs but less common in cats. Canine RAP is often associated with grade II or higher RT-induced dermatitis or oral mucositis, which is characterized by moist desquamation and edema. In a prospective study of 80 dogs undergoing RT for head and neck cancer, 80% of dogs undergoing definitive-intent RT developed grade II radiation-induced mucositis, with 44% progressing to grade III lesions.[22]

The treatment of RAP is empirical. Whereas many dogs with RAP once were treated with glucocorticoids, practice patterns have shifted, and patients with non–round cell neoplasms that have RAP now often are managed with NSAIDs instead. This is due in part to the expectation of enhanced analgesia, but it is also influenced by the hope for additive antineoplastic effects.[197–199] Other systemic and topical therapies are frequently used; complete discussion of this topic is beyond the scope of this chapter but has been summarized elsewhere.[200] Because that review focused on management of radiation-induced dermatitis, it is also worth noting that some veterinary radiation oncologists use "magic mouthwash" to manage radiation-induced oral mucositis. Magic mouthwash is a term used to describe lidocaine-based rinses. Several formulations are used in clinical practice, and many include ingredients such as diphenhydramine, corticosteroids, antifungals, and antibiotics. In a recent phase III clinical trial, the severity of RAP was significantly lower in humans with oral mucositis that had been treated with magic mouthwash versus placebo.[201] The methods included a rinse and spit technique. Unfortunately, rinsing and gargling cannot be used in dogs. Thus it is unclear whether there is sufficient distribution or contact time to promote a clinically advantageous effect in dogs with oral mucositis. Furthermore, because of the risk of promoting multidrug-resistant infections via exposure to prophylactic antibiotics, clinicians are strongly cautioned against prescribing antibiotic-containing formulations for patients that have oral mucositis without clear evidence of a superimposed bacterial infection.[202]

Pharmacologic Desensitization Strategy

Many of the aforementioned treatments have been formulated to target both peripheral and central mechanisms, mainly designed as long-term therapies. However, a large number of cancer patients must undergo surgical procedures that can exacerbate the signs of pain. In this context the perioperative management of pain is a critical step in avoiding upregulation of peripheral and central components that contribute to pain hypersensitivity syndromes.[203–205] Meta-analyses have been performed to evaluate the efficacy of various systemically administered drugs for the prevention of chronic pain after soft tissue surgery in human adults. The most common pharmacologic interventions include perioperative use of oral gabapentin, pregabalin, mexiletine, venlafaxine, NSAIDs, and IV steroids, ketamine, fentanyl, and lidocaine.[206]

In veterinary medicine a multimodal approach is most often applied in small animal medicine, with apparent improvement in acute postoperative pain.[207–214] Fentanyl, hydromorphone, morphine, medetomidine, ketamine, and lidocaine are the most common drug infusions used both intraoperatively and postoperatively (Table 16.6); however, no study has evaluated the effect of such an approach on the incidence, severity, and/or character of chronic pain after surgery (whether associated with nociceptive, neuropathic, or cancer pain).

Acupuncture

Acupuncture can be provided through simple needle placement or by needle placement combined with electrical stimulation (of high or low frequency, although most types of pain respond to low-frequency stimulation). Results of a study in normal experimental dogs demonstrated a weak analgesic effect of electroacupuncture in anesthetized patients, as evaluated by a reduction in the minimum alveolar concentration of an inhaled anesthetic agent.[215] Recent data from a rodent model suggests that electroacupuncture may have beneficial effects in the treatment of pain associated with bone cancer.[216,217] As yet, no evidence indicates that acupuncture provides pain relief in veterinary patients, but the authors do encourage its use along with known analgesics.

Future Analgesic Therapies

Over the past few years, evidence has shown that the pain transmission system is plastic (i.e., it alters in response to inputs). This plasticity results in a unique neurobiologic signature within the PNS and CNS for each painful disease. Understanding the individual neurobiologic signatures for different disease processes should allow novel, targeted, and more effective treatments to be established.[218] This approach should also allow for a more informed choice to be made on which of the currently available drugs might be most effective.

Several new approaches to pain treatment revolve around the use of mechanisms to destroy or "exhaust" neurons involved in pain transmission. One approach is to use targeted neurotoxins to cause neuronal death.[219] An example of this is the combination of a neurotoxin (saporin) and a conjugate of substance P, called substance P saporin (SP-SAP). Substance P binds to the neurokinin receptor (NKR), and the conjugate is internalized (a normal phenomenon of the receptor-ligand interaction), resulting in cell

TABLE 16.6	Dosages of Selected Analgesic Drugs for Constant Rate Infusions in Dogs and Cats		
Drug	**Dog Dosage**	**Cat Dosage**	**Notes**
Fentanyl	2–5 µg/kg loading dose, followed by 2–6 µg/kg/hr (10–30 µg/kg/hr for surgical analgesia)	1–3 µg/kg loading dose, followed by 2–6 µg/kg/hr (10–30 µg/kg/hr for surgical analgesia)	Appears to result in significant anorexia, especially at higher doses. Can become expensive for larger dogs. Cats do not always "look happy" on this. Cats can become hyperthermic.
Hydromorphone	0.05 mg/kg loading dose followed by 0.01–0.02 mg/kg/hr	0.05 mg/kg loading dose followed by 0.005–0.01 mg/kg/hr	Appears to be very effective in cats, but hyperthermia can be seen.
Morphine	0.5 mg/kg loading dose followed by 0.1 mg/kg/hr (often need to reduce this when other analgesics are administered concurrently because of excessive sedation)	0.2 mg/kg loading dose followed by 0.05 mg/kg/hr	Morphine may not be as effective in cats as in dogs and humans because of their inability to form an active metabolite. This seems to vary from cat to cat. Avoid in GI surgery because of induced stasis.
Dexmedetomidine	1 µg/kg loading dose followed by 0.5–2.5 µg/kg/hr	0.5 µg/kg loading dose followed by 0.5 µg/kg/hr	Caution needed in heart disease patients; increase in systemic vascular resistance can be significant.
Ketamine	0.5 mg/kg bolus followed by 10 µg/kg/min intraoperatively, then 0.002 mg/kg/min postoperatively	0.5 mg/kg bolus followed by 10 µg/kg/min intraoperatively, then 0.002 mg/kg/min postoperatively	Small doses are thought to provide analgesia by virtue of NMDA antagonism.
Lidocaine	1 mg/kg bolus followed by 30 µg/kg/min	Best avoided because of tendency for cardiotoxicity	Provides analgesia (when given in small quantities) probably by interaction with aberrantly expressed sodium channels. Intravenous CRI should not be used with "analgesic" catheters using local anesthetics or other intermittent dosing of local anesthetics.

CRI, Constant rate infusion; *GI,* gastrointestinal; *NMDA,* N-methyl D-aspartate.

death as a result of the neurotoxin.[220,221] Because sensory neurons are rich in NKRs, if the conjugate is targeted appropriately (e.g., given intrathecally), sensory neurons are killed. Research indicates that in models of chronic pain, general sensory function is left intact, whereas hyperalgesia associated with chronic pain is reduced. Some toxicity work has been performed in dogs,[222] and clinical trials in pet dogs with naturally occurring OSA have been performed. In this model of pain SP-SAP significantly reduced experimental pain behaviors within 6 weeks. However, signs of motor dysfunctions were observed over 5 to 7 weeks after injection in some cases.[223] The current status of development of this therapeutic is unknown. A phase I study currently is underway in humans.[224]

Chemokine CCL2 and its receptor, CCR2, are involved in neuropathic pain. The exact mechanism by which CCR2 induces pain it is not completely defined, but overexpression of CCR2 has been observed in DRG and microglial cells after nerve or spinal injury, suggesting both peripheral and central mechanisms.[225] In a rat model of bone cancer, spinal cord expression of CCR2 was significantly increased, and central neuronal excitation, in addition to mechanical and thermal hyperalgesia, was attenuated after spinal administration of a selective CCR2 antagonist, AZ889.[226] Additional studies are needed to develop an effective and safe pharmacologic formulation for use in humans. Furthermore, CCR2 antagonists have not been evaluated for potential usefulness in veterinary pain management and/or oncology, and thus can be considered only as a putative therapeutic target.

Another approach uses Transient Receptor Potential Vanilloid 1 (TRPV1) to target neurons involved in pain. If the activation of TRPV1 by drugs such as capsaicin or resiniferatoxin occurs for long enough or is intense enough, the resulting calcium influx can cause neuronal degeneration. Capsaicin is used in humans for neuropathic pain and is being developed for long-term management of OA pain in humans.[227] Resiniferatoxin has been evaluated through preliminary studies in both rodents and dogs.[228–231] Short-lived and self-limiting side effects were reported by pet owners, including lethargy, lack of interaction with the family, and inappetance[223,229]; nonetheless, these studies provide encouraging evidence that intrathecal administration of resiniferatoxin can be associated with prolonged pain relief in dogs with OSA-associated pain.

Nerve growth factor also represents an attractive druggable target for preventing chronic pain. Experimental and clinical studies indicate that NGF is a key component in the establishment and maintenance of pain.[232–234] NGF is expressed by several cell types, including structural, tumor, inflammatory and immune cells.[235,236] Increased levels of this protein have been described in inflammatory, neuropathic, and cancer models of pain, and this overexpression appears to induce long-lasting pain in animals and humans.[237–240] In cancer models NGF induces sensory and sympathetic nerve sprouting and neuroma formation.[241,242] In mouse models preemptive and sustained administration of anti-NGF monoclonal antibodies significantly attenuated tumor-induced nerve sprouting and nociceptive behaviors in bone cancer models.[242] The anti-NGF tanezumab currently is being evaluated in phase III human trials for its usefulness in OA management.[243] NGF inhibition appears to produce substantial improvements in pain and function; some studies indicate that it is superior to either NSAIDs or opioid monotherapy.[240,244] In veterinary medicine the potential participatory role of NGF in cancer pain has been supported by its active secretion by canine OSA cells.[245] Furthermore, anti-NGF monoclonal antibody therapy has been tested in clinical pilot studies in both dogs and cats with OA; analgesic relief without associated side effects was achieved.[70] Nevertheless, more preclinical and clinical evaluations need to be performed to provide a better understanding of the potential role of such a targeted agent in small animal clinical practice.

SECTION B: NUTRITIONAL MANAGEMENT OF THE CANCER PATIENT

JOSEPH WAKSHLAG

Over the past 80 years the examination of nutrients and their relationship to cancer and cancer prevention has led to a better understanding of how nutrition may play a role in the management of the disease. The paucity of well-controlled studies in companion animals and the extrapolation of data derived from humans studies in the investigation of uncommon tumor types in companion animals (colon, prostate, pancreas) are frustrating and make general recommendations for nutritional interventions challenging. However, owners often wish to alter their pets' feeding regimen, regardless of proven efficacy. That said, three areas of nutrition often are discussed with clients: modification of tumor metabolism; adjustment of nutritional risk factors that may affect outcomes; and nutritional intervention during therapy. All of these are addressed in this section.

Metabolism of Cancer

Substrate Utilization

Numerous neoplastic cell lines have been propagated successfully in cell culture, allowing examination of cellular behavior. One fundamental finding from cell culture is that most neoplastic cells propagate better in a high-glucose media. This likely is due to limited fatty acid metabolism coupled with increases in metabolic pathways that utilize glucose; this traditionally has been termed the "Warburg effect," after Otto Warburg's seminal work suggesting that glycolysis is the primary pathway for energy production in neoplastic cells.[246,247] Studies in humans have shown that certain cancer patients liberate excessive lactate from solid tumors,[248,249] providing evidence that glycolysis and pyruvate production are critical to neoplastic cell metabolism. This has led to the Cori cycle hypothesis of neoplasia; that is, neoplastic tissue, much like skeletal muscle tissue, appears to undergo regeneration of glucose from lactate through hepatic resynthesis of glucose.[250] Unfortunately, this regeneration of glucose is an energy-costly cycle and is thought to contribute to increases in resting energy requirements.

In veterinary medicine a significant body of work has examined metabolism and cancer, often through the application of indirect calorimetry assessments to study whole body metabolism. Such studies investigate oxygen consumption and carbon dioxide liberation; the ratios of carbon dioxide production to oxygen consumption can provide estimates of energy consumption (resting energy expenditure [REE]) and substrate utilization (respiratory quotient [RQ]). In one study healthy dogs displayed a higher REE than dogs with stage III or stage IV lymphoma.[251] RQ values between the groups were no different, suggesting that the dogs were all burning similar substrate and that the dogs with lymphoma were not preferentially burning more glucose than their control counterparts.[251] Dogs with lymphoma that were fed either a high-fat or a high-carbohydrate diet during doxorubicin chemotherapy did not differ in remission times,

survival times (STs), or tumor burden, suggesting that lymphoma was not sensitive to this basic dietary alteration.[252] During this study the REE and RQ assessed during treatment did not change significantly when the tumor burden was eliminated through chemotherapy, suggesting that no significant changes occurred in energy expenditure or metabolism. These data collectively indicate that removal of the tumor burden does not alter the resting energy requirement (RER) and that no fundamental differences were observed between normal healthy dogs and dogs with lymphoma.

Canine nonhematopoietic malignancies were also examined in this context before and 4 to 6 weeks after excision of the primary tumors (including mammary carcinoma, OSA, high-grade mast cell tumors [MCTs], and lung carcinoma). As in dogs with lymphoma, the REE was no different from that of control dogs, and no difference in REE was seen before and after excision of the primary tumor, suggesting no futile cycling of energy in these patients.[253] Interestingly, the RQ values were above 0.8 for all control and tumor-bearing dogs, suggesting that the resting energy was not from lipolysis; this was contradictory to a follow-up study performed in dogs with OSA. In dogs with OSA, a difference was observed in the REE; affected dogs had a higher REE than control dogs, and the RQ was closer to 0.7 in both affected and control dogs.[254] This increased REE was still present after excision of the primary lesion, suggesting that the modest increase in REE was due to factors other than the primary neoplasia and could possibly be associated with micrometastasis, inflammation associated with neoplastic disease, or heightened pain response associated with the primary tumor and surgical procedure.[254] These findings were surprising in light of the previously mentioned studies but likely were more valid considering that the REE calculations were based on lean mass rather than total kilograms of body weight in the OSA study.[254] In general, fat mass is considered to be metabolically inert; therefore an REE based on lean body mass is more appropriate. The previous studies in nonhematopoietic malignancies and lymphoma did not adjust for body condition or lean body mass in tumor-bearing or normal populations,[252,253] and the inability to document differences in REE noted in these two studies may have been at least partly due to a lack of body condition assessment.

Metabolic changes were observed in dogs with OSA in addition to an increased REE. Alterations in glucose metabolism (potentially higher glucose turnover), increased protein turnover, and urinary protein losses in affected dogs were also observed.[254] Studies in dogs with lymphoma identified alterations in carbohydrate metabolism, such as increased serum lactate, and insulin concentrations during glucose tolerance testing suggesting insulin resistance.[251,255,256] This may be partially explained by aberrant interleukin-6 (IL-6) cytokine influences on glucose metabolism resulting in insulin resistance in dogs with lymphoma.[257] Insulin insensitivity and serum lactate did not change once remission was achieved in one of the previously mentioned studies.[251] Additionally, mild alterations in lipid metabolism in dogs with lymphoma were seen as higher basal triglyceride and cholesterol concentrations compared with control dogs,[258] and treatment with doxorubicin lowered serum cholesterol, perhaps as a result of hepatic effects of the chemotherapy[258]; however, the dyslipidemia was not ameliorated once the primary tumor burden was eliminated, which is logical in light of the insulin resistance observed.

Anorexia and Cachexia

Anorexia is common in cancer patients. In some patients this may be partially explained by adverse events associated with the use of chemotherapy. Chemotherapeutics can cause a variety of alterations in olfactory and taste senses.[258] Because dogs and cats rely heavily on olfactory cues, the loss of olfactory bulb stimulus diminishes the palatability of foods.[258,259] Additionally, the loss or alteration of taste (ageusia or dysgeusia) can further complicate anorexia and may last for several months before neuronal regeneration can take place at the olfactory bulb and tongue.[258,259]

Cachexia, on the other hand, although identified in many human cancer patients, does not appear to be common in dogs with nonhematopoietic malignancies.[251,255,260,261] Evidence in humans and mouse models suggests that the most prominent influence inciting the cachectic phenomenon may be excessive cytokine stimulation, which leads to insulin resistance, extensive lipolysis, and proteolysis of tissue stores.[262,263] The three primary cytokines thought to be involved in promoting enhanced proteolysis are tumor necrosis factor-alpha (TNF-α), interleukin-1β (IL-1β), and IL-6.[262,263] TNF-α and IL-1β have both been directly associated with anorexia and upregulation of the mitochondrial uncoupling protein, whereas IL-6 and TNF-α have been observed to increase myofibrillar degradation machinery—all of which may play a role in the anorexia/cachexia syndrome associated with neoplasia.[264,265] IL-6 and C-reactive protein, both markers of inflammation, are increased in canine lymphoma patients.[257,266,267] Yet it does not appear that cachexia is a common occurrence in dogs diagnosed with neoplasia, because dogs examined 6 months before diagnosis of cancer showed no difference in body weight or body condition than when presenting with various neoplasias.[260] This may be partially explained by differences in common tumor types between species. Cachexia in humans is often associated with epithelial cancers, such as pancreatic, colon, mammary, and prostate cancer. Additionally, human patients undergo dramatically different and more aggressive treatment protocols over lengthy periods, which we typically do not encounter in veterinary medicine because of owners' financial constraints and quality of life decisions.

Cats may show a more typical cachectic response involving excessive lean body mass wasting. Approximately 56% of cats with lymphoma and other solid tumors have body condition scores less than 5 out of 9.[268] More intriguing is that the ST for cats with lymphoma with a body condition score of 5 or greater was 16.9 months, compared with 3.3 months for cats with lower scores.[268] This warrants monitoring of caloric intake and aggressive implementation of nutritional interventions in feline oncology patients.

These sensitivities should be taken into consideration during radiation therapy, for which cats often stay overnight and are fasted for multiple days in a row. Providing ample time to consume calorie-dense foods should be considered for the hospitalized cat to ensure that food is offered often enough for the cat to maintain a normal caloric intake. Anecdotally, 19 of 20 cats undergoing RT at the author's (JJW) facility for a month lost weight during treatment, suggesting that feeding patterns and weight loss should be monitored and ameliorated when possible.

Metronomic feeding surrounding chemotherapy protocols may be beneficial to tumor growth and progression. The exact nature of how this would be implemented in dogs and cats is in its infancy; however, the concept of starving the tumor during chemotherapy may be beneficial for chemotherapeutic efficacy.[269,270] The typical protocols involve either not feeding the patient or limiting feeding in the 24 to 72 hours before chemotherapy to help sensitize the tumor cells to a more stressful environment and dampen the inflammation associated with the tumor. Many clinical trials are underway in humans to achieve a better understanding of this phenomenon.

Epidemiology, Prevention, and Risk Factors

In humans the two major nutritional factors associated with the relative risk of developing cancer are body weight (obesity) and fruit and vegetable consumption.[271–274] Although these parameters may be interrelated, both appear to play a role in carcinogenesis. Convincing data indicate that the westernized diet and lack of fruit and vegetable matter are linked to an increased relative risk of nearly all types of neoplasia, including prostate, colon, and breast cancers, lymphomas, and leukemias.[275–277] It is not yet clear whether this increased relative risk is due to a decreased dietary intake of fiber, carotenoids, and flavonoids or to an increased intake of saturated fat and protein. In people consuming higher amounts of fruits and vegetables, it is apparent that combined factors may be involved, in addition to confounding lifestyle differences, that may be important.

Few studies in veterinary medicine have examined the effects of dietary substrate (protein, fat, and carbohydrate) and plant-based dietary intake and cancer incidence. Two epidemiologic studies used validated food frequency questionnaires to examine the calories coming from fat, protein, and carbohydrate for 1 year before diagnosis of mammary carcinoma and after diagnosis and compared this with survival data.[278,279] This data was contradictory to human findings because dogs with an increased protein intake had increased STs after diagnosis, and fat and carbohydrate intake did not play a role in progression of the disease.[278,279] In another study the risk of neoplasia was increased in dogs fed nontraditional, poorly balanced diets (i.e., table foods as primary consumption).[280] Further examination showed no association between blood selenium concentration and mammary carcinomas compared with healthy, age-matched and hospitalized control dogs; however, tissue retinol status was decreased in dogs with mammary carcinoma.[280] Whether the lower serum retinol resulted from the dogs being fed a commercial diet with inadequate retinol or was a manifestation of the disease was not determined. Because feeding an incomplete diet was associated with an increased risk, feeding a complete and balanced commercial diet is highly recommended. These results are not surprising considering that food stuffs and methods of feeding are dramatically different between dogs and people. In many cases a high-protein food may be evaluated as higher quality because protein is an expensive ingredient; therefore many confounding variables—such as ingredient inclusion, ingredient quality, digestibility, and owner socioeconomic-associated health provisions—should be considered in studies of this nature, and such studies cannot be directly compared with human studies.

A study that examined nutritional risk factors in Scottish terriers, which have a genetic predisposition to developing transitional cell carcinoma (TCC), found that the addition of vegetables to the diet resulted in a lower incidence of the disease[281]; however, there were confounding lifestyle factors that cannot be accounted for in this epidemiologic investigation, including better health care, variation in nutrition supplied as commercial food, and other associated environmental exposures. Nevertheless, the findings of this study are provocative and suggest that further study is warranted.

Recent investigations of specific nutrients and cancer treatment primarily have focused on oxidative damage in tumors and antioxidants (addressed in a later section of the chapter). Specific vitamins and their relationship to cancer development have received significant attention, including retinol, ascorbic acid, vitamin E, selenium, and vitamin D. In veterinary medicine these nutrients have not been studied in a prospective or retrospective fashion. The findings in human meta-analyses examining oral supplementation for single nutrients (e.g., ascorbate, selenium, vitamin E) have been inconclusive or negative with regard to protective antineoplastic effects.[282] β-Carotene, the precursor to retinol, currently is thought to be ineffective as an antineoplastic agent, and in some instances has proven to be harmful in certain populations (i.e., smoking populations).[283–285] Currently vitamin D status and supplementation have been an area of intense epidemiologic investigation because of the relative risks of various neoplastic diseases being higher for individuals with low serum vitamin D.[286–288] Unlike in humans, vitamin D status in dogs and cats directly depends on dietary intake because they cannot convert 7-OH-dehydrocholesterol to pre–vitamin D. One would expect that serum vitamin D concentrations would not fluctuate tremendously in dogs fed commercial dog food.[289] Multiple investigations suggest that dogs with lymphoma and MCT (but not OSA) have lower serum vitamin D levels than healthy, breed- and age-matched dogs, which makes vitamin D status an interesting area of investigation.[290,291] Part of the conundrum in dogs is that the serum concentrations are about double normal human values, and it is possible that the supplementation of pet foods ensures adequate serum concentrations. The lower limit of normal ranges from 60 to 100 ug/mL.[291] The lack of uniformity in laboratory testing, such as methods involving high-performance liquid chromatography versus mass spectroscopy are examples of differences in methodology and applied reference ranges.[292,293] More interestingly, when dogs with serum concentrations of less than 100 ug/mL are supplemented with oral cholecalciferol at the safe upper limit established by the National Research Council, serum 25-OH-cholecalciferol serum concentrations do not increase.[294] This suggests that there may be inherent pathways in individuals to eliminate vitamin D from the body which may just represent metabolic differences between dogs. These findings further corroborate that serum 25-OH-cholecalciferol status may be a marker for hepatic and renal cytochrome activity that makes individual dogs more prone to develop cancer based on each individual dog's inherited metabolism. Whether this is a direct reflection of dietary intake or a reflection of the biochemical disposition in affected dogs with cancer remains to be determined.

In humans obesity has been associated with an increased risk of many cancers, including breast, prostate, colon, and pancreatic cancers; leukemias; and lymphomas.[270–272] Studies examining this association in companion animals are limited. The largest retrospective study in dogs showed no association between body condition and cancer,[260] whereas other epidemiologic studies suggest obese cats and dogs may have a slightly higher rate of neoplastic diseases.[295,296] Two other investigations revealed a more definitive link between obesity in female dogs and mammary carcinoma.[278–280] The risk of mammary carcinoma was greater in obese spayed dogs in one study, whereas obesity was an increased risk independent of spay status in another study.[278,280] Both studies suggested an increased risk when obesity is present at 1 year of age and one suggested that obesity at 1 year before diagnosis also was associated with an increased risk.[280] The question of whether early-onset obesity, much like early spaying, epigenetically predisposes mammary glands to an altered risk of cancer remains to be addressed.

Implementing a Nutritional Plan for the Oncology Patient

Nutritional Assessment

To fully assess the cancer patient, information about body weight, the body condition score, and a dietary history are crucial. The dietary history, before and during treatment, should be obtained to assess kilocaloric intake appropriately. This information allows the practitioner to feed the patient appropriately during hospitalization and, more importantly, to recognize hypophagic behaviors, allowing for interventions. A typical diet history should include the forms of food (wet or dry), amounts fed daily, and treats, human table foods, and additional supplements provided.

Serial assessment of body weight is important, particularly when malnutrition is a consideration. Malnutrition often is associated with cachexia and/or anorexia. Anorexic behavior can be deduced from the dietary history and can be treated aggressively with nutritional and/or pharmacologic intervention; however, if cachexia is suspected, then alternative treatments can be sought. The difficulty in clinically differentiating cachexia from anorexia is our inability to measure loss of lean versus fat mass. The loss of fat mass is typical during anorexia, whereas equal loss of lean and fat mass suggests cachexia. Although this cannot be deciphered efficiently in veterinary practice, overall weight loss guidelines have been offered in the human literature; that is, body weight loss of 5% in 1 month or 10% in 3 months without conscientious dieting suggests cancer cachexia.[297] This approach may be difficult in veterinary species because routine loss and gain of weight may be seasonal, and the burden of gastrointestinal (GI) parasites potentially confounds weight loss issues. Two body condition scoring systems have been adopted as a means of nutritional assessment in companion species; however, the 1 to 9 body condition scoring system (see Fig. 16.2) is better validated in the literature.[469, 470] Modest differences in body condition scoring between dogs and cats exist because of preferential deposition of body fat along the inguinal and abdominal areas in cats, whereas dogs tend to have no preferential deposition. These differences may justify a muscle condition scoring system in cats (Table 16.7).[268]

The final component of nutritional assessment consists of a routine physical examination, complete blood cell count, and chemistry evaluation. Physical exam findings consistent with malnutrition include poor hair coat, chronic GI disturbance, seborrhea, lethargy, and pallor. The first signs of chronic nutrient deficiency are often manifested in areas of rapid cellular anorexia/cachexia syndrome turnover, leading to skin, GI, and hematologic signs, and should be considered in cases of prolonged anorexia. Chronic malnutrition can result in low hemoglobin and red blood cell counts, in addition to hypoproteinemia and hypoalbuminemia. Additionally, with the trend toward nontraditional feeding practices, diets may lack sufficient mineral content, including calcium, iron, and copper, resulting in bone and hematologic manifestations. Many homemade diets lacking supplementation with bone meal can lead to secondary hyperparathyroidism and clinical osteopenia.[298,299] Clients using nontraditional diets should be educated through consultation with a veterinary nutritionist.

In dogs, excess body condition (i.e., obesity) may be more of a concern than malnutrition or deficiency. Treatment of obesity is not a priority in many cancer patients, considering the metabolic changes that may occur during chemotherapy and the potential for treatment-related changes in eating patterns. In one study body condition did not change from 6 months before diagnosis to

☒ Nestlé PURINA

BODY CONDITION SYSTEM

TOO THIN

1 Ribs visible on shorthaired cats; no palpable fat; severe abdominal tuck; lumbar vertebrae and wings of ilia easily palpated.

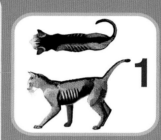

2 Ribs easily visible on shorthaired cats; lumbar vertebrae obvious with minimal muscle mass; pronounced abdominal tuck; no palpable fat.

3 Ribs easily palpable with minimal fat covering; lumbar vertebrae obvious; obvious waist behind ribs; minimal abdominal fat.

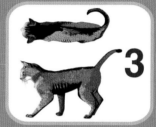

4 Ribs palpable with minimal fat covering; noticeable waist behind ribs; slight abdominal tuck; abdominal fat pad absent.

IDEAL

5 **Well-proportioned; observe waist behind ribs; ribs palpable with slight fat covering; abdominal fat pad minimal.**

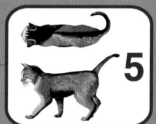

TOO HEAVY

6 Ribs palpable with slight excess fat covering; waist and abdominal fat pad distinguishable but not obvious; abdominal tuck absent.

7 Ribs not easily palpated with moderate fat covering; waist poorly discernible; obvious rounding of abdomen; moderate abdominal fat pad.

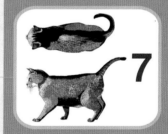

8 Ribs not palpable with excess fat covering; waist absent; obvious rounding of abdomen with prominent abdominal fat pad; fat deposits present over lumbar area.

9 Ribs not palpable under heavy fat cover; heavy fat deposits over lumbar area, face and limbs; distension of abdomen with no waist; extensive abdominal fat deposits.

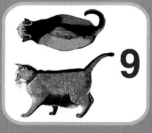

Call 1-800-222-VETS (8387), weekdays, 8:00 a.m. to 4:30 p.m. CT

☒ Nestlé PURINA

• **Fig. 16.2** One to nine body condition score for dogs and cats.

TABLE 16.7	Muscle Mass Scoring System
Score	Muscle Mass[a]
0	Severely wasted
1	Moderately wasted
2	Mildly wasted
3	Normal

[a]Results detected from palpation over the spine.

TABLE 16.8	Maintenance Energy Requirement Equations for Adult Cats and Dogs	
Animal	MER Equation	
Neutered adult dog	$(70 + 30[BW_{kg}]) \times 1.6$	
Intact adult dog	$(70 + 30[BW_{kg}]) \times 1.8$	
Obesity-prone adult dog	$(70 + 30[BW_{kg}]) \times 1.2$ to 1.4	
Neutered adult cat	$(70 + 30[BW_{kg}]) \times 1.2$ to 1.4	
Intact adult cat	$(70 + 30[BW_{kg}]) \times 1.4$ to 1.6	
Inactive obesity-prone adult cat	$(70 + 30[BW_{kg}]) \times 1$	

BW, Body weight; *MER*, maintenance energy requirement.

the day of diagnosis.[260] Another study showed that 68% of dogs lost weight during treatment[300]; however, in this study the loss was less than 5% of body weight, and nearly 30% of dogs were scored as obese before treatment. The occurrence of obesity in dogs with neoplasia appears to follow the national trends in canine obesity.

Feeding the Hospitalized Oncology Patient

Hospitalization during RT is common. Repeated radiation treatments or complications associated with chemotherapy treatment are frequent reasons for overnight or extended hospitalization. The provision of more than the RER often is unnecessary except in extreme circumstances, such as when extensive tissue repair is ongoing (e.g., epithelial sloughing or mucositis). This increased energy requirement, known as the *illness energy requirement* (IER), often is considered to be 1.1 to 2 times the RER, particularly when transudates or exudates are involved with the repair process and protein losses are excessive. Table 16.8 presents the calculations for the RER and IER used in veterinary patients based on activity status. Exponential equations are preferred in dogs and cats under 2 kg or over 30 kg to derive a more accurate estimate of the RER:

$$RER \doteq 70 \times (\text{Body weight [kg]})^{0.75}$$

The exponent of the equation may be different for cats (e.g., 0.67).[301] Once a patient returns home, the RER typically increases slightly as a result of increased activity. Therefore clinicians should adjust the energy intake after discharge.

Coax Feeding and Pharmacologic Appetite Stimulation

Ensuring full energy requirement intake enterally may be difficult because of a diminished appetite in cancer patients. Many considerations are involved in trying to promote adequate intake, and these may be different in dogs and cats. Hand feeding in dogs and cats that enjoy this approach should be considered, rather than putting a bowl in the cage and leaving it there. Hand feeding may be best achieved during owner visits, when the animal is most comfortable and often away from the busy atmosphere of most intensive care units or oncology wards.[302,303] For cats, having a quiet place away from distractions that create a fearful environment may be helpful to achieving adequate intake. Making one cage an eating cage that is covered and located away from the litter box is ideal, because some cats will not eat near the litter box during hospitalization.[302,303]

Addition of flavorings may also be helpful. Dogs have salt and sweet receptors, and the addition of sugar, syrups, or other sweeteners sometimes can improve appetite.[302,303] Cats do not have the sweet receptors; salt can be used to entice cats to eat, but they tend to be more averse to oversalted foods.[302,303] Adding protein to the diet of both dogs and cats can improve appetite and enhance intake, because dogs appear to prefer higher protein diets, and cats have an increased density of lingual amino acid receptors, which makes high-protein choices logical.[302,303] Supplementing with fat through the use of animal- or vegetable-based fat may increase palatability but must be monitored, because additional fat can dilute the nutrient content of the food. If the animal has nausea, introducing multiple foods can create long-term aversions, limiting choices of form and texture once the nausea has resolved.[302,303] Using one or two foods to coax feed, rather than an entire array of products from the kitchen, is the ideal approach.

Pharmacologic approaches to improve enteral support may be attempted. Human interventions have not been proven successful in veterinary patients, including pharmacologic alterations in serotonergic stimulation in the brain, decreased cytokine stimulation, and the promotion of hypothalamic satiety center signaling.[303,304] Approaches in veterinary medicine have revolved around use of the antiserotonergic drug mirtazapine which does appear to increase appetite and reduce vomiting in cats.[305] Equally promising, if not more so, is the recent release of the ghrelin agonist, capromorelin, which has been shown to promote short-term food intake in hospitalized dogs.[306] Capromorelin appears to be moderate to good at improving appetite in the author's (JJW) experience, and trials are ongoing to examine the effects in cats. In addition, propofol can be used to induce eating behavior in dogs. It has been used as an appetite stimulant on a single-time basis to see if eating induces ill effects (i.e., vomiting) when the enteral status is uncertain.[307]

Assisted Enteral Support

In many instances the use of assisted enteral nutrition should be considered, particularly if the animal is not consuming appropriate kilocaloric requirements. In the hypophagic cancer patient, it may be essential to provide assisted feeding through various techniques, including syringe, nasogastric, esophagostomy, or gastrostomy feeding. Syringe feeding is the easiest and requires the least attention to detail by owners and clinicians. In the nauseous and anosmic patient, this can be difficult to implement because of patient resistance. Nasogastric tubes can be easily placed without anesthesia and can be useful in hospitalized animals; however, they often are problematic to manage at home and are limited to the use of liquid enteral products because of the small tube diameter. The two most widely accepted means of implementing long-term enteral support involve placement of an esophagostomy tube or a gastrostomy tube. The esophagostomy tube typically is placed under light anesthesia (techniques for placement have been described elsewhere).[308] Once secured the tube site typically is wrapped, and the insertion site should be examined every 24 to 48 hours for signs of cellulitis and discharge. These tubes typically are recommended for intermediate- to long-term feeding (2 weeks to 3 months).

Gastrostomy tube placement should be considered when supplemental feeding is required for longer than 6 to 8 weeks.[308,309] Advantages include direct gastric delivery of nutrients, and the fact that emesis does not cause tube eversion. Anesthesia is required for placement, which can be performed via surgical or percutaneous endoscopic approaches. The endoscopic approaches are generally safe and effective but are associated with a higher risk of complications.[309] The author (JJW) prefers surgical placement in large breed dogs because they may be predisposed to separation of the stomach from the body wall after endoscopic placement, increasing the risk of cellulitis, and/or peritonitis. Peritonitis is the most serious complication after tube placement, because the peritoneum is disturbed with this approach, which also leads to a permanent stoma from the stomach to the outside of the body.[308,309] After successful placement the gastrostomy tube can be used within 24 hours; it should not be removed before 2 weeks to allow adhesion and fibrosis of the gastric wall to develop. Once a stoma has formed, the original surgically placed tube may be replaced with a low-profile or "button" feeding device. Owners should be aware that these low-profile devices need replacing every 6 to 8 months and require mild sedation for replacement.[310]

Esophagostomy and gastrostomy tubes allow for a diverse number of products to be used for feeding, beyond the liquid veterinary diets. Many over-the-counter and veterinary therapeutic diets can be blended for feeding; however, when some products are blended with water, they result in less than 1 kcal per milliliter. Table 16.9 list some diets that provide higher caloric density and can be passed through a 7 French or greater diameter catheter. These products tend to be higher in protein and fat and can be fed at reduced volumes and rates when nausea or food volume is an issue. In addition, a typical dog or cat receiving a slurry of food at 1 kcal/mL is meeting its fluid requirements.[311] Similarly, dogs and cats that are not actively consuming water at home should be provided 1 kcal/mL.

Parenteral Support

If enteral support is not an option, then parenteral nutrition (PN) support should be considered. Parenteral support can be either partial (PPN) or total (TPN). PPN has also been termed *peripheral PN* because it is typically delivered through peripheral veins. Prospective clinical studies examining outcomes after parenteral support have not been performed in veterinary medicine, and only a handful of retrospective investigations characterize complication rates.[312–317] In veterinary patients, particularly cats, the metabolic complication most often encountered is hyperglycemia. Mechanical complications also are prevalent, such as feeding line problems and inadvertent removal. A common misconception is that sepsis is a common complication, when in fact it is quite rare.[312–317] Parenteral support should be considered only when enteral support is not an option because of medical complications; enteral support is considered superior because it prevents transmigration of bacteria to the portal blood and improves the patient's immunologic status.[318]

Parenteral support is not well studied in veterinary medicine and the relative use and utility of the three main substrates (glucose, amino acid, and lipid) differ, depending on the source of information.[319–321] Some advocate using glucose and lipid to meet the energy requirements and then add in amino acids to the formulation based on the protein needs per kilogram of body weight. Others advocate adding just above the minimal protein requirement as amino acids making up part of the RER. The protein requirements for ill cats and dogs currently is unknown, and we can only assume that the requirement is similar to that of healthy normal animals. Extrapolation from human data suggests that protein turnover may be higher during catabolic illness, and we often add slightly more protein than required. An elegantly designed study found that approximately 2.3 grams of protein per kilogram of body weight is sufficient for an IV amino acid solution in dogs.[322] This suggests that adding 2.5 to 3 g/kg of amino acid solution for a dog appears sufficient, and 4 g/kg often is used as a starting point for cats. Amino acids come in several different formulations and strengths (e.g., 5.5%, 8.5%, and 10%). Additionally, amino acid solutions come with and without electrolytes. Amino acids with electrolytes typically provide basal sodium, chloride, magnesium, phosphorus, and potassium when used at 1.5 to 2.5 g/kg body weight of protein; however, these are used less often in cats and dogs, particularly in cats whose protein requirement may be higher. When amino acids are used with electrolytes, the electrolytes provided should be considered before additional electrolytes are supplemented in fluids. Fig. 16.3 describes a typical

TABLE 16.9	Selected High Protein/Calorie Products for Tube Feeding of Cancer Patients and the Amount of Water Needed to Make a 1 Kcal/mL Mixture to Meet Daily Fluid Requirements			
Product	Calories (kcal/mL)	Protein (g/100 kcal)	Fat (g/100kcal)	Water needed for 1 kcal/mL
Royal Canin Recovery RS (5.8 oz)	1.1	9.9	6.4	18
Hill's a/d (5.5 oz)	1.2	9.2	6.3	30
Purina CN (5.5 oz)	1.4	8.0	7.5	53
Carnivore Care (2 oz.; 56 gr.)[a]	2.6	9.0	6.2	220

[a]For dry powder products, 50 cc of water and thorough mixing are required for preparation before the product is administered.

RER = 30(kg BW) + 70 or 70(kg BW)$^{0.75}$ RER = _____

A. Protein requirement:
DOGS: 3 grams/kg BW   CATS: 4 grams/kg/BW

     Protein requirement (gm/day) = _____ gm/kg × W kg = _____ gm/day

     Protein calories (gm/day) × 4 kcal/gm = _____ kcal/day

     Total kcal − protein calories = _____ nonprotein calories

B. Nonprotein calories (NPC)

     Glucose (40-60%) NPC = _____ × _____ NPC = _____kcal glucose

     Lipid (40-60%) NPC = _____ × _____ NPC = _____ kcal lipid

C. Volumes of substrates

     10% amino acid solution = 0.10 gm/mL

     Protein gm req _____ / 0.10 gm = _____ mL of AA solution. (½ volume day 1_____)

     50% dextrose (kcals) _____ / 1.7 kcal/mL = _____ mL of 50% dextrose. (½ volume day 1_____)

     20% Lipid (kcals) _____ / 2.0 kcal/mL = _____ mL of 20% lipid. (½ volume day 1_____)

     Total volume of TPN solution = _____ mL/24 hrs / 24 hrs = _____ mL/hr. (½ rate day 1_____)

     Fluid req _____ mL − TPN volume _____ mL = Remaining fluid req _____ mL

     Remaining fluid requirement/24 hours = _____ mL/hr of fluids

• **Fig. 16.3** Small animal total parenteral nutrition (TPN) formulation sheet.

TPN feeding program using a 10% amino acid solution without electrolytes. It is typically recommended that, during the first day of TPN, only half of the calorie requirement should be provided, particularly if the animal has a history of anorexia. This recommendation is due to the potential for refeeding syndrome, in which rapid glucose metabolism can lead to hypophosphatemia, hypokalemia, and hypomagnesemia. This also illustrates the need to assess electrolyte status every 12 to 24 hours for the first 48 to 72 hours when implementing TPN.

PN formulation should be done in a laminar flow hood with appropriate aseptic procedures to prevent contamination of solutions. A sterile catheter should be used, and PN should be administered through its own port in a multilumen catheter, with the most distal port reserved for PN. The addition of other medications or treatments should be avoided because some medications are not compatible with PN. The typical osmolality and pH of a TPN solution is far different from plasma osmolality (around 1000–1300 mOsm and a pH less than 7). This may be irritating to the vascular endothelium and requires a large vessel for administration.[321] Such high osmolar solutions cannot be used in a peripheral vein because they may induce thrombophlebitis; this is the reason 5% glucose is used to dilute PPN, rather than the 50% glucose solution used in TPN solutions.[313–319] Using 5% dextrose creates an osmolality of less than 700 mOsm, which is a guideline from human medicine that has been adopted by many veterinary nutritionists and internists.[323] Fig. 16.4 describes guidelines for PPN formulation for dogs and cats.[313,319] The addition of B-complex vitamins should also be considered when TPN or PPN is used. Most preparations do not include folate and

cobalamin, and supplementation should be considered separately if long-term IV support is required. Furthermore, if chronic use of TPN is required, calcium should be added separately to TPN, and the use of amino acids with electrolytes and trace mineral additions to the TPN should be considered.

The proportions of glucose and lipids in parenteral solutions have become the subject of much debate, particularly in the cancer patient because neoplastic tissue may utilize glucose more readily, as well as the potential for mild insulin resistance.[255,256] However, increasing the use of lipid to meet energy requirements also has been met with some trepidation because of lipids' potential to mildly suppress the immune system.[324] Lipid also has been incriminated as causing microemboli[325]; however, lipid particles remain well emulsified in a typical veterinary-formulated TPN solution, and no bacterial growth was evident for 3 days after formulation when the solution was kept refrigerated.[326] PPN, with its lower osmolality, is at an increased risk of sequestering microbial growth.

Nutritional Support in the Cancer Patient

Substrate

Based on our present understanding, the use of specific dietary regimens in cancer patients is premature. Because of the glycolytic nature of neoplastic cell growth, altering the substrates to hypothetically "starve the tumor" by eliminating some carbohydrates may be indicated[246,247,255,256]; however this argument falls short for a number of reasons. If carbohydrates are limited, energy

RER = [30(kg BW) + 70] or 70 (kg BW)$^{0.75}$ RER = _____ × 0.50 = _____ Partial Energy Req

A. Nutrient Distributions:

　　1) Cats and Dogs 2-10 kg

　　　　PER = _____ × 0.25 = _____ kcal/day from carbohydrates

　　　　PER = _____ × 0.25 = _____ kcal/day protein

　　　　PER = _____ × 0.50 = _____ kcal/day lipid

　　2) Dogs 10-25 kg

　　　　PER = _____ × 0.33 = _____ kcal/day from carbohydrates

　　　　PER = _____ × 0.33 = _____ kcal/day protein

　　　　PER = _____ × 0.33 = _____ kcal/day lipid

　　3) Dogs > 25 kg

　　　　PER = _____ × 0.50 = _____ kcal/day from carbohydrates

　　　　PER = _____ × 0.25 = _____ kcal/day protein

　　　　PER = _____ × 0.25 = _____ kcal/day lipid

B. Volumes of solutions required

　　1) 5% dextrose solution = 0.17 kcal/mL

　　　　_____ kcals from carbohydrate/ 0.17 kcal = _____ mL/day

　　2) 10% amino acid solution = 0.1 gm/mL = 0.4 kcal/mL

　　　　_____ kcals from protein/0.4 kcal/mL = _____ mL/day

　　3) 20% lipid solution = 2 kcal/mL

　　　　_____ kcals from lipid/2 kcal = _____ mL/day

　　　　　　Total volume = _____ mL/day/ 24 hours = _____ mL/hr

C. _____ mL osmolarity of solutions 5% dextrose × 0.252 (mOsm/mL)　　　 = _____ mOsm

　　_____ mL 10% amino acid soln without electrolytes × 1.0 (mOsm/mL)　 = _____ mOsm

　　_____ mL 20% lipid solution × 0.25 (mOsm/mL)　　　 = _____ mOsm

　　_____ mL Total volume of PPN solution　　　 = _____ mOsm

　　(Total mOsm/Total volume) × 1000 =_____ mOsm/L (MUST BE LESS THAN 700 mOsm)

• **Fig. 16.4** Small animal partial parenteral nutrition (PPN) formulation sheet.

sources are replaced with additional fat and/or protein. Added protein leads to increased transaminase and deaminase activity, causing conversion of the protein to glucose and carbon precursors for glucose or fatty acid synthesis, and serum glucose and delivery of glucose to the tumor tissue may remain constant. If appetite is diminished, choosing a higher protein and higher fat food may enhance palatability and caloric density, making these foods appropriate for long-term management during treatment.[305] Previous sections have discussed the discordance of the results of studies investigating advantages of low-carbohydrate, high-fat, and modified-fat diets.[252] One study documented slight increases in remission and STs when a diet high in polyunsaturated fat (high in omega-3 fatty acids) and arginine was used.[257]

Cats appear more prone to weight loss during hospitalization. Many cats receive inadequate caloric intake, particularly during RT, when food availability is limited each day because of repeated induction of anesthesia. Many cats eat 12 to 20 small meals throughout the day and night, based on observed feeding patterns.[327] The use of higher protein diets may be worthwhile, because recent rodent data showed that a high-protein, low-carbohydrate diet reduced tumor growth in a variety of different xenografted tumors.[328] In this diet, dietary calories were met with approximately 50% protein, implying that high protein may be the benefit, rather than low carbohydrate.[328] The use of high-protein diets also may have benefits in cats with lean body mass wasting issues.[329,330] Although the studies conducted were small,

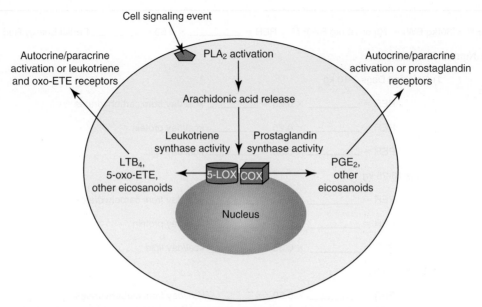

• **Fig. 16.5** Arachidonic acid (AA) is released from the cell membrane as a result of cell signaling events that lead to nuclear translocation of AA. Cyclooxygenase and lipoxygenase activity, coupled with leukotriene synthase or prostaglandin synthase, allows the formation of bioactive eicosanoids; when released, these can have autocrine or paracrine cell proliferation signaling activities, depending on receptor presence.

skeletal muscle in cats may respond to a higher protein intake by increasing lean mass slightly. With these ideas in mind, we often recommend feeding cats higher protein (>35% dry matter) and fat (>20% dry matter); dogs can be fed similarly, even though many commercial dog foods have lower protein levels (typically >30% dry matter is recommended) than cat food.

Amino Acids

The benefits of additional protein to the diet of cancer patients may result from increased circulating amino acids as inhibitory molecules in neoplastic cell proliferation.[328] Arginine has received considerable attention, because low millimolar concentrations of arginine can inhibit various neoplastic cell lines by altering cell cycle progression.[331–334] A diet higher in arginine and omega-3 fatty acids improved remission and STs in dogs with lymphoma[257]; however, the practicality of using an amino acid supplement such as arginine leaves much to be desired, because the required dose is in excess of 100 mg/kg body weight. Additionally, the bitter taste of arginine and the potential for creating amino acid imbalance prevent its use in long-term feeding regimens. The benefits of glutamine also have been touted because of its abilities to preserve lean body mass and enhance mucosal barrier function[335,336]; however, enterocytes' ability to utilize glutamine and first-pass hepatic metabolism do not allow glutamine to have any pronounced effects on lean mass. The use of high-protein mixed meals to support enterocyte health and mucosal barrier function often is recommended anyway.

Polyunsaturated Fats

Using fat in diets is helpful for increasing palatability and energy density, but in many instances the fatty acid constituents can influence neoplastic cell growth. Human and rodent model studies suggest that consumption of high concentrations of omega-3 fatty acids, namely eicosapentaenoic acid (EPA) and docosahexaenoic acid (DHA), in the form of marine oils may perturb loss of

lean body mass and possibly reduce the tumor growth rate.[337–344] These fatty acids may transform into inert eicosanoids (PGE$_3$, LTB$_5$, 12-HEPE, and 5-HEPE) rather than proinflammatory eicosanoids (PGE$_2$, LTB$_4$, 12-HETE and 5-HETE). The pathways and eicosanoids liberated are highly dependent on the enzymatic machinery present in the cells. Although the addition of fatty acids into the cell membrane may affect intracellular signaling events, the intracellular enzymatic machinery that modifies the primary fatty acid into promitogenic, or inert, eicosanoids may be more important.[343–346] Cell signaling events that lead to the release of arachidonic acid from the cell membrane can be converted to eicosanoids which, when released from the cell, can have local or paracrine effects on cell growth through interactions with eicosanoid receptors (Fig. 16.5). The two enzymes that have received the most attention are cyclooxygenase and 5-lipoxygenase because of the promitogenic mechanisms of action observed by their respective eicosanoids, PGE$_2$ (COX) and 5-oxoETE/LTB$_4$ (5-LOX).[343–346] Although this may be relevant to many types of human cancers, little data is available on companion animals; the most intriguing studies focused on the use of COX inhibition in TCC.[347,348]

A study in dogs with cancer that were fed a fish-based omega-3 fatty acid–enhanced diet showed a small improvement in STs; however, there were multiple changes in the dietary trial, including arginine and energy substrate differences, which may have played a role.[257] The increased EPA may inhibit promitogenic eicosanoid formation[346]; but it is unclear to what tumor types this may apply. Some neoplastic tissues use the proinflammatory cytokine milieu to promote proliferation or upregulate pathways that may promote metastasis.[349] The benefits of fish oils may go beyond mild suppression of tumor cell proliferation, because the antiinflammatory effects of fish oil may also quench the inflammatory reactions associated with certain cancers.[350–352] Hence, there is little downside to increasing dietary omega-3 fatty acid consumption in cancer patients. The lack of clinical studies in this area precludes an optimal dosing regimen, and the findings of a recent meta-analysis of human trials using fish oils for quality of life issues were inconclusive.[353] Additionally, cats seem to be more sensitive to fish oil supplementation than dogs because of greater effects on platelet reactivity, resulting in alterations of clotting times.[354] A safe and tolerable dose for fatty acids in dogs can be extrapolated from studies in cardiac cachexia in dogs,[355,356] in which the dosage used was 45 mg EPA and 25 mg DHA per kilogram of body weight (e.g., 1 teaspoon per 20 kg body weight). Unpublished data from our laboratory suggests that the same dosing schedule did not alter thromboelastography results in cats.

During RT the paradigm may be altered, because RT has the effect of causing irreparable damage to tumor cellular microstructure, resulting in apoptosis of cells and negative effects on surrounding tissues. Polyunsaturated fats, the longest being the omega-3 fatty acid DHA, may be oxidized to a greater extent during RT, and this may lead to increased membrane compromise and cellular death.[357] Surrounding tissues may not exhibit as aggressive of an inflammatory action because of the hastened eicosanoid response with EPA and other essential fatty acids quenching this proinflammatory response, which may lead to less surrounding tissue damage.[358] This principle has not been studied in veterinary patients but has proven to diminish radiation-induced tissue damage in pig models.[359]

Vitamins and Minerals

Essential vitamin and mineral supplementation is an interesting area of investigation in human cancer, with nutrients such as vitamin A, vitamin D, and selenium receiving attention.[286,288,359–363] Much of the research has centered on cancer prevention rather than cancer treatment. That being said, certain vitamins and minerals are being used in therapeutic clinical trials in humans because of their ability to reduce tumor cell proliferation in preclinical models. Vitamin A, in the form of retinoic acid and synthetic derivatives, has been used to treat certain cancers; however, discordant effects on nuclear signaling occur with different heterodimers.[361–363] Some heterodimers drive the proliferative response, whereas others diminish cell proliferation.[364] Their use cannot be recommended at this time.

Low concentrations of vitamin D in people may promote tumorigenesis, and treatment with active vitamin D may cause tumor regression in some cases[286–288,365]; however, the antiproliferative form, calcitriol, can be toxic at high levels, and the repercussions of vitamin D toxicity can lead to calcification of soft tissue and hypercalcemia, resulting in low margins of safety. This was illustrated in a recent trial in dogs with MCTs, in which many patients developed clinical signs of hypercalcemia, inappetence, and vomiting.[365,366]

Selenium has generated considerable interest in certain human neoplastic diseases, such as lung, dermal squamous cell, and prostatic carcinomas.[367–370] Low serum concentrations have been associated with an increased risk of prostatic cancer in humans[367,369]; however, meta-analysis of human intervention studies suggests no definitive benefits from selenium supplementation in the treatment or prevention of neoplastic diseases.[282]

B-vitamins of interest include folate and vitamin B_{12} (cobalamin). The interest once again derives from human literature, which has shown that the effects of these two vitamins on epigenetic alterations may affect tumor suppressor and oncogene expression over time.[371–373] Considering the consistent intake of folate and cobalamin in the pet population, a considerable gap exists in applying these paradigms of subclinical deficiency to pet populations. Furthermore, the lack of clinical or in vitro investigation prevents any postulation as to their effects on cancer cells.

Antioxidants/Supplements

The use of supplements, most commonly substances termed "antioxidants," has grown tremendously in the past 15 years. Approximately 65% of pet owners are using some sort of alternative treatments; more than 30% of owners are giving their pets oral supplements, and more than 50% say their veterinarian approves of this use.[374] More recent epidemiologic data on conventional diets and supplementation shows that more than 50% of owners incorporate some sort of nontraditional feeding pattern after cancer diagnosis, and 39% supplement the diet of their dog.[375] This is a concern, because most oncology referral centers generally recommend that clients refrain from using antioxidants or herbal supplements, and from feeding raw and home-prepared foods because of the lack of clinical data to support their use.[376]

It is clear that antioxidant and oxidative balance is altered in tumor tissue. Canine mammary cancer tissue has an increased presence of lipid peroxidation coupled with an increase in upregulated antioxidant mechanisms, including glutathione peroxidase, glutathione, superoxide dismutase, and catalase.[377] In one study of dogs with lymphoma, reductions in serum antioxidants (tocopherols) and increased lipid peroxidation were observed, whereas total oxygen radical absorption capacity and glutathione peroxidase were increased, suggesting an increase in antioxidant capability.[378] Therefore the addition of an antioxidant is unlikely to have a dramatic effect on the overall antioxidant capability of tumor cells compared with normal tissue.

Further complicating this issue, many substances given as antioxidants may be considered pro-oxidants in some environments.[379] Many isothiocyanates, flavonoids, and carotenoids actually may cause alteration of cell signaling or depletion of specific antioxidant systems.[379,380] Furthermore, the evidence increasingly indicates that many of these compounds upregulate or downregulate specific cell signaling systems to alter the proliferative cycle from activities such as cell cycle disruption (CDKs, p16, p21), prosurvival signals (nuclear factor-κB [Nf-κB], AKT), mitochondrial-induced apoptosis (Bcl and Bax family proteins), and proliferative signaling pathways (i.e., mitogen-activated protein [MAP] kinase, tyrosine kinase [TK] activity).[381–383] Primary cancer cell culture data in lymphoma and OSA supports these principles. Astaxanthin and lycopene, two carotenoids, showed limited antioxidant capability in canine OSA cells lines, and when coupled with doxorubicin or irradiation, no protective effects were seen on cell proliferation indices or cell death.[384,385] Isoflavones appear to induce mitochondrial apoptosis in canine lymphoma cells.[386] Further examination of the flavonoid baicalein from *Scutellaria* root, shows mitochondrial-induced apoptosis.[387] Rosemary and curcumin extracts supplemented at slightly higher than presumed physiologic doses have antineoplastic activity and act synergistically in round, spindle, and epithelial canine cancer cells to promote cell death; they do not hinder chemotherapeutic cell death and may augment it.[388] These in vitro data must be interpreted with caution because another recent study examining the isothiocyanate sulforaphane, which has been touted to protect cells during cisplatin chemotherapy, may also augment cell growth in the canine OSA cell culture environment.[389]

Even if some of these compounds have little to no detrimental effect on current chemotherapy or RT protocols, the limiting factor to their effective use is absorption, hepatic metabolism, and the attainment of tissue concentrations that recapitulate what has been used in vitro.[381] Pharmacokinetic data has been collected on three nutraceuticals: genistein in cats (an isoflavone), epigallocathecin gallate (EGCG, a flavone from green tea), and lycopene in dogs (carotenoids).[390–392] All of these nutraceuticals required dosing at very high concentrations, which may preclude their clinical use. There is tremendous disconnect between what is available and what may be required, in addition to a lack of clinical trial investigations to assess the efficacy and safety of these compounds. Furthermore, metabolism of these compounds may be different in cats and dogs; therefore caution is advised. Dosages over 150 mg/kg of EGCG in dogs caused hepatic necrosis, and the use of lipoic acid (an antioxidant thought to help salvage glutathione) has potential for toxicity and hepatic damage in cats when used at dosages thought safe in dogs and humans.[393,394]

In conclusion, set nutritional requirements during neoplasia do not exist in companion animals. In part this is due to the variety of neoplastic diseases involved and the danger of trying to extrapolate data generated in human cancers. Many aspects remain to be addressed, including nutritional interventions for anorexia/cachexia during treatment and remission, and nutrition recommendations based on specific disease processes. Therefore no one dietary recommendation can be made for cancer patients; rather each case should be evaluated based on the patient's body condition, the specific neoplastic process, and the treatment protocol initiated by the oncologist. The topics discussed are merely guidelines for interested clients and clinicians – the most important factor in nutritional intervention is to supply a complete and balanced ration that meets the patient's energy requirements to prevent weight loss.

SECTION C: RELATIONSHIP-CENTERED APPROACH TO CANCER COMMUNICATION

JANE R. SHAW

Recognition of the relationships that people develop with their companion animals brings an awareness of the impact of animal illness on pet caregivers and the veterinary team.[395,397] Increasing acknowledgment of pets as family members is associated with greater expectations by pet owners for the highest quality medical care for their companion animals, in addition to compassionate care and respectful communication for themselves.[395,396,398–400] The human-animal bond is particularly stressed and fragile when an animal is sick, and even more so after a diagnosis of cancer. Appreciating the effect of animal companionship on the health and well-being of humans creates a new dimension in public health. Today, the responsibilities of veterinary professionals include the emotional health and well-being of clients and their pets.[398]

Communication about the diagnosis, treatment, and prognosis of cancer presents challenges both for veterinarians and for clients. From the veterinarian's perspective, a number of factors may contribute to discomfort with this conversation, including lack of training, insufficient time, practice culture, feeling responsible for the patient's illness, perceptions of failure, unease with death and dying, lack of comfort with uncertainty, the effect on the veterinarian-client-patient relationship, worry about the patient's quality of life, concerns about the client's emotional response, and the veterinarian's own emotional response to the circumstances.[400,402] Some of these same reasons may account for clients' anxiety during difficult conversations; these include self-blame, unease with death and dying, anticipatory grief, effect on the human-animal bond, effect on the veterinarian-client-patient relationship, pet's QOL, and concerns about their emotional response to the

situation. Research in human medicine indicates that breaking bad news, discussions of the prognosis, and end-of-life discussions often are suboptimal because of many of these barriers and a lack of specific training in communication.[401–404]

The content, duration, and methods of communication training in veterinary curricula are highly diverse and variable. Many practitioners have not received formal communication training and may feel unprepared to engage in difficult conversations.[405–407] The veterinary profession identified a skills gap between the content of the veterinary school curriculum and the actual skills required to be a successful veterinarian.[408] Using experiential techniques, defining key skills, and creating practice opportunities enhance effective communication.[409–412] In accreditation standards, the American Veterinary Medical Association's Council on Education recognizes communication as a core clinical competency for success.[413]

Several aspects of cancer care make it a unique communication context.[414] The initial diagnosis frequently is made by the primary care veterinarian, who may refer the client and patient to a specialist. Therefore the first visit with the specialist often occurs after the patient receives at least a tentative diagnosis, and the focus of the conversation is on confirming the diagnosis, treatment and prognostic information, and decision making. In this setting tough conversations occur on the back of a newly formed veterinarian-client-patient relationship. Cancer is an emotionally laden diagnosis, and clients often have high levels of uncertainty, anxiety, fear, frustration, and guilt, which heightens the stakes for both parties. Fortunately today we can offer clients a menu of sophisticated diagnostic and therapeutic options for treating their pet's cancer. This also presents the challenge of navigating complex information sharing and the decision-making processes of making the "right choice" for their pet without overwhelming clients. The initial visit may require as much listening as talking to hear what is most important to clients to address these challenges.

Cancer communication is a process that occurs over time, starting with delivering the diagnosis (i.e., often delivering bad news); making decisions about treatment options; discussing the prognosis; assessing the QOL; transitioning to palliative, supportive, or hospice care when required; and ending with preparing families for euthanasia, dying, and/or natural death. These difficult conversations are spread throughout multiple visits over time; during this time, the relationship grows and a partnership develops, making it more comfortable to address end-of-life conversations when appropriate.

Another special consideration is that cancer conversations frequently are managed by a team of veterinarians, including the referring veterinarian and multiple specialists. Most pets with cancer are treated with a combination of therapies involving different types of expertise (i.e., medical oncology, surgical oncology, or radiation oncology) or different disciplines (i.e., cardiology, neurology, or internal medicine). For example, the medical oncologist may determine the diagnosis and conduct the clinical staging; a surgical oncologist may remove the tumor; and a medical and/or radiation oncologist presents the efficacy of adjunct therapies after surgery. Each of these experts layers on information for the client about potential treatment options and the effect on the pet's QOL and prognosis. Then a medical oncologist might discuss palliative, supportive, or hospice care and facilitate end-of-life decisions. Referring veterinarians are involved throughout, because they share the closest bond with the client, who often trusts their opinions and seeks their guidance. This shared case management model underscores the importance of continuity of communication among all care providers. Given the team approach to cancer care, the inclusive term "veterinarian" is used in this section to encompass the roles of the referring veterinarian and specialists in conducting cancer conversations.

The purpose of this section is to present best practices for cancer communication. Only limited empiric studies are available in the veterinary literature concerning cancer communication,[400,415] and information is based largely on clinical experience.[447,479,460] In contrast, the literature on human medical communication contains a large number of empiric studies; however, in relation to cancer communication, what is available is based on expert opinion, case studies, reviews, and predominantly descriptive studies.[414,416] The objectives of this section are to describe relationship-centered care, define core cancer communication skills, and highlight communication approaches to difficult discussions. The medical cancer communication literature[402,404,416–420] and clinical experience provide the foundation for communication techniques presented here.

Before moving on we should address one of the most common concerns expressed in communication training: there is not enough time in the clinical interview. It seems as if the conversational approach of relationship-centered care takes more time; however, it was found in veterinary general practice visits that relationship-centered care appointments were shorter because the veterinarian and the client achieved common ground early in the appointment.[419] In human medicine, when patients are left to tell their story uninterrupted, their average talking time was 92 seconds, and they provided key clues to the diagnosis.[444] Empathy also can be expressed without prolonging the appointment time; in one study as little as 40 seconds of empathy reduced the patient's anxiety level.[421] Although it seems counterintuitive, evidence suggests that using the core communication skills actually saves time and allows for a more efficient veterinarian-client-patient interaction. In addition, spending time to build a relationship at the beginning of the appointment creates trust, and this will pay off when diagnostic and treatment recommendations are made.

Paradigm Shift: Paternalism to Partnership

Recent societal changes caused a paradigm shift in the veterinarian-client-patient relationship. Growing client expectations, the strong attachment between people and their pets, and increasing consumer knowledge demand a swing in communication style from the traditional paternalistic approach to a collaborative partnership.[399,400,419,281] Many clients are no longer content with taking a passive role in the healthcare of their animal, preferring to take an active role in the decision-making process.[399,400,419,422]

Paternalism is characterized as a relationship in which the veterinarian sets the agenda for the appointment, assumes that the client's values are the same as the veterinarian's, and takes on the role of a guardian for the patient.[419,423–425] Traditionally, paternalism is the most common approach to medical and veterinary visits. In a quantitative study published in 2006, companion animal practitioners used a paternalistic approach in 31% of wellness visits and 85% of problem visits.[419] In a qualitative study published in 2017, livestock practitioners used a directive communication style reflective of a paternalistic approach.[422] The topic of conversation was primarily biomedical in nature, focusing on the medical condition, diagnosis, treatment, and prognosis.[419]

In a paternalistic relationship the veterinarian does most of the talking and the client plays a passive role. This approach often is referred to as the *data dump* and symbolized by a shot-put.[412]

Throwing a shot-put is unidirectional, the intent is on the delivery, the information to be presented is large in mass and scale, and it is challenging to receive the message. Intuitively, it seems as if this "take charge" approach enhances efficiency and promotes time management. The challenge is that the agenda and subsequent diagnostic or treatment plan may not be shared by the veterinarian and client, compromising the ability to reach agreement and achieve adherence to recommendations or, moving forward too quickly may lead to client regrets. This could result in a roadblock and the need to take steps backward to recover and regain client understanding, commitment, and trust.

In contrast, partnership or relationship-centered care represents a balance of power between veterinarian and client and is based on mutuality.[419,423–425] In the relationship-centered model the relationship between veterinarian and client is characterized by negotiation between partners, resulting in creation of a joint venture, with the veterinarian taking on the role of advisor for the client and advocate for the patient. Respect for the client's perspective and values and recognition of the role the animal plays in the client's life are incorporated into all aspects of care. In companion animal practice, 69% of wellness visits and 15% of problem visits were characterized as relationship-centred.[419]

The conversation content of relationship-centered visits is broad; it includes biomedical topics, lifestyle discussion of the pet's daily activities (e.g., exercise regimen, environment, travel, diet, and sleeping habits), and social interactions (e.g., personality or temperament, behavior, human-animal interaction, and animal-animal interactions) that are key indicators of the patient's QOL.[419] In addition, a relationship-centered approach encompasses building rapport, establishing a partnership, and encouraging client participation in the animal's care, all of which have the potential to enhance clinical outcomes.

This collaborative relationship is a dialog and is symbolized by a Frisbee.[412] In playing Frisbee, the interaction is reciprocal; the intent is on the exchange of information, small pieces of information are delivered, the client responds, and the message is adjusted to target the individual. The emphasis of the Frisbee analogy[412] is on eliciting client feedback to assess how the client perceives, processes, and understands the information presented.

Relationship-Centered Care

Combining several frameworks Mead and Bower[426] identified five distinct dimensions of relationship or patient-centered care in the human medical setting.

1. The biopsychosocial perspective—A perspective on illness that includes social, psychological, lifestyle, and biomedical factors.
2. The "patient/client as a person"—Understanding the personal meaning of the illness for each individual patient or the personal meaning of the animal's illness for the client.
3. Sharing power and responsibility—Sensitivity to preferences of the patient and/or client for information and shared decision making.
4. The therapeutic alliance—Developing common therapeutic goals and enhancing the physician-patient or veterinarian-client-patient relationship.
5. The "doctor as person"—Awareness of the influence of the subjectivity of the doctor on the practice of medicine.

Incorporating these dimensions, cancer communication strives to balance exchanging information, making decisions, fostering healing relationships, enabling clients to provide patient care, managing uncertainty, and responding to emotions.[414]

These principles translate readily to the veterinary context.[419,427,428] Expanding data gathering to explore the broader lifestyle of the client and pet enhances the veterinarian's understanding of the animal's cancer. Discussing unique details, such as financial resources, the role of the primary caregiver, feasibility of implementing a plan, and recent life events (e.g., new birth, death, new job, or moving) promotes adherence to recommendations. With increased recognition of the human-animal bond, it is important to assess the level of attachment and the effect of the animal's cancer on the family. Eliciting information on the client's expectations, thoughts, feelings, and fears about the pet's cancer fosters client participation and satisfaction and promotes shared decision making.

Studies found potential missed opportunities for eliciting client perspectives during euthanasia discussions. In a quantitative study investigating the use of client-centered communication in euthanasia discussions with undisclosed standardized clients (USC) (i.e., "secret shopper" in the marketing setting), veterinarians did not fully explore clients' feelings, ideas, and expectations, or the effect of the illness on the animal's function.[428] Veterinarian and client perceptions of the client-centeredness of the euthanasia discussions differed—veterinarians perceived that client-centeredness components were addressed more thoroughly than was perceived by the USC.[427] For both euthanasia scenarios, the veterinarian and client agreed that discussion of personal and family issues was lacking.[428] Identifying clients' background, experiences, perspectives, and preferences is critical to shared decision making, and working toward consensus is important to achieve significant clinical outcomes for the veterinarian, client, and patient.

Relationship-centered communication can be learned and taught. Communication interventions conducted in the practice setting focused on relationship-centered care, and effective communication resulted in a more client-centered approach.[410,411] After a 1-year training, veterinarians gathered more lifestyle-social data and used more partnership-building and positive rapport-building communication; clients provide more lifestyle-social information and emotional statements.[410] After a 6-month communication program veterinarians used more facilitative and emotional rapport communication; clients felt more involved in the appointment and veterinarians expressed greater interest in their opinions.[411]

Clinical Outcomes

Based on medical communication studies, relationship-centered care is associated with significant improvements in clinical outcomes. Broadening the explanatory perspective of disease beyond the biomedical to include lifestyle and social factors is related to expanding the field of inquiry and improved diagnostic reasoning and accuracy.[420] Building a strong relationship is associated with increased accuracy of data gathering,[420] patient satisfaction,[429–431] and physician satisfaction.[432,433] Encouraging participation, negotiation, and shared decision making promotes patient satisfaction,[429–431] adherence to recommendations,[434] and improved health.[435]

Veterinarian-client communication also is correlated with clinical outcomes. In a study in which closed- and open-ended solicitation of client concerns were compared, open-ended inquiry elicited more concerns and client dialog, with decreased odds of a new concern arising at the close of the interview.[436] Investigation of the relationship between veterinarian-client communication and adherence to dentistry and surgical recommendations revealed

that enhanced adherence was associated with clear recommendations, relationship-centered care, client satisfaction, an empathetic and unhurried atmosphere, longer appointment time, and use of positive rapport-building statements.[437] Moreover, evaluation of the association between veterinarian-client communication and veterinarian satisfaction with the visit revealed that veterinarian positive talk (e.g., compliments, laughter, statements of approval and agreement) was correlated with veterinarian satisfaction with wellness visits (i.e., pets brought to the veterinarian for routine examination), and client rapport building and veterinarian-to-pet talk were associated with veterinarian satisfaction with problem visits (i.e., pets brought to the veterinarian because of a health problem).[438] In a detailed analysis of the use of communication skills by companion animal veterinarians, the veterinarian's expressions of empathy resulted in higher levels of client satisfaction.[439]

Client Uncertainty

Uncertainty is at the core of the illness experience and the practice of medicine. During in-depth interviews of oncology clients at a tertiary referral center, client uncertainty arose as a dominant client psychological experience during oncology appointments.[440] Traditionally veterinarians focus on treating the animal's disease, and the results of this study highlighted the importance of the veterinarian's role in managing the client's experience of the animal's illness. The diagnosis of cancer and its association with death shifted clients' worldviews from orderly, predictable, and reliable to one of chaos, unpredictability, and ambiguity. Client experiences of uncertainty were greatest in the early stages and again in the late stages of cancer treatment. For many clients uncertainty was seen as danger, although some saw opportunity expressed through optimism, hope, and living in the present. Veterinarians can facilitate adaptive uncertainty management by supporting clients' efforts to reduce uncertainty; this can be done by meeting the client's informational and relational needs.

Client informational needs[440] include orientation to the oncology appointment provided by the primary care veterinarian and the oncology service, such as new client information packages, service websites, conversations with a client liaison, walking clients through the hospital processes and protocols, hospital tours, and meeting members of the oncology team, all of which prepare clients for the initial visit. For some clients, providing information can be empowering, but for others this can be incapacitating; for a few clients avoidance, denial, or minimizing may be vital coping mechanisms. Therefore it is critical to tailor the approach to giving information and identifying clients' background and experiences, need for information, and information preferences (e.g., presenting the big picture or a highly-detailed discussion). It is equally important to discuss with clients the efficacy and success of treatment approaches, in addition to potential adverse effects, so clients are prepared for all treatment outcomes. Provide warnings when necessary when delivering test results or progress reports to reduce unnecessary client distress. Set the course of cancer ahead of time, if required, so clients anticipate transitions from focusing on treatment to conversations addressing QOL, palliative, hospice, or end-of-life care.

Client relational support plays an equally critical role in reducing client uncertainty.[440] The foremost relationship is that with the veterinarian or nurse, and continued, established, and trusting relationships are paramount. Another source of relational support is timeliness of service, including booking appointments, returning client's phone calls, conducting diagnostic tests, providing test results, and starting treatment. Providing 24-hour information support in case of an unexpected event or complication, allowing clients to seek advice and guidance, manages uncertainty by addressing the client's questions and concerns and unexpected outcomes in a timely manner. In addition, peer support, waiting room interactions, social communities (i.e., family, friends, or neighbors), and formal Internet groups offer opportunities to share and normalize the client's experiences.

Veterinarian Expressions of Uncertainty

As much as is known today about cancer, much is still unknown, and veterinarians need to express uncertainty to their clients. Studies in human medicine contradict each other on whether a clinician's expressions of uncertainty enhance or undermine a patient's confidence and satisfaction. A qualitative survey study in veterinary medicine explored veterinarian and client expressions of clinical uncertainty.[441] All clients wanted to know about clinical uncertainties related to diagnostic accuracy and treatment appropriateness, and expressions of uncertainty did not erode clients' confidence. Behavioral expressions of uncertainty (e.g., consulting with or referring to a specialist) were less damaging to client confidence than verbal expressions (e.g., *"I need to find our more"* or *"This might be…"*).

Client Expectations

In a survey study of members of the online Pet Cancer Support group 77% of respondents were satisfied with their veterinarian, 71% with the information the veterinarian provided about treatment options, and 70% with the support they received from their veterinarian.[442] In a study of in-depth interviews of oncology clients at tertiary referral center, clients identified important aspects of veterinarian-client communication.[400,415] These client comments can be divided into those related to communication content (i.e., what is said[415]) and process (i.e., how it is said[400]). Interweaving communication content and process ensures effective sharing of information.

Regarding the content of information delivery,[415] the central theme was that clients wanted the truth about all aspects of their animal's cancer and treatment. In particular they expected the veterinarian to share information in relation to the client's background, previous experiences, and information preferences (i.e., presenting the big picture or a highly-detailed discussion), in other words, tailored to each client. This information was empowering for clients and enabled them to make treatment decisions, granted a sense of control, and fostered hope and overall ability to cope with their pet's cancer diagnosis and treatment process.

From a process perspective,[400] clients wanted information to be delivered upfront in a forthright manner, in lay language, and using multiple formats, such as oral, written, and visual client education tools (e.g., discharge instructions, brochures, handouts, diagrams, drawings, models, images, and websites). It was important to clients that the oncologists take time to listen, address their questions, and repeat information as needed, facilitating understanding of their pet's disease. Survey respondents of the Pet Cancer Support group identified problem-focused support (i.e., sharing information, engaging in open discussion, and considering options) as a common source of support provided by their veterinarians.[443] Clients appreciated an established relationship with the oncologist or nurse, and having 24-hour information support in case of an unexpected event or complication, allowing them

to seek advice and guidance. Likewise, survey respondents of the Pet Cancer Support group stated that problem-focused tangible support (i.e., veterinarian investment in animal care and being available and accessible to clients) was the other customary source of support provided by their veterinarians.[443] It was supportive to clients when information was conveyed in a positive, compassionate, empathetic, and nonjudgmental manner, which provided much needed emotional support. In contrast, emotional-focused support was not expected of their veterinarians.[443] Meeting informational needs and creating a humanistic environment helped clients cope with their pet's cancer.[400]

Core Communication Skills for Cancer Communication

The Calgary-Cambridge Guide[412] is an evidence-based communication model that provides structure to the clinical interview, describing the tasks and identifying key communication skills to help veterinarians achieve clinical outcomes. Defining and demonstrating specific skills and behaviors are instrumental first steps to enhancing communication approaches.[409–412] The communication tools described in the following discussions were identified as core communication skills in human cancer communication literature[402,409,414,416] and are highly applicable to veterinarian-client-patient interactions.[442,446]

Gathering Information

Identify the Client's Full Agenda[442]
Eliciting the client's full agenda through open-ended inquiry promotes early detection of problem(s) and sets a plan for the rest of the visit.[437] This includes exploring the client's reasons for the visit, concerns, goals, expectations, and priorities. An open-ended question is designed to draw out a full response from the client rather than a brief one; it usually begins with "how," "what," "tell me," "describe for me," or "explain to me." In a quantitative study of soliciting client concerns, the use of open-ended solicitations resulted in significantly more client concerns being revealed than with closed-ended solications.[437]

"Your referring veterinarian diagnosed Mandy with [disease]. What specific questions would you like me to address today?" [reasons for visit]

"I see that your veterinarian referred you for [disease]. What else would you like to discuss?" [reasons]

"What are your greatest concerns about Mandy's cancer?" [concerns]

"What other worries do you have about Mandy?" [concerns]

"What are your goals for our time together?" [goals]

"How can I best help you today?" [expectations]

"What is the most important thing for us to address today?" [priorities]

This process of questioning may seem redundant, but clients often bring a laundry list (i.e., three to four[444]) of concerns, questions, or topics that they would like to discuss with their veterinarian. Given the overwhelming nature of cancer conversations, these steps help identify the key questions and information sought by the client. Helping generate the client's list of concerns and melding it with your agenda sets the structure for the remainder of the appointment and optimizes efficient use of the visit time.

Elicit the Client's Perspective[415,442]

Invite clients to share their thoughts, beliefs, opinions, ideas, feelings, and perceptions.[427,428] Again, a client's perspectives are best obtained by asking open-ended questions. How the client perceives the pet's cancer can have a major effect on the decision-making process and adherence to recommendations. Many clients have had previous experiences with cancer, and it is helpful to hear these stories to address the client's concerns, provide reassurance, and identify misconceptions or barriers to patient care. Pick up on the client's verbal cues (*"I am not sure how she will do with chemotherapy."* or *"I am really concerned about her loss of appetite."* or *"My big fear is that we won't get quality time."*) and invite the client to share his or her worries. Knowing the client's expectations enables you to get on the same page and customize the message to the client's concerns and meet the individual's needs.

"I am wondering what experiences you have had with cancer in your life, because they may affect decisions we make for Mandy."
"How are you coping with all of this?"
"What are your greatest hopes in caring for Mandy?"

Explaining and Planning

Assess the Client's Starting Knowledge[415,442]

Assessing the client's prior knowledge allows you to evaluate his or her understanding and determine at what level to deliver the information. Each client brings his or her own knowledge, background, experiences, and ideas to the table. Assessing the client's starting knowledge through open-ended questions allows you to gauge the entry point to the conversation and enables the veterinary team to meet the client where the person is.

"What do you know about cancer in general?"
"What have you heard or read about osteosarcoma?"
"I am wondering what your veterinarian told you about Mandy's cancer."

Ascertain the Client's Information Preferences[415,442]

An equally important goal is to ascertain the type and kind of information the client desires, because not all clients may want the same degree of information. Client preferences for information may change over time; initially, overwhelmed clients may want just the big picture; as they absorb and process the information, they may produce a list of detailed questions for follow-up discussions. Open-ended inquiry is a key technique for evaluating the client's information preferences.

"Some clients prefer the big picture and for others it is important to get into the details. What is your preference?"
"What additional information would be helpful to you?"
"Let me know if you would like me to go into greater detail."

Give Information in Manageable Chunks and Checks[442]

Chunk-and-check consists of giving information in small pieces (i.e., chunks), followed by checking for understanding before proceeding further (i.e., check)—the Frisbee approach in action.[412] Sharing small pieces of information, one to three sentences at a time, allows your client time to absorb the news, and checking-in encourages client participation in the discussion and ensures that the client stays with you to achieve shared

understanding. This approach to giving information avoids lecturing to the client and aims to increase recall, understanding, and commitment to plans. In this manner the process of giving information is responsive to the client's needs and provides an opportunity for the client to participate in the conversation, provide feedback, or ask for clarification. The check takes the form of an open-ended question.

"What questions do you have at this point?"
"What needs more explanation?"
"What part will be most difficult for you and Mandy?"

Building Relationships

Offer Partnership[442]

Partnership is inclusive language (e.g., let's, we, together, our, or us), which reflects that you and the client are working as a team toward mutual goals. Offering partnership informs clients that they are not alone and that they have a working partner in their veterinarian, who will guide and advise them at each stage. Often clients may arrive at the appointment on their own, and it may be helpful to assess their support system and offer to include other key decision makers in the conversations.

"We'll work together to determine the best treatment plan for Mandy."
"I'm here for you. Take your time. We have a few days to decide how to proceed."
"Who else will take part in making decisions in Mandy's care?"

Ask Permission[442]

Asking permission is a gentle approach to assess the client's readiness to take the next step. This act of respect allows the client to ready his or her mind, be receptive to what you have to say, and pace the conversation with you. Asking permission is a method of structuring the conversation by proposing a transition to the client and to determine whether the client would like to move on.

"Would it be alright if we sit down and I asked you some questions about Mandy?"
"I am wondering if we could talk more about pain management."
"Are you okay with talking about how we can reduce the tumor size?"
"Maybe you could write down your specific questions before our next visit."

Express Empathy[442]

The stress of cancer can result in intense emotions: sadness, fear, anxiety, uncertainty, and guilt, and acknowledging these emotions reduces client distress.[421] Empathy is an affective response resulting from perceiving the situation of another, vicariously experiencing what it might be like, and paying deep attention to another person's emotions. As a result, three tasks are involved in expressing empathy.[445] The first is to appreciate the client's situation, perspective, and feelings, and the attached meanings. The second is to communicate that understanding to the client and check its accuracy. The third is to move forward in the clinical interview and act on that understanding with the client and patient in a helpful way. Simply, empathy is putting yourself in clients' shoes and communicating that you understand where they are coming from. Expressing empathy acknowledges, validates, and normalizes the client's emotional response and is essential to establishing a trusting veterinarian-client-patient relationship.

"I'm so sorry to tell you this. I know it was <u>not what you were expecting</u>."
"I can only imagine <u>how hard</u> this is to hear. Mandy has been your companion for so long."
"I can see that you are <u>agonizing</u> over the right decision for Mandy."

Demonstrate Appropriate Nonverbal Behavior[442]

Expression of all of the verbal core communication skills is strengthened when accompanied by complementary nonverbal communication. As much as 80% of communication is nonverbal in nature, whereas 20% is based on verbal content.[446] When verbal and nonverbal communication are incongruent, the nonverbal behaviors reveal the truth. There are two areas of focus for nonverbal communication: the first is to increase your sensitivity to picking up on client cues, and the second is enhanced awareness of the nonverbal messages you are sending out. Tune in closely to the client's nonverbal behaviors, such as breaking eye contact, nervous body movements, or tone of voice, because nonverbal behaviors often reflect the client's true underlying feelings and responses. Out of respect for their relationship with their veterinarian, clients often express hesitation indirectly through their nonverbal behaviors and may not feel comfortable with directly verbalizing their concerns, doubts or criticisms. It is important to pick up on these client clues and follow-up on them with the client to explore the concerns (*"I sensed some <u>hesitation</u> when I mentioned chemotherapy as a treatment option."* or *"You seem <u>worried</u> about taking Mandy to surgery; what are you most <u>scared</u> about?"*)

Veterinarian nonverbal cues include attentive body posture, appropriate distance from the client, turning your body toward the client, sitting at the same level, maintaining good eye contact, and complementary gestures. Display your compassion through nonverbal cues, such as sitting at a comfortable distance with your client; using a gentle, calm tone and soft volume; slowing your pace of speech; and leaning forward and reaching out through touch when appropriate. Use silence to create time for clients to examine their thoughts and feelings. It can be difficult at times to find the right words to say, and simply being a caring presence can provide just as much comfort to the client as any spoken words. Being mindful of the non-verbal messages sent is important because when veterinarians are triggered or feeling judgmental, these sentiments can be leaked to the client through nonverbal behaviors.

Providing Structure

Provide a Warning Shot[442,446,447]

A warning shot forewarns of difficult discussions or decisions ahead. It warns clients of bad news and allows them to prepare themselves for what they are about to hear. This approach reduces the chances of blind-siding and enhances the client's ability to process versus react to the information.

"This may be <u>difficult</u> for you to hear."
"<u>Unfortunately</u>, we do not have effective treatments for this kind of cancer."
"<u>I am sorry to tell you</u> that Mandy's cancer is growing and no longer responding to the chemotherapy."
"<u>I have disappointing news</u>. Mandy's cancer has spread to her lungs."

Summarize[442]

Summarizing is an explicit review of the information that has been discovered and discussed with the client. Multiple opportunities arise to present a summary: reflect back what you heard and learned at several stages during information gathering, take time to repeat the key aspects of the diagnostic and treatment plan, and finally provide a full and complete summary at the end of the clinical interview. Summarizing helps structure the conversation by reviewing what has been discussed, identifying data that needs further clarification, providing an opportunity for reflection on where the interview could go next, and managing effective use of time during the visit. The skill of summarizing creates a window to inform clients that they have been heard and time for clinicians to gather their thoughts, synthesize and integrate the data, and work through the diagnostic reasoning process.

"<u>So, if I understand it correctly</u>, your referring veterinarian felt the large lymph nodes, took a sample, and diagnosed lymphoma. You were sent here for further testing to determine if the lymphoma has spread to other organs. What other tests did your referring veterinarian perform?"
"<u>What we talked about doing today</u> is requesting a second opinion from our pathologist on the tumor sample, and taking chest x-rays and conducting an ultrasound exam to look at the abdominal lymph nodes, liver, and spleen for spread of the tumor. What further questions do you have about those diagnostic tests?"

"I Don't Have Time for This..."

The concern about how veterinarians find the time to elicit the client's agenda, perspectives, starting knowledge, and information preferences, and managing client emotions, may still remain. But contrary to popular belief the skills just discussed enhance appointment efficiency. More time with the client may be needed upfront, but this will pay dividends in time savings by streamlining decision making during diagnostic and treatment planning.

1. *Eliciting clients' full agenda, goals, and expectations* early in the appointment is critical to optimizing appointment time.[436] Clients often bring a laundry list of issues, topics, or questions they would like to discuss with their veterinarian.[444] Exploring this list and melding it with your agenda determines the structure and tasks for the remainder of the appointment. If you are unable to fully meet the client's agenda, it allows you to reset client expectations and consider alternatives, such as a drop-off, recheck visit, follow-up phone call, further discussion with a veterinary nurse, or counseling support or referral.
2. *Identifying clients' perspectives* is important, because these can act as either promoters or inhibitors of clients' decision-making process in considering diagnostic and treatment options. Identifying concerns a client brings to the visit enables the veterinarian to tailor a care plan that aligns with the client's needs, enabling the client to move forward more quickly.[415]
3. *Assessing what clients already know* helps veterinary professionals deliver information that is appropriate to the individual's level, enhancing understanding and recall.[415] This step also helps identify gaps, misunderstandings, or misinformation that can be addressed in the moment before confusion arises. Also, appointment efficiency can be enhanced by identifying clients who are already well informed and need less education.
4. *Assessing clients' information preferences* enables you to gauge what information the client desires and how much detail is preferred.[415] This promotes explanations that are on target on initial delivery, reducing the need to revisit material or to start over again and provide the big picture or more in-depth details.

5. *Defusing clients' emotions* (e.g., frustration, sadness, anxiety) can be accomplished by building rapport; expressing empathy; creating a safe, nonjudgmental space and providing opportunities to be heard; and posing questions. This puts clients at ease and enhances their ability to process, understand, and recall information; it also prepares them to make decisions.[421,447]

Approaches to Cancer Conversations

As presented in the introduction, cancer communication is a series of conversations over time, starting with delivering the diagnosis (i.e., delivering bad news); discussing the prognosis; making decisions about treatment options; assessing the patient's QOL; transitioning to palliative, supportive, or hospice care; and ending with preparing families for euthanasia, dying, or natural death. These difficult conversations are spread throughout multiple visits. This step-by-step approach is guided by the veterinarian's expertise, the client's agenda and perspective, and the patient's condition, response to treatment, and QOL.

Conduct these conversations in an appropriate setting to ensure privacy, client and patient comfort, lack of distractions, ability to sit down together, and place to include multiple individuals (e.g., examination, consultation, or comfort room). Start by creating a safe space for clients by taking time to establish initial rapport, checking in on their well-being, and demonstrating interest in the client. (*"How are you doing? Thank you for bringing Mandy in so that we could address this problem. Sounds like it's a stressful time for you all."*) Identify the client's support system and extend an invitation for key decision makers, family members, and friends to track information and provide emotional support (*"I am wondering who makes decisions regarding Mandy's care"* or *"Who else may want to participate in this discussion?"*) Because these are emotionally laden discussions loaded with complex information and associated with decision making, compose and center yourself beforehand, pace yourself with your client, and offer some time for reflection. Allow for silence or offer a break to create space for clients and yourself to work through emotions and process the information exchanged.

Delivering Bad News

Bad news is defined as any news that drastically and negatively alters the person's views of her or his future with their pet, such as a cancer diagnosis.[402] Clients interpret bad news on an individual basis, and their response is related to their relationship with their companion animal, the severity of the diagnosis, past experiences, other stressors in their lives, and their support system. Grief often accompanies change, and clients may express a wide range of emotions that are largely unpredictable. One useful model for delivering bad news is the SPIKES six-step model developed by Buckman[402] and used in many medical school curricula. The SPIKES model[402] (i.e., *s*etting, *p*erception, *i*nvitation, *k*nowledge, *e*mpathize, and *s*ummarize) provides guidelines on how to present information, structure the conversation, and create a supportive environment.[447, 479]

Explore clients' perspectives by asking open-ended questions about their concerns, ideas, thoughts, beliefs, previous experiences, and the effect of the pet's illness on their lives (*"What worries you most about Mandy's cancer?"* or *"What types of treatment did you have in mind?"*). Assess what the client knows about the pet's cancer or cancer in general (*"Tell me what you understand about Mandy's cancer?"* or *"Share with me your experiences with cancer or those of others in your life."*). Determine the client's information

preferences to tailor your discussion to the individual client's needs (*"Some clients like to know all the details about their pet's cancer, and others prefer the basic facts. What would you prefer?"*).

Provide a warning shot to forewarn the client of information that may be difficult to hear (*"Unfortunately, we do not have good options for treating this cancer."*). Then deliver the bad news in stages, giving information in small, easily understandable pieces and checking for the client's understanding before moving on (*"This is going to be difficult to hear. The cancer has spread to Mandy's lungs, making it hard for her to breathe. What concerns would you like to discuss at this point?"*). To pace the conversation with your client, ask permission to proceed to the next step in the conversation (*"Would it be alright if I went over Mandy's prognosis?"* or *"Is it alright if we talk about what this will mean for Mandy?"*). Avoid use of technical jargon and define medical terms. Use supplemental educational tools, such as written materials (e.g., client handouts, information sheets, or discharge statements), website resources, whiteboard notes, or audiotape recordings, so clients can review the information at a later date.

Empathize throughout the conversation to acknowledge, validate, and normalize the client's emotional responses (*"This is not what you were hoping to hear."*; *"This is overwhelming."*; or *"I can feel your sadness."*). Allow for silence and display compassionate and caring nonverbal cues (e.g., sit close to the client; mirror facial expressions; use a gentle, calm, and caring tone of voice; use a slow pace of speech; lean forward; reach out with touch if appropriate) (*"I'm here for you. Take your time."*). Offer partnership so the client does not feel alone in processing the information and making decisions (*"I will talk you through this, and we will make decisions for Mandy together."*). Summarize what was discussed, negotiate a plan for treatment, palliative or hospice care, and a timeline for follow-up (*"Today, we talked about the cancer spreading to Mandy's lungs. Unfortunately, it will be more and more difficult for Mandy to breathe. We discussed ways to monitor Mandy's quality of life. I am going to talk to your veterinarian about Mandy's supportive care. What questions do you have?"*).

Discussing the Prognosis

Three different approaches have been described in the medical communication literature for presenting prognostic information—realism, optimism, and avoidance.[404] The challenge with realism in human medicine is that approximately 20% of patients do not want full information about their prognosis.[448–451] In veterinary medicine, clients wanted the truth and information about all aspects of their pet's cancer and its treatment.[443] The drawback of optimism is that clients may lose opportunities to fulfill last wishes, prepare themselves and their family, and spend quality time with their pet. Finally, the shortcoming of avoidance is appearing evasive or dishonest, risking the trust that has been built between the veterinarian and client and potentially compromising the pet's care.

Based on recommendations in human[404,415,416] and veterinary medicine,[443] information should be tailored to the client's background, previous experiences, and information preferences (*"How much would you like to know about the course of Mandy's cancer?"* or *"Some clients would like all the details and others would like the big picture. What works best for you?"*). Provide a warning shot, so the client can prepare to hear the information (*"Unfortunately, the prognosis is serious for Mandy."* or *"This is the next difficult step in our conversation."*) Break the information into small pieces (i.e., chunks) and then check for client understanding and how the prognostic information is affecting the client (*"This is hard to talk about."* or *"I am wondering if this is the kind of information you need."*). Asking permission is a key skill in this conversation to assess the client's readiness to hear more information (*"What questions do you have at this point?"* or *"Would you like me to continue?"*).

Read the client's nonverbal cues to assess how clients are processing the information (*"I notice that you seem hesitant when I was talking about survival time with chemotherapy. Could you tell me more about this?"*). To balance sustaining hope and maintaining reality, it may be helpful to frame the prognosis using both positive and negative language (*"Median survival time means that half the patients live longer than 2 years and half the patients live less than 2 years."*).[452] Given the overwhelming nature of this discussion, take time to empathize with the client (*"This is a lot of information to take in. How are you doing?"* or *"I can see how sad this is for you."*). Offer partnership to walk beside the client during this conversation (*"This is really difficult to talk about, and we can take it one step at a time."*).

Assessing Quality of Life

In human medicine a spectrum of hopes lies from the initial cancer diagnosis to preparing for death.[453] In veterinary medicine a cancer diagnosis means a client's initial expectations may center around curing the cancer and the pet living longer, and then move toward spending special time with their pet and then seeking a peaceful death. This breakpoint discussion is a crucial conversation that signals the transition from striving for quantity of time to embracing QOL.[452] It can be challenging for clients who have been working so hard to treat the cancer to shift their energy to living the fullest life with their pet right now and preparing to let go (*"It seems like it may be helpful to focus on what time Mandy has left with you."* or *"Just because we can do something does not mean that we should."*). Warn clients of the difficulty in making the transition from treating cancer to focusing on QOL (*"It can be difficult to switch gears from fighting the cancer to preserving Mandy's quality of life."*).

Ask permission to ready the client to enter into a quality of life discussion (*"Would it be alright if we took some time to talk about Mandy's quality of life?"*) Pose open-ended questions to elicit the client's perspective of the pet's quality of life (*"What do you think Mandy's quality of life is like now?"*; *"What makes life worth living for Mandy?"* or *"Under what circumstances would life not be worth living for Mandy?"*). Obtain the client and patient goals to move the conversation forward (*"Can we create a plan together to ensure Mandy's quality of life?"* or *"What is most important to you in caring for Mandy at the end of life?"*). A supportive way to acknowledge the client's desire to do more is through expressions of "I hope" or "I wish" statements (*"I wish there was something we could do to cure Mandy's cancer."* or *"I hope that Mandy has many good weeks ahead."*).[454] At this stage it is equally important to reflect on the veterinarian's conversational emphasis and what influence the presentation of information may have on the client's decision making,[455] such as how much time is spent talking about anticancer therapy compared with QOL; supportive, palliative, or hospice care; or euthanasia. The veterinarian inadvertently can influence the client's decisions through the prioritization of the options for care.[456]

Educate the client on how to monitor the pet's condition and assess the pet's QOL. Clients often wonder aloud "how they are going to know when it is time?" Anticipating that the end of life care can be intimidating, overwhelming, and anxiety provoking

for clients. Concrete information about what to watch for and what to do may make the decisions feel more manageable (*"Things to watch for in Mandy are a decrease in appetite or interest in drinking water; reduced activity level; difficulty breathing, such as panting or increased effort; and change in personality, a lack of interest or responsiveness to you and her daily activities."*)

To validate and support clients, veterinarians may need to reassure their clients that they did everything they could for their pet (*"You have given Mandy every chance possible."*).[456] Words of empathy, reassurance, and partnership can be highly supportive (*"All along you have made your decisions with Mandy's best interests in mind."* or *"We will do this together, just as we have done everything that got us to this point."*).[456] Clients often are overwhelmed and feel alone, and it is comforting to know that their veterinarian will guide, advise, and inform them through this process.

Transitioning to Palliative Care or Hospice Care

Fortunately much can be done for a veterinary cancer patient's comfort, despite the inability to effect a cure; this includes symptom management, supportive care, enrichment, and pain management to ease suffering. Depending on the resources in your region, it may be appropriate to provide palliative care or refer the client and patient to a veterinary hospice service.[457,458] Palliative care begins at the cancer diagnosis and is incorporated into the treatment plan. Hospice care begins after treatment of the cancer is stopped. Veterinary hospice is the care provided after a terminal diagnosis of weeks to months has been given; it includes providing supportive care for the animal and emotional support for the family to prepare for the imminent death of the animal and to help clients focus on spending quality time with their pet. At-home patient care entails administering medications, assessing and monitoring pain management, emotional well-being and social enrichment, evaluating proper hydration and nutrition, and educating families about euthanasia, the grief process, and death and dying.[458] Today, statements such as "There is nothing more we can do" can be replaced with words of encouragement and offers of partnership to comfort clients (*"There is still much that we can do to make sure that Mandy is content and comfortable."*).[454]

Client and patient abandonment may be a concern that arises during this stage of care. The value placed by the client on the relationship with the veterinarian may increase as the patient's cancer progresses, as the desire for information lessens, and the need for support grows.[459] The relationship with the veterinarian or nurse is foremost in reducing client uncertainty at the late stages.[400] With the change in the care provided from cancer treatment to palliative care, the client may perceive that the veterinarian's relationship with the client and patient has ended. Offering partnership helps create a sense of support for the client (*"We will work through these decisions together."* or *"I will be here to help you and Mandy whatever your decisions may be."*) Clients may want to hear explicitly that their veterinarian will still be taking care of their pet, even if they decide to discontinue treatment. Depending on the client's relationship with the specialist and the referring veterinarian, it may be critical to determine the client's expectations and offer to maintain the relationship to provide end-of-life care. Caring for clients and patients at the end of life can be a source of meaning and fulfillment for the specialist, in addition to an opportunity to recognize the special relationships formed during this difficult time.

Euthanasia Decision Making

Clients may be waiting for the veterinarian to raise the option of euthanasia to give permission to consider euthanasia as a valid and supported option (*"One of the options that is important to discuss is euthanasia."*). Clients may be worried that the oncologist may perceive them as "giving up" if they bring up the option of euthanasia, therefore clients may need your validation (*"It is a valid and caring decision to consider euthanasia at this time."* or *"Euthanasia is a humane option for Mandy given how the cancer has spread."*). Client anxiety results from the uncertainty that lies ahead, and a large part of these conversations is helping clients cope with the unknown.[440] Previously clients had a clear plan for how to treat the cancer, and it may be helpful to have a designated path for how to care for their animal at the end of life. Discussing end-of-life wishes for the patient is crucial to preparing the client for euthanasia decision making, and creating a euthanasia plan often eases the client's discomfort and anxiety.[447] Once completed, it can be put on the shelf until it is needed, and the client can focus his or her energies on being present with the pet during these final precious days, weeks, or months. Being prepared ensures that the client's needs are met, minimizes regrets, and reduces uncertainty during this difficult time of grief.[440]

Use the communication skills to walk a client through euthanasia decision making; discuss the procedure and present options for location, body care, memorializing, and family presence.[447,460,479] Begin by asking the client about previous experiences with euthanasia (*"Could you share with me your previous experiences with euthanasia?"* or *"I am wondering whether you have been present at a euthanasia procedure in the past. Tell me about that situation."*). If appropriate, explore the client's religious or spiritual beliefs, which may affect a decision about euthanasia. (*"Some clients have religious or spiritual beliefs that guide the euthanasia decision. I am interested in how these beliefs might guide your decision-making process."*)

Provide a warning shot (*"This is one of the most difficult decisions in caring for your pet."* or *"There is a lot to consider, and the decision-making process can feel overwhelming."*)

Give information in small, easily understandable pieces, pause, and check for the client's understanding before proceeding (*"Max is probably feeling like you do when you have a bad flu. It probably hurts just to move, and it is difficult for him to get comfortable. What questions do you have about his condition?"*). Ask permission throughout to move from one topic to the next (e.g., timing, location, body care, being present, and memorializing [e.g., paw prints, hair clippings, pictures, videos, readings, or songs]) (*"I am wondering if it would be alright with you if I were to walk you through the euthanasia procedure we use at our clinic."* or *"There are a few options and decisions in relation to the euthanasia procedure and body care, and I am wondering if you would like to discuss them now."*) During the conversation, avoid use of technical jargon and define medical terms.

Empathize throughout the conversation; acknowledge, validate, and normalize the client's emotions (*"You have taken such good care of Mandy throughout his illness. I can tell how much you love her."*; *"These are difficult decisions. It feels like an enormous responsibility."*; or *"It is normal to feel sad. Mandy means so much to you."*). Use silence and display compassionate and caring nonverbal cues. Offer partnership so the client feels you by his or her side (*"We will talk through each step together."* or *"I want you to know that I fully support your decision, and will do my best to honor your wishes for Mandy"*). At the end, summarize what has been discussed and the decisions made, and outline the next steps for the client.

Providing Support for Grief and Loss

Research indicates that 70% of clients are affected emotionally by the death of their pet, and as many as 30% of clients experience severe grief in anticipation of or after the death of their pet.[397] In addition, approximately 50% of clients studied reported feeling guilty about their decision to euthanize their pet.[397] One of the factors contributing to client grief was the perception of the professional support provided by the veterinarian. A qualitative interview study described the emotional, informational, and instrumental social support veterinarians provide to grieving clients; the study revealed that these skills were often learned on the job, and little or no training was provided in veterinary school.[461] A qualitative ethnographic study documented the emotional work of veterinarians in attending to the death of their patients and managing the guilt and grief of their clients as a gratifying experience for clients and a fulfilling part of being a veterinarian.[462]

The manner in which the veterinarian provides care for a client whose pet has died has the potential to alleviate or aggravate grief. Use your communication toolbox to acknowledge, validate, and normalize client grief responses and provide emotional support.[460] Offer written materials and verbal grief education to help clients understand their grief experiences (*"Grief is hard. You may find it difficult to sleep; you may feel disoriented, restless, or exhausted, and unable to focus or concentrate; you may gain or lose your appetite. It can be crazy making."*). Send condolences in a timely manner after euthanasia (e.g., a card, memorial gift, or flowers) or place a phone call to check in with the client to see how she or he is doing (*"I wanted to call to see how you are doing. I know that you miss Mandy terribly."*). Assess the client's support system and identify at-risk clients who may need more active grief support (*"Who will you speak with about losing Mandy?"* or *"Who do you turn to during difficult times?"*). Provide information on support services (e.g., grief counseling, pet loss support hotlines and groups, and websites) (*"We have a grief counselor who works with our practice and hosts regular pet loss support groups. Our clients share that it is helpful to them."* or *"I have a list of pet loss support hotlines, if it would be helpful to speak with someone who understands how difficult it is to lose a pet."*).

Caring for Yourself

The health and wellness of veterinary professionals is a current and poignant issue in the veterinary profession. Veterinarians' risk of suicide is four times that of the general population and twice that of other health professionals,[79] and attitudes toward and involvement in death and euthanasia are possible influences.[463,464] One in 11 veterinarians have reported serious psychological distress, and 1 in 6 veterinarians have experienced suicidal ideation since graduating from veterinary school.[465]

Compassion fatigue is deep physical, emotional, and spiritual exhaustion that can result from working day to day in an intense caregiving environment.[466,467] The natural response to this downward spiral is to work harder until there is nothing left to give, which is counter to the adaptive response of taking a break. The symptoms are the same as those of chronic stress and are a consequence of caring for the needs of others before caring for your own needs.[466,467] Compassion fatigue results from a lack of daily self-care practices that create opportunities to reflect, refuel, and rejuvenate.

The good news is that compassion fatigue results from being a deeply caring person. When veterinarians care for themselves, they can care for others from a place of abundance, not scarcity. By developing healthy self-care routines, practitioners can continue to successfully provide compassionate care to others. This includes asking for help, using the expertise of colleagues (i.e. client service coordinators, veterinary nurses or client liaisons) to address clients' concerns, to answer out-of-hours calls, and to provide support or counseling if available to care for clients. Recognizing the signs of compassion fatigue is the first step toward positive change, and the second step is making a daily, firm commitment to choices that lead to resiliency. The American Veterinary Medical Association provides resources for veterinary well-being on their website https://www.avma.org/ProfessionalDevelopment/PeerAndWellness/Pages/default.aspx.[468]

Conclusion

Given the growing expectations of clients, the strength of the human-animal relationship, and the resultant emotional impact of cancer communication on pet caregivers and the veterinary team, relationship-centered care is integral to providing quality cancer care.[399,400,418,427,428] Compassionate cancer communication is related to significant clinical outcomes for the veterinarian, client, and patient, including enhancing client[439] and veterinarian satisfaction,[438] improving adherence to recommendations,[437] and working through emotions.[400,440] Effective techniques for cancer communication can be taught and are a series of learned skills.[409–412] Through supportive approaches, cancer communication can be made less distressing to the client, fostering client relationships and optimizing patient care while promoting professional fulfillment for the veterinarian.

References

1. Honore P, Rogers SD, Schwei MJ, et al.: Murine models of inflammatory, neuropathic and cancer pain each generates a unique set of neurochemical changes in the spinal cord and sensory neurons, *Neuroscience* 98:585–598, 2000.
2. Falk S, Dickenson AH: Pain and nociception: mechanisms of cancer-induced bone pain, *J Clin Oncol* 32:1647–1654, 2014.
3. Lam DK, Schmidt BL: Serine proteases and protease-activated receptor 2-dependent allodynia: a novel cancer pain pathway, *Pain* 149:263–272, 2010.
4. Schmidt BL: The neurobiology of cancer pain, *J Oral Maxillofac Surg* 73:S132–S135, 2015.
5. Grivennikov SI, Greten FR, Karin M: Immunity, inflammation, and cancer, *Cell* 140:883–899, 2010.
6. Yan L, Anderson GM, DeWitte M, et al.: Therapeutic potential of cytokine and chemokine antagonists in cancer therapy, *Eur J Cancer* 42:793–802, 2006.
7. Song XJ, Lamotte RH, Xie Z: Regulation of cytokines in cancer pain, *Mediators Inflamm* 2–4, 2016.
8. Descalzi G, Ikegami D, Ushijima T, et al.: Epigenetic mechanisms of chronic pain, *Trends Neurosci* 38:237–246, 2015.
9. McMahon SB, Cafferty WBJ, Marchand F: Immune and glial cell factors as pain mediators and modulators, *Exp Neurol* 192:444–462, 2005.
10. Donovan-Rodriguez T, Dickenson AH, Urch CE: Superficial dorsal horn neuronal responses and the emergence of behavioural hyperalgesia in a rat model of cancer-induced bone pain, *Neurosci Lett* 360:29–32, 2004.
11. Hald A, Nedergaard S, Hansen RR, et al.: Differential activation of spinal cord glial cells in murine models of neuropathic and cancer pain, *Eur J Pain* 13:138–145, 2009.
12. Yao M, Chang XY, Chu YX, et al.: Antiallodynic effects of propentofylline elicited by interrupting spinal glial function in a rat model of bone cancer pain, *J Neurosci Res* 89:1877–1886, 2011.
13. Wang LN, Yang JP, Zhan Y, et al.: Minocycline-induced reduction of brain-derived neurotrophic factor expression in relation to cancer-induced bone pain in rats, *J Neurosci Res* 90:672–681, 2012.
14. Hanisch UK, Kettenmann H: Microglia: active sensor and versatile effector cells in the normal and pathologic brain, *Nat Neurosci* 10:1387–1394, 2007.
15. Zhou YQ, Liu Z, Liu HQ, et al.: Targeting glia for bone cancer pain, *Expert Opin Ther Targets* 20:1365–1374, 2016.
16. Huang ZX, Lu ZJ, Ma WQ, et al.: Involvement of RVM-expressed P2X7 receptor in bone cancer pain: mechanism of descending facilitation, *Pain* 155:783–791, 2014.
17. Mogil JS: Animal models of pain: progress and challenges, *Nat Rev Neurosci* 10:283–294, 2009.
18. Dib-Hajj SD, Waxman SG: Translational pain research: lessons from genetics and genomics, *Sci Transl Med* 6;249sr4-249sr4, 2014.
19. Klinck MP, Mogil JS, Moreau M, et al.: Translational pain assessment: could natural animal models be the missing link? *Pain* 158:1633–1646, 2017.
20. Mogil JS: Laboratory environmental factors and pain behavior: the relevance of unknown unknowns to reproducibility and translation, *Lab Anim (NY)* 46:136–141, 2017.
21. Lascelles BDX: Surgical pain: pathophysiology, assessment and treatment strategies. In Tobias KMJS, editor: *Veterinary surgery small animal*, St. Louis, 2012, Elsevier, pp 237–247.
22. Brown DC, Nolan MW: Radiation therapy induced pain in dogs, *PAWS Abstr* 187, 2017.
23. Nolan MW, Long CT, Marcus KL, et al.: Nocifensive behaviors in mice with radiation-induced oral mucositis, *Radiat Res* 187:397–403, 2017.
24. Venable RO, Saba CF, Endicott MM, et al.: Dexrazoxane treatment of doxorubicin extravasation injury in four dogs, *J Am Vet Med Assoc* 240:304–307, 2012.
25. Marker BA, Barber LG, Clifford CA, et al.: Extravasation reactions associated with the administration of pamidronate: 11 cases (2008–2013), *Vet Comp Oncol* 15:470–480, 2017.
26. Bennett MI, Rayment C, Hjermstad M, et al.: Prevalence and aetiology of neuropathic pain in cancer patients: a systematic review, *Pain* 153:359–365, 2012.
27. Giglio P, Gilbert MR: Neurologic complications of cancer and its treatment, *Curr Oncol Rep* 12:50–59, 2010.
28. Peters CM, Jimenez-Andrade JM, Jonas BM, et al.: Intravenous paclitaxel administration in the rat induces a peripheral sensory neuropathy characterized by macrophage infiltration and injury to sensory neurons and their supporting cells, *Exp Neurol* 203:42–54, 2007.
29. Zhang H, Yoon SY, Zhang H, et al.: Evidence that spinal astrocytes but not microglia contribute to the pathogenesis of paclitaxel-induced painful neuropathy, *J Pain* 13:293–303, 2012.
30. Di Cesare Mannelli L, Pacini A, Bonaccini L, et al.: Morphologic features and glial activation in rat oxaliplatin-dependent neuropathic pain, *J Pain* 14:1585–1600, 2013.
31. Warwick RA, Hanani M: The contribution of satellite glial cells to chemotherapy-induced neuropathic pain, *Eur J Pain (United Kingdom)* 17:571–580, 2013.
32. Flatters SJL, Bennett GJ: Studies of peripheral sensory nerves in paclitaxel-induced painful peripheral neuropathy: evidence for mitochondrial dysfunction, *Pain* 122:245–257, 2006.
33. Joseph EK, Chen X, Bogen O, et al.: Oxaliplatin acts on IB4-positive nociceptors to induce an oxidative stress-dependent acute painful peripheral neuropathy, *J Pain* 9:463–472, 2008.
34. Xiao W, Boroujerdi A, Bennett GJ, et al.: Chemotherapy-evoked painful peripheral neuropathy: analgesic effects of gabapentin and effects on expression of the alpha-2-delta type-1 calcium channel subunit, *Neuroscience* 144:714–720, 2007.
35. Materazzi S, Fusi C, Benemei S, et al.: TRPA1 and TRPV4 mediate paclitaxel-induced peripheral neuropathy in mice via a glutathione-sensitive mechanism, *Pflugers Arch Eur J Physiol* 463:561–569, 2012.
36. Sittl R, Lampert A, Huth T, et al.: Anticancer drug oxaliplatin induces acute cooling-aggravated neuropathy via sodium channel subtype NaV1.6-resurgent and persistent current, *Proc Natl Acad Sci* 109:6704–6709, 2012.

37. Esin E, Yalcin S: Neuropathic cancer pain: what we are dealing with? how to manage it? *Onco Targets Ther* 7:599–618, 2014.

38. Hamilton TA, Cook JJ, Braund KG, Morrison WB MJ: Vincristine-induced peripheral neuropathy in a dog, *J Am Vet Med Assoc* 198:635–638, 1991.

39. Martins B de C, Martins G de C, Horta R dos S, et al.: Sensory-motor neuropathy due to vincristine treatment in a dog, *Acta Sci Vet* 42:1–4, 2014.

40. Lynch S, Savary-Bataille K, Leeuw B, et al.: Development of a questionnaire assessing health-related quality-of-life in dogs and cats with cancer, *Vet Comp Oncol* 9:172–182, 2011.

41. Hamilton MJ, Sarcornrattana O, Illiopoulou M, et al.: Questionnaire-based assessment of owner concerns and doctor responsiveness: 107 canine chemotherapy patients, *J Small Anim Pract* 53:627–633, 2012.

42. Giuffrida MA, Farrar JT, Brown DC: Psychometric properties of the Canine Symptom Assessment Scale, a multidimensional owner-reported questionnaire instrument for assessment of physical symptoms in dogs with solid tumors, *J Vet Intern Med* 251(12):1405–1414, 2014.

43. Fleming JM, Creevy KE, Promislow DEL: Mortality in North American dogs from 1984 to 2004: an investigation into age-, size-, and breed-related causes of death, *J Vet Intern Med* 25:187–198, 2011.

44. Greco MT, Roberto A, Corli O, et al.: Quality of cancer pain management: an update of a systematic review of undertreatment of patients with cancer, *J Clin Oncol* 32:4149–4154, 2014.

45. Biller B, Berg J, Garrett L, et al.: AAHA Oncology guidelines for dogs and cats, *J Am Anim Hosp Assoc* 52:181–204, 2016.

46. Arpinelli F, Bamfi F: The FDA guidance for industry on PROs: the point of view of a pharmceutical company, *Health Qual Life Outcomes* 4(1–5), 2006.

47. Apolone G, De CG, Brunetti M, et al.: Health-related quality of life (HR-QOL) and regulatory issues. An assessment of the European Agency for the Evaluation of Medicinal Products (EMEA) recommendations on the use of HR-QOL measures in drug approval, *Pharmacoeconomics* 19:187–195, 2001.

48. Muller C, Gaines B, Gruen M, et al.: Evaluation of clinical metrology instrument in dogs with osteoarthritis, *J Vet Intern Med* 30:836–846, 2016.

49. Hercock CA, Pinchbeck G, Giejda A, et al.: Validation of a client-based clinical metrology instrument for the evaluation of canine elbow osteoarthritis, *J Small Anim Pract* 50:266–271, 2009.

50. Walton MB, Cowderoy E, Lascelles D, et al.: Evaluation of construct and criterion validity for the "Liverpool osteoarthritis in dogs" (LOAD) clinical metrology instrument and comparison to two other instruments, *PLoS One* 8, 2013

51. Brown DC, Boston RC, Coyne JC, et al.: Development and psychometric testing of an instrument designed to measure chronic pain in dogs with osteoarthritis, 68:631–637, 2007.

52. Brown C: Ability of the canine brief pain inventory to detect response to treatment in dogs with osteoarthritis, *J Am Vet Med Assoc* 233:1278–1283, 2008.

53. Hielm-Björkman AK, Rita HTR: Psychometric testing of the Helsinki chronic pain index by completion of a questionnaire in Finnish by owners of dogs with chronic signs of pain caused by osteoarthritis, *Am J Vet Res* 70:727–734, 2009.

54. Benito J, DePuy V, Hardie E, et al.: Reliability and discriminatory testing of a client-based metrology instrument, feline musculoskeletal pain index (FMPI) for the evaluation of degenerative joint disease-associated pain in cats, *Vet J* 196:368–373, 2013.

55. Benito J, Hansen B, Depuy V, et al.: Feline musculoskeletal pain index: responsiveness and testing of criterion validity, *J Vet Intern Med* 27:474–482, 2013.

56. Gruen ME, Griffith E, Thomson A, et al.: Detection of clinically relevant pain relief in cats with degenerative joint disease associated pain, *J Vet Intern Med* 28:346–350, 2014.

57. Gruen ME, Griffith EH, Thomson AE, et al.: Criterion validation testing of clinical metrology instruments for measuring degenerative joint disease associated mobility impairment in cats, *PLoS One* 10:1–22, 2015.

58. Giuffrida MA, Brown DC, Ellenberg SSFJ: Development and psychometric testing of the canine owner-reported quality of life questionnaire, an instrument designed to measure quality of life in dogs with cancer, *J Am Vet Med Assoc* 252:1073–1083, 2018.

59. Mellanby RJ, ME H, JM D: Owners' assessments of their dog's quality of life during palliative chemotherapy for lymphoma, *J Small Anim Pract* 44:100–103, 2003.

60. Yazbek KVB, Fantoni DT: Validity of a health-related quality-of-life scale for dogs with signs of pain secondary to cancer, *J Am Vet Med Assoc* 226:1354–1358, 2005.

61. Tzannes S, Hammond MF, Murphy S, et al.: Owners "perception of their cats" quality of life during COP chemotherapy for lymphoma, *J Feline Med Surg* 10:73–81, 2008.

62. Brown DC, Boston R, Coyne JC, et al.: A novel approach to the use of animals in studies of pain: validation of the canine brief pain inventory in canine bone cancer, *Pain Med* 10:133–142, 2009.

63. Crawford AH, Tivers MS, Adamantos SE: Owner assessment of dogs' quality of life following treatment of neoplastic haemoperitoneum, *Vet Rec* 170:566, 2012.

64. Iliopoulou MA, Kitchell BE, Yuzbasiyan-Gurkan V: Development of a survey instrument to assess health-related quality of life in small animal cancer patients treated with chemotherapy, *J Am Vet Med Assoc* 242:1679–1687, 2013.

65. Mullan S: Assessment of quality of life in veterinary practice: developing tools for companion animal carers and veterinarians, *Vet Med Res Reports* 6:203–210, 2015.

66. Hansen BD, Lascelles BDX, Keene BW, et al.: Evaluation of an accelerometer for at-home monitoring of spontaneous activity in dogs, *Am J Vet Res* 68:468–475, 2007.

67. Lascelles BDX, Hansen BD, Roe S, et al.: Evaluation of client-specific outcome measures and activity monitoring to measure pain relief in cats with osteoarthritis, *J Vet Intern Med* 21:410–416, 2007.

68. Brown DC, Boston RC, Farrar JT: Use of an activity monitor to detect response to treatment in dogs with osteoarthritis, *J Am Vet Med Assoc* 237:66–70, 2010.

69. Wernham BGJ, Trumpatori B, Hash J, et al.: Dose reduction of meloxicam in dogs with osteoarthritis-associated pain and impaired mobility, *J Vet Intern Med* 25:1298–1305, 2011.

70. Lascelles BD, Knazovicky D, Case B, et al.: A canine-specific anti-nerve growth factor antibody alleviates pain and improves mobility and function in dogs with degenerative joint disease-associated pain, *BMC Vet Res* 11:1–12, 2015.

71. Corbee RJ, Barnier MMC, van de Lest CHA, et al.: The effect of dietary long-chain omega-3 fatty acid supplementation on owner's perception of behaviour and locomotion in cats with naturally occurring osteoarthritis, *J Anim Physiol Anim Nutr (Berl)* 97:846–853, 2013.

72. Lascelles BDX, Court MH, Hardie EM, et al.: Nonsteroidal anti-inflammatory drugs in cats: a review, *Vet Anaesth Analg* 34:228–250, 2007.

73. Gruen ME, Thomson AE, Griffith EH, et al.: A feline-specific anti-nerve growth factor antibody improves mobility in cats with degenerative joint disease-associated pain: a pilot proof of concept study, *J Vet Intern Med* 30:1138–1148, 2016.

74. Brown DC, Michel KE, Love M, et al.: Evaluation of the effect of signalment and body conformation on activity monitoring in companion dogs, *Am J Vet Res* 71:322–325, 2010.

75. Wolvers MDJ, Bussmann JBJ, Bruggeman-Everts FZ, et al.: Physical behavior profiles in chronic cancer-related fatigue, *Int J Behav Med* 25:30–37, 2018.

76. Briley JD, Williams MD, Freire M, et al.: Feasibility and repeatability of cold and mechanical quantitative sensory testing in normal dogs, *Vet J* 199:245–250, 2014.

77. Williams MD, Kirkpatrick AE, Griffith E, et al.: Feasibility and repeatability of thermal quantitative sensory testing in normal dogs and dogs with hind limb osteoarthritis-associated pain, *Vet J* 199:63–67, 2014.

78. Bergh MS, Budsberg SC: The coxib NSAIDs: potential clinical and pharmacologic importance in veterinary medicine, *J Vet Intern Med* 19:633–643, 2005.

79. Papich MG: An Update on nonsteroidal anti-inflammatory drugs (NSAIDs) in small animals, *Vet Clin North Am Small Anim Pract* 38:1243–1266, 2008.

80. Innes JF, Clayton J, Lascelles BDX: Review of the safety and efficacy of long-term NSAID use in the treatment of canine osteoarthritis, *Vet Rec* 166:226–230, 2010.

81. Kukanich B, Bidgood T, Knesl O: Clinical pharmacology of nonsteroidal anti-inflammatory drugs in dogs, *Vet Anaesth Analg* 39:69–90, 2012.

82. Belshaw Z, Asher L, Dean RS: The attitudes of owners and veterinary professionals in the United Kingdom to the risk of adverse events associated with using non-steroidal anti-inflammatory drugs (NSAIDs) to treat dogs with osteoarthritis, *Prev Vet Med* 131:121–126, 2016.

83. Duncan B, Lascelles X, McFarland JM, et al.: Guidelines for safe and effective use of NSAIDs in dogs, *Vet Ther* 6:237–251, 2005.

84. Monteiro-Steagall BP, Steagall PVM, Lascelles BDX: systematic review of nonsteroidal anti-inflammatory drug-induced adverse effects in dogs, *J Vet Intern Med* 27:1011–1019, 2013.

85. Robertson SA: Osteoarthritis in cats: what we now know about recognition and treatment, *Vet Med* 103:611–616, 2008.

86. Adrian D, Papich M, Baynes R, et al.: Chronic maladaptive pain in cats: a review of current and future drug treatment options, *Vet J* 230:52–61, 2017.

87. Hunt JR, Dean RS, Davis GND, et al.: An analysis of the relative frequencies of reported adverse events associated with NSAID administration in dogs and cats in the United Kingdom, *Vet J* 206:183–190, 2015.

88. Budsberg SC, Torres BT, Kleine SA, et al.: Lack of effectiveness of tramadol hydrochloride for the treatment of pain and joint dysfunction in dogs with chronic osteoarthritis, *J Am Vet Med Assoc* 252:427–432, 2018.

89. Nakao K, Murase A, Ohshiro H, et al.: CJ-023, 423, a novel, potent and selective prostaglandin EP4 receptor antagonist with antihyperalgesic properties, *Pharmacology* 322:686–694, 2007.

90. Okumura T, Murata Y, Taniguchi K, et al.: Effects of the selective EP4 antagonist, CJ-023,423 on chronic inflammation and bone destruction in rat adjuvant-induced arthritis, *J Pharm Pharmacol* 60:723–730, 2008.

91. Rausch-Derra LC, Rhodes L, Freshwater L, et al.: Pharmacokinetic comparison of oral tablet and suspension formulations of grapiprant, a novel therapeutic for the pain and inflammation of osteoarthritis in dogs, *J Vet Pharmacol Ther* 39:566–571, 2016.

92. Nagahisa A, Okumura T: Pharmacology of grapiprant, a novel EP4 antagonist: receptor binding, efficacy in a rodent postoperative pain model, and a dose estimation for controlling pain in dogs, *J Vet Pharmacol Ther* 40:285–292, 2017.

93. Rausch-Derra LC, Rhodes L: Safety and toxicokinetic profiles associated with daily oral administration of grapiprant, a selective antagonist of the prostaglandin E2EP4 receptor, to cats, *Am J Vet Res* 77:688–692, 2016.

94. Rozic JG, Chakraborty C, Lala PK: Cyclooxygenase inhibitors retard murine mammary tumor progression by reducing tumor cell migration, invasiveness and angiogenesis, *Int J Cancer* 93:497–506, 2001.

95. Timoshenko AV, Xu G, Chakrabarti S, et al.: Role of prostaglandin E2 receptors in migration of murine and human breast cancer cells, *Exp Cell Res* 289:265–274, 2003.

96. Timoshenko AV, Lala PK, Chakraborty C: PGE2-mediated upregulation of iNOS in murine breast cancer cells through the activation of EP4 receptors, *Int J Cancer* 108:384–389, 2004.

97. Timoshenko AV, Chakraborty C, Wagner GF, et al.: COX-2-mediated stimulation of the lymphangiogenic factor VEGF-C in human breast cancer, *Br J Cancer* 94:1154–1163, 2006.

98. Xin X, Majumder M, Girish GV, et al.: Targeting COX-2 and EP4 to control tumor growth, angiogenesis, lymphangiogenesis and metastasis to the lungs and lymph nodes in a breast cancer model, *Lab Investig* 92:1115–1128, 2012.

99. Smith HS: Potential analgesic mechanisms of acetaminophen, *Pain Physician* 12:269–280, 2009.

100. Mburu DN: Evaluation of the anti−inflammatory effects of a low dose of acetaminophen following surgery in dogs, *J Vet Pharmacol Ther* 14(109–111), 1991.

101. Klinger RY, Habib AS: Acetaminophen and ondansetron: the central serotonergic connection, *J Clin Anesth* 40:101–102, 2017.

102. Saliba SW, Marcotegui AR, Fortwängler E, et al.: AM404, paracetamol metabolite, prevents prostaglandin synthesis in activated microglia by inhibiting COX activity, *J Neuroinflammation* 14:246, 2017.

103. Pickering G, Loriot M, Libert F, Eschalier A, Beaune PDC: Analgesic effect of acetaminophen in humans: first evidence of a central serotonergic mechanism, *Clin Pharmacol Ther* 79:371–378, 2006.

104. Ottani A, Leone S, Sandrini M, et al.: The analgesic activity of paracetamol is prevented by the blockade of cannabinoid CB1 receptors, *Eur J Pharmacol* 531:280–281, 2006.

105. Mallet C, Barrière DA, Ermund A, et al.: TRPV1 in brain is involved in acetaminophen-induced antinociception, *PLoS One* 5:1–11, 2010.

106. Andersson DA, Gentry C, Alenmyr L, et al.: TRPA1 mediates spinal antinociception induced by acetaminophen and the cannabinoid Δ9-tetrahydrocannabiorcol, *Nat Commun* 2:551, 2011.

107. Mburu DN, Mbugua SW, Skoglund LA, et al.: Effects of paracetamol and acetylsalicylic acid on the post−operative course after experimental orthopaedic surgery in dogs, *J Vet Pharmacol Ther* 11:163–171, 1988.

108. Kukanich B, Papich MG: Pharmacokinetics of tramadol and the metabolite O-desmethyltramadol in dogs, *J Vet Pharmacol Ther* 27:239–246, 2004.

109. Kukanich B, Lascelles BDX, Aman AM, et al.: The effects of inhibiting cytochrome P450 3A, p-glycoprotein, and gastric acid secretion on the oral bioavailability of methadone in dogs, *J Vet Pharmacol Ther* 28:461–466, 2005.

110. Kukanich B, Lascelles BDX, Papich MG: Pharmacokinetics of morphine and plasma concentrations of morphine-6-glucuronide following morphine administration to dogs, *J Vet Pharmacol Ther* 28:371–376, 2005.

111. Kukanich B: Pharmacokinetics of acetaminophen, codeine, and the codeine metabolites morphine and codeine-6-glucuronide in healthy Greyhound dogs, *Vet Pharmacol Ther* 33:15–21, 2009.

112. Egger CM, Glerum LE, Allen SW, et al.: Plasma fentanyl concentrations in awake cats and cats undergoing anesthesia and ovariohysterectomy using transdermal administration, *Vet Anaesth Analg* 30:229–236, 2003.

113. Egger CM, Glerum L, Haag KM, et al.: Efficacy and cost-effectiveness of transdermal fentanyl patches for the relief of postoperative pain in dogs after anterior cruciate ligament and pelvic limb repair, *Vet Anaesth Analg* 34:200–208, 2007.

114. Lascelles BDX, Robertson SA, Taylor PM, et al.: Comparison of the pharmacokinetics and thermal antinociceptive pharmacodynamics of 20 μg kg-1 buprenorphine administered sublingually or intravenously in cats, *Vet Anaesth Analg* 30:99–119, 2003.

115. Dayer P, Desmeules J, Collart L: Pharmacologie du tramadol, *Drugs* 53:18–24, 1997.

116. Oliva P, Aurilio C, Massimo F, et al.: The antinociceptive effect of tramadol in the formalin test is mediated by the serotonergic component, *Eur J Pharmacol* 445:179–185, 2002.

117. Leppert W: Tramadol as an analgesic for mild to moderate cancer pain, *Pharmacol Reports* 61:978–992, 2009.

118. McMillan CJ, Livingston A, Clark CR, et al.: Pharmacokinetics of intravenous tramadol in dogs, *Can J Vet Res* 72:325–331, 2008.

119. Giorgi M, Saccomanni G, Łebkowska-Wieruszewska B, et al.: Pharmacokinetic evaluation of tramadol and its major metabolites after single oral sustained tablet administration in the dog: a pilot study, *Vet J* 180:253–255, 2009.

120. Giorgi M, Del Carlo S, Saccomanni G, et al.: Pharmacokinetics of tramadol and its major metabolites following rectal and intravenous administration in dogs, *NZ Vet J* 57:146–152, 2009.

121. Giorgi M, Del Carlo S, Saccomanni G, et al.: Pharmacokinetic and urine profile of tramadol and its major metabolites following oral immediate release capsules administration in dogs, *Vet Res Commun* 33:875–885, 2009.

122. Giorgi M, De Carlo S, Saccomanni G, et al.: Biopharmaceutical profile of tramadol in the dog, *Vet Res Commun* 33:189–192, 2009.

123. Perez TE, Mealey KL, Grubb TL, et al.: Tramadol metabolism to o-desmethyl tramadol (M1) and n-desmethyl tramadol (M2) by dog liver microsomes: species comparison and identification of responsible canine cytochrome P450s, *Drug Metab Dispos* 44:1963–1972, 2016.

124. Pypendop BH, Ilkiw JE: Pharmacokinetics of tramadol, and its metabolite O-desmethyl-tramadol, in cats, *Pharmacetical Sci* 2:52–59, 2007.

125. Pypendop BH, Siao KT, Ilkiw JE: Effects of tramadol hydrochloride on the thermal threshold in cats, *Am J Vet Res* 70:1465–1470, 2009.

126. Monteiro BP, Klinck MP, Moreau M, et al.: Analgesic efficacy of tramadol in cats with naturally occurring osteoarthritis, *PLoS One* 12:1–13, 2017.

127. Woolf CJ, Thompson SWN: The induction and maintenance of central sensitization is dependent on N-methyl-d-aspartic acid receptor activation; implications for the treatment of post-injury pain hypersensitivity states, *Pain* 44:293–299, 1991.

128. Graven-Nielsen T, Arendt-Nielsen L: Peripheral and central sensitization in musculoskeletal pain disorders: an experimental approach, *Curr Rheumatol Rep* 4:313–321, 2002.

129. Wagner AE, Walton JA, Hellyer PW, et al.: Use of low doses of ketamine administered by constant rate infusion as an adjunct for postoperative analgesia in dogs, *J Am Vet Med Assoc* 221:72–75, 2002.

130. Slingsby LS, Waterman-Pearson AE: The post-operative analgesic effects of ketamine after canine ovariohysterectomy - a comparison between pre- or post-operative administration, *Res Vet Sci* 69:147–152, 2000.

131. Eisenberg E, Pud D: Can patients with chronic neuropathic pain be cured by acute administration of the NMDA receptor antagonist amantadine? *Pain* 74:337–339, 1998.

132. Lascelles BDX, Hansen BD, Thomson A, et al.: Evaluation of a digitally integrated accelerometer-based activity monitor for the measurement of activity in cats, *Vet Anaesth Analg* 35:173–183, 2008.

133. Vernier VG, Harmon JB, Stump JM, et al.: The toxicologic and pharmacologic properties of amantadine hydrochloride, *Toxicol Appl Pharmacol* 15:642–665, 1969.

134. KuKanich B, Papich MG: Plasma profile and pharmacokinetics of dextromethorphan after intravenous and oral administration in healthy dogs, *J Vet Pharmacol Ther* 27:337–341, 2004.

135. Vollmer KO KE: Pharmacokinetics and metabolism of gabapentin in rat, dog and man, *Arzneimittelforschung* 36:830–839, 1986.

136. Radulovic LL, Türck D, von Hodenberg AL, et al.: Disposition of gabapentin (neurontin) in mice, rats, dogs, and monkeys, *Drug Metab Dispos* 23:441–448, 1995.

137. Pypendop BH, Siao KT, Ilkiw JE: Thermal antinociceptive effect of orally administered gabapentin in healthy cats, *Am J Vet Res* 71:1027–1032, 2010.

138. Siao KT, Pypendop BHIJ: Pharmacokinetics of gabapentin in cats, *Am J Vet Res* 71:817–821, 2010.

139. Platt SR, Adams V, Garosi LS, et al.: Treatment with gabapentin of 11 dogs with refractory idiopathic epilepsy, *Vet Rec* 159:881–884, 2006.

140. Verdu B, Decosterd I, Buclin T, et al.: Antidepressants for the treatment of chronic pain, *Drugs* 68:2611–2632, 2008.

141. Kautio AL, Haanpää M, Saarto TKE: Amitriptyline in the treatment of chemotherapy-induced neuropathic symptoms, *Anticancer Res* 29:2601–2606, 2008.

142. Kautio AL, Haanpää M, Leminen A, et al.: Amitriptyline in the prevention of chemotherapy-induced neuropathic symptoms, *Anticancer Res* 29:2601–2606, 2009.

143. Chew DJ, Buffington CA, Kendall MS, et al.: Amitriptyline treatment for severe recurrent idiopathic cystitis in cats, *J Am Vet Med Assoc* 213:1282–1286, 1998.

144. Cashmore RG, Harcourt-Brown TR, Freeman PM, et al.: Clinical diagnosis and treatment of suspected neuropathic pain in three dogs, *Aust Vet J* 87:45–50, 2009.

145. Norkus C, Rankin D, Kukanich B: Pharmacokinetics of intravenous and oral amitriptyline and its active metabolite nortriptyline in Greyhound dogs, *Vet Anaesth Analg* 42:580–589, 2015.

146. Challapalli V, Tremont-Lukats IW, McNicol ED, et al.: Systemic administration of local anesthetic agents to relieve neuropathic pain, *Cochrane Database Syst Rev* 4, 1996.

147. Ann Fleming J, David O' Connor B: Use of lidocain patches for neuropathic pain in a comprehensive cancer centre, *Pain Ress Manag* 14:381–388, 2009.

148. Weiland L, Croubels S, Baert K, et al.: Pharmacokinetics of a lidocaine patch 5% in dogs, *J Vet Med Ser A Physiol Pathol Clin Med* 53:34–39, 2006.

149. Ko JCH, Maxwell LK, Abbo LA, et al.: Pharmacokinetics of lidocaine following the application of 5% lidocaine patches to cats, *J Vet Pharmacol Ther* 31:359–367, 2008.

150. Ko J, Weil A, Maxwell L, Kitao THT: Plasma concentrations of lidocaine in dogs following lidocaine patch application, *J Vet Pharmacol Ther* 43:280–283, 2007.

151. Weil AB, Ko J, Inoue T: The use of lidocaine patches, *Compend Contin Educ Vet* 29: 208–210, 212, 214–216, 2007.

152. Firestein G, Paine M, Littman B: Gene expression (collagenase, tissue inhibitor of metalloproteinases, complement, and hla-dr) in rheumatoid arthritis and osteoarthritis synovium, *Arthritis Rheum* 34:1094–1105, 1991.

153. Fakih M, Johnson CS, Trump DL: Glucocorticoids and treatment of prostate cancer: a preclinical and clinical review, *Urology* 60:553–561, 2002.

154. Sibilia J: Corticosteroids and inflammation, *Rev Prat* 53:495–501, 2003.

155. Mensah-Nyagan AG, Meyer L, Schaeffer V, et al.: Evidence for a key role of steroids in the modulation of pain, *Psychoneuroendocrinology* 34, 2009

156. Melcangi RC: Neuroprotective effects of neuroactive steroids in the spinal cord and peripheral nerves, *J Mol Neurosci* 28:1–2, 2006.

157. Jones JS, Brown MD, Bermingham M, et al.: Efficacy of parenteral dexamethasone to prevent relapse after emergency department treatment of acute migraine, *Acad Emerg Med* 10:542, 2003.

158. Rowe BH, Blitz S, Coleman IEM: Dexamethasone in migraine relapse: a randomized, placebo-controlled clinical trial, *Acad Emerg Med* 13:S16, 2006.

159. Fiesseler FW, Shih R, Szucs P, et al.: Steroids for migraine headaches: a randomized double-blind, two-armed, placebo-controlled trial, *J Emerg Med* 40:463–468, 2011.

160. Wareham D: Postherpetic neuralgia, *Clin Evid* 12:1182–1193, 2004.

161. Takeda K, Sawamura S, Sekiyama H, et al.: Effects of methylprednisolone on neuropathic pain and spinal glial activation in rats, *Medscape* 100:1249–1257, 2004.

162. Maranzano E, Latini P, Beneventi S, et al.: Radiotherapy without steroids in selected metastatic spinal cord compression patients: a phase II trial, *Am J Clin Oncol* 19:179–183, 1996.

163. Serafini AN: Therapy of metastatic bone pain, *J Nucl Med* 42:895–906, 2001.
164. Patchell RA, Tibbs PA, Regine WF, et al.: Direct decompressive surgical resection in the treatment of spinal cord compression caused by metastatic cancer: a randomised trial, *Lancet* 366:643–648, 2005.
165. Chow E, Fan G, Hadi S, et al.: Symptom clusters in cancer patients with brain metastases, *Clin Oncol* 20:76–82, 2008.
166. Mantyh PW: Bone cancer pain: from mechanism to therapy, *Curr Opin Support Palliat Care* 8:83–90, 2014.
167. Sabino MAMP: Pathophysiology of bone cancer pain, *J Support Oncol* 3:15–24, 2005.
168. Jimenez-Andrade JM: Pathological sprouting of adult nociceptors in chronic prostate cancer-induced bone pain: editorial comments, *J Urol* 186:342, 2011.
169. Jimenez–Andrade JM, Mantyh WG, Bloom AP, et al.: Bone cancer pain, *Ann NY Acad Sci* 1198:173–181, 2010.
170. Fan TM, de Lorimier L-P, Charney SC, et al.: Evaluation of IV pamidronate administration in 33 cancer-bearing dogs with primary or secondary bone involvement, *J Vet Intern Med* 19:74–80, 2005.
171. Mashiba T, Turner CH, Hirano T, et al.: Effects of suppressed bone turnover by bisphosphonates on microdamage accumulation and biomechanical properties in clinically relevant skeletal sites in beagles, *Bone* 28:524–531, 2001.
172. Burr DB, Allen MR: Mandibular necrosis in beagle dogs treated with bisphosphonates, *Orthod Craniofacial Res* 12:221–228, 2009.
173. Lundberg AP, Roady PJ, Somrak AJ, et al.: Zoledronate-associated osteonecrosis of the jaw in a dog with appendicular osteosarcoma, *J Vet Intern Med* 30:1235–1240, 2016.
174. Fan TM, Lorimier LP De, Garrett LD, et al.: The bone biologic effects of zoledronate in healthy dogs and dogs with malignant osteolysis, *J Vet Intern Med* 380–387, 2008.
175. Milner RJ, Farese J, Henry CJ, et al.: Bisphosphonates and cancer, *J Vet Intern Med* 18:597–604, 2004.
176. Fan TM: Intravenous aminobisphosphonates for managing complications of malignant osteolysis in companion animals, *Top Companion Anim Med* 24:151–156, 2009.
177. Berenson J, Hirschberg R: Safety and convenience of a 15-minute infusion of zoledronic acid, *Oncologist* 9:319–329, 2004.
178. Farese JP, Ashton J, Milner R, et al.: The effect of the bisphosphonate alendronate on viability of canine osteosarcoma cells in vitro, *Vet Comp Oncol* 40:113–117, 2004.
179. Ashton JA, Farese JP, Milner RJ, et al.: Investigation of the effect of pamidronate disodium on the in vitro viability of osteosarcoma cells from dogs, *Am J Vet Res* 66:885–891, 2005.
180. Wolfe TD, Pillai SPS, Hildreth BE, et al.: Effect of zoledronic acid and amputation on bone invasion and lung metastasis of canine osteosarcoma in nude mice, *Clin Exp Metastasis* 28:377–389, 2011.
181. Piperno-Neumann S, Le Deley MC, Rédini F, et al.: Zoledronate in combination with chemotherapy and surgery to treat osteosarcoma (OS2006): a randomised, multicentre, open-label, phase 3 trial, *Lancet Oncol* 17:1070–1080, 2016.
182. Milner RJ, Dormehl I, Louw WKA, et al.: Targeted radiotherapy with Sm-153-EDTMP in nine cases of canine primary bone tumours, *J S Afr Vet Assoc* 69:12–17, 1998.
183. Barnard SM, Zuber RM, Moore AS: Samarium Sm 153 lexidronam for the palliative treatment of dogs with primary bone tumors: 35 cases (1999-2005), *J Am Vet Med Assoc* 230:1877–1881, 2007.
184. Lutz S, Balboni T, Jones J, et al.: Palliative radiation therapy for bone metastases: update of an ASTRO evidence-based guideline, *Pr Radiat Oncol* 7:4–12, 2017.
185. Bregazzi VS, LaRue SM, Powers BE, et al.: Response of feline oral squamous cell carcinoma to palliative radiation therapy, *Vet Radiol Ultrasound* 42:77–79, 2001.
186. Fidel JL, Sellon RK, Houston RK, et al.: A nine-day accelerated radiation protocol for feline squamous cell carcinoma, *Vet Radiol Ultrasound* 48:482–485, 2007.
187. Fidel J, Lyons J, Tripp C, et al.: Treatment of oral squamous cell carcinoma with accelerated radiation therapy and concomitant carboplatin in cats, *J Vet Intern Med* 25:504–510, 2011.
188. Bateman KE, Catton PA, Pennock PW, et al.: 0–7–21 radiation therapy for the treatment of canine oral melanoma, *J Vet Intern Med* 8:267–272, 1994.
189. Blackwood LDJ: Radiotherapy of oral malignant melanomas in dogs, *J Am Vet Med Assoc* 209:98–102, 1996.
190. Freeman KP, Hahn KA, Harris FD, et al.: Treatment of dogs with oral melanoma by hypofractionated radiation therapy and platinum based chemotherapy, *J Vet Intern Med* 17:96–101, 2003.
191. Proulx DR, Ruslander DM, Dodge RK, et al.: A retrospective analysis of 140 dogs with oral melanoma treated with external beam radiation, *Vet Radiol US* 44:352–359, 2003.
192. Murphy S, Hayes AM, Blackwood L, et al.: Oral malignant melanoma - the effect of coarse fractionation radiotherapy alone or with adjuvant carboplatin therapy, *Vet Comp Oncol* 3:222–229, 2005.
193. Kawabe M, Baba Y, Tamai R, et al.: Profiling of plasma metabolites in canine oral melanoma using gas chromatography-mass spectrometry, *J Vet Med Sci* 77:1025–1028, 2015.
194. Weinstein JI, Payne S, Poulson JM, et al.: Use of force plate analysis to evaluate the efficacy of external beam radiation to alleviate osteosarcoma pain, *Vet Radiol Ultrasound* 50:673–678, 2009.
195. Knapp-Hoch HM, Fidel JL, Sellon RK, et al.: An expedited palliative radiation protocol for lytic or proliferative lesions of appendicular bone in dogs, *J Am Anim Hosp Assoc* 45:24–32, 2009.
196. Green EM, Adams WM, Forrest LJ: Four fraction palliative radiotherapy for osteosarcoma in 24 dogs, *J Am Anim Hosp Assoc* 38:445–451, 2002.
197. Sonzogni-Desautels K, Knapp DW, Sartin E, et al.: Effect of cyclooxygenase inhibitors in a xenograft model of canine mammary tumours, *Vet Comp Oncol* 9:161–171, 2011.
198. Knapp DW, Henry CJ, Widmer WR, et al.: Randomized trial of cisplatin versus firocoxib versus cisplatin/firocoxib in dogs with transitional cell carcinoma of the urinary bladder, *J Vet Intern Med* 27:126–133, 2013.
199. Kleiter M, Malarkey DE, Ruslander DE, et al.: Expression of cyclooxygenase-2 in canine epithelial nasal tumors, *Vet Radiol Ultrasound* 45:255–260, 2004.
200. Flynn AK, Lurie D: Canine acute radiation dermatitis, a survey of current management practices in North America, *Vet Comp Oncol* 5:197–207, 2007.
201. Miller RC, Le-Rademacher J, Sio TTW, et al.: A phase III, randomized double-blind study of doxepin rinse versus magic mouthwash versus placebo in the treatment of acute oral mucositis pain in patients receiving head and neck radiotherapy with or without chemotherapy (Alliance A221304), *Int J Radiat Oncol* 96:938, 2016.
202. Keyerleber MA, Ferrer L: Effect of prophylactic cefalexin treatment on the development of bacterial infection in acute radiation-induced dermatitis in dogs: a blinded randomized controlled prospective clinical trial, *Vet Dermatol* 29:18–37, 2018.
203. Kopf A: Managing a chronic pain patient in the perioperative period, *J Pain Palliat Care Pharmacother* 27:394–396, 2013.
204. Reddi D: Preventing chronic postoperative pain, *Anaesthesia* 71:64–71, 2016.
205. Horne CE, Engelke MK, Schreier A, et al.: Effects of tactile desensitization on postoperative pain after amputation surgery, *J Perianesthesia Nurs* 1–10, 2017.
206. Chaparro LE, Smith SA, Moore RA, et al.: Pharmacotherapy for the prevention of chronic pain after surgery in adults, *Cochrane Database Syst Rev* 7, 2013.
207. Mathews KA, Pettifer G, Foster R, et al.: Safety and efficacy of preoperative administration of meloxicam, compared with that of ketoprofen and butorphanol in dogs undergoing abdominal surgery, *Am J Vet Res* 62:882–888, 2001.
208. Budsberg SC, Cross AR, Quandt JE, et al.: Evaluation of intravenous administration of meloxicam for perioperative pain management following stifle joint surgery in dogs, 63:1557–1563, 2002.

209. Acosta ADP, Gomar C, Correa-Natalini C, et al.: Analgesic effects of epidurally administered levogyral ketamine alone or in combination with morphine on intraoperative and postoperative pain in dogs undergoing ovariohysterectomy, *Am J Vet Res* 66:54–61, 2005.

210. Sarrau S, Jourdan J, Dupuis-Soyris F, et al.: Effects of postoperative ketamine infusion on pain control and feeding behaviour in bitches undergoing mastectomy, *J Small Anim Pract* 48:670–676, 2007.

211. Kongara K, Chambers JP, Johnson CB: Effects of tramadol, morphine or their combination in dogs undergoing ovariohysterectomy on peri-operative electroencephalographic responses and postoperative pain, *NZ Vet J* 60:129–135, 2012.

212. Kalchofner Guerrero KS, Reichler IM, Schwarz A, et al.: Alfaxalone or ketamine-medetomidine in cats undergoing ovariohysterectomy: a comparison of intra-operative parameters and post-operative pain, *Vet Anaesth Analg* 41:644–653, 2014.

213. Crociolli GC, Cassu RN, Barbero RC, et al.: Gabapentin as an adjuvant for postoperative pain management in dogs undergoing mastectomy, *J Vet Med Sci* 77:1011–1015, 2015.

214. Gutierrez-Blanco E, Victoria-Mora JM, Ibancovichi-Camarillo JA, et al.: Postoperative analgesic effects of either a constant rate infusion of fentanyl, lidocaine, ketamine, dexmedetomidine, or the combination lidocaine-ketamine-dexmedetomidine after ovariohysterectomy in dogs, *Vet Anaesth Analg* 42:309–318, 2015.

215. Culp LB, Skarda RT, Muir WW: Comparisons of the effects of acupuncture, electroacupuncture, and transcutaneous cranial electrical stimulation on the minimum alveolar concentration of isoflurane in dogs, *Am J Vet Res* 66:1364–1370, 2005.

216. Zhang RX, Li A, Liu B, et al.: Electroacupuncture attenuates bone cancer pain and inhibits spinal interleukin-1β expression in a rat model, *Anesth Analg* 105:1482–1488, 2007.

217. Zhang RX, Li A, Liu B, et al.: Electroacupuncture attenuates bone cancer-induced hyperalgesia and inhibits spinal preprodynorphin expression in a rat model, *Eur J Pain* 12:870–878, 2008.

218. Mantyh PW: Neurobiology of substance P and the NK1 receptor, *J Clin Psychiatry* 63:6–10, 2002.

219. Wiley RGLDA: Targeted toxins in pain, *Adv Drug Deliv Rev* 55:1043–1054, 2003.

220. Wiley RG, Kline IVRH, Vierck CJ: Anti-nociceptive effects of selectively destroying substance P receptor-expressing dorsal horn neurons using [Sar9,Met(O2)11]-substance P-saporin: behavioral and anatomical analyses, *Neuroscience* 146:1333–1345, 2007.

221. Wiley RG: Substance P receptor-expressing dorsal horn neurons: lessons from the targeted cytotoxin, substance P-saporin, *Pain* 136:7–10, 2008.

222. Allen JW, Horais KA, Tozier NA, et al.: Intrathecal substance P-saporin selectively lesions NK-1 receptor bearing neurons in dogs, *J Pain* 3:51, 2002.

223. Brown DC, Agnello K, Iadarola MJ: Intrathecal resiniferatoxin in a dog model: efficacy in bone cancer pain, *Pain* 156:1018–1024, 2015.

224. Nymeyer H, Lappi DA, Higgins D, et al.: Substance P–saporin for the treatment of intractable pain. In Grawunder UBS, editor: *milestones in drug therapy*, Cham, 2017, Springer, pp 107–130.

225. Huang ZJ, Li HC, Cowan AA, et al.: Chronic compression or acute dissociation of dorsal root ganglion induces cAMP-dependent neuronal hyperexcitability through activation of PAR2, *Pain* 153:1426–1437, 2012.

226. Serrano A, Paré M, McIntosh F, et al.: Blocking spinal CCR2 with AZ889 reversed hyperalgesia in a model of neuropathic pain, *Mol Pain* 6:1–14, 2010.

227. Stevens R, Hanson P, Wei N, et al.: Safety and tolerability of CNTX-4975 in subjects with chronic, moderate to severe knee pain associated with osteoarthritis: a pilot study, *J Pain* 18:S70, 2017.

228. Karai L, Brown DC, Mannes AJ, et al.: Deletion of vanilloid receptor 1–expressing primary afferent neurons for pain control, *J Clin Invest* 113:1344–1352, 2004.

229. Brown DC, Iadarola MJ, Perkowski SZ, et al.: Physiologic and antinociceptive effects of intrathecal resiniferatoxin in a canine bone cancer model, *Anesthesiology* 103:1052–1059, 2005.

230. Brown DC, Agnello K: Intrathecal substance P-saporin in the dog: efficacy in bone cancer pain, *Anesthesiology* 19:1178–1185, 2013.

231. Sapio MR, Neubert JK, Lapaglia DM, et al.: Pain control through selective chemo-axotomy of centrally projecting TRPV1+ sensory neurons, *J Clin Invest* 128:1657–1670, 2018.

232. Lewin GR, Ritter AM, Mendell LM: Nerve growth factor-induced hyperalgesia in the neonatal and adult rat, *J Neurosci* 13:2136–2148, 1993.

233. Lane NE, Schnitzer TJ, Birbara CA, et al.: Tanezumab for the treatment of pain from osteoarthritis of the knee, *N Engl J Med* 363:1521–1531, 2010.

234. Sanga P, Katz N, Polverejan E, et al.: Efficacy, safety, and tolerability of fulranumab, an anti-nerve growth factor antibody, in the treatment of patients with moderate to severe osteoarthritis pain, *Pain* 154:1910–1919, 2013.

235. Bannwarth B, Kostine M: Biologics in the treatment of chronic pain: a new era of therapy? *Clin Pharmacol Ther* 97:122–124, 2015.

236. Malfait AM, Miller RJ: Emerging targets for the management of osteoarthritis pain, *Curr Osteoporos Rep* 14:260–268, 2016.

237. Malik-Hall M, Dina OA, Levine JD: Primary afferent nociceptor mechanisms mediating NGF-induced mechanical hyperalgesia, *Eur J Neurosci* 21:3387–3394, 2005.

238. Cirillo G, Cavaliere C, Bianco MR, et al.: Intrathecal NGF administration reduces reactive astrocytosis and changes neurotrophin receptors expression pattern in a rat model of neuropathic pain, *Cell Mol Neurobiol* 30:51–62, 2010.

239. Eibl JK, Strasser BC, Ross GM: Structural, biological, and pharmacological strategies for the inhibition of nerve growth factor, *Neurochem Int* 61:1266–1275, 2012.

240. Schnitzer TJ, Marks JA: A systematic review of the efficacy and general safety of antibodies to NGF in the treatment of osteoarthritis of the hip or knee, *Osteoarthr Cartil* 23:S8–S17, 2015.

241. Kryger GS, Kryger Z, Zhang F, et al.: Nerve growth factor inhibition prevents traumatic neuroma formation in the rat, *J Hand Surg Am* 26:635–644, 2001.

242. Jimenez-Andrade JM, Ghilardi JR, Castañeda-Corral G, et al.: Preventive or late administration of anti-NGF therapy attenuates tumor-induced nerve sprouting, neuroma formation, and cancer pain, *Pain* 152:2564–2574, 2011.

243. Miller RE, Block JA, Malfait AM: Nerve growth factor blockade for the management of osteoarthritis pain, *Curr Opin Rheumatol* 29:110–118, 2017.

244. Schnitzer TJ, Ekman EF, Spierings ELH, et al.: Efficacy and safety of tanezumab monotherapy or combined with non-steroidal anti-inflammatory drugs in the treatment of knee or hip osteoarthritis pain, *Ann Rheum Dis* 74:1202–1211, 2015.

245. Shor S, Fadl-Alla BA, Pondenis HC, et al.: Expression of nociceptive ligands in canine osteosarcoma, *J Vet Intern Med* 29:268–275, 2015.

246. Koppenol WH, Bounds PL, Dang CV: Otto Warburg's contributions to current concepts of cancer metabolism, *Nat Rev* 11:325–337, 2011.

247. Cairns RA, Harris IS, Mak TW: Regulation of cancer cell metabolism, *Nat Rev* 11:85–95, 2011.

248. Walenta S, Schroeder T, Mueller-Klieser W: Lactate in solid malignant tumors: potential basis of a metabolic classification in clinical oncology, *Curr Med Chem* 11:2195–2204, 2004.

249. Vaupel P: Metabolic microenvironment of tumor cells: a key factor in malignant progression, *Exp Oncol* 32:125–127, 2010.

250. Ogilvie GK, Vail DM: Nutrition and cancer - recent developments, *Vet Clin North Am Small Anim Pract* 20:969–985, 1990.

251. Ogilvie GK, Vail DM, Wheeler SL, et al.: Effects of chemotherapy and remission on carbohydrate metabolism in dogs with lymphoma, *Cancer* 69:233–238, 1992.

252. Ogilvie GK, Walters LM, Fettman MJ, et al.: Energy expenditure in dogs with lymphoma fed two specialized diets, *Cancer* 71:3146–3152, 1993.

253. Ogilvie GK, Walters LM, Salman MD, et al.: Resting energy expenditure in dogs with nonhematopoietic malignancies before and after excision of tumors, *Am J Vet Res* 57:1463–1467, 1996.

254. Mazzaferro EM, Hackett TB, Stein TP, et al.: Metabolic alterations in dogs with osteosarcoma, *Am J Vet Res* 62:1234–1239, 2001.

255. Ogilvie GK, Walters L, Salman MD, et al.: Alterations in carbohydrate metabolism in dogs with non hematopoietic malignancies, *Am J Vet Res* 58:277–2281, 1997.

256. Vail DM, Ogilvie GK, Wheeler SL, et al.: Alterations in carbohydrate metabolism in canine lymphoma, *J Vet Int Med* 4:8–11, 1990.

257. Ogilvie GK, Fettman MJ, Mallinckrodt CH, et al.: Effect of fish oil, arginine, and doxorubicin chemotherapy on remission and survival time for dogs with lymphoma: a double-blind, randomized placebo-controlled study, *Cancer* 88:1916–1928, 2000.

258. Ogilvie GK, Ford RB, Vail DM, et al.: Alterations in lipoprotein profiles in dogs with lymphoma, *J Vet Intern Med* 8:62–66, 1994.

259. Ackerman BH, Kasbekar N: Disturbances of taste and smell induced by drugs, *Pharmacotherapy* 17:482–496, 1997.

260. Weeth LP, Fascetti AJ, Kass PH, et al.: Prevalence of obese dogs in a population of dogs with cancer, *Am J Vet Res* 68:389–398, 2007.

261. Tisdale MJ: Are tumoral factors responsible for host tissue wasting in cancer cachexia? *Future Oncol* 6:503–513, 2010.

262. Penna F, Minero VG, Costamagna D, et al.: Anti-cytokine strategies for the treatment of cancer-related anorexia and cachexia, *Expert Opin Biol Ther* 10:1241–1250, 2010.

263. Seruga B, Zhang H, Bernstein LJ, et al.: Cytokines and their relationship to the symptoms and outcome of cancer, *Nat Rev Cancer* 8:887–899, 2008.

264. Pajak B, Orzechowska S, Pijet B, et al.: Crossroads of cytokine signaling--the chase to stop muscle cachexia, *J Physiol Pharmacol* 59(Suppl 9):251–264, 2008.

265. Fearon KC: Cancer cachexia and fat-muscle physiology, *N Engl J Med* 365:565–567, 2011.

266. Merlo A, Rezende BC, Franchini ML, et al.: Serum C-reactive protein concentrations in dogs with multicentric lymphoma undergoing chemotherapy, *J Am Vet Med Assoc* 230:522–526, 2007.

267. Tecles F, Caldín M, Zanella A, et al.: Serum acute phase protein concentrations in female dogs with mammary tumors, *J Vet Diagn Invest* 21:214–219, 2009.

268. Baez JL, Michel KE, Sorenmo K, Shofer FS: A prospective investigation of the prevalence and prognostic significance of weight loss and changes in body condition in feline cancer patients, *J Feline Med Surg* 9:411–417, 2007.

269. Caccialanza R, Cereda E, De Lorenzo F, Farina G, Pedrazzoli P, AIOM-SINPE-FAVO Working Group: To fast, or not to fast before chemotherapy, that is the question, *BMC Cancer* 18:337, 2018.

270. Simone BA, Palagani A, Strickland K, et al.: Caloric restriction counteracts chemotherapy-induced inflammation and increases response to therapy in a triple negative breast cancer model, *Cell Cycle* 7:1536–1544, 2018.

271. Wolin KY, Carson K, Colditz GA: Obesity and cancer, *Oncologist* 15:556–565, 2010.

272. Roberts DL, Dive C, Renehan AG: Biological mechanisms linking obesity and cancer risk: new perspectives, *Ann Rev Med* 61:301–316, 2010.

273. Calle EE, Rodriguez C, Walker-Thurmond K, et al.: Overweight, obesity, and mortality from cancer in a prospectively studied cohort of U.S. adults, *N Eng J Med* 348:1625–1638, 2003.

274. Lichtman MA: Obesity and the risk for a hematological malignancy: leukemia, lymphoma, or myeloma, *Oncologist* 15:1083–1101, 2010.

275. de Boer EJ, Slimani N, van 't Veer P, et al.: The European Food Consumption Validation Project: conclusions and recommendations, *Eur J Clin Nutr* 65(Suppl 1):S102–S107, 2011.

276. Jansen RJ, Robinson DP, Stolzenberg-Solomon RZ, et al.: Fruit and vegetable consumption is inversely associated with having pancreatic cancer, *Cancer Causes Control* 22:1613–1625, 2011.

277. Magalhães B, Peleteiro B, Lunet N: Dietary patterns and colorectal cancer: systematic review and meta-analysis, *Eur J Cancer Prev* 21:15–23, 2012.

278. Sonnenschein EG, Glickman LT, Goldschmidt MH, et al.: Body conformation, diet, and risk of breast cancer in pet dogs: a case-control study, *Am J Epidemiol* 133:694–703, 1991.

279. Shofer FS, Sonnenschein EG, Goldschmidt MH, et al.: Histopathologic and dietary prognostic factors for canine mammary carcinoma, *Breast Cancer Res Treat* 13:49–60, 1989.

280. Pérez Alenza D, Rutteman GR, Peña L, et al.: Relation between habitual diet and canine mammary tumors in a case-control study, *J Vet Intern Med* 12:132–139, 1998.

281. Raghavan M, Knapp DW, Bonney PL, et al.: Evaluation of the effect of dietary vegetable consumption on reducing risk of transitional cell carcinoma of the urinary bladder in Scottish Terriers, *J Am Vet Med Assoc* 227:94–100, 2005.

282. Dennart G, Zwahlen M, Vinceti M, et al.: Selenium for preventing cancer, *Cochrane Database Syst Rev* 11:CD005195, 2011.

283. Wu K, Erdman JW, Schwartz SJ: Plasma and dietary carotenoids, and the risk of prostate cancer: a nested case-control study, *Cancer Epidemiol Biomarkers Prev* 13:260–269, 2004.

284. Bendich A: From 1989 to 2001: what have we learned about the "biological actions of beta-carotene"? *J Nutr* 134:225S–230S, 2004.

285. Cooper DA: Carotenoids in health and disease: recent scientific evaluations, research recommendations and the consumer, *J Nutr* 134:221S–224S, 2004.

286. Deeb KK, Trump DL, Johnson CS: Vitamin D signaling pathways in cancer: potential for anticancer therapeutics, *Nature Rev Canc* 7:684–700, 2007.

287. Abbas S, Linseisen J, Slanger T, et al.: Serum 25- hydroxyvitamin D and risk of post-menopausal breast cancer-results of a large case-control study, *Carcinogenesis* 29:93–99, 2007.

288. Yin L, Grandi N, Raum E, et al.: Meta-analysis: longitudinal studies of serum vitamin D and colorectal cancer risk, *Aliment Pharmacol Ther* 30:113–125, 2009.

289. How KL, Hazewinkel HA, Mol JA: Dietary vitamin D dependence of cat and dog due to inadequate cutaneous synthesis of vitamin D, *Gen Comp Endocrinol* 96:12–18, 1994.

290. Wakshlag JJ, Rassnick KM, Malone EK, et al.: Cross sectional study to investigate the association between serum vitamin D and cutaneous mast cell tumours in Labrador retrievers, *Br J Nutr* 106:S60–S63, 2011.

291. Selting KA, Sharp CR, Ringold R, et al.: Serum 25-hydroxyvitamin D concentrations in dogs - correlation with health and cancer risk, *Vet Comp Oncol* 14:295–305, 2016.

292. Binkley N, Carter GD: Toward clarity in clinical vitamin D status assessment: 25(OH)D assay standardization, *Endocrinol Metab Clin North Am* 46:885–899, 2017.

293. Sempos CT, Heijboer AC, Bikle DD, et al.: Vitamin D assays and the definition of hypovitaminosis D: results from the First International Conference on Controversies in Vitamin D, *Br J Clin Pharmacol* 84:2194–2207, 2018.

294. Young LR, Backus RC: Oral vitamin D supplementation at five times the recommended allowance marginally affects serum 25-hydroxyvitamin D concentrations in dogs, *J Nutr Sci* 5:e31, 2016.

295. Lund EM, Armstrong PJ, Kirk CA, et al.: Prevalence and risk factors for obesity in adult cats from private US veterinary practices, *Int J Appl Res Vet Med* 3:88–96, 2005.

296. Lund EM, Armstrong PJ, Kirk CA, et al.: Prevalence and risk factors for obesity in adult dogs from private US veterinary practices, *Int J Appl Res Vet Med* 4:177–186, 2006.

297. Inui A: Cancer anorexia-cachexia syndrome: current issues in research and management, *CA Cancer J Clin* 52:72–91, 2002.

298. de Fornel-Thibaud P, Blanchard G, Escoffier-Chateau L, et al.: Unusual case of osteopenia associated with nutritional calcium and vitamin D deficiency in an adult dog, *J Am Anim Hosp Assoc* 43:52–60, 2007.

299. Taylor MB, Geiger DA, Saker KE, et al.: Diffuse osteopenia and myelopathy in a puppy fed a diet composed of an organic premix and raw ground beef, *J Am Vet Med Assoc* 234:1041–1048, 2009.

300. Michel KE, Sorenmo K, Shofer FS: Evaluation of body condition and weight loss in dogs presented to a veterinary oncology service, *J Vet Intern Med* 18:692–695, 2004.

301. Kienzle E: Energy. In Beitz DC, editor: *National Research Council nutrient requirements of dogs and cats*, ed 1, Washington DC, 2006, National Academies Press, pp 28–48.

302. Remillard RL, Saker KE: Critical care nutrition and enteral-assisted feeding. In Hand MS, Thatcher CD, Remillard RL, et al.: *Small animal clinical nutrition*, ed 5, Topeka, 2010, Mark Morris Institute, pp 441–476.

303. Delaney SJ: Management of anorexia in dogs and cats, *Vet Clin North Am Small Anim Pract* 36:1243–1249, 2006.

304. Fox CB, Treadway AK, Blaszczyk AT, et al.: Megestrol acetate and mirtazapine for the treatment of unplanned weight loss in the elderly, *Pharmacotherapy* 29:383–397, 2009.

305. Zollers B, Wofford JA, Heinen E, et al.: A prospective, randomized, masked, placebo-controlled clinical study of capromorelin in dogs with reduced appetite, *J Vet Intern Med* 30:1851–1857, 2016.

306. Quimby JM, Lunn KF: Mirtazapine as an appetite stimulant and anti-emetic in cats with chronic kidney disease: a masked placebo-controlled crossover clinical trial, *Vet J* 197:651–655, 2013.

307. Long JP, Greco SC: The effect of propofol administered intravenously on appetite stimulation in dogs, *Contemp Top Lab Anim Sci* 39:43–46, 2000.

308. Salinardi BJ, Harkin KR, Bulmer BJ, et al.: Comparison of complications of percutaneous endoscopic versus surgically placed gastrostomy tubes in 42 dogs and 52 cats, *J Am Anim Hosp Assoc* 42:51–56, 2006.

309. Yoshimoto SK, Marks SL, Struble AL, et al.: Owner experiences and complications with home use of a replacement low profile gastrostomy device for long-term enteral feeding in dogs, *Can Vet J* 47:144–150, 2006.

310. Hill RC: Physical activity and environment. In Beitz DC, editor: *National Research Council nutrient requirements of dogs and cats*, ed 1, Washington DC, 2006, National Academies Press, pp 258–312.

311. Wakshlag JJ: Nutritional management of megaesophagus, *Clin Brief* Aug 59–62, 2009.

312. Chandler ML, Payne-James JJ: Prospective evaluation of a peripherally administered three-in-one parenteral nutrition product in dogs, *J Am An Hosp Assoc* 47:518–523, 2006.

313. Chan DL, Freeman LM, Labata MA, et al.: Retrospective evaluation of partial parenteral nutrition in dogs and cats, *J Vet Int Med* 16:440–445, 2002.

314. Pyle SC, Marks SL, Kass PH: Evaluation of complications and prognostic factors associated with administration of total parenteral nutrition in cats: 75 cases (1994-2001), *J Am Vet Med Assoc* 225:242–250, 2004.

315. Crabb SE, Freeman LM, Chan DL, et al.: Retrospective evaluation of total parenteral nutrition in cats: 40 cases (1991-2003), *J Vet Emer Crit Care* 16:S1–S26, 2006.

316. Lippert AC, Fulton RB, Parr RB: A retrospective study of the use of total parenteral nutrition in dogs and cats, *J Vet Int Med* 7:52–64, 1993.

317. Queau Y, Larsen JA, Kass PH, et al.: Factors associated with adverse outcomes during parenteral nutrition administration in dogs and cats, *J Vet Intern Med* 25:446–452, 2011.

318. Qin HL, Su ZD, Hu LG, et al.: Effect of early intrajejunal nutrition on pancreatic pathological features and gut barrier function in dogs with acute pancreatitis, *Clin Nutr* 21:469–472, 2002.

319. Chan DL: Parenteral nutritional support. In Ettinger SL, Feldman EC, editors: *Textbook of veterinary internal medicine*, ed 6, St. Louis, 2005, Elsevier Saunders, pp 586–591.

320. Remillard RL, Saker KE: Critical care nutrition and enteral-assisted feeding. In Hand MS, Thatcher CD, Remillard RL, et al.: *Small animal clinical nutrition*, ed 5, Topeka, 2010, Mark Morris Institute, pp 477–491.

321. Wakshlag J, Schoeffler GL, Russell DS, et al.: Extravasation injury associated with parenteral nutrition in a cat with presumptive gastrinomas, *J Vet Emerg Crit Care* 21:375–381, 2011.

322. Mauldin GE, Reynolds AJ, Mauldin GN, et al.: Nitrogen balance in clinically normal dogs receiving parenteral nutrition solutions, *Am J Vet Res* 62:912–920, 2001.

323. ASPEN Board of Directors and the Clinical Guidelines Task Force: Guidelines for the use of parenteral and enteral nutrition in adult and pediatric patients, *JPEN J Parenter Enteral Nutr* 26(Suppl 1):1SA–138SA, 2002.

324. Gogos CA, Kalfarentzos F: Total parenteral nutrition and immune system activity: a review, *Nutrition* 11:339–344, 1995.

325. Kitchell CC, Balogh K: Pulmonary lipid emboli in association with long-term hyperalimentation, *Hum Pathol* 17:83–85, 1986.

326. Thomovsky EJ, Backus RC, Mann FA, et al.: Effects of temperature and handling conditions on lipid emulsion stability in veterinary parenteral nutrition admixed during simulated intravenous administration, *Am J Vet Res* 69:652–658, 2008.

327. Martin GJ, Rand JS: Food intake and blood glucose in normal and diabetic cats fed ad libitum, *J Feline Med Surg* 1:241–251, 1999.

328. Ho VW, Leung K, Hsu A, et al.: A low carbohydrate, high protein diet slows tumor growth and prevents cancer initiation, *Cancer Res* 71:4484–4493, 2011.

329. Nguyen P, Lerray V, Dumon H, et al.: High protein intake affects lean body mass but not energy expenditure in nonobese neutered cats, *J Nutr* 134:2084S–2086S, 2004.

330. Hannah SS, LaFlamme DP: Effect of dietary protein on nitrogen balance and lean body mass in cats, *Vet Clin Nutr* 3:30, 1996.

331. Burns RA, Milner JA: Effects of arginine on the carcinogenicity of 7,12-dimethylbenz(a)-anthracene and N-methyl-N-nitrosurea, *Carcinogenesis* 5:1539–1542, 1984.

332. Brittenden J, Heys SD, Ross J, et al.: Natural cytotoxicity in breast cancer patients receiving neoadjuvant chemotherapy: effects of L-arginine supplementation, *Eur J Surg Onc* 20:467–472, 1994.

333. Reynolds JV, Daly JM, Shou J, et al.: Immunologic effects of arginine supplementation in tumor-bearing and non-tumor-bearing hosts, *Ann Surg* 211:202–210, 1990.

334. Wakshlag JJ, Kallfelz FA, Wakshlag RR, et al.: The effects of branched-chain amino acids on canine neoplastic cell proliferation and death, *J Nutr* 136:2007S–2010S, 2006.

335. Kaufmann Y, Kornbluth J, Feng Z, et al.: Effect of glutamine on the initiation and promotion phases of DMBA-induced mammary tumor development, *J Parenter Enteral Nutr* 27:411–418, 2003.

336. Yoshida S, Kaibara A, Ishibashi N, et al.: Glutamine supplementation in cancer patients, *J Nutr* 17:766–768, 2001.

337. Wigmore SJ, Barber MD, Ross JA, et al.: Effect of oral eicosapentaenoic acid on weight loss in patients with pancreatic cancer, *Nutr Cancer* 36:177–184, 2000.

338. Togni V, Ota CC, Folador A, et al.: Cancer cachexia and tumor growth reduction in Walker 256 tumor-bearing rats supplemented with N-3 polyunsaturated fatty acids for one generation, *Nutr Cancer* 46:52–58, 2003.

339. Fearon KC, Von Meyenfeldt MF, Moses AG, et al.: Effect of a protein and energy dense N-3 fatty acid enriched oral supplement on loss of weight and lean tissue in cancer cachexia: a randomized double blind trial, *Gut* 52:1479–1486, 2003.

340. Colas S, Paon L, Denis F, et al.: Enhanced radiosensitivity of rat autochthonous mammary tumors by dietary docosahexaenoic acid, *Int J Cancer* 109:449–454, 2004.

341. Senzaki H, Iwamoto S, Ogura E, et al.: Dietary effects of fatty acids on growth and metastasis of KPL-1 human breast cancer cells in vivo and in vitro, *Anticancer Res* 18:1621–1627, 1998.

342. Noguchi M, Earashi M, Minami M, et al.: Effects of eicosapentaenoic and docosahexaenoic acid on cell growth and prostaglandin

E and leukotriene B production by a human breast cancer cell line (MDA-MB-231), *Oncology* 52:458–464, 1995.

343. Hawcroft G, Loadman PM, Belluzzi A, et al.: Effect of eicosapentaenoic acid on E-type prostaglandin synthesis and EP4 receptor signaling in human colorectal cancer cells, *Neoplasia* 12:618–627, 2010.

344. Hayashi T, Nishiyama K, Shirahama T: Inhibition of 5-lipoxygenase pathway suppresses the growth of bladder cancer cells, *Int J Urol* 13:1086–1091, 2006.

345. Schley PD, Brindley DN, Field CJ: (n-3) PUFA alter raft lipid composition and decrease epidermal growth factor receptor levels in lipid rafts of human breast cancer cells, *J Nutr* 137:548–553, 2007.

346. Furstenberger G, Krieg P, Muller-Decker K, et al.: What are cyclooxygenases and lipoxygenases doing in the driver's seat of carcinogenesis, *Int J Cancer* 119:2247–2254, 2006.

347. Mohammed SI, Bennett PF, Craig BA, et al.: Effects of the cyclooxygenase inhibitor, piroxicam, on tumor response, apoptosis and angiogenesis in a canine model of human invasive urinary bladder cancer, *Cancer Res* 62:356–358, 2002.

348. McMillan SK, Boria P, Moore GE, et al.: Antitumor effects of deracoxib treatment in 26 dogs with transitional cell carcinoma of the urinary bladder, *J Am Vet Med Assoc* 239:1084–1089, 2011.

349. Hanahan D, Weinberg RA: Hallmarks of cancer: the next generation, *Cell* 144:646–674, 2011.

350. Weylandt KH, Krause LF, Gomolka B, et al.: Suppressed liver tumorigenesis in fat-1 mice with elevated omega-3 fatty acids is associated with increased omega-3 derived lipid mediators and reduced TNF-α, *Carcinogenesis* 32:897–903, 2011.

351. Endres S, Ghorbani R, Kelley VE, et al.: The Effect of dietary supplementation with n-3 polyunsaturated fatty acids on the synthesis of interleukin-1 and tumor necrosis factor by mononuclear cells, *N Engl J Med* 320:265–271, 1989.

352. Purasiri P, Murray A, Richardson S, et al.: Modulation of cytokine production in vivo by dietary essential fatty acids in patients with colorectal cancer, *Clin Sci* 87:711–717, 1994.

353. Dewey A, Baughan C, Dean T, et al.: Eicosapentaenoic acid (EPA, an omega-3 fatty acid from fish oils) for the treatment of cancer cachexia, *Cochrane Database Syst Rev* 24:CD004597, 2007.

354. Saker KE, Eddy AL, Thatcher CD, et al.: Manipulation of dietary (n-6) and (n-3) fatty acids alters platelet function in cats, *J Nutr* 128:2645s–2647s, 1998.

355. Freeman LM, Rush JE, Kehayias JJ, et al.: Nutritional alterations and the effect of fish oil supplementation in dogs with heart failure, *J Vet Intern Med* 12:440–448, 1998.

356. Freeman LM, Rush JE: Cardiovascular diseases: nutritional modulation. In Pibot P, Ellliot D, Biourge V, editors: *Encyclopedia of canine clinical nutrition*, ed 1, Paris, 2006, Aniwa SAS, pp 316–347.

357. Kikawa KD, Herrick JS, Tateo RE, et al.: Induced oxidative stress and cell death in the A549 lung adenocarcinoma cell line by ionizing radiation is enhanced by supplementation with docosahexaenoic acid, *Nutr Cancer* 62:1017–1024, 2010.

358. Hopewell JW, van den Aardweg GJ, et al.: Amelioration of both early and late radiation-induced damage to pig skin by essential fatty acids, *Int J Radiat Oncol Biol Phys* 30:1119–1125, 1994.

359. Fulan H, Changxing J, Baina WY, et al.: Retinol, vitamins A, C, and E and breast cancer risk: a meta-analysis and meta-regression, *Cancer Causes Control* 22:1383–1396, 2011.

360. Arain MA, Abdul Qadeer A: Systematic review on "vitamin E and prevention of colorectal cancer", *Pak J Pharm Sci* 23:125–130, 2010.

361. Paik J, Blaner WS, Sommer KM, et al.: Retinoids, retinoic acid receptors, and breast cancer, *Cancer Invest* 21:304–312, 2003.

362. Tang XH, Gudas LJ: Retinoids, retinoic acid receptors, and cancer, *Annu Rev Pathol* 6:345–364, 2011.

363. Bushue N, Wan YJ: Retinoid pathway and cancer therapeutics, *Adv Drug Deliv Rev* 62:1285–1298, 2010.

364. Hayes KC: Nutritional problems in cats: taurine deficiency and vitamin A excess, *Can Vet J* 23:2–5, 1982.

365. Rassnick KM, Muindi JR, Johnson CS, et al.: Oral bioavailability of DN101, a concentrated formulation of calcitriol, in tumor-bearing dogs, *Cancer Chemother Pharmacol* 67:165–171, 2011.

366. Malone EK, Rassnick KM, Wakshlag JJ, et al.: Calcitriol enhances mast cell tumour chemotherapy and receptor tyrosine kinase inhibitor activity in-vitro and has single agent activity against spontaneously occurring canine mast cell tumours, *Vet Comp Oncol* 8:209–220, 2010.

367. Nelson MA, Porterfield BW, Jacobs ET, et al.: Selenium and prostate cancer prevention, *Semin Urol Oncol* 17:91–96, 1999.

368. Reid ME, Duffield-Lillico AJ, Garland L, et al.: Selenium supplementation and lung cancer incidence: an update of the nutritional prevention of cancer trial, *Cancer Epidemiol Biomarkers Prev* 11:1285–1291, 2002.

369. Duffield-Lillico AJ, Dalkin BL, Reid ME, et al.: Selenium supplementation, baseline plasma selenium status and incidence of prostate cancer: an analysis of the complete treatment period of the Nutritional Prevention of Cancer Trial, *BJU Int* 91:608–612, 2003.

370. Clark LC, Comb Jr GF, Turnbull BW, et al.: Effects of selenium supplementation for cancer prevention in patients with carcinoma of the skin. A randomized controlled trial. Nutritional Prevention of Cancer Study Group, *J Am Med Aassoc* 276:1957–1963, 1996.

371. Xiao SD, Meng XJ, Shi Y, et al.: Interventional study of high dose folic acid in gastric carcinogenesis in beagles, *Gut* 50:61–64, 2002.

372. Jhaveri MS, Wagner C, Trepel JB: Impacts of extracellular folate levels on global gene expression, *Mol Pharmacol* 60:1288–1295, 2001.

373. Friso S, Choi SW: The potential cocarcinogenic effect of vitamin B12 deficiency, *Clin Chem Lab Med* 43:1158–1163, 2005.

374. Lana SE, Kogan LR, Crump KA, et al.: The use of complementary and alternative therapies in dogs and cats with cancer, *J Am An Hosp Assoc* 42:361–365, 2006.

375. Rajagopaul S, Parr JM, Woods JP, et al.: Owners' attitudes and practices regarding nutrition of dogs diagnosed with cancer presenting at a referral oncology service in Ontario, Canada, *J Small Anim Pract* 57:484–490, 2016.

376. Seifried HE, McDonald SS, Anderson DE, et al.: The antioxidant conundrum in cancer, *Cancer Res* 63:4295–4298, 2003.

377. Szczubial M, Kankofer M, Lopuszynski W, et al.: Oxidative stress parameters in bitches with mammary gland tumors, *J Vet Med* 51:336–340, 2004.

378. Winter JL, Barber LG, Freeman TM, et al.: Antioxidant status and biomarkers of oxidative stress in dogs with lymphoma, *J Vet Int Med* 23:311–316, 2009.

379. Chandhok D, Saha T: Redox regulation in cancer: a double-edged sword with therapeutic potential, *Oxid Med Cell Longev* 3:23–34, 2010.

380. Zhao CR, Gao ZH, Qu XJ: Nrf2-ARE signaling pathway and natural products for cancer chemoprevention, *Cancer Epidemiol* 34:523–533, 2010.

381. Crozier A, Jaganath IB, Clifford MN: Dietary phenolics: chemistry, bioavailability and the effects on health, *Nat Prod Rep* 26:1001–1043, 2009.

382. Khan N, Afaq F, Mukhtar H: Cancer chemoprevention through dietary antioxidants: progress and promise, *Antioxidants Redox Signal* 10:1–36, 2008.

383. Shanmugam MK, Kannaiyan R, Sethi G: Targeting cell signaling and apoptotic pathways by dietary agents: role in the prevention and treatment of cancer, *Nutr Cancer* 63:161–173, 2011.

384. Wakshlag JJ, Balkman CA, Morgan SK, et al.: Evaluation of the protective effects of all-trans-astaxanthin on canine osteosarcoma cell lines, *Am J Vet Res* 71:89–96, 2010.

385. Wakshlag JJ, Balkman CE: Effects of lycopene on proliferation and death of canine osteosarcoma cells, *Am J Vet Res* 71:1362–1370, 2010.

386. Jamadar-Shroff V, Papich MG, Suter SE: Soy-derived isoflavones inhibit the growth of canine lymphoid cell lines, *Clin Cancer Res* 15:1269–1276, 2009.

387. Helmerick EC, Loftus JP, Wakshlag JJ: The effects of baicalein on canine osteosarcoma cell proliferation and death, *Vet Comp Oncol* 12:299–309, 2014.

388. Levine CB, Bayle J, Biourge V, et al.: Effects and synergy of feed ingredients on canine neoplastic cell proliferation, *BMC Vet Res* 12:159–168, 2016.

389. Rizzo VL, Levine CB, Wakshlag JJ: The effects of sulforaphane on canine osteosarcoma proliferation and invasion, *Vet Comp Oncol* 15:718–730, 2017.

390. McClain RM, Wolz E, Davidovich A, et al.: Subchronic and chronic safety studies with genistein in dogs, *Food and Chem Tox* 43:1461–1482, 2005.

391. Korytko PJ, Rodvold KA, Crowell JA, et al.: Pharmacokinetics and tissue distribution of orally administered lycopene in male dogs, *J Nutr* 133:2788–2792, 2003.

392. Serisier S, Leray V, Poudroux W, et al.: Effects of green tea on insulin sensitivity, lipid profile and expression of PPAR-γ and PPAR-α and their target genes in dogs, *Br J Nutr* 99:1208–1216, 2008.

393. Kapetanovic IM, Crowell JA, Krishnaraj R, et al.: Exposure and toxicity of green tea polyphenols in fasted and non-fasted dogs, *Toxicology* 260:28–36, 2009.

394. Hill AS, Werner JA, Rogers QR, et al.: Lipoic acid is 10 times more toxic in cats than reported in humans, dogs or rats, *J An Phys An Nutr* 88:150–156, 2004.

395. Brown JP, Silverman JD: The current and future market for veterinarians and veterinary medical services in the United States, *J Am Vet Med Assoc* 225:161–183, 2004.

396. Lue TW, Patenburg DB, Crawford PM: Impact of the owner-pet and client-veterinarian bond on the care that pets receive, *J Am Vet Med Assoc* 232:531–540, 2008.

397. Adams CL, Bonnett BN, Meek AH: Predictors of owner response to companion animal death in 177 clients from 14 practices in Ontario, *J Am Vet Med Assoc* 217:1303–1309, 2000.

398. Blackwell MJ: The 2001 Iverson Bell Symposium keynote address: beyond philosophical differences: the future training of veterinarians, *J Vet Med Educ* 28:148–152, 2001.

399. Coe JB, Adams CL, Bonnett BN: A focus group study of veterinarians' and pet owners' perceptions of veterinarian-client communication in companion animal practice, *J Am Vet Med Assoc* 233:1072–1080, 2008.

400. Stoewen DL, Coe JB, MacMartin C, et al.: Qualitative study of the communication expectations of clients accessing oncology care at tertiary referral center for dogs with life-limiting cancer, *J Am Vet Med Assoc* 245:785–795, 2014.

401. Gorman TE, Ahern SP, Wiseman J, et al.: Residents' end-of-life decision making with adult hospitalized patients: a review of the literature, *Acad Med* 80:622–633, 2005.

402. Buckman R: *Practical plans for difficult conversations in medicine: strategies that work in breaking bad news*, Baltimore, 2010, Johns Hopkins University Press.

403. Girgis A, Sanson-Fisher RW: Breaking bad news: current best advice for clinicians, *Behav Med* 24:53–60, 1998.

404. Back AL, Arnold RM: Discussing prognosis: "how much do you want to know?" talking to patients who are prepared for explicit information, *J Clin Oncol* 24:4209–4213, 2006.

405. Tinga CE, Adams CL, Bonnett BN, et al.: Survey of veterinary technical and professional skills in students and recent graduates of a veterinary college, *J Am Vet Med Assoc* 219:924–931, 2001.

406. Butler C, William S, Koll S: Perceptions of fourth-year veterinary students regarding emotional support of clients in veterinary practice and in veterinary college curriculum, *J Am Vet Med Assoc* 221:360–363, 2002.

407. Meehan MP, Menniti MF: Final-year veterinary students' perceptions of their communication competencies and a communication skills training program delivering in a primary care setting

408. NAVMEC Board of Directors: The North American Veterinary Medical Education Consortium (NAVMEC) looks to veterinary medical education for the future: roadmap for veterinary medical education in the 21st century: responsive, collaborative, flexible, *J Vet Med Educ* 38:320–327, 2011.

409. Bylund CL, Brown R, Gueguen JA, et al.: The implementation and assessment of a comprehensive communication skills training curriculum for oncologists, *Psychooncology* 19:583–593, 2010.

410. Shaw JR, Barley GE, Hill AE, et al.: Communication skills education onsite in a veterinary practice, *Patient Educ Couns* 80:337–344, 2010.

411. Shaw JR, Barely GE, Broadfoot K, et al.: Communication assessment of on-site communication skills education in a companion animal practice, *J Am Vet Med Assoc* 249:419–432, 2016.

412. Adams CL, Kurtz SM: *Skills for communicating in veterinary medicine*, New York, 2017, Dewpoint Publishing.

413. *COE Accreditation Policies and Procedures – Standards*: Available at: https://www.avma.org/ProfessionalDevelopment/Education/Accreditation/Programs/Pages/cvtea-pp-standards.aspx. Accessed Aug 8, 2018.

414. Venetis MK, Robinson JD, LaPlant Turkiewics K, et al.: An evidence base for patient-centered cancer care: a meta-analysis of studies of observed communication between cancer specialists and their patients, *Patient Educ Couns* 77:379–383, 2009.

415. Stoewen DL, Coe JB, MacMartin C, et al.: Qualitative study of the information expectations of clients accessing oncology care at tertiary referral center for dogs with life-limiting cancer, *J Am Vet Med Assoc* 245:773–783, 2014.

416. Epstein RM, Street RL: *Patient-centered communication in cancer care: promoting healing and reducing suffering*, Bethesda, MD, 2007, National Institutes of Health.

417. Back AL, Anderson WG, Bunch L, et al.: Communication about cancer near the end of life, *Cancer* 113:1897–1910, 2008.

418. Back AL, Arnold RM: Discussing prognosis: "how much do you want to know?" talking to patients who do not want information or who are ambivalent, *J Clin Oncol* 24:4214–4217, 2006.

419. Shaw JR, Bonnett BN, Adams CL, et al.: Veterinarian-client-patient communication patterns used during clinical appointments in companion animal practice, *J Am Vet Med Assoc* 228:714–721, 2006.

420. Roter DL, Larson S, Rischer GS, et al.: Experts practice what they preach: a descriptive study of best and normative practices in end-of-life discussions, *Arch Intern Med* 160:3477–3485, 2000.

421. Roter DL, Hall JA, Kern DE, et al.: Improving physicians' interviewing skills and reducing patients' emotional distress: a randomized clinical trial, *Arch Intern Med* 155:1877, 1995.

422. Bard AM, Main DCJ, Haase AM, et al.: The future of veterinary communication: partnership or persuasion? A qualitative investigation of veterinary communication in the pursuit of client behavior change, *PLoS One* 12:1–17, 2017.

423. Emanual EJ, Emanual LG: Four models of the physician-patient relationship, *J Am Med Assoc* 267:2221–2226, 1992.

424. Roter DL: The enduring and evolving nature of the patient-physician relationship, *Patient Educ Couns* 39:5–15, 2000.

425. Tresolini C, Pew-Fetzer Task Force: *Health professional education and relationship-centered care*, San Francisco, 1994, The Pew-Fetzer Task Force on Advancing Psychosocial Health Education.

426. Mead N, Bower P: Patient-centredness: a conceptual framework and review of the empirical literature, *Soc Sci Med* 51:1087–1110, 2000.

427. Nogueira Borden LJ, Adams CL, Bonnett BN, et al.: Use of the measure of patient-centered communication to analyze euthanasia discussions in companion animal practice, *J Am Vet Med Assoc* 237:1275–1286, 2010.

428. Nogueira Borden LJ, Adams CL, Bonnett BN, et al.: Euthanasia discussions: a comparison of veterinarian and standardized client perceptions of veterinarian-client communication, *J Am Vet Med Assoc* 254:1073-1085, 2019.

and based on Kolb's experiential learning theory, *J Vet Med Educ* 41:317–382, 2014.

429. Bertakis KD, Roter DL, Putnam SM: The relationship of physician medical interview style to patient satisfaction, *J Fam Pract* 32:175–181, 1991.

430. Buller MK, Buller DB: Physicians' communication style and patient satisfaction, *J Health Soc Behav* 28:375–388, 1987.

431. Hall JA, Dornan MC: Meta-analyses of satisfaction with medical care: description of research domain and analysis of overall satisfaction levels, *Soc Sci Med* 27:637–644, 1988.

432. Levinson W, Stiles WB, Inui TS, et al.: Physician frustration in communicating with patients, *Med Care* 1:285–295, 1993.

433. Roter DL, Stewart M, Putnam SM, et al.: Communication patterns of primary care physicians, *J Am Med Assoc* 277:350–356, 1997.

434. DiMatteo MR, Sherbourne CD, Hays RD: Physicians' characteristics influence patient's adherence to medical treatments: results from the medical outcomes study, *Health Psychol* 12:93–102, 1993.

435. Stewart MA: Effective physician-patient communication and health outcomes: a review, *Can Med Assoc J* 152:1423–1433, 1995.

436. Dysart LM, Coe JB, Adams CL: Analysis of solicitation of client concerns in companion animal practice, *J Am Vet Med Assoc* 238:1609–1615, 2011.

437. Kanji N, Coe JB, Adams CL, et al.: Effect of veterinarian-client-patient interactions on client adherence to dentistry and surgery recommendations in companion-animal practice, *J Am Vet Med Assoc* 240:427–436, 2012.

438. Shaw JR, Adams CL, Bonnett BN, et al.: Veterinarian satisfaction with companion animal visits, *J Am Vet Med Assoc* 240:832–841, 2012.

439. McArthur ML, Fitzgerald JR: Companion animal veterinarians' use of clinical communication skills, *Aust Vet J* 91:374–380, 2013.

440. Stoewen DL, Coe JB, MacMartin C, Stone E, Dewey C: Identification of illness uncertainty in veterinary oncology: implications for service. *Front Vet Sci,* in press.

441. Mellanby RG, Crisp J, DePalma G, et al.: Perceptions of veterinarians and clients to expressions of clinical uncertainty, *J Sm Anim Prac* 48:26–31, 2007.

442. Adams CL, Kurtz SM: *Skills for communicating in veterinary medicine,* Parsippany, NJ, 2017, Dewpoint Publishing.

443. Kedrowicz AA: Clients and veterinarians as partners in problem solving during cancer management: implications for veterinary education, *J Vet Med Educ* 42:373–381, 2015.

444. Beckman HB, Frankel RM: The effect of physician behavior on the collection of data, *Ann Intern Med* 101:692–696, 1984.

445. Neumann M, Bensing J, Mercer S, et al.: Analyzing the "nature" and "specific effectiveness" of clinical empathy: a theoretical overview and contribution towards a theory-based research agenda, *Patient Educ Couns* 74:339–346, 2009.

446. Shaw JR: Four core communication skills of highly effective practitioners, *Vet Clin North Am Small Anim Pract* 36:385–396, 2006.

447. Allen E, Shaw JS: Delivering bad news: a crucial conversation, *Vet Team Brief* 2:17–19, 2010.

448. Fogarty LA, Curbow BA, Wingard JR, et al.: Can 40 seconds of compassion reduce patient anxiety? *J Clin Oncol* 17:371–379, 1999.

449. Fried TR, Bradley EH, O'Leary J: Prognosis communication in serious illness: perceptions of older patients, caregivers and clinicians, *J Am Geriatr Soc* 51:1398–1403, 2003.

450. Leydon GM, Boulton M, Moynihan C, et al.: Faith, hope and charity: an in-depth interview study of cancer patients' information needs and information-seeking behavior, *West J Med* 173:26–31, 2000.

451. Jenkins V, Fallowfield L, Poole K: Information needs of patients with cancer: results from a large study in UK cancer centres, *Br J Cancer* 84:322–331, 2001.

452. Cassileth BR, Zupkis RV, Sutton-Smith K, et al.: Information and participation preferences among cancer patients, *Ann Intern Med* 92:832–836, 1980.

453. Clayton JM, Butow PN, Arnold RM, et al.: Fostering coping and nurturing hope when discussing the future with terminally ill cancer patients and their caregivers, *Cancer* 103:1965–1975, 2005.

454. Gawande A: Letting go: what should medicine do when it can't save your life? *The New Yorker,* August 2, 2010.

455. Pantilat SZ: Communication with seriously ill patients: better words to say, *J Am Med Assoc* 301:1279–1281, 2009.

456. Yeates JW, Main DC: The ethics of influencing clients, *J Vet Med Assoc* 237:263–267, 2010.

457. Bishop GA, Long CC, Carlsten KS, et al.: The Colorado State University pet hospice program: end-of-life care for pets and their families, *J Vet Med Educ* 35:525–531, 2008.

458. Johnson CL, Patterson-Kane E, Lamison A, et al.: Elements of and factors important in veterinary hospice, *J Vet Med Assoc* 238:148–150, 2011.

459. Graugaard PK, Holgersen K, Eide H, et al.: Changes in physician-patient communication from initial to return visits: a prospective study in a haematology outpatient clinic, *Patient Educ Couns* 57:22–29, 2005.

460. Lagoni L: Bond-centered cancer care: an applied approach to euthanasia and grief support for your clients, your staff, and yourself. In Withrow SJ, Vail DM, editors: *Withrow and McEwen's small animal clinical oncology,* ed 4, St. Louis, 2007, Saunders Elsevier, pp 333–346.

461. Pilgram MD: Communicating social support to grieving clients: the veterinarians' view, *Death Stud* 34:699–714, 2010.

462. Morris P: Managing pet owners' guilt and grief in veterinary euthanasia encounters, *J Contemp Ethnogr* 41:337–365, 2012.

463. Bartram DJ, Baldwin DS: Veterinary surgeons and suicide: a structured review of possible influences on increased risk, *Vet Rec* 166:388–397, 2010.

464. Nett RJ, Witte TK, Holzbauer SM, et al.: Risk factors for suicide, attitudes toward mental illness, and practice-related stressors among US veterinarians, *J Am Vet Med Assoc* 247:945–955, 2015.

465. Platt B, Hawton K, Simkin S, et al.: Suicidal behavior and psychosocial problems in veterinary surgeons: a systematic review, *Soc Psychiatry Psychiatr Epidemiol* 47:223–240, 2012.

466. Pfifferling JH, Gilley K: Overcoming compassion fatigue, *Fam Pract Manag* 7:39–44, 2000.

467. Figley CR, Roop RG: *Compassion fatigue in the animal-care community,* Washington, DC, 2006, Humane Society Press.

468. Wellbeing and Peer Assistance. Available at: https://www.avma.org/ProfessionalDevelopment/PeerAndWellness/Pages/default.aspx. Accessed Aug 8, 2018.

469. Laflamme DP: Development and validation of a body condition score system for cats: a clinical tool, *Fel Pract* 25:5–6, 1997.

470. Mawby DI, Bartges JW, d'Avignon A, et al.: Comparison of various methods for estimating body fat in dogs, *J Am Anim Hosp Assoc* 40:109–111, 2004.

471. Shaw JR, Lagoni L: End-of-life communication in veterinary medicine: delivering bad news and euthanasia decision making, *Vet Clin North Am Small Anim Pract* 37:95–108, 2007.

17

Integrative Oncology

NARDA G. ROBINSON

What *Is* "Integrative Oncology"?

Integrative oncology constitutes a diverse approach to the treatment of patients with cancer that encompasses both conventional and unconventional approaches. The term "integrative" medicine has largely replaced the longer designation, "complementary and alternative medicine" (CAM). Several National Cancer Institute (NCI)-designated comprehensive cancer centers have formally established integrative medicine centers within their hospitals, offering integrative approaches such as acupuncture, oncology massage, music therapy, meditation consultations, physical therapy, nutrition counseling, health psychology, and more. Patients and families who consult these centers are typically seeking to improve survival, manage side effects of conventional care, and take a proactive approach to treatment. Although many of these methods, such as acupuncture and massage, translate readily to veterinary care, others (e.g., botanical medicine and dietary supplements) require more caution because of physiologic differences in xenobiotic metabolism. That said, more research focusing on integrative oncologic approaches is necessary in veterinary oncology, as limited data exist at present for the target species. Consequently, the topics and techniques presented in the text that follows rely heavily on human and laboratory animal findings.

Looking for an "All Natural" Cure for Cancer

One of the most frequently asked questions clients raise is whether any "natural" approach exists that can replace more conventional cancer therapies such as surgery, chemotherapy, or radiation therapy (RT). Unfortunately, there is no reliable nonconventional cancer "cure." However, as research sheds light on the ability of botanical products to halt tumor progression in certain tumors, the incorporation of integrative approaches may become more important in the overall care of cancer patients. Furthermore, pursuing integrative medicine during and after chemotherapy and/or radiation may boost host defenses, reduce conventional treatment side effects, accelerate healing, and promote resumption of normal daily living. Clients want and need factual, science-based guidance on which therapies offer the most help and the least harm, and veterinarians that scientifically assess the benefits and risks of integrative medicine will occupy a central role and responsibility in providing vital education for those that depend on them.

Integrative Medicine Inroads into Oncology

Nearly 40% of adults and 12% of children in the United States access integrative medicine, and more than 50% of human cancer patients include some form of integrative medicine in their treatment.[1,2] They do so to improve quality of life and treatment outcomes and to fill gaps left by conventional medicine, especially in the areas of physical and emotional pain. Integrative medicine may cushion the effect of treatments that can be otherwise frightening and painful, allowing patients to relax and, at least for humans, maintain hope.

A survey of clients at the Colorado State University Flint Animal Cancer Center found that 76% accessed integrative approaches. Most did so to support the well-being of their animal. Others were seeking pain control, reduction in treatment toxicity, and appetite support.[3] The study also found that most clients had not discussed these treatments with their primary care veterinarian. What would have happened if they had done so? Would their veterinarian have challenged them and attempt to talk them out of pursuing additional options? Or, would their veterinarian have been able to provide clear and appropriate guidance on the pros and cons of various integrative medicine approaches? Until more veterinary schools offer science-based education to students in integrative therapeutics, most veterinarians will graduate and enter practice lacking a full understanding of the pharmacologic basis of botanical medicine, the neuromodulatory benefits of acupuncture and massage, the restorative effect of photobiomodulation, and the risks not only of folkloric approaches but also scientifically scrutinized care. The goal of this chapter is to elucidate the pros and cons and also the promises and pitfalls of integrative medicine for cancer patients.

Where to Begin?

No "one size fits all" approach exists. As conventional care strategies become increasingly tailored to the individual (so called *personalized medicine*), so should integrative care strategies.

Identify Treatment Goals

Before embarking on an integrative approach, clearly defining goals will help develop the initial plan. Discussions should include methods (e.g., metrics) to monitor comfort, mobility, pain control, appetite, and the activities of daily living along with strategies to achieve those goals. Revisiting and revising preliminary goals as treatment proceeds will keep the integrative approach focused and tailored to current needs and challenges.

See the Big Picture

By definition, integrative oncology includes both conventional and complementary medical treatment methods; this may translate into multiple health care providers participating in the patient's treatment care. Communication becomes vital to avoid unnecessary, duplicative, or counterproductive approaches. Sometimes, excessive treatment can be taxing on both the patient and client, and a frank discussion about what is working and what is not may streamline care and place fewer burdens on both. Exploring the pros and cons in this broader context with the client may help alleviate family members' feelings of guilt and the fear of "not doing enough," when in reality they might be doing more than indicated or warranted.

Recognize Patient Comorbidities

The advanced age of patients with cancer raises the likelihood that those individuals will be harboring medical and/or physical problems in addition to neoplasia. Attending to the "whole patient" embodies a cornerstone of integrative oncology care. Introducing acupuncture and massage to alleviate pain and stress carries the side benefit of homeostatic regulation and stronger host defenses (i.e., robust immunologic protection and the ability to recover after injury). Evidence suggests that patients who feel better overall will more likely complete their planned course of chemotherapy and/or RT and have more positive results.[4,5]

Fully evaluating a patient with myofascial palpation[6] before chemotherapy and/or RT with respect to general well-being may provide practitioners insight into ways to address preexisting pain and dysfunction even before conventional treatment commences.

Common Approaches in Integrative Oncology

Acupuncture

Nearly two-thirds of human cancer patients experience pain.[7,8] Negative side effects from opioid analgesics or other concerns regarding conventional pain medications often prompt clients to request drug-free alternatives. Acupuncture, which uses the insertion of thin, sterile needles into certain sites (called "acupuncture points") on the body is one such alternative.

Acupuncture points correspond to influential neurovascular or myofascial zones that, when activated, promote analgesia, recovery of normal circulation and immune function, physiologic restoration, and homeostasis.[9,10] In addition to needling, other forms of somatic afferent stimulation include acupressure, laser acupuncture, and electroacupuncture, wherein one clips electrode wires to the needles to augment the stimulation and neurologic response. Research supports that patients who receive acupuncture require less medication to control pain.[11,12]

Specifically, nerve fiber stimulation begins at the needle–tissue interface, where local alterations in cytokines and inflammatory mediators lead to modulation (i.e., normalization) of circulation and immune function in the immediate area surrounding the site around the needle.[13,14] From there, agitation of the connective tissue and subsequent tugging of the collagen fibers, fibroblasts, and myofascia in the region produce activation of sensory somatic and autonomic nerve fibers. When excited, afferent pathways ferry action potentials along large nerve axons that underlie and

often define the trajectory of acupuncture channels. A cascade of responses follows in the central nervous system (CNS) and autonomic nervous system (ANS), generating somatosomatic, somatoautonomic, and somatovisceral reflexes in spinal cord segments related to the excited nerve(s). In addition to propriospinal signaling, acupuncture induces changes in the neuronal firing patterns in the limbic system, cerebellum, cortex, and brainstem. Functional brain imaging research shows, by reflecting alterations in neuronal metabolism, which centers process pain, regulate autonomic function, and affect moods in response to acupuncture.[15] This aids in the ever-deepening awareness of the neurophysiologic underpinnings of acupuncture.

How Might Acupuncture Benefit a Veterinary Patient with Cancer?

Although acupuncture provides repeatable and measurable benefits for patients with advanced cancer, the treatment is underutilized.[16–22] Human integrative oncology clinics have found acupuncture to be a safe, inexpensive, and effective intervention for problems that cancer patients often encounter, including leukopenia, gastrointestinal upset, and systemic reactions.[23,24] Acupuncture may reduce the emetic effects of chemotherapy and opioids.[25,26] For pain management, many studies on acupuncture show improvement, though more rigorous studies are needed.[27] Acupuncture has also been used to treat fatigue, hot flashes, immune system support, neuropathy, anxiety, depression, xerostomia,[28-30] and sleep disturbances in humans.[31] Even for human patients with advanced, incurable cancer, acupuncture has been shown to alleviate a wide range of symptoms with no significant or unexpected adverse effects.[32]

Risks of Acupuncture

Studies indicate that acupuncture performed by a medical professional for patients with cancer poses little risk of injury.[33–35] That said, one should obviously avoid penetrating the tumor or seeding local tissues with cancer cells. Owing to the complexity of treatment and patient considerations for animals with cancer, any acupuncturist treating animals should have a thorough understanding of animal health and disease, and acupuncture anatomy and physiology, to minimize risk of injury.

Botanical Medicine

Considering their diverse and documented anticancer benefits, plant-based medicines offer some of the greatest hope for an actual cure for cancer. After all, nearly half of cancer drugs used over the past two decades arose directly as derivatives from plants or indirectly, as chemically altered derivatives.[36] Classes of plant-associated chemotherapeutics include the vinca alkaloids (vinblastine, vincristine, and vindesine), the taxanes (paclitaxel and docetaxel), camptothecin derivatives (irinotecan and camptothecin), and the epipodophyllotoxins (etoposide and teniposide).[37] The search for new and better drugs continues; to date, the NCI has screened tens of thousands of plant species for anticancer value. Of these, nearly 9% have demonstrated reproducible activity against cancer.[37]

Many natural products from both Eastern (most notably, Asian) and Western herbs have demonstrated anticancer benefits through in vitro analysis of their effects on human cancer cell lines.[38] For example, extracts and pure compounds derived from the Chinese herb *Euphorbia fischeriana* Steud exhibit antitumor, antimicrobial, antiviral, immune stimulating, and analgesic activities.[39] Research on mice has shown *E. fischeriana* extracts to be effective against malignant melanoma, ascitic hepatoma, and Lewis lung carcinoma. Other research on mice has demonstrated the ability of a mixture of botanical extracts made from fermented soybeans, grape seed, green tea, and more to enhance the effectiveness of chemotherapy while limiting adverse effects.[40]

Botanical products frequently encountered in veterinary integrative oncology include Asian mushrooms (immune-enhancing), curcumin from the spice turmeric, *Boswellia* from the frankincense tree (antitumor and antiinflammatory), and bloodroot (escharotic), though the latter has fallen out of favor in recent years because of its potential for causing injury and pain, as described in the text that follows. Veterinarians who decide to introduce botanical agents into a patient's care should do so with the same degree of caution and critical evaluation as one would employ with any chemotherapy drug. The tendency to overlook the potential for intrinsic toxicity or risk of herb–drug interactions could lead to unforeseen problems such as a heightened bleeding risk or alterations in serum concentrations of prescribed drugs. Furthermore, little research exists on veterinary botanical products and their pharmacokinetics and pharmacodynamics remain mostly a mystery, as do safe and effective dosing levels.

Supplement Questions and Quality Control Issues

In contrast to the more tightly regulated pharmaceutical industry, products comprising dietary supplements and herbal products raise far-reaching concerns about manufacturing quality, purity, and reliability. Contamination with microbes, heavy metals, and dirt from manufacturing, combined with undisclosed adulteration with pharmaceuticals complicate the picture and can obscure the actual risk or benefit from the listed ingredients. Chinese mixtures raise even more red flags, ranging from US Food and Drug Administration (FDA) import bans[41] on the importation of veterinary Chinese herbal products to the potential inclusion of endangered plant and animal species. Plant substitution, misidentification, and proprietary (secret) ingredients leave additional gaps in health care providers' trust in Chinese remedies.

Risk of Treatment Interactions

Scrutinizing a patient's entire integrative oncology treatment plan should help diminish the client's reliance on redundant, superfluous, and/or counterproductive concurrent approaches. In particular, the risk/benefit ratio of adding or omitting a botanical product should take into account the potential for herb-drug interactions. Pharmacologic interplay between medications and supplements could change circulating drug concentrations and render a chemotherapy, analgesic, or anesthetic compound ineffective or toxic. Herbs that have anticancer effects but contain phytoestrogens such as *Angelica sinensis* may adversely affect patients with hormone-sensitive cancer.[42]

Herb-drug interactions in oncology occur through a number of pharmacodynamic and pharmacokinetic pathways, and much more remains to be learned about specific herbs, drugs, and clinical significance through research in veterinary target species. Often ignored among herbalists and oncologists alike, herb-drug interactions pose a clinically relevant problem in oncology, due to the narrow therapeutic index of most cytotoxic drugs.[43] In fact, induction of drug-metabolizing enzymes and transporters may lower plasma levels of anticancer drugs and result in subsequent treatment failure. Inhibition of these detoxification pathways could also contribute to enhanced chemotherapy drug toxicity. Several popular herbal products have been identified as likely to contribute to herb-drug interactions under certain conditions.[44]

These include, but are not limited to, St. John's wort,[45] kava-kava, ginseng, garlic, milk thistle (silybin), evening primrose oil, green tea, Echinacea,[46] vitamin E, beta-carotene, and quercetin[47] supplements.

Some plant mixtures both induce and inhibit drug-metabolizing enzymes because of the complexity of their biochemically active constituents. Many plant-based substances act as antioxidants. The antioxidant activity of some phytotherapeutics such as green tea is potent enough that clinicians should consider the risk of abrogating the benefits of chemotherapy if the two are coadministered.

Another concern involves the potential for immune system stimulation by plant products that promote lymphocyte proliferation. Although immune-enhancing herbs may help a patient fight some immunogenic cancers, adding these products (e.g., burdock root, astragalus, medicinal mushrooms, Echinacea) could prove counterproductive for conditions such as lymphoma.

Finally, several botanical ingredients can increase the risk of hemorrhage through inhibition of platelet activity and aggregation.[48] This could negatively affect patients with hemangiosarcoma, those undergoing biopsies or surgery, and individuals receiving concurrent anticoagulant or antiplatelet medications. Cancer patients may already have thrombocytopenia from chemotherapy or bone marrow infiltration (myelopthisis) that could compromise their capacity to clot.

A study of a standardized extract of Maitake mushroom in dogs with lymphoma reported no objective value, although two dogs did develop hyphema and one developed petechiae.[49] These agents can inhibit platelet function; whether the bleeding noted in this study related to the Maitake mushroom or the lymphoma was unclear.

The "4 G's" mnemonic (i.e., ginkgo, ginseng, ginger, and garlic) helps one remember which herbs most notably inhibit coagulation.[50] Many Chinese herbal formulations contain one or more of these ingredients. That said, proprietary mixtures that fail to disclose the amounts of their ingredients to keep the mixture a "trade secret" make it impossible for practitioners to ascertain the level of risk that that supplement poses.

For more information on specific plant compounds and their interaction risk, the reader is referred to Memorial Sloan-Kettering Cancer Center's website or their free app entitled "About Herbs."[51]

Additional Issues with Chinese Herbs

Recommending traditional Chinese herbal medicine (TCHM) based on rigorously derived discoveries in botanical research allows practitioners to discard untestable, abstract mechanisms of action such as claiming that they "resolve stagnation, invigorate Qi, and remove phlegm/damp accumulation."[52] Computerized databases may assist oncologists by enabling determination of relevant, potential interactions between anticancer drugs and Chinese herbs.[53] Even oncologists in China are encouraging their colleagues to maintain a watchful eye for surprise sequelae. For example, one paper warned: "[P]rofessional complacency about TCM [Traditional Chinese Medicine] use is becoming less acceptable as the knowledge base of TCM-induced toxicities and interactions expands. Being rich sources of bioactive xenobiotics, TCMs are frequent causes of puzzling complications, including hepatotoxicity, nephrotoxicity, and hematologic disorders."[54]

Some TCHMs are chemosensitizing or radiosensitizing and thus may cause conventional treatment to have more robust activity, whereas others directly antagonize medication through one or more mechanisms. Toxicity from Chinese herbs coadministered with chemotherapy may lead to diagnostic dilemmas when clinicians misattribute problems to the drug rather than the TCHM product, thereby delaying discontinuation of the appropriate compound. In fact, Chinese herbalists in Taiwan who work directly with herbs in the raw form are at increased risk of liver and bladder cancer, possibly owing to heavy metal contamination of TCHMs and/or the intrinsic toxicity of some ingredients.[55] This heightened risk for urologic cancers, chronic and unspecified nephritis, renal failure, and renal sclerosis "highlights the urgent need for safety assessments of Chinese herbs."[56]

Public perception holds that TCHMs may protect cancer patients' health and well-being during chemotherapy. A double-blind, randomized, placebo-controlled study questioned this assumption, showing that TCHMs did not significantly reduce hematologic toxicities (leukopenia, neutropenia, and thrombocytopenia) associated with adjuvant chemotherapy for breast and colon cancer.[57] Three licensed, experienced TCHM practitioners from China prescribed herbal formulas to patients on an individualized basis, as many believe this approach yields superior benefits. Even the myth that individualizing TCHMs produces more significant improvement could be more folklore than fact. According to some critics, "[A]lmost all individualized herbal medicine is practiced without the support of any rigorous evidence about effectiveness whatsoever."[58] They continue,

> The lack of standardisation and use of multiple herbs in a single prescription also greatly multiply the safety risks. There are additional risks associated with variability in the diagnostics skills of the practitioner, their awareness or lack of awareness of potential interactions, and their ability or inability to identify red flag symptoms indicating serious diseases requiring immediate mainstream medical treatment. Given the risks and lack of supporting evidence, the use of individualised herbal medicine cannot be recommended in any indication.

Examples of Herbs Suggested for Patients with Cancer

The botanical agents covered in the text that follows appear because of their popularity, not as a means of advocacy for their inclusion in veterinary oncologic care. The responsibility of prescribing or recommending herbal products lies with the practitioner handling each case and should be approached with the same critical mindset and scientific rationale as any chemotherapeutic drug or other conventional intervention.

Asian/Medicinal Mushrooms

Medicinal mushrooms and fungi display more than a hundred medicinal functions potentially relevant to the treatment of cancer.[59] These activities include antitumor, immunomodulatory, antioxidant, radical scavenging, and hepatoprotective effects that enhance humoral and cell-mediated immune responses. A variety of medicinal mushrooms and extracts have proved beneficial, improving immune parameters such as natural killer (NK) cell activity and cytokine expression, without significant toxicity.

Mushroom mixtures and mushroom-derived polysaccharide preparations modify tumor response and improve immune function in patients with solid tumors.[60] The active agents in Asian mushrooms, polysaccharides, also possess antitumor effects through inhibition of cellular proliferation and tumor growth, invasion, and angiogenesis.[61]

Enthusiasm for the use of medical mushrooms in dogs with cancer followed the publication of a 2012 study in the journal *Evidence-Based Complementary and Alternative Medicine*.[62] This research investigated the ability of an extract of turkey tail mushroom (*Coriolus versicolor*) containing standardized amounts of the bioactive agent polysaccharopeptide (PSP), to affect the survival and quality of life of a small number (*n* = 15) of dogs with hemangiosarcoma. Results suggested that the median time to developing abdominal metastases or finding progression was lengthened in five dogs taking 100 mg/kg/day of the commercially available preparation called "I'm-Yunity" compared with lower doses of I'm-Yunity. No differences were noted in survival times, however. Of note, the survival time of nearly 200 days for five dogs in the highest dose treatment group was numerically longer than that reported for dogs on doxorubicin-based chemotherapeutic treatment protocols, which typically falls between 141 and 179 days. These findings raise important questions. Could this product demonstrate survival effects similar to or beyond that provided by standard of care chemotherapy in larger scale studies? Could research such as this lead to changes in standard of care from cytotoxic drugs to botanical medicine? The answers to these questions are yet unanswered. No direct statistical comparison was made between this very small (*n* = 5) group of dogs and dogs receiving standard of care chemotherapy. The "randomization" in this trial was between I'm-Yunity dosing groups, not between I'm-Yunity and standard of care. Although these results suggest activity, a randomized trial with sufficient statistical power would be necessary to confirm activity either equivalent or superior to standard of care chemotherapy.

Human trials have found benefit with turkey tail mushroom as well. A proprietary, protein-bound polysaccharide extract of *Coriolus versicolor* reduced serum levels of immunosuppressive acidic protein in stage II and III colorectal cancer patients, increased 5-year disease-free survival, and decreased relative risk of regional metastases.[63] A meta-analysis of three trials involving more than a thousand subjects with colorectal cancer confirmed these results.[64] Moreover, a systematic review and meta-analysis of the efficacy of *Coriolus versicolor* on survival in cancer patients revealed that this mushroom confers survival benefit for patients with breast, stomach, and colorectal carcinoma.[65]

Bloodroot

Bloodroot extract acts as an escharotic when topically applied in a salve or destructive agent when injected directly into tumors.[66,67] The "black salve" version of bloodroot (*Sanguinaria canadensis*) may come admixed with mineral agents such as zinc chloride, chromium chloride, or arsenic trisulfide and possibly other herbs. Bloodroot pastes became popular in the midtwentieth century and have persisted despite risks of serious injury. It causes strong and rapid apoptotic responses through several modes of cell death, including an early and severe glutathione-depleting effect.

Sanguinarine, the active ingredient in bloodroot, supposedly targets only cancer cells, according to its enthusiastic supporters. Sanguinarine does appear to selectively target cancer cells over normal cells *in vitro*, and it may sensitize these cells to chemotherapy-mediated growth inhibition and apoptosis.[68] Sanguinarine has also been reported to exert dose-dependent differential antiproliferative and apoptotic effects on cancer and normal cells.[69] How tissue levels in vivo would compare with those tested in vitro is unknown, although high concentrations of sanguinarine can cause normal keratinocytes to necrose.

Websites selling black salves for veterinary cancer patients have, over the years, posted pictures showing tumor elimination for patients that were purportedly deemed untreatable by conventional practitioners. Even Dr. Andrew Weil, the author of the bestseller *Spontaneous Healing* and director of the Program in Integrative Medicine (PIM) at the University of Arizona in Tucson, reportedly claimed that black salve cured a tumor on his dog, though his own post is no longer available on this topic.[70] Instead, he now cautions on www.DrWeil.com that the use of bloodroot can cause excruciating pain and tissue degradation. It may also leave residual tumor.[71] Over time, the toxicity of bloodroot in dogs with cancer has come into focus and their use in cancer patients is now discouraged.[67]

Boswellia

Boswellic acids exhibit potent antiinflammatory properties in vitro and in vivo. Triterpenes in boswellic acid reduce the synthesis of leukotrienes in intact neutrophils by inhibiting 5-lipoxygenase, the key enzyme involved in the biosynthesis of leukotrienes, which mediate inflammation.[72,73] *Boswellia* extracts exert immunomodulatory effects by simultaneously inhibiting T-helper 1 (Th1) and promoting Th2 cytokine production.[74] They regulate vascular responses to inflammation and stabilize mast cells.[75] In cases of intestinal inflammation, boswellic acids may modulate the adhesive interactions between leukocytes and endothelial cells by countering the activation of leukocytes and/or downregulating the expression of endothelial cell-adhesion molecules.[76,77]

Side effects of boswellic acids may include abdominal discomfort, nausea, epigastric pain, and diarrhea.[78]

The presence of food in the stomach, and the type of food eaten, dramatically alters the bioavailability of boswellic acids, and bile acids significantly affect their absorption. When human subjects ingest boswellic acids along with a high-fat meal, the area under the plasma concentration—time curves and peak concentrations were several times greater than when the herbal preparations are taken in the fasting condition. A human study showed that the elimination half-life for boswellic acid was approximately 6 hours, suggesting that oral administration would require dosing every 6 to 8 hours.[79]

Frankincense extracts, and boswellic acids themselves, display moderate-to-potent inhibition of human drug-metabolizing CYP450 enzymes, but the potential to cause clinically relevant drug—herb interactions is unclear.[80]

Curcumin

Cancer cells have various methods to evade host defenses. Intuitively, this implies that a drug or herb would work best against cancer when it has more than one mechanism of action against the disease. Curcumin, a bioactive component of the spice turmeric, has been shown to have several mechanisms of action.[81,82] It induces phase II detoxification enzymes, suppresses tumor cell proliferation in several cancer cell lines, and downregulates transcription factors (nuclear factor κB [NFκB], activator protein 1 [AP-1], and early growth response 1 [EGR-1]).[83,84] Curcumin also downregulates enzymes such as cyclooxygenase-2 (COX-2), lipoxygenase (LOX), nitric oxide synthase (NOS), matrix metalloproteinase 9 (MMP9), and urokinase-type plasminogen activator; it also limits production of tumor necrosis factor, chemokines, cell surface adhesion molecules, and growth factor receptors (e.g., epidermal growth factor receptor [EGFR], human EGFR 2 [HER2]).[85] Curcumin may have antiangiogenic effects[86] and may alter the cytotoxicity of certain chemotherapy drugs.[87,88]

Curcumin causes cell death in several human cancer cell lines, including breast, lung, prostate, colon, melanoma, kidney, hepatocellular, ovarian, and leukemia.[89] Curcumin produces cell death through both apoptotic mechanisms and alternative means.

When resistance develops to apoptosis-inducing factors, curcumin can overcome this impediment through alternative cell-signaling pathways, such as mitotic catastrophe.[84] Curcumin may also counteract the induction of prosurvival factors in cells generated by RT and chemotherapy.

Human clinical trials demonstrate no dose-limiting toxicity for pure curcumin when given at up to 10 g daily, whether orally (in human studies) or by means of intraperitoneal or intravenous administration in rodent-based experimental animal research.[84] The amount of curcumin contained in turmeric averages only about 3% by weight; concentrated curcumin supplements therefore supposedly provide higher levels of the active constituent, provided that the label and actual contents agree. The hurdles of maintaining adequate blood levels of curcumin pertain to its low bioavailability, although absorption varies between species. One way to overcome delivery challenges could include coupling it with compounds that focus curcumin's activity toward specific target cells.

Curcumin could hypothetically negate some of the effects of chemotherapy because it affects so many pathways. Research suggests that curcumin can inhibit chemotherapy-induced apoptosis in breast cancer cells, specifically in combination with camptothecin, mechlorethamine, or doxorubicin.[90] The potential benefits of certain herbs should be considered and compared against the risks. For example, a synthetic analog of curcumin helped reduce doxorubicin-induced cardiotoxicity through an anticancer–antioxidant dual function in vitro.[91] In addition, curcumin and catechin (from green tea) may work synergistically against cancer through cytotoxicity, nuclear fragmentation, and antiproliferative and proapoptotic effects.[92]

Yunnan Baiyao

Yunnan Baiyao (also known as Yunnan Paiyao) is a Chinese herbal mixture consisting primarily of notoginseng that has become a popular product among veterinary clients, particularly those caring for animals with hemangiosarcoma. This popularity is the result of claims that Yunnan Baiyao regulates bleeding. Therefore patients with a high risk of hemorrhage might be less likely to bleed if Yunnan Baiyao was indeed effective.

Westerners first learned of the Chinese herbal mixture "Yunnan Baiyao," meaning "the white medicine of Yunnan," during the Vietnam War. Members of the US military discovered that prisoners from North Vietnam often carried with them a tiny bottle of this product to take in the event that they were injured and bleeding, either internally or externally.[93] Over the ensuing decades, Yunnan Baiyao has grown in popularity among complementary medical practitioners and even in some conventional medicine practices for its hemostatic and thrombolytic properties.[94]

The Chinese doctor Qu Huangzhang developed Yunnan Baiyao in the Yunnan province of China in the early 1900s. The Yunnan province is known as "the Kingdom of Fauna and Flora" for its vast supply of plants and animals used in Chinese medicinals. Although the capsule's contents were kept secret until relatively recently, suspicion grew that its main active ingredient consisted of pseudoginseng root, now called *Panax notoginseng*, notoginseng, "tien chi," or "san qi." Notoginseng is a type of ginseng that offers the highest concentration of hemostatic constituents among all seven major ginseng types.[95] Notoginseng from the Yunnan outperforms that grown elsewhere in terms of crop yield and quality.[96] Other substances in Yunnan Baiyao formulations vary between manufacturers and may include myrrh, ox bile, Chinese yam, sweet geranium, lesser galangal root, and possibly other antiseptics or astringent substances in a starch base. Some preparations of Yunnan Baiyao contain a different colored "hit pill" among the regular pills; however, the contents of this pill do not specifically appear on the label, although some suspect that it may contain either a concentrated dose of notoginseng or the more troublesome herb, aconite, which has both cardiotoxic and neurotoxic effects.

That there is no formal "recipe" for Yunnan Baiyao and the fact that some manufacturers still refuse to disclose their ingredients means that many unknowns persist with currently available products and caution is warranted.

Despite the many questions regarding the contents and manufacturing quality of Yunnan Baiyao, some research has emerged that may validate its hemostatic potential.[97] For example, a prospective, randomized, double-blind, placebo-controlled study on Yunnan Baiyao for human patients undergoing bimaxillary orthognathic surgery found significant reduction in intraoperative blood loss when Yunnan Baiyao was administered preoperatively for 3 days.[98] No thrombolic events or other side effects were noted during this short-term administration. A prospective study of the effects of oral Yunnan Baiyao on thromboelastographic parameters in apparently healthy dogs showed that the product was well tolerated and increased the strength of blood clotting.[99]

On the other hand, a 2017 report of the effects of Yunnan Baiyao on blood coagulation in beagle dogs found no clinically significant effects on the coagulation parameters under study.[100]

Additional indications in the future may arise for cancer treatment because of the cytotoxic effects of notoginseng,[101] which also exhibits the capacity to specifically sensitize tumor cells to ionizing radiation. An in vitro analysis of Yunnan Baiyao on canine hemangiosarcoma (HSA) cell lines revealed a dose- and time-dependent HAS cell death by means of caspase-mediated apoptosis.[101a] That said, high doses of notoginseng could also be toxic to bone marrow stem cells.[102] Furthermore, a retrospective case-controlled study of Yunnan Baiyao administration in dogs with right atrial masses and pericardial effusion did not show a significantly delayed recurrence of clinical signs or improved survival.[103]

In summary, although Yunnan Baiyao may reduce the risk of bleeding, one must weigh the strength of its anecdotal acclaim against the unknowns regarding dosage, purity, and long-term benefits or risks.

Homeopathy

Homeopathy constitutes an alternative type of health care based on an irrational premise that the more dilute a remedy is, the more potent it is. Homeopathic remedies are produced with low to extremely low concentrations of the substance from which it was derived. This means that the amount of active pharmacologic ingredients in the solution may range from a weak extract of plant, animal, or mineral contents to barely undetectable amounts. That said, even small amounts of toxic substances, especially when ingested over long periods of time, can still induce injury or death.

Homeopathic practitioners claim that they prescribe their remedies to stimulate an individual's natural healing response. According to homeopathic principles and the "like cures like" doctrine, a natural substance that causes symptoms of illness in a healthy person can, when prepared correctly, cure that same set of symptoms in an unhealthy person. Thus when selecting a remedy for a patient, the homeopath determines which substance would most closely cause an identical "symptom picture" if given in larger quantities. She or he then recommends the homeopathic dilution to alleviate those issues based on the aforementioned "like cures like" principle.

Contrary to conventional medical pharmacotherapeutic methodology, homeopathic lore asserts that remedies are more powerful as they become more dilute. As difficult as homeopathic theory is to believe, the remedies are as easy to administer as sugar pills because, for many remedies, the pills are just that: lactose tablets impregnated on the outer surface with a diluted homeopathic mixture. Most remedies are available over the counter. Although most states consider the practice of homeopathy on animals as part of veterinary medicine, clients can and do self-prescribe and self-administer the medication to their animals. Several do-it-yourself books on veterinary homeopathy are available.

How Does Homeopathy Work?

First, there is the question of whether homeopathy does, in fact, work. Most systematic reviews and meta-analyses find that the effects of homeopathy resemble the strength of placebos. The benefits seen in humans receiving homeopathy may be due to the lengthy interviewing process itself rather than the homeopathic remedies per se.[104] Currently, there is no repeatable, rigorous evidence that homeopathy works for veterinary patients. Similarly, there is no rational mechanism of action.

In human homeopathy, evidence for the incorporation of homeopathy for symptom control in cancer patients is weak and burdened with methodological flaws, uncontrolled trials, and/or small subject numbers. Positive benefits shown in smaller studies frequently disappear when the study is repeated with larger numbers and controls.

The most reliable benefit from homeopathy may be its placebo effects on the client (i.e., bolstering a feeling that they are doing something safe and supportive for their animal with cancer). This false sense of assurance could work against the animal's best interests if it delays meaningful diagnosis and effective care, as illustrated in a human study on the effect of antecedent use of CAM in delaying medical advice sought for breast cancer.[105]

Can Homeopathy Cause Direct Harm?

Scrutiny of homeopathic claims is growing in both human and veterinary medicine. Serious adverse events and deaths in children consuming homeopathic teething pills finally came to light as a US FDA investigation became public into homeopathic products that had a 10-year track record of serious adverse effects.[106] As it turned out, dilutions assumed to be safe were not. Similarly, concerns are mounting in the veterinary community about the dangers of homeopathy for animals, whether due to intrinsic toxicity of improperly produced remedies or the ethical infractions of treating animals with substances indistinguishable from placebo.[107] Owing to its unlikelihood of helping and risk of harm, homeopathy has no place in cancer care for animals.

Massage

Massage incorporates several methods of hands-on, low-force techniques that target restrictions and pain, mostly in the soft tissues of the body. The benefits that massage may hold for cancer patients encompass quality of life, control of postoperative or postprocedural pain and stress, and support of improved mobility and functional recovery after amputation.

Cancer and its standard control measures can make people and animals physically uncomfortable. A 2011 study of patients with metastatic bone cancer, reported in the journal *Pain*, found that "[T]he reduction in pain with massage was both statistically and clinically significant, and the massage-related effects on relaxation were sustained for at least 16–18 hours postintervention."[108] Massage also showed benefit in terms of mood, muscle relaxation, and sleep quality.

A 2017 systematic review of controlled clinical trials on massage for children with cancer found that patients experienced less pain, nausea, stress, anxiety, and immune suppression.[109] These findings comport with assessments of the effects of massage in adults both with and without cancer.

How Does Massage Work?

Based on the rapidly expanding paradigm of autonomic neuromodulation and the desire by medical massage therapists to explain how their treatments work, a unifying theory is beginning to emerge that helps explain the effects of massage on diverse bodily activities, such as digestion, emotional states, sleep, weight regulation, pain control, and immune function.[110] Ordinarily, animals suffering from acute and chronic illness exhibit heightened sympathetic tone that can cause maladaptive changes. The complementary, dualistic reciprocity encoded within the ANS dictates that as parasympathetic tone increases, sympathetic (fight-or-flight) activity diminishes. Consequently, reducing sympathetic hyperactivity by means of massage can benefit patients by countering peripheral vasoconstriction, inflammation, muscle tension, spinal cord windup, and pain. For older veterinary patients suffering from cancer and those recovering from surgery and experiencing postoperative ileus, regulation of digestive function through massage may provide much-needed parasympathetic support.

The relaxing benefits of medical massage assist veterinary oncology patients in counteracting stress during minimally invasive procedures, although it should never be relied on to replace conventional anesthesia and analgesia for more painful events. Facial massage calms patients at least in part by activating trigeminal-vagal reflexes.[111] Veterinary technicians can include certain techniques while assisting with gentle restraint; slow, up-and-down moderate pressure massage along the midline between the nose and forehead can sometimes induce a quasihypnotic state.

What Are the Risks of Massage for Cancer Patients?

Patients with osteosarcoma, skeletal metastasis, spinal instability, low platelet count, or osteopenia should avoid deep massage. Light or moderate pressure, delivered through skilled hands after informed palpation, would not be contraindicated, except over painful regions or areas that have undergone recent surgery, demonstrate instability, or harbor infection. Massage should be avoided over implantations to deliver chemotherapy or other drugs. Massage to sites containing stents or prostheses may cause displacement. Tissues subjected to prior surgery or RT may be fragile, and massage to these areas should either be avoided or be done gently. Hypercoagulable patients may experience emboli subsequent to deep pressure over a thrombus; patients who are prone to bleeding may develop hematomas secondary to pressures that in normal patients would not cause problems. Deep abdominal massage has caused internal bleeding even in the absence of bleeding disorders. Although no evidence exists to indicate that massage promotes the likelihood of tumor metastasis, one should avoid massage directly over known tumors or predictable metastasis sites.

Photobiomodulation (Laser Therapy)

Photobiomodulation (PBM), formerly known as low-level laser therapy (LLLT) or simply laser therapy (LT), involves exposing tissues to photons from laser units or light-emitting diodes (LEDs)

in a manner that stimulates cellular function and produces clinical benefits. It contrasts with laser surgery, which destroys tissue.

In contrast to acupuncture, in which input begins with the microtraumatic mechanical effects of the needle on local tissue, LT relies on the absorption and scattering of light within tissue. LT imparts a monochromatic, narrow-band, coherent light source. Photons from the laser support endogenous processes that involve cell division and proliferation; this is one of the main reasons why cancer has been considered a relative contraindication for PBM.

Physiologic responses from LT's PBM include increased phagocytosis; vasodilation; increased rate of regeneration of lymphatic and blood vessels; stimulation of enzyme activity at the wound edges; fibroblast stimulation; keratinocyte and fibroblast proliferation; scar and keloid reduction; increased adenosine triphosphate (ATP) and DNA synthesis; and stimulation of muscle, tendon, and nerve regeneration.[112] Clinically, PBM provides safe and cost-effective treatment for wound healing, neurologic recovery, pain reduction, and lymphedema control.[113]

With respect to oncologic care, a growing body of evidence suggests that LT may help alleviate oral mucositis. A 2007 Phase III, randomized, double-blind, placebo-controlled clinical trial that evaluated the efficacy of LLLT for the prevention of oral mucositis (OM) indicated that laser with a 650-nm wavelength reduced the severity of OM and pain scores.[114] No adverse effects were noted in this study. In 2011 a systematic review of studies on this topic concluded that although sample sizes were low, overall data were consistently in favor of LLLT both preventing and diminishing the severity of OM in patients receiving chemotherapy or RT.[115] PBM for the prevention of oral mucositis not only lowers morbidity; it also may save thousands of dollars per case prevented.[116]

Human patients with advanced head and neck cancer experience many complications after receiving RT or chemoradiotherapy. These interventions may cause loss of function and negatively affect quality of life. In the acute phase, complications include OM, pain, dysphagia, dysgeusia, dermatitis, changes in salivary function, and infection. Over time, patients may develop neuropathies, tooth demineralization and caries, periodontitis, soft tissue and/or bone necrosis, mucocutaneous and muscular fibrosis, trismus, lymphedema, and voice or speech changes.[116] Biologically, PBM has the potential to control pain, improve tissue health, maintain organ function and prevent or mitigate these complications. PBM has demonstrated the ability to enhance wound repair and tissue regeneration as it proceeds from the inflammatory, to the proliferative, and finally to the remodeling phases of injury resolution, resulting in significantly less inflammation and fibrosis.[117]

How Might Laser Therapy Harm Cancer Patients?

Little in vivo research is currently available pertaining to the risk of LT stimulating cancer growth. However, prudent practice warrants avoiding LT in cancer patients or at least, tumor sites. Questions remain about the safe distance from a tumor at which one can deliver light therapy and appropriate and nonproliferative wavelengths and doses of light. Until more is known about the specific effects of PBM on tumors and circulating lymphocytes, LT may be considered contraindicated for patients with lymphoma.

Conclusion

Cancer patients face a multiplicity of challenges, as both the treatment and the disease can make them miserable. Fortunately, medical research is revealing ways in which integrative options can lessen cancer patients' suffering and even improve survivorship.[118]

Considering the growing popularity of integrative medicine, oncology clients are eager to learn about nondrug, noninvasive options. With the appropriate, science-based education, veterinarians can guide clients toward legitimate, effective, and rational approaches that will make a positive difference and yield better outcomes.

References

1. National Center for Complementary and Integrative Health Web site: The use of complementary and alternative medicine in the United States. Available at: https://nccih.nih.gov/research/statistics/2007/camsurvey_fs1.htm. Accessed 18.06.18.
2. Zappa SB, Cassileth BR: Complementary approaches to palliative oncological care, *J Nurs Care Qual* 18:22–26, 2003.
3. Lana SE, Kogan LR, Crump KA, et al.: The use of complementary and alternative therapies in dogs and cats with cancer, *J Am Anim Hosp Assoc* 42:361–365, 2006.
4. Ben-Arye E, Samuels N, Schiff E, et al.: Quality-of-life outcomes in patients with gynecologic cancer referred to integrative oncology treatment during chemotherapy, *Support Care Cancer* 23:3411–3419, 2015.
5. Greenlee H, Balneaves LG, Carlson LE, et al.: Society for Integrative Oncology. Clinical practice guidelines on the use of integrative therapies as supportive care in patients treated for breast cancer, *J Natl Cancer Inst Monogr* 346–358, 2014.
6. Shah JP, Thaker N: Myofascial Pain Syndrome. In Cheng J, Rosenquist R, editors: *Fundamentals of pain medicine*, Cham, 2018, Springer, pp 177–184.
7. Lu W, Dean-Clower E, Doherty-Gilman A, et al.: The value of acupuncture in cancer care, *Hematol Oncol Clin North Am* 22:631–648, 2008. viii.
8. Lu W, Rosenthal DS: Acupuncture for cancer pain and related symptoms, *Curr Pain Headache Rep* 17:321, 2013.
9. Xu Y, Guo Y, Song Y, et al.: A new theory for acupuncture: Promoting robust regulation, *J Acupunct Meridian Stud* 11:39–43, 2018.
10. Robinson NG: *Interactive medical acupuncture anatomy*, New York, 2016, Teton NewMedia.
11. Cassileth BR, Deng GE, Gomez JE, et al.: Complementary therapies and integrative oncology in lung cancer: ACCP evidence-based clinical practice guidelines (2nd edition), *Chest* 132:340S–354S, 2007.
12. Dean-Clower E, Doherty-Gilman AM, Keshaviah A, et al.: Acupuncture as palliative therapy for physical symptoms and quality of life for advanced cancer patients, *Integr Cancer Ther* 9:158–167, 2010.
13. Langevin HM, Yandow JA: Relationship of acupuncture points and meridians to connective tissue planes, *Anat Rec* 269:257–265, 2002.
14. Kavoussi B, Ross BE: The neuroimmune basis of anti-inflammatory acupuncture, *Integr Cancer Ther* 6:251–257, 2007.
15. Hui KKS, Napadow V, Liu J, et al.: Monitoring acupuncture effects on human brain by fMRI, *J Vis Exp* 38:e1190, 2010.
16. Junqin Z, Zhihua L, Jin Pule: A clinical study on acupuncture for prevention and treatment of toxic side-effects during radiotherapy and chemotherapy, *J Trad Chin Med* 19:16–21, 1999.
17. He XR, Want Q, Li PP: Acupuncture and moxibustion for cancer-related fatigue: a systematic review and meta-analysis, *Asian Pac J Cancer Prev* 14:3067–3074, 2018.
18. Liu YH, Dong GT, Ye Y, et al.: Effectiveness of acupuncture for early recovery of bowel function in cancer: a systematic review and meta-analysis, *Evid Based Complement Alternat Med* 2504021, 2017.
19. Zhang Y, Lin L, Li H, et al.: Effects of acupuncture on cancer-related fatigue: a meta-analysis, *Support Care Cancer* 26:415–425, 2018.
20. Chien TJ, Hsu CH, Liu CY, et al.: Effect of acupuncture on hot flush and menopause symptoms in breast cancer – a systematic review and meta-analysis, *PLoS One* 12:e0180918, 2017.
21. Chen L, Lin CC, Huang TW, et al.: Effect of acupuncture on aromatase inhibitor-induced arthralgia in patients with breast cancer: a meta-analysis of randomized controlled trials, *Breast* 33:132–138, 2017.
22. Hu C, Zhang H, Wu W, et al.: Acupuncture for pain management in cancer: a systematic review and meta-analysis, *Evid Based Complement Alternat Med* 1720239, 2016.
23. Johnstone PAS, Polston GR, Niemtzow RC, et al.: Integration of acupuncture into the oncology clinic, *Palliat Med* 16:235–239, 2002.
24. Wong R, Sagar CM, Sagar SM: Integration of Chinese medicine into supportive cancer care: a modern role for an ancient tradition, *Cancer Treat Rev* 27:235–246, 2001.
25. Vickers AJ: Can acupuncture have specific effects on health? a systematic review of acupuncture antiemesis trials, *J R Soc Med* 89:303–311, 1996.
26. Garcia MK, McQuade J, Haddad R, et al.: Systematic review of acupuncture in cancer care: a synthesis of the evidence, *J Clin Oncol* 31:952–960, 2013.
27. National Cancer Institute Web site: Acupuncture (PDQ®) – Health Professional Version. Available at: www.cancer.gov/about-cancer/treatment/cam/hp/acupuncture-pdq#link/_147_toc. Accessed 18.06.18.
28. Braga FP, Lemos Junior CA, Alves FA, et al.: Acupuncture for the prevention of radiation-induced xerostomia in patients with head and neck cancer, *Braz Oral Res* 25:180–185, 2011.
29. Blom M, Dawidson I, Fernberg JO, et al.: Acupuncture treatment of patients with radiation-induced xerostomia, *Oral Oncol* 32B:182–190, 1996.
30. Wong RKW, Jones GW, Sagar SM, et al.: A Phase I-II study in the use of acupuncture-like transcutaneous nerve stimulation in the treatment of radiation-induced xerostomia in head-and-neck cancer patients treated with radial radiotherapy, *Int J Radiat Oncol Biol Phys* 57:472–480, 2003.
31. Dean-Clower E, Doherty-Gilman AM, Keshaviah A, et al.: Acupuncture as palliative therapy for physical symptoms and quality of life for advanced cancer patients, *Integr Cancer Ther* 9:158–167, 2010.
32. Lim JT, Wong ET, Aung SK: Is there a role for acupuncture in the symptom management of patients receiving palliative care for cancer? a pilot study of 20 patients comparing acupuncture with nurse-led supportive care, *Acupunct Med* 29:173–179, 2011.
33. Wu X, Chung VC, Hui EP, et al.: Effectiveness of acupuncture and related therapies for palliative care of cancer: overview of systematic reviews, *Sci Rep* 5:16776, 2015.
34. Cybularz PA, Brothers K, Singh GM, et al.: The safety of acupuncture in patients with cancer therapy-related thrombocytopenia, *Med Acupunct* 27:224–229, 2015.
35. Shen J, Glaspy J: Acupuncture: evidence and implications for cancer supportive care, *Cancer Pract* 9:147–150, 2001.
36. Amin A, Gali-Muhtasib H, Ocker M, et al.: Overview of major classes of plant-derived anticancer drugs, *Int J Biomed Sci* 5:1–11, 2009.
37. Desai AG, Qazi GN, Ganju RK, et al.: Medicinal plants and cancer chemoprevention, *Curr Drug Metab* 9:581–591, 2008.
38. Tan W, Lu J, Huang M, et al.: Anti-cancer natural products isolated from Chinese medicinal herbs, *Chin Med* 6(27), 2011.
39. Jian B, Zhang H, Han C, et al.: Anti-cancer activities of diterpenoids derived from *Euphorbia fischeriana* Steud, *Molecules* 23:287, 2018.
40. Chen WT, Yang TS, Chen HC, et al.: Effectiveness of a novel herbal agent MB-6 as a potential adjunct to 5-fluoracil-based chemotherapy in colorectal cancer, *Nutr Res* 34:585–594, 2014.
41. US Food & Drug Administration Web site: Import alert 68-19. Available at: https://www.accessdata.fda.gov/cms_ia/importalert_1147.html. (Accessed 11.02.18).

42. Piersen CE: Phytoestrogens in botanical dietary supplements: Implications for cancer, *Integr Cancer Ther* 2:120–136, 2003.

43. Meijerman I, Beijnen JH, Schellens JHM: Herb-drug interactions in oncology: focus on mechanisms of induction, *The Oncologist* 11:742–752, 2006.

44. He SM, Yang AK, Li XT, et al.: Effects of herbal products on the metabolism and transport of anticancer agents, *Expert Opin Drug Metab Toxicol* 6:1195–1213, 2010.

45. Chrubasik-Hausmann S, Vlachojannis J, McLachlan AJ: Understanding drug interactions with St. John's wort (*Hypericum perforatum* L.): impact of hyperforin content, *J Pharm Pharmcol*, 2018. [Epub ahead of print].

46. Haefeli WE, Carls A: Drug interactions with phytotherapeutics in oncology, *Expert Opin Drug Metab Toxicol* 10:359–377, 2014.

47. Zhao Q, Wei J, Zhang H: Effects of quercitin on the pharmacokinetics of losartan and its metabolite EXP3174 in rats, *Xenobiotica* 1–6, 2018. [Epub ahead of print].

48. Andersen MR, Sweet E, Zhou M, et al.: Complementary and alternative medicine use by breast cancer patients at time of surgery which increases the potential for excessive bleeding, *Integr Cancer Ther* 14:119–124, 2015.

49. Griessmayr PC, Gautheir M, Barber LG, et al.: Mushroom-derived maitake PET fraction as a single agent for the treatment of lymphoma in dogs, *J Vet Intern Med* 21:1409–1412, 2007.

50. Peck P: ACP: Garlic, ginseng, ginkgo biloba, and ginger all bad actors with coumadin, *MedPage Today*, 2006. Available at: https://www.medpagetoday.com/meetingcoverage/acp/3050. (Accessed 17.07.18).

51. Memorial Sloan Kettering Cancer Center Web site: About Herbs, Botanicals, and Other Products. Available at: https://www.mskcc.org/cancer-care/diagnosis-treatment/symptom-management/integrative-medicine/herbs. (Accessed 11.02.18).

52. DiNatale C: Clinical application of Chinese herbal medicine for companion animals. In Xie H, Preast V, editors: *Xie's Chinese veterinary herbology*, Ames, 2010, Blackwell Publishing.

53. Yap KY, Kuo EY, Lee JJ, et al.: An onco-informatics database for anticancer drug interactions with complementary and alternative medicines used in cancer treatment and supportive care: an overview of the OncoRx project, *Support Care Cancer* 18:883–891, 2010.

54. Chiu J, Yau T, Epstein RJ: Complications of traditional Chinese/herbal medicines (TCM)—a guide for perplexed oncologists and other cancer caregivers, *Support Care Cancer* 17:231–240, 2009.

55. Liu SH, Liu YF, Liou SH, et al.: Mortality and cancer incidence among physicians of traditional Chinese medicine: a 20 year national follow-up study, *Occup Environ Med* 67:166–169, 2010.

56. Yang HY, Wang JD, Lo TC, et al.: Increased mortality risk for cancers of the kidney and other urinary organs among Chinese herbalists, *J Epidemiol* 19:17–23, 2009.

57. Mok TSK, Yeo W, Johnson PJ, et al.: A double-blind placebo-controlled randomized study of Chinese herbal medicine as complementary therapy for reduction of chemotherapy-induced toxicity, *Ann Oncol* 18:768–774, 2007.

58. Guo R, Canter PH, Ernst E: A systematic review of randomized clinical trials of individualized herbal medicine in any indication, *Postgrad Med J* 83:633–637, 2007.

59. Wasser SP: Medicinal mushroom science: current perspectives, advances, evidences, and challenges, *Biomed J* 37:345–356, 2014.

60. Hardy ML: Dietary supplement use in cancer care: help or harm, *Hematol Oncol Clin North Am* 22:581–617, 2008.

61. Song KS, Kim JS, Jing K, et al.: Protein-bound polysaccharide from *Phellinus linteus* inhibits tumor growth, invasion, and angiogenesis and alters Wnt/beta-catenin in SW480 human colon cancer cells, *BMC Cancer* 11:307, 2011.

62. Brown DC, Reetz J: Single agent polysaccharopeptide delays metastases and improves survival in naturally occurring hemangiosarcoma, *Evid Based Complement Alternat Med* 8, 2012. Article ID 384301.

63. Ohwada S, Ikeya T, Yokomori T: Adjuvant immunochemotherapy with oral Tegafur/Uracil plus PSK in patients with stage II or III colorectal cancer: a randomised controlled study, *Br J Cancer* 90:1003–1010, 2004.

64. Sakamoto J, Morita S, Oba K, et al.: Efficacy of adjuvant immunochemotherapy with polysaccharide K for patients with curatively resected colorectal cancer: a meta-analysis of centrally randomized controlled clinical trials, *Cancer Immunol Immunother* 55:404–411, 2006.

65. Wong LYE, Fai CK, Leung PC: Efficacy of *Yun Zhi (Coriolus versicolor)* on survival in cancer patients: systematic review and meta-analysis, *Recent Pat Inflamm Allergy Drug Discov* 6:78–87, 2012.

66. Cienki JJ, Zaret L: An internet misadventure: bloodroot salve toxicity, *J Alt Comp Med* 16:1125–1127, 2010.

67. Childress MO, Burgess RC, Holland CH, et al.: Consequences of intratumoral injection of a herbal preparation containing blood root (*Sanguinaria canadensis*) extract in two dogs, *J Am Vet Med Assoc* 239:374–379, 2011.

68. Sun M, Lou W, Chun JY, et al.: Sanguinarine suppresses prostate tumor growth and inhibits survivin expression, *Genes Cancer* 1:283–292, 2010.

69. Ahmad N, Gupta S, Husain MM, et al.: Differential antiproliferative and apoptotic response of sanguinarine for cancer cells versus normal cells, *Clin Cancer Res* 6:1524–1528, 2000.

70. Dee R: *Dr. Andrew Weil Treats His Dog's Tumor.* June 18, 2015. Available at: https://www.bloodrootsalve.com/andrew-weil/. (Accessed 11.02.18).

71. Dr.Weil.com: Web site Bloodroot for skin cancer? January 9, 2006. Available at: https://www.drweil.com/health-wellness/body-mind-spirit/cancer/bloodroot-for-skin-cancer/. Accessed 11.02.18.

72. Hostanska K, Daum G, Saller R: Cytostatic and apoptosis-inducing activity of boswellic acids toward malignant cell lines in vitro, *Anticancer Res* 22:2853–2862, 2002.

73. Roy S, Khanna S, Krishnaraju AV, et al.: Regulation of vascular responses to inflammation: inducible matrix metalloproteinase-3 expression in human microvascular endothelial cells is sensitive to anti-inflammatory *boswellia*, *Antioxid Redox Signal* 8:653–660, 2006.

74. Chevrier MR, Ryan AE, Lee DYW, et al.: *Boswellia carterii* extract inhibits TH1 cytokines and promotes TH2 cytokines in vitro, *Clin Diagn Lab Immunol* 12:575–580, 2005.

75. Pungle P, Banayalikar M, Suthar A, et al.: Immunomodulatory activity of boswellic acids of *Boswellia serrata* Roxb, *Indian J Exp Biol* 41:1460–1462, 2003.

76. Anthoni C, Laukoetter MG, Rijcken E, et al.: Mechanisms underlying the anti-inflammatory actions of boswellic acid derivatives in experimental colitis, *Am J Physiol Gastro Liver Physiol* 290:G1131–G1137, 2006.

77. Krieglstein CE, Anthoni C, Rijcken EJM, et al.: Acetyl-11-keto-beta-boswellic acid, a constituent of a herbal medicine from *Boswellia serrata* resin, attenuates experimental ileitis, *Int J Colorectal Dis* 16:88–95, 2001.

78. Kimmatkar N, Thawani V, Hingorani L, et al.: Efficacy and tolerability of *Boswellia serrata* extract in treatment of osteoarthritis of knee—a randomized double-blind placebo-controlled trial, *Phytomedicine* 10:3–7, 2003.

79. Sharma S, Thawani V, Hingorani L, et al.: Pharmacokinetic study of 11-keto beta-boswellic acid, *Phytomedicine* 11:255–260, 2004.

80. Frank A, Unger M: Analysis of frankincense from various *Boswellia* species with inhibitory activity on human drug metabolizing cytochrome P450 enzymes using liquid chromatography mass spectrometry after automated on-line extraction, *J Chromatogr A* 1112:255–262, 2006.

81. Zhu HL, Ji JL, Huang XF: Curcumin and its formulations: Potential anti-cancer agents, *Anticancer Agents Med Chem* 12:210–218, 2011.

82. Schaffer M, Schaffer PM, Zidan J, et al.: Curcuma as a functional food in the control of cancer and inflammation, *Curr Opin Clin Nutr Metab Care* 14:588–597, 2001.

83. Salvioli S, Sikora E, Cooper EL, et al.: Curcumin in cell death processes: a challenge for CAM of age-related pathologies, *eCAM* 4:181–190, 2007.

84. Aggarwal BB, Kumar A, Bharti AC: Review. Anticancer potential of curcumin: preclinical and clinical studies, *Anticancer Res* 23:363–398, 2003.

85. He Y, Yue Y, Zheng X, et al.: Curcumin, inflammation, and chronic diseases: how are they linked? *Molecules* 20:9183–9213, 2015.

86. Koo HJ, Shin S, Choi JY, et al.: Introduction of methyl groups at C2 and C6 positions enhances the antiangiogenesis activity of curcumin, *Sci Rep* 5:14205, 2015.

87. Ramayanti O, Brikkemper M, Verkuijlen S, et al.: Curcuminoids as EBV lytic activators for adjuvant treatment in EBV-positive carcinomas, *Cancers (Basel)* 10, 2018.

88. Ferguson JE, Orlando RA: Curcumin reduces cytotoxicity of 5-fluorouracil treatment in human breast cancer cells, *J Med Food* 18:497–502, 2015.

89. Ravindran J, Prasad S, Aggarwal BB: Curcumin and cancer cells: how many ways can curry kill tumor cells selectively? *AAPS J* 11:495–510, 2009.

90. Somasundaram S, Edmund NA, Moore DT, et al.: Dietary curcumin inhibits chemotherapy-induced apoptosis in models of human breast cancer, *Cancer Res* 62:3868–3875, 2002.

91. Dayton A, Selvendiran K, Meduru S, et al.: Amelioration of doxorubicin-induced cardiotoxicity by an anticancer-antioxidant dual-function compound, HO-3867, *J Pharmacol Exp Ther* 339:350–357, 2011.

92. Manikandan R, Beulaja M, Arulvasu C, et al.: Synergistic anticancer activity of curcumin and catechin: an in vitro study using human cancer cell lines, *Microsc Res Tech* 75:112–116, 2012.

93. Bergner P: *Panax notoginseng* (Yunnan bai yao): a must for the first aid kit, *Medical Herbalism* 31:12, 1994.

94. Fratkin J: *Chinese herbal patent formulas: a practical guide*, Santa Fe, 1986, Shya Publications.

95. Zheng YN: Comparative analysis of the anti-haemorrhagic principle in ginseng plants, *Acta Agri Univ Jilin* 11:24–27, 102, 1989. Article in Chinese.

96. Jin H, Cui XM, Zhu Y, et al.: Effects of meteorological conditions on the quality of radix Notoginseng, *Southwest China, J Agri Sci* 8:825–828, 2005.

97. Yang B, Xu Z-Q, Xu F-Y, et al.: The efficacy of Yunnan Baiyao on haemostasis and antiulcer: a systematic review and meta-analysis of randomized controlled trials, *Int J Clin Exp Med* 7:41–462, 2014.

98. Tang ZL, Wang X, Yi B, et al.: Effects of the preoperative administration of Yunnan Baiyao capsules on intraoperative blood loss in bimaxillary orthognathic surgery: a prospective, randomized, double-blind, placebo-controlled study, *Int J Oral Maxillofac Surg* 38:261–266, 2009.

99. Tansey C, Wieve ML, Hybki GC, et al.: A prospective evaluation of oral Yunnan Baiyao therapy on thromboelastographic parameters in apparently healthy dogs, *J Vet Emerg Crit Care (San Antonio)* 28:221–225, 2018.

100. Frederick J, Boysen S, Wagg C, et al.: The effects of oral administration of Yunnan Baiyao on blood coagulation in beagle dogs as measured by kaolin-activated thromboelastography and buccal mucosal bleeding times, *Can J Vet Res* 81:41–45, 2017.

101. Chung VQ, Tattersall M, Cheung HTA: Interactions of a herbal combination that inhibits growth of prostate cancer cells, *Cancer Chemo Pharmcol* 53:384–390, 2004.

101a Wirth KA, Kolbw K, Salute ME, et al.: In vitro effects of Yunnan Baiyao on canine hemangiosarcoma cell lines, *Vet Comp Oncol* 14:281–294, 2016.

102. Chen FD, Wu MC, Wang HE, et al.: Sensitization of a tumor, but not normal tissue, to the cytotoxic effect of ionizing radiation using *Panax* notoginseng extract, 29:517–524, 2001.

103. Murphy LA, Panek CM, Bianco D, et al.: Use of Yunnan Baiyao and epsilon aminocaproic acid in dogs with right atrial masses and pericardial effusion, *J Vet Emerg Crit Care (San Antonio)* 27:121–126, 2017.

104. Rostock M, Naumann J, Guethlin C, et al.: Classical homeopathy in the treatment of cancer patients—a prospective observational study of two independent cohorts, *BMC Cancer* 11:19, 2011.

105. Malik IA, Gopalan S: Use of CAM results in delay in seeking medical advice for breast cancer, *Eur J Epidemiol* 18:817–822, 2003.

106. Kaplan S: Homeopathic remedies harmed hundreds of babies, families say, as FDA investigated for years, *STAT News*, 2017. Retrieved from: https://www.statnews.com/2017/02/21/hylands-homeopathic-teething-fda/.

107. Knapton S: Homeopathy can kill pets and should be banned, say vets, *The Telegraph*, 2016. Retrieved from: http://www.telegraph.co.uk/science/2016/06/24/homeopathy-can-kill-pets-and-should-be-banned-say-vets/.

108. Jane SW, Chen SL, Wilkie DJ, et al.: Effects of massage on pain, mood status, relaxation, and sleep in Taiwanese patients with metastatic bone pain: a randomized clinical trial, *Pain* 152:2432–2442, 2011.

109. Rodriguez-Mansilla J, Gonzalez-Sanchez B, Torres-Piles S, et al.: Effects of the application of therapeutic massage in children with cancer: a systematic review, *Rev Lat Am Enfermagem* 25:e2903, 2017.

110. Diego MA, Field T: Moderate pressure massage elicits a parasympathetic nervous system response, *Int J Neurosci* 119:630–638, 2009.

111. Hatayama T, Kitamura S, Tamura C, et al.: The facial massage reduced anxiety and negative mood status, and increased sympathetic nervous activity, *Biomed Res* 29:317–320, 2008.

112. Chung H, Dai T, Sharma SK, et al.: The nuts and bolts of low-level laser (light) therapy, *Ann Biomed Eng* 40:516–533, 2012.

113. Baxter GD, Liu L, Petrich S, et al.: Low level laser therapy (Photobiomodulation therapy) for breast cancer-related lymphedema: a systematic review, *BMC Cancer* 17:833, 2017.

114. Schubert MM, Eduardo FP, Guthrie KA, et al.: A phase III randomized double-blind placebo-controlled clinical trial to determine the efficacy of low level laser therapy for the prevention of oral mucositis in patients undergoing hematopoietic cell transplantation, *Support Care Cancer* 15:1145–1154, 2007.

115. Antunes HS, Schluckebier LF, Herchenhorn D, et al.: Cost-effectiveness of low-level laser therapy (LLLT) in head and neck cancer patients receiving concurrent chemoradiation, *Oral Oncol* 52:85–90, 2016.

116. Zecha JAEM, Raber-Durlacher JE, Nair JG, et al.: Low level laser therapy/photobiomodulation in the management of side effects of chemoradiation therapy in head and neck cancer: part 1: mechanisms of action, dosimetric, and safety considerations, *Support Care Cancer* 24:2781–2792, 2016.

117. Kuffler DP: Photobiomodulation in promoting wound healing: a review, *Regen Med* 11:107–122, 2016.

118. Frenkel M, Sierpina V, Sapire K: Effects of complementary and integrative medicine on cancer survivorship, *Curr Oncol Rep* 17:445, 2015.

18

Clinical Trials and Developmental Therapeutics

AMY K. LEBLANC, DOUGLAS H. THAMM, AND DAVID M. VAIL

Clinical research is essential to improving patient outcome and quality of life (QOL). Clinical trials in veterinary oncology have gained interest and focus over the past decade, with a growing number of consortia and cooperative groups that support multiinstitutional efforts, advocating for veterinary clinical trials and emphasizing the synergy between basic science and clinical progress. Clients who are motivated to seek advanced care for their pets and to enroll them in investigational trials that offer new therapies are key to ongoing advancement of clinical research in veterinary oncology.

Oncology clinical trials attempt to find better ways to prevent, diagnose, and treat cancer. Their model is different from trials involving infectious or nonneoplastic chronic diseases because the risks of morbidity and mortality can be greater, but the rewards, particularly for aggressive cancers lacking in highly efficacious standards of care, can be high. The culture of oncology care, whether physician-based or veterinary-based, should be on continued improvement in survival and QOL, and thus the option of entry into a clinical trial should be available. For example, the majority of children with aggressive childhood cancers are offered and entered into clinical trials that provide investigational therapies in addition to standard of care treatments; and the National Comprehensive Cancer Network recommends human patient participation in clinical trials as the "gold standard" for aggressive nonindolent T-cell lymphomas. In veterinary oncology, a similar trial-centric culture should be applied to patients with aggressive cancers (e.g., hemangiosarcoma, osteosarcoma, nonindolent T-cell lymphoma, feline squamous cell carcinoma, etc.) where cures are rare and outcomes are still generally poor with current standards of care.

During the years since the late 1970s, in investigations of standard cytotoxic chemotherapy agents in clinical trial settings, a "traditional" drug development approach using fairly rigid phases (I, II, III) and adherence to "rule-based" methods was advocated and employed. Since approximately 2008, however, a major shift in cancer drug development, both in human and veterinary medicine, has concerned a move from traditional cytotoxic agents to molecular targeted agents (MTAs). With many and varied MTAs entering the development pipeline, clinical trial methodologies employed for cytotoxic agents may not be ideal or appropriate. Although a clear dose–response relationship exists for most cytotoxic agents, this may not be the case for many MTAs. Thus a

paradigm shift in clinical trial methodology, referred to as "model-based" methods, has been proposed.

This chapter considers clinical trial design and implementation, and not statistical analysis of generated data or in-depth biostatistical considerations in trial design. For the reader seeking more thorough reviews on trial design and statistical methods, recent references are listed throughout the chapter. It cannot be stressed enough that knowledgeable biostatisticians should be consulted to ensure statistical design and power are appropriate before study implementation.

Traditional Drug Development Phases

Traditional first-in-species drug development follows a strict, stepwise paradigm that begins with a phase I dose-finding trial, followed by a phase II efficacy/activity trial, and concludes with a phase III "pivotal" trial that pits a novel agent against or with the current standard of care (Table 18.1).[1,2] Veterinary oncology trials sometimes combine these concepts. Clinical trial designs, pertinent endpoints and analyses, the process for drug approval, and clinical trial ethics are explored in the sections that follow.

Phase I Trials (Dose Finding)

Phase I trials are the first step in the evaluation of a new agent or biologic.[3-5] The primary goal is to determine a tolerable dose to be used in future studies by evaluating adverse event (AE) profile, tolerability, and dose-limiting toxicities (DLTs). Typically, safety is determined in dosing cohorts that escalate toward the goal of a maximum tolerated dose (MTD) or, for targeted therapies, a biologically effective dose (BED). Activity/efficacy is not a primary goal. In fact, response rates in phase I trials for classic cytotoxic agents are seldom more than 10%. Secondary goals of phase I trials may include exploration of various drug administration schedules, response rates, pharmacokinetic (PK) information (absorption, distribution, metabolism, and elimination [ADME]), biomarker development, and effects on molecular targets or pathways (pharmacodynamics [PD]). These biologic endpoints are increasingly important components of phase I trials as dose determinants are inherently linked to drug exposure and effect, especially as we move away from more indiscriminant cytotoxic agents and toward study of MTAs. These biologic questions

TABLE 18.1 Goals of Phase I–III Clinical Trials

Characteristic	PHASE OF CLINICAL TRIAL		
	Phase I (Dose Finding)	Phase II (Activity/Efficacy)	Phase III (Pivotal)
Primary Goals	• Determine MTD or BED • Define DLT • Characterize type and severity of adverse events	• Determine activity/efficacy in defined populations • Inform the decision to move to a phase III trial	• Compare a new drug or combination with therapy currently regarded as standard of care
Secondary Goals	• PK/PD issues • Scheduling issues • Target modulation effects • Preliminary efficacy data • Investigate surrogate biomarkers of response	• Estimate therapeutic index • Expand adverse event data • Evaluate additional dosing groups • Expand target modulation and biomarker data • QOL measures • Explore predictors of outcome	• QOL comparisons • Comparative costs

BED, Biologically effective dose; *DLT*, dose-limiting toxicity; *MTD*, maximum tolerated dose; *PK/PD*, pharmacokinetic/pharmacodynamics; *QOL*, quality of life.

are also the basis of comparative oncology modeling of drug development and are emphasized in their design.[6–8] In the growing field of cancer immunotherapy, the same guiding principles apply for phase I trials, but with the added nuance of determining relationships between biologic agent exposure and the host immune response. This is yet another example of how clinical trials carried out in immune-competent tumor-bearing companion dogs offer a distinct advantage over xenograft models in early development of novel immunotherapeutic agents.

Human oncology phase I trials are typically small, open-label, single-arm trials that include patients who have failed standard therapies. As such, subjects are generally heavily pretreated with advanced disease. In veterinary medicine, the phase I patient may have failed standard of care or have a condition for which no effective standard of care exists, the standard of care is beyond the client's financial means, or the client is interested in investigational therapy. In addition, because failure of the standard of care is not a necessary prerequisite, phase I veterinary trials can proceed in patients with naïve disease. Many veterinary oncology trials provide financial support and/or include the provision of funds for traditional therapies if investigational agents fail. Incentivization enhances accrual.

Phase I starting dose selection is typically based on preclinical PK/PD/AE data in nontarget species exist to inform starting dose.[1,3–5,9] Different options include starting with one-third of the "no observable adverse event level" (NOAEL), or one-tenth of the severe toxicity dose in the most sensitive species, or if normal dog data are available, one-half of the MTD in laboratory dogs as they seem to be less sensitive to AEs than are tumor-bearing companion dogs owing to differences in age, comorbidity, or monitoring/observation practices.

As with starting dose, escalation strategies greatly affect the number of patients treated at a potentially ineffective dose, the length of the trial, the use of resources, and the risk of AEs.[9] The traditional method of escalation, outlined in Table 18.2, uses a "3 × 3" cohort design wherein dose escalations are made with three patients per dose level and the MTD is set based on the number of patients experiencing a DLT. A DLT is defined as grade III or greater toxicity in any category (except hematologic) according to predefined AE categories, such as those in the Veterinary Cooperative Oncology Group—Common Terminology Criteria for Adverse Events (VCOG-CTCAE version 1.1).[10] Grade IV

TABLE 18.2 Standard Phase I Dose Escalation Scheme

Number of Patients with DLT at a Given Dose Level	Escalation Decision Rule
0 out of 3	Enter three patients at the next dose level.
≥2	Dose escalation will be stopped. This dose level will be declared the maximally administered dose (highest dose administered). Three additional patients will be entered at the next lowest dose level if only three patients were treated previously at that dose.
1 out of 3	Enter at least three more patients at this dose level. • If none of these three patients experiences DLT, proceed to the next dose level. • If one or more of this group suffer DLT, then dose escalation is stopped, and this dose is declared the maximally administered dose. Three additional patients will be entered at the next lowest dose level if only three patients were treated previously at that dose.
≤1 out of 6 at highest dose level below the maximally administered dose	This is generally the recommended phase II dose (MTD). At least six patients must be entered at the recommended phase II dose.

DLT, dose-limiting toxicity; *MTD*, maximum tolerated dose.

From National Cancer Institute: Cancer Therapy Evaluation Program: http://ctep.cancer.gov/protocolDevelopment/templates_applications.htm.

is often the preferred cutoff for myelosuppression-related DLTs because these events are usually considered manageable with supportive care, generally transient, and often clinically silent. Additional DLTs are defined on an agent-by-agent basis because of expected toxicities. These can include or exclude some grade III events from being DLTs, again if transient and clinically silent in nature and are prospectively defined in the study protocol. The MTD is defined as the highest dose level in which no more than one of six dogs develops a DLT. Traditionally, a fixed-dose modified Fibonacci method of dose escalation is used wherein the dose is escalated 100%, 67%, 50%, 40%, and then 33% of the previous dose as the dosing cohorts increase.[9] If the escalation increments are too conservative, more patients receive a suboptimal dose; conversely, if the escalations are too rapid, more patients are at risk for significant toxicity and the accuracy of the MTD is compromised. Interdosing cohorts can be added during the study period if more refined escalation or deescalation is found to be necessary.

Alternative, "accelerated titration" dose-escalation strategies have been suggested.[3–5,9,11,12] These include (1) two-stage designs in which initially single-patient cohorts are used and the dose is increased by a factor of two until a grade II toxicity occurs; then the second stage involves more traditional three-patient cohorts and acceleration strategies; (2) within-patient escalation in which the same patient receives a higher dose on subsequent treatments until a DLT is observed; however, this may mask cumulative toxicity; (3) escalations based on PK parameters, e.g., to achieve a target level of drug exposure; (4) escalations based on target modulation (if known); and (5) continual reassessment strategies using Bayesian methods.[11–14] In the end, it is always a trade-off of risk versus benefit; however, accelerated titration designs are generally associated with both a reduction in total patient number and a reduction in the number of patients receiving a suboptimal dose.

Although the phase I MTD approach works well for traditional cytotoxic drugs, phase I trials designed to determine the BED may be more relevant for MTAs.[15–19] Trials evaluating the BED require validated assays that measure an effect on the target in serial tumor samples and/or a surrogate tissue or fluid that documents activity at the molecular level. Examples of early incorporation of PD markers in tumor and surrogate tissue (peripheral blood) include canine phase I trials of the KIT kinase inhibitor toceranib,[20] the Btk inhibitor ibrutinib,[21] the histone deacetylase inhibitor sodium valproate,[22] and the putative autophagy modulator hydroxychloroquine.[23] Such PD modulation studies are increasingly important endpoints of phase I and II designs and are now commonly required as proof of mechanism for drug approval.

Phase II Trials (Activity/Efficacy Trials)

Several good reviews have outlined phase II trial designs.[4,24–27] The primary goal of phase II trials is, using the MTD or BED established in phase I, to identify the clinical or biologic activity in defined patient populations (e.g., tumors with a particular histology or particular molecular target) and inform the decision to embark on a larger pivotal phase III trial. The traditional phase II design (phase IIA) is a single-arm, open-label activity assessment of a novel drug or therapeutic modality that lacks a control group or uses historical controls, which are prone to bias (selection, population drift, and stage migration bias). The number of patients to be enrolled is variable depending on the "minimal useful response rate" and the rate of spontaneous regression (usually <5%). Multiple references discuss the statistical underpinnings of these power calculations, and there are several online resources for performing them. Often, "two-stage min-max" designs are employed where enrollment is halted if the response rate falls below a predetermined minimum level in an initial, small group of patients.[28] If

the response rate is higher, a second stage of enrollment continues to establish an approximate response rate. For example, at least 9 to 14 patients with the same histology or molecular target are treated to test the null hypothesis of insufficient efficacy. If no responses are observed in this group, the study ends. If a response is noted in one of the cases, the accrual is increased to 31 patients to establish a more accurate response rate. If a less robust response rate is expected (e.g., 20%), then the initial accrual number must be increased. Sample-size effect on study power calculations will be outlined in a subsequent section. Some have opined that the leading cause of drug failure in later phase development is our overdependence on these unpredictable single-arm, uncontrolled phase II trials and that, as such, they should be avoided to ensure phase III trial resources are not wasted because of the results of poorly designed phase II trials.[27] It used to be considered that the consequence of type I error (false positive) was less deleterious than that of type II error (false negative) because false-positive trials are likely to be repeated, whereas false-negative trials would result in the abandonment of a potentially active treatment.[29] The goals of comparative oncology modeling can help minimize type II error by mechanistically defining activity of novel agents through more detailed PK–PD studies. In today's environment, however, with an abundance of novel drugs to be evaluated, false-positive results are just as serious because they tie up patient and financial resources. With this in mind, the ideal phase II design would be randomized across several potential investigational drugs, blinded, and controlled; modifications of this type applied to standard phase II design are discussed subsequently (controlled phase II or phase IIB trials).[30]

Endpoints of Activity/Efficacy

As the primary goal of phase II trials is assessment of activity/efficacy, endpoints used to evaluate response are critical to the design. Median survival time is the ultimate "gold standard" primary endpoint that may be objectively measured to determine whether a drug is beneficial; however, this endpoint requires too great a length of time for early phase trials to be meaningful and can be affected in veterinary patients by decisions to euthanize or seek alternative or rescue therapies. Therefore most early phase trials utilize interim or secondary endpoints that are reasonably likely to predict clinical benefit. These surrogate endpoints may allow for shorter, less expensive, and technically simpler trials, which allow for early termination if an interim outcome reaches a prespecified positive or negative level. It is important that the validity of the surrogate outcome actually correlates with lower mortality (or improved QOL)—this is often validated in larger later phase trials. With traditional cytotoxic chemotherapeutics, response is assessed based on criteria that describe changes in size or volume according to several published methodologies (e.g., Response Evaluation Criteria in Solid Tumors [RECIST], World Health Organization [WHO]).[31–33] Veterinary consensus modifications of RECIST have been published.[34] It is readily evident that such criteria may not be appropriate for MTAs that are more likely to be cytostatic rather than cytotoxic, thus resulting in disease stabilization rather than measurable regression.[35,36] In such cases, it is critical that a designation of "stable disease" persist for a clinically relevant period of time, generally not less than 6 to 8 weeks, to avoid reflection of slow progression rather than a true treatment effect. Alternatively, temporal measures such as progression-free survival (PFS) or time to progression (TTP) may be appropriate endpoints; however, these often take too long to mature for timely phase II trials.[37] Alternatively, an adequate compromise could be progression-free rate (PFR) at predetermined time points. Again, comparative oncology models may more expediently define TTP or PFR because of compressed progression times in veterinary patients. These measures can also more accurately define efficacy in the minimal residual disease (MRD) setting such as trials interrogating novel adjuvant therapies for canine osteosarcoma (OSA) in the postamputation setting. For gauging response to immunotherapeutics, expanded response criteria have been published that help define methods of capturing unique response patterns observed in patients receiving these agents, which can be used in conjunction with RECIST or WHO methods.[38,39]

Secondary endpoints that may be evaluated in phase II trials include QOL assessments, comparative cost of therapy, days of hospitalization, validated surrogate biomarkers or measures of a molecular effect such as dephosphorylation of a growth factor receptor,[20,21] changes in microvessel density or regulatory T-cell number,[40] or target modulation that is linked to clinical outcome.[25] Importantly, phase II trials serve to expand knowledge of cumulative or long-term toxicities associated with new agents that may not be observed in short-term phase I trials designed to elucidate acute toxicity. An example of this in the veterinary literature involved a combined phase I/II trial simultaneously investigating the safety of liposome-encapsulated doxorubicin (LED) while comparing its activity with native doxorubicin in cats with vaccine-associated sarcomas.[41] Unexpectedly, the MTD established for LED in the acute phase I component of the trial was found to result in delayed and dose-limiting nephrotoxicity after long-term follow-up in the phase II component of the trial. Such discoveries are key to defining an agent's therapeutic window with repeated administrations.

New clinical trial concepts have entered into use in great part because of a recent initiative of the US Food and Drug Administration (FDA) to allow for "preclinical studies to provide evidence necessary to support the safety of administering new compounds to humans."[42] These are known as phase 0 trials, and they precede the traditional trials defined previously.[43,44] The role of phase 0 trials in cancer drug development is for biomarker and assay development/validation and evaluation of target modulation. Phase 0 trials allow for the systematic deprioritization of investigational agents that exhibit excessive toxicity or fail to show expected biologic effects and are used to direct dose selection for future studies. They represent first-in-species trials, usually of a small number of patients, and utilize lower and likely subtherapeutic drug doses. Comparative oncology trials allow the unique opportunity to answer the preclinical questions necessary to advance an agent. Phase 0 trials are "proof of concept" studies, wherein PK parameters are measured along with PD effects within target tissues, such as the tumor itself. These trials can also define surrogate markers of target effect, therapeutic response, or metabolites in surrogate tissues or fluids, such as blood or urine. Assessment of PK/PD relationships allow for a much broader understanding of new drug mechanism, therefore informing phase I/II trial design.

Controlled Phase II Trials

Sometimes referred to as phase IIB trials, these tend to be controlled, blinded, and randomized investigations of two or more novel regimens that identify promising agents to send to phase III trials for additional evaluation. Randomized phase II trials can be as simple as randomizing standard-of-care plus or minus the addition of a new drug. Another approach is to randomize subjects into multiple treatment arms or schedules with only enough power to make inferences as to which is the best drug to take

forward into phase III trials; so called "pick-the-winner" trials.[26] Although often not sufficiently powered for direct comparisons, they may use a less rigorous statistical assessment, such as setting the p-value at 10% and using 1-tailed analyses.

Phase III Trials (Pivotal/Confirming Trials)

It has been suggested that if phase II trials are "learning" trials, phase III trials are "confirming" trials.[45] These larger, randomized, blinded, and controlled trials have the goal of comparing a new drug or combination with standard-of-care therapies. They are often performed by large cooperative groups, which ensures greater case accrual, and FDA pivotal trials require multiinstitutional involvement. An example of a multicenter phase III trial would be the randomized comparison of liposome-encapsulated cisplatin (SPI-77) versus standard-of-care carboplatin in dogs with appendicular OSA.[46] No difference was observed between treatment groups, despite SPI-77 allowing five times the MTD of native cisplatin to be delivered in a liposome-encapsulated form. True phase III trials are not common in veterinary oncology because of their size and expense, with the exception of multicenter "registration" trials that have formed the basis for New Animal Drug Applications with the FDA Center for Veterinary Medicine (FDA-CVM).[47–49] Pivotal trials have included the registration of the first approved veterinary oncology agents, two tyrosine kinase inhibitors (TKIs; Palladia, Zoetis; Kinavet, AB Sciences) for the treatment of mast cell tumors.[47,48] TKIs showed improvement in PFS over placebo controls, and these trials define the process for expanding future efforts in veterinary oncology drug approval.

Sample Size and Power

The overriding function of clinical research is to provide a definitive answer to a clinical question. However, it is possible that, once complete, clinical trial conclusions may be incorrect based on chance or design error. Chance error results when an erroneous inference is drawn from a study sample group that is not actually representative of an entire patient population. Accounting for this potential error is essential in prospective clinical trial design, and its first critical step is to articulate the study hypothesis.[50] Type I or α error (false positive) occurs if an investigator rejects the null hypothesis when it is actually true.[45,50] This is also referred to as the study's level of significance. Type II or β error (false negative) occurs when one fails to reject the null hypothesis when it is actually incorrect. Type I and II errors are due to chance and cannot be avoided completely, although steps can be taken to reduce their potential effect by increasing sample size and augmenting study design or measurements.

Power is the ultimate measure of a clinical trial's results and also must be prospectively controlled. Power is defined as $1 - \beta$, the probability of correctly rejecting the null in the sample if the actual effect in the population is equal to (or greater than) the effect size.[45,50] Power is governed by sample size, with the goal being to enroll enough patients to accurately allow for a difference to be seen between groups. Power is irrelevant if the results are statistically significant, but if not, it is important to ensure the study had adequate numbers to detect a difference between groups. If a study to detect the difference between two cancer treatments is designed with an α of 0.05, then the principal investigator (PI) has set 5% as the maximum chance of incorrectly rejecting the null hypothesis if it is true. This is the level of doubt the PI is willing to accept when statistical tests are used to compare the two treatments. If β is set at 0.10, the PI is willing to accept a 10% chance of missing an association of a given effect if it exists. This represents a power of 0.90 (1 − β), or a 90% chance of finding an association of that size or greater. The α and β levels are determined before trial initiation, and their set points are based on the importance of avoiding either a false-positive or a false-negative result.

Randomization

Bias is introduced error in clinical research. One of the main ways to minimize bias is through the use of randomization, wherein research participants are assigned to a group within a clinical trial by chance instead of choice.[1] Groups include either the investigational group, those to receive the study drug, or the control group, those to receive a placebo (or comparator drug). Each participant enrolling in a trial has an equal chance of receiving the study drug, and the goal is to balance the groups based on participant characteristics (e.g., age, stage of disease, previous treatments) that may influence a response to therapy. At the end of the study, if bias is reduced by randomization, then the result (positive or negative) is more likely to be true. Unfortunately, in veterinary medicine, historical rather than active controls have been used for comparison of new therapies all too often. It is common in oncology trials to also blind participants so that patients or, in our case, clients do not know which treatment group their pet is in. Blinded or true active comparator trials are becoming more frequent as regulatory registration trials ultimately require them.

Reducing bias in clinical trials is an integral concept within trial design. Stratification is a concept used often in human oncology trials and is gaining headway in veterinary oncology trial design as well.[45,51] This allows for grouping of patients based on known prognostic factors. For example, this might include the stratification of dogs with lymphoma by clinical stage or immunophenotype with the goal of creating equal numbers of each within a treatment group. One of the main benefits of stratification is that it can prevent potential bias from *known* prognostic factors. For example, a treatment cohort may be doing comparatively poorly because the majority of dogs in that cohort had T-cell lymphoma. However, a difficulty with stratification is that the more prognostic factors are controlled, the less power the study has, and thus the need to increase sample size. Randomization to treatment groups should be performed after stratification.

Phase IV Trials (Postregistration Trials)

Once a drug has been granted a license or registered for a specific label use by the appropriate regulatory body (e.g., the FDA), postregistration phase IV trials may be performed to gain more information on AEs, long-term risks, off-label benefits, and the economic effect of the agent in the marketplace.[52] Phase IV trials may also involve treatment of special populations (e.g., the elderly, pediatric patients, or individuals with renal or hepatic dysfunction). The body of data on PK generated from postregistration trials is used to inform decisions on dose in special populations. Alternatively, phase IV trials may assess the benefit of the new drug for activity against diseases not included in the current approved regulatory label.

Good Manufacturing Practice/Good Clinical Practice Criteria

Provisions that create uniformity and consistency are key in clinical research implementation. Their primary intent is to ensure the safety of trial materials and participants and the integrity of clinical data. Such provisions determine good manufacturing

practice (GMP) and good clinical practice (GCP). GMP principles ensure the safe manufacture and testing of pharmaceutical drugs, biologics, and medical devices by outlining aspects of production that can affect the quality of a product. GCP guidelines were devised by the International Conference on Harmonization (ICH) to protect the rights and safety of human patients in clinical trials.[53]

GCP includes standards on how clinical trials should be designed and conducted, defines the roles and responsibilities of trial sponsors and clinical research investigators, and monitors the reporting of trial data.[53] It requires the use of a standardized clinical protocol and strict documentation of procedures and adherence to that protocol. GCP also establishes guidelines for oversight by external bodies, such as the Institutional Review Board (IRB) and the Data Safety and Monitoring Board (DSMB). The IRB serves as an independent ethics committee that has the power to approve, disapprove, or ask for modifications to planned study protocols. IRBs must include at least one nonscientist and a noninstitutional member known as a *community member*. If a clinical trial includes a vulnerable population, then the IRB must include an expert in the needs and specialties of this group. The IRB reviews protocol ethics, informed consent, and possible conflicts of interest, and provides scientific review of study protocol and results.

The DSMB (sometimes called a Data Monitoring Committee) is a third-party panel of experts consisting of at least one statistician, and is populated by clinicians who are experts in the field of research or drug of study.[54] In long-term and high-impact studies, an ethicist and/or a patient advocate representative may also serve on the DSMB. The purpose of the DSMB is to ensure the safety of participants through oversight and management of serious AEs (SAE). This group also ensures validity of data, and appropriate termination of studies for which significant benefits or risks have been uncovered or if it appears that the trial cannot be concluded successfully. However, the DSMB also reviews interim study results to determine whether an overwhelming benefit is evident in either the study or the control arm or if it is unlikely the study will answer the proposed study aim and thus should be terminated prematurely. It is important for all safety monitoring to be contemporaneous, including disclosure to the FDA of SAEs in real time. GCP compliance is necessary for FDA registration trials in both veterinary and human oncology drug development. Oversight of GMP and GCP provisions are provided by the FDA (http://www.fda.gov) and, in the European Union, oversight is provided by the European Medicines Agency (EMA; http://www.ema.europa.eu).

Effectiveness versus Efficacy Definitions

A key distinction in phase III trials is that data may be obtained within the context of randomized clinical trials (RCTs) or from effectiveness studies in the "real world." Because RCTs are designed to assess safety and efficacy of pharmaceuticals with an emphasis on study validity over generalizability, the applicability of data collected from them may be limited. The data may not be valid in more heterogeneous patients encountered in actual clinical practice and may be inaccurate because of strict protocol requirements or inclusion/exclusion criteria. Effectiveness studies, in which treatments are studied under real-world conditions, remedy some of these limitations. An efficacy study asks the question, "Does the drug work?" Whereas an effectiveness study asks the question "Does the drug help the targeted general population?" Some refer to this efficacy research as type I research (bench to bedside) and effectiveness research as type II (bedside to curbside) research. Generally, an RCT that determines efficacy occurs under ideal conditions whereas long-term effectiveness studies, which can be prospective or, on occasion, either meta-analyses or retrospective, define the overall effect of a drug. Also important to consider are the pharmacoeconomics of a drug, wherein a cost/benefit analysis weighs factors such as actual cost of medication, number or lives saved, minimization or exacerbation of hospital stays or doctor visits, and QOL measures, and computes their individual and societal expense. Once these outcome measures are studied and calculated, then comparisons between agents, new and old, can be made.[55-57]

Regulatory Oversight

The FDA is the regulatory body of the US government that oversees the activities of the drug and pharmaceutical industry. The FDA provides oversight for drug development primarily through written guidance, which describes rules and requirements for quality control and conduct. FDA guidance include oversight of drug standards, including chemistry, manufacturing, and control (CMC); preclinical animal toxicology; documentary requirements for investigational new drug (INDs) and new drug applications (NDAs); and ethics of clinical trials. In 1997 the FDA moved beyond its traditional approval paradigm by creating the FDA Modernization Act.[58] It necessitates PK bridging studies for new populations (e.g., pediatric PK studies) and allows for one adequate and well-controlled clinical investigation by "confirmatory evidence" comprising PK or PK/PD data to lead to drug approval. This emphasizes the importance of exposure and mechanism studies to more accurately determine the safety and effectiveness of novel drugs, especially targeted agents or ones evaluated in special populations.[59]

FDA drug development is a multistep process that defines interaction between the FDA, the drug sponsor, and their discovery and clinical teams with a shared goal of FDA approval. It involves a preclinical testing phase (IND requirements for CMC, animal testing, design of phase I clinical studies), IND evaluation, and NDA review, and marketing. FDA is attempting to improve and expedite the process of drug development through a number of initiatives. The most innovative are the Critical Path Initiative (2004), end-of-phase 2a (EOP2a) meeting (2004), and model-based drug development (2005) (physiologically based PK [PBPK], 2009).[60] In January 2017, the FDA formed the Oncology Center of Excellence (OCE), which leverages the combined skills of regulatory scientists and reviewers with expertise in drugs, biologics, and devices. This initiative will help expedite the development of oncology and hematology medical products and support an integrated approach in the clinical evaluation of such agents for treatment of cancer. In addition, the FDA is working to implement provisions of the Cancer Moonshot initiative and 21st Century Cures Act through the formation of the OCE, and has recently published a perspective on oncology drug development that explores concepts geared toward an approach that could provide earlier access to highly effective therapeutic drugs, thus complementing existing expedited programs such as breakthrough designation and accelerated approval.[61] The OCE also supports the use of common control trials, which share a common control arm, involve multiple different drugs for the same indication, and may involve different companies and/or sponsors. The Morris Animal Foundation's Osteosarcoma Project trials, currently underway through the National Cancer Institute (NCI) Comparative Oncology Trials Consortium (COTC), are emblematic of this approach, and are focused on providing advances for both humans and dogs to combat metastatic progression in the MRD setting.

Veterinary Registration Trials

Veterinary drug development follows the same critical regulatory steps described earlier but oversight is provided by the FDA–CVM and, in the case of biologics, by the US Department of Agriculture (USDA). Before 2007 with the conditional approval of ONCEPT (Canine Melanoma Vaccine, DNA, Boehringer-Ingelheim), all cancer drugs used in veterinary medicine were originally developed for humans and not approved for use in animals. Cancer chemotherapeutics are used in an "extralabel" manner as allowed by the Animal Medicinal Drug Use Clarification Act of 1994. Significant gains have occurred recently in veterinary oncology product development with full approval of toceranib phosphate (Palladia, Zoetis), masitinib (Masivet, AB Science), and ONCEPT (Boehringer-Ingelheim). Palladia and Masivet are both receptor TKIs and are approved for treatment of recurrent or inoperable grade II or III mast cell tumors with or without regional lymph node involvement.[20,47,48,62] Palladia was developed by SUGEN as SU11654, a sister compound to SU11248 later approved for human patients as Sutent.[63] ONCEPT is a xenogeneic tyrosinase DNA vaccine indicated for dogs with stage II or stage III oral canine melanoma.[64,65] Registration trials for these agents involved safety and efficacy assessments in multicenter clinical trials under GCP conditions.

Consortia

One of the most exciting achievements in veterinary oncology since 2008 has been the development of successful and collaborative consortia that are purposed to perform multicenter clinical trials and prospective tumor biospecimen repository collections. Consortium infrastructures allow larger scale clinical trials and provide the voice for collective advocacy in veterinary and comparative oncology.

Comparative Oncology Trials Consortium

The COTC is an active network of 24 academic comparative oncology centers (https://ccrod.cancer.gov/confluence/display/CCRCOPWeb/Comparative+Oncology+Trials+Consortium), centrally managed by the National Institutes of Health–NCI's Comparative Oncology Program that functions to design and execute clinical trials in dogs with cancer to assess novel therapies.[66,67] The goal of this effort is to answer biologic questions geared to inform the development path of these agents for use in human cancer patients. COTC trials are pharmacokinetically and pharmacodynamically rich, with the product of this work directly integrated into the design of current human early and late phase clinical trials. They are focused to answer mechanistic questions and define dose–toxicity and dose–response relationships. They can be designed to compare varying schedules and routes of drug administration, validate target biology, model clinical standard operating procedures (SOPs), and assess biomarkers. In addition, within this effort, the COTC PD Core was created. The COTC PD Core is a virtual laboratory of assays and services, including pathology, immunohistochemistry, immunocytochemistry, flow cytometry, genomics, proteomics, cell culture, PK, and cell biology designed to support COTC clinical trial biologic endpoints.[68] As of 2018, the COTC has completed 13 clinical trials and has been successful in promoting the utility of comparative oncology modeling within the drug development community.

Veterinary Contract Research Organizations

Contract research organizations (CROs) are generally privately organized and run specialty networks of veterinary hospitals that design, conduct, and report clinical studies for the animal health industry. Examples include Animal Clinical Investigation (ACI; www.animalci.com), The One Health Company (www.theonehealthcompany.com), and VetPharm (www.vetpharm.com). Although oncology drug development is within their portfolios, other medical conditions, including inflammatory and metabolic disease, cardiovascular disease, and arthritis, are also managed. CROs provide multisite, pivotal, or nonpivotal studies and commercialization support to help define effective novel veterinary therapeutics.

Current Challenges and Opportunities in Oncology Drug Development

Oncology drug development is a difficult and costly process. It is estimated that only 5% to 10% of drugs entering phase I oncology clinical trials ultimately are approved by the FDA, with a cost of between 0.8 and 1.7 billion dollars per drug accrued through the development process.[55,69] The most prevalent cause of cancer drug failure is toxicity or inactivity. For every 1000 oncology agents in development, only 40% transition from preclinical studies to phase I, 75% from phase I to phase II, 60% from phase II to phase III, and 55% from phase III to approval. This means that for every 1000 preclinical candidates, only 99 new drugs will reach the clinic.

Model-Based (Adaptive) Drug Development

Adaptive Trial Designs and Stopping Rules

Adaptive trial designs[70–74] allow investigators to modify trials while they are ongoing based on newly acquired data and, in some cases, taking into account data generated in other trials or past trials. In adaptive trial designs, interim data from a trial is used to modify and improve the study design, in a preplanned manner and without undermining its validity or integrity. In the exploratory setting, an adaptive trial can assign a larger proportion of the enrolled subjects to the treatment arms that are performing well, drop arms that are performing poorly, and investigate a wider range of doses so as to more effectively select doses that are most likely to succeed in the confirmatory phase. In the confirmatory phase, adaptive design can facilitate the early identification of efficacious treatments, decisions to drop poorly performing trial arms, determining whether the trial should be terminated for futility, and making sample-size adjustments at interim time points to ensure that the trial is adequately powered. In some cases, it might even be possible to enrich the patient population by altering the eligibility criteria at an interim time point. These also include biomarker-based adaptive designs which enable adaptations based on the response of biomarkers, biomarker/target screening designs (e.g., enrichment designs such as "basket" or "umbrella" trials).[73]

Potential benefits of adaptive designs include[72] (1) they allow the investigator to correct wrong assumptions made at the beginning of the trial; (2) they help the investigator select the most promising option early; (3) they make use of information that emerges outside of the trial; (4) they enable the investigator to react earlier to surprises (either positive or negative); and (5) they may shorten the development time and consequently speed up the development process. However, adaptive designs may undermine validity and integrity of the trial if not managed appropriately.

That being said, adaptations based on blinded analyses at interim, if the blinding is strictly maintained, can largely reduce or completely avoid bias.

Stopping Rules

Stopping rules, which are rules that terminate a clinical trial earlier than originally projected or within a predetermined adaptive trial design, can be applied to randomized phase II or phase III trials. Several methods and variations have been extensively reviewed.[75–77] Stopping rules are designed to protect treatment subjects from unsafe drugs, to hasten the general availability of superior drugs as soon as sufficient evidence has been collected, and to help ensure the transfer of resources and patients to alternative trials. Trials are stopped for three reasons: the investigational treatment is clearly better than the control, the investigational treatment is clearly worse than the control (less activity or more toxicity), or the investigational therapy is not likely to be better (so-called "stopping for futility" or "futility analysis"). The methods by which stopping rules are applied usually involve some type of interim analysis that evaluates the data (by a blinded individual or DSMB) generated to date and makes a determination based on predetermined rules. The interim data are often analyzed for conditional power, which is the probability of the final study result demonstrating statistical significance in the primary efficacy endpoint, conditional on the current data observed, and a specific assumption about the pattern of the data to be observed in the remainder of the study. If a study is designed a priori to involve conditional power calculations of interim data, the rules for early termination are sometimes referred to as *stochastic curtailing*.

Bayesian (Continuous Learning) Adaptive Designs

Adaptive trial designs can also be used to change the randomization weight to better performing treatment arms, add new treatment arms, drop poorly performing arms, or extend accrual beyond the original target when more information is needed. With the availability of advanced computational techniques, a new statistical methodology, the Bayesian approach, was developed that makes statistical inferences that focus on the probability that a hypothesis is true given the available evidence.

In contrast, Bayesian trials differ from the *frequentist* approach to statistics by using available patient outcome information, including biomarkers that accumulate data related to outcome (if available and validated), and even historic information or results from other relevant trials to adapt the current trial design continually based on newly informed probabilities.[78–80] An example that illustrates the utility of the Bayesian approach involves interim analysis applied to a randomized phase II trial of neoadjuvant trastuzumab, paclitaxel, and epirubicin in epidermal growth factor receptor 2 (HER2/neu)–positive breast cancer.[81] In this trial initially designed to enter 164 patients (based on the frequentist approach to power), a Bayesian approach was used to perform an interim analysis after 34 patients were enrolled; 67% of patients in the investigational treatment arm experienced complete responses compared with 25% in the standard treatment arm. The Bayesian predictive probability of statistical significance if 164 patients were accrued, based on the data available from these 34 patients, was calculated to be 95%, and the trial was stopped and the drug moved to phase III early because of these promising results. The very first Bayesian response adaptive trial involving companion animals was recently published.[82] In this trial comparing toceranib versus vinblastine therapy for canine mast cell tumors, patients were randomized based on the "play-the-winner" rule;

as more information regarding efficacy and KIT localization and c-*kit* mutation status became available, newly accrued dogs were randomized proportional to the predicted response probability.

Randomized Discontinuation Trials

This phase II design was proposed for evaluating the efficacy of newer targeted agents that are thought to have disease-stabilizing activity (cytostatic) in contrast to disease-regressing activity of more traditional cytotoxic chemotherapeutics. Several reviews of this trial design are recommended.[83–85] Trials that evaluate growth-inhibiting agents in tumors with a variable natural history seem ideally suited for randomized discontinuation trials (RDTs) because the "no treatment effect" is hard to control in these cases. In essence, these trials serve to enrich and homogenize the static agent for those patients likely to benefit from it. RDTs involve a two-stage trial design, wherein the first stage involves a "run-in" phase in which all patients receive the cytostatic agent under investigation. At the end of the run-in phase, assessment of disease response is made. If a response is noted, the subject continues on the investigational drug, whereas if progression (or excess toxicity) is noted, the subject is removed from trial and allowed to receive alternative treatment. Those patients who meet stable disease criteria enter the second stage of the RDT and are randomized to continue on the investigational drug or placebo (the discontinuation arm). Then, at predetermined times, follow-up determinations are made. Endpoints in stage II of the trial at these follow-up intervals are "stable or better" versus "progression." Time-to-event measures may be applied as well (e.g., PFS, TTP), although this takes more time to complete. If a subject progresses in the second stage, the code can be broken, and if that subject is in the placebo group, the investigational drug can be reinstituted. Therefore there are two ways for RDTs to be stopped: there are a substantial number of objective responses noted in the run-in phase making a second stage unnecessary, or the number of subjects progressing in the second stage differs statistically between the treatment and placebo groups. It becomes intuitive that the length of the run-in phase is critical to RDTs: if it is too long, some initially responding patients progress during the late stage of the run-in and are missed (therefore increasing subject numbers); if it is too short, insufficient enrichment occurs (not enough time for nonresponders to progress) and the randomization might as well have been done at the outset. The two major advantages of RDTs are that all subjects receive the drug up front so that every patient is given a chance to respond to the drug (something that is popular with patients [or companion animal owners]) and enrichment of likely responders may increase power and decrease subject numbers. Potential disadvantages of RDTs include the ethics of discontinuation (but the design can allow reinstitution), the potential for a carryover effect of the drug after discontinuation (unlikely for most targeted agents), and failure to detect short duration activity (but this would likely be a clinically irrelevant duration anyway). RDTs can be improved by combining other modifications of clinical trials, such as interim analysis and Bayesian analysis, and by using active controls. For purposes of illustration, an RDT in veterinary medicine that the authors have considered would be the investigation of a cytostatic agent in dogs with pulmonary metastatic OSA. All dogs would enter the run-in phase, receive the cytostatic drug for 4 weeks, and then be evaluated for response. From what we already know about the natural history of OSA in dogs, most (probably 80%) of dogs that did not receive treatment would progress in that period. Those that were stable at 4 weeks, however, would be randomized to drug continuation or discontinuation (placebo) and followed with monthly reevaluations. This would ensure all dogs had a chance to respond to the drug and enrich the population likely to respond, and a positive result would be clinical response noted in the run-in phase or a statistical difference in PFR between groups in the second stage.

Personalized Medicine

Advancements in genomic, proteomic, and epigenetic profiling have created new opportunities to tailor cancer treatments to individual patient and tumor molecular characteristics; this field is known as personalized or molecular-based medicine. The goals of personalized medicine approaches include improving outcomes by revealing disease drivers, toxicity, susceptibilities, and resistance profiles unique to the individual patient. Molecular profiling approaches have been employed to stratify and prescribe therapies for human oncology patients. The most successful examples to date have been in the identification of HER2 overexpression in breast cancer and the oncogenic *bcr–abl* translocation in chronic myelogenous leukemia and the prescription of monoclonal antibodies (trastuzumab, Herceptin) and TKIs (imatinib, Gleevec) against these key pathways (also the basis for Bayesian approaches previously mentioned).[86–88] Veterinary oncology has also benefited from molecular-based approaches, most notably in the targeting of c-*kit* mutations in canine mast cell tumors.[48,89] TKIs (toceranib and masitinib) have shown clinical utility against macroscopic disease and have been approved by the FDA for use in this setting. Although both agents are nonselective inhibitors that also have activity against other key pathways (e.g., vascular endothelial growth factor receptor 2 [VEGFR2] for toceranib), their approval marks an important step forward in veterinary tumor biology-based therapeutics and sets the stage for future directed research in other tumor types.

The field of personalized medicine expands beyond patient prescription to also include the study of patient pharmacogenomics and pharmacometabolics, the genetic variation of response and metabolism of novel agents or medications. These include the study of individual patient single nucleotide polymorphisms (SNPs) in key metabolic pathways (cytochrome p450) and the measurement of metabolites in blood and urine. An example of this in veterinary oncology is the use of multidrug resistance gene 1 (*MDR1*) mutation analysis in certain herding breeds (e.g., collies and shelties) before initiating *MDR1* substrate chemotherapeutic agents (e.g., doxorubicin and vincristine).

Newer personalized medicine approaches based on complex mathematical algorithms have been created that include a broader base of tumor characteristics to define potential treatments. The use of pretreatment biopsies to create prospective molecular profiles has been modeled by the COTC in veterinary patients and found to be achievable in a practical clinical window.[90] More recently, so called "liquid biopsy" techniques have been developed whereby tumor DNA in blood is used to detect, track, and develop personalized treatment protocols in cancer patients.[91] The publication of the canine genome and the advent of high-throughput technologies have enabled the field of veterinary oncology to describe canine cancer biology and characterize potential therapeutic targets more globally.[92] This creates the opportunity for personalized medicine investigations in the dog to inform novel therapy development for both veterinary and human oncology patients using these algorithmic approaches. In addition, strong cancer breed predilections support "breed-based" genetic approaches that may uncover oncogenic pathways and targets more easily and inform discovery and application of personalized medicine strategies.

Clinical Trial Ethics

There are key ethical standards employed in clinical trial design, and the goal of all clinicians is to ensure standards are met when offering a trial to a client or enrolling a patient within a clinical trial. Many clinical trials provide partially or fully funded care for eligible pets with cancer. This is important because traditional veterinary oncology treatments, surgery, chemotherapy, and radiation therapy, are expensive and costs are prohibitive for some clients. Clinical trial enrollment may present an opportunity to help some clients who may not have the financial means to pursue treatment or receive care for their pet, or provide treatment to those pets that have progressed in the face of traditional therapies. When all medical options are described to clients as far as care for their pet's disease, some may choose clinical trials to make an impact for future pets or people with cancer. This altruism (by proxy) drives the decision-making process for many caregivers.

Informed consent defines a trial's purpose and the requirements for the client to return with their pet for future follow-up procedures/appointments, and is required for all patients to enroll in a clinical trial. This consent is a written acknowledgment, created by a trial's PIs and signed by a client, of the possible positive and conversely AEs (known or unknown) of an investigational agent. Goals for clinical trials must be clearly outlined so true informed consent can be obtained. Although AEs outside of those described are always possible, informed consent ensures that clients understand that in many trials the outcome/side effects are as yet unknown. Ethical considerations also require rigorous informed consent of study procedures, especially in biologically intensive trials, because repeated invasive procedures or even serial imaging may result in the false perception of a stronger therapeutic intent.[93]

As the treatment of companion animals with cancer is purely a client-driven choice, there are no true "standards of care" in veterinary oncology. Although there are proven active regimes for the care of common cancers in dogs (i.e., *c*yclophosphamide, *h*ydroxydaunorubicin (doxorubicin), vincristine [*O*ncovin], and *p*rednisone [CHOP]-based chemotherapy in lymphoma, platinum or anthracyclines in OSA), these therapies are not required. Therefore veterinary and comparative oncology trials can offer investigational therapies in naïve disease. Clinical trials can randomize patients to placebo arms if there is an interest in comparing a novel therapy to no therapy. Although, as in human trials, informed consent must clearly state the inclusion of a placebo arm, the protocol design may include an allowance for crossover to study drug or traditional therapies either at a defined interval or in documented progressive disease. Requirements for early stopping rules can also alleviate some of these ethical concerns when overt drug inactivity or activity is evident.[94] Box 18.1 defines the suggested elements that should be included in any clinical trial informed consent document.[1]

Many regulatory safeguards have been put in place to promote the welfare and interests of animals used in biomedical and clinical research. Protocols to use animal subjects in clinical research must be approved by Institutional Animal Care and Use Committees (IACUCs), and these bodies are also involved in oversight of research study conduct to ensure ethical standards are maintained.

• BOX 18.1 Suggested "Elements of Consent" to Include in Informed Client Consent Documents

1. Purpose of research
2. Expected duration of participation
3. Description of procedures
4. Possible discomforts and risks
5. Possible benefits
6. Alternative treatment (or alternative to participation)
7. Extent of confidentiality of records
8. Compensation or therapy for injuries or adverse events
9. Contact person for the study
10. Voluntary participation and right to withdraw
11. Termination of participation by the principal investigator
12. Unforeseen risks
13. Financial obligations
14. Hospital review committee contact person

Modified with permission from Morris Animal Foundation: www.morrisanimalfoundation.org.

Some veterinary hospitals also have Clinical Review Boards that function similarly to human IRBs as described previously. In some cases, pet dogs are receiving "first in dog" drugs and AEs are expected, with grade V events (fatality) possible. Although this would be predicted to reflect what is seen in an aged and ill cancer population, it is an important element to be detailed in informed consent. The grading and reporting of AEs in clinical trials include uniform common toxicity criteria for AEs (e.g., VCOG-CTCAE version 1.1) and ethical care includes treatment for any such events.[10] Clients also have the option to withdraw their pets from a clinical trial at any time without penalty. All of these provisions are designed to ensure safety for trial participants and the ethical conduct of clinical research.

Trial Reporting

The transparent reporting of clinical trials has received considerable attention in the past several years. For randomized trials, the current "gold standard" guidelines for reporting of data is the Consolidated Standards of Reporting Trials (CONSORT; www.consort-statement.org). In these guidelines, logical and stepwise guides to the reporting of patient enrollment, patient allocation (between and within treatment groups), patient follow-up, and data analysis are clearly spelled out. Anyone devising, performing, and indeed critically appraising clinical trials should be well versed in these guidelines.

Conclusions

Clinical trials are an important research discipline to improve care and outcome for cancer patients in both human and veterinary oncology. Steps should be made to ensure study aims are achievable within a crafted study design and protocol. Rules governing design are prospective and involve questions of dose and schedule selection, toxicity, activity, and comparison to known effective therapies. Statistical expertise is also necessary to ensure appropriate clinical trial design. Regulatory oversight of veterinary oncology trials is increasing, and new approval of veterinary oncology agents will emphasize these processes over the next decade. Comparative oncology trials also are key to the inclusion of pet animals in the evaluation of novel anticancer therapeutics, imaging strategies, and medical devices. Consortia groups will continue to advocate and advance the use and utility of veterinary oncology clinical trials. The field of veterinary oncology will continue to grow through the proper use and design of both traditional and novel clinical trial designs.

References

1. Thamm DH, Vail DM: Veterinary oncology clinical trials: design and implementation, *Vet J* 205:226–232, 2015.
2. Vail DM: Cancer clinical trials: development and implementation, *Vet Clin North Am Small Anim Pract* 37:1033–1057, 2007.
3. Potter DM: Phase I studies of chemotherapeutic agents in cancer patients: a review of the designs, *J Biopharm Stat* 16:579–604, 2006.
4. Kummar S, Gutierrez M, Doroshow JH, et al.: Drug development in oncology: classical cytotoxics and molecularly targeted agents, *Br J Clin Pharmacol* 62:15–26, 2006.
5. Acevedo PV, Topmeyer DL, Rubin EH: Phase I trial design and methodology for anticancer drugs. In Teicher BA, Andrews PA, editors: *Anticancer Drug Development Guide*, ed 2, Totowa, NJ, 2004, Humana Press, pp 351–362.
6. Khanna C, Lindblad-Toh K, Vail D, et al.: The dog as a cancer model, *Nat Biotechnol* 24:1065–1066, 2006.
7. Paoloni M, Khanna C: Translation of new cancer treatments from pet dogs to humans, *Nat Rev Cancer* 8:147–156, 2008.
8. LeBlanc AK, Mazcko CN, Khanna C: Defining the value of a comparative approach to cancer drug development, *Clin Cancer Res* 22:2133–2138, 2016.
9. Le Tourneau C, Lee JJ, Siu LL: Dose escalation methods in phase I cancer clinical trials, *J Natl Cancer Inst* 101:708–720, 2009.
10. Vail D: Veterinary Co-operative Oncology Group—Common Terminology Criteria for Adverse Events (VCOG-CTCAE) following chemotherapy or biological antineoplastic therapy in dogs and cats v1.1, *Vet Comp Oncol* 10:1–30, 2011.
11. Ishizuka N, Ohashi Y: The continual reassessment method and its applications: a Bayesian methodology for phase I cancer clinical trials, *Stat Med* 20:2661–2681, 2001.
12. Zohar S, Chevret S: Phase I (or phase II) dose-ranging clinical trials: proposal of a two-stage Bayesian design, *J Biopharm Stat* 13:87–101, 2003.
13. Hanson AR, Graham DM, Pond GR, et al.: Phase 1 trial design: is 3+3 best? *Cancer Control* 21:200–208, 2014.
14. Wong KM, Capasso A, Eckhardt SG: The changing landscape of phase I trials in oncology, *Nat Rev Clin Oncol* 13:106–117, 2016.
15. Bria E, Di Maio M, Carlini P, et al.: Targeting targeted agents: open issues for clinical trial design, *J Exp Clin Cancer Res* 28:66, 2009.
16. Brunetto AT, Kristeleit RS, de Bono JS: Early oncology clinical trial design in the era of molecular-targeted agents, *Future Oncol* 6:1339–1352, 2010.
17. Hoekstra R, Verweij J, Eskens FA: Clinical trial design for target specific anticancer agents, *Invest New Drugs* 21:243–250, 2003.
18. Parulekar WR, Eisenhauer EA: Phase I trial design for solid tumor studies of targeted, non-cytotoxic agents: theory and practice, *J Natl Cancer Inst* 96:990–997, 2004.
19. Dowlati A, Manda S, Gibbons J, et al.: multi-institutional phase I trials of anticancer agents, *J Clin Oncol* 26:1926–1931, 2008.
20. Pryer NK, Lee LB, Zadovaskaya R, et al.: Proof of target for SU11654: inhibition of KIT phosphorylation in canine mast cell tumors, *Clin Cancer Res* 9:5729–5734, 2003.
21. Honigberg LA, Smith AM, Sirisawad M, et al.: The Bruton tyrosine kinase inhibitor PCI-32765 blocks B-cell activation and is efficacious in models of autoimmune disease and B-cell malignancy, *Proc Natl Acad Sci USA* 107:13075–13080, 2010.
22. Wittenburg LA, Gustafson DL, Thamm DH: Phase I pharmacokinetic and pharmacodynamic evaluation of combined valproic acid/doxorubicin treatment in dogs with spontaneous cancer, *Clin Cancer Res* 16:4832–4842, 2010.
23. Barnard RA, Wittenburg LA, Amaravadi RK, et al.: Phase I clinical trial and pharmacodynamic evaluation of combination hydroxychloroquine and doxorubicin treatment in pet dogs treated for spontaneously occurring lymphoma, *Autophagy* 10:1415–1425, 2014.
24. Gray R, Manola J, Saxman S, et al.: Phase II clinical trial design: methods in translational research from the Genitourinary Committee at the Eastern Cooperative Oncology Group, *Clin Cancer Res* 12:1966–1969, 2006.
25. Lee JJ, Feng L: Randomized phase II designs in cancer clinical trials: current status and future directions, *J Clin Oncol* 23:4450–4457, 2005.
26. Brown SR, Gregory WM, Twelves CJ, et al.: Designing phase II trials in cancer: a systematic review and guidance, *Br J Cancer* 105:194–199, 2011.
27. Michaelis LC, Ratain MJ: Phase II trials published in 2002: a cross-specialty comparison showing significant design differences between oncology trials and other medical specialties, *Clin Cancer Res* 13:2400–2405, 2007.
28. Simon R: Optimal two-stage designs for phase II clinical trials, *Control Clin Trials* 10:1–10, 1989.
29. Ocana A, Tannock IF: When are "positive" clinical trials in oncology truly positive?, *J Natl Cancer Inst* 103:16–20, 2011.
30. Mandrekar SJ, Sargent DJ: Randomized phase II trials: time for a new era in clinical trial design, *J Thorac Oncol* 5:932–934, 2010.
31. Eisenhauer EA, Therasse P, Bogaerts J, et al.: New response evaluation criteria in solid tumours: revised RECIST guideline (version 1.1), *Eur J Cancer* 45:228–247, 2009.
32. Jaffe CC: Measures of response: RECIST, WHO, and new alternatives, *J Clin Oncol* 24:3245–3251, 2006.
33. Gomez-Roca C, Koscielny S, Ribrag V, et al.: Tumour growth rates and RECIST criteria in early drug development, *Eur J Cancer* 47:2512–2516, 2011.
34. Nguyen SM, Thamm DH, Vail DM, et al.: Response evaluation criteria for solid tumours in dogs (v1.0): a Veterinary Cooperative Oncology Group (VCOG) consensus document, *Vet Comp Onc* 13:176–183, 2015.
35. Rasmussen F: RECIST and targeted therapy, *Acta Radiol* 50:835–836, 2009.
36. Rosen MA: Use of modified RECIST criteria to improve response assessment in targeted therapies: challenges and opportunities, *Cancer Biol Ther* 9:20–22, 2010.
37. Gutierrez ME, Kummar S, Giaccone G: Next generation oncology drug development: opportunities and challenges, *Nat Rev Clin Oncol* 6:259–265, 2009.
38. Hoos A, Wolchok JD, Humphrey RW, et al.: CCR 20th Anniversary commentary: immune-related response criteria – capturing clinical activity in immune-oncology, *Clin Cancer Res* 21:4989–4991, 2015.
39. Wolchok JD, Hoos A, O'Day S, et al.: Guidelines for the evaluation of immune therapy activity in solid tumors: immune-related response criteria, *Clin Cancer Res* 15:7412–7420, 2009.
40. Burton JH, Mitchell L, Thamm DH, et al.: Low-dose cyclophosphamide selectively decreases regulatory T cells and inhibits angiogenesis in dogs with soft tissue sarcoma, *J Vet Intern Med* 25:920–926, 2011.
41. Poirier VJ, Thamm DH, Kurzman ID, et al.: Liposome-encapsulated doxorubicin (Doxil) and doxorubicin in the treatment of vaccine-associated sarcoma in cats, *J Vet Intern Med* 16:726–731, 2002.
42. Kinders R, Parchment RE, Ji J, et al.: Phase 0 clinical trials in cancer drug development: from FDA guidance to clinical practice, *Mol Interv* 7:325–334, 2007.
43. Kummar S, Kinders R, Rubinstein L, et al.: Compressing drug development timelines in oncology using phase '0' trials, *Nat Rev Cancer* 7:131–139, 2007.
44. Murgo AJ, Kummar S, Rubinstein L, et al.: Designing phase 0 cancer clinical trials, *Clin Cancer Res* 14:3675–3682, 2008.
45. Hulley SB, Cummings SR, Browner WS, et al.: *Designing Clinical Research*, Philadelphia, 2007, Lippincott Williams & Wilkins.

46. Vail DM, Kurzman ID, Glawe PC, et al.: STEALTH liposome-encapsulated cisplatin (SPI-77) versus carboplatin as adjuvant therapy for spontaneously arising osteosarcoma (OSA) in the dog: a randomized multicenter clinical trial, *Cancer Chemother Pharmacol* 50:131–136, 2002.

47. London CA, Malpas PB, Wood-Follis SL, et al.: Multi-center, placebo-controlled, double-blind, randomized study of oral toceranib phosphate (SU11654), a receptor tyrosine kinase inhibitor, for the treatment of dogs with recurrent (either local or distant) mast cell tumor following surgical excision, *Clin Cancer Res* 15:3856–3865, 2009.

48. Hahn KA, Ogilvie G, Rusk T, et al.: Masitinib is safe and effective for the treatment of canine mast cell tumors, *J Vet Intern Med* 22:1301–1309, 2008.

49. Vail DM, von Euler H, Rusk AW, et al.: A randomized trial investigating the efficacy and safety of water soluble micellar paclitaxel (Paccal Vet) for treatment of nonresectable grade 2 or 3 mast cell tumors in dogs, *J Vet Intern Med* 26:598–607, 2012.

50. Gallo C, Perrone F: Clinical trial design in oncology: statistical power, *Lancet Oncol* 5:760–761, 2004.

51. Fey MF: Clinical trial design in oncology: selection of patients, *Lancet Oncol* 5:760, 2004.

52. Lonning PE: Strength and weakness of phase I to IV trials, with an emphasis on translational aspects, *Breast Cancer Res* 10(suppl 4):S22, 2008.

53. Zon R, Meropol NJ, Catalano RB, et al.: American Society of Clinical Oncology Statement on minimum standards and exemplary attributes of clinical trial sites, *J Clin Oncol* 26:2562–2567, 2008.

54. McLemore MR: The role of the data safety monitoring board: why was the Avastin phase III clinical trial stopped? *Clin J Oncol Nurs* 10:153–154, 2006.

55. DiMasi JA, Grabowski HG: Economics of new oncology drug development, *J Clin Oncol* 25:209–216, 2007.

56. Milne CP, Kaitin KI, Dimasi JA: Mandatory comparator trials for therapeutically similar drugs: an assessment of the facts, *Am J Ther* 14:231–234, 2007.

57. Biotechnology Industry Organization (BIO): Late-stage clinical success rates, New York, 2011, *BIO CEO & Investor Conference*. February 15.

58. Rossen BR: FDA's proposed regulations to expand access to investigational drugs for treatment use: the status quo in the guise of reform, *Food Drug Law J* 64:183–223, 2009.

59. Karsdal MA, Henriksen K, Leeming DJ, et al.: Biochemical markers and the FDA Critical Path: how biomarkers may contribute to the understanding of pathophysiology and provide unique and necessary tools for drug development, *Biomarkers* 14:181–202, 2009.

60. Woodcock J, Woosley R: The FDA critical path initiative and its influence on new drug development, *Annu Rev Med* 59:1–12, 2008.

61. Prowell TM, Theoret MR, Pazdur R: Seamless oncology-drug development, *N Eng J Med* 374:2001–2003, 2016.

62. Hahn KA, Legendre AM, Shaw NG, et al.: Evaluation of 12- and 24-month survival rates after treatment with masitinib in dogs with nonresectable mast cell tumors, *Am J Vet Res* 71:1354–1361, 2010.

63. Pryer NK, Lee LB, Zadovaskaya R, et al.: Proof of target for SU11654: inhibition of KIT phosphorylation in canine mast cell tumors, *Clin Cancer Res* 9:5729–5734, 2003.

64. Bergman PJ, McKnight J, Novosad A, et al.: Long-term survival of dogs with advanced malignant melanoma after DNA vaccination with xenogeneic human tyrosinase: a phase I trial, *Clin Cancer Res* 9:1284–1290, 2003.

65. Liao JC, Gregor P, Wolchok JD, et al.: Vaccination with human tyrosinase DNA induces antibody responses in dogs with advanced melanoma, *Cancer Immun* 6(8), 2006.

66. Gordon I, Paoloni M, Mazcko C, et al.: The comparative oncology trials consortium: using spontaneously occurring cancers in dogs to inform the cancer drug development pathway, *PLoS Med* 6:e1000161, 2009.

67. Paoloni MC, Tandle A, Mazcko C, et al.: Launching a novel preclinical infrastructure: comparative oncology trials consortium directed therapeutic targeting of TNFalpha to cancer vasculature, *PLoS One* 4:e4972, 2009.

68. Paoloni M, Lana S, Thamm D, et al.: The creation of the Comparative Oncology Trials Consortium Pharmacodynamic Core: infrastructure for a virtual laboratory, *Vet J* 185:88–89, 2010.

69. Steensma DP, Kantarijian HM: Impact of cancer research bureaucracy on innovation, costs and patient care, *J Clin Oncol* 32:376–378, 2014.

70. Freidlin B, Korn EL: Biomarker enrichment strategies: matching trial design to biomarker credentials, *Nat Rev Clin Oncol* 11:81–90, 2014.

71. Sharma MR, Schilsky RL: Role of randomized phase III trials in an era of effective targeted therapies, *Nat Rev Clin Oncol* 9:208–214, 2012.

72. Chow SC: Adaptive clinical trial design, *Annu Rev Med* 65:405–415, 2014.

73. Menis J, Hasan B, Besse B: New clinical research strategies in thoracic oncology: clinical trial design, adaptive, basket and umbrella trials, new end-points and new evaluations of response, *Eur Respir Rev* 23:367–378, 2014.

74. Sargent DJ, Korn EL: Sifting paradigms in cancer clinical trial design, *Nat Rev Clin Oncol* 11:625–626, 2014.

75. Whitehead J: Stopping clinical trials by design, *Nat Rev Drug Discov* 3:973–977, 2004.

76. Betensky RA: Conditional power calculations for early acceptance of H0 embedded in sequential tests, *Stat Med* 16:465–477, 1997.

77. Lachin JM: A review of methods for futility stopping based on conditional power, *Stat Med* 24:2747–2764, 2005.

78. Berry DA: Decision analysis and Bayesian methods in clinical trials, *Cancer Treat Res* 75:125–154, 1995.

79. Biswas S, Liu DD, Lee JJ, et al.: Bayesian clinical trials at the University of Texas M. D. Anderson Cancer Center, *Clin Trials* 6:205–216, 2009.

80. Rosner GL, Berry DA: A Bayesian group sequential design for multiple arm randomized clinical trials, *Stat Med* 14:381–394, 1995.

81. Buzdar AU, Ibrahim NK, Francis D, et al.: Significantly higher pathologic complete remission rate after neoadjuvant therapy with trastuzumab, paclitaxel, and epirubicin chemotherapy: results of a randomized trial in human epidermal growth factor receptor 2-positive operable breast cancer, *J Clin Oncol* 23:3676–3685, 2005.

82. Weishaar KM, Ehrhart EJ, Avery AC, et al.: Kit mutation and localization status as response predictors in mast cell tumors in dogs treated with prednisone and toceranib or vinblastine, *J Vet Intern Med* 32:394–405, 2018.

83. Stadler W: Other paradigms: randomized discontinuation trial design, *Cancer J* 15:431–434, 2009.

84. Stadler WM: The randomized discontinuation trial: a phase II design to assess growth-inhibitory agents, *Mol Cancer Ther* 6:1180–1185, 2007.

85. Rosner GL, Stadler W, Ratain MJ: Randomized discontinuation design: application to cytostatic antineoplastic agents, *J Clin Oncol* 20:4478–4484, 2002.

86. Kindler T, Breitenbuecher F, Marx A, et al.: Sustained complete hematologic remission after administration of the tyrosine kinase inhibitor imatinib mesylate in a patient with refractory, secondary AML, *Blood* 101:2960–2962, 2003.

87. McKeage K, Perry CM: Trastuzumab: a review of its use in the treatment of metastatic breast cancer overexpressing HER2, *Drugs* 62:209–243, 2002.

88. Sawyers CL, Hochhaus A, Feldman E, et al.: Imatinib induces hematologic and cytogenetic responses in patients with chronic myelogenous leukemia in myeloid blast crisis: results of a phase II study, *Blood* 99:3530–3539, 2002.

89. London CA, Galli SJ, Yuuki T, et al.: Spontaneous canine mast cell tumors express tandem duplications in the proto-oncogene c-kit, *Exp Hematol* 27:689–697, 1999.

90. Paoloni M, Webb C, Mazcko C, et al.: Prospective molecular profiling of canine cancers provides a clinically relevant comparative model for evaluating personalized medicine (PMed) trials, *PLoS One* 9(3):e90028, 2014.
91. Husain H, Velculescu VE: Cancer DNA in the circulation: the liquid biopsy, *JAMA* 318:1272–1273, 2017.
92. Lindblad-Toh K, Galli SJ, Yuuki T, et al.: Genome sequence, comparative analysis and haplotype structure of the domestic dog, *Nature* 438:803–819, 2005.
93. Kimmelman J, Nalbantoglu J: Faithful companions: a proposal for neurooncology trials in pet dogs, *Cancer Res* 67:4541–4544, 2007.
94. Pater J, Goss P, Ingle J, et al.: The ethics of early stopping rules, *J Clin Oncol* 23:2862–2863, 2005.

19

Tumors of the Skin and Subcutaneous Tissues

MARLENE L. HAUCK AND MICHELLE L. OBLAK

Incidence

The overall incidence of tumors of the skin and subcutaneous tissues of dogs and cats is difficult to determine because of inconsistency of reporting, particularly with tumors of the subcutaneous tissues. If tumors determined to be of "skin" origin are considered, the percentage of biopsy specimens has been reported to be 26% to 43%.[1–6] Of these, between 20% and 40% are malignant.[3,4] In a survey of neoplasms in Alameda and Contra Costa counties performed from 1963 to 1966, the estimated incidence of skin and connective tissue tumors in dogs was 150.4/100,000; this decreased to 90.4/100,000 when melanocytic skin tumors were excluded.[5] The incidence of skin and connective tissue tumors in cats was 51.7/100,000.[5] In one report, skin tumors represented 10% of all feline biopsy or necropsy accessions, but skin tumors accounted for 30% of all cancer cases.[6] Other studies report a similar percentage of tumors arising from the skin, ranging from 19%[2] to 21%.[7] Disregarding basal cell tumors (BCTs), the percentage of malignant skin tumors is higher in cats than dogs, ranging from 70%[2] to 82%.[6]

The relative prevalence of the most common tumor types in dogs and cats can be determined from prevalence studies. In dogs, the numbers are based on a large number of surveys of skin tumor types from across the globe, totaling almost 9000 skin tumor submissions to various pathology services.[1,3,7–14] The data for the prevalence of the most common tumors of dogs are presented in Table 19.1. The overall prevalence of lipomas and sebaceous adenomas is likely higher than reported because of the bias present in samples submitted for histopathologic evaluation. The data on the prevalence of feline tumors is compiled from four studies with a total of 1225 skin tumors and is presented in Table 19.2.[2,6,9,15] In cats, the top four tumor types of the skin and subcutaneous tissues are consistently BCTs, mast cell tumors (MCTs), squamous cell carcinoma (SCC), and fibrosarcoma; these account for approximately 70% of all feline skin tumors.

The remainder of this chapter focuses on SCC, BCTs, glandular skin tumors, and additional assorted primary tumors of the skin, ears, and digits. Other tumor types are discussed in specific chapters: melanomas (Chapter 20), MCTs (Chapter 21), soft tissue sarcomas (Chapter 22), cutaneous lymphoma (Chapter 33, Sections A and B), and hemangiosarcoma (Chapter 34, Section A).

Etiology

Physical Factors

Ionizing radiation and thermal injury are reported to increase the risk of skin cancer in many species; however, a recent epidemiologic study on the incidence of cancer in human burn victims demonstrated no increased risk of the development of skin cancer compared with the general population.[16] Ultraviolet (UV) radiation has long been known to cause neoplastic transformation in the skin and is a major contributor to rising rates of skin cancer of all subtypes in people.[17] Evidence for the role of UV irradiation in the development of skin tumors in cats and dogs is primarily epidemiologic[18–20] and supported by case reports on dogs diagnosed with a spectrum of sunlight-induced lesions.[21,22]

The association of SCC development with solar exposure of skin in light-colored cats has been established epidemiologically. White cats in California had a 13.4-fold increased risk of developing SCC, and 143 of the 149 cases of nonoral SCC occurred on the head or neck.[18] Similar results were found in a case series of nasal planum or pinnal SCC in cats; 58 of the 61 cats were white or partially white in color, and all but three cats spent time outdoors.[23]

Viral Factors

The ability to induce neoplastic transformation in mucosal infections of papillomaviruses (PPVs) of people is well-established. PPVs are only able to replicate in terminally differentiated cells, therefore infection of the keratinocyte can stimulate increased proliferation and terminal differentiation.[24] Neoplastic transformation arises from the viral effects on cell proliferation, integration into the genome, and interaction of papilloma viral proteins with cellular proteins, particularly the destabilization of p53 by viral protein E6 and the inhibition of pRB by viral protein E7.[25] This disruption in p53 can result in increased levels of p16 protein, which is detectable with immunohistochemistry (IHC).[26] The association of PPV infection with cutaneous SCC in people is primarily epidemiologic: organ transplant recipients and immunosuppressed individuals have an increased rate of cutaneous PPV infection and an increased risk of SCC development.[27,28]

TABLE 19.1	Most Common Canine Skin Tumors[a]	
SKIN TUMOR INCIDENCE IN DOGS N = 8901 SKIN TUMORS		
Tumor Type	Overall (No.)	Overall (%)
Mast cell tumor	1494	16.8
Lipoma	758	8.5
Histiocytoma	752	8.4
Perianal gland adenoma	692	7.8
Sebaceous gland hyperplasia/ adenoma	577	6.5
Squamous cell carcinoma	531	6.0
Melanoma	500	5.6
Fibrosarcoma	478	5.4
Basal cell tumor	445	5.0
Malignant peripheral nerve sheath tumor	381	4.3
Papilloma	251	2.8
Sweat gland adenocarcinoma	101	1.1
Sebaceous adenocarcinoma	42	0.5
Miscellaneous	1899	21.3
Total	8901	100

[a]Overall incidence of the most common canine skin tumors as determined from the collation of 10 worldwide studies.[1,3,7–14]

TABLE 19.2	Most Common Skin Tumors in Cats[a]	
SKIN TUMOR INCIDENCE IN CATS N = 1,225 SKIN TUMORS		
Tumor	Overall (No.)	Overall (%)
Basal cell tumor	282	23.02
Mast cell tumor	202	16.49
Squamous cell carcinoma	127	10.37
Fibrosarcoma	219	17.88
Apocrine adenoma	41	3.35
Lipoma	40	3.27
Hemangiosarcoma	35	2.86
Sebaceous adenoma	34	2.78
Fibroma	33	2.69
Hemangioma	21	1.71
Melanoma	21	1.71
Malignant fibrous histiocytoma	9	0.73
Miscellaneous	124	10.12
Total	1225	100

[a]Relative incidence of the most common skin tumors in cats collated from four studies.[2,6,7,15]

The association of canine oral PPV with the development of oral papillomas has been studied since the 1950s.[29,30] The association of viral infection with the development of SCC has evolved from a combination of evidence, including the detection of canine PPV in oral and cutaneous SCCs and the induction of cutaneous SCC in 10 beagles out of 4500 vaccinated with a live oral PPV vaccine.[31–33] Canine oral PPV has also been detected in multiple cases of cutaneous SCC.[32] A novel PPV with malignant potential was cloned from a dog with footpad papillomas.[34] Dogs persistently infected with this novel virus developed invasive and metastatic SCC.[35] Several additional novel canine PPVs were detected in SCC from a variety of locations, including four dogs with cutaneous tumors.[36]

Case reports support the correlation between PPV infection and the development of invasive SCC, including lesions of mixed histology.[33,37,38] Similar to the epidemiologic studies in immunosuppressed people, a case report of a patient on ongoing chemotherapy developing cutaneous PPV infection and multiple papillomas supports the concept of immunosuppression allowing persistent infection of PPV.[39] Susceptibility to infection may also be breed dependent.[40,41] Recently a dog with multiple viral plaques developed more than 20 invasive cutaneous SCCs over a 3-year period, with no evidence of underlying immunosuppression.[42] A novel PPV was sequenced from these lesions.

In cats, PPVs are associated with viral plaques and feline fibropapillomas (also known as *feline sarcoids*).[43,44] PPV can be detected with IHC in most feline viral plaques; as these plaques progress to SCC, the ability to detect PPV antigens decreases.[45] However, when polymerase chain reaction (PCR) is used to amplify PPV DNA, up to 76% of "UV-protected" SCCs are positive, compared with 42% of SCC in regions exposed to UV irradiation.[26] In people, it has been suggested that UV exposure and PPV infection may act as cofactors in the development of SCC.[46] In a large retrospective study that tested for the presence of PPV in SCCs, SCCs in situ, or Bowen's in situ carcinomas (BISCs) in 84 cats, no correlation was found with PPV infection and UV exposure.[47] A novel feline PPV has been sequenced from three feline BISC lesions.[48] Twenty-five percent of the 73 cutaneous lesions were positive for PPV by PCR. Human PPVs 5, 21, and 38 were identified in approximately half of the virus-positive cats.

A second study evaluated the levels of p16 in 60 cats; tissues tested included 14 viral plaques, 14 BISCs, 18 invasive SCCs, and 14 trichoblastomas (controls).[26] Eleven of the invasive SCCs were solar induced, and seven were classified as non–solar-induced tumors. P16 protein levels were compared with the trichoblastomas and solar-induced SCCs and were found to be elevated in all viral plaques, BISCs, and nonsolar invasive SCCs, consistent with the presence of PPV infection.[26] Most recently, the presence of E6 and E7 RNA was demonstrated in preneoplastic and neoplastic feline cells in a pattern similar to that seen with PPV-induced SCC in people.[49] Taken together, this data supports the possibility of a role for PPV in the development of SCC in cats.

Immune Status

Immunosuppressed people have a greatly increased risk of skin cancer; organ transplant recipients have up to a 100-fold increased risk for development of SCC.[50] Although this may reflect susceptibility to persistent PPV infection in some instances, it is also thought to reflect loss of normal immune surveillance, with resulting lack of an immune response against early neoplasia. A case report of the development of multiple cutaneous hamartomas and SCCs in situ in a dog receiving long-term immunosuppressive therapy with prednisone and cyclosporine also demonstrated positive staining for PPV antigens.[51] Interestingly, the lesions persisted and new lesions developed even after discontinuation of the drug therapy. The successful use of immune stimulants for early cancer lesions, such as imiquimod for carcinoma in situ, supports the role of the immune system in controlling skin cancer. The ability of the immune system of dogs to cause regression of histiocytomas and papillomas also illustrates the role of immune surveillance in veterinary patients.[52]

Genetic Abnormalities in Skin Cancer

Cancer is a genetic disease (see Chapter 1, Section A). The accumulation of multiple alterations in critical genes is usually necessary for full neoplastic transformation. An understanding of these genetic abnormalities, which can include both genetic and epigenetic modifications in a particular cancer type, allows for the formulation of therapeutics to circumvent these critical mutations and their pathways. The accumulation of such genetic data is only beginning in veterinary oncology. The discovery of activating mutations in the stem cell factor receptor, c-kit in canine MCTs, and the subsequent successful targeting of this mutation with tyrosine kinase inhibitors, is the first step in applying this approach in veterinary oncology. The current understanding of mutations in the most common forms of skin cancer and their role in either tumorigenesis or prognosis/response to treatment are presented according to tumor type.

Basal Cell Carcinomas

In people, basal cell carcinomas (BCCs) are thought to arise from critical mutations in the hedgehog signaling pathway.[53] Limited genetic evaluation of BCTs has been performed in veterinary medicine. One study demonstrated a reciprocal translocation in a canine BCT of t(10:35).[54] In the dog, chromosome 10 contains the gene GLI1, which is the effector transcription factor of the hedgehog signaling cascade. Two aberrant karyotypes were found in feline BCTs: trisomy E3 and monosomy E3, although the significance of these findings is unknown.[55,56] IHC for p53 in five feline BCTs were negative.[57] Likewise, IHC evaluation for the presence of the apoptotic regulatory proteins Bcl-2 and Bax showed 23 of 24 tumors expressed Bcl-2, but only seven of the BCTs expressed Bax.[58] Interestingly, Bcl-2 staining is considered fairly specific for human BCC.[59]

Squamous Cell Carcinoma

The genetic abnormalities responsible for the development of cutaneous SCC are incompletely understood in human oncology. One common finding is mutations in p53. A pathway of sequentially necessary mutations has been proposed.[60] In addition, several genetic changes in cutaneous SCC have been suggested to be of prognostic value in people with this disease.

A number of studies have evaluated p53 in canine and feline cutaneous SCC. When p53 is present in the wild-type form, its short half-life prevents detection of the protein with IHC. The presence of a detectable form of the p53 protein correlates with mutations within the coding sequence. Three IHC studies of p53 in canine cutaneous SCC revealed that 30% were positive for p53 overexpression.[32,57,61] Interestingly, two of six cutaneous papillomas were also positive for p53 expression by IHC.[32] Detectable expression is even more prevalent in feline cutaneous SCCs, with 19 of 40 cutaneous

SCCs (48%) positive for p53 expression in three studies.[56,57,62] In addition, feline actinic keratosis was found to be highly positive for p53 expression (79%), whereas BISC lesions were less commonly positive (18%).[63] These studies have raised questions about the relative roles of PPV infection and UV irradiation in the development of different subtypes of feline SCC, because both mechanisms of tumorigenesis can result in increased identification of p53.

Several studies have used IHC to evaluate changes in selected protein expression. For example, IHC staining of p27, a protein thought important in maintaining cells in G0, showed SCC to have much lower levels than benign cutaneous neoplasms.[64] β-Catenin is a protein that is responsible for normal skin homeostasis. When dysregulated, β-catenin can be oncogenic. A study of β-catenin expression in normal skin and in benign and malignant tumors demonstrated nuclear presence of this protein, representing pathway activation, in 100% of trichoepitheliomas and pilomatricomas; no nuclear expression was found in any of the other malignant tumors or normal skin.[65] This finding led the authors to suggest a role for aberrantly activated β-catenin in the formation of tumors of the hair follicle. Evaluation for the presence of cyclin D1 and cyclin A, proteins important in the regulation of the cell cycle, demonstrated that cyclin A was present in 90% of feline SCCs and 44% of canine SCCs.[57] Cyclin D1 was rarely expressed in skin tumors of any type.[57] Staining for these proteins in normal skin and benign tumors showed rare or weak staining. The investigators suggested a role for cyclin A in the regulation of proliferation and neoplastic transformation in cutaneous SCC.

The syndrome of renal cystadenocarcinoma and nodular dermatofibrosis deserves mention, because this disease often presents to the veterinarian as the result of manifestation of multiple firm, cutaneous nodules. The disorder was first described as a genetic disease in the mid-1980s, and it was not until 2003 that the causative mutation in the Birt-Hogg-Dubé (BHD) gene was described.[66,67] The BHD gene codes for the tumor suppressor protein folliculin and mutations in this gene are thought to lead to loss of function.[68] This disease is primarily seen in German shepherd dogs.[66,69]

Identification of the driver mutations underlying neoplastic transformation in the skin will be the key to optimizing the use of drugs that target these pathways and of avoiding unwanted cutaneous side effects. The use of pathway-specific drugs may have unanticipated effects in the skin. Sorafenib, a tyrosine kinase inhibitor of Raf and VEGF/PDGFR, has been associated with the rapid development of actinic keratosis and invasive SCC in people.[70,71] As understanding of these pathways and their role in normal skin homeostasis develops, preventing these types of unintended consequences may become possible.

Pathologic Classification of Skin Tumors

Skin tumors arise from the epidermis and associated structures. For ease of use, these tumors are categorized based on their differentiation into specific subelements of the skin.[72] Some histologies are divided into benign and malignant forms based on known clinical and histologic predictors of behavior. In other tumor types, such clear-cut division may not be possible.

The World Health Organization's classification system of tumor-node-metastasis (TNM) can be applied to skin tumors in the clinical setting.[73] Location is also prognostic for particular tumor types; for example, digit and oral melanomas are highly malignant tumors, whereas cutaneous melanomas are often benign. Therefore this information should be included in the clinical description of the tumor at presentation.

History and Clinical Signs

Tumors of the skin are often noticed by pet owners and brought to their veterinarian's attention. The biologic history of these masses can be quite variable. Self-trauma or secondary infection may cause a patient to be presented for evaluation. Ultimately, however, it is critical to remember that physical examination cannot definitively determine whether a lesion is benign or malignant – cytology or histopathology is necessary to diagnose any skin tumor.

Diagnostic Techniques and Workup

The evaluation of a skin tumor is generally similar to the evaluation for any solid tumor. A complete history can be very informative. Careful elucidation of the duration, rate of growth, and clinical signs associated with the tumor may be helpful in differentiating benign from malignant masses. The clinical evaluation of any patient with a mass involves two steps: diagnosis and staging. Many cutaneous and subcutaneous masses can be diagnosed with fine-needle aspiration and cytology or direct impression cytology of a lesion. Cytology is an inexpensive and relatively noninvasive means of diagnosing many common benign skin tumors, such as lipomas or sebaceous adenomas. For lesions that appear malignant or are nondiagnostic on cytology, histopathology may be necessary. In addition to confirming a diagnosis, histopathology yields useful information on the histologic grade of some tumors, such as MCTs, or the malignant behavior of a tumor, such as vascular and lymphatic invasion. Other characteristics, such as degree of differentiation, nuclear morphology, and percentage of necrosis, may be helpful with certain tumor types.

The type of biopsy performed usually is dictated by the location of the mass. Where wide surgical excision is feasible without undue morbidity, the biopsy can be combined with a therapeutic procedure (e.g., excisional biopsy), provided this approach does not affect definitive surgical excision if a malignant process is identified. However, in most instances the biopsy is a diagnostic test. The authors' preference for a biopsy of a skin or subcutaneous mass is multiple punch biopsies or an incisional biopsy. (See Chapter 9 for a more detailed discussion of biopsy techniques.) These techniques allow the procurement of a sufficiently large piece of tissue for an accurate diagnosis and, where applicable, grading of the tumor. In addition, the use of advanced histopathologic techniques, such as IHC for evaluation of prognostic markers, can be performed. Some molecular tests, such as PCR, can be carried out on formalin-fixed tissues.

Staging involves determination of the extent of disease locally, regionally, and distantly. Assessment of the primary tumor's size by measuring the longest diameter is the first step in the staging process. For large, infiltrative or fixed masses, local assessment may require advanced imaging, such as a computed tomography (CT) or magnetic resonance imaging (MRI), to accurately determine the tumor's size and extent. One study demonstrated that the use of advanced local imaging techniques increased the stage of the primary tumor in 69% of patients.[74] Regional staging involves the assessment of the draining lymph node(s) (LN). Determination of the draining node can be difficult for some locations, so evaluation of all LNs in the region may be necessary. Radiographic or CT lymphography may be helpful for determining the sentinel LN when drainage patterns are unclear (see Chapter 9).[75,76] LN palpation is a poor predictor of metastasis because metastatic LNs may be normal in size and consistency.[77,78] Conversely, large, firm LNs may be reactive in response to an infection or inflammatory process. Aspiration and cytologic examination by an experienced clinical pathologist is critical for the assessment of regional LNs for evidence of metastasis. IHC may also be more accurate for identifying metastasis, but

these techniques are still being developed in veterinary medicine.[79] Despite careful evaluation of a cytology sample, it is possible to underestimate metastatic disease. Because of the unreliable nature of LN cytology and the potential effect of LN metastasis on the prognosis and adjunctive therapy, histopathology should be considered in cases with a high risk of malignancy.[78,80]

Evaluation of the patient for distant metastatic disease before histopathologic confirmation of a neoplastic process is based on the degree of suspicion that the mass is malignant, in addition to the desires and financial limitations of the owner. After confirmation of a malignant process, additional staging for detection of distant metastatic disease and evaluation of overall suitability for proposed treatments are indicated. Such staging may include three-view thoracic radiographs, thoracic CT, abdominal ultrasound, and/or additional tests as indicated by the tumor type and clinical findings.

Treatment and Prognosis for Specific Tumor Types

Given the external location of most skin and subcutaneous tumors, the primary treatment option for achieving local control is surgery. For benign masses, marginal excision may be adequate to achieve long-term control. For malignant tumors, adequate surgical excision requires a margin of normal tissue around the neoplasm. For a pathologist to determine whether excision is complete, all surgical margins must be identified with surgical ink or sutures to ensure correct reporting of margins (see Chapter 10).[81] The surgeon must properly prepare the sample to allow the pathologist to report all critical information, including margin evaluation (see Chapter 3).[81]

Likewise, to report the tumor grade accurately in tumors for which a grading scheme has been validated, a pathologist needs a reasonably sized piece of tissue to evaluate. Needle-core or Tru-Cut biopsies often yield limited amounts of tissue and should be limited to tumors for which they are the only option.

The most common cutaneous and subcutaneous tumors, melanomas, MCTs, and soft tissue sarcomas (STSs) are discussed separately in Chapters 20, 21, and 22, respectively. The remainder of this chapter covers the additional skin tumors, focusing on those with malignant behavior.

Epithelial Tumors

Tumors of the Primitive Follicular Epithelium

The term *basal cell tumor* was used for many years to include BCCs, basal cell epithelioma, trichoblastoma, and solid-cystic ductular sweat gland adenomas and adenocarcinomas. Because of progress in the ability of pathologists to differentiate these tumors on the basis of keratin and other membrane markers, trichoblastomas and solid-cystic ductular sweat gland tumors are no longer considered BCTs. Consequently, older studies that reported high rates of BCT, particularly in cats, may not reflect diagnostic patterns today.[82] These related tumor types are believed to arise from stem cells in the outer follicular root sheath displaying variable differentiation, although the origin for all tumors in this category cannot be absolutely identified.

Basosquamous cell carcinoma is a tumor with characteristics of both BCC and SCC. Immunohistochemically basosquamous cell carcinomas are more closely related to BCCs and so are discussed in this section. Trichoepitheliomas are a more differentiated form of the trichoblastoma. The most appropriate nomenclature and classification schema for this group of tumors remains controversial. Tumor types are presented as categorized in the Armed Forces

Institute of Pathology publication on the histologic classification of skin tumors.[72]

Basal Cell Carcinoma

The true incidence of BCC in both dogs and cats is unknown. The different tumors previously categorized as BCTs are difficult to distinguish histologically and cytologically, both in determining the category of tumor and in differentiating benign lesions from malignant. On cytology BCTs can contain inflammatory cells, squamous cells, sebaceous epithelial cells, melanin, and melanophages, and these cells can express the criteria of malignancy. Well-differentiated fibroblasts, reactive fibroblasts, and mast cells may also be present on cytologic examination.[83] The inability to distinguish the subtypes on cytology has led to the suggestion that these tumors be called "cutaneous basilar epithelial neoplasms" when they are evaluated by cytology alone.[84]

In histopathologic evaluation, tumors sometimes can be grossly differentiated based on growth pattern.[85] The epithelial membrane glycoprotein BerEP4 is highly specific for BCC versus SCC or cystic-solid ductular tumors for the diagnosis of BCC in people.[59] Cytokeratin 8 (CAM5.2) is used in human tumors to identify tumors with sweat gland epithelial differentiation; it also has been used to differentiate a BCC from a solid-cystic ductular tumor in a dog.[84] However, validation of these IHC markers in a larger veterinary population remains to be performed.

BCC is rare in dogs. In two studies reporting BCC or basal cell epithelioma (benign variant), the incidence ranged from 6% to 8% of all skin tumors; however, it is unclear whether trichoblastomas were included in these studies.[10,11] Breeds reported to be at increased risk for BCC included cocker spaniel and poodle in one study, and spaniels were overrepresented in another study; however, no breed predispositions were identified in other studies.[9,10] Clinically, these tumors present as plaques or nodules, often darkly pigmented. The overlying skin may be alopecic and intact or ulcerated. In dogs the median age is 9 years; however, dogs of all ages may be affected.[10,11] The three recognized histologic subtypes are solid, keratinizing, and clear cell.[85]

In dogs BCC is considered a low-grade malignancy. Although local recurrence of this tumor after surgical excision has been reported, there are no reports of metastasis. Morphometric analysis of cell nuclei has been reported to be useful in differentiating BCC with the potential for local recurrence from BCC that is unlikely to recur.[86]

In cats BCCs are now thought to be rare, and many feline BCTs are being reclassified as either solid-cystic apocrine ductular adenomas (approximately 60%) or trichoblastomas (approximately 40%).[87] However, given the preponderance of the literature referring to BCTs in cats, this group of tumors is discussed here with the realization that the population is actually not homogenous. These tumors comprise some of the most common solid tumors in cats, second only to mammary tumors in one large study.[2] They represent 10% to 26% of feline skin tumors.[2,6,9,88] They are reported in middle-aged cats with a mean age of 9.6 to 10.8 years.[2,6,88] One study reported a predisposition to BCT in Siamese cats,[2] and a second study showed an increased number of these tumors in long-haired cats (Himalayans, domestic long-hair, and Persian cats)[88]; however, a third study did not find a breed predisposition.[6] BCC can appear anywhere on the body but may have a predilection for the head and neck.[6,88] BCC can appear pigmented and may clinically resemble melanoma.

Clinically most tumors classified as BCTs appear benign in behavior. Malignant BCTs have been described in 10 of 97 cats in one series based on the presence of stromal invasion, vascular invasion, necrosis, a high mitotic index, and LN metastasis.[2]

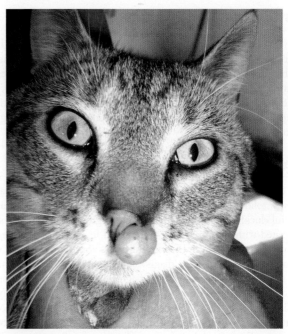

• **Fig. 19.1** Fibropapilloma (sarcoid) on the face of a cat. (From Miller WH Jr., Griffin CE, Campbell KL: *Muller & Kirk's small animal dermatology,* ed 7, St Louis, 2013, Saunders.)

Pulmonary metastasis has been documented in one cat with a BCC.[89] Nucleomorphometric analysis was able to predict local tumor recurrence in one study of 24 cats with BCC.[90] Overall, the likelihood of metastasis with BCC in cats appears low.

Treatment for BCC is wide surgical excision, which often results in long-term control. In people with masses less than 2 cm, surgical margins of 4 mm result in a high cure rate. However, surgical margins of 5 to 10 mm are recommended in cats and dogs, when possible, because intraoperative margin assessment cannot be performed.[91] The data is limited, but adjuvant radiation therapy (RT) and doxorubicin have been used to treat BCCs in two cats; although their contribution to tumor control and survival are unknown.[89]

Basosquamous Cell Carcinoma

Histologically basosquamous cell carcinoma has characteristics of both SCC and BCC. Clinically it is indistinguishable from both BCC and SCC. The true incidence and clinical behavior of this tumor in dogs and cats are unknown.

Papillomas

Papillomas are benign epidermal proliferative lesions that often are associated with PPV infection.[34] They are considered rare in the cat and dog.[92] Papillomas typically have an exophytic growth pattern. Another benign variant is the inverted papilloma, which grows into the subcutaneous tissue rather than externally. Cutaneous papillomas are typically found in younger dogs with an average age of 3.2 years.[38] Surgical excision is usually curative, but some of these lesions spontaneously regress.[93] In patients with multiple lesions, azithromycin has been shown to be effective.[94]

In cats a particular type of papilloma, the fibropapilloma, is seen. These tumors demonstrate a proliferation of mesenchymal cells covered by hyperplastic epithelium.[44] Evaluation for PPV demonstrated a nonproductive infection of the mesenchymal cells.[95] Feline fibropapillomas may be more similar to equine sarcoids than papillomas (Fig. 19.1).

Squamous Cell Carcinoma in Situ

SCC in situ is defined as a carcinoma that has not penetrated the basement membrane of the epithelium. In some cases it is thought to be caused by *Felis catus* papillomavirus infection.[30] When it appears in multiple sites, it is also known as *Bowen's carcinoma*, BISC, or multicentric PPV–induced SCC. This disease is seen primarily in cats, with only a few reports in dogs.[6,51,96–98] Actinic keratosis is the name typically used for SCC in situ that arises as a consequence of UV exposure.[85] Differentiation of actinic keratosis from BISC is based on location and histopathologic appearance.

Clinically SCC in situ can present as erosions of the epidermis, proliferations, or crusted plaques. They may be painful on palpation. BISC lesions can occur anywhere on the body, on both haired and unhaired skin, and in areas with and without sun exposure (Fig. 19.2). Solitary lesions are unusual.[6,97] Actinic keratosis, on the other hand, occurs in lightly haired skin with UV exposure, and these lesions are often solitary. Actinic keratosis typically is accompanied by solar elastosis and fibrosis of the skin, consistent with the effects of chronic UV exposure.[85] By definition, carcinoma in situ is not yet invasive and so metastasis has not occurred. However, left untreated, carcinoma in situ can progress to invasive carcinoma and put the patient at risk for metastasis. Patients with BISC typically continue to develop new lesions over time, but metastasis is uncommon.[6,51,96–98]

Many treatment approaches are effective for solitary SCC in situ. Surgical excision is the treatment of choice for most lesions. The median disease-free interval (DFI) and survival time (MST) in 39 cats treated with surgical excision for single nasal and pinna lesions were 594 days and 675 days, respectively.[23] Strontium-90 plesiotherapy in 14 cats with SCC in situ of the nasal planum resulted in 14 complete responses (CRs) with no recurrences and an overall survival time of >3000 days.[99] As expected, metastasis appears rare in cats with SCC in situ/actinic keratosis; in 61 cats with SCC of the nasal planum and pinnae, only one cat eventually developed metastasis to the regional LN.[23]

BISC lesions are often multifocal. As a result, marginal surgical resection is primarily indicated to improve comfort and local control when other therapies are no longer effective. Imiquimod cream (5%) has been reported to be effective in treating BISC in 12 cats, with five cats having at least one lesion undergo a complete response (CR).[97] Most cats were treated with daily application, although some were treated three times per week. One study on the use of 13-cis-retinoic acid for SCC in situ did not demonstrate clinical efficacy in cats with BISCs or SCCs.[100] Etretinate showed some promise for the treatment of SCC in situ and for invasive SCC, but this drug is no longer available.[101] Photodynamic therapy (PDT) is also effective in the treatment of BISC in people and cats, with reported response rates up to 100%.[102–104] With PDT, the clinical stage of the tumor was prognostic for survival. One author (MH) has treated a cat with BISC with palliative RT, and partial response/ stable disease was achieved for 8 months.

Squamous Cell Carcinoma

SCC is a malignant tumor of the epidermis in which the cells demonstrate differentiation to squamous cells (keratinocytes).[105]

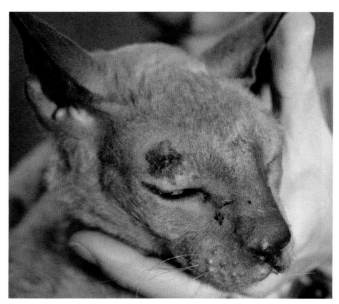

• **Fig. 19.2** Plaquelike lesion of Bowen's in situ carcinoma on the head of a cat. Multiple such lesions may be present on the patient. (Courtesy Dr. Rodney Rosychuk.)

These tumors typically occur in cats older than 10 years of age and at a median age of 10 to 11 years in dogs.[6,38,105] Cats have a predilection for developing these tumors on their heads, particularly in lightly haired areas of white cats.[6] This predilection reflects the role of UV light in the induction of many of these tumors. A decreased risk has been reported in Siamese, Himalayan, and Persian breeds.[6,92] Labrador and golden retrievers may have a predisposition for the development of nasal planum SCC.[106] Bloodhounds, basset hounds, and standard poodles may be predisposed to develop cutaneous SCC.[105]

The clinical presentation of cutaneous SCC can be highly variable. Cutaneous SCC can appear plaquelike to papillary and from crateriform to fungiform.[85] These lesions may be erythemic, ulcerated, or crusted.[92] Paraneoplastic hypercalcemia has been reported in three cats with cutaneous SCC, two with ear canal tumors, and one with multiple cutaneous tumors.[107,108] Metastasis at the time of death was present in 6 of 15 cats with invasive SCC of the nasal planum, with the most common metastatic sites being regional LNs and the lungs.[109] Metastasis in dogs with cutaneous SCC appears rare, with only four dogs described in the literature.[35,110] Four of 17 dogs with SCC of the nasal planum had regional metastasis to the mandibular LNs.[106] Metastasis to distant sites was not reported.

Treatment for cutaneous SCC is primarily surgical when feasible. Wide surgical excision results in long-term control in both dogs and cats. In a series of 61 cats treated with surgery, RT, and cryosurgery, surgery resulted in the longest median DFI at 594 days, although many of these cats may not have had invasive disease.[23] Complete surgical excision of nasal planum SCC in dogs resulted in long-term control in four of six dogs; two dogs with incomplete excision developed local recurrence (see Chapter 24, Section A, for further discussion of nasal planum tumors).[111]

Little data is available on the use of chemotherapy to treat cutaneous SCC in dogs and cats. Carboplatin compounded with sterile sesame oil injected into nasal planum SCCs in cats resulted in a CR rate of 73% and a 55% progression-free

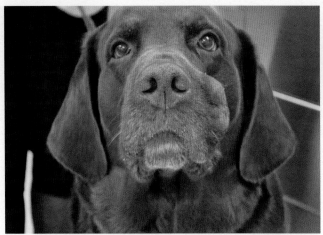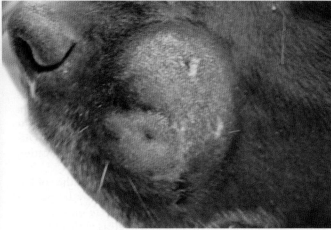

• **Fig. 19.3** Large trichoblastoma on the muzzle of a dog. Local surgical excision was curative.

survival (PFS) rate at 1 year.[112] Electrochemotherapy with intravenous bleomycin has shown an 82% CR rate for 2 months to 3 years in cats with cutaneous SCC; it may be a good option for the treatment of lesions for which surgical resection may be challenging.[113] Two dogs with metastatic SCC were treated with cisplatin.[114] One dog with cutaneous SCC metastatic to the axillary LN and lungs had a marked reduction in the number and size of lung nodules, in addition to a partial response (PR) of the axillary LN after cisplatin chemotherapy; however, the response duration was only 4.5 months. The other dog had a complete and durable response of multiple lesions (>22 months). Bleomycin has demonstrated short-lived clinical activity in the treatment of both dogs and cats with SCC.[115] Two dogs with SCC were treated with actinomycin-D; one dog had stable disease after a single dose, and the second dog had a PR after treatment with a total of six doses.[116] Mitoxantrone resulted in a response in four of nine dogs with SCC in one study, but only 4 of 32 cats with SCC.[117,118]

Tumors with Adnexal Differentiation

A number of tumors arise from the hair follicle, and most of them are benign. Treatment for these benign tumors is surgical excision. Characteristics unique to these tumors are discussed individually.

Infundibular Keratinizing Acanthoma

Infundibular keratinizing acanthoma (IKA) is a benign tumor. It is common in dogs but has not been reported in cats. Previous names for this tumor include intracutaneous cornifying epithelioma (ICE), intracutaneous keratinizing epithelioma, keratoacanthoma, and squamous papilloma.[92] Peak incidence is from 4 to 9 years of age, but IKAs can occur in younger dogs.[119] Nordic breeds (particularly Norwegian elkhounds), Belgian sheepdogs, Lhasa apso, German shepherd dogs, terriers, and other breeds appear to be at increased risk for the development of these tumors.[119–122] They occur most commonly on the back, neck, trunk, tail, and upper limbs, and they may appear as solitary or multiple lesions.[119–122] They may have a central pore that communicates with the surface. Rupture of these masses can allow keratinized tissue into the adjacent dermis and incite a marked inflammatory response.

When surgical excision is not feasible, treatment with isotretinoin (1.7–3.7 mg/kg/day) proved effective in three of seven dogs, with one CR and two PRs.[121]

Tricholemmoma

Tricholemmomas are rare, benign tumors in dogs.[123,124] They are well-encapsulated cutaneous or subcutaneous masses that may cause hair loss in the overlying skin. The most common location appears to be the head.[119] Surgical excision is the treatment of choice.

Trichoblastoma

Trichoblastoma is the new designation for what previously was called BCT in the dog and spindle cell variant of BCT in the cat.[92] Histologically this tumor shows differentiation to the hair germ of the developing hair follicle. Breeds at increased risk of developing trichoblastomas include poodles and setters.[119] Trichoblastomas are common in both dogs and cats. In a review of follicular tumors and tumorlike lesions, trichoblastomas comprised 26% of 308 canine follicular lesions and approximately 2% of all skin biopsies, and 26% of 50 feline follicular lesions (<2% of all skin biopsies).[119] The mean age at diagnosis was approximately 7 years for dogs and 10 years for cats.[119] The most common sites for trichoblastomas are the head and neck in dogs and the head, neck, limbs, and trunk in cats (Fig. 19.3). Although at least six subtypes have been described (ribbon, medusoid, trabecular, spindle, granular cell, and clear cell), trichoblastomas are benign and the subtype does not affect the prognosis. Surgical excision is the treatment of choice.[92,125]

Trichoepithelioma

Trichoepithelioma is an uncommon benign tumor in cats and dogs comprising approximately 4% of follicular tumors and tumorlike lesions.[119] These tumors demonstrate differentiation into all segments of the hair follicle[72]; they are dermal in origin but can extend into the subcutis. Their surface can be ulcerated or alopecic. Predisposed breeds include the basset hound, bullmastiff, standard poodle, soft-coated wheaten terrier, English springer spaniel, golden retriever, schnauzer, and setters.[92,119,126] Persian cats may or may not be predisposed.[92,126]

Common locations include the limbs, neck, and back, and multiple trichoepitheliomas have been reported in basset hounds and English springer spaniels. Surgical excision is the preferred treatment, except in cases with a multicentric presentation.[126]

Malignant Trichoepithelioma

Malignant trichoepithelioma is differentiated from its benign variant on the basis of invasion into the surrounding tissues and lymphatic involvement. It is also known as *matrical carcinoma,* and it may be difficult to differentiate from a malignant pilomatrixoma.[127] The mitotic index is usually higher in malignant trichoepithelioma compared with the benign counterpart.[72] The few described cases in the literature were highly metastatic to the regional LNs and lungs.[126] The locally invasive nature of some trichoepitheliomas may also represent a lower grade variant of malignant trichoepithelioma.[127] Wide surgical excision is recommended.[126] No information is available on response to adjuvant therapies.

Pilomatricoma

Pilomatricoma is a benign follicular tumor demonstrating only matrical differentiation.[72] Alternative names for this tumor include the necrotizing and calcifying epithelioma of Malherbe and pilomatrixoma. These tumors are uncommon, representing 13% of the follicular lesions in one study and approximately 1% of all skin biopsies.[119] They are rare in the cat, with only one case described in 1225 skin biopsies.[2,6,7,15] Breed predispositions include the Kerry blue terrier, soft-coated wheaten terrier, Bouvier des Flandres, standard poodle, old English sheepdog, bichon frise, and Airedale terrier, among others.[92,128] The mean age at presentation is 6.5 years.[128] The most common locations are the neck, back, and trunk. These tumors are typically well circumscribed and may be very firm as a result of ossification.[127,128] Surgical excision is the recommended treatment.

Malignant Pilomatricoma

Malignant pilomatricoma is thought to be a rare tumor, although a recent study suggests it may be more common than previously reported, with four malignant variants described from a total of 13 pilomatricomas.[129] Malignant pilomatricoma has not been reported in cats. Differentiating benign and malignant pilomatricomas can be difficult histologically.[130] Invasion into underlying tissues, particularly bone, may be an indicator of potential malignant behavior in the absence of a malignant histologic appearance.[129–131] A recent review of several published cases demonstrated a high metastatic potential with metastasis to the lungs, bone, LN, mammary gland, or skin in 11 of 12 dogs.[129] There is one report of a dog with recurrent malignant pilomatricoma being treated with surgery and RT; this dog was diagnosed with pulmonary metastasis 14 months after local treatment.[130] The efficacy of chemotherapy for the treatment of dogs with malignant pilomatricoma is unknown.

Tumors of Glandular Origin

Sebaceous Hyperplasia, Sebaceous Adenoma, Sebaceous Ductal Adenoma, and Sebaceous Epithelioma

Tumors of glandular origin are very common in the dog but rare in the cat, and divisions between these tumors may be arbitrary.[92] A review of 172 sebaceous gland tumors in dogs revealed a female predisposition for sebaceous hyperplasia and an over-representation of miniature schnauzers, beagles, poodles, and

cocker spaniels.[132,133] Coonhounds, Nordic breeds, and some terriers may also be predisposed to benign sebaceous tumors.[134] The limbs, trunk, and eyelids were the most common locations for these benign sebaceous tumors. Although these can occur even in young dogs, the peak occurrence is 7 to 13 years of age.[132–134]

Sebaceous epitheliomas may recur locally, and LN metastasis has been reported anecdotally.[135] Because lymphatic invasion occasionally may be found at the margin of sebaceous epitheliomas, these tumors sometimes are considered a low-grade malignancy rather than a benign tumor.[72] A recent report of distant metastasis in a dog with a recurrent sebaceous epithelioma confirms their malignant potential.[135] In general, adequate surgical excision is the preferred treatment.

Sebaceous Gland Carcinoma

Sebaceous gland carcinomas are uncommon in the dog and cat.[92] They are more common in intact male dogs, and the Cavalier King Charles spaniel, cocker spaniel, and terrier breeds are predisposed.[134] The tumors typically are found on the head and neck in dogs and on the head, thorax, and perineum in cats. Sebaceous carcinomas tend to be low-grade malignancies, with distant metastasis reported in one dog.[136,137] The most common finding of malignancy is local infiltration. Wide surgical excision is the recommended treatment.

Apocrine Gland Adenoma and Solid-Cystic Apocrine Ductal Adenoma

Apocrine gland adenomas are relatively common in dogs but uncommon in cats. The solid-cystic apocrine ductal adenoma previously was designated a BCT. Apocrine ductal adenomas are firm or fluid filled on palpation. Feline apocrine adenomas have a high predilection for the head.[138] Surgical excision is the recommended treatment.

Apocrine Gland Carcinoma

Apocrine sweat gland tumors are relatively uncommon in dogs (1% of all skin tumors) and cats (3% of all skin tumors) (see Tables 19.1 and 19.2). In a series of apocrine gland tumors, 40 of 44 dogs and 8 of 10 cats had malignant apocrine gland carcinomas.[139] In dogs the median age at diagnosis is 9 years, with most tumors occurring between 6 and 11 years of age.[140] Golden retrievers and the Treeing Walker coonhound may be predisposed.[138,139] The thoracic limbs are the most common site in dogs. Apocrine gland carcinomas were diagnosed in cats ranging from 6 to 17 years of age, and no breed or sex predilections were identified.[138,139] The most common locations for this tumor in cats include the head, limbs, and abdomen.[138] In both species most lesions are solitary. In addition to the nodular tumors, apocrine gland carcinomas may present as erosive and inflammatory skin disease, termed "inflammatory carcinoma."[138]

Local invasion is common, with 66% of tumors demonstrating invasion of the capsule and/or stroma, and 11% invading the vasculature.[140] In another series 23% had lymphatic invasion.[139] Grossly no features differentiated benign from malignant tumors. Despite the high incidence of local invasion, cure rates are high with surgery alone; only two dogs developed local recurrence (4%) and one dog developed distant metastasis (2%) in two case series.[139,140] Surgery is the recommended treatment.

Eccrine Adenoma and Carcinoma

Eccrine adenoma and carcinoma are benign and malignant tumors, respectively, of the sweat glands of the footpads. They are rare in dogs and cats, with only one report of a dog with involvement of multiple pads on one foot.[143] Wide surgical excision is the recommended treatment.[92]

Neuroendocrine Carcinoma

Neuroendocrine carcinoma is also known as *Merkel cell carcinoma*. Merkel cells are thought to be part of the mechanoreceptor in the skin. Recent studies have demonstrated a role for the Merkel cell polyomavirus in the development of human Merkel cell tumors.[144] Merkel cell tumors are highly malignant in humans; however, most case reports in cats and dogs suggest a more benign clinical course,[141,145] although distant metastasis has been reported in both species.[142,146,147] A recent evaluation of two canine neuroendocrine carcinomas demonstrated expression of β-catenin or E-cadherin, proteins whose loss predicts a more malignant behavior in humans.[148] There was also expression of chromogranin-A, neurone-specific enolase, S-100, and c-*kit* (which is also expressed in human neuroendocrine carcinomas). Current treatment recommendations reflect the generally benign behavior of these tumors and consist of wide surgical excision. The efficacy of chemotherapy for treatment of metastatic neuroendocrine carcinomas is unknown, as is the effect of c-*kit* targeted tyrosine kinase inhibition.

Renal Cystadenocarcinoma and Nodular Dermatofibrosis

Nodular dermatofibrosis is a pathognomonic cutaneous syndrome associated with renal cystadenocarcinomas, primarily described in German shepherd dogs.[66,69] These dogs have multiple firm, haired masses all over their bodies. On histopathologic examination these nodules are composed of dense, irregular collagen. They do not typically cause clinical problems unless they cause lameness or otherwise disrupt normal function. Surgical removal is indicated in these instances. Most of these dogs die as a result of renal failure or progressive renal cystadenocarcinoma (see Chapter 30), on average 3 years after initial detection of the dermatofibrosis.[149] There are no known effective treatments for the renal cysts or bilateral renal adenocarcinoma. A recent case report of nodular dermatofibrosis in an Australian cattle dog without any evidence of renal cysts or adenocarcinoma at necropsy suggests the possibility of a nonlethal version of this syndrome.[150]

Tumors of the Ear Canal

Ceruminous glands are modified apocrine glands found in the external ear canal. Benign and malignant tumors arising from these glands are the most common tumor types in the ear canal of dogs and cats. Additional tumor types that have been reported include SCC, undifferentiated carcinoma, BCC, hemangiosarcoma (HSA), MCT, melanoma, and benign fibroma, papilloma, sebaceous gland tumors, ceruminous gland cysts, and histiocytomas.[151–154] Inflammatory polyps also are found in dogs and more commonly in cats.

Most tumors of the ear canal are diagnosed as a result of the mass effect, which may cause clinical signs such as chronic otitis or partial deafness. Occasionally patients may present for pain on opening of the mouth or neurologic signs. This is more common with malignant tumors.[154] The role of chronic otitis in the development of these tumors is an area of ongoing discussion.

Ceruminous Gland Adenoma and Cyst

Ceruminous gland adenomas are benign tumors of the ceruminous gland. On gross appearance they are typically exophytic

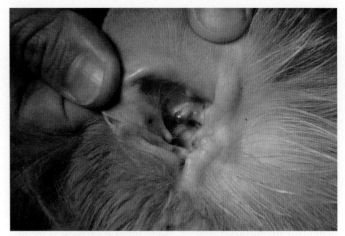

• **Fig. 19.4** Typical appearance of a ceruminous gland cyst in the ear of a cat.

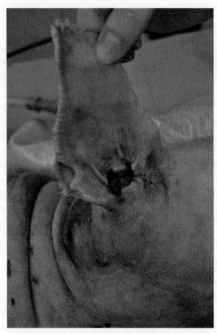

• **Fig. 19.5** Aural ceruminous gland carcinoma confined to the vertical ear canal in a cocker spaniel. (Courtesy Michelle Oblak.)

and pendunculated, although they can also be ulcerated.[155] Cats with ceruminous gland adenomas are slightly younger than those presenting with malignant tumors; in dogs both lesions present around 9 years of age.[154,155] Cocker spaniels and poodles are predisposed. Surgery is the treatment of choice.

Ceruminous gland cysts are found in cats. These are darkly pigmented, sessile masses that are usually <5 mm in diameter and can occur as multiple lesions (Fig. 19.4).[153] If necessary, these can be surgically excised.

Ceruminous Gland Adenocarcinoma

Ceruminous gland adenocarcinoma is the most common malignant tumor of the ear canal in both dogs and cats (Fig. 19.5). In dogs, cocker spaniels and German shepherd dogs are at increased risk .[155] Malignant ceruminous gland tumors are more common than benign tumors in cats; however, there is conflicting information on whether malignant or benign tumors are more common in the dog.[155,156]

Ceruminous gland adenocarcinomas have metastatic potential, and full staging is recommended before treatment. Local invasion, including through the cartilage of the ear canal, can occur. Advanced imaging (CT or MRI) is indicated to better delineate the extent of local disease before surgery. Skull radiographs revealed lysis of the bulla in 13 of 27 dogs with malignant tumors of the ear canal, and sclerosis of the bulla was evident in eight dogs.[154] LN and distant metastasis are uncommon, with LN metastasis diagnosed cytologically in 1 of 30 dogs and pulmonary metastasis in 3 of 35 dogs, in addition to one dog with a lytic bone lesion.[154] In cats with malignant ceruminous gland adenocarcinomas, 5 of 27 cats had lysis of the bulla on skull radiographs, and five cats had sclerosis of the bulla.[154] Five of 56 cats had cytologic evidence of regional LN metastasis, but none of 32 cats evaluated had evidence of distant metastasis.[154] A staging scheme adopted from the human ear canal tumors has been proposed for primary tumors of the ear canal in cats and dogs (Table 19.3).[157]

Surgery is recommended for excision of noninvasive ear canal tumors; total ear canal ablation and lateral bulla osteotomy (TECA-LBO) is most commonly indicated.[158,159] Local tumor recurrence was significantly decreased in both dogs and cats treated with TECA-LBO compared with those treated with a lateral ear canal resection.[158,159] The MST for cats and dogs with malignant ear canal tumors treated with TECA-LBO was 42 to 50.3 months and not reached at 36 months, respectively.[158–160] RT also appears effective for the treatment of ceruminous gland adenocarcinoma[157]; six cats and five dogs treated with orthovoltage RT (12 4-Gy fractions for a total dose of 48 Gy) had an estimated mean PFS of 39.5 months and a 1-year PFS rate of 56%.

Several prognostic factors have been identified for ceruminous gland adenocarcinomas (Table 19.4). In cats a proposed grading scheme was not prognostic for survival, but a mitotic index ≤2 predicted improved survival.[160] A correlation between mitotic index and tumor grade was also noted in a series of cats and dogs treated with RT, although the small sample size precluded further evaluation for prognostic significance.[157] The overriding conclusion from the series of studies regarding treatment for ceruminous gland adenocarcinoma is that, with appropriate local therapy, long-term survival is possible.

Tumors of the Digit

The most common malignant digit tumors of dogs include SCC (47%), melanoma (24%), STS (13%), MCT (8%), osteosarcoma (OSA, 3%), round cell sarcoma, adenocarcinoma, malignant adnexal tumor, HSA, lymphoma, chondrosarcoma, giant cell tumor of bone, and synovial cell sarcoma. Benign and nonneoplastic diseases of the canine digits include pyogranulomatous inflammation, epithelial inclusion cysts, IKA, benign adnexal tumors, histiocytoma, hemangioma, BCT, intraosseous epidermoid cyst, infiltrating lipoma, fibroma, papilloma, hamartoma, trichoblastoma, keratoma, and plasmacytoma.[161,162] The median age at diagnosis is 10 years.[161,163] Approximately 3% of dogs with digital SCC have involvement of multiple digits. These dogs are typically large breed dogs with a black hair coat.[164,165] Predisposed breeds for multiple digit SCCs include standard poodles, black Labrador retrievers, giant schnauzers, Gordon setters, rottweilers, Beaucerons, and Briards.[165] Additional breeds that may be predisposed to digital SCC include dachshunds and flat-coated retrievers.[162] The thoracic limbs are more commonly affected than the pelvic limbs.[165] Scottish terriers were overrepresented in dogs with digital malignant melanomas.[162]

The definitive diagnosis of a digital mass can be difficult in both cats and dogs. A review of pathologists demonstrated a 20% rate of disagreement in the diagnosis of digital tumors, with 75% of the changes in diagnosis being clinically significant.[166] The differentiation between SCC and IKA was most difficult.

The most common digital tumors in cats include SCC (25%), fibrosarcoma (23%), adenocarcinoma (22%), OSA (8%), HSA

TABLE 19.3	Proposed Staging Scheme for Primary Tumors of the Ear Canal[165]
T_1	Tumor confined to the external or horizontal ear canal
T_2	Tumor extending beyond the tympanic membrane
T_3	Tumor extending beyond the middle ear/bone destruction

TABLE 19.4 Prognostic Factors for Primary Tumors of the Ear Canal				
Prognostic Factor		Species	Median Survival (Months)	Reference
Mitoses per high power field	≤2	Feline	≈180	160
	≥3		≈24	
Extension beyond the ear canal	No	Canine	30	154
	Yes		5.9	
Presence of neurologic signs	No	Feline	15.5	154
	Yes		1.5	
Histology	Ceruminous gland adenocarcinoma	Feline	49	154
	Squamous cell carcinoma		3.8	
	Carcinoma of unknown origin		5.7	
Extension beyond the ear canal	No	Feline	21.7	154
	Yes		4	

(8%), MCT (7%), giant cell tumor of bone, malignant fibrous histiocytoma, sarcoma, and melanoma; nonneoplastic masses included inflammatory masses, hemangioma, and BCT.[167,168] Thoracic limb digits may be more commonly affected than pelvic limb digits. Multiple digit involvement has been reported in cats with fibrosarcoma, adenocarcinoma, and SCC.[167,169] Acrometastasis, or lung-digit syndrome, is common in cats with primary pulmonary carcinomas. In a series of 64 cats with digital carcinomas, 88% of cats had acrometastasis from primary lung tumors, whereas only 13% of cats had primary SCC of the digit.[169] Primary digital SCC and metastatic pulmonary carcinoma were differentiated based on histopathologic staining characteristics and cell morphology. In this series the MSTs of cats with acrometastasis and primary digital SCC were 4.9 weeks and 29.5 weeks, respectively.[169]

The most common clinical signs in dogs and cats with digital tumors are the presence of a mass and/or lameness. Digital tumors can metastasize, so appropriate clinical staging is recommended before definitive therapy, including regional LN evaluation and three-view thoracic radiographs or thoracic CT.[161–163,170] Regional radiographs are recommended to assess for bone involvement because this may have prognostic significance, especially for dogs with digital melanoma.[176] Bone lysis was noted in 80% of dogs with digital SCC and in 5% to 100% of dogs with digital melanoma.[161,163,171] In dogs with digital SCC, 6% to 13% had evidence of metastasis at the time of presentation, and an additional 9% to 17% subsequently developed metastasis.[161,163] A subungual location may carry a better prognosis than other sites in the digit with digital SCC.[161] In dogs with digital malignant melanoma, 32% to 40% had either regional LN or distant metastasis at the time of diagnosis, and an additional 10% to 26% developed metastatic disease after definitive treatment.[161,163] Little information is available on cats with primary digital tumors. For cats with digital SCC, three of six cats had evidence of bone invasion, one of eight had regional LN metastasis, and none of three had pulmonary metastasis.[169] Among cats with digital malignant melanoma, four of five developed metastasis to the regional LN, lung, bone, and/or vertebrae.[168]

The recommended treatment for most cats and dogs with digital tumors is digital or partial foot amputation (Fig. 19.6).[163]

Limb function is very good to excellent in most dogs after either procedure, regardless of the digit(s) amputated.[172] The roles of RT and chemotherapy remain to be elucidated for the treatment of malignant digital tumors in the dog and cat. The high metastatic rate of digital malignant melanoma in dogs clearly suggests that adjuvant treatment should be considered.

For SCC of the digit treated with surgery alone, 1- and 2-year survival rates range from 50% to 83% and 18% to 62%, respectively.[161–163] When the tumors are categorized by the site of origin, dogs with SCC arising from the subungual epithelium had a significantly improved survival compared with dogs with SCC from other sites on the digit. Dogs with a subungual SCC had 1- and 2-year survival rates of 95% and 74%, respectively, whereas dogs with SCC at other digital sites had 60% and 40% 1- and 2-year survival rates, respectively.[161] MSTs for cats with digital SCC ranged from 73 days to 29.5 weeks.[167,169]

Dogs with digital malignant melanoma have 1- and 2-year survival of 42% to 57% and 13% to 36%, respectively, after treatment with surgery alone.[161–163,170,171] A more recent retrospective study that evaluated the effect of carboplatin chemotherapy on the survival of dogs with digital melanomas treated with surgery found no difference with the inclusion of chemotherapy; these dogs had 1- and 2-year survival rates of 89% and 67%, respectively, and an MST of 1350 days.[173] In a study of 58 dogs treated with an adjuvant xenogenic (murine) tyrosinase vaccine,[174] 57 dogs were treated with digital amputation, two dogs were treated with RT, and three dogs had received adjuvant chemotherapy. Sixteen dogs (28%) had either regional LN or distant metastasis at the time of presentation. The overall MST from the time of digital amputation was 476 days, with 1- and 2-year survival rates of 63% and 32%, respectively. Metastatic disease was identified as a negative prognostic factor, and distant metastatic disease was associated with a worse prognosis than metastasis to the regional LNs. For five cats diagnosed with digital malignant melanoma, survival times ranged from 0 to >577 days, with four cats developing metastatic disease.[168]

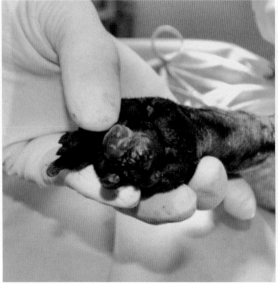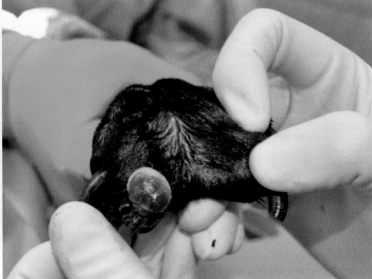

• **Fig. 19.6** Digital melanoma on a dog before digit amputation.

References

1. Pakhrin B, Kang MS, Bae IH, et al.: Retrospective study of canine cutaneous tumors in Korea, *J Vet Sci* 8:229–236, 2007.

2. Carpenter JL, Andrews LK, Holzworth J: Tumors and tumor-like lesions. In Holzworth J, editor: *Diseases of the cat: medicine and surgery*, Philadephia, 1987, W.B. Saunders Company, pp 406–428.

3. Priester WA: Skin tumors in domestic animals. Data from 12 United States and Canadian colleges of veterinary medicine, *J Natl Cancer Instit* 50:457–466, 1973.

4. MacVean DW, Monlux AW, Anderson PS, et al.: Frequency of canine and feline tumors in a defined population, *Vet Pathol* 15:700–715, 1978.

5. Dorn CR, Taylor DO, Schneider R, et al.: Survey of animal neoplasms in alameda and contra costa counties, california. II, Cancer morbidity in dogs and cats from alameda county, *J Natl Cancer Instit* 40:307–318, 1968.

6. Miller MA, Nelson SL, Turk JR, et al.: Cutaneous neoplasia in 340 cats, *Vet Pathol* 28:389–395, 1991.

7. Brodey RS: Canine and feline neoplasia, *Adv Vet Sci Comp Med* 14:309–354, 1970.

8. Finnie JW, Bostock DE: Skin neoplasia in dogs, *Aust Vet J* 55:602–604, 1979.

9. Bostock DE: Neoplasia of the skin and mammary glands in dogs and cats. In Kirk RW, editor: *Current veterinary therapy small animal practice*, Philadelphia, 1977, W.B. Saunders, pp 493–505.

10. Rothwell TL, Howlett CR, Middleton DJ, et al.: Skin neoplasms of dogs in Sydney, *Aust Vet J* 64:161–164, 1987.

11. Kaldrymidou H, Leontides L, Koutinas AF, et al.: Prevalence, distribution and factors associated with the presence and the potential for malignancy of cutaneous neoplasms in 174 dogs admitted to a clinic in northern Greece, *J Vet Med A Physiol Pathol Clin Med* 49:87–91, 2002.

12. Ladds PW, Kraft H, Sokale A, et al.: Neoplasms of the skin of dogs in tropical Queensland, *Aust Vet J* 60:87–88, 1983.

13. Mukaratirwa S, Chipunza J, Chitanga S, et al.: Canine cutaneous neoplasms: prevalence and influence of age, sex and site on the presence and potential malignancy of cutaneous neoplasms in dogs from Zimbabwe, *J Sth Afr Vet Med Assoc* 76:59–62, 2005.

14. Er JC, Sutton RH: A survey of skin neoplasms in dogs from the Brisbane region, *Aust Vet J* 66:225–227, 1989.

15. Jorger K: Skin tumors in cats. Occurrence and frequency in the research material (biopsies from 1984-1987) of the institute for veterinary pathology, zurich, *Schweiz Arch Tierheilkd* 130:559–569, 1988.

16. Mellemkjaer L, Holmich LR, Gridley G, et al.: Risks for skin and other cancers up to 25 years after burn injuries, *Epidemiology* 17:668–673, 2006.

17. Narayanan DL, Saladi RN, Fox JL: Ultraviolet radiation and skin cancer, *Int J dermatol* 49:978–986, 2010.

18. Dorn CR, Taylor DO, Schneider R: Sunlight exposure and risk of developing cutaneous and oral squamous cell carcinoma in white cats, *J Natl Cancer Inst* 46:1073–1078, 1971.

19. Nikula KJ, Benjamin SA, Angleton GM, et al.: Ultraviolet radiation, solar dermatosis, and cutaneous neoplasia in beagle dogs, *Radiat Res* 129:11–18, 1992.

20. Hargis AM, Thomassen RW, Phemister RD: Chronic dermatosis and cutaneous squamous cell carcinoma in the beagle dog, *Vet Pathol* 14:218–228, 1977.

21. Madewell BR, Conroy JD, Hodgkins EM: Sunlight-skin cancer association in the dog: a report of three cases, *J Cutan Pathol* 8:434–443, 1981.

22. Knowles DP, Hargis AM: Solar elastosis associated with neoplasia in two dalmations, *Vet Pathol* 23:512–514, 1986.

23. Lana SE, Ogilvie GK, Withrow SJ, et al.: Feline cutaneous squamous cell carcinoma of the nasal planum and the pinnae: 61 cases, *J Am Anim Hosp Assoc* 33:329–332, 1997.

24. Munday JS, Kiupel M: Papillomavirus-associated cutaneous neoplasia in mammals, *Vet Pathol* 47:254–264, 2010.

25. zur Hausen H: Human papillomavirus & cervical cancer, *Ind J Med Res* 130:209, 2009.

26. Munday JS, Gibson I, French AF: Papillomaviral DNA and increased p16CDKN2A protein are frequently present within feline cutaneous squamous cell carcinomas in ultraviolet-protected skin, *Vet Dermatol* 22:360–366, 2011.

27. Stockfleth E, Ulrich C, Meyer T, et al.: Skin diseases following organ transplantation—risk factors and new therapeutic approaches, *Transplant Proc* 33:1848–1853, 2001.

28. Stockfleth E, Nindl I, Sterry W, et al.: Human papillomaviruses in transplant-associated skin cancers, *Dermatol Surg* 30:604–609, 2004.

29. Chambers VC, Evans CA: Canine oral papillomatosis. i. Virus assay and observations on the various stages of the experimental infection, *Cancer Res* 19:1188–1195, 1959.

30. Munday JS, Thomson NA, Luff JA: Papillomaviruses in dogs and cats, *Vet J* 225:23–31, 2017.

31. Bregman CL, Hirth RS, Sundberg JP, et al.: Cutaneous neoplasms in dogs associated with canine oral papillomavirus vaccine, *Vet Pathol* 24:477–487, 1987.

32. Teifke JP, Lohr CV, Shirasawa H: Detection of canine oral papillomavirus-DNA in canine oral squamous cell carcinomas and p53 overexpressing skin papillomas of the dog using the polymerase chain reaction and non-radioactive in situ hybridization, *Vet Microbiol* 60:119–130, 1998.

33. Stokking LB, Ehrhart EJ, Lichtensteiger CA, et al.: Pigmented epidermal plaques in three dogs, *J Am Anim Hosp Assoc* 40:411–417, 2004.

34. Yuan H, Ghim S, Newsome J, et al.: An epidermotropic canine papillomavirus with malignant potential contains an E5 gene and establishes a unique genus, *Virology* 359:28–36, 2007.

35. Goldschmidt MH, Kennedy JS, Kennedy DR, et al.: Severe papillomavirus infection progressing to metastatic squamous cell carcinoma in bone marrow-transplanted X-linked SCID dogs, *J Virol* 80:6621–6628, 2006.

36. Zaugg N, Nespeca G, Hauser B, et al.: Detection of novel papillomaviruses in canine mucosal, cutaneous and in situ squamous cell carcinomas, *Vet Dermatol* 16:290–298, 2005.

37. Watrach AM, Small E, Case MT: Canine papilloma: progression of oral papilloma to carcinoma, *J Natl Cancer Inst* 45:915–920, 1970.

38. Schwegler K, Walter JH, Rudolph R: Epithelial neoplasms of the skin, the cutaneous mucosa and the transitional epithelium in dogs: an immunolocalization study for papillomavirus antigen, *Zentralbl Veterinarmed A* 44:115–123, 1997.

39. Lucroy MD, Hill FI, Moore PF, et al.: Cutaneous papillomatosis in a dog with malignant lymphoma following long-term chemotherapy, *J Vet Diagn Invest* 10:369–371, 1998.

40. Campbell KL, Sundberg JP, Goldschmidt MH, et al.: Cutaneous inverted papillomas in dogs, *Vet Pathol* 25:67–71, 1988.

41. Shimada A, Shinya K, Awakura T, et al.: Cutaneous papillomatosis associated with papillomavirus infection in a dog, *J Comp Pathol* 108:103–107, 1993.

42. Munday JS, O'Connor KI, Smits B: Development of multiple pigmented viral plaques and squamous cell carcinomas in a dog infected by a novel papillomavirus, *Vet Dermatol* 22:104–110, 2011.

43. Sundberg JP, Van Ranst M, Montali R, et al.: Feline papillomas and papillomaviruses, *Vet Pathol* 37:1–10, 2000.

44. Schulman FY, Krafft AE, Janczewski T: Feline cutaneous fibropapillomas: clinicopathologic findings and association with papillomavirus infection, *Vet Pathol* 38:291–296, 2001.

45. Wilhelm S, Degorce-Rubiales F, Godson D, et al.: Clinical, histological and immunohistochemical study of feline viral plaques and bowenoid in situ carcinomas, *Vet Dermatol* 17:424–426, 2006.

46. Bouwes Bavinck JN, Plasmeijer EI, Feltkamp MC: Beta-papillomavirus infection and skin cancer, *J Invest Dermatol* 128:1355–1358, 2008.

47. O'Neill SH, Newkirk KM, Anis EA, et al.: Detection of human papillomavirus DNA in feline premalignant and invasive squamous cell carcinoma, *Vet Dermatol* 22:68–74, 2011.

48. Lange CE, Tobler K, Markau T, et al.: Sequence and classification of FdPV2, a papillomavirus isolated from feline Bowenoid in situ carcinomas, *Vet Microbiol* 137:60–65, 2009.

49. Hoggard N, Munday JS, Luff J: Localization of *Felis catus* Papillomavirus Type 2 E6 and E7 RNA in feline cutaneous squamous cell carcinoma, *Vet Pathol* 55:409–416, 2018.

50. Moloney FJ, Comber H, O'Lorcain P, et al.: A population-based study of skin cancer incidence and prevalence in renal transplant recipients, *Br J Dermatol* 154:498–504, 2006.

51. Callan MB, Preziosi D, Mauldin E: Multiple papillomavirus-associated epidermal hamartomas and squamous cell carcinomas in situ in a dog following chronic treatment with prednisone and cyclosporine, *Vet Dermatol* 16:338–345, 2005.

52. Cockerell GL, Slauson DO: Patterns of lymphoid infiltrate in the canine cutaneous histiocytoma, *J Comp Pathol* 89:193–203, 1979.

53. Epstein EH: Basal cell carcinomas: attack of the hedgehog, *Nat Rev Cancer* 8:743–754, 2008.

54. Mayr B, Wallner A, Reifinger M, et al.: Reciprocal translocation in a case of canine basal cell carcinoma, *J Small Anim Pract* 39:96–97, 1998.

55. Ortner BM, Reifinger GL: Monosomy E3 in a feline basal cell tumour, *J Small Anim Pract* 36:400–401, 1995.

56. Mayr B, Ortner W: Trisomy E3 in a feline basal cell tumour, *J Small Anim Pract* 36:400–401, 1995.

57. Murakami Y, Tateyama S, Rungsipipat A, et al.: Immunohistochemical analysis of cyclin A, cyclin D1 and P53 in mammary tumors, squamous cell carcinomas and basal cell tumors of dogs and cats, *J Vet Med Sci* 62:743–750, 2000.

58. Madewell BR, Gandour-Edwards R, Edwards BF, et al.: Bax/bcl-2: cellular modulator of apoptosis in feline skin and basal cell tumours, *J Comp Pathol* 124:115–121, 2001.

59. Swanson PE, Fitzpatrick MM, Ritter JH, et al.: Immunohistologic differential diagnosis of basal cell carcinoma, squamous cell carcinoma, and trichoepithelioma in small cutaneous biopsy specimens, *J Cutan Pathol* 25:153–159, 1998.

60. Burnworth B, Arendt S, Muffler S, et al.: The multi-step process of human skin carcinogenesis: a role for p53, cyclin D1, hTERT, p16, and TSP-1, *Eur J Cell Biol* 86:763–780, 2007.

61. Teifke JP, Lohr CV: Immunohistochemical detection of P53 overexpression in paraffin wax-embedded squamous cell carcinomas of cattle, horses, cats and dogs, *J Comp Pathol* 114:205–210, 1996.

62. Nasir L, Krasner H, Argyle DJ, et al.: Immunocytochemical analysis of the tumour suppressor protein (p53) in feline neoplasia, *Cancer Lett* 155:1–7, 2000.

63. Favrot C, Welle M, Heimann M, et al.: Clinical, histologic, and immunohistochemical analyses of feline squamous cell carcinoma in situ, *Vet Pathol* 46:25–33, 2009.

64. Sakai H, Yamane T, Yanai T, et al.: Expression of cyclin kinase inhibitor p27(Kip1) in skin tumours of dogs, *J Comp Pathol* 125:153–158, 2001.

65. Bongiovanni L, Malatesta D, Brachelente C, et al.: beta-catenin in canine skin: immunohistochemical pattern of expression in normal skin and cutaneous epithelial tumours, *J Comp Pathol* 145:138–147, 2011.

66. Lium B, Moe L: Hereditary multifocal renal cystadenocarcinomas and nodular dermatofibrosis in the German shepherd dog: macroscopic and histopathologic changes, *Vet Pathol* 22:447–455, 1985.

67. Lingaas F, Comstock KE, Kirkness EF, et al.: A mutation in the canine BHD gene is associated with hereditary multifocal renal cystadenocarcinoma and nodular dermatofibrosis in the German Shepherd dog, *Hum Mol Genet* 12:3043–3053, 2003.

68. Hasumi H, Baba M, Hong SB, et al.: Identification and characterization of a novel folliculin-interacting protein FNIP2, *Gene* 415:60–67, 2008.

69. Suter M, Lott-Stolz G, Wild P: Generalized nodular dermatofibrosis in six Alsatians, *Vet Pathol* 20:632–634, 1983.

70. Hong DS, Reddy SB, Prieto VG, et al.: Multiple squamous cell carcinomas of the skin after therapy with sorafenib combined with tipifarnib, *Arch Dermatol* 144:779–782, 2008.

71. Kwon EJ, Kish LS, Jaworsky C: The histologic spectrum of epithelial neoplasms induced by sorafenib, *J Am Acad Dermatol* 61:522–527, 2009.

72. Goldschmidt MH, Dunstan RW, Stannard AA, et al.: Histological classification of epithelial and melanocytic tumors of the skin. In Schulman FY, editor: *worldwide reference for comparative oncology*, ed 2, Washington, 1998, Armed Forces Institute for Pathology, 104.

73. Owen LN: *TNM Classification of Tumors in Domestic Animals*, Geneva, 1980, World Health Organization.

74. Hahn KA, Lantz GC, Salisbury SK, et al.: Comparison of survey radiography with ultrasonography and x-ray computed tomography for clinical staging of subcutaneous neoplasms in dogs, *J Am Vet Med Assoc* 196:1990, 1795–1798.

75. Brissot HN, Edery EG: Use of indirect lymphography to identify sentinel lymph node in dogs: a pilot study in 30 tumours, *Vet Comp Oncol* 15:740–753, 2017.

76. Grimes JA, Secrest SA, Northrup NC, et al.: Indirect computed tomography lymphangiography with aqueous contrast for evaluation of sentinel lymph nodes in dogs with tumors of the head, *Vet Radiol Ultrasound* 58:559–564, 2017.

77. Williams LE, Packer RA: Association between lymph node size and metastasis in dogs with oral malignant melanoma: 100 cases (1987–2001), *J Am Vet Med Assoc* 222:1234–1236, 2003.

78. Baginski H, Davis G, Bastian RP: The prognostic value of lymph node metastasis with grade 2 mcts in dogs: 55 cases (2001–2010), *J Am Anim Hosp Assoc* 50:89–95, 2014.

79. Matos AJF, Faustino AMR, Lopes C, et al.: Detection of lymph node micrometastases in malignant mammary tumours in dogs by cytokeratin immunostaining, *Vet Rec* 158:626–630, 2006.

80. Grimes JA, Matz BM, Christopherson PW, et al.: Agreement between cytology and histopathology for regional lymph node metastasis in dogs with melanocytic neoplasms, *Vet Pathol* 54:579–587, 2017.

81. Kamstock DA, Ehrhart EJ, Getzy DM, et al.: Recommended guidelines for submission, trimming, margin evaluation, and reporting of tumor biopsy specimens in veterinary surgical pathology, *Vet Pathol* 48:19–31, 2011.

82. Gross TL, Ihrke PJ, Walder EJ, et al.: *Skin diseases of the dog and cat: clinical and histopathologic diagnosis*, ed 2, Ames, 2005, Blackwell Science.

83. Stockhaus C, Teske E, Rudolph R, et al.: Assessment of cytological criteria for diagnosing basal cell tumours in the dog and cat, *J Small Anim Pract* 42:582–586, 2001.

84. Bohn AA, Wills T, Caplazi P: Basal cell tumor or cutaneous basilar epithelial neoplasm? Rethinking the cytologic diagnosis of basal cell tumors, *Vet Clin Pathol* 35:449–453, 2006.

85. Gross TL, Ihrke PJ, Walder EJ, et al.: Epidermal tumors. In Gross TL, Ihrke PJ, Walder EJ, et al.: *Skin diseases of the dog and cat: clinical and histopathologic diagnosis*, ed 2, Ames, 2005, Blackwell Science, pp 562–603.

86. Simeonov R, Simeonova G: Comparative morphometric analysis of recurrent and nonrecurrent canine basal cell carcinomas: a preliminary report, *Vet Clin Pathol* 39:96–98, 2010.

87. Gross TL, Ihrke PJ, Walder EJ, et al.: Sweat gland tumors. In Gross TL, Ihrke PJ, Walder EJ, et al.: *Skin diseases of the dog and cat: clinical and histopathologic diagnosis*, ed 2, Ames, 2005, Blackwell Science, pp 665–694.

88. Diters RW, Walsh KM: Feline basal cell tumors: a review of 124 cases, *Vet Pathol* 21:51–56, 1984.

89. Day DG, Couto CG, Weisbrode SE, et al.: Basal cell carcinoma in two cats, *J Am Anim Hosp Assoc* 30:265–269, 1994.

90. Simeonov R, Simeonova G: Nucleomorphometric analysis of feline basal cell carcinomas, *Res Vet Sci* 84:440–443, 2008.

91. Gulleth Y, Goldberg N, Silverman RP, et al.: What is the best surgical margin for a basal cell carcinoma: a meta-analysis of the literature, *Plast Reconst Surg* 126:1222–1231, 2010.

92. Goldschmidt MH, Hendrick MJ: Tumors of the skin and soft tissues. In Meuten DJ, editor: *Tumors in domestic animals*, ed 4, Ames, 2002, Iowa State Press, pp 45–117, 2002.

93. Debey BM, Bagladi-Swanson M, Kapil S, et al.: Digital papillomatosis in a confined Beagle, *J Vet Diagn Invest* 13:346–348, 2001.

94. Yagci BB, Ural K, Ocal N, et al.: Azithromycin therapy of papillomatosis in dogs: a prospective, randomized, double-blinded, placebo-controlled clinical trial, *Vet Dermatol* 19:194–198, 2008.

95. Teifke JP, Kidney BA, Lohr CV, et al.: Detection of papillomavirus-DNA in mesenchymal tumour cells and not in the hyperplastic epithelium of feline sarcoids, *Vet Dermatol* 14:47–56, 2003.

96. Baer KE, Helton K: Multicentric squamous cell carcinoma in situ resembling Bowen's disease in cats, *Vet Pathol* 30:535–543, 1993.

97. Gill VL, Bergman PJ, Baer KE, et al.: Use of imiquimod 5% cream (Aldara) in cats with multicentric squamous cell carcinoma in situ: 12 cases (2002-2005), *Vet Comp Oncol* 6:55–64, 2008.

98. Gross TL, Brimacomb BH: Multifocal intraepidermal carcinoma in a dog histologically resembling Bowen's disease, *Am J Dermatopathol* 8:509–515, 1986.

99. Hammond GM, Gordon IK, Theon AP, et al.: Evaluation of strontium Sr 90 for the treatment of superficial squamous cell carcinoma of the nasal planum in cats: 49 cases (1990-2006), *J Am Vet Med Assoc* 231:736–741, 2007.

100. Evans AG, Madewell BR, Stannard AA: A trial of 13-cis-retinoic acid for treatment of squamous cell carcinoma and preneoplastic lesions of the head in cats, *Am J Vet Res* 46:2553–2557, 1985.

101. Marks SL, Song MD, Stannard AA, et al.: Clinical evaluation of etretinate for the treatment of canine solar-induced squamous cell carcinoma and preneoplastic lesions, *J Am Acad Dermatol* 27:11–16, 1992.

102. Braathen LR, Szeimies RM, Basset-Seguin N, et al.: Guidelines on the use of photodynamic therapy for nonmelanoma skin cancer: an international consensus. International Society for Photodynamic Therapy in Dermatology, 2005, *J Am Acad Dermatol* 56:125–143, 2007.

103. Buchholz J, Wergin M, Walt H, et al.: Photodynamic therapy of feline cutaneous squamous cell carcinoma using a newly developed liposomal photosensitizer: preliminary results concerning drug safety and efficacy, *J Vet Intern Med* 21:770–775, 2007.

104. Peaston AE, Leach MW, Higgins RJ: Photodynamic therapy for nasal and aural squamous cell carcinoma in cats, *J Am Vet Med Assoc* 202:1261–1265, 1993.

105. Goldschmidt MH, Shofer FS: Squamous cell carcinoma. In Goldschmidt MH, Shofer FS, editors: *Skin tumors of the dog and cat*, ed 2, Oxford, 1998, Reed Educational and Professional Publishing, pp 37–49.

106. Lascelles BD, Parry AT, Stidworthy MF, et al.: Squamous cell carcinoma of the nasal planum in 17 dogs, *Vet Rec* 147:473–476, 2000.

107. Klausner JS, Bell FW, Hayden DW, et al.: Hypercalcemia in two cats with squamous cell carcinomas, *J Am Vet Med Assoc* 196:103–105, 1990.

108. Savary KC, Price GS, Vaden SL: Hypercalcemia in cats: a retrospective study of 71 cases (1991-1997), *J Vet Intern Med* 14:184–189, 2000.

109. Theon AP, Madewell BR, Shearn VI, et al.: Prognostic factors associated with radiotherapy of squamous cell carcinoma of the nasal plane in cats, *J Am Vet Med Assoc* 206:991–996, 1995.

110. Jonsson L, Gustafsson PO: Bone-metastasizing squamous-cell carcinoma of the skin in a dog, *J Small Anim Pract* 14:159–165, 1973.

111. Lascelles BD, Henderson RA, Seguin B, et al.: Bilateral rostral maxillectomy and nasal planectomy for large rostral maxillofacial neoplasms in six dogs and one cat, *J Am Anim Hosp Assoc* 40:137–146, 2004.

112. Theon AP, VanVechten MK, Madewell BR: Intratumoral administration of carboplatin for treatment of squamous cell carcinomas of the nasal plane in cats, *Am J Vet Res* 57:205–210, 1996.

113. Tozon N, Pavlin D, Sersa G, et al.: Electrochemotherapy with intravenous bleomycin injection: an observational study in superficial squamous cell carcinoma in cats, *J Fel Med Surg* 16:291–299, 2014.

114. Himsel CA, Richardson RC, Craig JA: Cisplatin chemotherapy for metastatic squamous cell carcinoma in two dogs, *J Am Vet Med Assoc* 189:1575–1578, 1986.

115. Buhles WC, Theilen GH: Preliminary evaluation of bleomycin in feline and canine squamous cell carcinoma, *Am J Vet Res* 34:289–291, 1973.

116. Hammer AS, Couto CG, Ayl RD, et al.: Treatment of tumor-bearing dogs with actinomycin D, *J Vet Intern Med* 8:236–239, 1994.

117. Ogilvie GK, Obradovich JE, Elmslie RE, et al.: Efficacy of mitoxantrone against various neoplasms in dogs, *J Am Vet Med Assoc* 198:1618–1621, 1991.

118. Ogilvie GK, Moore AS, Obradovich JE, et al.: Toxicoses and efficacy associated with administration of mitoxantrone to cats with malignant tumors, *J Am Vet Med Assoc* 202:1839–1844, 1993.

119. Abramo F, Pratesi F, Cantile C, et al.: Survey of canine and feline follicular tumours and tumour-like lesions in central Italy, *J Small Anim Pract* 40:479–481, 1999.

120. Stannard AA, Pulley LT: Intracutaneous cornifying epithelioma (keratoacanthoma) in the dog: a retrospective study of 25 cases, *J Am Vet Med Assoc* 167:385–388, 1975.

121. White SD, Rosychuk RA, Scott KV, et al.: Use of isotretinoin and etretinate for the treatment of benign cutaneous neoplasia and cutaneous lymphoma in dogs, *J Am Vet Med Assoc* 202:387–391, 1993.

122. Goldschmidt MH, Schofer FS: Intracutaneous cornigying epithelioma. In Goldschmidt MH, Shofer FS, editors: *Skin tumors of the dog and cat*, ed 2, Oxford, 1998, Reed Educational and Professional Publishing Ltd, pp 109–114.

123. Diters RW, Goldschmidt MH: Hair follicle tumors resembling tricholemmomas in six dogs, *Vet Pathol* 20:123–125, 1983.

124. Walsh KM, Corapi WV: Tricholemmomas in three dogs, *J Comp Pathol* 96:115–117, 1986.

125. Sharif M, Reinacher M: Clear cell trichoblastomas in two dogs, *J Vet Med A Physiol Pathol Clin Med* 53:352–354, 2006.

126. Goldschmidt MH, Schofer FS: Trichoepithelioma. In Goldschmidt MH, Shofer FS, editors: *Skin tumors of the dog and cat*, ed 2, Oxford, 1998, Reed Educational and Professional Publishing Ltd, pp 115–124.

127. Gross TL, Ihrke PJ, Walder EJ, et al.: *Follicular tumors, skin diseases of the dog and cat: clinical and histopathologic diagnosis*, ed 2, Ames, 2005, Blackwell Science Ltd, pp 604–640.

128. Goldschmidt MH, Schofer FS: Pilomatrixoma. In Goldschmidt MH, Shofer FS, editors: *Skin tumors of the dog and cat*, ed 2, Oxford, 1998, Reed Educational and Professional Publishing, pp 125–130.

129. Carroll EE, Fossey SL, Mangus LM, et al.: Malignant pilomatricoma in 3 dogs, *Vet Pathol* 47:937–943, 2010.

130. Johnson RP, Johnson JA, Groom SC, et al.: Malignant pilomatrixoma in an old english sheepdog, *Can Vet J* 24:392–394, 1983.

131. Jackson K, Boger L, Goldschmidt M, et al.: Malignant pilomatricoma in a soft-coated wheaten terrier, *Vet Clin Pathol* 39:236–240, 2010.

132. Scott DW, Anderson WI: Canine sebaceous gland tumors: a retrospective analysis of 172 cases, *Can Pract* 15:19–27, 1990.

133. Strafuss AC: Sebaceous gland adenomas in dogs, *J Am Vet Med Assoc* 169:640–642, 1976.

134. Goldschmidt MH, Schofer FS: Sebaceous tumors. In Goldschmidt MH, Shofer FS, editors: *Skin tumors of the dog and cat*, ed 2, Oxford, 1998, Reed Educational and Professional Publishing, pp 50–65.

135. Bettini G, Morini M, Mandrioli L, et al.: CNS and lung metastasis of sebaceous epithelioma in a dog, *Vet Dermatol* 20:289–294, 2009.

136. Case MT, Bartz AR, Bernstein M, et al.: Metastasis of a sebaceous gland carcinoma in the dog, *J Am Vet Med Assoc* 154:661–664, 1969.

137. Strafuss AC: Sebaceous gland carcinoma in dogs, *J Am Vet Med Assoc* 169:325–326, 1976.

138. Goldschmidt MH, Schofer FS: Apocrine gland tumors. In Goldschmidt MH, Shofer FS, editors: *Skin tumors of the dog and cat*, ed 2, Oxford, 1998, Reed Educational and Professional Publishing, pp 80–95.

139. Kalaher KM, Anderson WI, Scott DW: Neoplasms of the apocrine sweat glands in 44 dogs and 10 cats, *Vet Red* 127:400–403, 1990.

140. Simko E, Wilcock BP, Yager JA: A retrospective study of 44 canine apocrine sweat gland adenocarcinomas, *Can Vet J* 44:38–42, 2003.

141. Bagnasco G, Properzi R, Porto R, et al.: Feline cutaneous neuroendocrine carcinoma (Merkel cell tumour): clinical and pathological findings, *Vet Dermatol* 14:111–115, 2003.

142. Patnaik AK, Post GS, Erlandson RA: Clinicopathologic and electron microscopic study of cutaneous neuroendocrine (Merkel cell) carcinoma in a cat with comparisons to human and canine tumors, *Vet Pathol* 38:553–556, 2001.

143. Whitley DB, Mansell JE: Multiple eccrine poromas in the paw of a dog, *Vet Dermatol* 23:167–170, 2012.

144. Chang Y, Moore PS: Merkel cell carcinoma: a virus-induced human cancer, *Annu Rev Pathol* 7:123–144, 2012.

145. Konno A, Nagata M, Nanko H: Immunohistochemical diagnosis of a Merkel cell tumor in a dog, *Vet Pathol* 35:538–540, 1998.

146. Glick AD, Holscher MA, Crenshaw JD: Neuroendocrine carcinoma of the skin in a dog, *Vet Pathol* 20:761–763, 1983.

147. Joiner KS, Smith AN, Henderson RA, et al.: Multicentric cutaneous neuroendocrine (Merkel cell) carcinoma in a dog, *Vet Pathol* 47:1090–1094, 2010.

148. Gil da Costa RM, Rema A, Pires MA, et al.: Two canine Merkel cell tumours: immunoexpression of c-KIT, E-cadherin, beta-catenin and S100 protein, *Vet Dermatol* 21:198–201, 2010.

149. Moe L, Lium B: Hereditary multifocal renal cystadenocarcinomas and nodular dermatofibrosis in 51 German shepherd dogs, *J Small Anim Pract* 38:498–505, 1997.

150. Gardiner DW, Spraker TR: Generalized nodular dermatofibrosis in the absence of renal neoplasia in an Australian Cattle Dog, *Vet Pathol* 45:901–904, 2008.

151. Scott DW: External ear disorders, *J Am Anim Hosp Assoc* 16:426–433, 1980.

152. Legendre AM, Krahwinkel DJ: Feline ear tumors, *J Am Anim Hosp Assoc* 17:1035–1037, 1981.

153. Rogers KS: Tumors of the ear canal, *Vet Clin Nth Am Small Anim Pract* 18:859–868, 1988.

154. London CA, Dubilzeig RR, Vail DM, et al.: Evaluation of dogs and cats with tumors of the ear canal: 145 cases (1978-1992), *J Am Vet Med Assoc* 208:1413–1418, 1996.

155. Goldschmidt MH, Schofer FS: Ceruminous gland tumors. In Goldschmidt MH, Shofer FS, editors: *Skin tumors of the dog and cat*, ed 2, Oxford, 1998, Reed Educational and Professional Publishing, pp 96–102.

156. Moisan PG, Watson GL: Ceruminous gland tumors in dogs and cats: a review of 124 cases, *J Am Anim Hosp Assoc* 32:448–452, 1996.

157. Theon AP, Barthez PY, Madewell BR, et al.: Radiation therapy of ceruminous gland carcinomas in dogs and cats, *J Am Vet Med Assoc* 205:566–569, 1994.

158. Marino DJ, MacDonald JM, Mattiesen DT, et al.: Results of surgery and long-term follow-up in dogs with ceruminous gland adenocarcinoma, *J Am Anim Hosp Assoc* 29:560–563, 1993.

159. Marino DJ, MacDonald JM, Mattiesen DT, et al.: Results of surgery in cats with ceruminous gland adenocarcinoma, *J Am Anim Hosp Assoc* 30:54–58, 1994.

160. Bacon NJ, Gilbert RL, Bostock DE, et al.: Total ear canal ablation in the cat: indications, morbidity and long-term survival, *J Small Anim Pract* 44:430–434, 2003.

161. Marino DJ, Matthiesen DT, Stefanacci JD, et al.: Evaluation of dogs with digit masses: 117 cases (1981-1991), *J Am Vet Med Assoc* 207:726–728, 1995.

162. Wobeser BK, Kidney BA, Powers BE, et al.: Diagnoses and clinical outcomes associated with surgically amputated canine digits submitted to multiple veterinary diagnostic laboratories, *Vet Pathol* 44:355–361, 2007.

163. Henry CJ, Brewer WG, Whitley EM, et al.: Canine digital tumors: a veterinary cooperative oncology group retrospective study of 64 dogs, *J Vet Intern Med* 19:720–724, 2005.

164. Madewell BR, Pool RR, Theilen GH, et al.: Multiple subungual squamous cell carcinomas in five dogs, *J Am Vet Med Assoc* 180:731–734, 1982.

165. Belluco S, Brisebard E, Watrelot D, et al.: Digital squamous cell carcinoma in dogs: epidemiological, histological, and imunohistochemical study, *Vet Pathol* 50:1078–1082, 2013.

166. Wobeser BK, Kidney BA, Powers BE, et al.: Agreement among surgical pathologists evaluating routine histologic sections of digits amputated from cats and dogs, *J Vet Diagn Invest* 19:439–443, 2007.

167. Wobeser BK, Kidney BA, Powers BE, et al.: Diagnoses and clinical outcomes associated with surgically amputated feline digits submitted to multiple veterinary diagnostic laboratories, *Vet Pathol* 44:362–365, 2007.

168. Luna LD, Higginbotham ML, Henry CJ, et al.: Feline non-ocular melanoma: a retrospective study of 23 cases (1991-1999), *J Fel Med Surg* 2:173–181, 2000.

169. van der Linde-Sipman JS, van den Ingh tSGAM: Primary and metastatic carcinomas in the digits of cats, *Vet Quart* 22:141–145, 2000.

170. Aronsohn MG, Carpenter JL: Distal extremity melanocytic nevi and malignant melanoma in dogs, *J Am Anim Hosp Assoc* 26:605–612, 1990.

171. Schultheiss PC: Histologic features and clinical outcomes of melanomas of lip, haired skin, and nail bed locations of dogs, *J Vet Diagn Invest* 18:422–425, 2006.

172. Kaufman KL, Mann FA: Short- and long-term outcomes after digit amputation in dogs: 33 cases (1999-2011), *J Am Vet Med Assoc* 242:1249–1254, 2013.

173. Brockley LK, Cooper MA, Bennett PF: Malignant melanoma in 63 dogs (2001-2011): the effect of carboplatin chemotherapy on survival, *NZ Vet J* 61:25–31, 2013.

174. Manley CA, Leibman NF, Wolchok JD, et al.: Xenogeneic murine tyrosinase DNA vaccine for malignant melanoma of the digit of dogs, *J Vet Intern Med* 25:94–99, 2011.

20
Melanoma

PHILIP J. BERGMAN, LAURA E. SELMIC, AND MICHAEL S. KENT

Melanoma is a relatively common cancer of dogs, especially those with significant amounts of skin pigmentation. Melanomas are relatively rare in cats. The most common location for canine melanoma is the haired skin, where they grossly appear to be small brown to black masses, but they can also appear as large, flat, and/or wrinkled masses.[1,2] Primary melanomas can also occur in the oral cavity, nailbed, footpad, eye, gastrointestinal tract, nasal cavity, anal sac, or mucocutaneous junction.[3-6] Metastatic sites are numerous including lymph nodes (LNs), lungs, liver, meninges, and adrenal glands.[3]

Melanoma arises from melanocytes, which are the cells that generate pigment through the melanosome by a number of melanosomal glycoproteins. In humans, cutaneous melanoma can arise as a result of mutations induced by repeated, intense exposure to ultraviolet light (for example, frequent tanning or working outdoors). Melanoma is currently the most rapidly increasing incident human cancer.[7,8] Significant recent research into the etiology of human melanoma suggests multiple causes independent of the aforementioned UV-associated mutagenesis.[9,10] Because most breeds of dogs have a significant hair coat that likely affords them protection from sunlight, UV-associated melanoma is less likely to be a primary causative agent in the dog. However, risk factors for canine melanoma are not well established.

The most common oral malignancy in the dog is melanoma.[2,3,11,12] Oral melanoma is most commonly diagnosed in Scottish terriers, golden retrievers, Chow Chows, poodles, and dachshunds.[2,13-16] Oral melanoma is more commonly seen in heavily pigmented breeds and is primarily a disease of older dogs without gender predilection, but may also be seen in younger dogs.[13,17,18] Differential diagnoses for oral tumors include squamous cell carcinoma, fibrosarcoma, osteosarcoma, acanthomatous ameloblastoma, and peripheral odontogenic fibroma.[2,3,12,19-21] Canine oral melanomas are found in the following locations by order of decreasing frequency: gingiva, lips, tongue, and hard palate.[2,3,11,13,16] Feline melanoma is relatively rare, but appears to be malignant in most cases.[3,22-29]

Melanomas in dogs have extremely diverse biologic behaviors depending on a large variety of factors. A greater understanding of these factors helps the clinician to determine the appropriate staging, treatment options, and prognosis. The primary factors that determine the biologic behavior of an oral melanoma in a dog are site, size, stage, and histologic parameters.[13,17,18,30,31] Unfortunately, even with a comprehensive understanding of all of these factors, there are melanomas that have an unreliable biologic behavior, hence the need for additional research into this relatively common, heterogeneous, but frequently aggressive tumor.

Pathology and Molecular Biology

Melanomas can be difficult to diagnose pathologically in some situations, especially anaplastic amelanotic melanomas, which can masquerade as soft tissue sarcomas.[32-34] Numerous investigators have attempted to increase the precision of identifying melanomas, predominantly through immunohistochemical (IHC) means.[16,33,35-37] This has been accomplished through the use of multiple IHC assays or use of an IHC cocktail of antibodies. The use of PNL2 and tyrosinase beyond the typical use of Melan A and S-100 appears to hold particular promise.[38-40]

The molecular characterization of canine and feline melanomas is significantly limited compared with the more comprehensive evaluation of human melanomas.[41] BRAF is a member of the MAPK signaling pathway that is commonly mutated in human cutaneous melanoma, but not in human oral melanoma.[42] Interestingly, BRAF mutations are also uncommon in canine oral malignant melanomas (MMs).[43] However, downstream constitutive activation of ERK has been identified in both human and canine MMs,[44] supporting the idea that certain canine and feline malignancies can have molecular signatures similar to those of human malignancies in addition to their already well known clinical similarities in the context of resistance to chemotherapy and/or radiation therapy (RT) and similar atypical sites of metastasis. A number of other investigators have reported a variety of molecular abnormalities and/or associations in canine and feline melanoma.[44-85]

Transcriptome analysis has recently uncovered a variety of possible new therapeutic targets in canine melanoma.[86] The melanoma-associated genes clustered in the areas of focal adhesion and PI3K-Akt (phosphoinositide 3-kinase/protein kinase B) signaling pathways, extracellular matrix–receptor interactions, and protein digestion and absorption. A small subset of dogs with malignant melanoma have exon 11 c-kit gene mutations,[62,87] and therefore the more routine use of c-kit mutation analysis by polymerase chain reaction (PCR) of canine MMs, and subsequent use of KIT small molecule inhibitors (particularly in dogs with advanced stage disease and/or lack of response to Oncept), should be considered. Furthermore, with somatic mutations in NRAS and PTEN being found in canine MM,[88] similar to human melanoma hotspot sites, these may represent logical therapeutic targets in the future.

Biologic Behavior and Prognostic Factors

The biologic behavior of canine oral melanoma is extremely variable and best characterized based on anatomic site, size, stage, and histologic parameters. On divergent ends of the malignancy spectrum, a low-grade 0.5-cm haired-skin melanocytoma is highly likely to be cured with simple surgical excision whereas a 5.0-cm high-grade oral MM has a poor to grave prognosis regardless of treatment options. Similar to the development of a rational staging, prognostic, and therapeutic plan for any tumor, two primary questions must be answered: what is the local invasiveness of the tumor and what is the metastatic potential? These will determine the prognosis and appropriate therapies.

The anatomic site of melanoma is highly, although not completely, predictive of local invasiveness and metastatic propensity. Melanomas involving the haired skin, which are not in proximity to mucosal margins, often behave in a benign manner.[1,3] Surgical excision is often curative, but histopathologic examination is imperative for delineation of margins as well as a description of cytologic features. The use of Ki67 IHC has been reported previously to more reliably predict potential malignant behavior than classical histology for cutaneous melanoma.[89]

Oral and mucosal melanoma has been routinely considered an extremely malignant tumor with a high degree of local invasiveness and high metastatic potential.[2,13,17,18,30,90] This biologic behavior is similar to that of human oral and mucosal melanoma.[3,91] Two recent studies have called this dogma into question and suggest benign oral melanomas can occur more frequently than previously thought.[92,93] Extreme caution is necessary when one receives a histopathology report suggesting a benign course with an oral melanoma, as this author (PJB) has seen approximately 30 dogs over the past 12 years presenting with florid systemic metastases despite an original histopathology report suggesting benign disease. Similar to cutaneous melanoma, Ki67 appears to hold prognostic importance in canine oral melanoma as well.[94]

The anatomic sites that split the opposite ends of the prognostic spectrum of generally benign acting, haired skin versus often malignant and metastatic oral/mucosal melanomas in dogs include melanomas of the digit and foot pad. Dogs with melanoma of the digits without LN or distant metastasis treated with digit amputation have reported median survival times (MSTs) of approximately 12 months with 1- and 2-year survival rates of 42% to 57% and 11% to 13%, respectively.[95,96] Metastasis at presentation is reported in approximately 30% to 40% of dogs,[95,97] and the majority of dogs with digit melanoma will develop regional or distant metastatic disease.[95–97] The prognosis for dogs with melanoma of the foot pad has not been previously reported; the first author (PJB) has found this anatomic site to be anecdotally similar in metastatic potential and prognosis to digit melanoma. Interestingly, human acral lentiginous melanoma (plantar surface of the foot, palms of the hand, and digit) also has an increased potential for metastasis.[98]

The most exhaustive review of prognostic factors in canine melanocytic neoplasms took a regimented, systematic approach to analyze the studies published to date in order to identify factors that appear to be repeatable, statistical, and therefore likely real, while also identifying areas where additional work is necessary because of incomplete data.[99] For veterinary clinicians and/or researchers interested in canine melanoma, this publication is strongly recommended. A flurry of recent investigations has given us a much greater understanding of feline ocular melanoma and iridociliary cysts that are grossly similar to melanoma.[6,100–103] The use of all this information by clinicians and pathologists will allow for the best determination of prognosis for a specific patient that then allows for identification of the most logical treatment plans.

Size and Stage

For dogs with oral melanoma, primary tumor size has been found to be extremely prognostic. The World Health Organization staging scheme for dogs with oral melanoma is based on local tumor size and regional and distant metastasis, with stage I being a nonmetastatic tumor less than 2 cm in diameter, stage II being a nonmetastatic tumor 2 cm to 4 cm in diameter tumor, stage III being a tumor greater than 4 cm in diameter and/or LN metastasis, and stage IV being a melanoma with distant metastasis (Fig. 20.1).[104] The MSTs for dogs with oral melanoma treated with surgery are 511 to 874 days, 160 to 818 days, and 168 to 207 days with stage I, II, and III disease, respectively.[17,105] More recent reports suggest dogs with stage I oral melanoma treated with standardized therapies, including surgery, RT, and/or chemotherapy, have an MST of approximately 12 to 14 months, with most dogs dying of distant metastatic disease and not local recurrence.[106,107] Other investigators have found dogs with stage I oral melanoma have a median progression-free survival (PFS) time of 19 months.[108]

Diagnostic Workup and Clinical Staging

The diagnosis and clinical staging of dogs with melanoma is relatively straightforward. A minimum database should include a thorough history and physical examination, complete blood count, biochemical profile, and urinalysis.

Gross characteristics of melanomas, such as pigmentation of mass, should raise the suspicion for a diagnosis of melanoma. Pigmented melanomas can be easily confirmed via fine-needle aspiration (FNA) and cytology. In dogs, small (<2 cm), mobile, well-circumscribed, slow-growing cutaneous melanomas tend to be benign and easily excisable, whereas large, poorly defined,

T:	Primary Tumor	
	T1	Tumor ≤ 2 cm in diameter
	T2	Tumor 2–4 cm in diameter
	T3	Tumor >4 cm in diameter
N:	Regional Lymph Nodes	
	N0	No evidence of regional node involvement
	N1	Histologic/Cytologic evidence of regional node involvement
	N2	Fixed nodes
M:	Distant Metastasis	
	M0	No evidence of distant metastasis
	M1	Evidence of distant metastasis

Stage I = T1 N0 M0

Stage II = T2 N0 M0

Stage III = T2 N1 M0 or T3 N0 M0

Stage IV = Any T, Any N and M1

• **Fig. 20.1** Traditional World Health Organization TNM-based staging scheme for dogs with oral melanoma. (From Owen LN. *TNM Classification of Tumors in Domestic Animals.* 1st ed. Geneva, Switzerland; 1980.)

ulcerated, and rapidly growing tumors can make surgical excision challenging. In the latter example, incisional biopsy and IHC can be an important part of the diagnostic workup, particularly if the mass is nonpigmented, to allow other tumor types to be ruled out and a diagnosis of melanoma confirmed.

Clinical staging tests routinely include evaluation of the regional LNs and assessment of the thoracic cavity with either three-view thoracic radiographs or thoracic CT scan. The regional LNs should be assessed whether lymphadenomegaly is present or not. LN metastasis is present in approximately 70% of dogs with lymphadenomegaly (Fig. 20.2) but, more importantly, in approximately 40% with normal sized LNs.[109] FNA cytology of the ipsilateral regional LNs has been recommended to assess for nodal metastasis; however, the only accessible regional LN is the mandibular LN. This may provide misleading information, as the lymphatic drainage of the head is complex and metastases to contralateral LNs has been documented. Furthermore, the mandibular LN can be normal when other LNs, such as the medial retropharyngeal or parotid LN, are metastatic.[110,111] Although earlier studies showed a high concordance of cytology and histopathology in dogs with melanomas,[111] a recent study highlighted discordance between cytology findings and histopathology, with a low correlation between the final cytology and histopathology reports in dogs with melanocytic neoplasia.[112] As a result, histologic examination of the LN is recommended either through excision of the major LNs of the head and neck or sentinel LN (SLN) mapping.

Nondiscriminate extirpation of the regional LNs of the head and neck has been described in dogs with and cats with malignant oral tumors.[113,114] One approach describes ipsilateral extirpation of the parotid, mandibular, and retropharyngeal LNs, but this requires an extensive dissection and does not investigate the contralateral LNs.[113] A second approach involves extirpation of the left and right mandibular and medial retropharyngeal LNs through a single incision, but does not investigate the parotid LNs.[114] The limitations of both approaches include more extensive dissections and incomplete testing of the regional LNs, and hence there is a risk of postoperative complications and missed metastatic LNs.

SLN mapping allows identification of the direct lymphatic drainage pathway from the tumor to the first draining LN. This LN can then be targeted for selective lymphadenectomy and histopathologic testing. Selective lymphadenectomy avoids the indiscriminate extirpation of multiple LNs and, because it is a less extensive surgical dissection, reduces the risk of postoperative complications. The use of SLN mapping and lymphadenectomy has been proven to be of diagnostic, prognostic, and clinical benefit in human melanoma.[115] Relatively few investigations have been reported to date for SLN mapping and/or excision for dogs with malignancies,[116–123] and the authors strongly encourage additional investigation and clinical adoption in this area.

Although not commonly described, abdominal ultrasonography or CT scans should be considered in dogs with melanomas arising from the oral cavity, digits, or pads because of the risk of metastasis to the abdominal LNs, liver, adrenal glands, and other intraabdominal sites. The use of novel staging modalities, such as gallium citrate scintigraphy, requires further investigation.[124]

Cross-sectional imaging (i.e., computed tomography [CT] scans or magnetic resonance imaging [MRI]) is critical for surgical planning for oral melanoma, especially melanomas involving the maxilla and caudal mandible. This allows for assessment of the extent of tumor, invasion into soft tissues, bone and the nasal cavity, and assessment of regional LNs, particularly the nonpalpable medial retropharyngeal, parotid, and buccal LNs.

Treatment

Surgery

Surgery continues to be the most effective local treatment modality for melanoma. There are few objective data available to guide decision making for appropriate surgical margin width for resection of melanomas. Benign cutaneous tumors are typically completely excised with 1-cm skin margins (and ideally one fascial plane for deep margins). Given the invasive nature of MMs, wide margins (2–3 cm) are ideal whenever possible; however, for oral melanomas, wide margins may not possible because of the limited amount of adjacent normal tissues. In these cases, surgery may need to be combined with RT for adequate local tumor control. In the authors' experience, 1- to 2-cm margins are usually adequate for complete histologic excision of MMs with well-defined borders (Fig. 20.3). Wide margins are usually possible with cutaneous and digit melanomas.

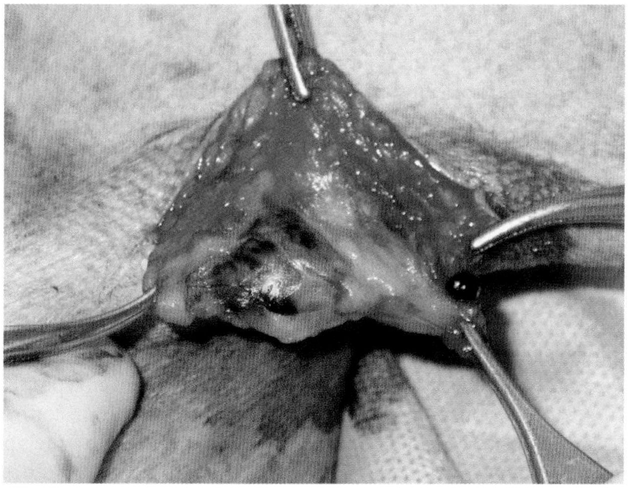

• **Fig. 20.2** Extirpation of a popliteal lymph node from the dog in Fig. 20.7. Note the effaced node overtaken with pigmented cells and the smaller nodule within the lymphatic vessel slightly distal to the node.

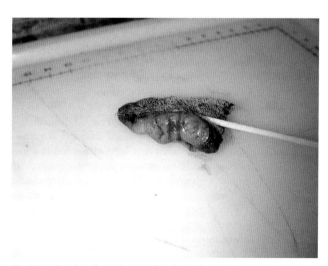

• **Fig. 20.3** Amelanotic melanoma involving the rostral aspect of the right lip; 1- to 2-cm lateral margins resulted in complete histologic excision.

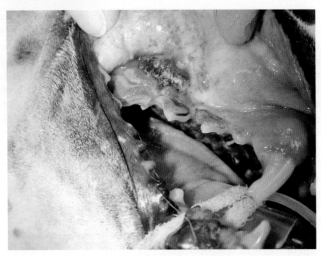

• **Fig. 20.4** Local tumor recurrence after incomplete histologic excision and postoperative radiation of a gingival melanoma dorsal to the right carnassial tooth (caudal is to the left and the right canine tooth can be seen in the lower right-hand corner). When first treated, the mass was reportedly less than 1 cm in diameter and wide resection (i.e., partial maxillectomy) was not performed.

Partial mandibulectomy or maxillectomy is often required for resection of oral melanomas arising from the gingiva or mucosa in close proximity to the bone.[125] A common error is to resect a gingival mass without taking underlying bone simply because bone invasion is not observed. Owing to the proximity of the gingiva to the underlying bone, this approach typically leaves residual microscopic disease that leads to local recurrence (Fig. 20.4). Occasionally, tumors do occur in mucosal areas that are not adjacent to bone (e.g., buccal mucosa) or originate in the lip or tongue (Fig. 20.5) and are amenable to excision of the soft tissues only. Complete histologic excision of oral tumors has been shown to significantly affect prognosis in some studies (Fig. 20.6).[126–128] Dogs with incomplete histologic excision are 3.6 times more likely to die of tumor-related causes compared with dogs with complete histologic excision.[128] In this study, dogs with tumors caudal to the third premolar tooth (PM3) were 4.3 times more likely to die of tumor-related causes compared with dogs with tumors located rostral to PM3. For more specific surgical approaches to oral melanoma please see Chapter 23, Section A on oral tumors.

With the widespread access to cross-sectional imaging, improvements in surgical techniques (e.g., combined dorsal and intraoral approach for caudal maxillary tumors), and increased availability of surgical oncologic training, complete histologic excisions are more likely to be achieved than previously reported. The surgical goals should be driven by tumor location, clinical stage, owner preferences, and the ability of the surgeon to perform a wide resection in locations where surgery is difficult (e.g., large caudal tumors). Unplanned or limited attempts at excision should not be made, as these will often leave either residual gross or microscopic disease and result in rapid tumor recurrence. The first chance to operate with undisrupted anatomy is often the best chance to achieve tumor-free margins. For patients that undergo surgical excision with either a mandibulectomy or maxillectomy, quality of life is usually very good, and most dogs resume eating within 3 days of surgery. Furthermore, owner satisfaction with functional and cosmetic results after mandibulectomy and maxillectomy is high.[129] The functional outcome of single digit amputation is excellent and partial foot amputations (requiring excision

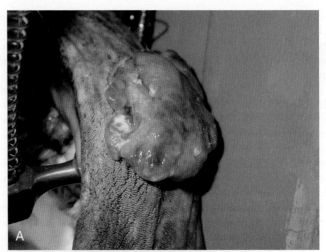

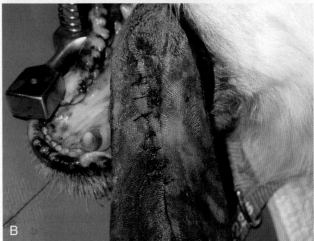

• **Fig. 20.5** (A) Lingual melanoma near the midline of the tongue of a dog. These masses are often superficial and can be easily excised with 1- to 2-cm lingual mucosal margins and a layer of muscle fibers deep to the mass. (B) Closure results in little disruption of the lingual architecture and postoperative function is excellent.

of more than one digit; see Fig. 20.7) are also tolerated very well and result in a good functional outcome.[130,131]

For tumors that are not amenable to wide resection or for which resection results in incomplete histologic margins, the combination of surgery with RT or other adjuvant therapies should be considered. Historically, surgery has not been recommended in the presence of metastatic disease (e.g., a positive LN is discovered during tumor staging); however, the role of adjuvant therapy (chemotherapy or immunotherapy) in conjunction with cytoreductive surgery is being investigated for metastatic melanoma in people and such approaches are now being explored in dogs.[132–134]

Radiation Therapy

RT plays an important role in the management and treatment of canine and feline oral melanomas. As with most tumor types, RT is used for the purpose of achieving locoregional tumor control. RT has been described as both a primary and adjuvant therapy, and both hypofractionated and definitive protocols have been described (Table 20.1).[26,106–108, 135–141]

Melanoma is thought to be a relatively radioresistant tumor type necessitating a higher dose in each fraction to achieve local

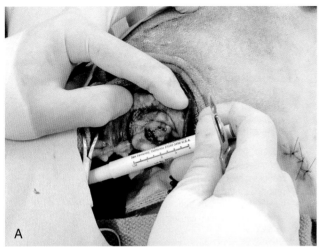

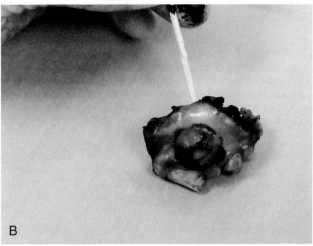

• **Fig. 20.6** (A) Intraoperative photograph of a melanoma confined to the lateral aspect of the caudal dental arcade. Surgical margins in this case were approximately 1.5 cm around the rostral, dorsal, and caudal borders of the tumor. The incision along the hard palate was made just medial to the dental arcade. (B) Surgical margins are inked with a green surgical ink and histopathologic assessment showed complete histologic excision.

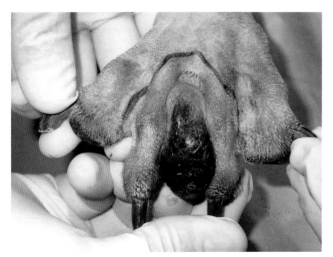

• **Fig. 20.7** Malignant melanoma in the interdigital webbing between digits 3 and 4 (same dog as in Fig. 20.2). Surgical margins were between 1 and 2 cm. Complete histologic excision was achieved in this case after partial foot amputation.

control, although this is somewhat controversial.[142] Most published protocols in dogs and cats have used higher dose per fraction protocols, although the relative radiosensitivity of melanoma in companion animal species has not been determined and nor has the ideal dose per fraction in hypofractionated protocols been determined.

Hypofractionated protocols have the advantage of fewer treatments with fewer anesthetic episodes, lower cost, and less time commitment for the owner. These protocols also result in less severe acute effects. The main disadvantage of hypofractionated protocols is a lower overall and biologic equivalent dose, which theoretically results in lower rates of local control and an increased risk for late side effects. For dogs with a better prognosis, lower dose per fraction protocols can be used to decrease the risk of late effects. For a discussion of radiation effects, see the section on radiation side effects in Chapter 13.

When planning for RT, most radiation oncologists will treat both the primary tumor and the regional LN, including the mandibular and medial retropharyngeal LNs (Fig. 20.8). These LNs are included because, as noted earlier in this chapter, normal sized LNs do not preclude the possibility of metastasis.[109]

The reported range of partial and complete responses to RT are 25% to 67% and 19% to 69%, respectively, yielding an overall response rate of 82% to 94%, although one recent study reported a 0% complete and partial response rates and a 73% overall response rate when including stable disease in this measure.[107,136–138,140,141] When treating gross disease, responses are generally rapid and dramatic decreases in tumor volume can be seen within several weeks of starting therapy (Fig. 20.9). The PFS ranges from 3.6 to 8.6 months.[107,108,135,136] Interestingly, the longest reported PFS was from a study in which all dogs had surgery as part of their treatment protocol.[135] Local recurrence rates after RT vary and are confounded by different radiation protocols and adjuvant therapies used in these studies: local recurrence rates of 26% and 27% have been reported after the treatment of microscopic disease, whereas local progression was reported in 45% of dogs after the irradiation of macroscopic disease.[107,135]

The reported MSTs for dogs treated with RT range from 4.5 to 14.7 months (see Table 20.1).[106–108,135–138,139–141] The majority of these studies are retrospective and use different RT equipment, protocols, and adjuvant therapies, making it difficult to determine an ideal treatment regimen. Reported protocols include 2 to 4 Gy fractions daily for 12 to 19 treatments (45.6–57 Gy),[107,108] 4 Gy per fraction three times weekly for 4 weeks (48 Gy), 6 Gy per fraction twice weekly for 2.5 (30 Gy) or 3 weeks (36 Gy),[135,136,141] 6 Gy per fraction once weekly for 4 weeks (24 Gy),[135] 6 Gy once weekly for 6 fractions (36 Gy),[106,141] 8 Gy per fraction once weekly for 3 (24 Gy) or 4 fractions (32 Gy),[135,137,141] 9 Gy per fraction once weekly for 4 fractions (36 Gy),[107,138,139] and 10 Gy per fraction once weekly for 3 fractions (30 Gy).[107]

Five cats with oral melanoma and treated with RT have been reported.[26] There was one complete response and two partial responses with an MST of 146 days. Three cats were treated adjuvantly: one cat with carboplatin, one cat with carboplatin and mitoxantrone, and one cat with a DNA-based vaccine as an adjuvant to RT.

Chemotherapy may have a role in the management of dogs and cats with MMs treated with RT, either as a radiation sensitizer and/or because of the risk of metastatic disease. In one study, 39 dogs with incompletely excised oral melanomas were treated with either cisplatin (10–30 mg/m² IV) or carboplatin (90 mg/m² IV) once weekly approximately 1 hour before receiving RT.[106] The

TABLE 20.1   Published Studies on the Treatment of Oral Melanoma with Radiation Therapy

Study, Study Type (Year Published)	Species (No.)	Source and Dose/Protocol of Radiation	Outcomes	Chemotherapy
Bateman et al, Prospective single-arm trial (1994)[137]	Canine (18)	Cobalt-60; 24 Gy in three once-weekly fractions of 8 Gy.	One dog died during treatment, 9/18 had a complete response, 5/18 had a partial response, 3/18 had no response, MST: 7.9 months.	
Blackwood et al, Prospective single-arm trial (1996)[138]	Canine (36)	4 MV linear accelerator ($n = 29$), 250 kVp orthovoltage unit ($n = 1$), combination of the two machines ($n = 4$) 36 Gy in four once-weekly fractions of 9 Gy.	25/36 dogs had a complete response, 9/36 had a partial response, overall MST not reported (range, 5–213 weeks), MST for dogs that died of tumor-related causes: 21 weeks.	
Theon et al, Prospective single-arm trial (1997)[108]	Canine (38)	Cobalt-60; 48 Gy in 12 4-Gy fractions on a Monday–Wednesday–Friday schedule.	PFS 7.9 months, MST not reported.	
Proulx et al, Retrospective case series (2003)[107]	Canine (140)	Cobalt-60: 36 Gy in four once weekly 9-Gy fractions ($n = 54$); 30 Gy in 3 once-weekly 10-Gy fractions ($n = 69$), or 45.6–57 Gy in 12 to 19 2–4 Gy fractions ($n = 17$).	45/86 dogs had a complete response and 27/86 dogs had a partial response. Median time to first event (metastasis, local recurrence, or death): 5.0 months, MST: 7.0 months.	80 dogs received chemotherapy (carboplatin [$n = 60$], cisplatin [$n = 3$], melphalan [$n = 17$]). Chemotherapy did not affect time to first event or survival.
Freeman et al, Retrospective case series (2003)[106]	Canine (39)	Cobalt-60 and 4 MV linear accelerator: 36 Gy in 6 once-weekly 6-Gy fractions.	MST: 363 days.	Dogs received cisplatin (10–30 mg/m² IV) or carboplatin (90 mg/m² IV) chemotherapy 60 minutes before radiation delivery.
Farrelly et al, Retrospective case series (2004)[26]	Feline (5)	Cobalt-60: 24 Gy in three once-weekly 8-Gy fractions.	One complete response, two partial responses, MST: 146 days.	Two cats received chemotherapy, one received carboplatin, one carboplatin and mitoxantrone, and one was treated with a DNA-based vaccine. One cat had additional radiation after initial failure.
Murphy et al, Retrospective two-arm study (2005)[139]	Canine (28)	4 MV linear accelerator: 36 Gy in four once weekly 9-Gy fractions.	No chemotherapy group, MST 307 days. Chemotherapy group, MST 286 days.	No chemotherapy, 13 dogs. Chemotherapy group, 15 dogs treated with carboplatin (planned dose: 300 mg/m² IV every 21 days).
Dank et al, Retrospective case series (2012)[135]	Canine (17); 11 dogs treated with surgery, chemotherapy, and radiation; 6 dogs treated with surgery and chemotherapy	Radiotherapy sources not indicated. 32 Gy in four once-weekly 8-Gy fractions ($n = 5$), 36 Gy in six twice-weekly 6-Gy fractions ($n = 4$), 30 Gy in three once-weekly 10-Gy fractions ($n = 1$), and 24 Gy in four once-weekly 6-Gy fractions ($n = 1$).	PFS radiotherapy group, 259 days; PFS no radiotherapy group, 210 days. MST radiotherapy group, 440 days; MST no radiotherapy group, 387 days. No significant difference between groups.	Carboplatin (median dose of 300 mg/m² IV).
Kawabe et al, Retrospective case series (2015)[140]	Canine (111)	Orthovoltage 300 Kvp ($n = 68$), 4 MV linear accelerator ($n = 34$) or combined ($n = 5$); electron therapy, energy not reported ($n = 4$). The median total radiation dose was 37.8 Gy (range, 6.3–74.3 Gy).	38/87 dogs had a complete response and 36/87 dogs had a partial response. MST: 171 days; MST for orthovoltage-treated dogs, 122 days; MST for megavoltage-treated dogs, 233 days. This was statistically different.	66 dogs had chemotherapy: either intralesional cisplatin (0.5mg/dog q1–2wks; $n = 26$), carboplatin IV (180–250 mg/m² q3wks; $n = 26$), or both ($n = 14$).

TABLE 20.1	Published Studies on the Treatment of Oral Melanoma with Radiation Therapy—cont'd			
Study, Study Type (Year Published)	Species (No.)	Source and Dose/Protocol of Radiation	Outcomes	Chemotherapy
Cancedda et al, Prospective multicenter, non-randomized, two-arm clinical trial (2016)[136]	Canine (27)	Linear accelerator using photons or electrons. Energy not specified. 30 Gy in five fractions over 2.5 weeks.	Radiation therapy alone group: 3/15 dogs had a complete response and 10/15 dogs had a partial response; PFS 110 days; MST: 192 days. RT and temozolamide group: 2/15 dogs had a complete response and 8/15 dogs had a partial response. PFS of 205 days. MST: 401. Statistically significant difference for PFS but not MST.	No chemotherapy given to 15. 12 received temozolomide at 60 mg/m² PO once daily for 5 days every 4 weeks.
Tollett et al, Retrospective case series (2016)[141]	Canine (11)	6 MV linear accelerator. 32 Gy in four once-weekly 8-Gy fractions (*n* = 9) or 36 Gy in six once- or twice-weekly 6-Gy fractions (*n* = 2).	0/11 dogs had a complete or partial response. MST: 134 days.	

IV, Intravenous; *MST*, median survival time; *PFS*, progression-free survival; *PO*, per os.

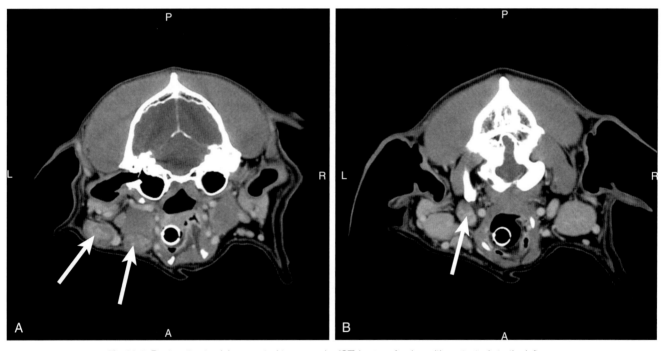

• **Fig. 20.8** Postcontrast axial computed tomography (CT) image of a dog with metastasis to the left mandibular lymph nodes (A, *arrows*) and the enlarged left medial retropharyngeal lymph node (B, *arrow*). Note the heterogeneous contrast enhancement in both lymph nodes.

radiation protocol consisted of six once-weekly 6 Gy fractions. Local recurrence was reported in 15% of dogs, the median time to metastasis was 10.2 months, and the MST was 11.9 months. These results may have been favorably biased because the majority of dogs had either T1 (56.4%) or T2 (35.9%) stage melanomas.

Several studies have looked at using adjuvant chemotherapy in addition to RT. Administered drugs included carboplatin, cisplatin, or melphalan. Adding chemotherapy to the radiation protocol did not improve outcomes.[107] However, two studies suggest that there may be a role for chemotherapy in the treatment of oral melanoma in combination with RT. In a multicenter retrospective study of 17 dogs with oral melanoma treated with surgery and carboplatin, including 11 dogs also treated with RT, the overall median PFS (259 days) and MST (440 days) for dogs did not significantly change when RT was added to the treatment protocol.[135] The proportion of dogs with local recurrence, however, was lower in the RT group (27%) compared with dogs not treated with RT (67%). The authors concluded that there may be a role

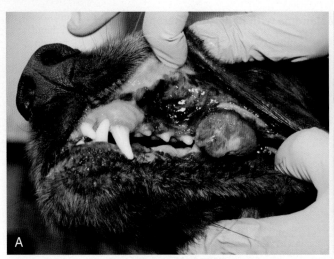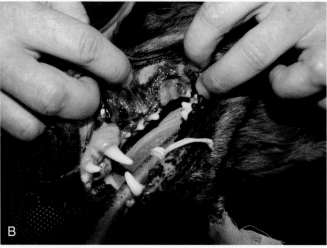

• **Fig. 20.9** A dog with an oral melanoma treated with a hypofractionated protocol of 8 Gy per fraction once weekly on the first day of therapy (A) and before the fourth and final fraction of radiotherapy (B). This dog went on to have a complete response.

for carboplatin in the multimodal treatment of dogs with oral melanomas because of the relatively long PFS and MST in this study. This may be related to the dose intensity of carboplatin used in this study with the majority of dogs not having dose reductions from the intended 300 mg/m^2 dose of carboplatin.

In a prospective study of 27 dogs with malignant melanoma in oral and nonoral sites, 15 dogs were treated with RT only and 12 dogs were treated with RT and adjuvant temozolomide.[136] The RT protocol used in all dogs was 5 fractions of 6 Gy delivered over 2.5 weeks; temozolomide was administered at 60 mg/m^2 PO once daily for 5 days and repeated every 28 days for dogs in the chemotherapy group. Both groups had similar overall response rates of 86.7% and 81.1%, respectively. The median time to progression (TTP) was significantly longer in dogs treated with RT and temozolomide (205 days) compared with dogs treated with RT alone (110 days). The MSTs, however, were not statistically significant different with MSTs of 192 days and 402 days for dogs treated with RT alone and RT and temozolomide, respectively.[136] Given the small number of dogs, it is possible that temozolomide may have an effect on MST and further clinical trials will be necessary to evaluate this.

Radiation-Associated Prognostic Factors

Several prognostic factors have been identified in dogs with oral melanoma treated with RT. These factors must be viewed with caution because some of the data are conflicting and most are derived from retrospective case series without the use of control groups.

Similar to the situation after surgery, the size of the irradiated oral melanoma is prognostic in several studies. In one study of 105 dogs with oral tumors, 38 of which were MM, treated with 4 Gy per fraction on a Monday–Wednesday–Friday schedule to a total dose of 48 Gy, the overall median PFS was 7.9 months.[108] Dogs with T1 lesions had a median PFS of 11.3 months whereas dogs with T2 and T3 lesions had median PFSs of 6.0 and 6.7 months, respectively. The most common cause of failure in this study was distant metastasis rather than local tumor recurrence. In another study of dogs with oral melanomas treated with a 9 Gy per fraction once weekly for 4 weeks, dogs with tumors less than 5 cm^3 were more likely to achieve a complete response and

have significantly better MST than dogs with larger tumors.[138] The MSTs were 86 weeks, 16 weeks, and 21 weeks for dogs with tumors less than 5 cm^3, 5 to 15 cm^3, and greater than 15 cm^3, respectively. Tumor size also affects times to first event, pulmonary metastasis, and death. In a study in which dogs were treated with a variety of different radiation protocols and adjuvant treatments, dogs with stage I disease had a significantly longer MST (758 days) compared with dogs with stage II (278 days), stage III (163 days), and stage IV (80 days) disease; however, these results contrast with other studies in which tumor size was not found to be prognostic.[137]

In one study, dogs without radiographic evidence of bone invasion had significantly longer times to first event and overall survival times than dogs with radiographic evidence of bone changes.[107] However, bony involvement has been reported in up to 92% of dogs with melanoma (Fig. 20.10).[106]

The role of vascular endothelial growth factor (VEGF) in the response and clinical outcome of melanomas to RT has been investigated, although its clinical effect has not been completely elucidated.[143] Several studies have found that dogs with oral melanoma have higher plasma VEGF concentrations than normal control dogs.[53,144] In a preliminary study investigating plasma VEGF levels in a variety of tumor types treated with hypofractionated RT, four dogs diagnosed with melanoma had the highest mean plasma VEGF levels of all tumor types, although no significant changes in VEGF levels were noted over the course of treatment.[145] The effect of VEGF levels had on patient outcome has also been investigated in 39 dogs, six of which were diagnosed with melanoma.[145,146] VEGF levels did not significantly increase over the course of RT in these dogs; however, dogs with higher plasma VEGF levels treated with hypofractionated protocols had a shorter time to treatment failure and a shorter MST.

Chemotherapy and Immunotherapy

Systemic therapy is indicated in dogs with a moderate to high metastatic risk, such as dogs with oral, digit or pad melanomas, and dogs with cutaneous MM with a high tumor score and/or increased proliferation index through increased Ki67 expression. Chemotherapy does not seem to have a role in the management

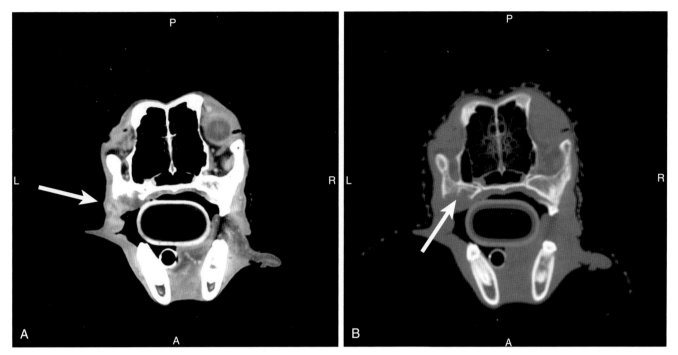

• **Fig. 20.10** (A) Postcontrast axial CT image of a dog with a maxillary oral melanoma. Note the heterogeneously contrast enhancing soft tissue mass *(arrow)*. Precontrast axial image at the same level as the image in (A). (B) Note the bone destruction of the maxillary bone and the invasion of the soft tissue mass into the nasal cavity *(arrow)*.

of dogs with MM. Overall response rates for dogs with measurable disease are largely disappointing, especially with single-agent dacarbazine, melphalan, vinorelbine, or doxorubicin,[147–150] with the highest reported response rates response being 18% for dogs treated with cisplatin and piroxicam[151] and 28% for dogs treated with carboplatin.[152] Furthermore, the majority of responses are short lived. More recently and importantly, five retrospective studies investigating the role of chemotherapy in the adjuvant setting after either surgery or RT found no significant differences in outcomes with the addition of chemotherapy to the treatment protocol.[104,107,127,139,153] Other nonimmunologic antiproliferative and/or prodifferentiation approaches have included lupeol or targeting SET/I2PP2A, proteasomes, and SINE (selective inhibitor of nuclear export).[154–158] Although it can be effectively argued that the studies performed to date to evaluate the activity of chemotherapy in an adjuvant setting for canine melanoma have been suboptimal for a variety of reasons, the human literature is extensive and this suggests melanoma is an extremely chemotherapy-resistant tumor.[135,159] It is clear that new approaches to the systemic treatment of this disease are desperately needed.

One potential clinical therapy avenue that has been minimally reported on to date in canine or feline melanoma is the use of cyclooxygenase (COX)-2 inhibitors. A number of authors have investigated the expression of COX-2 and neurokinin-1 (NK-1) in canine melanoma and/or melanoma cell lines and found positive correlations of expression to proliferation and survival.[79,160–165] Studies investigating the clinical responsiveness of canine melanoma to COX-2 inhibitors (and potential correlation to COX-2 expression) and/or NK-1 antagonists, such as maropitant, are required. Other modalities reported for local tumor control as case reports and/or case series include intralesional cisplatin implants, intralesional bleomycin with electronic pulsing, and many others, but widespread use has not been reported to date.[166–168]

Immunotherapy represents one potential systemic therapeutic strategy for the adjuvant treatment of malignant melanoma. A variety of immunotherapeutic strategies for the treatment of human melanoma have been reported with typically poor outcomes because of a lack of breaking tolerance. Immunotherapy targets and strategies to date in canine melanoma have used autologous tumor cell vaccines (with or without transfection with immunostimulatory cytokines and/or melanosomal differentiation antigens); allogeneic tumor cell vaccines transfected with interleukin-2 (IL-2) or granulocyte macrophage colony-stimulating factor (GM-CSF); liposomal-encapsulated nonspecific immunostimulators (e.g.. L-MTP-PE); intralesional Fas ligand DNA; siRNA (small interfering) against the *survivin* and/or *Bcl-2* genes; bacterial superantigen approaches with GM-CSF or IL-2 as immune adjuvants; polyethylene glycol (PEG) ylated TNF-no suicide gene therapy; adenovector CD40 ligand; chondroitin sulfate proteoglycan 4 (CSPG4); IL-12; interferon-beta (IFN-beta); and lastly canine dendritic cell vaccines loaded with melanosomal differentiation antigens.[17,158,169–189] Although these approaches have produced some clinical antitumor responses, the methodologies for the generation of these products are often expensive, time consuming, sometimes dependent on patient tumor samples being established into cell lines, and fraught with the difficulties of consistency, reproducibility, and other quality control issues, and none are currently commercially available. Furthermore, we now more fully understand the native immune dysregulation potentially induced by the malignancy through increased T regulatory (Treg) cells that suppress antitumor responses.[190–193]

The advent of DNA vaccination circumvents many of the previously encountered hurdles in vaccine development. DNA is relatively inexpensive and simple to purify in large quantities. The antigen of interest is cloned into a bacterial expression plasmid with a constitutively active promoter. The plasmid is introduced into the skin or muscle with an intradermal or intramuscular injection. Once in the skin or muscle, professional antigen-presenting cells, particularly dendritic cells, are able to present the transcribed and translated antigen in the proper context of major histocompatibility complex and costimulatory molecules. Although DNA vaccines have induced immune responses to viral proteins, vaccinating against tissue-specific self proteins on cancer cells is clearly a more difficult problem. One way to induce immunity against a tissue-specific differentiation antigen on cancer cells is to vaccinate with xenogeneic antigen or DNA that is homologous to the cancer antigen. Vaccination with DNA encoding cancer differentiation antigens is ineffective when self DNA is used, but tumor immunity can be induced by orthologous DNA from another species.[194]

A xenogeneic DNA vaccine program for melanoma was developed in collaboration with human investigators from Memorial Sloan-Kettering Cancer Center.[195,196] Preclinical and clinical studies showed that xenogeneic DNA vaccination with tyrosinase family members (e.g., tyrosinase, GP100, GP75) produced immune responses resulting in tumor rejection or protection with prolonged survival times, whereas syngeneic vaccination with orthologous DNA did not induce an immune response.[197] Although tyrosinase may not appear to be a preferred target in amelanotic canine melanoma because of poor expression when assessed by IHC,[32] more appropriate and/or sensitive PCR-based studies and other IHC-based studies document significant tyrosinase overexpression in melanotic and amelanotic melanomas across species.[16,39,198–201] These studies provided the impetus for development of a xenogeneic tyrosinase DNA vaccine program in canine MM. The antibody and T-cell responses in dogs vaccinated biweekly for a total of four vaccinations with human tyrosinase (huTyr) demonstrated antigen-specific IFN-γ T-cells with 2- to 5-fold increases in circulating antibodies to huTyr which can cross react to canine tyrosinase, suggesting the breaking of tolerance.[202,203] The clinical results with prolongation in survival have been reported previously.[195,196]

The results of these trials demonstrate that xenogeneic DNA vaccination in canine MM: (1) is safe; (2) leads to the development of antityrosinase antibodies and T cells; (3) is potentially therapeutic; and (4) is an attractive candidate for further evaluation in an adjuvant, minimal residual disease phase II setting for canine MM. Based on these studies, a multiinstitutional safety and efficacy trial compared 58 prospectively enrolled dogs with surgically resected stage II and III oral melanomas treated with adjuvant HuTyr-based canine melanoma vaccine (Oncept, Merial, Inc.) to a historical control group of 53 dogs.[204] Dogs treated with Oncept had a significantly better outcome; the MST for dogs in the historical group was 324 days compared with an MST that was not reached in the vaccinated group because only 26% of vaccinated dogs died as a result of their disease.[204] A number of clinical case series have not found a significant difference in outcome with the addition of Oncept after surgical resection of oral MMs.[104,126,205–208] Compared with the aforementioned prospective study, conclusions are more difficult to make from these studies, as they are retrospective, noncontrolled, include a high proportion of stage I oral melanomas, include a wide variety of other treatments utilized in both the nonvaccinate and vaccinate groups, had small numbers of patients investigated, and/or the cause of death and/or progression of disease was not reported.

The concurrent use of RT and Oncept has been investigated in dogs with oral MM.[209] This pilot study determined that concurrent use was well tolerated with no unexpected toxicities. Oncept also appears to be safe for use in cats.[210] Human clinical trials

utilizing various xenogeneic melanosomal antigens as DNA (or peptide with adjuvant) vaccination have begun and the preliminary results look favorable.[197,211,212]

Further evidence for the efficacy of immunotherapy for the treatment of canine oral melanoma has been shown in clinical trials with the CSPG4 vaccination.[184,213] In a controlled prospective study of dogs with stage II or III oral MM, 19 dogs were treated with surgical resection only and 23 dogs were treated with surgical resection and adjuvant CSPG4 vaccination. The outcomes were significantly better in the vaccinated group. The median disease-free interval, MST, and 1- and 2-year survival rates in the vaccinated group were 477 days, 684 days, and 73.9% and 30.4%, respectively, compared with 180 days, 200 days, and 26.3% and 5.3%, respectively, in the nonvaccinated group.[184]

The role of xenogeneic DNA vaccination in the adjuvant management of dogs with digit MM has also been investigated.[214] A staging scheme was developed based on tumor size, tumor depth, bone involvement, and presence of nodal and distant metastatic disease. A T1 digit melanoma was defined as less than 2 cm diameter and superficial or exophytic; a T2 tumor was defined as 2 to 5 cm in diameter with minimal invasion; a T3 digit melanoma was defined as greater than 5 cm or invading the subcutaneous tissue; and a T4 tumor was defined as invading into fascia or bone. Stage I was defined as nonmetastatic T1 digit melanoma; stage II as nonmetastatic T2 digit melanoma; stage III as nonmetastatic T3 or T4 digit melanoma and/or LN metastasis; and stage IV was defined as distant metastasis.[214] Treatment of dogs with digit melanoma with digit amputation and adjuvant Oncept resulted in significantly improved outcomes compared with historical outcomes with digit amputation only.[214] Dogs presenting with metastatic disease had a significantly worse MST (105 days) than dogs without evidence of metastatic disease at presentation (533 days), with a 3-year survival rate of 48% in the latter group. The clinical staging scheme was also prognostic, with MSTs of greater than 952 days, greater than 1093 days, 321 days, and 76 days for dogs with stage I, II, III, and IV disease, respectively.[214]

References

1. Goldschmidt MH: Pigmented lesions of the skin, *Clin Dermatol* 12:507–514, 1994.
2. Goldschmidt MH: Benign and malignant melanocytic neoplasms of domestic animals, *Am J Dermatopathol* 7(Suppl):203–212, 1985.
3. Smith SH, Goldschmidt MH, McManus PM: A comparative review of melanocytic neoplasms, *Vet Pathol* 39:651–678, 2002.
4. Lemetayer J, Al-Dissi A, Tryon K, et al.: Primary intranasal melanoma with brain invasion in a dog, *Can Vet J* 58:391–396, 2017.
5. Vinayak A, Frank CB, Gardiner DW, et al.: Malignant anal sac melanoma in dogs: eleven cases (2000–2015), *J Small Anim Pract* 58:231–237, 2017.
6. Wang AL, Kern T: Melanocytic ophthalmic neoplasms of the domestic veterinary species: a review, *Top Companion Anim Med* 30:148–157, 2015.
7. Leiter U, Garbe C: Epidemiology of melanoma and nonmelanoma skin cancer—the role of sunlight, *Adv Exp Med Biol* 624:89–103, 2008.
8. Erdmann F, Lortet-Tieulent J, Schuz J, et al.: International trends in the incidence of malignant melanoma 1953–2008—are recent generations at higher or lower risk? *Int J Cancer* 132:385–400, 2013.
9. Ragnarsson-Olding BK: Spatial density of primary malignant melanoma in sun-shielded body sites: a potential guide to melanoma genesis, *Acta Oncol* 50:323–328, 2011.
10. Gillard M, Cadieu E, De BC, et al.: Naturally occurring melanomas in dogs as models for non-UV pathways of human melanomas, *Pigment Cell Melanoma Res* 27:90–102, 2014.

11. Todoroff RJ, Brodey RS: Oral and pharyngeal neoplasia in the dog: a retrospective survey of 361 cases, *J Am Vet Med Assoc* 175:567–571, 1979.

12. Wallace J, Matthiesen DT, Patnaik AK: Hemimaxillectomy for the treatment of oral tumors in 69 dogs, *Vet Surg* 21:337–341, 1992.

13. Hahn KA, DeNicola DB, Richardson RC, et al.: Canine oral malignant melanoma: prognostic utility of an alternative staging system, *J Small Anim Pract* 35:251–256, 1994.

14. Dobson JM: Breed-predispositions to cancer in pedigree dog, *Vet Sci* 941275, 2013.

15. Boerkamp KM, Teske E, Boon LR, et al.: Estimated incidence rate and distribution of tumours in 4,653 cases of archival submissions derived from the Dutch golden retriever population, *BMC Vet Res* 10(34), 2014.

16. Ramos-Vara JA, Beissenherz ME, Miller MA, et al.: Retrospective study of 338 canine oral melanomas with clinical, histologic, and immunohistochemical review of 129 cases, *Vet Pathol* 37:597–608, 2000.

17. MacEwen EG, Patnaik AK, Harvey HJ, et al.: Canine oral melanoma: comparison of surgery versus surgery plus Corynebacterium parvum, *Cancer Invest* 4:397–402, 1986.

18. Harvey HJ, Macewen EG, Braun D, et al.: Prognostic criteria for dogs with oral melanoma, *J Am Vet Med Assoc* 178:580–582, 1981.

19. Bradley RL, Macewen EG, Loar AS: Mandibular resection for removal of oral tumors in 30 dogs and 6 cats, *J Am Vet Med Assoc* 184:460–463, 1984.

20. Harvey HJ: Oral tumors, *Vet Clin North Am Small Anim Pract* 15:493–500, 1985.

21. Kosovsky JK, Matthiesen DT, Marretta SM, et al.: Results of partial mandibulectomy for the treatment of oral tumors in 142 dogs, *Vet Surg* 20:397–401, 1991.

22. Schobert CS, Labelle P, Dubielzig RR: Feline conjunctival melanoma: histopathological characteristics and clinical outcomes, *Vet Ophthalmol* 13:43–46, 2010.

23. Planellas M, Pastor J, Torres MD, et al.: Unusual presentation of a metastatic uveal melanoma in a cat, *Vet Ophthalmol* 13:391–394, 2010.

24. Munday JS, French AF, Martin SJ: Cutaneous malignant melanoma in an 11-month-old Russian blue cat, *NZ Vet J* 59:143–146, 2011.

25. Morges MA, Zaks K: Malignant melanoma in pleural effusion in a 14-year-old cat, *J Fel Med Surg* 13:532–535, 2011.

26. Farrelly J, Denman DL, Hohenhaus AE, et al.: Hypofractionated radiation therapy of oral melanoma in five cats, *Vet Radiol Ultrasound* 45:91–93, 2004.

27. Grahn BH, Peiffer RL, Cullen CL, et al.: Classification of feline intraocular neoplasms based on morphology, histochemical staining, and immunohistochemical labeling, *Vet Ophthalmol* 9:395–403, 2006.

28. Patnaik AK, Mooney S: Feline melanoma: a comparative study of ocular, oral, and dermal neoplasms, *Vet Pathol* 25:105–112, 1988.

29. Luna LD, Higginbotham ML, Henry CJ, et al.: Feline non-ocular melanoma: a retrospective study of 23 cases (1991-1999), *J Fel Med Surg* 2:173–181, 2000.

30. Bostock DE: Prognosis after surgical excision of canine melanomas, *Vet Pathol* 16:32–40, 1979.

31. Spangler WL, Kass PH: The histologic and epidemiologic bases for prognostic considerations in canine melanocytic neoplasia, *Vet Pathol* 43:136–149, 2006.

32. Smedley RC, Lamoureux J, Sledge DG, et al.: Immunohistochemical diagnosis of canine oral amelanotic melanocytic neoplasms, *Vet Pathol* 48:32–40, 2011.

33. Choi C, Kusewitt DF: Comparison of tyrosinase-related protein-2, S-100, and Melan A immunoreactivity in canine amelanotic melanomas, *Vet Pathol* 40:713–718, 2003.

34. Przezdziecki R, Czopowicz M, Sapierzynski R: Accuracy of routine cytology and immunocytochemistry in preoperative diagnosis of oral amelanotic melanomas in dogs, *Vet Clin Pathol* 44:597–604, 2015.

35. Berrington AJ, Jimbow K, Haines DM: Immunohistochemical detection of melanoma-associated antigens on formalin-fixed, paraffin-embedded canine tumors, *Vet Pathol* 31:455–461, 1994.

36. Koenig A, Wojcieszyn J, Weeks BR, et al.: Expression of S100a, vimentin, NSE, and melan A/MART-1 in seven canine melanoma cells lines and twenty-nine retrospective cases of canine melanoma, *Vet Pathol* 38:427–435, 2001.

37. Sandusky GEJ, Carlton WW, Wightman KA: Immunohistochemical staining for S100 protein in the diagnosis of canine amelanotic melanoma, *Vet Pathol* 22:577–581, 1985.

38. Giudice C, Ceciliani F, Rondena M, et al.: Immunohistochemical investigation of PNL2 reactivity of canine melanocytic neoplasms and comparison with Melan A, *J Vet Diagn Invest* 22:389–394, 2010.

39. Ramos-Vara JA, Miller MA: Immunohistochemical identification of canine melanocytic neoplasms with antibodies to melanocytic antigen PNL2 and tyrosinase: comparison with Melan A, *Vet Pathol* 48:443–450, 2011.

40. Grandi F, Rocha RM, Miot HA, et al.: Immunoexpression of S100A4 in canine skin melanomas and correlation with histopathological parameters, *Vet Q* 34:98–104, 2014.

41. Palmieri G, Capone M, Ascierto ML, et al.: Main roads to melanoma, *J Transl Med* 7:86, 2009.

42. Bollag G, Hirth P, Tsai J, et al.: Clinical efficacy of a RAF inhibitor needs broad target blockade in BRAF-mutant melanoma, *Nature* 467:596–599, 2010.

43. Shelly S, Chien MB, Yip B, et al.: Exon 15 BRAF mutations are uncommon in canine oral malignant melanomas, *Mamm Genome* 16:211–217, 2005.

44. Fowles JS, Denton CL, Gustafson DL: Comparative analysis of MAPK and PI3K/AKT pathway activation and inhibition in human and canine melanoma, *Vet Comp Oncol* 13:288–304, 2015.

45. Roels S, Tilmant K, Ducatelle R: p53 expression and apoptosis in melanomas of dogs and cats, *Res Vet Sci* 70:19–25, 2001.

46. Roels SL, Van Daele AJ, Van Marck EA, et al.: DNA ploidy and nuclear morphometric variables for the evaluation of melanocytic tumors in dogs and cats, *Am J Vet Res* 61:1074–1079, 2000.

47. Modiano JF, Ritt MG, Wojcieszyn J: The molecular basis of canine melanoma: pathogenesis and trends in diagnosis and therapy, *J Vet Intern Med* 13:163–174, 1999.

48. Ritt MG, Mayor J, Wojcieszyn J, et al.: Sustained nuclear localization of p21/WAF-1 upon growth arrest induced by contact inhibition, *Cancer Lett* 158:73–84, 2000.

49. Han JI, Kim DY, Na KJ: Dysregulation of the Wnt/beta-catenin signaling pathway in canine cutaneous melanotic tumor, *Vet Pathol* 47:285–291, 2010.

50. Stell AJ, Dobson JM, Scase TJ, et al.: Evaluation of variants of melanoma-associated antigen genes and mRNA transcripts in melanomas of dogs, *Am J Vet Res* 70:1512–1520, 2009.

51. Thamm DH, Huelsmeyer MK, Mitzey AM, et al.: RT-PCR-based tyrosine kinase display profiling of canine melanoma: IGF-1 receptor as a potential therapeutic target, *Melanoma Res* 20:35–42, 2010.

52. Kent MS, Collins CJ, Ye F: Activation of the AKT and mammalian target of rapamycin pathways and the inhibitory effects of rapamycin on those pathways in canine malignant melanoma cell lines, *Am J Vet Res* 70:263–269, 2009.

53. Taylor KH, Smith AN, Higginbotham M, et al.: Expression of vascular endothelial growth factor in canine oral malignant melanoma, *Vet Comp Oncol* 5:208–218, 2007.

54. Murua EH, Gunther K, Richter A, et al.: Absence of ras-gene hotspot mutations in canine fibrosarcomas and melanomas, *Anticancer Res* 24:3027–3028, 2004.

55. Dincer Z, Jasani B, Haywood S, et al.: Metallothionein expression in canine and feline mammary and melanotic tumours, *J Comp Pathol* 125:130–136, 2001.

56. Stiles J, Bienzle D, Render JA, et al.: Use of nested polymerase chain reaction (PCR) for detection of retroviruses from formalin-fixed, paraffin-embedded uveal melanomas in cats, *Vet Ophthalmol* 2:113–116, 1999.

57. Mayr B, Eschborn U, Schleger W, et al.: Cytogenetic studies in a canine malignant melanoma, *J Comp Pathol* 106:319–322, 1992.

58. Mayr B, Schaffner G, Reifinger M, et al.: N-ras mutations in canine malignant melanomas, *Vet J* 165:169–171, 2003.

59. Mayr B, Reifinger M, Grohe D, et al.: Cytogenetic alterations in feline melanoma, *Vet J* 159:97–100, 2000.

60. Mayr B, Wilhelm B, Reifinger M, et al.: Absence of p21 WAF1 and p27 kip1 gene mutations in various feline tumours, *Vet Res Commun* 24:115–124, 2000.

61. Sulaimon SS, Kitchell BE: The basic biology of malignant melanoma: molecular mechanisms of disease progression and comparative aspects, *J Vet Intern Med* 17:760–772, 2003.

62. Murakami A, Mori T, Sakai H, et al.: Analysis of KIT expression and KIT exon 11 mutations in canine oral malignant melanomas, *Vet Comp Oncol* 9:219–224, 2011.

63. Abou AS: Immunohistochemical expression of MCAM/CD146 in canine melanoma, *J Comp Pathol* 157:27–33, 2017.

64. Heishima K, Ichikawa Y, Yoshida K, et al.: Circulating microRNA-214 and -126 as potential biomarkers for canine neoplastic disease, *Sci Rep* 7:2301, 2017.

65. Starkey MP, Compston-Garnett L, Malho P, et al.: Metastasis-associated microRNA expression in canine uveal melanoma, *Vet Comp Oncol* 18:81–89, 2017.

66. Lee BH, Neela PH, Kent MS, et al.: IQGAP1 is an oncogenic target in canine melanoma, *PLoS One* 12:e0176370, 2017.

67. Ogasawara S, Honma R, Kaneko MK, et al.: Podoplanin expression in canine melanoma, *Monoclon Antib Immunodiagn Immunother* 35:304–306, 2016.

68. Finotello R, Monne Rodriguez JM, Vilafranca M, et al.: Immunohistochemical expression of MDR1-Pgp 170 in canine cutaneous and oral melanomas: pattern of expression and association with tumour location and phenotype, *Vet Comp Oncol* 15:1393–1402, 2016.

69. Zoroquiain P, Mayo-Goldberg E, Alghamdi S, et al.: Melanocytoma-like melanoma may be the missing link between benign and malignant uveal melanocytic lesions in humans and dogs: a comparative study, *Melanoma Res* 26:565–571, 2016.

70. Wei BR, Michael HT, Halsey CH, et al.: Synergistic targeted inhibition of MEK and dual PI3K/mTOR diminishes viability and inhibits tumor growth of canine melanoma underscoring its utility as a preclinical model for human mucosal melanoma, *Pigment Cell Melanoma Res* 29:643–655, 2016.

71. Lin W, Modiano JF, Ito D: Stage-specific embryonic antigen: determining expression in canine glioblastoma, melanoma, and mammary cancer cells, *J Vet Sci* 18:101–104, 2017.

72. Abou AS, Anwar S, Yanai T, et al.: Immunohistochemical analysis of CD146 expression in canine skin tumours, *Histol Histopathol* 31:453–459, 2016.

73. Noguchi S, Mori T, Nakagawa T, et al.: DNA methylation contributes toward silencing of antioncogenic microRNA-203 in human and canine melanoma cells, *Melanoma Res* 25:390–398, 2015.

74. Bongiovanni L, D'Andrea A, Porcellato I, et al.: Canine cutaneous melanocytic tumours: significance of beta-catenin and survivin immunohistochemical expression, *Vet Dermatol* 26:270–e59, 2015.

75. Kawabe M, Baba Y, Tamai R, et al.: Profiling of plasma metabolites in canine oral melanoma using gas chromatography-mass spectrometry, *J Vet Med Sci* 77:1025–1028, 2015.

76. Poorman K, Borst L, Moroff S, et al.: Comparative cytogenetic characterization of primary canine melanocytic lesions using array CGH and fluorescence in situ hybridization, *Chromosome Res* 23:171–186, 2015.

77. Noguchi S, Kumazaki M, Mori T, et al.: Analysis of microRNA-203 function in CREB/MITF/RAB27a pathway: comparison between canine and human melanoma cells, *Vet Comp Oncol* 14:384–394, 2016.

78. Guth AM, Deogracias M, Dow SW: Comparison of cancer stem cell antigen expression by tumor cell lines and by tumor biopsies from dogs with melanoma and osteosarcoma, *Vet Immunol Immunopathol* 161:132–140, 2014.

79. Borrego JF, Huelsmeyer MK, Pinkerton ME, et al.: Neurokinin-1 receptor expression and antagonism by the NK-1R antagonist maropitant in canine melanoma cell lines and primary tumour tissues, *Vet Comp Oncol* 14:210–224, 2016.

80. Seo KW, Coh YR, Rebhun RB, et al.: Antitumor effects of celecoxib in COX-2 expressing and non-expressing canine melanoma cell lines, *Res Vet Sci* 96:482–486, 2014.

81. Teixeira TF, Gentile LB, da Silva TC, et al.: Cell proliferation and expression of connexins differ in melanotic and amelanotic canine oral melanomas, *Vet Res Commun* 38:29–38, 2014.

82. Greene VR, Wilson H, Pfent C, et al.: Expression of leptin and iNOS in oral melanomas in dogs, *J Vet Intern Med* 27:1278–1282, 2013.

83. Campagne C, Jule S, Alleaume C, et al.: Canine melanoma diagnosis: RACK1 as a potential biological marker, *Vet Pathol* 50:1083–1090, 2013.

84. Chon E, Thompson V, Schmid S, et al.: Activation of the canonical Wnt/beta-catenin signalling pathway is rare in canine malignant melanoma tissue and cell lines, *J Comp Pathol* 148:178–187, 2013.

85. Han JI, Kim Y, Kim DY, et al.: Alteration in E-cadherin/beta-catenin expression in canine melanotic tumors, *Vet Pathol* 50:274–280, 2013.

86. Brachelente C, Cappelli K, Capomaccio S, et al.: Transcriptome analysis of canine cutaneous melanoma and melanocytoma reveals a modulation of genes regulating extracellular matrix metabolism and cell cycle, *Sci Rep* 7:6386, 2017.

87. Chu PY, Pan SL, Liu CH, et al.: KIT gene exon 11 mutations in canine malignant melanoma, *Vet J* 196:226–230, 2012.

88. Gillard M, Cadieu E, De BC, et al.: Naturally occurring melanomas in dogs as models for non-UV pathways of human melanomas, *Pigment Cell Melanoma Res* 27:90–102, 2014.

89. Laprie C, Abadie J, Amardeilh MF, et al.: MIB-1 immunoreactivity correlates with biologic behaviour in canine cutaneous melanoma, *Vet Dermatol* 12:139–147, 2001.

90. Millanta F, Fratini F, Corazza M, et al.: Proliferation activity in oral and cutaneous canine melanocytic tumours: correlation with histological parameters, location, and clinical behaviour, *Res Vet Sci* 73:45–51, 2002.

91. Vail DM, Macewen EG: Spontaneously occurring tumors of companion animals as models for human cancer, *Cancer Invest* 18:781–792, 2000.

92. Esplin DG: Survival of dogs following surgical excision of histologically well-differentiated melanocytic neoplasms of the mucous membranes of the lips and oral cavity, *Vet Pathol* 45:889–896, 2008.

93. Spangler WL, Kass PH: The histologic and epidemiologic bases for prognostic considerations in canine melanocytic neoplasia, *Vet Pathol* 43:136–149, 2006.

94. Bergin IL, Smedley RC, Esplin DG, et al.: Prognostic evaluation of Ki67 threshold value in canine oral melanoma, *Vet Pathol* 48:41–53, 2011.

95. Henry CJ, Brewer Jr WG, Whitley EM, et al.: Canine digital tumors: a Veterinary Cooperative Oncology Group retrospective study of 64 dogs, *J Vet Intern Med* 19:720–724, 2005.

96. Wobeser BK, Kidney BA, Powers BE, et al.: Diagnoses and clinical outcomes associated with surgically amputated canine digits submitted to multiple veterinary diagnostic laboratories, *Vet Pathol* 44:355–361, 2007.

97. Marino DJ, Matthiesen DT, Stefanacci D, et al.: Evaluation of dogs with digit masses: 117 cases (1981-1991), *J Am Vet Med Assoc* 207:726–728, 1995.

98. Piliang MP: Acral lentiginous melanoma, *Clin Lab Med* 31:281–288, 2011.

99. Smedley RC, Spangler WL, Esplin DG, et al.: Prognostic markers for canine melanocytic neoplasms: a comparative review of the literature and goals for future investigation, *Vet Pathol* 48:54–72, 2011.

100. Wiggans KT, Reilly CM, Kass PH, et al.: Histologic and immunohistochemical predictors of clinical behavior for feline diffuse iris melanoma, *Vet Ophthalmol* 19(Suppl 1):44–55, 2016.

101. Rushton JG, Ertl R, Klein D, et al.: Mutation analysis and gene expression profiling of ocular melanomas in cats, *Vet Comp Oncol* 15:1403–1416, 2017.

102. Fragola JA, Dubielzig RR, Bentley E, et al.: Iridociliary cysts masquerading as neoplasia in cats: a morphologic review of 14 cases, *Vet Ophthalmol* 21:125–131, 2017.

103. Chamel G, Abadie J, Albaric O, et al.: Non-ocular melanomas in cats: a retrospective study of 30 cases, *J Feline Med Surg* 19:351–357, 2017.

104. Tuohy JL, Selmic LE, Worley DR, et al.: Outcome following curative-intent surgery for oral melanoma in dogs: 70 cases (1998-2011), *J Am Vet Med Assoc* 245:1266–1273, 2014.

105. Owen LN: *TNM classification of tumours in domestic animals*, ed 3, 1980. Geneva, Switzerland.

106. Freeman KP, Hahn KA, Harris FD, et al.: Treatment of dogs with oral melanoma by hypofractionated radiation therapy and platinum-based chemotherapy (1987-1997), *J Vet Intern Med* 17:96–101, 2003.

107. Proulx DR, Ruslander DM, Dodge RK, et al.: A retrospective analysis of 140 dogs with oral melanoma treated with external beam radiation, *Vet Radiol Ultrasound* 44:352–359, 2003.

108. Theon AP, Rodriguez C, Madewell BR: Analysis of prognostic factors and patterns of failure in dogs with malignant oral tumors treated with megavoltage irradiation, *J Am Vet Med Assoc* 210:778–784, 1997.

109. Williams LE, Packer RA: Association between lymph node size and metastasis in dogs with oral malignant melanoma: 100 cases (1987-2001), *J Am Vet Med Assoc* 222:1234–1236, 2003.

110. Skinner OT, Boston SE, Souza CHM: Patterns of lymph node metastasis identified following bilateral mandibular and medial retropharyngeal lymphadenectomy in 31 dogs with malignancies of the head, *Vet Comp Oncol* 15:881–889, 2017.

111. Herring ES, Smith MM, Robertson JL: Lymph node staging of oral and maxillofacial neoplasms in 31 dogs and cats, *J Vet Dent* 19:122–126, 2002.

112. Grimes JA, Matz BM, Christopherson PW, et al.: Agreement between cytology and histopathology for regional lymph node metastasis in dogs with melanocytic neoplasms, *Vet Pathol* 54:579–587, 2017.

113. Smith MM: Surgical approach for lymph node staging of oral and maxillofacial neoplasms in dogs, *J Vet Dent* 19:170–174, 2002.

114. Green K, Boston SE: Bilateral removal of the mandibular and medial retropharyngeal lymph nodes through a single ventral midline incision for staging of head and neck cancers in dogs: a description of surgical technique, *Vet Comp Oncol* 15:208–214, 2017.

115. Leong SP, Accortt NA, Essner R, et al.: Impact of sentinel node status and other risk factors on the clinical outcome of head and neck melanoma patients, *Arch Otolaryngol Head Neck Surg* 132:370–373, 2006.

116. Herring ES, Smith MM, Robertson JL: Lymph node staging of oral and maxillofacial neoplasms in 31 dogs and cats, *J Vet Dent* 19:122–126, 2002.

117. Nwogu CE, Kanter PM, Anderson TM: Pulmonary lymphatic mapping in dogs: use of technetium sulfur colloid and isosulfan blue for pulmonary sentinel lymph node mapping in dogs, *Cancer Invest* 20:944–947, 2002.

118. Yudd AP, Kempf JS, Goydos JS, et al.: Use of sentinel node lymphoscintigraphy in malignant melanoma, *Radiographics* 19:343–353, 1999.

119. Wells S, Bennett A, Walsh P, et al.: Clinical usefulness of intradermal fluorescein and patent blue violet dyes for sentinel lymph node identification in dogs, *Vet Comp Oncol* 4:114–122, 2006.

120. Suga K, Karino Y, Fujita T, et al.: Cutaneous drainage lymphatic map with interstitial multidetector-row computed tomographic lymphography using iopamidol: preliminary results, *Lymphology* 40:63–73, 2007.

121. Majeski SA, Steffey MA, Fuller M, et al.: Indirect computed tomographic lymphography for iliosacral lymphatic mapping in a cohort of dogs with anal sac gland adenocarcinoma: technique description, *Vet Radiol Ultrasound* 58:295–303, 2017.

122. Brissot HN, Edery EG: Use of indirect lymphography to identify sentinel lymph node in dogs: a pilot study in 30 tumours, *Vet Comp Oncol* 15:740–753, 2017.

123. Worley DR: Incorporation of sentinel lymph node mapping in dogs with mast cell tumours: 20 consecutive procedures, *Vet Comp Oncol* 12:215–226, 2014.

124. Liuti T, de VJ, Bosman T, et al.: 67Gallium citrate scintigraphy to assess metastatic spread in a dog with an oral melanoma, *J Small Anim Pract* 50:31–34, 2009.

125. Wallace J, Matthiesen DT, Patnaik AK: Hemimaxillectomy for the treatment of oral tumors in 69 dogs, *Vet Surg* 21:337–341, 1992.

126. Sarowitz BN, Davis GJ, Kim S: Outcome and prognostic factors following curative-intent surgery for oral tumours in dogs: 234 cases (2004 to 2014), *J Small Anim Pract* 58:146–153, 2017.

127. Boston SE, Lu X, Culp WT, et al.: Efficacy of systemic adjuvant therapies administered to dogs after excision of oral malignant melanomas: 151 cases (2001-2012), *J Am Vet Med Assoc* 245:401–407, 2014.

128. Schwarz PD, Withrow SJ, Curtis CR, et al.: Partial maxillary resection as a treatment for oral cancer in 61 dogs, *J Am Anim Hosp Assoc* 27:617–624, 1991.

129. Fox LE, Geoghegan SL, Davis LH, et al.: Owner satisfaction with partial mandibulectomy or maxillectomy for treatment of oral tumors in 27 dogs, *J Am Anim Hosp Assoc* 33:25–31, 1997.

130. Liptak JM, Dernell WS, Rizzo SA, et al.: Partial foot amputation in 11 dogs, *J Am Anim Hosp Assoc* 41:47–55, 2005.

131. Kaufman KL, Mann FA: Short- and long-term outcomes after digit amputation in dogs: 33 cases (1999-2011), *J Am Vet Med Assoc* 242:1249–1254, 2013.

132. Bergman PJ: Immunotherapy in veterinary oncology, *Vet Clin North Am Small Anim Pract* 44:925–939, 2014.

133. Grosenbaugh DA, Leard AT, Bergman PJ, et al.: Safety and efficacy of a xenogeneic DNA vaccine encoding for human tyrosinase as adjunctive treatment for oral malignant melanoma in dogs following surgical excision of the primary tumor, *Am J Vet Res* 72:1631–1638, 2011.

134. Morton DL: Cytoreductive surgery and adjuvant immunotherapy in the management of metastatic melanoma, *Tumori* 87:S57–S59, 2001.

135. Dank G, Rassnick KM, Sokolovsky Y, et al.: Use of adjuvant carboplatin for treatment of dogs with oral malignant melanoma following surgical excision, *Vet Comp Oncol* 12:78–84, 2014.

136. Cancedda S, Rohrer BC, Aresu L, et al.: Efficacy and side effects of radiation therapy in comparison with radiation therapy and temozolomide in the treatment of measurable canine malignant melanoma, *Vet Comp Oncol* 14:e146–e157, 2016.

137. Bateman KE, Catton PA, Pennock PW, et al.: 0-7-21 radiation therapy for the treatment of canine oral melanoma, *J Vet Intern Med* 8:267–272, 1994.

138. Blackwood L, Dobson JM: Radiotherapy of oral malignant melanomas in dogs, *J Am Vet Med Assoc* 209:98–102, 1996.

139. Murphy S, Hayes AM, Blackwood L, et al.: Oral malignant melanoma - the effect of coarse fractionation radiotherapy alone or with adjuvant carboplatin therapy, *Vet Comp Oncol* 3:222–229, 2005.

140. Kawabe M, Mori T, Ito Y, et al.: Outcomes of dogs undergoing radiotherapy for treatment of oral malignant melanoma: 111 cases (2006-2012), *J Am Vet Med Assoc* 247:1146–1153, 2015.

141. Tollett MA, Duda L, Brown DC, et al.: Palliative radiation therapy for solid tumors in dogs: 103 cases (2007-2011), *J Am Vet Med Assoc* 248:72–82, 2016.

142. Khan N, Khan MK, Almasan A, et al.: The evolving role of radiation therapy in the management of malignant melanoma, *Int J Radiat Oncol Biol Phys* 80:645–654, 2011.

143. Flickinger I, Rutgen BC, Gerner W, et al.: Radiation up-regulates the expression of VEGF in a canine oral melanoma cell line, *J Vet Sci* 14:207–214, 2013.

144. Wergin MC, Ballmer-Hofer K, Roos M, et al.: Preliminary study of plasma vascular endothelial growth factor (VEGF) during low- and high-dose radiation therapy of dogs with spontaneous tumors, *Vet Radiol Ultrasound* 45:247–254, 2004.

145. Wergin MC, Roos M, Inteeworn N, et al.: The influence of fractionated radiation therapy on plasma vascular endothelial growth factor (VEGF) concentration in dogs with spontaneous tumors and its impact on outcome, *Radiother Oncol* 79:239–244, 2006.

146. Wergin MC, Kaser-Hotz B: Plasma vascular endothelial growth factor (VEGF) measured in seventy dogs with spontaneously occurring tumours, *Vivo* 18:15–19, 2004.

147. Page RL, Thrall DE, Dewhirst MW, et al.: Phase I study of melphalan alone and melphalan plus whole body hyperthermia in dogs with malignant melanoma, *Int J Hyperthermia* 7:559–566, 1991.

148. Ogilvie GK, Reynolds HA, Richardson RC, et al.: Phase II evaluation of doxorubicin for treatment of various canine neoplasms, *J Am Vet Med Assoc* 195:1580–1583, 1989.

149. Aigner K, Hild P, Breithaupt H, et al.: Isolated extremity perfusion with DTIC. An experimental and clinical study, *Anticancer Res* 3:87–93, 1983.

150. Wouda RM, Miller ME, Chon E, et al.: Clinical effects of vinorelbine administration in the management of various malignant tumor types in dogs: 58 cases (1997-2012), *J Am Vet Med Assoc* 246:1230–1237, 2015.

151. Boria PA, Murry DJ, Bennett PF, et al.: Evaluation of cisplatin combined with piroxicam for the treatment of oral malignant melanoma and oral squamous cell carcinoma in dogs, *J Am Vet Med Assoc* 224:388–394, 2004.

152. Rassnick KM, Ruslander DM, Cotter SM, et al.: Use of carboplatin for treatment of dogs with malignant melanoma: 27 cases (1989-2000), *J Am Vet Med Assoc* 218:1444–1448, 2001.

153. Brockley LK, Cooper MA, Bennett PF: Malignant melanoma in 63 dogs (2001-2011): the effect of carboplatin chemotherapy on survival, *NZ Vet J* 61:25–31, 2013.

154. Enjoji S, Yabe R, Fujiwara N, et al.: The therapeutic effects of SET/I2PP2A inhibitors on canine melanoma, *J Vet Med Sci* 77:1451–1456, 2015.

155. Breit MN, Kisseberth WC, Bear MD, et al.: Biologic activity of the novel orally bioavailable selective inhibitor of nuclear export (SINE) KPT-335 against canine melanoma cell lines, *BMC Vet Res* 10(160), 2014.

156. London CA, Bernabe LF, Barnard S, et al.: Preclinical evaluation of the novel, orally bioavailable selective inhibitor of nuclear export (SINE) KPT-335 in spontaneous canine cancer: results of a phase I study, *PLoS One* 9:e87585, 2014.

157. Ito K, Kobayashi M, Kuroki S, et al.: The proteasome inhibitor bortezomib inhibits the growth of canine malignant melanoma cells in vitro and in vivo, *Vet J* 198:577–582, 2013.

158. Yokoe I, Azuma K, Hata K, et al.: Clinical systemic lupeol administration for canine oral malignant melanoma, *Mol Clin Oncol* 3:89–92, 2015.

159. O'Day S, Boasberg P: Management of metastatic melanoma 2005, *Surg Oncol Clin North Am* 15:419–437, 2006.

160. Martinez CD, Penafiel-Verdu C, Vilafranca M, et al.: Cyclooxygenase-2 expression is related with localization, proliferation, and overall survival in canine melanocytic neoplasms, *Vet Pathol* 48:1204–1211, 2011.

161. Pires I, Garcia A, Prada J, et al.: COX-1 and COX-2 expression in canine cutaneous, oral and ocular melanocytic tumours, *J Comp Pathol* 143:142–149, 2010.

162. Paglia D, Dubielzig RR, Kado-Fong HK, et al.: Expression of cyclooxygenase-2 in canine uveal melanocytic neoplasms, *Am J Vet Res* 70:1284–1290, 2009.

163. Yoshitake R, Saeki K, Watanabe M, et al.: Molecular investigation of the direct anti-tumour effects of nonsteroidal anti-inflammatory drugs in a panel of canine cancer cell lines, *Vet J* 221:38–47, 2017.

164. Gregorio H, Raposo TP, Queiroga FL, et al.: Investigating associations of cyclooxygenase-2 expression with angiogenesis, proliferation, macrophage and T-lymphocyte infiltration in canine melanocytic tumours, *Melanoma Res* 26:338–347, 2016.

165. Seo KW, Coh YR, Rebhun RB, et al.: Antitumor effects of celecoxib in COX-2 expressing and non-expressing canine melanoma cell lines, *Res Vet Sci* 96:482–486, 2014.

166. Kitchell BE, Brown DM, Luck EE, et al.: Intralesional implant for treatment of primary oral malignant melanoma in dogs, *J Am Vet Med Assoc* 204:229–236, 1994.

167. Theon AP, Madewell BR, Moore AS, et al.: Localized thermocisplatin therapy: a pilot study in spontaneous canine and feline tumours, *Int J Hyperthermia* 7:881–892, 1991.

168. Spugnini EP, Dragonetti E, Vincenzi B, et al.: Pulse-mediated chemotherapy enhances local control and survival in a spontaneous canine model of primary mucosal melanoma, *Melanoma Res* 16:23–27, 2006.

169. Alexander AN, Huelsmeyer MK, Mitzey A, et al.: Development of an allogeneic whole-cell tumor vaccine expressing xenogeneic gp100 and its implementation in a phase II clinical trial in canine patients with malignant melanoma, *Cancer Immunol Immunother* 55:433–442, 2006.

170. Hogge GS, Burkholder JK, Culp J, et al.: Preclinical development of human granulocyte-macrophage colony-stimulating factor-transfected melanoma cell vaccine using established canine cell lines and normal dogs, *Cancer Gene Ther* 6:26–36, 1999.

171. Macewen EG, Kurzman ID, Vail DM, et al.: Adjuvant therapy for melanoma in dogs: results of randomized clinical trials using surgery, liposome-encapsulated muramyl tripeptide, and granulocyte macrophage colony-stimulating factor, *Clin Cancer Res* 5: 4249–4258.

172. Bianco SR, Sun J, Fosmire SP, et al.: Enhancing antimelanoma immune responses through apoptosis, *Cancer Gene Ther* 10:726–736, 2003.

173. Dow SW, Elmslie RE, Willson AP, et al.: In vivo tumor transfection with superantigen plus cytokine genes induces tumor regression and prolongs survival in dogs with malignant melanoma, *J Clin Invest* 101:2406–2414, 1998.

174. Gyorffy S, Rodriguez-Lecompte JC, Woods JP, et al.: Bone marrow-derived dendritic cell vaccination of dogs with naturally occurring melanoma by using human gp100 antigen, *J Vet Intern Med* 19:56–63, 2005.

175. Helfand SC, Soergel SA, Modiano JF, et al.: Induction of lymphokine-activated killer (LAK) activity in canine lymphocytes with low dose human recombinant interleukin-2 in vitro, *Cancer Biother* 9:237–244, 1994.

176. Mayayo SL, Prestigio S, Maniscalco L, et al.: Chondroitin sulfate proteoglycan-4: a biomarker and a potential immunotherapeutic target for canine malignant melanoma, *Vet J* 190:e26–e30, 2011.

177. Moriyama M, Kano R, Maruyama H, et al.: Small interfering RNA (siRNA) against the survivin gene increases apoptosis in a canine melanoma cell line, *J Vet Med Sci* 72:1643–1646, 2010.

178. Watanabe Y, Kano R, Maruyama H, et al.: Small interfering RNA (siRNA) against the Bcl-2 gene increases apoptosis in a canine melanoma cell line, *J Vet Med Sci* 72:383–386, 2010.

179. Thamm DH, Kurzman ID, Clark MA, et al.: Preclinical investigation of PEGylated tumor necrosis factor alpha in dogs with spontaneous tumors: phase I evaluation, *Clin Cancer Res* 16:1498–1508, 2010.

180. Finocchiaro LM, Fiszman GL, Karara AL, et al.: Suicide gene and cytokines combined nonviral gene therapy for spontaneous canine melanoma, *Cancer Gene Ther* 15:165–172, 2008.

181. Finocchiaro LM, Glikin GC: Cytokine-enhanced vaccine and suicide gene therapy as surgery adjuvant treatments for spontaneous canine melanoma, *Gene Ther* 15:267–276, 2008.

182. Gil-Cardeza ML, Villaverde MS, Fiszman GL, et al.: Suicide gene therapy on spontaneous canine melanoma: correlations between in vivo tumors and their derived multicell spheroids in vitro, *Gene Ther* 17:26–36, 2010.

183. von EH, Sadeghi A, Carlsson B, et al.: Efficient adenovector CD40 ligand immunotherapy of canine malignant melanoma, *J Immunother* 31:377–384, 2008.

184. Piras LA, Riccardo F, Iussich S, et al.: Prolongation of survival of dogs with oral malignant melanoma treated by en bloc surgical resection and adjuvant CSPG4-antigen electrovaccination, *Vet Comp Oncol* 15:996–1013, 2017.

185. Paoloni M, Mazcko C, Selting K, et al.: Defining the pharmacodynamic profile and therapeutic index of nhs-il12 immunocytokine in dogs with malignant melanoma, *PLoS One* 10:e0129954, 2015.

186. Rossi UA, Gil-Cardeza ML, Villaverde MS, et al.: Interferon-beta gene transfer induces a strong cytotoxic bystander effect on melanoma cells, *Biomed Pharmacother* 72:44–51, 2015.

187. Finocchiaro LM, Fondello C, Gil-Cardeza ML, et al.: Cytokine-enhanced vaccine and interferon-beta plus suicide gene therapy as surgery adjuvant treatments for spontaneous canine melanoma, *Hum Gene Ther* 26:367–376, 2015.

188. Riccardo F, Iussich S, Maniscalco L, et al.: CSPG4-specific immunity and survival prolongation in dogs with oral malignant melanoma immunized with human CSPG4 DNA, *Clin Cancer Res* 20:3753–3762, 2014.

189. Westberg S, Sadeghi A, Svensson E, et al.: Treatment efficacy and immune stimulation by AdCD40L gene therapy of spontaneous canine malignant melanoma, *J Immunother* 36:350–358, 2013.

190. Horiuchi Y, Tominaga M, Ichikawa M, et al.: Relationship between regulatory and type 1 T cells in dogs with oral malignant melanoma, *Microbiol Immunol* 54:152–159, 2010.

191. Tominaga M, Horiuchi Y, Ichikawa M, et al.: Flow cytometric analysis of peripheral blood and tumor-infiltrating regulatory T cells in dogs with oral malignant melanoma, *J Vet Diagn Invest* 22:438–441, 2010.

192. Fortuna L, Relf J, Chang YM, et al.: Prevalence of FoxP3(+) Cells in canine tumours and lymph nodes correlates positively with glucose transporter 1 expression, *J Comp Pathol* 155:171–180, 2016.

193. Pinheiro D, Chang YM, Bryant H, et al.: Dissecting the regulatory microenvironment of a large animal model of non-Hodgkin lymphoma: evidence of a negative prognostic impact of FOXP3+ T cells in canine B cell lymphoma, *PLoS One* 9:e105027, 2014.

194. Guevara-Patino JA, Turk MJ, Wolchok JD, et al.: Immunity to cancer through immune recognition of altered self: studies with melanoma, *Adv Cancer Res* 90:157–177, 2003.

195. Bergman PJ, Camps-Palau MA, McKnight JA, et al.: Development of a xenogeneic DNA vaccine program for canine malignant melanoma at the Animal Medical Center, *Vaccine* 24:4582–4585, 2006.

196. Bergman PJ, McKnight J, Novosad A, et al.: Long-term survival of dogs with advanced malignant melanoma after DNA vaccination with xenogeneic human tyrosinase: a phase I trial, *Clin Cancer Res* 9:1284–1290, 2003.

197. Wolchok JD, Yuan J, Houghton AN, et al.: Safety and immunogenicity of tyrosinase DNA vaccines in patients with melanoma, *Mol Ther* 15:2044–2050, 2007.

198. Phillips JC, Lembcke LM, Noltenius CE, et al.: Evaluation of tyrosinase expression in canine and equine melanocytic tumors, *Am J Vet Res* 73:272–278, 2012.

199. Cangul IT, van Garderen E, van der Poel HJ, et al.: Tyrosinase gene expression in clear cell sarcoma indicates a melanocytic origin: insight from the first reported canine case, *APMIS JID - 8803400* 107:982–988, 1999.

200. de Vries TJ, Smeets M, de GR, et al.: Expression of gp100, MART-1, tyrosinase, and S100 in paraffin-embedded primary melanomas and locoregional, lymph node, and visceral metastases: implications for diagnosis and immunotherapy. A study conducted by the EORTC Melanoma Cooperative Group, *J Pathol* 193:13–20, 2001.

201. Gradilone A, Gazzaniga P, Ribuffo D, et al.: Prognostic significance of tyrosinase expression in sentinel lymph node biopsy for ultra-thin, thin, and thick melanomas, *Eur Rev Med Pharmacol Sci* 16:1367–1376, 2012.

202. Liao JC, Gregor P, Wolchok JD, et al.: Vaccination with human tyrosinase DNA induces antibody responses in dogs with advanced melanoma, *Cancer Immun* 6(8), 2006.

203. Goubier A, Fuhrmann L, Forest L, et al.: Superiority of needle-free transdermal plasmid delivery for the induction of antigen-specific IFNgamma T cell responses in the dog, *Vaccine* 26:2186–2190, 2008.

204. Grosenbaugh DA, Leard AT, Bergman PJ, et al.: Safety and efficacy of a xenogeneic DNA vaccine encoding for human tyrosinase as adjunctive treatment for oral malignant melanoma in dogs following surgical excision of the primary tumor, *Am J Vet Res* 72:1631–1638, 2011.

205. Ottnod JM, Smedley RC, Walshaw R, et al.: A retrospective analysis of the efficacy of Oncept vaccine for the adjunct treatment of canine oral malignant melanoma, *Vet Comp Oncol* 11:219–229, 2013.

206. Verganti S, Berlato D, Blackwood L, et al.: Use of Oncept melanoma vaccine in 69 canine oral malignant melanomas in the UK, *J Small Anim Pract* 58:10–16, 2017.

207. Treggiari E, Grant JP, North SM: A retrospective review of outcome and survival following surgery and adjuvant xenogeneic DNA vaccination in 32 dogs with oral malignant melanoma, *J Vet Med Sci* 78:845–850, 2016.

208. McLean JL, Lobetti RG: Use of the melanoma vaccine in 38 dogs: the South African experience, *J South Afr V et Assoc* 86:1246, 2015.

209. Herzog A, Buchholz J, Ruess-Melzer K, et al.: Concurrent irradiation and DNA tumor vaccination in canine oral malignant melanoma: a pilot study, *Schweiz Arch Tierheilkd* 155:135–142, 2013.

210. Sarbu L, Kitchell BE, Bergman PJ: Safety of administering the canine melanoma DNA vaccine (Oncept) to cats with malignant melanoma - a retrospective study, *J Feline Med Surg* 19:224–230, 2017.

211. Perales MA, Yuan J, Powel S, et al.: Phase I/II study of GM-CSF DNA as an adjuvant for a multipeptide cancer vaccine in patients with advanced melanoma, *Mol Ther* 16:2022–2029, 2008.

212. Yuan J, Ku GY, Gallardo HF, et al.: Safety and immunogenicity of a human and mouse gp100 DNA vaccine in a phase I trial of patients with melanoma, *Cancer Immun* 9(5), 2009.

213. Riccardo F, Iussich S, Maniscalco L, et al.: CSPG4-specific immunity and survival prolongation in dogs with oral malignant melanoma immunized with human CSPG4 DNA, *Clin Cancer Res* 20:3753–3762, 2014.

214. Manley CA, Leibman NF, Wolchok JD, et al.: Xenogeneic murine tyrosinase DNA vaccine for malignant melanoma of the digit of dogs, *J Vet Intern Med* 25:94–99, 2011.

21

Mast Cell Tumors

CHERYL A. LONDON AND DOUGLAS H. THAMM

The neoplastic proliferation of mast cells (MCs) referred to as mast cell tumor (MCT; mastocytoma, MC sarcoma) represents the most commonly encountered cutaneous tumor in the dog and the second most common cutaneous tumor in the cat.[1–5] Systemic forms of the disease are often referred to as *mastocytosis*. Canine and feline forms of the disease are considered separately in this chapter, as many differences exist with regard to histologic type, biologic behavior, therapy, and prognosis.

Canine Mast Cell Tumors

Biology of Canine Mast Cells

MC precursors leave the bone marrow and migrate to various tissues throughout the body where they undergo differentiation into mature MCs with their characteristic cytoplasmic granules, which stain metochromatically with Geimsa and toluidine blue.[6] These granules contain a number of bioactive substances including heparin, histamine, preformed tumor necrosis factor-alpha (TNF-α), and several proteases.[6] The nature and composition of MC granules is highly influenced by the microenvironment in which the MC mature. For example, in dogs, MCs in the gastrointestinal (GI) tract express primarily chymase whereas MCs in the skin express both chymase and tryptase.[7] On stimulation, MCs can rapidly produce a variety of proteases (chymase, tryptase), cytokines (TNF-α, interleukin-6 [IL-6]), chemokines (CCL2, CXCL1), growth factors (vascular endothelial growth factor [VEGF], basic fibroblast factor [bFGF]), and lipid mediators (prostaglandin D_2 [PGD_2], leukotriene C_4 [LTC_4]).[6] Through this process, MCs participate in several biologic activities, including wound healing, induction of innate immune responses, antiparasite activity, and modulation of reaction to insect and spider venoms.[6,8]

Normal canine MCs can be generated from bone marrow derived hematopoietic precursors.[9,10] These cells, known as canine bone marrow derived MCs (cBMMCs), have been used to characterize the functional properties of MCs in this species. As with normal human MCs, their differentiation requires the presence of the growth factor stem cell factor (SCF), and can be influenced by the presence of other cytokines.[9,10] On stimulation, these cells rapidly release histamine, monocyte chemoattractant protein-1 (MCP-1), TNF-α, and tryptase, and they produce several additional cytokines and chemokines including IL-3, IL-13, granulocyte-macrophage colony-stimulating factor (GM-CSF), and macrophage inflammatory protein-1 alpha (MIP-1α).[9,10]

Interestingly, the cBMMCs are extremely sensitive to chemical degranulation, which may help explain why dogs exhibit such a high degree of hypersensitivity to several chemical agents including polysorbate 80, cremaphor EL, and doxorubicin.[9] The function of cBMMCs can be modulated by cytokines, steroids, and nonsteroidal antiinflammatory drugs.[9–11]

Incidence and Risk Factors

MCT is the most common cutaneous tumor in the dog, accounting for between 16% and 21% of all cutaneous tumors.[1,3,5,12] Although MCTs are primarily a disease of older dogs (mean age approximately 8–9 years), they have also been reported in younger dogs and there is no apparent sex predilection.[1,3,5] Most occur in mixed breeds; however, several breeds are at increased risk for MCTs, including dogs of bulldog descent (boxer, Boston terrier, English bulldog, pug), Labrador and golden retrievers, cocker spaniels, schnauzers, Staffordshire terriers, beagles, Rhodesian ridgebacks, Weimaraners, and Chinese shar-pei.[1,5,13–15] The increased incidence of MCTs in certain breeds suggests the possibility of an underlying genetic cause.[14] A recent genome-wide association study in golden retrievers identified polymorphisms in the *GNAI2* gene and multiple genes associated with hyaluronic acid synthesis as risk factors for MCT development.[16] Interestingly, although dogs of bulldog ancestry are at higher risk for MCT development, it is generally accepted that MCTs in these dogs are likely to be less aggressive.[1,17] In contrast, anecdotal evidence suggests that Chinese shar-pei develop MCTs that may be more biologically aggressive (A. Avery, personal communication). Spontaneously regressing MCTs in young animals have been described in cats, pigs, horses, and humans. Multiple cutaneous MCT that all regressed within 27 weeks was reported in a 3-week-old Jack Russell terrier.[18] This syndrome of spontaneous regression in young animals may indicate a hyperplastic or dysplastic syndrome rather than a true neoplastic lesion.

The etiology of MCTs in dogs is for the most part unknown. Historically, MCTs have been associated with chronic inflammation or the application of skin irritants; however, the epidemiology of disease in dogs does not support the role of a topical carcinogen.[19–21] Unequivocal evidence is lacking for a viral etiology, although MCTs have been transplanted to very young or immunocompromised laboratory dogs using tumor cell tissues and rarely by cell-free extracts.[22–24] No C-type or other identifiable virus particles have been observed, and no epidemiologic evidence exists to suggest horizontal transmission. Chromosomal fragile site expression, a phenomenon thought to genetically predispose humans to develop certain tumors, was shown to be increased in boxer dogs with MCT[25]; however, the control population for this study was young, non–tumor-bearing boxers, and the increased expression of chromosomal fragile sites may be due to this age difference.

The genetic changes that predispose to canine MCTs are incompletely understood. Alterations in the p53 tumor suppressor pathway have been identified in some canine MCTs,[26–28] but p53 sequencing in a limited number of cases has revealed no mutations.[29] Perturbations in expression of the proteins p21 and p27, cyclin-dependent kinase inhibitors that contribute to regulation of the cell cycle, have been identified in many canine MCTs.[30] Cytosolic receptors for estrogen and progesterone have also been detected in canine MCTs,[31] but their role in the etiopathogenesis of MCTs is poorly understood. One European study reported that female dogs with MCTs had a more favorable prognosis with chemotherapy.[32] Although the majority of studies performed in North America have failed to detect such an association, the relatively higher frequency of intact females present in the European population may have allowed the effect of sex hormones to have a greater statistical effect on biologic behavior. Expression of the angiogenic growth factor VEGF and its receptor VEGFR2 has been demonstrated in many canine MCTs, and preliminary evidence suggests that VEGFR2 activation may be associated with inferior postsurgical outcomes.[33,34]

Perhaps the best-described molecular abnormality in canine MCTs involves the receptor tyrosine kinase (RTK) KIT. KIT is expressed normally on a variety of cells including hematopoietic stem cells, melanocytes, and MCs, among others.[35–37] The ligand for KIT, SCF, induces KIT dimerization, subsequent phosphorylation, and generation of intracellular signaling that promotes the proliferation, differentiation, and maturation of normal MCs.[35–37] SCF is essential for the differentiation of mature MC from CD34+ hematopoietic stem cells *in vitro*, and inhibition of KIT signaling induces apoptosis of cBMMCs.[10,36,37] KIT expression has been demonstrated on canine MCTs, and aberrant cytoplasmic localization and/or increased phosphorylation of KIT in MCTs may be associated with dysregulated KIT function.[38–42] A significant minority of canine MCTs possess somatic mutations in the c-*kit* gene involving either the juxtamembrane domain (exons 11–12) or extracellular domain (exons 8–9).[43–47] These mutations result in SCF-independent activation of KIT and subsequent unregulated KIT signal transduction.[45,46] In dogs, the c-*kit* mutations appear to be associated with 25% to 30% of intermediate- and high-grade MCTs, and evidence suggests that they are linked to increased risk of local recurrence, metastasis, and a worse prognosis.[43,46,48–50]

More recently, studies have been undertaken to better characterize copy number variation (CNV), gene expression profile, and proteomic profile of canine MCTs to identify those pathways that contribute to aggressive biologic behavior. In one study of CNVs found in MCTs from dogs that survived <6 and >12 months, regions of loss in phosphatase and tensin homolog (PTEN), FAS*, and regions of gains in MAPK3, WNT5B, FGF, FOXM1, and RAD51 were detected in those tumors with shorter survival times (STs).[51] In another study, CNVs were found to increase as tumor grade increased, and tumors with c-*kit* mutations showed genome-wide aberrant CNVs often involving genes in the p53 and rB pathways, whereas CNVs were very limited in tumors with wild-type c-*kit*.[52] Gene expression profiling comparing MCTs from dogs cured with surgery versus those that died of disease revealed differential expression of genes associated with drug metabolism and cell cycle pathways including members of solute carrier transporter and UDP glucuronosyltransferase gene families.[53] In contrast, another study found that expression of 13 specific transcripts divided samples into two categories (differentiated and undifferentiated), harboring a different prognosis. Among these, a significant association was found between expression of FOXM1, GSN, FEN1, and KPNA2 and MCT-related mortality.[54] Using proteomic profiling, four stress response proteins (HSPA9, PDIA3, TCP1A, and TCP1E) were found to be significantly upregulated in high-grade tumors, whereas proteins mainly associated with cell motility and metastasis had either increased (WDR1, ACTR3, ANXA6) or decreased (ANXA2, ACTB) expression levels.[55] Lastly, overexpression of micro-RNA-9 was associated with MCT metastasis, potentially through the induction of an invasive phenotype.[56] It is likely that future work to more definitely characterize the canine MCT genome will help clarify how the abnormalities described earlier influence tumor biologic behavior.

History and Clinical Signs

The vast majority of MCTs in dogs occur in the dermis and subcutaneous tissue,[5,57] and most are solitary in nature, although 11% to 14% of dogs present with multiple lesions.[58,59] Approximately 50% of cutaneous MCTs occur on the trunk and perineal region, 40% on the limbs, and 10% on the head and neck.[20,60] MCTs have also been reported to occur in other sites including the conjunctiva, salivary gland, nasopharynx, larynx, oral cavity, ureter, and spine.[61–65] A visceral form of MCT, often referred to as disseminated or systemic mastocytosis, has also been documented, although it is usually preceded by an aggressive primary lesion.[66–70] Infiltration of abdominal lymph nodes (LNs), spleen, liver, and bone marrow is commonly observed in dogs with visceral disease, and pleural/peritoneal effusions containing neoplastic MCs have been documented. A case series of dogs with primary GI MCT was reported in which most dogs presented for vomiting, diarrhea, and melena. Only 40% dogs were alive at 30 days after first admission and fewer than 10% were alive at 6 months.[28]

It is important to note that cutaneous MCTs have an extremely varied range of clinical appearances and they are sometimes inadvertently mistaken for nonneoplastic lesions. Well-differentiated MCTs tend to be solitary, small, slow-growing tumors that may have been present for several months. They are not typically ulcerated, but overlying hair may be lost. Undifferentiated MCT tend to be rapidly growing, ulcerated lesions that cause considerable irritation and attain a large size. Surrounding tissues may become inflamed and edematous. Small satellite nodules may develop in surrounding tissues. Tumors of intermediate differentiation fill the spectrum between these two extremes. A subcutaneous form of MCT that is soft and fleshy on palpation is often misdiagnosed clinically as a lipoma (Fig. 21.1).

The history and clinical signs of dogs with MCTs may be complicated by signs attributable to release of histamine, heparin, and other vasoactive amines from MC granules. Occasionally, mechanical manipulation during examination of the tumor results in degranulation and subsequent erythema and wheal formation in surrounding tissues. This phenomenon has been referred to as

---

*Fas or FasR, also known as apoptosis antigen 1 (APO-1 or APT), cluster of differentiation 95 (CD95) or tumor necrosis factor receptor superfamily member 6 (TNFRSF6) is a protein that is encoded by the *FAS* gene. Fas was first identified using a monoclonal antibody generated by immunizing mice with the FS-7 cell line. Thus, the name Fas is derived from FS-7-associated surface antigen.

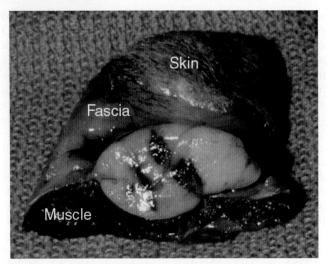

• **Fig. 21.1** Subcutaneous mast cell tumor from the shoulder of a dog. This mass was originally misdiagnosed as a lipoma based on palpation alone. Wide surgical excision to include the deep muscle layer was necessary to achieve complete surgical margins.

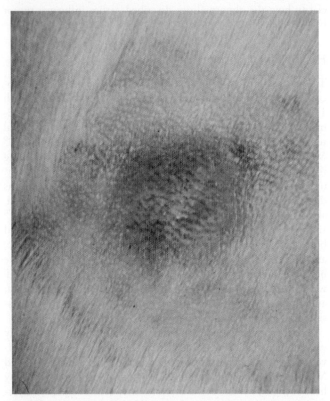

• **Fig. 21.2** Erythema and wheal formation occurred in surrounding skin after manipulation of this cutaneous mast cell tumor. This phenomenon resulting from release of vasoactive amines from mast cell granules is known as Darier's sign. (Courtesy D. Vail, University of Wisconsin–Madison.)

"Darier's sign" (Fig. 21.2).[71] This can also occur spontaneously, and dog owners may describe the tumor as periodically increasing and decreasing in size. GI ulceration has been documented in 35% to 83% of dogs with MCTs that underwent necropsy.[72,73] The incidence of GI ulceration may be overrepresented owing to the fact that more aggressive forms of the disease likely end up in necropsy surveys. Histamine released from MCT granules is thought to act on parietal cells via H_2 receptors, resulting in increased hydrochloric acid secretion. Plasma histamine concentrations have been shown to be high in dogs with measurable high-grade MCTs, and there is preliminary information that monitoring of plasma histamine concentrations may be useful in assessing disease progression.[74] These dogs also have decreased concentrations of plasma gastrin, which is normally released by antral G cells in response to increased gastric hydrochloric acid concentrations, acting as a negative feedback loop. Dogs with substantial MCT burden (i.e., large tumors, metastatic disease, systemic disease) are much more likely to present with clinical signs related to the release of MC mediators. These may include vomiting, diarrhea, fever, peripheral edema, and rarely collapse.

Perioperative degranulation of MCTs and subsequent release of histamine and other less characterized vasoactive substances may also result in potentially life-threatening hypotensive events during surgery. It is thought that prostaglandins in the D series secreted by tumor cells may mediate the hypotensive effects observed in humans with MC diseases.[75,76] Coagulation abnormalities, also reported in dogs with MCTs, are likely due to heparin release from MC granules.[68,77] Although clinical evidence of systemic hemorrhage is not typically associated with this phenomenon, localized excessive bleeding at the time of biopsy or surgery due to degranulation after tumor manipulation can be a complication, even in the presence of normal presurgical coagulation parameters.

Prognostic Factors

A discussion of prognostic factors associated with canine MCTs will precede sections on diagnosis and treatment, as steps followed in those sections are predicated on the presence or absence of these prognostic factors. Table 21.1 lists factors known to be predictive of biologic behavior and clinical outcome in dogs with MCTs. It is important to note that no one factor is entirely predictive of biologic behavior and, as such, all prognostic indicators should be taken into consideration when evaluating a patient.

Histologic grade is considered the most consistent and reliable prognostic factor available for dogs with MCTs, although it will not predict the behavior of every tumor.[13,57,78,79] Several investigators have applied histologic grading systems to canine MCTs based on degree of differentiation (Table 21.2). The number grades used in these studies are at odds. Therefore for the sake of clarity, the three differentiation groups should be simply referred to as undifferentiated (high) grade, intermediate grade, and well-differentiated (low) grade. Table 21.3 lists the relative distribution of MCT grades encountered in larger series. STs after surgical excision based on histologic grade are presented in Table 21.4. The vast majority of dogs with well-differentiated MCTs (80%–90%) and approximately 75% of dogs with intermediate-grade MCTs experience long-term survival after complete surgical excision.[58,78,80–83] Metastatic rates for undifferentiated MCT range from 55% to 96%, and most dogs with these tumors die of their disease within 1 year.[57,84] The majority disseminate first to local LNs, then to spleen and liver. Other visceral organs may be involved; however, lung involvement is rare. Neoplastic MCs may be observed in the bone marrow and peripheral blood in cases of widespread systemic dissemination.[68]

The current histopathologic grading system does not detect a small percentage of those well- or intermediately differentiated MCTs that result in death of affected dogs, and this is complicated by the fact that there is disagreement in tumor grading schemes among pathologists. In one study, there was significant variation among pathologists in grading a specific set of MCTs, although this was found to be less so if all pathologists strictly employed the system described by Patnaik.[13,85,86] Recently, an attempt was

TABLE 21.1 Prognostic Factors for Mast Cell Tumors in Dogs

Factor	Comment
Histologic grade	Strongly predictive of outcome. Dogs with undifferentiated tumors typically die of their disease after local therapy alone, whereas those with well-differentiated tumors are usually cured with appropriate local therapy.
Clinical stage	Stages 0 and 1, confined to the skin without local lymph node or distant metastasis, have a better prognosis than higher-stage disease.
Location	Subungual, oral, and other mucous membrane sites are associated with more high-grade tumors and worse prognosis. Preputial and scrotal tumors are also associated with a worse prognosis. Subcutaneous tumors have a better prognosis. Visceral or bone marrow disease usually carries a grave prognosis.
Cell proliferation rate	Mitotic index, relative frequency of AgNORs, and percent PCNA or Ki-67 immunopositivity are predictive of postsurgical outcome.
Growth rate	MCTs that remain localized and are present for prolonged periods of time (months or years) without significant change are usually benign.
Microvessel density	Increased microvessel density is associated with higher grade, a higher degree of invasiveness, and a worse prognosis.
Recurrence	Local recurrence after surgical excision may carry a more guarded prognosis.
Systemic signs	The presence of systemic illness (e.g., hyporexia, vomiting, melena, GI ulceration) may be associated with a higher stage of disease.
Age	Older dogs may have shorter median disease-free intervals when treated with radiation therapy than younger dogs.
Breed	MCTs in boxers (and potentially other brachycephalic breeds) tend to be of low or intermediate grade and are thus associated with a better prognosis.
Sex	Male dogs had a shorter survival time than female dogs when treated with chemotherapy.
Tumor size	Large tumors may be associated with a worse prognosis after surgical removal and/or radiation therapy.
c-kit mutation	The presence of an activating mutation in the c-kit gene is associated with a worse prognosis.
DNA copy number variation	Higher CNVs are observed in tumors of higher grade and those with a worse prognosis.

AgNORs, Argyrophilic nucleolar organizer regions; *CNV*, copy number variation; *GI*, gastrointestinal; *MCTs*, mast cell tumors; *PCNA*, proliferating cell nuclear antigen.

TABLE 21.2 Histologic Classification of Mast Cell Tumors in Dogs

Grade	Bostock Grading	Patnaik Grading	Microscopic Description
Anaplastic, undifferentiated (high grade)	1	3	Highly cellular, undifferentiated cytoplasmic boundaries, irregular size and shape of nuclei; frequent mitoses, sparse cytoplasmic granules
Intermediate grade	2	2	Cells closely packed with indistinct cytoplasmic boundaries; nucleus-to-cytoplasmic ratio lower than anaplastic; infrequent mitoses; more granules than anaplastic
Well differentiated (low grade)	3	1	Clearly defined cytoplasmic boundaries with regular, spherical or ovoid nuclei, mitoses rare or absent; cytoplasmic granules large, deep staining, and abundant

TABLE 21.3 Relative Frequency of Canine Mast Cell Tumors by Histologic Grade

Investigator	Number of Dogs	High Grade (%)	Intermediate Grade (%)	Low Grade (%)
Hottendorf[21]	300	19	27	54
Bostock[59]	114	39	26	34
Patnaik[14]	83	20	43	36
Simoes[85]	87	22	40	38

made to develop a new grading system that would separate tumors into "high" or "low" grade based on one of four features identified on histopathologic evaluation, in an attempt to minimize interpathologist disagreement and still provide useful prognostic information.[87] In this setting, tumors were classified as high grade if they possessed (1) at least 7 mitotic figures/10 HPF, (2) at least 3 multinucleated cells/10 HPF, (3) at least 3 bizarre nuclei/10 HPF, or (4) karyomegaly. In a series of 95 dogs evaluated by both the Patnaik and this alternative system, the alternative system was somewhat better at predicting which dogs would be more likely to die of disease[87]; at least one follow-up study has confirmed the utility of this two-tiered system.[88] There remains incomplete information to confirm whether two-tiered system is truly better than the Patnaik three-tiered system for predicting the biologic behavior of MCTs. The authors prefer to receive grades according to both schemes on MCT histopathology reports.

Several markers of proliferation have been evaluated to assist in determining whether an MCT is likely to behave in a more aggressive manner.[49,79,89–97] Ki-67 is a protein found in the nucleus, the levels of which appear to correlate with cell proliferation and patient survival.[90,91] Silver colloid staining of paraffin-embedded sections can be used to determine the relative presence

TABLE 21.4	**Survival Times of Dogs with Surgically Treated Mast Cell Tumors According to Histologic Grade[a]**			
Investigator	Number of Dogs	Percent Alive	Months Post Surgery	Median Survival Time (weeks)
Bostock[59]				
Low grade	39	79	7	NR
Intermediate grade	30	37	7	
High grade	45	15	7	
Patnaik[14]				
Low grade	30	83	48	NR
Intermediate grade	36	44	48	
High grade	17	6	48	
Bostock[104]				
Low grade	19	90	NR	>40[b]
Intermediate grade	16	75		>36
High grade	15	27		13
Murphy[84]				
Low grade	87	100	12	>80[b]
Intermediate grade	199	92	12	>80
High grade	54	46	12	40
Simoes[85]				
Low grade	33	91	20	NR
Intermediate grade	35	71	20	
High grade	19	42	20	

NR, Not reported.

[a]Unclear in these studies if death was due to metastasis or local recurrence.

[b]Medians not reached at the time of last follow-up (i.e., >50% alive).

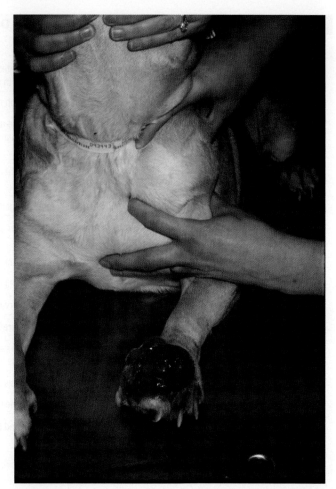

• **Fig. 21.3** Subungual undifferentiated mast cell tumor in an English bulldog. As with some mast cell tumors in this location, early lymph node metastasis has occurred. (Courtesy D. Vail, University of Wisconsin–Madison.)

of argyrophilic nucleolar organizer regions (AgNOR), another surrogate marker of proliferation. These have been correlated with histologic grade and postsurgical outcome.[79,98] Finally, proliferating cell nuclear antigen (PCNA), another indicator of cell proliferation, has been used to determine the biologic behavior of MCTs, although this is probably not as reliable as the other markers.[79,98,99] The previously discussed markers of proliferation all require the use of special stains. In contrast, mitotic index (MI, number of mitoses per 10 HPF) in hematoxylin and eosin–stained sections has been used to assess the biologic behavior of canine MCTs. In one study, those dogs with tumors possessing an MI <5 had a median ST (MST) of 80 months compared with 3 months for those possessing a MI >5, suggesting that MI is a strong predictor of overall survival for dogs with MCTs.[100] Additional studies have also found a role for MI in MCT prognosis.[87,97,101–103]

Other cellular assessments have been employed to evaluate the biologic behavior of MCTs. A study of DNA ploidy determined by flow cytometric analysis suggested a trend toward shorter survival and higher clinical stage of disease in aneuploid tumors compared with diploid tumors.[104] Complementary to this, increases in DNA CNV also appear to be associated with higher grade and shorter postsurgical ST.[51,52] Studies have found a correlation between intratumor microvessel density and invasiveness, MI, and prognosis,[89,105] and a correlation between nuclear characteristics (assessed by computerized morphometry) and outcome and grade.[106,107]

The potential role of KIT dysregulation in MCT prognosis was investigated by assessing KIT immunohistochemical staining patterns on histopathologic specimens.[108] Three distinct patterns were identified: membrane, focal/stippled, and diffuse cytoplasmic staining. Although there was some evidence that dogs with diffuse cytoplasmic KIT staining patterns did not live as long as those with other patterns, no group reached an MST and most dogs in each of the KIT staining groups evaluated experienced extremely long postoperative STs.[108] The presence of c-*kit* activating mutations has been associated with a higher rate of local recurrence, metastasis, and death from disease, suggesting that KIT dysregulation confers a more aggressive phenotype to MCT.[43,48,49] Finally, investigators have attempted to correlate histologic grading of MCT with a combined Ki67/PCNA/AgNOR/KIT immunohistochemical scoring.[109] No significant correlation was found for KIT staining and MCT grade, but high Ki67/PCNA/AgNOR scores all positively correlated with tumor grade (i.e., higher scores for higher grade). This suggests that proliferation indices increase with increasing grade and are ultimately reflected in the eventual biologic behavior of the tumor.

Tumor location has been investigated as a potential prognostic indicator.[58,110–114] Tumors in the preputial/inguinal area, subungual (nail bed) region (Fig. 21.3), and other mucocutaneous sites, including the oral cavity and perineum, historically have been associated with aggressive behavior. Two reports did not show a poorer prognosis for tumors occurring in the inguinal

TABLE 21.5	World Health Organization Clinical Staging System for Mast Cell Tumors
Stage	**Description**
0	One tumor incompletely excised from the dermis, identified histologically, without regional lymph node involvement a. Without systemic signs b. With systemic signs
I	One tumor confined to the dermis, without regional lymph node involvement a. Without systemic signs b. With systemic signs
II	One tumor confined to the dermis, with regional lymph node involvement a. Without systemic signs b. With systemic signs
III	Multiple dermal tumors; large, infiltrating tumors with or without regional lymph node involvement a. Without systemic signs b. With systemic signs
IV	Any tumor with distant metastasis, including blood or bone marrow involvement

and perineal region; however, when preputial and scrotal regions were specifically evaluated, they were indeed associated with worse outcomes.[111,112] Approximately 50% to 60% of dogs with MCTs located in the muzzle present with regional LN metastasis.[113,115] Interestingly, this does not necessarily indicate a worse long-term prognosis, as the MST for dogs with metastatic disease was 14 months.[113] MCTs that originate in the viscera (GI tract, liver, spleen) or bone marrow carry a grave prognosis.[67,68] Recent data indicate that MCTs arising in the subcutaneous tissues have a favorable prognosis with extended STs and low rates of recurrence and metastasis. In one study of 306 dogs with subcutaneous MCTs, metastasis occurred in 4% of dogs and 8% experienced local recurrence.[103] The estimated 2- and 5-year survival probabilities were 92% and 86%, respectively. Decreased survival was linked to MI >4, infiltrative growth pattern, and presence of multinucleation.[103] Lastly, conjunctival MCTs were found to have a good prognosis, with 15 of 32 dogs disease-free at a mean of 21.4 months postsurgery; no dogs in this study died of MCT-related disease.[116]

Clinical stage, represented in Table 21.5, is also predictive of outcome.[32,57,104,110,117,118] There is controversy regarding the effect of multiple MCTs on prognosis and, as such, this part of the staging scheme may not accurately correlate with outcome. Several studies indicate that there is no difference in outcome between patients with a single cutaneous MCTs and those with multiple MCTs,[58,114,119,120] whereas others have suggested an inferior outcome in dogs with multiple tumors.[102,121] It is uncertain whether this phenomenon represents an atypical form of metastasis or multiple, unrelated tumors arising independently, although one study demonstrated a clonal origin for two distant cutaneous tumors arising over years.[122] The effect of LN metastasis on prognosis is also somewhat controversial. In two studies, the presence of MCs in the regional LNs was a negative prognostic factor for disease-free interval (DFI) and survival[120,123]; however, an additional study revealed that dogs with intermediately differentiated MCTs and LN metastasis treated with postoperative radiation

therapy (RT) achieved long-term survival.[124] Other studies have shown that dogs with intermediately differentiated MCTs with LN metastasis may have a good prognosis if the affected LN is removed and adjuvant chemotherapy and/or RT is administered.[114,120,125] For poorly differentiated tumors, the presence of LN metastatic disease resulted in an MST of 194 days compared with 503 days for dogs with no metastasis.[84] For these dogs, treatment of the LN improved MST (240 days) compared with those dogs whose LNs were not treated (42 days).[84] As with all cases, clinical judgment regarding LN metastasis is probably important.

Several miscellaneous factors have been linked to prognosis in dogs with MCTs. Certain breeds of dogs such as boxers, pugs, and dogs of bulldog descent appear to develop MCTs that often behave in a more benign fashion.[1,17,57,126] Recent rapid growth has been associated with a worse outcome. For example, in one study, 83% of dogs with tumors present for longer than 28 weeks before surgery survived for at least 30 weeks compared with only 25% of dogs with tumors present for less than 28 weeks.[57] Systemic signs of hyporexia, vomiting, melena, widespread erythema, and edema associated with vasoactive substances from MC degranulation are more commonly associated with visceral forms of MCT and, as such, carry a more guarded prognosis.[58,68,127] In recent retrospective studies of visceral or disseminated MCT, STs were short and nearly all dogs with follow-up died of their disease.[69,70,128] Local tumor ulceration, erythema, or pruritus has been associated with a worse prognosis in some studies.[58,120] Lastly, recurrence of MCTs after surgical excision has also been associated with a more guarded prognosis.[92,118,120,129] Thus appropriate aggressive therapy at the time of first presentation, rather than at the time of recurrence, may improve the long-term prognosis in patients with MCTs.

Diagnostic Technique and Workup

MCTs are initially diagnosed on the basis of fine-needle aspiration (FNA) cytology. Rowmanovsky's or rapid hematologic-type stains used in most practices will suffice. MCs appear as small- to medium-sized round cells with abundant, small, uniform cytoplasmic granules that stain purplish red (metachromatic) (see Figs. 7.2 and 7.5 of Chapter 7).[1,130] A small percentage of MCTs have granules that do not stain readily, giving them an epithelial or macrophage-like appearance that has often been referred to as giving a "fried-egg" impression (Fig. 7.2, Chapter 7). In these cases, a Wright–Giemsa or toluidine blue stain will often reveal granules; however, histologic assessment may ultimately be necessary. Highly anaplastic, agranular MCTs can sometimes be challenging to definitively diagnose by routine light microscopy. Immunohistochemical techniques have been applied in an attempt to differentiate these from other anaplastic round cell tumors. MCTs are vimentin positive and the majority are tryptase and CD117 (KIT) positive.[38,131–133] Other markers that could potentially be useful include chymase, MCP-1, and IL-8.[9,10]

Historically, preoperative diagnostic tests have included a minimum database (complete blood count [CBC], serum biochemistry profile), a buffy coat smear to document peripheral mastocytosis, cytologic assessment of regional LNs, abdominal ultrasound (US) with cytologic assessment of spleen or liver if warranted, thoracic radiographs, and a bone marrow aspirate. It is now likely that an extensive workup is unnecessary for dogs with MCTs that do not exhibit the previously discussed negative prognostic factors. Fig. 21.4 illustrates the diagnostic steps and the order in which they are pursued in the authors' practice.

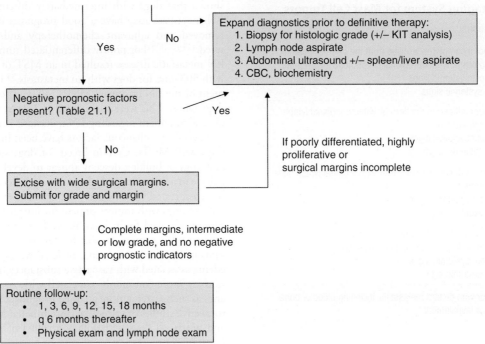

Anatomic site amenable to wide surgical excision?

```
                                                          ┌─────────────────────────────────────────────────────┐
                                                          │ Expand diagnostics prior to definitive therapy:     │
                   No                                     │  1. Biopsy for histologic grade (+/– KIT analysis)  │
   Yes ──────────────────────►                            │  2. Lymph node aspirate                              │
    │                                                     │  3. Abdominal ultrasound +/– spleen/liver aspirate  │
    │                                                     │  4. CBC, biochemistry                                │
    ▼                                                     └─────────────────────────────────────────────────────┘
┌──────────────────────────┐              Yes
│ Negative prognostic       │──────────────►
│ factors present?          │
│ (Table 21.1)              │
└──────────────────────────┘
    │
    │  No                              If poorly differentiated, highly
    ▼                                  proliferative or
┌──────────────────────────┐          surgical margins incomplete
│ Excise with wide surgical │
│ margins.                  │
│ Submit for grade and      │
│ margin                    │
└──────────────────────────┘
    │
    │  Complete margins, intermediate
    │  or low grade, and no negative
    │  prognostic indicators
    ▼
┌──────────────────────────┐
│ Routine follow-up:        │
│  • 1, 3, 6, 9, 12, 15,    │
│    18 months              │
│  • q 6 months thereafter  │
│  • Physical exam and      │
│    lymph node exam        │
└──────────────────────────┘
```

• **Fig. 21.4** Suggested diagnostic steps for canine cutaneous mast cell tumors.

If the MCT is in a location amenable to wide surgical excision and no negative prognostic indicators are present (see Table 21.1), no further tests other than minimum database and FNA of the regional LN (if possible) are performed before wide surgical excision. If there is ambiguity regarding the location of the regional LNs, sentinel LN mapping may be performed to facilitate identification (see Chapter 9 for more information). Although cytologic methods for assigning a grade have been recently described,[134–136] histologic assessment after excision remains critical to provide guidance regarding necessary further diagnostics and therapeutics.

If the tumor presents at a site that is not amenable to wide surgical excision or primary closure (e.g., distal extremity) or if negative prognostic factors exist in the history or physical examination, ancillary diagnostics to further stage the disease are recommended before definitive therapy. An incisional/needle biopsy may be performed at this point for determination of histologic grade. The minimum staging that is advisable in those cases requiring presurgical staging consists of a minimum database, FNA cytology of the regional LN (even if normal in size), and abdominal US. With respect to cytologic evaluation of LNs, definitive criteria for metastatic disease can be challenging if MCs are present in low numbers; this is because MCs are normally found in LNs and their numbers can be increased in the presence of infection and ulceration, which are sometimes observed in MCTs. For example, in 56 healthy beagle dogs, approximately 24% of LN aspirates contained MCs (range of 1–16 MCs/slide, mean of 6.4/slide).[137] Therefore an occasional solitary MC is not indicative of metastasis; rather, clustering and aggregates are more worrisome (Fig. 21.5).[117] Surgical removal of a cytologically suspicious LN for histologic assessment may be necessary to accurately determine whether MCs present in the LN truly represent metastatic disease. A histologic grading scheme has been described for "degree of LN metastasis" to account for the varying levels of LN involvement that can be observed histologically (from scattered, isolated MCs to complete

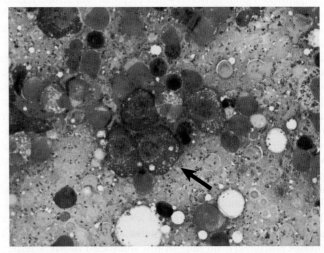

• **Fig. 21.5** Regional lymph node aspirate from a dog with a cutaneous mast cell tumor. Note clustering of mast cells in a background of lymphocytes more indicative of true metastasis.

effacement with tumor cells).[138] Dogs with high histologic node (HN) scores had shorter STs than dogs with low HN scores.[138] Abdominal US is now considered an important diagnostic test for the evaluation of dogs with potentially aggressive MCT. Although FNA cytology of structurally normal livers or spleens is generally unrewarding,[139,140] the presence of negative prognostic indicators (metastatic LN, clinical signs, etc.) is sufficient justification to perform cytologic evaluation of these organs even if they appear ultrasonographically normal.[141]

Thoracic radiographs rarely demonstrate metastasis; however, it is reasonable to procure them before an expensive or invasive procedure to rule out occult cardiopulmonary disease that could complicate anesthesia or unrelated disease processes (primary lung tumor, etc.). Occasionally, thoracic lymphadenomegaly may be observed as a result of MCT metastasis. Knowledge of the extent of MCT margins before surgery, usually accomplished by digital palpation, can be enhanced with the use of diagnostic US or computed tomography (CT). In dogs with cutaneous MCT or soft tissue sarcomas the extent of local tumor margins was upgraded in 19% and 65% of cases when imaged by US and CT, respectively.[142] Such information allows more appropriate planning of definitive surgery or RT. The cost-effectiveness of such a study depends on the location of the tumor and whether wide excision is technically simple or difficult.

With respect to evaluation of buffy coat smears for evidence of systemic MC disease, peripheral mastocytosis (1–90 MCs/μL) is reported in dogs with acute inflammatory disease (in particular parvoviral infections), inflammatory skin disease, regenerative anemias, neoplasia other than MCT, and trauma.[143–145] One study revealed that peripheral mastocytosis is actually more likely to occur and may be more dramatic in dogs with diseases other than MCT.[144] Therefore this test is no longer routinely performed in the staging of MCT patients. In a report evaluating 157 dogs with MCT, the incidence of bone marrow infiltration at initial staging was only 2.8%.[146] Although the presence of bone marrow involvement is indicative of systemic MC disease, it is usually easier to find evidence of systemic involvement in other organs (liver, spleen).[68] This is in contrast to dogs that present with visceral MCT, in which 37% of buffy coat smears are positive for MC and 56% of bone marrow aspirates reveal MC dissemination[128]; however, these constitute a small minority of all MCT cases. Therefore with the exception of the extremely rare case of primary mastocytic leukemia,[147,148] involvement of bone marrow or peripheral blood in the absence of disease in regional LN or abdominal organs is unlikely and the routine performance of bone marrow aspirates for clinical staging has fallen out of favor.[146]

Treatment

Treatment decisions are predicated on the presence or absence of negative prognostic factors and on the clinical stage of disease. In tumors localized to the skin in areas amenable to wide excision, surgery is the treatment of choice. Historically, surgical excision to include a 3-cm margin of surrounding normal tissue has been recommended. However, this recommendation was largely anecdotal. More recently, surgical margins have been evaluated for the excision of low- and intermediate-grade MCTs less than 5 cm diameter, and two different approaches have been described. The metric approach uses a prescribed metric distance, with lateral margins of 1 cm and 2 cm for low- and intermediate-grade MCTs, respectively.[149,150] The proportional approach uses lateral margins proportional to the maximum dimension of the MCT.[151] For both approaches, deep margins include removal of one uninvolved fascial plane in continuity with the tumor. If necessary, muscle layers may also be removed deep to the tumor. In 100 dogs with 115 resectable MCT (primarily low- and intermediate-grade), no local recurrence or metastasis was noted for greater than 2 years after excision with lateral histologic margins 10 mm or greater and deep histologic margins 4 mm or greater,[83] although the "quality" of the margin (e.g., fascia vs loose connective tissue vs fat) needs to be considered for deep margin evaluation. It should be noted that these microscopic, formalin-fixed margin parameters may not accurately reflect margin size at surgery; tissue shrinkage (up to 30% for cutaneous tissues) can occur subsequent to formalin fixation.[152–154] Considering that the majority of naïve dermal MCTs encountered in practice are of low or intermediate grade, it can be

said that most MCTs can be adequately treated with surgery alone provided the site is amenable to adequate surgical resection. All surgical margins should be evaluated histologically for completeness of excision. For tumors in which wide surgical excision is not possible because of size, geographic constraints, or owner concerns, a biopsy to determine histologic grade maybe helpful before definitive therapy to determine whether smaller lateral margins may be sufficient for complete histologic excision (i.e., 1 cm lateral margins for a low-grade MCTs).

The management of MCTs in locations where primary closure after wide excision is difficult to impossible, such as the distal extremities, can be challenging. Options include tailoring the surgical approach according to preoperative determination of histologic grade, wide excision followed by reconstruction of the subsequent defect, limb amputation, and primary closure of a marginally excised MCTs followed by either RT or chemotherapy. Histologic grade can be accurately diagnosed based on preoperative biopsies,[155] and histologic grade can be used to determine the lateral margins required for complete histologic excision of low- to intermediate-grade MCTs; 1-cm and 2-cm lateral margins are usually sufficient for grade I and grade II MCTs, respectively.[149] If primary closure is not possible regardless of the width of the lateral margins, then the two basic options include wide excision, with or without chemotherapy depending on histologic grading, or marginal excision followed by adjuvant therapy. Wide excision with 2-cm lateral margins,[149,150] or proportional lateral margins[151] is still feasible despite an inability to close the resultant defect primarily. Options for management of these defects include closure with random or axial pattern flaps or free-meshed skin grafts, or healing by second intention. In one study of 31 dogs managed with second-intention healing after excision of soft tissue sarcomas with 2-cm lateral margins, 93.5% of resulting wounds healed completely after a median time of 53 days.[156] Limb amputation is the most aggressive option; however, although wide margins are guaranteed, it results in the least functional outcome and is generally not recommended given the availability of other effective therapies.

Marginal excision of low- to intermediate-grade MCTs is also an acceptable approach if followed by treatment with RT. In this situation, the MCT must be able to be excised with no evidence of gross residual disease and the wound closed primarily. If this is possible, then adjuvant RT is associated with long-term tumor control. Two-year control rates of 85% to 95% can be expected for stage 0 tumors of low- or intermediate-grade MCTs.[110,123,157–159] If RT is either not available or declined, then two studies have demonstrated a low rate of recurrence in dogs with incompletely excised MCTs that receive some form of postoperative chemotherapy[160,161]; however, both studies were single-arm retrospective studies with low case numbers and hence these results should be regarded with caution. There is also information to suggest that some low- or intermediate-grade MCTs will not recur even if no adjuvant therapy is employed.[162] Although this approach is not considered optimal, it can be used in cases in which RT is unavailable or unaffordable. Regardless of the local therapy chosen, dogs with low- and intermediate-grade tumors should be reevaluated regularly (so-called *active surveillance*) for local recurrence and regional and distant metastasis. Local site and regional LN evaluation, complete physical examination, and FNA of any new cutaneous masses or enlarged LNs are performed at these intervals. More complete staging, including abdominal US, should be included if the dog has an MCT with negative prognostic factors.

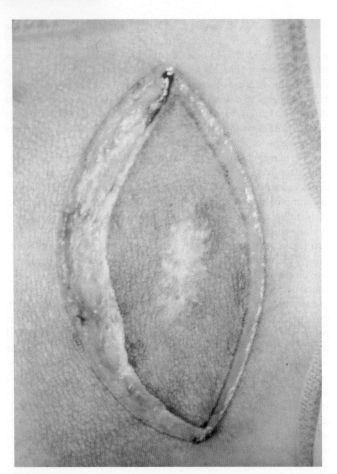

• **Fig. 21.6** Reexcision of a mast cell tumor from the skin of a golden retriever. The first surgery resulted in incomplete surgical margins. Three-cm margins are taken around and deep to the previous incision and the entire sample is again submitted for margin analysis by the pathologist.

Some authors advocate prophylactic irradiation of cytologically negative regional LNs (prophylactic nodal irradiation [PNI]).[114,123,124,163] Owing to the generally low risk of postsurgical metastasis in low- to intermediate-grade tumors, PNI is probably unwarranted in this group of patients, and at least one study has demonstrated no advantage in terms of disease-free or overall survival when PNI is employed[159]; however, in MCTs at high risk for metastasis, PNI may provide improvement in outcome over local site irradiation only.[114,163]

For cases in which planned curative excisional surgery is unsuccessful and histologic margins are incomplete, further local therapy is generally warranted. If possible, a second excision of the surgical scar with additional wide margins should be performed (Fig. 21.6); however, some evidence suggests that marginal, "staging" reexcision of dirty surgical scars may be associated with an acceptable likelihood of achieving tumor-free margins.[78,162,164] Alternatively, adjuvant RT can be used in cases in which reexcision is not an option. Not all MCTs with surgically incomplete margins will recur; in some studies only 10% to 30% of MCTs with histologically confirmed incomplete margins did so.[92,162,165] One study suggests that measurement of proliferation indices (Ki67 and PCNA) via IHC may be useful in predicting likelihood of recurrence after incomplete resection of intermediate-grade MCTs.[92] Although recurrence rates vary by study, several studies have demonstrated increased local recurrence rates and/or decreased overall STs in dogs with incompletely resected MCTs.[28,78,80,120] Fig. 21.7 summarizes the treatment recommendations for clinical stage 0 and I, histologically low- or intermediate-grade MCTs.

Alternative local therapies for MCTs have been reported and include hyperthermia in combination with RT,[166] intralesional brachytherapy,[167] photodynamic therapy,[168,169] intralesional corticosteroids,[170,171] cryotherapy, and electrochemotherapy.[172–175] Although some have advocated the use of intralesional deionized water at the site of an incompletely excised MCT, clinical data indicate that this approach is not effective at preventing local

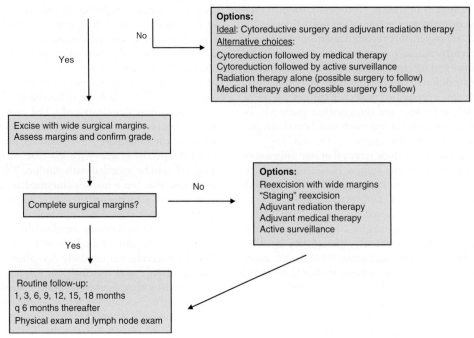

• **Fig. 21.7** Suggested treatment approach for clinical stage 0 and 1 canine mast cell tumors of low or intermediate grade.

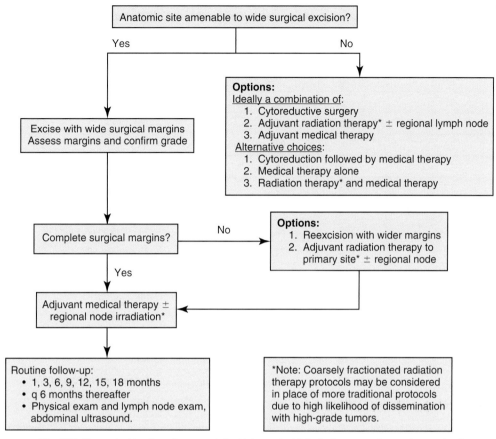

• **Fig. 21.8** Suggested treatment approach for high-grade, biologically aggressive canine mast cell tumors.

recurrence and therefore should not be used.[176–181] It is important to note that none of these alternative local therapies are as thoroughly investigated, clinically effective, or practical as surgery, RT, or a combination of the two. Lastly, despite its common use, there are no published studies to suggest that adjuvant corticosteroid or antihistamine therapy is of benefit in cases of individual intermediate-grade MCTs that have been either excised completely or treated with postoperative RT.

The treatment of anaplastic or undifferentiated MCTs remains frustrating. This designation includes dogs with intermediate-grade tumors with regional or distant metastasis, high-grade tumors, MCTs with high proliferative activity as assessed by special stains, and mucous membrane or mucocutaneous junction MCTs. There is some evidence to suggest that intermediate-grade tumors with only regional LN involvement have a better prognosis than high-grade tumors.[113,114] In the authors' opinion, until convincing evidence exists, such tumors should still be treated as if they have a high potential for metastasis. Fig. 21.8 summarizes the treatment recommendations for high-grade MCTs. The long-term prognosis for such dogs is less favorable, as regional and distant metastasis is more likely.

Poorly differentiated and metastatic MCT will, in most instances, progress to kill the dog in the absence of effective postsurgical intervention. Systemic adjuvant therapy should be offered in such cases in an attempt to decrease the likelihood of systemic involvement, or at least potentially improve DFIs. Corticosteroids, such as prednisone, have been reported for many years in preclinical or anecdotal settings to be of some benefit.[182–186] Although

corticosteroids can inhibit canine MCT proliferation and induce tumor cell apoptosis in vitro,[187] they may also contribute to apparent antitumor response by decreasing peritumoral edema and inflammation. The Veterinary Cooperative Oncology Group (VCOG) studied the efficacy of single-agent systemic prednisone therapy for intermediate- and high-grade canine MCTs.[186] Of 21 dogs receiving 1 mg/kg daily PO, only one complete response (CR) and four partial responses (PRs) were noted, and these were short lived, lasting only a few weeks in the majority of cases. More recent studies have reported 70% to 75% response rates; however, tumors were excised or irradiated after short-term prednisone treatment and thus duration of response was not evaluable.[185,188] One report found that response of MCTs to corticosteroids was dependent on expression of the glucocorticoid receptor; those dogs with tumors that expressed low levels of receptor had MCTs that were resistant to prednisolone therapy.[189] These data suggest that a subset of MCTs may indeed benefit from corticosteroid therapy if there is adequate expression of the glucocorticoid receptor.

Recently a number of studies have evaluated the response rates of measurable canine MCTs to various cytotoxic chemotherapy drugs and protocols (see Table 21.6).[32,120,125,190–196] Objective response rates as high as 64% have been reported, and accumulating evidence suggests that multiagent protocols may confer a higher response rate than single-agent therapy.[32,120,125,193,195,197] It is important to note that, in most instances, the response of bulky MCT to any chemotherapy protocol tends to be short lived, stressing the need for local control of disease before the institution of adjuvant therapy.

TABLE 21.6   Responses to Available Agents in Measurable Canine Mast Cell Tumors

Agent(s)	Number Treated	% CR	% PR	% ORR	Median Response Duration	Reference
Prednisone	25	4	16	20	NR	195
Vincristine	27	0	7	7	NR	198
CCNU	21	6	38	44	79 days[a]	199
Pred/VBL	17	33	13	47	154 days	128
Pred/VBL	28	4	39	43	NR	292
P/C/V	11	18	45	63	74 days	134
COP-HU	17	23	35	59	53 days	34
Pred/VBL/CCNU	37	24	32	57	52 weeks	201
Pred/VBL/CCNU	17	29	35	64	141 days/66 days (CR/PR)	204
Hydroxyurea	46	4	24	28	46 days (for PRs)	200
Pred/chlorambucil	21	14	24	38	533 days	203
Toceranib	60	17	46	63	NR	292
Toceranib	145	14	28	43	12 weeks	214
Masitinib	39	38	44	82	NR	293
Masitinib	161	26	29	55	NR	216
Toceranib/CCNU	41	10	36	46	Not reached/132 days (CR/PR)	222
Toceranib/VBL	14	14	57	71	NR	224

CCNU, Lomustine; *COP-HU*, cyclophosphamide/vincristine/prednisone/hydroxyurea; *CR*, complete response; *NR*, not reported; *ORR*, overall response rate; *P/C/V*, prednisone/cyclophosphamide/vinblastine; *PR*, partial response; *Pred*, prednisone; *VBL*, vinblastine.

[a]Excludes patient that experienced a CR; euthanized without evidence of disease after 440 days.

A few single-arm studies have attempted to evaluate the efficacy of chemotherapy for "high-risk" MCT in the postsurgical setting. One study evaluated the use of postoperative prednisone and vinblastine (VBL) for dogs with MCTs considered to be at high risk for metastasis (LN positive, mucous membrane origin, or high histologic grade). In this study, dogs with high-grade MCTs had an MST of 1374 days.[114] A second study reported 70% 1- and 2-year disease-free survival rates after prednisone–VBL in dogs with high-grade MCTs.[198] A combination of prednisone, lomustine, and VBL has been used for residual microscopic disease in dogs at high risk for dissemination. Dogs with microscopic disease had a median progression-free ST of 35 weeks and an overall ST of 48 weeks.[193] Combination therapy using cyclophosphamide, VBL, and prednisone also yielded promising results in the microscopic residual disease setting for dogs considered at high risk of recurrence or metastasis. The reported progression-free and overall STs were 865 days and >2092 days, respectively.[125] Most studies described earlier used a dose of 2 mg/m² of VBL. There is now information suggesting that dogs may tolerate higher doses[199–202]; however, it remains to be seen if dose-escalation of VBL will translate into improved efficacy.

As previously discussed, virtually all canine MC neoplasms express the KIT RTK, and a large minority of canine MCT (20%–40%) possess a mutation in the c-*kit* gene, which renders the KIT protein constitutively active.[43,46,50,203] Orally available molecules have been developed that inhibit signaling through KIT called small molecule tyrosine kinase inhibitors (TKIs). The two veterinary-approved TKIs in this class are toceranib (TOC;

Palladia, Zoetis) and masitinib (MAS; Masivet, AB Science), and limited studies have also been performed with the human KIT inhibitor imatinib (Gleevec, Novartis).

After encouraging in vitro and early-phase clinical trials,[47,204,205] a multicenter, placebo-controlled, double-blind, randomized study of TOC was performed in dogs with recurrent or metastatic intermediate- or high-grade MCTs.[206] During the blinded phase of the study, the objective response rate in TOC-treated dogs (n = 86) was 37.2% (7 CRs and 25 PRs) versus 7.9% (5 PRs) in placebo-treated dogs. When all 145 dogs that received TOC were analyzed, including those in which placebo was switched to TOC, the objective response rate was 42.8% (21 CRs and 41 PRs) with an additional 16 dogs experiencing stable disease for an overall biologic activity of 60%.[206] The median duration of objective response and time to tumor progression were 12.0 and 18.1 weeks, respectively.[206] Interestingly, dogs whose MCT harbored activating mutations in the c-*kit* gene were roughly twice as likely to respond to TOC than those with wild-type c-*kit* (69% vs 37%), although more recent studies have failed to confirm a higher response rate to TOC in c-*kit* mutant MCT.[129,207] In fact, TOC-treated c-*kit* mutant MCTs had an inferior PFS time compared with *c-kit* wild-type MCT (hazard ratio = 2.34) in one study.[207] GI toxicity, in the form of hyporexia, weight loss, diarrhea, and occasionally vomiting or melena, were the most common adverse effects and were generally manageable with symptomatic therapy, drug holidays, and dosage reductions as necessary. Hypertension, generally manageable with standard hypertensive agents (e.g., enalapril, amlodipine), has also been reported after initiation of TOC therapy in dogs and blood pressure monitoring and intervention is advised.[208] Other adverse effects reported include mild to moderate leukopenia, proteinuria (with or without hypertension), and muscle pain.[206,208] Recent clinical experience with TOC suggests that equivalent antitumor activity and reduced adverse effects may be observed if dosages lower than the label dosage are employed. A dosage of 2.5 to 2.75 mg/kg every other day or 3 days per week (Monday, Wednesday, Friday) is currently used by many oncologists.[209]

A clinical trial of similar design was completed with MAS in dogs with recurrent or unresectable MCT.[210] This study demonstrated significantly improved time to progression in MAS-treated dogs versus placebo-treated dogs, and, again, outcome was improved in dogs with MCT harboring activating c-kit mutations. Subsequent follow-up of patients treated with long-term MAS identified an increased number of patients with long-term disease control compared with those treated with placebo (40% vs 15% alive at 2 years),[211] underscoring the potential for long-term disease stabilization with TKIs. GI adverse effects (vomiting or diarrhea) were most common but were mild and self-limiting in the majority of cases. Myelosuppression was also observed and was mild in most cases. A small percentage of dogs developed a protein-losing nephropathy leading to edema. Increases in urea and creatinine were observed in some dogs, and hemolytic anemia was also observed rarely.[210]

Lastly, small studies have evaluated the efficacy of imatinib for the treatment of measurable canine MCT.[212-214] Imatinib was well tolerated and objective antitumor responses were observed in dogs with both c-kit mutant and wild-type MCTs. It is important to note that no studies have yet been performed in dogs with MCTs to assess the pharmacokinetics of imatinib, and thus current dosing recommendations are based on observed clinical activity, not pharmacokinetic and pharmacodynamic relationships.

There are now several published studies regarding the safety and efficacy of combination therapy with KIT inhibitors and standard forms of therapy, such as RT or cytotoxic chemotherapy; however, evidence of benefit when used in the postoperative setting has yet to be demonstrated. Combinations of continuously or intermittently administered TOC with lomustine and VBL have been evaluated.[215-218] In all of these studies, significant reductions in chemotherapy drug dosage and/or frequency were required to avoid additive myelosuppression. Another study investigated the combination of TOC, prednisone, and hypofractionated RT in dogs with unresectable and/or metastatic MCTs. The overall response rate was 76.4%, with 58.8% of dogs achieving CRs and 17.6% PRs. The overall MST was not reached with a median follow-up of 374 days. The combination of hypofractionated RT and TOC was well tolerated and demonstrated efficacy in the majority of dogs, indicating that this may be a viable treatment option for dogs with unresectable MCTs.[219]

Novel medical approaches that may hold promise for the future treatment of MCT include JAK2/STAT5 inhibitors,[220] histone deacetylase inhibitors,[221-223] HSP90 inhibitors,[224,225] retinoids,[226-228] TRAIL,[229] and polo-like kinase-1 inhibitors.[230] A recent study evaluated a KIT-targeting monoclonal antibody for the treatment of canine MCT; KIT protein activation was blocked in vivo and multiple objective responses were observed.[231]

Ancillary therapy to address the systemic effects of MC mediators is sometimes warranted in dogs with MCT. Minimizing the effects of histamine release can be accomplished by administering the H_1 blockers diphenhydramine (2–4 mg/kg PO q12hrs) or chlorpheniramine (0.22–0.5 mg/kg q8hrs) and the H_2 blockers

cimetidine (4–5.5 mg/kg PO q8hrs), famotidine (0.5–1 mg/kg q12hrs), or ranitidine (2 mg/kg q12hrs). Omeprazole (0.5–1 mg/kg q12–24hrs), a proton pump inhibitor, may be more effective, particularly in the setting of bulky MC disease. These agents are generally used in the setting of gross disease, particularly those cases in which (1) systemic signs are present; (2) the tumor is likely to be entered or manipulated at surgery (i.e., cytoreductive surgery); or (3) treatment is undertaken where gross disease will remain and degranulation is likely to occur in situ (e.g., RT or medical therapy for tumors that are not surgically cytoreduced). For cases with active evidence of GI ulceration, the addition of sucralfate (0.5–1.0 g PO q8hrs) and occasionally misoprostol (2–4 µg/kg PO q8hrs) to histamine blockers is prudent. Some experimental data suggest that the use of H_1 and H_2 blockers could also be beneficial for the prevention or resolution of histamine-mediated wound breakdown,[232-234] but this has not been systematically evaluated. The use of protamine sulfate, a heparin antagonist, has been mentioned by some for use in cases of severe hemorrhage.[128]

Feline Mast Cell Tumors

Unlike MCTs in the dog, which are primarily cutaneous/subcutaneous in nature, MCTs in the cat typically occur in three distinct syndromes, although there is some overlap among them. These are cutaneous MCT, splenic/visceral MC disease, and intestinal MCT. The etiology of feline MCT is currently unknown and appears unrelated to viral infection[235]; however, it is now evident that feline MCTs also possess somatic activating mutations in c-kit.[175,236-238] In one study, 42 of 62 (67%) of cutaneous and splenic/visceral MCT had c-kit mutations that were primarily present in exons 8 (28/62) and 9 (15/62), both of which encode the fifth immunoglobulin domain of KIT.[239] Similar to the canine juxtamembrane domain mutations, these feline c-kit mutations induce ligand independent activation of KIT, which can be inhibited by imatinib in vitro.[238]

The granules present in feline MCTs stain blue with Giemsa and purple with toluidine blue.[1,2,4] As in the dog, granules present in feline MCs contain vasoactive substances such as heparin and histamine.[2,240] In culture, feline MCs express surface-bound immunoglobulins and are capable of secreting histamine, heparin, and probably other vasoactive compounds when appropriately stimulated.[240] Feline MCs also have phagocytic capability and can endocytose erythrocytes in both experimental models and in clinical samples.[241] Complications associated with degranulation of MCTs can also occur in the cat, including coagulation disorders, GI ulceration, and anaphylactoid reactions.[2,242,243] Given that the biologic behaviors of the three feline MCT syndromes are different, they will be described individually.

Cutaneous Feline Mast Cell Tumors

MCTs represent the second most common cutaneous tumors in the cat, accounting for approximately 20% of cutaneous tumors in cats in the United States.[2,4,12] The incidence of MCTs in cats appears to have increased dramatically since 1950.[2] Interestingly, MCTs appear to occur much less frequently in the United Kingdom than in the United States, accounting for only 8% of all cutaneous tumors.[1] The typical feline cutaneous MCT is a solitary, raised, firm, well-circumscribed, hairless, dermal nodule between 0.5 and 3.0 cm in diameter.[2,4,244,245] They are often white in appearance, although a pink erythematous form is occasionally

TABLE 21.7	Histologic Classification of Mast Cell Tumors in Cats	
Type	Subtype	Microscopic Description
Mastocytic	Compact (well-differentiated)	Homogeneous cords and nests of slightly atypical mast cells with basophilic round nuclei, ample eosinophilic cytoplasm and distinct cell borders. Eosinophils conspicuous in only half of cases.
	Diffuse (anaplastic)	Less discrete, infiltrated into subcutis. Larger nuclei (>50% cell diameter), 2–3 mitoses/high-power field. Marked anisocytosis, including mononuclear and multinucleated giant cells. Eosinophils more commonly observed.
Histiocytic		Sheets of histiocyte-like cells with equivocal cytoplasmic granularity. Accompanied by randomly scattered lymphoid aggregates and eosinophils. Granules lacking in some reports, others report granules readily demonstrable.

encountered. Approximately 20% are multiple, although one series reported multiple lesions in the majority of cases.[1] Superficial ulceration is present in approximately 25% of cases. Other clinical forms that have been described include a flat pruritic plaque-like lesion, similar in appearance to eosinophilic plaques, and discrete subcutaneous nodules.

Two distinct types of cutaneous MCTs in the cat have been reported (Table 21.7): (1) the more typical mastocytic MCT, histologically similar to MCT in dogs; and (2) the less common histiocytic MCT, with morphologic features characteristic of histiocytic MC and that may regress spontaneously over a period of 4 to 24 months.[239,245] An overall mean age of 8 to 9 years is reported for cats with MCTs; however, the mastocytic and histiocytic forms occur at mean ages of 10.0 and 2.4 years, respectively.[2,4,244] Siamese cats appear to be predisposed to development of MCT of both histologic types.[2,4,239,244,245] The histiocytic form of MCT in cats is reported to occur primarily in young (<4 years of age) Siamese cats, including two related litters.[239] In contrast to these reports, Siamese cats were not more likely to develop the histiocytic form of MCT than the mastocytic form in another series of cases.[4] Earlier studies reported a male predilection for development of MCT[243,244]; however, larger, more recent series have failed to confirm this predilection.[2,4]

The mastocytic form can be further subdivided on histologic appearance into two categories, previously referred to as compact (representing 50%–90% of all cases) and diffuse (histologically anaplastic), which may have prognostic significance.[2,239,246] Well-differentiated compact tumors tend to behave in a benign manner and metastasis is uncommon.[244,247,248] In contrast, anaplastic tumors may have a high MI, marked cellular and nuclear pleomorphism, and infiltration into the subcutaneous tissues.[245] Although these have been reported to behave in a more malignant manner with metastasis to LNs and the abdomen, a more recent study evaluating pleomorphic cutaneous MCTs from 15 cats found that the majority were behaviorally benign, with only one cat euthanized because of disease progression.[249]

Unlike in the dog, the head and neck are the most common site for MCTs in the cat, followed by the trunk, limbs, and miscellaneous sites (Fig. 21.9A, B).[2,4,244] Those on the head often involve the pinnae near the base of the ear. They rarely occur in the oral cavity. Intermittent pruritus and erythema are common, and self-trauma or vascular compromise may result in ulceration. Darier's sign, the erythema and wheal formation after mechanical manipulation of the tumor, has been reported in the cat.[243] Affected cats are usually otherwise healthy. The spontaneously regressing histiocytic form of cutaneous MCT usually presents as multiple, nonpruritic, firm, hairless, pink, and sometimes ulcerated subcutaneous nodules (Fig. 21.10).[4,239]

As with canine tumors, most feline MCTs are usually easily diagnosed by cytologic examination of FNAs. In contrast, the uncommon histiocytic form of feline MCT is more challenging to diagnose both by FNA and histopathology.[239,245] MCs may comprise only 20% of the cells present, with the majority being sheets of histiocytes that lack distinct cytoplasmic granules and are accompanied by randomly scattered lymphoid aggregates and eosinophils. In contrast, one report readily demonstrated metachromatic granules in seven cases of the histiocytic subtype. These tumors can be initially misdiagnosed as granulomatous nodular panniculitis or deep dermatitis.

Cats with cutaneous MCTs should be evaluated for evidence of additional cutaneous and splenic tumors, as one study found that 3 of 41 cats with cutaneous MCTs also had splenic disease.[247] In addition, a minimum database is recommended along with careful examination of regional LNs for evidence of lymphadenopathy. Interestingly, unlike dogs, cats rarely exhibit evidence of circulating MCs on buffy coat smears when healthy or ill from non–MCT-related causes.[250] In contrast, one study demonstrated that 43% of cats with MC disease had positive buffy coats, although most of these cats tended to have splenic/visceral MCTs.[251]

Feline MCT are usually positive for vimentin, α-1 antitrypsin, and KIT.[252,253] Although the histologic grading system described for canine MCTs has provided no prognostic information for cats in several series and is not used,[243,254] tumors with a high MI appear to be at greatest risk for local recurrence and metastasis, suggesting that this histopathologic feature may be useful for predicting biologic behavior, and as in dogs, a cutoff of 5/10 HPF has been suggested.[245,249,255,256] In recent studies evaluating the prognostic value of histologic and immunohistochemical features in feline cutaneous MCT, MI, and KIT immunoreactivity score/localization were the strongest predictive variables.[255,257,258]

The definitive treatment for cutaneous feline MCT is surgical excision. In a series of 32 cats with cutaneous MCT, five cats developed local recurrence after surgical excision, although none of the cats in this study died of their disease. In this study, completeness of excision and histopathologic factors, such as nuclear pleomorphism and MI, were not associated with tumor recurrence.[248] In a more recent series of cats with MCT of the eyelids, local tumor control in 19 of 23 (83%) cats was achieved with surgery alone and another three cats had local tumor control with surgery and adjuvant RT or cryotherapy; the MST was 945 days.[259] Despite the fact that only 50% of the tumors were completely excised, no cats developed either local tumor recurrence or metastatic disease and only one cat developed disseminated cutaneous tumors.[259] Other reports have demonstrated local recurrence rates after excision between 0% and 24%.[2,244,245,247,249] These data suggest that most cutaneous feline MCTs are behaviorally benign and wide

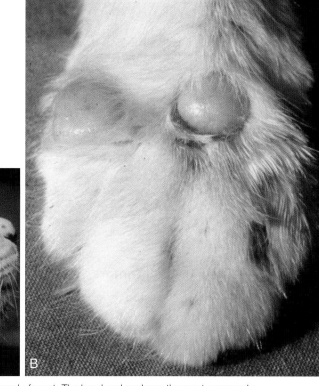

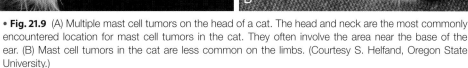

• **Fig. 21.9** (A) Multiple mast cell tumors on the head of a cat. The head and neck are the most commonly encountered location for mast cell tumors in the cat. They often involve the area near the base of the ear. (B) Mast cell tumors in the cat are less common on the limbs. (Courtesy S. Helfand, Oregon State University.)

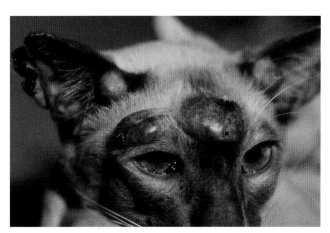

• **Fig. 21.10** Histiocytic mast cell tumors on the head of a young Siamese cat. This form of mast cell tumors in cats typically regress spontaneously, as was the case in the cat pictured here. (Courtesy Dr. K. Moriello, University of Wisconsin–Madison.)

surgical margins may not be as critical as in the dog. Frequency of systemic spread after surgical excision varies from 0% to 22%, although those that metastasize are more likely to be anaplastic tumors.[244,245,247–249] Therefore for histologically anaplastic tumors or those with a high MI more likely recur postoperatively or metastasize, a more aggressive approach similar to that used for canine MCT may be prudent.[249,260] After biopsy confirmation, conservative resection or active surveillance may be taken with the histiocytic form in young cats with multiple masses, as these may spontaneously regress.[2,4,239]

RT may be considered for tumors that are incompletely excised. In one study of feline cutaneous MCT, a 98% control rate was achieved with strontium-90 irradiation with an MST greater than 3 years.[261] Limited information exists concerning the utility of chemotherapy in cats with MCT. It is generally believed that feline MCTs are less responsive to prednisone than dogs; biologic activity of corticosteroids in cats with the histiocytic variant was found to be equivocal.[239] Objective responses to lomustine (CCNU) have been reported in cats.[262,263] Of 20 cats with cutaneous MCTs, two had a CR and eight cats had a PR with lomustine.[263] The authors have observed evidence of clinical activity in cats treated with prednisone and VBL. Some investigators have utilized a combination of prednisone and chlorambucil to treat metastatic or multiple tumors. This is generally well tolerated, although its effectiveness is not known.

Biologic activity of imatinib has been observed in cats with MCT expressing activating mutations in *c-kit,* although the responses were all partial.[237,238,264] Studies in healthy cats have demonstrated that MAS may be safe to administer to clinically normal cats, and plasma concentrations associated with MCT inhibitory activity are likely achievable.[265] Cats should be monitored very closely for neutropenia, proteinuria, and increases in creatinine.[266,267] TOC has been evaluated in multiple feline tumor types, including MCT. Tolerability appears good at the canine label dose and objective responses have been observed in some cats with MCTs.[268,269]

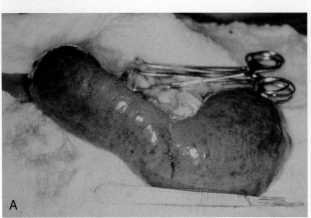 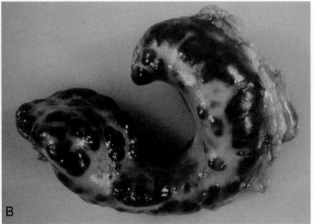

• **Fig. 21.11** (A) Diffuse massive splenomegaly in a cat with splenic mast cell disease. (B) The less common nodular form of splenic mast cell tumor in a cat. (Courtesy D. Vail, University of Wisconsin–Madison.)

Splenic/Visceral Feline Mast Cell Tumors

MCT represents the most common differential for splenic disease in cats, accounting for 15% of submissions in a series of 455 pathologic specimens.[270] This disease affects primarily older animals (mean age, 10 years), with no sex or breed predilection.[2,247,270] The majority of cats with splenic MCTs do not have a history of cutaneous MCT, although recent evidence suggests that some cats with multiple cutaneous MCTs may also have splenic involvement.[247] Although the spleen is the primary site, other organs may also be involved.[2,242] Necropsy data on 30 cats with splenic MCT revealed dissemination in the following organs in decreasing order of frequency: liver (90%), visceral LN (73%), bone marrow (40%), lung (20%), and intestine (17%).[2] Up to one-third of cases have peritoneal and pleural effusions rich in eosinophils and MCs.[2,242] Peripheral blood mastocytosis has been reported in 40% to 100% of cats with peripheral MC counts up to 32,000 cells/μL.[2,251] In one clinical report of 43 cats with splenic MCT, 23% had bone marrow involvement.[242]

Cats with splenic MCTs may present with signs of systemic illness including vomiting, hyporexia, and weight loss.[2,242] Dyspnea may be evident if pleural effusion is present. Abdominal palpation usually reveals a markedly enlarged spleen and/or liver. Other common differential diagnoses for splenomegaly in the cat include lymphoma, myeloproliferative disease, accessory spleen, hemangiosarcoma, hyperplastic nodules, and splenitis.[270] Clinical signs associated with the release of MC mediators, such as GI ulceration, hemorrhage, hypotensive shock, and labored breathing may also be noted. Cats with suspected splenic MCTs should undergo a standard workup including minimum database, abdominal US, and thoracic radiographs. FNA cytology is usually diagnostic for splenic MCT, as is cytologic evaluation of thoracic or abdominal fluid. Anemia is a common hematologic finding, with eosinophilia less likely to be observed.[2,242] In one report of 43 cats with splenic MCTs, 90% had an abnormal coagulation profile, although this did not appear to be of clinical significance.[242]

Splenectomy is the treatment of choice for cats with splenic MCTs, even if involvement of other organs is noted. Pretreatment with H_1 and H_2 blockers before surgery may be indicated to avoid possible anesthetic complications associated with the release of MC mediators. Two gross forms of splenic involvement are possible: a diffuse smooth form and a less common nodular form (Fig. 21.11).[139,271] Surprisingly, even in the face of significant bone marrow and peripheral blood involvement, long-term survival with good quality of life is the norm after splenectomy, with MSTs from 12 to 19 months reported,[2,242,265,272–275] although one study reported an MST of only 132 days after splenectomy.[276] Hyporexia, significant weight loss, and male sex were found to be negative prognostic indicators in one study.[242] Peripheral mastocytosis often declines significantly and may completely resolve after therapy.[274] Cats should be followed postoperatively with complete blood cell counts (CBCs) and peripheral blood smears because an increase in the number of circulating MCs may indicate disease progression. Adjunctive chemotherapy with prednisone, VBL, lomustine, and/or chlorambucil has been attempted in a limited number of cases, but it is not clear if postoperative chemotherapy improves postsplenectomy outcome.[274,275] As discussed earlier, recent data indicate that cats with MCTs may respond to the KIT inhibitors imatinib and TOC.[237,238,268,269]

Feline Intestinal Mast Cell Tumors

Intestinal MCT is the third most common primary intestinal tumor in cats after lymphoma and adenocarcinoma.[2] No breed or sex predilection is known. Older cats appear to be at risk, with a mean age of 13 years; however, cats as young as 3 years have been reported.[277] Most cats have a history of vomiting, diarrhea, and hyporexia, and a solitary palpable abdominal mass is usually evident on physical examination.[2,277] Intestinal MCT more commonly involves the small intestine (equally divided among duodenum, jejunum, and ileum), with colonic involvement reported in fewer than 15% of cases; lesions can be solitary or multiple.[2,277,278] Diarrhea, with or without hematochezia, is commonly observed with the intestinal form, and fever may be present. Affected cats may be ill for several months before diagnosis. As metastasis is common with intestinal MCT, enlarged mesenteric LNs and/or hepatosplenomegaly may be noted. A peritoneal effusion may be present, and this often contains MCs and eosinophils. Diagnosis is usually made by FNA cytology of the mass or involved organs; MCs from intestinal lesions are often less differentiated than those of skin MCTs, and cytoplasmic granules may be less prominent, making diagnosis challenging in certain cases. Cats with intestinal MCT should be staged with a minimum database, thoracic radiographs, and abdominal US, which may be required to determine the extent of intestinal involvement and presence of visceral dissemination. Buffy coat smear may also be performed although, unlike in splenic MCT, peripheral mastocytosis is rarely associated with intestinal MCT and only two reports of peripheral eosinophilia exist in the literature.[277]

Intestinal MCT in cats often carries a poor prognosis because metastasis is common at the time of diagnosis and many cats either die or are euthanized soon after diagnosis.[2,277–279] However, two recent reports totaling 48 cats suggest a more favorable outcome for cats with intestinal MCT.[279,280] MSTs after surgical and/or medical (TKIs/corticosteroids) management were approximately 1.5 years. Histologic differentiation and MI were found to be prognostic, whereas c-*kit* mutation was not prognostic.[279] Surgery is the treatment of choice and wide surgical margins are necessary (5–10 cm), as the tumor typically extends histologically well beyond the gross disease.[2,277] Undifferentiated tumors and those with a MI >2 may have worse postsurgical outcomes.[279] Recently, a variant of feline intestinal MCT, termed sclerosing MCT, was described in 50 cats.[278] Metastatic disease to the LN and/or liver was present in 23 of 36 cats evaluated. Of the 25 cases with clinical follow-up information, 23 died or were euthanized within 2 months of diagnosis.[278] Limited information exists regarding the use of chemotherapy and/or TKIs for the treatment of feline intestinal MCT, although responses to lomustine and TOC have been reported.[263,268]

Comparative Aspects of Mast Cell Tumors

Neoplastic diseases of MCs are rare in people and present as three main clinical entities.[281–285] Cutaneous mastocytosis, also known as urticaria pigmentosa, is a benign disease in which MC infiltration is confined to the skin. It occurs primarily in young children and usually regresses spontaneously before progression into adulthood. Systemic mastocytosis (SM) occurs primarily in adults and includes four major subtypes: (1) indolent SM, the most common form involving mainly skin and bone marrow that does not progress to aggressive disease; (2) a unique subcategory termed SM with an associated non-MC clonal hematologic disease; (3) aggressive SM usually presenting without skin lesions; and (4) MC leukemia, probably representing the rarest variant of human leukemias. Lastly, rare localized extracutaneous MCT (either benign or malignant) have been reported. Dysregulation of KIT is also found commonly in human neoplastic MC diseases and is primarily driven by a point mutation in exon 17 of c-*kit* that induces ligand-independent activation.[282,286] More recently, mutations have also been identified in exons 8 to 11, most of which are also activating.[282,286]

Treatment of the benign human MC disorders is focused primarily on supportive therapy, including H_1 and H_2 antagonists, and topical or systemic therapy with corticosteroids. Unfortunately, an effective treatment protocol for people with aggressive mastocytosis or MC leukemia has not been identified. Treatment with interferon-alpha and/or cladribine is often used, although response rates are typically low.[281,286] Most of the currently available small molecule KIT inhibitors, including imatinib, nilotinib, and dasatinib, have been ineffective in treating human mastocytosis.[286] This may in part be due to the fact that inhibiting phosphorylation of KIT expressing activating exon 17 mutations is extremely challenging. More recently, the protein kinase C inhibitor midostaurin has demonstrated activity in human MC disease.[286]

References

1. Bostock DE: Neoplasms of the skin and subcutaneous tissues in dogs and cats, *Br Vet J* 142:1–19, 1986.
2. Carpenter JL, Andrews LK, Holzworth J: Tumors and tumor-like lesions. In Holzworth J, editor: *Diseases of the cat: medicine and surgery*, Philadelphia, 1987, WB Saunders, pp 406–596.
3. Finnie JW, Bostock DE: Skin neoplasia in dogs, *Aust Vet J* 55:602–604, 1979.
4. Miller MA, Nelson SL, Turk JR, et al.: Cutaneous neoplasia in 340 cats, *Vet Pathol* 28:389–395, 1991.
5. Rothwell TL, Howlett CR, Middleton DJ, et al.: Skin neoplasms of dogs in Sydney, *Aust Vet J* 64:161–164, 1987.
6. Kumar V, Sharma A: Mast cells: emerging sentinel innate immune cells with diverse role in immunity, *Mol Immunol* 48:14–25, 2010.
7. Noviana D, Mamba K, Makimura S, et al.: Distribution, histochemical and enzyme histochemical characterization of mast cells in dogs, *J Mol Histol* 35:123–132, 2004.
8. Metz M, Piliponsky AM, Chen CC, et al.: Mast cells can enhance resistance to snake and honeybee venoms, *Science* 313:526–530, 2006.
9. Lin TY, London CA: A functional comparison of canine and murine bone marrow derived cultured mast cells, *Vet Immunol Immunopathol* 114:320–334, 2006.
10. Lin TY, Rush LJ, London CA: Generation and characterization of bone marrow-derived cultured canine mast cells, *Vet Immunol Immunopathol* 113:37–52, 2006.
11. Lin TY, London CA: Characterization and modulation of canine mast cell derived eicosanoids, *Vet Immunol Immunopathol* 135:118–127, 2010.
12. Brodey RS: Canine and feline neoplasia, *Adv Vet Sci Comp Med* 14:309–354, 1970.
13. Patnaik AK, Ehler WJ, MacEwen EG: Canine cutaneous mast cell tumor: morphologic grading and survival time in 83 dogs, *Vet Pathol* 21:469–474, 1984.
14. Peters JA: Canine mastocytoma: excess risk as related to ancestry, *J Natl Cancer Inst* 42:435–443, 1969.
15. White CR, Hohenhaus AE, Kelsey J, et al.: Cutaneous MCTs: associations with spay/neuter status, breed, body size, and phylogenetic cluster, *J Am Anim Hosp Assoc* 47:210–216, 2011.
16. Arendt ML, Melin M, Tonomura N, et al.: Genome-wide association study of golden retrievers identifies germ-line risk factors predisposing to mast cell tumours, *PLoS Genet* 11:e1005647, 2015.
17. McNiel EA, Prink AL, O'Brien TD: Evaluation of risk and clinical outcome of mast cell tumours in pug dogs, *Vet Comp Oncol* 4:2–8, 2004.
18. Davis BJ, Page R, Sannes PL, et al.: Cutaneous mastocytosis in a dog, *Vet Pathol* 29:363–365, 1992.
19. Dunn TB, Patter H: A transplantable mast cell neoplasm in the mouse, *J Natl Cancer Inst* 18:587–601, 1957.
20. Hottendorf GH, Nielsen SW: Pathologic survey of 300 extirpated canine mastocytomas, *Zentralbl Veterinarmed A* 14:272–281, 1967.
21. Peterson SL: Scar-associated canine mast cell tumor, *Canine Pract* 12:23–29, 1985.
22. Bowles CA, Kerber WT, Rangan SRS, et al.: Characterization of a transplantable, canine, immature mast cell tumor, *Cancer Res* 32:1434–1441, 1972.
23. Lombard LS, Moloney JB: Experimental transmission of mast cell sarcoma in dogs, *Fed Proc* 18:490–495, 1959.
24. Nielson SW, Cole CR: Homologous transplantation of canine neoplasms, *Am J Vet Res* 27:663–672, 1961.
25. Stone JM, Jacky PB, Prieur DJ: Chromosomal fragile site expression in boxer dogs with mast cell tumors, *Am J Med Genetics* 40:223–229, 1991.
26. Ginn PE, Fox LE, Brower JC, et al.: Immunohistochemical detection of p53 tumor-suppressor protein is a poor indicator of prognosis for canine cutaneous mast cell tumors, *Vet Pathol* 37:33–39, 2000.

27. Jaffe MH, Hosgood G, Taylor HW, et al.: Immunohistochemical and clinical evaluation of p53 in canine cutaneous mast cell tumors, *Vet Pathol* 37:40–46, 2000.

28. Ozaki K, Yamagami T, Nomura K, et al.: Mast cell tumors of the gastrointestinal tract in 39 dogs, *Vet Pathol* 39:557–564, 2002.

29. Mayr B, Reifinger M, Brem G, et al.: Cytogenetic, ras, and p53: studies in cases of canine neoplasms (hemangiopericytoma, mastocytoma, histiocytoma, chloroma), *J Hered* 90:124–128, 1999.

30. Wu H, Hayashi T, Inoue M: Immunohistochemical expression of p27 and p21 in canine cutaneous mast cell tumors and histiocytomas, *Vet Pathol* 41:296–299, 2004.

31. Elling H, Ungemach FR: Sexual hormone receptors in canine mast cell tumour cytosol, *J Comp Pathol* 92:629–630, 1982.

32. Gerritsen RJ, Teske E, Kraus JS, et al.: Multi-agent chemotherapy for mast cell tumours in the dog, *Vet Q* 20:28–31, 1998.

33. Da Silva L, Fonseca-Alves CE, Thompson JJ, et al.: Pilot assessment of vascular endothelial growth factor receptors and trafficking pathways in recurrent and metastatic canine subcutaneous mast cell tumours, *Vet Med Sci* 3:146–155, 2017.

34. Thompson JJ, Morrison JA, Pearl DL, et al.: Receptor tyrosine kinase expression profiles in canine cutaneous and subcutaneous mast cell tumors, *Vet Pathol* 53:545–558, 2016.

35. Galli SJ, Zsebo KM, Geissler EN: The kit ligand, stem cell factor, *Adv Immunol* 55:1–95, 1994.

36. Roskoski Jr R: Structure and regulation of Kit protein-tyrosine kinase—the stem cell factor receptor, *Biochem Biophys Res Commun* 338:1307–1315, 2005.

37. Roskoski Jr R: Signaling by Kit protein-tyrosine kinase—the stem cell factor receptor, *Biochem Biophys Res Commun* 337:1–13, 2005.

38. Kiupel M, Webster JD, Kaneene JB, et al.: The use of KIT and tryptase expression patterns as prognostic tools for canine cutaneous mast cell tumors, *Vet Pathol* 41:371–377, 2004.

39. London CA, Kisseberth WC, Galli SJ, et al.: Expression of stem cell factor receptor (c-kit) by the malignant mast cells from spontaneous canine mast cell tumours, *J Comp Pathol* 115:399–414, 1996.

40. Morini M, Bettini G, Preziosi R, et al.: C-kit gene product (CD117) immunoreactivity in canine and feline paraffin sections, *J Histochem Cytochem* 52:705–708, 2004.

41. Reguera MJ, Rabanal RM, Puigdemont A, et al.: Canine mast cell tumors express stem cell factor receptor, *Am J Dermatopathol* 22:49–54, 2000.

42. Halsey CHC, Thamm DH, Weishaar KM, et al.: Expression of phosphorylated KIT in canine mast cell tumor, *Vet Pathol* 54:387–394, 2017.

43. Downing S, Chien MB, Kass PH, et al.: Prevalence and importance of internal tandem duplications in exons 11 and 12 of c-kit in mast cell tumors of dogs, *Am J Vet Res* 63:1718–1723, 2002.

44. Jones CL, Grahn RA, Chien MB, et al.: Detection of c-kit mutations in canine mast cell tumors using fluorescent polyacrylamide gel electrophoresis, *J Vet Diagn Invest* 16:95–100, 2004.

45. Letard S, Yang Y, Hanssens K, et al.: Gain-of-function mutations in the extracellular domain of KIT are common in canine mast cell tumors, *Mol Cancer Res* 6:1137–1145, 2008.

46. London CA, Galli SJ, Yuuki T, et al.: Spontaneous canine mast cell tumors express tandem duplications in the proto-oncogene c-kit, *Exp Hematol* 27:689–697, 1999.

47. London CA, Hannah AL, Zadovoskaya R, et al.: Phase I dose-escalating study of SU11654, a small molecule receptor tyrosine kinase inhibitor, in dogs with spontaneous malignancies, *Clin Cancer Res* 9:2755–2768, 2003.

48. Webster JD, Yuzbasiyan-Gurkan V, Kaneene JB, et al.: The role of c-KIT in tumorigenesis: evaluation in canine cutaneous mast cell tumors, *Neoplasia* 8:104–111, 2006.

49. Webster JD, Yuzbasiyan-Gurkan V, Thamm DH, et al.: Evaluation of prognostic markers for canine mast cell tumors treated with vinblastine and prednisone, *BMC Vet Res* 4:32, 2008.

50. Zemke D, Yamini B, Yuzbasiyan-Gurkan V: Mutations in the juxtamembrane domain of c-KIT are associated with higher grade mast cell tumors in dogs, *Vet Pathol* 39:529–535, 2002.

51. Jark PC, Mundin DB, de Carvalho M, et al.: Genomic copy number variation associated with clinical outcome in canine cutaneous mast cell tumors, *Res Vet Sci* 111:26–30, 2017.

52. Mochizuki H, Thomas R, Moroff S, et al.: Genomic profiling of canine mast cell tumors identifies DNA copy number aberrations associated with KIT mutations and high histological grade, *Chromosome Res* 25:129–143, 2017.

53. Giantin M, Baratto C, Marconato L, et al.: Transcriptomic analysis identified up-regulation of a solute carrier transporter and UDP glucuronosyltransferases in dogs with aggressive cutaneous mast cell tumours, *Vet J* 212:36–43, 2016.

54. Giantin M, Granato A, Baratto C, et al.: Global gene expression analysis of canine cutaneous mast cell tumor: could molecular profiling be useful for subtype classification and prognostication? *PLoS One* 9:e95481, 2014.

55. Schlieben P, Meyer A, Weise C, et al.: Differences in the proteome of high-grade versus low-grade canine cutaneous mast cell tumours, *Vet J* 194:210–214, 2012.

56. Fenger JM, Bear MD, Volinia S, et al.: Overexpression of miR-9 in mast cells is associated with invasive behavior and spontaneous metastasis, *BMC Cancer* 14:84, 2014.

57. Bostock DE: The prognosis following surgical removal of mastocytomas in dogs, *J Small Anim Pract* 14:27–41, 1973.

58. Mullins MN, Dernell WS, Withrow SJ, et al.: Evaluation of prognostic factors associated with outcome in dogs with multiple cutaneous mast cell tumors treated with surgery with and without adjuvant treatment: 54 cases (1998-2004), *J Am Vet Med Assoc* 228:91–95, 2006.

59. Van Pelt DR, Fowler JD, Leighton FA: Multiple cutaneous mast cell tumors in a dog: a case report and brief review, *Can Vet J* 27:259–263, 1986.

60. Cohen D, Reif SS, Brodey RS: Epidemiological analysis of the most prevalent sites and types of canine neoplasia observed in a veterinary hospital, *Cancer Res* 34:2859–2868, 1974.

61. Crowe DT, Goodwin MA, Greene CE: Total laryngectomy for laryngeal mast cell tumor in a dog, *J Am Anim Hosp Assoc* 22:809–816, 1986.

62. Iwata N, Ochiai K, Kadosawa T, et al.: Canine extracutaneous mast-cell tumours consisting of connective tissue mast cells, *J Comp Pathol* 123:306–310, 2000.

63. Patnaik AK, MacEwen EG, Black AP, et al.: Extracutaneous mast-cell tumor in the dog, *Vet Pathol* 19:608–615, 1982.

64. Steffey M, Rassnick KM, Porter B, et al.: Ureteral mast cell tumor in a dog, *J Am Anim Hosp Assoc* 40:82–85, 2004.

65. Moore TW, Bentley RT, Moore SA, et al.: Spinal mast cell tumors in dogs: imaging features and clinical outcome of four cases, *Vet Radiol Ultrasound* 58:44–52, 2017.

66. Davies AP, Hayden DW, Klausner JS, et al.: Noncutaneous systemic mastocytosis and mast cell leukemia in a dog: case report and literature review, *J Am An Hosp Assoc* 17:361–368, 1981.

67. Takahashi T, Kadosawa T, Nagase M, et al.: Visceral mast cell tumors in dogs: 10 cases (1982-1997), *J Am Vet Med Assoc* 216:222–226, 2000.

68. O'Keefe DA, Couto CG, Burke-Schwartz C, et al.: Systemic mastocytosis in 16 dogs, *J Vet Intern Med* 1:75–80, 1987.

69. Moirano SJ, Lima SF, Hume KR, et al.: Association of prognostic features and treatment on survival time of dogs with systemic mastocytosis: a retrospective analysis of 40 dogs, *Vet Comp Oncol* 16:E194–E201, 2018.

70. Pizzoni S, Sabattini S, Stefanello D, et al.: Features and prognostic impact of distant metastases in 45 dogs with de novo stage IV cutaneous mast cell tumours: a prospective study, *Vet Comp Oncol* 16:28–36, 2018.

71. Tams TR, Macy DW: Canine mast cell tumors, *Comp Cont Ed Pract Vet* 27:259–263, 1981.

72. Fox LE, Rosenthal RC, Twedt DC, et al.: Plasma histamine and gastrin concentrations in 17 dogs with mast cell tumors, *J Vet Intern Med* 4:242–246, 1990.

73. Howard EB, Sawa TR, Nielsen SW, et al.: Mastocytoma and gastroduodenal ulceration. Gastric and duodenal ulcers in dogs with mastocytoma, *Pathol Vet* 6:146–158, 1969.

74. Ishiguro T, Kadosawa T, Takagi S, et al.: Relationship of disease progression and plasma histamine concentrations in 11 dogs with mast cell tumors, *J Vet Intern Med* 17:194–198, 2003.

75. Roberts II LJ, Sweetman BJ, Lewis RA, et al.: Increased production of prostaglandin D2 in patients with systemic mastocytosis, *N Engl J Med* 303:1400–1484, 1980.

76. Scott HW, Parris WCV, Sandidge PC, et al.: Hazards in operative management of patients with systemic mastocytosis, *Ann Surg* 197:507–514, 1983.

77. Hottendorf GH, Nielsen SW, Kenyon AJ: Canine mastocytoma: I. Blood coagulation time in dogs with mastocytoma, *Pathol Vet* 2:129–141, 1965.

78. Murphy S, Sparkes AH, Smith KC, et al.: Relationships between the histological grade of cutaneous mast cell tumours in dogs, their survival and the efficacy of surgical resection, *Vet Rec* 154:743–746, 2004.

79. Simoes JP, Schoning P, Butine M: Prognosis of canine mast cell tumors: a comparison of three methods, *Vet Pathol* 31:637–647, 1994.

80. Michels GM, Knapp DW, DeNicola DB, et al.: Prognosis following surgical excision of canine cutaneous mast cell tumors with histopathologically tumor-free versus nontumor-free margins: a retrospective study of 31 cases, *J Am Anim Hosp Assoc* 38:458–466, 2002.

81. Seguin B, Leibman NF, Bregazzi VS, et al.: Clinical outcome of dogs with grade-II mast cell tumors treated with surgery alone: 55 cases (1996-1999), *J Am Vet Med Assoc* 218:1120–1123, 2001.

82. Weisse C, Shofer FS, Sorenmo K: Recurrence rates and sites for grade II canine cutaneous mast cell tumors following complete surgical excision, *J Am Anim Hosp Assoc* 38:71–73, 2002.

83. Schultheiss PC, Gardiner DW, Rao S, et al.: Association of histologic tumor characteristics and size of surgical margins with clinical outcome after surgical removal of cutaneous mast cell tumors in dogs, *J Am Vet Med Assoc* 238:1464–1469, 2011.

84. Hume CT, Kiupel M, Rigatti L, et al.: Outcomes of dogs with grade 3 mast cell tumors: 43 cases (1997-2007), *J Am Anim Hosp Assoc* 47:37–44, 2011.

85. Northrup NC, Harmon BG, Gieger TL, et al.: Variation among pathologists in histologic grading of canine cutaneous mast cell tumors, *J Vet Diagn Invest* 17:245–248, 2005.

86. Northrup NC, Howerth EW, Harmon BG, et al.: Variation among pathologists in the histologic grading of canine cutaneous mast cell tumors with uniform use of a single grading reference, *J Vet Diagn Invest* 17:561–564, 2005.

87. Kiupel M, Webster JD, Bailey KL, et al.: Proposal of a 2-tier histologic grading system for canine cutaneous mast cell tumors to more accurately predict biological behavior, *Vet Pathol* 48:147–155, 2011.

88. Sabattini S, Scarpa F, Berlato D, et al.: Histologic grading of canine mast cell tumor: is 2 better than 3? *Vet Pathol* 52:70–73, 2015.

89. Preziosi R, Sarli G, Paltrinieri M: Prognostic value of intratumoral vessel density in cutaneous mast cell tumors of the dog, *J Comp Pathol* 130:143–151, 2004.

90. Abadie JJ, Amardeilh MA, Delverdier ME: Immunohistochemical detection of proliferating cell nuclear antigen and Ki-67 in mast cell tumors from dogs, *J Am Vet Med Assoc* 215:1629–1634, 1999.

91. Scase TJ, Edwards D, Miller J, et al.: Canine mast cell tumors: correlation of apoptosis and proliferation markers with prognosis, *J Vet Intern Med* 20:151–158, 2006.

92. Seguin B, Besancon MF, McCallan JL, et al.: Recurrence rate, clinical outcome, and cellular proliferation indices as prognostic indicators after incomplete surgical excision of cutaneous grade II mast cell tumors: 28 dogs (1994-2002), *J Vet Intern Med* 20:933–940, 2006.

93. Webster JD, Yuzbasiyan-Gurkan V, Miller RA, et al.: Cellular proliferation in canine cutaneous mast cell tumors: associations with c-KIT and its role in prognostication, *Vet Pathol* 44:298–308, 2007.

94. Maglennon GA, Murphy S, Adams V, et al.: Association of Ki67 index with prognosis for intermediate-grade canine cutaneous mast cell tumours, *Vet Comp Oncol* 6:268–274, 2008.

95. Ozaki K, Yamagami T, Nomura K, et al.: Prognostic significance of surgical margin, Ki-67 and cyclin D1 protein expression in grade II canine cutaneous mast cell tumor, *J Vet Med Sci* 69:1117–1121, 2007.

96. Sakai H, Noda A, Shirai N, et al.: Proliferative activity of canine mast cell tumours evaluated by bromodeoxyuridine incorporation and Ki-67 expression, *J Comp Pathol* 127:233–238, 2002.

97. Thompson JJ, Yager JA, Best SJ, et al.: Canine subcutaneous mast cell tumors: cellular proliferation and KIT expression as prognostic indices, *Vet Pathol* 48:169–181, 2011.

98. Bostock DE, Crocker J, Harris K, et al.: Nucleolar organiser regions as indicators of post-surgical prognosis in canine spontaneous mast cell tumours, *Br J Cancer* 59:915–918, 1989.

99. Kravis LD, Vail DM, Kisseberth WC, et al.: Frequency of argyrophilic nucleolar organizer regions in fine-needle aspirates and biopsy specimens from mast cell tumors in dogs, *J Am Vet Med Assoc* 209:1418–1420, 1996.

100. Romansik EM, Reilly CM, Kass PH, et al.: Mitotic index is predictive for survival for canine cutaneous mast cell tumors, *Vet Pathol* 44:335–341, 2007.

101. Elston L, Sueiro FA, Cavalcanti J, et al.: The importance of the mitotic index as a prognostic factor for canine cutaneous mast cell tumors - a validation study, *Vet Pathol* 46:362–365, 2009.

102. Preziosi R, Sarli G, Paltrinieri M: Multivariate survival analysis of histological parameters and clinical presentation in canine cutaneous mast cell tumours, *Vet Res Commun* 31:287–296, 2007.

103. Thompson JJ, Pearl DL, Yager JA, et al.: Canine subcutaneous mast cell tumor: characterization and prognostic indices, *Vet Pathol* 48:156–168, 2011.

104. Ayl RD, Couto CG, Hammer AS, et al.: Correlation of DNA ploidy to tumor histologic grade, clinical variables, and survival in dogs with mast cell tumors, *Vet Pathol* 29:386–390, 1992.

105. Patruno R, Arpaia N, Gadaleta CD, et al.: VEGF concentration from plasma-activated platelets rich correlates with microvascular density and grading in canine mast cell tumour spontaneous model, *J Cell Mol Med* 13:555–561, 2009.

106. Strefezzi Rde F, Xavier JG, Catao-Dias JL: Morphometry of canine cutaneous mast cell tumors, *Vet Pathol* 40:268–275, 2003.

107. Strefezzi Rde F, Xavier JG, Kleeb SR, et al.: Nuclear morphometry in cytopathology: a prognostic indicator for canine cutaneous mast cell tumors, *J Vet Diagn Invest* 21:821–825, 2009.

108. Webster JD, Kiupel M, Kaneene JB, et al.: The use of KIT and tryptase expression patterns as prognostic tools for canine cutaneous mast cell tumors, *Vet Pathol* 41:371–377, 2004.

109. Bergman PJ, Craft DM, Newman SJ, et al.: Correlation of histologic grading of canine mast cell tumors with Ki67/PCNA/AgNOR/c-Kit scores: 38 cases (2002-2003), *Vet Comp Oncol* 2:98–98, 2004.

110. Turrel JM, Kitchell BE, Miller LM, et al.: Prognostic factors for radiation treatment of mast cell tumor in 85 dogs, *J Am Vet Med Assoc* 193:936–940, 1988.

111. Cahalane AK, Payne S, Barber LG, et al.: Prognostic factors for survival of dogs with inguinal and perineal mast cell tumors treated surgically with or without adjunctive treatment: 68 cases (1994-2002), *J Am Vet Med Assoc* 225:401–408, 2004.

112. Sfiligoi G, Rassnick KM, Scarlett JM, et al.: Outcome of dogs with mast cell tumors in the inguinal or perineal region versus other cutaneous locations: 124 cases (1990-2001), *J Am Vet Med Assoc* 226:1368–1374, 2005.

113. Hillman LA, Garrett LD, de Lorimier LP, et al.: Biological behavior of oral and perioral mast cell tumors in dogs: 44 cases (1996-2006), *J Am Vet Med Assoc* 237:936–942, 2010.

114. Thamm DH, Turek MM, Vail DM: Outcome and prognostic factors following adjuvant prednisone/vinblastine chemotherapy for high-risk canine mast cell tumour: 61 cases, *J Vet Med Sci* 68:581–587, 2006.

115. Gieger TL, Theon AP, Werner JA, et al.: Biologic behavior and prognostic factors for mast cell tumors of the canine muzzle: 24 cases (1990-2001), *J Vet Intern Med* 17:687–692, 2003.

116. Fife M, Blocker T, Fife T, et al.: Canine conjunctival mast cell tumors: a retrospective study, *Vet Ophthalmol* 14:153–160, 2011.

117. Krick EL, Billings AP, Shofer FS, et al.: Cytological lymph node evaluation in dogs with mast cell tumours: association with grade and survival, *Vet Comp Oncol* 7:130–138, 2009.

118. Horta RS, Lavalle GE, Monteiro LN, et al.: Assessment of canine mast cell tumor mortality risk based on clinical, histologic, immunohistochemical, and molecular features, *Vet Pathol* 55:212–223, 2018.

119. Murphy S, Sparkes AH, Blunden AS, et al.: Effects of stage and number of tumours on prognosis of dogs with cutaneous mast cell tumours, *Vet Rec* 158:287–291, 2006.

120. Thamm DH, Mauldin EA, Vail DM: Prednisone and vinblastine chemotherapy for canine mast cell tumor—41 cases (1992-1997), *J Vet Intern Med* 13:491–497, 1999.

121. Kiupel M, Webster JD, Miller RA, et al.: Impact of tumour depth, tumour location and multiple synchronous masses on the prognosis of canine cutaneous mast cell tumours, *J Vet Med A Physiol Pathol Clin Med* 52:280–286, 2005.

122. Zavodovskaya R, Chien MB, London CA: Use of kit internal tandem duplications to establish mast cell tumor clonality in 2 dogs, *J Vet Intern Med* 18:915–917, 2004.

123. LaDue T, Price GS, Dodge R, et al.: Radiation therapy for incompletely resected canine mast cell tumors, *Vet Radiol Ultrasound* 39:57–62, 1998.

124. Chaffin K, Thrall DE: Results of radiation therapy in 19 dogs with cutaneous mast cell tumor and regional lymph node metastasis, *Vet Radiol Ultrasound* 43:392–395, 2002.

125. Camps-Palau MA, Leibman NF, Elmslie R, et al.: Treatment of canine mast cell tumours with vinblastine, cyclophosphamide and prednisone: 35 cases (1997-2004), *Vet Comp Oncol* 5:156–167, 2007.

126. Mochizuki H, Motsinger-Reif A, Bettini C, et al.: Association of breed and histopathological grade in canine mast cell tumours, *Vet Comp Oncol* 15:829–839, 2017.

127. Pollack MJ, Flanders JA, Johnson RC: Disseminated malignant mastocytoma in a dog, *J Am Anim Hosp Assoc* 27:435–440, 1991.

128. O'Keefe DA: Canine mast cell tumors, *Vet Clin North Amer - Sm Anim Pract* 20:1105–1115, 1990.

129. Horta RDS, Giuliano A, Lavalle GE, et al.: Clinical, histological, immunohistochemical and genetic factors associated with measurable response of high-risk canine mast cell tumours to tyrosine kinase inhibitors, *Oncol Lett* 15:129–136, 2018.

130. Clinkenbeard KD: Diagnostic cytology: mast cell tumors, *Comp Cont Ed Pract Vet* 13:1697–1704, 1991.

131. Mederle O, Mederle N, Bocan EV, et al.: VEGF expression in dog mastocytoma, *Rev Med Chir Soc Med Nat Iasi* 114:185–188, 2010.

132. Rabanal RH, Fondevila DM, Montane V, et al.: Immunocytochemical diagnosis of skin tumours of the dog with special reference to undifferentiated types, *Res Vet Sci* 47:129–133, 1989.

133. Sandusky GE, Carlton WW, Wightman KA: Diagnostic immunohistochemistry of canine round cell tumors, *Vet Pathol* 24:495–499, 1987.

134. Camus MS, Priest HL, Koehler JW, et al.: Cytologic criteria for mast cell tumor grading in dogs with evaluation of clinical outcome, *Vet Pathol* 53:1117–1123, 2016.

135. Hergt F, von Bomhard W, Kent MS, et al.: Use of a 2-tier histologic grading system for canine cutaneous mast cell tumors on cytology specimens, *Vet Clin Pathol* 45:477–483, 2016.

136. Scarpa F, Sabattini S, Bettini G: Cytological grading of canine cutaneous mast cell tumours, *Vet Comp Oncol* 14:245–251, 2016.

137. Bookbinder PF, Butt MT, Harvey HJ: Determination of the number of mast cells in lymph node, bone marrow, and buffy coat cytologic specimens from dogs, *J Am Vet Med Assoc* 200:1648–1650, 1992.

138. Weishaar KM, Thamm DH, Worley DR, et al.: Correlation of nodal mast cells with clinical outcome in dogs with mast cell tumour and a proposed classification system for the evaluation of node metastasis, *J Comp Pathol* 151:329–338, 2014.

139. Sato AF, Solano M: Ultrasonographic findings in abdominal mast cell disease: a retrospective study of 19 patients, *Vet Radiol Ultrasound* 45:51–57, 2004.

140. Stefanello D, Valenti P, Faverzani S, et al.: Ultrasound-guided cytology of spleen and liver: a prognostic tool in canine cutaneous mast cell tumor, *J Vet Intern Med* 23:1051–1057, 2009.

141. Book AP, Fidel J, Wills T, et al.: Correlation of ultrasound findings, liver and spleen cytology, and prognosis in the clinical staging of high metastatic risk canine mast cell tumors, *Vet Radiol Ultrasound* 52:548–554, 2011.

142. Hahn KA, Lantz GC, Salisbury SK: Comparison of survey radiography with ultrasonography and X-ray computed tomography for clinical staging of subcutaneous neoplasms in dogs, *J Am Vet Med Assoc* 196:1795–1798, 1990.

143. Cayatte SM, McManus PM, Miller WH, et al.: Identification of mast cells in buffy coat preparations from dogs with inflammatory skin diseases, *J Am Vet Med Assoc* 206:325–326, 1995.

144. McManus PM: Frequency and severity of mastocytemia in dogs with and without mast cell tumors: 120 cases (1995-1997), *J Am Vet Med Assoc* 215:355–357, 1999.

145. Stockham SL, Basel DL, Schmidt DA: Mastocytemia in dogs with acute inflammatory diseases, *Vet Clin Pathol* 15:16–21, 1986.

146. Endicott MM, Charney SC, McKnight JA, et al.: Clinicopathological findings and results of bone marrow aspiration in dogs with cutaneous mast cell tumours: 157 cases (1999-2002), *Vet Comp Oncol* 5:31–37, 2007.

147. Plier ML, MacWilliams PS: Systemic mastocytosis and mast cell leukemia. In Feldman BF, Zinkl JG, Jain NC, editors: *Schalm's veterinary hematology*, ed 5, Philadelphia, 2000, Lippincott Williams & Wilkins, pp 747–754.

148. Hikasa Y, Morita T, Futaoka Y, et al.: Connective tissue-type mast cell leukemia in a dog, *J Vet Med Sci* 62:187–190, 2000.

149. Simpson AM, Ludwig LL, Newman SJ, et al.: Evaluation of surgical margins required for complete excision of cutaneous mast cell tumors in dogs, *J Am Vet Med Assoc* 224:236–240, 2004.

150. Fulcher RP, Ludwig LL, Bergman PJ, et al.: Evaluation of a two-centimeter lateral surgical margin for excision of grade I and grade II cutaneous mast cell tumors in dogs, *J Am Vet Med Assoc* 228:210–215, 2006.

151. Pratschke KM, Atherton MJ, Sillito JA, et al.: Evaluation of a modified proportional margins approach for surgical resection of mast cell tumors in dogs: 40 cases (2008-2012), *J Am Vet Med Assoc* 243:1436–1441, 2013.

152. Johnson RE, Sigman JD, Funk GF, et al.: Quantification of surgical margin shrinkage in the oral cavity, *Head Neck* 19:281–286, 1997.

153. Kerns MJ, Darst MA, Olsen TG, et al.: Shrinkage of cutaneous specimens: formalin or other factors involved? *J Cutan Pathol* 35:1093–1096, 2008.

154. Reimer SB, Seguin B, DeCock HE, et al.: Evaluation of the effect of routine histologic processing on the size of skin samples obtained from dogs, *Am J Vet Res* 66:500–505, 2005.

155. Shaw T, Kudnig ST, Firestone SM: Diagnostic accuracy of pretreatment biopsy for grading cutaneous mast cell tumours in dogs, *Vet Comp Oncol* 16:214–219, 2018.

156. Prpich CY, Santamaria AC, Simcock JO, et al.: Second intention healing after wide local excision of soft tissue sarcomas in the distal aspects of the limbs in dogs: 31 cases (2005-2012), *J Am Vet Med Assoc* 244:187–194, 2014.

157. al-Sarraf R, Mauldin GN, Patnaik AK, et al.: A prospective study of radiation therapy for the treatment of grade 2 mast cell tumors in 32 dogs, *J Vet Intern Med* 10:376–378, 1996.

158. Frimberger AE, Moore AS, LaRue SM, et al.: Radiotherapy of incompletely resected, moderately differentiated mast cell tumors in the dog: 37 cases (1989-1993), *J Am Anim Hosp Assoc* 33:320–324, 1997.
159. Poirier VJ, Adams WM, Forrest LJ, et al.: Radiation therapy for incompletely excised grade II canine mast cell tumors, *J Am Anim Hosp Assoc* 42:430–434, 2006.
160. Hosoya K, Kisseberth WC, Alvarez FJ, et al.: Adjuvant CCNU (lomustine) and prednisone chemotherapy for dogs with incompletely excised grade 2 mast cell tumors, *J Am Anim Hosp Assoc* 45:14–18, 2009.
161. Davies DR, Wyatt KM, Jardine JE, et al.: Vinblastine and prednisolone as adjunctive therapy for canine cutaneous mast cell tumors, *J Am Anim Hosp Assoc* 40:124–130, 2004.
162. Vincenti S, Findji F: Influence of treatment on the outcome of dogs with incompletely excised grade-2 mast cell tumors, *Schweiz Arch Tierheilkd* 159:171–177, 2017.
163. Hahn KA, King GK, Carreras JK: Efficacy of radiation therapy for incompletely resected grade-III mast cell tumors in dogs: 31 cases (1987-1998), *J Am Vet Med Assoc* 224:79–82, 2004.
164. Kry KL, Boston SE: Additional local therapy with primary re-excision or radiation therapy improves survival and local control after incomplete or close surgical excision of mast cell tumors in dogs, *Vet Surg* 43:182–189, 2014.
165. Misdorp W: Incomplete surgery, local immunostimulation, and recurrence of some tumour types in dogs and cats, *Vet Q* 9:279–286, 1987.
166. Lagoretta RA, Denman DL, Kelley MC, et al.: Use of hyperthermia and radiotherapy in treatment of a large mast cell sarcoma in a dog, *J Am Vet Med Assoc* 193:1545–1548, 1988.
167. Northrup NC, Roberts RE, Harrell TW, et al.: Iridium-192 interstitial brachytherapy as adjunctive treatment for canine cutaneous mast cell tumors, *J Am Anim Hosp Assoc* 40:309–315, 2004.
168. Frimberger AE, Moore AS, Cincotta L, et al.: Photodynamic therapy of naturally occurring tumors in animals using a novel benzophenothiazine photosensitizer, *Clin Cancer Res* 4:2207–2218, 1998.
169. Tanabe S, Yamaguchi M, Iijima M, et al.: Fluorescence detection of a new photosensitizer, PAD-S31, in tumour tissues and its use as a photodynamic treatment for skin tumours in dogs and a cat: a preliminary report, *Vet J* 167:286–293, 2004.
170. Rogers KS: Common questions about diagnosing and treating canine mast cell tumors, *Vet Med* 88:246–250, 1993.
171. Case A, Burgess K: Safety and efficacy of intralesional triamcinolone administration for treatment of mast cell tumors in dogs: 23 cases (2005-2011), *J Am Vet Med Assoc* 252:84–91, 2018.
172. Spugnini EP, Vincenzi B, Baldi F, et al.: Adjuvant electrochemotherapy for the treatment of incompletely resected canine mast cell tumors, *Anticancer Res* 26:4585–4589, 2006.
173. Spugnini EP, Vincenzi B, Citro G, et al.: Evaluation of cisplatin as an electrochemotherapy agent for the treatment of incompletely excised mast cell tumors in dogs, *J Vet Intern Med* 25:407–411, 2011.
174. Kodre V, Cemazar M, Pecar J, et al.: Electrochemotherapy compared to surgery for treatment of canine mast cell tumours, *In Vivo* 23:55–62, 2009.
175. Lowe R, Gavazza A, Impellizeri JA, et al.: The treatment of canine mast cell tumors with electrochemotherapy with or without surgical excision, *Vet Comp Oncol* 15:775–784, 2017.
176. Neyens IJ, Kirpensteijn J, Grinwis GC, et al.: Pilot study of intraregional deionised water adjunct therapy for mast cell tumours in dogs, *Vet Rec* 154:90–91, 2004.
177. Grier RL, Di Guardo G, Schaffer CB, et al.: Mast cell tumor destruction by deionized water, *Am J Vet Res* 51:1116–1120, 1990.
178. Grier RL, DiGuardo G, Myers R, et al.: Mast cell tumour destruction in dogs by hypotonic solution, *J Sm An Pract* 36:385–388, 1995.
179. Jaffe MH, Hosgood G, Kerwin SC, et al.: The use of deionized water for the treatment of canine cutaneous mast cell tumors, *Vet Cancer Soc Newsl* 22:9–10, 1998.
180. Jaffe MH, Hosgood G, Kerwin SC, et al.: Deionised water as an adjunct to surgery for the treatment of canine cutaneous mast cell tumours, *J Small Anim Pract* 41:7–11, 2000.
181. Brocks BA, Neyens IJ, Teske E, et al.: Hypotonic water as adjuvant therapy for incompletely resected canine mast cell tumors: a randomized, double-blind, placebo-controlled study, *Vet Surg* 37:472–478, 2008.
182. Asboe-Hanson G: The mast cell: cortisone action on connective tissue, *Proc Soc Exp Biol Med* 80:677–679, 1952.
183. Bloom F: Effect of cortisone on mast cell tumors (mastocytoma) of the dog, *Proc Soc Exp Biol Med* 80:651–654, 1952.
184. Brodey RS, McGrath JT, Martin JE: Preliminary observations on the use of cortisone in canine mast cell sarcoma, *J Am Vet Med Assoc* 123:391–393, 1953.
185. Stanclift RM, Gilson SD: Evaluation of neoadjuvant prednisone administration and surgical excision in treatment of cutaneous mast cell tumors in dogs, *J Am Vet Med Assoc* 232:53–62, 2008.
186. McCaw DL, Miller MA, Ogilvie GK, et al.: Response of canine mast cell tumors to treatment with oral prednisone, *J Vet Intern Med* 8:406–408, 1994.
187. Takahashi T, Kadosawa T, Nagase M, et al.: Inhibitory effects of glucocorticoids on proliferation of canine mast cell tumor, *J Vet Med Sci* 59:995–1001, 1997.
188. Dobson J, Cohen S, Gould S: Treatment of canine mast cell tumours with prednisolone and radiotherapy, *Vet Comp Oncol* 2:132–141, 2004.
189. Matsuda A, Tanaka A, Amagai Y, et al.: Glucocorticoid sensitivity depends on expression levels of glucocorticoid receptors in canine neoplastic mast cells, *Vet Immunol Immunopathol* 144:321–328, 2011.
190. McCaw DL, Miller MA, Bergman PJ, et al.: Vincristine therapy for mast cell tumors in dogs, *J Vet Intern Med* 11:375–378, 1997.
191. Rassnick KM, Moore AS, Williams LE, et al.: Treatment of canine mast cell tumors with CCNU (lomustine), *J Vet Intern Med* 13:601–605, 1999.
192. Rassnick KM, Al-Sarraf R, Bailey DB, et al.: Phase II open-label study of single-agent hydroxyurea for treatment of mast cell tumours in dogs, *Vet Comp Oncol* 8:103–111, 2010.
193. Cooper M, Tsai X, Bennett P: Combination CCNU and vinblastine chemotherapy for canine mast cell tumours: 57 cases, *Vet Comp Oncol* 7:196–206, 2009.
194. Grant IA, Rodriguez CO, Kent MS, et al.: A phase II clinical trial of vinorelbine in dogs with cutaneous mast cell tumors, *J Vet Intern Med* 22:388–393, 2008.
195. Taylor F, Gear R, Hoather T, et al.: Chlorambucil and prednisolone chemotherapy for dogs with inoperable mast cell tumours: 21 cases, *J Small Anim Pract* 50:284–289, 2009.
196. Rassnick KM, Bailey DB, Russell DS, et al.: A phase II study to evaluate the toxicity and efficacy of alternating CCNU and high-dose vinblastine and prednisone (CVP) for treatment of dogs with high-grade, metastatic or nonresectable mast cell tumours, *Vet Comp Oncol* 8:138–152, 2010.
197. Malone EK, Rassnick KM, Wakshlag JJ, et al.: Calcitriol (1,25-dihydroxycholecalciferol) enhances mast cell tumour chemotherapy and receptor tyrosine kinase inhibitor activity in vitro and has single-agent activity against spontaneously occurring canine mast cell tumours, *Vet Comp Oncol* 8:209–220, 2010.
198. Hayes A, Adams V, Smith K, et al.: Vinblastine and prednisolone chemotherapy for surgically excised grade III canine cutaneous mast cell tumours, *Vet Comp Oncol* 5:168–176, 2007.
199. Rassnick KM, Bailey DB, Flory AB, et al.: Efficacy of vinblastine for treatment of canine mast cell tumors, *J Vet Intern Med* 22:1390–1396, 2008.
200. Vickery KR, Wilson H, Vail DM, et al.: Dose-escalating vinblastine for the treatment of canine mast cell tumour, *Vet Comp Oncol* 6:111–119, 2008.
201. Singh J, Rana JS, Sood N, et al.: Clinico-pathological studies on the effect of different anti-neoplastic chemotherapy regimens on transmissible venereal tumours in dogs, *Vet Res Commun* 20:71–81, 1996.

202. Serra Varela JC, Pecceu E, Handel I, et al.: Tolerability of a rapid-escalation vinblastine-prednisolone protocol in dogs with mast cell tumours, *Vet Med Sci* 2:266–280, 2016.

203. Ma Y, Longley BJ, Wang X, et al.: Clustering of activating mutations in c-KIT's juxtamembrane coding region of canine mast cell neoplasms, *J Invest Dermatol* 112:165–170, 1999.

204. Liao AT, Chien MB, Shenoy N, et al.: Inhibition of constitutively active forms of mutant kit by multitargeted indolinone tyrosine kinase inhibitors, *Blood* 100:585–593, 2002.

205. Pryer NK, Lee LB, Zadovaskaya R, et al.: Proof of target for SU11654: inhibition of KIT phosphorylation in canine mast cell tumors, *Clin Cancer Res* 9:5729–5734, 2003.

206. London CA, Malpas PB, Wood-Follis SL, et al.: Multi-center, placebo-controlled, double-blind, randomized study of oral toceranib phosphate (SU11654), a receptor tyrosine kinase inhibitor, for the treatment of dogs with recurrent (either local or distant) mast cell tumor following surgical excision, *Clin Cancer Res* 15:3856–3865, 2009.

207. Weishaar KM, Ehrhart EJ, Avery AC, et al.: c-Kit mutation and localization status as response predictors in mast cell tumors in dogs treated with prednisone and toceranib or vinblastine, *J Vet Intern Med* 32:394–405, 2018.

208. Tjostheim SS, Stepien RL, Markovic LE, et al.: Effects of toceranib phosphate on systolic blood pressure and proteinuria in dogs, *J Vet Intern Med* 30:951–957, 2016.

209. London C, Mathie T, Stingle N, et al.: Preliminary evidence for biologic activity of toceranib phosphate (Palladia((R))) in solid tumours, *Vet Comp Oncol* 10:194–205, 2012.

210. Hahn KA, Ogilvie G, Rusk T, et al.: Masitinib is safe and effective for the treatment of canine mast cell tumors, *J Vet Intern Med* 22:1301–1309, 2008.

211. Hahn KA, Legendre AM, Shaw NG, et al.: Evaluation of 12- and 24-month survival rates after treatment with masitinib in dogs with nonresectable mast cell tumors, *Am J Vet Res* 71:1354–1361, 2010.

212. Isotani M, Ishida N, Tominaga M, et al.: Effect of tyrosine kinase inhibition by imatinib mesylate on mast cell tumors in dogs, *J Vet Intern Med* 22:985–988, 2008.

213. Marconato L, Bettini G, Giacoboni C, et al.: Clinicopathological features and outcome for dogs with mast cell tumors and bone marrow involvement, *J Vet Intern Med* 22:1001–1007, 2008.

214. Yamada O, Kobayashi M, Sugisaki O, et al.: Imatinib elicited a favorable response in a dog with a mast cell tumor carrying a c-kit c.1523A>T mutation via suppression of constitutive KIT activation, *Vet Immunol Immunopathol* 142:101–106, 2011.

215. Bavcar S, de Vos J, Kessler M, et al.: Combination toceranib and lomustine shows frequent high grade toxicities when used for treatment of non-resectable or recurrent mast cell tumours in dogs: a European multicentre study, *Vet J* 224:1–6, 2017.

216. Burton JH, Venable RO, Vail DM, et al.: Pulse-administered toceranib phosphate plus lomustine for treatment of unresectable mast cell tumors in dogs, *J Vet Intern Med* 29:1098–1104, 2015.

217. Pan X, Tsimbas K, Kurzman ID, et al.: Safety evaluation of combination CCNU and continuous toceranib phosphate (Palladia((R))) in tumour-bearing dogs: a phase I dose-finding study, *Vet Comp Oncol* 14:202–209, 2016.

218. Robat C, London C, Bunting L, et al.: Safety evaluation of combination vinblastine and toceranib phosphate (Palladia(R)) in dogs: a phase I dose-finding study, *Vet Comp Oncol* 10:174–183, 2012.

219. Carlsten KS, London CA, Haney S, et al.: Multicenter prospective trial of hypofractionated radiation treatment, toceranib, and prednisone for measurable canine mast cell tumors, *J Vet Intern Med* 26:135–141, 2012.

220. Keller A, Wingelhofer B, Peter B, et al.: The JAK2/STAT5 signaling pathway as a potential therapeutic target in canine mastocytoma, *Vet Comp Oncol* 16:55–68, 2018.

221. Kisseberth WC, Murahari S, London CA, et al.: Evaluation of the effects of histone deacetylase inhibitors on cells from canine cancer cell lines, *Am J Vet Res* 69:938–945, 2008.

222. Lin TY, Fenger J, Murahari S, et al.: AR-42, a novel HDAC inhibitor, exhibits biologic activity against malignant mast cell lines via down-regulation of constitutively activated Kit, *Blood* 115:4217–4225, 2010.

223. Nagamine MK, Sanches DS, Pinello KC, et al.: In vitro inhibitory effect of trichostatin A on canine grade 3 mast cell tumor, *Vet Res Commun* 35:391–399, 2011.

224. Lin TY, Bear M, Du Z, et al.: The novel HSP90 inhibitor STA-9090 exhibits activity against Kit-dependent and -independent malignant mast cell tumors, *Exp Hematol* 36:1266–1277, 2008.

225. London CA, Bear MD, McCleese J, et al.: Phase I evaluation of STA-1474, a prodrug of the novel HSP90 inhibitor ganetespib, in dogs with spontaneous cancer, *PLoS One* 6:e27018, 2011.

226. Pinello KC, Nagamine M, Silva TC, et al.: In vitro chemosensitivity of canine mast cell tumors grades II and III to all-trans-retinoic acid (ATRA), *Vet Res Commun* 33:581–588, 2009.

227. Ohashi E, Miyajima N, Nakagawa T, et al.: Retinoids induce growth inhibition and apoptosis in mast cell tumor cell lines, *J Vet Med Sci* 68:797–802, 2006.

228. Miyajima N, Watanabe M, Ohashi E, et al.: Relationship between retinoic acid receptor alpha gene expression and growth-inhibitory effect of all-trans retinoic acid on canine tumor cells, *J Vet Intern Med* 20:348–354, 2006.

229. Elders RC, Baines SJ, Catchpole B: Susceptibility of the C2 canine mastocytoma cell line to the effects of tumor necrosis factor-related apoptosis-inducing ligand (TRAIL), *Vet Immunol Immunopathol* 130:11–16, 2009.

230. Peter B, Gleixner KV, Cerny-Reiterer S, et al.: Polo-like kinase-1 as a novel target in neoplastic mast cells: demonstration of growth-inhibitory effects of small interfering RNA and the Polo-like kinase-1 targeting drug BI 2536, *Haematologica* 96:672–680, 2011.

231. London CA, Gardner HL, Rippy S, et al.: KTN0158, a humanized anti-KIT monoclonal antibody, demonstrates biologic activity against both normal and malignant canine mast cells, *Clin Cancer Res* 23:2565–2574, 2017.

232. Macy DW: Canine and feline mast cell tumors: biologic behavior, diagnosis, and therapy, *Sem Vet Med Surg (Sm An)* 1:72–83, 1986.

233. Kenyon AJ, Ramos L, Michaels EB: Histamine-induced suppressor macrophage inhibits fibroblast growth and wound healing, *Am J Vet Res* 44:2164–2166, 1983.

234. Huttunen M, Hyttinen M, Nilsson G, et al.: Inhibition of keratinocyte growth in cell culture and whole skin culture by mast cell mediators, *Exp Dermatol* 10:184–192, 2001.

235. Saar C, Opitz M, Lange W, et al.: Mastzellenreitkulose bei katzen, *Berl Munch Tierarztl Wochenschr* 82:438–444, 1969.

236. Hadzijusufovic E, Peter B, Rebuzzi L, et al.: Growth-inhibitory effects of four tyrosine kinase inhibitors on neoplastic feline mast cells exhibiting a Kit exon 8 ITD mutation, *Vet Immunol Immunopathol* 132:243–250, 2009.

237. Isotani M, Tamura K, Yagihara H, et al.: Identification of a c-kit exon 8 internal tandem duplication in a feline mast cell tumor case and its favorable response to the tyrosine kinase inhibitor imatinib mesylate, *Vet Immunol Immunopathol* 114:168–172, 2006.

238. Isotani M, Yamada O, Lachowicz JL, et al.: Mutations in the fifth immunoglobulin-like domain of kit are common and potentially sensitive to imatinib mesylate in feline mast cell tumours, *Br J Haematol* 148:144–153, 2009.

239. Chastain CB, Turk MA, O'Brien D: Benign cutaneous mastocytomas in two litters of Siamese kittens, *J Am Vet Med Assoc* 193:959–960, 1988.

240. Mohr FC, Dunston SK: Culture and initial characterization of the secretory response of neoplastic cat mast cells, *Am J Vet Res* 53:820–828, 1992.

241. Antognoni MT, Spaterna A, Lepri E, et al.: Characteristic clinical, haematological and histopathological findings in feline mastocytoma, *Vet Res Commun* 27(suppl 1):727–730, 2003.

242. Feinmehl R, Matus R, Mauldin GN, et al.: Splenic mast cell tumors in 43 cats (1975-1992), *Proc Annu Conf Vet Cancer Soc* 12:50(abstract) 1992.
243. Macy DW, Reynolds HA: The incidence, characteristics, and clinical management of skin tumors of cats, *J Am An Hosp Assoc* 17:1026–1034, 1981.
244. Buerger RG, Scott DW: Cutaneous mast cell neoplasia in cats: 14 cases (1975-1985), *J Am Vet Med Assoc* 190:1440–1444, 1987.
245. Wilcock BP, Yager JA, Zink MC: The morphology and behavior of feline cutaneous mastocytomas, *Vet Pathol* 23:320–324, 1986.
246. Holzinger EA: Feline cutaneous masocytomas, *Cornell Vet* 63:87–93, 1973.
247. Litster AL, Sorenmo KU: Characterisation of the signalment, clinical and survival characteristics of 41 cats with mast cell neoplasia, *J Feline Med Surg* 8:177–183, 2006.
248. Molander-McCrary H, Henry CJ, Potter K, et al.: Cutaneous mast cell tumors in cats: 32 cases (1991-1994), *J Am Anim Hosp Assoc* 34:281–284, 1998.
249. Johnson TO, Schulman FY, Lipscomb TP, et al.: Histopathology and biologic behavior of pleomorphic cutaneous mast cell tumors in fifteen cats, *Vet Pathol* 39:452–457, 2002.
250. Garrett LD, Craig CL, Szladovits B, et al.: Evaluation of buffy coat smears for circulating mast cells in healthy cats and ill cats without mast cell tumor-related disease, *J Am Vet Med Assoc* 231:1685–1687, 2007.
251. Skeldon NC, Gerber KL, Wilson RJ, et al.: Mastocytaemia in cats: prevalence, detection and quantification methods, haematological associations and potential implications in 30 cats with mast cell tumours, *J Feline Med Surg* 12:960–966, 2010.
252. Rodriguez-Carino C, Fondevila D, Segales J, et al.: Expression of KIT receptor in feline cutaneous mast cell tumors, *Vet Pathol* 46:878–883, 2009.
253. Fondevila D, Rabanal R, Ferrer L: Immunoreactivity of canine and feline mast cell tumors, *Schweiz Arch Tierheilk* 132:409–484, 1990.
254. Buss MS, Mollander H, Potter K, et al.: Predicting survival and prognosis in cats with cutaneous mastocytomas of varying histological grade, *Proc Annu Conf Vet Cancer Soc* 16:56–57(abstract), 1996.
255. Dobromylskyj MJ, Rasotto R, Melville K, et al.: Evaluation of minichromosome maintenance protein 7 and c-kit as prognostic markers in feline cutaneous mast cell tumours, *J Comp Pathol* 153:244–250, 2015.
256. Melville K, Smith KC, Dobromylskyj MJ: Feline cutaneous mast cell tumours: a UK-based study comparing signalment and histological features with long-term outcomes, *J Feline Med Surg* 17:486–493, 2015.
257. Sabattini S, Bettini G: Prognostic value of histologic and immunohistochemical features in feline cutaneous mast cell tumors, *Vet Pathol* 47:643–653, 2010.
258. Sabattini S, Guadagni Frizzon M, Gentilini F, et al.: Prognostic significance of Kit receptor tyrosine kinase dysregulations in feline cutaneous mast cell tumors, *Vet Pathol* 50:797–805, 2013.
259. Montgomery KW, van der Woerdt A, Aquino SM, et al.: Periocular cutaneous mast cell tumors in cats: evaluation of surgical excision (33 cases), *Vet Ophthalmol* 13:26–30, 2010.
260. Lepri E, Ricci G, Leonardi L, et al.: Diagnostic and prognostic features of feline cutaneous mast cell tumours: a retrospective analysis of 40 cases, *Vet Res Commun* 27(suppl 1):707–709, 2003.
261. Turrel JM, Farrelly J, Page RL, et al.: Evaluation of strontium 90 irradiation in treatment of cutaneous mast cell tumors in cats: 35 cases (1992-2002), *J Am Vet Med Assoc* 228:898–901, 2006.
262. Rassnick KM, Gieger TL, Williams LE, et al.: Phase I evaluation of CCNU (lomustine) in tumor-bearing cats, *J Vet Intern Med* 15:196–199, 2001.
263. Rassnick KM, Williams LE, Kristal O, et al.: Lomustine for treatment of mast cell tumors in cats: 38 cases (1999-2005), *J Am Vet Med Assoc* 232:1200–1205, 2008.
264. Lachowicz JL, Post GS, Brodsky E: A phase I clinical trial evaluating imatinib mesylate (Gleevec) in tumor-bearing cats, *J Vet Intern Med* 19:860–864, 2005.
265. Schulman A: Splenic mastocytosis in a cat, *California Vet* 17:17–18, 1987.
266. Bellamy F, Bader T, Moussy A, et al.: Pharmacokinetics of masitinib in cats, *Vet Res Commun* 33:831–837, 2009.
267. Daly M, Sheppard S, Cohen N, et al.: Safety of masitinib mesylate in healthy cats, *J Vet Intern Med* 25:297–302, 2011.
268. Berger EP, Johannes CM, Post GS, et al.: Retrospective evaluation of toceranib phosphate (Palladia) use in cats with mast cell neoplasia, *J Feline Med Surg* 20:95–102, 2018.
269. Harper A, Blackwood L: Toxicity and response in cats with neoplasia treated with toceranib phosphate, *J Feline Med Surg* 19:619–623, 2017.
270. Spangler WL, Culbertson MR: Prevalence and type of splenic diseases in cats: 455 cases (1985-1991), *J Am Vet Med Assoc* 201:773–776, 1992.
271. Hanson JA, Papageorges M, Girard E, et al.: Ultrasonographic appearance of splenic disease in 101 cats, *Vet Radiol Ultrasound* 42:441–445, 2001.
272. Guerre R, Millet P, Groulade P: Systemic mastocytosis in a cat: remission after splenectomy, *J Small Anim Pract* 20:769–772, 1979.
273. Liska WD, MacEwen EG, Zaki FA, et al.: Feline systemic mastocytosis: a review and results of splenectomy in seven cases, *J Am An Hosp Assoc* 15:589–597, 1979.
274. Evans BJ, O'Brien D, Allstadt SD, et al.: Treatment outcomes and prognostic factors of feline splenic mast cell tumors: a multi-institutional retrospective study of 64 cases, *Vet Comp Oncol* 16:20–27, 2018.
275. Kraus KA, Clifford CA, Davis GJ, et al.: Outcome and prognostic indicators in cats undergoing splenectomy for splenic mast cell tumors, *J Am Anim Hosp Assoc* 51:231–238, 2015.
276. Gordon SS, McClaran JK, Bergman PJ, et al.: Outcome following splenectomy in cats, *J Feline Med Surg* 12:256–261, 2010.
277. Bortnowski HB, Rosenthal RC: Gastrointestinal mast cell tumors and eosinophilia in two cats, *J Am An Hosp Assoc* 28:271–275, 1992.
278. Halsey CH, Powers BE, Kamstock DA: Feline intestinal sclerosing mast cell tumour: 50 cases (1997-2008), *Vet Comp Oncol* 8:72–79, 2010.
279. Sabattini S, Giantin M, Barbanera A, et al.: Feline intestinal mast cell tumours: clinicopathological characterisation and KIT mutation analysis, *J Feline Med Surg* 18:280–289, 2016.
280. Barrett LE, Skorupski K, Brown DC, et al.: Outcome following treatment of feline gastrointestinal mast cell tumours, *Vet Comp Oncol* 16:188–193, 2018.
281. Arock M: Valent P: Pathogenesis, classification and treatment of mastocytosis: state of the art in 2010 and future perspectives, *Expert Rev Hematol* 3:497–516, 2010.
282. Bodemer C, Hermine O, Palmerini F, et al.: Pediatric mastocytosis is a clonal disease associated with D816V and other activating c-KIT mutations, *J Invest Dermatol* 130:804–815, 2010.
283. Valent P, Arock M, Akin C, et al.: The classification of systemic mastocytosis should include mast cell leukemia (MCL) and systemic mastocytosis with a clonal hematologic non-mast cell lineage disease (SM-AHNMD), *Blood* 116:850–851, 2010.
284. Horny HP, Sotlar K: Valent P: Mastocytosis: state of the art, *Pathobiology* 74:121–132, 2007.
285. Valent P, Akin C, Escribano L, et al.: Standards and standardization in mastocytosis: consensus statements on diagnostics, treatment recommendations and response criteria, *Eur J Clin Invest* 37:435–453, 2007.
286. Ustun C, Deremer DL, Akin C: Tyrosine kinase inhibitors in the treatment of systemic mastocytosis, *Leuk Res* 35:1143–1152, 2011.

22

Soft Tissue Sarcomas

JULIUS M. LIPTAK AND NEIL I. CHRISTENSEN

Incidence and Risk Factors

Soft tissue sarcomas (STSs) are a heterogeneous population of mesenchymal tumors that comprise 15% and 7% of all skin and subcutaneous tumors in the dog and cat, respectively.[1] The annual incidence of STSs in companion animals is about 35 per 100,000 dogs at risk and 17 per 100,000 cats at risk.[2] In dogs, sarcomas have been associated with radiation, trauma, foreign bodies, orthopedic implants, and the parasite *Spirocerca lupi*.[3–9]

Most STSs are solitary tumors in middle-aged to older dogs and cats, except for rhabdomyosarcomas which occur in young dogs.[10,11] There is no specific breed or sex predilection for STSs. STSs tend to be overrepresented in large-breed dogs.[10]

Pathology and Natural History

STSs are typically regarded as a heterogeneous group of tumors whose classification is based on similar pathologic appearance and clinical behavior; however, this may be an overly simplistic interpretation. Sarcomas arise from mesenchymal tissues and have features similar to those of the cell type of origin. These tumors originate in connective tissues, including muscle, adipose, neurovascular, fascial, and fibrous tissue, and can give rise to benign and malignant entities. STSs can arise at any anatomic location, but they most commonly involve the skin and subcutaneous tissues. For simplicity and consistency, a number of sarcomas arising from soft tissue are excluded from the umbrella term of cutaneous and subcutaneous STSs because of differences in anatomic location, biologic behavior (such as a higher metastatic rate and/or a different distribution of metastasis), and histologic features.[12] These include histiocytic sarcoma (HS), synovial cell sarcoma (SCS), hemangiosarcoma (HSA), lymphangiosarcoma, rhabdomyosarcoma, oral fibrosarcoma (FSA), and peripheral nerve sheath tumors (PNSTs) of the brachial and lumbar plexi.[12] HS, SCS, HSA, and oral FSA are covered in other chapters, with this chapter concentrating primarily on malignant STSs.

The majority of cutaneous and subcutaneous STSs have a similar biologic behavior. This is characterized by a locally expansile mass growing between fascial planes, but STSs can also be infiltrative. STSs are often surrounded by a pseudocapsule formed by the compression of peritumoral connective tissue, which may contain or be confluent with neoplastic tissue.[12,13] Overall, cutaneous and subcutaneous STSs have a low to moderate local recurrence rate after surgical excision, with or without adjuvant radiation therapy (RT), and a low metastatic rate. The likelihood of local recurrence is dependent on tumor size, degree of infiltration, completeness of histologic excision, and histologic grade; the likelihood of metastasis is dependent primarily on histologic grade.

STS is a general term encompassing a heterogenous group of tumors, but STSs can be subclassified according to the tissue of origin or phenotype.[12] These include FSA, perivascular wall tumor (PWT), PNST (nonbrachial plexus), liposarcoma, myxosarcoma, pleomorphic sarcoma (or malignant fibrous histiocytoma), malignant mesenchymoma, and undifferentiated sarcoma.[12,14,15] These can be difficult to differentiate histologically because common components include an intercellular collagen matrix and spindle or fusiform mesenchymal cells forming bundles, streams, and whorls.[12] STSs may be characterized histologically by areas of mature tissue or via immunohistochemistry (IHC) by the expression of certain cellular markers to determine phenotype (Table 22.1).[12,16–21] However, STSs may display more than one histologic pattern, and histologic patterns and IHC features may not be exclusive to a single cell type of origin or phenotype.[12] STSs are sometimes referred to by alternate names such as spindle cell tumors of soft tissue because of the complexity of phenotypic differentiation, the use of the term "sarcoma" for tumors that have a low metastatic potential, and the difficulty in differentiating benign from low-grade malignant variants of some mesenchymal tumors of soft tissue (Table 22.2).[12,22–25] Histologic distinction of tumor type may not be clinically important because most STSs have a similar biologic behavior (i.e., locally aggressive with a low to moderate risk of distant metastasis); however, this may be an overly simplistic approach as there is increasing evidence that discernible differences in presentations and outcomes may exist between different types of STSs.

Specific Tumor Types

Tumors of Fibrous Tissue

Nodular Fasciitis (Fibromatosis, Pseudosarcomatous Fibromatosis)

Nodular fasciitis is a benign nonneoplastic lesion arising from the subcutaneous fascia or superficial portions of the deep fascia in dogs. These lesions are usually nodular, poorly circumscribed, and very invasive.[26] Histologically, nodular fasciitis is characterized by large plump or spindle-shaped fibroblasts in a stromal network of variable amounts of collagen and reticular fibers with scattered lymphocytes, plasma cells, and macrophages.[26] The morphologic and pathologic characteristics of nodular fasciitis can result in these lesions being misdiagnosed as FSA. Infantile desmoid-type

TABLE 22.1	Types of Cutaneous and Subcutaneous Soft Tissue Sarcomas with Distinctions Based on Histogenesis, Phenotype, Histologic Features, and Immunohistochemistry			
Type	Tissue of Origin	Phenotype	Histologic Features	Immunohistochemistry
Fibrosarcoma	Fibrous tissue	Fibroblast, fibrocyte	Interwoven bundles, herringbone pattern, pronounced collagenous stroma	
Myxosarcoma	Fibrous tissue	Fibroblast, fibrocyte	Stellate- or spindle-shaped cells in mucinous stroma	
Pleomorphic sarcoma (malignant fibrous histiocytoma)	Fibrous tissue	Primitive mesenchymal cells (fibroblast or myofibroblast)	Mixture of fibroblastic cells and karyomegalic, cytomegalic, or multinucleate histiocytoid cells in storiform patterns with variable inflammatory infiltrate	Positive: lysozyme (29%–100%), MHC II (70%), desmin (86%), vimentin Negative: S-100, CD18
Perivascular wall tumor	Perivascular wall cells	Pericyte, myopericyte, smooth myocyte	Vascular growth patterns including staghorn, placentoid, perivascular whirling, and bundles from tunica media	Positive: calponin, pan actin, smooth muscle actin (50%) Negative: S-100, NSE, GFAP, myoglobin
Peripheral nerve sheath tumor	Peripheral nerve	Schwann cell, neurofibroblast	Interwoven bundles, whorls around collagen bundles, Antoni A and B patterns	Positive: NSE (45%–82%), S-100 (50%–100%), neurofilament (82%), NGFR (47%), myoglobin (64%), GFAP (0%–35%)
Liposarcoma	Adipose tissue	Lipoblast, lipocyte	Polygonal cells with distinctly vacuolated cytoplasm	Positive: MDM2 (67% of well-differentiated and 75% of dedifferentiated), CDK4 (88% well-differentiated, 71% myxoid, 67% pleomorphic, and 100% dedifferentiated)[84]
Rhabdomyosarcoma	Skeletal muscle	Skeletal myoblast, skeletal mycoyte	Cytoplasmic striation, racket and strap cells	Positive: desmin, S-100 (75%), NSE (50%), GFAP (50%)
Lymphangiosarcoma	Lymph tissue		Irregular, anastomosing, and arborizing vascular channels and trabeculae lined by a single layer of flattened, elongate to plump spindle-shaped cells with scant cytoplasm supported on a collagenous stroma; with lumina characterized by a paucity of erythrocytes.[91]	Positive: *PROX-1* (80%–88%),[90,91] Factor VIII-related antigen (100%), LYVE-1 (80%)[91]
Mesenchymoma	Any mesenchymal tissue	Multiple cell types	Multiple soft tissue mesenchymal cell types and matrix components including osteoid, chondroid, and collagen	

GFAP, Glial fibrillary acidic protein; *LYVE-1*, lymphatic vessel endothelial receptor-1; *MDM2*, mouse double minute 2 homolog; *MHC*, major histocompatibility complex; *NGFR*, nerve growth factor receptor; *NSE*, neuron specific enolase; *PROX-1*, prospero-related homeobox gene 1.
Modified from Dennis et al, *Vet Pathol*, 2011.[12,84,90,91]

TABLE 22.2	Soft Tissue Sarcoma Grading System		
Score	Differentiation	Mitosis[a]	Necrosis
1	Resembles normal adult mesenchymal tissue	0–9	None
2	Specific histologic subtype	10–19	<50% necrosis
3	Undifferentiated	>20	>50% necrosis

Grade I: Cumulative score of ≤4 for the 3 categories.
Grade II: Cumulative score of 5–6.
Grade III: Cumulative score of ≥7.
[a]Mitosis is calculated as the number of mitotic figures/10 HPF.

fibromatosis is a variant of nodular fasciitis and is characterized by fibroblast proliferation with a dense reticular fiber network and mucoid material.[27] Wide excision of both nodular fasciitis and infantile desmoid-type fibromatosis lesions is usually curative.[28] Local recurrence is possible with incomplete resection. These tumors do not metastasize.[26]

Fibrosarcoma

FSAs arise from malignant fibroblasts in any location, but most commonly in the skin, subcutaneous tissue, and oral cavity. Similar to other STSs, FSAs can range from well differentiated to anaplastic.[29] FSAs tend to occur in older dogs and cats with no breed or sex predilection; however, a there was higher predilection in golden retrievers and Doberman pinschers in one study[30] and dogs with FSAs were significantly younger than dogs with other histologic subtypes of STSs in another study.[31] FSAs are more likely to recur after incomplete histologic excision and have higher mitotic rates than other histologic subtypes of STSs[32–35] but, conversely, are more likely to be low grade.[31]

Pleomorphic Sarcoma (or Malignant Fibrous Histiocytoma)

Malignant fibrous histiocytoma (MFH) is a tumor with histologic characteristics resembling histiocytes and fibroblasts.[36] According to the World Health Organization classification of soft tissue tumors, the preferred term for MFH is undifferentiated pleomorphic sarcoma because electron microscopic and IHC analyses of these tumors have shown that the term "fibrohistiocytic" is a misnomer.[37] Pleomorphic sarcomas are typically diagnosed in middle-aged to older dogs. There is no sex predilection, although in one report 70% of dogs with the giant cell variant of pleomorphic sarcoma were female.[38] Flat-coated retrievers, Rottweilers, and golden retrievers are overrepresented.[38,39] Pleomorphic sarcomas is most commonly diagnosed in the subcutaneous tissues of the trunk and pelvic limbs and the spleen in dogs. Computed tomography (CT) and magnetic resonance imaging (MRI) characteristics of pleomorphic sarcomas have been described in humans but not in dogs.[40] In people, pleomorphic sarcomas are typically characterized as a large lobulated inhomogeneous hypo- to isodense mass with inhomogeneous enhancement on CT and hypo- to isointense on T1-weighted images, with inhomogeneous enhancement, hyperintensity, and hypointense areas on T2-weighted images on MRI.[40] Four histologic subtypes of pleomorphic sarcoma are described: storiform–pleomorphic, myxoid, giant cell, and inflammatory.[40] Definitive IHC staining patterns have not been established, but pleomorphic sarcomas will typically be vimentin positive and CD18 negative.[39] Histologic subtype has prognostic significance in people, with the giant cell subtype having a higher local recurrence rate than storiform–pleomorphic subtype and a higher metastatic rate than the inflammatory subtype.[41] Giant cell pleomorphic sarcomas have been described in 10 dogs: they were highly metastatic to subcutaneous tissue, lymph nodes (LNs), liver, and lungs; and the median survival time (MST) in these dogs was only 61 days.[38] Canine pleomorphic sarcomas are significantly more likely to be high grade and have metastases at the time of diagnosis compared with other histologic subtypes of STSs.[31]

Myxosarcoma

Myxosarcomas are neoplasms of fibroblast origin with an abundant myxoid matrix composed of mucopolysaccharides. These rare tumors occur in middle-aged or older dogs and cats. The majority are subcutaneous tumors of the trunk or limbs,[29] but there are reports of myxosarcomas arising from the heart, eye, and brain.[42–44] These tumors tend to be infiltrative growths with ill-defined margins.[29]

Tumors of the Vascular Wall

Perivascular Wall Tumor

PWTs are derived from the different cellular components of the vascular wall, excluding the endothelial lining.[45] The components of the vascular wall depend on the type of vessel. Capillaries are composed of endothelium, pericytes, and basement membrane; large veins and arteries are composed of endothelium, subendothelial lining cells, basement membrane, a medial layer of smooth muscle cells, and an adventitial layer of myofibroblasts and fibroblasts.[45] PWTs are characterized by the amounts and types of cytoplasmic contractile proteins, which progressively increase from pericytes in capillaries to myopericytes and smooth muscle myocytes in the vascular subendothelial lining of larger vessels.[45] PWTs have a characteristic cytologic appearance with moderate to high cellularity, cohesion of spindle cells, presence of capillaries, and multinucleate cells.[45] They are diagnosed histologically based on vascular growth patterns (e.g., staghorn, placentoid, perivascular whirling, bundles of media) and are further characterized by IHC staining patterns.[45] Pericytes express vimentin and variable amounts of pan and α-smooth muscle actin; myopericytes are characterized by the additional expression of desmin and calponin; and smooth muscle cells express smoothelin and heavy caldesmon.[45] Based on IHC staining, canine PWTs have been classified similarly to human PWTs, with the following being recognized: myopericytoma, angioleiomyoma, angioleiomyosarcoma, hemangiopericytoma, angiofibroma, and adventital tumor.[45,46] PWTs are differentiated from PNSTs by both histology and IHC.[45,47] PWTs are characterized by a less aggressive biologic behavior, with significantly lower rates of local recurrence than other histologic subtypes.[34]

Tumors of Peripheral Nerves

Peripheral Nerve Sheath Tumor

PNSTs are tumors of nerve sheath origin, arising from Schwann cells, perineural cells, or perineural or endoneural fibroblasts.[47] Benign and malignant variants have been described.[48] The most common benign PNSTs are schwannomas and neurofibromas, and these tend to be well circumscribed, located in the skin and subcutaneous tissue, with an equal distribution of Antoni A and B histologic patterns.[48] Malignant PNSTs are often subcutaneous, poorly circumscribed, and invasive into deeper tissues, and associated with high local tumor recurrence rates and relatively poor survival times.[47,48] Malignant PNSTs can be differentiated from PWTs based on IHC staining; malignant PNSTs stain positive with S-100, vimentin, glial fibrillary acidic protein (GFAP), nerve growth factor receptor, and neuron-specific enolase.[47–49] In additional, PNSTs have significantly higher Ki67 index than PWTs.[49]

Regardless of nomenclature, these tumors can occur anywhere in the body. Despite appearing encapsulated at surgery, they are similar to FSAs and are usually poorly defined without histologic encapsulation.[48] Most are adherent to deeper tissues and may infiltrate underlying fascia, muscle, and skin.[48] Although PNSTs are considered malignant, they have a modest metastatic rate. Local recurrence is common after conservative surgery.[48] PNSTs tend to grow slowly and can range in size from 0.5 cm to greater than 12 cm in diameter. In some cases, they can easily be confused with lipomas on initial clinical examination.[29]

PNSTs of macroscopic nerves, which are not considered part of the conventional classification of STSs in dogs, are classified as peripheral, root, or plexus.[50] Peripheral PNSTs involve macroscopic nerves distant to either the brain or spinal cord, and this form is much more amenable to treatment than either the root or plexus PNSTs. Plexus PNSTs can involve either the brachial or lumbrosacral plexus.[50] The vast majority of cases will show signs of unilateral lameness, muscle atrophy, paralysis, and pain.[50] They can invade the spinal cord, especially high-grade root and plexus PNSTs.[50] Treatment options include surgery, surgery with adjuvant RT, or RT alone. Surgical excision typically involves forequarter amputation,[50] although limb-sparing nerve-specific compartmental resection is occasionally possible.[51]

In one study of 16 dogs with brachial plexus PNSTs treated with limb-sparing compartmental resection, the overall MST was 1303 days and was significantly better for dogs with complete histologic excision (MST 2227 days) compared with dogs with incomplete excision (MST 487 days).[51] For peripheral nerve tumors extending through the foramen, hemilaminectomy may be required in addition to forequarter amputation for adequate tumor excision.[50] Stereotactic RT has been described in 10 dogs with brachial plexus tumors with partial or complete resolution of neurologic signs in all dogs.[52] The mean progression-free survival (PFS) and overall survival times (OSTs) were 240 days and 371 days, respectively, with progression reported in 90% of dogs.[52] Regardless of histologic grade, local disease usually limits survival before metastasis occurs.[50,52]

Tumors of Adipose Tissue

Lipoma

Lipomas are benign tumors of adipose tissue, and can be differentiated from liposarcomas based on morphologic, CT, and histologic appearance.[53] There are three morphologic types of lipomas: regular, infiltrative, and intermuscular.[53–59] Histologically, lipomas have indistinct nuclei and cytoplasm resembling normal fat, whereas liposarcomas are characterized by increased cellularity, distinct nuclei, and abundant cytoplasm with one or more droplets of fat.[60] Histologic variants of lipomas have been reported and include angiolipoma and angiofibrolipoma.[61]

Regular lipomas are relatively common in older dogs, especially in subcutaneous locations, and are rarely symptomatic. They have been reported in the thoracic cavity, abdominal cavity, spinal canal, and vulva and vagina of dogs, and can cause clinical abnormalities secondary to either compression or strangulation.[60,62–69] Marginal excision is recommended for lipomas that interfere with normal function; however, the majority are asymptomatic and do not require surgical intervention. Liposuction and intralesional triamcinolone have also been reported with variable results.[70,71] Surgical resection is usually curative, but local recurrence has been reported.[68]

Intermuscular Lipoma

Intermuscular lipomas are a variant of the subcutaneous lipoma and are located between muscle bellies. The most common location is the caudal thigh of dogs, particularly between the semitendinosus and semimembranosus muscles (Fig. 22.1), but they have also been reported in the axilla.[72,73] Clinically, intermuscular lipomas appear as a slow-growing, firm, and fixed mass in either the axillary or caudal thigh region and may occasionally cause lameness.[72,73] Cytologic analysis of fine-needle aspirates is usually diagnostic. The recommended treatment is surgical resection, involving blunt dissection and digital extrusion, and placement of a negative-suction drain. Seromas are a common complication in dogs in which a drain is not used.[72] The prognosis is excellent with no recurrence reported after surgical excision in two published papers totaling 27 dogs.[72,73]

Infiltrative Lipoma

Infiltrative lipomas are uncommon tumors composed of well-differentiated adipose cells without evidence of anaplasia. These tumors cannot be readily distinguished from the more common simple lipoma by cytology or small biopsy specimens. They are considered "benign" and do not metastasize; however, infiltrative lipomas are locally aggressive and commonly invade adjacent muscle,

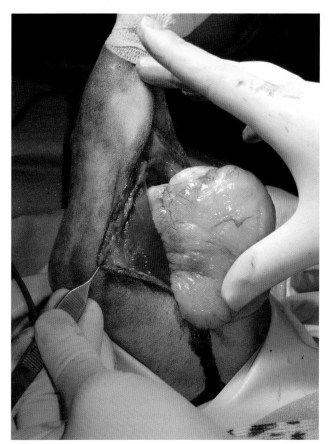

• **Fig. 22.1** An intermuscular lipoma arising from between the semitendinosus and semimembranosus muscles. Surgical dissection and removal was curative.

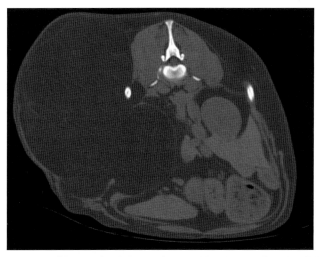

• **Fig. 22.2** A CT scan of an infiltrative lipoma of the chest wall in a dog. Differentiating an infiltrative lipoma from normal fat can be difficult on CT, but extension of the lipoma through the chest and body wall into the thoracic and abdominal (pictured) cavities is characteristic of an infiltrative lipoma.

fascia, nerve, myocardium, joint capsule, and even bone.[55,74,75] CT is used to better delineate these tumors and they can be differentiated from regular lipomas based on differences in shape, margins, and type of attenuation[53]; however, they do not contrast enhance and differentiating infiltrative lipomas from normal fat can be problematic (Fig. 22.2).[72] One retrospective analysis of 16

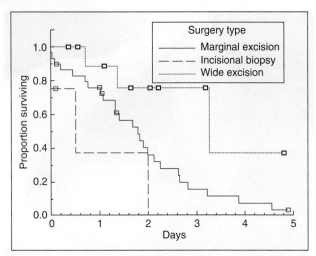

• **Fig. 22.3** Kaplan–Meier survival curve of 56 dogs with liposarcoma treated with either incisional biopsy, marginal resection, or wide excision. The median survival time is significantly longer, at 1188 days, after wide surgical resection than less aggressive techniques. (Reprinted with permission from Baez JL, Hendrick MJ, Shofer FS, et al: Liposarcomas in dogs: 56 cases (1989–2000), *J Am Vet Med Assoc* 224:887, 2004.)

cases reported a 4:1 female-to-male ratio.[57] Aggressive treatment, including amputation, may be necessary for local control. RT can be considered either alone or in combination with surgical excision. Complete and partial responses have been reported in the gross disease setting after external beam RT.[59]

Liposarcoma

Liposarcomas are uncommon malignant tumors originating from lipoblasts and lipocytes in older dogs.[76] Liposarcomas are usually firm and poorly circumscribed. They are locally invasive with a low metastatic potential. Metastatic sites include the lungs, liver, spleen, and bone.[29,76] Liposarcomas do not arise from malignant transformation of lipomas. Specific causes are not known, but foreign body–associated liposarcoma has been reported in one dog.[5] There is no breed or sex predilection.[76] They are commonly reported in subcutaneous locations, especially along the ventrum and extremities, but can also occur in other primary sites such as bone, spleen, and the abdominal cavity.[76–78] Liposarcomas are differentiated from lipomas based on morphologic appearance, cytologic findings, and CT characteristics. Staining cytologic samples with Oil Red O can be useful to differentiate liposarcomas from other soft tissue saromas by staining lipid.[79] Liposarcomas appear as mixed-attenuating, heterogeneous, multinodular, contrast-enhancing masses on precontrast CT images, and these features can be used to differentiate liposarcomas from regular and infiltrative lipomas.[53,80]

The prognosis for liposarcoma is good with appropriate surgical management. The MST after wide surgical excision is 1188 days; this is significantly better than either marginal excision or incisional biopsy, which have MSTs of 649 days and 183 days, respectively (Fig. 22.3).[76] Liposarcoma is histologically classified as well-differentiated, myxoid, round cell (or poorly differentiated), pleomorphic, or dedifferentiated. This classification scheme has clinical and prognostic importance in humans because pleomorphic liposarcomas have a high metastatic rate, myxoid liposarcomas are more likely to metastasize to extrapulmonary soft tissue structures, and well-differentiated liposarcomas are unlikely to metastasize.[81–83] In a retrospective study in dogs, histologic

subtype was not prognostic, but metastatic disease was more common in dogs with pleomorphic liposarcomas.[76] A revised classification scheme has been proposed on the basis of IHC expression of MDM2 and CDK4. In one study, MDM2 and CDK4 were expressed in 67% and 88% of well-differentiated liposarcomas, 14% and 71% of myxoid liposarcomas, 0% and 67% of pleomorphic liposarcomas, and 75% and 100% of dedifferentiated liposarcomas.[84] Furthermore, Ki67 index also correlated with histotype and was lowest in well-differentiated liposarcomas and highest in dedifferentiated liposarcomas.[84] These results parallel the human data to some degree and suggest that not only are well-differentiated and dedifferentiated liposarcomas distinct entities, but that this classification scheme may have prognostic significance.[84]

Tumors of Skeletal Muscle

Rhabdomyosarcoma

Rhabdomyosarcomas are rare malignant tumors originating from myoblasts or primitive mesenchymal cells capable of differentiating into striated muscle cells.[85] In dogs, rhabdomyosarcomas are most frequently reported to arise from skeletal muscle of the urinary bladder, retrobulbar musculature (Fig. 22.4), larynx, tongue, and myocardium.[86,87] They are locally invasive with a low to moderate metastatic potential. Metastatic sites include the lungs, liver, spleen, kidneys, and adrenal glands.[85]

Rhabdomyosarcomas are histologically classified as embryonal, botryoid, alveolar, and pleomorphic.[86] The histologic diagnosis of rhabdomyosarcoma is difficult (see Fig. 22.4C), and IHC staining for vimentin, skeletal muscle actin, myoglobin, myogenin, and myogenic differentiation (MyoD) may be required for definitive diagnosis.[88] Embryonal rhabdomyosarcomas have a predilection for the head and neck region, such as the tongue, oral cavity, larynx, and retrobulbar musculature.[86,87] In contrast, botryoid rhabdomyosarcoma commonly arises in the urinary bladder of young, female large-breed dogs, with Saint Bernard dogs possibly being overrepresented in one data set.[85] Botryoid tumors are characterized by their grapelike appearance. The histologic classification scheme for rhabdomyosarcoma has prognostic significance in humans.[85,89] In humans, botryoid rhabdomyosarcoma has a good prognosis, embryonal rhabdomyosarcoma has an intermediate prognosis, and alveolar rhabdomyosarcoma has a poor prognosis.[85,89] In dogs, botryoid rhabdomyosarcomas have a 27% metastatic rate whereas embryonal and alveolar rhabdomyosarcomas have a 50% metastatic rate.[86] Metastatic disease is more common in younger dogs, with the majority of dogs with metastatic disease being less than 2 years of age in one study[86] and, in another study, all dogs less than 4 years of age died of metastatic disease or local tumor recurrence (with an MST of 2.5 months), whereas no dog older than 4 years of age died of tumor-related reasons.[87]

Tumors of Lymphatic Tissue

Lymphangiosarcoma

Lymphangiosarcoma is a rare tumor arising from lymphatic endothelial cells.[29,90] They are usually soft, cystic-like, and edematous, usually occurring in the subcutis (Fig. 22.5).[29] In most cases, clinical signs are associated with extensive edema and drainage of lymph through the skin or a cystic mass, or nonhealing, discharging wounds.[90] Lymphangiosarcoma and HSA can be difficult to differentiate using histopathology and immunohistochemical markers for vascular endothelium, such

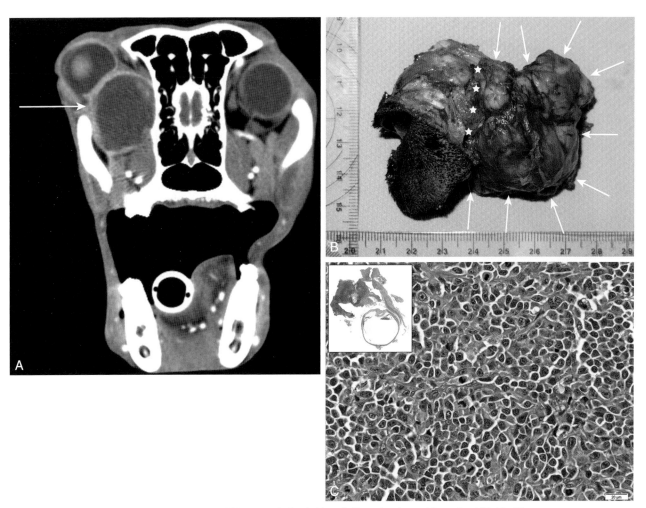

• **Fig. 22.4** (A) Postcontrast axial CT image at the level of the cribriform plate from a 12-month-old Belgian Turvuren. A hypoattenuating mass with a contrast enhancing rim (*arrow*) is causing significant dorsal displacement of the right eye. The dog developed local recurrence and pulmonary metastatic disease despite surgery and postoperative radiation therapy within 2 months after diagnosis. (B) A postoperative specimen image of a retrobulbar rhabdomyosarcoma resected from a 6-year-old Labrador retriever (*arrows*). An en bloc enucleation was performed because of adhesion of the rhabdomyosarcoma into the caudal aspect of the globe (*stars*). (C) Histopathology of the rhabdomyosarcoma in Fig. 4A reveals rafts of highly pleomorphic and haphazardly arranged polygonal to spindle cells with multiple mitotic figures. H&E, bar = 20 μm. Inset: Photomicrographs showing a basophilic mass expanding and partially effacing orbital and subconjunctival tissues, H&E. (Image courtesy Dr. L. Teixeira.)

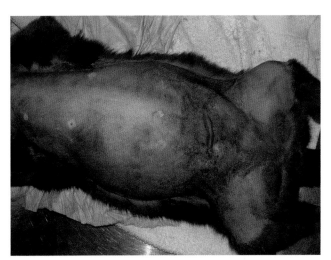

• **Fig. 22.5** Lymphangiosarcoma of the ventral abdomen in a male cat. These tumors are often subcutaneous, soft, and edematous, and with poorly defined margins.

as factor VIII–related antigen and CD31.[29,91] IHC staining with the lymphatic endothelial cell-specific markers lymphatic vessel endothelial receptor-1 (LYVE-1) and propsero-related homeobox gene-1 (*PROX-1*) successfully differentiated lymphangiosarcoma from HSA in the majority of dogs.[91] In one series of 12 dogs with lymphangiosarcoma, the MST was 168 days (range, 60–876 days) for three dogs with no treatment and 487 days (range, 240–941 days) for five dogs treated with surgery alone; one dog treated with surgery, RT, and chemotherapy had an ST of 574 days.[90] All dogs treated surgically had incomplete histologic excision and all dogs were euthanized because of recurrent or progressive local disease.[90]

Tumors of Uncertain Histogenesis

Malignant Mesenchymoma

Malignant mesenchymomas are rare STSs comprising a fibrous component with two or more different varieties of other types of sarcoma.[26] Malignant mesenchymomas have been reported in the heart, lungs, thoracic wall, liver, spleen, kidney, digits, and soft

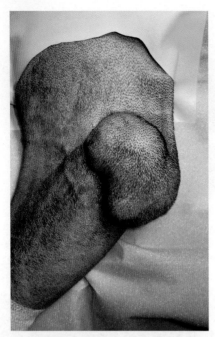

• **Fig. 22.6** The typical gross appearance of a canine soft tissue sarcoma with a firm, well-circumscribed, expansile subcutaneous mass.

tissue.[92–101] They have a slow rate of growth and can grow very large. Metastasis has been reported.[96–100] The outcome for dogs with splenic mesenchymomas is better than for those with other types of splenic sarcomas, with a MST of 12 months and a 1-year survival rate of 50%.[96]

History and Clinical Signs

STSs generally present as slow-growing expansile masses. Rapid tumor growth, intratumoral hemorrhage, or necrosis can be seen in some cases. Symptoms are directly related to site of involvement and tumor invasiveness, with the vast majority of subcutaneous and cutaneous STSs causing no clinical signs. There is marked variability in the physical features of STS, but they are generally firm and well circumscribed (Fig. 22.6). They can be either mobile or adherent (fixed) to skin, muscle, or bone. STSs can also be soft and lobulated, mimicking lipomas.

Diagnostic Techniques and Workup

Fine-needle aspiration (FNA) is recommended for a cytologic diagnosis; however, cytologic evaluation may not be sufficient for a definitive diagnosis because variable degrees of necrosis and poor exfoliation of cells may result in a nondiagnostic sample.[26] The cytologic accuracy of correctly diagnosing an STS varies from 63% to 97%.[32,102] Cytologic preparations should be assessed by a board-certified cytopathologist because a disproportionate number of false-negative cytologic results were associated with in-house cytologic assessments compared with evaluation by a board-certified cytopathologist in one study.[33] Even in the absence of a definitive diagnosis, FNA cytology can exclude the diagnosis of readily exfoliating tumors such as epithelial and round cell tumors, and this may be sufficient for the suspected diagnosis of an STS by exclusion.[102,103]

Biopsy methods for definitive preoperative diagnosis of STSs include needle-core, punch, incisional, or excisional biopsies.

The biopsy should be planned and positioned so that the biopsy tract can be included in the curative-intent treatment without increasing the surgical dose or size of the radiation field. Although needle-core and incisional biopsies will typically provide sufficient tissue for a definitive diagnosis of STS, the determination of histologic grade from preoperative biopsies was incorrect in 41% of dogs compared with the definitive surgical sample, with histologic grade underestimated in 29% of dogs and overestimated in 12% of dogs.[104] Excisional biopsies are *not* recommended because they may not be curative and the subsequent surgery required to achieve complete histologic margins is often more aggressive than surgery after core or incisional biopsies, resulting in additional morbidity and treatment costs. Furthermore, multiple attempts at resection, including excisional biopsy, before definitive therapy have a negative effect on ST in dogs with STSs.[105]

Diagnostic tests performed for workup and clinical staging include routine hematologic and serum biochemical blood tests, three-view thoracic radiographs, abdominal ultrasonography or advanced imaging, FNA or biopsy of the regional LNs, and regional imaging of the STS. Three-view thoracic radiographs should be performed before definitive treatment because the lungs are the most common metastatic site for typical STSs.[35] Although LN metastasis is uncommon, FNA or biopsy of regional LNs should be performed in dogs with clinically abnormal LNs, grade III STSs, or suspected nonconventional STSs with a high rate of metastasis to regional LNs (e.g., HS).[106] Abdominal imaging is recommended for the assessment of metastasis to intraabdominal organs in animals with high-grade pelvic limb STS. Imaging studies of the local tumor may be required for planning of the surgical approach or RT if the tumor is fixed to underlying structures or located in an area that may make definitive treatment difficult, such as the pelvic region. Three-dimensional (3D) imaging techniques such as CT and MRI are particularly useful for staging local disease.[107] Other imaging modalities for staging of the local tumor include survey radiographs and ultrasonography.[108]

Clinical Staging

A modified staging system has been described for STSs in dogs.[26] The American Joint Committee on Cancer (AJCC) staging system currently used in humans with STSs has been substantially modified from the original staging system, on which the modified animal staging system is based. The most important change to AJCC staging is categorization of local disease, with less emphasis on tumor size, which is an arbitrary assignment, and greater emphasis on depth of invasion.[81,109] A superficial tumor is defined as an STS located above the superficial fascia and that does not invade the fascia, whereas a deep tumor is located deep to the superficial fascia, invades the fascia, or both.[109]

Treatment

The predominant challenge in the management of cutaneous and subcutaneous STSs is local tumor control. As such, surgical resection is the principal treatment for dogs with STSs. RT may also play a significant role in local tumor control, especially for incompletely resected and unresectable STSs. However, definitive treatment options depend on tumor location, clinical stage, histologic grade, and completeness of histologic margins.[10,26,110] A suggested algorithm for managing dogs with STSs is presented in Fig. 22.7.

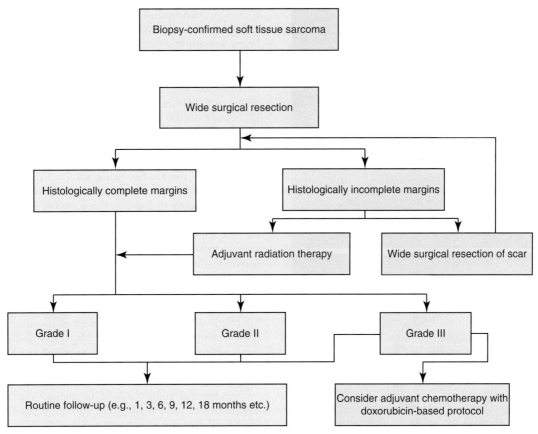

• **Fig. 22.7** Suggested algorithm for the treatment of soft tissue sarcomas in dogs.

Surgery

The surgical options for management of STSs include marginal resection, wide resection, or radical resection, and the preferred surgical approach can be tailored to each individual patient depending on location, size, degree of infiltration, histologic grade of the STS, and the outcome goals of the client. The majority of STSs are characterized by a locally expansile mass, but they can also be infiltrative.[111] This was supported by a histologic study showing that grade I and II STSs were significantly less invasive than low-grade mast cell tumors in both circumferential and deep directions.[112] STSs are often surrounded by a pseudocapsule formed by the compression of peritumoral connective tissue that may contain or be confluent with neoplastic tissue.[12,26] The pseudocapsule can give the false impression of a well-encapsulated tumor; however, surgical removal of the encapsulated mass without adequate margins may result in incomplete histologic margins and a higher risk of local tumor recurrence.[35] The minimum recommended margins for wide surgical resection of STSs are 2 to 3 cm lateral and one fascial layer deep to the tumor (Fig. 22.8),[10,13,103,110,113,114] although this is an arbitrary recommendation and does not account for tumor size, patient size, tumor location, or local tumor characteristics.[10,103,110,113,114] In one study of 22 dogs with 24 subcutaneous STSs, all STSs were completely excised with mean lateral and deep margins of 22.23 mm (range, 6–50 mm) and 7 mm (1–24 mm), respectively, with all deep margins including an uninvolved fascial plane (Fig. 22.9).[113] A proportional margin system, where the lateral surgical margins are equal to the maximal diameter of the tumor as validated for the resection of low-grade mast cell tumors,[115] may also be appropriate

for the resection of STSs in dogs because incomplete histologic excision is significantly more likely after surgical resection of larger tumors and tumors in smaller patients.[46,116] Biopsy tracts and any areas of fixation, including bone and fascia, should be resected en bloc with the tumor using the recommended surgical margins. Radical surgery such as limb amputation or hemipelvectomy may be required to achieve adequate histologic margins and local tumor control, especially for fixed and invasive STSs. Wide excision of STSs is associated with a significantly increased likelihood of complete histologic excision,[32] and dogs with complete histologic excision are 10.5 times less likely to have local tumor recurrence compared with dogs with incompletely excised STSs.[35]

Marginal excision may be an acceptable treatment option for well-circumscribed, noninfiltrative STSs less than 5 cm in diameter, and located on the limbs at or below the elbow or stifle. STSs in these locations tend to be less infiltrative and more well-circumscribed than STSs in other locations, such as the upper limbs and trunk (Fig. 22.10).[46,117] In one study of 236 dogs with subcutaneous STSs treated with excisional biopsy, the local recurrence rate was 0% for completely excised tumors and dependent on histologic grade for incompletely excised tumors, with 7% of grade I and 34% of grade II incompletely excised STSs developing local tumor recurrence.[118] Similar results have been reported in other studies after marginal excision of STSs from nonreferral practices and low-grade PWTs. In a study of 35 dogs with marginal excision of 37 low-grade STSs, the local recurrence rate was 11% and no prognostic factors for local recurrence were identified.[117] In a study of 104 canine STSs managed with surgery alone in nonreferral practices, which did not include undifferentiated

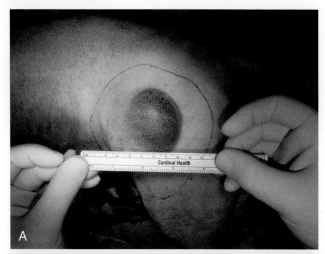

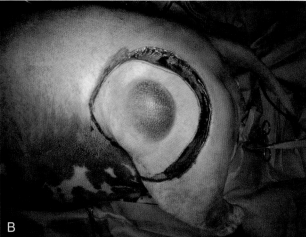

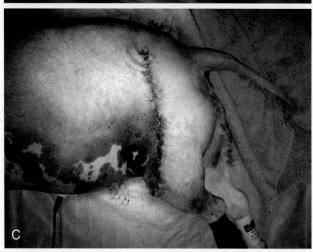

• **Fig. 22.8** Wide resection of a grade II soft tissue sarcoma from the craniolateral thigh of a dog. (A) Planned lateral surgical margins are indicated with a sterile marker pen 3 cm in all directions around the soft tissue sarcoma. (B) An incision is then performed along the marked margins, and continued deeply to include an uninvolved fascial layer. (C) Primary closure after wide resection of the soft tissue sarcoma.

STSs and liposarcomas, fewer than 10% were excised with 3 cm lateral margins, and local tumor recurrence was reported in 28% of dogs (29% of marginal excisions, 17% of narrow excisions, and 5% of wide excisions); local tumor recurrence was significantly more likely to occur with fixed and invasive

STSs.[25] In two studies of dogs with PWTs, the local recurrence rate was 18% to 20.0% despite 60% to 63% of these tumors being incompletely excised.[46,111] The only prognostic factor for local recurrence in both studies was tumor size, with local recurrence up to 7.0 times more likely for PWTs greater than 5 cm diameter with the risk of local tumor recurrence increasing by up to 1.3 times for every 1 cm increase in tumor size.[46,111] In a study of 350 canine STSs treated surgically in nonreferral practices, the local recurrence rate was 21% despite only 5% of these STSs being excised with wide surgical margins.[34] Histologic grade was the only prognostic factor for local tumor recurrence in this study, with grade III STSs having a 5.8-fold increased risk for local recurrence compared with grade I and II STSs.[34] Taken in totality, these studies suggest that acceptable local tumor control rates are achievable with less aggressive surgical approaches; however, they also illustrate that the traditional consideration of STSs having a similar biologic behavior is overly simplistic. The ideal treatment for dogs with cutaneous and subcutaneous STSs should not necessarily be standardized but rather tailored to each individual case according to location, tumor size, degree of infiltration, histologic subtype, histologic grade, and completeness of excision. If insufficient information is available before surgery to individualize treatment options, then wide surgical resection (with 2–3 cm lateral margins and one fascial layer for deep margins) is the preferred surgical approach.

The resected tumor should be pinned out to the original dimensions to prevent shrinkage during formalin fixation[119]; the lateral and deep margins should be inked to aid in histologic identification of surgical margins; and any areas of concern should be tagged with suture material, inked in a different color, or submitted separately for specific histologic assessment. Histologic margins and histologic grade are important in determining the need and type of further treatment.

There are a number of limitations with our current ability to assess the adequacy of the completeness of the excision and risk of local tumor recurrence, and thus our ability to determine which patients require further therapy and which patients may benefit from monitoring. These include sample shrinkage after excision and during formalin fixation, the techniques used to assess margins histologically, the lack of information on the definition of a "narrow" histologic margin, and the significance of narrow margins on the risk of local tumor recurrence.[13,120] Perhaps most important is that histopathology is an examination of excised tissue ex vivo and not residual tissue in vivo, and that this assessment is made days after surgery rather than in real time. A number of advancements are being made in both veterinary and human surgical oncology in the real-time assessment of the wound bed after excision of STSs for residual neoplastic disease.[121–125] Hopefully, as these real-time in vivo assessment methods are validated and become available for clinical use, there will be an improvement in the rate of complete histologic excision and local tumor control.

The treatment options for incompletely excised STSs include active surveillance (i.e., frequent observation for local tumor recurrence and appropriate treatment if the tumor recurs), staging surgery, wide excision (i.e., revision surgery), RT, metronomic chemotherapy, and electrochemotherapy. The first surgery provides the best opportunity for local tumor control, as the management of incompletely resected tumors increases patient morbidity and treatment costs, increases the risk of further local tumor recurrence, and potentially decreases ST.[10,31,34,35,105,110,126–130] Active surveillance may be appropriate

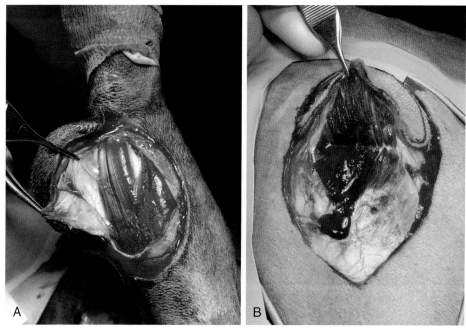

• **Fig. 22.9** (A) Wide and marginal resection of soft tissue sarcomas should include an uninvolved fascial layer for deep margins or, (B) if a defined anatomic fascia layer is not present, then either partial or full thickness muscle.

for dogs with grade I and possibly grade II STSs with favorable local characteristics, such as well-circumscribed tumors, less than 5 cm in diameter, and located on either the thoracic or pelvic limb at or below the elbow or stifle.[25,34,46,110,111,117,118] Active surveillance may be appropriate in these cases because, as discussed earlier, local recurrence rates are relatively low (7% and 34% for incompletely excised grade I and II STSs, respectively)[118] and further aggressive treatment may be unnecessary in up to 93% of dogs (with incompletely grade I STSs), with an associated increased risk in morbidity and costs.

Staging surgery is a decision-making surgery. The surgical scar is excised with minimal margins (<1 cm), with the aim being to determine whether there is histologic evidence of residual tumor cells.[33] In one study in which the surgical scar was excised with 0.5- to 3.5-cm lateral margins, histologic evidence of residual tumor was identified in only 22% of 39 dogs with incompletely excised STSs.[33] If there is no evidence of tumor cells, then no further treatment is required and these dogs should be monitored regularly for local tumor recurrence. If there is evidence of residual tumor cells, then wide resection of the surgical scar should be performed with the same margins recommended for primary STSs (2–3 cm lateral to the tumor and one fascial layer deep to the tumor[10,13,103,110,113,114]) or the entire surgical scar should be irradiated.[128,129] Surgery is preferred to RT for the management of incompletely resected STSs in humans because local tumor control is better with repeat surgical resection than adjunctive RT alone.[128,129]

Metronomic (or low-dose) chemotherapy is another option for the management of dogs with incompletely excised STSs. The administration of piroxicam and low-dose cyclophosphamide in 30 dogs with incompletely excised STSs resulted in a significantly prolonged disease-free interval (DFI) compared with a nonrandomized control group of 55 dogs with incompletely excised STSs and no metronomic chemotherapy.[131] Of note, the control population used in this study experienced recurrence rates much greater than what is expected in the general population based on

the preponderance of current data, perhaps weakening the generalizability of this study. Metronomic chemotherapy has been much less thoroughly studied than wide excision or postoperative RT, and should not be considered an equivalent substitute for these other modalities at this time. Additional studies are needed to confirm the efficacy of metronomic chemotherapy in the management of dogs with incompletely excised STSs.

Electrochemotherapy has also been investigated in the management of incompletely excised high-grade STSs in 22 dogs.[132] Bleomycin was injected into the tumor bed followed by sequential application of trains of biphasic electrical pulses. The local recurrence rate was 36% with a mean time to recurrence of 730 days.[132] Wound dehiscence was reported in 14% of dogs.

Surgery and Radiation Therapy

RT is often recommended in the management of dogs with STSs, particularly after incomplete histologic excision, and adjuvant RT has a documented role in improving local tumor control in people with STSs.[103,114,128,129] The evidence is less robust in veterinary medicine because all published studies of adjuvant RT in the management of dogs with incompletely excised STSs are retrospective and, more importantly, lack a control group. Local recurrence rates are similar in studies of dogs treated with marginal resection alone, compared with recurrence rates occurring in dogs with either marginal resection or incomplete histologic excision treated with adjuvant RT (fractionated or hypofractionated) or intralesional chemotherapy (Table 22.3); however, it is important to recognize that study results cannot be compared because of differences in study populations and methodologies. Furthermore, because canine STSs have a biologic behavior similar to that of low-grade STSs in people and because RT significantly improves local tumor control in people with incompletely excised STSs, RT should still be considered in the management of dogs with STSs.[114,128,129] RT can be used as an adjunct to surgery after either planned marginal resection or unplanned incomplete histologic excision. Marginal surgical

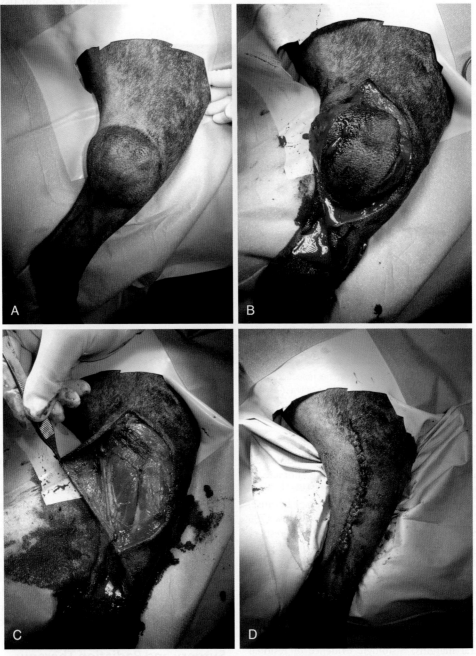

• **Fig. 22.10** (A) Marginal resection of a well-circumscribed, noninfiltrative, grade I soft tissue sarcoma below the level of the stifle in a dog. (B) Freely movable skin over the soft tissue sarcoma is carefully dissected away from the mass to avoid iatrogenic penetration of the tumor capsule and (C, D) permit primary closure of the subsequent wound defect. This soft tissue sarcoma was resected with complete histologic margins and the dog remains tumor-free 2 years postoperatively.

TABLE 22.3	Comparison of Local Tumor Control Outcomes for Dogs with Cutaneous and Subcutaneous Soft Tissue Sarcomas Between Different Treatment Modalities				
	Local Recurrence Rate	Median Disease-Free Interval	1-Year Disease-Free Rate	2-Year Disease-Free Rate	3-Year Disease-Free Rate
Surgery[25,32,34,46,111,113,117,118]	Wide: 0%–5% Marginal: 11%–29%	368 days to not reached	89%–93%	78%–82%	66%–76%
Surgery[a] and fractionated radiation therapy[135–138]	17%–39%	412 days to not reached	71%–84%	60%–81%	57%–81%
Surgery[a] and hypofractionated Radiation therapy[140,141]	18%–21%	698 days to not reached	81%	73%	73%
Marginal surgical resection and intralesional chemotherapy[162–164]	17%–31%	264 days to not reached	81%–100%	69%–89%	59%–84%

[a]Incomplete histologic excision.

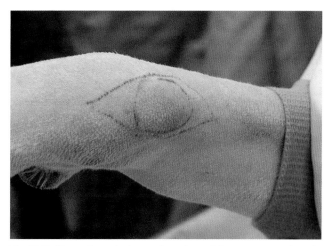

• **Fig. 22.11** Planned marginal resection of a soft tissue sarcoma in a dog. Marginal resection followed by full-course postoperative radiation therapy provides excellent local tumor control and preserves both the limb and limb function. Radiation therapy should not involve the limb circumferentially to preserve both lymphatic and venous drainage of the distal extremity. If close but clean margins were obtained for a grade I soft tissue sarcoma, observation alone may be an acceptable alternative.

resection combined with full-course postoperative RT is an attractive alternative to limb amputation for extremity STS (Fig. 22.11). This multimodality approach requires additional planning and costs, but preserves the limb and limb function. Surgery involves completely removing all grossly visible tumor and then marking the lateral, proximal, and distal extents of the surgical field with radiopaque clips to assist in planning of RT.[133] Migration of the radiopaque clips has been reported but does not significantly influence the planned radiation field.[133]

RT should be started a minimum of 7 days postoperatively to minimize the risk of radiation-induced complications with the surgical wound, such as delayed healing and dehiscence.[134] Full-course fractionated protocols are recommended, with reported schedules including 3.0- to 4.2-Gy fractions on a Monday-to-Friday or Monday–Wednesday–Friday schedule for a total dose of 42 to 63 Gy.[135-138] The optimal fractionation and total dose schemes for canine STS have not been determined, but cumulative doses greater than 50 Gy are recommended because local tumor control is better with higher cumulative doses.[135] Acute side effects of RT, such as moist desquamation, are relatively mild and transient.[136]

Local tumor control and ST are very good when incompletely resected STSs are treated with postoperative, definitively fractionated RT with local tumor recurrence reported in 16.7% to 36.8% of dogs,[135-137] and 1-, 2-, 3-, and 4-year local control rates of 71% to 84%, 60% to 81%, 57% to 81%, and up to 81%, respectively.[135,136,138] The local tumor recurrence rates may have been adversely affected by the inclusion of incompletely excised oral FSAs in one study.[135] The median time to local recurrence is 412 days to more than 798 days.[105,135-137] The median time to recurrence was significantly shorter in dogs with grade III STSs (78 days) compared with dogs with grade I and II STSs (>1416 days) in one study.[135] The overall MST for incompletely resected nonoral STSs treated with postoperative RT is 2270 days, with survival rates ranging from 80% to 87% at 1 year, 72% to 87% at 2 years, 92% at 3 years, and 76% at 5 years.[135-139] In one study, dogs with STSs with a mitotic index greater than 9 per 10 high-power fields (HPFs) were more likely to have local recurrence and shorter ST.[139]

Hypofractionated RT after either incomplete or close complete (<3 mm) histologic excision of STSs has also been reported with encouraging results.[140,141] Protocols reported have utilized weekly fractions of 6 to 9 Gy to a total dose of 24 to 36 Gy.[140] An 18% to 21% local recurrence rate was reported in these studies; however, the majority of STSs were initially small (median size 3.6 cm) and either grade I or II (83%).[140,141] Acute toxicity was mild, but late toxicities, although uncommon, were noted in both studies.[140,141] An increased risk of late toxicity generally occurs with larger radiation doses per fraction and this risk must be considered in a group of patients who are expected to survive for prolonged periods after RT. Progression-free intervals (PFIs) in these studies were 698 days to not reached, and the probability of being free of local tumor recurrence at 1, 2, and 3 years was 81%, 73%, and 73%, respectively.[140,141] In one study, delaying hypofractionated RT for more than 4 weeks after surgery was associated with an improved outcome, with local recurrence nine times more likely in dogs in which RT was started less than 4 weeks after surgical excision.[140] Histologic grade was prognostic for both median PFS and OST in one study.[141] Median PFS times were 1904 days, 582 days, and 292 days for dogs with grade I, II, and III STSs, respectively; the median tumor-specific OST was not reached for dogs with grade I and II STSs, but was 940 days for dogs with grade III STSs.[141]

Radiation Therapy for Gross Disease

RT can also be used a single modality, usually for palliation of clinical signs. RT alone, using a cumulative dose of 50 Gy, resulted in 1- and 2-year tumor control rates of 50% and 33%, respectively.[142] Measurable and palpable (i.e., macroscopic) STSs are resistant to long-term control with conventional doses of radiation alone (40–48 Gy).[143,144] Although one study reported a 30% complete response rate with RT alone,[145] these tumors do not rapidly regress after RT and, if there is significant tumor shrinkage, it is not usually a durable response.

Hypofractionated RT has been reported for the treatment of macroscopic STSs using a number of different protocols, including 3 to 4 fractions of 8 Gy once weekly for a total dose of 24 to 32 Gy, 5 to 6 fractions of 6 Gy once to twice weekly for a total dose of 30 to 36 Gy, and 5 fractions of 4 Gy for a total dose of 20 Gy.[146-150] The results of hypofractionated RT are similar to those of full-course RT in the gross disease setting. In two studies, the overall response rate was 46% to 50%,[146,148] whereas stable disease was more common in two other studies.[147,149] The median PFI ranged from 155 to 419 days.[146-150] Prognostic factors for median PFI include tumor location and previous surgeries. The median PFI is significantly better for limb STSs (466 days) than STSs located on the head or trunk (110 days), and dogs treated with more than one surgery had a significantly decreased median PFI (105 days) compared with dogs treated with one or no surgery (420 days).[148] The MST after hypofractionated RT for macroscopic STS is 206 to 513 days.[146-150] STS location has a significant effect on MST, with STSs located on the limbs (579 days) having a better outcome than those on the head (195 days) or trunk (190 days).[148] In this study, 40% of dogs were also treated with metronomic chemotherapy. Metronomic chemotherapy did not improve median PFIs, but this adjunctive treatment did significantly improve MSTs (757 days compared with 518 days for dogs not treated with metronomic chemotherapy).[148]

Preoperative RT is becoming commonplace in veterinary oncology. The rationale and advantage of administering RT before surgery are that (1) the radiation field is smaller because, after surgery, the entire surgical site must be included in the field plus a margin of normal tissue and this may contribute to local toxicity; (2) a large number of peripheral tumor cells are inactivated (with reduced contamination of the surgical site); and (3) tumor volume reduction may make surgical resection less difficult.[15,151–153] In a randomized phase III human trial of preoperative compared with postoperative RT, wound complications were found to be higher in people treated with preoperative RT (35% vs 17%); however, OST was found to be marginally improved in patients treated with preoperative RT.[154] Other studies, including a meta-analysis of 1098 patients, have confirmed these findings and further suggested that both local recurrence rates and ST may be improved in patients treated with preoperative RT.[155] Lower doses of preoperative RT (<50 Gy) are generally used to reduce the risk of surgical complications.

Chemotherapy

The role of chemotherapy in the management of dogs with STS is controversial. The metastatic rates for dogs with grade I, II, and III cutaneous STSs are 0% to 13%, 7% to 27%, and 22% to 44%, respectively.[31,35,156] Metastasis often occurs late in the course of disease, with a median time to metastasis of up to 365 days,[35] and this may minimize the beneficial effects of postoperative chemotherapy on the development of metastatic disease. In one retrospective study of 39 dogs with grade III STSs arising from various locations, including noncutaneous and subcutaneous sites, treated with either surgery alone (n = 18) or surgery and doxorubicin (DOX) (n = 21), there was no significant difference in survival outcomes with the addition of DOX to the treatment protocol.[156] An alternating protocol of DOX and ifosfamide was reported in 12 dogs with various STSs after surgical excision, but survival outcomes were not investigated because of low case numbers.[157] DOX and ifosfamide are the most effective single agents in the management of STS in humans, but meta-analyses show that single- and multiple-agent chemotherapy protocols do not significantly increase OST compared with surgery alone in people.[158,159]

Although adjuvant chemotherapy has not shown the same effect on local tumor control in dogs with STSs as it does in people,[158] metronomic and local chemotherapy protocols may be effective in decreasing the rate of local tumor recurrence and improving DFIs in dogs with STSs. Metronomic chemotherapy improves local tumor control in experimental and human studies by inhibiting tumor angiogenesis and suppressing regulatory T cells, and a similar effect was demonstrated in dogs with STSs treated with low-dose cyclophosphamide at a dose of 15.0 mg/m^2/day, but not 12.5 mg/m^2/day.[160] Clinically, metronomic chemotherapy improved ST in dogs with macroscopic STSs treated with hypofractionated RT.[148] Although not investigated clinically, there may be a role for tyrosine kinase inhibitors in the management of STS because increased vascular endothelial growth factor (VEGF) and VEGF receptor expression has been demonstrated in the peri- and intratumoral regions of canine STSs.[161–163] Furthermore, VEGF has been postulated to have a role in the angiogenesis of canine STSs because serum VEGF levels decrease after STS excision.[164]

The effect of the local release of chemotherapy on local tumor recurrence rates after marginal excision of STSs has been investigated in dogs. Intralesional chemotherapy agents include cisplatin, released locally from either a biodegradable polymer or calcium sulfate and dextran sulfate beads implanted into the surgical bed, and 5-fluorouracil, injected weekly for a minimum of

six treatments.[165–168] Local recurrence was reported in 17% to 31%, and this was significantly more likely for dogs with grade III STSs.[162–164] Wound complications are common after treatment with intralesional chemotherapy and are reported in 47% to 84% of dogs.[163–167]

Prognosis

Local Tumor Recurrence

Local tumor control is often the most challenging aspect of managing STSs, but this is dependent on a number of factors including tumor size, local tumor characteristics such as well-circumscribed or infiltrative, tumor location, histologic grade, completeness of histologic excision, and treatment methods. The overall local recurrence rates are 0% to 5% after wide resection,[25,113] 11% to 29% after marginal resection,[25,34,46,111,117,118] 17% to 37% after incomplete histologic excision and fractionated RT,[135–137] and 18% to 21% after incomplete histologic excision and hypofractionated RT (see Table 22.2).[140,141] The DFIs and local tumor control rates are also similar between the different treatment options, with a median DFI of 368 to 637 days to not reached and disease-free rates of 89% to 93%, 78% to 82%, and 66% to 76% at 1, 2, and 3 years, respectively, after surgery alone[32,34,35,46,113]; a median DFI of 412 to more than 798 days and disease-free rates of 71% to 84%, 60% to 81%, 57% to 81%, and up to 81% at 1, 2, 3, and 4 years, respectively, for incomplete excision and fractionated RT[135,136,138]; and a median DFI of 698 days to not reached and disease-free rates of 81%, 73%, and 73% at 1, 2, and 3 years, respectively, after incomplete excision and hypofractionated RT.[140,141] Poor prognostic factors for local tumor control include large tumor size (>5 cm), infiltrative tumors, tumors in locations other than the limbs at or below the elbow or stifle, histologic subtypes, grade III STSs, and incomplete surgical margins.

In one study of 75 dogs, the local tumor recurrence rate after incomplete histologic excision was 28% and 11 times more likely compared with STSs resected with complete histologic margins (Fig. 22.12).[35] Complete histologic excision is significantly more likely when STSs are treated with wide resection rather than more conservative approaches,[31,32] and complete histologic excision is associated with long-term survival in up to 98% of dogs with STSs.[31,32,35,113] Despite the importance of complete histologic excision in the management of dogs with STSs, incomplete excision has infrequently been identified as a prognostic factor for local tumor recurrence after marginal resection,[25,118] with the majority of studies showing no significant association between incomplete histologic excision and local tumor recurrence.[34,46,111,117]

Histologic grade has an effect on local tumor recurrence both overall and after incomplete histologic excision. Grade III STSs have a six-fold greater risk for local recurrence compared with low-grade tumors.[34] In one study of 236 dogs with subcutaneous STSs treated with excisional biopsy, the local recurrence rate was 0% for STSs excised with complete histologic margins and 19% overall for incompletely excised STSs.[118] The recurrence rate for incompletely excised grade I, II, and III STSs was 7%, 34%, and 75% (three of four) respectively.[118]

Histologic subtype may also be associated with local tumor recurrence; however, it is important to recognize that differentiating histologic subtypes of STSs can be problematic, even with IHC.[12,114] PWTs are often associated with a low risk of local tumor recurrence,[12,34] whereas FSAs have been associated with a higher local recurrence rate.[32–34]

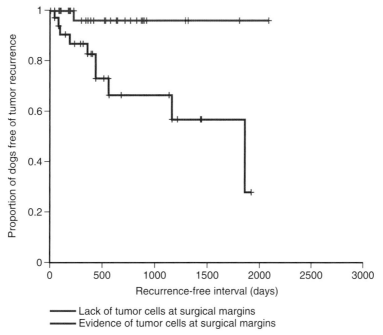

• **Fig. 22.12** Kaplan–Meier curve for disease-free interval in 39 dogs with complete surgical removal of soft tissue sarcomas and 36 dogs with incomplete surgical margins. (Reprinted with permission from Kuntz CA, Dernell WS, Powers BE, et al: Prognostic factors for surgical treatment of soft-tissue sarcomas in dogs: 75 cases (1986–1996), *J Am Vet Med Assoc* 211:1147, 1997.)

Local tumor characteristics also influence local tumor control. Tumor size has been reported to have a negative effect on local tumor control, especially for incompletely excised STSs.[35,46,111] Local tumor recurrence is up to 7.0 times more likely after marginal resection of PWTs greater than 5 cm diameter and the risk of local tumor recurrence increases by up to 1.3 times for every 1 cm increase in tumor size.[46,111] This may be because a large tumor size influences the ability to achieve complete histologic excision or because a larger tumor size may indicate a more aggressive biologic behavior.[46,116] Tumor size has not been identified as a prognostic factor in other studies,[32,33,139,169] and does not influence local tumor control in dogs treated with surgery and adjuvant RT or RT alone.[142,169,170] Dogs with fixed or invasive STSs have significantly decreased DFIs and STs.[34] Invasive or fixed tumors are associated with a two-fold increased risk for local recurrence compared with well-circumscribed STSs after marginal resection,[25] and PWTs invasive into muscle were eight times more likely to recur after marginal resection.[32,111]

Local tumor recurrence has been associated with an increased risk of tumor-related death and decreased STs in some studies.[31,34] In one study of 350 dogs with STSs managed in nonreferral practices, local tumor recurrence was associated with a 5-fold risk of death.[34] Although many dogs can live with recurrent STSs, local recurrence is more difficult to manage and may result in owners electing euthanasia rather than pursuing further treatment. The median postrecurrence ST for dogs euthanized because of their local tumor recurrence is 256 days and this is significantly worse than the 945 days median postrecurrence ST for dogs with local recurrence that die of unrelated reasons.[34] This underscores the importance of wide excision of STSs initially, as the management of recurrent STSs is usually more difficult with curative-intent treatment of recurrent STSs requiring a more aggressive approach, resulting in increased treatment-related morbidity with the potential for shorter DFIs, higher metastatic rates, and

poorer STs.[32,113,126–130] Local tumor recurrence is still possible after either complete resection or incomplete resection combined with adjunctive RT.[35,135–138] Consequently, examination of the treatment site is recommended at regular intervals, such as monthly for the first 3 months, then every 3 months for the first 12 months, and then every 6 months thereafter.[10,110] The median time to local tumor recurrence varies from 368 to greater than 798 days, which emphasizes the need for long-term follow-up in these cases.[32,34,35,46,113,135–137,140,141]

Metastasis

The overall metastatic rate in dogs with STS varies from 0% to 31%, with a median time to metastasis of 230 to 365 days.[31–34,35,46,113,135–138,141] Factors that increase the risk of metastatic disease include histologic grade, number of mitotic figures, percentage of tumor necrosis, and local tumor recurrence. The metastatic rates for dogs with grade I, II, and III STSs are 0% to 13%, 7% to 27%, and 22% to 44%, respectively.[31,35,156] Metastasis is significantly more likely in dogs with pleomorphic and undifferentiated sarcomas compared with FSAs, PNSTs, myxosarcomas, and liposarcomas.[31] Metastasis is five times more likely when tumors have a mitotic rate of 20 or more mitotic figures/10 HPF compared with fewer than 20 mitotic figures/10 HPF.[35] In one study, no dog with a STS at or below the level of the elbow or stifle developed metastatic disease.[35]

Survival

The MST for dogs with STS ranges from 1013 to 1796 days after surgery alone to 2270 days with surgery and adjunctive RT for nonoral STSs.[25,34,35,135,136] However, the majority of studies report MSTs that cannot be calculated because only 9% to 33% of dogs eventually die of tumor-related causes after curative-intent treatment.[25,31–35,113,117,118,136,140,141] The 1-, 2-, 3-, 4-, and 5-year survival probabilities are 80% to 94%, 72% to 87%, 61% to 81%, 81%, and 76% respectively.[34,141]

Clinical factors associated with decreased ST include tumor invasiveness, surgical approach, completeness of excision, and local tumor recurrence, all of which may be related to some degree. Dogs with grossly invasive and fixed STSs have a 5-fold increased risk of tumor-related deaths,[25,34] presumably because of greater difficulty in achieving complete excision of their STSs. Dogs treated with wide surgical resection have a MST of greater than 1306 days compared with 264 days for dogs treated with non–curative-intent surgeries.[31] The MST for dogs with incompletely excised STSs is 657 days, and this is significantly worse than the MST of greater than 1306 days for dogs with completely excised STSs.[31] Dogs with local tumor recurrence have a 5-fold risk of tumor-related death.[34]

Histologic and IHC features associated with survival include tumor necrosis, mitotic rate, histologic grade, argyrophilic nucleolar organizer region (AgNOR) score, and Ki67 score.[31,34,35] Tumor-related deaths are three times more likely with greater than 10% tumor necrosis and three times more likely with a mitotic rate of 20 or more mitotic figures/10 HPFs.[35] The MSTs for dogs with 10 or fewer, 10 to 19, and 20 or more mitotic figures/10 HPFs are 1444 days, 532 days, and 236 days, respectively.[35] Histologic grade was prognostic in two adjuvant RT studies with an MST not reached and greater than 1461 days for dogs with grade I and II STSs compared with 78 days for dogs with grade III STSs in one study of incompletely excised STSs treated with fractionated RT,[135] and a 940-day MST for dogs with grade III STSs compared with an MST not reached for dogs with grade I and II MSTs in dogs treated with incomplete excision and hypofractionated RT.[141] The MSTs and survival rates for dogs with STSs with AgNORs below and above the median AgNOR scores were greater than 1188 days and 76% versus greater than 1306 days and 53%, and dogs with an increased AgNOR score are 77 times more likely to die as a result of their disease.[31] Similarly, MSTs and survival rates for dogs with STSs with Ki67 scores below and above the median AgNOR scores were MST greater than 1188 days with 94% survival versus 657 days, and dogs with an increased Ki67 score are 12 times more likely to die as a result of their disease.[31]

Feline Sarcomas and Injection-Site Sarcomas

Epidemiology and Risk Factors

The following events are linked to the development of postvaccinal sarcomas in the cat. The prevalence of feline rabies led to the enactment of a law in Pennsylvania in 1987 requiring rabies vaccinations for cats.[171] In addition, two changes in vaccines occurred in the mid-1980s: development of a killed rabies vaccine licensed for subcutaneous administration and a killed vaccine for feline leukemia virus (FeLV). Epidemiologic studies have shown a strong association between the administration of inactivated feline vaccines, such as rabies and FeLV, and subsequent development of STSs at vaccination sites.[172–179] This is further supported by the significant decrease in interscapular injection-site sarcomas (ISSs) and significant increase in body wall and left and right pelvic limb ISSs since the recommendations of the Vaccine-Associated Feline Sarcoma Task Force (VAFSTF) were published in 2001.[180,181] Some authors report the reaction to vaccines was additive and this increased the likelihood of sarcoma development with multiple vaccines given at the same site simultaneously.[175] The prevalence

of sarcoma development of at sites of vaccine administration has been estimated between 1 to 4/10,000 cases,[176,182,183] but as high as 13 to 16/10,000 cases.[177,184,185] The ratio of ISSs to non-ISSs has increased from 0.5 in 1989 to 4.3 in 1994.[186]

The time to tumor development postvaccination has been reported to be 4 weeks to 10 years, and is associated with a robust inflammatory reaction around the tumor.[176] Adjuvant-containing vaccines have been proposed to be more likely to cause a vaccine site reaction and/or develop into an ISS[176]; however, three large epidemiologic studies did not provide evidence that aluminum-containing vaccines pose a greater risk,[175,178,187] and thus it remains unclear whether nonadjuvanted vaccines are safer.[180,187,188] A multicenter study of cats in the United States and Canada found that no single vaccine manufacturer or vaccine type had a higher association with the development of ISSs.[178] Cats with pelvic limb ISSs are significantly more likely to have been vaccinated with an inactivated rabies vaccine than a recombinant rabies vaccine, and cats with interscapular ISSs were more likely to have received long-acting corticosteroid injections.[187] Vaccination practices such as needle gauge, syringe reuse, use and shaking of multidose vials, mixing vaccines in a single syringe, and syringe type had no role in the development of tumors.[178]

Although no vaccine type has been associated with a higher risk of ISS development, nonadjuvanted vaccines are associated with less tissue inflammation compared with adjuvanted vaccines.[180] ISSs are hypothesized to develop from an inflammatory reaction induced by injectable medications that leads to uncontrolled fibroblast and myofibroblast proliferation and eventual tumor formation, either alone or in association with immunologic factors.[189–193] The thought that inflammation precedes tumor development is supported by histologic identification of transition zones from inflammation to sarcoma and microscopic foci of sarcoma located in areas of granulomatous inflammation (Fig. 22.13). A similar phenomenon of intraocular sarcoma development exists in cats after trauma or chronic uveitis.[194–197] ISSs have also been reported to arise at sites of injections other than vaccines such as lufenuron, long-acting steroids, nonsteroidal antiinflammatory drugs, cisplatin, vascular access ports, deep nonabsorbable sutures, and microchips,[187,198–204] and for this reason the term ISS is preferred to vaccine-associated sarcoma.

Growth factors regulate the cellular events involved in granulation tissue formation and wound healing. When these factors are added to fibroblast cultures, the cells develop a neoplastic phenotype. IHC identification and localization of growth factors and their receptors are being investigated in ISSs. ISSs are immunoreactive for platelet-derived growth factor (PDGF), epidermal growth factor and its receptors, and transforming growth factor (TGF)-β. Conversely, non–injection-site FSAs are negative or faintly positive for these factors and their receptors.[205,206] Lymphocytes in ISSs are positive for PDGF, but lymphocytes in non–injection-site FSAs and normal LNs are negative for PDGF.[205] Regional macrophages also stain positively for PDGF receptor (PDGFR). Neoplastic cells that are closest to lymphocytes in these tumors have the strongest staining for PDGFR, which has led to a hypothesis that lymphocytes in ISSs may secrete PDGF, recruit macrophages, and lead to fibroblast proliferation.[205,206] The expression of c-jun, a proto-oncogene coding for the transcriptional protein AP-1, has also been examined in ISSs. c-jun was found to be strongly positive in ISSs and not expressed in non–injection-site FSAs.[205,206] FeLV and the feline sarcoma virus are not involved in the pathogenesis of feline ISSs.[207]

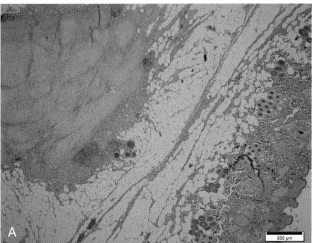

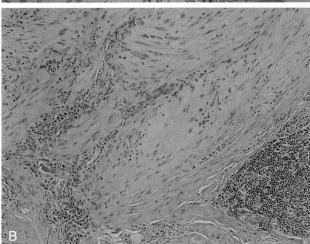

• **Fig. 22.13** Histologic image of a feline subcutaneous injection-site myxosarcoma. (A) A poorly delineated, highly cellular, neoplastic mass composed of streams and bundles of spindle cells supported by a myxomatous extracellular matrix expands the subcutaneous adipose tissue. Peripheral lymphoplasmacytic nodules are characteristic for this entity. H&E, 4×. (B) Lymphoplasmacytic infiltrates in perivascular regions in the absence of tumor necrosis. H&E, 20×. (Image courtesy Dr. J. Dreyfus.)

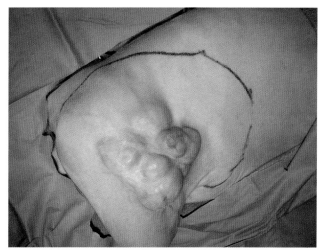

• **Fig. 22.14** The typical gross appearance of a feline injection-site sarcoma with a firm, large, multilobulated subcutaneous or cutaneous mass arising at a location consistent with the administration of a vaccine or other injections, such as the interscapular region, body wall, or pelvic limbs (pictured).

Studies have attempted to link growth factors with development of ISSs in cats. Continued immunohistochemical probing of feline ISSs documents expression of growth-regulating proteins: p53 protein, basic fibroblast growth factor, and TGF-α.[208] Researchers recently concluded that PDGF and PDGFR play an important role in the in vitro growth of ISS cell lines, both alone and in the presence of chemotherapeutic agents.

Pathology

There are many similarities between histologic subtypes and biologic behavior of STSs in cats and dogs. The three principal exceptions in cats are ISSs, virally induced multicentric FSA, and the relative rarity of PNST, SCS, and HS.[192,209] There are significant differences between ISSs and non-ISSs. Clinically, ISSs are usually large with a rapid growth rate and typically arise from the subcutis at sites consistent with the administration of vaccines and other injections, such as the interscapular region, body wall, and pelvic limbs (Fig. 22.14), whereas non-ISSs are smaller, slower growing, and will often arise from the skin rather than

subcutaneous tissue.[174,210,211] ISSs are typically mesenchymal in origin and include FSAs, rhabdomyosarcomas, MFHs, undifferentiated sarcomas, and extraskeletal osteosarcomas and chondrosarcomas.[205,212,213] ISSs have histologic features consistent with a more aggressive biologic behavior than non–ISSs, such as marked nuclear and cellular pleomorphism, increased tumor necrosis, high mitotic activity, multinucleate giant cells, and the presence of a peripheral inflammatory cell infiltrate consisting of lymphocytes and macrophages.[172,185,186,193,205] In a series of 91 cats with histologically confirmed and graded ISSs, the prevalence of high-grade lesions was substantially higher than reported in dogs,[35] with 59% of cats diagnosed with grade III tumors and only 5% with grade I tumors.[214] Microscopically, areas of transition between inflammation and tumor development are frequently observed in cats with ISS.[205,215] The macrophages in these peripheral inflammatory cell infiltrates often contain a bluish-gray foreign material that has been identified as aluminum and oxygen by electron probe x-ray microanalysis.[192] Aluminum hydroxide is one of several adjuvants used in currently available feline vaccines.[192] Although nonadjuvanted vaccines are currently available for FeLV and rabies, it is unknown if these vaccines are less likely to result in sarcoma formation, especially as studies have shown that all vaccines have the potential to cause ISSs.[180,187,188] ISSs are histologically similar to mesenchymal tumors arising in the traumatized eyes of cats, which suggests a common pathogenesis of inflammation and the development of STSs in these cats.[196,197,206] The presence of inflammatory cells, fibroblasts, and myofibroblasts in and adjacent to ISSs supports this hypothesis.[26,216,217]

Diagnosis and Workup

The diagnostic techniques and clinical staging tests recommended for cats with suspected ISSs are similar to those described in dogs earlier in this chapter. Advanced imaging, such as contrast-enhanced CT or MRI, is recommended for local staging of the tumor because these 3D imaging modalities provide essential information for proper planning of surgery and/or RT (Fig. 22.15).[192,218–223] The volume of tumor based on contrast-enhanced CT is larger than the volume measured using calipers during physical examination.[191,223] Furthermore, the presence

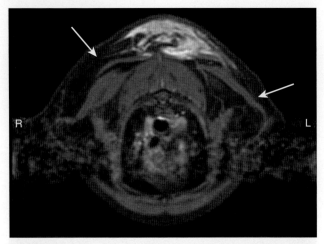

• **Fig. 22.15** Contrast-enhanced magnetic resonance imaging of a cat with an injection-site sarcoma. Note the fingerlike projections of the tumor (*arrows*).

of skip metastases on CT scans was significantly associated with local tumor recurrence.[222] Although CT and MRI are both very sensitive for the detection of the peritumoral extent of disease in cats with suspected ISSs, up to 59% of these peritumoral lesions are nonneoplastic when examined histologically.[221] Moreover, the low-field MRI characteristics of ISSs can vary and this may be influenced by previous incisional or excisional biopsies.[218] For interscapular ISSs, it is important to perform postcontrast CT scans with the thoracic limbs extended cranially and caudally along the body to permit better evaluation of the relationship between the ISS and the adjacent tissue.[219] Accurate pretreatment knowledge of the extent of disease is important because ISSs are very invasive, are frequently located in areas in which regional anatomy can complicate an aggressive surgical approach (e.g., interscapular area, body wall, and proximal pelvic limb), and have a high rate of local tumor recurrence, especially if incompletely excised. Excisional biopsy of a suspected ISS is not recommended because the risk of local tumor recurrence is increased, and DFI and ST are significantly decreased.[224,225]

Treatment

Surgery

ISSs are poorly encapsulated tumors with extension and infiltration along fascial planes.[215,216] The VAFSTF has recommended surgical resection with a minimum of 2 cm margins both lateral and deep to the tumor[192]; however, this recommendation is now considered inadequate. The preferred approach is based on how the extent of the ISS is assessed, with 5-cm lateral margins and two fascial layers for deep margins recommended when the extent of disease is based on gross palpation, whereas 3-cm lateral margins and one fascial layer for deep margins are recommended when the extent of disease is based on contrast-enhanced CT scans.[214,226,227] Only 50% of ISSs are completely excised when resected with 2- to 3-cm lateral margins compared with 95% to 97% when excised with 4- to 5-cm lateral margins.[214,224–226] Marginal resection or excisional biopsy should not be attempted. The median DFI and MST are significantly decreased with marginal resection, with more than one attempt at surgical resection, and if surgery is performed by nonreferral surgeons.[214,224,225] The median time to first recurrence after marginal resection is 79 days compared with 325 to 419 days

for wide resection or radical surgery.[224] In addition, the median time to first recurrence is only 66 days when the first surgery is performed at a nonreferral institution compared with 274 days at referral institutions.[224] Inadequate biopsy planning, preoperative staging, and/or attempts at first surgery will result in an increase in tumor margins and may make further surgical treatment more difficult to impossible. The first attempt at surgical management of cats with ISSs should be performed by a referral surgeon with experience in aggressive resection, especially in the interscapular, body wall, or pelvic regions, to increase the chance of a successful outcome.[214,224–228] Similar to dogs with STSs, biopsy tracts and any areas of fixation, including bone and fascia, should be resected en bloc with the tumor. In cats with ISSs, wide surgical resection of tumors located in the interscapular region will often involve excision of dorsal spinous processes (Fig. 22.16), whereas thoracic or body wall resection is often required for truncal tumors (Fig. 22.17).[224,225] Limb amputation or hemipelvectomy is usually required to achieve adequate surgical margins and local tumor control for ISSs located on the extremity.[214]

Local tumor control is very good if the ISS is treated aggressively with 5-cm lateral margins and one to two fascial layers for deep margins, or compartmental resections. When the VAFSTF recommendations of 2- to 3-cm lateral margins and one fascial layer for deep margins are used, complete resection is achieved in fewer than 50% of cats and overall 1- and 2-year disease-free rates are only 35% and 9%, respectively.[224,225] In comparison, the complete excision rate is 97% and the local recurrence rate is 14% at 3 years when ISSs are resected with 5-cm lateral margins and two fascial layers for deep margins, including ISSs located in the interscapular region, body wall, and extremities.[214] These findings are supported by an earlier study of 57 cats treated with 4- to 5-cm lateral margins and one fascial layer for deep margins, in which complete histologic excision was achieved in 95% of cats.[226] Chest wall and body resection, using a minimum of 3-cm margins, was well tolerated in six cats and local tumor recurrence was not reported in any of these cats at a minimum of 12 months postoperatively.[228] Compartmental resections of interscapular ISSs, in combination with neoadjuvant epirubicin, resulted in a local recurrence rate of 14% in 21 cats after a median follow-up time of 1072 days.[229] Despite these aggressive approaches, major wound healing complications are relatively uncommon, with wound dehiscence reported in 11% to 17% of cats.[214,227] Wound dehiscence is more common after wide resection of interscapular ISSs compared with other locations[214] and in overweight cats, cats with larger tumors, ISSs that required longer anesthetic and surgical times for surgical resection, and wound defects which were closed in an X-shape rather than linearly.[227] Real-time in vivo assessment of residual tumor in the wound bed has been investigated with good initial results in 12 cats with ISSs,[230] and local tumor control rates may be improved when this technology becomes commercially available.

Neoadjuvant chemotherapy or RT may have benefits when combined with surgery. In people, both preoperative chemotherapy and RT have resulted in the conversion of the tumor pseudocapsule into a thick, collagenized capsule with no viable tumor cells.[114] Clinically, this may result in a better defined tumor that is more amenable to complete histologic excision. In one study, there was no difference in local recurrence rates or STs in 49 cats treated with neoadjuvant DOX and surgery compared with 20 cats treated with surgery alone.[231] However, in another study,

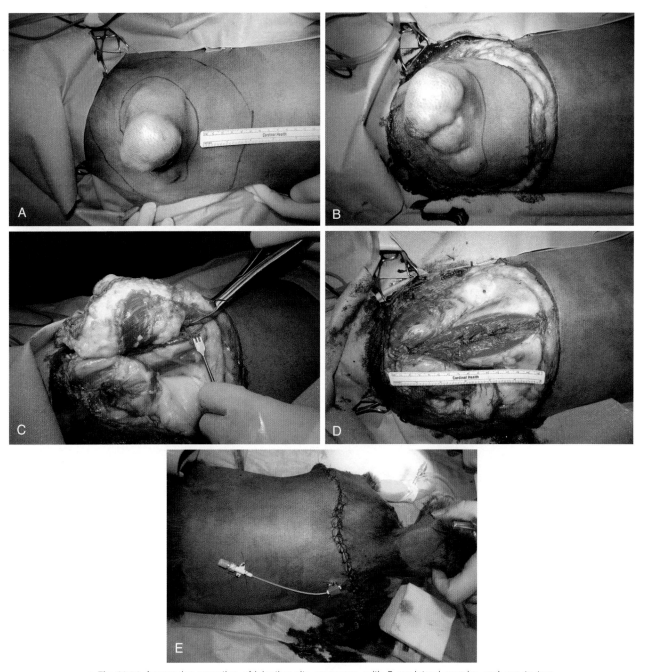

• **Fig. 22.16** Aggressive resection of injection-site sarcomas, with 5-cm lateral margins and one to two uninvolved fascial layers for deeps margins, is required for the best opportunity for complete histologic excision and local tumor control. (A) Planned lateral surgical margins are indicated with a sterile marker pen 5 cm in all directions around an interscapular injection-site sarcoma. (B) An incision is then performed along the marked margins, and continued deeply to include two uninvolved fascial layers. (C) In this cat, ostectomy of the dorsal spinous processes was performed with bone cutters to achieve deep surgical margins and compartmental resection of the injection-site sarcoma. (D) The wound defect after these aggressive wide resections can be large, but primary closure is almost always achievable (E).

neoadjuvant chemotherapy with three doses of epirubicin followed by compartmental resection of interscapular ISSs resulted in an overall local recurrence rate of 14% in 21 cats after a median follow-up time of 1072 days.[229]

Surgery and Radiation Therapy

Although aggressive surgical resection is recommended for the management of cats with ISSs, this may not always be feasible. In these cases, multimodality therapy with either preoperative or postoperative RT results in better rates of local tumor control than more conservative surgical approaches alone.[213,232–236]

In two studies investigating preoperative RT, local tumor recurrence was reported in 40% to 45% of cats at a median of 398 to 584 days postoperatively.[232,234] In both studies, complete resection significantly improved the time to local recurrence, with a 700- to 986-day median DFI for completely excised tumors and 112- to 292-day median DFI for tumors resected with incomplete margins.[232,234] However, complete resection after preoperative RT does

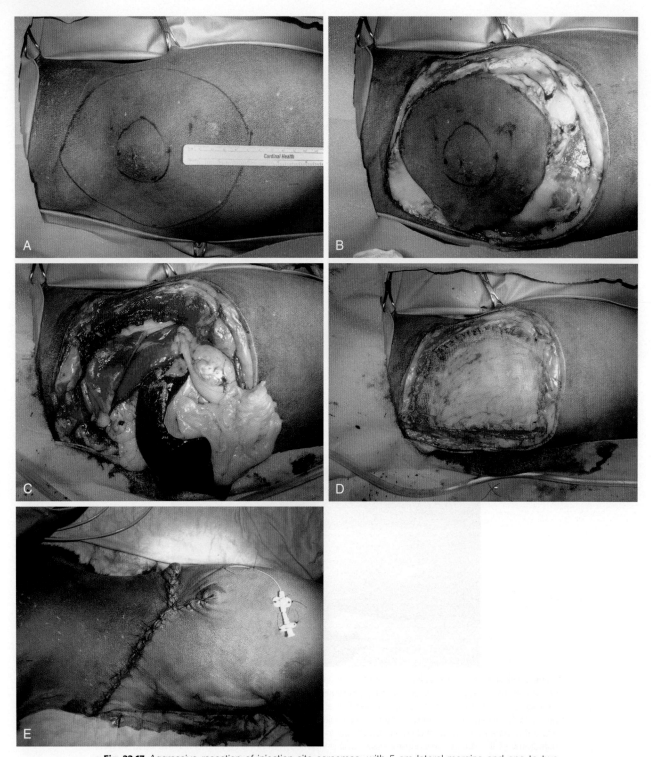

• **Fig. 22.17** Aggressive resection of injection-site sarcomas, with 5-cm lateral margins and one to two uninvolved fascial layers for deeps margins, is required for the best opportunity for complete histologic excision and local tumor control. (A) Planned lateral surgical margins are indicated with a sterile marker pen 5 cm in all directions around a body wall injection-site sarcoma. (B) An incision is then performed along the marked margins. (C) Deep margins of two uninvolved fascial layers included chest (seven ribs) and body wall. (D) After caudal lung lobectomy and diaphragmatic advancement, the body wall defect was reconstructed with an omental pedicle graft and prosthetic mesh. (E) The wound defect was closed primarily.

not appear to improve local control rates because local tumor recurrence was reported in 42% of 59 cats with complete histologic excision and 32% of 28 cats with incomplete histologic excision.[234]

The outcome after postoperative RT is similar to preoperative RT. In one study of 79 cats treated with surgery and curative-intent RT, the MST was significantly longer in cats treated with postoperative rather than preoperative RT; however, the practice at this institution was to treat larger tumors with preoperative RT and hence this finding may be due to a selection bias.[236] In one study, local tumor recurrence was reported in 41% of 76 cats at a median of 405 days postoperatively.[232] In another study investigating the effects of chemotherapy in cats treated with surgery and postoperative RT, local tumor recurrence occurred in 28% of 25 cats with a median time to first recurrence not reached in cats treated with surgery and RT alone and 661 days in cats also treated with DOX.[233] In a study of 46 cats treated with surgery and curative-intent postoperative RT, the median PFI was 37 months, with 1- and 2-year progression-free rates of 63% and 60%, respectively.[235] In comparison, 27 cats treated with postoperative palliative hypofractioned protocols had a median PFI of 10 months and a MST of 24 months.[235] Importantly, RT should start 10 to 14 days postoperatively as DFI and ST decreases as the interval between surgery and starting RT increases.[213] Local tumor recurrence does not influence ST and, regardless of the timing of RT relative to surgery, survival data are encouraging with MSTs of 600 to 1307 days and 1-, 2-, and 3-year survival rates of 86%, 44% to 71%, and 28% to 68%, respectively.[213,232–235]

Local tumor control is still disappointing with 28% to 45% of tumors recurring after multimodality treatment with surgery using 2- to 3-cm lateral margins and RT.[213,232–236] The radiation field used in these studies typically included a minimum of 3-cm margins around the tumor or surgical scar. The majority of tumors recur within the radiation field, although tumors have been reported to recur outside the radiation field.[234] Similar to surgery alone, a more aggressive approach may be warranted to improve local tumor control, such as higher radiation doses, larger radiation fields, and more aggressive surgical resections.

Radiation Therapy for Gross Disease

Although RT alone is rarely effective for the management of cats and dogs with measurable STSs, RT may have a role in the palliative setting for cats with large and unresectable ISSs. In a pilot study of 10 cats with ISSs, 7 cats achieved partial responses and 2 cats had complete responses after treatment with liposomal DOX as a radiation sensitizer and irradiation with a median of 5 fractions of 4 Gy for a total dose of 20 Gy; however, PFIs were not durable (median of 117 days).[237] Similar findings were reported in 17 cats with gross disease treated with 4 fractions of 8 Gy for a total dose of 32 Gy in which the median PFI was 4 months and MST was 7 months.[235] Stereotactic RT (SRT) has also been reported in a series of 11 cats.[238] These cats were treated with variable protocols (most commonly 3 fractions of 10 Gy) with three complete and five partial responses documented. The median PFI was 242 days and the MST was 301 days.[238] A margin for subclinical microscopic disease was not utilized in these patients and thus the intent of SRT alone cannot be considered definitive; however, it may facilitate surgical resection or result in palliation of clinical signs.

Chemotherapy

The role of chemotherapy in the management of cats with ISS remains undefined. Metastasis has been reported in 0% to 26% of cats with ISSs, despite the aggressive histologic appearance and prevalence of high-grade lesions in these tumors, with a median time to metastasis of 265 to 309 days.[209,210,220–222,228,230] ISS cell lines have shown in vitro sensitivity at clinically relevant doses to DOX, mitoxantrone, vincristine, lomustine, and paclitaxel.[239–241] Clinically, partial and complete responses to DOX, either alone or in combination with cyclophosphamide, or lomustine have been reported in 25% to 50% of cats with gross tumors, but these responses are often short-lived with a median duration of 83 to 125 days.[242–244] However, MSTs are significantly prolonged in cats that respond to chemotherapy: 242 days for responders and 83 days for nonresponders.[242] Furthermore, MSTs are significantly increased for cats with gross residual disease after surgical

excision and treated with postoperative RT and chemotherapy with an MST of 29 months compared with 5 months for cats treated with surgery and postoperative RT.[235]

Postoperative chemotherapy has minimal effect on survival in cats treated with curative-intent surgery and RT.[214,226,232,233,243] Chemotherapy may, however, have beneficial effects on local tumor control and time to local tumor recurrence. DOX and liposome-encapsulated DOX significantly prolonged DFI after surgery, with a median DFI of 393 days for cats receiving chemotherapy and 93 days for those in which chemotherapy was not administered.[243] The completeness of surgical margins may be a confounding factor in this analysis because the median DFI was greater than 449 days in cats with complete surgical margins compared with 281 days after incomplete resection.[243] Chemotherapy has also been reported to affect MST but not DFI in cats treated with hypofractionated RT for gross disease.[235] Carboplatin was associated with an insignificant but numerically superior median DFI of greater than 986 days in cats treated with preoperative RT and surgery.[234] Other studies have shown no effect of adjunctive chemotherapy on either local tumor control or ST.[232,233]

The tyrosine kinase inhibitors toceranib phosphate (Palladia), masitinib mesylate (Kinavet/Masivet), and imatinib mesylate (Gleevec) have also been investigated for the therapy of ISSs in cats based on dysregulation of PDGFR in feline ISS cell lines.[245,246,247,248] Imatinib has been shown to result in inhibition of the PDGF/PDGFR pathway and results in chemosensitization of feline ISS cells.[245] Masitinib also resulted in inhibition of PDGFR and cellular proliferation in feline ISS cell lines, but at doses that were higher than those readily achievable clinically.[246] Masitinib was also investigated as a radiation sensitizer in feline ISS cell lines, but was not found to result in sensitization in vitro.[247] Finally, toceranib was administered to 18 cats with unresectable ISSs and, although well tolerated at doses commonly administered in dogs, responses were not documented.[248]

Novel treatments such as electrochemotherapy and immunotherapy are also being investigated with some encouraging results. In one study, cats with high-grade STSs were treated either intraoperatively or postoperatively with intratumoral bleomycin followed by eight biphasic pulses of up to 1300 V/cm.[249] The median time to local tumor recurrence in the control (surgery only) group was 4 months compared with 12 months for cats treated intraoperatively and 19 months for cats treated postoperatively. Of further interest, the metastatic rate was only 1.7%.[249] In a second study, 64 cats with FSA were treated postoperatively with two rounds of electrochemotherapy utilizing cisplatin.[250] The local recurrence rate was 29%. Minimal systemic toxicity, including pulmonary, renal, or cutaneous toxicity, was documented in these cats.[250] It should be noted that cisplatin cannot be administered systemically in cats because cisplatin causes fatal pulmonary edema even at relatively low doses.[251]

Immunotherapy, using recombinant viruses expressing interleukin-2 (IL-2), has shown some promise in improving local tumor control rates in cats with ISSs. After surgical resection and iridium-based brachytherapy, the 1-year local tumor recurrence rate was 61% in cats receiving no adjunctive treatment, 39% in cats administered human IL-2 using a vaccinia virus vector, and 28% with feline IL-2 using a canary pox virus vector.[252] In a randomized trial by the same group comparing surgery and brachytherapy with surgery and brachytherapy combined with high- and low-dose IL-2 vaccine, the frequency of relapse was significantly reduced in the groups receiving the IL-2 vaccine at both 12 (52% vs 28%) and 24 months (59% vs 28%).[253] This product is now commercially available in the United States and European Union for the postoperative treatment of feline ISSs. In a phase I trial, two doses of intratumoral feline IL-2, interferon-gamma

(IFN-γ), and granulocyte-macrophage colony-stimulating factor (GM-CSF) followed by magnetofection before surgical resection resulted in a 1-year local recurrence rate of 24%.[254] In another phase I trial by the same research group, two doses of intratumoral GM-CSF followed by magnetofection before surgical resection resulted in a 1-year local recurrence rate of 50% and minimal treatment-related toxicities.[255] Other immunotherapeutic agents such as IL-12 and acemannan have been investigated with less favorable results.[256–258]

Prognosis

Local Recurrence

Local tumor control is the most challenging aspect of managing cats with ISS. The best results are achieved after complete histologic excision, and complete histologic excision is more likely after aggressive surgical resection. The rate of complete histologic excision is less than 50% when ISSs are excised with 2- to 3-cm lateral margins,[224,225] compared with 95% to 97% when excised with 4- to 5-cm lateral margins.[214,226] The local tumor recurrence rate is 14% to 22% after complete histologic excision compared with 58% to 69% after incomplete excision.[214,229,243,259] Incomplete histologic excision of ISSs is associated with a 10-fold increased risk of local tumor recurrence.[259] Overall, the 1- and 2-year disease-free rates are 35% and 9%, respectively, after wide resection with 2- to 3-cm lateral margins,[224,225] compared with a 3-year disease-free rate of 86% after wide resection with 5-cm lateral margins or compartmental resections.[214,229]

When surgical resection is combined with either preoperative or postoperative RT, the local recurrence rates are 28% to 45% with median DFIs of 13 to 37 months.[213,226,228,232–234,260] Similar to surgical management of ISSs, complete histologic excision results in a significant improvement in time to local recurrence for cats treated with surgery and RT, with a 700- to 986-day median DFI for completely excised tumors and 112- to 292-day median DFI for tumors resected with incomplete margins.[232,234] However, complete excision after preoperative RT does not appear to improve local control rates because local tumor recurrence was reported in 42% of 59 cats with complete histologic excision and 32% of 28 cats with incomplete histologic excision.[234]

Prognostic factors for local recurrence include tumor size, surgical dose or aggressiveness, completeness of histologic excision, and histologic grade. In one study of 24 cats with ISSs, local recurrence was significantly more likely after wide resection of larger tumors; and for each unit increase in tumor size, cats were two times more likely to develop local recurrence and two times more likely to have a tumor-related death.[261] A number of studies have shown the importance of an aggressive surgical approach in the management of cats with ISSs, but this most likely is related to the ability to achieve complete histologic excision rather than the surgical approach specifically. The median time to first recurrence after marginal resection is 79 days compared with 325 to 419 days for wide resection or radical surgery.[225] In addition, the median time to first recurrence is only 66 days when the first surgery is performed at a nonreferral institution compared with 274 days at referral institutions.[224,225] In another study of 57 cats with wide resection of ISSs, the local recurrence rate was 39% and significantly more likely with grade III ISSs compared with either grade I or II ISSs.[226]

Metastasis

Metastasis is relatively uncommon in cats with ISSs. The metastatic rate varies from 0% to 24%.[209,213–215,225,226,232,234,261,262] Metastasis is significantly more likely in cats with grade III ISSs[226]; and the metastatic rates for cats with grade I, II, and III ISSs are 0% to 17%, 15% to 19%, and 22% to 100%.[214,226] The lungs are the most common site of metastasis, with other sites including regional lymph nodes, kidney, liver, spleen, intestines, and epidural and ocular infiltration.[214,215,225,226,232]

Survival

The overall prognosis for cats with ISSs is often very good despite their propensity for local tumor recurrence. The overall MST is 804 to 901 days to not reached for cats treated with wide surgical resection of 4-cm to 5-cm lateral margins and one to two fascial layers for deep margins.[214,226,229] For cats treated with less aggressive surgery, the overall MST varies from greater than 395 days to 608 days.[224,225,262] For cats treated with surgery and RT, regardless of the timing of RT, the overall MSTs range from 520 to 1307 days with 1-, 2-, and 3-year survival rates of 62% to 86%, 42% to 71%, and 28% to 68%, respectively.[213,232–236,260]

Prognostic factors associated with survival in cats with ISSs include anemia, tumor size, treatment type, histologic subtype, mitotic rate, local tumor recurrence, and metastatic disease. For cats treated with surgery and either preoperative or postoperative RT, anemia with a packed cell volume (PCV) less than 25% was associated with decreased ST.[236] The MSTs for cats with a PCV less than and greater than or equal to 25% were 308 days and 760 days, respectively, with a 2-fold increased risk of tumor-related death for cats with a PCV less than 25%.[236] The 1- and 2-year survival rates for cats treated with a PCV less than 25% were 40% and 24%, respectively, whereas the 1- and 2-year survival rates for cats with a PCV greater than or equal to 25% were 72% and 50%, respectively.[236] Tumor size was associated with prognosis in two studies of cats treated with surgery alone. Cats with STSs smaller than 2 cm in diameter had an MST of 643 days, which was significantly longer than the MSTs of 558 days for cats with tumors 2 to 5 cm in diameter and 394 days for cats with STSs larger than 5 cm in diameter.[262] In another study, cats with ISSs greater than 3.75 cm had a significantly decreased ST.[261] Although most studies do not show differences in outcomes between cats treated with surgery and either preoperative or postoperative RT, the outcome was significantly worse for cats treated with preoperative RT (MST 310 days) than postoperative RT (MST 705 days) in one study, and cats treated with preoperative RT had a 2-fold increased risk of tumor-related death.[236] The 1- and 2-year survival rates for cats treated with preoperative and postoperative RT were 42% and 29%, and 70% and 47%, respectively.[236] In another study of 52 cats treated with surgery alone, including eight cats with presumed ISSs, histologic subtype was prognostic with MSTs for cats with FSA (640 days) and PNST (645 days) significantly better than for cats with MFH (290 days).[262] Survival was significantly associated with mitotic rate in one study of 24 cats with a 994-day MST for cats with mitotic count greater than 20 mitoses per 10 HPFs compared with an MST that was not reached in cats with a mitotic rate less than or equal to 20 mitoses per 10 HPFs.[261] The MST for cats with local tumor recurrence was 327 to 499 days compared with 1098 to 1461 days to not reached for cats without local tumor recurrence.[214,226,261] The estimated 2-year survival rates for cats without and with local recurrence are 75% and 37%, respectively.[261] The MST for cats without distant metastasis was 929 to 1528 days compared with 165 to 388 days for the 20% to 21% of cats that developed distant metastasis.[214,226] Distant metastasis increased the risk of tumor-related death by three times.[226]

Prevention

The recommendations on preventing ISSs in cats are controversial. These include changing the sites of vaccine administration, decreasing the use of polyvalent vaccines, using nonadjuvanted vaccines, avoiding the use of aluminum-based adjuvants, and increasing the interval between vaccinations.[26,177,263,264]

The VAFSTF has recommended that no vaccine be administered in the interscapular region, rabies vaccines be administered in the distal aspect of the right pelvic limb, FeLV vaccines be administered in the distal aspect of the left pelvic limb, and all other vaccines be administered in the right shoulder.[26,192] The location of each injection, the type of vaccine, and the manufacturer and serial number of the vaccine should be documented in the patient records. These recommendations are intended to provide epidemiologic information rather than prevent ISSs. Vaccines should be administered into the distal, rather than mid to proximal, aspects of the limb to aid in earlier detection and increase the chance of achieving complete resection. Subcutaneous and intramuscular administration can both cause local inflammatory reactions and result in the development of ISSs.[26] Subcutaneous administration is preferred to intramuscular injection because ISSs developing from subcutaneous sites are more readily palpable and diagnosed earlier in the course of disease. The VAFSTF has recommended that masses at vaccination sites be interrogated if the mass is evident 3 or more months after vaccination, is larger than 2 cm in diameter, or is increasing in size more than 1 month after vaccine administration (3–2–1 Rule).[191,192] Unfortunately, feline ISSs are still occurring at sites not recommended by the VAFSTF.[178,179,181,185] Vaccination in the tail has been recommended by some investigators because masses are more readily visible and palpable in the tail than other sites and the tail is relatively simple to amputate with good margins and minimal effect on the function and quality of life of cats, especially compared with other locations such as interscapular resections, body wall resections, and limb amputations or hemipelvectomies.[265] In a pilot study, vaccination in the tip of the tail was well tolerated and did not require sedation or restraint.[265]

Traditionally, annual boosters have been recommended for most vaccines in cats. The U.S. Department of Agriculture–Animal Plant Health Inspection Service (USDA-APHIS) does not require duration of immunity studies for licensing of vaccines; however, if a duration of immunity study has not been performed, the USDA-APHIS requires that vaccine labels include a recommendation for annual revaccination.[192] Vaccine practices have been questioned by the profession and this has been supported by duration of immunity studies. The duration of immunity for a single commercially available inactivated, adjuvanted combination of feline panleukopenia, herpesvirus, and calicivirus is greater than 7 years, with persistent antibodies against all three viruses for more than 3 years.[266–268] Local and state requirements often mandate annual rabies boosters, despite a duration of immunity of at least 3 years, because of the significant public health concern of rabies infection.[192] The VAFSTF has recommended that the administration of vaccines is a medicinal procedure and vaccination protocols should be customized for individual cats.[192] A vaccine should not be administered until the medical importance and zoonotic potential of the infectious agent, risk of exposure, and legal requirements have been considered and balanced against the risk of ISSs and other adverse effects.[192]

Comparative Aspects

In general, STSs have a similar pathologic appearance, clinical presentation, and behavior in humans and animals. However, a higher incidence is seen in young people as opposed to young companion animals, with the exception of rhabdomyosarcoma,

which is seen in young dogs. The distribution of STS in humans is similar to animals. In humans, 43% are in the extremities, with two-thirds occurring in the lower limb, and 34% are intraperitoneal, with 19% visceral in origin and 15% retroperitoneal. STSs of the trunk occur in 10% of human patients, and the remaining 13% occur at other sites. Metastasis is generally hematogenous and appears to be more common in human STS than in dogs, which may partially be explained by the higher numbers of nerve sheath tumors (with lower metastatic rate) seen in the dog.

Most sarcomas recognized in humans are also diagnosed in animals, although the specific incidences may vary markedly. There are many more histologic subtypes recognized in humans, which are often site dependent. With the exception of benign smooth muscle tumors and subcutaneous lipomas, there is little evidence that these lesions arise from their mature (differentiated) tissue counterparts. One current theory is that switching on a set of genes that programs mesenchymal differentiation in any mesenchymal cell may give rise to any type of mesenchymal tumor. Common subtypes of STSs seen in the extremities of humans are liposarcomas, MFHs, SCS, and FSAs. In the retroperitoneal location, liposarcomas and leiomyosarcomas are the most common histotypes noted in humans. The most common subtype noted viscerally are gastrointestinal stromal tumors (GISTs). Overall, leiomyosarcoma is the most common genitourinary sarcoma. Up to 15% of all sarcomas occur in children, and the subtypes most commonly represented are rhabdomyosarcomas, Ewing's sarcomas, and primitive neuroectodermal tumors.

Prognostic variables in humans include clinical stage, histologic grade, necrosis, site, size, LN involvement, and aggressiveness of surgery or RT. The histopathologic grading system used and shown to be predictive for metastasis in dogs is a grading system adopted from human pathology that is also predictive for survival.[26] In addition, it appears that histologic grade is the predominant predictor of early recurrence, whereas tumor size plays a more important role for late recurrence. It is unclear whether age plays a prognostic role in human STS.

Surgical treatment is the mainstay of therapy for STS in the control of local disease. The definition of the surgical approach varies between different organizations, with 1- to 4-cm lateral margins considered a wide resection and those 5 cm or greater termed a curative resection; however, tissue barriers are also taken into account in determining surgical margins, with thin and thick tissue barriers being considered equivalent to 2 cm and 3 cm of margins, respectively.[13] Surgery can be combined with neoadjuvant chemotherapy, neoadjuvant RT, and/or adjuvant RT to improve local tumor control.[114] Amputation is reserved for patients with unresectable tumors, no evidence of metastasis, and the potential for good long-term rehabilitation. Local recurrence is greater in those patients undergoing limb-sparing therapies compared with amputation; however, there is no difference in disease-free survival between the two groups. Distant metastasis is more common in people with STS; however, chemotherapy is not routinely used because of either a lack of or small but significant improvements in tumor control and survival outcomes with adjuvant chemotherapy.[114] Ifosfamide is currently the most active salvage agent for patients who have failed DOX-based protocols, but tyrosine kinase inhibitors are also used. Permanent local control with the first treatment is related to long-term survival. High-risk STS patients are treated with combined chemoradiation before surgical resection. The chemotherapy protocol often used is DOX, ifosfamide, mesna, and dacarbazine. In human patients with metastatic disease, combination chemotherapy produces response rates of 20%, and most of these patients are candidates for investigational agents.

References

1. Theilen GH, Madewell BR: Tumors of the skin and subcutaneous tissues. In Theilen GH, Madewell BR, editors: *Veterinary cancer medicine*, Philadelphia, 1979, Lea & Febiger, pp 123–191.

2. Dorn ER: Epidemiology of canine and feline tumors, *J Am Anim Hosp Assoc* 12:307–312, 1976.

3. Hardy WD: The etiology of canine and feline tumors, *J Am Anim Hosp Assoc* 12:313–334, 1976.

4. Madewell BR, Theilen GH: Etiology of cancer in animals. In Theilen GH, Madewell BR, editors: *Veterinary cancer medicine*, Philadelphia, 1979, Lea & Febiger, pp 13–25.

5. McCarthy PE, Hedlund CS, Veazy RS, et al.: Liposarcoma associated with a glass foreign body in a dog, *J Am Vet Med Assoc* 209:612–614, 1996.

6. Thrall DE, Goldschmidt MH, Biery DN: Malignant tumor formation at the site of previously irradiated acanthomatous epulides in four dogs, *J Am Vet Med Assoc* 178:127–132, 1981.

7. Johnstone PA, Laskin WB, DeLuca AM, et al.: Tumors in dogs exposed to experimental intraoperative radiotherapy, *Int J Radiat Oncol Biol Phys* 34:853–857, 1996.

8. Barnes M, Duray P, DeLuca A, et al.: Tumor induction following intraoperative radiotherapy: late results of the National Cancer Institute canine trials, *Int J Radiat Oncol Biol Phys* 19:651–660, 1990.

9. Sinibaldi K, Rosen H, Liu SK, et al.: Tumors associated with metallic implants in animals, *Clin Orthop* 118:257–266, 1976.

10. Ehrhart N: Soft–tissue sarcomas in dogs: a review, *J Am Anim Hosp Assoc* 41:241–246, 2005.

11. Kim DY, Hodgin EC, Cho DY, et al.: Juvenile rhabdomyosarcomas in two dogs, *Vet Pathol* 33:447–450, 1996.

12. Dennis MM, McSporran KD, Bacon NJ, et al.: Prognostic factors for cutaneous and subcutaneous soft tissue sarcomas in dogs, *Vet Pathol* 48:73–84, 2011.

13. Bray JP: Soft tissue sarcoma in the dog – part 2: surgical margins, controversies, and a comparative review, *J Small Anim Pract* 58:63–72, 2017.

14. Duda RB: Review: biology of mesenchymal tumors, *Cancer J* 7:52–62, 1994.

15. Thrall DE, Gillette EL: Soft-tissue sarcomas, *Semin Vet Med Surg Small Anim* 10:173–179, 1995.

16. Ordonez NG: Immunocytochemistry in the diagnosis of soft-tissue sarcomas, *Cancer Bull* 45:13–23, 1993.

17. Madewell BR, Munn RJ: The soft tissue sarcomas: immunohistochemical and ultrastructural distinctions, *ACVIM Proc* 9:717–720, 1991.

18. Ciekot P, Powers B, Withrow S, et al.: Histologically low-grade, yet biologically high-grade, fibrosarcoma of the mandible and maxilla in dogs: 25 cases (1982–1991), *J Am Vet Med Assoc* 204:610–615, 1994.

19. Zhang P, Brooks JS: Modern pathological evaluation of soft tissue sarcoma specimens and its potential role in soft tissue sarcoma research, *Curr Treat Options Oncol* 5:441–450, 2004.

20. Hogendoorn PC, Collin F, Daugaard S, et al.: Pathology and Biology Subcommittee of the EORTC Soft Tissue and Bone Sarcoma Group. Changing concepts in the pathological basis of soft tissue and bone sarcoma treatment, *Eur J Cancer* 40:1644–1654, 2004.

21. Nilbert M, Engellau J: Experiences from tissue microarray in soft tissue sarcomas, *Acta Orthop Scand Suppl* 75:29–34, 2004.

22. Perez J, Bautista MJ, Rollon E, et al.: Immunohistochemical characterization of hemangiopericytomas and other spindle cell tumors in the dog, *Vet Pathol* 33:391–397, 1996.

23. Williamson MM, Middleton DJ: Cutaneous soft tissue tumours in dogs: classification, differentiation, and histogenesis, *Vet Dermatol* 9:43–48, 1998.

24. Gaitero L, Anor S, Fondevila D, et al.: Canine cutaneous spindle cell tumours with features of peripheral nerve sheath tumours: a histopathological and immunohistochemical study, *J Comp Pathol* 139:16–23, 2008.

25. Chase D, Bray J, Ide A, et al.: Outcome following removal of canine spindle cell tumours in first opinion practice: 104 cases, *J Small Anim Pract* 50:568–574, 2009.

26. MacEwen EG, Powers BE, Macy D, et al.: Soft tissue sarcomas. In Withrow SJ, MacEwen EG, editors: *Small animal clinical oncology*, ed 3, Philadelphia, 2001, Saunders, pp 283–304.

27. Cook JL, Turk JR, Pope ER, et al.: Infantile desmoid-type fibromatosis in an Akita puppy, *J Am Anim Hosp Assoc* 34:291–294, 1998.

28. Gwin RM, Gelatt KN, Peiffer RL: Ophthalmic nodular fasciitis in the dog, *J Am Vet Med Assoc* 170:611–614, 1977.

29. Goldschmidt MH, Hendrick MJ: Tumors of the skin and soft tissue. In Meuten DJ, editor: *Tumors in domestic animals*, ed 4, Ames, IA, 2002, Iowa State Press, pp 45–117.

30. Goldschmidt MH, Shofer FS: *Skin tumors of the dog and cat*, Oxford, 1998, Butterworth Heinemann.

31. Ettinger SN, Scase TJ, Oberthaler KT, et al.: Association of argyrophilic nucleolar organizing regions, Ki-67, and proliferating cell nuclear antigen scores with histologic grade and survival in dogs with soft tissue sarcomas: 60 cases (1996–2002), *J Am Vet Med Assoc* 228:1053–1062, 2006.

32. Baker-Gabb M, Hunt GB, France MP: Soft tissue sarcomas and mast cell tumours in dogs: clinical behaviour and response to surgery, *Aust Vet J* 81:732–738, 2003.

33. Bacon NJ, Dernell WS, Ehrhart N, et al.: Evaluation of primary re-excision after inadequate resection of soft tissue sarcomas in dogs: 41 cases (1999-2004), *J Am Vet Med Assoc* 230:548–554, 2007.

34. Bray JP, Polton GA, McSporran KD, et al.: Canine soft tissue sarcoma managed in first opinion practice: outcome in 350 cases, *Vet Surg* 43:774–782, 2014.

35. Kuntz CA, Dernell WS, Powers BE, et al.: Prognostic factors for surgical treatment of soft-tissue sarcomas in dogs: 75 cases (1986-1996), *J Am Vet Med Assoc* 21:1147–1151, 1997.

36. Fulmer AK, Mauldin GE: Canine histiocytic neoplasia: an overview, *Can Vet J* 48:1041–1050, 2007.

37. Fletcher CDM, Unni KK, Mertens F: *World Health Organization classification of tumors: pathology and genetics of tumors of soft tissue and bone*, Lyon, 2002, IARC Press.

38. Waters CB, Morrison WB, DeNicola DB, et al.: Giant cell variant of malignant fibrous histiocytoma in dogs: 10 cases (1986-1993), *J Am Vet Med Assoc* 205:1420, 1994.

39. Morris JS, McInnes EF, Bostock DE, et al.: Immunohistochemical and histopathologic features of 14 malignant fibrous histiocytomas from flat-coated retrievers, *Vet Pathol* 39:473–479, 2002.

40. Choi H, Kwon Y, Chang J, et al.: Undifferentiated pleomorphic sarcoma (malignant fibrous histiocytoma) of the head in a dog, *J Vet Med Sci* 73:235–239, 2011.

41. Weiss SW, Enzinger FM: Malignant fibrous histiocytoma: an analysis of 200 cases, *Cancer* 41:2250–2266, 1978.

42. Foale RD, White RA, Harley R, et al.: Left ventricular myxosarcoma in a dog, *J Small Anim Pract* 44:503–507, 2003.

43. Briggs OM, Kirberger RM, Goldberg NB: Right atrial myxosarcoma in a dog, *J S Afr Vet Assoc* 68:144–146, 1997.

44. Richter M, Stankeova S, Hauser B, et al.: Myxosarcoma in the eye and brain in a dog, *Vet Ophthalmol* 6:183–189, 2003.

45. Avallone G, Helmbold P, Caniatti M, et al.: Spectrum of canine perivascular wall tumors: morphologic, phenotypic and clinical characterization, *Vet Pathol* 44:607–620, 2007.

46. Stefanello D, Avallone G, Ferrari R, et al.: Canine cutaneous perivascular wall tumors at first presentation: clinical behavior and prognostic factors in 55 cases, *J Vet Intern Med* 25:1398–1405, 2011.

47. Chijiwa K, Uchida K, Tateyama S: Immunohistochemical evaluation of canine peripheral nerve sheath tumors and other soft tissue sarcomas, *Vet Pathol* 41:307–318, 2004.

48. Boos GS, Bassuino DM, Wurster F, et al.: Retrospective canine skin peripheral nerve sheath tumors data with emphasis on histologic, immunohistochemical and prognostic factors, *Pesq Vet Bras* 35:965–974, 2015.

49. Teixeira S, Amorim I, Rema A, et al.: Molecular heterogeneity of canine cutaneous peripheral nerve sheath tumors: a drawback in the diagnosis refinement, *Vivo* 30:819–827, 2016.

50. Brehm D, Steinberg H, Haviland J, et al.: A retrospective evaluation of 51 cases of peripheral nerve sheath tumors in the dog, *J Am Anim Hosp Assoc* 31:349–359, 1995.

51. Van Stee L, Boston S, Teske E, et al.: Compartmental resection of peripheral nerve tumors with limb preservation in 16 dogs (1995-2011), *Vet Surg* 26:40–45, 2017.

52. Dolera M, Malfassi L, Bianch C, et al.: Frameless stereotactic volumetric modulated arc radiotherapy of brachial plexus tumours in dogs: 10 cases, *Br J Radiol* 90:20160617, 2017.

53. Spoldi E, Schwarz T, Sabattini S, et al.: Comparisons among computed tomographic features of adipose masses in dogs and cats, *Vet Radiol Ultrasound* 58:29–37, 2017.

54. Gleiser CA, Jardine JH, Raulston GL, et al.: Infiltrating lipomas in the dog, *Vet Pathol* 16:623–624, 1979.

55. McChesney AE, Stephens LC, Lebel J, et al.: Infiltrative lipoma in dogs, *Vet Pathol* 17:316–322, 1980.

56. Doige CE, Farrow CS, Presnell KR: Parosteal lipoma in a dog, *J Am Anim Hosp Assoc* 16(87), 1980.

57. Bergman PJ, Withrow SJ, Straw RC, et al.: Infiltrative lipoma in dogs: 16 cases (1981-1992), *J Am Vet Med Assoc* 205:322–324, 1994.

58. McEntee MC, Page RL, Mauldin GN, et al.: Results of irradiation of infiltrative lipoma in 13 dogs, *Vet Radiol Ultrasound* 41:554–556, 2000.

59. McEntee MC, Thrall DE: Computed tomographic imaging of infiltrative lipoma in 22 dogs, *Vet Radiol Ultrasound* 42:221–225, 2001.

60. Head KW, Else RW, Dubielzig RR: Tumors of the alimentary tract. In Meuten DJ, editor: *Tumors in domestic animals*, Ames, IA, 2002, Iowa State Press, pp 401–481.

61. Liggett AD, Frazier KS, Styler EL: Angiolipomatous tumors in dogs and a cat, *Vet Pathol* 39:286–289, 2002.

62. Brodey RS, Rozel JF: Neoplasms of the canine uterus, vagina, vulva: a clinicopathologic survey of 90 cases, *J Am Vet Med Assoc* 151:1294–1307, 1967.

63. Woolfson JM, Dulisch ML, Tams TR: Intrathoracic lipoma in a dog, *J Am Vet Med Assoc* 185:1007–1009, 1984.

64. Anderson SM, Lippincott CL: Intrathoracic lipoma in a dog, *Calif Vet* 43(9), 1989.

65. Umphlet RC, Vicini DS, Godshalk CP: Intradural-extramedullary lipoma in a dog, *Compend Contin Educ Pract Vet* 11:1192, 1989.

66. McLaughlin R, Kuzma AB: Intestinal strangulation caused by intra-abdominal lipomas in a dog, *J Am Vet Med Assoc* 199:1610–1611, 1991.

67. Plummer SB, Bunch SE, Khoo LH, et al.: Tethered spinal cord and an intradural lipoma associated with a meningocele in a Manx-type cat, *J Am Vet Med Assoc* 203:1159–1161, 1993.

68. Mayhew PD, Brockman DJ: Body cavity lipomas in six dogs, *J Small Anim Pract* 43:177–181, 2002.

69. Gibbons SE, Straw RC: Intra-abdominal lipoma in a dog, *Aust Vet Pract* 33:86, 2003.

70. Hunt GB, Wong J, Kuan S: Liposuction for removal of lipomas in 20 dogs, *J Small Anim Pract* 52:419–425, 2011.

71. Lamagna B, Greco A, Guardascione A, et al.: Canine lipomas treated with steroid injections: clinical findings, *PLoS One* 7:e50234, 2012.

72. Thomson MJ, Withrow SJ, Dernell WS, et al.: Intermuscular lipomas of the thigh region in dogs: 11 cases, *J Am Anim Hosp Assoc* 35:165–167, 1999.

73. Case JB, MacPhail CM, Withrow SJ: Anatomic distribution and clinical findings of intermuscular lipomas in 17 dogs (2005-2010), *J Am Anim Hosp Assoc* 48:245–249, 2012.

74. Kramek BA, Spackman CJA, Hayden DW: Infiltrative lipoma in three dogs, *J Am Vet Med Assoc* 186:81–82, 1985.

75. Frazier KS, Herron AJ, Dee JF, et al.: Infiltrative lipoma in a stifle joint, *J Am Anim Hosp* 29:81–83, 1993.

76. Baez JL, Hendrick MJ, Shofer FS, et al.: Liposarcomas in dogs: 56 cases (1989-2000), *J Am Vet Med Assoc* 224:887–891, 2004.

77. Forlani A, Roccabianca P, Palmieri C, et al.: Pathological characterization of primary splenic myxoid liposarcomas in three dogs, *Vet Q* 35:181–184, 2015.

78. Gower KL, Liptak JM, Culp WT, et al.: Splenic liposarcoma in dogs: 13 cases (2002-2012), *J Am Vet Med Assoc* 247:1404–1407, 2015.

79. Masserdotti C, Bonfanti U, De Lorenzi D, et al.: Use of Oil Red O stain in the cytologic diagnosis of canine liposarcoma, *Vet Clin Pathol* 35:37–41, 2006.

80. Fuesrt JA, Reichle JK, Szabo D, et al.: Computed tomographic findings in 24 dogs with liposarcoma, *Vet Radiol Ultrasound* 58:23–28, 2017.

81. Brennan MF, Singer S, Maki RG, et al.: Soft tissue sarcoma. In DeVita RT, Hellman S, Rosenberg SA, editors: *Cancer: principles and practice of oncology*, ed 8, Philadelphia, 2008, Lippincott Williams & Wilkins, pp 1741–1789.

82. Chang HR, Hajdu SI, Collin C, et al.: The prognostic value of histologic subtypes in primary extremity liposarcoma, *Cancer* 64:1514–1520, 1989.

83. Choong PFM, Pritchard DJ: Common malignant soft-tissue tumors. In Simon MA, Springfield D, editors: *Surgery for bone and soft-tissue tumors*, Philadelphia, 1998, Lippincott-Raven, pp 539–551.

84. Avallone G, Roccabianca P, Crippa L, et al.: Histologic classification and immunohistochemical evaluation of MDM2 and CDK4 expression in canine liposarcoma, *Vet Pathol* 53:773–780, 2016.

85. Cooper BJ, Valentine BA: Tumors of muscle. In Meuten DJ, editor: *Tumors in domestic animals*, Ames, IA, 2002, Iowa State Press, pp 319–363.

86. Caserto BG: A comparative review of canine and human rhabdomyosarcoma with emphasis on classification and pathogenesis, *Vet Pathol* 50:806–826, 2013.

87. Scott EM, Teixeira LB, Flanders DJ, et al.: Canine orbital rhabdomyosarcoma: a report of 18 cases, *Vet Ophthalmol* 19:130–137, 2016.

88. Kobayashi M, Sakai H, Hirata A, et al.: Expression of myogenic regulating factors, myogenin and MyoD, in two canine botryoid rhabdomyosarcomas, *Vet Pathol* 41:275–277, 2004.

89. Russell HV, Pappo AS, Nuchtern JG, et al.: Solid tumors of childhood. In DeVita RT, Hellman S, Rosenberg SA, editors: *Cancer: principles and practice of oncology*, ed 8, Philadelphia, 2008, Lippincott Williams & Wilkins, pp 2043–2074.

90. Curran KM, Halsey CH, Worley DR: Lymphangiosarcoma in 12 dogs: a case series (1998-2013), *Vet Comp Oncol* 14:181–190, 2016.

91. Halsey CH, Worley DR, Curran K, et al.: The use of novel lymphatic endothelial-cell specific immunohistochemical markers to differentiate cutaneous angiosarcomas in dogs, *Vet Comp Oncol* 14:236–244, 2016.

92. Spangler WL, Culbertson MR, Kass PH: Primary mesenchymal (nonangiomatous/nonlymphomatous) neoplasms occurring in the canine spleen: anatomic classification, immunohistochemistry, and mitotic activity correlated with patient survival, *Vet Pathol* 31:37–47, 1994.

93. McDonald RK, Helman RG: Hepatic malignant mesenchymoma in a dog, *J Am Vet Med Assoc* 188:1052–1053, 1986.

94. Hahn KA, Richardson RC: Use of cisplatin for control of metastatic malignant mesenchymoma and hypertrophic osteopathy in a dog, *J Am Vet Med Assoc* 195:351–353, 1989.

95. Carpenter JL, Dayal Y, King NW, et al.: Distinctive unclassified mesenchymal tumor of the digit of dogs, *Vet Pathol* 28:396–402, 1991.

96. Watson AD, Young KM, Dubielzig RR, et al.: Primary mesenchymal or mixed-cell-origin lung tumors in four dogs, *J Am Vet Med Assoc* 202:968–970, 1993.

97. Robinson TM, Dubielzig RR, McAnulty JF: Malignant mesenchymoma associated with an unusual vasoinvasive metastasis in a dog, *J Am Anim Hosp Assoc* 34:295–299, 1998.
98. Murphy S, Blunden AS, Dennis R, et al.: Intermandibular malignant mesenchymoma in a crossbreed dog, *J Small Anim Pract* 47:550–553, 2006.
99. Gomez-Laguna J, Barranco I, Rodriguez-Gomez IM, et al.: Malignant mesenchymoma of the heart base in a dog with infiltration of the pericardium and metastasis to the lung, *J Comp Pathol* 147:195–198, 2012.
100. Weishaar KM, Edmonson EF, Thamm DH, et al.: Malignant mesenchymoma with widespread metastasis including bone marrow involvement in a dog, *Vet Clin Pathol* 43:447–452, 2014.
101. Machida N, Kobayashi M, Tanaka R, et al.: Primary malignant mixed mesenchymal tumour of the heart in a dog, *J Comp Pathol* 128:71–74, 2003.
102. Ghisleni G, Roccabianca P, Ceruti R, et al.: Correlation between fine-needle aspiration cytology and histopathology in the evaluation of cutaneous and subcutaneous masses from dogs and cats, *Vet Clin Pathol* 35:24–30, 2006.
103. Hohenhaus AE, Kelsey JL, Haddad J, et al.: Canine cutaneous and subcutaneous soft tissue sarcoma: an evidence-based review of case management, *J Am Anim Hosp Assoc* 52:77–89, 2016.
104. Perry JA, Culp WT, Dailey DD, et al.: Diagnostic accuracy of pretreatment biopsy for grading soft tissue sarcoma in dogs, *Vet Comp Oncol* 12:106–113, 2014.
105. Postorino NC, Berg RJ, Powers BE, et al.: Prognostic variables for canine hemangiopericytoma: 50 cases (1979-1984), *J Am Anim Hosp Assoc* 24:501–509, 1988.
106. Affolter VK, Moore PF: Localized and disseminated histiocytic sarcoma of dendritic cell origin in dogs, *Vet Pathol* 39:74–83, 2002.
107. Sugiura H, Takahashi M, Katagiri H, et al.: Additional wide resection of malignant soft tissue tumors, *Clin Orthop* 394:201–210, 2002.
108. Loh ZH, Allan GS, Nicoll RG, et al.: Ultrasonographic characteristics of soft tissue tumours in dogs, *Aust Vet J* 87:323–329, 2009.
109. Greene FL, Page DL, Fleming ID, et al.: *AJCC cancer staging manual*, New York, 2002, Springer.
110. Dernell WS, Withrow SJ, Kuntz CA, et al.: Principles of treatment for soft tissue sarcoma, *Clin Tech Small Anim Pract* 13:59–64, 1998.
111. Avallone G, Boracchi P, Stefanello D, et al.: Canine perivascular wall tumors: high prognostic impact of site, depth, and completeness of margins, *Vet Pathol* 51:713–721, 2014.
112. Russell DS, Townsend KL, Gorman E, et al.: Characterizing microscopical invasion patterns in canine mast cell tumours and soft tissue sarcomas, *J Comp Path* 157:231–240, 2017.
113. Banks T, Straw R, Thomson M, et al.: Soft tissue sarcomas in dogs: a study correlating optimal surgical margin with tumour grade, *Aust Vet Pract* 34:158–163, 2004.
114. Bray JP: Soft tissue sarcoma in the dog – part 1: a current review, *J Small Anim Pract* 57:510–519, 2016.
115. Pratschke KM, Atherton MJ, Sillito JA, et al.: Evaluation of a modified proportional margins approach for surgical resection of mast cell tumors in dogs: 40 cases (2008-2012), *J Am Vet Med Assoc* 243:1436–1441, 2013.
116. Monteiro B, Boston S, Monteith G: Factors influencing complete tumor excision of mast cell tumors and soft tissue sarcomas: a retrospective study in 100 dogs, *Can Vet J* 52:1209–1214, 2011.
117. Stefanello D, Morello E, Roccabianca P, et al.: Marginal excision of low-grade spindle cell sarcoma of canine extremities: 35 dogs (1996-2006), *Vet Surg* 37:461–465, 2008.
118. McSporran KD: Histologic grade predicts recurrence for marginally excised canine subcutaneous soft tissue sarcomas, *Vet Pathol* 46:928–933, 2009.
119. Reimer SB, Séguin B, DeCock HE, et al.: Evaluation of the effect of routine histologic processing on the size of skin samples obtained from dogs, *Am J Vet Res* 66:500–505, 2005.
120. Kamstock DA, Ehrhart EJ, Getzy DM, et al.: Recommended guide-lines for submission, trimming, margin evaluation, and reporting of tumor biopsy specimens in veterinary surgical pathology, *Vet Pathol* 48:19–31, 2011.
121. Eward WC, Mito JK, Eward CA, et al.: A novel imaging system permits real-time in vivo tumor bed assessment after resection of naturally occurring sarcomas in dogs, *Clin Orthop Relat Res* 471:834–842, 2013.
122. Holt D, Parthasarathy AB, Okusanya O, et al.: Intraoperative near-infrared fluorescence imaging and spectroscopy identifies residual tumor cells in wounds, *J Biomed Opt* 20:76002, 2015.
123. Fidel J, Kennedy KC, Dernell WS, et al.: Preclinical validation of the utility of BLZ-100 in providing fluorescence contrast for imaging spontaneous solid tumors, *Cancer Res* 75:4283–4291, 2015.
124. DeWitt SB, Eward WC, Eward CA, et al.: A novel imaging system distinguishes neoplastic from normal tissue during resection of soft tissue sarcomas and mast cell tumors in dogs, *Vet Surg* 45:715–722, 2016.
125. Cabon Q, Sayag D, Texier I, et al.: Evaluation of intraoperative fluorescence imaging-guided surgery in cancer-bearing dogs: a prospective proof-of-concept phase II study in 9 cases, *Transl Res* 170:73–88, 2016.
126. Ramanathan RC, A'Hern R, Fisher C, et al.: Prognostic index for extremity soft tissue sarcomas with isolated local recurrence, *Ann Surg Oncol* 8:278–289, 2011.
127. Stojadinovic A, Leung DHY, Hoos A, et al.: Analysis of the prognostic significance of microscopic margins in 2,084 localized primary adult soft tissue sarcomas, *Ann Surg* 235:424–434, 2002.
128. Zagars GK, Ballo MT, Pisters PWT, et al.: Prognostic factors for patients with localized soft-tissue sarcoma treated with conservative surgery and radiation therapy: an analysis of 1225 patients, *Cancer* 97:2530–2543, 2003.
129. Zagars GK, Ballo MT, Pisters PWT, et al.: Surgical margins and reresection in the management of patients with soft tissue sarcoma using conservative surgery and radiation therapy, *Cancer* 97:2544–2553, 2003.
130. Eilber FC, Rosen G, Nelson SD, et al.: High-grade extremity soft tissue sarcomas: factors predictive of local recurrence and its effect on morbidity and mortality, *Ann Surg* 237:218–226, 2003.
131. Elmslie RE, Glawe P, Dow SW: Metronomic chemotherapy with cyclophosphamide and piroxicam effectively delays tumor recurrence in dogs with incompletely resected soft tissue sarcomas, *J Vet Intern Med* 22:1373–1379, 2008.
132. Spugnini EP, Vincenzi B, Citro G, et al.: Adjuvant electrochemotherapy for the treatment of incompletely excised spontaneous canine sarcomas, *Vivo* 21:819–822, 2007.
133. McEntee MC, Samii VF, Walsh P, et al.: Postoperative assessment of surgical clip position in 16 dogs with cancer: a pilot study, *J Am Anim Hosp Assoc* 40:300–308, 2004.
134. Henry CJ, Stoll MR, Higginbotham ML, et al.: Effect of timing of radiation initiation on post-surgical wound healing in dogs, *Proc Vet Cancer Soc* 23:52, 2003.
135. Forrest LJ, Chun R, Adams WM, et al.: Postoperative radiotherapy for canine soft tissue sarcoma, *J Vet Intern Med* 14:578–582, 2000.
136. McKnight JA, Mauldin GN, McEntee MC, et al.: Radiation treatment of incompletely resected soft-tissue sarcomas in dogs, *J Am Vet Med Assoc* 217:205–210, 2000.
137. Heller D, Stebbins ME, Reynolds T, et al.: A retrospective study of 87 cases of canine soft tissue sarcoma 1986–2001, *Int J Appl Res Vet Med* 3:81–87, 2005.
138. Simon D, Ruslander DM, Rassnick KM, et al.: Orthovoltage radiation and weekly low dose of doxorubicin for the treatment of incompletely resected soft-tissue sarcomas in 39 dogs, *Vet Rec* 160:321–326, 2007.
139. Graves GM, Bjorling DE, Mahaffey E: Canine hemangiopericytoma: 23 cases (1967-1984), *J Am Vet Med Assoc* 192:99–102, 1988.

140. Demetriou JL, Brearley MJ, Constantino-Casas F, et al.: Intentional marginal excision of canine limb soft tissue sarcomas followed by radiotherapy, *J Small Anim Pract* 53:174–181, 2012.
141. Kung MBJ, Poirier VJ, Dennis MM, et al.: Hypofractionated radiation therapy for the treatment of microscopic canine soft tissue sarcoma, *Vet Comp Oncol* 14:135–145, 2016.
142. McChesney SL, Withrow SJ, Gillette EL, et al.: Radiotherapy of soft tissue sarcomas in dogs, *J Am Vet Med Assoc* 194:60–63, 1989.
143. Hilmas DE, Gillett EL: Radiotherapy of spontaneous fibrous connective-tissue sarcomas in animals, *J Natl Cancer Inst* 56:365–368, 1976.
144. Banks WC, Morris E: Results of radiation treatment of naturally occurring animal tumors, *J Am Vet Med Assoc* 166:1063–1064, 1975.
145. Richardson RC, Anderson VL, Voorhees WD, et al.: Irradiation-hyperthermia in canine hemangiopericytomas: large-animal model for therapeutic response, *J Natl Cancer Inst* 73:1187–1194, 1984.
146. Lawrence J, Forrest L, Adams W, et al.: Four-fraction radiation therapy for macroscopic soft tissue sarcomas in 16 dogs, *J Am Anim Hosp Assoc* 44:100–108, 2008.
147. Plavec T, Kessler M, Kandel B, et al.: Palliative radiotherapy as treatment for non-resectable soft tissue sarcomas in the dog – a report of 15 cases, *Vet Comp Oncol* 4:98–103, 2006.
148. Cancedda S, Marconato L, Meier V, et al.: Hypofractionated radiotherapy for macroscopic canine soft tissue sarcoma: a retrospective study of 50 cases treated with a 5 x 6 Gy protocol with or without metronomic chemotherapy, *Vet Radiol Ultrasound* 57:75–83, 2016.
149. Tollett MA, Duda L, Brown DC, et al.: Palliative radiation therapy for solid tumors in dogs: 103 cases (2007-2011), *J Am Vet Med Assoc* 248:72–82, 2016.
150. McDonald C, Looper J, Greene S: Response rate and duration associated with a 4 Gy 5 fraction palliative radiation protocol, *Vet Radiol Ultrasound* 53:358–364, 2012.
151. Kalnicki S, Bloomer W: *Radiation therapy in the treatment of bone and soft tissue sarcomas*, Philadelphia, 1992, Saunders.
152. MacLeod DA, Thrall DE: The combination of surgery and radiation in the treatment of cancer. A review, *Vet Surg* 18:1–6, 1989.
153. Cheng EY, Dusenbery KE, Winters MR, et al.: Soft tissue sarcomas: preoperative versus postoperative radiotherapy, *J Surg Oncol* 61:90–99, 1996.
154. O'Sullivan B, Davis AM, Turcotte R, et al.: Preoperative versus postoperative radiotherapy in soft-tissue sarcoma of the limbs: a randomised trial, *Lancet* 359:2235–2241, 2002.
155. Al-Absi E, Farrokhyar F, Sharma R, et al.: A systematic review and meta-analysis of oncologic outcomes of pre- versus postoperative radiation in localized resectable soft-tissue sarcoma, *Ann Surg Oncol* 17:1367–1374, 2010.
156. Selting KA, Powers BE, Thompson LJ, et al.: Outcome of dogs with high-grade soft tissue sarcomas treated with and without adjuvant doxorubicin chemotherapy: 39 cases (1996-2004), *J Am Vet Med Assoc* 227:1442–1448, 2005.
157. Payne SE, Rassnick KM, Northrup NC, et al.: Treatment of vascular and soft-tissue sarcomas in dogs using an alternating protocol of ifosfamide and doxorubicin, *Vet Comp Oncol* 1:171–179, 2003.
158. Sarcoma Meta-Analysis Collaboration: Adjuvant chemotherapy for localised resectable soft-tissue sarcoma of adults: meta-analysis of individual data, *Lancet* 350:1647–1654, 1997.
159. Komdeur R, Hoekstra HJ, van den Berg E, et al.: Metastasis in soft tissue sarcomas: prognostic criteria and treatment perspectives, *Cancer Metastasis Rev* 21:167–183, 2002.
160. Burton JH, Mitchell L, Thamm DH, et al.: Low-dose cyclophosphamide selectively decreases regulatory T cells and inhibits angiogenesis in dogs with soft tissue sarcomas, *J Vet Intern Med* 25:920–926, 2011.
161. de Queiroz GF, Dagli ML, Fukumasu H, et al.: Vascular endothelial growth factor expression and microvascular density in soft tissue sarcomas in dogs, *J Vet Diagn Invest* 22:105–108, 2010.
162. Al-Dissi AN, Haines DM, Singh B, et al.: Immunohistochemical expression of vascular endothelial growth factor and vascular endothelial growth factor receptor in canine cutaneous fibrosarcoma, *J Com Pathol* 141:229–236, 2009.
163. Avallone G, Stefanello D, Boracchi P, et al.: Growth factors and COX2 expression in canine perivascular wall tumors, *Vet Pathol* 52:1034–1040, 2015.
164. de Queiroz GF, Dagli MLZ, Meira SA, et al.: Serum vascular endothelial growth factor in dogs with soft tissue sarcomas, *Vet Comp Oncol* 11:230–235, 2013.
165. Dernell WS, Withrow SJ, Straw RC, et al.: Intracavitary treatment of soft tissue sarcomas in dogs using cisplatin in a biodegradable polymer, *Anticancer Res* 17:4499–4505, 1997.
166. Havlicek M, Straw RC, Langova V, et al.: Intra-operative cisplatin for the treatment of canine extremity soft tissue sarcomas, *Vet Comp Oncol* 7:122–129, 2009.
167. Bergman NS, Urie BK, Pardo AD, et al.: Evaluation of local toxic effects and outcomes for dogs undergoing marginal tumor excision with intralesional cisplatin-impregnated bead placement for treatment of soft tissue sarcomas: 62 cases (2009-2012), *J Am Vet Med Assoc* 248:1148–1156, 2016.
168. Marconato L, Comastri S, Lorenzo MR, et al.: Postsurgical intra-incisional 5-fluorouracil in dogs with incompletely resected, extremity malignant spindle cell tumours: a pilot study, *Vet Comp Oncol* 5:239–249, 2007.
169. Bostock DE, Dye MT: Prognosis after surgical excision of canine fibrous connective tissue sarcomas, *Vet Pathol* 17:581–588, 1980.
170. Evans SM: Canine hemangiopericytoma: a retrospective analysis of response to surgery and orthovoltage radiation, *Vet Radiol* 28:13–16, 1987.
171. Hauck M: Feline injection site sarcomas, *Vet Clin North Am Small Anim Pract* 33:553–557, 2003.
172. Hendrick MJ, Goldschmidt MH, Shofer FS, et al.: Postvaccinal sarcomas in the cat: epidemiology and electron probe microanalytical identification of aluminum, *Cancer Res* 52:5391–5394, 1992.
173. Hendrick MJ, Goldschmidt MH: Do injection site reactions induce fibrosarcomas in cats? *J Am Vet Med Assoc* 199:968, 1991.
174. Hendrick MJ, Shofer FS, Goldschmidt MH, et al.: Comparison of fibrosarcomas that developed at vaccination sites and at nonvaccination sites in cats: 239 cases (1991-1992), *J Am Vet Med Assoc* 205:1425–1429, 1994.
175. Kass PH, Barnes WG, Spangler WL, et al.: Epidemiologic evidence for a causal relation between vaccination and fibrosarcoma tumorigenesis in cats, *J Am Vet Med Assoc* 203:396–405, 1993.
176. Macy DW, Hendrick MJ: The potential role of inflammation in the development of postvaccinal sarcomas in cats, *Vet Clin North Am Small Anim Pract* 26:103–109, 1996.
177. Hendrick MJ, Kass PH, McGill LD, et al.: Postvaccinal sarcomas in cats, *J Natl Cancer Inst* 86:341–343, 1994.
178. Kass PH, Spangler WL, Hendrick MJ, et al.: Multicenter case-control study of risk factors associated with development of injection-site sarcomas in cats, *J Am Vet Med Assoc* 223:1283–1292, 2003.
179. Dean R, Adams V, Whitbread T, et al.: Study of feline injection site sarcomas, *Vet Rec* 159:641–642, 2006.
180. Day MJ, Schoon HA, Magnol JP, et al.: A kinetic study of histopathological changes in the subcutis of cats injected with non-adjuvanted and adjuvanted multi-component vaccines, *Vaccine* 25:4073–4084, 2007.
181. Shaw SC, Kent MS, Gordon IK, et al.: Temporal changes in characteristics of injection-site sarcomas in cats: 392 cases (1990-2006), *J Am Vet Med Assoc* 234:376–380, 2009.
182. Coyne MJ, Reeves NCP, Rosen DK, et al.: Estimated prevalence of injection sarcomas in cats during 1992, *J Am Vet Med Assoc* 210:249–251, 1997.
183. Gober GM, Kass PH: World Wide Web-based survey of vaccination practices, postvaccinal reactions, and vaccine site-associated sarcomas in cats, *J Am Vet Med Assoc 2002* 220:1477–1482, 2002.

184. Lester S, Clemett T, Burt A: Vaccine site-associated sarcomas in cats: clinical experience and a laboratory review (1982-1993), *J Am Anim Hosp Assoc* 32:91–95, 1996.

185. Kliczkowska K, Jankowska U, Jagielski D, et al.: Epidemiological and morphological analysis of feline injection site sarcomas, *Pol J Vet Sci* 18:313–322, 2015.

186. Doddy FD, Glickman LT, Glickman NW, et al.: Feline fibrosarcomas at vaccination sites and nonvaccination sites, *J Comp Pathol* 114:165–174, 1996.

187. Srivastav A, Kass PH, McGill LD, et al.: Comparative vaccine-specific and other injectable-specific risks of injection-site sarcomas in cats, *J Am Vet Med Assoc* 241:595–602, 2012.

188. Wilcock B, Wilcock A, Bottoms K: Feline postvaccinal sarcoma: 20 years later, *Can Vet J* 53:430–434, 2012.

189. Dubielzig RR, Hawkins KL, Miller P: Myofibroblastic sarcoma originating at the site of rabies vaccination in a cat, *J Vet Diagn Invest* 5:637–638, 1993.

190. Hendrick MJ: Feline injection-site sarcomas, *Cancer Invest* 17:273–274, 1999.

191. McEntee MC, Page RL: Feline injection-site sarcomas, *J Vet Intern Med* 15:176–182, 2001.

192. McNiel EA: Vaccine-associate sarcomas in cats: a unique cancer model, *Clin Orthop* 382:21–27, 2001.

193. Morrison WB, Starr RM: Injection-site feline sarcoma task force: injection-site feline sarcomas, *J Am Vet Med Assoc* 218:697–702, 2011.

194. Séguin B: Injection site sarcomas in cats, *Clin Tech Small Anim Pract* 17:168–173, 2002.

195. Peiffer RL, Monticello T, Bouldin TW: Primary ocular sarcomas in the cat, *J Small Anim Pract* 29:105, 1988.

196. Dubielzig RR, Everitt J, Shadduck JA, et al.: Clinical and morphologic features of post-traumatic ocular sarcomas in cats, *Vet Pathol* 27:62–65, 1990.

197. Hakanson N, Forrester SD: Uveitis in the dog and cat, *Vet Clin North Am Small Anim Pract* 20:715–735, 1990.

198. Esplin DG, Bigelow M, McGill LD, et al.: Fibrosarcoma at the site of a lufenuron injection in a cat, *Vet Cancer Soc Newsletter* 23(8), 1999.

199. Buracco P, Martano M, Morello E, et al.: Vaccine-associated-like fibrosarcoma at the site of a deep nonabsorbable suture in a cat, *Vet J* 163:105–107, 2002.

200. Daly MK, Saba CF, Crochik SS, et al.: Fibrosarcoma adjacent to the site of microchip implantation in a cat, *J Feline Med Surg* 10:202–205, 2008.

201. Carminato A, Vascellari M, Marchioro W, et al.: Microchip-associated fibrosarcoma in a cat, *Vet Dermatol* 22:565–569, 2011.

202. Munday JS, Banyay K, Aberdein D, et al.: Development of an injection-site sarcoma shortly after meloxicam injection in an unvaccinated cat, *J Feline Med Surg* 13:988–991, 2011.

203. Martano M, Morello E, Iussich S, et al.: A case of feline injection-site sarcoma at the site of cisplatin injections, *J Feline Med Surg* 14:751–754, 2012.

204. McLeland SM, Imhoff DJ, Thomas M, et al.: Subcutaneous fluid port-associated soft tissue sarcoma in a cat, *J Feline Med Surg* 15:917–920, 2013.

205. Hendrick MJ, Brooks JJ: Postvaccinal sarcomas in the cat: histology and immunohistochemistry, *Vet Pathol* 31:126–129, 1994.

206. Hendrick MJ: Feline injection-site sarcomas: current studies on pathogenesis, *J Am Vet Med Assoc* 213:1425–1426, 1998.

207. Ellis JA, Jackson ML, Bartsch RC, et al.: Use of immunohistochemistry and polymerase chain reaction for detection of oncornaviruses in formalin-fixed, paraffin-embedded fibrosarcomas from cats, *J Am Vet Med Assoc* 209:767–771, 1996.

208. Nieto A, Sánchez MA, Martínez E, et al.: Immunohistochemical expression of p53, fibroblast growth factor-b and transforming growth factor-α in feline injection-site sarcomas, *Vet Pathol* 40:651–658, 2003.

209. Moore PF, Affolter VK: Canine and feline histiocytic diseases. In Ettinger SJ, Feldman EC, editors: *Textbook of veterinary internal medicine*, ed 6, St Louis, 2005, Elsevier Saunders, pp 779–782.

210. Ladlow J: Injection site-associated sarcoma in the cat: treatment recommendations and results to date, *J Feline Med Surg* 15:409–418, 2013.

211. Hartmann K, Day MJ, Thiry E, et al.: Feline injection-site sarcoma: ABCD guidelines on prevention and management, *J Feline Med Surg* 17:606–613, 2015.

212. Heldmann E, Anderson MA, Wagner-Mann C: Feline osteosarcoma: 145 cases (1990-1995), *J Am Anim Hosp Assoc* 36:518–521, 2000.

213. Cohen M, Wright JC, Brawner WR, et al.: Use of surgery and electron beam irradiation, with or without chemotherapy, for treatment of injection-site sarcomas in cats: 78 cases (1996-2000), *J Am Vet Med Assoc* 219:1582–1589, 2001.

214. Phelps HA, Kuntz CA, Milner RJ, et al.: Radical excision with five-centimeter margins for treatment of feline injection-site sarcomas: 91 cases (1998-2002), *J Am Vet Med Assoc* 239:97–106, 2011.

215. Esplin DG, McGill LD, Meininger AC, et al.: Postvaccination sarcomas in cats, *J Am Vet Med Assoc* 202:1245–1247, 1993.

216. Madewell BR, Griffey SM, McEntee MC, et al.: Feline injection-site fibrosarcoma: an ultrastructural study of 20 tumors (1996-1999), *Vet Pathol* 38:196–202, 2001.

217. Couto SS, Griffey SM, Duarte PC, et al.: Feline injection-site fibrosarcoma: morphologic distinctions, *Vet Pathol* 39:33–41, 2002.

218. Rousset N, Holmes MA, Caine A, et al.: Clinical and low-field characteristics of injection site sarcomas in 19 cats, *Vet Radiol Ultrasound* 54:623–629, 2013.

219. Travetti O, di Giancamillo M, Stefanello D, et al.: Computed tomography characteristics of fibrosarcoma – a histological subtype of feline injection-site sarcoma, *J Feline Med Surg* 15:488–493, 2013.

220. Longo M, Modina SC, Bellotti A, et al.: Advances in the anatomic study of the interscapular region of the cat, *BMC Vet Res* 11:249, 2015.

221. Nemanic S, Milovancev M, Terry JL, et al.: Microscopic evaluation of peritumoral lesions of feline injection site sarcomas identified by magnetic resonance imaging and computed tomography, *Vet Surg* 45:392–401, 2016.

222. Zardo KM, Damiani LP, Matera JM, et al.: Recurrent and nonrecurrent feline injection-site sarcoma: computed tomographic and ultrasonographic findings, *J Feline Med Surg* 18:773–782, 2016.

223. Ferrari R, Di Giancamillo M, Stefanello D, et al.: Clinical and computed tomography tumour dimension assessments for planning wide excision of injection-site sarcomas in cats: how strong is the agreement, *Vet Comp Oncol* 15:374–382, 2017.

224. Davidson EB, Gregory CR, Kass PH: Surgical excision of soft tissue fibrosarcomas in cats, *Vet Surg* 26:265–269, 1997.

225. Hershey AE, Sorenmo KU, Hendrick MJ, et al.: Prognosis for presumed feline injection-site sarcoma after excision: 61 cases (1986-1996), *J Am Vet Med Assoc* 216:58–61, 2000.

226. Romanelli G, Marconato L, Olivero D, et al.: Analysis of prognostic factors associated with injection-site sarcomas in cats: 57 cases (2001-2007), *J Am Vet Med Assoc* 232:1193–1199, 2008.

227. Cantatore M, Ferrari R, Boracchi P, et al.: Factors influencing wound healing complications after wide excision of injection site sarcomas of the trunk of cats, *Vet Surg* 43:783–790, 2014.

228. Lidbetter DA, Williams FA, Krahwinkel DJ, et al.: Radical lateral body-wall resection for fibrosarcoma with reconstruction using polypropylene mesh and a caudal superficial epigastric axial pattern flap: a prospective clinical study of the technique and results in 6 cats, *Vet Surg* 31:57–64, 2002.

229. Bray J, Polton G: Neoadjuvant and adjuvant chemotherapy combined with anatomical resection of feline injection-site sarcoma: results in 21 cats, *Vet Comp Oncol* 14:147–160, 2016.

230. Wenk CHF, Ponce F, Guillermet S, et al.: Near-infrared optical guided surgery of highly infiltrative fibrosarcomas in cats using an anti-$\alpha_v\beta_3$ integrin molecular probe, *Cancer Lett* 334:188–195, 2013.

231. Martano M, Morello E, Ughetto M, et al.: Surgery alone versus surgery and doxorubicin for the treatment of feline injection-site sarcomas: a report on 69 cases, *Vet J* 170:84–90, 2005.
232. Cronin K, Page RL, Spodnick G, et al.: Radiation therapy and surgery for fibrosarcoma in 33 cats, *Vet Radiol Ultrasound* 39:51–56, 1998.
233. Bregazzi VS, LaRue SM, McNiel E, et al.: Treatment with a combination of doxorubicin, surgery, and radiation versus surgery and radiation alone for cats with injection-site sarcomas: 25 cases (1995-2000), *J Am Vet Med Assoc* 218:547–550, 2001.
234. Kobayashi T, Hauck ML, Dodge R, et al.: Preoperative radiotherapy for injection-site sarcoma in 92 cats, *Vet Radiol Ultrasound* 43:473–479, 2002.
235. Eckstein C, Guscetti F, Roos M, et al.: A retrospective analysis of radiation therapy for treatment of feline vaccine-associated sarcoma, *Vet Comp Oncol* 7:54–68, 2009.
236. Mayer MN, Treuil PL, LaRue SM: Radiotherapy and surgery for feline soft tissue sarcoma, *Vet Radiol Ultrasound* 50:669–672, 2009.
237. Kleiter M, Tichy A, Willmann M, et al.: Concomitant liposomal doxorubicin and daily palliative radiation therapy in advanced feline soft tissue sarcomas, *Vet Radiol Ultrasound* 51:349–355, 2010.
238. Nolan MW, Griffin LR, Custis JT, et al.: Stereotactic body radiation therapy for treatment of injection-site sarcomas in cats: 11 cases (2008-2012), *J Am Vet Med Assoc* 15:526–531, 2013.
239. Williams LE, Banerji N, Klausner JS, et al.: Establishment of two injection-site feline sarcoma cell lines and determination of in vitro chemosensitivity to doxorubicin and mitoxantrone, *Am J Vet Res* 62:1354–1357, 2001.
240. Banerji N, Li X, Klausner JS, et al.: Evaluation of in vitro chemosensitivity of injection-site feline sarcoma cell lines to vincristine and paclitaxel, *Am J Vet Res* 63:728–732, 2002.
241. Hill J, Lawrence J, Saba C, et al.: In vitro efficacy of doxorubicin and etoposide against a feline injection-site sarcoma cell line, *Res Vet Sci* 97:348–356, 2014.
242. Barber LG, Sorenmo KU, Cronin KL, et al.: Combined doxorubicin and cyclophosphamide chemotherapy for nonresectable feline fibrosarcoma, *J Am Anim Hosp Assoc* 36:416–421, 2000.
243. Poirier VJ, Thamm DH, Kurzman ID, et al.: Liposome-encapsulated doxorubicin (Doxil) and doxorubicin in the treatment of injection-site sarcomas in cats, *J Vet Intern Med* 16:726–731, 2002.
244. Saba CF, Vail DM, Thamm DH: Phase II clinical evaluation of lomustine chemotherapy for feline vaccine-associated sarcoma, *Vet Comp Oncol* 10:283–291, 2012.
245. Katayama R, Huelsmeyer MK, Marr AK, et al.: Imatinib mesylate inhibits platelet-derived growth factor activity and increases chemosensitivity in feline injection-site sarcoma, *Cancer Chemother Pharmacol* 54:25–33, 2004.
246. Lawrence J, Saba C, Gogal R, et al.: Mastinib demonstrates antiproliferative and pro-apoptotic activity in primary and metastatic feline injection-site sarcoma cells, *Vet Comp Oncol* 10:143–154, 2012.
247. Turek M, Gogal R, Saba C, et al.: Masitinib mesylate does not enhance sensitivity to radiation in three feline injection-site sarcoma cell lines under normal growth conditions, *Res Vet Sci* 96:304–307, 2014.
248. Holtermann N, Kiupel M, Hirschberger J: The tyrosine kinase inhibitor toceranib in feline injection-site sarcomas: efficacy and side effects, *Vet Comp Oncol* 15:632–640, 2017.
249. Spugnini EP, Baldi A, Vincenzi B, et al.: Intraoperative versus postoperative electrochemotherapy in high grade soft tissue sarcomas: a preliminary study in a spontaneous feline model, *Cancer Chemother Pharmacol* 59:375–381, 2007.
250. Spugnini EP, Renaud SM, Buglioni S, et al.: Electrochemotherapy with cisplatin enhances local control after surgical ablation of fibrosarcoma in cats: an approach to improve the therapeutic index of highly toxic chemotherapy drugs, *J Transl Med* 9:152, 2011.
251. Knapp DW, Richardson RC, DeNicola DB, et al.: Cisplatin toxicity in cats, *J Vet Intern Med* 1:29–35, 1987.
252. Jourdier TM, Moste C, Bonnet MC, et al.: Local immunotherapy of spontaneous feline fibrosarcomas using recombinant poxviruses expressing interleukin 2 (IL2), *Gene Ther* 10:2126–2132, 2003.
253. Jas D, Soyer C, De Fornel-Thibaud P, et al.: Adjuvant immunotherapy of feline injection-site sarcomas with the recombinant canarypox virus expressing feline interleukine-2 evaluated in a controlled monocentric clinical trial when used in association with surgery and brachytherapy, *Trials Vaccinol* 4:1–8, 2015.
254. Jahnke A, Hirschberger J, Fischer C, et al.: Intra-tumoral gene delivery of feIL-2, feIFN-gamma and feGM-CSF using magnetofection as a neoadjuvant treatment option for feline fibrosarcoma: a phase I trial, *J Vet Med A Physiol Pathol Clin Med* 54:599–606, 2007.
255. H007.A Physiol Pathberger J, Jahnke A, et al: Neoadjuvant gene delivery of feline granulocyte-macrophage colony-stimulating factor using magnetofection for the treatment of feline fibrosarcomas: a phase I trial, *J Gene Med* 10:655–667, 2008.
256. Kent EM: Use of an immunostimulant as an aid in treatment and management of fibrosarcoma in three cats, *Fel Pract* 21(13), 1993.
257. King GK, Yates KM, Greenlace PG, et al.: The effect of acemannan immunostimulant in combination with surgery and radiation therapy on spontaneous canine and feline fibrosarcomas, *J Am Anim Hosp Assoc* 31:439–447, 1995.
258. Quintin-Colonna F, Devauchelle P, Fradelizi D, et al.: Gene therapy of spontaneous canine melanoma and feline fibrosarcoma by intratumoral administration of histoincompatible cells expressing human interleukin-2, *Gene Ther* 3:1104–1112, 1996.
259. Giudice C, Stefanello D, Sala M, et al.: Feline injection-site sarcoma: recurrence, tumour grading and surgical margin status evaluated using the three-dimensional histological technique, *Vet J* 186:84–88, 2010.
260. Hahn KA, Endicott MM, King GK, et al.: Evaluation of radiotherapy alone or in combination with doxorubicin chemotherapy for the treatment of cats with incompletely excised soft tissue sarcomas: 71 cases (1989–1999), *J Am Vet Med Assoc* 231:742–745, 2007.
261. Porcellato I, Menchetti L, Brachelente C, et al.: Feline injection-site sarcoma: matrix remodeling and prognosis, *Vet Pathol* 54:204–211, 2017.
262. Dillon CJ, Mauldin GN, Baer KE: Outcome following surgical removal of nonvisceral soft tissue sarcomas in cats: 42 cases (1992-2000), *J Am Vet Med Assoc* 227:1955–1957, 2005.
263. Macy DW: Current understanding of vaccination site-associated sarcomas in the cat, *J Feline Med Surg* 1:15–21, 1999.
264. Martano M, Morello E, Buracco P: Feline injection-site sarcoma: past, present and future perspectives, *Vet J* 1888:136–141, 2011.
265. Hendricks CG, Levy JK, Tucker SJ, et al.: Tail vaccination in cats: a pilot study, *J Feline Med Surg* 16:275–280, 2014.
266. Scott FW, Geissinger CM: Duration of immunity in cats vaccinated with an inactivated feline panleukopenia, herpesvirus, and calicivirus vaccine, *Fel Pract* 25(12), 1997.
267. Scott FW, Geissinger CM: Long-term immunity in cats vaccinated with an inactivated trivalent vaccine, *Am J Vet Res* 60:652–658, 1999.
268. Jas D, Frances-Duvert V, Vernes D, et al.: Three-year duration of immunity for feline herpesvirus and calicivirus evaluated in a controlled vaccination-challenge laboratory trial, *Vet Microbiol* 177:123–131, 2015.

23

Cancer of the Gastrointestinal Tract

JULIUS M. LIPTAK

Incidence and Risk Factors

Oral tumors are common in both cats and dogs, with cancers of the oral cavity accounting for 3% to 12% and 6% of all tumors in these species, respectively.[1–5] Oropharyngeal cancer is 2.6 times more common in dogs than in cats, and male dogs have a 2.4 times greater risk of developing oropharyngeal malignancy compared with female dogs.[6,7] A male sex predisposition has also been reported for dogs with malignant melanoma (MM), tonsillar squamous cell carcinoma (SCC), and peripheral odontogenic fibromas,[8,9] and a female sex predisposition has been reported for dogs with axial osteosarcoma (OSA).[10] Dog breeds with the highest risk of developing oropharyngeal cancer include the cocker spaniel, German shepherd dog, German shorthaired pointer, Weimaraner, golden retriever, Gordon setter, miniature poodle, Chow Chow, and boxer.[3,8,11] In one study, German shepherd dogs and boxers had a decreased risk of developing oral melanoma.[11]

In dogs, the most common malignant oral tumors are, in descending order, MM, SCC, and fibrosarcoma (FSA),[12–24] although in other studies SCC is more common than MM.[25] SCC is the most common oropharyngeal cancer in cats, followed by FSA, which accounts for 13% of feline oral tumors.[5] Other malignant oral tumors in dogs include OSA, chondrosarcoma, anaplastic sarcoma, multilobular osteochondrosarcoma (MLO), intraosseous carcinoma, myxosarcoma, hemangiosarcoma, lymphoma, mast cell tumor, and transmissible venereal tumor.[12–28] Tumors or tumor-like lesions of unusual sites, types, and biologic behavior (e.g., peripheral odontogenic fibroma, acanthomatous ameloblastoma [AA], odontogenic tumors, tonsillar SCC, tongue tumors, malignancy of young dogs, viral papillomatosis, canine and feline eosinophilic granuloma complex, and nasopharyngeal polyps) will be covered at the end of this chapter. A general summary of the common oral tumors is found in Table 23.1.

Pathology and Natural Behavior

The oral cavity is a very common site for a wide variety of malignant and benign cancers. Although most cancers are fairly straightforward histologically, some have confusing nomenclature or extenuating circumstances that warrant discussion.

Malignant Melanoma

In comparison to other malignant oral tumors, MM tends to occur in smaller body weight dogs. Cocker spaniel, miniature poodle, Anatolian sheepdog, Gordon setter, Chow Chow, and golden retriever are overrepresented breeds.[11] The mean age at presentation is 11.4 years.[11] MM occurs in cats, but is uncommon.[29]

MM can present a confusing histopathologic picture if the tumor or the biopsy section does not contain melanin (Fig. 23.1A), and amelanotic melanomas (see Fig. 23.1B) represent up to 38% of cases.[30] A histopathologic diagnosis of undifferentiated or anaplastic sarcoma or even epithelial cancer should be viewed with suspicion for possible reclassification as melanoma. Several immunohistochemical antibodies can be applied to biopsy specimens to help differentiate melanoma from other poorly differentiated tumors and an immunodiagnostic cocktail using antibodies against PNL2, Melan A, TRP-1, and TRP-2 was found to have 100% specificity and 94% sensitivity and may be helpful in differentiation.[11,31]

Melanoma of the oral cavity is a highly malignant tumor with frequent metastasis to the regional lymph nodes (LNs) and then the lungs.[9,30–68] There is a small subset of dogs with well-differentiated oral melanomas and these may have a more benign biologic behavior.[41,69] The metastatic rate is site, size, and stage dependent and reported in up to 80% of dogs.[12,20,30–68] The World Health Organization (WHO) clinical staging system for oral tumors in dogs may have prognostic significance in dogs with oral melanoma (Table 23.2).[30–68,70] MM is a highly immunogenic tumor, and molecular and immunomodulatory approaches to treatment are active areas of research and treatment.[56–68] A review of the biology and molecular mechanisms of canine melanoma development and progression is provided in Chapter 20.[71,72]

Squamous Cell Carcinoma

SCC is the most common oral tumor in cats (Fig. 23.2) and the second most common in dogs.[1,4,5,20–24] There are five different histologic subtypes of SCC in dogs: conventional, papillary, basaloid, adenosquamous, and spindle cell.[73] Papillary SCCs typically occur in the rostral oral cavity of dogs less than 9 months old, although cases in older dogs have also been reported.[73–77] The metastatic rate for nontonsillar SCC in dogs is 5% to 29%,[43,76–85] but the metastatic risk is site dependent, with the rostral oral cavity having a low metastatic rate and the caudal tongue and tonsil having a high metastatic potential.[77]

TABLE 23.1   Summary of Common Oral Tumors in the Dog and Cat[a]

	CANINE				FELINE	
	Malignant Melanoma	SCC	Fibrosarcoma	Acanthomatous Ameloblastoma	SCC	Fibrosarcoma
Frequency	30%–40%	17%–25%	8%–25%	5%	70%–80%	13%–17%
Median age (years)	12	8–10	7–9	8	10–12	10
Sex predisposition	None to male	None	Male	None	None	None
Animal size	Smaller	Larger	Larger	None	—	—
Site predilection	Gingival, buccal, and labial mucosa	Rostral mandible	Maxillary gingiva and hard palate	Rostral mandible	Tongue, pharynx, and tonsils	Gingiva
Lymph node metastasis	Common (41%–74%)	Rare (<40%) Tonsil SCC up to 73%	Occasional (9%–28%)	None	Rare	Rare
Distant metastasis	Common (14%–92%)	Rare (<36%)	Occasional (0%–71%)	None	Rare	Rare (<20%)
Gross appearance	Pigmented (67%) or amelanotic (33%), ulcerated	Red, cauliflower, ulcerated	Flat, firm, ulcerated	Red, cauliflower, ulcerated	Proliferative, ulcerated	Firm
Bone involvement	Common (57%)	Common (77%)	Common (60%–72%)	Common (80%–100%)	Common	Common
Surgery response	Fair to good	Good	Fair to good	Excellent	Poor	Fair
Local recurrence	0%–59%	0%–50%	31%–60%	0%–11%		
MST	5–17 months	9–26 months	10–12 months	>28–64 months	45 days	
1-Year survival rate	21%–35%	57%–91%	21%–50%	72%–100%	<10%	
Radiation response	Good	Good	Poor to fair	Excellent	Poor	Poor
Response rate	83%–94%	—	—	—		
Local recurrence	11%–27%	31%–42%	32%	8%–18%		
MST	4–12 months	16–36 months	7–26 months	37 months	90 days	
1-Year survival rate	36%–71%	72%	76%	>85%		
Best treatment	Surgery and/ or radiation ± chemotherapy ± immunotherapy	Surgery and/or radiation	Surgery and/or radiation	Surgery	Surgery and radiation ± sensitizer	Surgery and/or radiation
Prognosis	Fair to good	Good to excellent	Good	Excellent	Poor to fair	Fair
MST	<36 months	26–36 months	18–26 months	>64 months	14 months	
Cause of death	Distant disease	Local or distant disease	Local disease	Rarely tumor related	Local disease	Local disease

MST, Mean survival time; *SCC*, squamous cell carcinoma.
[a]References 11–21, 28–32, 37, 53, 57–60, 78, 84–86, 104–111.

In cats, the risk of developing oral SCC is significantly increased by 4-fold with the use of flea collars and high intake of either canned food in general or canned tuna fish specifically.[86] Exposure to household tobacco smoke increases the risk of oral SCC by 2-fold in cats,[86] and although this was not statistically significant, smoke exposure is associated with a significant increase in expression of *p53* in SCC lesions compared with cats with oral SCC not exposed to environmental smoke.[87] For this reason, mutations of *p53* may be involved in the development and progression of smoke-related oral SCC in cats.

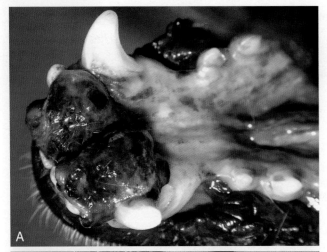

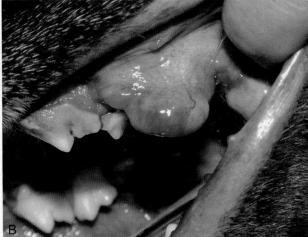

• **Fig. 23.1** (A) A malignant melanoma arising from the rostral mandible. (B) An amelanotic malignant melanoma arising from the caudal maxilla.

TABLE 23.2	Clinical Staging (TNM) of Oral Tumors in Dogs and Cats[70]		

Clinical Staging System for Oral Tumors

Primary Tumor (T)
Tis Tumor in situ
T1 Tumor <2 cm in diameter at greatest dimension
T1a Without evidence of bone invasion
T1b With evidence of bone invasion
T2 Tumor 2–4 cm in diameter at greatest dimension
T2a Without evidence of bone invasion
T2b With evidence of bone invasion
T3 Tumor >4 cm in diameter at greatest dimension
T3a Without evidence of bone invasion
T3b With evidence of bone invasion

Regional Lymph Nodes (N)
N0 No regional lymph node metastasis
N1 Movable ipsilateral lymph nodes
N1a No evidence of lymph node metastasis
N1b Evidence of lymph node metastasis
N2 Movable contralateral lymph nodes
N2a No evidence of lymph node metastasis
N2b Evidence of lymph node metastasis
N3 Fixed lymph nodes

Distant Metastasis (M)
M0 No distant metastasis
M1 Distant metastasis [specify site(s)]

Stage Grouping	Tumor (T)	Nodes (N)	Metastasis (M)
I	T1	N0, N1a, N2a	M0
II	T2	N0, N1a, N2a	M0
III	T3	N0, N1a, N2a	M0
IV	Any T	N1b	M0
	Any T	N2b, N3	M0
	Any T	Any N	M1

SCC frequently invades bone in both cats and dogs, and bone invasion is usually severe and extensive in the cat. Increased tumor expression of parathyroid hormone–related protein in cats with oral SCC may play a role in bone resorption and tumor invasion.[88] Control of local disease is the most challenging aspect in cats with oral SCC because of the extent of the local tumor[89–112]; [not superscript] however, metastasis has been reported to the mandibular LNs and lungs in 31% and 10% of cats, respectively,[95] and hence treatment for this metastatic potential may be warranted for cats in which local tumor control is achieved.

Fibrosarcoma

Oral FSA is the second most common oral tumor in cats and the third most common in dogs.[2,5, 20–24,90] In dogs, oral FSA tends to occur in large breed dogs, particularly golden and Labrador retrievers.[20–24,113–117] The median age at diagnosis is 7.3 to 8.6 years and there may be a male predisposition.[113–116] Oral FSA may look surprisingly benign histologically and, even with large biopsy samples, the pathologist can find it difficult to differentiate fibroma from low-grade FSA.[113] This syndrome, which is common on the hard palate (Fig. 23.3) and maxillary arcade between the canine and carnassial teeth

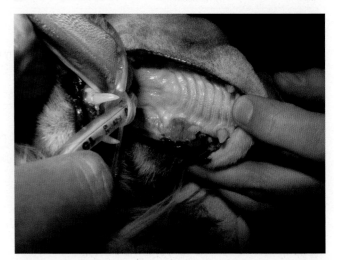

• **Fig. 23.2** Typical appearance of an oral squamous cell carcinoma in a cat. Although these can be proliferative and firm, ulceration is more common.

of large-breed dogs, has been termed *histologically low-grade but biologically high-grade FSA*.[113] Even with a biopsy result suggesting fibroma or low-grade FSA, the treatment should be aggressive, especially if the cancer is rapidly growing, recurrent,

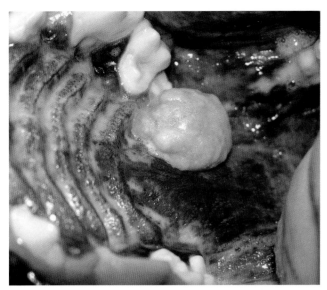

• **Fig. 23.3** Typical appearance of a biologically high-grade but histologically low-grade fibrosarcoma. These often appear histologically benign or low-grade, but have an aggressive local behavior. Wide surgical resection and possibly postoperative radiation therapy are required for adequate local tumor control.

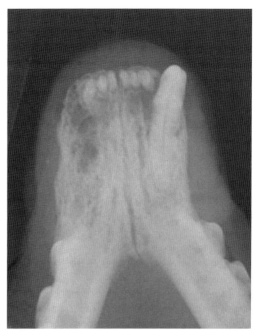

• **Fig. 23.4** An intraoral radiograph of the rostral mandible of a cat with a squamous cell carcinoma. Note the extensive bone lysis resulting in tooth loss, which is very common in cats with this type of tumor.

or invading bone. FSA is locally invasive, but metastasis to the lungs and occasionally regional LNs occurs in fewer than 30% of dogs.[12,20–24,43,113–117]

Osteosarcoma

OSA of axial sites is less common than appendicular OSA and represents approximately 25% of all cases.[10] Of the axial OSA, the mandible and maxilla are involved in 27% and 16% to 22% of cases, respectively.[10,118] OSA is the fourth most common malignant oral tumor in dogs. The metastatic potential for axial OSA is less than appendicular OSA.[10,119–122] A female sex predisposition has been reported.[10]

Peripheral Odontogenic Fibroma

Peripheral odontogenic fibroma is the preferred term for a group of benign tumors previously known as epulides.[123] Four types of epulides have been described in the dog: acanthomatous, fibromatous, ossifying, and giant cell.[123–135] Acanthomatous epulis has been renamed acanthomatous ameloblastoma, and the fibromatous and ossifying epulides have been renamed peripheral odontogenic fibroma.[123] Peripheral odontogenic fibromas are relatively common in dogs, but rare in cats.[135] Multiple epulides have been described in cats, with 50% of cases occurring in cats younger than 3 years.[135] They are benign gingival proliferations arising from the periodontal ligament and appear similar to focal fibrous hyperplasia of the gingiva.[123] Unlike AAs, they do not invade into underlying bone. The mean age at presentation for dogs with peripheral odontogenic fibromas is 8 to 9 years, and a male predisposition has been reported.[123–127] Peripheral odontogenic fibromas are slow-growing, firm masses and usually are covered by intact epithelium. They have a predilection for the maxilla rostral to the third premolar teeth.[123–127]

Acanthomatous Ameloblastoma

AA is a benign tumor, but has an aggressive local behavior and frequently invades bone of the underlying mandible or maxilla. Medium- to large-breed dogs are most commonly affected, and Shetland sheepdogs, Old English sheepdogs, and golden retrievers are overrepresented.[123–130] The mean age at presentation is 7 to 10 years, and a sex predisposition is unlikely, with three studies reporting conflicting results.[125,128–130] The rostral mandible is the most common site, representing 51% of all cases in one study of 263 dogs with AA, with other sites being the caudal mandible (22%), rostral maxilla (22%), and caudal maxilla (6%).[128,129] They do not metastasize. AA is the preferred term, but some pathologists will refer to these tumors by their previous terminology of *acanthomatous epulis* or *adamantinoma*.[124]

History and Clinical Signs

Most cats and dogs with oral cancer present with a mass in the mouth noticed by the owner. Cancer in the caudal pharynx, however, is rarely seen by the owner and the animal will present with signs of increased salivation, exophthalmos or facial swelling, epistaxis, weight loss, halitosis, bloody oral discharge, dysphagia or pain on opening the mouth, or occasionally cervical lymphadenopathy (especially SCC of the tonsil).[20–24,91] Loose teeth, especially in an animal with generally good dentition, should alert the clinician to possible underlying neoplastic bone lysis (Fig. 23.4), particularly in the cat. Although paraneoplastic syndromes associated with oral tumors are rare, hypercalcemia has been reported in two cats with oral SCC[87] and hyperglycemia in a cat with a gingival vascular hamartoma.[136]

Diagnostic Techniques and Workup

The diagnosis and clinical staging of animals with oropharyngeal masses is imperative before definitive surgical excision. A biopsy is required for definitive diagnosis and this will assist the clinician in determining biologic behavior and prognosis. Clinical staging consists of evaluating the extent of the local tumor and the presence of metastatic disease. The regional LNs and lungs are the two most common sites of metastasis in cats and dogs with oral tumors.[30–68,76–85,89–122] The procedures required for the diagnosis and clinical staging of animals with oral cancer can usually be performed under a short general anesthesia.

Diagnosis

A large incisional biopsy is often required for a definitive diagnosis. Fine-needle aspirate (FNA) or impression smear cytology has traditionally been considered unrewarding because many oral tumors are associated with a high degree of necrosis and inflammation; however, one prospective study of 114 cats and dogs with oral masses showed that, in comparison to definitive histopathologic results, FNA cytology had a diagnostic accuracy rate of 98% in dogs and 96% in cats, and impressions smear cytology had a diagnostic accuracy rate of 92% in dogs and 96% in cats.[137] Dogs with exophytic or ulcerated masses will generally tolerate a deep wedge or core punch biopsy without general anesthesia. Biopsy is recommended in the diagnostic workup of cats and dogs with an oral mass to differentiate benign from malignant disease, for owners basing their treatment options on prognosis, and when other treatment modalities, such as radiation therapy (RT), may be preferable. Oral cancers are commonly infected, inflamed, or necrotic, and it is important to obtain a large representative specimen. Cautery may distort the specimen and should be used for hemostasis only after blade incision or punch biopsy. Large samples of healthy tissue at the edge and center of the lesion will increase the diagnostic yield, but care must be taken not to contaminate normal tissue, which cannot be removed with surgery or included in the radiation field. Biopsies should always be performed from within the oral cavity and not through the lip to avoid seeding tumor cells in normal skin and compromising curative-intent surgical resection. For small lesions (e.g., epulides, papillomas, or small labial mucosal melanoma), curative-intent resection (excisional biopsy) may be undertaken at the time of initial evaluation. However, accurate notes should be included in the medical records, and/or photographic evidence, to detail the size and anatomic location of the mass if excision is incomplete and further treatment is required. For more extensive disease, waiting for biopsy results is recommended so that appropriate treatment plans can be formulated.

Clinical Staging: Local Tumor

Tumor size is an important prognostic factor for some types of oral tumors, such as MM, SCC, and tongue tumors,[40,41,78,138–142] and hence an accurate measurement of tumor size should be recorded. Cancers that are adherent to or arising from bones of the mandible, maxilla, or palate should be imaged under general anesthesia to determine the presence of bone lysis and the extent of local disease. Regional radiographs include open mouth, intraoral, oblique lateral, and ventrodorsal or dorsoventral projections. Bone lysis is not radiographically evident until 40% or more of

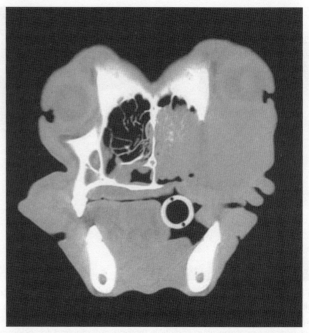

• **Fig. 23.5** A computed tomography image of a dog with a maxillary fibrosarcoma. Advanced imaging allows better planning of surgery and radiation therapy, as the extent of bone involvement and extension into the nasal cavity is often much greater than can be appreciated grossly.

the cortex is destroyed and hence apparently normal radiographs do not exclude bone invasion. Advanced imaging modalities are now widely available and these are recommended for imaging of oral tumors, particularly tumors arising from the maxilla, palate, and caudal mandible (Fig. 23.5).[143–145] Computed tomography (CT) scans are generally preferred to magnetic resonance imaging (MRI) because of superior bone detail, but both CT or MRI scans will provide more information on the local extent of the tumor than regional radiographs. In one study, invasion into adjacent structures was noted in only 30% of dogs imaged with radiographs compared with more than 90% of dogs imaged with contrast-enhanced CT.[145] In another study, MRI provided more accurate information on invasion into adjacent structures, MRI and CT showed similar accuracy in assessing bone invasion, and calcification and cortical bone erosion were better assessed with CT scan.[144] Although not widely available, positron emission tomography (PET)/CT provided valuable information on the extent of soft tissue infiltration and presence of LN metastasis in cats with oral SCC in comparison to CT.[146,147] This information is important for planning the definitive surgical procedure (or RT if indicated).

Clinical Staging: Regional Lymph Nodes

Regional LNs should be carefully palpated for enlargement or asymmetry. However, caution should be exercised when making clinical judgments based on palpation alone because LN size is not an accurate predictor of metastasis. In one study of 100 dogs with oral MM, 40% of dogs with normal sized LNs had metastasis and 49% of dogs with enlarged LNs did not have metastasis.[34] Furthermore, the regional LNs include the mandibular, parotid, and medial retropharyngeal LNs; but the parotid and medial retropharyngeal LNs are not externally palpable.[148–151] In addition, only 55% of 31 cats and dogs with metastasis to the regional LNs had metastasis to the mandibular LNs.[149] CT and PET/CT can be useful to determine LN metastasis and guide further diagnostics.[143,147,148] LN aspiration should be performed in all animals with oral tumors, regardless of the size or degree of fixation of the LNs.[34,149] The accuracy of LN aspirates for the detection of metastatic cancer in cats and dogs is 77%.[152] Resection of some or all of the regional LNs has been described and, although the therapeutic benefit of this approach is unknown, it may provide valuable staging information.[148–151] The major concerns with nontargeted LN resection are the possibility of missing a metastatic lesion and the potential morbidity associated with excision of multiple LNs. Lymphatic drainage of the oral cavity is highly variable in humans and likely in dogs and cats,[151] and the first draining LN can be ipsilateral or contralateral to the tumor and include any one of the mandibular, medial retropharyngeal, parotid, or minor LNs, such as the buccal LN.[149,151] For these reasons, sentinel LN (SLN) mapping and biopsy is becoming the preferred technique for LN staging of oral tumors.

SLN mapping and biopsy is the assessment of LN metastasis without more aggressive en bloc surgical excisions of the regional LNs. The SLN is the first draining LN and the status of this LN is representative of the entire LN bed. Furthermore, the SLN is not necessarily the regional anatomic LN. In one study of dogs with cutaneous mast cell tumors, the SLN was different from the regional anatomic LN in 40% of dogs.[153] Methods to detect SLN in people with head and neck cancer include lymphoscintigraphy, intraoperative blue dyes, and intraoperative gamma probes.[154] Lymphoscintigraphy, intraoperative dyes, and contrast-enhanced ultrasonography have been described in dogs with various tumors, including head and neck cancer.[154,155] The use of lipid-soluble and water-soluble contrast agents has also been reported as methods of detecting the location of the SLN preoperatively, and then combining this with methylene blue to aide in the identification of the SLN intraoperatively (Fig. 23.6).[156] The advantage of this latter technique is that radioactive materials are not required and hence this is a more widely applicable SLN mapping technique.

Clinical Staging: Distant Metastasis

The final step in the clinical staging of animals with oral tumors is imaging of the thoracic cavity for metastasis to the lungs. Three-view thoracic radiographs (right and left lateral projections, and either dorsoventral or ventrodorsal projection) are generally recommended. CT scans should be considered for animals with highly metastatic tumor types, such as oral MM, as they are significantly more sensitive in detecting pulmonary metastatic lesions compared with radiographs.[157–160] Based on these diagnostic steps, oral tumors are then clinically staged according to the WHO staging scheme (see Table 23.2).[70]

Treatment

Surgery

Surgery and RT are the most common treatments used for the local control of oral tumors. Surgical resection is the most economic, expeditious, and curative treatment. The type of oral surgery depends on tumor histology and location. Except for peripheral odontogenic fibromas, most oral tumors have some underlying bone involvement and surgical resection should include bony margins to increase the likelihood of local tumor control. More aggressive surgeries such as mandibulectomy, maxillectomy, and orbitectomy are generally well tolerated by cats and dogs. These procedures are indicated for all aggressive and/or invasive oral tumors, particularly lesions with extensive bone invasion, with poor sensitivity to RT (Tables 23.3 and 23.4).[13–24,161–164] Margins of at least 2 cm are generally necessary for malignant cancers such as SCC, MM, FSA, and OSA in the dog. If possible, FSA in the dog and SCC in the cat should be treated with surgical margins greater than 2 cm because of high local recurrence rates. Bone reconstruction after bony resection has been described,[165–172] but is rarely necessary in dogs because of good postoperative function and cosmetic appearance with mandibulectomy alone.[13–24] Furthermore, a high complication rate has been reported after reconstruction and these complications often require revision surgeries for their management.[24,172] In contrast to dogs, cats frequently have poor postoperative function after mandibulectomy[90] and hence mandibular reconstruction may improve postoperative functional outcome in cats.[173] Rostral and segmental resections (e.g., mandibulectomy and maxillectomy) may be sufficient for benign lesions and rostral SCC in dogs. Rim resections, in which the ventral cortex of the mandible is preserved, may be possible for small benign tumors localized to the alveolar margin of the mandible (Fig. 23.7).[174–176] Larger resections, including hemimandibulectomy, hemimaxillectomy, orbitectomy, and radical maxillectomy, are necessary for more aggressive tumors, especially FSA, and malignant tumors with a more caudal location.[13–24,161–164] Although these large resections carry some morbidity, owner satisfaction with the cosmetic and functional outcomes is in excess of 85%.[13–24,90,161–164] Cosmesis is usually very good after most mandibulectomy and maxillectomy procedures (Fig. 23.8), but can be challenging with aggressive bilateral rostral mandibulectomies and radical maxillectomies.[13–24,161–164,177] Blood loss and hypotension are the most common intraoperative complications, particularly during caudal or aggressive maxillectomy procedures.[21,162,177] Postoperative complications include incisional dehiscence and oronasal fistula formation, epistaxis, increased salivation, mandibular drift and malocclusion, lip trauma, infection, and difficulty prehending food, particularly after bilateral rostral mandibulectomy caudal to the second premolar teeth.[13–24,161–164,177] Elastic training, consisting of an orthodontic elastic rubber chain between an orthodontic button on the lingual aspect of the intact mandible tooth and buccal aspect of the maxillary fourth premolar tooth, has been described to maintain occlusion and prevent mandibular drift after mandibulectomy in dogs.[178] Enteral feeding tubes are not usually required after oral surgery in dogs; however, they are recommended for cats treated with any type of mandibulectomy because eating can be difficult for 2 to 4 months after surgery and 12% of cats never eat voluntarily after mandibulectomy.[89,90]

Local disease control is the goal of treatment for most animals with oral tumors. Regional LN resection has been described in cats and dogs; although it adds to clinical staging information, its effectiveness in controlling local and metastatic disease is unknown.[148–151]

Radiation Therapy

RT can be effective for locoregional control of oral tumors. RT can be used as a primary treatment, with either palliative or curative intent, as an adjunct for incompletely resected tumors, or as an adjunct for locally aggressive tumors regardless of the completeness of excision, such as oral FSA. MM,[42–49] canine oral SCC,[80,81,179]

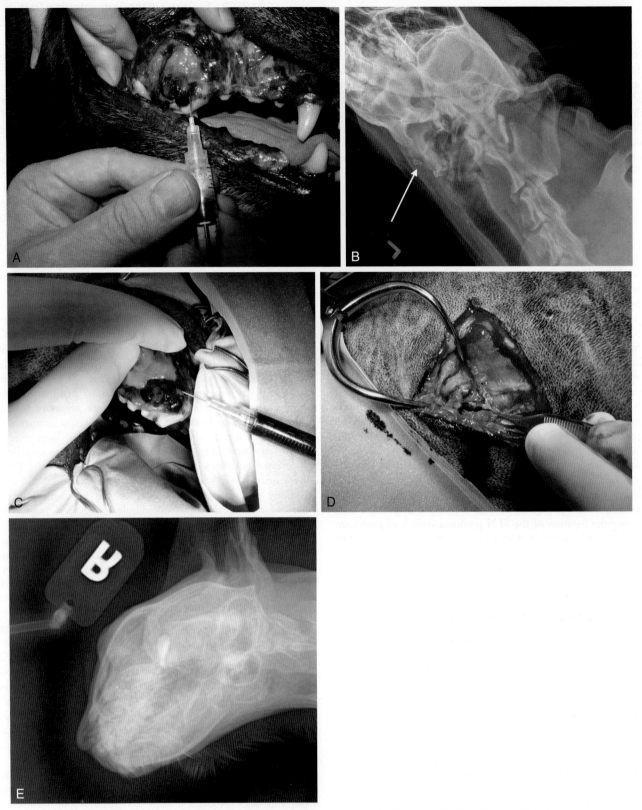

• **Fig. 23.6** Indirect lymphography for sentinel lymph node mapping. (A) A lipid-soluble, radio-opaque contrast agent is being injected peritumorally in four quadrants around a malignant melanoma in a dog. (B) The lipid-soluble contrast agent is taken up slowly into the lymphatics. A regional radiograph is taken 24 hours postinjection to identify the sentinel lymph node, which was the ipsilateral mandibular lymph node in this case (arrow). (C) To confirm the sentinel lymph node, methylene blue is injected in four quadrants peritumorally during surgery. (D) Methylene blue is rapidly taken up into the lymphatics. A surgical approach is made to the sentinel lymph node identified radiographically. Blue discoloration of the afferent lymphatics and lymph node assist in identifying this node as the sentinel lymph node. The sentinel lymph node is submitted for histopathologic assessment to determine whether there is evidence of metastatic disease. (E) Regional radiograph of a cat with a malignant melanoma of the lip 24 hours after peritumoral injection of a lipid-soluble contrast agent. The sentinel lymph node is the buccal lymph node. Note that the mandibular lymph nodes are the only palpable regional lymph nodes; however, malignant oral tumors can metastasize the ipsilateral or contralateral mandibular, medial retropharyngeal, parotid, and minor lymph nodes. Aspiration or excision of only the mandibular lymph node may result in metastatic lymph nodes being missed.

TABLE 23.3	**Various Mandibulectomies**	

Mandibulectomy Procedure	Indications	Comments	
Unilateral rostral	Lesions confined to rostral hemimandible; not crossing midline	Most common tumor types are squamous cell carcinoma and adamantinoma that do not require removal of entire affected bone; tongue may lag to resected side.	
Bilateral rostral	Bilateral rostral lesions crossing the symphysis	Tongue will be "too long," and some cheilitis of chin skin will occur; has been performed as far back as PM4 but preferably at PM1.	
Vertical ramus	Low-grade bony or cartilaginous lesions confined to vertical ramus	These tumors are variously called *chondroma rodens* or *multilobular osteosarcoma*; temporomandibular joint may be removed; cosmesis and function are excellent.	
Complete unilateral	High-grade tumors with extensive involvement of horizontal ramus or invasion into medullary canal of ramus	Usually reserved for aggressive tumors; function and cosmesis are good.	
Segmental	Low-grade midhorizontal ramus cancer, preferably not into medullary cavity	Poor choice for highly malignant cancer in medullary cavity because growth along mandibular artery, vein, and nerve is common.	

TABLE 23.4	**Various Maxillectomies**	

Maxillectomy Procedure	Indications	Comments	
Unilateral rostral	Lesions confined to hard palate on one side	One-layer closure.	
Bilateral rostral	Bilateral lesions of rostral hard palate	Needs viable buccal mucosa on both sides for flap closure.	
Lateral	Laterally placed midmaxillary lesions	Single-layer closure if small defect, two-layer if large.	
Bilateral	Bilateral palatine lesions	High rate of closure dehiscence because lip flap rarely reaches from side to side; may result in permanent oronasal fistula.	

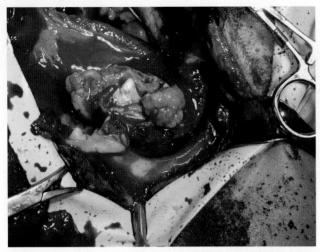

• **Fig. 23.7** Rim resection of an acanthomatous ameloblastoma in a dog. The rim resection has been performed with a 24-mm biradial saw to preserve the ventral cortex of the mandibular body and hence prevent postoperative mandibular drift.

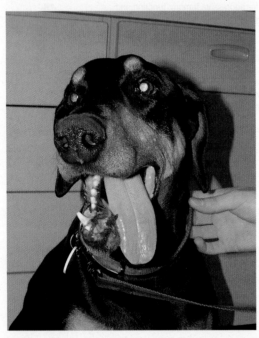

• **Fig. 23.8** The typical appearance of a dog 6 months postoperatively after subtotal unilateral mandibulectomy for an osteosarcoma. The tongue will often hang out and the remaining hemimandible will drift toward the resected side.

and some benign tumors, such as AA,[130–132] are known to be radiation responsive, and RT should be considered in the primary treatment of these tumors. RT can also be used for the palliation of oral SCC in cats and a variety of hypofractionated, accelerated, and stereotactic RT protocols have been described.[96–106]

Acute effects are common but self-limiting. These include alopecia and moist desquamation, oral mucositis, dysphagia, and ocular changes, such as blepharitis, conjunctivitis, keratitis, and uveitis.[43,80,81,116,117,130] The acute effects of coarse fractionation are less than experienced with the full-course protocols used for oral SCC and dental tumors and usually resolve rapidly.[44–49,96–104] Late complications are rare, occurring in fewer than 5% of cases,

but can include permanent alopecia, skin fibrosis, bone necrosis and oronasal fistula formation, development of a second malignancy within the radiation field, keratoconjunctivitis sicca, cataract formation, xerostomia, and retinal atrophy.[43,130–132] Orthovoltage radiation may be associated with a higher incidence of second malignancies and bone necrosis than megavoltage irradiation.[32,130,131]

Chemotherapy

The major problem with most oral tumors is control of local disease; however, chemotherapy may be indicated for some tumors with higher metastatic potential, especially oral MM in dogs,[9,30–68] tonsillar SCC in cats and dogs, OSA in dogs,[122] and possibly oral SCC in cats.[89–112]

Prognosis

Clinical series of more than 750 dogs with various oral malignancies treated with either mandibulectomy or maxillectomy have been described.[13–24,161–164] The majority of cases were treated with surgery alone. Unfortunately, the methods of reporting and outcome results vary with each paper. Overall, the lowest rates of local tumor recurrence and best survival times (STs) are reported in dogs with AA and SCC, whereas FSA and MM are associated with the least favorable results.[13–24] Most of these reports suggest that histologically complete resection, smaller diameter, and a rostral location are favorable prognostic factors.[24] In two studies of 142 dogs treated with either mandibulectomy or maxillectomy, tumor-related deaths were 10 to 21 times more likely with malignant tumors, up to five times more likely with tumors located caudal to the canine teeth, and two to four times more likely after incomplete resection.[22,23] Rostral locations are usually detected at an earlier stage and are more likely to be resectable with complete surgical margins. Local tumor recurrence is more frequent after incomplete resection with 15% to 22% and 62% to 65% of tumors recurring after complete and incomplete excision, respectively.[22,23] Recurrent disease negatively affects ST because further treatment is more difficult and the response to treatment is poorer.[31] FSA continues to have high local recurrence rates in most studies, and more aggressive surgical approaches or adjuvant therapies, such as postoperative RT, should be considered.[24,115] On the other hand, MM is controlled locally in 75% of cases, but metastatic disease requires more effective systemic adjuvant therapy.

Malignant Melanoma

The prognosis for dogs with oral MM is guarded. Metastatic disease is the most common cause of death, with metastasis to the lungs reported in 14% to 67% of dogs.[9,13–24, 30–68] Surgery or RT can provide good local control, but the majority of dogs will fail treatment because of metastatic disease and hence the search for effective adjuvant immunotherapy holds the most promise to ultimately improve outcomes.

Surgery is the most common treatment for management of the local tumor. The median survival time (MST) for untreated dogs with oral MM is 65 days,[31] whereas tumor control and STs are significantly better when surgery is included in the treatment plan.[32] The overall local tumor recurrence rate after surgery is up to 45%,[24,40,41] with local tumor recurrence rates of 22% after mandibulectomy and 48% after maxillectomy.[7,18,19] The median ST (MST) for dogs with MM treated with surgery alone varies

TABLE 23.5	Prognostic Factors for Dogs with Oral Malignant Melanoma Treated with Surgery, with or without Radiation Therapy, Chemotherapy, and/or Immunotherapy		
Prognostic Factor	**Median Progression-Free Survival**	**Median Survival Time**	
Age[40]	—	630 days if <12 years 224 days if ≥12 years	
Tumor size[56]	—	511 days if >2 cm 164 days if >2 cm	
Tumor size[40]	—	630 days if <2 cm 240 days if 2–4 cm 173 days if >4 cm	
Tumor size[41]	>567 days if <3 cm 245 days if >3 cm	874 days if <3 cm 396 days if >3 cm	
Metastasis at diagnosis[41]	567 days if no metastasis 187 days if metastasis	818 days if no metastasis 131 days if metastasis	
Clinical stage[40,41]	>567 days for stage I >187 days for stage II 245 days for stage III	874 days for stage I 818 days for stage II 207 days for stage III	
PDGFRs-α and -β coexpression[30]	239 days if no coexpression 159 days if no coexpression	335 days if no coexpression 183 days if no coexpression	
Ki67[30]	484 days if Ki67 <19.5% 188 days if Ki67 >19.5%	484 days if Ki67 <19.5% 224 days if Ki67 >19.5%	

PDGFR, Platelet-derived growth factor receptor.

considerably from 150 to 874 days with 1-year survival rates less than 35%.[9,13–24,30–68] In a recent study, the median progression-free interval (PFI) and MST after surgery alone for oral MM were greater than 567 days and 874 days, respectively.[41] Variables which are known to have prognostic significance in dogs treated with surgery alone or in combination with other modalities include age, tumor size, clinical stage, the ability of the first treatment to achieve local control, and histologic and immunohistochemical criteria such as the degree of differentiation, mitotic index, nuclear atypia score, pigment quantification, COX-2 expression, PDGFR expression, Ki67 expression, and *c-kit* expression (Table 23.5).[9,13–24,30–68] In some studies, tumor location has prognostic importance with rostral mandibular and caudal maxillary sites having a better prognosis than other sites.[32,37,53] MSTs are significantly shorter for dogs with recurrent oral MM compared with dogs with previously untreated oral MM.[31] In one study, dogs treated with adjunctive RT had significantly longer STs, but this result may have been confounded by age, which was also prognostic in this study.[40] In 64 dogs with surgically treated well-differentiated melanomas of the lips and oral cavity, 95% of dogs were either alive or had died of unrelated causes at the end of the study period.[69] Prognostic information for melanocytic tumors in dogs has recently been reviewed.[39]

Oral melanoma is responsive to hypofractionated RT protocols. A number of different hypofractionated RT protocols have been described: (1) 3 weekly 8 to 10 Gy fractions for a total dose of 24 to 30 Gy,[44,47] (2) 4 weekly fractions of 9 Gy for a total dose of 36 Gy,[45,47] (3) 6 weekly 6 Gy fractions for a total dose of 36 Gy,[46] (4) 5 fractions of 6 Gy over 2.5 weeks,[49] and (5) 8 weekly 6 Gy fractions for a total dose of 48 Gy.[42] Response rates are excellent, with 81% to 100% of tumors responding and a complete response observed in up to 70% of melanomas.[42–49] Local recurrence is reported in 15% to 26% of dogs experiencing a complete response with a median

time to local recurrence of 139 days.[44–49] In one study progressive local disease was observed in all dogs that did not achieve a complete response.[44] The most common cause of death is metastasis, and this is reported in 58% of dogs with a median time of metastasis of 311 days.[46] The MST for dogs treated with RT is 192 to 401 days, with a 1-year survival rate of 36% to 48% and a 2-year survival rate of 21%.[44–49] Local tumor control and ST are significantly improved with rostral tumor location, smaller tumor volume, no radiographic evidence of bone lysis, postoperative irradiation of microscopic disease, and megavoltage irradiation.[43,45,47,48] In one series of 140 dogs with oral MM, the MST was 21 months if none of these risk factors were present compared with an MST of 11 months with one risk factor, 5 months with two risk factors, and three months with all three risk factors.[47]

Tumor size is important with median PFS for dogs with T1 oral melanomas of 19 months compared with less than 7 months for T2 and T3 tumors.[43] In one study of 111 dogs treated with either orthovoltage or megavoltage hypofractionated protocols, tumor size and clinical stage had a significant effect on outcome with MSTs for dogs with stage I, II, III, and IV oral malignant melanoma of 758, 278, 163, and 80 days, respectively.[48] In this study, there was a greater risk of death and decreased STs overall (MSTs of 233 days compared with 122 days) and for dogs with stage III melanoma (MSTs of 210 days compared with 99 days) when treated with orthovoltage rather than megavoltage RT.[48] The median PFI was significantly prolonged in one study of 27 dogs when hypofractionated RT was combined with adjuvant oral temozolomide compared with hypofractionated RT alone.[49] Hypofractionated RT has also been described in five cats with oral melanoma, resulting in a 60% response rate and MST of 146 days (range: 66–224 days).[29]

Effective systemic adjuvant therapies (e.g., immunotherapy, chemotherapy) are ultimately necessary for successful management of dogs with oral MM owing to the high metastatic risk. Unfortunately, these tumors, in dogs and people, are generally poorly responsive to cytotoxic chemotherapy and effective immunotherapies that result in meaningful immunologic responses in the majority of patients are currently lacking.

In a small study of 17 dogs treated with surgery and adjuvant carboplatin, the median PFS was 259 days (with 41% of dogs developing local tumor recurrence and 41% of dogs developing metastasis) and the MST was 440 days.[52] However, two recent studies have shown no benefit in STs with the use of adjunctive chemotherapy,[40,41] with overall MSTs of 335 days and 352 days in dogs that were and were not treated with systemic adjuvant therapy.[41]

Immunotherapy holds the most promise for effective management in dogs with MM and this is an area of very active research in both veterinary and physician-based oncology. The use of DNA vaccinations with either murine or human tyrosinase in dogs with advanced stages of oral MM (clinical stage II–IV) results in MSTs of 224 to 389 days.[61–66] In one study of nine dogs treated with DNA vaccine encoded for human tyrosinase, complete response was observed in one dog with lung metastasis, two dogs with stage IV disease and bulky metastasis lived for greater than 400 days, and two dogs with stage II or III disease died of other causes approximately 500 days after treatment with no evidence of tumor at necropsy.[61] The MST is significantly improved to 589 days when the primary oral site and regional LNs are controlled with surgery or RT.[61] In a prospective study of dogs with surgically excised stage II or III oral MM that compared 58 dogs treated with DNA vaccine encoded for human tyrosinase with a historical control of 53 unvaccinated dogs, the MST was significantly longer for dogs in the vaccinated group (not reached compared with 324 days) with tumor-related deaths in only 26% of vaccinated dogs compared with 64% of unvaccinated dogs.[62] In two prospective studies investigating human recombinant chondroitin sulfate proteoglycan-4 DNA–based electrovaccination after surgical resection in dogs with stage II or III oral MMs, the survival outcomes were significantly longer in vaccinated dogs.[67,68] For vaccinated and unvaccinated dogs, respectively, the local recurrence rates were 21% to 35% and 39% to 42%; the metastatic rates were less than 36% and 79% to 90%; the 6-month survival rates were 96% to 100% and 63% to 69%; the 12-month survival rates were 64% to 74% and 15% to 26%; the 24-month survival rates were 30% and 5%; the median disease-free intervals (DFIs) were 477 days and 180 days; and the MSTs were 653 to 684 days and 200 to 220 days.[67,68] For vaccinated dogs, outcomes were significantly better for dogs weighing less than 20 kg.[68] A thorough discussion of MM and its prognosis after definitive treatment with surgery, RT, chemotherapy, and/or immunomodulatory agents is provided in Chapter 20.

The location of MM may also have some prognostic significance. Melanomas of the lip and tongue may have a lower metastatic rate, with survival more dependent on local control of the tumor. In one series of 60 dogs with oral MMs at various sites treated with combinations of surgery, RT, chemotherapy, and immunotherapy, the MST for dogs with lip and tongue MMs was 580 days and was greater than 551 days, respectively.[9] In comparison, the MST was 319 days for maxillary MMs and 330 days for MMs of the hard palate.[9] In another study, the MST was significantly longer for dogs with labial mucosal MMs (310 days) than mandibular and maxillary MMs (123 days).[38]

In another study, only 5% of 64 dogs with well-differentiated melanomas of the mucous membranes of the lips and oral cavities treated with surgery alone had died from tumor-related causes,

with an overall MST of 34 months.[69] This improved prognosis may reflect the location of these lesions (lip compared with oral cavity) or the degree of differentiation. Nuclear atypia and mitotic index have also been shown to be prognostic in dogs with oral MM.[35]

Canine Oral Squamous Cell Carcinoma

The prognosis for dogs with oral SCC is good, particularly for rostral tumor locations. Local tumor control is usually the most important challenge, although metastasis to the regional LNs is reported in up to 10% of dogs and to the lungs in 3% to 36% of dogs.[24,43,76–85,179] In contrast, SCC of the tonsils and base of the tongue are highly metastatic, with metastasis reported in up to 73% of dogs, and locoregional recurrence is common.[138–141,180,181] Surgery and RT can both be used for locoregional control of oral SCC in dogs. Photodynamic therapy has also been reported with fair-to-good results in 11 dogs with smaller oral SCC.[182]

Surgery is the most common treatment for nontonsillar SCC.[13–24,74,78,79,179] Overall local recurrence rates vary from 18% to 23%[24,179] and, in one study, local recurrence was significantly associated with incomplete histologic excision.[24] After mandibulectomy, the local recurrence rate is 0% to 10% and the MST varies from 19 to 43 months with 88% to 100%, 79%, and 58% 1-, 2-, and 3-year STs, respectively.[20,74,78,79] In comparison, the local recurrence rate is 14% to 29% after maxillectomy, with an MST of 10 to 39 months and a 1-, 2- and 3-year survival rates of 57% to 94%, 69%, and 38%, respectively.[21,78,79] The reason for the higher local control and survival rates with mandibular resections is probably that the rostral mandible is the most common location for oral SCC in dogs and complete surgical resection is more likely for these rostral tumors. However, tumor location (both mandibular vs. maxillary and location within the oral cavity) was not prognostic after surgical excision in three recent studies.[77–79] In one study, the MST for untreated dogs was 54 days, with a 0% 1-year survival rate.[78] In comparison, the 1-year survival rate for dogs with surgically excised oral SCC was 94%, with MSTs not reached for dogs with stage I oral SCC and 420, 365, and 50 days for dogs with stage II, III, and IV oral SCC, respectively.[78] The presence of tumor-associated inflammation and risk score of 2 or ≥3 (combination of tumor-associated inflammation, lymphatic or vascular invasion, and peripheral nerve invasion) were associated with a significantly worse prognosis.[78] In two studies of dogs with surgically resected mandibular and maxillary SCC, overall median disease-free STs were not reached with 1- and 2-year disease-free survival rates of 75% to 79% and 61% to 76%, respectively.[76,179] The median disease-free survival was significantly shorter for dogs with grade III SCCs (138 days) and SCCs with a proliferating cell nuclear antigen expression greater than 65% (155 days) compared with dogs with grade II SCCs and SCCs with a proliferating cell nuclear antigen expression ≤65% (not reached).[77] In one study, incomplete histologic margins were associated with a significantly worse outcome (MST 1140 days compared with not reached for dogs with complete histologic excision), but dogs with incomplete histologic margins treated with adjuvant hypofractionated RT were significantly less likely to die of tumor-related reasons than dogs not treated with adjuvant RT.[179]

Full-course RT, either alone or as an adjunct after incomplete surgical resection, is also a successful treatment modality for the management of oral SCC in dogs.[43,80,81,179] The local tumor recurrence rate is 31%.[80,81] The MST for RT alone is 15 to 16 months and increases to 34 months when combined with surgery.[80,81]

In one series of 39 dogs with oral SCC, the overall median PFS time was 36 months, with 1- and 3-year PFS rates of 72% and 55%, respectively.[43] Local tumor control was more successful with smaller lesions; the median PFS time for T1 tumors (<2 cm diameter) was not reached and greater than 68 months compared with 28 months for T2 tumors (2–4 cm diameter) and 8 months for dogs with T3 tumors (>4 cm diameter).[43] Other favorable prognostic factors for dogs receiving orthovoltage irradiation include rostral tumor location, maxillary SCC, and young age.[80] Rostral tumors (MST of 28 months compared with 2–10 months for caudal to extensive tumors), nonrecurrent tumors (MST 29 months compared with 7 months for recurrent SCC), portal size less than 100 cm^2/m^2 (MST 24 months compared with 7 months), and age less than 6 years (MST of 39 months compared with 10 months) are good prognostic factors for dogs treated with orthovoltage RT.[80] Younger age is also prognostic for dogs treated with megavoltage RT, as the MST of 315 days for dogs with oral SCC and older than 9 years is significantly shorter than the 1080 day MST for dogs younger than 9 years.[81]

Chemotherapy is indicated for dogs with metastatic disease, dogs with bulky disease, and when owners decline surgery and RT; however, although responses are noted in the macroscopic (gross disease) setting, durability of response is expected to be short (2–3 months). As the metastatic potential of oral SCC in dogs is relatively low, the role of adjuvant chemotherapy in minimizing the risk of metastatic disease is unknown. In a series of 17 dogs treated with piroxicam alone, the response rate was 17%, with one complete response and two partial responses.[82] The median PFI for dogs responding to piroxicam was 180 days and significantly longer than the 102 days for dogs with stable disease.[82] The outcome is better when piroxicam is combined with either cisplatin or carboplatin. In a series of nine dogs treated with piroxicam and cisplatin, the overall MST was 237 days, with the 56% of dogs responding to this chemotherapy protocol having a significantly better MST (272 days) than nonresponders (116 days).[83] However, renal toxicity was reported in 41% of dogs in this study and such toxicities limit the clinical usefulness of this protocol. In another small series of seven dogs with T3 oral SCC treated with piroxicam and carboplatin, a complete response was observed in 57% of dogs and this response was sustained in all dogs at the median follow-up time of 534 days.[84] Novel therapies under investigation include the combination of intralesional bleomycin and feline interleukin-12 (IL-12) DNA with translesional electroporation.[54]

Feline Oral Squamous Cell Carcinoma

The prognosis for cats with oral SCC is poor. There is no known effective treatment that consistently results in durable control or survival. Local control is the most challenging problem. In one series of 52 cats, the 1-year survival rate was less than 10%, with MSTs of 3 months or less for surgery alone, surgery and RT, RT and low-dose chemotherapy, or RT and hyperthermia.[91] However, 42% of these cats had SCC involving the tongue, pharynx, or tonsils. In another series of 54 cats treated in general practice, the MST was 44 days, with a 10% 1-year survival rate.[94] The oncologic outcome may be better for cats with mandibular SCC. The MST for seven cats treated with a combination of mandibulectomy and RT was 14 months, with a 1-year survival rate of 57%.[89] Local recurrence was the cause of failure in 86% of these cats between 3 and 36 months after therapy. In another series of 22 cats treated with mandibulectomy alone, the median DFI was 340 days.[90] Tumor location and extent of resection had prognostic importance, with an MST of 911 days for rostral mandibulectomies,

217 days after hemimandibulectomy, and 192 days when more than 50% of the mandible was resected.[90] Expansile, blastic, and discrete lesions are often more resectable than invasive, lytic, and ill-defined lesions. The use of esophagostomy or gastrostomy tubes may be necessary to provide supplemental nutrition in these cats for up to 4 months postoperatively.[90]

RT alone is generally considered ineffective in the management of cats with oral SCC. In nine cats treated with an accelerated radiation protocol (14 fractions of 3.5 Gy delivered twice daily for 9 days), the overall MST was 86 days and, although not significant, the MST for cats with a complete response was 298 days.[100] The combination of RT with radiation sensitizers or chemotherapy improves response rates and STs. Using the same accelerated radiation protocol with carboplatin resulted in a 52% complete and 22% partial response rate at 30 days with a MST of 163 days in 31 cats.[101] Intratumoral etanidazole, a hypoxic cell sensitizer, resulted in a 100% partial response rate in nine cats completing the RT course, with a median decrease in tumor size of 70% and a MST of 116 days.[96] Gemcitabine was used at low doses as a radiation sensitizer in eight cats with oral SCC, with an overall response rate of 75%, including two cats with complete responses, for a median duration of 43 days and an MST of 112 days.[98] However, gemcitabine is not recommended as a radiosensitizer in cats because of significant hematologic and local tissue toxicities.[99] The combination of RT with mitoxantrone holds some promise; in two series of 18 cats, a complete response was observed in 73%, with a median duration of response of 138 to 170 days and an MST of 184 days.[97,107] Tumor location, clinical stage, and the completeness of response are reported prognostic factors.[101,103] Location was a prognostic factor in this study, with significantly longer MSTs in cats with SCC of the tonsils (not reached, mean 724 days) and cheek (not reached) than other locations.[101] A complete response at 30 days was also associated with a significantly longer ST (379 days) than non- or partial responders (115 days).[101]

Hypofractionated RT has also been reported in cats with oral SCC. An overall response rate of 81%, with an MST of 174 days, was reported in 21 cats treated with an accelerated hypofractionated RT protocol consisting of 10 daily fractions of 4.8 Gy for a total dose of 48 Gy.[103] In 54 cats treated with 8 to 10 Gy weekly fractions for a total dose of 24 Gy to 40 Gy, the radiation-induced adverse effects were considered mild, with the majority of owners reporting a subjectively improved quality of life.[104] The overall MST was 92 days and cats with sublingual SCCs had a longer MST (135 days) than cats with mandibular SCC (80 days).[104]

Palliative stereotactic RT has been investigated in 20 cats with a 39% overall response rate and a median PFI and MST of 87 and 106 days, respectively; however, there was a high complication rate with mandibular fracture in 6 of 11 cats, fibrosis in three of six cats with lingual SCC, and oronasal fistula in one of three cats with maxillary SCC.[105,106] In this study, cats with a low *Bmi-1* percentage, which is an oncogene responsible for suppression of cell-cycle inhibitors and confers resistance to both chemotherapy and RT, had a significantly better outcome with longer median PFI than cats with a higher *Bmi-1* percentage.[106] Other prognostic factors for cats with oral SCC treated with stereotactic RT include sex, tumor microvascular density, and degree of keratinization.[105]

Localized irradiation with strontium-90 may be effective for selected cats with very superficial disease.[183]

Chemotherapy appears to be largely ineffective in the management of cats with oral SCC. No responses were observed in 18 cats treated with liposome-encapsulated cisplatin or 13 cats treated with piroxicam.[108,110] However, nonsteroidal antiinflammatory drugs (NSAIDs) and toceranib have been shown to significantly improved outcomes in cats with measureable oral SCC.[94,111] In one study of 23 cats with oral SCC with no previous treatments, toceranib and/or an NSAID resulted in a biologic response rate of 57%, with a complete response in 4% of cats, partial response in 9% of cats, and stable disease in 43% of cats.[111] The MST of cats treated with toceranib and/or an NSAID (123 days) was significantly longer than the 45-day MST for cats not treated with toceranib.[111] Cats with a biologic response to treatment with toceranib and/or an NSAID had significantly better median PFS (112 days) and overall MSTs (202 days) than cats that did not respond to treatment (29 days and 73 days, respectively).[111] Cats treated with an NSAID also had a significantly improved MST (169 days) than cats not treated with an NSAID (55 days).[111] As most of these small case series are retrospective in nature, caveats as to the true efficacy of these therapeutic approaches await conformation in controlled, randomized trial settings.

Pamidronate, a bisphosphonate drug with antiosteoclastic activity, has been shown to reduce proliferation of feline cancer cells in vitro and palliate cats with bone-invasive tumors, including oral SCC.[112] In a pilot study of five cats with oral SCC treated with pamidronate, some of which were treated with other modalities including NSAIDs, the median PFS time and overall MST were 71 days and 170 days, respectively.[112]

Fibrosarcoma

The prognosis for dogs with oral FSA is guarded. These are locally aggressive tumors and local control is more problematic than metastasis. Metastasis is reported to the regional LNs in 19% to 22% of dogs and to the lungs in up to 27% of dogs.[12,20–24,43,113–117,179] Multimodality treatment of local disease appears to afford the best survival rates, with combinations of surgery and RT or RT and hyperthermia.[115]

Surgery is the most common treatment for oral FSA. Local recurrence has been reported in up to 54% of dogs overall,[24,179] up to 59% of dogs after mandibulectomy,[20] and up to 40% of dogs after maxillectomy.[21] However, a recent retrospective series reported local recurrence in 24% of 29 dogs with mandibular and maxillary FSA.[114] Local tumor recurrence was significantly associated with incomplete excision and breed (golden retriever or golden retriever mixed breed dogs).[114] Two of the seven dogs with local tumor recurrence developed recurrence after incomplete excision and adjunctive RT.[114] In older reports, the 1-year survival rates rarely exceed 50% with surgery alone;[13–23] however, the MST in a recent retrospective series was 743 days with a median PFI of greater than 653 days and 1- and 2-year survival rates of 88% and 58%, respectively.[114] The median DFI for five cats treated with mandibulectomy was 859 days.[90] The combination of surgery and RT may provide the best opportunity to control local disease in dogs regardless of completeness of excision.[115]

Oral FSAs are considered radiation resistant in the macroscopic (gross) disease setting.[116] The mean ST of 17 dogs treated with RT alone was only 7 months.[116] When RT is used as an adjunct to surgical resection, local tumor recurrence was reported in 32% of dogs overall and the MST increased to 18 to 26 months with a 1-year PFS rate of 76%.[43,117] In one study, 17 of 48 dogs with oral FSA were treated with adjuvant hypofractionated RT and RT did not provide a protective effect with significantly poorer STs in dogs treated with RT.[179] However, in another study, the addition of RT to surgery resulted in significantly longer median PFS

(301 days compared with 138 days) and overall MSTs (505 days compared with 220 days) than mandibulectomy or maxillectomy alone.[115] A smaller tumor size improves the outcome after RT, with a median PFS time of 45 months for dogs with T1 tumors compared with 31 months and 7 months for T2 and T3 tumors, respectively.[43]

Osteosarcoma

OSA of axial sites is less common than appendicular OSA and represents approximately 25% of all cases.[10] Of the axial OSA, the mandible and maxilla are involved in 27% and 16% to 22% of cases, respectively.[10,118] The prognosis for dogs with oral OSA is better than for those with appendicular OSA because of an apparent lower metastatic potential.[10,119–122] In one study, only 4% of 183 dogs with maxillary, mandibular or calvarial OSA had evidence of metastasis at the time of diagnosis,[12] with distant metastasis reported in 32% to 46% of dogs after definitive treatment.[12,24]

The outcome after mandibulectomy alone is variable, with MSTs of 14 to 18 months and 1-year survival rates of 35% to 71%.[10,20,119] After mandibulectomy, local recurrence and metastasis has been reported in 15% to 28% and 35% to 58% of dogs, respectively.[20,121,122] The median metastasis-free interval and MST were 627 days and 525 days, respectively, in one study of 50 dogs.[122] After maxillectomy, local recurrence and metastasis were reported in 58% and 32% of 69 dogs, respectively.[121] The MST for dogs with maxillary OSA varies from 5 to 10 months, with a 1-year survival rate of 17% to 27% and with local tumor recurrence rather than distant metastasis being the most common cause of death.[10,21,118,121]

Local tumor control is the most challenging problem and resecting oral OSAs with complete surgical margins is imperative. The completeness of excision was prognostic for both local tumor recurrence and survival in multivariate analyses in one study.[121] The combination of surgery with either RT or chemotherapy has not resulted in improved outcomes in dogs with incompletely resected tumors, highlighting the necessity for an aggressive surgical approach.[120,121] These results are supported by another study of 45 dogs with axial OSA in which favorable prognostic factors included complete surgical excision, mandibular location, and smaller body weight dogs.[118] Other poor prognostic factors for dogs with mandibular, maxillary, and/or calvarial OSA include serum alkaline phosphatase levels greater than 140 units/L, increased monocyte counts, telangiectatic histologic subtype, mitotic index, histologic grade, and local tumor recurrence.[121,122] The role of chemotherapy in the management of dogs with oral OSA was considered controversial because local tumor recurrence was the most common cause of tumor-related deaths; however, adjuvant chemotherapy results in significantly longer metastasis-free intervals and STs in dogs with mandibular OSA.[122]

Peripheral Odontogenic Fibroma

The prognosis for dogs with peripheral odontogenic fibromas is excellent after treatment with either surgery or RT. These are benign tumors, and metastasis has not been reported; hence, local tumor control is the principal goal of therapy. The local tumor recurrence rate after surgical resection without bone removal varies from 0% to 17%,[125,126] whereas a 4% local recurrence rate was reported in one study of dogs treated with either mandibulectomy or maxillectomy.[24] RT is also effective, with an 3-year PFS rate of 86%.[131] However, definitive RT is usually not required, as these tumors can be adequately managed with simple surgical resection.[127] Local recurrence is common in cats with multiple peripheral odontogenic fibromas and is reported in 73% of 11 cats 3 months to 8 years after surgical resection.[135]

Acanthomatous Ameloblastoma

Surgery or RT is also used in the management of dogs with AA. Mandibulectomy or maxillectomy is required for surgical resection of AAs because of frequent bone invasion by this benign tumor. In one study, 91% of AAs recurred at a mean of 32 days after marginal excision.[127] Local recurrence rates after either mandibulectomy or maxillectomy with appropriate margins are less than 5%.[13–24,125,128,129] In one study of 263 dogs with AA, complete histologic excision was reported in 67%, 75%, and 100% of dogs with 1.0 cm, 1.5 cm, or 2.0 cm surgical margins, respectively. Despite incomplete histologic excision, the local recurrence rate was 0%, with a mean follow-up of 33 months.[129]

Megavoltage RT, consisting of an alternate day protocol of 4 Gy per fraction to a total of 48 Gy, results in a 3-year PFS rate of 80% in dogs with AAs.[131] The overall local recurrence rate with RT varies from 8% to 18% in two studies of 39 dogs and recurrence was eight times more likely with T3 tumors compared with T1 and T2 tumors.[130,131] The majority of tumors recur within the radiation field, which suggests a higher radiation dose may be required to achieve higher rates of local tumor control, particularly for tumors greater than 4 cm in diameter.[131] Other complications associated with RT include malignant transformation in 5% to 18% of dogs and bone necrosis in 6% of dogs.[130–132]

Intralesional bleomycin has been reported in two studies of dogs with AA.[133,134] In total, 10 dogs were treated with curative-intent intralesional bleomycin and all had complete responses. In one study of six dogs,[134] 1 to 16 (median, 5) intralesional injections were administered before a complete response was achieved. The median time to complete response was 1.5 months. There was no evidence of recurrence at 1 year in one study and after a median follow-up of 842 days in another study.[134]

Selected Sites or Cancer Conditions in the Oral Cavity

Tonsillar Squamous Cell Carcinoma

Tonsillar SCC is 10 times more common in animals living in urban versus rural areas, implying an etiologic association with environmental pollutants.[184] The most common tonsillar tumor is SCC.[185,186] Tonsillar SCC has a significantly higher proportion of grade III lesions and metastatic disease at diagnosis compared with oral SCC at other sites.[77] Lymphoma can affect the tonsils, but bilateral tonsillar involvement is more common and this is usually accompanied by generalized lymphadenopathy.[185,186] Other cancers, especially MM, can metastasize to the tonsils.[185,186] Cervical lymphadenopathy is a common presenting sign, even with very small primary tonsillar cancers. FNA of the regional LNs or excisional biopsy of the tonsil are required for definitive diagnosis. Up to 20% of cases have evidence of pulmonary metastasis at presentation. In spite of disease apparently confined to the tonsil, this disease is considered systemic at diagnosis in more than 90% of cats and dogs.[185,186] The CT features of pharyngeal neoplasia have been described, and these are useful in determining the extent of local disease and the presence of LN

and distant metastasis.[185,186] If disease is localized to the tonsils and not infiltrative, then surgery should be considered as part of a multimodal treatment protocol. Simple tonsillectomy is almost never curative, but probably should be done bilaterally because of the high percentage of bilateral disease.[10] Cervical lymphadenectomy, especially if the regional LNs are large and fixed, is rarely curative and should be considered diagnostic only. Regional RT of the pharyngeal region and cervical LNs can achieve locoregional control in more than 75% of cases; however, survival still remains poor with 1-year survival rates of only 10%.[180,181] Local tumor control and STs were significantly improved in one study of 22 dogs with tonsillar SCC when RT was combined with a variety of different chemotherapy drugs.[181] Cause of death is local disease early and systemic disease (usually lung metastasis) later. To date, no known effective chemotherapeutic agents exist for canine or feline SCC, although cisplatin, carboplatin, doxorubicin, vinblastine, and bleomycin have been used with limited success.[85,181] In one study of 44 dogs with tonsillar SCC treated with surgery, RT, and/or chemotherapy, the MST was 179 days and dogs presenting with either anorexia or lethargy had significantly shorter STs.[187]

Lingual

Lingual tumors are uncommon in cats and dogs. In dogs, tongue tumors account for up to 4% of all oropharyngeal neoplasms.[188] Neoplasia accounts for up to 54% of canine lingual lesions with 64% of these being malignant tumors.[138,140,188] The majority of these tumors are located on the dorsal surface of the tongue, and are evenly distributed between the rostral, mid, and caudal portions of the tongue.[138,141] For unknown reasons, 16% of dogs and up to 29% of people with tongue tumors have a second primary tumor.[189] Hence, thorough physical examination and clinical staging are important in animals with tongue tumors. White dogs appear to be at higher risk for SCC, even though lack of pigment would not be intuitive as an etiologic contributor as it is in other more sunlight-exposed areas of the body (e.g., nose, eyelids, and ears).[139] Other reported breed predilections include Chow Chow and Chinese Shar-Pei for MM; poodle, Labrador retriever, and Samoyed for SCC; border collie and golden retriever for hemangiosarcoma and FSA; and cocker spaniel for plasma cell tumors.[188] The most common cancer of the canine tongue is SCC, accounting for up to 50% of cases, followed by MM, mast cell tumor, hemangiosarcoma and hemangioma, granular cell myoblastoma, FSA, adenocarcinoma, neurofibrosarcoma, leiomyosarcoma, rhabdomyoma and rhabdomyosarcoma, myxoma, and lipoma.[139,141,188,190] Feline tongue tumors are usually SCCs, and most are located on the ventral surface near the frenulum. Presenting signs are similar to those of other oral tumors. Ulceration is common with SCC.

An incisional biopsy, such as a punch or wedge biopsy, is recommended for the diagnosis of tongue lesions in cats and dogs. A biopsy is necessary to differentiate malignant tumors from nonneoplastic lesions, such as eosinophilic granuloma and calcinosis circumscripta, and because a knowledge of the definitive diagnosis may change treatment options (i.e., surgical dose or multimodality therapy with either RT and/or chemotherapy) or the willingness of the owner to pursue curative-intent treatment. Ultrasonography can be useful in delineating the margins of tongue masses to determine surgical resectability.[191] Regional LNs should be aspirated for staging purposes and three-view thoracic radiographs evaluated for lung metastasis.

Surgical resection is recommended,[141] whereas RT is reserved for MMs, inoperable cancer, or tumors metastatic to the regional LNs. Surgical resection, involving either marginal excision, subtotal glossectomy, or total glossectomy, was well tolerated in one study of 97 dogs.[141] Complications included postoperative bleeding (10%), partial tongue paralysis (2%), and incisional dehiscence (2%); and no dog had long-term prehension difficulties.[141] Resection of 50% to 100% of the tongue or avulsion of the tongue was reported in five dogs with minimal postoperative problems, which suggests that more aggressive resections may be possible without compromising quality of life.[189] Feeding tubes are recommended for enteral nutrition during postoperative recovery after total glossectomy but, in the long term, eating and drinking are usually only mildly impaired and good hydration and nutrition can be maintained postoperatively.[139,189] Hypersalivation is the most common complaint after aggressive resections.[189] Thermoregulation can be a problem in hot and humid environments. Grooming in cats will be compromised and may result in poor hair-coat hygiene.

The prognosis for tongue tumors depends on the site, size, type, and grade of cancer, completeness of excision, local tumor recurrence, and metastasis.[139–141] Cancer in the rostral tongue has a better prognosis, possibly because rostral lesions are detected at an earlier stage, the caudal tongue may have richer lymphatic and vascular channels to allow metastasis, and rostral tumors are easier to resect with wide margins.[139] Tumor size was prognostic in two studies. In one study, dogs with tongue tumors greater than 4 cm^2 were 10 times more likely to develop local recurrence and/or distant metastasis and up to 19 times more likely to die of their tongue tumor than dogs with tumors ranging from 1 cm^2 to 4 cm^2.[140] In another study, tumor size was the only variable prognostic on multivariate analysis; dogs with tumors less than 2 cm had a MST of 818 days compared with 207 days for dogs with tumors 2 cm or greater.[141]

Complete surgical excision was significantly more likely with smaller tumors and tumors located in the rostral free portion of the tongue.[139,140] Furthermore, complete surgical excision was significantly associated with increased STs and dogs with incomplete histologic margins were significantly more likely to develop local recurrence and/or distant metastasis and die of their tumor.[139,140] Local tumor recurrence has been reported in 26% to 28% of dogs after glossectomy, and is more likely with incomplete histologic excision, large tumors, and malignant tumors.[140,141] Dogs with local tumor recurrence were 33 times more likely to die as a result of their tumor than dogs without local recurrence.[140]

Dogs with benign tongue tumors have a significantly longer DFI and MST than dogs with malignant tongue tumors.[140] In one study, the MST for dogs with benign tongue tumors was not reached and greater than 1607 days compared with 286 days for dogs with malignant tongue tumors.[140] Dogs with malignant tongue tumors were eight times more likely to have local recurrence and/or distant metastasis and 15 times more likely to die of their tumor than dogs with benign tongue tumors.[140] Dogs with metastatic disease have a significantly worse outcome, with an MST of 241 days compared with a MST of 661 days for dogs without metastatic disease.[141]

Tongue SCCs in dogs are graded from I (least malignant) to III (most malignant) based on histologic features such as degree of differentiation and keratinization, mitotic rate, tissue and vascular invasion, nuclear pleomorphism, and scirrhous reaction.[139] The MST for dogs with grade I tongue SCC is 16 months after surgical resection, which is significantly better than the MSTs

of 4 and 3 months reported for grade II and III SCC, respectively.[139] The 1-year survival rate is 50% after complete surgical resection and approaches 80% with complete histologic excision of low-grade SCCs.[139] Long-term control of feline tongue tumors is rarely reported with 1-year survival rates for tongue SCC less than 25%.

The MST for dogs with tongue MM is variable, with 222 days reported in one study,[140] but not reached and was greater than 551 days in another study.[9] The metastatic rate ranges from 29% to 45%.[9,138,140,141]

The overall MST for 20 dogs with surgically treated lingual hemangiosarcoma was 553 days.[142] Lingual hemangiosarcomas are typically small, located on the ventral aspect of the tongue, and low to intermediate histologic grade.[142] Prognostic factors included tumors causing clinical signs and larger tumors. Dogs with clinical signs associated with their lingual hemangiosarcoma had a significantly shorter MST (159 days) than asymptomatic dogs (633 days).[142] The MST for dogs with lingual hemangiosarcomas less than 2 cm (633 days) was significantly longer than for dogs with tumors 2 cm to 4 cm (150 days).[142]

Granular cell myoblastoma is a curable cancer.[192] These cancers may look large and invasive, but are almost always removable by conservative and close margins (Fig. 23.9). Permanent local control rates exceed 80%.[192] They may recur late, but serial surgeries are usually possible. Metastasis is rare with this cancer.

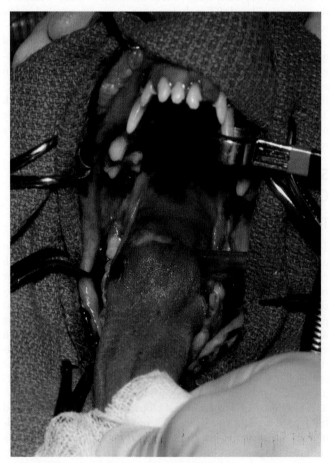

• **Fig. 23.9** This large granular cell myoblastoma was easily removed surgically. The dog had a recurrence 2 years postoperatively, which was resected again, and the dog is tumor free 3 years after the second surgery.

Undifferentiated Malignancy of Young Dogs

Undifferentiated malignancy is seen in dogs under 2 years of age (range, 6–22 months).[193] Most dogs are large breeds and there is no sex predilection. The disease is manifest by a rapidly growing mass in the area of the hard palate, upper molar teeth, maxilla, and/or orbit.[193] Biopsies reveal an undifferentiated malignancy of undetermined histiogenesis. The majority of dogs present with metastasis to the regional LNs and distant sites. An effective treatment has not been identified, although chemotherapy would be necessary considering the high metastatic rate. Most dogs are euthanatized within 30 days of diagnosis because of progressive and uncontrolled tumor growth.[193]

Papillary SCC has been reported to occur in the oral cavity of young dogs (mean age, 3.9 years).[74] The most common location is the rostral maxilla, and bone invasion is frequently noted on CT.[74] Treatment recommendations include complete surgical resection or surgical cytoreduction and curettage followed by RT (40 Gy in 20 fractions). In two studies, no dogs developed either local tumor recurrence or regional or distant metastasis after treatment with either surgery alone or cytoreductive surgery and RT.[74,194]

Multilobular Osteochondrosarcoma

MLO is an infrequently diagnosed bony and cartilaginous tumor that usually arises from the canine skull, including the mandible, maxilla, hard palate, orbit, and calvarium.[27,28] Histologically, these tumors are characterized by multiple lobules with a central cartilaginous or bone matrix surrounded by a thin layer of spindle cells.[27,28] On imaging, MLO is characterized by a typical "popcorn" appearance (Fig. 23.10). Surgery is recommended for management of the local tumor. The overall rate of local recurrence after surgical resection is 47% to 58% and depends on completeness of surgical resection and histologic grade.[27,28] The median DFI for completely resected MLO is 1332 days and significantly better than the 330 days reported for incompletely

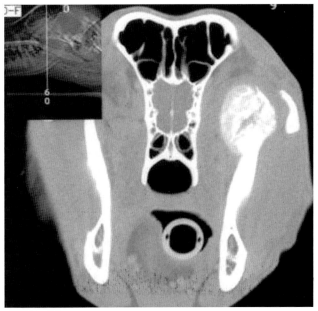

• **Fig. 23.10** A computed tomography image of a multilobular osteochondrosarcoma of the vertical ramus of the mandible. Note the characteristic "popcorn" appearance of the mass. After resection of the vertical ramus, this dog was tumor free 3 years after surgery.

excised tumors.[28] In terms of tumor grade, the local recurrence rate for grade III tumors is 78% and significantly worse than the recurrence rates of 30% and 47% for grade I and II MLO, respectively.[28] This tumor has a moderate metastatic potential (usually to the lung), which is grade dependent, but usually occurs late in the course of disease. Metastasis is reported in up to 58% of dogs with the median time to metastasis of 426 to 542 days.[27,28] Metastasis is significantly more likely after incomplete surgical resection with a 25% metastatic rate in completely excised tumors and 75% after incomplete resection.[28] Tumor grade also has a significant effect on metastatic rate with metastasis reported in 78% of grade III MLO compared with 30% of grade I and 60% of grade II tumors.[28] There is no known effective chemotherapy treatment for metastatic disease, but STs greater than 12 months have been reported with pulmonary metastasectomy because of the slow-growing nature of this tumor.[28] The overall MST is 21 months and is grade dependent, with reported MSTs of 50 months, 22 months, and 11 months for grade I, II, and III tumors, respectively.[27,28] Tumor location also has prognostic significance because the outcome for dogs with mandibular MLO is significantly better, with an MST of 1487 days compared with 587 days for these tumors at other sites.[28]

Odontogenic Tumors

Odontogenic tumors originate from epithelial cells of the dental lamina. They account for up to 2.4% of all feline oral tumors,[5] but are rare in dogs. They are broadly classified into two groups depending on whether the tumors are able to induce a stromal reaction.[195,196] Inductive odontogenic tumors include ameloblastic fibroma, feline inductive odontogenic tumor, and complex and compound odontomas.[196] Ameloblastomas, AAs, and amyloid-producing odontogenic tumors are examples of noninductive odontogenic tumors.[195,196] Additional odontogenic tumor groups include tumors composed primarily of odontogenic ectomesenchyme (cementoma and cementifying fibroma), tumors derived from the periodontal ligament (peripheral odontogenic fibroma), cysts of the jaw (dentigerous cyst and radicular cyst), and tumorlike lesions (giant cell epulis and gingival hyperplasia.[196]

Inductive fibroameloblastoma is the most common odontogenic tumor in cats, usually occurs in cats less than 18 months of age, and has a predilection for the region of the upper canine teeth and maxilla.[5,124,195–197] Radiographically the tumor site shows variable degrees of bone destruction, production, and expansion of the mandibular or maxillary bones (Fig. 23.11). Teeth deformity is common. Smaller lesions are treated with surgical debulking and cryosurgery or premaxillectomy. Larger lesions will respond to RT. Local treatment needs to be aggressive, but control rates are good and metastasis has not been reported.[5,124]

Odontomas are benign tumors arising from the dental follicle during the early stages of tooth development.[198] Odontomas induce both enamel and dentin within the tumor. Odontomas have a biologic behavior similar to ameloblastomas.

Dentigerous cysts are nonneoplastic, circumscribed cystic lesions originating from islands of odontogenic epithelium.[195] They contain one or more teeth embedded in the cyst wall. Radiographs show a characteristic radiolucent halo surrounding the nonerupted tooth originating at the cementoenamel junction and enveloping the crown of the tooth.[199] Odontogenic cysts may represent an early stage of malignant epithelial tumors.[195] Surgical treatment is recommended, consisting of surgical removal of nonerupted teeth and the cyst lining with possible cancellous bone grafting, to prevent local tumor recurrence.[199]

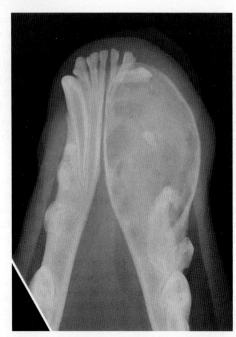

• **Fig. 23.11** An intraoral radiograph of the rostral mandible in a dog with an ameloblastoma. Note the expansile mandibular mass. The tumor was curetted and filled with cancellous bone graft and the dog was tumor free 1 year after surgery.

Osteomas

Osteomas have been described in both dogs and cats.[200,201] Osteomas are benign tumors of histologically normal mature compact and/or trabecular bone.[201] They are slow growing and rarely cause clinical signs unless the mass interferes with adjacent structures or prevents occlusion.[200,201] Radiographically, osteomas are typically proliferative masses with no evidence of bone lysis.[200,201] They are classified as peripheral, central, or extraskeletal in people, and peripheral and central osteomas have been described in dogs.[200,201] Surgical excision is usually curative.[200,201]

Comparative Aspects[202]

SCC accounts for the vast majority of oral cancer in humans. Oral tumors are associated with alcohol and tobacco use and usually occur in patients more than 40 years old. Patients with oral cancer have an increased risk of developing esophageal and lung cancer. Tumors are staged similar to animals and clinical stage influences both treatment options and prognosis.

Surgery and RT are the only options that provide the opportunity for a cure. Surgery and radiation are occasionally combined, especially because neither modality is likely to achieve a cure rate greater than 70% when used as sole therapy. Chemotherapy has a limited role for control of local disease but has shown promise, often in combination with radiation, for advanced stage cancer.

Prognosis is strongly correlated to histologic grade, stage, and site. Metastasis, particularly to the regional LNs, is more frequent with tonsillar and pharyngeal SCC and larger sized tumors. Tumors of the pharynx and caudal tongue are associated with a worse prognosis than cancers of the rostral tongue and oral cavity because of the higher incidence of nodal metastasis and difficulty in controlling disease once it has spread beyond the primary site.

SECTION B: SALIVARY GLAND NEOPLASIA

SARAH E. BOSTON

Incidence and Risk Factors

Salivary gland neoplasia in dogs and cats is rare; however, it is a significant cause of salivary disease. In a study of the histopathologic diagnosis of salivary gland biopsies in dogs and cats, 30% were diagnosed with neoplasia.[203] The second most common diagnosis in that study was sialadenitis (26%).

Pathology

Salivary gland neoplasms are primarily malignant epithelial tumors. Simple adenocarcinoma is the most common histopathologic diagnosis, with other types of carcinomas being represented second most commonly.[204] Other reported tumors in this location include oncocytoma[205] and carcinosarcoma in cats[206]; and pleomorphic adenoma,[207] myoepithelioma,[208] OSA,[209] and mast cell tumor in dogs[210]; however, these are single case reports and are rare.

History and Clinical Signs

Clinical signs of salivary neoplasia and sialadenitis may be similar. The most common presenting complaint in a retrospective of salivary gland neoplasia in dogs and cats was the presence of a mass.[204] Other presenting complaints included halitosis, weight loss, anorexia, dysphagia, exophthalmos, Horner's syndrome, sneezing, and dysphonia.[204] In one retrospective study of dogs and cats, there appeared to be a predilection for male sex and Siamese breed in cats.[204] In that study, the mandibular salivary gland was most commonly affected in cats and the parotid salivary gland was most commonly affected in dogs.[204]

Diagnostic Techniques and Workup

An FNA for cytology should be performed as a first step in attempting to distinguish between benign and malignant disease.[211] If this is not successful, a needle-core, incisional, or possibly an excisional biopsy can be considered for histopathology. Salivary gland adenocarcinoma is both locally aggressive and has metastatic potential, and hence local and distant staging should be considered before definitive treatment. Thoracic radiographs or CT can be performed to assess the lungs for metastatic disease. An ultrasound of the affected area can also be performed for initial staging and possibly to obtain an ultrasound-guided aspirate of the mass and/or regional LNs.[212] The medial retropharyngeal LNs are the primary lymphatic drainage center of the salivary glands and should be evaluated cytologically and/or biopsied for histopathology.[213] Ultimately, a CT scan of the head and thorax is recommended for staging and surgical planning.[212] In cases where surgery may not be possible, the patient should be positioned for a concurrent radiation planning CT for potential RT alone. In one retrospective study, cats presented at a more advanced stage of disease than dogs, suggesting that this disease may be more aggressive in cats.[204]

Therapy

Surgery is the mainstay of therapy. Using a CT scan for surgical planning, the affected salivary gland is removed. By definition, this is a marginal excision. However, the degree of tumor encapsulation will help guide whether or not adjunctive RT is indicated. Regional LNs should be sampled for staging purposes.

The surgical approach to the affected mandibular or parotid salivary gland is generally straightforward. If the parotid salivary gland is removed, care must be taken to identify and protect the facial nerve. If this is not possible, facial nerve paralysis may occur. In rare cases of zygomatic salivary neoplasia,[214,215] the zygomatic salivary gland is approached via an orbitotomy and removal of the zygomatic arch.[214]

Prognosis

In one retrospective study of dogs and cats with salivary gland neoplasia, the median survival times were 550 days and 516 days for dogs and cats, respectively.[204] In that study, patients were treated with surgery alone or in combination with RT or chemotherapy.[204] The small number of patients treated with adjunctive therapy in that study makes it difficult to make a general recommendation for adjunctive therapy. Postoperative RT is generally recommended, especially in cases where the tumor is invasive and has extended beyond the capsule.[216] Recommendations for chemotherapy are less defined due to the paucity of information in the literature, but may be indicated in cases with evidence of metastatic disease and with highly malignant histopathology.

Comparative Aspects

Salivary gland adenocarcinoma has been reported in many other mammalian species other than dogs and cats.[217–225]

Treatment of salivary carcinoma in humans is commonly surgery followed by RT.[226–229] Factors that have been associated with a negative prognosis in one study included male sex, perineural invasion, high risk pathology, and late stage.[226] Another study found that age, sex, stage, site, and skin or bone invasion were significantly associated with survival.[227] The use of postoperative RT has been shown to improve locoregional control.[227] Local control has been shown to be significantly associated with tumor stage and treatment type, with the combination of RT and surgery being superior to surgery alone.[228] Tumor stage was significantly associated with survival.[228]

Five- and 10-year survival rates are 68%[229] and 50%, respectively.[227] A 20-year actuarial rate of local control of 57% was reported in one study with a 12-year probability of distant metastasis of 40%.[227]

SECTION C: ESOPHAGEAL TUMORS

PIERRE M. AMSELLEM AND JAMES P. FARESE

Incidence and Risk Factors

Esophageal neoplasia is rare in dogs and cats. Esophageal sarcomas have been reported in association with infestation by the nematode *Spirocerca lupi*.[230–237] Although this parasite has been reported worldwide (South Africa, Kenya, India, Israel, the southeastern United States), *Spirocerca lupi*–associated esophageal granulomas and sarcomas are reported mainly in Israel.[230–237] Leiomyomas may have a genetic component, as a high incidence was reported in a colony of laboratory beagle dogs.[238] Most animals with esophageal tumors are middle-aged or older and there does not seem to be a gender predisposition.

Pathology and Behavior

It is postulated that with spirocercosis-associated sarcomas, a parasitic esophageal granuloma undergoes malignant transformation leading to the development of an esophageal sarcoma, typically in the caudal thoracic portion of the esophagus.[234] Histologic types of spirocercosis-associated sarcomas include OSAs, fibrosarcomas, and undifferentiated sarcomas.[239] Metastasis to the lungs was reported in 5 of 11 dogs at necropsy.[234] Additional metastatic sites included kidneys, adrenals, stomach, regional LNs, tongue, and the heart.[234] Complicating factors include the presence of megaesophagus and hypertrophic osteopathy.[234]

Plasmocytoma,[240] adenomatous polyp,[241] leiomyosarcoma,[242] carcinoma,[243] adenocarcinoma,[243] adenosquamous carcinoma,[244] and squamous cell carcinoma[245] have also been reported in dogs, but these are rare. Squamous cell carcinoma is the most common esophageal tumor in cats, typically occurring in the middle third of the esophagus just caudal to the thoracic inlet.[246,247]

Leiomyomas are benign tumors of the muscularis of the esophagus. They have been reported in the distal esophagus near the gastroesophageal junction in dogs.[238,248] In some cases, multiple leiomyomas can occur in the distal esophagus and the stomach.[232,233] Leiomyomas do not invade the esophageal mucosa. In contrast, low-grade leiomyosarcomas occasionally penetrate the esophageal mucosa.[242]

Paraesophageal tumors, such as thyroid, thymic, or heart base tumors, can invade the esophagus.[249,250]

History and Clinical Signs

Clinical signs are usually related to obstruction of the esophagus, leading to regurgitation and weight loss. The presence of ulceration of the mass can cause melena and secondary anemia.

Respiratory signs can occur if aspiration pneumonia or metastatic disease develops.

Leiomyomas often are an incidental finding but can occasionally cause signs associated with esophageal obstruction.[232,233,243]

Diagnostic Tests and Workup

Diagnostic tests for esophageal masses usually include survey thoracic radiographs, contrast esophagram, esophagoscopy (Fig. 23.12), and CT scan (Fig. 23.13).[242] Survey radiographs may show retention of gas within the esophageal lumen, a mass, or esophageal dilatation proximal to the mass (Fig. 23.14). Spondylitis on the ventral aspect of the vertebral body T6 to T12 was detected radiographically in 12 of 15 dogs with spirocercosis-associated esophageal sarcoma.[234] A positive-contrast esophagram may show a stricture or mass lesion in the esophageal lumen. Ultrasound- or CT-guided aspirates can be performed for cytologic evaluation. Endoscopic biopsies of esophageal masses are possible; however, for smooth muscle tumors, such as leiomyomas and leiomyosarcomas, they are usually unrewarding, as these tumors do not penetrate the esophageal mucosa.[242,248] A surgical approach may be needed in these cases to obtain an incisional biopsy; however, given the invasive nature of the surgical approach, most biopsies are excisional.

A fecal flotation test may be performed in dogs with esophageal masses to test for *Spirocerca lupi* eggs, particularly in areas where the parasite is endemic. This is a poorly sensitive test; eggs were detected in only two of eight dogs in one study of spirocercosis-associated sarcomas.[234]

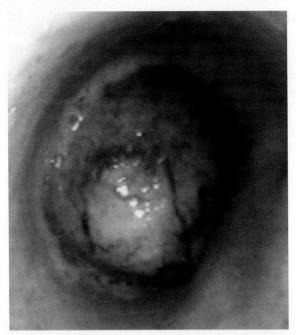

• **Fig. 23.12** Esophagoscopic view of an esophageal leiomyosarcoma in a dog. (From Farese JP, Bacon NJ, Ehrhart NP, et al. Oesophageal leiomyosarcoma in dogs: surgical management and clinical outcome of four cases. *Vet Comp Oncol.* 2008;6(1):31–38)

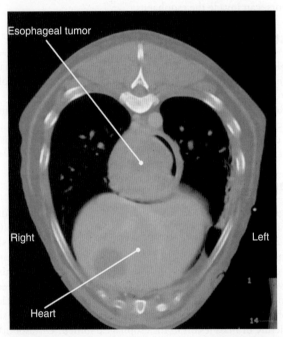

• **Fig. 23.13** Computed tomographic image of an esophageal leiomyosarcoma in a dog. (From Farese JP, Bacon NJ, Ehrhart NP, et al. Oesophageal leiomyosarcoma in dogs: surgical management and clinical outcome of four cases. *Vet Comp Oncol.* 20089;6(1):31–38.)

Treatment Options

Most esophageal cancers have extensive local involvement that typically precludes curative-intent therapy. In dogs with esophageal sarcomas, partial esophagectomy has been reported.[251] The authors' preferred approach is to perform an esophagotomy opposite to the esophageal mass to visualize the mass from

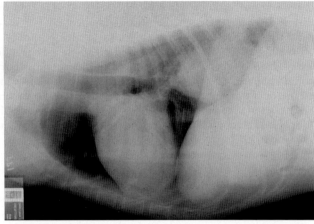

• **Fig. 23.14** Lateral thoracic radiographic image of a large (8 cm long × 6 cm wide) leiomyosarcoma in the caudal esophagus, just cranial to the diaphragm. (From Farese JP, Bacon NJ, Ehrhart NP, et al. Oesophageal leiomyosarcoma in dogs: surgical management and clinical outcome of four cases. *Vet Comp Oncol.* 2008;6(1):31–38.)

within the esophageal lumen.[251] A full-thickness esophagectomy can then be performed to resect the mass with a minimum of 1-cm margins.[251] Endoscopic laser or electrocautery debulking of esophageal sarcomas has also been reported.[236] In one study, there was no difference in survival times between dogs treated with surgery and dogs treated with endoscopic ablation.[233]

Leiomyomas and low-grade leiomyosarcomas can be marginally excised via an intercostal thoracotomy or laparotomy.[248] Marginal excision appears to provide good long-term local tumor control for most dogs with esophageal leiomyomas. In contrast, marginal excision resulted in incomplete histologic excision in three of four dogs with esophageal leiomyosarcomas; however, local tumor recurrence was confirmed in only one dog and clinical signs of recurrence may not develop because of the slow-growing nature of this tumor.[242]

More aggressive excision with end-to-end resection of esophageal tumors can be curative,[240] but this is often not possible because of the extent of the resection required and/or the location of the mass. Resection of caudal esophageal masses is possible with gastric advancement through the diaphragm,[243] but persistent gastroesophageal reflux and esophagitis can occur.[250]

Nonsurgical treatment options for esophageal tumors have not been established. There are no published reports in dogs or cats documenting successful treatment with either chemotherapy or radiation therapy, either alone or as an adjuvant therapy.

Successful palliative treatment by placement of esophageal stents has been reported in the management of a squamous cell carcinoma[252] and of a leiomyoma in dogs.[253]

Prognosis

Except for leiomyoma and low-grade leiomyosarcomas, the overall prognosis for dogs and cats with esophageal tumors is guarded to poor because of the extent of local disease and/or the presence of metastasis at the time of diagnosis. In one study on 17 dogs with spirocercosis-associated esophageal sarcomas, five dogs treated with partial esophagectomy and adjuvant doxorubicin survived a median of 267 days.[234]

The prognosis for dogs and cats with esophageal carcinomas seems to be poor, as most tumors are unresectable.[243,250] The prognosis for dogs with esophageal leiomyomas after marginal excision appears to be good in a small case series of three dogs[248] and an additional case report,[243] although local recurrence was reported in one dog. Similarly, dogs with low-grade leiomyosarcomas had good long-term resolution of clinical signs after marginal excision, despite incomplete histologic margins in three of four dogs.[242]

Comparative Aspects

A high mortality rate is associated with esophageal cancers in humans.[254] The American Cancer Society predicts that 17,290 new cases of esophageal cancers will occur in 2018, causing 15,850 deaths.[254] The most common esophageal cancer in the United States of America is adenocarcinoma followed by squamous cell carcinoma.[254] Adenocarcinoma has a predilection for the distal esophagus.[255] Risk factors include obesity, male gender, alcohol and tobacco consumption, gastroesophageal reflux, and Barrett esophagus.[255] Barrett esophagus consists of metaplasia of the esophageal mucosa secondary to severe gastroesophageal reflux and may be a preneoplastic lesion.[255]

SECTION D: EXOCRINE PANCREATIC CANCER

LAURA E. SELMIC

Incidence and Risk Factors

Cancer of the exocrine pancreas is very rare (<0.5% of all cancers) in the dog and the cat.[256,257] Incidence rates of pancreatic cancer have been estimated at 17.8 per 100,000 patient years for dogs and 12.6 per 100,000 patient years for cats.[258] Older female dogs and spaniels have been described as being at higher risk.[259–261] Experimentally, N-ethyl-N′-nitro-N-nitrosoguanidine has been shown to induce pancreatic duct adenocarcinoma when administered intraductally in dogs.[262]

Pathology and Natural Behavior

Almost all cancers of the pancreas are epithelial and most are malignant adenocarcinoma of ductular or acinar origin. Nodular hyperplasia is a common asymptomatic finding in older dogs and cats. Benign pancreatic pseudocysts and adenomas have been diagnosed by ultrasonography or surgery in dogs and cats.[256,263] In the vast majority of cases, malignant pancreatic cancer has metastasized to regional or distant sites before a diagnosis can be made.[260,264]

History and Clinical Signs

The history and clinical signs of exocrine pancreatic cancer are vague and nonspecific and may mimic or be accompanied by pancreatitis. Weight loss and anorexia (marked in cats),[265] paraneoplastic alopecia in cats,[266,267] vomiting, rare associated diabetes mellitus,[265,268] abdominal distension due to a mass effect or abdominal effusions secondary to tumor implantation on the peritoneum (i.e., carcinomatosis; common in cats), icterus (with common bile duct obstruction), and lethargy are common symptoms.[265] Alternatively, patients may present for symptoms of metastatic disease.

Diagnostic Techniques and Workup

Most hematologic and biochemical evaluations are nonspecific, but may include mild anemia, hyperglycemia, neutrophilia, and bilirubinemia (if occluding the common bile duct).[256] Elevations of serum amylase and lipase are inconsistent.[269] In extreme cases, signs of pancreatic insufficiency may be exhibited.[270]

In the dog, most tumors are not palpable through the abdominal wall. In the cat, late-stage, large palpable masses may be present.

Positive-contrast upper GI radiographs may reveal slowed gastric emptying and occasionally compression or invasion of the duodenum. Ultrasonography should be a useful diagnostic tool for localization of the primary tumor, documentation, and aspiration of fluid, as well as metastasis to liver and regional LNs.[271] Ascites may be a clinical sign and, when present, may reveal malignant cells on cytologic examination (carcinomatosis). A large (>2 cm) solitary mass is suggestive of pancreatic cancer rather than nodular hyperplasia in cats.[272] Contrast ultrasound has been assessed for distinguishing between pancreatic adenocarcinoma or insulinoma in four dogs.[273] In B-mode ultrasound, a hypoechoic nodule was present in the pancreas in three dogs, whereas heterogeneous pancreatic tissue was evident in the other dog. Contrast ultrasound could differentiate between the two tumors: adenocarcinomas appeared as hypoechoic and hypervascular lesions whereas insulinomas showed uniformly hypervascular lesions.[273] The utility of advanced imaging such as CT and MRI has not been documented for exocrine pancreatic tumors in veterinary patients. At present, most diagnoses are made at exploratory celiotomy. Immunohistochemical markers have been evaluated for aiding diagnosis of pancreatic carcinoma in dogs. More specifically, the expression patterns of claudin-4, a tight junction molecule, and claudin-5, an endothelium specific tight junction protein, were compared between well-differentiated and poorly differentiated pancreatic acinar cell carcinomas and normal pancreatic tissues.[274,275] Claudin-4 was present laterally in normal pancreatic acinar cells and intense apical lateral position in cells from a well-differentiated exocrine pancreatic carcinoma. Poorly differentiated exocrine pancreatic adenocarcinomas demonstrated a loss of claudin-4 expression.[274] The authors concluded claudin-4 immunohistochemistry may be useful to distinguish well-differentiated and undifferentiated exocrine pancreatic carcinomas.[274] Claudin-5 has also been evaluated in this manner with expression documented in lateral membranes of exocrine acinar cells and the endothelial cells of vessels and lymphatics within the stroma of the intact pancreas. The well- and poorly differentiated carcinomas showed loss of claudin-5 expression.[275]

Therapy

Most non–islet cell carcinomas of the pancreas are locally invasive and metastatic to regional LNs and liver at diagnosis. If liver, peritoneal cavity, or draining LNs are positive for tumor, aggressive surgery should generally not be performed. Total pancreatectomy or pancreaticoduodenectomy (Whipple's procedure) have been described in humans and dogs,[276] but carries a high operative morbidity and mortality without significant cure rates and is not recommended. Bypass procedures, such as gastrojejunostomy or cholecystoduodenostomy, are short-term palliative options for patients with imminent or present gastrointestinal or common bile duct obstruction, respectively. Radiation therapy and chemotherapy have shown limited value in humans and animals. Occasionally, uncomfortable effusions from carcinomatosis can be diminished with systemic or intracavitary chemotherapy (see Chapter 12); however, the palliative response tends to be short lived.

Prognosis

The outlook for this disease in companion species is very poor because of its critical location and advanced stage at diagnosis. In a recent study evaluating the outcome for 34 cats with pancreatic carcinoma, the overall median survival time was 97 days and, for cats treated with either chemotherapy or surgery, the median survival time was 165 days.[265] Cats with abdominal effusion at diagnosis survived a median of 30 days.[265] Only three cats survived greater than 1 year.[265]

Comparative Aspects[277–279]

Pancreatic exocrine carcinoma accounted for an estimated 53,670 new cases and 43,090 deaths in the United States in 2017.[278] Several risk factors have been identified, including older age, inherited susceptibility, cigarette smoking, obesity, and diabetes mellitus. Most patients have disease progression beyond the pancreas at the time of initial diagnosis. Seventy-five percent are located in the head of the pancreas and the remainder in the body and tail of the pancreas. Direct extension to duodenum, bile duct, and stomach, as well as common metastasis to LNs and liver, make treatment difficult.

Treatments that are currently used include surgery (curative or palliative), radiotherapy (as an adjuvant or for treatment of advanced local disease), and systemic chemotherapy. Surgical resection is the mainstay of treatment for pancreatic carcinoma in humans, especially if the patient has a small tumor localized to the pancreas. Depending on the extent of disease within the pancreas, other surgical procedures include pancreaticoduodenectomy (Whipple's procedure) or total pancreatectomy. With recent advances in surgical technique, the mortality associated with these procedures has decreased; however, considerable patient morbidity still exists. Removal of the entire pancreas necessitates management of the patient for exocrine pancreatic insufficiency and diabetes mellitus. After surgery, chemotherapy is recommended to improve survival, but there is no superior single chemotherapeutic approach. In patients whose tumors are determined to be borderline resectable, chemotherapy is administered for 2 to 4 months and then, if the patient is still free from metastases, surgery or chemoradiation can be considered. Treatments for locally advanced or widely metastatic disease are palliative, but include chemotherapy alone or chemoradiation. If biliary outflow is obstructed, several procedures may be indicated including surgical bypass, endoscopic biliary stenting, or percutaneous biliary decompression. Palliative bypass of gastric outflow obstruction can be performed by open gastrojejunostomy, laparoscopic gastrojejunostomy, duodenal stenting, or decompressive gastrostomy tube. Despite recent developments and research into treatment of this disease, the prognosis remains poor, with overall 5-year survival rates for all patients less than 6%.[280]

OWEN T. SKINNER

Incidence and Risk Factors

Gastric cancer is rare in small animals, comprising 0.16% of cancers in one large study.[281] The causes of gastric cancers have not been identified in dogs.[281–284] Gastric carcinoma has been experimentally induced in dogs with nitrosamines; however, the clinical relevance of these findings is unclear.[285] Hypergastrinemia is a risk factor in humans, typically associated with atrophic gastritis caused by *Helicobacter pylori*.[286] Although gastrin levels have not been reported to be increased in small populations of dogs with gastric carcinoma, individual dogs have been noted with substantial increases in serum gastrin.[287,288] *H. pylori* infection is rare in dogs.[289] Non–*H. pylori* *Helicobacter* species are highly prevalent in dogs, although the clinical significance of these organisms is uncertain, with both mild gastritis and asymptomatic presentations reported.[289–291]

Gastric carcinoma is the most common nonhematopoietic gastric tumor in dogs.[292–294] Breeds at higher risk of gastric carcinoma include the Tervueren, Bouvier des Flandres, Groenendael, collie, standard poodle, Norwegian elkhound, and Norwegian lundehund.[281,287,295–297] Mean age at presentation is typically 8 to 10 years.[281,283,284,293,294] Male dogs are consistently overrepresented, with a male-to-female ratio of approximately 1.5:1.[281,292–294,298] The most common mesenchymal tumors of the stomach are smooth muscle tumors (leiomyomas and leiomyosarcomas) and gastrointestinal stromal tumors (GISTs). These occur with similar frequency in male and female dogs, with a mean age at diagnosis of approximately 11 years.[299] Other reported canine gastric tumors include mast cell tumor (MCT),[300] histiocytic sarcoma,[301,302] plasmacytoma,[303] and undifferentiated sarcoma.[304]

Lymphoma is the most common primary gastric malignancy in cats.[305] Gastric carcinoma is rare in cats, representing fewer than 5% of feline gastrointestinal carcinoma cases.[306–308] Gastritis and *Helicobacter* have been proposed as risk factors for feline gastric carcinoma and lymphoma.[309,310] Other reported feline gastric tumors include MCT,[311] carcinoid,[312] hamartoma,[313] and polyps.[314]

Pathology and Natural Behavior

Gastric carcinoma is classified as either "intestinal" (with papillary, acinar, or solid subtypes) or "diffuse" (with undifferentiated or glandular subtypes).[298,315] Intestinal type tumors in humans are thought to arise from sequential progression through gastritis, metaplasia, and dysplasia, whereas diffuse type tumors may be associated with mutation or methylation of CDH1.[316] The diffuse histologic type is more common in dogs.[283,287,298] Canine gastric carcinoma commonly arises in the pylorus or lesser curvature, although some carcinomas may lead to diffuse, firm thickening of the stomach (*linitis plastica*).[281,293,296,298,317] Ulceration is common and may progress to full-thickness perforation and peritonitis.[294] Metastasis to regional LNs is common (32% at presentation and 77% at postmortem), with liver and lungs less frequently affected.[292,298]

Many mesenchymal tumors previously diagnosed as leiomyosarcomas have been reclassified as GISTs.[299,304] Gastric leiomyoma and leiomyosarcoma are typically focal, with or without cavitating ulceration, and are most often found at the cardia or pylorus.[293,318–321] Paraneoplastic hypoglycemia has been reported with leiomyoma and leiomyosarcoma, possibly due to excessive release of IGF-2.[320,321] Although smooth muscle tumors are more common in the stomach, approximately 10% to 20% of GISTs arise at this site.[299,304,322] GISTs arise from the interstitial cells of Cajal, which normally express c-Kit (CD117) and may also express CD34, and hence immunohistochemistry (IHC) is required to differentiate leiomyosarcomas from GISTs.[322,323] Mutations in exon 11 of the *c-kit* gene are common in canine GIST and mutations in exon 9 have been reported.[299,324–327] GISTs are rare in cats.[328]

Gastric involvement of feline alimentary lymphoma is relatively uncommon.[329,330] Readers should refer to Chapter 33, Section B (Feline Lymphoma and Leukemia) for further information regarding gastric lymphoma.

History and Clinical Signs

Vomiting is the most common clinical sign, with or without associated hematemesis, in cats and dogs with gastric tumors.[284,292] Weight loss, anorexia, melena, diarrhea, and abdominal pain may also be encountered. Gastric cancer should be considered as a potential cause of septic peritonitis or pneumoperitoneum. Duration of clinical signs may vary widely, but is commonly in the order of 1 to 2 months.[292,294]

Diagnostic Techniques and Workup

Routine blood tests are not expected to be diagnostic, but may reveal anemia, hypoalbuminemia, thrombocytopenia, or thrombocytosis in patients with hemorrhage associated with ulceration.[284,292] Hepatocellular leakage enzymes may be increased with liver metastasis. Abdominal radiographs may identify changes such as a cranial abdominal mass, loss of serosal detail, or apparent thickening of the gastric wall. Contrast radiography may be helpful to identify delayed gastric emptying. Given the limited detail typically observed on radiographs, this modality has been largely superseded by abdominal ultrasound and, increasingly, CT (Fig. 23.15).[292,331–333] Gastric carcinomas tend to be broad-based on imaging, whereas mesenchymal tumors and benign lesions may be more focal or pedunculated.[314,334] Intraluminal gas can make ultrasonography challenging.[335] Thoracic imaging, whether radiographs or CT, should be assessed as part of the clinical staging protocol, but pulmonary metastasis at presentation is rare in patients with gastric cancer.[292,304] Gastroscopy can provide complementary information to the findings of diagnostic imaging (Fig. 23.16).[335] Multiple biopsies of any gastric lesions should be obtained, given the potential for acquisition of nondiagnostic samples in dogs and cats with gastric pathology.[336] If the disease process does not involve the mucosa, diagnosis from endoscopic biopsies can be challenging. Surgical biopsies may be considered if a diagnosis cannot be obtained with gastroscopy. Histopathology is the gold standard for diagnosis; however, squash preparation cytology, with assessment for the presence of signet ring cells and/or cytoplasmic microvacuolation, is sensitive (94%) and specific (94%) for gastric carcinoma.[337] IHC should be considered if there is doubt regarding tumor type.[299,304] FNA cytology of gastric masses has poor agreement (50%) with definitive histopathology in dogs and cats.[308]

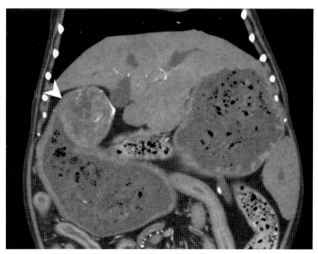

• **Fig. 23.15** Dorsal plane computed tomography image of a dog with an ulcerated and cavitated pyloric leiomyosarcoma *(white arrowhead)*.

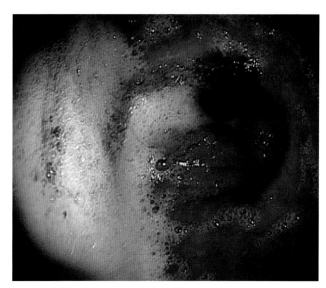

• **Fig. 23.16** Ulcerated gastric carcinoma seen at gastroscopy in a dog.

Treatment

Resection of local disease may be considered in patients with solid tumors without evidence of either diffuse disease or distant metastasis. Surgery, if feasible, typically consists of various partial gastrectomy procedures. For tumors located in the pyloric region, surgical resection often requires a gastroduodenostomy (Billroth I).[293,338] Gastrojejunostomy (Billroth II) has been performed for patients with more extensive disease; however, outcomes are guarded because of persistent vomiting, poor appetite, and progressive disease with poor survival times of only 4 to 5 weeks.[293,339] Partial gastrectomy is recommended for tumors located in the gastric body. If surgery is pursued, complete abdominal exploration should be performed to assess for metastasis, with particular attention paid to all abdominal LNs and the liver. Benign lesions, such as leiomyomas, can be excised with a marginal approach.[319]

Adjuvant RT is used in humans after resection of gastric carcinomas, but RT has played a minimal role in dogs because of the proximity of sensitive tissues.[340]

The role of chemotherapy for animals with solid gastric tumors is unclear. Response of carcinomas to chemotherapy has typically been poor, although multiple protocols have been attempted.[284,292,293] Expression of HER-2 is common in canine gastric carcinoma (58%), and this may represent a therapeutic target in dogs; however, clinical data are not available.[341] Responses to imatinib have been reported in dogs with GISTs, but large-scale studies are lacking.[324,325]

Prognosis

Gastric carcinoma typically carries a poor prognosis because of the difficulty in achieving local tumor control and a moderate-to-high metastatic rate. Long-term survival is possible after partial gastrectomy, but survival times are usually less than 6 months.[292–294,297,338,342,343] Given the challenges with controlling systemic disease, few dogs with gastric carcinoma are good surgical candidates and careful case selection is critical. Improvements in systemic therapies may increase the number of animals considered candidates for surgery. The median survival times for dogs with GIST, leiomyosarcoma, and undifferentiated sarcoma, provided they survive the perioperative period, are 37.4 months, 8 to 12 months, and 2.9 months, respectively.[304,318] The prognosis is excellent after surgical resection of leiomyoma, with the majority of dogs cured.[319,344] The median survival times for dogs and cats with gastrointestinal MCTs are less than 1 month[300] and 531 days, respectively.[311]

Comparative Aspects

In 2012 gastric cancer was the third most common cause of cancer-related death in men worldwide and the fifth most common cause of cancer-related death in women.[345] Men are approximately twice as likely to be affected as women.[346] Approximately 89% of noncardia gastric cancer in humans is associated with *H. pylori*.[347] Significant geographic differences are observed in the incidence of gastric carcinoma and this may be a result of *H. pylori* prevalence, socioeconomic status, and likely genetic susceptibility.[316,347] Mortality rates are approximately 60% to 80%, reflecting advanced disease at presentation and an aggressive disease course.[348] Treatment of local gastric tumors varies from endoscopic mucosal resection for superficial lesions to partial or total gastrectomy for more infiltrative and advanced lesions.[349,350] Adjuvant therapy, particularly chemoradiotherapy, is common in patients with advanced gastric cancer, although improvements in survival are often limited.[340,351] Targeted therapies, including trastuzumab targeting of HER-2, have shown promise, but improvements in outcome are still small for most patients.[352]

SECTION F: HEPATOBILIARY TUMORS

JULIUS M. LIPTAK

Incidence and Risk Factors

Primary hepatic tumors are uncommon and account for fewer than 1.5% of all canine tumors and 1.0% to 2.9% of all feline tumors, but up to 6.9% of nonhematopoietic tumors in cats.[353–356] Metastasis to the liver from nonhepatic neoplasia is more common and occurs 2.5 times more frequently than primary liver

TABLE 23.6	Morphologic Types of Canine Hepatic Tumors		
	Massive (%)	Nodular (%)	Diffuse (%)
Hepatocellular carcinoma	53–84	16–25	0–19
Bile duct carcinoma	37–46	0–46	17–54
Neuroendocrine tumor	0	33	67
Sarcoma	36	64	0

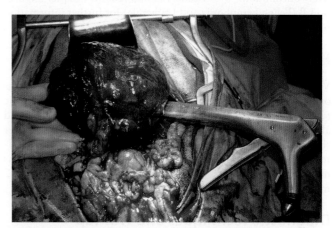

• **Fig. 23.17** A solitary hepatocellular carcinoma with classic massive liver tumor morphology. A liver lobectomy is being performed using a thoracoabdominal surgical stapling device.

tumors in dogs, particularly from primary cancer of the spleen, pancreas, and GI tract.[353,354] Primary hepatobiliary tumors are more common than metastatic disease in cats.[356] The liver can also be involved in other malignant processes, such as lymphoma, malignant histiocytosis, and systemic mastocytosis.[354,355] Nodular hyperplasia is a relatively common diagnosis in older dogs but is benign and probably does not represent a preneoplastic lesion.[356]

There are four basic categories of primary malignant hepatobiliary tumors in cats and dogs: hepatocellular, bile duct, neuroendocrine (or carcinoid), and mesenchymal.[356] Malignant tumors are more common in dogs, whereas benign tumors occur more frequently in cats.[354–360] There are three morphologic types of these primary hepatic tumors: massive, nodular, and diffuse (Table 23.6).[357] Massive liver tumors are defined as a large, solitary mass confined to a single liver lobe (Fig. 23.17); nodular tumors are multifocal and involve several liver lobes (Fig. 23.18); and diffuse involvement may represent the final spectrum of neoplastic disease with multifocal or coalescing nodules in all liver lobes or diffuse effacement of the hepatic parenchyma (Fig. 23.19).[356,357]

The prognosis for cats and dogs with liver tumors is determined by histology and morphology. The prognosis is good for massive hepatocellular carcinomas (HCC) and benign tumors because complete surgical resection is usually achievable and their biologic behavior is relatively nonaggressive with an indolent growth rate.[359–363] In contrast, the prognosis is poor for cats with any type of malignant tumor, dogs with malignant tumors other than massive HCC, and cats and dogs with nodular and diffuse liver tumors because resection is less feasible and/or metastasis is more common.[354–366]

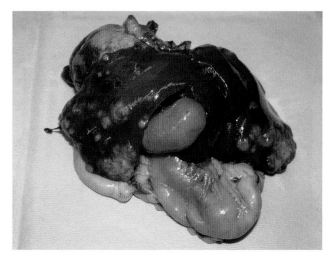

• **Fig. 23.18** Nodular morphologic appearance of a bile duct carcinoma in a cat.

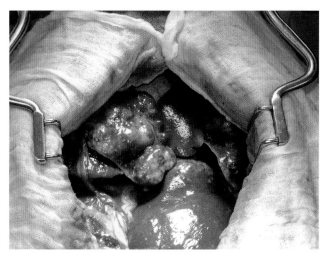

• **Fig. 23.19** Diffuse morphologic appearance in a dog with a bile duct carcinoma.

In people, primary liver tumors have been reclassified according to the presence of hepatic progenitor cells and immunohistochemical markers to differentiate hepatocytic and cholangiocytic lineages.[367] Liver tumors with hepatic progenitor cell characteristics are typically more poorly differentiated and biologically aggressive, resulting in a poorer prognosis.[367] Primary liver tumors in dogs and cats have also been reclassified according to these criteria.[367,368] Based on histologic findings and the degree of immunoreactivity to keratin 19, hepatocellular tumors were divided into well-differentiated, scirrhous, and poorly differentiated tumors.[367] HCCs expressing less than 5% of keratin 19 were more likely to be derived from mature hepatocytes with minimal evidence of cellular pleomorphism, infiltrative growth, and rare metastasis,[367] and this accounted for 79% of canine HCCs and all feline HCCs.[367,368] In contrast, primary liver tumors with keratin 19 expression, which included poorly differentiated HCCs and cholangiosarcomas, were characterized by a high grade of cellular pleomorphism, infiltrative growth, vascular invasion, and intra- or extrahepatic metastasis.[367,368] These tumors were probably derived from either hepatic progenitor cells or dedifferentiation of mature hepatocytes.[367]

Pathology and Natural Behavior

Hepatocellular Tumors

Hepatocellular tumors include HCC, hepatocellular adenoma (or hepatoma), and hepatoblastoma.[356] Hepatoblastoma is a rare tumor of primordial hepatic stem cells and has only been reported in one dog.[369] Hepatocellular adenoma is usually an incidental finding and rarely causes clinical signs.[354] Of the hepatocellular tumors, hepatocellular adenoma is more common in cats and HCC occurs more frequently in dogs.[354,357,358]

HCC is the most common primary liver tumor in dogs, accounting for up to 77% of cases, and the second most common in cats.[354–360,367] Etiologic factors implicated in the development of HCC in humans include infection with hepatitis virus B or C and cirrhosis.[370] A viral etiology has also been demonstrated in woodchucks but not in cats or dogs, and cirrhosis is rare in dogs with HCC.[358–361] A link between progressive vacuolar hepatopathy and HCC has been proposed in Scottish terriers, with HCC diagnosed in 34% of Scottish terriers with progressive vacuolar hepatopathy.[371] In one study, 20% of dogs with HCC were diagnosed with additional tumors although most were benign and endocrine in origin.[357]

A breed and sex predisposition has not been confirmed in dogs with HCC, but miniature schnauzers and male dogs are overrepresented in some studies.[357,361,363,372] Morphologically, 53% to 83% of HCCs are massive (see Fig. 23.17), 16% to 25% are nodular, and up to 19% are diffuse.[354,357] The left liver lobes, which include the left lateral and medial lobes and papillary process of the caudate lobe, are involved in more than two-thirds of dogs with massive HCC,[357,361–363] but tumors are equally distributed between the left and right liver lobes in cats.[373] Metastasis to regional LNs, peritoneum, and lungs is more common in dogs with nodular and diffuse HCC.[354,357,361] Other metastatic sites include the heart, kidneys, adrenal glands, pancreas, intestines, spleen, and urinary bladder.[354,357,361] The metastatic rate varies from 0% to 37% for dogs with massive HCCs and 93% to 100% for dogs with nodular and diffuse HCCs.[354,357–363]

Bile Duct Tumors

Bile Duct Adenoma (Biliary Cystadenoma)

There are two types of bile duct tumors in cats and dogs: bile duct adenoma and carcinoma.[354,357–360,364,365,374–378] Bile duct adenomas are common in cats, accounting for more than 50% of all feline hepatobiliary tumors, and are also known as biliary or hepatobiliary cystadenomas because of their cystic appearance (Fig. 23.20).[358–360,374–376] Male cats may be predisposed.[374,376] Bile duct adenomas usually do not cause clinical signs until they reach a large size and compress adjacent organs.[374–376] There is an even distribution between single and multiple lesions.[358–360,374–376] Malignant transformation has been reported in humans, and anaplastic changes have been observed in some feline adenomas.[358,374]

Bile Duct Carcinoma (Cholangiocarcinoma)

Bile duct carcinoma is the most common malignant hepatobiliary tumor in cats and the second most common in dogs.[354,357–360] Bile duct carcinomas account for 9% to 41% of all malignant liver tumors in dogs.[357,368,379] In humans, trematode infestation, cholelithiasis, and sclerosing cholangitis are known risk factors for bile duct carcinoma.[380] Trematodes may also be involved in the etiology of bile duct carcinoma in cats and dogs, but they are

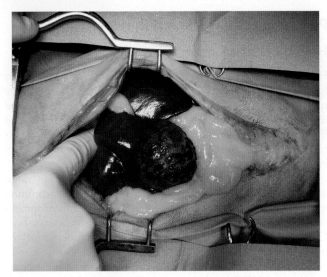

• **Fig. 23.20** Intraoperative image of a bile duct cystadenoma in a cat. Surgical resection was curative in this cat.

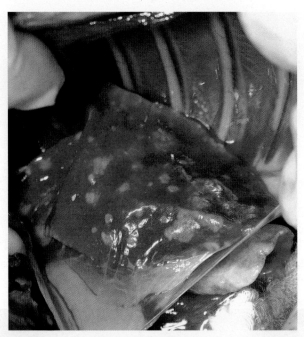

• **Fig. 23.21** Lung metastasis in the cat with bile duct carcinoma depicted in Fig. 23.18. This cat also had diffuse peritoneal metastasis.

unlikely to be a major contributor because bile duct carcinomas also occur in geographic regions outside the normal distribution of trematodes.[356,360,365]

A predilection for Labrador retrievers has been proposed.[365] A sex predisposition has been reported for female dogs.[357,364,372] In cats, however, the sex predisposition is conflicting.[358-360] The distribution of morphologic types of bile duct carcinoma is similar to HCC, with 37% to 46% massive, up to 54% nodular (see Fig. 23.18), and 17% to 54% diffuse.[354,357,364,365] Bile duct carcinomas can be intrahepatic, extrahepatic, or within the gall bladder.[354,357-360,364,365] Intrahepatic carcinomas are more common in dogs,[357,364,365] whereas an equal distribution of intrahepatic and extrahepatic tumors to extrahepatic predominance has been reported in cats.[358-360] Solid and cystic (or cystadenocarcinoma) bile duct carcinomas have been reported, but this distinction does not influence either treatment or prognosis.[364] Bile duct carcinoma of the gall bladder is rare in both species.[354,357-360,364,365]

Bile duct carcinomas have an aggressive biologic behavior. Metastasis is common in dogs, with up to 88% metastasizing to the regional LNs and lungs (Fig. 23.21); other sites include the heart, spleen, adrenal glands, pancreas, kidneys, and spinal cord.[354,357,364,365] In cats, diffuse intraperitoneal metastasis and carcinomatosis occur in 67% to 80% of cases.[358-360]

Neuroendocrine Tumors

Neuroendocrine tumors, also known as carcinoids, are rare in cats and dogs.[354,357-360,367,368] These tumors arise from neuroectodermal cells and are histologically differentiated from carcinomas with the use of silver stains.[355,366] Neuroendocrine hepatobiliary tumors are usually intrahepatic, although extrahepatic tumors have been reported in the gall bladder.[366,377,378,381] Carcinoids tend to occur at a younger age than other primary hepatobiliary tumors.[357,366] Morphologically, carcinoids are nodular in 33% and diffuse in the remaining 67% of cases.[357,366] Primary hepatic neuroendocrine tumors have an aggressive biologic behavior with frequent involvement of more than one liver lobe and metastasis to the regional LNs, peritoneum, and lungs in cats and dogs.[357,366,381] Other metastatic sites include the heart, spleen, kidneys, adrenal glands, and pancreas.[366]

Sarcomas

Primary and nonhematopoietic hepatic sarcomas are rare in cats and dogs.[354,357-360,380] The most common primary hepatic sarcomas are hemangiosarcoma (HSA), leiomyosarcoma, and fibrosarcoma, with HSA the most frequently diagnosed primary hepatic sarcoma in cats and leiomyosarcoma the most common in dogs.[354,357-360,380,382-385] The liver is a common site for metastatic HSA in dogs, whereas only 4% to 6% of HSA occur primarily in the liver.[384,385] Other primary hepatic sarcomas include rhabdomyosarcoma, liposarcoma, OSA, and malignant mesenchymoma.[354-360] The liver, with lungs, LNs, spleen, and bone marrow, is commonly involved in dogs with disseminated histiocytic sarcoma (HS).[386,387] Benign mesenchymal tumors such as hemangiomas are rare.[354-360] There are no known breed predispositions, although a male predilection has been reported.[357] Diffuse morphology has not been reported, with massive and nodular types accounting for 36% and 64% of sarcomas, respectively.[357,380] Hepatic sarcomas have an aggressive biologic behavior, with metastasis to the spleen and lungs reported in 86% to 100% of dogs.[357,380]

Other Primary Hepatic Tumors

Myelolipoma is a benign hepatobiliary tumor in cats.[355,356] Histologically, myelolipomas are composed of well-differentiated adipose tissue intermixed with normal hematopoietic elements.[356] Chronic hypoxia has been proposed as an etiologic factor because myelolipomas have been reported in liver lobes entrapped in diaphragmatic herniae.[356] Myelolipomas can be either single or multifocal.[356]

History and Clinical Signs

Hepatobiliary tumors are symptomatic in approximately 50% of cats and 75% of dogs, especially in animals with malignant tumors.[353-366,373] With respect to the massive form of HCC, most clinical signs are related to the mechanical mass effect of the tumor and only rarely to any systemic effects of the tumor or hepatic insufficiency. The most common presenting signs are nonspecific, such as inappetence, weight loss, lethargy, vomiting, polydipsia–polyuria, and ascites.[353-366,373] Weakness, ataxia, and seizures are uncommon and may be caused by hepatic encephalopathy, paraneoplastic hypoglycemia, or central nervous system metastasis.[357,361,388] Icterus is more common in dogs with extrahepatic bile duct carcinomas and diffuse neuroendocrine tumors.[354,357,364] Hemoperitoneum secondary to rupture of massive HCC has been reported in two dogs.[389] Physical examination findings are often unrewarding. A cranial abdominal mass is palpable in up to 75% of cats and dogs with liver tumors, although palpation can be misleading because hepatic enlargement may be either absent in nodular and diffuse forms of liver tumors or missed because of the location of the liver in the cranial abdominal cavity deep to the costal arch.[353-366]

Diagnostic Techniques and Workup

Laboratory Tests

Hematologic and serum biochemical abnormalities are usually nonspecific. Leukocytosis, anemia, and thrombocytosis are common in dogs with liver tumors.[353-366] Anemia is usually mild and nonregenerative.[357,363] Thrombocytosis is seen in approximately 50% of dogs with massive HCC.[363] Anemia and thrombocytopenia are relatively common in dogs with primary and metastatic hepatic HSAs.[355] Prolonged coagulation times (e.g., increased prothrombin time, thrombin time, and activated partial thromboplastin time) and specific clotting factor abnormalities (e.g., decreased factor VIII:C and increased factor VIII:RA and fibrinogen degradation products) have been identified in dogs with hepatobiliary tumors, although these are rarely clinically relevant.[390]

Liver enzymes are commonly elevated in dogs with hepatobiliary tumors (Table 23.7). Increased activity of liver enzymes probably reflects hepatocellular damage or biliary stasis and is not specific for hepatic neoplasia.[356] There is also no correlation between the degree of hepatic involvement and magnitude of liver enzyme alterations.[356,363] The type of liver enzyme abnormalities may provide an indication of the type of tumor and differentiate primary and metastatic liver tumors.[391] Alkaline phosphatase (ALP) and alanine transferase (ALT) are commonly increased in dogs with primary hepatic tumors, whereas aspartate aminotransferase (AST) and bilirubin are more consistently elevated in dogs with metastatic liver tumors.[353,391] Furthermore, an AST-to-ALT ratio less than one is consistent with HCC or bile duct carcinoma, whereas a neuroendocrine tumor or sarcoma is more likely when the ratio is greater than one.[357] In general, however, liver enzyme elevations are not specific for the diagnosis of hepatobiliary diseases.[392] Other changes in the serum biochemical profile in dogs with hepatic tumors may include hypoglycemia, hypoalbuminemia, hyperglobulinemia, and increased preprandial and postprandial bile acids.[353,354,357,361-366] Hypoglycemia is a paraneoplastic syndrome reported secondary to hepatic adenoma and management is described in more detail in Chapter 5. In contrast to dogs, azotemia is often present in cats with hepatobiliary tumors and may be the only biochemical abnormality, although liver enzyme abnormalities, especially ALT, AST, and total bilirubin, are also common and are significantly higher in cats with malignant tumors.[358-360]

TABLE 23.7	Common Clinicopathologic Abnormalities in Cats and Dogs with Hepatobiliary Tumors	
Parameter	Cat (%)	Dog (%)
Leukocytosis		54–73
Anemia		27–51
Hypoalbuminemia		52–83
Increased ALP	10–64	61–100
Increased ALT	10–78	44–75
Increased AST	15–78	56–100
Increased GGT	78	39
Increased total bilirubin	33–78	18–33
Increased serum bile acids	67	50–75

ALP, Alkaline phosphatase; *ALT,* alanine transferase; *AST,* aspartate aminotransferase; *GGT,* γ-glutamyltransferase.

α-Fetoprotein, an oncofetal glycoprotein, is used in the diagnosis, monitoring response to treatment, and prognostication of HCC in humans.[370] In dogs, serum levels of α-fetoprotein are increased in 75% of HCC and 55% of bile duct carcinomas.[393,394] However, α-fetoprotein has limited value in the diagnosis and treatment monitoring of canine HCC, as serum levels of α-fetoprotein are also increased in other types of liver tumors, such as bile duct carcinoma and lymphoma, and nonneoplastic hepatic disease.[394,395] Hyperferritinemia is common in dogs with HS and immune-mediated hemolytic anemia (IMHA); thus, once IMHA has been excluded, serum ferritin levels may be useful in differentiating HS from other causes of liver disease.[396]

Imaging

Radiographs, ultrasonography (US), and advanced imaging can be used for the diagnosis, staging, and surgical planning of cats and dogs with hepatobiliary tumors. A cranial abdominal mass, with caudal and lateral displacement of the stomach, is frequently noted on abdominal radiographs of cats and dogs with massive liver tumors.[362,363,372] Mineralization of the biliary tree is a rare finding in dogs with bile duct carcinoma.[356] Sonographic or CT examination is recommended because these radiographic findings are not specific for the diagnosis of a hepatic mass and do not provide information on the relationship of the hepatic mass with regional anatomic structures.

Abdominal US or triphasic (arterial, venous, and delayed contrast phases) CT are preferred for identifying and characterizing hepatobiliary tumors in cats and dogs.[397] US examination is useful in determining the presence of a hepatic mass and defining the tumor as massive, nodular, or diffuse[398-402] and, in the case of cats, whether the tumor is cystic or not.[372] If focal, the size and location of the mass and its relationship with adjacent anatomic structures, such as the gall bladder or caudal vena cava, can be assessed.[376,398-402] Tumor vascularization can be determined using Doppler imaging techniques or triphasic CT, although the latter is superior.[356,402] The US appearance of hepatobiliary tumors varies and does not correlate with histologic tumor type.[376,397-406] However, US-guided FNA or needle-core biopsy of hepatic masses is a useful, minimally invasive technique to obtain cellular or tissue samples for diagnostic purposes.[398–401] A coagulation profile is recommended before hepatic biopsy because mild-to-moderate hemorrhage is the most frequent complication, occurring in approximately 5% of cases.[398–401] A correct diagnosis is obtained in up to 60% of hepatic aspirates and 90% of needle-core biopsies.[398–401,407] The most useful cytologic features for the diagnosis of well-differentiated HCCs include dissociation of hepatocytes, acinar or palisading arrangement of neoplastic cells, and the presence of naked nuclei and capillaries, together with mild anisocytosis, anisokaryosis, multinuclearity, and increased N:C ratios.[408,409] More invasive techniques, such as laparoscopy and open keyhole approaches, can also be used for the biopsy and staging of cats and dogs with suspected liver tumors. In humans, laparoscopy is recommended for local staging, as up to 20% of cases do not proceed with open surgery because of either nodular or diffuse tumors or unresectable disease.[410] However, for solitary and massive hepatic masses, surgical resection can be performed without a preoperative biopsy because both diagnosis and treatment can be achieved in a single procedure.

Advanced imaging techniques, such as triphasic CT and MRI, are preferred in humans for the diagnosis and staging of liver tumors and many veterinary centers also use this methodology.[370,397] Unlike US, imaging appearance may provide an indication of tumor type.[370] Furthermore, CT and MRI are more sensitive for the detection of small hepatic lesions and determining the relationship of liver masses with adjacent vascular and soft tissue structures.[370] In dogs, there are CT features that can be used to differentiate nodular hyperplasia, hepatic adenomas, and HCCs based on enhancement patterns during arterial and portal venous phases.[411,412] However, in another study, there were no features on dual-phase CT scans that differentiated benign and malignant hepatic lesions.[413] Triphasic CT was reported to be more than 90% accurate in differentiating benign from malignant masses in 44 dogs and was superior to color-flow, power, and pulse-wave Doppler US, but could not differentiate the histologic type of malignant tumor.[397] MRI with a liver-specific contrast agent, gadoxetate disodium, has been described in seven dogs with HCC, but imaging findings were variable.[414]

Imaging is also important for the staging of cats and dogs with liver tumors. Local extension and regional metastasis can be assessed with abdominal US, CT, MRI, or laparoscopy. The sonographic and sometimes gross appearance of nodular hyperplasia and metastatic disease is similar. In two studies, 25% to 36% of dogs with ultrasonographically detectable focal hepatic lesions were diagnosed with nodular hyperplasia.[415,416] Biopsy of such lesions is recommended before definitively diagnosing metastatic disease and excluding animals from curative-intent surgery.[417] Although rare at the time of diagnosis, three-view thoracic radiographs or advanced imaging techniques should be assessed for evidence of lung metastasis before treatment.

Therapy and Prognosis

Hepatocellular Tumors

Liver lobectomy is recommended for cats and dogs with any hepatic tumor that has a massive morphologic appearance, particularly HCC. Surgical techniques for liver lobectomy include finger fracture, mass ligation, mattress sutures, bipolar vessel sealant devices, and surgical stapling.[417] Mass ligation is not recommended for large dogs, tumors involving either the central or right

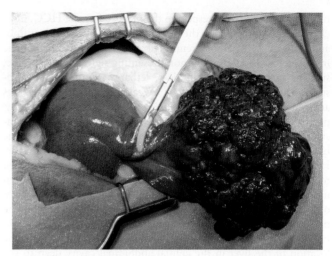

• **Fig. 23.22** Liver lobectomy using a bipolar vessel sealing device.

liver divisions, or tumors with a wide base.[417] The finger-fracture technique, involving blunt dissection through hepatic parenchyma and individual ligation of bile ducts and vessels, is acceptable for smaller lesions. Surgical staplers or bipolar vessel sealant devices are preferred for liver lobectomy because operative time is shorter with fewer complications (see Fig. 23.17; and 23.22).[363,417] A hilar dissection technique may be required for larger tumors extending to the hilus of the liver lobe because adequate margins may not be achievable with a surgical stapler.[418] Complete histologic excision of massive HCCs is associated with significantly better local tumor control and survival times,[419] and the use of real-time fluorescent imaging has been described to assess the completeness of excision intraoperatively in dogs with massive HCCs.[420] Advanced imaging and intraoperative US may provide information on the relationship of right-sided and central liver tumors with the caudal vena cava before liver lobectomy. Right-sided liver tumors can be excised even if intimately associated with the caudal vena cava, with or without an ultrasonic aspirator, but the surgeon should be familiar with the course of the caudal vena cava through the hepatic parenchyma. En bloc resection of the caudal vena cava with a right-sided HCC has been reported.[421] In one report of 42 dogs with massive HCC treated with liver lobectomy, the intraoperative mortality rate was 4.8% and the complication rate was 28.6%.[363] Complications include hemorrhage, vascular compromise to adjacent liver lobes, and transient hypoglycemia and reduced hepatic function.[356,363,417] In one single institution study, blood transfusions were required in 17% of dogs and 44% of cats treated with liver lobectomy for various hepatic conditions,[422] which highlights the importance of preoperative cross-matching or blood typing before liver lobectomy to be more adequately prepared to manage intraoperative bleeding.

The prognosis for dogs and cats with massive HCC is good (Fig. 23.23). Local tumor recurrence is reported in 0% to 13% of dogs with massive HCC after liver lobectomy.[362,363] In a recent study investigating the effect of the completeness of histologic excision in 37 dogs with massive HCC, local tumor recurrence was reported in 12% of dogs with complete histologic excision and 58% of dogs with incomplete histologic excision.[419] The median progression-free and overall survival times were significantly longer in dogs with complete histologic excision (1000 days and greater than 1836 days, respectively) than incomplete histologic excision (521 days and 765 days, respectively) although both groups enjoyed durable postsurgical

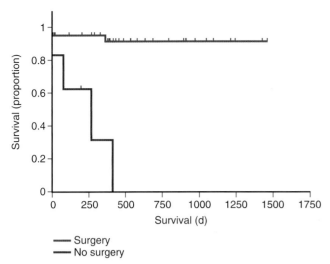

• **Fig. 23.23** Kaplan–Meier survival curve for dogs with massive hepatocellular carcinoma. The median survival time for dogs with surgically resected tumors is significantly better than dogs not treated with curative-intent liver lobectomy. (Reprinted with permission from Liptak JM, Dernell WS, Monnet E, et al. Massive hepatocellular carcinoma in dogs: 48 cases (1992–2002). *J Am Vet Med Assoc*. 2004;225:1225–1230.)

survival.[419] Metastasis to other regions of the liver and lungs has been documented in 0% to 37% of dogs, but metastasis is rare in recent clinical reports and most deaths are unrelated to HCC.[357,362,363,419] The MST for dogs with massive HCC after liver lobectomy are greater than 1460 to 1836 days,[363,419] and the MST was 2.4 years for six cats with HCC treated with liver lobectomy.[373] In comparison, the MST of 270 days was significantly decreased for six dogs managed conservatively, and these dogs were 15.4 times more likely to die of tumor-related causes than dogs treated surgically.[363] Prognostic factors in dogs with massive HCC include surgical treatment, side of liver involvement, ALT and AST activity, ratios of ALP-to-AST and ALT-to-AST, and completeness of histologic excision.[363,419] Right-sided liver tumors, involving either the right lateral lobe or caudate process of the caudate lobe, had a poorer prognosis because intraoperative death was more likely due to caudal vena cava trauma during surgical dissection.[363] There was no difference in survival time if dogs with right-sided massive HCC survived surgery.[363] Increased ALT and AST were associated with a poor prognosis in one study, which may reflect more severe hepatocellular injury secondary to either large tumor size or more aggressive biologic behavior.[363]

In contrast, the prognosis for dogs with nodular and diffuse HCC is poor. Surgical resection is usually not possible because of involvement of multiple liver lobes. Treatment options for nodular and diffuse HCC in humans include liver transplantation or minimally invasive procedures for regional control, such as ablation or embolization.[370] Bland embolization and chemoembolization have been reported with moderate success in the palliation of four dogs and one cat with HCC,[423–425] and microwave ablation has been described in five dogs with diffuse hepatic neoplasia, including one dog with HCC.[426] The role of RT and chemotherapy in the management of HCC is largely unknown.

Traditional RT is ineffective in the management of liver tumors, as the canine liver cannot tolerate cumulative doses greater than 30 Gy[356,370]; however, three-dimensional (3-D) conformal RT, which enables targeted high-dose RT to the tumor while sparing adjacent normal hepatic tissue, has been described in 6 dogs with nonresectable HCC.[427] In this study, 3-D conformal RT was delivered at 6 to 10 Gy per fraction to a total dose of 18 to 42 Gy with 1 to 2 fractions per week for a total of 3 to 7 fractions.[427] This RT protocol resulted in partial responses in five of the six dogs, and an MST of 567 days.[427]

HCC is considered chemoresistant in humans because response rates are usually less than 20%.[356,370] The poor response to systemic chemotherapy is probably a result of rapid development of drug resistance due to either the role of hepatocytes in detoxification or expression of P-glycoprotein, a cell membrane efflux pump associated with multidrug resistance.[356] However, single-agent gemcitabine has been investigated in dogs with unresectable HCC with encouraging results.[428] In one this study, 18 dogs with mostly nodular and diffuse well-differentiated HCCs were treated with gemcitabine for 5 weeks.[428] The overall MST was 983 days, but depended on the morphology and resectability of the tumor.[428] The MSTs were 1339 days for dogs with massive HCC, 983 days for dogs with nodular HCC, and 113 days for dogs with diffuse HCC; and the MSTs were 1339 days for dogs with incompletely excised HCC, which included all four dogs with massive HCC and 9 of 10 dogs with nodular HCC, and 197 days for dogs with nonresectable HCC, including all four dogs with diffuse HCC.[428] Novel treatment options currently being investigated in human medicine include immunotherapy, hormonal therapy with tamoxifen, and antiangiogenic agents.[370]

Bile Duct Tumors

Bile duct adenomas can present as either single (e.g., massive) or multifocal lesions. Liver lobectomy is recommended for cats with single bile duct adenoma (cystadenoma) or multifocal lesions confined to one to two lobes.[358–360,374–376] The prognosis is very good after surgical resection with resolution of clinical signs and no reports of local recurrence or malignant transformation.[360,374,375]

Liver lobectomy is also recommended for cats and dogs with massive bile duct carcinoma. However, survival time has been poor in cats and dogs treated with liver lobectomy because the majority have died within 6 months as a result of local recurrence and metastatic disease.[360,429] There is no known effective treatment for cats and dogs with nodular or diffuse bile duct carcinomas because these lesions are not amenable to surgical resection and other treatments are often not successful.

Neuroendocrine Tumors

Carcinoids have an aggressive biologic behavior and are usually not amenable to surgical resection because solitary lesions and massive morphology are rare.[357,366] The efficacy of RT and chemotherapy is unknown. Prognosis is poor because metastasis to the regional LNs, peritoneum, and lungs occurs in 93% of dogs and usually early in the course of disease.[357,366]

Sarcomas

Liver lobectomy can be attempted for solitary and massive sarcomas. However, the prognosis is poor because metastatic disease is often present at the time of surgery.[357,380] Chemotherapy has not been investigated in the treatment of primary hepatic sarcomas, although, similar to other solid sarcomas, response rates are likely to be poor. Doxorubicin-based protocols and ifosfamide have shown some promise with sarcomas in other locations and warrant consideration for cats and dogs with primary hepatic sarcomas.[430,431]

Other Primary Hepatic Tumors

Surgical resection with liver lobectomy is recommended for cats with primary hepatic myelolipoma, and the prognosis is excellent with prolonged survival time and no reports of local recurrence.[356]

Comparative Aspects

HCC is one of the most common malignancies in humans as a result of viral infections with hepatitis viruses B and C and cirrhosis induced by alcohol consumption and other disease.[370] A number of paraneoplastic syndromes have been described including hypoglycemia, erythrocytosis, and hypercalcemia.[368] US is considered a good screening imaging modality, but advanced imaging with contrast-enhanced CT or MRI is preferred to determine the location, size, and extent of hepatic lesions.[368] Other tests include serum α-fetoprotein, serologic tests for hepatitis B and C viruses, and histologic confirmation with core liver biopsies.[368] Unlike HCC in dogs, the morphology of HCC in humans is often nodular or diffuse, which makes definitive treatment more problematic. Treatment options depend on the stage of disease and include surgery (e.g., liver lobectomy and liver transplantation), local ablative therapies (e.g., cryosurgery, ethanol or acetic acid injection, and microwave or radiofrequency ablation), regional therapies (e.g., transarterial chemotherapy, embolization, chemoembolization, or RT), and systemic treatment with chemotherapy or immunotherapy.[368] Response rates to single- and multiple-agent chemotherapy protocols are less than 25%, and chemotherapy is no longer recommended for human patients with HCC.[370]

Bile duct carcinomas are rare and, similar to those in cats and dogs, often associated with a poor prognosis.[382] Risk factors include primary sclerosing cholangitis, the liver flukes *Opisthorchis viverrini* and *Clonorchis sinensis* in endemic areas of Southeast Asia and China, and cholelithiasis.[382] Surgical resection is preferred but, because of the high rate of local or regional recurrence, adjuvant treatment with RT or chemotherapy is recommended.[382] However, because of the rarity of this tumor, studies supporting the efficacy of these adjuvant treatments are lacking. Papillary histology, extrahepatic location, and complete resection are favorable prognostic factors in humans with bile duct carcinomas.[432]

SECTION G: INTESTINAL TUMORS

LAURA E. SELMIC, KIM A. SELTING AND JENNIFER K. REAGAN

Incidence and Risk Factors

Intestinal tumors are rare in dogs and cats.[433–435] In a survey of insured dogs in the United Kingdom, a standardized incidence rate of 210/100,000 dogs was reported for alimentary tumors and this accounted for 8% of all tumor submissions.[436] Incidence of feline digestive neoplasia in a South African survey comprised 13.5% of all tumors, which likely included oral tumors.[437] In the United States, a query of more than 300,000 cat submissions to the Veterinary Medical Database found 8% to relate to cancer and less than 1% (13% of the cancer cases) to be intestinal neoplasia.[438] Regarding specific tumor types, lymphoma comprises nearly 30% of all feline tumors and 6% of all canine tumors and is the most common intestinal tumor in most reports.[434,439–441] In 163 cases of feline lymphoma, the intestine was the most commonly affected site.[442] Adenocarcinoma is the second most frequent tumor in both species, with mast cell tumors (MCTs) in cats and leiomyosarcomas or gastrointestinal stromal tumors (GISTs) in dogs the third most common tumors.

As with many cancers, the incidence of intestinal neoplasia increases in older dogs and cats. Mean ages of affected cats for small and large intestinal neoplasia generally range between 10 and 12 years, and increasing risk after 7 years of age has been reported.[434,438,442–448] Dogs are also usually middle aged or older, with mean ages most often between 6 and 9 years and possibly older (12 years) for dogs with leiomyosarcoma.[443,448–452]

Overall, there may be a slight sex predilection for males to develop intestinal tumors. Many studies report a near equal incidence among male and female dogs,[452–455] although one study did find 76% of dogs with intestinal adenocarcinoma to be male.[456] Males also appear overrepresented for smooth muscle tumors,[448] comprising 82% of gastrointestinal (GI) leiomyomas[457] and 76% of dogs with leiomyosarcoma.[451] In addition, 90% of dogs with GI lymphoma were male[448] and there was a slight male predominance in nonlymphomatous tumors.[441,458,459] In cats, males have greater representation in some studies,[446,460] while only slightly exceeding or equaling females in other studies.[445,446,460–462]

Siamese cats are 1.8 times more likely to develop intestinal neoplasia[438] and are overrepresented in studies of intestinal adenocarcinoma, up to eight times greater than other breeds.[434,438,444,458,461] Although small numbers of Siamese cats are included in many series of feline intestinal lymphoma, one study did show a significant overrepresentation.[443] Otherwise, there is no breed predilection for intestinal lymphoma in cats. In dogs, few studies of intestinal neoplasia report an overrepresentation of specific breeds. Large-breed dogs in general constituted most cases in a series of smooth muscle tumors.[454] Collies and German shepherd dogs are overrepresented in some reports for intestinal tumors, especially adenocarcinoma, rectal carcinoma, and rectal polyps.[449,463] In a recent Czech necropsy study, breed predispositions were identified in the pug, Leonberger, and English setter for intestinal adenoma; in the English setter and Hovawart for intestinal adenocarcinoma; and the Doberman and Hovawart for intestinal lymphoma.[448] MCTs have been reported primarily in Maltese. Although these reports came from Japan, where small breeds are popular, more than 50% of reported cases in two series were in Maltese dogs with a male predominance.[464,465]

With the exception of retroviral influence on the development of feline lymphoma, there are no known etiologic organisms or chemical agents that reliably contribute to the development of spontaneously occurring intestinal neoplasia in dogs and cats. A recent retrospective study in 55 cats with intestinal carcinoma showed significant association between the presence of *Helicobacter* species and development of poorly differentiated large intestinal mucinous adenocarcinoma.[466] The findings of this study suggest *Helicobacter* spp. may play a possible role in intestinal carcinoma formation and determining site of development in cats.[466] However, it has also been suggested *Helicobacter* species in the feces may represent normal flora rather than pathogens.[467]

Pathology and Natural Behavior

Epithelial, mesenchymal, neuroendocrine, and discrete/round cell neoplasias can all be found in the intestinal tract. Although most small intestinal tumors are malignant in dogs, most rectal tumors are benign polyps, adenomas, or carcinomas in situ (Fig. 23.24).[455,468]

When tumors of the GI system metastasize, sites of predilection in decreasing frequency include mesenteric LNs (especially adenocarcinoma), liver (especially leiomyosarcoma), mesentery, omentum, spleen, kidney, bone, peritoneum (e.g., carcinomatosis), and lung.[441,458,462,469] Interestingly, metastasis from intestinal adenocarcinoma was discovered in three dogs initially presented for testicular masses.[470] One dog was presented for multiple cutaneous masses that IHC confirmed were epithelial in origin and a primary small intestinal adenocarcinoma with additional visceral metastasis was diagnosed at necropsy.[471] GI

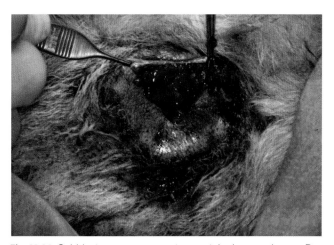

• **Fig. 23.24** Cobblestone appearance to a rectal adenocarcinoma. Dogs with this tumor type live an average of 12 months after surgical excision. (Courtesy Dr. Eric Pope, Ross University, College of Veterinary Medicine.)

lymphoma is often a systemic disease; 25% of dogs and 80% of cats will have concurrent involvement of other organs.[443,450]

Lymphoma

Lymphoma is the most common type of small intestinal neoplasia in cats and dogs. For feline intestinal lymphoma, subtypes include lymphocytic, lymphoblastic, epitheliotropic, and large granular lymphocyte (LGL) types. Intestinal lymphoma in dogs occurs in the stomach and small intestine equally and more often in both of these sites than in the large intestine. For additional information regarding canine and feline lymphoma the reader is referred to Chapter 33, Sections A and B.

Adenomatous Polyps and Adenocarcinoma

Most alimentary adenocarcinoma in cats is found in the small intestine[433,456,462]; however, the colon and rectum are more common sites in dogs.[472,473] For colorectal adenocarcinomas, the rectum is a more common site than the colon.[474] The cecum is more likely to develop leiomyosarcomas or GISTs than adenocarcinoma.[451,473] Histologic descriptors for carcinoma of the intestine include adeno- (forming glands), mucinous (>50% mucin), signet ring (>50% of cells have intracellular mucin), and undifferentiated or solid (no evidence of gland formation).[472] Grossly, colorectal adenocarcinomas may demonstrate a pedunculated (especially in the distal rectum), cobblestone (middle rectum), or annular (middle rectum) appearance, which may relate to behavior and prognosis (Fig. 23.25).[469,473,474]

Adenomatous polyps are found in the rectum of dogs and carcinomas in situ are found in both the colon and rectum. Most lesions are solitary, although multiple and diffuse lesions can be seen and are associated with increased recurrence rates.[455] A case series of 31 dogs with colorectal carcinoma found that most were B-cell, high-grade, and caused hematochezia.[475] Miniature dachshunds are overrepresented for inflammatory colorectal polyps, suggesting a breed predisposition in multiple case series from Japan.[476,477] The

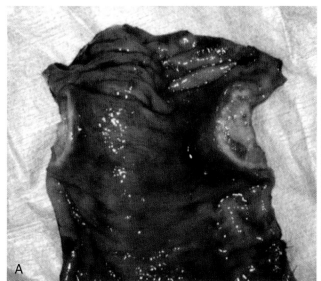
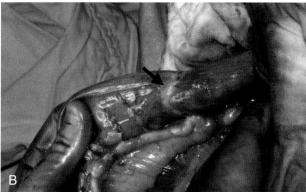

• **Fig. 23.25** An annular form of colonic adenocarcinoma causing a structure. The thick band of tissue (B) creating the stricture is seen on cross-section (A). In one study, dogs with this type of tumor survived an average of only 1.6 months. (Courtesy Dr. Eric Pope, Ross University, College of Veterinary Medicine.)

inflammatory polyps presented as multiple small polyps, whereas other colorectal polyps generally presented as either solitary or multiple lesions.[476,477] In cats, polyps are more common in the duodenum and intestinal obstruction resulting from a duodenal Brunner's gland adenoma has been reported in a dog.[478]

Leiomyomas, Leiomyosarcomas, and GISTs

Leiomyomas occur more commonly in the stomach, but have also been reported in the esophagus, small intestine, and colorectum.[457] GISTs are well documented in humans and have been reported in dogs and cats.[479–481] These nonlymphoid tumors of mesenchymal origin were originally diagnosed as leiomyosarcomas and some, but not all, were leiomyomas. Histologically, GISTs are highly cellular mesenchymal tumors that do *not* show ultrastructural characteristics consistent with smooth muscle differentiation. GISTs are thought to arise from multipotential stem cells phenotypically similar to interstitial cells of Cajal, driven by activating mutations of c-*Kit* (a proto-oncogene). Although these cells can differentiate into smooth muscle cells if deprived of KIT (a receptor tyrosine kinase), GISTs are a discrete clinical entity from leiomyosarcoma.[482] Leiomyosarcomas are positive for smooth muscle actin and desmin and negative for KIT. GISTs are distinguished by high vimentin immunoreactivity, low alpha smooth muscle actin reactivity, and CD117 (KIT) reactivity, and arise primarily in the small and large intestine.[457,483,484] c-*Kit* exon 11 mutations have been found to occur frequently in canine GISTs, which is similar to human GISTs, where exon 11 mutations occur in 60% to 70% of cases and mutations in exon 9 occur in 5% to 10% of cases.[457,485] To date, only one dog with an exon 9 mutation has been reported.[486] CD117 (KIT) reactivity is considered a major diagnostic criterion and is used to distinguish GISTs from leiomyosarcomas in many studies.[487,488] When stratified as such, 28 of 42 leiomyosarcomas in dogs were reclassified as GISTs and only 2 of the 28 cases of GIST metastasized (7%), with those dogs living longer than dogs with leiomyosarcoma.[487] These investigators also found that GISTs were significantly more likely to occur in the large intestine, specifically the cecum, and leiomyosarcomas in the stomach and small intestine,[487] yet a recent study contradicted this finding with GISTs occurring primarily in the small intestine.[484] Considering these findings, the incidence of true leiomyosarcoma is likely low because many previously reported cases may have actually been GISTs. The inclusion of GISTs as leiomyosarcomas will also have caused confounding of clinical behavior in these studies. In addition to the effect on incidence, conflicting reports of biologic behavior are problematic. Although the study cited earlier found a 7% rate of metastasis for dogs with GISTs and a worse prognosis for dogs with leiomyosarcoma, a recent study reported a higher rate of metastasis (27%) in GISTs and no metastasis in dogs with leiomyosarcomas.[484]

Mast Cell Tumors

Intestinal MCTs are the third most common tumor after lymphoma and adenocarcinoma in cats, but their incidence and behavior are poorly reported. For further details, the reader is referred to Chapter 21.

Other Tumor Types

The term *carcinoid* refers to tumors that arise from the diffuse endocrine system rather than the intestinal epithelium, despite histologic similarity to carcinomas. Carcinoid cells arise from enterochromaffin cells of the intestinal mucosa and contain secretory granules that may contain substances such as 5-hydroxytryptamine (serotonin), secretin, somatostatin, and gastrin, among others.[472] IHC for cytokeratin and for secretory substances, such as serotonin, may be positive, and serum concentration of serotonin has been documented at 10 times the normal range in one dog with a carcinoid.[489] Carcinoids have been described in many species and may occur in both the large and the small intestines and frequently metastasize to the liver.[434,473,489] Carcinoids may follow an aggressive and debilitating clinical course.[489]

Extramedullary plasmacytomas (EMPs) are solitary tumors with no evidence of systemic multiple myeloma and the reader is referred to Chapter 33, Section D , where they are covered in detail. Another uncommon tumor type is extraskeletal OSA, which has been reported in the duodenum of a cat.[490] This cat had no evidence of metastasis at diagnosis and did well for 4 months after surgery when clinical signs recurred and the cat died.[490] Three of 55 extraskeletal and 145 total cases of feline OSA were of intestinal origin.[491] A series of four cats was reported with intestinal hemangiosarcoma arising from four different locations within the intestines; no cat survived greater than 1 week.[492] Finally, one dog was diagnosed with ganglioneuroma of the rectum and experienced long-term survival after surgical resection.[493] Small intestinal ganglioneuromatosis has also been reported in a dog with a similar good outcome after surgical resection.[494]

Molecular Aspects

With an increasing armamentarium of molecular diagnostics, insights into the pathogenesis, progression, and prognosis of tumors are constantly emerging. Cellular adhesion and invasion (e.g., Tenascin-C,[463,495] versica, hyaluronan,[496] β-catenin, and E-cadherin[497–499]), stromal remodeling, and alterations in tumor suppressor genes (e.g., *p53*[497,499–501]) may play a role in the development and progression of intestinal neoplasia. The importance of the relationship between a tumor cell and its stroma should not be underestimated. Although molecular markers/targets likely play an important role in intestinal tumors, the utility of these in diagnostics, prognostication, and therapy in companion animal species, with the exception of GIST and CD117 expression, is limited.[481]

COX enzymes are responsible for prostaglandin synthesis and COX-2 is overexpressed in many head/neck and genitourinary tumors, creating a possible therapeutic target. COX-2 has been identified in both benign and malignant small intestinal and colorectal epithelial tumors in dogs, although the number of positive cells varies and was very low in some studies.[502,503] In addition, one study found no COX-2 staining in 13 intestinal tumors in cats.[504] COX inhibitors are thus of questionable value in treating intestinal tumors.

History and Clinical Signs

The duration of clinical signs before presentation typically averages 6 to 8 weeks, but can range from less than 1 day to several months.[441,450,451] Clinical signs include (in varying order of frequency): weight loss, diarrhea, vomiting, and anorexia, and, less frequently, melena, anemia, and hypoglycemia (with smooth muscle tumors).[434,441,444,453,460,461,505–508] Clinical signs often relate to location of the tumor within the GI tract. Proximal lesions more commonly result in vomiting;

small intestinal lesions in weight loss; and large bowel lesions in hematochezia and tenesmus.[456,458] Although carcinoids may secrete endocrine substances, clinical signs do not always reflect hypersecretion.[472] Dogs and cats may present with clinical signs relating to intestinal obstruction, such as anorexia, weight loss, and vomiting. In dogs with cecal GISTs, 25% to 32% cause perforation which results in a localized peritonitis and clinical signs of an acute abdomen.[487,488] Smooth muscle tumors are located within the muscular layer of the intestines and not within the lumen and evidence of GI bleeding is often absent, but anemia and melena have been reported.[451,452] Clinical signs of chronic small bowel disease should not be ignored in cats, as 96% to 99% had abnormalities on biopsy consistent with inflammatory bowel disease (IBS) or neoplasia (lymphoma, MCT, adenocarcinoma).[507,508]

Paraneoplastic Syndromes

One dog was presented for alopecia and *Cheyletiella* infection within 2 months of euthanasia for abdominal carcinomatosis from intestinal carcinoma. The neoplasia was not identified with abdominal US at the original workup, but immunosuppression resulting from an underlying neoplasia was thought to lead to opportunistic *Cheyletiella* infection. Although pruritus resolved with ivermectin therapy, alopecia persisted, suggesting a paraneoplastic origin.[509] Alopecia has also been reported as a paraneoplastic syndrome secondary to a metastasizing colonic carcinoma in a cat.[510] Neutrophilic leukocytosis (in one dog associated with monocytosis and eosinophilia) has been reported in dogs with rectal tumors. Resolution or improvement of hematologic abnormalities occurred after treatment for adenomatous rectal polyps.[502,511] Hypereosinophilia and eosinophilic tumor infiltrates have been reported in a cat and several dogs with intestinal T-cell lymphoma; the suggested cause was IL-5 secretion by the neoplastic lymphocytes.[512–514] EMP may lead to a hyperviscosity syndrome resulting from overproduction of immunoglobulin.[515] Erythrocytosis managed with periodic phlebotomy was related to a cecal leiomyosarcoma in a 14-year-old dog. The diagnosis was made at postmortem 2 years later; erythropoietin mRNA and protein were isolated from tumor cells, suggesting ectopic erythropoietin production as the cause of the erythrocytosis.[516] Hypoglycemia has also reported with intestinal smooth muscle tumors as a paraneoplastic syndrome.[517] Nephrogenic diabetes insipidus has also been documented in one dog with intestinal leiomyosarcoma.[518]

Diagnostic Techniques and Workup

Physical Examination

An abdominal mass may be palpated on initial examination in approximately 20% to 40% of dogs with lymphoma[450,453] and 20% to 50% of dogs with nonlymphomatous solid intestinal tumors.[441,456,458] Pain and fever were reported in 20% of dogs with lymphoma in one report.[450] Digital rectal examination may identify masses or annular strictures due to rectal tumors or polyps in as high as 63% of dogs.[456,474] Abdominal masses are also often readily palpated in cats with both lymphoma and adenocarcinoma.[444,445,458,460] Dehydration is also common and occurs in 30% to 60% of cats with nonlymphomatous tumors.[444,458]

Clinical Pathology

Complete Blood Count

Anemia is common in dogs and cats with intestinal tumors and is often not characterized, but may occur in conjunction with melena and elevated blood urea nitrogen (BUN). Anemia affects nearly 40% of dogs in most studies and as low as 15% but up to 70% of cats.[441,445,451,452,456,458,460] Leukogram changes are also common including leukocytosis in 25% to 70% of dogs and 40% of cats.[441,444,452,458] A left shift may be seen as well as monocytosis in some patients.[458,460]

Chemistry Profile

Biochemical abnormalities are similar between dogs and cats with intestinal tumors. As a result of malabsorption, hypoproteinemia may be present in one-fourth to one-third of patients.[441,444,445,452,453,456] Other common abnormalities include elevated liver enzymes, specifically alkaline phosphatase in 15% to 33% of dogs and up to 85% of cats with nonlymphomatous neoplasia.[441,452,456,458,460] In one series, high cholesterol was seen in 41% of cats with nonlymphomatous tumors.[458] An elevated BUN has been reported in 13% of dogs and 30% of cats with intestinal adenocarcinoma.[441,444] This may be a result of concurrent renal insufficiency, intestinal bleeding due to the tumor, or dehydration. Although some cats may have hyperglycemia,[458] smooth muscle tumors can cause up to 55% of patients to be hypoglycemic as a result of insulin-like growth factor secretion.[451] Dogs may also have increased amylase and electrolyte disturbances,[456] and patients with lymphoma may be hypercalcemic.[445] Serum alpha 1-acid glycoprotein, an acute-phase reactant protein, may be increased in cats with cancer, but this lacks specificity and prognostic relevance.[519,520]

Cytology and Histopathology

As with other anatomic sites, cytology of the intestinal tract can help differentiate major tumor types. In addition, lymphocyte accumulations can be tested using polymerase chain reaction (PCR) for antigen receptor rearrangement (PARR) for clonality (see Chapter 33, Section A and B for further details). In cats, mucosal biopsies of the upper GI tract are commonly obtained in a minimally invasive fashion using endoscopy. Despite the superiority of full thickness biopsies (because submucosal and muscularis infiltration can be characterized), the ease of endoscopic biopsy has resulted in rigorous evaluation of ancillary diagnostics to improve accuracy on these samples. Because of reported eosinophilia with intestinal lymphoma and reports of MCT with concurrent small T-cell lymphoma in cats, it may be challenging to distinguish between the two tumor types.[512,521,522]

Imaging

Abdominal Radiographs and Ultrasound

In dogs and cats with intestinal lymphoma, concurrent enlargement of liver, spleen, and/or mesenteric LNs may be seen.[450] Plain abdominal radiographs may reveal an abdominal mass in approximately 40% of both dogs and cats, although some reports are higher for solid tumor types and lower for lymphoma.[441,444,445,450,452,458] An obstructive pattern may also be seen on plain radiographs in 10% to 75% of cats and dogs.[441,452,456,458] Other abnormalities may include poor serosal detail and thickened stomach wall.[445]

Contrast radiography, although used less after advances in US, has often been used to evaluate patients with signs of primary GI disease. US can help facilitate noninvasive localization of the tumor and identification of other sites of metastasis or involvement. It also can guide needle aspiration or needle biopsy or assist in treatment planning. US is a more sensitive diagnostic test than radiographs for identifying a mass.[441,451,454,523] US is also less time consuming than contrast radiography, and the increased use, availability, and operator skill for the former has diminished the need for the latter.

US findings in dogs and cats with intestinal neoplasia most consistently include bowel wall thickening and loss of normal wall layering.[456,523,524] Intestinal lymphoma in dogs more often results in long segments of involved bowel and either a solitary mass or diffusely thickened bowel loops with thickening of the muscularis propria in cats.[506,524,525] However, the normal appearance of intestine does not rule out the presence of lymphoma, as one study showed 26% of dogs diagnosed with GI lymphoma did not have sonographic abnormalities.[526] Adenocarcinoma in cats has been described as having mixed echogenicity and was asymmetric in three of five cats.[523] In one study, two-thirds of dogs with intestinal adenocarcinoma had hypoechoic tumors and most had decreased motility.[456] These masses averaged 4 cm long with a median wall thickness of 1.2 cm.[456,473] MCTs have an eccentric appearance with alteration, but not loss of wall layering, commonly involving the muscularis propria.[522] Smooth muscle tumors are characteristically large (median diameter 4.8 cm) and anechoic/hypoechoic, and a muscular layer origin may be identified. Leiomyomas may have a smooth contour.[454] One report of metastatic mammary carcinoma to the small intestine described the appearance as multiple, hypoechoic, well-defined or marginated nodules within the muscularis layer of the jejunum that did not disrupt the intestinal layering.[527]

Degree of thickening, distribution of lesion(s), and symmetry are used to help differentiate neoplastic from nonneoplastic disease.[528] In one study, 99% of dogs with neoplasia had a loss of wall layering and this was associated with a 50 times greater likelihood of neoplasia than enteritis (Fig. 23.26).[524] In addition, dogs with

walls thicker than 1 cm are nearly four times as likely to have a tumor and those with focal lesions are nearly 20 times as likely to have a tumor.[524] Nevertheless, possible differential diagnoses include fungal (pythiosis and histoplasmosis) masses, as these can mimic neoplasia.[528] In general, neoplasia exhibits more dramatic thickening with loss of wall layering and greater LN enlargement, as well as more frequent focal lesions than nonneoplastic intestinal disease.[528] Similar changes (thickened muscularis propria, and ratio of muscularis to mucosa >1) can be seen in cats with intestinal lymphoma, but do not reliably distinguish neoplasia from IBD.[529] In a series of 14 cats with carcinomatosis, three of which were a result of small intestinal tumors (two carcinomas and one lymphoma), the hallmark ultrasonographic finding was the presence of masses in the double sheet portion of peritoneum that connects the visceral and parietal portions (100% of cats); all cats also had free peritoneal fluid.[530]

Thoracic Radiographs

Thoracic radiographs are critical to the complete evaluation of the cancer patient. For dogs with nonlymphomatous intestinal tumors, yield is low, with very few patients presenting with pulmonary metastasis.[441] This may be due to a bias in reporting because many reports detail outcome of treatment and patients with metastatic disease may not receive treatment. In fact, many case series report no evidence of metastasis on initial evaluation for solid tumors of the intestine in dogs.[441,451,452,456,458] Two of 14 cats in one series and no cats in another series had pulmonary nodules at initial evaluation.[444,458] For cats and dogs with lymphoma, enlarged sternal or perihilar LNs, pleural effusion, or diffuse interstitial changes may be seen.[445,450]

Endoscopy, Colonoscopy, and Laparoscopy

Minimally invasive methods of collecting tissues to aid in diagnosis are increasingly used. Endoscopic findings in dogs with intestinal lymphoma include an irregular cobblestone or patchy erythematous appearance to the duodenal mucosa and poor distensibility and elasticity of the duodenal wall.[453] Colonoscopy can be considered to evaluate for multiple colorectal masses as well as

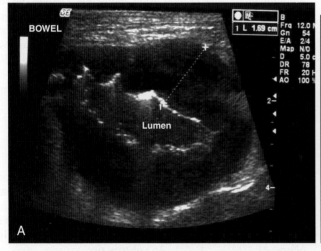
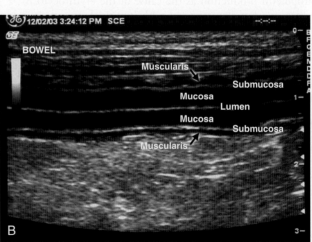

• **Fig. 23.26** A cross-sectional ultrasound image of a segment of small intestine with lymphoma (A) is compared with a longitudinal view of a segment of normal small intestine (B). Note that the clearly defined intestinal layers in the normal tissue are completely effaced in the tumor tissue. A loss of layering is strongly supportive of neoplasia. The diseased bowel is also markedly thickened, suggesting neoplasia. (Courtesy Dr. Stephanie Essman, University of Missouri, College of Veterinary Medicine.)

obtain biopsy samples; however, single rectal masses appear to be more common in dogs and these masses were not present beyond the colorectal border.[531] Therefore proctoscopy or transanal single laparoscopic port evaluation may provide information regarding mass number and characteristics without the need for extensive bowel preparation and surgical delay.[531] Of note, 5 of 16 dogs (31%) had different colonoscopy biopsy results compared with the final histopathology results with a tendency to underdiagnose malignancy.[531] Interobserver variation is likely to be more pronounced with small tissue samples and this is a limitation of these less invasive approaches.

Exploratory Laparotomy

When noninvasive or minimally invasive diagnostics fail to confirm a diagnosis, an exploratory laparotomy may be indicated for dogs and cats with persistent signs of GI disease. Benefits include direct visualization of all abdominal viscera and the ability to collect full-thickness biopsies of all segments of intestines and other viscera. Patients with resectable solid tumors may be both diagnosed and treated in a single procedure with intestinal resection and anastomosis. In a series of dogs with GI lymphoma, endoscopic biopsies were sometimes difficult to interpret because of lymphoplasmacytic infiltrate, but surgical biopsies obtained by laparotomy confirmed the diagnosis in all cases.[450] In a study evaluating 367 dogs and cats undergoing GI biopsies, the risk of GI dehiscence was found to be very low (1% dogs, <3% cats) with possible risk factors in cats being neoplasia and hypoalbuminemia, although these had wide confidence intervals.[532] It should be noted that carcinomatosis should not always be seen as an indication for euthanasia (Fig. 23.27). After removal of the primary intestinal adenocarcinoma, two cats with malignant effusion lived 4.5 and 28 months after surgery.[444]

Therapy and Prognosis

Surgery

With the exception of lymphoma, surgical resection is the primary treatment for intestinal tumors. Lymphoma is treated primarily with chemotherapy except when intestinal perforation or the need for a biopsy necessitates surgery (Fig. 23.28). As long as severe extraserosal invasion and/or adhesions do not complicate the surgical approach, complete excision of intestinal tumors is often possible. For dogs and cats without evidence of local or distant metastasis, long-term survival is possible, although some tumors may later metastasize. Overall, the 1-year survival rate is approximately 40% for dogs with solid small intestinal tumors.[441] For cats with adenocarcinoma, approximately 50% will metastasize to the local LNs, 30% to the peritoneal cavity (carcinomatosis), and 20% or less to the lungs.[434,458,462] Dogs have similar rates of metastasis to LNs for both adenocarcinoma and leiomyosarcoma, although the liver is usually the second most frequent site.[441,458,473] Perioperative mortality can approach 30% to 50% as a result of sepsis, peritonitis, or owner decision for euthanasia when nonresectable tumors are present.[441,451]

Small Intestine

Intestinal resection and anastomosis is the most common surgical technique for tumors of the small intestine. Stapling techniques have been shown to be equivalent to hand suturing in both the large and small intestine.[533,534] Canine small intestinal adenocarcinoma has a guarded prognosis with a mean survival time (ST) of only 12 days without treatment and a mean ST of 114 days after surgical resection, though others report median STs (MSTs) of 7 and 10 months.[441,456,458] Dogs with leiomyosarcoma who survive the perioperative period have MSTs of 1.1 to almost 2 years.[451,452] One case series found the MST for 28 dogs with GIST to be approximately 38 months (1 year if postoperative deaths were included) versus an MST of 8 months for 10 dogs with leiomyosarcoma, although this difference was not statistically significant.[487] Another study found no difference in survival between dogs with GIST and leiomyosarcoma with 1-year survival rates of approximately 80% for both tumor types (Fig. 23.29).[488] The benefit of surgery is questionable for dogs with intestinal MCTs. In two case series, most dogs died within the first month. Only 2 of 49 dogs (combined total for two series with almost all being GI MCTs) lived past 180 days and prednisone was not helpful in most cases.[465,466]

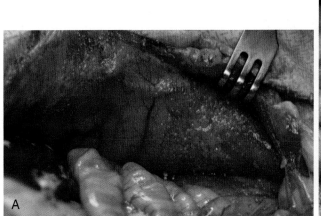
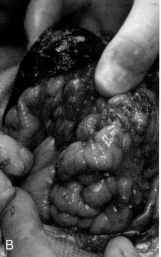

• **Fig. 23.27** Carcinomatosis discovered at exploratory laparotomy. Note the irregular peritoneal surface instead of a normal glossy appearance (A) and the multiple serosal implants (B). (Courtesy Dr. F. A. Mann, University of Missouri, College of Veterinary Medicine.)

In cats with small intestinal adenocarcinoma, there is significant perioperative risk, but cats that live beyond 2 weeks may experience long-term control with surgery alone (Fig. 23.30). In two series, all cats that did not have their tumors resected were euthanized or died within 2 weeks of surgery.[444,458] After surgical resection, one-half of cats in one report and all cats in another study died within 2 weeks of surgery, and 4 of 11 cats surviving beyond 2 weeks died within 2 months of complications or other nontumor causes.[444,458,462] For eleven of the 12 cats that survived 2 weeks beyond surgery, mean ST was 15 months, although in another report the MST was 2.5

months.[444,461] For details about outcome after treatment for alimentary lymphoma see Chapter 33, Sections A and B.

Large Intestine

There are various approaches for removal of tumors from the large intestine based on the size, location, and depth of penetration of the mass. Generally, for rectal mucosal masses suspected to be benign polyps, the masses can be removed via mucosal eversion and submucosal resection.[535] Transrectal endoscopic removal of benign canine rectal tumors can be considered if more extensive surgery is required because of the location of the tumor. Using this technique, five of six dogs showed significant improvement in quality of life and three dogs were cured; however, one dog died due to rectal perforation, which is a known complication of this procedure.[536] The other disadvantage of this technique is there is often incomplete removal of the mass, as it is usually removed piecemeal. In a recent case report, this technique was modified to inject saline to separate the mucosa from the submucosa to improve visibility and the ability to completely remove

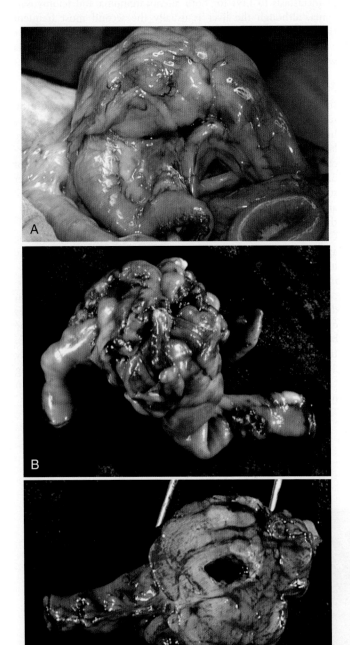

• **Fig. 23.28** Intestinal lymphoma in a dog (A). The specimen is shown after resection and anastomosis (B) and on cross-section (C) to illustrate the marked thickening of the bowel wall. (Courtesy Dr. Eric Pope, Ross University, College of Veterinary Medicine.)

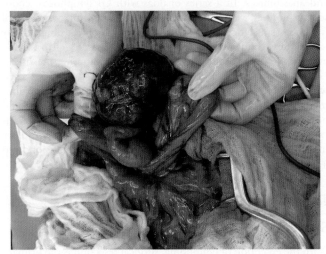

• **Fig. 23.29** Cecal gastrointestinal stromal tumor seen at exploratory laparotomy. Note the darkly colored perforated area of the tumor that led to septic peritonitis in this dog. (Courtesy Dr. E. A. Maxwell, University of Illinois, College of Veterinary Medicine.)

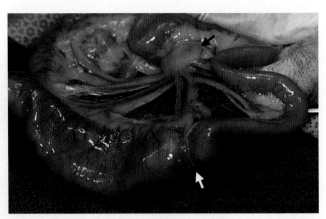

• **Fig. 23.30** Intestinal obstruction as a result of adenocarcinoma (*white arrow*). Note the distention of the jejunum oral to the mass compared with the normal diameter aboral to the mass. There is also an enlarged lymph node (*black arrow*). (Courtesy Dr. Eric Pope, Ross University, College of Veterinary Medicine.)

the mass.[537] For malignant rectal tumors, full-thickness removal of the rectum is generally indicated. Rectal-pull through is commonly performed for rectal adenocarcinomas. This can be performed through either a perineal or combined perineal-abdominal approach.[538,539] Complications are relatively common, including fecal incontinence (57% total with 40% permanent fecal incontinence), diarrhea (43%), tenesmus (31%), stricture formation (21%), rectal bleeding (11%), dehiscence (8%), and infection (5%).[538] Colostomy use has been reported to aid in management of dogs with nonresectable rectal tumors. In one report, skin excoriation was the most common complication, but colostomy bags were managed for up to 7 months.[540]

For rectal polyps and carcinomas in situ, depending on the surgical technique used for resection, local recurrence of clinical signs is reported in up to 41% of dogs and 18% of dogs had malignant transformation associated with tumor recurrence.[455] Surgical removal of duodenal polyps in cats is typically curative.[446] For dogs with colorectal adenocarcinoma, local excision results in MSTs of 2 to more than 4 years compared with 15 months for stool softeners alone;[474,475,539,541] colorectal EMPs and polyps also fare well with MSTs of 15 months and 2 years or more, respectively, after surgical excision.[464,542]

In cats with large intestinal neoplasia, STs after surgery alone are approximately 3.5 months for lymphoma, 4.5 months for adenocarcinoma, and 6.5 months for MCT. Subtotal colectomy has been recommended for cats with colonic adenocarcinoma.[447,543] Adjuvant chemotherapy has improved STs for cats with adenocarcinoma, but not for lymphoma.[447]

Chemotherapy

No randomized studies exist to investigate the efficacy of adjuvant chemotherapy after resection of epithelial intestinal tumors in dogs and cats. The benefit of adjuvant chemotherapy in humans is questionable, although current fluorouracil-based regimens are often considered to be the standard of care. When attempted, adjuvant chemotherapy typically includes doxorubicin in veterinary medicine. One retrospective study in cats with colonic adenocarcinoma treated with subtotal colectomy did show a significant survival advantage for cats receiving adjuvant doxorubicin; MSTs were 280 days with and 56 days without chemotherapy.[447] In another retrospective study using adjuvant carboplatin, the MST was 269 days, but no controls were included to evaluate treatment without chemotherapy.[543] Distant and nodal metastases were found to be negative prognostic indicators, with an MST of 200 days versus 340 days and 178 days versus 328 days, respectively.[543] For carcinomatosis, intracavitary therapy may be helpful with carboplatin for cats or cisplatin or 5-fluorouracil (5-FU) for dogs.[544] For further details about treatment of alimentary lymphoma please see Chapter 33, Sections A and B.

Individual case reports in dogs using receptor tyrosine kinase inhibitors (TKIs, imatinib and toceranib phosphate) to treat GISTs in the setting of metastatic disease, nonresectable disease, or recurrent disease have shown good responses with partial (PR, n = 1) or complete responses (n = 2) for greater than 140 days, greater than 9 months, and greater than 4 years, respectively.[486,545,546] The only toxicity seen was in one dog, and this manifested as an increase in ALT resulting in dose reduction of imatinib.[546] After this dose decrease, the PR ceased, which could have been due to the lower dose or emergence of resistance as has been documented in human GISTs due to a second site mutation in c-kit.[546] Imatinib has also been reported in the treatment of canine intestinal

MCT with metastasis to the spleen. A strong PR was seen but was brief in duration.[547]

A reduction in the size and clinical signs of rectal polyps in 8 dogs was noted after piroxicam therapy, either orally or in suppository form. Clinical response did not relate to whether there was inflammation associated with the tumor.[502]

Radiation Therapy

RT is seldom used in the treatment of intestinal tumors because of the concern regarding toxicity to surrounding abdominal viscera, the ability to often obtain adequate local control via surgery, and the inability to reliably irradiate the same tissue each day because of the mobility of the intestine.

Prognostic Factors

Intestinal perforation does not appear to be a negative prognostic factor for leiomyosarcoma because dogs surviving the perioperative period had prolonged STs in one series.[451] For colorectal tumors, treatment is prognostic, with local excision resulting in significantly better outcomes than palliative care. Gross appearance, although not statistically examined, may determine outcome because dogs with annular, obstructing masses survived a mean ST of 1.6 months whereas dogs nodular/cobblestone masses or single pedunculated masses had mean STs of 12 and 32 months, respectively.[474]

For nonlymphomatous small intestinal tumors in dogs, metastasis at the time of surgery resulted in significantly shorter STs (3 months vs. 15 months). The 1-year survival rates for dogs with and without LN metastasis were 20% and 67%, respectively.[441] In another study, however, dogs with and without visceral metastasis from leiomyosarcoma survived equally as long after surgical resection (21 months).[451] Male dogs with small intestinal adenocarcinoma had a significantly better outcome; however, the number of female dogs in that study was low.[456] Cats with adenocarcinoma, however, survived significantly longer if they were treated with subtotal colectomy (138 days vs. 68 days with mass excision), received postoperative doxorubicin (280 days with vs. 56 days without doxorubicin), and had no LN metastasis at surgery (259 days for no LN metastasis vs. 49 days with LN metastasis).[447] For further details about prognosis for dogs and cats with intestinal MCT see Chapter 21. For prognostic factors for canine and feline alimentary lymphoma see Chapter 33, Sections A and B.

Comparative Aspects

Although cancer of the large intestine and rectum is well characterized in humans, small intestinal neoplasia is rare. Theories for this discrepancy include more rapid small intestinal transit time compared with the large intestine (creating less contact time for carcinogens), dilution of carcinogens with fluid compared with solid stool, differences in pH, relative lack of bacteria to allow transformation of procarcinogens, presence of detoxifying enzymes, and increased presence of immunoglobulin A promoting local immunosurveillance of damaged cells as a result of increased lymphocytes in the small intestine. This is in contrast to veterinary medicine where in cats and sometimes dogs, malignant neoplasia is more common in the small intestine than the large intestine. This may reflect differences in physiology, diet, or genetics. As in animals, tumors of the small intestine of humans are usually malignant. Diagnostic evaluation is similar to that described in animals, although advanced imaging modalities, such as CT, are more often used. Most diagnoses are made at surgery and 5-year survival rates average approximately 20%.[548]

Large bowel/colorectal cancer is one of the most frequently diagnosed cancers in both men and women. Risk factors include genetic predisposition/familial history, tobacco and alcohol intake, advanced age, and predisposing medical conditions, among others. Colorectal cancer development may further be influenced by intake of red meat (especially fried), low-fiber and/or high-fat diets, obesity, fecal pH, and fecal mutagens. Among genetic risk factors, polymorphism in colonic enzymes and mutations leading to familial adenomatous syndromes are uncommon but are important as models of carcinogenesis. In most familial polyposis syndromes, the adenomatous polyposis coli (APC) gene is mutated. The multistage progression from benign polyp to carcinoma is well understood and underscores the importance of early detection.[549] Recently, the APC gene was found to be altered in about 70% of tested canine colorectal tumor samples, suggesting a similar molecular pathogenesis.[550] In contrast, hereditary nonpolyposis colon cancer develops without known premalignant polyps; this is inherited via autosomal dominance with high penetration and is characterized by microsatellite instability.[551]

In human medicine, GISTs are also subcategorized by the histopathologic morphology, a recent publication on canine intestinal tumor classification divided canine GISTs into 2 morphologic groups: spindlyloid/storiform and epitheloid, with the majority of GISTs in this study being spindlyloid.[484] In addition, it has been suggested in humans there may be a subset of GISTs that are KIT negative.[484] A recent study evaluated the use of protein 1 (DOG1) IHC marker to identify GISTs and it was found to have an increased specificity and sensitivity compared with KIT IHC.[552] In this study, 2 tumors were negative for KIT and positive for DOG1. This may indicate there is a subpopulation of GISTs in dogs that are also KIT negative. The authors concluded that utilizing diagnostic panels with KIT and DOG1 markers would improve the accuracy of diagnosis.[552]

The most clinically important aspects of comparative oncology when considering intestinal neoplasia in humans are the use of COX inhibitors in the treatment and prevention of colorectal neoplasia, and the use of TKIs. In people, KIT mutations in GISTs have led to the use of imatinib mesylate, a TKI that inhibits KIT.[553] This illustrates the notion of therapy directed at the molecular defect rather than the histologic diagnosis. KIT is mutated in some canine GISTs and thus TKIs may benefit this population as well. COX inhibition byNSAIDs decrease the incidence of colorectal cancer and mortality by 40% to 50%.[554] Among the proposed mechanisms of action, prostaglandin production may be related to tumor progression and therefore inhibition leads to cancer prevention. In addition, non-COX pathways include inhibition of transcription factors and induction of nuclear hormone receptors that lead to cellular differentiation.[554] Interestingly, a retrospective study found a significantly reduced incidence of cancer in dogs with a history of NSAID use (71% reduced risk).[555]

Therapy in humans is similar to that in companion animals. Surgical resection is the primary mode of therapy with adjuvant targeted or traditional chemotherapy in many cases, especially if patients present with LN metastasis or unresectable disease. TKIs may improve prognosis for unresectable and metastatic GISTs.[556] Adjuvant chemotherapy is used in colon cancer, with oxaliplatin in combination with capecitabine or with leukovorin and 5-FU,

but without a convincing increase in overall STs.[557] RT is used primarily for areas of the GI tract that are not very mobile, such as the stomach and rectum.

SECTION H: PERIANAL TUMORS

JULIUS M. LIPTAK AND MICHELLE M. TUREK

The perianal area of dogs contains several glands and structures from which tumors may develop. Perianal, or circumanal, glands are located in the dermis in a circular fashion around the anus and are also scattered in areas on the prepuce, tail, pelvic limbs, and trunk.[558] These are commonly referred to as hepatoid glands as a result of their cellular morphologic resemblance to hepatocytes and are considered nonsecretory sebaceous glands in the adult dog.[558,559] The anal sacs represent blind cutaneous diverticula that are located on each side of the anus at the 4 o'clock and 8 o'clock positions. Located in the connective tissue surrounding these diverticula are distinct apocrine sweat glands that empty their secretions into the lumen of the anal sacs. The most frequently observed tumors of this region in dogs include perianal sebaceous adenoma, perianal sebaceous adenocarcinoma, and apocrine gland anal sac adenocarcinoma (AGASAC). Other tumors arising from the anal sacs include squamous cell carcinoma (SCC) and malignant melanoma,[560–563] but benign tumors of the anal sac are rare.[564] Any cutaneous or subcutaneous tumor can affect the perianal region, including mast cell tumor, soft tissue sarcoma, squamous cell carcinoma, hemangiosarcoma, lymphoma, melanoma, leiomyoma, and transmissible venereal tumor.

Because cats do not have glands analogous to the perianal sebaceous glands in the dog, perianal adenoma and perianal adenocarcinoma are uncommonly recognized in this species. Apocrine gland adenocarcinoma of the anal sac occurs rarely in the cat.[565–567]

Perianal Adenoma and Adenocarcinoma

Incidence and Risk Factors

Perianal adenomas (circumanal, hepatoid tumors) represent the majority of canine perianal tumors (58%–96%).[558,568] Development and progression of these benign tumors appear to be sex hormone–dependent, with growth stimulated by androgenic hormones and supressed by estrogenic hormones.[558,569,570] Older, intact male dogs are at higher risk.[558,568,569] The mean reported age is 10 years.[568] A high incidence of associated testicular interstitial cell tumors has been reported for males with perianal adenomas, supporting testosterone production as a cause[569]; however, a true cause-and-effect relationship has not been clarified because interstitial cell tumors are also a common incidental finding in non–adenoma-bearing, older intact males. Perianal adenomas in the female occur almost exclusively in ovariohysterectomized animals in which low levels of estrogen do not suppress tumor growth. Rarely, androgenic steroid secretion from the adrenal glands, occasionally accompanied by signs of hyperadrenocorticism, may stimulate perianal adenoma formation in female dogs.[571,572] Cocker spaniels, beagles, bulldogs, and Samoyeds may be predisposed.[558,569] Some authors have proposed the term epithelioma to describe a subset of perianal sebaceous gland tumors.[573] Epitheliomas are considered low-grade malignancies with a greater tendency to be locally invasive and to recur after surgical excision.[574,575] To date, there is little clinical information to support a distinction between adenoma and epithelioma.

Perianal adenocarcinoma, a malignant tumor of the perianal glands, occurs much less frequently than its benign counterpart, representing only 3% to 21% of all tumors in this region.[558,568] The mean age of affected dogs is 11 years.[568,576] Tumors occur in castrated or intact males, as well as in females, implying no hormonal dependency; however, this does not preclude earlier hormonal initiation.[569,576] Large-breed male dogs appear to be overrepresented.[576]

Pathology and Natural Behavior

Perianal adenoma is benign. These are slow-growing tumors and, although local disease may be extensive, metastasis does not occur.[558,576]

Perianal adenocarcinoma is generally associated with a low rate of metastasis (<15%) at the time of diagnosis.[576] Metastasis may be more likely to develop later in the course of disease as the primary tumor becomes larger and more invasive.[576] The most frequent site of metastasis is the regional LNs.[558,576] Distant metastasis is rare, but has been reported in the lungs, liver, kidney, and bone.[569,576] This tumor tends to be more rapidly growing, fixed, and firmer than the more common benign perianal adenoma.

The pathogenesis of canine perianal tumors is not known. In a large study evaluating tumor growth characteristics of 240 perianal gland tumors, cell proliferation and apoptosis were quantified by proliferating cell nuclear antigen (PCNA) IHC and microscopic detection of apoptotic corpuscles.[577] Increases in both parameters were observed in perianal adenocarcinomas compared with perianal adenomas.[577] Ki67 immunoreactivity has also been evaluated and was found to increase from benign to malignant lesions, being highest in perianal adenocarcinomas and recurrent tumors.[574,575,578] Collectively, these results suggest that a high proliferative index may be related to tumor aggressiveness. Other IHC studies have attempted to elucidate possible molecular mechanisms involved in canine perianal gland tumorigenesis. Nuclear p53 accumulation was detected in 50% of perianal sebaceous gland adenocarcinomas in one study, suggesting that expression of a mutated p53 tumor suppressor protein may play a role.[579] Discordant results were reported in another study in which p53 reactivity was found in none of 11 perianal gland adenocarcinomas and in only a small percentage of adenomas.[580] In the same tumor samples, Mdm2 expression was observed in both adenomas and adenocarcinomas.[580] A study that evaluated androgen receptor expression found no difference between perianal adenomas and adenocarcinomas; the authors concluded that the mechanism by which androgens influence carcinogenesis is still unknown.[581] Vascular endothelial growth factor (VEGF) may also be involved in tumorigenesis. Serum VEGF levels corresponded with tumor aggressiveness and tumor burden in one study.[575] The same study suggested a correlation between serum 17-β-estradiol and VEGF levels, supporting the role of hormones in carcinogenesis in some perianal tumors.[575] Another proposed mediator of tumor development is growth hormone. Growth hormone was detected with IHC in 96% of perianal adenomas and 100% of perianal sebaceous gland adenocarcinomas.[582] Finally, serum magnesium levels were found to be higher in dogs with malignant perianal tumors than in those with benign tumors.[583]

History and Clinical Signs

Benign perianal adenomas tend to be slow-growing (over months to years) masses that are nonpainful and usually asymptomatic.

They may be single, multiple, or diffuse (similar to generalized hyperplasia or hypertrophy of the perianal tissue).[558] Most occur on the hairless skin around the anus, although they may extend to haired regions and can develop on the prepuce, scrotum, or tail head (stud tail or "caudal tail gland").[558] Benign lesions may ulcerate and become infected but are rarely adherent or fixed to deeper structures.[558] They are usually fairly well circumscribed, on average 0.5 to 3 cm in diameter, and elevated from the perineum.[558]

Perianal adenocarcinoma may have a similar gross appearance to perianal adenoma; however, they tend to have a faster growth rate, present more commonly as a larger and firmer mass with some degree of ulceration and fixation to deeper tissues, and they are more likely to recur after conservative surgical resection.[576] Perianal adenocarcinomas can be multiple.[573] Obstipation, dyschezia, or perianal pain or irritation can be seen with larger masses.[576] Rarely, clinical signs are related to obstruction of the pelvic canal by LN metastasis. Castrated male dogs with a new or recurrent perianal tumor may have an increased risk for malignant rather than benign disease because, unlike perianal adenoma, perianal adenocarcinomas are not hormonally dependent.

Diagnostic Techniques and Workup

Signalment, history, and physical examination findings will assist in developing a preliminary suspicion of tumor type as well as treatment planning. The mass should be palpated and a rectal examination performed to assess the degree of fixation and extent of the mass as well as the presence of enlarged LNs. Physical examination findings may provide some indication of whether a perianal mass is benign or malignant; however, there is a degree of overlap in the gross appearance of perianal adenoma and adenocarcinoma. FNA cytology to differentiate benign from malignant tumors can be unrewarding, although it is helpful in ruling out other tumor types. Incisional biopsy is recommended for definitive diagnosis and to better direct clinical staging tests and treatment options.[584] Malignant disease is more likely in tumors showing invasiveness into surrounding tissue, disorderly arrangement of cells, increased nuclear pleomorphism, and increased numbers of mitotic figures.[584] In some cases, a definitive diagnosis may not be possible histologically, and IHC with monoclonal antibodies against carcinoma-associated antigens 4A9, 1A10, as well as PCNA, and Ki67 may assist in differentiating perianal adenoma from adenocarcinoma.[573–578,585] In the rare event that differentiation from AGASAC is needed, cytokeratin expression patterns may be helpful.[586] Clinical validation is needed to confirm the utility of these IHC approaches.

For dogs with perianal adenocarcinoma, abdominal and thoracic imaging is recommended to investigate for the presence of metastatic disease. Up to 15% of dogs with perianal adenocarcinoma have evidence of metastatic disease at the time of diagnosis, and the regional LNs and lungs are the most common sites of metastasis.[558,569,576] Based on studies of canine AGASAC, advanced imaging modalities, such as CT and MRI, are superior to abdominal ultrasonography for the detection of enlarged LNs, particularly those within the pelvic canal. Although distant metastasis is uncommon, three-view thoracic radiographs or thoracic CT is recommended for the detection of pulmonary metastasis.

Treatment

Surgical resection is the recommended treatment for dogs with perianal adenomas and adenocarcinomas. Perianal adenomas can be excised with minimal margins of less than 1 cm, whereas larger margins are recommended for perianal adenocarcinomas because of their propensity for local recurrence after more conservative resections.[574] Castration is also recommended in intact male dogs with perianal adenomas because of the role of testosterone in the tumorigenesis of these tumors.[569,587] For diffuse or large perianal adenomas located on or in the anal sphincter, staged surgery may be preferable with castration initially to decrease tumor volume followed by surgical resection when the perianal adenoma is small enough that it can be more easily and safely resected. More than 90% of male dogs will be cured with castration and local resection of the perianal adenoma.[558,569]

Cryosurgery and carbon dioxide laser ablation are possible alternative treatment options for perianal adenomas, especially if small,[588,589] but the major limitation of these techniques is an inability to assess the surgical margins for the completeness of excision. Hyperthermia and RT have also been used successfully.[590,591] The cost, added morbidity, and limited availability of these modalities make them a poor alternative to standard surgical resection.

Electrochemotherapy has been described in dogs with perianal adenoma and consists of intratumoral injections of chemotherapy followed by local delivery of electric pulses to potentiate drug uptake by tumor cells.[587,592] Treatments are delivered in 1 or 2 weekly sessions. Based on limited studies, the reported overall response rate is greater than 90%, with 65% complete responses.[587,592] Smaller tumors (<5 cm) generally respond better than larger tumors.[587,592] Larger tumors are more likely to develop local complications, including focal necrosis, erythema, and inflammation.[587,592] Systemic effects are not reported.[587,592] Perianal adenoma may also regress after estrogen therapy[575]; however, its use is associated with a risk of myelosuppression. Cyclosporin is reported to have had a palliative effect in one dog with multiple ulcerated perianal adenomas and a measurable reduction in tumor size was observed.[593]

Perianal sebaceous gland adenocarcinoma is more locally invasive and generally does not respond to castration.[569] Aggressive surgical resection with a minimum of 1-cm lateral margins is recommended. Removal of one-half or more of the anal sphincter is possible with only rare transient loss of fecal continence. Preoperative incisional biopsy is recommended to differentiate perianal adenoma from adenocarcinoma because this differentiation may not be possible based on history, gross tumor characteristics, or cytology. If an excisional biopsy is performed, then there is a risk of incomplete histologic excision and local tumor recurrence. The rate of local tumor recurrence is unknown after incomplete histologic excision, but further surgery is complicated by the regional anatomy with a greater risk of treatment-associated morbidity. Adjuvant RT may improve local tumor control after incomplete excision; however, data for this approach are lacking. The use of electrochemotherapy has been reported in a small series of dogs.[587,592] Favorable outcomes have been reported, but additional clinical studies are needed to validate the efficacy of electrochemotherapy.[587,592]

Prognosis

The vast majority of dogs with perianal adenoma are cured with surgical resection and, if indicated, castration.[558,561] Serum VEGF levels may correlate with biologic behavior of this tumor type.[576]

In a series of 41 dogs with perianal adenocarcinoma, stage of tumor had a significant influence on DFI and overall survival times (OSTs).[576] Tumors less than 5 cm in diameter (T2) were associated with 2-year tumor control rates in excess of 60%,[576] suggesting that surgical removal of these masses at an early stage

is relatively successful with respect to disease control. The rate of metastasis at diagnosis is 15% and is a poor prognostic factor for survival.[576] The MST for dogs with LN or distant metastasis was 7 months; however, aggressive treatment was not attempted in five of six dogs.[576] In a smaller study, tumor recurrence occurred in 75% of dogs; however, tumor size, surgical approach, and completeness of excision were not reported.[574]

If present, regional LN metastasis may be resected and this may result in improved ST. The use of RT and/or chemotherapy, including actinomycin D, has been reported anecdotally, but their role in local or distant control is undefined.[576,594,595] Nuclear size, as measured by computer-assisted image analysis in cytologic tumor samples, and Ki67 expression may correlate with biologic behavior of perianal adenocarcinoma.[574,596]

Apocrine Gland Anal Sac Adenocarcinoma and Other Tumors of the Anal Sac

Incidence and Risk Factors

AGASAC accounts for 17% of perianal malignancies and 2% of all skin and subcutaneous tumors.[568,597] Spaniels, particularly English cocker spaniels, German shepherds, Alaskan malamutes, and dachshunds have been reported to have an increased risk of AGASAC.[598–601] A female predilection was reported in earlier studies[601–604]; however, an approximately equal sex distribution has been shown in multiple larger series.[598–601,605] Neutering may be associated with increased incidence of AGASAC in male dogs.[598] The mean age of dogs at diagnosis of AGASAC is 9 to 11 years.[568,599–606] Tumors in dogs as young as 5 years have been reported, suggesting that evaluation of the perineum and palpation of the anal sacs should be a routine part of the physical examination of every adult dog.

AGASAC is a rare tumor in the cat, representing 0.5% of all feline skin and subcutaneous neoplasms.[565] The median age of affected cats is 13 years, although animals as young as 6 years have been reported.[565,566] Siamese cats may be at higher risk.[565,566]

Pathology and Natural Behavior

AGASACs are distinct from perianal gland adenocarcinomas histologically and clinically. Histologic patterns of tumor cell arrangement in AGASAC have been classified as solid (closely packed neoplastic cells in lobules or nests with minimal stroma), tubules/rosettes/pseudorosettes (cells are radially arranged around a central tubule or a collection of cytoplastic processes or a small blood vessel), and papillary (elongated tree-like projections with a fibrovascular stalk).[607,608] The solid and tubules/rosettes/pseudorosettes patterns occur in about 95% of cases.[607,608]

AGASACs are usually unilateral, although bilateral AGASACs have been reported.[564,603–606,609–611] The overall incidence of bilateral AGASACs, either simultaneously or temporally separated, is up to 14%.[603,604,606,611,612]

Paraneoplastic hypercalcemia is reported in 16% to 53% of dogs with AGASAC.[564,581–602,605–607,609,613–617] Hypercalcemia is caused by the synthesis and secretion of parathyroid hormone–related peptide from neoplastic tissue.[618–620] Hypertrophic osteopathy in association with pulmonary involvement has been reported in two dogs.[621,622] Metastasis is common in dogs with AGASAC. Overall, metastasis is reported in 26% to 96% of dogs at the time of diagnosis, with 26% to 89% of dogs having metastasis to the regional LNs and 0% to 42% with metastasis to distant sites.[564,568,599–602,605,606,610,616] Metastasis can be present even when the primary tumor is small (<1 cm).[607] The medial iliac and internal iliac LNs (collectively called sublumbar LNs) and sacral LNs are the most common sites of metastasis,[564,599–601,605,606,609] whereas distant sites include lungs, liver, spleen, bone, and, less commonly, heart, adrenal glands, stomach, omentum, pancreas, kidneys, urinary bladder, and the mediastinum.[564,568,599–604] AGASAC micrometastases were detected incidentally in the bone marrow in one of four dogs in one study.[623] Tumor behavior can vary, because some dogs with large primary tumors may present without metastatic disease, whereas others may have a small primary tumor that has already metastasized.[607] In one study, dogs with clinical signs were more likely to have LN metastasis at diagnosis compared with dogs whose tumors were detected incidentally.[607] Histologic features including marked peripheral infiltration into surrounding tissue (neoplastic aggregates separated from the main tumor nodule), lymphovascular invasion, and solid pattern of cell arrangement were also associated with nodal metastasis at diagnosis, whereas mitotic index and presence of necrosis were not.[607] In another study, E-cadherin, a protein that mediates adhesion and communication between cells and the extracellular matrix, was evaluated as a prognostic marker in dogs with AGASAC.[624] A positive relationship between survival and the proportion of cells expressing E-cadherin immunoreactivity was observed, suggesting that loss of E-cadherin expression may play a role in tumor progression.[624] *p53* expression has been detected via IHC in a low-to-moderate proportion of AGASAC samples; however, no clinical implications have come from these findings.[579] A genetic analysis study in English cocker spaniels showed a higher frequency of AGASAC in dogs with the major histocompatibility complex DLA–DBQ1 allele, suggesting that a genetic factor may play a role in tumor development in this breed.[625] COX-2 expression also has been evaluated in AGASAC.[626] All tumor samples evaluated in one study showed positive immunoreactivity, as did ductal cells in normal anal sacs.[626] Neuroendocrine differentiation, suggested by expression of markers including synaptophysin, chromogranin A, and neuron-specific enolase, was detected via IHC in 30% of AGASAC.[608,627]

To further dissect the molecular basis of AGASAC and its reported sensitivity to the tyrosine kinase inhibitor toceranib phosphate (Palladia), expression of key toceranib targets has been evaluated.[628,629] In one study, mRNA for vascular endothelial growth factor receptor (VEGFR)-2, platelet-derived growth factor receptor (PDGFR)-α and -ß, and KIT was detected in all 24 tumors evaluated, but protein expression assessed by IHC was less consistent.[629] Protein expression of VEGFR-2 and PDGFR-α was present in most tumors; however, only one third expressed KIT. PDGFR-ß was strongly expressed in stroma.[629] Interestingly, RET expression was observed at both the mRNA and phosphorylated protein levels.[629] Phosphorylation of other receptor tyrosine kinases, including EGFR, Dtk/TYRO3, ROR-1, ROR-2, Tie-1, insulin-R, and RON, was observed in more than half of the tumors, suggesting that these may also have a role in AGASAC tumorigenesis.[629]

A case series of 11 dogs with anal sac melanoma suggests a moderate to aggressive biologic behavior.[560] Primary tumors were unilateral in all cases with a mean diameter of 3.4 cm. At the time of diagnosis, four of eight dogs had confirmed or suspected sublumbar LN metastasis, and 1 of 11 dogs had pulmonary metastasis.[560] The median mitotic index of the primary tumors was 50 per 10 high-power fields. Ten of 11 dogs died due to tumor progression.[560] Squamous cell carcinoma has also been reported arising

from the anal sac in nine dogs, all with unilateral disease.[561–563] Four of these dogs were clinically staged and none had evidence of regional LN or distant metastasis. Tumors recurred in four of five dogs after surgical excision.[561–563]

The biologic behavior of feline AGASAC has not been clearly defined. Most reports suggest that it is a locally invasive disease associated with a moderate-to-high risk of tumor recurrence after surgery.[565–567] The rate of metastasis is variable between studies.[565–567] Metastasis to the regional LNs was suspected at the time of diagnosis in 20% of surgically treated cats with AGASAC.[566] Metastatic sites include regional LNs, liver, diaphragm, and lungs.[565,567] Paraneoplastic hypercalcemia is relatively rare in cats with AGASAC, being reported in 11% of cats in one series.[565,566] Bilateral tumors have not been reported.

History and Clinical Signs

Clinical signs in dogs with AGASAC are often referable to either the presence of the primary mass (perianal discomfort, swelling [Fig. 23.31A], discharge, bleeding, scooting, perianal licking), obstruction of the pelvic canal by LN metastasis (tenesmus, abnormal stool shape, constipation, lethargy, anorexia), or to hypercalcemia (polyuria, polydipsia, hyporexia, lethargy, vomiting).[599,600,607] The primary tumor is an incidental finding on physical examination in up to 47% of reported dogs.[600,603] Rarely, dogs present with pain or lameness as a result of bone metastasis or direct extension of metastatic LNs into the lumbar or sacral vertebrae. In one study, presence of clinical signs was associated with the size of the primary tumor.[616]

Dogs with anal sac melanoma or SCC present with clinical signs related to the primary tumor.[561–563] Common signs include hemorrhagic discharge and perineal licking.[561–563] Tenesmus and constipation may be less common than in dogs with AGASAC.[561–563] In one study, all dogs with anal sac melanoma presented with clinical signs; none of the tumors were detected incidentally.[560] Of nine dogs with anal sac SCC, one dog was diagnosed incidentally.[561–563]

In cats with AGASAC, the most common clinical sign is perineal ulceration or discharge and this is present in up to 85% of cats (see Fig. 23.31B).[566] Other clinical signs include tenesmus, constipation, scooting, and excessive grooming of the perineal area.[565–567] Lethargy and/or hyporexia may be secondary to severe constipation. Not all cats present with clinical signs, and tumors can be detected incidentally during a routine physical examination, although this is rare.[565] It is not uncommon for an AGASAC to be misdiagnosed as an anal sac abscess based on the presence of ulceration and discharge in the perineal region.[565,566]

Diagnostic Techniques and Workup

Because dogs with AGASAC may present with signs unrelated to perianal disease (i.e., polyuria and polydipsia due to hypercalcemia), assessment of animals with suspicious clinical signs requires a careful rectal examination, including palpation of both anal sacs and evaluation for possible regional lymphadenomegaly. Although a definitive diagnosis requires either an FNA or biopsy, the likelihood of AGASAC is high in animals with a firm and discrete mass in the anal sac. AGASAC has a characteristic "neuroendocrine" cytologic appearance consisting of polyhedral to roundish epithelial cells with uniform round nuclei and light blue-gray, slightly granular cytoplasm (see Fig. 7.18). Cytologic criteria of malignancy are often subtle or absent. FNA cytology

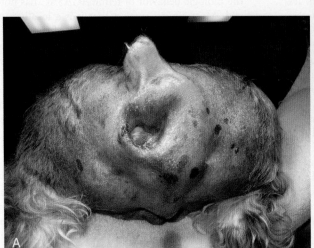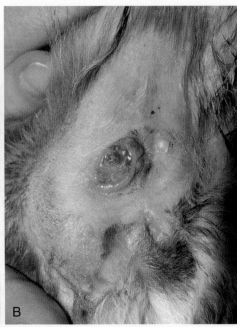

• **Fig. 23.31** (A) The typical appearance of a large apocrine gland anal sac adenocarcinoma in a dog. (B) The typical appearance of an apocrine gland anal sac adenocarcinoma in a cat. Ulceration with an associated discharge is the most common finding in cats with apocrine gland anal sac adenocarcinomas.

is valuable for ruling out impaction, infection, or inflammatory disease of the anal sac, although AGASAC can become secondarily infected or inflamed. Although special stains are almost never needed to confirm the diagnosis, a small study of cytokeratin immunoreactivity in perianal tumors showed a repeatable pattern of expression (CK7+/CK14–) in AGASAC.[586]

Clinical staging in dogs and cats with AGASAC includes assessing the size of the anal sac mass, evaluating for hypercalcemia, and investigating the abdomen and thorax for metastatic disease. Serum ionized calcium levels are preferred to total calcium concentrations for the assessment of hypercalcemia.

Accurate tumor staging in the abdomen and pelvic canal is important, because presence of metastasis affects prognosis and treatment decisions. Abdominal radiographs may reveal regional lymphadenomegaly in advanced cases, but are inadequate for the assessment of smaller metastatic LNs and metastasis to other abdominal organs such as the liver and spleen. Abdominal ultrasonography is commonly used to evaluate the abdomen and is more sensitive than radiography.[630] Despite its superiority to radiography, ultrasound has limitations. In one study, the only sonographic feature that separated benign from malignant LNs was LN size.[631] Changes in shape, contour, cavitation, echogenicity, and parenchymal uniformity did not reliably distinguish metastatic LNs.[631] Identification of nodal metastasis by ultrasound is further limited by anatomy, because the pelvic floor precludes visualization of LNs in the pelvic canal. Advanced imaging, including CT and MRI, allows for evaluation of LNs in the pelvic canal and can detect lymphadenomegaly in dogs deemed normal by ultrasound (Fig. 23.32).[632] Furthermore, studies have shown that advanced imaging detects a greater number of enlarged LNs than ultrasonograpy.[632–634] Sentinel LN mapping, using indirect CT lymphography, has been described in 18 dogs with AGASAC.[635] This study, along with the advanced imaging studies, suggests that patterns of LN metastasis can vary, and do not always follow lymphatic drainage linearly from the perineum.[633–635]

Lymphadenopathy related to AGASAC can involve any of the three LN centers (medial iliac, internal iliac, or sacral), and often skips LNs. The sacral LN was deemed the sentinel LN in only 25% of cases.[635] Collectively, these findings suggest that advanced imaging is necessary for optimal treatment planning to thoroughly assess the extent of disease. Importantly, these studies also bring to light that outcomes of treatment studies can be significantly affected by choice of staging tests. Three-view thoracic radiographs or thoracic CT are recommended for detection of pulmonary metastasis or rare mediastinal involvement.

In rare instances, pulmonary metastasis can be present without obvious regional LN disease. Lameness or bone pain should be evaluated with radiography, advanced imaging, and/or nuclear scintigraphy to rule out bone metastasis. Workup should also include complete blood count, serum biochemistry panel, and urinalysis. Hypercalcemia of malignancy can result in renal damage, which may modify prognosis and anesthetic risk. Medical management of hypercalcemia or impaired renal function may be necessary before surgery or for nonresectable disease (see Chapter 5).

Diagnosis of anal sac melanoma or SCC requires a tissue biopsy for histopathologic confirmation; however, cytology can be highly suggestive.[560] Although the biologic behavior of these less common anal sac tumors is not clearly defined, abdominal and thoracic imaging are recommended for complete tumor staging.[561–563] Metastasis appears common in dogs with anal sac melanoma, but not with SCC.[560–563]

Treatment

Surgery is considered the mainstay of treatment for dogs with nonmetastatic AGASAC or AGASAC metastatic to the regional LNs.[564,600,605,606,612] Excision of the primary tumor can be daunting because of the location of the anal sacs relative to the rectum, external anal sphincter, and perineal neurovascular structures;

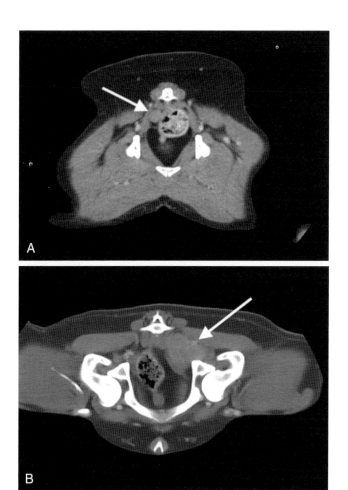

• **Fig. 23.32** Transverse computed tomography (CT) images at the level of the pelvic canal in two dogs with apocrine gland anal sac adenocarcinoma. Small (A) and large (B) ipsilateral sacral lymphadenomegaly is noted *(arrow)*, and both of these were not detected during abdominal ultrasonography. Three-dimensional advanced imaging, such as CT or magnetic resonance imaging, is preferred for tumor staging because it allows better visualization of the sacral lymph nodes within the pelvic canal.

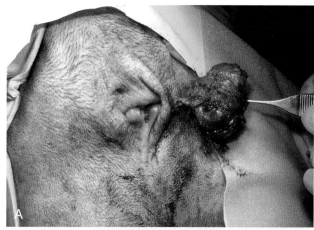

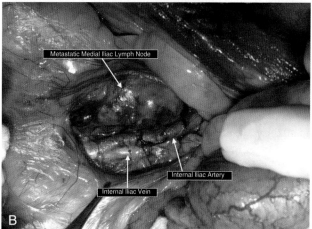

• **Fig. 23.33** Surgical management of dogs with apocrine gland anal sac adenocarcinoma depends on the stage of disease. (A) Closed anal sacculectomy for excision of an apocrine gland anal sac adenocarcinoma in a dog. (B) View of the dorsal aspect of the caudal abdomen during surgical extirpation of a metastatic sublumbar lymph node. Resection of metastatic lymph nodes can be complicated by regional vasculature *(pictured)*, deep location within the abdominal cavity and pelvic canal, and the nature of the metastatic lymph nodes (such as invasion into regional musculature or being cystic).

however, the majority of AGASACs can be resected with a closed anal sacculectomy and a low risk of postoperative complications (Fig. 23.33A).[605] The complication rate after local AGASAC excision is 5% to 24%, with the most common complications being wound dehiscence, rectal perforation, rectocutaneous fistulation, incisional infection, and transient fecal incontinence.[605,606,610] Risk of complications may be related to tumor size.[610] In an older study, mild to severe fecal incontinence was reported in 19% of dogs, and this incontinence was transient in 40% and permanent in 60%[603]; however, the surgical approach used in this study was more aggressive than what is currently recommended, with resections involving 120° to 270° anoplasties.[603] Local resection of AGASAC is almost always marginal because of the location of these masses within the perineal space.[616] As a result, the completeness of histologic excision is determined by tumor biology rather than the surgical approach; incomplete histologic excisions are expected when tumors have ruptured through their capsule either microscopically or macroscopically.

Lymphadenectomy is recommended for excision of metastatic sublumbar and sacral LNs because STs appear to be significantly improved when metastatic LNs are removed.[601] When nodal enlargement is obstructing the pelvic canal or contributing to hypercalcemia, lymphadenectomy relieves clinical signs and improves quality of life. The sublumbar LNs include the paired medial and internal iliac LNs.[630,631] These LNs are located in close proximity to the terminal branches of the aorta and caudal vena cava in the dorsal aspect of the caudal abdomen (see Fig. 23.33B). The majority of metastatic sublumbar and sacral LNs are solid, although occasionally they can be cystic.[636] Excision can be complicated by their location, regional anatomic structures, invasion into lumbar vertebrae, and if they are cystic. Omentalization of an unresectable cystic nodal metastasis was reported in one dog with good results.[636] Iatrogenic trauma to the terminal branches of the aorta or, more commonly, the thin-walled caudal vena cava, can result in significant intraoperative bleeding and the need for blood products. As a result, cross-matching is recommended before surgery in dogs treated with surgical excision of metastatic LNs. The complication rate after LN extirpation varies from 0% to 12%, with the most commonly reported complications being intraoperative hemorrhage, unresectable metastatic LNs, LN rupture, and abdominal wall dehiscence.[605,606,612] Sacral LNs are more difficult to expose, but can usually by extirpated with careful digital dissection. Pelvic osteotomies are rarely required to provide additional exposure for removal of metastatic sacral LNs. Multiple studies have shown that there is a survival advantage associated with treatment of progressive disease in dogs with AGASAC.[605,606,612,637] Therefore excision of recurrent tumors or progressive nodal metastasis is recommended, especially when it can be done with low morbidity. Although surgery rarely has a role in the management of distant metastatic disease, particularly at the time of diagnosis, splenectomy may be considered in dogs with splenic metastasis in the context of slowly progressive disease when there is no evidence of metastasis to other distant sites.[607]

The roles for adjuvant chemotherapy and RT are controversial and not fully defined. Chemotherapy has traditionally been recommended for the treatment of canine AGASAC because of the risk of metastasis. Drugs with demonstrated antitumor activity in the gross disease setting include carboplatin, cisplatin, and actinomycin D.[594,598,599] Other drugs reported in the postoperative setting include mitoxantrone and melphalan.[564,609] However, no controlled study has shown a survival advantage with the use of adjuvant chemotherapy in dogs with AGASAC.[600,601,605,606] In one study of 113 dogs with AGASAC, there was no significant difference in outcome between dogs treated with surgery alone and dogs treated with surgery and chemotherapy, with MSTs of 500 days and 540 days, respectively.[600] Similarly, in another study of 74 dogs, there was no significant difference in either MST or time to progression for dogs treated with surgery alone (581 days and 402 days, respectively) and surgery and carboplatin (723 days and 384 days, respectively).[606] In fact, in another study, the use of adjuvant chemotherapy had a negative effect on DFI and no effect on ST.[605] In these retrospective studies, it is possible chemotherapy was more often offered or chosen in patients with more advanced disease, which could have resulted in a bias against chemotherapy effectiveness. Until controlled clinical trials are performed to definitively define the role of chemotherapy in the management of dogs with AGASAC, there is little evidence to support its use in the adjuvant setting.

Toceranib has been associated with modest tumor responses in canine AGASAC.[638] In a retrospective study of 32 dogs with multiple prior failed therapies, use of toceranib resulted in tumor response durations of 10 to 47 weeks.[638] A 25% partial response rate was noted and an additional 63% of dogs maintained stable disease, for a total clinical benefit rate of 88%. Resolution of hypercalcemia has also been reported with toceranib treatment.[638] The antitumor effect of toceranib may be mediated through inhibition of the PDGFR-β or vascular endothelial growth factor receptor 2, both of which are expressed in canine AGASAC.[628,629] Controlled clinical trials are needed to determine the role of toceranib in the treatment of dogs with AGASAC. COX-2 is expressed in the glandular epithelial cells of AGASAC,[626] and this may suggest a potential role for COX-2 inhibitors in the management of dogs with AGASAC. Adjuvant electrochemotherapy using cisplatin has been reported in a single dog after an incomplete primary tumor excision.[639]

RT has been described for both palliation and multimodal, curative-intent treatment of dogs with AGASAC.[600,601,609,611,617] Measurable response rates of 38% to 75% have been observed in dogs with bulky disease treated with hypofractionated or fractionated protocols, suggesting radiosensitivity in the gross disease setting[609,611,617,640]; however, the role of RT for tumor control in the microscopic setting after surgical resection of primary or nodal AGASAC remains poorly defined. In a study of 113 variably treated dogs, the use of adjuvant RT did not result in a significant improvement in STs in 15 dogs.[600] This may have been due to low statistical power, as the MST of these dogs was longest among the

treatment groups at 742 days.[600] Radiation protocols, treatment intent, and tumor stage were not described.[600] In the only report of standardized curative-intent adjuvant RT, the MST of 15 dogs was 956 days.[609] Dogs received 15 daily fractions of 3.2 Gy (total dose of 48 Gy) to the primary site and regional LN beds using a nonconformal technique in combination with mitoxantrone chemotherapy. Although STs were favorable, late complications developed in half of the dogs.[609] Subsequent radiation toxicity studies showed that late radiation effects such as rectal stricture, rectal perforation, and chronic colitis are more likely to occur when radiation doses per fraction of 3 Gy or greater are used.[641,642] Therefore future curative-intent protocols should include pelvic irradiation at doses less than 3 Gy per fraction.[641,642] Use of conformal radiation technology, such as intensity-modulated RT, should further reduce the risk of toxicity by optimizing avoidance of critical structures. Dose-dependent, self-limiting acute effects reported in the study of nonconformal curative-intent irradiation of this region included mild to severe moist desquamation of the perianal area and colitis resulting in perianal discomfort lasting 1 to 4 weeks.[609,642]

The role of palliative-intent RT for relief of clinical signs associated with bulky AGASAC is better defined. Various hypofractionated protocols have been described including 5 daily fractions of 4 Gy, 3 to 4 weekly fractions of 6 to 9 Gy, 8 fractions of 3.8 Gy on a Monday–Wednesday–Friday schedule, and 5 biweekly fractions of 5 Gy.[601,611,617,640] These palliative RT protocols resulted in an improvement in clinical signs in up to 63% of dogs, including resolution of obstipation in some dogs.[611,617,640] Hypercalcemia resolved with RT alone in 31% of dogs and in an additional 46% of dogs when RT was combined with prednisone and a bisphosphonate.[617,640] The reported median progression-free intervals (PFIs) for dogs treated with palliative-intent hypofractionated protocols were 10 to 11 months, and MSTs ranged from 8 to 15 months.[601,611,617,640] Acute effects were mild and infrequent with grade I–II acute colitis in 8% to 27% of dogs, and grade I–II acute skin effects in 17% to 21% of dogs.[611,617] Late effects were rare in one study and included suspected rectal stricture in 3% of dogs and grade I late skin effects in 6% of dogs; these occurred in dogs treated with fractions of 5 Gy or greater.[617] In contrast, late effects were not observed in dogs treated with 8 fractions of 3.8 Gy delivered on a Monday–Wednesday–Friday schedule.[611] Severely hypofractionated RT should be used cautiously because late effects, such as rectal stricture, rectal perforation and chronic colitis, are related to dose per fraction.[611,617,641,642]

When interpreting the results of RT studies, it is important to consider that tumor control probability and risk of RT complications are affected by radiation dose distributions in the patient. A radiation treatment planning study showed that computerized, CT-based, 3-D conformal RT planning results in improved radiation dose distributions, with greater dose homogeneity in neoplastic tissues and better control of exposure of critical normal structures compared with nongraphic manual RT planning.[643] This has important implications for the interpretation of tumor control and toxicity profiles of older studies in which manual treatment planning was used.[643] It is possible that contemporary and future studies that take advantage of sophisticated treatment planning systems and conformal radiation delivery techniques may achieve different tumor control rates and complication risks than those described in older reports. Radiation studies should also be evaluated in the context of the regions that are irradiated, with reported radiation fields including the perianal region alone, perianal region and enlarged LNs,[611,617] or perianal region and regional lymphatic chain regardless of the size of the regional LNs.[609,617] These differences could affect clinical outcomes and should be considered when studies are compared. There may be a role for RT in the curative-intent management of dogs with incompletely excised AGASAC or dogs with surgically excised regional LN metastasis, or in the palliative management of dogs with measureable disease[600,601,609,619]; however, further studies are required to determine how RT should be optimized.

The majority of published studies have not standardized therapy for AGASAC according to clinical stage, and there is some evidence that the treatment approach may be stage dependent.[601] In one study, a clinical stage system and treatment algorithm were developed on the basis of a retrospective analysis of 80 dogs, and then these were evaluated in a prospective cohort of 50 dogs.[601] The proposed treatment algorithm included various combinations of surgery, carboplatin chemotherapy, and hypofractionated RT. However, this staging system has not been widely accepted, likely because it does not prioritize surgical excision on the basis of resectability. Surgery, according to the algorithm, is recommended only for primary tumors smaller than 2.5 cm and for metastatic LNs smaller than 4.5 cm when the primary tumor is smaller than 2.5 cm. In light of the increasing evidence of the importance of surgery in the treatment of AGASAC and its positive effect on survival,[600,601,605–607,612,637] surgical excision, including resection of recurrent disease, has become the mainstay of treatment for resectable AGASAC irrespective of size. Further studies are required to investigate the optimal combinations of surgery, chemotherapy, and RT in the management of dogs with various clinical stages of AGASAC.

Prognosis

Although dogs with metastatic AGASAC are rarely cured, long-term survival may be achieved in many cases after surgery-based treatments of the primary tumor and metastatic LNs both at presentation and in the face of recurrence. The reported DFIs for dogs treated surgically, with or without adjuvant therapy, range from 262 to 443 days.[605–607] Local recurrence rates vary widely from 5% to 44%.[603,605–607,612] Local recurrence is not associated with completeness of excision,[603,607] and this highlights the difficulty in using the completeness of excision to determine whether adjuvant therapies, such as RT or revision surgery, are required after incomplete histologic excision. Metastasis to regional LNs and to distant sites after surgery has been reported in 31% to 69% and 14% to 18% of dogs, respectively.[603,606,607,612] Multiple studies have reported shorter median DFIs in dogs with LN metastasis at diagnosis (134–197 days) compared with dogs without LN metastasis (529–760 days).[603,606,607] Dogs with LN metastasis at the time of surgery have a 2.5-fold hazard of disease progression compared with dogs without LN metastasis.[603]

For dogs with either local recurrence or postoperative LN metastasis, further treatment can improve STs.[606,610,637] In one study of 74 dogs with AGASAC treated surgically, with or without adjuvant chemotherapy, 55% developed either local recurrence and/or LN metastasis.[606] Of these dogs, 68% were treated with additional surgery, RT, and/or chemotherapy. The MST for dogs in which recurrent or metastatic disease was treated was 374 days after treatment for progressive disease, compared with 47 days for dogs in which the recurrent or metastatic disease was not treated.[606] In another study, the additional MST associated with a second surgical intervention was 283 days.[612]

Overall, the reported MSTs for dogs with AGASAC range from 386 to 960 days,[564,599–603,605–607,609–611,615,616] with estimated 1- and 2-year survival rates of 65% and 29%, respectively.[600] Tumor-related deaths vary widely between studies, with 41% to 81% of dogs dying as a result of AGASAC.[600,601,605,606]

The prognosis for dogs with AGASAC is dependent on a number of factors, especially clinical stage. In one study, dogs with no metastasis and primary tumor size less than 2.5 cm treated with surgery alone had overall favorable outcomes with the MST not reached and with only 9% of dogs experiencing tumor-related deaths.[601] In other studies, dogs with LN metastasis treated surgically, with or without adjuvant chemotherapy, had significantly shorter OSTs compared with dogs without metastasis.[605–607] OST was 293 to 448 days in dogs with LN metastasis and 529 to 925 days in dogs without metastasis.[605–607] In a study of 28 dogs with advanced LN metastasis (larger than 4.5 cm), treatment with hypofractionated RT resulted in a better median PFI and MST (347 days and 447 days, respectively) than did surgery with extirpation of metastatic LNs (159 days and 182 days, respectively).[611] Based on these collective findings, the role of a stage-dependent treatment algorithm is attractive and may become a future direction in the treatment of dogs with AGASAC.

Poor prognostic factors reported in various studies include primary tumor size,[600,601,607,617] presence of clinical signs,[607] presence of LN metastasis,[601,605–607] size of LN metastasis,[601] presence of distant metastasis,[600,601,624] nonpursuit of surgery,[600,601] treatment with chemotherapy alone,[600] lack of any therapy at all,[601] histologic features of the primary tumor,[607,608] E-cadherin immunoreactivity,[624] and, in some studies, hypercalcemia.[600,602,607]

Tumor size is prognostic for survival in a number of studies, but the threshold varies.[600,601,606,615,616] In one study of 113 dogs, dogs with tumors less than 10 cm^2 had a better MST (584 days) than dogs with AGASAC greater than 10 cm^2 (292 days).[600] In another study, a maximal tumor dimension of 2.5 cm was found to be prognostic.[601] In the retrospective arm of this study, the MSTs were 1205 and 722 days for dogs with non-metastatic AGASAC less and greater than 2.5 cm, respectively.[601] In a study of 77 dogs treated with palliative-intent hypofractionated RT, the only negative predictor for survival was tumor size greater than 2.5 cm.[617] In another study, a tumor size of 2.5 cm was not predictive of survival in 39 dogs, but a 4-cm cutoff was prognostic.[607] Dogs with AGASAC smaller than 4 cm had a longer PFI and MST (518 and 773 days, respectively) than dogs whose tumors were greater than 4 cm (251 and 433 days, respectively). These discrepancies in prognostic tumor size could reflect differences in how tumors are measured, the difficulty in using an absolute metric measurement across a wide range of dog sizes and body weights, and/or the inherent difficulty in identifying consistent prognostic factors using nonstandardized cohorts. Tumor size was associated with the presence of clinical signs in one study.[607] Dogs with clinical signs were more likely to have local recurrence after surgery and shorter OSTs compared with dogs diagnosed incidentally.[607] Compared with asymptomatic dogs or dogs with local signs, dogs with systemic clinical signs (e.g., anorexia, polyuria/polydipsia, abnormal stool shape, tenesmus, constipation, and/or lethargy) had significantly shorter PFIs and OSTs.[607]

Metastatic disease, both to the regional LNs and distant sites, is associated with a worse prognosis in dogs with AGASAC (Fig. 23.34).[600,601,605–607,624] The reported MSTs for dogs with LN metastasis at diagnosis treated with various modalities

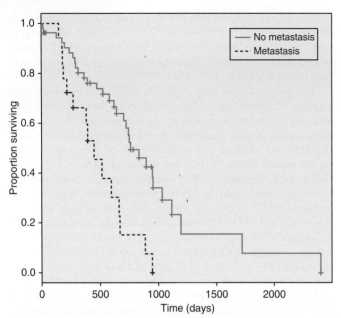

• **Fig. 23.34** Estimated Kaplan–Meier survival curves for overall survival times in dogs with apocrine gland anal sac adenocarcinoma with *(dashed)* and without *(solid)* metastasis at the time of diagnosis. The median overall survival times for dogs with metastasis (448 days) was significantly shorter than for dogs without metastasis (761 days, *p* = 0.042). (Reprinted with permission from Wouda RM, Borrego J, Keuler NS, et al. Evaluation of adjuvant carboplatin chemotherapy in the management of surgically excised anal sac apocrine gland adenocarcinoma in dogs. *Vet Comp Oncol.* 2016;14:67–80.)

range from 293 to 448 days and this is significantly worse than the MSTs of 529 to 1205 days for dogs without LN metastasis.[601,605,606] Dogs with LN metastasis at the time of diagnosis have a 2.3-fold increased risk of tumor-related death.[605] Although the prognosis is worse for dogs with LN metastasis,[601] MSTs improve after excision of the metastatic LNs.[601] The role of chemotherapy in dogs with LN metastasis disease remains undefined. The MST for dogs with distant metastasis ranges from 71 to 82 days in one study to 219 days in another study, and this is significantly worse than the MST in dogs without distant metastasis.[600,601]

Treatment also has an effect on STs in dogs with AGASAC. Overall, when considering all dogs with AGASAC, those treated with surgery have a significantly better outcome (MST 548 days) than those treated with either chemotherapy (MST 202 days) or those for which surgery was not part of the treatment protocol (MST 402 days).[600] However, when dogs with advanced LN metastasis (>4.5 cm) were expressly evaluated, treatment with hypofractionated RT resulted in significantly better outcomes compared with surgical extirpation.[611]

AGASAC has been classified histologically according to its tumor cell arrangement, including solid, rosette, tubular, papillary, and mixed patterns.[607,608] In one study of 39 dogs, dogs with a predominantly solid pattern had shorter PFIs and OSTs compared with dogs with other histologic patterns, corroborating a prior study that also associated tumor-related death with solid histologic pattern.[607,608] Other histologic features of the primary tumor that have been associated with shorter PFIs and OSTs include increased peripheral infiltration into surrounding tissue, presence of necrosis, and lymphovascular invasion.[607] In an IHC study, the expression of E-cadherin in greater than 75%

of AGASAC cells was associated with a longer MST (1168 days) than in dogs whose AGASAC expressed E-cadherin in fewer than 75% of cells (448 days).[624]

In a study of 113 dogs with AGASAC, MSTs for dogs with and without hypercalcemia were 256 days and 584 days, respectively.[600] Although hypercalcemia is a poor prognostic factor in some studies,[600,602,607] other studies have found no difference in survival between hypercalcemic and normocalcemic dogs.[599,605,606,609] Dogs with hypercalcemia require complete or near-complete removal of the tumor burden, including metastatic disease, to resolve the hypercalcemia.[603,613,637] Tumor responses to hypofractionated RT and toceranib have resulted in resolution of hypercalcemia in some dogs.[611,617,640] Medical management with corticosteroids and/or bisphosphonates may be needed to improve control of hypercalcemia. Recurrence of hypercalcemia after tumor-ablating treatment is typically associated with recurrent or metastatic disease.[600,603,614]

In 11 dogs with anal sac melanoma treated with various combinations of surgery, RT, chemotherapy, immunotherapy, and supportive medical management, the median PFI and OST were only 3 months and 3.5 months, respectively.[560] Ten of 11 dogs died due to local or distant tumor progression.[560] One dog with a small, 1.5 cm primary tumor survived at least 58 months after surgery and adjuvant chemotherapy.[560] Six of nine dogs with anal SCC survived 0 to 7 months after diagnosis.[561–563] Two dogs were lost to follow-up 7 months after diagnosis and one dog was disease-free 1 year after treatment with hypofractionated RT and carboplatin for a recurrent SCC.[561–563] Of five dogs that underwent surgical resection of the primary tumor, four dogs had recurrence within 1 to 5 months of surgery.[561,563]

The MST for 30 cats treated surgically, with or without adjunctive chemotherapy and/or RT, is 260 days.[566] The 1-, 2-, and 3-year survival rates were 42%, 27%, and 18%, respectively, with a tumor-related mortality rate of 53%.[566] Poor prognostic factors for survival in treated cats with AGASAC include local tumor recurrence and increased nuclear pleomorphic score. The risk of tumor-related death increased by 8 times for cats with local tumor recurrence and 10 times for cats with increased nuclear pleomorphic score.[566] The MSTs for cats with a nuclear pleomorphic score of 2 and 3 were 909 days and 187 days, respectively, and this was significantly different.[566] The role of chemotherapy and RT are unknown, but RT would theoretically be indicated because of the high rate of local tumor recurrence, especially after incomplete histologic excision. A short-lived partial response to carboplatin was reported in one cat with recurrent AGASAC.[644] In another report, adjuvant curative-intent RT (48 Gy) and carboplatin resulted in local recurrence and/or metastasis within 6 months of treatment in two cats.[567] In both cats, RT was well tolerated with minimal acute effects.[567]

Comparative Aspects[645–648]

No similar hormonally dependent perianal disease state exists in humans. The most common cancer of the anal margin is squamous cell (epidermoid) carcinoma. These tumors arise from the junction of haired skin and mucous membrane of the anal canal. Risk of developing cancer in this location is positively correlated with sexual activity, and most tumors are associated with human papillomavirus infection. Precancerous changes (dysplasia) in the epithelium of the anal canal may precede tumor development. Regional LNs are the most common site of metastasis. Previously considered a surgical disease requiring a permanent colostomy, improved outcomes have been achieved with definitive chemoradiation. The standard approach to therapy is concomitant RT and chemotherapy using 5-FU and mitomycin C. Surgery is reserved for locally recurrent or persistent disease. The mean 5-year disease-free survival and overall survival rates are 60% and 75%, respectively. Size and degree of invasion of the primary tumor, regional LN involvement, and presence of distant metastases are important prognostic factors. Identification of biomarkers that may serve as predictors of outcome or targets for therapy is being explored.

References

1. Patnaik AK, Liu SK, Hurvitz AI, et al.: Nonhematopoietic neoplasms in cats, *J Natl Cancer Inst* 54:855–860, 1975.
2. Hoyt RF, Withrow SJ: Oral malignancy in the dog, *J Am Anim Hosp Assoc* 20:83–92, 1984.
3. Dorn CR, Priester WA: Epidemiologic analysis of oral and pharyngeal cancer in dogs, cats, horses and cattle, *J Am Vet Med Assoc* 169:1202–1206, 1976.
4. Vos JH, van der Gaag I: Canine and feline oral-pharyngeal tumours, *Zentralbl Veterinarmed A* 34:420–427, 1987.
5. Stebbins KE, Morse CC, Goldschmidt MH: Feline oral neoplasia: a ten year survey, *Vet Pathol* 26:121–128, 1989.
6. Dorn CR, Taylor DON, Frye FL, et al.: Survey of animal neoplasms in Alameda and Contra Costa Counties, California. I. Methodology and description of cases, *J Natl Cancer Inst* 40:295–305, 1968.
7. Dorn CR, Taylor DON, Schneider R, et al.: Survey of animal neoplasms in Alameda and Contra Costa Counties, California. II. Cancer morbidity in dogs and cats from alameda county, *J Natl Cancer Inst* 40:307–318, 1968.
8. Cohen D, Brodey RS, Chen SM: Epidemiologic aspects of oral and pharyngeal neoplasms in the dog, *Am J Vet Res* 25:1776–1779, 1964.
9. Kudnig ST, Ehrhart N, Withrow SJ, et al.: Survival analysis of oral melanoma in dogs, *Vet Cancer Soc Proc* 23:39, 2003.
10. Heyman SJ, Diefenderfer DL, Goldschmidt MH, et al.: Canine axial skeletal osteosarcoma: a retrospective study of 116 cases (1986 to 1989), *Vet Surg* 21:304–310, 1992.
11. Ramos-Vara JA, Beissenherz ME, Miller MA, et al.: Retrospective study of 338 canine oral melanomas with clinical, histologic, and immunohistochemical review of 129 cases, *Vet Pathol* 37:597–608, 2000.
12. Todoroff RJ, Brodey RS: Oral and pharyngeal neoplasia in the dog: a retrospective survey of 361 cases, *J Am Vet Med Assoc* 175:567–571, 1979.
13. Withrow SJ, Holmberg DL: Mandibulectomy in the treatment of oral cancer, *J Am Anim Hosp Assoc* 19:273–286, 1983.
14. Withrow SJ, Nelson AW, Manley PA, et al.: Premaxillectomy in the dog, *J Am Anim Hosp Assoc* 21:49–55, 1985.
15. White RAS, Gorman NT, Watkins SB, et al.: The surgical management of bone-involved oral tumours in the dog, *J Small Anim Pract* 26:693–708, 1985.
16. Bradley RL, MacEwen EG, Loar AS: Mandibular resection for removal of oral tumors in 30 dogs and 6 cats, *J Am Vet Med Assoc* 184:460–463, 1984.
17. Salisbury SK, Richardson DC, Lantz GC: Partial maxillectomy and premaxillectomy in the treatment of oral neoplasia in the dog and cat, *Vet Surg* 15(16), 1986.
18. Salisbury SK, Lantz GC: Long-term results of partial mandibulectomy for treatment of oral tumors in 30 dogs, *J Am Anim Hosp Assoc* 24:285–294, 1988.
19. White RAS: Mandibulectomy and maxillectomy in the dog: long-term survival in 100 cases, *J Small Anim Pract* 32:69–74, 1991.
20. Kosovsky JK, Matthiesen DT, Marretta SM, et al.: Results of partial mandibulectomy for the treatment of oral tumors in 142 dogs, *Vet Surg* 20:397–401, 1991.
21. Wallace J, Matthiesen DT, Patnaik AK: Hemimaxillectomy for the treatment of oral tumors in 69 dogs, *Vet Surg* 21:337–341, 1992.
22. Schwarz PD, Withrow SJ, Curtis CR, et al.: Mandibular resection as a treatment for oral cancer in 81 dogs, *J Am Anim Hosp Assoc* 27:601–610, 1991.
23. Schwarz PD, Withrow SJ, Curtis CR, et al.: Partial maxillary resection as a treatment for oral cancer in 61 dogs, *J Am Anim Hosp Assoc* 27:617–624, 1991.
24. Sarowitz BN, Davis GJ, Kim S: Outcome and prognostic factors following curative-intent surgery for oral tumours in dogs: 234 cases (2004 to 2014), *J Small Anim Pract* 58:146–153, 2017.
25. Bronden LB, Eriksen T, Kristensen AT: Oral malignant melanomas and other head and neck neoplasms in Danish dogs: data from the danish veterinary cancer registry, *Acta Vet Scand* 51:54, 2009.
26. Richardson RC: Canine transmissible venereal tumor, *Compend Contin Educ Pract Vet* 3:951–956, 1981.
27. Straw RC, LeCouteur RA, Powers BE, et al.: Multilobular osteochondrosarcoma of the canine skull: 16 cases (1978-1988), *J Am Vet Med Assoc* 195:1764–1769, 1989.
28. Dernell WS, Straw RC, Cooper MF, et al.: Multilobular osteochondrosarcoma in 39 dogs: 1979-1993, *J Am Anim Hosp Assoc* 34:11–18, 1998.
29. Farrelly J, Denman DL, Hohenhaus AE, et al.: Hypofractionated radiation therapy of oral melanoma in five cats, *Vet Radiol Ultrasound* 45:91–93, 2004.
30. Iussich S, Maniscalco L, Di Sciuva A, et al.: PDGFRs expression in dogs affected by malignant oral melanomas: correlation with prognosis, *Vet Comp Oncol* 15:462–469, 2017.
31. Smedley RC, Lamoureux J, Sledge DG, et al.: Immunohistochemical diagnosis of canine oral amelanotic melanocytic neoplasms, *Vet Pathol* 48:32–40, 2011.
32. Harvey HJ, MacEwen GE, Braun D, et al.: Prognostic criteria for dogs with oral melanoma, *J Am Vet Med Assoc* 178:580–582, 1981.
33. Hahn KA, DeNicola DB, Richardson RC, et al.: Canine oral malignant melanoma: prognostic utility of an alternative staging system, *J Small Anim Pract* 35:251–256, 1994.
34. William LE, Packer RA: Association between lymph node size and metastasis in dogs with oral malignant melanoma: 100 cases (1987-2001), *J Am Vet Med Assoc* 222:1234–1236, 2003.
35. Spangler WL, Kass PH: The histologic and epidemiologic bases for prognostic considerations in canine melanocytic neoplasia, *Vet Pathol* 43:136–149, 2006.
36. Sánchez J, Ramirez GA, Buendia AJ, et al.: Immunohistochemical characterization and evaluation of prognostic factors in canine oral melanomas with osteocartilaginous differentiation, *Vet Pathol* 44:676–682, 2007.
37. Bergin IL, Smedley RC, Esplin DG, et al.: Prognostic evaluation of Ki67 threshold value in canine oral melanoma, *Vet Pathol* 48:41–53, 2011.
38. Newman SJ, Jankovsky JM, Rohrbach BW, et al.: C-kit expression in canine mucosal melanomas, *Vet Pathol* 49:760–765, 2012.
39. Smedley RC, Spangler WL, Esplin DG, et al.: Prognostic markers for canine melanocytic neoplasms: a comparative review of the literature and goals for future investigations, *Vet Pathol* 48:54–72, 2011.
40. Boston SE, Lu X, Culp WTN, et al.: Efficacy of systemic adjuvant therapies administered to dogs after excision of oral malignant melanomas: 151 cases (2001–2012), *J Am Vet Med Assoc* 245:401–407, 2014.
41. Tuohy JL, Selmic LE, Worley DR, et al.: Outcome following curative-intent surgery for oral melanoma in dogs: 70 cases (1998–2011), *J Am Vet Med Assoc* 245:1266–1273, 2014.
42. Turrel JM: Principles of radiation therapy. In Thielen GH, Madewell BR, editors: *Veterinary cancer medicine*, ed 2, Philadelphia, 1987, Lea & Febiger.
43. Théon AP, Rodriguez C, Madewell BR: Analysis of prognostic factors and patterns of failure in dogs with malignant oral tumors treated with megavoltage irradiation, *J Am Vet Med Assoc* 210:778–784, 1997.

44. Bateman KE, Catton PA, Pennock PW, et al.: Radiation therapy for the treatment of canine oral melanoma, *J Vet Intern Med* 8:267–272, 1994.

45. Blackwood L, Dobson JM: Radiotherapy of oral malignant melanomas in dogs, *J Am Vet Med Assoc* 209:98–102, 1996.

46. Freeman KP, Hahn KA, Harris FD, et al.: Treatment of dogs with oral melanoma by hypofractionated radiation therapy and platinum-based chemotherapy (1987-1997), *J Vet Intern Med* 17:96–101, 2003.

47. Proulx DR, Ruslander DM, Dodge RK, et al.: A retrospective analysis of 140 dogs with oral melanoma treated with external beam radiation, *Vet Radiol Ultrasound* 44:352–359, 2003.

48. Kawabe M, Mori T, Ito Y, et al.: Outcomes of dogs undergoing radiotherapy for treatment of oral malignant melanoma: 111 cases (2006–2012), *J Am Vet Med Assoc* 247:1146–1153, 2015.

49. Cancedda S, Bley CR, Aresu L, et al.: Efficacy and side effects of radiation therapy in comparison with radiation therapy and temozolomide in the treatment of measurable canine malignant melanoma, *Vet Comp Oncol* 14:146–157, 2016.

50. Page RL, Thrall DE, Dewhirst MW, et al.: Phase I study of melphalan alone and melphalan plus whole body hyperthermia in dogs with malignant melanoma, *Int J Hyperthermia* 7:559–566, 1991.

51. Rassnick KM, Ruslander DM, Cotter SM, et al.: Use of carboplatin for treatment of dogs with malignant melanoma: 27 cases (1989-2000), *J Am Vet Med Assoc* 218:1444–1448, 2001.

52. Dank G, Rassnick KM, Sokolovsky Y, et al.: Use of adjuvant carboplatin for treatment of dogs with oral malignat melanoma following surgical excision, *Vet Comp Oncol* 12:78–84, 2012.

53. Kitchell BE, Brown DM, Luck EE, et al.: Intralesional implant for treatment of primary oral malignant melanoma in dogs, *J Am Vet Med Assoc* 204:229–236, 1994.

54. Reed SD, Fulmer A, Buckholz J, et al.: Bleomycin/interleukin-12 electrochemogenetherapy for treating naturally occurring spontaneous neoplasms in dogs, *Cancer Gene Ther* 17:571–578, 2010.

55. Spugnini EP, Dragonetti E, Vincenzi B, et al.: Pulse-mediated chemotherapy enhances local control and survival in a spontaneous canine model of primary mucosal melanoma, *Melanoma Res* 16:23–27, 2006.

56. MacEwen EG, Patnaik AK, Harvey HJ, et al.: Canine oral melanoma: comparison of surgery versus surgery plus Corynebacterium parvum, *Cancer Invest* 4:397–402, 1986.

57. Quintin-Colonna F, Devauchelle P, Fradelizi D, et al.: Gene therapy of spontaneous canine melanoma and feline fibrosarcoma by intratumoral administration of histoincompatible cells expressing human interleukin-2, *Gene Ther* 3:1104–1112, 1996.

58. Dow SW, Elmslie RE, Willson AP, et al.: In vivo tumor transfection with superantigen plus cytokine genes induces tumor regression and prolongs survival in dogs with malignant melanoma, *J Clin Invest* 101:2406–2414, 1998.

59. Hogge G, Burkholder J, Culp J, et al.: Development of human granulocyte-macrophage colony-stimulating factor-transfected tumor cell vaccines for the treatment of spontaneous cancer, *Human Gene Ther* 9:1851–1861, 1998.

60. MacEwen EG, Kurzman ID, Vail DM, et al.: Adjuvant therapy for melanoma in dogs: results of randomized clinical trials using surgery, liposome-encapsulated muramyl tripeptide and granulocyte-macrophage colony-stimulating factor, *Clin Cancer Res* 5:4249–4258, 1999.

61. Bergman PJ, McKnight J, Novosad A, et al.: Long-term survival of dogs with advanced malignant melanoma after DNA vaccination with xenogeneic human tyrosinase: a phase I trial, *Clin Cancer Res* 9:1284–1290, 2003.

62. Grosenbaugh DA, Leard AT, Bergman PJ, et al.: Safety and efficacy of a xenogeneic DNA vaccine encoding for human tyrosinase as adjunctive treatment for oral malignant melanoma in dogs following surgical excision of the primary tumor, *Am J Vet Res* 72:1631–1638, 2011.

63. Ottnod JM, Smedley RC, Walshaw R, et al.: A retrospective analysis of the efficacy of Oncept vaccine for the adjunct treatment of canine oral malignant melanoma, *Vet Comp Oncol* 11:219–229, 2013.

64. Treggiari E, Grant JP, North SM: A retrospective review of outcome and survival following surgery and adjuvant xenogeneic DNA vaccination in 32 dogs with oral malignant melanoma, *J Vet Med Sci* 78:845–850, 2016.

65. Verganti S, Berlato D, Blackwood L, et al.: Use of oncept melanoma vaccine in 69 canine oral malignant melanomas in the UK, *J Small Anim Pract* 58:10–16, 2017.

66. McLean JL, Lobetti RG: Use of the melanoma vaccine in 38 dogs: the South African experience, *J S Afr Vet Assoc* 86:1246, 2015.

67. Riccardo F, Iussich S, Maniscalco L, et al.: CSPG4-specific immunity and survival prolongation in dogs with oral malignant melanoma immunized with human CSPG4 DNA, *Clin Cancer Res* 20:3753–3762, 2014.

68. Piras LA, Riccardo F, Iussich S, et al.: Prolongation of survival of dogs with oral malignant melanoma treated by en bloc surgical resection and adjuvant CSPG4-antigen electrovaccination, *Vet Comp Oncol* 15:996–1013, 2017.

69. Esplin DG: Survival of dogs following surgical excision of histologically well-differentiated melanocytic neoplasms of the mucous membranes of the lips and oral cavity, *Vet Pathol* 45:889–896, 2008.

70. Owen LN: *TNM classification of tumors in domestic animals*, ed 1, Geneva, 1980, WHO.

71. Modiano JF, Ritt MG, Wojcieszyn J: The molecular basis of canine melanoma: pathogenesis and trends in diagnosis and therapy, *J Vet Intern Med* 13:163–174, 1999.

72. Sulaimon SS, Kitchell BE: The basic biology of malignant melanoma: molecular mechanisms of disease progression and comparative aspects, *J Vet Intern Med* 17:760–772, 2003.

73. Nemec A, Murphy B, Kass PH, et al.: Histologic subtypes of oral non-tonsillar squamous cell carcinoma in dogs, *J Comp Path* 147:111–120, 2012.

74. Soukup JW, Snyder CJ, Simmons BT, et al.: Clinical, histologic, and computed tomographic features of oral papillary squamous cell carcinoma in dogs: 9 cases (2008–2011), *J Vet Dent* 30:18–24, 2013.

75. Nemec A, Murphy BG, Jordan RC, et al.: Oral papillary squamous cell carcinoma in twelve dogs, *J Comp Path* 150:155–161, 2014.

76. Mestrinho LA, Faísca P, Peleteiro MC, et al.: PCNA and grade in 13 canine oral squamous cell carcinomas: association with prognosis, *Vet Comp Oncol* 15:18–24, 2017.

77. Mestrinho LA, Pissarra H, Carvalho S, et al.: Comparison of histological and proliferation features of canine oral squamous cell carcinoma based on intraoral location: 36 cases, *J Vet Dent* 34:92–99, 2017.

78. Fulton AJ, Nemec A, Murphy BG, et al.: Risk factors associated with survival in dogs with nontonsillar oral squamous cell carcinoma: 31 cases (1990–2010), *J Am Vet Med Assoc* 243:696–702, 2013.

79. Kühnel S, Kessler M: Prognosis of canine oral (gingival) squamous cell carcinoma after surgical therapy. A retrospective analysis of 40 patients, *Tierarztl Prax* 42:359–366, 2014.

80. Evans SM, Shofer F: Canine oral nontonsillar squamous cell carcinoma, *Vet Radiol* 29:133–137, 1988.

81. LaDue-Miller T, Price S, Page RL, et al.: Radiotherapy for canine non-tonsillar squamous cell carcinoma, *Vet Radiol Ultrasound* 37:74–77, 1996.

82. Schmidt BR, Glickman NW, DeNicola DB, et al.: Evaluation of piroxicam for the treatment of oral squamous cell carcinoma in dogs, *J Am Vet Med Assoc* 218:1783–1786, 2001.

83. Boria PA, Murry DJ, Bennett PF, et al.: Evaluation of cisplatin combined with piroxicam for the treatment of oral malignant melanoma and oral squamous cell carcinoma in dogs, *J Am Vet Med Assoc* 224:388–394, 2004.

84. Vos JP, Burm AGD, Focker BP, et al.: Piroxicam and carboplatin as a combination treatment of canine oral non-tonsillar squamous cell carcinoma: a pilot study and a literature review of a canine model of human head and neck squamous cell carcinoma, *Vet Comp Oncol* 3:16–24, 2005.

85. Buhles WC, Theilan GH: Preliminary evaluation of bleomycin in feline and canine squamous cell carcinomas, *Am J Vet Res* 34: 289–291, 1973.

86. Bertone ER, Snyder LA, Moore AS, et al.: Environmental and lifestyle risk factors for oral squamous cell carcinoma in domestic cats, *J Vet Intern Med* 17:557–562, 2003.

87. Snyder LA, Bertone ER, Jakowski RM, et al.: p53 expression and environmental tobacco smoke exposure in feline oral squamous cell carcinoma, *Vet Pathol* 41:209–214, 2004.

88. Martin CK, Tannehill-Gregg SH, Wolfe TD, et al.: Bone-invasive oral squamous cell carcinoma in cats: pathology and expression of parathyroid hormone-related protein, *Vet Pathol* 48: 302–312, 2011.

89. Hutson CA, Willauer CC, Walder EJ, et al.: Treatment of mandibular squamous cell carcinoma in cats by use of mandibulectomy and radiotherapy: seven cases (1987-1989), *J Am Vet Med Assoc* 201:777–781, 1992.

90. Northrup NC, Selting KA, Rassnick KM, et al.: Outcomes of cats with oral tumors treated with mandibulectomy, *J Am Anim Hosp Assoc* 42:350–360, 2006.

91. Reeves NCP, Turrel JM, Withrow SJ: Oral squamous cell carcinoma in the cat, *J Am Anim Hosp Assoc* 29:438–441, 1993.

92. Bostock DE: The prognosis in cats bearing squamous cell carcinoma, *J Small Anim Pract* 13:119–125, 1972.

93. Cotter SM: Oral pharyngeal neoplasms in the cat, *J Am Anim Hosp Assoc* 17:917–920, 1981.

94. Hayes AM, Adams VJ, Scase TJ, et al.: Survival of 54 cats with oral squamous cell carcinoma in United Kingdom general practice, *J Small Anim Pract* 48:394–399, 2007.

95. Soltero-Rivera MM, Krick EL, Reiter AM, et al.: Prevalence of regional and distant metastasis in cats with advanced oral squamous cell carcinoma: 49 cases (2005–2011), *J Feline Med Surg* 16:164–169, 2014.

96. Evans SM, LaCreta F, Helfand S, et al.: Technique, pharmacokinetics, toxicity, and efficacy of intratumoral etanidazole and radiotherapy for treatment of spontaneous feline oral squamous cell carcinoma, *Int J Radiat Oncol Biol Phys* 20:703–708, 1991.

97. LaRue SM, Vail DM, Ogilvie GK, et al.: Shrinking-field radiation therapy in combination with mitoxantrone chemotherapy for the treatment of oral squamous cell carcinoma in the cat, *Vet Cancer Soc Proc* 11:99, 1991.

98. Jones PD, de Lorimier LP, Kitchell BE, et al.: Gemcitabine as a radiosensitizer for nonresectable feline oral squamous cell carcinoma, *J Am Anim Hosp Assoc* 39:463–467, 2003.

99. LeBlanc AL, LaDue TA, Turrel JM, et al.: Unexpected toxicity following use of gemcitabine as a radiosensitizer in head and neck carcinomas: a Veterinary Radiation Therapy Oncology Group pilot study, *Vet Radiol Ultrasound* 45:466–470, 2004.

100. Fidel JL, Sellon RK, Houston RK, et al.: A nine-day accelerated radiation protocol for feline squamous cell carcinoma, *Vet Radiol Ultrasound* 48:482–485, 2007.

101. Fidel J, Lyons J, Tripp C, et al.: Treatment of oral squamous cell carcinoma with accelerated radiation therapy and concomitant carboplatin in cats, *J Vet Intern Med* 25:504–510, 2011.

102. Bregazzi VS, LaRue SM, Powers BE, et al.: Response of feline oral squamous cell carcinoma to palliative radiation therapy, *Vet Radiol Ultrasound* 42:77–79, 2001.

103. Poirier VJ, Kaser-Hotz B, Vail DM, et al.: Efficacy and toxicity of an accelerated hypofractionated radiation therapy protocol in cats with oral squamous cell carcinoma, *Vet Radiol Ultrasound* 54:81–88, 2013.

104. Sabhlok A, Ayl R: Palliative radiation therapy outcomes for cats with oral squamous cell carcinoma (1999–2005), *Vet Radiol Ultrasound* 55:565–570, 2014.

105. Yoshikawa H, Ehrhart EJ, Charles JB, et al.: Assessment of predictive molecular variables in feline oral squamous cell carcinoma treated with stereotactic radiation therapy, *Vet Comp Oncol* 14: 39–57, 2016.

106. Yoshikawa H, Maranon DG, Battaglia CLR, et al.: Predicting clinical outcome in feline oral squamous cell carcinoma: tumour initiating cells, telomeres and telomerase, *Vet Comp Oncol* 14: 371–383, 2016.

107. Ogilvie GK, Moore AS, Obradovich JE, et al.: Toxicoses and efficacy associated with administration of mitoxantrone to cats with malignant tumor, *J Am Vet Med Assoc* 202:1839–1844, 1993.

108. Fox LE, Rosenthal RC, King RR, et al.: Use of cis-bis-neodecanoato-trans-R,R-1,2-diaminocyclohexane platinum (II), a liposomal cisplatin analogue, in cats with oral squamous cell carcinoma, *Am J Vet Res* 61:791–795, 2000.

109. Hayes A, Scase T, Miller J, et al.: COX-1 and COX-2 expression in feline oral squamous cell carcinoma, *J Comp Pathol* 135:93–99, 2006.

110. DiBernardi L, Dore M, Davis JA, et al.: Study of feline oral squamous cell carcinoma: potential target for cyclooxygenase inhibitor treatment, *Prostaglandins Leukot Essent Fatty Acids* 76:245–250, 2007.

111. Wiles V, Hohenhaus A, Lamb K, et al.: Retrospective evaluation of toceranib phosphate (Palladia) in cats with oral squamous cell carcinoma, *J Feline Med Surg* 19:185–193, 2017.

112. Wypij JM, Heller DA: Pamidronate disodium for palliative therapy of feline bone-invasive tumors, *Vet Med Int* 2014: 675172, 2014.

113. Ciekot PA, Powers BE, Withrow SJ, et al.: Histologically low grade yet biologically high grade fibrosarcomas of the mandible and maxilla of 25 dogs (1982-1991), *J Am Vet Med Assoc* 204: 610–615, 1994.

114. Frazier SA, Johns SM, Ortega J, et al.: Outcome in dogs with surgically resected oral fibrosarcoma (1997–2008), *Vet Comp Oncol* 10:33–43, 2011.

115. Gardner H, Fidel J, Haldorson G, et al.: Canine oral fibrosarcomas: a retrospective analysis of 65 cases (1998–2010), *Vet Comp Oncol* 13:40–47, 2013.

116. Thrall DE: Orthovoltage radiotherapy of oral fibrosarcomas in dogs, *J Am Vet Med Assoc* 172:159–162, 1981.

117. Forrest LJ, Chun R, Adams WM, et al.: Postoperative radiation therapy for canine soft tissue sarcoma, *J Vet Intern Med* 14:578–582, 2000.

118. Hammer AS, Weeren FR, Weisbrode SE, et al.: Prognostic factors in dogs with osteosarcomas of the flat and irregular bones, *J Am Anim Hosp Assoc* 31:321–326, 1995.

119. Straw RC, Powers BE, Klausner J, et al.: Canine mandibular osteosarcoma: 51 cases (1980-1992), *J Am Anim Hosp Assoc* 32:257–262, 1996.

120. Kazmierski KJ, Dernell WS, Lafferty MH, et al.: Osteosarcoma of the canine head: a retrospective study of 60 cases, *Vet Cancer Soc Proc* 22:30, 2002.

121. Selmic LE, Lafferty MH, Kamstock DA, et al.: Outcome and prognostic factors for osteosarcoma of the maxilla, mandible, or calvarium in dogs: 183 cases (1986–2012), *J Am Vet Med Assoc* 245:930–938, 2014.

122. Coyle VJ, Rassnick KM, Borst LB, et al.: Biological behaviour of canine mandibular osteosarcoma. A retrospective study of 50 cases (1999–2007), *Vet Comp Oncol* 13:89–97, 2015.

123. Fiani N, Vertstraete FJ, Kass PH, et al.: Clinicopathologic characterization of odontogenic tumors and focal fibrous hyperplasia in dogs: 152 cases (1995-2005), *J Am Vet Med Assoc* 238:495–500, 2011.

124. Dubielzig RR: Proliferative dental and gingival disease of dogs and cats, *J Am Anim Hosp Assoc* 18:577–584, 1982.

125. Bjorling DE, Chambers JN, Mahaffey EA: Surgical treatment of epulides in dogs: 25 cases (1974-1984), *J Am Vet Med Assoc* 190:1315–1318, 1987.

126. Bostock DE, White RAS: Classification and behaviour after surgery of canine epulides, *J Comp Pathol* 97:197–206, 1987.

127. Yoshida K, Yanai T, Iwasaki T, et al.: Clinicopathological study of canine oral epulides, *J Vet Med Sci* 61:897–902, 1999.

128. White RAS, Gorman NT: Wide local excision of acanthomatous epulides in the dog, *Vet Surg* 18:12–14, 1989.

129. Goldschmidt SL, Bell CM, Hetzel S, et al.: Clinical characterization of canine acanthomatous ameloblastoma in 263 dogs and the influence of postsurgical histopathological margins on local recurrence, *J Vet Dent* 34:241–247, 2017.

130. Thrall DE: Orthovoltage radiotherapy of acanthomatous epulides in 39 dogs, *J Am Vet Med Assoc* 184:826–829, 1984.

131. Théon AP, Rodriguez C, Griffey S, et al.: Analysis of prognostic factors and patterns of failure in dogs with periodontal tumors treated with megavoltage irradiation, *J Am Vet Med Assoc* 210:785–788, 1997.

132. Thrall DE, Goldschmidt MH, Biery DN: Malignant tumor formation at the site of previously irradiated acanthomatous epulides in four dogs, *J Am Vet Med Assoc* 178:127–132, 1981.

133. Yoshida K, Watarai Y, Sakai Y, et al.: The effect of intralesional bleomycin on canine acanthomatous epulis, *J Am Anim Hosp Assoc* 34:457–461, 1998.

134. Kelly JM, Belding BA, Schaefer AK: Acanthomatous ameloblastoma in dogs treated with intralesional bleomycin, *Vet Comp Oncol* 8:81–86, 2010.

135. Colgin LMA, Schulman FY, Dubielzig RR: Multiple epulides in 13 cats, *Vet Pathol* 38:227–229, 2001.

136. Padgett SL, Tillson DM, Henry CJ, et al.: Gingival vascular hamartoma with associated paraneoplastic hyperglycemia in a kitten, *J Am Vet Med Assoc* 210:914–915, 1997.

137. Bonfanti U, Bertazzolo W, Gracis M, et al.: Diagnostic value of cytological analysis of tumours and tumour-like lesions of the oral cavity in dogs and cats: a prospective study on 114 cases, *Vet J* 205:322–327, 2015.

138. Beck ER, Withrow SJ, McChesney AE, et al.: Canine tongue tumors: a retrospective review of 57 cases, *J Am Anim Hosp Assoc* 22:525–532, 1986.

139. Carpenter LG, Withrow SJ, Power BE, et al.: Squamous cell carcinoma of the tongue in 10 dogs, *J Am Anim Hosp Assoc* 29:17–24, 1993.

140. Syrcle JA, Bonczynski JJ, Monnette S, et al.: Retrospective evaluation of lingual tumors in 42 dogs: 1999-2005, *J Am Anim Hosp Assoc* 44:308–319, 2008.

141. Culp WTN, Ehrhart N, Withrow SJ, et al.: Results of surgical excision and evaluation of factors associated with survival time in dogs with lingual neoplasia: 97 cases (1995–2008), *J Am Vet Med Assoc* 242:1392–1397, 2013.

142. Burton JH, Powers BE, Biller BJ: Clinical outcome in 20 cases of lingual hemangiosarcoma in dogs: 1996–2011, *Vet Comp Oncol* 12:198–204, 2014.

143. Gendler A, Lewis JR, Reetz JA, et al.: Computed tomographic features of oral squamous cell carcinoma in cats: 18 cases (2002–2008), *J Am Vet Med Assoc* 236:319–325, 2010.

144. Kafka UCM, Carstens A, Steenkamp G, et al.: Diagnostic value of magnetic resonance imaging and computed tomography for oral masses in dogs, *J S Afr Vet Assoc* 75:163–168, 2004.

145. Ghirelli CO, Villamizar LA, Carolina A, et al.: Comparison of standard radiography and computed tomography in 21 dogs with maxillary masses, *J Vet Dent* 30:72–76, 2013.

146. Yoshikawa H, Randall EK, Kraft SL, et al.: Comparison between 2-^{18}fluoro-2-deoxy-D-glucose positron emission tomography and contrast-enhanced computed tomography for measuring gross tumor volume in cats with oral squamous cell carcinoma, *Vet Radiol Ultrasound* 54:307–313, 2013.

147. Randall EK, Kraft SL, Yoshikawa H, et al.: Evaluation of 18F–FDG PET/CT as a diagnostic imaging and staging tool for feline oral squamous cell carcinoma, *Vet Comp Oncol* 14:28–38, 2016.

148. Smith MM: Surgical approach for lymph node staging of oral and maxillofacial neoplasms in dogs, *J Am Anim Hosp Assoc* 31:514–518, 1995.

149. Herring ES, Smith MM, Robertson JL: Lymph node staging of oral and maxillofacial neoplasms in 31 dogs and cats, *J Vet Dent* 19:122–126, 2002.

150. Green K, Boston SE: Bilateral removal of the mandibular and medial retropharyngeal lymph nodes through a single ventral midline incision for staging of head and neck cancers in dogs: a description of surgical technique, *Vet Comp Oncol* 15:208–214, 2017.

151. Skinner OT, Boston SE, Souza CH de M: Patterns of lymph node metastasis identified following bilateral mandibular and medial retropharyngeal lymphadenectomy in 31 dogs with malignancies of the head, *Vet Comp Oncol* 15:881–889, 2017.

152. Ku CK, Kass PH, Christopher MM: Cytologic-histologic concordance in the diagnosis of neoplasia in canine and feline lymph nodes: a retrospective study of 367 cases, *Vet Comp Oncol* 15:1206–1217, 2017.

153. Worley DR: Incorporation of sentinel lymph node mapping in dogs with mast cell tumours: 20 consecutive procedures, *Vet Comp Oncol* 12:215–226, 2014.

154. Balogh L, Thuróczy J, Andócs G, et al.: Sentinel lymph node detection in canine oncological patients, *Nucl Med Rev Cent East Eur* 5:139–144, 2002.

155. Lurie DM, Seguin B, Verstraete FJ, et al.: Contrast-assisted ultrasound for sentinel node detection in canine head and neck neoplasia, *Invest Radiol* 41:415–421, 2006.

156. Brissot HN, Edery EG: Use of indirect lymphography to identify sentinel lymph node in dogs: a pilot study in 30 tumours, *Vet Comp Oncol* 15:740–753, 2017.

157. Waters DJ, Coakley FV, Cohen MD, et al.: The detection of pulmonary metastases by helical CT: a clinicopathologic study in dogs, *J Comput Assist Tomogr* 22:235–240, 1998.

158. Nemanic S, London CA, Wisner ER: Comparison of thoracic radiographs and single breath-hold hemical CT for detection of pulmonary nodules in dogs with metastatic neoplasia, *J Vet Intern Med* 20:508–515, 2006.

159. Eberle N, Fork M, von Babo V, et al.: Comparison of examination of thoracic radiographs and thoracic computed tomography in dogs with appendicular osteosarcoma, *Vet Comp Oncol* 9:131–140, 2011.

160. Armbrust LJ, Biller DS, Bamford A: Comparison of three-view thoracic radiography and computed tomography for detection of pulmonary nodules in dogs with neoplasia, *J Am Vet Med Assoc* 240:1088–1094, 2012.

161. Kirpensteijn J, Withrow SJ, Straw RC: Combined resection of the nasal planum and premaxilla in three dogs, *Vet Surg* 23:341–346, 1994.

162. Lascelles BD, Thomson MJ, Dernell WS, et al.: Combined dorsolateral and intraoral approach for the resection of tumors of the maxilla in the dog, *J Am Anim Hosp Assoc* 39:294–305, 2003.

163. Lascelles BDX, Henderson RA, Seguin B, et al.: Bilateral rostral maxillectomy and nasal planectomy for large rostral maxillofacial neoplasms in six dogs and one cat, *J Am Anim Hosp Assoc* 40:137–146, 2004.

164. Fox LE, Geoghegan SL, Davis LH, et al.: Owner satisfaction with partial mandibulectomy or maxillectomy for treatment of oral tumors in 27 dogs, *J Am Anim Hosp Assoc* 33:25–31, 1997.

165. Boudrieau RJ, Tidwell AS, Ullman SL, et al.: Correction of mandibular nonunion and malocclusion by plate fixation and autogenous cortical bone grafts in two dogs, *J Am Vet Med Assoc* 204, 1994. 774–750.

166. Bracker KE, Trout NJ: Use of a free cortical ulnar autograft following en bloc resection of a mandibular tumor, *J Am Anim Hosp Assoc* 36:76–79, 2000.

167. Boudrieau RJ, Mitchell SL, Seeherman H: Mandibular reconstruction of a partial hemimandibulectomy in a dog with severe malocclusion, *Vet Surg* 33:119–130, 2004.

168. Spector DI, Keating JH, Boudreau RJ: Immediate mandibular reconstruction of a 5cm defect using rhBMP–2 after partial mandibulectomy in a dog, *Vet Surg* 36:752–759, 2007.

169. Jégoux F, Goyenvalle E, Cognet R, et al.: Mandibular segmental defect regenerated with macroporous biphasic calcium phosphate, collagen membrane, and bone marrow graft in dogs, *Arch Otolaryngol Head Neck Surg* 136:971–978, 2010.

170. Arzi B, Cissell DD, Pollard RE, et al.: Regenerative approach to bilateral rostral mandibular reconstruction in a case series of dogs, *Front Vet Sci* 2:4, 2015.

171. Arzi B, Verstraete FJM, Huey DJ, et al.: Regenerating mandibular bone using rhBMP–2: part 1 – immediate reconstruction of segmental mandibulectomies, *Vet Surg* 44: 403–409, 2015.

172. Boudrieau RJ: Initial experience with rhBMP–2 delivered in a compressive resistant matrix for mandibular reconstruction in 5 dogs, *Vet Surg* 44:443–458, 2015.

173. Liptak JM, Thatcher GP, Bray JP: Reconstruction of a mandibular segmental defect with a customized 3-dimensional-printed titanium prosthesis in a cat with a mandibular osteosarcoma, *J Am Vet Med Assoc* 250:900–908, 2017.

174. Reynolds D, Fransson B, Preston C: Cresentic osteotomy for resection of oral tumours in four dogs, *Vet Comp Orthop Traumatol* 22:412–416, 2009.

175. Arzi B, Verstraete FJ: Mandibular rim excision in seven dogs, *Vet Surg* 39:226–231, 2010.

176. Linden D, Matz BM, Farag R, et al.: Biomechanical comparison of two ostectomy configurations for partial mandibulectomy, *Vet Comp Orthop Traumatol* 30:15–19, 2017.

177. MacLellan RH, Rawlinson JE, Rao S, et al.: Intraoperative and postoperative complications of partial maxillectomy for the treatment of oral tumors in dogs, *J Am Vet Med Assoc* 252: 1538–1547, 2018.

178. Bar-Am Y, Verstraete FJM: Elastic training for the prevention of mandibular drift following mandibulectomy in dogs: 18 cases (2005-2008), *Vet Surg* 39:574–580, 2010.

179. Riggs J, Adams VJ, Hermer JV, et al.: Outcomes following surgical excision or surgical excision combined with adjunctive, hypofractionated radiotherapy in dogs with oral squamous cell carcinoma or fibrosarcoma, *J Am Vet Med Assoc* 253:73–83, 2018.

180. MacMillan R, Withrow SJ, Gillette EL: Surgery and regional irradiation for treatment of canine tonsillar squamous cell carcinoma: retrospective review of eight cases, *J Am Anim Hosp Assoc* 18:311–314, 1982.

181. Brooks MB, Matus RE, Leifer CE, et al.: Chemotherapy versus chemotherapy plus radiotherapy in the treatment of tonsillar squamous cell carcinoma in the dog, *J Vet Intern Med* 2: 206–211, 1988.

182. McCaw DL, Pope ER, Payne JT, et al.: Treatment of canine oral squamous cell carcinoma with photodynamic therapy, *Br J Cancer* 82:1297–1299, 2000.

183. Nagata K, Selting KA, Cook CR, et al.: 90Sr therapy for oral squamous cell carcinoma in two cats, *Vet Radiol Ultrasound* 52:114–117, 2011.

184. Reif JS, Cohen D: The environmental distribution of canine respiratory tract neoplasms, *Arch Environ Health* 22:136–140, 1971.

185. Carozzi G, Zotti A, Alberti M, et al.: Computed tomographic features of pharyngeal neoplasia in 25 dogs, *Vet Radiol Ultrasound* 56:628–637, 2015.

186. Thierry F, Longo M, Pecceu E, et al.: Computed tomographic appearance of canine tonsillar neoplasia: 14 cases, *Vet Radiol Ultrasound* 59:54–63, 2018.

187. Mas A, Blackwood L, Cripps P, et al.: Canine tonsillar squamous cell carcinoma: a multicentre retrospective review of 44 clinical cases, *J Small Anim Pract* 52:359–364, 2011.

188. Dennis MM, Ehrhart N, Duncan CG, et al.: Frequency of and risk factors associated with lingual lesions in dogs: 1,196 cases (1995-2004), *J Am Vet Med Assoc* 228:1533–1537, 2006.

189. Dvorak LD, Beaver DP, Ellison GW, et al.: Major glossectomy in dogs: a case series and proposed classification system, *J Am Anim Hosp Assoc* 40:331–337, 2004.

190. Brodey RS: A clinical and pathologic study of 130 neoplasms of the mouth and pharynx in the dog, *Am J Vet Res* 21:787–812, 1960.

191. Solano M, Penninck DG: Ultrasonography of the canine, feline and equine tongue: normal findings and case history reports, *Vet Radiol Ultrasound* 37:206–213, 1996.

192. Turk MAM, Johnson GC, Gallina AM: Canine granular cell tumour (myoblastoma): a report of four cases and review of the literature, *J Small Anim Pract* 24:637–645, 1983.

193. Patnaik AK, Lieberman PH, Erlandson RA, et al.: A clinicopathologic and ultrastructural study of undifferentiated malignant tumors of the oral cavity in dogs, *Vet Pathol* 23:170–175, 1986.

194. Ogilvie GK, Sundberg JP, O'Banion MK, et al.: Papillary squamous cell carcinoma in three young dogs, *J Am Vet Med Assoc* 192:933–936, 1988.

195. Poulet FM, Valentine BA, Summers BA: A survey of epithelial odontogenic tumors and cysts in dogs and cats, *Vet Pathol* 29:369–380, 1992.

196. Bell CM, Soukup JW: Nomenclature and classification of odontogenic tumors – part II: clarification of specific nomenclature, *J Vet Dent* 31:234–243, 2014.

197. Dubielzig RR, Adams WM, Brodey RS: Inductive fibroameloblastoma, an unusual dental tumor of young cats, *J Am Vet Med Assoc* 174:720–722, 1979.

198. Figueiredo C, Barros HM, Alvares LC, et al.: Composed complex odontoma in a dog, *Vet Med Small Anim Clin* 69:268–270, 1974.

199. Dhaliwal RS, Kitchell BE, Marretta SM: Oral tumors in dogs and cats. Part I. Diagnosis and clinical signs, *Compend Contin Educ Pract Vet* 20:1011–1021, 1998.

200. Fiani N, Arzi B, Johnson EG, et al.: Osteoma of the oral and maxillofacial regions in cats: 7 cases (1999–2009), *J Am Vet Med Assoc* 238:1470–1475, 2011.

201. Volker MK, Luskin IR: Oral osteoma in 6 dogs, *J Vet Dent* 32:88–91, 2014.

202. Mendenhall WM, Riggs CE, Cassisi NJ: Treatment of head and neck cancers. In DeVita RT, Hellman S, Rosenberg SA, editors: *Cancer: principles and practice of oncology*, ed 7, Philadelphia, 2005, Lippincott Williams & Wilkins, pp 679–682.

203. Spangler WL, Culbertson MR: Salivary gland disease in dogs and cats: 245 cases(1985-1988), *J Am Vet Med Assoc* 198:465–469, 1991.

204. Hammer A, Getzy D, Ogilvie G, et al.: Salivary gland neoplasia in the dog and cat: survival times and prognostic factors, *J Am Anim Hosp Assoc* 37:478–482, 2001.

205. Brocks BA, Peeters ME, Kimpfler S: Oncocytoma in the mandibular salivary gland of a cat, *J Feline Med Surg* 10:188–191, 2008.

206. Kim H, Nakaichi M, Itamoto K, et al.: Malignant mixed tumor in the salivary gland of a cat, *J Vet Sci* 9:331–333, 2008.

207. Shimoyama Y, Yamashita K, Ohmachi T, et al.: Pleomorphic adenoma of the salivary gland in two dogs, *J Comp Pathol* 134:254–259, 2006.

208. Faustino AM, Dias Pereira P: A salivary malignant myoepithelioma in a dog, *Vet J* 173:223–226, 2007.

209. Thomsen BV, Myers RK: Extraskeletal osteosarcoma of the mandibular salivary gland in a dog, *Vet Pathol* 36:71–73, 1999.

210. Carberry CA, Flanders JA, Anderson WI, Harvey HJ: Mast cell tumor in the mandibular salivary gland in a dog, *Cornell Vet* 77:362–366, 1987.

211. Militerno G, Bazzo R, Marcato PS: Cytological diagnosis of mandibular salivary gland adenocarcinoma in a dog, *J Vet Med A Physiol Pathol Clin Med* 52:514–516, 2005.

212. Lenoci D, Ricciardi M: Ultrasound and multidetector computed tomography of mandibular salivary gland adenocarcinoma in two dogs, *Open Vet J* 5:173–178, 2015.

213. Belz GT, Heath TJ: Lymph pathways of the medial retropharyngeal lymph node in dogs, *J Anat* 186:517–526, 1995.

214. Boland L, Gomes E, Payen G, et al.: Zygomatic salivary gland diseases in the dog: three cases diagnosed by MRI, *J Am Anim Hosp Assoc* 49:333–337, 2013.

215. Buyukmihci N, Rubin LF, Harvey CE: Exophthalmos secondary to zygomatic adenocarcinoma in a dog, *J Am Vet Med Assoc* 167:162–165, 1975.

216. Evans SM, Thrall DE: Postoperative orthovoltage radiation therapy of parotid salivary gland adenocarcinoma in three dogs, *J Am Vet Med Assoc* 182(1):993–994, 1983.

217. Bundza A, Charlton KM, Becker SA: Adenocarcinoma of the salivary gland in a white Swiss mouse, *Can J Vet Res* 53:363–365, 1989.

218. Dorso L, Risi E, Triau S, et al.: High-grade mucoepidermoid carcinoma of the mandibular salivary gland in a lion (Panthera leo), *Vet Pathol* 45:104–108, 2008.

219. Girard C, Lagacé A, Higgins R, et al.: Adenocarcinoma of the salivary gland in a beluga whale (Delphinapterus leucas), *J Vet Diagn Invest* 3:264–265, 1991.

220. Nishikawa S, Sano F, Takagi K, et al.: Spontaneous poorly differentiated carcinoma with cells positive for vimentin in a salivary gland of a young rat, *Toxicol Pathol* 38:315–318, 2010.

221. Salgado BS, Monteiro LN, Grandi F, et al.: Adenocarcinoma of the parotid salivary gland in a cow, *Vet Clin Pathol* 41:424–428, 2012.

222. Shimada Y, Yoshida T, Takahashi N, et al.: Poorly differentiated salivary gland carcinoma with prominent squamous metaplasia in a pregnant Wistar Hannover rat, *J Vet Med Sci* 78:859–862, 2016.

223. Smith JL, Campbell-Ward M, Else RW, et al.: Undifferentiated carcinoma of the salivary gland in a chinchilla (Chinchilla lanigera), *J Vet Diagn Invest* 22:152–155, 2010.

224. Stackhouse LL, Moore JJ, Hylton WE: Salivary gland adenocarcinoma in a mare, *J Am Vet Med Assoc* 172:271–273, 1978.

225. Yamate J, Yamamoto E, Nabe M, et al.: Spontaneous adenocarcinoma immunoreactive to cyclooxygenase-2 and transforming growth factor-beta1 in the buccal salivary gland of a Richardson's ground squirrel (Spermophilus richardsonii), *Exp Anim* 56:379–384, 2007.

226. Gutschenritter T, Machiorlatti M, Vesely S, et al.: outcomes and prognostic factors of resected salivary gland malignancies: examining a single institution's 12-year experience, *Anticancer Res* 37:5019–5025, 2017.

227. Terhaard CH, Lubsen H, Van der Tweel I, et al.: Dutch Head and Neck Oncology Cooperative Group. Salivary gland carcinoma: independent prognostic factors for locoregional control, distant metastases, and overall survival: results of the Dutch head and neck oncology cooperative group, *Head Neck* 26:681–693, 2004.

228. Al-Mamgani A, van Rooij P, Verduijn GM, et al.: Long-term outcomes and quality of life of 186 patients with primary parotid carcinoma treated with surgery and radiotherapy at the daniel den hoed cancer center, *Int J Radiat Oncol Biol Phys* 84:189–195, 2012.

229. Parsons JT, Mendenhall WM, Stringer SP, et al.: Management of minor salivary gland carcinomas, *Int J Radiat Oncol Biol Phys* 35:443–454, 1996.

230. Aroch I, Markovics A, Mazaki-Tovi M, et al.: Spirocercosis in dogs in Israel: a retrospective case-control study (2004-2009), *Vet Parasitol* 211:234–240, 2015.

231. Dvir E, Kirberger RM, Mukorera V, et al.: Clinical differentiation between dogs with benign and malignant spirocercosis, *Vet Parasitol* 155:80–88, 2008.

232. Kirberger RM, Cassel N, Stander N, et al.: Triple phase dynamic computed tomographic perfusion characteristics of spirocercosis induced esophageal nodules in non-neoplastic versus neoplastic canine cases, *Vet Radiol Ultrasound* 56:257–263, 2015.

233. Pazzi P, Kavkovsky A, Shipov A, et al.: Spirocerca lupi induced oesophageal neoplasia: predictors of surgical outcome, *Vet Parasitol* 250:71–77, 2018.

234. Ranen E, Lavy E, Aizenberg I, et al.: Spirocercosis-associated esophageal sarcomas in dogs. A retrospective study of 17 cases (1997-2003), *Vet Parasitol* 119:209–221, 2004.

235. Sasani F, Javanbakht J, Javaheri A, et al.: The evaluation of retrospective pathological lesions on spirocercosis (Spirocerca lupi) in dogs, *J Parasit Dis* 38:170–173, 2014.

236. Shipov A, Kelmer G, Lavy E, et al.: Long-term outcome of transendoscopic oesophageal mass ablation in dogs with Spirocerca lupi-associated oesophageal sarcoma, *Vet Rec* 177:365, 2015.

237. Yas E, Kelmer G, Shipov A, et al.: Successful transendoscopic oesophageal mass ablation in two dogs with Spirocerca lupi associated oesophageal sarcoma, *J Small Anim Pract* 54:495–498, 2013.

238. Culbertson R, Branam JE, Rosenblatt LS: Esophageal/gastric leiomyoma in the laboratory Beagle, *J Am Vet Med Assoc* 183:1168–1171, 1983.

239. Ranen E, Dank G, Lavy E, et al.: Oesophageal sarcomas in dogs: histological and clinical evaluation, *Vet J* 178:78–84, 2008.

240. Hamilton TA, Carpenter JL: Esophageal plasmacytoma in a dog, *J Am Vet Med Assoc* 204:1210–1211, 1994.

241. Gibson CJ, Parry NM, Jakowski RM, et al.: Adenomatous polyp with intestinal metaplasia of the esophagus (Barrett esophagus) in a dog, *Vet Pathol* 47:116–119, 2010.

242. Farese JP, Bacon NJ, Ehrhart NP, et al.: Oesophageal leiomyosarcoma in dogs: surgical management and clinical outcome of four cases, *Vet Comp Oncol* 6:31–38, 2008.

243. Arnell K, Hill S, Hart J, et al.: Persistent regurgitation in four dogs with caudal esophageal neoplasia, *J Am Anim Hosp Assoc* 49:58–63, 2013.

244. Okanishi H, Shibuya H, Miyasaka T, et al.: Adenosquamous carcinoma of the oesophagus in a dog, *J Small Anim Pract* 56:521–523, 2015.

245. McCaw D, Pratt M, Walshaw R: Squamous cell carcinoma of the esophagus in a dog, *J Am Anim Hosp Assoc* 16:561–563, 1980.

246. Gualtieri M, Monzeglio MG, Di Giancamillo M: Oesophageal squamous cell carcinoma in two cats, *J Small Anim Pract* 40:79–83, 1999.

247. Berube D, Scott-Moncrieff JC, Rohleder J, et al.: Primary esophageal squamous cell carcinoma in a cat, *J Am Anim Hosp Assoc* 45:291–295, 2009.

248. Rolfe DS, Twedt DC, Seim HB: Chronic regurgitation or vomiting caused by esophageal leiomyoma in three dogs, *J Am Anim Hosp Assoc* 30:425–430, 1994.

249. Ridgway RL, Suter PF: Clinical and radiographic signs in primary and metastatic esophageal neoplasms of the dog, *J Am Vet Med Assoc* 174:700–704, 1979.

250. Withrow SJ: Esophageal cancer. In Withrow SJ, Vail DM, Page RL, editors: *Withrow and macewen's small animal clinical oncology*, ed 5, St Louis, MO, 2013, Elsevier Saunders, pp 399–401.

251. Ranen E, Shamir MH, Shahar R, et al.: Partial esophagectomy with single layer closure for treatment of esophageal sarcomas in 6 dogs, *Vet Surg* 33:428–434, 2004.

252. Hansen KS, Weisse C, Berent AC, et al.: Use of a self-expanding metallic stent to palliate esophageal neoplastic obstruction in a dog, *J Am Vet Med Assoc* 240:1202–1207, 2012.

253. Robin EM, Pey PB, de Fornel-Thibaud P, et al.: Esophageal leiomyoma in a dog causing esophageal distension and treated by transcardial placement of a self-expanding, covered, nitinol esophageal stent, *J Am Vet Med Assoc* 252:330–335, 2018.

254. American cancer society. https://www.cancer.org/cancer/esophagus-cancer/.

255. Chen X, Yang CS: Esophageal adenocarcinoma: a review and perspectives on the mechanism of carcinogenesis and chemoprevention, *Carcinogenesis* 22:1119–1129, 2001.

256. Seaman RL: Exocrine pancreatic neoplasia in the cat: a case series, *J Am Anim Hosp Assoc* 40:238–245, 2004.

257. Knecht C, Priester W: Osteosarcoma in dogs: a study of previous trauma, fracture and fracture fixation, *J Am Anim Hosp Assoc* 14:82–84, 1978.

258. Priester WA: Data from eleven United States and Canadian colleges of veterinary medicine on pancreatic carcinoma in domestic animals, *Cancer Res* 34:1372–1375, 1974.

259. Kircher CH, Nielsen SW: Tumours of the pancreas, *Bull World Health Organ* 53:195–202, 1976.
260. Anderson NV, Johnson KH: Pancreatic carcinoma in the dog, *J Am Vet Med Assoc* 150:286–295, 1967.
261. Brown PJ, Mason KV, Merrett DJ, et al.: Multifocal necrotising steatites associated with pancreatic carcinoma in three dogs, *J Small Anim Pract* 35:129–132, 1994.
262. Kamano T, Azuma N, Katami A, et al.: Preliminary observation on pancreatic duct adenocarcinoma induced by intraductal administration of N-ethyl-N'-nitro-N-nitrosoguanidine in dogs, *Jpn J Cancer Res* 79:1–4, 1988.
263. VanEnkevort BA, O'Brien RT, Young KM: Pancreatic pseudocysts in 4 dogs and 2 cats: ultrasonographic and clinicopathologic findings, *J Vet Intern Med* 13:309–313, 1999.
264. Chang SC, Liao JW, Lin YC, et al.: Pancreatic acinar cell carcinoma with intracranial metastasis in a dog, *J Vet Med Sci* 69:91–93, 2007.
265. Linderman MJ, Brodsky EM, de Lorimier LP, et al.: Feline exocrine pancreatic carcinoma: a retrospective study of 34 cases, *Vet Comp Oncol* 11:208–218, 2013.
266. Tasker S, Griffon DJ, Nuttall TJ, et al.: Resolution of paraneoplastic alopecia following surgical removal of a pancreatic carcinoma in a cat, *J Small Anim Pract* 40:16–19, 1999.
267. Brooks DG, Campbell KL, Dennis JS, et al.: Pancreatic paraneoplastic alopecia in three cats, *J Am Anim Hosp Assoc* 30:557–563, 1994.
268. Kipperman BS, Nelson RW, Griffey SM, et al.: Diabetes mellitus and exocrine pancreatic neoplasia in two cats with hyperadrenocorticism, *J Am Anim Hosp Assoc* 28:415–418, 1992.
269. Quigley KA, Jackson ML, Haines DM: Hyperlipasemia in 6 dogs with pancreatic or hepatic neoplasia: evidence for tumor lipase production, *Vet Clin Pathol* 30:114–120, 2001.
270. Bright JM: Pancreatic adenocarcinoma in a dog with a maldigestion syndrome, *J Am Vet Med Assoc* 187:420–421, 1985.
271. Bennett PF, Hahn KA, Toal RL, et al.: Ultrasonographic and cytopathological diagnosis of exocrine pancreatic carcinoma in the dog and cat, *J Am Anim Hosp Assoc* 37:466–473, 2001.
272. Hecht S, Penninck DG, Keating JH: Imaging findings in pancreatic neoplasia and nodular hyperplasia in 19 cats, *Vet Radiol Ultrasound* 48:45–50, 2007.
273. Vanderperren K, Haers H, Van der Vekens E, et al.: Description of the use of contrast-enhanced ultrasonography in four dogs with pancreatic tumours, *J Small Anim Pract* 55:164–169, 2014.
274. Jakab CS, Rusvai M, Demeter Z, et al.: Expression of claudin-4 molecule in canine exocrine pancreatic acinar cell carcinomas, *Histol Histopathol* 26:1121–1126, 2011.
275. Jakab C, Rusvai M, Galfi P, et al.: Expression of claudin-5 in canine pancreatic acinar cell carcinoma - An immunohistochemical study, *Acta Vet Hung* 59:87–98, 2011.
276. Cobb LF, Merrell RC: Total pancreatectomy in dogs, *J Surg Res* 37:235–240, 1984.
277. Winter JM, Brody JR, Abrams RA, et al.: Cancers of the gastrointestinal tract. In DeVita VT, Lawrence TS, Rosenberg SA, editors: *Devita, hellman, and rosenberg's cancer: principles & practice of oncology*, ed 10, Philadephia, 2015, Wolters Kluwer, pp 657–684.
278. American Cancer Society: *Cancer facts and 2017*, Atlanta, 2017, American Cancer Society.
279. Neoptolemos JP, Urrutia R, Abbruzzese J, Buechler MW, editors: *Pancreatic cancer*, ed 1, Verlag, 2010, Springer.
280. Siegel R, Naishadham D, Jemal A: Cancer statistics, 2013, *CA Cancer J Clin* 63:11–30, 2013.
281. Seim-Wikse T, Jörundsson E, Nødtvedt A, et al.: Breed predisposition to canine gastric carcinoma - a study based on the Norwegian canine cancer register, *Acta Vet Scand* 55:25, 2013.
282. Patnaik AK, Hurvitz AI, Johnson GF: Canine gastrointestinal neoplasms, *Vet Pathol* 14:547–555, 1977.
283. Gualtieri M, Monzeglio MG, Scanziani E: Gastric neoplasia, *Vet Clin North Am Small Anim Pract* 29:415–440, 1999.
284. Hugen S, Thomas RE, German AJ, et al.: Gastric carcinoma in canines and humans, a review, *Vet Comp Oncol* 15:692–705, 2017.
285. Kurihara M, Shirakabe H, Izumi T, et al.: Adenocarcinomas of the stomach induced in beagle dogs by oral administration of N-ethyl-N'-nitro-N-nitrosoguanidine, *Z Krebsforsch Klin Onkol Cancer Res Clin Oncol* 90:241–252, 1977.
286. Smith JP, Nadella S, Osborne N: Gastrin and gastric cancer, *Cell Mol Gastroenterol Hepatol* 4:75–83, 2017.
287. Qvigstad G, Kolbjørnsen Ø, Skancke E, et al.: Gastric neuroendocrine carcinoma associated with atrophic gastritis in the Norwegian lundehund, *J Comp Pathol* 139:194–201, 2008.
288. Seim-Wikse T, Kolbjørnsen Ø, Jörundsson E, et al.: Tumour gastrin expression and serum gastrin concentrations in dogs with gastric carcinoma are poor diagnostic indicators, *J Comp Pathol* 151:207–211, 2014.
289. Kubota-Aizawa S, Ohno K, Fukushima K, et al.: Epidemiological study of gastric Helicobacter spp. in dogs with gastrointestinal disease in Japan and diversity of Helicobacter heilmannii sensu stricto, *Vet J* 225:56–62, 2017.
290. Haesebrouck F, Pasmans F, Flahou B, et al.: Gastric Helicobacters in domestic animals and nonhuman primates and their significance for human health, *Clin Microbiol Rev* 22:202–223, 2009.
291. Strauss-Ayali D, Simpson KW: Gastric Helicobacter infection in dogs, *Vet Clin North Am Small Anim Pract* 29:397–414, 1999.
292. von Babo V, Eberle N, Mischke R, et al.: Canine non-hematopoietic gastric neoplasia. Epidemiologic and diagnostic characteristics in 38 dogs with post-surgical outcome of five cases, *Tierärztl Prax* 40:243–249, 2012.
293. Swann HM, Holt DE: Canine gastric adenocarcinoma and leiomyosarcoma: a retrospective study of 21 cases (1986-1999) and literature review, *J Am Anim Hosp Assoc* 38:157–164, 2002.
294. Sautter JH, Hanlon GF: Gastric neoplasms in the dog: a report of 20 cases, *J Am Vet Med Assoc* 166:691–696, 1975.
295. Lubbes D, Mandigers PJJ, Heuven HCM, et al.: Incidence of gastric carcinoma in Dutch Tervueren shepherd dogs born between 1991 and 2002, *Tijdschr Diergeneeskd* 134:606–610, 2009.
296. Scanziani E, Giusti AM, Gualtieri M, et al.: Gastric carcinoma in the Belgian shepherd dog, *J Small Anim Pract* 32:465–469, 1991.
297. Fonda D, Gualtieri M, Scanziani E: Gastric carcinoma in the dog: a clinicopathological study of 11 cases, *J Small Anim Pract* 30:353–360, 1989.
298. Patnaik AK, Hurvitz AI, Johnson GF: Canine gastric adenocarcinoma, *Vet Pathol* 15:600–607, 1978.
299. Frost D, Lasota J, Miettinen M: Gastrointestinal stromal tumors and leiomyomas in the dog: a histopathologic, immunohistochemical, and molecular genetic study of 50 cases, *Vet Pathol* 40:42–54, 2003.
300. Ozaki K, Yamagami T, Nomura K, et al.: Mast cell tumors of the gastrointestinal tract in 39 dogs, *Vet Pathol* 39:557–564, 2002.
301. Fant P, Caldin M, Furlanello T, et al.: Primary gastric histiocytic sarcoma in a dog—a case report, *J Vet Med* 51:358–362, 2004.
302. Lenz JA, Furrow E, Craig LE, et al.: Histiocytic sarcoma in 14 miniature schnauzers - a new breed predisposition? *J Small Anim Pract* 58:461–467, 2017.
303. Atherton MJ, Vazquez-Sanmartin S, Sharpe S, et al.: A metastatic secretory gastric plasmacytoma with aberrant CD3 expression in a dog, *Vet Clin Pathol* 46:520–525, 2017.
304. Russell KN, Mehler SJ, Skorupski KA, et al.: Clinical and immunohistochemical differentiation of gastrointestinal stromal tumors from leiomyosarcomas in dogs: 42 cases (1990-2003), *J Am Vet Med Assoc* 230:1329–1333, 2007.
305. Withrow SJ: Gastric cancer. In Withrow SJ, Vail DM, Page RL, editors: *Small animal clinical oncology*, ed 5, St. Louis, 2013, Elsevier, pp 402–404.
306. Turk MA, Gallina AM, Russell TS: Nonhematopoietic gastrointestinal neoplasia in cats: a retrospective study of 44 cases, *Vet Pathol* 18:614–620, 1981.

307. Cribb AE: Feline gastrointestinal adenocarcinoma: a review and retrospective study, *Can Vet J* 29:709, 1988.

308. Bonfanti U, Bertazzolo W, Bottero E, et al.: Diagnostic value of cytologic examination of gastrointestinal tract tumors in dogs and cats: 83 cases (2001-2004), *J Am Vet Med Assoc* 229:1130–1133, 2006.

309. Dennis MM, Bennett N, Ehrhart EJ: Gastric adenocarcinoma and chronic gastritis in two related Persian cats, *Vet Pathol* 43:358–362, 2006.

310. Bridgeford EC, Marini RP, Feng Y, et al.: Gastric Helicobacter species as a cause of feline gastric lymphoma: a viable hypothesis, *Vet Immunol Immunopathol* 123:106–113, 2008.

311. Barrett LE, Skorupski K, Brown DC, et al.: Outcome following treatment of feline gastrointestinal mast cell tumours, *Vet Comp Oncol* 16:188–193, 2018.

312. Rossmeisl JH, Forrester SD, Robertson JL, et al.: Chronic vomiting associated with a gastric carcinoid in a cat, *J Am Anim Hosp Assoc* 38:61–66, 2002.

313. Smith TJ, Baltzer WI, Ruaux CG, et al.: Gastric smooth muscle hamartoma in a cat, *J Feline Med Surg* 12:334–337, 2010.

314. Daure E, Jania R, Jennings S, et al.: Ultrasonographic and clinicopathological features of pyloroduodenal adenomatous polyps in cats, *J Feline Med Surg* 19:141–145, 2017.

315. Lauren P: The two histological main types of gastric carcinoma: diffuse and so-called intestinal-type carcinoma. An attempt at a histoclinical classification, *Acta Pathol Microbiol Scand* 64:31–49, 1965.

316. Wadhwa R, Song S, Lee J-S, et al.: Gastric cancer-molecular and clinical dimensions, *Nat Rev Clin Oncol* 10:643–655, 2013.

317. Pollock S, Wagner BM: Gastric adenocarcinoma or linitis plastica in a dog, *Vet Med Small Anim Clin* 68:139–142, 1973.

318. Kapatkin AS, Mullen HS, Matthiesen DT, et al.: Leiomyosarcoma in dogs: 44 cases (1983-1988), *J Am Vet Med Assoc* 201:1077–1079, 1992.

319. Kerpsack SJ, Birchard SJ: Removal of leiomyomas and other noninvasive masses from the cardiac region of the canine stomach, *J Am Anim Hosp Assoc* 30:500–504, 1994.

320. Beaudry D, Knapp DW, Montgomery T, et al.: Hypoglycemia in four dogs with smooth muscle tumors, *J Vet Intern Med* 9:415–418, 1995.

321. Bagley RS, Levy JK, Malarkey DE: Hypoglycemia associated with intra-abdominal leiomyoma and leiomyosarcoma in six dogs, *J Am Vet Med Assoc* 208:69–71, 1996.

322. Gillespie V, Baer K, Farrelly J, et al.: Canine gastrointestinal stromal tumors: immunohistochemical expression of CD34 and examination of prognostic indicators including proliferation markers Ki67 and AgNOR, *Vet Pathol* 48:283–291, 2011.

323. Sircar K, Hewlett BR, Huizinga JD, et al.: Interstitial cells of Cajal as precursors of gastrointestinal stromal tumors, *Am J Surg Pathol* 23:377–389, 1999.

324. Kobayashi M, Kuroki S, Ito K, et al.: Imatinib-associated tumour response in a dog with a non-resectable gastrointestinal stromal tumour harbouring a c-kit exon 11 deletion mutation, *Vet J* 198:271–274, 2013.

325. Irie M, Takeuchi Y, Ohtake Y, et al.: Imatinib mesylate treatment in a dog with gastrointestinal stromal tumors with a c-kit mutation, *J Vet Med Sci* 77:1535–1539, 2015.

326. Takanosu M, Amano S, Kagawa Y: Analysis of c-KIT exon 11 mutations in canine gastrointestinal stromal tumours, *Vet J* 207:118–123, 2016.

327. Gregory-Bryson E, Bartlett E, Kiupel M, et al.: Canine and human gastrointestinal stromal tumors display similar mutations in c-KIT exon 11, *BMC Cancer* 10:559, 2010.

328. Morini M, Gentilini F, Pietra M, et al.: Cytological, immunohistochemical and mutational analysis of a gastric gastrointestinal stromal tumour in a cat, *J Comp Pathol* 145:152–157, 2011.

329. Finotello R, Vasconi ME, Sabattini S, et al.: Feline large granular lymphocyte lymphoma: an Italian Society of Veterinary Oncology (SIONCOV) retrospective study, *Vet Comp Oncol* 16:159–166, 2018.

330. Pohlman LM, Higginbotham ML, Welles EG, et al.: Immunophenotypic and histologic classification of 50 cases of feline gastrointestinal lymphoma, *Vet Pathol* 46:259–268, 2009.

331. Yamada K, Morimoto M, Kishimoto M, et al.: Virtual endoscopy of dogs using multi–detector row CT, *Vet Radiol Ultrasound* 48:318–322, 2007.

332. Hoey S, Drees R, Hetzel S: Evaluation of the gastrointestinal tract in dogs using computed tomography, *Vet Radiol Ultrasound* 54:25–30, 2013.

333. Fitzgerald E, Lam R, Drees R: Improving conspicuity of the canine gastrointestinal wall using dual phase contrast-enhanced computed tomography: a retrospective cross-sectional study, *Vet Radiol Ultrasound* 58:151–162, 2017.

334. Lamb CR, Grierson J: Ultrasonographic appearance of primary gastric neoplasia in 21 dogs, *J Small Anim Pract* 40:211–215, 1999.

335. Marolf AJ, Bachand AM, Sharber J, et al.: Comparison of endoscopy and sonography findings in dogs and cats with histologically confirmed gastric neoplasia, *J Small Anim Pract* 56:339–344, 2015.

336. Willard MD, Mansell J, Fosgate GT, et al.: Effect of sample quality on the sensitivity of endoscopic biopsy for detecting gastric and duodenal lesions in dogs and cats, *J Vet Intern Med* 22:1084–1089, 2008.

337. Riondato F, Miniscalco B, Berio E, et al.: Diagnosis of canine gastric adenocarcinoma using squash preparation cytology, *Vet J* 201:390–394, 2014.

338. Eisele J, McClaran JK, Runge JJ, et al.: Evaluation of risk factors for morbidity and mortality after pylorectomy and gastroduodenostomy in dogs, *Vet Surg* 39:261–267, 2010.

339. Beaumont PR: Anastomotic jejunal ulcer secondary to gastrojejunostomy in a dog, *J Am Anim Hosp Assoc* 17:233–237, 1981.

340. Macdonald JS, Smalley SR, Benedetti J, et al.: Chemoradiotherapy after surgery compared with surgery alone for adenocarcinoma of the stomach or gastroesophageal junction, *N Engl J Med* 345:725–730, 2001.

341. Terragni R, Casadei Gardini A, Sabattini S, et al.: EGFR, HER-2 and KRAS in canine gastric epithelial tumors: a potential human model? *PLoS One* 9:e85388, 2014.

342. Sellon RK, Bissonnette K, Bunch SE: Long-term survival after total gastrectomy for gastric adenocarcinoma in a dog, *J Vet Intern Med* 10:333–335, 1996.

343. Walter MC, Matthiesen DT, Stone EA: Pylorectomy and gastroduodenostomy in the dog: technique and clinical results in 28 cases, *J Am Vet Med Assoc* 187:909–914, 1985.

344. Beck JA, Simpson DS: Surgical treatment of gastric leiomyoma in a dog, *Aust Vet J* 77:161–163, 1999.

345. Torre LA, Bray F, Siegel RL, et al.: Global cancer statistics, 2012, *CA Cancer J Clin* 65:87–108, 2015.

346. Torre LA, Siegel RL, Ward EM, et al.: Global cancer incidence and mortality rates and trends—an update, *Cancer Epidemiol Biomarkers Prev* 25:16–27, 2016.

347. Plummer M, Franceschi S, Vignat J, et al.: Global burden of gastric cancer attributable to Helicobacter pylori, *Int J Cancer* 136:487–490, 2015.

348. Guggenheim DE, Shah MA: Gastric cancer epidemiology and risk factors, *J Surg Oncol* 107:230–236, 2012.

349. Gotoda T, Iwasaki M, Kusano C, et al.: Endoscopic resection of early gastric cancer treated by guideline and expanded National Cancer Centre criteria, *Br J Surg* 97:868–871, 2010.

350. Halabi El HM, Lawrence W: Clinical results of various reconstructions employed after total gastrectomy, *J Surg Oncol* 97:186–192, 2008.

351. Ku GY, Ilson DH: Neoadjuvant and adjuvant treatment—strategies and clinical trials—Western perspective. In Strong VE, editor: *Gastric cancer*, ed 1, New York, 2015, Springer, pp 297–302.

352. Bang Y-J, Van Cutsem E, Feyereislova A, et al.: Trastuzumab in combination with chemotherapy versus chemotherapy alone for treatment of HER2-positive advanced gastric or gastro-oesophageal junction cancer (ToGA): a phase 3, open-label, randomised controlled trial, *Lancet* 376:687–697, 2010.

353. Strombeck DR: Clinicopathologic features of primary and metastatic neoplastic disease of the liver in dogs, *J Am Vet Med Assoc* 173:267–269, 1978.

354. Cullen JM, Popp JA: Tumors of the liver and gall bladder. In Meuten DJ, editor: *Tumors in domestic animals*, ed 4, Ames, 2002, Iowa State Press, pp 483–508.

355. Hammer AS, Sikkema DA: Hepatic neoplasia in the dog and cat, *Vet Clin North Am Small Anim Pract* 25:419–435, 1995.

356. Thamm DH: Hepatobiliary tumors. In Withrow SJ, MacEwen EG, editors: *Small animal clinical oncology*, ed 3, Philadelphia, 2001, WB Saunders, pp 327–334.

357. Patnaik AK, Hurvitz AI, Lieberman PH: Canine hepatic neoplasms: a clinicopathological study, *Vet Pathol* 17:553–564, 1980.

358. Patnaik AK: A morphologic and immunohistochemical study of hepatic neoplasms in cats, *Vet Pathol* 29:405–415, 1992.

359. Post G, Patnaik AK: Nonhematopoietic hepatic neoplasms in cats: 21 cases (1983–1988), *J Am Vet Med Assoc* 201:1080–1082, 1992.

360. Lawrence HJ, Erb HN, Harvey HJ: Nonlymphomatous hepatobiliary masses in cats: 41 cases (1972 to 1991), *Vet Surg* 23:365–368, 1994.

361. Patnaik AK, Hurvitz AI, Lieberman PH, et al.: Canine hepatocellular carcinoma, *Vet Pathol* 18:427–438, 1981.

362. Kosovsky JE, Manfra-Marretta S, Matthiesen DT, et al.: Results of partial hepatectomy in 18 dogs with hepatocellular carcinoma, *J Am Anim Hosp Assoc* 25:203–206, 1989.

363. Liptak JM, Dernell WS, Monnet E, et al.: Massive hepatocellular carcinoma in dogs: 48 cases (1992-2002), *J Am Vet Med Assoc* 225:1225–1230, 2004.

364. Patnaik AK, Hurvitz AI, Lieberman PH, et al.: Canine bile duct carcinoma, *Vet Pathol* 18:439–444, 1981.

365. Hayes HM, Morin MM, Rubenstein DA: Canine biliary carcinoma: epidemiological comparisons with man, *J Comp Pathol* 93:99–107, 1983.

366. Patnaik AK, Lieberman PH, Hurvitz AI, et al.: Canine hepatic carcinoids, *Vet Pathol* 18:445–453, 1981.

367. van Sprundel RGHM, van den Ingh TSGAM, Guscetti F, et al.: Classification of primary hepatic tumours in the dog, *Vet J* 197:596–606, 2013.

368. van Sprundel RGHM, van den Ingh TSGAM, Guscetti F, et al.: Classification of primary hepatic tumours in the cat, *Vet J* 202:255–266, 2014.

369. Shiga A, Shirota K, Shida T, et al.: Hepatoblastoma in a dog, *J Vet Med Sci* 59:1167–1170, 1997.

370. Bartlett DL, Carr BI, Marsh JW: Cancer of the liver. In DeVita VT, Hellman S, Rosenberg SA, editors: *Cancer: principles and practice of oncology*, ed 7, Philadelphia, 2005, Lippincott Williams & Wilkins, pp 986–1009.

371. Cortright CC, Center SA, Randolph JF, et al.: Clinical features of progressive vacuolar hepatopathy in Scottish terriers with and without hepatocellular carcinoma: 114 cases (1980–2013), *J Am Vet Med Assoc* 245:797–808, 2014.

372. Evans SM: The radiographic appearance of primary liver neoplasia in dogs, *Vet Radiol* 28:192–196, 1987.

373. Goussev SA, Center SA, Randolph JF, et al.: Clinical characteristics of hepatocellular carcinoma in 19 cats for a single institution (1980–2013), *J Am Anim Hosp Assoc* 52:36–41, 2016.

374. Adler R, Wilson DW: Biliary cystadenomas of cats, *Vet Pathol* 32:415–418, 1995.

375. Trout NJ, Berg J, McMillan MC, et al.: Surgical treatment of hepatobiliary cystadenomas in cats: five cases (1988-1993), *J Am Vet Med Assoc* 206:505–507, 1995.

376. Nyland TG, Koblik PD, Tellyer SE: Ultrasonographic evaluation of biliary cystadenomas in cats, *Vet Radiol Ultrasound* 40:300–306, 1999.

377. Willard MD, Dunstan RW, Faulkner J: Neuroendocrine carcinoma of the gall bladder in a dog, *J Am Vet Med Assoc* 192:926–928, 1988.

378. Morrell CN, Volk MV, Mankowski JL: A carcinoid tumor in the gallbladder of a dog, *Vet Pathol* 39:756–758, 2002.

379. Trigo FJ, Thompson H, Breeze RG, et al.: The pathology of liver tumors in the dog, *J Comp Pathol* 92:21–39, 1982.

380. Kapatkin AS, Mullen HS, Matthiesen DT, et al.: Leiomyosarcoma in dogs: 44 cases (1983-1988), *J Am Vet Med Assoc* 201:1077–1079, 1992.

381. Patnaik AK, Lieberman PH, Erlandson RA, et al.: Hepatobiliary neuroendocrine carcinoma in cats: a clinicopathologic, immunohistochemical, and ultrastructural study of 17 cases, *Vet Pathol* 42:331–337, 2005.

382. Bartlett DL, Ramanathan RK, Deutsch M: Cancer of the biliary tree. In DeVita VT, Hellman S, Rosenberg SA, editors: *Cancer: principles cxles and practice of oncology*, ed 7, Philadelphia, 2005, Lippincott Williams & Wilkins, pp 1009–1031.

383. Scavelli TD, Patnaik AK, Mehlhaff CJ, et al.: Hemangiosarcoma in the cat: retrospective evaluation of 31 surgical cases, *J Am Vet Med Assoc* 187:817–819, 1985.

384. Brown NO, Patnaik AK, MacEwen EG: Canine hemangiosarcoma: retrospective analysis of 104 cases, *J Am Vet Med Assoc* 186:56–58, 1985.

385. Srebernik N, Appleby EC: Breed prevalence and sites of haemangioma and haemangiosarcoma in dogs, *Vet Rec* 129:408–409, 1991.

386. Affolter VK, Moore PF: Canine cutaneous and systemic histiocytosis: reactive histiocytosis of dermal dendritic cells, *Am J Dermatopathol* 22:40–48, 2000.

387. Affolter VK, Moore PF: Localized and disseminated histiocytic sarcoma of dendritic cell origin in dogs, *Vet Pathol* 39:74–83, 2002.

388. Leifer CE, Peterson ME, Matus RE, et al.: Hypoglycemia associated with nonislet cell tumor in 13 dogs, *J Am Vet Med Assoc* 186:53–55, 1985.

389. Aronsohn MG, Dubiel B, Roberts B, et al.: Prognosis for acute nontraumatic hemoperitoneum in the dog: a retrospective analysis of 60 cases (2003-2006), *J Am Anim Hosp Assoc* 45:72–77, 2009.

390. Badylak SF, Dodds WJ, van Vleet JF: Plasma coagulation factor abnormalities in dogs with naturally occurring hepatic disease, *Am J Vet Res* 44:2336–2340, 1983.

391. McConnell MF, Lumsden JH: Biochemical evaluation of metastatic liver disease in the dog, *J Am Anim Hosp Assoc* 19:173–178, 1983.

392. Center SA, Slater MR, Manwarren T, et al.: Diagnostic efficacy of serum alkaline phosphatase and γ-glutamyltransferase in dogs with histologically confirmed hepatobiliary disease: 270 cases (1980-1990), *J Am Vet Med Assoc* 201:1258–1264, 1992.

393. Lowseth LA, Gillett NA, Chang IY, et al.: Detection of serum α-fetoprotein in dogs with hepatic tumors, *J Am Vet Med Assoc* 199:735–741, 1991.

394. Yamada T, Fujita M, Kitao S, et al.: Serum alpha-fetoprotein values in dogs with various hepatic diseases, *J Vet Med Sci* 61:657–659, 1999.

395. Hahn KA, Richardson RC: Detection of serum alpha-fetoprotein in dogs with naturally occurring malignant neoplasia, *Vet Clin Pathol* 24:18–21, 1995.

396. Friedrichs KR, Thomas C, Plier M, et al.: Evaluation of serum ferritin as a tumor marker for canine histiocytic sarcoma, *J Vet Intern Med* 24:904–911, 2010.

397. Feeney DA, Johnston GR, Hardy RM: Two-dimensional, grayscale ultrasonography for assessment of hepatic and splenic neoplasia in the dog and cat, *J Am Vet Med Assoc* 184:68–81, 1984.

398. Vörös K, Vrabély T, Papp L, et al.: Correlation of ultrasonographic and pathomorphological findings in canine hepatic diseases, *J Small Anim Pract* 32:627–634, 1991.

399. Newell SM, Selcer BA, Girard E, et al.: Correlations between ultrasonographic findings and specific hepatic disease in cats: 72 cases (1985-1997), *J Am Vet Med Assoc* 213:94–98, 1998.

400. Léveillé R, Partington BP, Biller DS, et al.: Complications after ultrasound-guided biopsy of abdominal structures in dogs and cats: 246 cases (1984-1991), *J Am Vet Med Assoc* 203:413–415, 1993.

401. Barr F: Percutaneous biopsy of abdominal organs under ultrasound guidance, *J Small Anim Pract* 36:105–113, 1995.

402. Grienie ER, David FH, Ober CP, et al.: Evaluation of canine hepatic masses by use of triphasic computed tomography and B-mode, color flow, power, and pulsed-wave Doppler ultrasonography and correlation with histopathologic classification, *Am J Vet Res* 78:1273–1283, 2017.

403. Warren-Smith CMR, Andrew S, Mantis P, et al.: Lack of associations between ultrasonographic appearance of parenchymal lesions of the liver and histological diagnosis, *J Small Anim Pract* 53:168–173, 2012.

404. O'Brien RT, Iani M, Matheson J, et al.: Contrast harmonic ultrasound of spontaneous liver nodules in 32 dogs, *Vet Radiol Ultrasound* 45:547–553, 2004.

405. Kutara K, Asano K, Kito A, et al.: Contrast harmonic imaging of canine hepatic tumors, *J Vet Med Sci* 68:433–438, 2006.

406. Nakamura K, Takagi S, Sasaki N, et al.: Contrast-enhanced ultrasonography for characterization of canine focal liver lesions, *Vet Radiol Ultrasound* 51:79–85, 2010.

407. Kanemoto H, Ohno K, Nakashima K, et al.: Characterization of canine focal liver lesions with contrast-enhanced ultrasound using a novel contrast agent – sonazoid, *Vet Radiol Ultrasound* 50:188–194, 2009.

408. Roth L: Comparison of liver cytology and biopsy diagnoses in dogs and cats: 56 cases, *Vet Clin Pathol* 30:35–38, 2001.

409. Masserdotti C, Drigo M: Retrospective study of cytologic features of well-differentiated hepatocellular carcinoma in dogs, *Vet Clin Pathol* 41:382–390, 2012.

410. D'Angelica M, Fong Y, Weber S, et al.: The role of staging laparoscopy in hepatobiliary malignancy: prospective analysis of 401 cases, *Ann Surg Oncol* 10:183–189, 2003.

411. Fukushima K, Kanemoto H, Ohno K, et al.: CT characteristics of primary hepatic mass lesions in dogs, *Vet Radiol Ultrasound* 53:252–257, 2012.

412. Kutara K, Seki M, Ishikawa C, et al.: Triple-phase helical computed tomography in dogs with hepatic masses, *Vet Radiol Ultrasound* 55:7–15, 2014.

413. Jones ID, Lamb CR, Drees R, et al.: Associations between dual-phase computed tomography features and histopathologic diagnoses in 52 dogs with hepatic or splenic masses, *Vet Radiol Ultrasound* 57:144–153, 2016.

414. Constant C, Hecht S, Craig LE, et al.: Gadoxetate disodium (Gd-EOB-DTPA) contrast enhanced magnetic resonance imaging characteristics of hepatocellular carcinoma in dogs, *Vet Radiol Ultrasound* 57:594–600, 2016.

415. Cuccovillo A, Lamb CR: Cellular features of sonographic target lesions of the liver and spleen in 21 dogs and a cat, *Vet Radiol Ultrasound* 43:275–278, 2002.

416. Stowater JL, Lamb CR, Schelling SH: Ultrasonographic features of canine hepatic nodular hyperplasia, *Vet Radiol* 31:268–272, 1990.

417. Martin RA, Lanz OI, Tobias KM: Liver and biliary system. In Slatter DH, editor: *Textbook of small animal surgery*, ed 3, Philadelphia, 2003, WB Saunders, pp 716–717.

418. Covey JL, Degner DA, Jackson AH, et al.: Hilar liver resection in dogs, *Vet Surg* 38:104–111, 2009.

419. Matsuyama A, Takagi S, Hosoya K, et al.: Impact of surgical margins on survival of 37 dogs with massive hepatocellular carcinoma, *NZ Vet J* 65:277–231, 2017.

420. Iida G, Asano K, Seki M, et al.: Intraoperative identification of canine hepatocellular carcinoma with indocyanine green fluorescent imaging, *J Small Anim Pract* 54:594–600, 2013.

421. Seki M, Asano K, Ishigaki K, et al.: En block resection of a large hepatocellular carcinoma involving the caudal vena cava in a dog, *J Vet Med Sci* 73:693–696, 2011.

422. Hanson KR, Pigott AM, Linklater AKJ: Incidence of blood transfusion requirement and factors associated with transfusion following liver lobectomy in dogs and cats: 72 cases (2007–2015), *J Am Vet Med Assoc* 251:929–934, 2017.

423. Weisse C, Clifford CA, Holt D, et al.: Percutaneous arterial embolization and chemoembolization for treatment of benign and malignant tumors in three dogs and a goat, *J Am Vet Med Assoc* 221:1430–1436, 2002.

424. Cave TA, Johnson V, Beths T, et al.: Treatment of unresectable hepatocellular adenoma in dogs with transarterial iodized oil and chemotherapy with and without an embolic agent: a report of two cases, *Vet Comp Oncol* 1:191–199, 2003.

425. Iwai S, Okano S, Chikazawa S, et al.: Transcatheter arterial embolization for treatment of hepatocellular carcinoma in a cat, *Vet Med Assoc* 247:1299–1302, 2015.

426. Yang T, Case BJ, Boston S, et al.: Microwave ablation for treatment of hepatic neoplasia in five dogs, *J Am Vet Med Assoc* 250:79–85, 2017.

427. Mori T, Ito Y, Kawabe M, et al.: Three-dimensional conformal radiation therapy for inoperable massive hepatocellular carcinoma in six dogs, *J Small Anim Pract* 56:441–445, 2015.

428. Elpiner A, Brodsky E, Hazzah T, et al.: Single-agent gemcitabine chemotherapy in dogs with hepatocellular carcinoma, *Vet Comp Oncol* 9:260–268, 2011.

429. Fry PD, Rest JR: Partial hepatectomy in two dogs, *J Small Anim Pract* 34:192–195, 1993.

430. Ogilvie GK, Powers BE, Mallinckrodt CH, et al.: Surgery and doxorubicin in dogs with hemangiosarcoma, *J Vet Intern Med* 10:379–384, 1996.

431. Rassnick KM, Frimberger AE, Wood CA, et al.: Evaluation of ifosfamide for treatment of various canine neoplasms, *J Vet Intern Med* 14:271–276, 2000.

432. Chung C, Bautista N, O'Connell TX: Prognosis and treatment of bile duct carcinoma, *Am Surg* 64:921–925, 1998.

433. Cotchin E: Some tumours of dogs and cats of comparative veterinary and human interest, *Vet Rec* 71:1040–1050, 1959.

434. Patnaik AK, Liu SK, Johnson GF: Feline intestinal adenocarcinoma. A clinicopathologic study of 22 cases, *Vet Pathol* 13:1–10, 1976.

435. Engle G, Brodey R: A retrospective study of 395 feline neoplasms, *J Am Anim Hosp Assoc* 5:21–31, 1969.

436. Dobson JM, Samuel S, Milstein H, et al.: Canine neoplasia in the UK: estimates of incidence rates from a population of insured dogs, *J Small Anim Pract* 43:240–246, 2002.

437. Demetriou JL, Brearley MJ, Constantino-Casas F, et al.: Intentional marginal excision of canine limb soft tissue sarcomas followed by radiotherapy, *J Small Anim Pract* 53:174–181, 2012.

438. Rissetto K, Villamil JA, Selting KA, et al.: Recent trends in feline intestinal neoplasia: an epidemiologic study of 1,129 cases in the veterinary medical database from 1964 to 2004, *J Am Anim Hosp Assoc* 47:28–36, 2011.

439. Dorn CR, Taylor DO, Schneider R, et al.: Survey of animal neoplasms in Alameda and Contra Costa Counties, California. II. Cancer morbidity in dogs and cats from alameda county, *J Natl Cancer Inst* 40:307–318, 1968.

440. Tamas MJ, Karlgren S, Bill RM, et al.: A short regulatory domain restricts glycerol transport through yeast Fps1p, *J Bio Chem* 278:6337–6345, 2003.

441. Crawshaw J, Berg J, Sardinas JC, et al.: Prognosis for dogs with nonlymphomatous, small intestinal tumors treated by surgical excision, *J Am Anim Hosp Assoc* 34:451–456, 1998.

442. Alroy J, Leav I, DeLellis RA, et al.: Distinctive intestinal mast cell neoplasms of domestic cats, *Lab Invest* 33:159–167, 1975.

443. Gabor LJ, Malik R, Canfield PJ: Clinical and anatomical features of lymphosarcoma in 118 cats, *Aust Vet J* 76:725–732, 1998.

444. Kosovsky JE, Matthiesen DT, Patnaik AK: Small intestinal adenocarcinoma in cats: 32 cases (1978-1985), *J Am Vet Med Assoc* 192:233–235, 1988.

445. Mahony OM, Moore AS, Cotter SM, et al.: Alimentary lymphoma in cats: 28 cases (1988-1993), *J Am Vet Med Assoc* 207:1593–1598, 1995.

446. MacDonald JM, Mullen HS, Moroff SD: Adenomatous polyps of the duodenum in cats: 18 cases (1985-1990), *J Am Vet Med Assoc* 202:647–651, 1993.

447. Slawienski MJ, Mauldin GE, Mauldin GN, et al.: Malignant colonic neoplasia in cats: 46 cases (1990-1996), *J Am Vet Med Assoc* 211:878–881, 1997.

448. Frgelecová L, Škorič M, Fictum P, et al.: Canine gastrointestinal tract tumours: a restrospective study of 74 cases, *Acta Vet Brno* 82:387–392, 2013.

449. Patnaik AK, Hurvitz AI, Johnson GF: Canine gastrointestinal neoplasms, *Vet Pathol* 14:547–555, 1977.

450. Couto CG, Rutgers HC, Sherding RG, et al.: Gastrointestinal lymphoma in 20 dogs. A retrospective study, *J Vet Intern Med* 3:73–78, 1989.

451. Cohen M, Post GS, Wright JC: Gastrointestinal leiomyosarcoma in 14 dogs, *J Vet Intern Med* 17:107–110, 2003.

452. Kapatkin AS, Mullen HS, Matthiesen DT, et al.: Leiomyosarcoma in dogs: 44 cases (1983-1988), *J Am Vet Med Assoc* 201:1077–1079, 1992.

453. Miura T, Maruyama H, Sakai M, et al.: Endoscopic findings on alimentary lymphoma in 7 dogs, *J Vet Med Sci* 66:577–580, 2004.

454. Myers NC, Penninck DG: Ultrasonographic diagnosis of gastrointestinal smooth muscle tumors in the dog, *Vet Radiol Ultrasound* 35:391–397, 1994.

455. Valerius KD, Powers BE, McPherron MA, et al.: Adenomatous polyps and carcinoma in situ of the canine colon and rectum: 34 cases (1982-1994), *J Am Anim Hosp Assoc* 33:156–160, 1997.

456. Paoloni MC, Penninck DG, Moore AS: Ultrasonographic and clinicopathologic findings in 21 dogs with intestinal adenocarcinoma, *Vet Radiol Ultrasound* 43:562–567, 2002.

457. Frost D, Lasota J, Miettinen M: Gastrointestinal stromal tumors and leiomyomas in the dog: a histopathologic, immunohistochemical, and molecular genetic study of 50 cases, *Vet Pathol* 40:42–54, 2003.

458. Birchard SJ, Couto CG, Johnson S: Nonlymphoid intestinal neoplasia in 32 dogs and 14 cats, *J Am Anim Hosp Assoc* 22:533–537, 1986.

459. Wolf JC, Ginn PE, Homer B, et al.: Immunohistochemical detection of p53 tumor suppressor gene protein in canine epithelial colorectal tumors, *Vet Pathol* 34:394–404, 1997.

460. Carreras JK, Goldschmidt M, Lamb M, et al.: Feline epitheliotropic intestinal malignant lymphoma: 10 cases (1997-2000), *J Vet Intern Med* 17:326–331, 2003.

461. Turk MA, Gallina AM, Russell TS: Nonhematopoietic gastrointestinal neoplasia in cats: a retrospective study of 44 cases, *Vet Pathol* 18:614–620, 1981.

462. Cribb AE: Feline gastrointestinal adenocarcinoma: a review and retrospective study, *Can Vet J* 29:709–712, 1988.

463. Seiler RJ: Colorectal polyps of the dog: a clinicopathologic study of 17 cases, *J Am Vet Med Assoc* 174:72–75, 1979.

464. Ozaki K, Yamagami T, Nomura K, et al.: Mast cell tumors of the gastrointestinal tract in 39 dogs, *Vet Pathol* 39:557–564, 2002.

465. Takahashi T, Kadosawa T, Nagase M, et al.: Visceral mast cell tumors in dogs: 10 cases (1982-1997), *J Am Vet Med Assoc* 216:222–226, 2000.

466. Swennes AG, Parry NM, Feng Y, et al.: Enterohepatic Helicobacter spp. in cats with non-haematopoietic intestinal carcinoma: a survey of 55 cases, *J Med Microbiol* 65:814–820, 2016.

467. Fox JG, Shen Z, Xu S, et al.: Helicobacter marmotae sp. nov. isolated from livers of woodchucks and intestines of cats, *J Clin Microbiol* 40:2513–2519, 2002.

468. Mukaratirwa S, de Witte E, van Ederen AM, et al.: Tenascin expression in relation to stromal tumour cells in canine gastrointestinal epithelial tumours, *J Comp Pathol* 129:137–146, 2003.

469. Prater MR, Flatland B, Newman SJ, et al.: Diffuse annular fusiform adenocarcinoma in a dog, *J Am Anim Hosp Assoc* 36:169–173, 2000.

470. Esplin DG, Wilson SR: Gastrointestinal adenocarcinomas metastatic to the testes and associated structures in three dogs, *J Am Anim Hosp Assoc* 34:287–290, 1998.

471. Juopperi TA, Cesta M, Tomlinson L, et al.: Extensive cutaneous metastases in a dog with duodenal adenocarcinoma, *Vet Clin Pathol* 32:88–91, 2003.

472. Head KW, Else RW, Dubielzig RR: Tumors of the intestines. In Meuten DJ, editor: *Tumors in domestic animals*, Ames, Iowa, 2002, Iowa State Press, pp 461–468.

473. Patnaik AK, Hurvitz AI, Johnson GF: Canine intestinal adenocarcinoma and carcinoid, *Vet Pathol* 17:149–163, 1980.

474. Church EM, Mehlhaff CJ, Patnaik AK: Colorectal adenocarcinoma in dogs: 78 cases (1973-1984), *J Am Vet Med Assoc* 191:727–730, 1987.

475. Desmas I, Burton JH, Post G, et al.: Clinical presentation, treatment and outcome in 31 dogs with presumed primary colorectal lymphoma (2001-2013), *Vet Comp Oncol* 15:504–517, 2017.

476. Uchida E, Chambers JK, Nakashima K, et al.: Pathologic features of colorectal inflammatory polyps in miniature dachshunds, *Vet Pathol* 53:833–839, 2016.

477. Ohmi A, Tsukamoto A, Ohno K, et al.: A retrospective study of inflammatory colorectal polyps in miniature dachshunds, *J Vet Med Sci* 74:59–64, 2012.

478. Bowen EJ, Mundy P, Tivers MS, et al.: Duodenal Brunner's gland adenoma causing chronic small intestinal obstruction in a dog, *J Small Anim Pract* 53:136–139, 2012.

479. Suwa A, Shimoda T: Intestinal gastrointestinal stromal tumor in a cat, *J Vet Med Sci* 79:562–566, 2017.

480. Morini M, Gentilini F, Pietra M, et al.: Cytological, immunohistochemical and mutational analysis of a gastric gastrointestinal stromal tumour in a cat, *J Comp Pathol* 145:152–157, 2011.

481. Gillespie V, Baer K, Farrelly J, et al.: Canine gastrointestinal stromal tumors: immunohistochemical expression of CD34 and examination of prognostic indicators including proliferation markers Ki67 and AgNOR, *Vet Pathol* 48:283–291, 2011.

482. Miettinen M, Majidi M, Lasota J: Pathology and diagnostic criteria of gastrointestinal stromal tumors (GISTs): a review, *Eur J Cancer* 38(Suppl 5):S39–51, 2002.

483. LaRock RG, Ginn PE: Immunohistochemical staining characteristics of canine gastrointestinal stromal tumors, *Vet Pathol* 34:303–311, 1997.

484. Hayes S, Yuzbasiyan-Gurkan V, Gregory-Bryson E, et al.: Classification of canine nonangiogenic, nonlymphogenic, gastrointestinal sarcomas based on microscopic, immunohistochemical, and molecular characteristics, *Vet Pathol* 50:779–788, 2013.

485. Takanosu M, Amano S, Kagawa Y: Analysis of c-KIT exon 11 mutations in canine gastrointestinal stromal tumours, *Vet J* 207:118–123, 2016.

486. Irie M, Takeuchi Y, Ohtake Y, et al.: Imatinib mesylate treatment in a dog with gastrointestinal stromal tumors with a c-kit mutation, *J Vet Med Sci* 77:1535–1539, 2015.

487. Russell KN, Mehler SJ, Skorupski KA, et al.: Clinical and immunohistochemical differentiation of gastrointestinal stromal tumors from leiomyosarcomas in dogs: 42 cases (1990-2003), *J Am Vet Med Assoc* 230:1329–1333, 2007.

488. Maas CP, ter Haar G, van der Gaag I, et al.: Reclassification of small intestinal and cecal smooth muscle tumors in 72 dogs: clinical, histologic, and immunohistochemical evaluation, *Vet Surg* 36:302–313, 2007.

489. Sako T, Uchida E, Okamoto M, et al.: Immunohistochemical evaluation of a malignant intestinal carcinoid in a dog, *Vet Pathol* 40:212–215, 2003.

490. Stimson EL, Cook WT, Smith MM, et al.: Extraskeletal osteosarcoma in the duodenum of a cat, *J Am Anim Hosp Assoc* 36:332–336, 2000.

491. Heldmann E, Anderson MA, Wagner-Mann C: Feline osteosarcoma: 145 cases (1990-1995), *J Am Anim Hosp Assoc* 36:518–521, 2000.

492. Sharpe A, Cannon MJ, Lucke VM, et al.: Intestinal haemangiosarcoma in the cat: clinical and pathological features of four cases, *J Small Anim Pract* 41:411–415, 2000.

493. Reimer ME, Leib MS, Reimer MS, et al.: Rectal ganglioneuroma in a dog, *J Am Anim Hosp Assoc* 35:107–110, 1999.

494. Paris JK, McCandlish IA, Schwarz T, et al.: Small intestinal ganglioneuromatosis in a dog, *J Comp Pathol* 148:323–328, 2013.

495. Mukaratirwa S, Gruys E, Nederbragt H: Relationship between cell proliferation and tenascin-C expression in canine gastrointestinal tumours and normal mucosa, *Res Vet Sci* 76:133–138, 2004.

496. Mukaratirwa S, van Ederen AM, Gruys E, et al.: Versican and hyaluronan expression in canine colonic adenomas and carcinomas: relation to malignancy and depth of tumour invasion, *J Comp Pathol* 131:259–270, 2004.

497. McEntee MF, Brenneman KA: Dysregulation of beta-catenin is common in canine sporadic colorectal tumors, *Vet Pathol* 36:228–236, 1999.

498. Restucci B, Martano M, DEV G, et al.: Expression of E-cadherin, beta-catenin and APC protein in canine colorectal tumours, *Anticancer Res* 29:2919–2925, 2009.

499. Aresu L, Pregel P, Zanetti R, et al.: E-cadherin and beta-catenin expression in canine colorectal adenocarcinoma, *Res Vet Sci* 89:409–414, 2010.

500. Gamblin RM, Sagartz JE, Couto CG: Overexpression of p53 tumor suppressor protein in spontaneously arising neoplasms of dogs, *Am J Vet Res* 58:857–863, 1997.

501. Mayr B, Reifinger M: Canine tumour suppressor gene p53 mutation in a case of anaplastic carcinoma of the intestine, *Acta Vet Hung* 50:31–35, 2002.

502. Knottenbelt C, Mellor D, Nixon C, et al.: Cohort study of COX-1 and COX-2 expression in canine rectal and bladder tumours, *J Small Anim Pract* 47:196–200, 2006.

503. McEntee MF, Cates JM, Neilsen N: Cyclooxygenase-2 expression in spontaneous intestinal neoplasia of domestic dogs, *Vet Pathol* 39:428–436, 2002.

504. Beam SL, Rassnick KM, Moore AS, et al.: An immunohistochemical study of cyclooxygenase-2 expression in various feline neoplasms, *Vet Pathol* 40:496–500, 2003.

505. Jeglum KA, Whereat A, Young K: Chemotherapy of lymphoma in 75 cats, *J Am Vet Med Assoc* 190:174–178, 1987.

506. Fondacaro JV, Richter KP, Carpenter JL, et al.: Feline gastrointestinal lymphoma: 67 cases (1988-1996), *Eur J Comp Gastroenterol* 4:5–11, 1999.

507. Norsworthy GD, Estep JS, Hollinger C, et al.: Prevalence and underlying causes of histologic abnormalities in cats suspected to have chronic small bowel disease: 300 cases (2008-2013), *J Am Vet Med Assoc* 247:629–635, 2015.

508. Norsworthy GD, Scot Estep J, Kiupel M, et al.: Diagnosis of chronic small bowel disease in cats: 100 cases (2008-2012), *J Am Vet Med Assoc* 243:1455–1461, 2013.

509. Muller A, Guaguere E, Degorce-Rubiales R: Cheyletiellosis associated with a bowel carcinoma in an old dog, *Prat Medic Chirurg* 37:405–406, 2002.

510. Grandt LM, Roethig A, Schroeder S, et al.: Feline paraneoplastic alopecia associated with metastasising intestinal carcinoma, *JFMS Open Rep* 1:2055116915621582, 2015.

511. Thompson JP, Christopher MM, Ellison GW, et al.: Paraneoplastic leukocytosis associated with a rectal adenomatous polyp in a dog, *J Am Vet Med Assoc* 201:737–738, 1992.

512. Barrs VR, Beatty JA, McCandlish IA, et al.: Hypereosinophilic paraneoplastic syndrome in a cat with intestinal T cell lymphosarcoma, *J Small Anim Pract* 43:401–405, 2002.

513. Ozaki K, Yamagami T, Nomura K, et al.: T-cell lymphoma with eosinophilic infiltration involving the intestinal tract in 11 dogs, *Vet Pathol* 43:339–344, 2006.

514. Marchetti V, Benetti C, Citi S, et al.: Paraneoplastic hypereosinophilia in a dog with intestinal T-cell lymphoma, *Vet Clin Pathol* 34:259–263, 2005.

515. Jackson MW, Helfand SC, Smedes SL, et al.: Primary IgG secreting plasma cell tumor in the gastrointestinal tract of a dog, *J Am Vet Med Assoc* 204:404–406, 1994.

516. Sato K, Hikasa Y, Morita T, et al.: Secondary erythrocytosis associated with high plasma erythropoietin concentrations in a dog with cecal leiomyosarcoma, *J Am Vet Med Assoc* 220(464): 486–490, 2002.

517. Bagley RS, Levy JK, Malarkey DE: Hypoglycemia associated with intra-abdominal leiomyoma and leiomyosarcoma in six dogs, *J Am Vet Med Assoc* 208:69–71, 1996.

518. Cohen M, Post GS: Nephrogenic diabetes insipidus in a dog with intestinal leiomyosarcoma, *J Am Vet Med Assoc* 215: 1818–1820, 1999.

519. Selting KA, Ogilvie GK, Lana SE, et al.: Serum alhpa 1-acid glycoprotein concentrations in healthy and tumor-bearing cats, *J Vet Intern Med* 14:503–506, 2000.

520. Correa SS, Mauldin GN, Mauldin GE, et al.: Serum alpha 1-acid glycoprotein concentration in cats with lymphoma, *J Am Anim Hosp Assoc* 37:153–158, 2001.

521. Takeuchi Y, Takahashi M, Tsuboi M, et al.: Intestinal T-cell lymphoma with severe hypereosinophilic syndrome in a cat, *J Vet Med Sci* 74:1057–1062, 2012.

522. Laurenson MP, Skorupski KA, Moore PF, et al.: Ultrasonography of intestinal mast cell tumors in the cat, *Vet Radiol Ultrasound* 52:330–334, 2011.

523. Rivers BJ, Walter PA, Feeney DA, et al.: Ultrasonographic features of intestinal adenocarcinoma in five cats, *Vet Radiol Ultrasound* 38:300–306, 1997.

524. Penninck D, Smyers B, Webster CR, et al.: Diagnostic value of ultrasonography in differentiating enteritis from intestinal neoplasia in dogs, *Vet Radiol Ultrasound* 44:570–575, 2003.

525. Zwingenberger AL, Marks SL, Baker TW, et al.: Ultrasonographic evaluation of the muscularis propria in cats with diffuse small intestinal lymphoma or inflammatory bowel disease, *J Vet Intern Med* 24:289–292, 2010.

526. Frances M, Lane AE, Lenard ZM: Sonographic features of gastrointestinal lymphoma in 15 dogs, *J Small Anim Pract* 54: 468–474, 2013.

527. Dominguez E, Anadon E, Espada Y, et al.: Imaging diagnosis—ultrasonographic appearance of small bowel metastasis from canine mammary carcinoma, *Vet Radiol Ultrasound* 55:208–212, 2014.

528. Gaschen L: Ultrasonography of small intestinal inflammatory and neoplastic diseases in dogs and cats, *Vet Clin North Am Small Anim Pract* 41:329–344, 2011.

529. Daniaux LA, Laurenson MP, Marks SL, et al.: Ultrasonographic thickening of the muscularis propria in feline small intestinal small cell T-cell lymphoma and inflammatory bowel disease, *J Feline Med Surg* 16:89–98, 2014.

530. Monteiro CB, O'Brien RT: A retrospective study on the sonographic findings of abdominal carcinomatosis in 14 cats, *Vet Radiol Ultrasound* 45:559–564, 2004.

531. Adamovich-Rippe KN, Mayhew PD, Marks SL, et al.: Colonoscopic and histologic features of rectal masses in dogs: 82 cases (1995-2012), *J Am Vet Med Assoc* 250: 424–430, 2017.

532. Swinbourne F, Jeffery N, Tivers MS, et al.: The incidence of surgical site dehiscence following full-thickness gastrointestinal biopsy in dogs and cats and associated risk factors, *J Small Anim Pract* 58:495–503, 2017.

533. Duell JR, Thieman Mankin KM, Rochat MC, et al.: Frequency of dehiscence in hand-sutured and stapled intestinal anastomoses in dogs, *Vet Surg* 45:100–103, 2016.

534. Coolman BR, Ehrhart N, Pijanowski G, et al.: Comparison of skin staples with sutures for anastomosis of the small intestine in dogs, *Vet Surg* 29:293–302, 2000.

535. Danova NA, Robles-Emanuelli JC, Bjorling DE: Surgical excision of primary canine rectal tumors by an anal approach in twenty-three dogs, *Vet Surg* 35:337–340, 2006.

536. Holt PE, Durdey P: Transanal endoscopic treatment of benign canine rectal tumours: preliminary results in six cases (1992 to 1996), *J Small Anim Pract* 40:423–427, 1999.

537. Coleman KA, Berent AC, Weisse CW: Endoscopic mucosal resection and snare polypectomy for treatment of a colorectal polypoid adenoma in a dog, *J Am Vet Med Assoc* 244:1435–1440, 2014.

538. Nucci DJ, Liptak JM, Selmic LE, et al.: Complications and outcomes following rectal pull-through surgery in dogs with rectal masses: 74 cases (2000-2013), *J Am Vet Med Assoc* 245: 684–695, 2014.

539. Morello E, Martano M, Squassino C, et al.: Transanal pull-through rectal amputation for treatment of colorectal carcinoma in 11 dogs, *Vet Surg* 37:420–426, 2008.

540. Hardie EM, Gilson SD: Use of colostomy to manage rectal disease in dogs, *Vet Surg* 26:270–274, 1997.

541. Swiderski J, Withrow S: A novel surgical stapling technique for rectal mass removal: a retrospective analysis, *J Am Anim Hosp Assoc* 45:67–71, 2009.

542. Kupanoff PA, Popovitch CA, Goldschmidt MH: Colorectal plasmacytomas: a retrospective study of nine dogs, *J Am Anim Hosp Assoc* 42:37–43, 2006.

543. Arteaga TA, McKnight J, Bergman PJ: A review of 18 cases of feline colonic adenocarcinoma treated with subtotal colectomies and adjuvant carboplatin, *J Am Anim Hosp Assoc* 48:399–404, 2012.

544. Moore AS, Kirk C, Cardona A: Intracavitary cisplatin chemotherapy experience with six dogs, *J Vet Intern Med* 5:227–231, 1991.

545. Elliott JW, Swinbourne F, Parry A, et al.: Successful treatment of a metastatic, gastrointestinal stromal tumour in a dog with toceranib phosphate (Palladia), *J Small Anim Pract* 58:416–418, 2017.

546. Kobayashi M, Kuroki S, Ito K, et al.: Imatinib-associated tumour response in a dog with a non-resectable gastrointestinal stromal tumour harbouring a c-kit exon 11 deletion mutation, *Vet J* 198:271–274, 2013.

547. Kobayashi M, Sugisaki O, Ishii N, et al.: Canine intestinal mast cell tumor with c-kit exon 8 mutation responsive to imatinib therapy, *Vet J* 193:264–267, 2012.

548. Coit DG: Cancer of the small intestine. In DeVita VT, Hellman S, Rosenberg SA, editors: *Cancer: principles and practice of oncology*, ed 6, Lippincott Williams & Wilkins, 2001.

549. Skibber JM, Minsky BD, Hoff PM: Cancer of the colon. In DeVita VT, Hellman S, Rosenberg SA, editors: *Cancer: principles and practice of oncology*, ed 6, Philadelphia, 2001, Lippincott Williams & Wilkins.

550. Youmans L, Taylor C, Shin E, et al.: Frequent alteration of the tumor suppressor gene APC in sporadic canine colorectal tumors, *PLoS One* 7:e50813, 2012.

551. Squire JA, Whitmore GF, Phillips RA: Genetic basis of cancer. In Tannock IF, Hill RP, editors: *The basic science of oncology*, ed 3, New York, 1998, McGraw-Hill.

552. Dailey DD, Ehrhart EJ, Duval DL, et al.: DOG1 is a sensitive and specific immunohistochemical marker for diagnosis of canine gastrointestinal stromal tumors, *J Vet Diagn Invest* 27:268–277, 2015.

553. Sawaki A, Yamao K: Imatinib mesylate acts in metastatic or unresectable gastrointestinal stromal tumor by targeting KIT receptors—a review, *Cancer Chemother Pharmacol* 54(Suppl 1): S44–49, 2004.

554. Peek Jr RM: Prevention of colorectal cancer through the use of COX-2 selective inhibitors, *Cancer Chemother Pharmacol* 54(Suppl 1):S50–56, 2004.

555. Oberthaler KT, Shofer FS, Bowden A: Chemoprevention using NSAIDs in dogs: A preliminary epidemiological survey. Proceeding 24th annual conference of the Veterinary Cancer Society, 3.

556. Nishida T, Doi T, Naito Y: Tyrosine kinase inhibitors in the treatment of unresectable or metastatic gastrointestinal stromal tumors, *Expert Opin Pharmacother* 15:1979–1989, 2014.

557. Meyers BM, Cosby R, Quereshy F, et al.: Adjuvant Chemotherapy for Stage II and III Colon Cancer Following Complete Resection: a cancer care ontario systematic review, *Clin Oncol (R Coll Radiol)* 29:459–465, 2017.

558. Nielsen SW, Aftosmis J: Canine perianal gland tumors, *J Am Vet Med Assoc* 144:127–135, 1964.

559. Maita K, Ishida K: Structure and development of the perianal gland of the dog, *Japan J Vet Sci* 37:349–356, 1975.

560. Vinayak A, Frank CB, Gardiner DW, et al.: Malignant anal sac melanoma in dogs: eleven cases (2000 to 2015), *J Small Anim Pract* 58:231–237, 2017.

561. Esplin DG, Wilson SR, Hullinger GA: Squamous cell carcinoma of the anal sac in five dogs, *Vet Pathol* 40:332–334, 2003.

562. Mellett S, Verganti S, Murphy S, et al.: Squamous cell carcinoma of the anal sacs in three dogs, *J Small Anim Pract* 56: 223–225, 2015.

563. Giuliano A, Dobson J, Mason S: Complete resolution of a recurrent canine anal sac squamous cell carcinoma with palliative radiotherapy and carboplatin chemotherapy, *Vet Sci* 43:E45, 2017.

564. Emms SG: Anal sac tumours of the dog and their response to cytoreductive surgery and chemotherapy, *Aust Vet J* 83: 340–343, 2005.

565. Shoieb AM, Hanshaw DM: Anal sac gland carcinoma in 64 cats in the United Kingdom (1995-2007), *Vet Pathol* 46: 677–683, 2009.

566. Amsellem PM, Cavanaugh RP, Chou PY, et al.: Apocrine gland anal sac adenocarcinoma in cats: 30 cases (1994-2015), *J Am Vet Med Assoc, in press*, 2018.

567. Elliott JW, Blackwood L: Treatment and outcome of four cats with apocrine gland carcinoma of the anal sac and review of the literature, *J Feline Med Surg* 13:712–717, 2011.

568. Berrocal A, Vos JH, van den Ingh TS, et al.: Canine perineal tumours, *J Vet Med Ser A* 36:739–749, 1989.

569. Wilson GP, Hayes HM: Castration for treatment of perianal gland neoplasms in the dog, *J Am Vet Med Assoc* 174:1301–1303, 1979.

570. Chaisiri N, Pierrpoint CG: Steroid-receptor interaction in a canine anal adenoma, *J Small Anim Pract* 20:405–416, 1979.

571. Dow SW, Olson PN, Rosychuk RA, et al.: Perianal adenomas and hypertestosteronemia in a spayed bitch with pituitary-dependent hyperadrenocorticism, *J Am Vet Med Assoc* 192: 1439–1441, 1988.

572. Hill KE, Scott-Montrieff CR, Koshko MA, et al.: Secretion of sex hormones in dogs with adrenal dysfunction, *J Am Vet Med Assoc* 226:556–561, 2005.

573. Goldschmidt MH, Dunstan RW, Stannard AA, et al.: Histological classification of epithelial and melanocytic tumors of the skin of domestic animals. In *WHO international histological classification of tumors of domestic animals*. 2nd Series, Vol. 3. Washington DC, 1998, Armed Forces Institute of Pathology, pp 38–40.

574. Pereira RS, Schweigert A, Dias de Melo GD, et al.: Ki-67 labeling in canine perianal glands neoplasms: a novel approach for immunohistological diagnostic and prognostic, *BMC Vet Res* 9: 83, 2013.

575. Sobczyńska-Rak A, Brodzki A: VEGF and 17-β-estradiol levels after tamoxifen administration in canine hepatoid gland adenomas and hepatoid gland epitheliomas, *In Vivo* 28:871–878, 2014.

576. Vail DM, Withrow SJ, Schwarz PD, et al.: Perianal adenocarcinoma in the canine male: a retrospective study of 41 cases, *J Am Anim Hosp Assoc* 26:329–334, 1990.

577. Martins AMCRPF, Vasques-Peyser A, Torres LN, et al.: Retrospective-systematic study and quantitative analysis of cellular proliferation and apoptosis in normal, hyperplastic and neoplastic perianal glands in dogs, *Vet Comp Oncol* 6:71–79, 2008.

578. Brodzki A, Lopuszyński W, Brodzki P, et al.: Diagnostic and prognostic value of cellular proliferation assessment with Ki-67 protein in dogs suffering from benign and malignant perianal tumors, *Folia Biol* 62:235–241, 2014.

579. Gamblin RM, Sagartz JE, Couto CG: Overexpression of p53 tumor suppressor protein in spontaneously arising neoplasms of dogs, *Am J Vet Res* 58:857–863, 1997.

580. Nakano M, Taura Y, Inoue M: Protein expression of Mdm2 and p53 in hyperplastic and neoplastic lesions of the canine circumanal gland, *J Comp Pathol* 132:27–32, 2005.

581. Pisani G, Millanta F, Lorenzi D, et al.: Androgen receptor expression in normal, hyperplastic and neoplastic hepatoid glands in the dog, *Res Vet Sci* 81:231–236, 2006.

582. Petterino C, Martini M, Castagnaro M: Immunohistochemical detection of growth hormone in canine hepatoid gland tumors, *J Vet Med Sci* 66:569–572, 2004.

583. Brodzki A, Tatara MR, Brodzki P: Serum concentrations of magnesium in dogs suffering from tumors of the perianal glands, *Magnes Res* 26:87–92, 2013.

584. Stannard AA, Pulley LT: Tumors of the skin and soft tissues. In Moulton JE, editor: *Tumors in domestic animals*, ed 2, Berkeley, 1978, University of California Press, pp 16–70.

585. Ganguly A, Wolfe LG: Canine perianal gland carcinoma-associated antigens defined by monoclonal antibodies, *Hybridoma* 25:10–14, 2006.

586. Pieper J, Stern A, LeClerc S: Coordinate expression of cytokeratin 7 and 14, vimentin and Bcl-2 in canine cutaneous epithelial tumors and cysts, *J Vet Diagn Invest* 27:497–503, 2015.

587. Tozon N, Kodre V, Sersa G, et al.: Effective treatment of perianal tumors in dogs with electrochemotherapy, *Anticancer Res* 25:839–845, 2005.

588. Liska WD, Withrow SJ: Cryosurgical treatment of perianal gland adenomas in the dog, *J Am Anim Hosp Assoc* 14:457–463, 1978.

589. Shelley BA: Use of the carbon dioxide laser for perianal and rectal surgery, *Vet Clin North Am Small Anim Pract* 32:621–637, 2002.

590. Grier RL, Brewer WG, Theilen GH: Hyperthermic treatment of superficial tumors in cats and dogs, *J Am Vet Med Assoc* 177:227–233, 1980.

591. Gillette EL: Veterinary radiotherapy, *J Am Vet Med Assoc* 157:1707–1712, 1970.

592. Spugnini EP, Dotsinsky I, Mudrov N, et al.: Biphasic pulses enhance bleomycin efficacy in a spontaneous canine perianal tumor model, *J Exp Clin Cancer Res* 26:483–487, 2007.

593. Park C, Yoo JH, Kim HJ, et al.: Cyclosporine treatment of perianal gland adenoma concurrent with benign prostatic hyperplasia in a dog, *Can Vet J* 51:1279–1282, 2010.

594. Hammer AS, Couto CG, Ayl RD, et al.: Treatment of tumor-bearing dogs with actinomycin D, *J Vet Intern Med* 8:236–239, 1994.

595. Bley CR, Stankeova S, Sumova A, et al.: Metastases of perianal gland carcinoma in a dog: palliative tumor therapy, *Schweiz Arch Tierheilkd* 145:89–94, 2003.

596. Simeonov R, Simeonova G: Computer-assisted nuclear morphometry in the cytological evaluation of canine perianal adenocarcinomas, *J Comp Path* 139:226–230, 2008.

597. Goldschmidt MH, Shofer FS: *Skin tumors of the dog and cat*, ed 1, Oxford, 1992, Pergamon Press.

598. Polton GA, Mowat V, Lee HC, et al.: Breed, gender and neutering status of British dogs with anal sac gland carcinoma, *Vet Comp Oncol* 4:125–131, 2006.

599. Bennett PF, DeNicola DB, Bonney P, et al.: Canine anal sac adenocarcinomas: clinical presentation and response to therapy, *J Vet Intern Med* 16:100–104, 2002.

600. Williams LE, Gliatto JM, Dodge RK, et al.: Carcinoma of the apocrine glands of the anal sac in dogs: 113 cases (1985-1995), *J Am Vet Med Assoc* 223:825–831, 2003.

601. Polton GA, Brearley MJ: Clinical stage, therapy, and prognosis in canine anal sac gland carcinoma, *J Vet Intern Med* 21:274–280, 2007.

602. Meuten DJ, Cooper BJ, Capen CC, et al.: Hypercalcemia associated with an adenocarcinoma derived from the apocrine glands of the anal sac, *Vet Pathol* 18:454–471, 1981.

603. Ross JT, Scavelli TD, Matthiesen DT, et al.: Adenocarcinoma of the apocrine glands of the anal sac in dogs: a review of 32 cases, *J Am Anim Hosp Assoc* 27:349–355, 1991.

604. Goldschmidt MH, Zoltowski C: Anal sac gland adenocarcinoma in the dog: 14 cases, *J Small Anim Pract* 22:119–128, 1981.

605. Potanas CP, Padgett S, Gamblin RM: Surgical excision of anal sac apocrine gland adenocarcinomas with and without adjunctive chemotherapy in dogs: 42 cases (2005–2011), *J Am Vet Med Assoc* 246:877–884, 2015.

606. Wouda RM, Borrego J, Keuler NS, et al.: Evaluation of adjuvant carboplatin chemotherapy in the management of surgically excised anal sac apocrine gland adenocarcinoma in dogs, *Vet Comp Oncol* 14:67–80, 2016.

607. Turek MM, Forrest LJ, Adams WM, et al.: Postoperative radiotherapy and mitoxantrone for anal sac adenocarcinoma in the dog: 15 cases (1991-2001), *Vet Comp Oncol* 1:94–104, 2003.

608. Bowlt KL, Friend EJ, Delisser P, et al.: Temporally separated bilateral anal sac gland adenocarcinomas in four dogs, *J Small Anim Pract* 54:432–436, 2013.

609. Meier V, Polton G, Cancedda S, et al.: Outcomes in dogs with advanced (stage 3b) anal sac gland carcinoma treated with surgery or hypofractionated radiation therapy, *Vet Comp Oncol* 15:1073–1086, 2017.

610. Barnes DC, Demetriou JL: Surgical management of primary, metastatic and recurrent anal sac adenocarcinoma in the dog: 52 cases, *J Small Anim Pract* 58:263–268, 2017.

611. White RAS, Gorman NT: The clinical diagnosis and management of rectal and pararectal tumours in the dog, *J Small Anim Pract* 28:87–107, 1987.

612. Hause WR, Stevenson S, Meuten DJ, et al.: Pseudohyperparathyroidism associated with adenocarcinomas of anal sac origin in four dogs, *J Am Anim Hosp Assoc* 17:373–379, 1981.

613. Meuten DJ, Segre GV, Capen CC, et al.: Hypercalcemia in dogs with adenocarcinoma derived from apocrine glands of the anal sac, *Lab Invest* 48:428–434, 1983.

614. Messinger JS, Windham WR, Ward CR: Ionized hypercalcemia in dogs: a retrospective study of 109 cases (1998-2003), *J Vet Intern Med* 23:514–519, 2009.

615. McQuown B, Keyerleber MA, Rosen K, et al.: Treatment of advanced canine anal sac adenocarcinoma with hypofractionated radiation therapy: 77 cases (1999–2013), *Vet Comp Oncol* 15:840–851, 2017.

616. Pradel J, Berlato D, Dobromylskyj M, et al.: Prognostic significance of histopathology in canine anal sac gland adenocarcinomas: preliminary results in a retrospective study of 39 cases, *Vet Comp Oncol, in press*, 2018.

617. Rosol TJ, Capen CC, Danks JA, et al.: Identification of parathyroid hormone-related protein in canine apocrine adenocarcinoma of the anal sac, *Vet Pathol* 27:89–95, 1990.

618. Gröne A, Werkmeister JR, Steinmeyer CL, et al.: Parathyroid hormone-related protein in normal and neoplastic canine tissues: immunohistochemical localization and biochemical extraction, *Vet Pathol* 31:308–315, 1994.

619. Mellanby RJ, Craig R, Evans H, et al.: Plasma concentrations of parathyroid hormone-related protein in dogs with potential disorders of calcium metabolism, *Vet Rec* 159:833–838, 2006.

620. Hammond TN, Turek MM, Regan J: What is your diagnosis? Metastatic anal sac adenocarcinoma with paraneoplastic hypertrophic osteopathy, *J Am Vet Med Assoc* 235:267–268, 2009.

621. Giuliano A, Salguero R, Dobson J: Metastatic anal sac carcinoma with hypercalcemia and associated hypertrophic osteopathy in a dog, *Open Vet J* 5:48–51, 2015.

622. Taylor B, Leibman N, Luong R, et al.: Detection of carcinoma micrometastases in bone marrow of dogs and cats using conventional and cell block cytology, *Vet Clin Pathol* 42:85–91, 2013.

623. Suzuki K, Morita R, Hojo Y, et al.: Immunohistochemical characterization of neuroendocrine differentiation of canine anal sac glandular tumours, *J Comp Pathol* 149:199–207, 2013.

624. Polton GA, Brearley MJ, Green LM, et al.: Expression of E-cadherin in canine anal sac gland carcinoma and its association with survival, *Vet Comp Oncol* 5:232–238, 2007.

625. Aguirre-Hernandez J, Polton G, Kennedy LJ, et al.: Association between anal sac gland carcinoma and dog leukocyte antigen-DQB1 in the english cocker spaniel, *Tissue Antigens* 76:476–481, 2010.

626. Knudsen CS, Williams A, Brearley MJ, et al.: COX-2 expression in canine anal sac adenocarcinomas and in non-neoplastic canine anal sacs, *Vet J* 197:782–787, 2013.

627. Ogawa B, Taniai E, Hayashi H, et al.: Neuroendocrine carcinoma of the apocrine glands of the anal sac in a dog, *J Vet Diagn Invest* 23:852–856, 2011.

628. Brown RJ, Newman SJ, Durtschi DC, et al.: Expression of PDGFR-β and kit in canine anal sac apocrine gland adenocarcinoma using tissue immunohistochemistry, *Vet Comp Oncol* 10:74–79, 2012.

629. Urie BK, Russell DS, Kisseberth WC, et al.: Evaluation of exporession and function of vascular endothelial growth factor receptor 2, platelet derived growth factor receptors-alpha and –beta, KIT, and RET in canine apocrine gland anal sac adenocarcinoma and thyroid carcinoma, *BMC Vet Res* 8:67, 2012.

630. Llabrés-Díaz FJ: Ultrasonography of the medial iliac lymph nodes in the dog, *Vet Radiol Ultrasound* 45:156–165, 2004.

631. De Swarte M, Alexander K, Rannou B, et al.: Comparison of sonographic features of benign and neoplastic deep lymph nodes in dogs, *Vet Radiol Ultrasound* 52:451–456, 2011.

632. Anderson CL, MacKay CS, Roberts GD, et al.: Comparison of abdominal ultrasound and magnetic resonance imaging for detection of abdominal lymphadenopathy in dogs with metastatic apocrine gland adenocarcinoma of the anal sac, *Vet Comp Oncol* 13:98–105, 2015.

633. Palladino S, Keyerleber M, King R, Burgess K: Utility of computed tomography versus abdominal ultrasound examination to identify iliosacral lymphadenomegaly in dogs with apocrine gland adenocarcinoma of the anal sac, *J Vet Intern Med* 30:1858–1863, 2016.

634. Pollard RE, Fuller MC, Steffey MA: Ultrasound and computed tomography of the iliosacral lymphatic centre in dogs with anal sac carcinoma, *Vet Comp Oncol* 15:299–306, 2017.

635. Majeski SA, Steffey MA, Fuller M, et al.: Indirect computed tomographic lymphography for iliosacral lymphatic mapping in a cohort of dogs with anal sac gland adenocarcinoma: technique description, *Vet Radiol Ultrasound* 58:295–303, 2017.

636. Hoelzler MG, Bellah JR, Donofro MC: Omentalization of cystic sublumbar lymph node metastases for long-term palliation of tenesmus and dysuria in a dog with anal sac adenocarcinoma, *J Am Vet Med Assoc* 219:1729–1731, 2001.

637. Hobson HP, Brown MR, Rogers KS: Surgery of metastatic anal sac adenocarcinoma in five dogs, *Vet Surg* 35:267–270, 2006.

638. London C, Mathie T, Stingle N, et al.: Preliminary evidence for biologic activity of toceranib phosphate (Palladia®) in solid tumours, *Vet Comp Oncol* 10:194–205, 2012.

639. Spugnini EP, Dotsinsky I, Mudrov N, et al.: Adjuvant electrochemotherapy for incompletely excised anal sac carcinoma in a dog, *In Vivo* 22:47–50, 2008.

640. McDonald C, Looper J, Greene S: Response rate and duration associated with 4Gy 5 fraction palliative radiation protocol, *Vet Radiol Ultrasound* 53:358–364, 2012.

641. Anderson CR, McNiel EA, Gillette EL, et al.: Late complications of pelvic irradiation in 16 dogs, *Vet Radiol Ultrasound* 43:187–192, 2002.

642. Arthur JJ, Kleiter MM, Thrall DE: Characterization of normal tissue complications in 51 dogs undergoing definitive pelvic region irradiation, *Vet Radiol Ultrasound* 49:85–89, 2008.

643. Keyerleber MA, Gieger TL, Erb HN, et al.: Three-dimensional conformal versus non-graphic radiation treatment planning for apocrine gland adenocarcinoma of the anal sac in 18 dogs (2002-2007), *Vet Comp Oncol* 4:237–245, 2012.

644. Wright ZM, Fryer JS, Calise DV: Carboplatin chemotherapy in a cat with recurrent anal sac apocrine gland adenocarcinoma, *J Am Anim Hosp Assoc* 46:66–69, 2010.

645. Lampejo T, Davanagh D, Clark J: Prognostic biomarkers in squamous cell carcinoma of the anus: a systematic review, *Br J Cancer* 103:1858–1869, 2010.

646. Chan E, Kachnic LA, Thomas CR: Anal cancer: progress on combined-modality and organ preservation, *Curr Prob Cancer* 33:302–326, 2009.

647. Shia J: An update on tumors of the anal canal, *Arch Pathol Lab Med* 134:1601–1611, 2010.

648. Causey MW, Steele SR, Maykel J: Surgical treatment for epidermoid carcinoma of the anal canal: an NSQIP assessment of short-term outcomes, *J Surg Res* 177:235–240, 2012.

24

Tumors of the Respiratory System

SECTION A: CANCER OF THE NASAL PLANUM

WILLIAM T.N. CULP

Anatomy

The nasal planum is considered the apical portion of the external nose. This region is flattened, generally hairless, and includes the nares and philtrum.[1] The nasal planum is located rostrally to the nasal cartilages, which is a mobile group of seven cartilages attached to the bony part of the nose via three ligaments (paired lateral nasal ligaments and a dorsal nasal ligament).[1]

Pathology, Behavior, and History

The vast majority of the literature dedicated to nasal planum neoplasia has focused on squamous cell carcinoma (SCC). Other reported tumors of the nasal planum include fibrosarcoma, melanoma, mast cell tumor (MCT), osteosarcoma, and desmoplastic ameloblastoma.[2] The biologic behavior of SCC of the nasal planum is similar to other locations in dogs and cats; these tumors rarely metastasize, but have the potential to be aggressive locally in some species.[3,4]

In general, SCC is a relatively common tumor in cats, but rare in dogs.[5] These tumors are thought to be sunlight-induced and may represent a malignant transformation from keratosis or carcinoma in situ to SCC;[6] many cats (95% in one study[3]) are white or partially white in color.[7] Labrador retrievers and golden retrievers may be overrepresented, accounting for 50% to 76% of cases in two studies.[4,8] These tumors occur in older dogs or cats, with ages at presentation generally greater than 10 years.[3,4]

Diagnostic Evaluation

Pretherapeutic evaluation of nasal planum tumors is important to direct diagnostics and eventual treatment. Although nasal planum SCC has a characteristic gross appearance, fine-needle aspiration (FNA) cytology and/or incisional biopsy should be considered to obtain a definitive diagnosis.

The nasal planum should be imaged to determine the extent of disease, especially in dogs. Radiographs, ultrasound, and rhinoscopy are of limited value; however, swelling of the nasal planum, occlusion of nasal passages, and increased opacity within the rostral portion of the nasal cavity has been noted on radiographs.[8] Advanced imaging with computed tomography (CT) or magnetic resonance imaging (MRI) is preferred, especially when tumors of the nasal planum are suspected to extend into the nasal cavity.[8] These diagnostics are also useful in determining the presence of bony invasion.[8]

Treatment

Surgery

Nasal planum resection is the most commonly described and performed technique for the management of dogs and cats with nasal planum SCC. The nasal planum can be removed alone (Fig. 24.1) or in combination with the incisive[9] or maxillary bones.[10] The latter is indicated for tumor types where larger surgical margins are required for complete histologic excision, such as MCTs or soft tissue sarcomas, or for tumors extending caudally beyond the nasal planum.

The postoperative appearance after nasal planum resection can be challenging, especially for owners. A thorough discussion with an owner regarding the treatment options, postoperative function, and postoperative cosmetic appearance is imperative to adequately prepare them for nasal planum resection, including the provision of images of the postoperative appearance of dogs postnasal planum resection.

The prognosis after nasal planum resection is generally good in dogs. Local recurrence was reported in two of six dogs treated with surgery alone in one study, both with incomplete histologic excision.[4] Seven dogs with more advanced tumors were treated with a combination of surgery and adjuvant radiation therapy (RT), and all seven dogs had local tumor recurrence with a median time to recurrence of 9 weeks.[4] Local recurrence was not reported in three dogs treated with combined nasal planum resection-incisivectomy[9] and five of six dogs treated with combined nasal planum resection-bilateral maxillectomy.[10]

The prognosis is very good in cats after surgery. In one study of 61 cats with SCC, local tumor recurrence (Fig. 24.2) was reported in less than 10% of cats, with median disease-free intervals (DFIs) of 594 days and 426 days for cats with isolated nasal planum SCC and SCC in multiple locations, respectively, when treated with

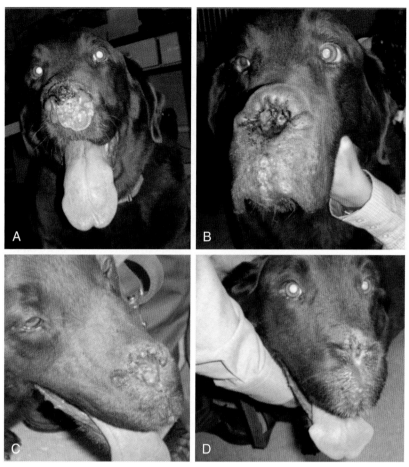

• **Fig. 24.1** (A) Preoperative image of nasal planum squamous cell carcinoma in a 10-year-old Labrador retriever. (B) Immediately after nasal planectomy; (C) 9 days postoperatively; and (D) 6 weeks postoperatively.

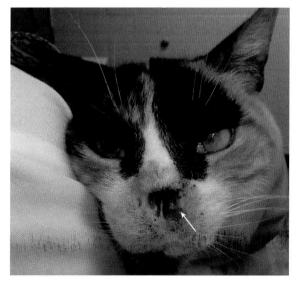

• **Fig. 24.2** Recurrence of a nasal planum squamous cell carcinoma (SCC) in a 13-year-old domestic shorthair cat 3 months after nasal planum resection. Recurrence of the tumor can be seen in the ventral aspect of the left neo-nare *(arrow)*.

surgery alone.[3] The median survival times (MSTs) for surgically treated cats in this study were 673 days and 530 days for cats with isolated nasal planum SCC and SCC in multiple locations, respectively.[3]

Conservative surgical approaches are not typically recommended as most nasal planum tumors are invasive and recurrence rates are high when an aggressive surgical approach is not utilized. However, surgical curettage and diathermy has been described in 34 cats with nasal planum tumors, including nine cats with carcinoma in situ and seven cats with SCC.[11] This technique resulted in better cosmesis and good local tumor control with a local tumor recurrence rate of 6% after a median follow-up time of 18 months.[11]

External Beam Radiation Therapy

External beam RT has been described for the treatment of nasal planum SCC in both dogs and cats, either for primary treatment or in the adjuvant setting. The results have been discouraging in dogs with local recurrence reported in virtually all patients with median times to recurrence of 2 to 3 months.[4,5]

RT has been described for the treatment of cats using either orthovoltage,[7] megavoltage,[3,12] or an accelerated protocol using protons.[13] For cats treated with orthovoltage, the 1-year progression-free survival (PFS) rate was 60%, and prognostic factors

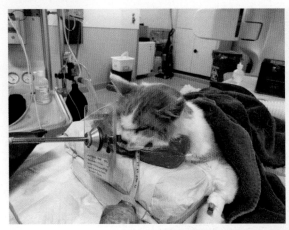

• **Fig. 24.3** Strontium plesiotherapy treatment of feline squamous cell carcinoma. (Image courtesy Dr. Michael Kent.)

included clinical stage and proliferative fraction.[7] The median DFIs for 55 cats treated with megavoltage in two studies was 361 to 916 days,[3,12] with a MST of 902 days.[12] Cats with larger tumors had 5.4 and 6.3 times greater risk of recurrence and dying, respectively, than cats with smaller tumors.[12] For 15 cats treated with an accelerated RT protocol using protons, the PFS rate was 64% and the MST was 946 days.[13] Side effects were considered minimal.[13]

Strontium Plesiotherapy

Strontium plesiotherapy is the application of a radioactive substance (strontium Sr90 or ^{90}Sr) directly to the nasal planum tumor (Fig. 24.3). When using this technique, less than 10% of the radiation dose penetrates to a depth of 3 mm, and hence this treatment is primarily indicated for cats with superficial and minimally invasive SCCs.[14] Strontium plesiotherapy allows for a large dose of radiation to be delivered to superficial lesions while avoiding radiation dosing of deeper nonneoplastic tissues.[15] In two studies totaling 64 cats treated with ^{90}Sr, the complete response (CR) rate was 88%; local recurrence was reported in 20% of cats, and 33% of cats developed new lesions in different locations.[15,16] The median progression-free interval was 1710 days, with 1- and 3-year disease-free rates of 89% and 82%, respectively.[15] The overall MST was 3076 days, and cats with a CR had significantly longer MSTs.[15]

Chemotherapy

The most common reported use for chemotherapy in cats with nasal planum SCC is intralesional, either alone or with electrochemotherapy. In one study of 23 cats treated with intratumoral administration of carboplatin to treat SCC of the nasal planum, there was no systemic toxicity and local side effects were minimal and self-limiting.[17] A CR was noted in 73% of cats, with a 30% local recurrence rate and a mean PFS time of 16 months.[17] Intralesional carboplatin was combined with superficial orthovoltage RT in six cats; all cats achieved a CR and five of six cats had local tumor control at 6 months posttreatment.[18]

Electrochemotherapy utilizing bleomycin has been described in two case series for a total of 15 cats with nasal planum SCC.[19,20] A CR was noted in 75% to 86% of cats with a DFI between 7 to 36 months.[19,20] No local or systemic side effects were noted.[20]

Photodynamic Therapy

Photodynamic therapy is the use of applied light after the administration of a photosensitizer. The photosensitizer is activated by the light to form free radicals, which results in the induction of cell death.[21] Due to the limited penetration of light into the tissue, the treatment depth is considered 5 mm or less.[21]

Photodynamic therapy has been described for the treatment of nasal planum SCC in cats.[21,22] In a large prospective study of 55 cats treated with photodynamic therapy using 5-aminolevulinic acid (5-ALA) as a photosensitizer,[23] the overall response rate was 96% with 85% of cats having a CR. Fifty-one percent of cats with a CR developed local recurrence with a median time to recurrence of 157 days. At a median follow-up time of 38 months, 45% of cats were alive without recurrence and 33% of cats were euthanized because of local recurrence.[23] In a study of 61 cats assessing response to photodynamic therapy based on tumor staging, 49%, 12%, and 39% of cats demonstrated complete, partial, and no responses, respectively.[22] The rate of CR was significantly associated with stage; CR was noted in 100% of noninvasive tumors measuring <1.5 cm in diameter, 56% of invasive tumors measuring <1.5 cm in diameter, and 18% of invasive tumors measuring >1.5 cm in diameter.[22]

Other Treatments

Cryosurgery, using liquid nitrogen to freeze SCC lesions, has been described in two studies totaling 101 cats,[3,24] and is primarily indicated for the treatment of small (<5 mm), superficial, and noninvasive SCC lesions.[3] The response rate for cats with nasal planum SCC was 81% after two to three treatments.[24] The local tumor recurrence rates are between 17%[24] and 73%[3] with a median DFI of 184 days[3] to 26.7 months.[24]

SECTION B: NASAL CAVITY AND SINUS TUMORS

SUSAN E. LANA AND MICHELLE M. TUREK

Canine Sinonasal Tumors

Incidence and Risk Factors

Tumors of the nasal cavity and paranasal sinuses account for approximately 1% of all neoplasms in dogs.[25] The average age of dogs with this disease is approximately 10 years, although canine patients as young as 9 months have been reported.[26,27,28] Medium-to-large breeds may be more commonly affected.[26,29] It has been speculated, but is unproved, that dolichocephalic breeds (long-nosed) or dogs living in urban environments, with resultant increased nasal filtering of pollutants, may be at higher risk for developing nasal cancer.[29–31] Exposure to environmental tobacco smoke has been associated with an increased risk of nasal cancer in a group of dogs in one study,[32] but the same was not true in another.[31] Evaluation of DNA damage in biopsy samples of the oropharyngeal region of dogs exposed to cigarette smoke showed higher levels compared with those not exposed, suggesting that dogs could be used as a sentinel for early DNA damage caused by exposure to environmental agents, although the numbers evaluated were small.[33] Indoor exposure to fossil fuel combustion products, such as those produced by coal or kerosene heaters, may contribute to the suggested environmental component of this cancer.[31]

Pathology and Natural Behavior

Carcinomas, including adenocarcinoma, SCC, and undifferentiated carcinoma represent nearly two-thirds of canine intranasal tumors.[34] Sarcomas (usually fibrosarcoma, chondrosarcoma, osteosarcoma, and undifferentiated sarcoma) comprise the bulk of the remaining cancers.[35] Both carcinomas and sarcomas are characterized by progressive local invasion. The metastatic rate is generally considered low at the time of diagnosis but may be as high as 40% to 50% at the time of death, which is usually attributable to the primary disease rather than metastatic lesions.[26] The most common sites of metastasis are the regional lymph nodes (LNs) and the lungs.[26,35,36] Less common sites include bones, kidneys, liver, skin, and brain.[37–40]

Rare tumors of the sinonasal region in dogs include round cell tumors (such as lymphoma), mast cell tumor (MCT), and transmissible venereal tumor. Other malignancies include hemangiosarcoma, melanoma, neuroendocrine carcinoma, nerve sheath tumor, neuroblastoma, fibrous histiocytoma, multilobular osteochondrosarcoma, hamartoma, rhabdomyosarcoma, and leiomyosarcoma.[26,41–58] The biologic behavior of these less common malignancies is not well defined, although small retrospective case series have been reported for lymphoma, intranasal MCT, and melanoma.[59–62] Benign, yet often locally invasive lesions such as polyps, fibromas, dermoid cysts, and angiofibroma can also be seen.[63,64]

A number of studies have attempted to elucidate possible molecular mechanisms associated with canine sinonasal tumorigenesis. In one study using a single polyclonal antihuman antibody, nuclear $p53$ accumulation was detected in nearly 60% of nasal adenocarcinomas (11 of 19), which suggests that overexpression of a mutated $p53$ tumor suppressor protein may play a role.[65] Cyclooxygenase-2 (COX-2) expression has been detected to varying degrees in most sinonasal epithelial tumors sampled[66–69] and in normal paratumoral respiratory epithelium and stromal tissue.[69] In one study, epidermal growth factor receptor (EGFR) expression and vascular endothelial growth factor (VEGF) expression were detected in over 50% and 90% of the 24 nasal carcinomas evaluated, respectively.[70] All tumors expressed either EGFR or VEGF, but there was no association between the immunoreactivity for each protein.[70] To evaluate expression of receptor tyrosine kinases (RTKs) with the intent to establish a rationale for use of TK inhibitors (TKIs), VEGFR2 and platelet derived growth factor receptor (PDGFR) α and β have been evaluated in 187 nasal carcinoma samples.[71] VEGFR was expressed in 84% of the samples and was predominantly cytoplasmic-membranous, similar to what is seen in high grade MCTs. PDGFRα was noted in 71% of cases and PDGFRβ in 40%, both with weak to moderate intensity. Coexpression of RTKs was common. The authors concluded that studies evaluating clinical utility of TKIs are warranted.[71] Expression of peroxisome proliferator-activated receptor γ (PPAR-γ), a nuclear receptor involved in glucose metabolism and fatty acid storage, has also been shown in canine nasal carcinomas.[72] The authors of that study suggested that expression patterns may differ in tumor tissue compared with normal nasal epithelium.[72] The role of these proteins in carcinogenesis is not clear, and further investigation is needed before clinical relevance can be determined. Evaluation of the inflammatory infiltrate in 31 canine nasal carcinomas revealed an abundance of neutrophils and macrophages, which were present in greater numbers than in normal canine mucosa.[73] Plasma cells and T lymphocytes were also detected; however, levels did not correlate with particular tumor subtype.

History and Clinical Signs

Although many intranasal diseases will have overlapping clinical signs, a strong suspicion of cancer is appropriate for older animals with an intermittent and progressive history of unilateral (initially) epistaxis or mucopurulent discharge (or both). The average duration of clinical signs before diagnosis is 2 to 3 months;[25,74] these most commonly include epistaxis, bloody or mucopurulent nasal discharge, facial deformity due to bone erosion and subcutaneous extension of tumor, unwillingness to open the mouth, sneezing, dyspnea or stertorous breathing, exophthalmos, and ocular discharge as a result of mechanical obstruction of the nasolacrimal duct.[25,34,74] Differential diagnoses for animals with these clinical signs include fungal (*Aspergillus* sp.) or bacterial rhinitis, idiopathic nonspecific rhinitis (usually lymphoplasmacytic), rare nasal parasites, bleeding disorders, hypertension, foreign body, trauma, and developmental anomalies (e.g., cystic Rathke's clefts).[75–77] If facial deformity is present, the diagnosis is almost always cancer;[78–79] however, aspergillosis, sporotrichosis, and a rare, benign condition, angiomatous proliferation of the nasal cavity or angiofibroma, also can cause facial deformity. In a retrospective study of 105 cases of dogs with intranasal disease, the characteristics of the nasal discharge were evaluated to determine whether they correlated with diagnosis.[80] In dogs with confirmed neoplasia ($n = 23$), the median duration of discharge was 60 days. Mucoid discharge in pure or mixed form was seen more frequently in neoplasia compared with fungal, nonspecific rhinitis and foreign body cases. When signs lasted more than 14 days, hemorrhagic discharge was seen more commonly in dogs with neoplasia compared with those with rhinitis or other causes. Nasal stridor was also noted more often in dogs with neoplasia.

Clinical signs can be temporarily alleviated by a variety of symptomatic treatments, including antibiotics, steroids, and nonsteroidal antiinflammatory drugs (NSAIDs).[74] An initial response to these treatments should not diminish the index of suspicion for neoplasia in older dogs with clinical signs consistent with cancer.[74]

On rare occasions, animals with tumors involving the caudal region of the nasal cavity may have only neurologic signs (e.g., seizures, acute blindness, behavior change, paresis, circling, and obtundation) caused by direct invasion of the cranial vault.[55,56,81] However, absence of neurologic signs does not rule out tumor extension into the cranial vault because most dogs with nasal tumors that extend beyond the cribriform plate do not exhibit neurologic signs.

Diagnosis and Staging

A definitive diagnosis of sinonasal cancer requires a tissue biopsy, even though diagnostic imaging and historic information can be highly suggestive. Coagulation disorders must be ruled out before biopsy because bleeding during the procedure is to be expected.

The superior imaging value of CT and MRI over conventional radiographs for canine nasal disease, including neoplasia, is well documented.[27,49,75,82–88] Cross-sectional imaging provides improved anatomic detail, which allows accurate determination of the extent of tumor (staging) and localization of nasal cavity abnormalities (Fig. 24.4).[27,49,75,82–88] It also facilitates evaluation of the integrity of the cribriform plate and identification of potential tumor extension into the cranial vault. Although, in general, MRI allows for better resolution of soft tissue structures, one report showed no clinically relevant benefit to using MRI over CT to evaluate nasal tumors that do not extend into the cranial

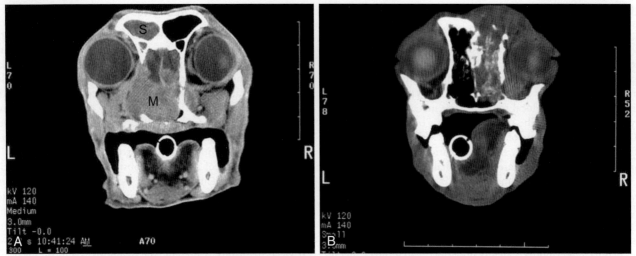

• **Fig. 24.4** (A) Contrast-enhanced computed tomography (CT) images of a dog with sinonasal cancer taken in the transverse plane at the level of the orbit and the olfactory bulb of the brain. Note the contrast-enhancing mass *(M)* in the nasopharynx, which is causing erosion of the frontal and palatine bones. The tumor has invaded the left retroorbital space and the cranial vault, resulting in deviation of the falx cerebri. Noncontrast-enhancing material in the left frontal sinus *(S)* suggests accumulation of the nasal exudates. (B) Noncontrast-enhanced CT images of a dog with sinonasal cancer taken in the transverse plane at the level of the orbit. Note the soft tissue attenuating mass in the right nasal cavity. Erosion of the frontal bone has allowed the tumor to extend into the subcutaneous tissues on the dorsum of the head; erosion of the palatine bone has allowed invasion of the right retroorbital space.

vault.[85] CT enables better visualization of lysis of bones bordering the nasal cavity, which is important for accurate RT planning. It has been proposed that tumor signal intensity on MRI may help distinguish sarcomas from carcinomas,[86] although this application requires further validation before it can be used clinically. Both modalities are useful for imaging nasal tumors, although CT is used more commonly than MRI due to its lower cost in most facilities, wider availability, and usefulness for computer planning of RT. A pilot study has evaluated tumor volume using bidimensional measurements and staging, comparing CT and MRI in six dogs with nasal tumors.[90] The authors concluded that determining extent of tumor margins on MRI resulted in a higher tumor volume (18%) in 5/6 dogs and greater likelihood of detecting meningeal involvement. However, 5/6 dogs were classified as the same stage whether determined by CT or MRI. Further research is needed to determine whether MRI will affect RT volumes, and ultimately total tumor dose and patient outcome.

Certain CT or MRI findings have been correlated with a diagnosis of cancer in dogs with nasal disease.[49,75,89] None of these, alone or in combination, is definitive for neoplasia.[49,75,89] These findings include bony destruction (e.g., ethmoid bones, cribriform plate, and the bones surrounding the nasal cavities), destruction of the sphenoid sinus, abnormal soft tissue in the retrobulbar space, nasopharyngeal invasion, hyperostosis of the lateral maxilla, and patchy areas of increased density within abnormal soft tissue opacity.[49,89] It is important to recognize that detection of a mass in the nasal cavity of a dog is not specific for a diagnosis of neoplasia.[49] Idiopathic inflammatory disease, polyps, and fungal infections can present in this manner.[49,64]

Conventional radiography can still have a place in the diagnostic workup of dogs suspected of having nasal tumors. Despite the inherent limitation of tissue superimposition, the sensitivity of radiography in detecting major nasal cavity abnormalities in dogs with nasal tumors is comparable to that of CT or MRI when tumors are sufficiently advanced to cause clinical signs.[88,91]

Certain radiographic signs have been correlated with a positive predictive value for neoplasia.[92] These include the presence of a soft tissue opacity, loss of turbinate detail affecting the entire ipsilateral nasal cavity, invasion of bones surrounding the nasal cavity, and soft tissue/fluid opacities within the ipsilateral frontal sinus (Fig. 24.5).[92] As is true for CT and MRI changes, no radiographic sign is definitively diagnostic for neoplasia.[88,92] PET/CT using ^{18}F-FDG as well as biomarkers of resistance to radiation, including ^{18}F-FLT for proliferation and ^{61}Cu-ATSM for hypoxia, has been used in a research setting for canine nasal carcinoma and sarcoma.[93–97] Changes in tracer uptake as a result of RT were observed; however, pretreatment PET/CT failed to reliably predict areas of residual tumor or recurrence that could be targeted with a boost dose of radiation to improve tumor control.[97] Relationships of glucose metabolism, proliferation, and hypoxia were heterogeneous across different tumor types.[94] Tumor volume measured by PET-CT and radiation-induced changes in tumor proliferation as shown by FLT uptake may be predictive of tumor behavior and clinical outcome.[96] Further validation of molecular imaging is needed before it can be used for treatment planning or prognostication. A tissue biopsy should be obtained while the patient is under anesthesia for diagnostic imaging. Suitable samples can be acquired by a variety of techniques.[98–100] These include vigorous nasal flushing to dislodge mass lesions, transnostril blind biopsy using cup forceps or a bone curette, rhinoscopic-guided biopsy, FNA or punch biopsy of facial deformities, transnostril core biopsy, CT-guided stereotactic biopsy, and surgical biopsy via rhinotomy (Fig. 24.6). Rhinoscopy can be used to visualize the nasal cavity and to guide biopsy, although this is often not necessary and samples collected in this manner risk being small and superficial.[101] With any nonimage guided transnostril technique, it is important to avoid penetrating the cribriform plate. The biopsy instrument should be marked with tape or cut off at a length that ensures that the instrument does not penetrate farther than the distance from the tip of the nares

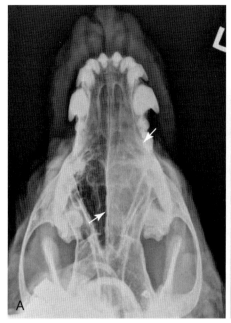
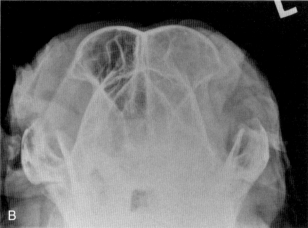

• **Fig. 24.5** Radiographs of a dog with an intranasal anaplastic carcinoma. (A) In this open mouth ventro-dorsal view of the maxilla, note the asymmetry from side to side. A soft tissue opacity in the left nasal cavity *(arrows)* suggest the presence of a space-occupying mass. (B) Rostral-caudal skyline view of the frontal sinuses. A soft tissue opacity in the left frontal sinus suggests extension of tumor or obstructive rhinitis. (Courtesy Dr. David Jimenez.)

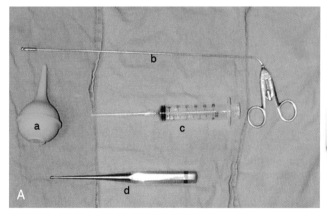
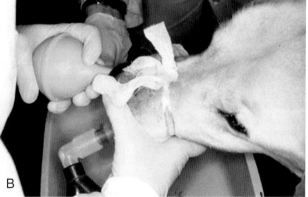

• **Fig. 24.6** (A) Several techniques can be used to procure tissue biopsy material from dogs with nasal tumors. A bulb syringe *(a)* can be used to flush out tumor material, or a biopsy forcep *(b)*, plastic cannula *(c)*, or bone curette *(d)* can be inserted through the nostril. (B) To flush biopsy tissue in an anesthetized dog with an endotracheal tube, the contralateral passage is occluded, and flushing pressure is created with a saline-filled bulb syringe; the tissue is flushed back through the nasopharynx and out the mouth into a collection bowl.

to the medial canthus of the eye (Fig. 24.7). Mild-to-moderate hemorrhage is to be expected and generally subsides within several minutes. Inadequate biopsy size or sampling outside the region of the tumor may preclude an accurate diagnosis. Further testing may be necessary when clinical and histologic findings are incongruent. In cases in which imaging results are suggestive of an aggressive process, yet histopathologic changes are consistent with nonspecific inflammatory disease, repeat biopsy may be needed for definitive diagnosis.[27,49] One study evaluated the diagnostic accuracy of three different biopsy techniques in 117 dogs with confirmed nasal neoplasia.[102] Techniques included blind biopsy, advanced image-guided biopsy to direct location of a blind biopsy, or rhinoscopy guided. For all patients, a diagnosis

of neoplasia was made in only 56% of the samples on the first attempt in spite of the presence of a mass lesion seen either on imaging or rhinoscopy. The proportion of first biopsies yielding accurate results did not differ between the techniques, indicating that blind biopsy may be as diagnostic as rhinoscopy guided. This study also found that in cases that had both advanced imaging and rhinoscopy (*n* = 54), imaging detected a mass in all cases compared with rhinoscopy, which identified a mass in 41% of the cases.[102]

Attempts at nasal washing and fluid retrieval for cytologic examination generally have been unrewarding and are not recommended as the sole means of diagnosis.[25] Brush cytology also has been described, but it often is not diagnostic.[103]

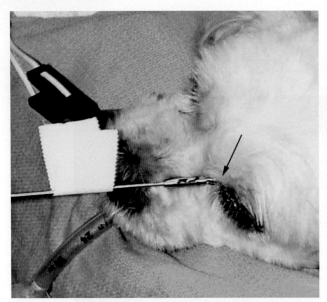

• **Fig. 24.7** Regardless of the biopsy technique chosen, any instrument that is passed through the naris must be measured; it also should be marked with tape or cut off at a length that ensures that the instrument does not penetrate farther than the distance from the tip of the naris to the medial canthus of the eye. This ensures that the instrument does not pass through a potentially compromised cribriform plate.

TABLE 24.1	Modified Adams Clinical Staging Method for Nasosinal Tumors[106]
Stage 1	Confined to one nasal passage, paranasal sinus or frontal sinus, with no bone involvement beyond turbinates
Stage 2	Any bone involvement (beyond turbinates), but with no evidence of orbit/subcutaneous/submucosal mass
Stage 3	Orbit involved, or nasopharyngeal, or subcutaneous, or submucosal mass
Stage 4	Tumor-causing lysis of the cribriform plate

Multiple staging systems for canine sinonasal neoplasia have been proposed on the basis of local tumor extent and bony erosion.[29,104–107] The most clinically relevant and commonly used system is the CT-based, modified Adams clinical staging method, which describes four clinical stages of local tumor extension (Table 24.1).[106] This staging system is based on a review of 94 dogs with nasal carcinoma or sarcoma treated with definitive-intent, nonconformal computer planned RT, which showed that CT evidence of cribriform plate involvement (stage 4) was associated with the shortest median survival time (MST, 6.7 months) and unilateral intranasal involvement without bone destruction beyond the turbinates (stage 1) had the longest MST (23.4 months).[106] Prognostic significance improved when CT findings were combined with histologic category.[106]

Regional LN cytology is positive for metastasis in as many as 10% to 24% of cases and is most commonly associated with carcinoma.[36,74,108–110] Enlarged regional (mandibular and retropharyngeal) LNs should be sampled for cytology to differentiate between a reactive process and metastasis. Thoracic imaging by radiography or CT should be performed but is usually negative for metastasis at initial presentation.[25,26,36,74,110] The reported risk of pulmonary metastasis at the time of diagnosis is 2% to 10%.[34,74,110] In a study evaluating the detection of comorbidities in a large cohort of dogs, 25 had a primary diagnosis of nasal tumor.[111] All dogs had thoracic radiographs and abdominal ultrasound done as part of routine staging. Two of 25 (8%) dogs had an unrelated intrathoracic abnormality detected, including thymoma in one and cardiac changes in the other. Twenty of 25 nasal tumor patients had abnormalities seen on abdominal ultrasound; however, all were considered clinically insignificant with the exception of two cases (8%): one dog had an intestinal foreign body and another had a bladder mass. Overall, 4 of the 25 dogs had treatment altered due to potentially serious comorbidities. Although it is a small number, the typical patient population with nasal tumors is older, and more thorough screening if treatment is being considered may be warranted.

Hematologic and biochemical findings generally are noncontributory in dogs with sinonasal tumors. In rare cases, paraneoplastic erythrocytosis and hypercalcemia have been documented.[112–114]

Treatment and Prognosis

Therapy for sinonasal carcinoma and sarcoma is directed primarily at control of local disease, which usually manifests in a relatively advanced stage in a critical location near the brain and eyes. Without treatment, the MST of dogs with nasal carcinoma is 95 days as reported in a retrospective case series of 139 dogs.[74] Prognosis of dogs with epistaxis appears worse than for dogs without epistaxis (MST 88 days vs. 224 days).[74] Bone invasion occurs early, and curative surgery is virtually impossible. Surgical removal by means of rhinotomy has been associated with a high rate of morbidity without significant extension of life, limiting the utility of this procedure as a sole form of treatment.[25,34,36,115,116] The MST after surgery alone is approximately 3 to 6 months, similar to that reported for no treatment.[25,36,115,116]

RT using high-energy megavoltage (MV) equipment as the sole treatment modality has become the therapy of choice for canine sinonasal tumors. It has the advantage of treating the entire nasal cavity, including bone, and its use has been associated with the greatest improvement in survival. Although surgical removal of the tumor before MV irradiation has not been shown to improve clinical outcome,[36,117,118] controlled studies have not been done for this combination. MSTs after standardly fractionated, definitive-intent MV irradiation alone range from 8 to 19.7 months.[104–106,110,118–125] The reported 1- and 2-year survival rates range from 43% to 68% (1 year) and 11% to 44% (2 years).[104,105,119–121,125] Doses of 42 to 54 Gy are usually delivered in 10 to 18 treatments of 3- to 4.2-Gy fractions over 2 to 4 weeks to the nasal cavity and frontal sinuses as dictated by imaging.[104–106,117,120–122] True statistical comparisons between reports are not possible because of inconsistencies in methodology (including within individual reports) with respect to total dose, fraction number, dose per fraction, treatment schedules, use of CT staging, use of computerized treatment planning, radiation dose distributions, response monitoring, and statistical assessment. Furthermore, differences in tumor type and tumor stage also affect patient outcome.[106] CT-based computerized RT planning greatly enhances normal tissue sparing while ensuring optimized dose distribution within the tumor.

RT can induce normal tissue complications in the radiation treatment field (see Chapter 13). Acute and late toxicities affect rapidly and slowly renewing tissues, respectively, and depend on daily dose to the tissue, total dose, overall treatment time, and volume of tissue treated.[126] The severity of side effects can therefore vary among protocols and also between individuals on the same treatment schedule, depending on the tissues included in the radiation field. Acute toxicities associated with irradiation of sinonasal tumors are dose- and schedule-dependent and can involve the oral cavity (oral mucositis), eye (keratoconjunctivitis and blepharitis), nasal cavity (rhinitis), and skin (desquamation) (Fig. 24.8).[104,105,119,122,127] Acute effects develop during the course of RT and resolve within 2 to 8 weeks after treatment.[104,105,119,127] Oral antibiotics, pain medications, and/or ocular medications including artificial tears may be needed to support the patient during this period. Rarely, temporary esophagostomy or gastrostomy tube feedings may be indicated if oral mucositis is severe to maintain adequate nutritional intake.

Late radiation effects, although less common than acute effects, are more detrimental and long lasting. Their development is also dose-dependent and should be prevented with thoughtful RT planning. Tissues that may be affected include the ocular lens (cataracts), cornea (keratitis, atrophy, keratoconjunctivitis sicca), anterior uvea (uveitis), retina (hemorrhage and degeneration), neuronal tissue (brain necrosis, causing neurologic changes and/or seizures, and optic nerve degeneration), bone (osteonecrosis), and skin (fibrosis).[104,105,119,122,127–130] Late complications develop months to years after therapy and are generally irreversible. The most commonly observed clinically relevant late effects in dogs treated with definitive RT for sinonasal tumors are those affecting ocular structures when it is not possible to spare the eyes using conformal radiation delivery.[104,119] Late ocular changes in the dog typically occur 6 to 9 months after RT and most often include keratoconjunctivitis sicca, cataract formation, and blindness in the irradiated eye if radiation doses are not limited.[122] The lens is particularly sensitive to radiation damage, with cataracts forming in people at doses as low as 2 to 5 Gy.[131] Other late effects are rare when standard radiation doses per fraction are used. In general, the risk of late effects increases when doses per fraction are increased. The use of highly conformal RT delivery techniques allows for avoidance of critical structures including the eyes and brain.[122]

Overall, although the majority dogs with sinonasal neoplasia experience a favorable tumor response to RT with resolution of clinical signs, the long-term prognosis is poor. Even when treated with a definitive RT protocol, most dogs die or are euthanized as a result of local disease progression. An investigation of treatment failure patterns after full-course MV irradiation showed that the median duration of local control in 24 dogs was 312 days.[132] Marked tumor regression (90% reduction in size) was observed using CT in 46% of cases and was associated with a longer duration of local control than that seen in dogs in which tumor response to radiation was less favorable (389 vs. 161 days).[132] Most of the dogs in that series experienced local progressive disease, which affirms the need for more effective treatment strategies.

The following approaches have been investigated to improve local control using conventionally fractionated RT.

1. Definitive-intent RT (4.2 Gy × 10 daily fractions) *followed* by surgical exenteration of residual or recurrent disease showed promise in a small series of dogs (*n* = 13), with a MST of 47 months, compared with 19 months for dogs treated with radiation alone.[121] In this study, complete exenteration of the nasal cavity involving removal of all turbinates and periosteal lining in the nasal cavity was performed. The combination treatment was associated with an increased incidence of late effects, including rhinitis (bacterial and fungal), osteomyelitis, and fistula formation, but MST was the longest reported for dogs with nonlymphomatous sinonasal tumors.[121] The risk of these complications may be reduced with a more limited and focused extirpation of intranasal tissue in the region of the tumor and with the use of highly conformal radiation delivery techniques that minimize dose to normal tissues. A larger group of dogs must be treated in this manner to confirm the safety and efficacy of this modified surgical approach. Another study (*n* = 16) evaluating exenteration after definitive-intent preoperative RT (median 3 Gy × 18 daily fractions) resulted in a MST of 457 days (15 months) with no long-term side effects observed.[133] The surgical approach used in these cases was not described and some dogs had advanced metastatic disease at the time of surgery, potentially contributing to the less favorable MST.

2. A logical and intuitive approach to improve local control is to increase radiation dose. This was investigated in an older study using a boost technique in which the total radiation dose was escalated to 57 Gy without an increase in overall treatment time. The treatment, delivered using nonconformal radiation and without the benefit of computerized treatment planning in most dogs, proved too toxic with respect to acute effects and

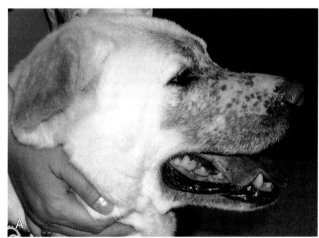

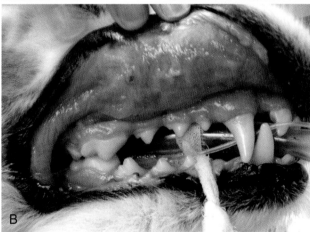

• **Fig. 24.8** Potential acute effects of radiation therapy (RT) in dogs. (A) Resolving desquamation 1 month after definitive RT for a nasal tumor. Note the hair loss in the radiation field. (B) Oral mucositis on the last day of a definitive radiation protocol. Note the yellowish material on the inner aspect of the upper lip. This represents dead epithelium that is being shed from the mucosa.

resulted in radiation-related deaths in one-third of evaluated dogs.[127] A recent investigation of a similar approach evaluated a simultaneously integrated boost using highly conformal intensity-modulated RT and led to clinically acceptable side effects in a small pilot study of nine dogs in which a 20% dose increase was delivered to gross disease.[134] These preliminary results suggest that modern conformal techniques may make dose escalation a feasible treatment strategy. Further evaluation is needed to confirm these findings and to assess effectiveness with respect to tumor control.

3. The use of radiosensitizers in conjunction with ionizing radiation has been reported. A Veterinary Radiation Therapy Oncology Group (VRTOG) pilot study described the use of gemcitabine as a radiosensitizer for sinonasal carcinoma.[135] Gemcitabine was given intravenously at a dosage of 50 mg/m^2 twice weekly before daily RT. The authors reported significant hematologic toxicity (neutropenia) and local acute tissue complications associated with this dose and schedule. In another report, low-dose cisplatin (7.5 mg/m^2 given intravenously every other day) administered in conjunction with definitive RT was well tolerated and did not appear to cause an increase in acute or late radiation effects.[123] The efficacy of this approach with respect to improvement of clinical outcome is not known. A combination of RT and cisplatin, administered intramuscularly throughout therapy using a slow-release polymer system (open cell polylactic acid polymer impregnated with platinum [OPLA-Pt]), was well tolerated; however, survival times were similar to those in other studies that used RT alone (MST: 474 days).[120] Use of firocoxib, a COX-2 inhibitor, was evaluated in combination with RT in a small, underpowered study. Quality of life was improved in the dogs receiving the nonsteroidal antiinflammatory drug, but there was no difference in progression-free interval or overall survival compared with RT alone.[136]

An important advancement in the treatment of sinonasal tumors has been the advent of intensity-modulated RT (IMRT), which is now widely available in veterinary medicine. IMRT achieves highly conformal distribution of radiation dose to the tumor while sparing sensitive normal tissues.[122,137–140] Multiple radiation fields of nonuniform beam intensity are delivered with the goal of distributing the radiation dose among larger volumes of normal tissue. The complex shape of sinonasal tumors and the surrounding critical structures, including eyes and brain, provide a strong rationale for application of IMRT with this tumor type. RT-related morbidity can be significantly reduced in dogs with sinonasal tumors when IMRT is used.[122,138] A clinical study compared radiation-induced ocular toxicity in dogs with nasal tumors treated with IMRT to that of historical controls treated with conventional 2D RT.[122] IMRT reduced the radiation dose delivered to the eyes and resulted in bilateral ocular sparing. This was in contrast to profound ocular morbidity observed in the historical control group. MSTs for both groups were similar. Paramount to the success of highly conformal RT is precise daily patient positioning.[137] Millimeter variation in patient setup can result in underdosing of the tumor and unintended irradiation of normal tissues. Daily setup inaccuracies associated with conventional (nonrigid) immobilization techniques used in veterinary RT reduce precision of IMRT delivery over a multiple-week course of treatment for nasal tumors.[140] Daily image guidance is often necessary to ensure daily setup precision.[140] This is referred to as image-guided IMRT (IGRT). Rigid immobilization techniques (head and cranial body fixation devices) have been developed for veterinary patients,[141–144,145] and, in conjunction with daily "on-board" image guidance, permit successful implementation of highly conformal therapy.[140,141,145,146] Also critical to the success of IMRT is the accuracy of radiation target and normal tissue delineation in the treatment planning process, as well as the choice of dose calculation algorithm in the treatment planning system.[147–149]

A newly emerging application of IMRT/IGRT is stereotactic RT (SRT). SRT refers to the delivery of high-dose (ablative) radiation in a single dose or a few fractions.[150] The treatment is delivered with extreme accuracy, and the dose is pinpointed to the tumor, minimizing the effect on nearby organs. The high degree of precision and sharp dose fall-off at the edge of the tumor target is achieved by delivering many (up to hundreds) irregular subfields. This is done using specialized software and sophisticated multileaf collimation to create a complex intensity pattern.[150] To achieve rapid dose fall off outside of the tumor target, dose heterogeneity in the tumor is allowed with the tumor target receiving as much as 30% to 40% above the prescribed dose (Fig. 24.9). SRT fractionation schedules usually involve a daily treatment for 1 to 3 days, which has obvious practical advantages compared with conventionally fractionated schedules that take weeks to complete. SRT requires precision throughout the treatment process: optimized imaging for treatment planning, thoughtful and accurate target and normal tissue delineation, highly reproducible patient immobilization, high-fidelity image guidance, and

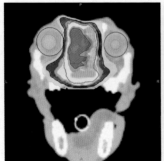
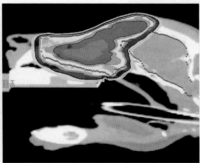
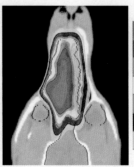

| 36.0 Gy |
| 33.0 Gy |
| 32.0 Gy |
| 30.0 Gy |
| 28.5 Gy |
| 24.0 Gy |
| 15.0 Gy |

• **Fig. 24.9** Stereotactic radiation therapy radiation dose distribution for a stereotactic treatment plan created for a dog with nasal carcinoma. The radiation prescription to the planning target volume (PTV, *red line*) is three daily fractions of 10 Gy for a total dose of 30 Gy. The various color wash regions show heterogeneity of dose within the PTV and rapid dose fall off outside the PTV. The eyes and brain receive minimal dose due to the conformity of the treatment plan.

an intensity modulated radiation beam to achieve extreme precision.[128] Initial SRT experiences in dogs with nasal tumors have been variable.[151–153] Published reports include radiation prescriptions with median doses ranging from 24 to 36 Gy delivered in three fractions (3 daily or every-other-day fractions of 10 Gy, or 3 daily treatments of 8–12 Gy)[152,153] or as a single fraction of up to 33 Gy.[151] In all of these studies, SRT improved clinical signs associated with sinonasal tumors. MST varied, however, ranging from 8.5 months to 19.5 months. Tumor control is dose-dependent, and thus will be contingent on the dose prescription, number of fractions, accuracy of target delineation in the treatment planning process, dose heterogeneity across the tumor, and accuracy of treatment delivery. Variation between studies in any of the factors can dramatically affect clinical outcome. Interestingly, tumor stage was not prognostic in any of these SRT studies,[151–153] which may reflect the ability of modern conformal RT techniques to deliver adequate radiation doses to regions of tumor that abut critical structures such as the brain. Acute effects associated with SRT at the doses delivered are reportedly rare and mild, although it is possible they were underreported.[151–153] Given the high dose per fraction used with SRT, the risk of late effects is higher than for conventionally fractionated protocols. With thoughtful treatment planning and use of normal tissue dose constraints during the treatment planning process, late effects can be minimized.[153] Severe late complications can include oronasal fistula formation, seizures, ocular changes, skin necrosis, and osteonecrosis.[151–153] Late effects are reported in 3% to 40% of dogs and depend on the degree of dose conformality achieved during the treatment process and the dose delivered to normal tissues.[151–153] The most favorable outcome reported to date both in terms of tumor control and toxicity is reported by Gieger et al. who prescribed three daily fractions of 10 Gy planned with well-defined and standardized contouring practices and normal tissue constraints.[153] In that study of 29 dogs, three developed fistulas within the radiation field 4 to 12 months after RT, two of which may have been related to tumor response or progression as opposed to radiation. Two dogs developed fungal rhinitis 1 year after RT. No information about ocular toxicity was provided. The MST was 586 days. Despite the multiple apparent advantages of SRT, the challenges associated with optimal use of this technology must be considered and treatment plan evaluation must be optimized. Controlled clinical trials that rigorously examine normal tissue effects and tumor responses are still needed to validate use of SRT over standardly fractionated conventional RT or IMRT/IGRT in veterinary medicine.

In contrast to curative-intent RT protocols, treatment schedules that are less intensive can be used to palliate tumor-related clinical signs. The goal of palliative RT is to improve quality of life without aiming to maximize tumor sterilization. Palliative protocols involve coarsely fractionated treatments (5–9 Gy per fraction) delivered weekly or biweekly, or daily treatments (4 Gy) for 5 days, or daily treatments (3 Gy) for 10 days.[69,109,110,136,154–158] The result of this approach is temporary improvement of clinical signs in 66% to 100% of dogs and limited morbidity associated with acute side effects.[109,136,154–158] The reported median duration of control of clinical signs ranges from 120 to 308 days.[109,155,157,158] Acute toxicities affecting the oral mucosa and skin are generally mild and short-lived.[109,154–158] Acute and chronic ocular toxicities can develop if the eye is not spared.[155,157,158] Reported MSTs range from 146 days to 512 days.[69,109,154–158] Tumor stage (stage 1) and duration of clinical signs (>90 days) have been correlated with longer survival in cases receiving this type of radiation.[109,155]

Although true statistical comparisons between studies are not possible because of inconsistencies in methodology, the best clinical outcomes in terms of survival (approximately 300–500 days) are reported in three studies in which RT planning was performed using CT and 3D-conformal computerized treatment planning software in most dogs.[109,133,158] Modernized RT planning in canine nasal tumor patients treated palliatively may result in more favorable clinical outcomes than for previously reported, less sophisticated approaches.[109,157,158] When lower doses per fraction are used, such as the five daily treatments of 4 Gy protocol described by Tan-Coleman, the radiation treatment course can be repeated upon return of clinical signs to prolong palliation.[157] The use of a nonsteroidal antiinflammatory drug can also help improve overall quality of life.[136]

A number of reports suggest that some dogs with recurrent nasal tumors can experience a second clinical remission after reirradiation.[157,159,160] One study evaluated a selected cohort of nine dogs in which the median time to tumor progression after a first definitive course of RT was 513 days. The first course of radiation delivered a median of 50 Gy in a median of 18 fractions. The median total dose used in the second protocol was 36 Gy, delivered in approximately 2-Gy fractions. The overall MST for this small, selection-biased cohort of dogs was 927 days (95% confidence interval [CI] 423 days to 1767 days). All dogs developed one or more late effects involving the skin, eyes, and nasal cavity. Late effects in seven of the nine dogs were considered mild and did not affect quality of life. Severe late effects were reported in two dogs, and both had sudden blindness that led to euthanasia. A second study reports a MST of 453 days in 37 dogs that were reirradiated after a coarsely fractionated radiation protocol.[159] The median dose for the first course of RT was 24 Gy (median dose per fraction, 7 Gy), and then 20 Gy for the second course (median dose per fraction, 8 Gy). The second course was initiated a median of 150 days after the first. All dogs responded clinically after the first course for a median of 114 days, and 70% responded after the second course for a median of 80 days. Acute toxicities were generally mild and included the skin, oral mucosa, and eye, although normal tissue doses are not described. Based on these reports, reirradiation for recurrent nasal tumors can result in improvement in clinical signs and potentially extend survival time. In a third study of dogs with sinonasal sarcoma, eight dogs that underwent reirradiation had a longer MST (654 days) than those that had a single course of RT (356 days).[28] Further work is needed to refine time-dose prescriptions to minimize radiation-induced late effects.[159,161] Conformal techniques such as IMRT could play a role in this setting to limit morbidity.[161]

Chemotherapy is used rarely as a sole therapy for canine sinonasal tumors. Treatment with cisplatin alone has been shown to benefit some dogs.[162] A clinical response rate of 27%, including one radiographically-confirmed complete remission, was reported in a small series of 11 dogs.[162] All of the dogs experienced alleviation of clinical signs, and the MST was 5 months. Another report evaluated a combination chemotherapy protocol of doxorubicin, carboplatin, and oral piroxicam in eight dogs with advanced nasal tumors.[163] A clinical response rate of 75% was observed, including 4 CRs confirmed by CT imaging. All dogs experienced resolution of clinical signs, and the protocol was well tolerated. The MST in these eight dogs was 210 days (range 150–960 days). These preliminary results are favorable, but the case number is small, and more dogs need to be treated in this manner to confirm these findings. Toceranib phosphate, a TKI, was associated with a clinical benefit in five of seven dogs (71%) with nasal carcinoma, including one complete tumor response and improvement of clinical signs in five dogs.[164] The median duration of treatment was 18 weeks. Use of toceranib in combination with RT has not yet been reported. In three dogs with SCC limited to the frontal sinus, tumor responses including two complete responses were observed with piroxicam and carboplatin. The third dog had a marked tumor response when toceranib was substituted for carboplatin.[165]

Electrochemotherapy has been described in dogs with nasal cavity tumors, consisting of an intravenous injection of bleomycin followed by local delivery of electric pulses using a custom single needle electrode to potentiate drug uptake.[166] The overall response rate in 11 dogs treated with electrochemotherapy alone was 90% with a MST of 16.9 months, compared with 5.3 months in 10 dogs treated with surgery followed by adjuvant carboplatin chemotherapy. Systemic effects were not reported. Adjuvant electrochemotherapy using a topical application of bleomycin in the nasal cavity is reported in a single dog after surgical extirpation of the tumor.[167]

Other therapeutic approaches to nasal tumors that have been investigated include proton-beam therapy, brachytherapy, immunotherapy, cryotherapy, and photodynamic therapy (PDT). Charged particles like protons have a well-defined tissue range and sharp dose fall off, which could potentially be exploited for conformal tumor targeting and normal tissue sparing.[168] A small clinical trial involving nine dogs with nasal tumors treated with proton-beam therapy resulted in tumor responses and survival times similar to those reported for MV irradiation.[168] Acute effects to the skin and eyes were pronounced in some dogs, and 50% of dogs developed radiation-induced cataracts. Due to limited availability of proton irradiators, this technology is unlikely to be optimized for use in dogs. Intracavitary RT using radioactive isotopes (brachytherapy) has been evaluated after surgical removal of sinonasal tumors in dogs.[169–170] Potential problems associated with this type of radiation include dose distribution and radiation exposure to personnel. The question of whether brachytherapy improves survival over traditional external-beam RT has not been answered. Immunotherapy and cryosurgery have not improved survival times.[25,171] A recent case report described the use of image-guided cryotherapy in the treatment of a rapidly recurrent nasal carcinoma that resulted in long-term tumor control and survival.[172] The authors suggested that further investigation of this technique may be warranted for the management of focal residual or recurrent nasal tumors. Reports evaluating PDT have been published, including in combination with surgery and RT; however, results are too preliminary to draw any conclusions.[173–175]

When all treatments fail to control epistaxis, unilateral or bilateral carotid artery ligation can palliate symptoms in dogs for up to 3 months or longer without damage to the brain.[99]

The importance of prognostic factors in the treatment of canine sinonasal tumors remains controversial. Negative predictors of survival from various studies include age (>10 years),[108] epistaxis,[74] duration of clinical signs,[155] advanced local tumor stage,[104–106,108,109] metastatic disease,[36,108,136] histologic subtype (carcinoma, particularly SCC or undifferentiated),[104,106,98] tumor expression of survivin,[176] and failure to achieve resolution of clinical signs.[155] An analysis of 94 dogs with varying subtypes of nasal carcinoma or sarcoma treated with curative-intent RT at three veterinary facilities was performed.[106] A correlation was demonstrated between clinical outcome and the original Adams tumor staging scheme,[105] as well as the modified Adams tumor staging method.[105] Based on these findings, dogs with cribriform

plate involvement as determined by CT imaging (stage 4) have the shortest disease-free survival (DFS) and overall survival time (OST). This subset of dogs had a median DFS of 3.8 months and a median OST of almost 7 months, compared with dogs with unilateral tumors without bone involvement (stage 1) in which DFS and OST were 6.5 and 23 months, respectively. In a recent study of 29 dogs with cribriform involvement (stage 4) treated with definitive-intent IMRT, the MST was 305 days.[177] Compared with the earlier studies that used nonconformal delivery techniques,[105–106] these favorable results suggest that IMRT, with its greater conformality and tumor dose homogeneity, may improve outcomes in dogs with stage 4 disease. Interestingly, intracranial tumor extension past the cribriform plate was not prognostic for survival.[177] This highlights the fact that prognostic indicators may change as technical advances in treatment develop. In most studies, sinonasal carcinomas and sarcomas are grouped together because of a similar biological behavior and clinical response to RT. In the multiinstitutional study of 94 dogs mentioned above,[106] there was no effect on clinical outcome when all carcinomas were compared with all sarcomas; however, when dogs with anaplastic carcinoma, undifferentiated carcinoma, and SCC were grouped together, they had a shorter DFS than dogs with other tumor types. A recent retrospective study limited to dogs with sinonasal sarcoma treated with RT ($n = 86$), the overall MST was 444 days (15 months), which is in line with previous studies.[28] Radiation protocols were not standardized, but dogs with sarcoma treated with definitive RT had more favorable outcomes compared with those treated in the palliative setting (MST 523 days vs. 305 days). Also, dogs treated daily Monday to Friday had an improved MST compared with dogs treated on a Monday, Wednesday, Friday schedule. Six dogs diagnosed with intracavitary nasal osteosarcoma had a significantly better MST at 624 days than dogs with other mesenchymal tumors. Interestingly, this is in contrast to seven dogs with nasal osteosarcoma treated with SRT that had a shorter OST than dogs with other carcinoma or sarcoma tumor types (MST 3 months vs. 10 months).[151] This difference may be due to chance, or variations in tumor stage, or tumor location, or treatment approaches in these small groups of dogs. The true prognosis of sinonasal osteosarcoma treated with RT is not clear. In a multiinstitutional study of 24 dogs with intranasal lymphoma treated with various RT protocols +/– adjuvant chemotherapy, the overall MST was 375 days for intermediate/large cell and 823 days for the small cell group.[59] There was no difference in MST for dogs treated with RT and chemotherapy versus chemotherapy alone. Eighty-five percent to 90% of dogs treated with RT improved clinically, suggesting that this is a radioresponsive tumor and that RT may play a role in its management. Angiofibroma is a histologically benign but locally aggressive vascular nasopharyngeal tumor characterized by a proliferation of irregular appearing blood vessels that are surrounded by a connective tissue stroma.[63] None of the 13 dogs reviewed retrospectively had metastasis. Prolonged survival of up to 4 years was reported in four dogs after surgical excision. Survival of 1 to 2 years was observed in some dogs with no treatment. A small series of four dogs with intranasal MCT receiving various chemotherapy agents has been reported.[60] Tumor response information was not provided. The survival times ranged from 27 to 134 days. Based on a case report of three dogs treated with RT, intranasal melanoma appears to be a radioresponsive tumor with two dogs experiencing a complete response after RT.[61] Finally, in a case series of five dogs with nasal polyps treated with surgery or nasal flushing, three dogs were alive without recurrence at 16 to 54 months.[64] Two dogs developed recurrence, one of which had nasal signs controlled for 10 months after definitive RT for polyp recurrence. The role of RT in the management of nasal polyps is not clear.

A major pitfall of many veterinary studies with respect to assessment of treatment efficacy in canine sinonasal cancer is the need for advanced imaging to assess tumor response. Tumor response and TTP are the most representative measures of treatment efficacy. Regular diagnostic imaging, ideally CT or MRI, is necessary for accurate determination of these endpoints. Due to high costs and the need for anesthesia, follow-up is rarely done in this manner. Analyzing the return of clinical signs as an indication of tumor recurrence is problematic because similar signs can result from rhinitis secondary to therapy (RT and/or surgery) or residual tumor.[178] Assessment of survival time may be biased by the use of additional treatments on suspicion of progressive disease and by the decision for euthanasia, which can vary greatly from one pet owner to another. Furthermore, inconsistencies in methodology between studies and even within individual reports, as well as a lack of controlled studies, have limited the informed development of the optimal treatment approach for sinonasal tumors in dogs.

Feline Sinonasal Tumors

Nasal and sinus cavity tumors in the cat are malignant in more than 90% of the histologically diagnosed cases. They occur in an older population of cats with a mean age reported between 9 and 10 years.[179–181] In general, these tumors are locally invasive and associated with a low metastatic rate at the time of diagnosis.[180,182]

Clinical signs related to sinonasal tumors in cats overlap with those of other causes of chronic nasal disease.[179,181] These include nasal discharge, upper respiratory tract dyspnea, sneezing, epistaxis, facial swelling, ocular discharge, and weight loss.[179–181,183–185] Although each of these signs can occur with both neoplasia and rhinitis, in some reports, certain signs are more commonly associated with neoplasia such as unilateral discharge or epistaxis,[179] whereas in others, the character of the clinical signs does not distinguish the underlying cause.[181] The median duration of clinical signs before diagnosis is several months, and many cats will experience temporary alleviation of clinical signs with use of antibiotics and or corticosteroids.[179–181] Differential diagnoses for chronic nasal signs include chronic rhinitis, infectious rhinitis, foreign body, nasal polyp, nasopharyngeal stenosis, and trauma.

Lymphoma is the most commonly diagnosed tumor type in the feline nasal cavity and sinuses, followed by epithelial neoplasms (carcinoma, adenocarcinoma, SCC). Less frequently reported tumor types include sarcomas (fibrosarcoma, osteosarcoma, chondrosarcoma), MCT, melanoma, plasmacytoma, olfactory neuroblastoma, and benign lesions such as nasal hamartoma, chondroma, and neurofibroma.[179–181,186,187]

Diagnostic principles are similar to those in the dog. A tissue sample is required to make a definitive diagnosis of cancer in most cases. DeLorenzi et al evaluated cytology from squash preparations obtained from endoscopic biopsies of nasopharyngeal masses in cats and found that cytologic results were in good agreement with histopathology with an overall accuracy of 90%.[188] However, distinguishing lymphoma from lymphoid inflammatory disease was not as accurate, and histopathologic confirmation was recommended.[188] Another study evaluated the histopathologic and cytologic features of nasal lymphoma in 50 cases. Ninety-one percent of cases were classified as immunoblastic lymphoma according to the National Institutes of Health Working Formulation.

The majority of cases were B-cell (68%) and 20% were T-cell, with 12% having a mixed population of B- and T-cells.[186] In another study of 39 cases, 28% were small cell and 87% were B cell.[189] In this study they also evaluated FeLV viral antigens (p27 and gp70) by immunohistochemistry (IHC) and found that 54% of samples were positive, although cases were not serologically tested. The majority of cases in this series did not receive therapy, so the effect of viral positivity on outcome is unknown. Because lymphoma makes up a high percentage of feline nasal tumor cases, special stains may be helpful in obtaining a correct diagnosis. In a retrospective study of 232 feline nasal tumor biopsies reviewed by two pathologists, disagreement in diagnosis was seen in 15 cases, 14 of which were originally diagnosed as carcinoma.[190] IHC with epithelial and lymphoid markers showed that the original diagnosis was incorrect 67% of the time, indicating the usefulness of IHC in establishing a correct diagnosis in feline nasal tumors.

Radiographs of the nasal cavity have been reported as a diagnostic tool in cats with both chronic rhinitis and nasal neoplasia. Although no radiographic sign is entirely specific for neoplasia, findings with the highest predictive value for cancer include displacement of midline structures, unilateral changes such as soft tissue opacity and loss of turbinate detail, and evidence of bone invasion.[191] Similarly, as CT scan becomes a common imaging tool, reports of the characteristic findings of scans from cats with sinonasal disease of all etiologies have been published.[192–194] One retrospective assessment of CT imaging in 62 cats with sinonasal disease showed that, although certain findings such as osteolysis of paranasal bones, extension of disease into the orbit of facial soft tissues, the presence of a space-occupying mass, and turbinate destruction may suggest a CT diagnosis of neoplasia over rhinitis, nasal biopsy is necessary for confirmation.[192] Another study evaluated the clinical characteristics and CT findings in 43 cats and found that those with neoplasia were significantly more likely to have unilateral lysis of the ethmoturbinates as well as dorsal and lateral maxilla, lysis of the vomer bone and ventral maxilla, and unilateral soft tissue or fluid in the sphenoid recess, frontal sinus, or retrobulbar space. Interestingly, in that study population, cribriform plate lysis was not significantly associated with neoplasia.[193] In another report describing CT findings in cats with confirmed fungal rhinitis, they found that some of the features overlap with those seen in neoplasia patients, including older age at the time of diagnosis, soft tissue mass, and osteolysis. Another study sought to determine whether CT characteristics of nasal passages and medial retropharyngeal LNs (MRPLNs) could be used to distinguish neoplasia from rhinitis.[195] Thirty-four cats with rhinitis and 22 cats with neoplasia were evaluated. These authors found that in addition to nasal passage findings typically sited in other studies, the MRPLN characteristics that were significantly associated with neoplasia included abnormal MRPLN hilus, height asymmetry, and decreased MRPLN precontrast heterogeneity. Although these studies confirm the utility of CT scan determining extent of disease, no one group of features replaces histopathology for definitive diagnosis.

Even though the metastatic rate of feline sinonasal cancer at the time of diagnosis is reportedly low, any enlarged regional LNs should be evaluated cytologically to differentiate a reactive process from metastasis. In a recent report of 123 cases of feline sinonasal cancer, 21 cats had regional lymphadenopathy. None showed cytologic evidence of metastasis.[180]

As in the dog, RT continues to be the predominant local therapy of choice for this disease. Reports of treatment for feline nonlymphoma sinonasal tumors are few, and case numbers are small.[182,196] In one study, 16 cats with nonlymphoproliferative neoplasms were treated using a definitive course of radiation to a total dose of 48 Gy. The therapy was well tolerated, and MST was 12 months with 44% and 16% of cats alive at 1 and 2 years, respectively.[182] In another report of RT for nonlymphoproliferative tumors, this time treated using a coarse fractionation regime, results showed that the protocol was well tolerated, with a MST of almost 13 months and a 63% 1-year survival rate reported.[196] A report of 65 cats receiving palliative hypofractionated RT also determined acute and late side effects in addition to outcome.[197] There were 29 high-grade lymphoma cases with the rest (n = 36) being a variety of carcinomas. Patients received RT weekly (6–8 Gy) for a median total dose of 32 Gy. Many patients also received chemotherapy. Acute complications occurred in 58% of the cases but were considered acceptable. Late effects, typically ocular, occurred in 20% of the cases. The MST in all 65 cats was 432 days. There was no significant difference in MST between cats with lymphoma versus those with other tumor types.

Recent reports of feline nasal and nasal pharyngeal lymphoma treated with RT and/or chemotherapy indicate the potential for long-term survival.[183–186,198] Although treatment protocols vary between reports, in general, overall response rate for feline nasal lymphoma is high, between 70% and 90%. The inclusion of RT appears to enhance overall survival, with MSTs for combination therapy ranging from 174 to 955 days.[184,185] Interestingly, systemic failure of disease at nonnasal sites is also reported in 13% to 16% of cases, indicating that a combination of RT and chemotherapy may be warranted in some patients. However, the timing of such treatment remains to be determined (concurrent vs. sequential), as does which patients are at highest risk for local failure. In an attempt to predict which feline nasal lymphoma cases would respond better to RT, a study was done evaluating pretreatment biopsies in 30 cats looking at apoptotic index and Ki-67 scores.[199] Cases with high proliferative scores were significantly more likely to have a response to RT and have prolonged survival compared with those with low scores. Furthermore, improved RT planning along with optimized RT schedules and doses may ultimately improve local control rates and reduce the risk of systemic failure without the addition of chemotherapy. Published reports of treatment of feline nasal tumors with SRT or more targeted treatment plans are lacking.

Comparative Aspects[200–205]

In humans, cancer of the nasal cavity and paranasal sinuses is classified with other cancers of the upper aerodigestive tract under the all-encompassing title of tumors of the head and neck. Head and neck cancers arise from a variety of sites within the head and neck region, which is divided into five basic areas: (1) oral cavity, (2) pharynx (oropharynx and nasopharynx), (3) larynx, (4) nasal cavity and paranasal sinuses, and (5) salivary glands. The majority of tumors affecting these sites are SCC (head and neck SCC [HNSCC]); however, a range of other malignancies can develop in the nasal cavity and paranasal sinuses, including adenocarcinoma, neuroblastoma, lymphoma, melanoma, angiosarcoma, and tumors of connective tissues. Benign but potentially invasive papillomas are also reported.

Tumors specifically of the nasal cavity and paranasal sinuses are rare in humans and represent less than 1% of all malignant tumors and only about 3% of head and neck cancers. The maxillary sinus is most commonly affected. Tumors of the ethmoid, sphenoid and frontal sinuses, the nasal vestibule and the nasal cavity are less common. Sinonasal cancers are more frequent in men than in women. Some data indicate that various industrial and environmental exposures may be related to sinonasal cancer, including exposure to wood, textile, and leather dusts, as well as formaldehyde. Air pollution and tobacco smoke are also related. Other factors associated with increased risk for all head and neck cancers include smoking and alcohol use, which may have an additive effect. Importantly, human papillomavirus (HPV), a sexually transmitted infection, may be involved in the pathogenesis of sinonasal cancer. HPV has been identified in 25% to 49% of oropharyngeal head and neck cancers and is associated with a significant survival difference compared with HPV-negative oropharyngeal cancers. There is striking evidence of improved outcomes in patients with HPV-positive oropharyngeal tumors. HPV status is the strongest independent determinant of local and regional control, disease specific survival, and overall survival in this group of head and neck cancers. Despite the dramatic influence of HPV in oropharyngeal cancer, its role in the etiology and prognosis of sinonasal head and neck tumors is less well defined.

Sinonasal head and neck tumors are locally invasive and cure rates are generally poor. They are typically advanced at the time of diagnosis because lesions in this area can go undetected for extended periods of time and clinical signs can mimic those of infectious or inflammatory disease. Nodal involvement and distant metastasis are infrequent at the time of diagnosis—reportedly between 10% and 15%. Locoregional recurrence accounts from the majority of cancer deaths.

Surgery and RT are the mainstay of treatment when considered possible, based on stage and location of disease. Chemotherapy can be useful in an adjuvant setting, but it is not curative when used alone. Both RT and surgery have advantages and disadvantages as primary therapies. The OST at 5 years is approximately 60% and 30% for nasal cavity and parasinal tumors, respectively. More favorable prognoses are associated with smaller lesions in which complete surgical resection is achievable. When adequate margins cannot be obtained, surgery and RT are often combined. Incomplete local control of advanced tumors leads to local tumor recurrence in many cases.

The role of chemotherapy in sinonasal head and neck cancer is not clear because these cases are usually reported in conjunction with other head and neck tumors. Active chemotherapy agents include the taxanes, 5-fluorouracil (5-FU), methotrexate, and the platinum drugs. Several studies have reported improved local control and, in some cases, improved OSTs in treatment protocols that combine traditional fractionated RT and chemotherapy; however, the toxicity may also be increased. The optimal case selection, chemotherapy agents, and radiation schedule has yet to be defined.

Multiple targeted and immunotherapies for head and neck cancer have been investigated in clinical trials, most involving EGFR and PD-1 antagonists. Other targeted therapies with potential benefits include VEGF or VEGFR inhibitors and PI3K/AKT/ mTOR pathway inhibitors. The U.S. Food and Drug Administration has granted approval to three monoclonal antibodies for use in certain patients with HNSCC. These include EGFR inhibitor cetuximab (Erbitux), and anti-PD-1 antagonists pembrolizumab (Keytruda) and nivolumab (Opdivo). Because of the rarity of sinonasal head and neck cancers, few molecular studies have been done to evaluate novel therapeutic strategies specifically for tumors in this location. In a study evaluating molecular markers in sinonasal SCC (SNSCC), including EGFR, HER2, p53, KIT, Bax, MMP-2, MMP-9 and VEGFR, only EGFR expression was associated with significantly worse DFS. If confirmed by further studies, EGFR expression may be a prognostic indicator for SNSCC, and targeted inhibition of EGFR may be a new approach to treatment of patients with this rare cancer.

SECTION C: CANCER OF THE LARYNX AND TRACHEA

NICHOLAS J. BACON

Incidence and Risk Factors

Primary tumors of the larynx and trachea are uncommon in domestic animals. Laryngeal tumors comprise 0.02% of all biopsy and necropsy specimens in dogs[206] and a literature review yielded less than 30 dogs with tumors specifically affecting the cartilaginous component of the larynx and trachea.[207] In a study of 2546 insured animals in the United Kingdom in a 12-month period, there were no reported cases of laryngeal or tracheal neoplasia.[208]

Dogs with tracheal masses are often under 2 years (benign cartilage dysplasias) or over 10 years (malignancies) of age. All sized dogs are susceptible with both males and females affected. Arctic breeds, such as the Alaskan malamute or Siberian husky, account for 27% of canine laryngo-tracheal tumors.[207]

Cats with laryngeal or tracheal masses are typically older with a median age of 12 years. Significant correlations have been found between Siamese and domestic long-haired cats and lymphoma, and domestic long-haired cats and adenocarcinoma.[209]

Pathology and Natural Behavior

The larynx is a musculocartilaginous organ lined internally by stratified squamous mucous epithelium. Nearly half of its length is occupied by the rostral epiglottic cartilage. The trachea runs from the larynx to its bifurcation at the carina, just cranial to the heart base. It is composed of approximately 35 C-shaped hyaline cartilages with the tracheal muscle running dorsally. The rings are interconnected by narrow fibro-elastic annular ligaments. The lumen is lined by epithelium.[210]

Benign lesions of the larynx are rare, and rhabdomyoma and oncocytoma make up the majority of these tumors. There is currently some uncertainty whether rhabdomyoma (striated muscle) and oncocytoma (epithelial origin) are in fact variants of the same tumor in the canine larynx.[211,212] Other benign diseases include chondroma, myxochondroma, congenital cysts in young dogs, and lymphoplasmacytic and eosinophilic masses.[207,213]

Rhabdomyosarcoma, SCC, adenocarcinoma, osteosarcoma (OSA), chondrosarcoma (CSA), fibrosarcoma, mast cell tumor (MCT), solitary extramedullary plasmacytoma, and granular cell tumor have been reported in the canine larynx.[214–217]

Young dogs, often 3 to 4 months of age, with active osteochondral ossification sites, are at a higher risk of benign tracheal chondromas, osteochondromas, and osteochondral dysplasia.[207,218–221] These benign osteocartilaginous tumors grow during development and stop growing at skeletal maturity. Leiomyoma has been infrequently reported in the dog.[222,223] Tracheal malignancies are more commonly located on the ventral wall, and adenocarcinoma, MCTs, extramedullary plasmacytoma, OSA, CSA, and lymphoma have all been reported in the canine trachea.[207,221,224–228]

Feline laryngeal tumors include SCC, lymphoma, adenocarcinoma, and poorly differentiated round cell tumors.[209,229–230] Benign laryngeal masses have also been reported, such as lymphoplasmacytic inflammation, lymphoid hyperplasia, and polypoid laryngitis.[209,231]

Primary masses of the trachea in cats include lymphoma, SCC, histiocytic sarcoma, neuroendocrine carcinoma, and adenocarcinoma.[209,232–238] Lymphoplasmacytic inflammation, lymphoid hyperplasia, and epithelial polyp have also been reported.[209,239]

The trachea can be secondarily invaded by adjacent tumors, such as thyroid carcinomas,[240] or the lumen can be narrowed by external compression from lymphomatous nodes.[241]

Distant metastasis from primary laryngo-tracheal tumors is very rare.

History and Clinical Signs

Symptoms may be vague and may include dyspnea, stridor, voice change, exercise intolerance, coughing, gagging, dysphagia, weight loss, wheezing, and anorexia. Some patients may present in acute respiratory distress, including open-mouth breathing in cats. Clinical findings may be unremarkable, although occasionally patients with extratracheal compression may present with a palpable growth in the neck.

Diagnostic Techniques and Workup

Hematology and biochemistry are likely to be unremarkable or show nonspecific changes.

Radiographs of the neck and thorax may identify a solitary soft tissue space-occupying lesion or luminal stenosis within the inherent negative contrast of the airway. Mineralization of tumors is possible for osteochondromas in dogs. Cats with laryngeal and tracheal masses have radiographic abnormalities in 88% of cases (Fig. 24.10).[209] Intraluminal tracheal masses may be able to be detected ultrasonographically.[238] MRI has also been used to identify neoplastic involvement of mucosal or submucosal layers.[216] CT will allow for precise localization of the mass within the lumen and determine whether it has crossed the wall to affect surrounding local tissues.

Direct access to the larynx allows for fine-needle aspirates or grab biopsies to be easily taken under light anesthesia. Superficial biopsies, however, may give a false diagnosis of inflammatory disease and normal squamous epithelium, when inflamed, can have many cytologic characteristics of malignancy. Rigid or flexible endoscopes allow for direct visualization of tracheal

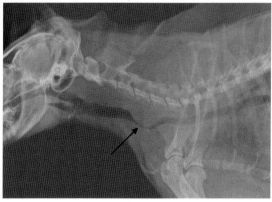

• **Fig. 24.10** Soft tissue mass visible within the air-filled trachea of a cat, later diagnosed as a tracheal carcinoma.

masses, and endoscopic brushings of masses often yield sufficient material for a cytologic diagnosis and immediate treatment (Fig. 24.11). Alternatively, tiny grab biopsies can be obtained through the instrument port for histopathology.[236] Care needs to be taken with larger-bore scopes as extubation must be performed in patients that may already suffer from respiratory compromise.

Excisional biopsy (intralesional or marginal excision, or resection and anastomosis) can be performed to obtain a diagnosis if earlier attempts at diagnosis have been unsuccessful.

Therapy

The relative infrequency and sporadic nature of laryngo-tracheal tumors mean definitive treatment guidelines are lacking. Recommendations are extrapolated from case reports, case series, or oncologic principles of treating similar tumors in other locations.

Larynx

Tube tracheostomy is a short-term measure to provide relief of obstructive symptoms by providing airflow bypass and can be surgically converted to a tracheostomy to allow time for therapies, such as chemotherapy or RT, to have an effect.

Small lesions may be removed by mucosal resection or partial laryngectomy through a transoral, ventral, or lateral laryngeal approach.[213,242,243] Larger lesions may require total laryngectomy incorporating a permanent tracheostomy, but this has been rarely described in dogs.[215,244] External beam RT can be used to treat radiosensitive tumors (e.g., lymphoma), but few reports exist.

Trachea

Surgical removal of the affected tracheal section is most likely to result in the longest disease-free intervals (DFIs) for solid tumors, although tracheal resection and anastomosis is a complex surgical procedure, especially if involving the intrathoracic trachea. Complications include dehiscence, tracheal stenosis, pneumothorax, and laryngeal paralysis.[244]

Endoscopic electrosurgical removal of a bronchial carcinoma in the right mainstem bronchus has been described in a cocker spaniel,[245] and a surgical diode laser has been used to endoscopically

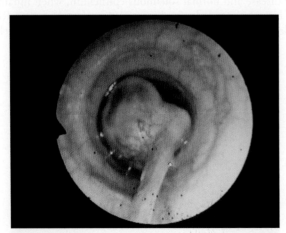

• **Fig. 24.11** Video tracheoscopy has significantly improved the ability to both diagnose and treat luminal masses in dogs and cats. This intraluminal tracheal mass was diagnosed by brush cytology as a poorly differentiated round cell tumor.

debulk an epiglottic CSA and a solid tracheal osteochondroma in dogs.[246,247] Similarly, an endoscopically guided wire snare has been used to debulk tracheal carcinomas in three cats.[248] Surgical debulking followed by cryotherapy has been described to treat an intratracheal adenoma in a cat.[249]

Palliative stenting of malignant tracheal obstructions should result in improvement in clinical signs in both dogs and cats. Endoluminal stents, such as stainless-steel self-expanding metallic stents, are placed minimally invasively under fluoroscopic guidance in anesthetized patients, and the procedure is rapid and low risk. Long sections of trachea that could not be resected surgically can be stented open with a stent greater than 2 cm longer than the tracheal segment affected.[238,250] Potential complications of stenting in dogs and cats include stent migration, fracture, granulation tissue formation, coughing, tumor growing through the stent open-weave, pneumonia, and death.[251]

Chemotherapy and/or RT are primarily reserved for round cell tumors of the trachea, especially lymphoma.

Prognosis

Surgical removal of laryngeal cysts should be curative with no reported long-term effect on function.[213] Likewise, benign osteochondromas in young dogs have an excellent prognosis after surgical resection. Intraoral diode laser total epiglottectomy for a laryngeal CSA resulted in a clinically normal dog 12 months postoperatively without any respiratory or digestive problem.[246] Another dog with a low-grade laryngeal CSA was still symptom free 12 months after surgical resection involving ventral laryngotomy and unilateral arytenoidectomy.[243] Three dogs with tracheal CSA underwent surgical excision, with two dogs having no recurrence.[207] One dog had local recurrence at 3 months; the recurrent disease was surgically resected, and the dog survived a further 8 months after the second excision.[207] Endoscopic removal of a bronchial carcinoma in one dog resulted in suspected local recurrence with respiratory difficulties 1 month postoperatively.[245] Macroscopic invasion of the trachea by thyroid carcinoma has been shown to be a significant negative predictor for DFI; this is seen in up to 24% of dogs with differentiated follicular cell thyroid carcinomas with a median survival time (MST) of 2.5 months.[240]

The prognosis for cats with tracheal carcinomas is poor as most historically have been euthanized immediately after or within a few days of diagnosis due to poor quality of life and rapid progression of disease. It is possible intraluminal stenting may improve this outcome in the future as this modality becomes more widely available.

Aggressive management in cats with solid laryngeal and tracheal tumors, including combinations of surgical resection, RT, and chemotherapy, have resulted in MSTs of 4 to 5 months with <10% of cats alive at 1 year.[209] More favorable prognoses with durable remission and survival times (STs) can be expected in cats with laryngeal and tracheal lymphoma after RT, chemotherapy, or combinations of these modalities; the reader is referred to Chapter 33B for a more thorough discussion. One cat with laryngeal SCC was treated with prednisolone and had a ST of 180 days.[230] A combination of local excision, RT, and melphalan and prednisolone was successful in long-term control of a feline laryngeal plasmacytoma.[216] Permanent tracheostomies in five cats with laryngeal carcinoma resulted in STs of 2 to 281 days, with two cats dying from tracheostomy occlusion and three cats from progressive disease.[252]

Comparative Aspects

Laryngeal cancer in humans is primarily related to smoking and alcohol consumption. The vast majority are SCCs. Initial management strategies were aimed at early laryngectomies with wide surgical margins for locoregional control, but this resulted in aphonia. The pendulum then swung toward chemoradiation to preserve the larynx and laryngeal function, but the quality of life and functional outcome did not correlate with an anatomically preserved larynx. Currently, the preferred treatment strategy has evolved into conservative laryngeal resections with preservation of laryngeal function, including good swallowing function without aspiration and speech production.[253] Early stage laryngeal cancer has overall survival rates of over 90%, but this falls to 27% to 39% in advanced cases treated with chemoradiotherapy.[254]

Intraluminal stenting of tracheal masses has been described in humans and is being performed increasingly commonly,[255] although primary tracheal cancer (unrelated to bronchial or lung cancer) is very uncommon.

SECTION D: PULMONARY NEOPLASIA

WILLIAM T.N. CULP AND ROBERT B. REBHUN

Incidence and Risk Factors

Lung cancer is the leading cause of cancer-related human deaths worldwide, but primary lung cancer remains relatively uncommon in pet dogs and cats. The incidence of primary lung cancer in dogs and cats presenting for necropsy is less than 1%.[256–258] Incidence rates in dogs range from 4.2 per 10,000 dogs per year in the United States to 15 per 100,000 dogs per year in the United Kingdom.[259,260] In contrast, the incidence of pulmonary neoplasia was 8.8% in a closed colony of beagles, with a high incidence of pulmonary tumors in dogs dying after the median lifespan of 13.6 years.[261]

The average age of dogs diagnosed with primary lung tumors is approximately 11 years,[256,262] with the exception of anaplastic carcinomas that occur at an average age of 7.5 years.[263] The Boxer, Doberman, Australian shepherd, Irish setter, and Bernese mountain dog breeds are possibly overrepresented.[256,262,264] The average age of cats with pulmonary tumors is 12 to 13 years.[258,263,265] Persian cats have been reported to be overrepresented.[266]

In people, the risk of developing primary lung cancer is strongly associated with environmental tobacco exposure, but no definitive risk factors have been identified in dogs and cats. Urban living and second-hand smoke exposure have both been implicated as potential causes of lung cancer in dogs but are yet to be clearly demonstrated.[267,268] An increased risk of lung cancer was found in dogs with increased amounts of anthracosis, suggesting an association between inhalation of polluted air and lung cancer.[269] Anthracosis has also been correlated to high EGFR expression in canine primary lung tumors.[270] Cytologic analysis of bronchoalveolar lavage fluid also revealed increased anthracosis in dogs exposed to passive tobacco smoke compared with dogs without a history of exposure.[271] In the experimental setting, laboratory dogs trained to smoke cigarettes through a tracheostoma (in the presence or absence of asbestos exposure) did develop lung cancer at a higher rate than control dogs.[272,273] Experimentally induced exposure to radiation, such as plutonium, also significantly increases the occurrence of lung cancer when inhaled as an aerosol in research dogs.[274,275]

Pathology and Natural Behavior

Pulmonary tumors can arise from any tissue in the lung, but most commonly they originate from the epithelium of the airways or alveolar parenchyma. Tumors derived from epithelium of large airways are typically located near the hilus, whereas parenchymally derived tumors tend to be peripherally located. However, in the most recent World Health Organization (WHO) guidelines on classification of pulmonary neoplasms, lung tumors of domestic animals are largely classified by histologic pattern and not by site of origin.[264]

Approximately 85% of canine primary epithelial lung tumors are bronchoalveolar in origin, whereas adenocarcinoma, adenosquamous carcinoma, and SCC collectively comprise the remaining 13% to 15% of primary epithelial lung tumors.[261,262] Primary pulmonary histiocytic sarcoma (HS) may also represent a significant percentage of diagnosed lung tumors, particularly in predisposed breeds such as miniature schnauzers.[276–278] Adenocarcinoma represents 60% to 70% of feline lung tumors, whereas bronchoalveolar carcinoma, SCC, and adenosquamous carcinoma are less common.[264,265] Small cell carcinoma represents approximately 25% of human pulmonary neoplasms, but rarely occurs in the dog or cat.

Lung tumors can spread by local invasion or via hematogenous and lymphatic routes, resulting in locoregional spread to other areas of the lung or LNs, or distant metastasis. Intrapulmonary metastases are believed to occur through vascular and lymphatic invasion or intraairway seeding. Local vascular or lymphatic invasion was present in 71% of canine pulmonary malignant tumors in one study, and 23% had distant metastasis beyond the tracheobronchial LNs.[262] SCC and anaplastic carcinomas have metastatic rates exceeding 50% and 90%, respectively, and are more likely to metastasize than adenocarcinoma or bronchoalveolar carcinoma.[258]

Metastasis is common in the cat with a reported metastatic rate of 76%.[265] The size of the largest mass has also been associated with metastatic potential in the cat.[266] Metastasis to bone or the nervous system is not uncommon in dogs or cats. Metastasis to the digits, otherwise known as acrometastasis or lung-digit syndrome, is a common and well-described clinical phenomenon in cats.[279,280]

Clinical Signs and Physical Examination Findings

Dogs and cats are often diagnosed with a primary pulmonary tumor incidentally during a routine geriatric screen.[256,261,281] Up to 30% of cases of primary pulmonary tumors will be diagnosed without the presence of clinical signs.[281] The most common clinical sign reported in dogs with pulmonary neoplasia is coughing, which is noted in 52% to 93% of dogs.[256,281–284] Other clinical signs include dyspnea (6%–24%), lethargy (12%–18%), hyporexia (13%), weight loss (7%–12%), hemoptysis (3%–9%), and lameness, likely secondary to hypertrophic osteopathy (HO, 4%).[281–283]

The clinical signs in cats are similar to dogs; however, the occurrence of these signs is variable and gastrointestinal signs may be noted as well.[285,286] As in dogs, signs referable to the respiratory tract are common with dyspnea (20%–65%), cough (29%–53%), tachypnea (9%–14%), and hemoptysis (10%) being noted regularly.[285–289] Recently, a study found that 5 of 35 cats with spontaneous pneumothorax had intrathoracic neoplasia and at least three of these cats had a primary pulmonary carcinoma.[290] Nonspecific signs, such as lethargy and hyporexia, can be seen in 14% to 43% and 19% to 71% of cats, respectively.[285–289] Vomiting/regurgitation and diarrhea are seen in approximately 19% of cats with primary pulmonary neoplasia.[285,286]

Abnormal physical examination findings consistent with pulmonary neoplasia are often not seen.[282] Increased bronchovesicular sounds may be auscultated in dogs with extensive pulmonary involvement.[282] As pleural effusion can occur in many cases, dull lung and heart sounds may also be noted.[281,285,286] Metastasis to the nervous system has been reported in several cases of primary pulmonary tumors and neurologic abnormalities can be diagnosed on physical examination.[291–294]

Lameness can occur in dogs and cats associated with primary pulmonary neoplasia for a variety of reasons. HO is a paraneoplastic syndrome commonly associated with primary and metastatic lung tumors, although other malignant and nonmalignant diseases have resulted in HO.[283,295–300] The disease is characterized by periosteal new bone formation at a site distant to the primary tumor. Dogs with HO tend to present with several clinical abnormalities including limb swelling, lameness, ocular signs, and lethargy.[300] The prevalence of ocular signs (occurring in 23 of 30 dogs) in a recent study evaluating HO was an interesting finding; an exact association between HO and ocular signs was not able to be determined retrospectively in that cohort, but it is important to evaluate for this in dogs with HO.[300] Lameness may improve with removal of the lung tumor.[295,298]

Several reports of cats with concurrent pulmonary neoplasia and digit metastasis can be found in the veterinary literature; this phenomenon has been noted with both pulmonary adenocarcinoma and SCC.[279,301–304] Cats naturally have significant blood flow to their digits to allow for heat loss and it has been theorized that this flow and the ability of pulmonary tumors to metastasize hematologically may work together to produce this unique metastatic pattern;[301] however, other factors contributing to a favorable metastatic microenvironment are likely to be involved. Of 36 cats with metastatic bronchogenic carcinoma to the digit in one study, all presented for lameness and none had respiratory signs.[304] The authors of that study concluded that thoracotomy with lung lobectomy and digital amputation should not be recommended as nonrespiratory disease often progressed and metastatic lesions in other digits resulted in continued lameness.[304] The MST for cats undergoing digit amputation was only 67 days.[304]

Diagnostics

Clinical Laboratory Findings

A complete blood count and serum chemistry panel are unlikely to signal the presence of a pulmonary mass.[265,304] These diagnostics, however, are essential to the preanesthetic and overall evaluation of a patient undergoing treatment for a pulmonary neoplasm. In one study, neutrophilia was noted in 50% of dogs with HO.[300]

The presence of pleural effusion at diagnosis is less common in dogs than cats. When pleural effusion is noted, a sample should be obtained via thoracocentesis. The pleural fluid tends to be a clear or blood-tinged modified transudate.[281,285] Fourteen percent to 30% of cats with primary pulmonary tumors have concurrent pleural effusion.[265,287–289] In one study, 13 of 26 cats underwent thoracocentesis to obtain fluid for analysis; fluid was diagnostic for a primary lung tumor in 12 of these cats.[265] However, in a separate study, fluid analysis was diagnostic for a malignant neoplasm in only one of eight cats.[285] Of three dogs with pleural effusion in one study, one dog was diagnosed with carcinoma based on evaluation of fluid obtained by thoracocentesis.[281]

Bronchoalveolar lavage (BAL) and transtracheal washes have been advocated as a method of diagnosing pulmonary neoplasia.[281,305–307] In a series of dogs that underwent BAL to aid in the diagnosis of respiratory tract diseases, carcinomas were identified in 14 dogs. Of those 14 cases, the BAL was definitive, supportive, or not helpful in eight, four, and two dogs, respectively.[306] Transtracheal washes have been less successful; of six dogs in one study with confirmed primary pulmonary neoplasia, none of the washes yielded neoplastic cells.[281]

Thoracic Radiographs

The majority of pulmonary tumors are diagnosed on thoracic radiographs (Fig. 24.12) and (Fig. 24.13). When evaluating 277 dogs from two large case series, 83% of pulmonary tumors were visible on thoracic radiographs.[281,283] Radiographic evidence of solitary or multiple pulmonary masses are present in 67% to 91% of cats with primary pulmonary tumors.[265,286]

Several studies have evaluated tumor location and number within the lungs.[256,282,283] Single and multiple masses were found in 54% to 87% and 13% to 37% of dogs, respectively, in two studies.[282,283] A side predilection has not been reported with the

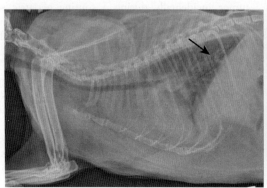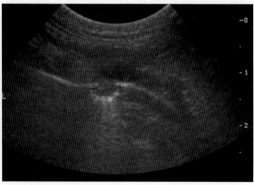

• **Fig. 24.12** Right lateral radiograph and ultrasound image of a pulmonary carcinoma (noted by *black arrow*) in the left caudal lung lobe of a cat.

left and right lung lobes affected in 24% to 50% and 50% to 76% of dogs, respectively.[256,282] Clinical signs were not noted until the pulmonary tumor grew to at least 3 cm in size in another study.[261]

In a study of 86 cats with primary pulmonary neoplasia, the location was determined radiographically in all cases.[265] Tumors were left-sided in 26 cats, right-sided in 27 cats, and bilateral in 33 cats.[265] In 45 cats, the tumors were found in a single lung lobe and the right and left caudal lung lobes were more commonly involved (34) than the right and left cranial (9) or right middle lung lobes (2).[265] In one study, 19 cats had a single lung lobe affected whereas two cats had multiple lesions.[286] Of 17 cats in a separate study, all single lesions were left-sided; however, 10 of these cats had multiple lesions (both right and left-sided).[285]

The radiographic pattern of primary pulmonary neoplasia has been variably reported in dogs and cats. Three radiographic patterns were described in a study evaluating 41 cats with primary pulmonary tumors: focal (nodules or masses), localized

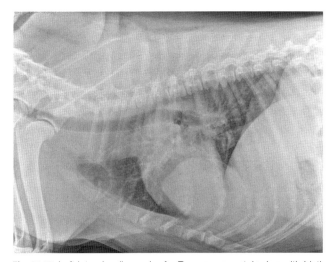

• **Fig. 24.13** Left lateral radiograph of a Bernese mountain dog with histiocytic sarcoma. A large soft tissue mass in the region of the ventral right middle lung lobe and tracheobronchial lymphadenomegaly are observed.

(lobar or segmental consolidations involving one or more lobes), and diffuse (involved most of both lungs).[308] In the focal group, 65% demonstrated solitary masses and 35% demonstrated multiple masses.[308] Recently, a study in dogs aimed to use radiographic features to distinguish between tumor types and compared pulmonary adenocarcinoma, bronchoalveolar carcinoma, and HS.[309] In this study, HSs were significantly larger than carcinomas and were more commonly found in the right middle (43%) and left cranial (38%) lung lobes.[309] Additionally, 57% of dogs with HS had internal air bronchograms. Adenocarcinomas were more often diagnosed in the left caudal lung lobe (29%).[309] Another study noted that in 19 of 29 dogs with pulmonary HS, the mass was located in the right middle lung lobe and this was significantly more common than other locations.[310]

Thoracic Ultrasound

Thoracic ultrasound may be employed to assess pulmonary neoplasia or to obtain a sample of tissue via FNA or pretreatment biopsy. The ultrasonographic appearance of pulmonary neoplasia has been described in several studies.[311–313] Pulmonary masses may be hypoechoic or exhibit variable echogenicity, and tumors are generally considered to have both a lack of discernable bronchi and normal branching vessels.[311,312]

Thoracic Computed Tomography

Thoracic CT scans are gaining popularity for the preoperative assessment of patients with pulmonary neoplasia (Fig. 24.14). Recently the CT findings of primary lung tumors were described in dogs and cats.[287,288,314] Several characteristics of solitary lung tumors were noted with CT in a majority of canine cases; 17 of 18 were well circumscribed, 16 of 19 were located in a cranial or caudal lobe, and 14 of 18 were located in the center to periphery of the lobe.[314] Internal mineralization was an uncommon finding being diagnosed in only 3 of 19 cases.[314] In one study, no association between the features

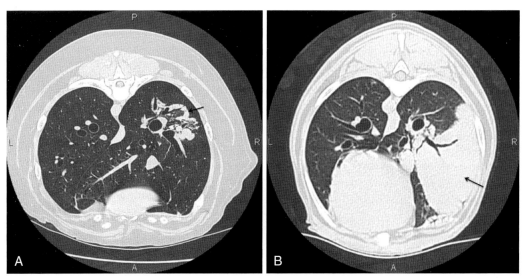

• **Fig. 24.14** Transverse computed tomography scan images of (A) a right caudal lung lobe histiocytic sarcoma (black arrow) in a 9-year-old Bernese mountain dog; and (B) a right caudal lung lobe pulmonary carcinoma (black arrow) in a 10-year-old fox terrier.

noted on CT and tumor type was identified, but intrapulmonary metastasis detected by CT was common, being noted in 53% of cats.[288]

Thoracic CT has been shown to be more accurate than thoracic radiographs in the assessment of tracheobronchial LN metastasis.[284] In 14 dogs with primary pulmonary tumors, the accuracy of CT to determine tracheobronchial LN metastasis was 93% compared with 57% for thoracic radiography.[284] Additionally, five dogs deemed to be free of pulmonary metastasis with thoracic radiographs were found to have pulmonary metastasis with CT.[284] In a separate study evaluating CT characteristics of tracheobronchial LN metastasis, 16 of 18 dogs were diagnosed with primary pulmonary tumors and these dogs were compared with 10 normal dogs.[315] Metastatic disease to LN was significantly more likely when a transverse maximum LN diameter of 12 mm or LN-to-thoracic body ratio of 1.05 were used as cutoffs.[315] Additionally, LN heterogenous and/or ring contrast enhancement patterns were significantly related to metastatic disease.[315]

In a study evaluating the assessment of pulmonary metastatic disease in 18 dogs (two of which had bronchoalveolar carcinoma) by thoracic radiography and CT, only 9% of CT-detected pulmonary nodules were noted on thoracic radiographs.[316] CT was able to detect pulmonary nodules as small as 1 mm, whereas the smallest lesions detected with thoracic radiography were 7 to 9 mm.[316] Overall, CT was significantly more sensitive than thoracic radiography in the identification of pulmonary nodules.[316] In a separate study, CT was able to detect a greater amount of nodules compared with computed and film-screen radiography.[317] Additionally, CT was better at identifying smaller nodules and was associated with greater diagnostic confidence and observer accuracy and agreement.[317]

Other Imaging Modalities

The use of positron emission tomography (PET) is uncommon in veterinary patients, but some early data regarding its use are available.[318–320] In one report, [18]fluorodeoxyglucose ([18]FDG) was administered as a radiotracer to evaluate a dog with pulmonary nodules. Increased [18]FDG uptake was noted in four nodules and these were identified as pulmonary adenocarcinoma at necropsy.[319]

Near-infrared (NIR) imaging was recently evaluated in eight dogs with primary pulmonary tumors.[321] In this study, pulmonary tumors and normal lung were both imaged. In situ, the tumor was easily pinpointed with NIR imaging and all eight tumors appeared equally fluorescent to the surgeon.[321] An additional interesting finding was that NIR imaging was able to accurately distinguish normal lung parenchyma from neoplastic tissue, but could not distinguish peritumoral inflammation from neoplastic tissue.[321] The intraoperative use of NIR imaging modality may better facilitate tumor resection.

Fine-Needle Aspiration

FNA of a pulmonary mass may be performed before lung lobectomy to attempt to obtain a cytologic diagnosis. FNA is often performed with ultrasound- or CT-guidance; however, blind aspirates have been reported.[265,313,322,323] Sedation is generally required to prevent iatrogenic trauma during the aspiration process. In dogs, preoperative FNA with cytology has resulted in a diagnosis in

38% to 90% of cases.[281–283] Diagnosis of primary pulmonary neoplasia in cats is reportedly higher with 80% to 100% of cases being diagnosed by FNA and cytology.[265,286,322]

Pretreatment Biopsy

A pretreatment biopsy (biopsy performed before definitive therapy) can be performed before lung lobectomy, although the clinical relevance is questionable.[324] A pretreatment biopsy may be considered if histologic grade or degree of differentiation is required before an owner is willing to consider lung lobectomy or there is suspicion that a pulmonary neoplasm is not a primary tumor (i.e., either metastatic or systemic neoplasia such as lymphoma). However, if the eventual goal is to remove the pulmonary tumor with a lung lobectomy, then a pretreatment biopsy is unnecessary because the biopsy result will not change the surgical recommendation or the owner's willingness to treat. Multiple techniques for performing a pretreatment biopsy have been described, including utilizing a biopsy needle, bronchoscopic biopsy, keyhole incision with staple application, and thoracoscopy.[265,281,283,307,323–325]

Sedation or anesthesia is required to perform a pretreatment needle-core biopsy. The use of ultrasound-, fluoroscopic- or CT-guidance is recommended to improve targeting of the lesion and decrease the risk of iatrogenic trauma to normal structures.[313,323,324] In a study of dogs and cats undergoing CT-guided tissue-core biopsies of intrathoracic lesions (including pulmonary tumors), the diagnostic accuracy was 92% and the sensitivity for diagnosing neoplasia was 80%.[323] A procedural complication rate of 43% was reported with pulmonary hemorrhage (30%) and pneumothorax (27%) the most common complications.[323]

Bronchoscopic biopsy has been performed in dogs and cats with pulmonary neoplasia with mixed success.[265,283] Bronchoscopic findings in patients with primary pulmonary neoplasia include narrowing of bronchi, mucosal erosions, and mucosal swelling and hyperemia.[326] In one series of seven cats, five cats were successfully diagnosed by means of endoscopic bronchiolar brushing.[265]

A keyhole lung biopsy technique has been described for nonneoplastic lung disease.[307] For this technique, a lung biopsy is obtained via a small thoracotomy (3–7 cm) with a surgical stapler applied across the lung lobe to seal vessels and small airways.[307] Thoracoscopy is a minimally invasive surgical option to obtain a pretreatment biopsy.[327] In a study describing the use of thoracoscopy to determine the cause of pleural effusion in 18 cats and dogs, biopsies of several suspicious intrathoracic lesions were performed.[328] In eight cases, neoplasia was the cause of the pleural effusion, although the number of primary pulmonary tumors resulting in pleural effusion was unknown.[328] Thoracoscopy provided a means to both biopsy lung lesions and explore the thoracic cavity.[328]

Differentiating poorly differentiated primary lung tumors from metastatic lesions can occasionally provide a diagnostic challenge, particularly when evaluating cytology. Immunohistochemistry or possibly immunocytochemistry using antibodies directed against thyroid transcription factor-1, cytokeratin, vimentin, or others may be useful in differentiating primary lung tumors from metastatic disease.[329–332] Antibodies against CD18 and CD204 may also be useful for differentiating pulmonary tumors of histiocytic origin.[333–335]

Treatment

Surgery

Surgery is the treatment of choice for dogs and cats with primary pulmonary tumors. The surgical approach to a pulmonary tumor is dependent on the clinician and tumor location, but certain overarching criteria exist. For unilateral tumors, a lateral thoracotomy is preferred, but a median sternotomy approach can also be used. Thoracoscopic lung lobectomy is feasible if the mass is peripherally located and in a suitable location; however, this surgery requires advanced training in minimally invasive procedures. If nodules in multiple lobes are found bilaterally and the goal is to remove all gross disease, then a median sternotomy should be performed.

Both partial and complete lung lobectomies have been described and the elected technique is based on the location of the tumor. In general, a complete lung lobectomy should be performed; however, partial lung lobectomy may be an option for small tumors located in a peripheral position on the lung lobe or for pulmonary metastatectomy. A cuff of normal tissue should be removed with the tumor to increase the chance of obtaining a wide margin.

Partial and complete lung lobectomies are generally performed with either a suturing method or the use of a surgical stapler. When performing a partial lung lobectomy with the suture method, the area to be removed is delineated by placing crushing forceps proximal to the lesion.[336] A continuous overlapping suture can then be placed proximal to the clamps.[336] The pulmonary artery and vein are individually ligated, and the bronchi are oversewn to prevent air leakage.[334]

Several studies have evaluated the use of stapling equipment for lung lobectomy.[282,337,338] In a study of 37 dogs and cats undergoing resection of pulmonary lesions (67% were neoplastic) with surgical staplers, complications were minimal and the technique was considered safe, fast, and efficient.[337] Use of surgical staplers is widely considered to be the technique of choice for partial and complete lung lobectomy.

Two recent studies evaluated outcomes after pneumonectomy, which is defined as the removal of the entire left or right lung fields.[339,340] In total, 33 dogs and 17 cats had a pneumonectomy performed and, of these, 18 dogs and 4 cats were diagnosed with pulmonary neoplasia.[339,340] Perioperative mortality rates were low with 94% of dogs and 86% of cats surviving to discharge in one study.[340] The partial pressure of oxygen was significantly higher and alveolar-arterial gradient was significantly lower postpneumonectomy compared with dogs treated with single lung lobectomy.[340]

Thoracoscopy can be used to explore the thoracic cavity, obtain biopsies (Fig. 24.15),[327,328] and perform thoracoscopic or thoracoscopic-assisted lung lobectomy.[341–345] In the largest study to date, 22 medium-to-large breed dogs underwent video-assisted thoracoscopic surgery (VATS) for lobectomy of primary lung tumors, and this group was compared with a cohort of dogs treated with lung lobectomy via an open thoracotomy.[345] In this study, an endoscopic stapler was used for lung lobectomy via either a three- or four-port technique.[345] Short-term complications were similar between the two approaches, and all VATS patients survived to discharge. Surgery time for VATS was significantly longer than open thoracotomy (120 vs. 95 minutes, respectively).[345] In a second study of nine dogs with either primary or metastatic pulmonary neoplasia, thoracoscopic lung lobectomy was performed

successfully in five dogs.[341] Cases that were deemed to be good candidates for thoracoscopic removal in this study included dogs with small masses located distant to the hilus. Caudal lung lobectomy was easier than cranial lung lobectomy; however, both were performed successfully.[341] Conversion rates for thoracoscopic lung lobectomy are between 9% to 23% and conversion is most commonly performed due to poor visualization.[341,344,345] One-lung ventilation should be considered in cases of thoracoscopic lung lobectomy to improve visualization.[341,342,346,347]

Biopsy of tracheobronchial LN is recommended in dogs and cats as a staging tool, as metastatic disease to the LN significantly affects prognosis.[284,287] The LNs are located dorsally along the trachea and bronchi, and hence exposure may be better via a lateral thoracotomy compared with a median sternotomy. Thoracoscopic LN biopsy is performed regularly in human lung cancer patients,[341,348] and this was recently described in dogs.[349] In this report, seven of eight purpose-bred research dogs successfully underwent tracheobronchial LN extirpation. Complications were minor, although further study is needed to determine the use of this technique in clinical patients.[349]

Chemotherapy

Cisplatin-based chemotherapy protocols are considered the standard of care for human lung cancer patients, either in the adjuvant or palliative setting.[350] Relatively little is known about the efficacy of chemotherapy for pulmonary tumors in domestic animals; however, chemotherapy has been largely unrewarding in the gross disease setting. Early clinical trials evaluating the safety and efficacy of doxorubicin in cancer-bearing pet dogs included one dog with papillary pulmonary adenocarcinoma, and this dog had progressive disease.[351] No responses were seen in three dogs with lung adenocarcinoma treated with mitoxantrone.[352] Minimal responses were reported in two dogs treated with vindesine, whereas two dogs treated with the combination of vindesine and cisplatin both experienced greater than 50% reduction in measurable disease.[282] Treatment with vinorelbine resulted in partial responses in two of seven dogs with measurable bronchoalveolar carcinoma.[353] Three additional dogs with microscopic disease were treated with adjuvant vinorelbine in the microscopic disease setting, and these dogs had individual survival times (STs) of 113, 169, and greater than 730 days.[353] Pharmacokinetic studies in humans have concluded that vinorelbine treatment results in 300-fold higher concentration in the lung compared with plasma, which is 3.4- and 13.8-fold higher than lung concentrations of vindesine and vincristine, respectively.[354] Based on observed partial responses in dogs and pharmacokinetic data in people, treatment with vinorelbine or cisplatin appears to hold the most promise for dogs with primary lung carcinoma. CCNU (lomustine) is recommended for dogs with localized pulmonary HS.[355]

Delivery of aerosolized chemotherapy or cytokines has been described and appears well tolerated in dogs with primary or metastatic pulmonary neoplasia. Complete and partial responses have been described in dogs treated with inhalational therapy for metastatic tumors, whereas stable or progressive disease was reported in dogs with primary lung tumors.[356,357]

Treatment with monoclonal antibodies or small-molecule tyrosine kinase inhibitors (TKIs) directed against cell signaling pathways have been shown to be beneficial in distinct subpopulations of human patients with nonsmall cell lung cancer (NSCLC). Such targeted therapies have yet to be thoroughly examined in dogs with primary lung tumors. In a phase I study, monotherapy with

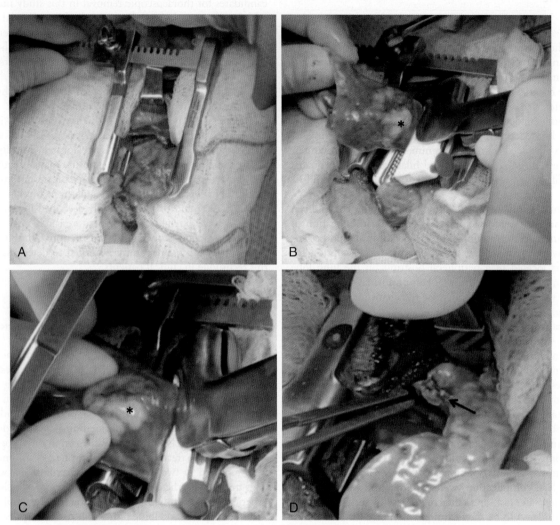

• **Fig. 24.15** (A) A lateral thoracotomy is being performed to allow for removal of a primary pulmonary carcinoma. (B) The lung lobe containing the tumor *(asterisk)* has been exteriorized and a surgical stapler is being positioned. (C) After placement of the surgical staples, the affected lung lobe is being transected to allow for removal. (D) The staple line *(black arrow)* can be seen after removal of the tumor. The line of resection is examined closely for leaks.

toceranib resulted in stable disease >10 weeks in one dog with a primary lung carcinoma.[358] Further research is warranted to determine the clinical efficacy of TKIs in the management of cats and dogs with primary lung tumors.

Malignant pleural effusions can be responsive to systemic chemotherapy, intrapleural chemotherapy, or a combination of both routes. Cisplatin, carboplatin, and mitoxantrone have been used successfully for this purpose, resulting in temporary palliation of clinical signs.[359–362] Sclerosing agents, such as talc or tetracyclines, have been also been used in a palliative setting.[363]

Radiation Therapy

Radiation therapy in physician-based medicine is most often reserved for locally advanced tumors.[364] Technologies such as intensity-modulated radiation therapy, stereotactic radiation therapy, or TomoTherapy can now be used to provide more precise delivery of radiation while sparing unaffected tissues, especially when used together with respiratory gating or breath hold

techniques. The use of such modalities in veterinary patients is now becoming more accessible but remains to be systematically investigated in dogs and cats with lung tumors.

Interventional Therapy

Interventional oncologic techniques for the treatment of primary pulmonary neoplasia have not been described in the veterinary literature; however, several treatment options exist in human medicine for pulmonary neoplasia.[365–368] These options are generally reserved for cases of pulmonary metastatic disease, nonresectable pulmonary tumors, or patients for which surgery is contraindicated due to existing comorbidities.[366–369] Research into this field in veterinary patients is ongoing and some of these techniques are currently being investigated.

Thermal ablation (radiofrequency and microwave) and regional chemotherapy administration are two interventional oncology techniques that have been reported in the treatment of pulmonary neoplasia. Radiofrequency ablation (RFA) is performed by placing an electrode within a tumor and generating heat; the heat results in coagulative necrosis in a defined region.[365,367,368] The goal is to produce a 360-degree region of necrosis around the tumor with a 1 cm thick margin of normal tissue included.[365,367] RFA has been performed in dogs with experimentally induced transmissible venereal tumor of the lung.[370] In five dogs, RFA was applied percutaneously with CT guidance to 14 tumors. Upon harvest of the affected lung lobes, gross and histopathologic evaluations demonstrated complete thermal coagulation necrosis of all treated lesions, and viable tumor was not identified in any dogs.[370]

Regional chemotherapy has been developed with the goal of increasing the efficacy of chemotherapy agents and decreasing systemic side effects.[371] Regional delivery allows for increased concentrations of chemotherapy to be delivered to the tumor by selective catheterization of the tumoral arterial supply.[371] Regional techniques involving the administration of chemotherapy into the bronchial arteries and pulmonary arteries have been described in several human studies.[369,371,372] Recently, in an experimental model study, significantly higher concentrations of chemotherapy agents (gemcitabine and carboplatin) were noted in pulmonary tissue treated with regional techniques (selective pulmonary artery perfusion) than intravenous administration.[372] The indications and clinical use of these treatments, while developing, still remains to be determined in veterinary patients.

Prognosis

In one clinical study of 67 dogs undergoing removal of primary lung tumors, the overall MST was 361 days.[281] Prognostic factors included the presence of clinical signs, clinical stage, tumor type, and histologic grade. Dogs with clinical signs associated with a primary lung tumor had an MST of 240 days compared with 545 days for asymptomatic dogs. Dogs with single solitary lung tumors (T1 clinical stage) had an MST of 790 days, which was significantly longer than dogs with multiple lung tumors (T2 clinical stage, 196 days) and dogs with lung tumors invading into adjacent structures (T3 clinical stage, 81 days). Finally, the MST for dogs with grade I lung carcinomas was 790 days, and this was significantly longer than the MSTs of 251 days and 5 days for dogs with grade II and III lung carcinomas, respectively.[281]

One study evaluated the effect of several variables on remission and survival in dogs with primary lung tumors.[373] Dogs for which surgery was successful in rendering them free of macroscopic disease lived significantly longer than dogs that had gross disease postoperatively.[373] Factors significantly associated with remission included limited degree of primary tumor involvement, normal sized LNs, and lack of metastatic disease.[373] In a separate study of 15 dogs, trends for longer STs were noted in dogs with adenocarcinoma versus SCC, dogs with peripheral lesions versus lesions that involved an entire lobe, and dogs with tumor volume <100 cm^3 compared with dogs with tumor volume >100 cm^3.[282]

The MST for dogs with no evidence of LN (N0) was 452 days, and this was significantly longer than the MST of 26 days for dogs with tracheobronchial LN metastasis (N1).[281] In another study, dogs with LN enlargement diagnosed before surgery survived for a median time of 60 days, whereas dogs without LN enlargement had a MST of 285 days.[373] A similar finding was noted in a more recent study where dogs with lymphadenomegaly had MSTs of 126 days versus a MST that had not been reached in the dogs without lymphadenomegaly.[284] In dogs for which a surgical remission could be achieved, MST is 330 days versus 28 days in dogs that could not be rendered free of visible disease.[373] Although

not statistically significant, the mean ST of dogs with SCC was 8 months and the mean ST of dogs with adenocarcinoma was 19 months in one study.[282]

A recent study evaluated 42 dogs with primary lung tumors and based the prognostic evaluation on the WHO classification scheme.[374] In these cases, 34 tumors were carcinomas (26 papillary adenocarcinomas) and eight were sarcomas. Fourteen of the carcinomas and two of the sarcomas were T1N0M0. Dogs with papillary adenocarcinomas and a clinical stage of T1N0M0 had the best overall prognosis with an MST of 555 days; this ST was significantly longer than dogs with any other tumor type or dogs with a worse clinical stage.[374] Dogs with other tumor types had an MST of 72 days.[374]

In regard to localized HS, one retrospective study reported that surgical excision and adjuvant therapy with CCNU resulted in an MST of 568 days.[355] Interestingly, five out of 16 dogs within that study had localized pulmonary lesions.

The prognosis is guarded to poor for cats with primary lung carcinomas. In one retrospective study of 21 cats treated with lung lobectomy,[286] the overall MST was 115 days. The only prognostic factor in this study was histologic grade; the MST for cats with moderately differentiated carcinomas was 698 days compared with only 75 days for cats with poorly differentiated carcinomas. In a separate study, cats with low-grade tumors had an MST of 730 days compared with 105 days for cats with high-grade tumors.[287] Similar to dogs, LN enlargement in cats significantly decreased MST to 65 days from 498 days for cats with no evidence of lymphadenomegaly.[287] The TNM staging scheme also correlated with ST in cats; cats staged T1N0M0 live significantly longer than cats with higher stages.[286] In this same study, the MST in cats with clinical signs was 4 days compared with 578 days in asymptomatic cats.[289] Pleural effusion has been identified as a negative prognostic factor; in two studies, the MST were less than 3 days and 31 to 467 days in cats with and without pleural effusion, respectively.[287,289]

Comparative Aspects

Lung cancer is the leading cause of cancer deaths in the United States and worldwide.[375] Approximately 85% of human lung cancers are NSCLC, with the remainder being small-cell lung cancer. NSCLC are composed of three distinct histologic subtypes: SCC, adenocarcinoma, and large-cell lung cancer. Large airway origin tumors predominated in humans through the 1960s and were commonly associated with smoking cigarettes. Adenocarcinoma arising from the smaller airways now predominates in human patients, likely a result of changes to tobacco blends and the use of cigarette filters.[376]

If curative-intent resection can be performed, prognosis for human patients with NSCLC is largely dependent on clinical stage with 5-year survival rates greater than 60% to 70% for patients with stage I disease. Five-year survival rates are approximately 30% to 40%, 10% to 30%, and less than 5% for patients with stage II, stage III, and stage IV disease, respectively.[350]

Inherited cancer syndromes caused by germ-line p53 mutations, retinoblastoma (Rb), EGFR, and other genes have been reported to increase the risk of lung cancer. Furthermore, associations between single-nucleotide polymorphism variations have been linked to lung carcinogenesis and may be associated with nicotine exposure. DNA synthesis and repair genes may also play a role in the development and prognosis of lung cancer. Commonly acquired molecular abnormalities in human lung cancer include, but are not limited to, microsatellite instability, EGFR mutations, P53 inactivation, Rb inactivation, P16INK4a inactivation, allelic loss, and high telomerase activity. K-*ras* mutations have been found in up to 30% of human NSCLC.[377] Close homology exists between canine and human K-*ras*. Interestingly, K-*ras* mutations were detected in five of 21 canine NSCLC specimens by direct sequencing.[262] Further studies concluded that the frequency and type of mutations in canine NSCLC tissues more matched those for tumors from human nonsmokers with K-*ras* mutations than those for smokers.[262]

Recent developments in biomarker driven targeted therapies of lung tumors have improved survival rates for NSCLC patients, including those with EGFR mutations or anaplastic lymphoma kinase (ALK) rearrangements. The FDA has approved the use of several TKIs based on large prospective trials, and these drugs are considered part of first-line standard-of-care in certain molecularly defined subsets of patients with advanced NSCLC. Unfortunately, this pertains to only a minority of patients with NSCLC, and acquired resistance to such therapies is commonplace. EGFR expression has recently been associated with anthracosis and a trend toward shortened STs in dogs with primary lung tumors; however, mutational status of canine primary lung tumors has not been extensively performed.[270] An increased expression of PDGFR-α and ALK receptor phosphorylation has been found in canine pulmonary adenocarcinomas compared with normal lung tissue, but no increases in expression or activity of EGFR and no EGFR mutations were identified. EGFR mutant protein expression is present in 20% of cats with lung tumors, but this has not been evaluated in regard to prognosis or response to therapy.[266]

Even more recently, excitement has been centered around a series of accelerated FDA approvals for immune checkpoint inhibitors such as pembrolizumab (Keytruda), atezolizumab, and nivolumab for the treatment of NSCLC. Some of these approvals are based on tumor expression of PD-L1, but such biomarkers are continuing to be refined. Although PD-L1 expression in lung tumors appears to correlate with response to checkpoint inhibition, there is additional evidence showing that mutational load, neoantigen density, and tumor infiltration by cytotoxic T-cells may also predict response in other tumor histologies. Ongoing research is focused on refining biomarkers to better understand and predict which patients will respond to checkpoint inhibitors in addition to identifying which patients may be more at risk of severe adverse events.[378] Several groups have reported on the potential importance of checkpoint inhibition in naturally occurring canine tumors, and work is ongoing to develop canine checkpoint inhibitors.[379-383] However, to date, no studies have thoroughly evaluated PD-1 or PD-L1 in canine lung tumors.

Miscellaneous Lung Condition: Canine Pulmonary Lymphomatoid Granulomatosis

Canine pulmonary lymphomatoid granulomatosis is a poorly understood disease occurring most commonly in young-to-middle aged dogs with no breed or gender predilection.[384] The most common laboratory abnormalities, as reported in seven dogs, were basophilia and leukocytosis. Lung lobe consolidation or large pulmonary granulomas and tracheobronchial LN enlargement are typically seen on thoracic radiographs. Transthoracic FNAs are not diagnostically rewarding. Differential diagnoses include heartworm granulomas, metastatic neoplasia, lymphoma, HS, and primary lung tumors. Traditionally, a definitive diagnosis requires biopsy and histopathology. Characteristic histopathology often demonstrates angiocentric and angiodestructive infiltration of the pulmonary parenchyma by large lymphoreticular and plasmacytoid cells in addition to normal appearing lymphocytes, eosinophils, and plasma cells. This infiltrate is typically centered around small to medium arteries and veins.

The etiology of this disease is unknown but is suspected to be neoplastic or preneoplastic. Clonality has been identified on PARR, but this finding needs to be investigated in a larger series of cases.[385] Additional molecular diagnostics, such as immunohistochemistry in combination with clonality testing, may eventually result in a better understanding of this disease.[386] It is not known whether flow cytometry or PARR testing may possibly improve the diagnostic power of fine-needle aspirates.

In a very limited number of cases, the response to chemotherapy has been quite variable.[387] Of five dogs that were treated with cyclophosphamide, vincristine, and prednisone, three dogs achieved a complete response. The remaining two dogs either showed worsening clinical signs or progressed to lymphoid leukemia within months. Dogs achieving a complete response were alive at 7, 12, and 32 months.

References

1. Al-Bagdadi F: *Miller's Anatomy of the do*, ed 4, St. Louis, Missouri, 2013, Elsevier Saunders.
2. Withrow SJ, Straw RC: Resection of the nasal planum in nine cats and five dogs, *J Am Anim Hosp Assoc* 26:219–222, 1990.
3. Lana SE, Ogilvie GK, Withrow SJ, et al.: Feline cutaneous squamous cell carcinoma of the nasal planum and the pinnae: 61 cases, *J Am Anim Hosp Assoc* 33:329–332, 1997.
4. Lascelles BD, Parry AT, Stidworthy MF, et al.: Squamous cell carcinoma of the nasal planum in 17 dogs, *Vet Rec* 147:473–476, 2000.
5. Thrall DE, Adams WM: Radiotherapy of squamous cell carcinoma of the canine nasal plane, *Vet Radiol* 23:193–195, 1982.
6. Hargis AM: A Review of solar-induced lesions in domestic animals, *Compend Contin Educ* 3:287–293, 1981.
7. Theon AP, Madewell BR, Shearn VI, et al.: Prognostic factors associated with radiotherapy of squamous cell carcinoma of the nasal plane in cats, *J Am Vet Med Assoc* 206:991–996, 1995.
8. Rogers KS, Helman RG, Walker MA: Squamous cell carcinoma of the canine nasal planum: eight cases (1988-1994), *J Am Anim Hosp Assoc* 31:373–378, 1995.
9. Kirpensteijn J, Withrow SJ, Straw RC: Combined resection of the nasal planum and premaxilla in three dogs, *Vet Surg* 23:341–346, 1994.
10. Lascelles BD, Henderson RA, Seguin B, et al.: Bilateral rostral maxillectomy and nasal planectomy for large rostral maxillofacial neoplasms in six dogs and one cat, *J Am Anim Hosp Assoc* 40:137–146, 2004.
11. Jarrett RH, Norman EJ, Gibson IR, et al.: Curettage and diathermy: a treatment for feline nasal planum actinic dysplasia and superficial squamous cell carcinoma, *J Small Anim Pract* 54:92–98, 2013.
12. Gasymova E, Meier V, Guscetti F, et al.: Retrospective clinical study on outcome in cats with nasal planum squamous cell carcinoma treated with an accelerated radiation protocol, *BMC Vet Res* 13:86, 2017.
13. Fidel JL, Egger E, Blattmann H, et al.: Proton irradiation of feline nasal planum squamous cell carcinomas using an accelerated protocol, *Vet Radiol Ultrasound* 42:569–575, 2001.
14. Menon G, Sloboda R: Measurement of relative output for 90Sr ophthalmic applicators using radiochromic film, *Med Dosim* 25:171–177, 2000.

15. Hammond GM, Gordon IK, Theon AP, et al.: Evaluation of strontium Sr 90 for the treatment of superficial squamous cell carcinoma of the nasal planum in cats: 49 cases (1990-2006), *J Am Vet Med Assoc* 231:736–741, 2007.

16. Goodfellow M, Hayes A, Murphy S, et al.: A retrospective study of (90)Strontium plesiotherapy for feline squamous cell carcinoma of the nasal planum, *J Feline Med Surg* 8:169–176, 2006.

17. Theon AP, VanVechten MK, Madewell BR: Intratumoral administration of carboplatin for treatment of squamous cell carcinomas of the nasal plane in cats, *Am J Vet Res* 57:205–210, 1996.

18. de Vos JP, Burm AG, Focker BP: Results from the treatment of advanced stage squamous cell carcinoma of the nasal planum in cats, using a combination of intralesional carboplatin and superficial radiotherapy: a pilot study, *Vet Comp Oncol* 2:75–81, 2004.

19. Spugnini EP, Vincenzi B, Citro G, et al.: Electrochemotherapy for the treatment of squamous cell carcinoma in cats: a preliminary report, *Vet J* 179:117–120, 2009.

20. Tozon N, Pavlin D, Sersa G, et al.: Electrochemotherapy with intravenous bleomycin injection: an observational study in superficial squamous cell carcinoma in cats, *J Feline Med Surg* 16:291–299, 2014.

21. Buchholz J, Wergin M, Walt H, et al.: Photodynamic therapy of feline cutaneous squamous cell carcinoma using a newly developed liposomal photosensitizer: preliminary results concerning drug safety and efficacy, *J Vet Intern Med* 21:770–775, 2007.

22. Magne ML, Rodriguez CO, Autry SA, et al.: Photodynamic therapy of facial squamous cell carcinoma in cats using a new photosensitizer, *Lasers Surg Med* 20:202–209, 1997.

23. Bexfield NH, Stell AJ, Gear RN, et al.: Photodynamic therapy of superficial nasal planum squamous cell carcinomas in cats: 55 cases, *J Vet Intern Med* 22:1385–1389, 2008.

24. Clarke RE: Cryosurgical treatment of feline cutaneous squamous cell carcinoma, *Australian Vet Pract* 21:148–153, 1991.

25. MacEwen EG, Withrow SJ, Patnaik AK: Nasal tumors in the dog: retrospective evaluation of diagnosis, prognosis, and treatment, *J Am Vet Med Assoc* 170:45–48, 1977.

26. Patnaik AK: Canine sinonasal neoplasms: clinicopathological study of 285 cases, *J Am Anim Hosp Assoc* 25:103–114, 1989.

27. Lefebvre J, Kuehn NJ, Wortinger A: Computed tomography as an aid in the diagnosis of chronic nasal disease in dogs, *J Small Anim Pract* 46:280–285, 2005.

28. Sones E, Smith A, Schleis S, et al.: Survival times for canine intranasal sarcomas treated with radiation therapy: 86 cases (1996-2011), *Vet Radiol Ultrasound* 54:194–201, 2013.

29. Strunzi H, Hauser B: Tumors of the nasal cavity, *Bull World Health Organ* 53:257–263, 1976.

30. Reif JS, Cohen D: The environmental distribution of canine respiratory tract neoplasms, *Arch Environ Health* 22:136–140, 1971.

31. Bukowski JA, Wartenberg D: Environmental causes for sinonasal cancers in pet dogs, and their usefulness as sentinels of indoor cancer risk, *J Toxicol Environ Health* 54:579–591, 1998.

32. Reif JS, Bruns C, Lower KS: Cancer of the nasal cavity and paranasal sinuses and exposure to environmental tobacco smoke in pet dogs, *Am J Epidemiol* 147:488–492, 1998.

33. Perez N, Berrio A, Jaramillo JE, et al.: Exposure to cigarette smoke causes DNA damage in oropharyngeal tissue in dogs, *Mut Res* 769:13–19, 2014.

34. Madewell BR, Priester WA, Gillette EL, et al.: Neoplasms of the nasal passages and paranasal sinuses in domesticated animals as reported by 13 veterinary colleges, *Am J Vet Res* 37:851–856, 1976.

35. Patnaik AK, Lieberman PH, Erlandson RA, et al.: Canine sinonasal skeletal neoplasms: chondrosarcomas and osteosarcomas, *Vet Pathol* 21:475–482, 1984.

36. Henry CJ, Brewer WG, Tyler JW, et al.: Survival in dogs with nasal adenocarcinoma: 64 cases (1981-1995), *J Vet Intern Med* 12:436–439, 1998.

37. Hahn KA, Matlock CL: Nasal adenocarcinoma metastatic to bone in two dogs, *J Am Vet Med Assoc* 197:491–494, 1990.

38. Hahn KA, McGavin MD, Adams WH: Bilateral renal metastases of nasal chondrosarcoma in a dog, *Vet Pathol* 34:352–355, 1997.

39. Northrup NC, Etue SM, Ruslander DM, et al.: Retrospective study of orthovoltage radiation therapy for nasal tumors in 42 dogs, *J Vet Intern Med* 15:183–189, 2001.

40. Snyder MK, Lipitz L, Skorupski KA, et al.: Secondary intracranial neoplasia in the dog: 177 cases (1986-2003), *J Vet Intern Med* 22:172–177, 2008.

41. Kaldrymidou E, Papaioannou N, Poutahidis T, et al.: Malignant lymphoma in nasal cavity and paranasal sinuses of a dog, *J Vet Med A Physiol Pathol Clin Med* 47:457–462, 2000.

42. Naganobu K, Ogawa H, Uchida K, et al.: Mast cell tumor in the nasal cavity of a dog, *J Vet Med Sci* 62:1009–1011, 2000.

43. Weir EC, Pond MJ, Duncan JR, et al.: Extragenital occurrence of transmissible venereal tumor in the dog: literature review and case reports, *J Am Anim Hosp Assoc* 14:532–536, 1978.

44. Perez J, Bautista MJ, Carrasco L, et al.: Primary extragenital occurrence of transmissible venereal tumors: three case reports, *Can Pract* 19:7–10, 1994.

45. Ginel PJ, Molleda JM, Novales M, et al.: Primary transmissible venereal tumour in the nasal cavity of a dog, *Vet Rec* 136:222–223, 1995.

46. Papazoglou LG, Koutinas AF, Plevraki AG, et al.: Primary intranasal transmissible venereal tumour in the dog: a retrospective study of six spontaneous cases, *J Vet Med A Physiol Pathol Clin Med* 48:391–400, 2001.

47. Patnaik AK: Canine sinonasal neoplasms: soft tissue tumors, *J Am Anim Hosp Assoc* 25:491–497, 1989.

48. Patnaik AK, Ludwig LL, Erlandson RA: Neuroendocrine carcinoma of the nasopharynx in a dog, *Vet Pathol* 39:496–500, 2002.

49. Miles MS, Dhaliwal RS, Moore MP, et al.: Association of magnetic resonance imaging findings and histologic diagnosis in dogs with nasal disease: 78 cases (2001-2004), *J Am Vet Med Assoc* 232:1844–1849, 2008.

50. Hicks DG, Fidel JL: Intranasal malignant melanoma in a dog, *J Am Anim Hosp Assoc* 42:472–476, 2006.

51. Ueno H, Kobayashi Y, Yamada K: Olfactory esthesioneuroblastoma treated with orthovoltage radiotherapy in a dog, *Aust Vet J* 85:271–275, 2007.

52. Kitagawa M, Okada M, Yamamura H, et al.: Diagnosis of olfactory neuroblastoma in a dog by magnetic resonance imaging, *Vet Rec* 159:288–289, 2006.

53. LeRoith T, Binder EM, Graham AH, et al.: Respiratory epithelial adenomatoid hamartoma in a dog, *J Vet Diagn Invest* 21:918–920, 2009.

54. Fujita M, Takaishi Y, Yasuda D, et al.: Intranasal hemangiosarcoma in a dog, *J Vet Med Sci* 70:525–528, 2008.

55. Siudak K, Klingler M, Schmidt MJ, et al.: Metastasizing esthesioneuroblastoma in a dog, *Vet Pathol* 52:692–695, 2015.

56. Gumpel E, Moore AS, Simpson DJ, et al.: Long-term control of olfactory neuroblastoma in a dog treated with surgery and radiation therapy, *Aust Vet J* 95:227–231, 2017.

57. Brosinski K, Janik D, Polkinghorne A, et al.: Olfactory neuroblastoma in dogs and cats – a histological and immunohistochemical analysis, *J Comp Path* 146:152–159, 2012.

58. McGhie JA, FitzGerald L, Hosgood G, et al.: Angioleiomyosarcoma in the nasal vestibule of a dog: surgical excision via a modified lateral approach, *J Am Anim Hosp Assoc* 51:130–135, 2015.

59. George R, Smith A, Schleis S, et al.: Outcome of dogs with intranasal lymphoma treated with various radiation and chemotherapy protocols: 24 Cases, *Vet Radiol Ultrasound* 57:306–312, 2016.

60. Khoo A, Lane A, Wyatt K: Intranasal mast cell tumor in the dog: a case series, *Can Vet J* 58:851–854, 2017.

61. Davies O, Spencer S, Necova S, et al.: Intranasal melanoma treated with radiation therapy in three dogs, *Vet Q* 37:274–281, 2017.

62. Lemetayer J, Al-Dissi A, Tryon et al.: Primary intranasal melanoma with brain invasion in a dog, *Can Vet J* 58:391–396, 2017.

63. Burgess KE, Green EM, Wood RD, et al.: Angiofibroma of the nasal cavity in 13 dogs, *Vet Comp Oncol* 9:304–309, 2011.

64. Holt DE, Goldschmidt MH: Nasal in dogs: five cases (2005-2011), *J Small Anim Pract* 52:660–663, 2011.

65. Gamblin FM, Sagartz JE, Couto CG: Overexpression of p53 tumor suppressor protein in spontaneously arising neoplasms of dogs, *Am J Vet Res* 58:857–863, 1997.

66. Kleiter MK, Malarkey DE, Ruslander DE, et al.: Expression of cyclooxygenase-2 in canine epithelial nasal tumors, *Vet Radiol Ultrasound* 45:255–260, 2004.

67. Borzacchiello G, Paciello O, Papparella S: Expression of cyclooxygenase-1 and -2 in canine nasal carcinomas, *J Comp Pathol* 131:70–76, 2004.

68. Impellizeri JA, Esplin DG: Expression of cyclooxygenase-2 in canine nasal carcinomas, *Vet J* 176:408–410, 2008.

69. Belshaw Z, Constantio-Casas F, Brearley MJ, et al.: COX-2 expression and outcome in canine nasal carcinomas treated with hypofractionated radiotherapy, *Vet Comp Oncol* 9:141–148, 2010.

70. Shiomitsu K, Johnson CL, Malarkey DE, et al.: Expression of epidermal growth factor receptor and vascular endothelial growth factor in malignant canine epithelial nasal tumours, *Vet Comp Oncol* 7:106–114, 2009.

71. Gramer I, Killick D, Scase T, et al.: Expression of VEGFR and PDGFR-α/-β in 187 canine nasal carcinomas, *Vet Comp Oncol* 15:1041–1050, 2017.

72. Paciello O, Borzacchiello G, Varricchio E, et al.: Expression of peroxisome proliferator-activated receptor gamma (PPAR-γ) in canine nasal carcinomas, *J Vet Med A Physiol Pathol Clin Med* 54:406–410, 2007.

73. Vanherberghen M, Day MJ, Delvaux F, et al.: An Immunohistochemical study of the inflammatory infiltrate associated with nasal carcinoma in dogs and cats, *J Comp Pathol* 141:17–26, 2009.

74. Rassnick KM, Goldkamp CE, Erb HN, et al.: Evaluation of factors associated with survival in dogs with untreated nasal carcinomas: 139 cases (1993-2003), *J Am Vet Med Assoc* 229:401–406, 2006.

75. Saunders JH, Van Bree H, Gielen I, et al.: Diagnostic value of computed tomography in dogs with chronic nasal disease, *Vet Radiol Ultrasound* 44:409–413, 2003.

76. Burrow RD: A nasal dermoid sinus in an English bull terrier, *J Small Anim Pract* 45:572–574, 2004.

77. Beck JA, Hunt GB, Goldsmid SE, et al.: Nasopharyngeal obstruction due to cystic Rathke's clefts in two dogs, *Aust Vet J* 77:94–96, 1999.

78. Lobetti RG: A retrospective study of chronic nasal disease in 75 dogs, *J S Afr Vet Assoc* 80:224–228, 2009.

79. Strasser JL, Hawkins EC: Clinical features of epistaxis in dogs: a retrospective study of 35 cases (1999-2002), *J Am Anim Hosp Assoc* 41:179–184, 2005.

80. Plickert HD, Tichy A, Hirt RA: Characteristics of canine nasal discharge related to intranasal diseases: a retrospective study of 105 cases, *J Sm Anim Prac* 55:145–152, 2014.

81. Smith MO, Turrel JM, Bailey CS, et al.: Neurologic abnormalities as the predominant signs of neoplasia of the nasal cavity in dogs and cats: seven cases (1973-1986), *J Am Vet Med Assoc* 195:242–245, 1989.

82. Thrall DE, Robertson ID, McLeod DA, et al.: A comparison of radiographic and computed tomographic findings in 31 dogs with malignant nasal cavity tumors, *Vet Radiol* 30:59–66, 1989.

83. Park RD, Beck ER, LeCouteur RA: Comparison of computed tomography and radiography for detecting changes induced by malignant nasal neoplasia in dogs, *J Am Vet Med Assoc* 201:1720–1724, 1992.

84. Codner EC, Lurus AG, Miller JB, et al.: Comparison of computed tomography with radiography as a noninvasive diagnostic technique for chronic nasal disease in dogs, *J Am Vet Med Assoc* 202:1106–1110, 1993.

85. Drees R, Forrest LJ, Chappell R: Comparison of computed tomography and magnetic resonance imaging for the evaluation of canine intranasal neoplasia, *J Small Anim Pract* 50:334–340, 2009.

86. Avner A, Dobson JM, Sales JI, et al.: Retrospective review of 50 canine nasal tumours evaluated by low-field magnetic resonance imaging, *J Small Anim Pract* 49:233–239, 2008.

87. Agthe P, Caine AR, Gear RNA, et al.: Prognostic significance of specific magnetic resonance imaging features in canine nasal tumours treated by radiotherapy, *J Small Anim Pract* 50:641–648, 2009.

88. Petite AFB, Dennis R: Comparison of radiography and magnetic resonance imaging for evaluating the extent of nasal neoplasia in dogs, *J Small Anim Pract* 47:529–536, 2006.

89. Burk RL: Computed tomographic imaging of nasal disease in 100 dogs, *Vet Radiol Ultrasound* 33:177–180, 1992.

90. Lux CN, Culp WT, Johnson LR, et al.: Prospective comparison of tumor staging using computed tomography versus magnetic resonance imaging findings in dogs with nasal neoplasia: a pilot study, *Vet Radiol Ultrasound* 58:315–325, 2017.

91. Gibbs C, Lane JG, Denny HR: Radiological features of intranasal lesions in the dog: a review of 100 cases, *J Small Anim Pract* 20:515–535, 1979.

92. Russo M, Lamb CR, Jakovljevic S: Distinguishing rhinitis and nasal neoplasia by radiography, *Vet Radiol Ultrasound* 41:118–124, 2000.

93. Bowen SR, Chappell RJ, Bentzen SM, et al.: Spatially resolved regression analysis of pre-treatment FDG, FLT and Cu-ATSM PET from post-treatment FDG PET: an exploratory study, *Radiother Oncol* 105:41–48, 2012.

94. Bradshaw TJ, Bowen SR, Jallow N, et al.: Heterogeneity in intratumor correlations of ^{18}F-FDG, ^{18}F-FLT, and ^{61}Cu-ATSM PET in canine sinonasal tumors, *J Nucl Med* 54:1931–1937, 2013.

95. Bradshaw TJ, Yip S, Jallow N, et al.: Spatiotemporal stability of Cu-ATSM and FLT positron emission tomography distributions during radiation therapy, *Int J Radiation Oncol Biol Phys* 89:399–405, 2014.

96. Bradshaw TK, Bowen SR, Deveau MA, et al.: Molecular imaging biomarkers of resistance to radiation therapy for spontaneous nasal tumors in canines, *Int J Radiation Oncol Biol Phys* 91:787–795, 2015.

97. Bradshaw T, Fu R, Bowen S, et al.: Predicting location of recurrence using FDG, FLT and Cu-ATSM PET in canine sinonasal tumors treated with radiotherapy, *Phys Med Biol* 60:5211–5224, 2015.

98. Withrow SJ, Susaneck SJ, Macy DW, et al.: Aspiration and punch biopsy techniques for nasal tumors, *J Am Anim Hosp Assoc* 21:551–554, 1985.

99. Rudd RG, Richardson DC: A diagnostic and therapeutic approach to nasal disease in dogs, *Compend Contin Educ Pract Vet* 7:103–112, 1985.

100. Kuhlman GM, Taylor AR, Thieman-Mankin KM, et al.: Use of a frameless computed tomography guided stereotactic biopsy system for nasal biopsy in five dogs, *J Am Vet Med Assoc* 248:929–934, 2016.

101. Lent SEF, Hawkins EC: Evaluation of rhinoscopy and rhinoscopy-assisted mucosal biopsy in diagnosis of nasal disease in dogs: 199 cases (1985-1989), *J Am Vet Med Assoc* 201:1425–1429, 1992.

102. Harris BJ, Lourenco BN, Dobson JM, et al.: Diagnostic accuracy of three biopsy techniques in 117 dogs with intra-nasal neoplasia, *J Sm Anim Prac* 55:219–224, 2014.

103. Clercx C, Wallon J, Gilbert S, et al.: Imprint and brush cytology in the diagnosis of canine intranasal tumours, *J Small Anim Pract* 37:423–427, 1996.

104. Theon AP, Madewell BR, Harb MF, et al.: Megavoltage irradiation of neoplasms of the nasal and paranasal cavities in 77 dogs, *J Am Vet Med Assoc* 202:1469–1475, 1993.

105. Adams WM, Miller PE, Vail DM, et al.: An accelerated technique for irradiation of malignant canine nasal and paranasal sinus tumors, *Vet Radiol Ultrasound* 39:475–481, 1998.

106. Adams WM, Kleiter MM, Thrall DE, et al.: Prognostic significance of tumor histology and computed tomographic staging for radiation treatment response of canine nasal tumors, *Vet Radiol Ultrasound* 50:330–335, 2009.

107. Kondo Y, Matsunaga S, Mochizuki M, et al.: Prognosis of canine patients with nasal tumors according to modified clinical stages based on computed tomography: a retrospective study, *J Vet Med Sci* 70:207–212, 2008.
108. LaDue TA, Dodge R, Page RL, et al.: Factors influencing survival after radiotherapy of nasal tumors in 130 dogs, *Vet Radiol Ultrasound* 40:312–317, 1999.
109. Buchholz J, Hagen R, Leo C, et al.: 3D conformal radiation therapy for palliative treatment of canine nasal tumors, *Vet Radiol Ultrasound* 50:679–683, 2009.
110. Mason SL, Maddox TW, Lillis SM, et al.: Late presentation of canine nasal tumours in a UK referral hospital and treatment outcomes, *J Small Anim Pract* 54:347–353, 2013.
111. Marcello A, Gieger TL, Jimenez DA, et al.: Detection of comorbidities and synchronous primary tumours via thoracic radiography and abdominal ultrasonography and their influence on treatment outcome in dogs with soft tissue sarcomas, primary brain tumours and intranasal tumours, *Vet Comp Oncol* 13:433–442, 2015.
112. Couto CF, Boudrieau RJ, Zanjani ED: Tumor-associated erythrocytosis in a dog with nasal fibrosarcoma, *J Vet Intern Med* 3:183–185, 1989.
113. Wilson RB, Bronstad DC: Hypercalcemia associated with nasal adenocarcinoma in a dog, *J Am Vet Med Assoc* 182:1246–1247, 1983.
114. Anderson GM, Lane I, Fischer J, et al.: Hypercalcemia and parathyroid hormone-related protein in a dog with undifferentiated nasal carcinoma, *Can Vet J* 40:341–342, 1999.
115. Laing EJ, Binnington AG: Surgical therapy of canine nasal tumors: a retrospective study (1982-1986), *Can Vet J* 29:809–813, 1988.
116. Holmberg DL, Fries C, Cockshutt J, et al.: Ventral rhinotomy in the dog and cat, *Vet Surg* 18:446–449, 1989.
117. Adams WM, Withrow SJ, Walshaw R, et al.: Radiotherapy of malignant nasal tumors in 67 dogs, *J Am Vet Med Assoc* 191:311–315, 1987.
118. Morris JS, Dunn KJ, Dobson JM, et al.: Effects of radiotherapy alone and surgery and radiotherapy on survival of dogs with nasal tumours, *J Small Anim Pract* 35:567–573, 1994.
119. McEntee MC, Page RL, Heidner GL, et al.: A retrospective study of 27 dogs with intranasal neoplasms treated with cobalt radiation, *Vet Radiol Ultrasound* 32:135–139, 1991.
120. Lana SE, Dernell WS, Lafferty MS, et al.: Use of radiation and a slow-release cisplatin formulation for treatment of canine nasal tumors, *Vet Radiol Ultrasound* 45:1–5, 2004.
121. Adams WM, Bjorling DE, McAnulty JF, et al.: Outcome of accelerated radiotherapy alone or accelerated radiotherapy followed by exenteration of the nasal cavity in dogs with intranasal neoplasia: 53 cases (1993-2002), *J Am Vet Med Assoc* 227:936–941, 2005.
122. Lawrence JA, Forrest LJ, Turek MM, et al.: Proof of principle of ocular sparing in dogs with sinonasal tumors treated with intensity-modulated radiation therapy, *Vet Radiol Ultrasound* 51:561–570, 2010.
123. Nadeau M, Kitchell BE, Rooks RL, et al.: Cobalt radiation with or without low-dose cisplatin for treatment of canine naso-sinus carcinomas, *Vet Radiol Ultrasound* 45:362–367, 2004.
124. Yoon JH, Feeney DA, Jessen CR, et al.: External-beam Co-60 radiotherapy for canine nasal tumors: a comparison of survival by treatment protocol, *Res Vet Sci* 84:140–149, 2008.
125. Hunley DW, Mauldin GN, Shiomitsu K, et al.: Clinical outcome in dogs with nasal tumors treated with intensity-modulated radiation therapy, *Can Vet J* 51:293–300, 2010.
126. Hall EJ, Giaccia AJ: Time, dose, and fractionation in radiotherapy. In Hall EJ, et al.: *Radiobiology for the radiologist*, ed 7, Philadelphia, 2012, Lippincott Williams & Wilkins.
127. Thrall DE, McEntee MC, Novotney C: A boost technique for irradiation of malignant canine nasal tumors, *Vet Radiol Ultrasound* 34:295–300, 1993.
128. Jamieson VE, Davidson MG, Nasisse MP, et al.: Ocular complications following cobalt 60 radiotherapy of neoplasms in the canine head region, *J Am Anim Hosp Assoc* 27:51–55, 1991.
129. Ching SV, Gillette SM, Powers BE, et al.: Radiation-induced ocular injury in the dog: a histological study, *Int J Radiation Oncology Biol Phys* 19:321–328, 1990.
130. Roberts SM, Lavach JD, Severin GA, et al.: Ophthalmic complications following megavoltage irradiation of the nasal and paranasal cavities in dogs, *J Am Vet Med Assoc* 100:43–47, 1987.
131. Hall EJ, Giaccia AJ: Radiation cataractogenesis. In Hall EJ, et al.: *Radiobiology for the radiologist*, ed 7, Philadelphia, 2012, Lippincott Williams & Wilkins.
132. Thrall DE, Heidner GL, Novotny CA, et al.: Failure patterns following cobalt irradiation in dogs with nasal carcinoma, *Vet Radiol Ultrasound* 34:126–133, 1993.
133. Bowles K, DeSandre-Robinson D, Kubicek L, et al.: Outcome of definitive fractionated radiation followed by exenteration of the nasal cavity in dogs with sinonasal neoplasia: 16 cases, *Vet Comp Oncol* 14:350–360, 2014.
134. Soukup A, Meier V, Pot S, et al.: A prospective pilot study on early toxicity of a simultaneous integrated boost technique for canine sinonasal tumors using image-guided intensity modulated radiation therapy, *Vet Comp Oncol,* epub ahead of print, 2018. https://doi.org/10.1111/vco.12399.
135. LeBlanc AK, LaDue TA, Turrel JM, et al.: Unexpected toxicity following use of gemcitabine as a radiosensitizer in head and neck carcinomas: a Veterinary Radiation Therapy Oncology Group pilot study, *Vet Radiol Ultrasound* 45:466–470, 2004.
136. Cancedda S, Sabattini S, Bettini G, et al.: Combination of radiation therapy and firocoxib for the treatment of canine nasal carcinoma, *Vet Radiol Ultrasound* 56:335–343, 2015.
137. Hong TS, Ritter MA, Tome WA, et al.: Intensity-modulated radiation therapy: emerging cancer treatment technology, *Br J Cancer* 92:1819–1824, 2005.
138. Vaudaux C, Schneider U, Kaser-Hotz B: Potential for intensity-modulated radiation therapy to permit dose escalation for canine nasal cancer, *Vet Radiol Ultrasound* 48:475–481, 2007.
139. Guttierez AN, Deveau M, Forrest LJ, et al.: Radiobiological and treatment planning study of a simultaneously integrated boost for canine nasal tumors using helical tomotherapy, *Vet Radiol Ultrasound* 48:594–602, 2007.
140. Deveau MA, Gutierrez AN, Mackie TR, et al.: Dosimetric impact of daily setup variations during treatment of canine nasal tumors using intensity-modulated radiation therapy, *Vet Radiol Ultrasound* 51:90–96, 2010.
141. Harmon J, Van Ufflen D, LaRue S: Assessment of a radiotherapy patient cranial immobilization device using daily on-board kilovoltage imaging, *Vet Radiol Ultrasound* 50:230–234, 2009.
142. Rohrer Bley C, Blattmann H, Roos M, et al.: Assessment of a radiotherapy patient immobilization device using single plane port radiographs and a remote computed tomography scanner, *Vet Radiol Ultrasound* 44:470–475, 2003.
143. Kippenes H, Gavin PR, Sande RD, et al.: Comparison of the accuracy of positioning devices for radiation therapy of canine and feline head tumors, *Vet Radiol Ultrasound* 41:371–376, 2000.
144. Kent MS, Gordon IK, Benavides I, et al.: Assessment of the accuracy and precision of a patient immobilization device for radiation therapy in canine head and neck tumors, *Vet Radiol Ultrasound* 50:550–554, 2009.
145. Kubicek L, Seo S, Chappell R, et al.: Helical tomotherapy setup variations in canine nasal tumor patients immobilized with a bite block, *Vet Radiol Ultrasound* 53:474–481, 2012.
146. Forrest LJ, Mackie TR, Ruchala K, et al.: The utility of megavoltage computed tomography images from a helical tomotherapy system for setup verification purposes, *Int J Radiat Oncol Biol Phys* 60:1639–1644, 2004.
147. Christensen NI, Forrest LJ, White PJ, et al.: Single institution variability in intensity modulated radiation target delineation for canine nasal neoplasia, *Vet Radiol Ultrasound* 57:639–645, 2016.

148. Jafry Z, Gal A, Fleck A, et al.: Proposed expansion margins for planning organ at risk volume for senses during variation therapy of the nasal cavity in dogs and cats, *Vet Radiol Ultrasound* 58:471–478, 2017.

149. Nagata K, Pethel T: A comparison of two dose calculation algorithms – anisotropic analytical algorithm and Acuros XB- for radiation therapy planning of canine intranasal tumors, *Vet Radiol Ultrasound* 58:479–485, 2017.

150. Martin A, Gaya A: Stereotactic body radiotherapy: a review, *Clin Oncol* 22:157–172, 2010.

151. Kubicek L, Milner R, An Q, et al.: Outcomes and prognostic factors associated with canine sinonasal tumors treated with curative intent cone-based stereotactic radiosurgery (1999-2013), *Vet Radiol Ultrasound* 57:331–340, 2016.

152. Glasser SA, Charney S, Dervisis NG, et al.: Use of an image-guided robotic radiosurgery system for the treatment of canine nonlymphomatous nasal tumors, *J Am Anim Hosp Assoc* 50:96–104, 2014.

153. Gieger TL, Nolan MW: Linac-based stereotactic radiation therapy for canine non-lymphmatous nasal tumours: 29 cases (2013-2016), *Vet Comp Oncol* 16:E68–75, 2018.

154. Mellanby RJ, Stevenson RK, Herrtage ME, et al.: Long-term outcome of 56 dogs with nasal tumours treated with four doses of radiation at intervals of seven days, *Vet Rec* 151:253–257, 2002.

155. Geiger T, Rassnick K, Siegel S, et al.: Palliation of clinical signs in 48 dogs with nasal carcinomas treated with coarse-fraction radiation therapy, *J Am Anim Hosp Assoc* 44:116–123, 2008.

156. Maruo T, Shida T, Fukuyama Y, et al.: Retrospective study of canine nasal tumor treated with hypofractionated radiotherapy, *J Vet Med Sci* 73:193–197, 2011.

157. Tan-Coleman B, Lyons J, Lewis C, et al.: Prospective evaluation of a 5 X 4 Gy prescription for palliation of canine nasal tumors, *Vet Radiol Ultrasound* 54:89–92, 2013.

158. Fujiwara A, Kobayashi T, Kazato Y, et al.: Efficacy of hypofractionated radiotherapy for nasal tumours in 38 dogs (2005-2008), *J Small Anim Pract* 54:80–86, 2013.

159. Gieger T, Siegel S, Rosen K, et al.: Reirradiation of canine nasal carcinomas treated with coarsely fractionated protocols: 37 cases, *J Am Anim Hosp Assoc* 49:318–324, 2013.

160. Bommarito DA, Kent MS, Selting KA, et al.: Reirradiation of recurrent canine nasal tumors, *Vet Radiol Ultrasound* 52:207–212, 2011.

161. Rancilio NJ, Custead MR, Poulson JM: Radiation therapy communication - Reirradation of a nasal tumor in a brachycephalic dog using intensity modulated radiation therapy, *Vet Radiol Ultrasound* 57:E46–E50, 2016.

162. Hahn KA, Knapp DW, Richardson RC, et al.: Clinical response of nasal adenocarcinoma to cisplatin chemotherapy in 11 dogs, *J Am Vet Med Assoc* 200:355–357, 1992.

163. Langova V, Mutsaers AJ, Phillips B, et al.: Treatment of eight dogs with nasal tumours with alternating doses of doxorubicin and carboplatin in conjunction with oral piroxicam, *Aust Vet J* 82:676–680, 2004.

164. London C, Mathie T, Stingle N, et al.: Preliminary evidence for biologic activity of toceranib phosphate (Palladia®) in solid tumours, *Vet Comp Oncol* 10:194–205, 2011.

165. De Vos J, Ramos Vega S, Noorman E, et al.: Primary frontal sinus squamous cell carcinoma in three dogs treated with piroxicam combined with carboplatin or toceranib, *Vet Comp Oncol* 10:206–213, 2011.

166. Maglietti F, Tellado M, Olaiz N, et al.: Minimally invasive electrochemotherapy procedure for treating nasal duct tumors in dogs using a single needle electrode, *Radiol Oncol* 51:422–430, 2017.

167. Suzuki D, Berkenbrock J, de Oliveira K, et al.: Novel application for electrochemotherapy: immersion of nasal cavity in dog, *Artif Organs* 41:767–784, 2017.

168. Mayer-Stankeova S, Fidel J, Wergin MC, et al.: Proton spot scanning radiotherapy of spontaneous canine tumors, *Vet Radiol Ultrasound* 50:314–318, 2009.

169. White R, Walker M, Legendre AM, et al.: Development of brachytherapy technique for nasal tumors in dogs, *Am J Vet Res* 51:1250–1256, 1990.

170. Thompson JP, Ackerman N, Bellah JR, et al.: 192 Iridium brachytherapy, using an intracavitary afterload device, for treatment of intranasal neoplasms in dogs, *Am J Vet Res* 53:617–622, 1992.

171. Withrow SJ: Cryosurgical therapy for nasal tumors in the dog, *J Am Anim Hosp Assoc* 18:585–589, 1982.

172. Murphy SM, Lawrence JA, Schmiedt CW, et al.: Image-guide transnasal cryoablation of a recurrent nasal adenocarcinoma in a dog, *J Small Anim Pract* 52:329–333, 2011.

173. Lucroy MD, Long KR, Blaik MA, et al.: Photodynamic therapy for the treatment of intranasal tumors in 3 dogs and 1 cat, *J Vet Intern Med* 17:727–729, 2003.

174. Osaki T, Takagi S, Hoshino Y, et al.: Efficacy of antivascular photodynamic therapy using benzoporphyrin derivative monoacid ring A (BPD-MA) in 14 dogs with oral and nasal tumors, *J Vet Med Sci* 71:125–132, 2009.

175. Maruo T, Nagata K, Fukuyama Y: Intraoperative acridine orange photodynamic therapy and cribriform electron-beam irradiation for canine intrasnasal tumors: a pilot study, *Can Vet J* 56:1232–1238, 2015.

176. Fu D, Kato D, Watabe A, et al.: Prognostic utility of apoptosis index, Ki-67 and survivin expression in dogs with nasal carcinoma treated with orthovoltage radiation therapy, *J Vet Med Sci* 76:1505–1512, 2014.

177. Personal Communication, Stevens A, Turek M, Vail D, et al.: Outcome of definitive-intent IMRT for stage 4 canine sinonasal tumors: 29 cases (2011-2017), *Vet Cancer Soc Proc*, 2018.

178. Thrall DE, Harvey CE: Radiotherapy of malignant nasal tumors in 21 dogs, *J Am Vet Med Assoc* 183:663–666, 1983.

179. Henderson SM, Bradley K, Day MJ, et al.: Investigation of nasal disease in the cat—a retrospective study of 77 cases, *J Feline Med Surg* 6:245–257, 2004.

180. Mukaratirwa S, van der Linde-Sipman JS, Gruys E: Feline nasal and paranasal sinus tumors: clinicopathological study, histomorphological description and diagnostic immunohistochemistry of 123 cases, *J Feline Med Surg* 3:235–245, 2001.

181. Demko JL, Cohn LA: Chronic nasal discharge in cats: 75 cases (1993-2004), *J Am Vet Med Assoc* 230:1032–1037, 2007.

182. Theon AP, Peaston AE, Madewell BR, et al.: Irradiation of nonlymphoproliferative neoplasms of the nasal cavity and paranasal sinuses in 16 cats, *J Am Vet Med Assoc* 204:78–83, 1994.

183. Taylor SS, Goodfellow MR, Browne WJ, et al.: Feline extranodal lymphoma: response to chemotherapy and survival in 110 cats, *J Small Anim Pract* 50:584–592, 2009.

184. Sfiligoi G, Theon AP, Kent MS: Response of nineteen cats with nasal lymphoma to radiation therapy and chemotherapy, *Vet Radiol Ultrasound* 48:388–393, 2007.

185. Haney SM, Beaver L, Turrel J, et al.: Survival analysis of 97 cats with nasal lymphoma: a multi institutional retrospective study (1986-2006), *J Vet Intern Med* 23:287–294, 2009.

186. Little L, Patel R, Goldschmidt M: Nasal and nasopharyngeal lymphoma in cats: 50 cases (1989-2005), *Vet Pathol* 44:885–892, 2007.

187. Greci V, Mortellaro CM, Olivero D, et al.: Inflammatory polyps of the nasal turbinates of cats: an argument for designation of feline mesenchymal nasal hamartoma, *J Feline Med Surg* 13:213–219, 2011.

188. DeLorenzi D, Bertoncello D, Bottero E: Squash preparation cytology from nasopharyngeal masses in the cat: cytological results and histological correlations in 30 cases, *J Feline Med Surg* 10:55–60, 2008.

189. Santagostino SF, Mortellaro CM, Boracchi P, et al.: Feline upper respiratory tract lymphoma: site, cyto-histology, phenotype, FeLV expression and prognosis, *Vet Pathol* 52:250–259, 2015.

190. Nagata K, Lamb M, Goldschmidt MH, et al.: The usefulness of immunohistochemistry to differentiate between nasal carcinoma and lymphoma in cats: 140 cases (1986-2000), *Vet Comp Oncol* 12:52–57, 2014.
191. Lamb CR, Richbell S, Mantis P: Radiographic signs in cats with nasal disease, *J Feline Med Surg* 5:227–235, 2003.
192. Schoenborn WC, Wisner ER, Kass PP, et al.: Retrospective assessment of computed tomographic imaging of feline sinonasal disease in 62 cats, *Vet Radiol Ultrasound* 44:185–195, 2003.
193. Tromblee TC, Jones JC, Etue AE, et al.: Association between clinical characteristics, computed tomography characteristics, and histologic diagnosis for cats with sinonasal disease, *Vet Radiol Ultrasound* 47:241–248, 2006.
194. Karnik K, Riechle JK, Fischetti AJ, et al.: Computed tomographic findings of fungal rhinitis and sinusitis in cats, *Vet Radiol Ultrasound* 50:65–68, 2009.
195. Nemanic S, Hollars K, Nelson NC, et al.: Combination of computed tomographic imaging characteristic of medial retropharyngeal lymph nodes and nasal passages aids discrimination between rhinitis and neoplasia in cats, *Vet Radiol Ultrasound* 56:617–627, 2015.
196. Mellanby RJ, Herrtage ME, Dobson JM: Long-term outcome of eight cats with non-lymphoproliferative nasal tumours treated by megavoltage radiotherapy, *J Feline Med Surg* 4:77–81, 2002.
197. Fujiwara-Igarashi A, Fujimori T, Oka M, et al.: Evaluation of outcomes and radiation complications in 65 cats with nasal tumors treated with palliative hypofractionated radiotherapy, *Vet J* 202:455–461, 2014.
198. Elmslie RE, Ogilvie GK, Gillette EL, et al.: Radiotherapy with and without chemotherapy for localized lymphoma in 10 cats, *Vet Radiol* 32:277–280, 1991.
199. Fu DR, Kato D, Endo Y, et al.: Apoptosis and Ki-67 as predictive factors for response to radiation therapy in feline nasal lymphomas, *J Vet Med Sci* 78:1161–1166, 2016.
200. Mendenhall WM, Werning JW, Pfister DG: Cancer of the head and neck. In DeVita VT, Lawrence TS, Rosenberg SA, editors: *Cancer: principles and practice of oncology*, Philadelphia, 2015, Wolters Kluwer.
201. PDQ Adult Treatment Editorial Board: *Paranasal sinus and nasal cavity cancer treatment (adult) (PDQ®): health professional version, PDQ cancer information summaries [internet]*, National Cancer Institute, 2002-2018 Feb 8.
202. Eriksen J, Lassen P: Human papilloma virus as a biomarker for personalized head and neck cancer radiotherapy, *Recent Results Cancer Res* 198:143–161, 2016.
203. Takahasi Y, Bell D, Agarwal G, et al.: Comprehensive assessment of prognostic markers for sinonasal squamous cell carcinoma, *Head Neck* 36:1094–1101, 2014.
204. Alos L, Moyano S, Nadal A, et al.: Human papillomaviruses are identified in a subgroup of sinonasal squamous cell carcinomas with favorable outcome, *Cancer* 115:2701–2709, 2009.
205. Kozakiewicz P, Grzybowska-Szatkowska L: Application of molecular targeted therapies in the treatment of head and neck squamous cell carcinoma, *Oncol Lett* 15:7497–7505, 2018.
206. Saik JE, Toll SL, Diters RW, et al.: Canine and feline laryngeal neoplasia: a 10-year survey, *J Am Anim Hosp Assoc* 22:359–365, 1986.
207. Ramirez GA, Altimira J, Vilafranca M: Cartilaginous tumors of the larynx and trachea in the dog: literature review and 10 additional cases (1995-2014), *Vet Pathol* 52:1019–1026, 2015.
208. Dobson JM, Samuel S, Milstein H, et al.: Canine neoplasia in the UK: estimates of incidence rates from a population of insured dogs, *J Small Anim Pract* 43:240–246, 2002.
209. Jacubiak MJ, Siedlecki CT, Zenger E, et al.: Laryngeal, laryngotracheal, and tracheal masses in cats: 27 cases (1998-2003), *J Am Anim Hosp Assoc* 41:310–316, 2005.
210. Evans HE, de LaHunta A: The respiratory system. In *miller's anatomy of the dog*, ed 4, St. Louis, 2013, Elsevier, pp 338–350.
211. Pass DA, Huxtable CR, Cooper BJ, et al.: Canine laryngeal oncocytomas, *Vet Pathol* 17:672–677, 1980.
212. Dunbar MD, Ginn P, Winter M: Laryngeal rhabdomyoma in a dog, *Vet Clin Path* 41:590–593, 2012.
213. Cuddy LC, Bacon NJ, Coomer AR, et al.: Excision of a congenital laryngeal cyst in a five-month-old dog via a lateral extraluminal approach, *J Am Vet Med Assoc* 236:1328–1333, 2010.
214. Caserto BG: A comparative review of canine and human rhabdomyosarcoma with emphasis on classification and pathogenesis, *Vet Pathol* 50:806–826, 2013.
215. Crowe DT, Goodwin MA, Greene CE: Total laryngectomy for laryngeal mast cell tumor in the dog, *J Am Anim Hosp Assoc* 22:809–816, 1986.
216. Hayes AM, Gregory SP, Murphy S, et al.: Solitary extramedullary plasmacytoma of the canine larynx, *J Small Anim Pract* 48:288–291, 2007.
217. Rossi G, Tarantino C, Taccini E, et al.: Granular cell tumour affecting the left vocal cord in a dog, *J Comp Path* 136:74–78, 2007.
218. Withrow SJ, Holmberg DL, Doige CE, et al.: Treatment of a tracheal osteochondroma with an overlapping end-to-end tracheal anastomosis, *J Am Anim Hosp Assoc* 14:469–473, 1978.
219. Carb A, Halliwell WH: Osteochondral dysplasias of the canine trachea, *J Am Anim Hosp Assoc* 17:193–199, 1981.
220. Dubielzig RR, Dickey DL: Tracheal osteochondroma in a young dog, *Vet Med Small Anim Clin* 73:1288–1290, 1978.
221. Carlisle CH, Biery DN, Thrall DE: Tracheal and laryngeal tumors in the dog and cat: literature review and 13 additional patients, *Vet Radiol* 32:229–235, 1991.
222. Bryan RD, Frame RW, Kier AB: Tracheal leiomyoma in a dog, *J Am Vet Med Assoc* 178:1069–1070, 1981.
223. Black AP, Liu S, Randolph JF: Primary tracheal leiomyoma in a dog, *J Am Vet Med Assoc* 179:905–907, 1981.
224. Chaffin K, Cross AR, Allen SW, et al.: Extramedullary plasmacytoma in the trachea of a dog, *J Am Vet Med Assoc* 212:1579–1581, 1998.
225. Brown MR, Rogers KS: Primary tracheal tumors in dogs and cats, *Comp Pract Vet* 25:854–860, 2003.
226. Brodey RS, O'Brien J, Berg P, et al.: Osteosarcoma of the upper airway in the dog, *J am Vet Med Assoc* 155:1460–1464, 1969.
227. Aron DN, DeVreis R, Short CE: Primary tracheal chondrosarcoma in a dog: a case report with description of surgical and anesthetic techniques, *J Am Anim Hosp Assoc* 16:31–37, 1980.
228. Harvey HJ, Sykes G: Tracheal mast cell tumor in a dog, *J Am Vet Med Assoc* 180:1097–1100, 1982.
229. Jelinek F, Vozkova D: Carcinoma of the trachea in a cat, *J Comp Path* 147:177–180, 2012.
230. Taylor SS, Harvey AM, Barr FJ, et al.: Laryngeal disease in cats: a retrospective study of 35 cases, *J Feline Med Surg* 11:954–962, 2009.
231. Costello MF, Keith D, Hendrick M, et al.: Acute upper airway obstruction due to inflammatory laryngeal disease in 5 cats, *J Vet Emerg Crit Care* 11:205–210, 2001.
232. Brown MR, Rogers KS, Mansell KJ, et al.: Primary intratracheal lymphosarcoma in four cats, *J Am Anim Hosp Assoc* 39:468–472, 2003.
233. Finotello R, Vasconi ME, Sabattini S, et al.: Feline large granular lymphocyte lymphoma: an Italian Society of Veterinary Oncology (SIONCOV) retrospective study, *Vet Comp Oncol* 1–8, 2017.
234. Veith LA: Squamous cell carcinoma of the trachea of a cat, *Feline Pract* 4:30–32, 1974.
235. Schneider PR, Smith CW, Feller DL: Histiocytic lymphosarcoma of the trachea in a cat, *J Am Anim Hosp Assoc* 15:485–487, 1979.
236. Rossi G, Magi GE, Tarantino C, et al.: Tracheobronchial neuroendocrine carcinoma in a cat, *J Comp Path* 137:165–168, 2007.
237. Cain GR, Manley P: Tracheal adenocarcinoma in a cat, *J Am Vet Med Assoc* 182:614–616, 1983.
238. Culp WT, Cole S, Weisse C: Intra-luminal tracheal stent placement in 3 cats, *Vet Surg* 36:107–113, 2007.

239. Hendricks JC, O'Brien JA: Tracheal collapse in two cats, *J Am Vet Med Assoc* 187:418–419, 1985.

240. Campos M, Ducatelle R, Rutteman G, et al.: Clinical, pathologic, and immunohistochemical prognostic factors in dogs with thyroid carcinoma, *J Vet Intern Med* 28:1805–1813, 2014.

241. Fujita M, Miura H, Yasuda D, et al.: Tracheal narrowing secondary to airway obstruction in two cats, *J Small Anim Pract* 45:29–31, 2004.

242. MacPhail C: Laryngeal disease in dogs and cats, *Vet Clin North Am Small Anim Pract* 44:19–31, 2014.

243. Muraro L, Apre F, White RAS: Successful management of an arytenoid chondrosarcoma in a dog, *J Small Anim Pract* 54:33–35, 2013.

244. Martano M, Boston S, Morello E, et al.: Respiratory tract and thorax. In Kudnig ST, Seguin B, editors: *veterinary surgical oncology*, ed 1, Wiley Blackwell, 2012, pp 273–328.

245. Mosing M, Iff I, Moens Y: Endoscopic removal of a bronchial carcinoma in a dog using one-lung ventilation, *Vet Surg* 37:222–225, 2008.

246. De Lorenzi D, Bertoncello D, Dentini A: Intraoral diode laser epiglottectomy for treatment of epiglottis chondrosarcoma in a dog, *J Small Anim Pract* 56:675–678, 2015.

247. Hawley MM, Johnson LR, Johnson EG, et al.: Endoscopic treatment of an intrathoracic tracheal osteochondroma in a dog, *J Am Vet Med Assoc* 247:1303–1308, 2015.

248. Queen E, Vaughan M, Johnson L: Bronchoscopic debulking of tracheal carcinoma in 3 cats using a wire snare, *J Vet Intern Med* 24:990–993, 2010.

249. Drynan EA, Moles AD, Raisis AL: Anaesthetic and surgical management of an intra-tracheal mass in a cat, *J Fel Med Surg* 13:460–462, 2011.

250. Weisse C: Veterinary interventional oncology: from concept to clinic, *Vet J* 205:198–203, 2015.

251. Sura PA, Krahwinkel DJ: Self-expanding nitinol stents for the treatment of tracheal collapse in dogs: 12 cases (2001-2004), *J Am Vet Med Assoc* 232:228–236, 2008.

252. Guenther-Yenke CL, Rozanski EA: Tracheostomy in cats: 23 cases (1998-2006), *J Fel Med Surg* 9:451–457, 2007.

253. Tomeh C, Holsinger FC: Laryngeal cancer, *Curr Opin Otolaryngol Head Neck Surg* 22:147–153, 2014.

254. Jenckel F, Kneckt R: State of the art in the treatment of laryngeal cancer, *Anticancer Res* 33:4701–4710, 2013.

255. Miyazawa T, Yamakido M, Ikeda S, et al.: Implantation of ultraflex nitinol stents in malignant tracheobronchial stenoses, *Chest* 118:959–969, 2000.

256. Brodey RS, Craig PH: Primary pulmonary neoplasms in the dog: a review of 29 cases, *J Am Vet Med Assoc* 147:1628–1643, 1965.

257. Nielsen SW, Horava A: Primary pulmonary tumors of the dog. A report of sixteen cases, *Am J Vet Res* 21:813–830, 1960.

258. Moulton JE, von Tscharner C, Schneider R: Classification of lung carcinomas in the dog and cat, *Vet Pathol* 18:513–528, 1981.

259. Dorn CR, Taylor DO, Frye FL, et al.: Survey of animal neoplasms in Alameda and Contra Costa Counties, California. I. Methodology and description of cases, *J Natl Cancer Inst* 40: 295–305, 1968.

260. Dobson JM, Samuel S, Milstein H, et al.: Canine neoplasia in the UK: estimates of incidence rates from a population of insured dogs, *J Small Anim Pract* 43:240–246, 2002.

261. Hahn FF, Muggenburg BA, Griffith WC: Primary lung neoplasia in a beagle colony, *Vet Pathol* 33:633–638, 1996.

262. Griffey SM, Kraegel SA, Madewell BR: Rapid detection of K-ras gene mutations in canine lung cancer using single-strand conformational polymorphism analysis, *Carcinogenesis* 19: 959–963, 1998.

263. Stunzi H, Head KW, Nielsen SW: Tumours of the lung, *Bull World Health Organ* 50:9–19, 1974.

264. Meuten DJ, editor: *Tumors in domestic animals*, ed 4, Ames, Iowa, 2002, Iowa State University Press.

265. Hahn KA, McEntee MF: Primary lung tumors in cats: 86 cases (1979-1994), *J Am Vet Med Assoc* 211:1257–1260, 1997.

266. D'Costa S, Yoon BI, Kim DY, et al.: Morphologic and molecular analysis of 39 spontaneous feline pulmonary carcinomas, *Vet Pathol* 49:971–978, 2012.

267. Reif JS, Cohen D: The environmental distribution of canine respiratory tract neoplasms, *Arch Environ Health* 22:136–140, 1971.

268. Reif JS, Dunn K, Ogilvie GK, et al.: Passive smoking and canine lung cancer risk, *Am J Epidemiol* 135:234–239, 1992.

269. Bettini G, Morini M, Marconato L, et al.: Association between environmental dust exposure and lung cancer in dogs, *Vet J* 186:364–369, 2009.

270. Sabattini S, Mancini FR, Marconato L, et al.: EGFR overexpression in canine primary lung cancer: pathogenetic implications and impact on survival, *Vet Comp Oncol* 12:237–248, 2014.

271. Roza MR, Viegas CA: The dog as a passive smoker: effects of exposure to environmental cigarette smoke on domestic dogs, *Nicotine Tob Res* 9:1171–1176, 2007.

272. Auerbach O, Hammond EC, Kirman D, et al.: Effects of cigarette smoking on dogs. II. Pulmonary neoplasms, *Arch Environ Health* 21:754–768, 1970.

273. Humphrey EW, Ewing SL, Wrigley JV, et al.: The production of malignant tumors of the lung and pleura in dogs from intratracheal asbestos instillation and cigarette smoking, *Cancer* 47:1994–1999, 1981.

274. Gillett NA, Stegelmeier BL, Kelly G, et al.: Expression of epidermal growth factor receptor in plutonium-239-induced lung neoplasms in dogs, *Vet Pathol* 29:46–52, 1992.

275. Wilson DA, Mohr LC, Frey GD, et al.: Lung, liver and bone cancer mortality after plutonium exposure in beagle dogs and nuclear workers, *Health Phys* 98:42–52, 2010.

276. Marlowe KW, Robat CS, Clarke DL, et al.: Primary pulmonary histiocytic sarcoma in dogs: a retrospective analysis of 37 cases (2000-2015), *Vet Comp Oncol*, epub ahead of print, 2018. https://doi.org/10.1111/vco.12437.

277. Lenz JA, Furrow E, Craig LE, et al.: Histiocytic sarcoma in 14 miniature schnauzers - a new breed predisposition? *J Small Anim Pract* 58:461–467, 2017.

278. Kagawa Y, Nakano Y, Kobayashi T, et al.: Localized pulmonary histiocytic sarcomas in Pembroke Welsh Corgi, *J Vet Med Sci* 77:1659–1661, 2016.

279. van der Linde-Sipman JS, van den Ingh TS: Primary and metastatic carcinomas in the digits of cats, *Vet Q* 22:141–145, 2000.

280. Goldfinch N, Argyle DJ: Feline lung-digit syndrome: unusual metastatic patterns of primary lung tumours in cats, *J Feline Med Surg* 14:202–208, 2012.

281. McNiel EA, Ogilvie GK, Powers BE, et al.: Evaluation of prognostic factors for dogs with primary lung tumors: 67 cases (1985-1992), *J Am Vet Med Assoc* 211:1422–1427, 1997.

282. Mehlhaff CJLC, Patnaik AK, et al.: Surgical treatment of primary pulmonary neoplasia in 15 dogs, *J Am Anim Hosp Assoc* 20:799–803, 1984.

283. Ogilvie GK, Haschek WM, Withrow SJ, et al.: Classification of primary lung tumors in dogs: 210 cases (1975-1985), *J Am Vet Med Assoc* 195:106–108, 1989.

284. Paoloni MC, Adams WM, Dubielzig RR, et al.: Comparison of results of computed tomography and radiography with histopathologic findings in tracheobronchial lymph nodes in dogs with primary lung tumors: 14 cases (1999-2002), *J Am Vet Med Assoc* 228:1718–1722, 2006.

285. Barr FG-JT, Brown PJ, Gibbs C: Primary lung tumours in the cat, *J Small Anim Pract* 28:1115–1125, 1987.

286. Hahn KA, McEntee MF: Prognosis factors for survival in cats after removal of a primary lung tumor: 21 cases (1979-1994), *Vet Surg* 27:307–311, 1998.

287. Nunley J, Sutton J, Culp W, et al.: Primary pulmonary neoplasia in cats: assessment of computed tomography findings and survival, *J Small Anim Pract* 56:651–656, 2015.

288. Aarsvold S, Reetz JA, Reichle JK, et al.: Computed tomographic findings in 57 cats with primary pulmonary neoplasia, *Vet Radiol Ultrasound* 56:272–277, 2015.

289. Maritato KC, Schertel ER, Kennedy SC, et al.: Outcome and prognostic indicators in 20 cats with surgically treated primary lung tumors, *J Feline Med Surg* 16:979–984, 2014.

290. Mooney ET, Rozanski EA, King RG, et al.: Spontaneous pneumothorax in 35 cats (2001-2010), *J Feline Med Surg* 14:384–391, 2012.

291. MacCoy DMTE, deLahunta A, MacDonald JM: Pelvic limb parealysis in a young miniature pinscher due to metastatic bronchogenic adenocarcinoma, *J Am Anim Hosp Assoc* 4, 1976.

292. Sorjonen DC, Braund KG, Hoff EJ: Paraplegia and subclinical neuromyopathy associated with a primary lung tumor in a dog, *J Am Vet Med Assoc* 180:1209–1211, 1982.

293. Moore JA, Taylor HW: Primary pulmonary adenocarcinoma with brain stem metastasis in a dog, *J Am Vet Med Assoc* 192:219–221, 1988.

294. Mori T, Yamagami T, Umeda M, et al.: Small cell anaplastic carcinoma of the lung with cerebral metastasis in a dog, *J Vet Med Sci* 53:1129–1131, 1991.

295. Brodey RS: Hypertrophic osteoarthropathy in the dog: a clinicopathologic survey of 60 cases, *J Am Vet Med Assoc* 159:1242–1256, 1971.

296. Halliwell WH, Ackerman N: Botryoid rhabdomyosarcoma of the urinary bladder and hypertrophic osteoarthropathy in a young dog, *J Am Vet Med Assoc* 165:911–913, 1974.

297. Caywood DD, Kramek BA, Feeney DA, et al.: Hypertrophic osteopathy associated with a bronchial foreign body and lobar pneumonia in a dog, *J Am Vet Med Assoc* 186:698–700, 1985.

298. Liptak JM, Monnet E, Dernell WS, et al.: Pulmonary metastatectomy in the management of four dogs with hypertrophic osteopathy, *Vet Comp Oncol* 2:1–12, 2004.

299. Grillo TP, Brandao CV, Mamprim MJ, et al.: Hypertrophic osteopathy associated with renal pelvis transitional cell carcinoma in a dog, *Can Vet J* 48:745–747, 2007.

300. Withers SS, Johnson EG, Culp WT, et al.: Paraneoplastic hypertrophic osteopathy in 30 dogs, *Vet Comp Oncol* 13:157–165, 2015.

301. Moore AS, Middleton DJ: Pulmonary adenocarcinoma in 3 cats with non-respiratory signs only, *J Small Anim Pract* 23:501–509, 1982.

302. Pollack M, Martin RA, Diters RW: Metastatic squamous cell carcinoma in multiple digits of a cat, *J Am Anim Hosp Assoc* 5, 1984

303. Scott-Moncrieff JC, Radovsky, Elliot GS, et al.: Pulmonary squamous cell carcinoma with multiple digitial metastases in a cat, *J Small Anim Pract* 30:696–699, 2008.

304. Gottfried SD, Popovitch CA, Goldschmidt MH, et al.: Metastatic digital carcinoma in the cat: a retrospective study of 36 cats (1992-1998), *J Am Anim Hosp Assoc* 36:501–509, 2000.

305. Hawkins EC, DeNicola DB, Kuehn NF: Bronchoalveolar lavage in the evaluation of pulmonary disease in the dog and cat. State of the art, *J Vet Intern Med* 4:267–274, 1990.

306. Hawkins EC, DeNicola DB, Plier ML: Cytological analysis of bronchoalveolar lavage fluid in the diagnosis of spontaneous respiratory tract disease in dogs: a retrospective study, *J Vet Intern Med* 9:386–392, 1995.

307. Norris CR, Griffey SM, Walsh P: Use of keyhole lung biopsy for diagnosis of interstitial lung diseases in dogs and cats: 13 cases (1998-2001), *J Am Vet Med Assoc* 221:1453–1459, 2002.

308. Koblik PD: Radiographic appearance of primary lung tumors in cats, *Vet Radiol* 27:66–93, 1986.

309. Barrett LE, Pollard RE, Zwingenberger A, et al.: Radiographic characterization of primary lung tumors in 74 dogs, *Vet Radiol Ultrasound* 55:480–487, 2014.

310. Tsai S, Sutherland-Smith J, Burgess K, et al.: Imaging characteristics of intrathoracic histiocytic sarcoma in dogs, *Vet Radiol Ultrasound* 53:21–27, 2012.

311. Schwarz LA, Tidwell A: Alternative imaging of the lung, *Clin Tech Small Anim Pract* 14:187–206, 1999.

312. Reichle JK, Wisner ER: Non-cardiac thoracic ultrasound in 75 feline and canine patients, *Vet Radiol Ultrasound* 41:154–162, 2000.

313. Larson MM: Ultrasound of the thorax (noncardiac), *Vet Clin North Am Small Anim Pract* 39:733–745, 2009.

314. Marolf AJ, Gibbons DS, Podell BK, et al.: Computed tomographic appearance of primary lung tumors in dogs, *Vet Radiol Ultrasound* 52:168–172, 2011.

315. Ballegeer EA, Adams WM, Dubielzig RR, et al.: Computed tomography characteristics of canine tracheobronchial lymph node metastasis, *Vet Radiol Ultrasound* 51:397–403, 2010.

316. Nemanic S, London CA, Wisner ER: Comparison of thoracic radiographs and single breath-hold helical CT for detection of pulmonary nodules in dogs with metastatic neoplasia, *J Vet Intern Med* 20:508–515, 2006.

317. Alexander K, Joly H, Blond L, et al.: A comparison of computed tomography, computed radiography, and film-screen radiography for the detection of canine pulmonary nodules, *Vet Radiol Ultrasound* 53:258–265, 2012.

318. Seiler SM, Baumgartner C, Hirschberger J, et al.: Comparative oncology: evaluation of 2-deoxy-2-[18F]fluoro-D-glucose (FDG) positron emission tomography/computed tomography (PET/CT) for the staging of dogs with malignant tumors, *PLoS One* 10:e0127800, 2015.

319. Kim J, Kwon SY, Cena R, et al.: CT and PET-CT of a dog with multiple pulmonary adenocarcinoma, *J Vet Med Sci* 76:615–620, 2014.

320. Song SH, Park NW, Eom KD: Positron emission tomography/computed tomography imaging features of renal cell carcinoma and pulmonary metastases in a dog, *Can Vet J* 55: 466–470, 2014.

321. Holt D, Okusanya O, Judy R, et al.: Intraoperative near-infrared imaging can distinguish cancer from normal tissue but not inflammation, *PLoS One* 9:e103342, 2014.

322. Wood EF, O'Brien RT, Young KM: Ultrasound-guided fine-needle aspiration of focal parenchymal lesions of the lung in dogs and cats, *J Vet Intern Med* 12:338–342, 1998.

323. Zekas LJ, Crawford JT, O'Brien RT: Computed tomography-guided fine-needle aspirate and tissue-core biopsy of intrathoracic lesions in thirty dogs and cats, *Vet Radiol Ultrasound* 46:200–204, 2005.

324. Bauer TG: Lung biopsy, *Vet Clin North Am Small Anim Pract* 30:1207–1225, 2000.

325. Norris CR, Griffey SM, Samii VF, et al.: Comparison of results of thoracic radiography, cytologic evaluation of bronchoalveolar lavage fluid, and histologic evaluation of lung specimens in dogs with respiratory tract disease: 16 cases (1996-2000), *J Am Vet Med Assoc* 218:1456–1461, 2001.

326. Venker-van Haagen AJVM, Heijn A, et al.: Bronchoscopy in small animal clinics: an analysis of the results of 228 bronchoscopies, *J Am Anim Hosp Assoc* 24:6, 1985.

327. Faunt KK, Jones BD, Turk JR, et al.: Evaluation of biopsy specimens obtained during thoracoscopy from lungs of clinically normal dogs, *Am J Vet Res* 59:1499–1502, 1998.

328. Kovak JR, Ludwig LL, Bergman PJ, et al.: Use of thoracoscopy to determine the etiology of pleural effusion in dogs and cats: 18 cases (1998-2001), *J Am Vet Med Assoc* 221:990–994, 2002.

329. Ramos-Vara JA, Miller MA, Johnson GC: Usefulness of thyroid transcription factor-1 immunohistochemical staining in the differential diagnosis of primary pulmonary tumors of dogs, *Vet Pathol* 42:315–320, 2005.

330. Bettini G, Marconato L, Morini M, et al.: Thyroid transcription factor-1 immunohistochemistry: diagnostic tool and malignancy marker in canine malignant lung tumours, *Vet Comp Oncol* 7:28–37, 2009.

331. Burgess HJ, Kerr ME: Cytokeratin and vimentin co-expression in 21 canine primary pulmonary epithelial neoplasms, *J Vet Diagn Invest* 21:815–820, 2009.

332. Beck J, Miller MA, Frank C, et al.: Surfactant protein A and napsin A in the immunohistochemical characterization of canine pulmonary carcinomas: comparison with thyroid transcription factor-1, *Vet Pathol* 54:767–774, 2017.

333. Affolter VK, Moore PF: Localized and disseminated histiocytic sarcoma of dendritic cell origin in dogs, *Vet Pathol* 39:74–83, 2002.

334. Kato Y, Murakami M, Hoshino Y, et al.: The class A macrophage scavenger receptor CD204 is a useful immunohistochemical marker of canine histiocytic sarcoma, *J Comp Pathol* 148:188–196, 2013.

335. Moore PF: A review of histiocytic diseases of dogs and cats, *Vet Pathol* 51:167–184, 2014.

336. Slatter DH, editor: *Textbook of small animal surgery*, ed 3, Philadelphia, PA, 2003, Saunders.

337. LaRue SM, Withrow SJ, Wykes PM: Lung resection using surgical staples in dogs and cats, *Vet Surg* 16:238–240, 1987.

338. Walshaw R: Stapling techniques in pulmonary surgery, *Vet Clin North Am Small Anim Pract* 24:335–366, 1994.

339. Wavreille V, Boston SE, Souza C, et al.: Outcome after pneumonectomy in 17 dogs and 10 cats: a Veterinary Society of Surgical Oncology case series, *Vet Surg* 45:782–789, 2016.

340. Majeski SA, Steffey MA, Mayhew PD, et al.: Postoperative respiratory function and survival after pneumonectomy in dogs and cats, *Vet Surg* 45:775–781, 2016.

341. Lansdowne JL, Monnet E, Twedt DC, et al.: Thoracoscopic lung lobectomy for treatment of lung tumors in dogs, *Vet Surg* 34:530–535, 2005.

342. Levionnois OL, Bergadano A, Schatzmann U: Accidental entrapment of an endo-bronchial blocker tip by a surgical stapler during selective ventilation for lung lobectomy in a dog, *Vet Surg* 35:82–85, 2006.

343. Dhumeaux MP, Haudiquet PR: Primary pulmonary osteosarcoma treated by thoracoscopy-assisted lung resection in a dog, *Can Vet J* 50:755–758, 2009.

344. Bleakley S, Duncan CG, Monnet E: Thoracoscopic lung lobectomy for primary lung tumors in 13 dogs, *Vet Surg* 44:1029–1035, 2015.

345. Mayhew PD, Hunt GB, Steffey MA, et al.: Evaluation of short-term outcome after lung lobectomy for resection of primary lung tumors via video-assisted thoracoscopic surgery or open thoracotomy in medium- to large-breed dogs, *J Am Vet Med Assoc* 243:681–688, 2013.

346. Mosing M, Iff I, Moens Y: Endoscopic removal of a bronchial carcinoma in a dog using one-lung ventilation, *Vet Surg* 37:222–225, 2008.

347. Mayhew PD, Pascoe PJ, Shilo-Benjamini Y, et al.: Effect of one-lung ventilation with or without low-pressure carbon dioxide insufflation on cardiorespiratory variables in cats undergoing thoracoscopy, *Vet Surg* 44:O15–O22, 2015.

348. Denlinger CE, Fernandez F, Meyers BF, et al.: Lymph node evaluation in video-assisted thoracoscopic lobectomy versus lobectomy by thoracotomy, *Ann Thorac Surg* 89:1730–1735, 2010.

349. Steffey MA, Daniel L, Mayhew PD, et al.: Video-assisted thoracoscopic extirpation of the tracheobronchial lymph nodes in dogs, *Vet Surg* 44:O50–O58, 2015.

350. DeVita VT, Lawrence TS, Rosenberg SA: *Devita, hellman, and rosenberg's cancer: principles & practice of oncolog*, 8th ed, Philadelphia, 2008, Wolters Kluwer/Lippincott Williams & Wilkins.

351. Ogilvie GK, Reynolds HA, Richardson RC, et al.: Phase II evaluation of doxorubicin for treatment of various canine neoplasms, *J Am Vet Med Assoc* 195:1580–1583, 1989.

352. Ogilvie GK, Obradovich JE, Elmslie RE, et al.: Efficacy of mitoxantrone against various neoplasms in dogs, *J Am Vet Med Assoc* 198:1618–1621, 1991.

353. Poirier VJ, Burgess KE, Adams WM, et al.: Toxicity, dosage, and efficacy of vinorelbine (Navelbine) in dogs with spontaneous neoplasia, *J Vet Intern Med* 18:536–539, 2004.

354. Chabner B, Longo DL: *Cancer chemotherapy and biotherapy: principles and practice*, ed 4, Philadelphia, 2006, Lippincott Williams & Wilkins.

355. Skorupski KA, Rodriguez CO, Krick EL, et al.: Long-term survival in dogs with localized histiocytic sarcoma treated with CCNU as an adjuvant to local therapy, *Vet Comp Oncol* 7:139–144, 2009.

356. Hershey AE, Kurzman ID, Forrest LJ, et al.: Inhalation chemotherapy for macroscopic primary or metastatic lung tumors: proof of principle using dogs with spontaneously occurring tumors as a model, *Clin Cancer Res* 5:2653–2659, 1999.

357. Khanna C, Vail DM: Targeting the lung: preclinical and comparative evaluation of anticancer aerosols in dogs with naturally occurring cancers, *Curr Cancer Drug Targets* 3:265–273, 2003.

358. London CA, Hannah AL, Zadovoskaya R, et al.: Phase I dose-escalating study of SU11654, a small molecule receptor tyrosine kinase inhibitor, in dogs with spontaneous malignancies, *Clin Cancer Res* 9:2755–2768, 2003.

359. Moore AS, Kirk C, Cardona A: Intracavitary cisplatin chemotherapy experience with six dogs, *J Vet Intern Med* 5:227–231, 1991.

360. Spugnini EP, Crispi S, Scarabello A, et al.: Piroxicam and intracavitary platinum-based chemotherapy for the treatment of advanced mesothelioma in pets: preliminary observations, *J Exp Clin Cancer Res* 27:6, 2008.

361. Kelly J, Holmes EC, Rosen G: Mitoxantrone for malignant pleural effusion due to metastatic sarcoma, *Surg Oncol* 2:299–301, 1993.

362. Sparkes A, Murphy S, McConnell F, et al.: Palliative intracavitary carboplatin therapy in a cat with suspected pleural mesothelioma, *J Feline Med Surg* 7:313–316, 2005.

363. Laing EJNA: Pleurodesis as a treatment for pleural effusion in the dog, *J Am Anim Hosp Assoc* 2(4), 1986.

364. Li R, Yu L, Lin S, et al.: Involved field radiotherapy (IFRT) versus elective nodal irradiation (ENI) for locally advanced non-small cell lung cancer: a meta-analysis of incidence of elective nodal failure (ENF), *Radiat Oncol* 11:124, 2016.

365. Rose SC, Thistlethwaite PA, Sewell PE, et al.: Lung cancer and radiofrequency ablation, *J Vasc Interv Radiol* 17:927–951, 2006.

366. Okuma T, Matsuoka T, Yamamoto A, et al.: Frequency and risk factors of various complications after computed tomography-guided radiofrequency ablation of lung tumors, *Cardiovasc Intervent Radiol* 31:122–130, 2008.

367. Crocetti L, Lencioni R: Radiofrequency ablation of pulmonary tumors, *Eur J Radiol* 75:23–27, 2010.

368. Duncan M, Wijesekera N, Padley S: Interventional radiology of the thorax, *Respirology* 15:401–412, 2010.

369. Grootenboers MJ, Schramel FM, van Boven WJ, et al.: Selective pulmonary artery perfusion followed by blood flow occlusion: new challenge for the treatment of pulmonary malignancies, *Lung Cancer* 63:400–404, 2009.

370. Ahrar K, Price RE, Wallace MJ, et al.: Percutaneous radiofrequency ablation of lung tumors in a large animal model, *J Vasc Interv Radiol* 14:1037–1043, 2003.

371. Muller H, Guadagni S: Regional chemotherapy for carcinoma of the lung, *Surg Oncol Clin North Am* 17:895–991, 2008.

372. van Putte BP, Grootenboers M, van Boven WJ, et al.: Selective pulmonary artery perfusion for the treatment of primary lung cancer: improved drug exposure of the lung, *Lung Cancer* 65:208–213, 2009.

373. Ogilvie GK, Weigel RM, Haschek WM, et al.: Prognostic factors for tumor remission and survival in dogs after surgery for primary lung tumor: 76 cases (1975-1985), *J Am Vet Med Assoc* 195:109–112, 1989.

374. Polton GA, Brearley MJ, Powell SM, et al.: Impact of primary tumour stage on survival in dogs with solitary lung tumours, *J Small Anim Pract* 49:66–71, 2008.

375. Jemal A, Center MM, DeSantis C, et al.: Global patterns of cancer incidence and mortality rates and trends, *Cancer Epidemiol Biomarkers Prev* 19:1893–1907, 2010.

376. Valaitis J, Warren S, Gamble D: Increasing incidence of adenocarcinoma of the lung, *Cancer* 47:1042–1046, 1981.

377. Westra WH, Slebos RJ, Offerhaus GJ, et al.: K-ras oncogene activation in lung adenocarcinomas from former smokers. Evidence that K-ras mutations are an early and irreversible event in the development of adenocarcinoma of the lung, *Cancer* 72:432–438, 1993.

378. Brahmer JR, Govindan R, Anders RA, et al.: The Society for Immunotherapy of Cancer consensus statement on immunotherapy for the treatment of non-small cell lung cancer (NSCLC), *J Immunother Cancer* 6:75, 2018.

379. Maekawa N, Konnai S, Ikebuchi R, et al.: Expression of PD-L1 on canine tumor cells and enhancement of IFN-gamma production from tumor-infiltrating cells by PD-L1 blockade, *PLoS One* 9:e98415, 2014.

380. Maekawa N, Konnai S, Okagawa T, et al.: Immunohistochemical analysis of PD-L1 expression in canine malignant cancers and PD-1 expression on lymphocytes in canine oral melanoma, *PLoS One* 11:e0157176, 2016.

381. Maekawa N, Konnai S, Takagi S, et al.: A canine chimeric monoclonal antibody targeting PD-L1 and its clinical efficacy in canine oral malignant melanoma or undifferentiated sarcoma, *Sci Rep* 7:8951, 2017.

382. Hartley G, Faulhaber E, Caldwell A, et al.: Immune regulation of canine tumour and macrophage PD-L1 expression, *Vet Comp Oncol* 15:534–549, 2017.

383. Shosu K, Sakurai M, Inoue K, et al.: Programmed cell death ligand 1 expression in canine cancer. *In Vivo* 30:195–204, 2016.

384. Postorino NC, Wheeler SL, Park RD, et al.: A syndrome resembling lymphomatoid granulomatosis in the dog, *J Vet Intern Med* 3:15–19, 1989.

385. Shimazaki T, Nagata M, Goto-Koshino Y, et al.: A case of canine lymphomatoid granulomatosis with cutaneous lesions, *J Vet Med Sci* 72:1061–1067, 2010.

386. Needle DB, Hollinger C, Singer LM, et al.: Pathology in practice. Lymphomatoid granulomatosis of lung tissue and mediastinal lymph node in a dog, *J Am Vet Med Assoc* 247:1113–1116, 2015.

387. Berry CR, Moore PF, Thomas WP, et al.: Pulmonary lymphomatoid granulomatosis in seven dogs (1976-1987), *J Vet Intern Med* 4:157–166, 1990.

25

Tumors of the Skeletal System

NICOLE P. EHRHART, NEIL I. CHRISTENSEN, AND TIMOTHY M. FAN

Osteosarcoma in Dogs

Incidence and Risk Factors

Osteosarcoma (OSA) is the most common primary bone tumor in dogs, accounting for up to 85% of malignancies originating in the skeleton.[1–5] OSA is estimated to occur in more than 10,000 dogs each year in the United States; however, this is probably an underestimation because not all cases are confirmed nor recorded.[6,7] The demographics of canine OSA have been well reported.[8–19] It is largely a disease of middle-aged to older dogs, with a median age of 7 years. There is a large range in age of onset, with a reported case in a 6-month-old pup and a small early peak in age incidence at 18 to 24 months.[13] Primary rib OSA tends to occur in younger adult dogs, with a mean age of 4.5 to 5.4 years.[20,21] OSA is classically a cancer of large and giant breeds. In a review of 1462 cases of canine OSA, dogs weighing more than 40 kg accounted for 29% of all cases and only 5% of their tumors occurred in the axial skeleton. Only 5% of OSA occurred in dogs weighing less than 15 kg, but 59% of their tumors originated in the axial skeleton. Increasing weight and, more specifically, height appear to be the most predictive factors for OSA in dogs.[22] The breeds most at risk for OSA are Saint Bernard, Great Dane, Irish Setter, Doberman Pinscher, Rottweiler, German Shepherd, and Golden Retriever; however, size seems to be a more important predisposing factor than breed.[1,2,4,8,9,13,17,19,22] A hereditary basis for the formation of OSA has been suspected based primarily on the breed prevalence of the disease as well as the subjective assessment of increased incidence in some related families. With regard to gender, males are slightly more frequently affected than females (1.1–1.5: 1)[2,3,9,12,13,16] with the exception of the Saint Bernard, Rottweiler, and Great Dane, and for dogs with primary OSA of the axial skeleton (except rib and spine), in which affected females outnumber males.[2,21] Intact males and females have an increased risk for OSA.[22] However, in Rottweilers, male and female dogs that underwent gonadectomy before 1 year of age had an approximate one in four lifetime risk for bone sarcoma and were significantly more likely to develop bone sarcoma than dogs that were sexually intact.[23] There was a highly significant inverse dose-response relationship between duration of lifetime gonadal exposure and incidence rate of bone sarcoma independent of adult height or body weight.

Approximately 75% of OSAs occur in the appendicular skeleton with the remainder occurring in the axial skeleton.[2,21] The metaphyseal region of long bones is the most common primary site, with thoracic limbs affected twice as often as pelvic limbs and the distal radius and proximal humerus as the two most common locations.[11] In the pelvic limbs, tumors are fairly evenly distributed between the distal femur, distal tibia, and proximal tibia, with the proximal femur a slightly less common site.[2] Primary OSA distal to the antebrachiocarpal and tarsocrural joints is relatively rare in dogs.[24] In 116 cases of canine primary OSA in the axial skeleton, 27% were located in the mandible, 22% in the maxilla, 15% in the spine, 14% in the cranium, 10% in ribs, 9% in the nasal cavity or paranasal sinuses, and 6% in the pelvis.[21] Clinically documentable multicentric OSA at the time of initial diagnosis occurs in less than 10% of all cases.[25] OSA of extraskeletal sites is rare, but primary OSA has been reported in mammary tissue, subcutaneous tissue, spleen, bowel, liver, kidney, testicle, vagina, eye, gastric ligament, synovium, meninges, and adrenal gland.[26–31]

Etiology

The etiology of canine OSA is generally unknown. Some have speculated a viral cause because OSA can occur in litter mates and may be experimentally induced by injecting OSA cells into canine fetii.[32] However, an etiologic virus has not been isolated.

Physical Factors

A simplistic theory based on circumstantial evidence is that, because OSA tends to occur in major weight-bearing bones adjacent to late closing physes and heavy dogs are predisposed, multiple minor trauma and subsequent injury to sensitive cells in the physeal region may occur. This may initiate the disease by inducing mitogenic signals increasing the probability for the development of a mutant lineage. One in vitro study comparing the incidence of microdamage in cadaver radii of small and large breed dogs found no difference between the two groups.[33] OSA has been associated with metallic implants used for fracture repair, chronic osteomyelitis, and fractures in which no internal repair was used.[34–37] OSA has also been reported at the site of a bone allograft used for fracture repair 5 years previously.[38] Exposure to ionizing radiation can induce OSA.[31,39–47] In plutonium-exposed people, 29% and 71% of the OSAs were in the appendicular and axial skeleton, respectively, with the spine having the most tumors (36%). An almost identical distribution of plutonium-induced OSA was reported for dogs injected with ^{239}Pu as young adults in experimental studies. This distribution of OSA is quite different from the distributions of naturally occurring OSA for both species and appears to be related to bone volume and turnover. Similar findings were seen for dogs injected with ^{226}R.[47]

A distribution favoring bone marrow volume was seen for dogs exposed to strontium-90.[46] OSA is a rare, late complication of radiation therapy (RT) in dogs, with an incidence of less than 5%.[39,41,43–45]

Genetic Factors

Ample evidence exists implicating the involvement of genetic and heritable factors for the development of OSA in dogs. Currently, the most thoroughly described gene mutation that contributes to OSA formation and/or progression in dogs is p53, which is supported by in vitro and in vivo studies.[48–55] In cell culture, missense point mutations within the DNA-binding domain of p53 have been identified in canine OSA cell lines with consequent loss of p53 functionality demonstrated by inappropriate downstream target gene transcription (p21 and MDM2) after genotoxic insult.[50] Similarly, p53 mutations have been identified in dogs with spontaneously arising OSA through various genetic techniques including single-strand conformational polymorphism (SSCP), polymerase chain reaction (PCR), or Southern blotting, followed by nucleotide sequence analysis, whereby missense mutations involving exons 4 to 8 of p53 have been identified in 24% to 47% of all spontaneously arising OSA samples.[48,52,54,55] In addition to exons 4 to 8, the entire gene sequence of p53 has also been assessed by PCR and SSCP from 59 spontaneously arising appendicular and axial OSA samples with missense point mutations affecting p53 identified as the most common gene abnormality.[49] Finally, through the implementation of targeted microarray-based comparative genomic hybridization analysis of 38 canine OSA cases, similar recurrent cytogenetic aberrations classically present in human OSA samples were also identified in OSA specimens collected from dogs, including loss of heterozygosity (LOH) of the p53 gene in 18% of tumors.[56]

Substantiation for the presence of p53 mutations in sporadic canine OSA has also been documented by immunohistochemical studies, as a hallmark of many p53 mutations is enhanced protein stability of this normally labile protein, enabling detection of protein with methodologies such as immunohistochemistry (IHC).[57] In one study of 106 osteogenic tumors, a greater percentage of appendicular (84%) OSAs overexpressed p53 protein in comparison with OSAs arising from the axial skeleton (56%) and other non-OSA bone tumors (20%).[53] Analogously, in a complementary study focusing on 103 OSA samples, 67% stained positively for p53 protein and associated staining intensity was significantly greater in OSAs derived from the appendicular versus axial skeleton.[51] Recently, a homolog within the p53 family of proteins, specifically ΔNp63, has been identified to be involved in canine OSA cellular survival and metastasis. The functionality of ΔNp63 in canine OSA cell lines contributed to apoptosis resistance through perturbations in the balance of proapoptotic Bcl-2 family members, Puma and Noxa, as well as STAT3 phosphorylation and modulation of angiogenesis and invasion through VEGF-A and IL-8 expressions.[58]

Another tumor suppressor gene likely contributing to OSA development is retinoblastoma (RB). Based upon investigations using five tumorigenic immortalized canine OSA cell lines, the RB gene signaling pathway was dysregulated with the persistence of hyperphosphorylated RB protein in the absence of mitogen stimulation. Despite apparent aberrant RB gene signaling, reduction in RB protein was only identified in one of five cells lines.[50] Corroborating these in vitro findings, the evaluation of

21 spontaneously arising OSAs failed to identify gross RB gene alterations by Southern blotting, and protein expressions of RB were identified in all OSA samples evaluated.[52]

Despite normal protein expression of RB in canine OSA samples, the observed translational normalcy does not exclude the possibility for allelic deletion of the RB gene as prior studies in human OSA samples have demonstrated that LOH at the RB gene locus does not absolutely correlate with inactivation of the RB gene at the protein level.[59] Substantiating the possibility that RB gene may have allelic deletion in spontaneously arising canine OSA, analysis of 38 OSA samples with comparative genomic hybridization techniques identified copy number loss in 29% of cases, resulting in a correlative reduction or absence of RB protein expression in 62% of OSA samples tested.[56] Most recently, the importance of RB functionality in OSA biologic behavior has been explored with aberrant RB-E2F transcriptional regulation contributing to aggressive OSA biologic behavior and worse clinical outcomes. Collectively, these findings support the functional role of the RB-E2F signaling pathway in OSA biology.[60] Based upon these investigative findings, it is likely that aberrations in the RB gene or transcriptional activities participate in sporadic OSA formation and/or progression in dogs.

In addition to p53 and RB gene abnormalities, the phosphatase and tensin homolog (PTEN) tumor suppressor gene is suspected to participate in the genetic pathogenesis of canine OSA. Original in vitro studies conducted with canine OSA cell lines demonstrated that most cell lines (60%) harbored mutations in PTEN. Corroborating the cell line findings, expression of PTEN was either absent (*n* = 6) or variable (*n* = 4) in 15 spontaneously arising OSA samples.[61] Further support for the loss of PTEN gene in canine OSA pathogenesis has been the identification of specific recurrent chromosome copy number aberrations through targeted microarray-based comparative genomic hybridization studies, with the identification of chromosomal region deletions and high recurrent copy number losses encompassing the PTEN gene locus.[56,62] In addition to the PTEN gene, other genes identified by high resolution comparative genome hybridization studies potentially involved in the genetic pathogenesis of OSA included overexpression of RHOC and RUNX2 and under expression of TUSC3.[62] Most recently, through a comparative approach utilizing high resolution oligonucleotide array comparative genomic hybridization, additional disease-associated DNA copy number aberrations have been identified as an ever expanding list of gene candidates that may have functional significance in the development of OSA, including ADAM15, CTC1, MEN1, and CDK7.[63]

A growing body of evidence in dogs supports breed-associated inheritance of OSA, especially in Scottish Deerhounds, Rottweilers, Greyhounds, Great Danes, Saint Bernards, and Irish Wolfhounds.[26,64–69] The presumed hereditary basis for OSA in specific canine breeds has been affirmed through genome-wide analyses whereby 33 genetic loci were identified to contribute to heritable OSA in Greyhounds, Rottweilers, and Irish Wolfhounds. These findings are highly significant and point to a polygenic spectrum of germline risk factors for OSA development in these three breeds with putative genes involved in OSA genesis connected with bone differentiation and growth pathways.[70] Another breed at risk is the Scottish Deerhound with a 15% incidence of OSA[65–67] and a narrow heritability of 0.69, which indicates that 69% of the cause for OSA development in Scottish Deerhounds is due to heritable trait, likely a Mendelian major gene with dominant expression.[67] A confirmatory study of familial OSA development in Scottish Deerhound litters further supports that the inheritance of OSA in this breed could be explained by a single genetic risk factor residing within an autosome.[71]

Although the putative contribution of specific genes in canine OSA development and biology has been more thoroughly explored, the role of microRNAs (miR) and their differential expression, which might contribute to OSA behavior, has recently been studied. In a comparative investigation with human and canine OSA tissue samples with clinically linked data, decreased expression of orthologous miR-134 and miR-544 in canine OSA samples imparted a reduced likelihood of survival and suggest that miR-134 and miR-544 might transcriptionally regulate target genes involved in aggressive behavior.[72] Similarly, the overexpression of miR-9 in canine OSA cell lines was shown to promote a metastatic phenotype through the upregulation of gelsolin, a protein involved in cytoskeletal remodeling.[73] Additionally, the loss of miR-34a in canine OSA cell lines resulted in the enrichment of genes responsible for cell invasion and motility, whereas the forced expression of miR-34a exerted potential anticancer effects through reduced expressions of KLF4, SEM3A, and VEGFA transcripts.[74] Collectively, these initial findings exploring the regulatory role of miRNAs demonstrate their likely contribution to canine OSA biology and pathogenesis.

Molecular Factors

Given the heterogeneous and chaotic nature of OSA, it has been difficult to definitively ascribe specific molecular derangements responsible for the etiopathogenesis of OSA.[75] Nonetheless, substantive progress has been achieved through experimental, preclinical, and comparative investigations to identify dysregulated intracellular signaling and cell survival pathways likely to participate in the pathogenesis of OSA. Significantly, the identification and tumorigenic consequences of several putative pathways have been characterized in immortalized OSA cell lines and spontaneously arising OSA tissue samples.

Tyrosine Protein Kinase MET

The MET protooncogene encodes a tyrosine kinase receptor which, upon ligation with hepatocyte growth factor (HGF), mediates multiple cellular functions including cell scattering, motility, and proliferation. Given its biologic activities, excessive or dysregulated MET signaling in canine OSA has been demonstrated to promote tumorigenic phenotypes in cell lines.[76-78] Furthermore, in a small pilot study with spontaneously arising OSA samples, the expression of MET protooncogene was identified in the majority (71%) of tumor specimens by northern blot analysis.[79] Additionally, a novel germline mutation resulting in enhanced receptor phosphorylation and aberrant MET signaling has been identified primarily in the Rottweiler breed.[80] In a larger study of 59 primary OSA samples, mRNA expression of MET and HGF was detected by real-time PCR (RT-PCR) in all specimens; this suggested the existence of a putative MET/HGF autocrine or paracrine feedback loop.[81]

Insulin-like Growth Factor

The cellular effects of growth hormone (GH) are mediated through the hepatic production of insulin-like growth factor 1 (IGF-1). In osteoblasts, IGF-1 induces cell mitogenesis and protection from apoptosis, as well as promotes angiogenesis. Derived from experimental and preclinical investigations, aberrant or excessive IGF-1 signaling likely participates in OSA pathogenesis. In three canine OSA cell lines, the expression and functionality of the IGF-1/IGF-1 receptor signaling cascade has been reported.[82] Recently, the activation and prognostic significance of the IGF pathway has been investigated in canine OSA cell lines and pet dogs, respectively. In cell lines, molecular studies demonstrated that IGF-1R is expressed and functionally activated by IGF-1 in a paracrine manner and leads to the activation of both MAPK and AKT signaling nodes. Importantly, the protein expression of IGF-1R in canine OSA tissue samples showed that most (71%) naturally occurring tumors express this receptor and that higher expression levels of IGF-1R correlated with a decreased survival time (ST).[83]

Epidermal Growth Factor

The protooncogene erbB-2 encodes human epidermal growth factor receptor 2 (HER2), which is a tyrosine kinase receptor capable of promoting cell transformation and growth. In both dogs and people, the overexpression of HER2 protein as a result of gene amplification is a negative prognostic factor in mammary carcinoma; however, less clarity exists for the role of HER2 overexpression in OSA.[84,85] To better characterize HER2 expressions in canine OSA, one study evaluated HER2 mRNA transcript and protein expression in seven cell lines and 10 OSA tumor specimens.[86] Based on RT-PCR, six of the OSA cell lines and 40% of primary OSA tumor samples overexpressed HER2; results of the study suggested the possibility of HER2 overexpression as a negative prognostic factor for survival.

Mammalian Target of Rapamycin

The mammalian target of rapamycin (mTOR) is an evolutionary conserved protein kinase downstream of AKT, which acts as a central hub for the integration of cellular signals induced by growth factors, nutrients, energy, and stress for the purposes of regulating cell cycle progression and growth. As such, aberrant signaling through the mTOR pathway contributes to growth, survival, and chemotherapy resistance in multiple tumor types. To characterize the functionality of the mTOR pathway in canine OSA, one study using three canine OSA cell lines investigated the expressions of mTOR and p70S6K, a downstream effector protein of mTOR, and demonstrated pathway activity and capacity to inhibit signaling with rapamycin.[87] In a complementary phase I dose-escalation study to assess the feasibility of mTOR inhibition as a treatment strategy, the pharmacokinetics and pharmacodynamics of rapamycin were investigated in dogs with primary OSAs and demonstrated that modulation of mTOR target proteins by rapamycin was achievable within the bone tumor microenvironment.[88]

Hedgehog and Notch

Hedgehog-GLI and Notch-HES1 signaling pathways have been linked to the growth, survival, and metastases of various human tumor histologies and recently have been investigated for their potential role in canine OSA biology. In one investigation, overexpression and functionality of the Hedgehog (HHG) pathway was confirmed in canine OSA cell lines by demonstrating elevated GLI1 and GLI2 transcription factors with correlative downstream target gene upregulation (PTCH1 and PAX6). Additionally, the functionality and biologic consequences of HHG signaling pathway blockade was assessed whereby inhibition of GLI transcription factors by GANT61 resulted in reduced proliferation and colony-forming capacity in canine OSA cell lines.[89] Analogous to HHG signaling, the involvement of the Notch pathway in canine OSA biology has been evaluated through the inclusion of a dichotomous outcome linked array of canine OSA tissues whereby dogs with OSA were categorized into unfavorable (disease-free interval [DFI] <100 days) versus favorable (DFI >300 days) responders. Gene array analysis of Notch/HES1 associated genes suggested

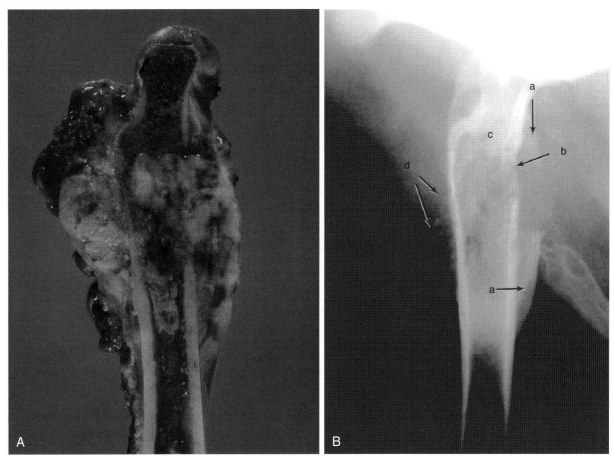

• **Fig. 25.1** (A) Gross, longitudinally split specimen of a proximal femoral osteosarcoma lesion in a dog showing cortical destruction, soft tissue, and osteoid neoplastic components. (B) Lateral radiograph of a proximal femoral osteosarcoma lesion from the case in part A. Radiographic features include *(a)* Codman triangle, *(b)* cortical lysis, *(c)* loss of trabecular pattern in the metaphases, and *(d)* tumor extension into the soft tissues in a sunburst pattern.

that upregulation of Notch signaling might contribute to OSA pathogenesis; however, an inverse relationship between Notch/HES1 with survival outcomes was identified, indicating that other mechanisms that do not alter HES1 expression might be responsible for driving OSA aggressive biology.[90]

Additional Pathways

In addition to various growth and survival pathways that potentially contribute to OSA pathogenesis, the ability of OSA cells to interact with their immediate microenvironment found in bone and lung tissues likely influences OSA progression and metastases. Tissue invasion and focal osteolysis are hallmark characteristics of OSA, and local disease progression is promoted by several OSA-associated proteins including matrix metalloproteinases, receptor activator of NF-κB ligand, lysosomal cathepsin K, endothelin-1, and transforming growth factor β.[91–97] Similar to the ability of OSA cells to invade local tissues, specific proteins have been identified to participate in the progression of canine OSA metastasis including ezrin,[98] a cytoskeletal linker protein, and CXCR4,[99,100] a chemokine receptor.

Pathology and Natural Behavior

OSA is a malignant mesenchymal tumor of primitive bone cells. These cells produce an extracellular matrix of osteoid, and the presence of tumor osteoid is the basis for the histologic diagnosis and differentiating OSAs from other sarcomas of bone. The

histologic pattern may vary between tumors or even within the same tumor. There are many histologic subclassifications of OSA, which are based on the type and amount of matrix and characteristics of the cells: osteoblastic, chondroblastic, fibroblastic, poorly differentiated, and telangiectatic. Alkaline phosphatase staining on histopathologic and aspiration cytology specimens has been shown to aid in differentiating OSA from other connective tissue tumors.[101–103] In dogs, it has not been well established that there is a difference in the biologic behavior of the different histologic subclassifications or histologic grades. Some investigations indicate that histologic grade is predictive of behavior, whereas other studies cast doubt on the predictive value of routine histologic grading.[104,105] Newer techniques designed to recognize molecular or genetic alterations are being evaluated to determine their potential use in predicting behavior of OSA.[106] The degree of aneuploidy of primary and metastatic tumors, as measured by flow cytometry, is potentially indicative of biologic behavior.[75] OSA has very aggressive local effects and causes lysis, bone production, or both (Fig. 25.1). Pathologic fracture at presentation in people and dogs with OSA does not preclude limb salvage surgery (LSS) and does not carry a worse prognosis than patients without fracture at presentation;[107–110] however, dogs presenting with pathologic fracture or high risk for pathologic fracture are poor candidates for treatment with stereotactic radiotherapy (SRT) and concurrent surgical stabilization given the high rate for major local complications such as infection and implant failure.[111,112]

Metastasis is very common and arises early in the course of the disease, although usually subclinically. Although less than 15% of dogs have radiographically detectable pulmonary or osseous metastasis at presentation, approximately 90% will die within 1 year (median ST [MST] of 19 weeks) with metastatic disease, usually to the lungs, when amputation is the only treatment.[2,16] Metastasis via the hematogenous route is most common; however, on rare occasions, metastasis to the regional lymph node (LN) may occur.[113] Although the lung is the most commonly reported site for metastasis, metastasis to bones or other soft tissue sites occurs with some frequency.[114] An increase in the incidence of bone metastasis after systemic chemotherapy has also been documented in humans and is suspected in dogs.[115,116] Suspected synchronous regional bone metastases (skip metastases) has also been reported.[117] Advanced imaging modalities, including bone scintigraphy, magnetic resonance imaging (MRI), computed tomography (CT), and positron emission tomography (PET)/CT scans, can aid in detection of occult skip metastases.[118,119] Some differences in metastatic behavior have been observed based on the anatomic location of the primary OSA site as well as anatomic skeletal size. For appendicular OSA arising from less common sites, including the ulna, retrospective investigations suggest that OSA behavior may be slightly less metastatic; however, more thorough studies are necessary to draw firmer conclusions.[120,121] Primary OSA arising from axial sites, such as mandible and calvarium, may have a less aggressive metastatic behavior too, although contradictory evidence exists as local tumor recurrence and subsequent regional disease failure might lead to early death and underestimation of the true metastatic potential of OSA arising from these sites.[122–125] In addition to primary tumor location, metastatic phenotype of OSA might be influenced by breed, size, or, more likely, genetics associated with small breed dogs. One recent investigation described the outcomes of 51 small breed dogs diagnosed with appendicular OSA and identified no difference in MSTs between dogs treated with amputation alone versus curative-intent therapy (local treatment and adjuvant chemotherapy).[126] Although preliminary in nature, these observational findings might suggest that the biologic behavior and associated metastatic potential of appendicular OSA is divergent between dogs of differing skeletal size.

History and Clinical Signs

Dogs with appendicular OSA generally present with a lameness and swelling at the primary site. There may be a history of mild trauma just before the onset of lameness. This history can often lead to misdiagnosis of an orthopedic or soft tissue injury. The lameness worsens and a moderately firm to soft, variably painful swelling may arise at the primary site. Dogs may present with acute, severe lameness associated with pathologic fractures, although pathologic fractures account for less than 3% of all fractures.[127] Up to 60% of these dogs are lame for a period before presentation.[107] Large and giant breed dogs that present with lameness or localized swelling at metaphyseal sites should be evaluated with OSA as a likely diagnosis. The pathophysiology of OSA pain is unclear but may be mediated by loss of mechanical bone strength resulting in microfractures, infiltration or compression of nerves, and the chemotaxis of immune cells with subsequent secretion of cytokines and proteases resulting in inflammatory pain. OSA cells have also been shown to secrete nociceptive ligands potentially resulting in pain generation.[97]

The signs associated with axial skeletal OSA are site dependent. Signs vary from localized swelling with or without lameness (scapular, pelvic, or rib sites) to dysphagia (oral sites), exophthalmos and pain on opening the mouth (caudal mandibular or orbital sites), facial deformity and nasal discharge (sinus and nasal cavity sites), and hyperesthesia with or without neurologic signs (spinal sites). Dogs with tumors arising from ribs usually present because of a palpable, variably painful mass. Respiratory signs are uncommon even when the lesions have large intrathoracic components; malignant pleural effusion is quite rare. Dogs rarely have respiratory signs as the first clinical evidence of pulmonary metastasis; rather, their first signs are usually nonspecific. With radiographically detectable pulmonary metastasis, dogs may remain asymptomatic for many months, but most dogs develop decreased appetite and nonspecific signs such as malaise within 1 month. Hypertrophic osteopathy may develop in dogs with pulmonary metastasis.

Systemic Alterations

Alterations in energy expenditure, protein synthesis, urinary nitrogen loss, and carbohydrate flux have been documented in dogs with OSA, similar to humans with neoplasia.[128] Changes in resting energy expenditure as well as protein and carbohydrate metabolism have been documented in dogs with OSA. These changes were evident even in dogs that did not have clinical signs of cachexia.[128] Although weight loss can occur during therapy for OSA, this has not been associated with worse outcomes.[129] Systemic metabolic derangements reported for dogs with OSA include lower chromium and zinc levels, lower iron and iron binding capacity, and increased ferritin levels compared with normal dogs.[130]

Diagnostic Techniques and Workup

Radiology

Initial evaluation of the primary site involves interpretation of good quality radiographs taken in lateral and craniocaudal projections. Special views may be necessary for lesions occurring in sites other than in the appendicular skeleton. The overall radiographic abnormality of bone varies from mostly bone lysis to almost entirely osteoblastic or osteogenic changes. There is an entire spectrum of changes between these two extremes, and the appearance of primary bone tumors can be quite variable. There are some features, however, that are commonly seen. Cortical lysis is a feature of primary bone tumors and may be severe enough to leave obvious areas of discontinuity of the cortex leading to pathologic fracture. There is often soft tissue extension with an obvious soft tissue swelling, and new bone (tumor or reactive bone) may form in these areas in a palisading pattern perpendicular or radiating from the axis of the cortex (i.e., sunburst). As the tumor invades the cortex, the periosteum is elevated, and new bone is laid down by the cambium layer providing a triangular appearing deposition of dense new bone on the cortex at the periphery of the lesion. This periosteal new bone has been called Codman triangle, but this is not pathognomonic for OSA. OSA rarely crosses articular cartilage, and primary lesions usually remain monostotic. The tumors may extend into periarticular soft tissues, however, and adjacent bones are at risk because of extension through adjacent soft tissue structures. Other radiographic changes associated with primary bone tumors include loss of the fine trabecular pattern in the metaphysis, a long transition zone at the periphery of the medullary extent of the lesion (rather than a sharp sclerotic margin), or areas of fine punctate lysis. Any one or combinations of these changes may be seen, depending on the size, histologic subtype, location, and duration of the lesion.

Differential diagnoses of lytic, proliferative, or mixed pattern aggressive bone lesions identified on radiographs include: other primary bone tumors (chondrosarcoma [CSA], fibrosarcoma [FSA], hemangiosarcoma [HSA]); metastatic bone cancer; multiple myeloma or lymphoma of bone; fungal osteomyelitis; bacterial osteomyelitis; and, albeit rare, bone cysts. Other primary bone tumors are far less common than OSA but may be suspected, especially in dogs with unusual signalment or tumor location. The radiographic appearance of primary bone tumors is similar to osteomyelitis, specifically fungal osteomyelitis.[131] In cases in which the travel or clinical history might support the possibility of osteomyelitis, a biopsy with submission for histology and culture may be warranted. Metastatic cancer can spread to bone from almost any malignancy, but is most commonly encountered from genitourinary carcinomas.[132] A careful physical examination is important, including a rectal examination, with special attention paid to the genitourinary system to help rule out the presence of a primary cancer. Common sites for metastatic bone cancer are lumbar and sacral vertebrae, pelvis, ribs, and diaphyses of long bones.[132] There are usually other clues for the diagnosis of multiple myeloma, such as hyperproteinemia, and both multiple myeloma and lymphoma of bone are usually associated with radiographic lesions that are almost entirely lytic.

Tissue Biopsy

A diagnosis of primary malignant bone tumor may be suggested by signalment, history, physical examination, and radiographic findings. Cytology has not been thought to be definitive for diagnosis; however, recent evidence indicates a high accuracy for diagnosis of sarcoma and, in combination with alkaline phosphatase staining, high specificity to support the diagnosis of OSA. Consistent cytologic criteria of OSA has recently been described; with repeated evaluations and dependent on experience, cytopathologists may be more definitive in making a diagnosis from cytology alone.[133,134] Alkaline phosphatase staining of cytologic samples has been shown to differentiate OSA from other vimentin-positive tumors;[101] however, in cases in which cytology is equivocal, a definitive diagnosis requires histopathologic assessment of a tissue sample. It is crucial that the biopsy procedure is planned and performed carefully with close attention to asepsis, hemostasis, and wound closure.[135] The skin incision for the biopsy must be small and placed such that it can be completely excised or included with the tumor if limb salvage surgery (LSS) or SRT is chosen. Poorly placed biopsy tracts can result in excessive normal tissue exposure (radiation) or difficulties in closure (LSS). Transverse or large incisions must be avoided. Ideally, the surgeon who is to perform the definitive surgical procedure (especially if this is LSS) should be the person to perform the preoperative bone biopsy.[136]

Bone biopsy may be performed as an open incisional, closed needle, or trephine biopsy (Fig. 25.2). The advantage of the open techniques is that a large sample of tissue is procured, which presumably improves the likelihood of establishing an accurate histologic diagnosis. Unfortunately, this advantage may be outweighed by the disadvantages of an involved operative procedure and risk of postsurgical complications such as hematoma formation, wound breakdown, infection, local seeding of tumor, and pathologic fracture.[137,138] Although biopsy with a trephine yields a diagnostic accuracy rate of 93.8%, there is increased risk of creating pathologic fracture than with a smaller gauge needle.[139] This underscores some of the advantages of a closed biopsy using a Jamshidi bone marrow biopsy needle or similar type of needle. Jamshidi

needle biopsy has an accuracy rate of 91.9% for detecting tumor versus other disorders and an 82.3% accuracy rate for diagnosis of specific tumor subtype.[140] Accuracy of diagnoses from needle core samples can be dependent on the experience of the pathologist and comfort level with examination of small samples. Histology reports indicating the presence of reactive bone should not rule out the presence of a primary bone tumor or other pathology, especially if the radiographic changes suggest tumor. In some cases, it can be very difficult to get the diagnosis by preoperative biopsy (i.e., repeated biopsy attempts yield "reactive bone"), and yet the pathologist has no trouble identifying tumor when the entire specimen is available for histopathologic analysis. This is likely because of the heterogeneity of the tumor tissue itself and the large amount of reactive bone present within the tumor.

The biopsy site is selected carefully. Radiographs (two projections) are reviewed and the center of the lesion chosen for biopsy. Biopsy at the lesion periphery will often result in sampling the reactive bone surrounding the tumor without a resulting diagnosis.[140] The skin incision is made so the biopsy tract and any potentially seeded tumor cells can be completely removed at the time of definitive surgery. Care is used to avoid major nerves, vessels, and joint spaces. A 4-inch, 8- or 11-gauge needle is used. With the dog anesthetized, prepared, and draped for surgery, a small stab incision (2–3 mm) is made in the skin with a #11 scalpel blade. The bone needle cannula, with the stylet locked in place, is pushed through the soft tissue to the bone cortex. The stylet is removed and the cannula is advanced through the bone cortex into the medullary cavity using a gentle twisting motion and firm pressure. The opposite cortex is not penetrated. The needle is removed and the specimen is gently pushed out of the base of the cannula by inserting the probe into the cannula tip. One or two more samples can be obtained by redirecting the needle through the same skin incision so that samples of the transition zone may also be obtained. Ideal specimens should be 1 or 2 cm in length and not fragmented. Biopsy is repeated until solid tissue cores are obtained. Material for culture and cytology may be taken from the samples before fixation in 10% neutral buffered formalin. Diagnostic accuracy is improved when samples are evaluated by a pathologist thoroughly familiar with bone cancer. Fluoroscopy or advanced imaging (CT) can assist in obtaining needle-core biopsy samples of suspected bone lesions, especially for axial sites.[141]

After tumor removal (amputation or limb sparing), histology should be performed on a larger specimen to confirm the preoperative diagnosis. If the clinical and radiographic features are typical for a primary bone tumor, especially when there is little possibility of fungal or bacterial infection, confirmation of histologic diagnosis after surgical treatment of local disease (amputation or limb sparing) can be considered. Few diseases causing advanced destruction of the bone can be effectively treated without removal of the local disease. If the owners are willing to treat aggressively, surgical removal of local disease with biopsy submission after surgery may be acceptable.

Staging and Patient Assessment

Systemic Staging

Examination for evidence of apparent spread of the disease is important. Regional LNs, although rarely involved, should be palpated and fine needle cytology performed on any enlarged LN.[113] Sites of bone metastasis may be detected by a careful orthopedic examination with palpation of long bones and the accessible axial skeleton. Organomegaly may be detected by abdominal palpation. Usually pulmonary metastases are undetectable by clinical

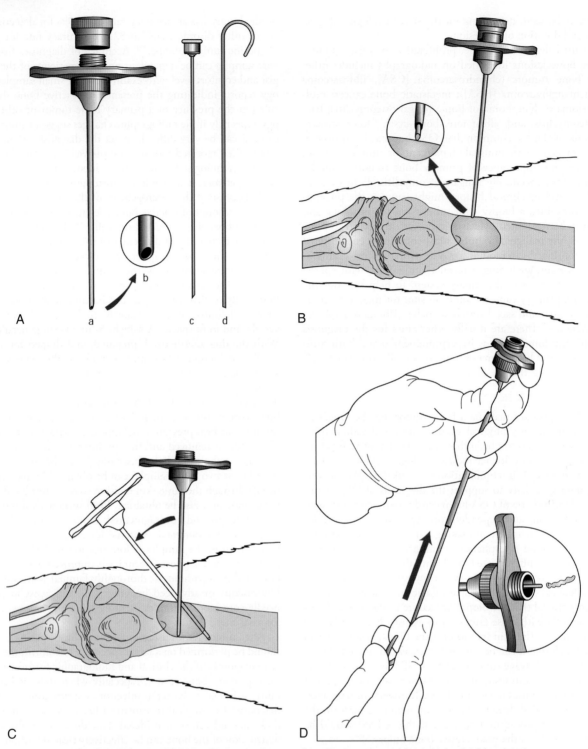

• **Fig. 25.2** (A) The Jamshidi bone biopsy needle: cannula and screw-on cap (d), tapered point (b), pointed stylet to advance cannula through soft tissues (c), and probe to expel specimen from cannula (d). (B) With the stylet locked in place, the cannula is advanced through the soft tissue until bone is reached. The inset is a close-up view showing stylet against bone cortex. (C) The stylet is removed and the bone cortex penetrated with the cannula. The cannula is withdrawn and the procedure repeated with redirection of the instrument to obtain multiple core samples. (D) The probe is then inserted retrograde into the tip of the cannula to expel the specimen through the base (inset). (Reprinted with permission from Powers BE, LaRue SM, Withrow SJ, et al. *J Am Vet Med Assoc.* 1988; 193(2):206–207.[140])

examination, but careful thoracic auscultation is important to detect concurrent cardiopulmonary disorders.

High detail thoracic radiographs should be taken during inspiration in a conscious patient. Although some controversy exists,[142] three-view thoracic radiographs are recommended for the assessment of pulmonary metastasis: a ventrodorsal or dorsoventral view and both right and left lateral views. OSA pulmonary metastases are generally soft tissue dense and cannot be detected radiographically until the nodules are 7 to 9 mm in diameter. Pulmonary metastasis is uncommon at the time of diagnosis

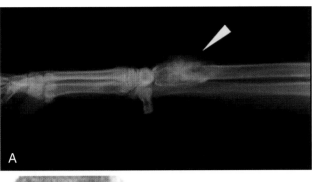
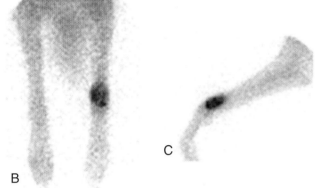

• **Fig. 25.3** Scintigraphic view of a distal radial osteosarcoma lesion in a dog after technetium-99M-hydroxymethylene diphosphonate injection. (A) Lateral radiograph demonstrating mixed osteolytic/osteoblastic bone lesion affecting distal radius (*yellow arrowhead*). (B) Anterior posterior and (C) lateral bone scintigraphy images 90 minutes postintravenous injection demonstrate preferential accumulation of technetium-99M at focal site of increased bone turnover.

(less than 10% of dogs). Advanced imaging (e.g., CT, MRI, PET/CT) may play a role in patient staging and is used to evaluate for pulmonary metastases and for evaluation of tumor vascularity, soft tissue and medullary involvement/tumor size, and response to treatment.[143–145] Multiple studies have demonstrated increased sensitivity of thoracic CT compared with thoracic radiography for the detection of pulmonary metastases;[118,119,146,147] however, published treatment and patient outcomes are generally based on patients staged by thoracic radiographs. As advanced imaging becomes more commonplace for staging dogs with OSA, comparisons to previous protocols will be subject to stage-migration and lead-time bias due to earlier detection of metastases.

Bone survey radiography may be useful for identifying second skeletal sites of OSA.[25] Bone survey radiographs include lateral radiographs of all bones in the body and a ventrodorsal projection of the pelvis using standard radiographic technique appropriate for the region radiographed. There are conflicting reports on the usefulness of nuclear scintigraphy (Fig. 25.3) for clinical staging of dogs with OSA.[148–152] Bone scintigraphy was used in one study to identify suspected second bone sites in 14 of 25 dogs with appendicular OSA;[149] seven of these lesions were biopsied and confirmed to be OSA. Another study of 70 dogs with appendicular primary bone tumors resulted in only one scintigraphically detectable occult bone lesion.[148] In a third report of 23 dogs with suspected skeletal neoplasia evaluated with scintigraphy and radiography, four dogs had second skeletal sites suspected to be neoplastic.[152] The suspicious site in one of these dogs was found on histologic evaluation to be normal bone. Another study found

secondary sites considered highly suspect of bony metastasis in 7.8% of (399) cases; however, most suspected lesions were not confirmed histologically.[150] A recent pilot study compared the utility of survey radiography, whole body CT, and nuclear scintigraphy for the detection of OSA metastasis in 15 dogs.[119] Nuclear scintigraphy was found to be the most useful modality for the detection of occult bone metastases; however, false positives did occur, and the diagnosis of metastasis was based on a gold standard reference constructed using all available imaging modalities, history, and signalment rather than histopathologic confirmation.

Abdominal ultrasound has been recommended by some veterinary oncologists to stage for visceral organ metastasis. Two recent retrospective studies documented abdominal metastases in 0% to 2.5% of cases, with sites of metastasis including the kidney, liver, and iliac LNs.[153,154] In four of 80 cases (5%), a second primary neoplasm was diagnosed, and in two of these cases, the mass was palpable on physical examination. Both studies suggest abdominal ultrasound is a low-yield diagnostic test but is warranted in patients with palpable abdominal abnormalities.

Surgical Staging

A surgical staging system for sarcomas of the skeleton has been devised for people.[155] This system is based on the histologic grade (G), the anatomic setting of the primary tumor (T), and regional or distant metastasis (M). There are three stages: stage I—low-grade (G_1) lesions without metastasis; stage II—high-grade (G_2) lesions without metastasis; and stage III—lesions with regional or distant metastasis regardless of histologic grade. The stages are subdivided by the anatomic setting with A being intracompartmental (T_1) and B being extracompartmental (T_2). According to this system, most dogs with OSA present with stage IIB disease. CT or PET/CT can be used to evaluate the degree of bone involvement from a primary bone tumor and distant metastasis.[145,156] Scintigraphy has also been used to determine extent of local disease, but in one study, scintigraphy overestimated the length of OSA disease in LSS patients by 30%.[157] CT may be useful to plan surgical margins, especially for tumors located in the axial skeleton; however, one study reported that survey radiographs were as accurate as advanced imaging (CT, MRI) in predicting true length of tumor involvement.[158] In contrast, it is anticipated that PET/CT, with its dual molecular and anatomic imaging capabilities, will have high sensitivity for assessing local tumor size, as well as detecting the presence of distant metastases.

Known or Suggested Prognostic Factors

Anatomic Location and Signalment

In a multiinstitutional study of 162 dogs with appendicular OSA treated with amputation alone, dogs younger than 5 years of age had shorter survival than older dogs; however, a recent large meta-analysis study did not identify age as being prognostic for the development of metastases.[16,159] Additional studies have found that large tumor size[13,160,161] and humeral location[162,163] are associated with a poor outcome, and a recent meta-analysis supports that proximal humeral OSA is a significant negative prognostic factor for both DFI and ST.[164] For OSA originating from flat bones, small dog size and completeness of excision were positive prognostic indicators.[124,165] Although strong conclusions cannot be made, a recent study suggested that small breed dogs with appendicular OSA may have improved STs compared with large breed dogs after the institution of curative-intent therapies.[126]

Higher histologic grade and mitotic index may be predictive for a poorer prognosis; however, the prognostic value of histologic grade for predicting biologic behavior remains controversial as study results are contradictory.[104,105]

The biologic behavior for less common appendicular (ulna) and nonappendicular sites of OSA appears to be similar (aggressive), with the exception of the mandible and possibly other calvarial sites.[120,122,123,166–168] OSA of the head (mandible, maxilla, and skull) is locally aggressive but has a lower metastatic rate than appendicular OSA.[124] In a study of 183 dogs, local recurrence or progression occurred in 51.3% of dogs, and 38.5% of dogs developed distant metastases; the overall MST was 239 days.[124] Dogs with OSA of the mandible treated with mandibulectomy alone had a 1-year survival rate of 71% in one study,[122] suggesting a less aggressive biologic behavior. A second study of 50 dogs with mandibular OSA also confirmed improved STs relative to appendicular OSA; however, the majority of dogs (58%) still developed metastatic disease, and the addition of adjuvant chemotherapy to mandibulectomy resulted in a significantly improved ST.[125] In contrast, maxillary OSA has a MST of 5 months after maxillectomy.[167,168] The MST for dogs with rib OSA lesions is 3 months after chest wall resection alone and 8 months after treatment with chest wall resection and adjuvant chemotherapy.[169–172] Scapular OSA has a guarded prognosis when treated with subtotal scapulectomy surgery and chemotherapy;[165,173,174] The DFI and MST in dogs diagnosed with scapular OSA were 210 days and 246 days, respectively.[121] Limb function after subtotal scapulectomy is good to excellent.[121] Survival of dogs with OSA distal to the antebrachiocarpal or tarsocrural joints was somewhat longer (MST 466 days) than survival of dogs with OSA of more common appendicular sites; however, OSA in these sites is aggressive with a high potential for metastasis.[24] Vertebral OSA is uncommon, but it is locally aggressive and local tumor recurrence or progressive disease is common after conservative surgical approaches.[21,175] In 15 dogs treated with a combination of surgery, RT, and chemotherapy, the MST was 4 months.[175] For dogs with pelvic OSA treated with hemipelvectomy, the local recurrence and metastatic rates were 21% and 46%, respectively, with a mean ST of 533 days and 1- and 2-year survival rates of 53% and 35%, respectively.[176] The biologic behavior of OSA in other nonappendicular bone sites has not been thoroughly evaluated.

Extraskeletal OSA is rare and most commonly affects visceral sites (gastrointestinal [GI] tract, spleen, liver, kidney, urinary bladder), skin or subcutaneous tissue, or mammary glands. Extraskeletal (soft tissue) OSA sites also appear to have aggressive systemic behavior with a high metastatic rate. In one report, dogs with extraskeletal OSA treated with surgery alone had a MST of only 1 month, and dogs treated with surgery and adjuvant chemotherapy had a MST of 5 months.[27] In a larger study, soft tissue and mammary OSAs were separated; the MST for dogs with nonmammary gland soft tissue OSA was 1 month and 3 months for dogs with mammary gland OSA after surgical resection alone.[28] The major cause of death was local recurrence (92%) in dogs with soft tissue OSA cases and pulmonary metastasis (62.5%) in dogs with mammary gland OSA.

Dogs presenting with stage III disease (measurable metastasis) have a very poor prognosis; however, improved survival may be achievable when appropriate metastasectomy (tumor control >300 days and <3 pulmonary nodules) is performed.[114,177] The MST for 90 dogs with stage III disease at presentation was 76 days. Dogs with bone metastasis (132 days) had a longer ST (132 days) than dogs with lung metastasis (59 days) or lung and other

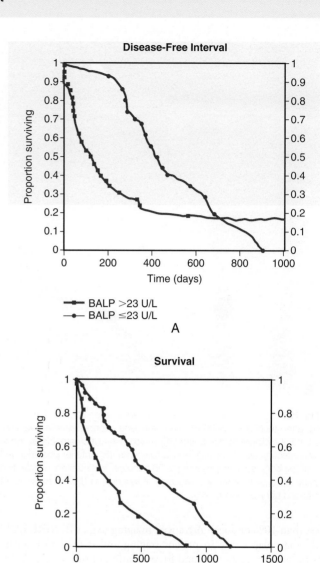

• **Fig. 25.4** (A) Disease-free interval outcome of dogs treated for osteosarcoma comparing preoperative bone alkaline phosphatase levels higher than and lower than 23 U/L. (B) Survival outcome of dogs treated for osteosarcoma comparing preoperative serum alkaline phosphatase levels higher than and lower than 110 U/L. (Reprinted with permission from Ehrhart N, Dernell WS, Hoffmann WE, et al. *J Am Vet Med Assoc*. 1998; 213:1002–1006.[178])

soft tissue metastases (19 days). Dogs with LN metastasis have a significantly shorter MST (59 days) than dogs without LN metastasis (318 days).[113,114] In dogs with stage III disease treated with metastasectomy, the MST (232 days) was significantly longer than for dogs not treated with metastasectomy (49 days).[177]

Serum Alkaline Phosphatase

Elevated alkaline phosphatase (ALP) has been clearly associated with a poorer prognosis for dogs with appendicular and rib OSA in several individual studies[113,162,178–181] and two recent large meta-analyses.[159,164] A preoperative elevation of either total (serum) or bone isoenzyme of ALP (greater than 110 U/L or 23 U/L, respectively) is associated with a shorter DFI and ST (Fig. 25.4).

The reasons for why serum ALP may impart a negative prognosis have been incompletely explored; however, two recent investigations postulate putative mechanisms. In one study of 96 dogs with appendicular OSA, a positive correlation between serum bone ALP and absolute tumor size was identified; in dogs with progressive OSA metastatic burden, serum bone ALP increased and coincided with the development of macroscopic metastases.[182] Based upon these findings, the association between increased pretreatment bone ALP and negative clinical prognosis may simply be attributed to a greater initial tumor burden and advanced clinical stage of disease.[182] In a second study, increased bone ALP was suggested as an epiphenomenon to active endothelin-1 signaling by malignant OSA cells whereby the secretion of endothelin-1 by OSA cells endowed a protumorigenic advantage and secondary "passenger" bone ALP production given the osteoblastic properties of endothelin-1 signaling.[96] These two studies suggesting that elevations in bone ALP may be an epiphenomenon of either tumor burden or osteoblastic signaling pathways are consistent with a third study demonstrating that canine OSA cell lines derived from dogs with differing bone ALP concentrations (normal versus high) do not differ in their in vitro protumorigenic potentials.[183]

Molecular, Genetic, and Immunologic Indices of Prognosis

The expression of several molecular proteins, including ezrin, recepteur d'origine Nantaise (RON), survivin, vascular endothelial growth factor (VEGF), cyclooxygenase-2 (COX-2), and heat shock protein (HSP), has been reported to influence DFIs and STs in dogs.[98,184–188] Ezrin is a cellular protein belonging to the ezrin-radixin-moesin family and serves as a physical and functional anchor site for cytoskeletal F-actin fibers. Given the involvement of ezrin in cytoskeletal remodeling, it has been demonstrated in murine preclinical models that ezrin is necessary for OSA metastases.[98] Through the use of a canine tissue microarray with known clinical outcome data, the presence of high ezrin staining in primary tumors was associated with a significantly shorter median DFI (116 days) compared with dogs with low primary tumor ezrin staining (188 days).

Hepatocyte growth factor receptor (MET) and RON are members of the MET protooncogene family of receptor tyrosine kinases, and signaling through MET or RON promotes tumorigenesis and the formation of metastases. MET and RON are capable of heterodimerization with one another, resulting in cellular crosstalk that may alter the strength and duration of signal transduction with resultant protumorigenic effects. Given the role of MET and RON in metastases, their expression in OSA has been evaluated in dogs.[184] Through the use of a canine OSA tissue array with linked outcome data, expression of RON, but not MET, was prognostic for survival. Dogs with high RON expression in their primary tumors had significantly decreased STs than dogs with absent, low, or intermediate RON expression.

Survivin is a small protein belonging to the inhibitor of apoptosis family and participates in the processes of cell division as well as apoptosis inhibition. As a dimer, survivin inhibits both caspase-dependent and -independent mediated apoptosis, and its expression can promote tumorigenesis. Given the antiapoptotic properties of survivin, its overexpression may provide a survival advantage to cancer cells and be associated with a negative prognosis. In one study, the expression of survivin was characterized in 67 primary OSA samples with known outcome data.[186] Survivin expression was detected in 65 tissue samples and expression intensity was associated with DFI. Dogs with primary tumors expressing low survivin immunoreactivity scores achieved a significantly

longer DFI (331 days) than dogs with high survivin immunoreactivity scores within the primary tumor (173 days).

VEGF and the enzymatic activities of COX-2 serve as potent regulators of angiogenesis, and their independent expressions have been associated with poorer prognosis for a variety of cancers. Given that angiogenesis is a necessary step for tumor growth and metastases, both VEGF and COX-2 have been investigated in dogs with OSA.[185,187,189] In one study of 25 dogs treated with definitive surgery and systemic chemotherapy, baseline platelet-corrected serum VEGF concentrations were associated with DFI, but not ST.[187] Dogs with VEGF concentration in the lower 50th percentile achieved a significantly longer DFI (356 days) than dogs with VEGF levels in the upper 50th percentile (145 days). In two studies, COX-2 expression was characterized in primary tumors derived from 44 dogs and 27 dogs, respectively, with positive COX-2 staining identified in 88% and 93% of tumors evaluated [185,189] In dogs treated with amputation and doxorubicin (DOX), COX-2 immunoreactivity score, a product of stain intensity and percentage of positive cells, was potentially correlated with disease outcome. Dogs with primary tumors demonstrating strong stain intensity had a significantly shorter MST (86 days) than dogs with tumors staining negative (MST 423 days), poor (MST 399 days), or moderate (MST 370 days) for COX-2. Recently, global gene expression analysis of canine OSA stem cells identified that COX-2 gene transcription was expressed 141-fold greater in canine OSA stem cells compared with nonstem cells; this suggests that COX-2 activity may play a role in tumor initiation and progression.[190]

HSPs play a critical role in cellular responses to stress and aid in appropriate protein folding and protection cells after endoplasmic reticulum stressors, which otherwise would induce programmed cell death. Cancer cells may deregulate HSP expression to favor survival and HSP gene expression has been investigated in canine OSA. In a study of dogs with OSA, a significantly increased expression of HSP60 was found to be associated with reduced DFIs and STs in a subset of patients achieving long-term disease control. Mechanistic studies demonstrated that knockdown of HSP60 reduced cell proliferative capacity and induced apoptosis. These collective findings suggest that HSP60 overexpression might be associated with poor prognosis in dogs with OSA.[188]

With the near complete sequencing of the canine genome and the commercial availability of canine-specific gene microarrays, it has become possible to characterize and validate specific tumor-associated genetic determinants associated with clinical outcomes and prognosis. In one gene expression profiling study, primary OSA tissues were analyzed from two groups of dogs with different clinical outcomes, specifically dogs achieving DFIs either less than 100 days or more than 300 days after uniform treatment with amputation and systemic chemotherapy.[106] Derived from microarray analysis and confirmed by RT-PCR, eight specific gene transcripts were significantly different between poor responders (<100 days) and good responders (>300 days). In dogs categorized as poor responders, six transcripts, including insulin-like growth factor II and alcohol dehydrogenase were downregulated, and two transcripts were upregulated in comparison to good responders. To better characterize the molecular pathways associated with the differentially expressed genes identified in microarray analysis, a broader systems approach was used to identify changes in groups of interacting genes or pathways that may contribute to metastatic progression or chemotherapy resistance. In general, pathway expression differences between good and poor responders involved oxidative phosphorylation, bone development, PKA signaling, cell adhesion, cytoskeletal remodeling, and immune response.[106]

In a similar expression profiling study, prognostic gene profiles were derived from 32 primary OSA tumors derived from two groups of dogs based upon ST.[191] Dogs surviving for less than 6 months or more than 6 months were categorized as either poor or good responders respectively. Gene profiling identified 51 gene transcripts to be differentially expressed. Within the poor responder group, genes uniformly overexpressed were associated with biologic pathways involved in proliferation, drug resistance, and metastases. In addition to identifying differentially expressed genes and associated pathways between dogs categorized as good and poor responders, the findings from the study further substantiated the molecular pathway similarities shared between humans and dogs, including Wnt, integrin, and chemokine/cytokine signaling.

Lastly, a highly influential study was conducted that leveraged the more homogeneous genetic background of dogs diagnosed with OSA to detect underlying and conserved gene expression patterns previously undetectable in historic canine and human gene microarray analysis.[192] By differential gene expression profiling of early passage immortalized OSA cell lines derived from primary tumors, the investigators were able to identify gene signatures associated with G2/M transition and DNA damage checkpoint, as well as microenvironment interactions, which permitted the unbiased segregation of OSA samples into distinct molecular subclassifications and predicted outcome. Most significantly, the same genetic signatures identified in dogs also allowed for prognostic molecular classification of human OSA, powerfully underscoring the scientific merit derived from comparative oncologic studies.

Perturbations of the immune system are common among cancer patients, and regulatory T cells (Tregs) and myeloid-derived suppressor cells have the capacity to attenuate effective antitumor immune responses with the potential to negatively affect prognosis. Tregs have been characterized in healthy and cancer-bearing dogs,[193–195] with some studies demonstrating that dogs with OSA have increases in the percentage and absolute counts of circulating Tregs.[196] The clinical significance of Tregs on OSA prognosis has recently been characterized in a study of 12 dogs treated with amputation and systemic chemotherapy.[196] Dogs with high (higher than the mean) versus low (lower than the mean) percentages of Tregs identified in blood or tumor tissue did not have differences in DFI or ST; however, high or low CD8/Treg ratio in the blood was associated with clinical outcomes as dogs with low CD8/Treg ratios had a significantly shorter ST than dogs with high CD8/Treg ratios.

In addition to Tregs and their potential prognostic value in OSA, one study has demonstrated that routine hemogram parameters—specifically lymphocyte and monocyte counts—can also predict clinical outcomes in dogs with OSA.[163] In 69 dogs treated with amputation and systemic chemotherapy, baseline lymphocyte and monocyte counts were associated with DFI. Shorter DFIs were observed in dogs initially presenting with relative lymphocytosis (≥1000 cell/uL) and relative monocytosis (≥400 cell/uL), and these original conclusions were further substantiated by a second population of OSA dogs treated in an identical manner. Mechanistically, it was hypothesized that the association of relative monocytosis and reduced DFI could be the presence of myeloid-derived suppressor cells, a population of cells characterized by their ability to suppress antitumor immune responses.

Recently, the putative role of monocyte and macrophage regulatory roles in dogs with OSA were evaluated in an attempt to understand how monocyte phenotype and chemotactic function might be perturbed in dogs with OSA.[197] In 18 dogs with OSA, the cell surface expression of multiple chemokine receptors, in particular CCR2 and CXCR2, were downregulated in peripheral blood monocytes, potentially leading to reduced directional migration and extravasation. Additionally, the monocytes from dogs with OSA were functionally impaired as exhibited by decreased chemotaxis ex vivo. These findings could explain why dogs with OSA may have elevations in circulating monocytes as well as provide potential mechanisms by which OSA cells might evade the innate immune system through the induction of monocyte chemotactic dysfunction.

Another study characterized the immune microenvironment of canine primary OSA through the association of macrophage (CD204+) and lymphocyte infiltrates (both effector CD3+ and regulatory Foxp3 T-cells) within the primary tumor with DFI and ST in 30 dogs treated with amputation and carboplatin therapy.[198] Although the extent and phenotype of primary tumoral lymphocyte infiltrates did not influence outcomes, the surface area of macrophage infiltration did have an effect on outcomes. Dogs with more than 4.7% surface area infiltrate with CD204+ macrophages experienced a significantly longer DFI. These findings suggest that tumor-infiltrating macrophages may contribute to inhibiting localized OSA metastatic progression.

Therapy Directed at the Primary Tumor

Surgery

Table 25.1 provides an overview of surgical options for primary bone tumors based on anatomic site.

Amputation

Amputation of the affected limb is the standard local treatment for canine appendicular OSA. Even large and giant breed dogs will usually function well after limb amputation, and most owners are pleased with mobility and quality of life of their pets after surgery; 88% of dogs have the same or near same quality of life after amputation, and 73% of dogs return to their preamputation activity levels after surgery.[199,200] Most dogs will readily compensate and, although the osteoarthritis may progress more rapidly in the three-legged dog, this rarely results in a clinical problem. Physical therapy and rehabilitation is an important adjunct to postamputation recovery and should be considered as part of the routine postoperative care for amputation patients. Severe preexisting orthopedic or neurologic conditions may cause poor results in some cases and careful preoperative examination is important. Complete forequarter amputation is recommended for thoracic limb tumors and coxofemoral disarticulation (amputation) for pelvic limb lesions. This level of amputation assures complete removal of the local tumor and also results in a more cosmetic and functional outcome. For proximal femoral tumors, complete amputation and en bloc acetabulectomy is recommended to obtain proximal soft tissue margins (Fig. 25.5).

Limb Salvage

Although most dogs function well with amputation, there are some dogs for which LSS would be preferred over amputation, such as dogs with severe preexisting orthopedic or neurologic disease or dogs whose owners absolutely will not permit amputation. Until relatively recently, only a few reports of LSS in dogs, with

TABLE 25.1	Treatment Options for Osteosarcoma by Site	
Site	Treatment Options	Comments
Humerus, femur, tibia	Limb amputation Limb salvage (stereotactic radiation therapy)	Generally high complication rate for limb salvage[162] Diaphyseal locations amenable to intercalary allografts[209] Total hip salvage possible for proximal femoral tumors[214,217] Intraoperative extracorporal radiation technique may apply[225]
Radius	Limb amputation Limb salvage (allograft,[201–206] endoprosthesis,[214] intercalary bone graft,[209] ulnar transposition,[223,224] bone transport osteogenesis,[218,219,221,222] intraoperative extracorporal radiation therapy[225])	-
Ulna	Limb amputation Ulnectomy[255]	Often does not require allograft reconstruction
Scapula	Limb amputation Scapulectomy[173,253,248]	Proximal lesions best; partial and total scapulectomy described
Pelvis	Pelvectomy with or without limb amputation[176,246]	Lateral portion of sacrum can be excised; may include body wall
Metacarpus/metatarsus	Digit amputation[250] Partial limb amputation with prosthesis	Limb function dependent on prosthetic design and patient tolerance
Mandible	Mandibulectomy[122]	Often requires total mandibulectomy Bilaterally limited to fourth premolar
Maxilla/orbit	Maxillectomy[256] Orbitectomy[260]	Limited by midline palate or cranial vault invasion Combined approach may assist exposure
Calvarium	Resection ± Radiation	Resection dependent on venous sinus involvement
Vertebrae	Decompression (palliative) ± Radiation ± Chemotherapy[175]	Vertebrectomy techniques not well developed; limited local disease control
Rib	Rib resection[170–172,181]	Requires removal of normal rib cranial and caudal to the tumor

limited follow-up, were published.[201–205] To date, more than 600 LSSs have been performed at Colorado State University's Flint Animal Cancer Center (CSU-FACC). Limb function has been fair to good in most dogs, and survival has not been adversely affected by removing the primary tumor with marginal resection.[206]

Suitable candidates for LSS include dogs with nonmetastatic OSA and when the primary tumor affects <50% of the bone (as determined radiographically). Other criteria for consideration include absence of pathologic fracture, less than 360-degree involvement of soft tissues, and a firm/definable soft tissue mass rather than an edematous lesion. Early on in the development of LSS procedures, many dogs treated at CSU-FACC received some form of preoperative treatment, (i.e., primary or neoadjuvant intraarterial [IA] cisplatin, intravenous [IV] cisplatin, RT to the tumor bone, or a combination of RT with IV or IA cisplatin). Results from 21 dogs treated with RT alone given in large doses per fraction before LSS were unsatisfactory for preservation of life or limb.[203] Many of the dogs treated with two preoperative IA cisplatin doses 21 days apart, with the last treatment 21 days before LSS, showed marked decrease in the degree of vascularization of the tumor. This represented a high degree of induced tumor necrosis in the resected specimen, especially when combined with RT, and facilitated LSS.[205,207] Most dogs at CSU-FACC receive systemic carboplatin, DOX, or combination therapy after surgery.[208]

The most suitable cases for LSS are dogs with tumors in the distal radius or ulna, as function after LSS and carpal arthrodesis is good. Arthrodesis of the scapulohumeral, coxofemoral, stifle, or tarsal joints after LSS generally results in only fair to poor function.[162] Resulting poor function, combined with a high complication rate, has generally led surgeons away from recommending LSS near these joints. LSS is a complicated process and requires a coordinated team effort between surgical and medical oncologists, radiologists, pathologists, and technical staff. Several methods of LSS have been described, each with unique advantages and limitations. The choice of LSS method depends on several factors, including owner choice, patient personality, and individual risk factors. At the CSU-FACC, owners are given a choice of LSS options and informed about the risks and benefits of each method compared with amputation. A brief description of the surgical options for a distal radial location (most common) follows. Meticulous aseptic technique is essential.

Allograft limb salvage surgery. For a distal radial site, the dog is placed in lateral or dorsal recumbency with the affected limb uppermost. A skin incision is made on the dorsolateral aspect of the antebrachium from a point just distal to the elbow to just proximal to the metacarpophalangeal joint. Any biopsy tracts are excised en bloc. Soft tissue is dissected to the level of the tumor pseudocapsule. Care is taken not to compromise the tumor capsule. The bone is osteotomized with an oscillating bone saw 3 to 5 cm proximal to the proximal radiographic (or scintigraphic) margin of the tumor. Extensor muscles attached to the tumor pseudocapsule are transected at this level to maintain 2- to 3-cm soft tissue margins. The joint capsule is incised, keeping close to the proximal row of carpal bones. For tumors of the mid diaphysis, tumor resection follows similar guidelines with the exception that the extensor and flexor muscle groups should be spared as the

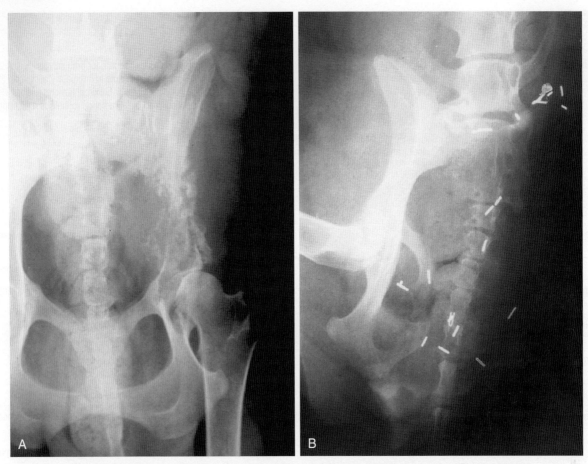

• **Fig. 25.5** (A) Ventrodorsal radiographic view of an osteosarcoma of the ilium of a dog. (B) Ventrodorsal radiographic view of the same dog 3 years after hemipelvectomy and amputation followed by cisplatin chemotherapy.

joint (above and below) may be spared.[209] The ulna is sectioned sagittally with an osteotome, and the medial ulnar cortex adjacent to the tumor is removed en bloc with the radius. For tumors that have extension to the ulna (rare), the ulna is also cut with a bone saw, and the distal one-third or more is removed with the tumor. Care is taken to preserve as much vasculature as possible, especially on the palmar surface.

Large vessels associated with the tumor are ligated or sealed and divided. The specimen is radiographed and then submitted for histologic evaluation, including assessment of completeness of surgical margins. In addition, a sample of bone marrow in the radius proximal to the resection level is obtained for histologic evaluation of marrow involvement. A fresh-frozen cortical allograft is thawed in 1 liter of an antibiotic in saline solution, the articular cartilage is removed, the graft is cut to fit, and the medullary cavity flushed to remove residual fat and cellular debris.[210,211] The articular cartilage of the proximal carpal bones is removed and the allograft is stabilized in compression using Association for the Study of Internal Fixation (ASIF/AO) principles. A locking compression plate with a minimum of three screws proximal and four screws distal to the graft is used; 3.5 mm broad locking plates of up to 22 holes or a custom-designed limb salvage plate are appropriate in most cases, but 4.5 mm narrow or broad plates may be required for very large breed dogs. The plate is fixed in the patient to the allograft with two or three screws, removed from the surgery site, and the medullary canal of the allograft is filled with polymethylmethacrylate bone cement containing amikacin

(1 g amikacin to 40 g of polymer powder). This provides support for the screws during revascularization of the graft and acts as a reservoir for antibiotics. The healing of the allograft is not significantly impeded by the presence of the bone cement and has been shown to significantly decrease the incidence of orthopedic failure, including allograft fracture and screw pullout.[212,213] The plate extends proximally on the remaining radius and distally to a level just proximal to the metacarpophalangeal joint (Fig. 25.6). For intercalary LSS the plate extends proximally and distally to meet or exceed ASIF standards with the intent to spare joint motion.

The wound is thoroughly lavaged with saline. A closed suction drain is inserted adjacent to the allograft, and the wound is closed. The limb is supported in a padded bandage. The drain is removed the day after surgery in most cases. An Elizabethan collar or other preventative measures should be used as necessary to prevent self-mutilation after surgery. No external coaptation is used, and most dogs use the limb relatively well by 10 days after surgery. Postoperative foot swelling can be considerable and should be carefully monitored but usually resolves by 2 weeks. Exercise restriction and physical therapy are recommended for 4 to 6 weeks. Thereafter, return to activity is recommended on a case-by-case basis.

The advantages of allograft LSS include the absence of external fixation, and minimal owner involvement is required in the postoperative period aside from bandage changes in the first several weeks. The disadvantages are the high infection rate and the need for permanent internal hardware. Canine LSS patients have an infection rate of approximately 40% to 50%. Once an infection

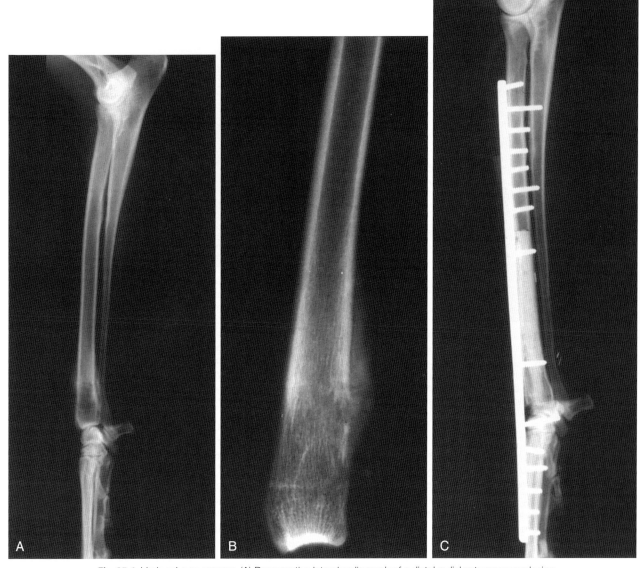

• **Fig. 25.6** Limb salvage surgery. (A) Preoperative lateral radiograph of a distal radial osteosarcoma lesion in a dog. (B) Craniocaudal specimen radiograph after tumor resection. (C) Lateral postoperative radiograph after allograft replacement and plate fixation.

occurs, it may be controlled with long-term antibiotic therapy, but infections are rarely resolved with antibiotics.[162] Infection may result in soft tissue defects from draining tracts, exposure of the plate or allograft, and hardware loosening. Revision surgeries, either for hardware complications or soft tissue reconstruction, are not uncommon. Additionally, amputation for catastrophic implant failure, local recurrence, or unmanageable infection is sometimes required.

Metal endoprosthesis. This technique utilizes a commercially available metal endoprosthesis with a modified bone plate (Fig. 25.7), 3D printed, or custom-designed endoprostheses. The surgery is nearly identical to the procedure described for cortical allografts with an endoprosthesis used instead of an allograft. A prospective comparison of complications between cortical allograft and commercially available endoprosthesis LSSs was

published in 2006.[214] No significant differences in the number of complications were noted between endoprostheses and allografts. In a recent study comparing clinical outcome in 45 dogs treated with either first or second generation endoprosthesis LSS, the overall complication rate was 96%, including infection in 78%, implant-related complications in 36%, and local recurrence in 24% of dogs.[215] An endoprosthesis is an attractive alternative to cortical allografts for LSS of the distal aspect of the radius in dogs because surgical and oncologic outcomes are similar. The commercially available endoprosthesis is an off-the-shelf implant with no need for tissue banking. Various patient-specific, 3D-printed endoprostheses have been utilized with good results.[216,217]

Longitudinal bone transport osteogenesis. Longitudinal bone transport osteogenesis (BTO) is a limb salvage technique reported in dogs (Fig. 25.8)[218–220] that utilizes Ilizarov (circular) fixators

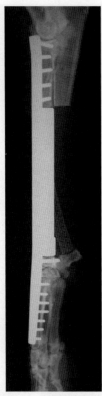

• **Fig. 25.7** Lateral radiographic projection of a limb salvage technique using a commercially available endoprosthesis with a modified bone plate in a dog with distal radial and ulnar osteosarcoma. A limb-sparing plate spans the radius and metacarpus, connected to the implant, which abuts the host radius proximally and the radial carpal bone distally. A negative suction drain has also been placed at the surgical site to decrease postoperative fluid accumulation.

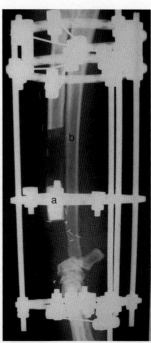

• **Fig. 25.8** Lateral radiographic projection of a limb salvage technique using longitudinal bone transport osteogenesis (BTO). In this case a distal radial osteosarcoma was removed, and BTO was accomplished using circular fixators and the principles of distraction osteogenesis to create bone in the defect remaining after tumor resection. Briefly, a longitudinal section of normal bone *(a, termed the "transport segment")* from the radius is osteotomized and attached to the transport ring and the osteotomized bone segment is slowly transported into the defect at a rate of 1 mm per day. Distraction osteogenesis occurs in the trailing distraction pathway *(b)*.

and the principles of distraction osteogenesis to create bone in the defect after tumor resection. Before surgery, a five- to six-ring circular fixator is constructed to allow one central ring (termed a transport ring) to move independently of the remainder of the fixator. Using the same procedure for removal of the tumor and preparation of the radiocarpal bone described earlier, the circular fixator is placed on the limb and attached to the remaining radius using tensioned, 1.6-mm diameter wires. A longitudinal section of normal bone (termed the transport segment) from the radius immediately proximal to the defect is osteotomized and attached to the transport ring with wires. After a 3- to 7-day delay period, the osteotomized bone segment is slowly transported into the defect at a rate of 1 mm per day. Distraction osteogenesis occurs in the trailing distraction pathway. New bone continues to form longitudinally within the defect proximal to the transport segment for as long as the steady, slow distraction continues. When the transport segment reaches the radiocarpal bone (docking), the transport segment is compressed to the radiocarpal bone and heals to create an arthrodesis. The circular fixator remains on the limb as the newly formed bone remodels and the arthrodesis occurs. This technique is compatible with adjuvant cisplatin, carboplatin, and combination chemotherapy.[219,221]

The advantages to BTO LSS are the low risk of infection due to the autologous, vascularized nature of the replacement bone and the ability of the new bone tissue to remodel over time. Patients are typically weight-bearing within the first 48 hours and, once the incision has healed, do not require exercise restriction. The disadvantages of the BTO procedure are the extensive client involvement required to perform the daily distractions on the fixator and the extended amount of time the fixator remains on the limb. Double level longitudinal BTO and translational transport of the ulna can significantly diminish the time required for distraction and has been used successfully in a case of limb salvage for a distal tibial OSA.[222]

Ulnar transposition. The vascularized ulnar transposition technique uses the ipsilateral distal ulna as an autograft to reconstruct the distal radial defect by rotating the graft into position while preserving the caudal interosseous artery and vein.[223,224] After excision of the tumor as described previously, two transverse osteotomies of the ulna are made. The distal osteotomy is performed at the level of the isthmus proximal to the facet that articulates with the radius. The proximal ulnar osteotomy is performed 1 to 2 mm distal to the level of the radial osteotomy. Direct visualization of the caudal interosseous artery and vein allows these structures to be preserved during dissection of the autograft. The ulnar graft is "rolled over" into the radial defect and fixed using a bone plate that extends from the proximal radius to the distal one-third of the fourth metacarpal bone (i.e., pancarpal arthrodesis).

Advantages to the ulnar transposition technique are that there is no distant donor site morbidity, the replacement bone is autologous, and the graft is vascularized, making it less likely to get infected and possibly more rapid healing. The disadvantages to this technique are that the ulnar transposition technique may be more prone to biomechanical complications in the postoperative period due to its smaller size relative to the radius and the need for permanent internal hardware.[223]

Nonsurgical Limb Salvage

Intracorporeal and Extracorporeal Intraoperative Radiation Therapy

Intraoperative RT (IORT), using either an intracorporeal or extra-corporeal approach, for limb sparing has been utilized in a small number of canine OSA patients[225,226] as well as human patients with extremity bone tumors.[227-229] This limb salvage technique involves a surgical approach to the bone with osteotomy proximal or distal to the affected site (depending on the anatomic location of the tumor) and reflection of normal soft tissues from the tumor affected bone. The neurovascular bundle, muscle, and skin are retracted away from the affected bone, and the tumor is pivoted from the site on the intact joint tissue. The patient is then transported to the radiation suite and a single dose of 70 Gy is then delivered to the tumor, taking care to spare the distracted neurovascular bundle. The irradiated bone is then anatomically replaced and surgical fixation of the osteotomy is achieved with either dynamic compression plating or an interlocking nail system. One advantage of IORT for limb salvage over LSS is that it can be used to preserve limb and joint function in anatomic sites that are not amenable to LSS with arthrodesis of the adjacent joint (e.g., proximal humerus).[162] Patients treated with IORT had good limb function in the immediate postoperative period; however, complications related to surgery or RT led to implant revisions in 69% of cases within 5 to 9 months of initial surgery, including four amputations. Pathologic fracture of the irradiated bone was the most common complication. Additionally, local tumor recurrence occurred in four dogs and infection in four dogs. A modification of this technique includes complete temporary removal of diaphyseal tumors, performing extracorporeal IORT, and then reimplantation and stabilization of the irradiated bone segment. In situ radiation of distal femur and any tibial tumors can be performed without osteotomy. The disease-free and overall limb and joint salvage rates for extracorporeal IORT as assessed at the time of death or data analysis were 46% and 54%, respectively. The MST for dogs with appendicular sarcoma treated with limb- and joint-sparing extracorporeal IORT was 298 days.

Stereotactic Radiation Therapy

SRT or stereotactic radiosurgery (SRS) offer the ability to deliver high dose RT to the tumor volume with relative sparing of the surrounding normal tissues by use of accurate patient immobilization, image guidance, and a rapid dose fall-off from the tumor margins (Fig. 25.9). In this respect, it is a refinement of the IORT technique that avoids the need for surgical exposure. A nonsurgical limb salvage technique using a single fraction SRS was developed at the University of Florida, and initial results were reported in 11 dogs.[230] Adjuvant carboplatin chemotherapy was used in six dogs immediately before RT for its potential radiosensitization action in addition to its conventional cytotoxic effects, and five dogs were treated with SRS alone. Four dogs developed pathologic fractures and one dog developed infection. Acute effects to the skin were generally mild to moderate; however, one dog developed an open skin wound 3 months after treatment, and another dog developed a full thickness skin wound under a splint used during the treatment of a pathologic fracture. Limb use in the dogs treated with SRS and chemotherapy was excellent. The overall MST was 363 days. In a follow-up retrospective study, the same group reported the outcome of 46 patients treated with a similar single fraction SRS technique (median prescribed dose 30 Gy).[231] Forty-five dogs received conventional maximal tolerated dose chemotherapy. The

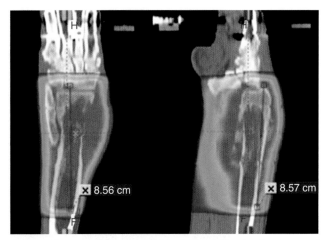

• Fig. 25.9 Dose color wash map of radiation distribution for stereotactic radiation therapy of distal radius osteosarcoma lesion showing a steep dose gradient drop off between tumor volume and normal tissues.

MST was 9.7 months. Of the patients with complete medical records, 63% developed pathologic fracture at a median of 5.9 months. Acute and late skin toxicities developed in 58% and 16% of dogs, respectively. Involvement of subchondral bone appeared to be predictive of shortened time to fracture.

Many veterinary radiation oncology facilities currently offer SRT for OSA. SRT protocols for the treatment of OSA typically involve two to three fractions with doses ranging from 8 to 13 Gy per fraction, and the most common protocol is three fractions of 10 Gy. These fractions are delivered daily or, less commonly, every other day.

In an orthotopic, athymic, rat model inoculated with canine OSA cells, three fractions of 12 Gy SRT was shown to induce complete tumor necrosis in 92% of rats treated.[232] Previous canine studies have indicated that therapies which induce more than 80% local tumor necrosis are associated with an increase in local tumor control.[233] The same athymic rat model also indicated that zoledronic acid combined with parathyroid hormone could increase bone volume after SRT. Many oncologists advocate the use of bisphosphonates before or after SRT. As SRT is a localized therapy, adjuvant chemotherapy is recommended to delay the onset of metastatic disease. Chemotherapy can also be considered as a radiation sensitizer as reported in the studies of single fraction SRS for canine OSA.[231] Radiation recall (recurrence of acute skin toxicities after initial resolution) has been observed in some patients treated with adjuvant DOX chemotherapy.

Pathologic fracture is the most frequent complication associated with SRT and SRS. Fracture is postulated to be due to the amount of preexisting tumor associated osteolysis and postirradiation bone necrosis resulting in loss of dynamic bone remodeling and healing capacity after SRT. Smaller, more blastic lesions may be better candidates for SRT limb salvage than larger, more lytic lesions. There is some evidence that lysis of subchondral bone may be associated with a higher rate of fracture.[231] Pathologic fracture has been treated by internal fixation, external coaptation, or amputation.[112] Preemptive stabilization has also been used for more concerning lesions or those with evidence of pathologic fracture at the time of SRT (Fig. 25.10).[111] In a recent study, seven dogs underwent surgical stabilization for fractures documented at the time of SRT, and 11 dogs were stabilized preemptively. Infection occurred in 15 dogs and was considered a major complication in 13 of these dogs and ultimately

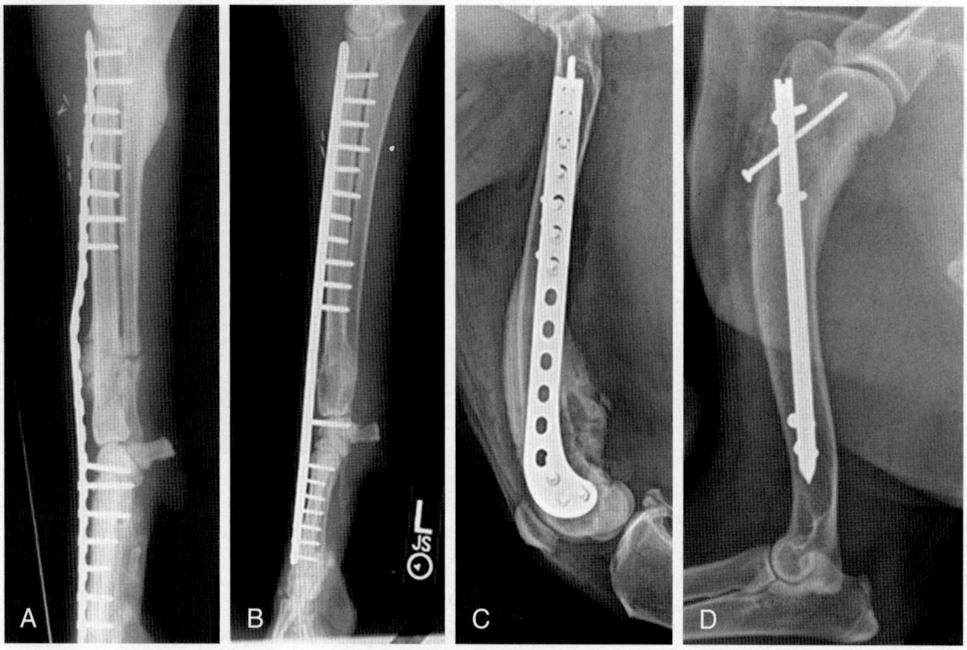

• **Fig. 25.10** Radiographs of internal fixation after fracture (A) and preemptive stabilization (B, C, and D) for stereotactic radiation therapy limb salvage cases with lytic lesions.

contributed to amputation or euthanasia. The high rate of complications in this study resulted in the authors not recommending stabilization concurrently with SRT.

Theoretically, fractionated SRT may offer a reduction in the rate of pathologic fracture in comparison to severely hypofractionated SRS, which results in pathologic fracture in 63% of patients. The rate of fracture after SRT has not been published to date. In a recent study of an accelerated palliative protocol, in which dogs were manually planned to receive two daily fractions of 10 Gy using parallel opposed geometry, the rate of fracture was 35.7% after RT.[234]

The advantages of SRS/SRT techniques include limb preservation in anatomic sites not amenable to LSS, the normal tissue-sparing effects of SRT compared with conventional RT, a lack of surgical alternatives, and good to excellent limb function. Disadvantages of the technique include limited but increasing access to equipment capable of delivering SRT and the high rate of postirradiation pathologic fracture.

Isolation of Limb Circulation and Perfusion

Isolated limb perfusion (ILP) with chemotherapy has been used in people and dogs with sarcomas and melanomas as a sole treatment or to downstage local disease to allow LSS.[235–237] ILP allows delivery of high concentrations of chemotherapy as well as delivery of compounds that are poorly tolerated systemically. Varying degrees of local toxicity are reported and these are dependent on the drugs used. Successful use of ILP in canine OSA has been reported.[235] One study determined that appendicular bone tumors have significantly higher interstitial fluid pressure and lower blood flow than do adjacent, unaffected soft tissues.[238] ILP may be a method to facilitate delivery of therapeutic drug concentrations to primary tumors for preoperative downstaging before LSS.

Systemic administration of [153]Samarium ethylenediamine-tetramethylene phosphonate ([153]Sm-EDTMP) is limited by systemic myelotoxicity. In a study at CSU-FACC, [153]Sm-EDTMP (37 MBq/kg) was administered via ILP through isolated limb circulation for 1 hour in nine dogs with primary appendicular

OSA 3 weeks before amputation to evaluate the potential for decreased systemic toxicity and to induce clinically meaningful tumor necrosis before primary tumor removal. No systemic toxicity was observed. Despite good dosimetry to the lesion, the mean percentage TN was 27.6%, which was similar to mean percentage TN of 26.8% in untreated OSA cases.[233] This low percentage TN may be due to incomplete perfusion of the [153]Sm-EDTMP, the heterogenous nature of OSA, and the inability of the beta particles to exert a cytotoxic effect on the noncalcified regions of the tumor due to their short track length (3 mm).

Summary of Outcome After Limb Salvage for Dogs with Osteosarcoma

There is no significant difference in survival rates for dogs treated with amputation and cisplatin compared with dogs treated with LSS and cisplatin.[206] Overall, limb function has been satisfactory with approximately 80% of dogs experiencing good to excellent limb function.[17] LSS requires a dedicated owner and clinical team. LSS is usually combined with some form of adjuvant therapy, and complications can arise in any or all phases of treatment (chemotherapy, RT, or surgery). High dose, external beam RT may complicate wound and bone healing and potentiate infection.[203] Moderate dose, external beam RT in combination with chemotherapy may, however, be useful for control of local disease, as indicated by tumor necrosis data.[205,239] The major complications related to LSS are infection, local recurrence, and implant complications. In a review of 220 LSSs performed at CSU-FACC, the 1-year local recurrence-free rate was 76% with 60% of dogs alive at 1 year.[206] Local disease control was improved with certain treatments such as pretreatment with moderate doses of RT and intra-arterial cisplatin or local implantation of biodegradable cisplatin polymer. The percentage of TN has been shown to be predictive of outcome.[7]

In two case series, 40% and 47.5% of dogs, respectively, developed allograft infections.[206,240] The majority had their infections adequately controlled with systemic antibiotics with or without local antibiotics (antibiotic-impregnated polymethylmethacrylate

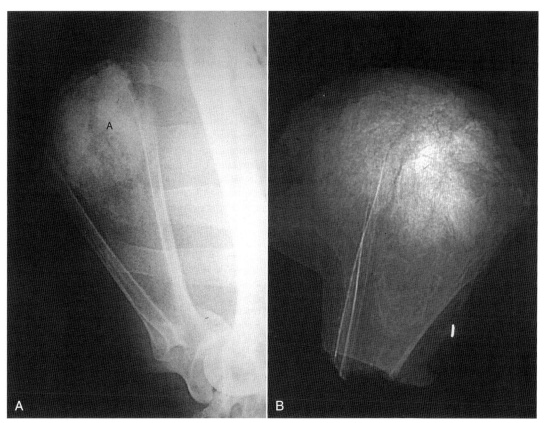

• **Fig. 25.11** (A) Preoperative radiograph of an osteosarcoma of the proximal scapula. (B) Specimen radiograph after partial scapulectomy.

beads).[162] Many of these dogs continued to have evidence of infection; however, their function was not severely affected. In severe and uncontrolled infections, allografts had to be removed, and a small number of dogs required amputation. An unexpected finding has been that dogs with LSS infections experienced a statistically significant prolongation of overall STs compared with dogs with LSS without infection.[214,241,242] This finding has also been reported in people with deep infections after LSS for OSA.[243] A mouse model of OSA examined the effects of infection on tumor angiogenesis and innate immunity and demonstrated that chronic localized bacterial infection could elicit significant systemic antitumor activity dependent on natural killer cells and macrophages.[244]

Surgery for Nonappendicular and Less Common Appendicular Sites of Osteosarcoma

Certain primary bone tumors of the pelvis can be removed by hemipelvectomy and, although these surgeries are difficult, function and cosmetic outcome are excellent.[245,246] Excellent reviews of the surgical techniques for hemipelvectomy and the surgical and oncologic factors to be considered with this surgery have been published.[245,247]

Vertebral OSAs are challenging to manage because of difficulty in adequately treating local disease. Total en bloc vertebrectomy techniques are not well established in veterinary medicine,[248,249] and surgery is often palliative to decompress dogs with neurologic deficits or intractable pain and to obtain a diagnosis.[175] Present recommendations are to perform surgery in cases that require decompression (with or without stabilization) and institute RT (discussed later) and chemotherapy.

A combination allograft and custom total joint arthroplasty has been described for successful LSS of a proximal femur OSA,[250]

and a patient-specific, 3D-printed endoprosthetic reconstruction of the proximal femur and hemipelvis has been reported in a dog with a histiocytic sarcoma.[217] An intraosseous transcutaneous amputation prosthesis (ITAP) for limb salvage has been described in four dogs with distal radial or tibial OSA lesions.[251] A case report using an ITAP prosthesis for a traumatic distal tibia injury has also been reported.[252] The success of an ITAP prostheses require a biologic seal to be formed between the skin and the prosthesis to minimize the risk of deep infection.

Bone tumors originating in the scapula can be successfully removed by partial or total scapulectomy (Fig. 25.11).[173,253,254] Significant gait abnormalities may occur after total scapulectomy by disarticulation at the scapulohumeral joint; however, lameness typically improves or resolves with rehabilitation and time.[254] Small primary tumors of the ulna can be removed by partial ulnectomy, and reconstruction is rarely needed.[255] Tumors located in the metatarsal and metacarpal bones can be treated with local resections or partial foot amputation.[250] Mandibulectomy and maxillectomy are appropriate surgeries for primary bone tumors of oral sites.[166,167,256–259] In a survey of owners of dogs undergoing partial mandibulectomy or maxillectomy, 85% were satisfied with the outcome despite 44% citing difficulty in eating as a complication.[257] Tumors of periorbital sites can be removed by orbitectomy.[260] Rib tumors can be removed by thoracic wall resection and the defect reconstructed with polypropylene mesh with plastic plates for large defects or by muscle flap techniques.[170–172,261] Diaphragmatic advancement can be used for caudally located defects.

Radiation Therapy

At present, the role of RT for curative-intent local tumor control is still evolving in veterinary medicine. The most common role of

RT in dogs with appendicular OSA is for palliation of bone pain. RT at relatively high total doses can cause considerable necrosis of primary OSA in dogs and people either before LSS to downstage the primary tumor to improve the success of local disease control after removal or as a primary therapy for unresectable tumors.[203,205,262-264] As a primary therapy, a MST of 209 days was reported in 14 dogs with appendicular OSA treated with fractionated high-dose RT (median dose of 57 Gy) to their primary tumor and systemic chemotherapy.[265] The introduction of SRT has allowed for delivery of high doses of radiation to the tumor volume with good local tumor control and relative sparing of the surrounding normal tissues.

Radioisotopes

A beta emitter radioisotope, ^{153}Sm-EDTMP, has been used to treat primary OSA and metastatic bone neoplasia in dogs and humans via systemic IV administration. ^{90}Yttrium-hydroxide (Y90) has been reported as an intralesional liquid brachytherapy in a dog with tibial OSA. ^{90}Y was deposited locally in the bone, bone marrow, and soft tissue components of the tumor using specialized cannulas. Localized, high-dose RT can be delivered in such a manner, and, in addition, a minor portion of the breakdown product of ^{90}Y can be imaged by PET/CT to confirm the presence of the agent at the tumor site.[266,267]

Systemic Adjuvant Therapy for Dogs with Osteosarcoma

For the most effective management of canine OSA, multimodality therapy is required to address both local and metastatic disease. Although amputation and LSSs, as well as nonsurgical techniques such as SRT, have proven highly effective for local OSA management, the ability to cure or durably control OSA metastases remains a clinical challenge; substantive improvements in DFIs and STs await advances in systemic antimetastatic treatment options.

Although systemic chemotherapy remains the backbone for the management of OSA metastases, it is improbable that the discovery of new chemotherapeutic agents or dose-intensification with existing agents will dramatically improve current clinical outcomes. Rather, the future of OSA management will likely depend on combining conventional cytotoxic agents with targeted molecular therapeutics or immunomodulatory agents. As such, considerable research focus has been committed to discovering and validating new combination therapies for improving the long-term prognosis of canine OSA.

Chemotherapy

Table 25.2 provides an abbreviated summary of conventional chemotherapeutic agents used in the adjuvant setting, evaluated as single agents or in combination. Table 25.2 is not an exhaustive description of all reported studies conducted to date, but rather presents findings from studies derived from sample populations of greater than 20 dogs per investigation.

Single-Agent Carboplatin Chemotherapy

Carboplatin is a second-generation platinum compound that is less nephrotoxic than cisplatin. Given its ease of administration, carboplatin has largely supplanted the use of cisplatin in the postoperative setting. In the first study reporting the tolerability and activity of carboplatin, 48 dogs with OSA were treated with amputation and intent-to-treat with four doses of carboplatin (300 mg/m^2 every 21 days).[160] Carboplatin was well-tolerated with neutropenia identified as the dose-limiting toxicity. For the entire study population, the median DFI and MST were 257 and 321 days, respectively. For dogs receiving the planned four doses of carboplatin, median DFI and MST were extended to 327 and 383 days, respectively.

Despite the initial report of carboplatin's comparable activity to cisplatin,[160] two prospective randomized studies using single-agent carboplatin as a comparator arm demonstrated less impressive antimetastatic effects.[268,269] In one study, dogs were treated with a single neoadjuvant dose of carboplatin and amputation 7 days later, then received two additional treatments with carboplatin (300 mg/m^2) every 21 days. Upon completion of carboplatin, dogs were then randomized to receive either placebo or a long-acting somatostatin analog.[268] For dogs treated with carboplatin and placebo, the median DFI and MST were 196 and 230 days, respectively. In a second study comparing the activity of a liposome-encapsulated cisplatin formulation (SPI-77) versus single-agent carboplatin, 40 dogs were treated with a single neoadjuvant dose of either SPI-77 (350 mg/m^2) or carboplatin (300 mg/m^2) 1 week before amputation and then received an additional three treatments of SPI-77 or carboplatin every 21 days.[269] No difference was identified between treatment groups; dogs treated with single-agent carboplatin had a median DFI and ST of 123 and 207 days, respectively.

Two relatively large retrospective studies have been conducted to substantiate the activity of carboplatin for managing pulmonary micometastases.[270,271] In a study initiated by the Veterinary Cooperative Oncology Group (VCOG), 155 dogs treated with amputation and carboplatin (variable dosage and schedule) had a median DFI and STs of 256 and 307 days, respectively.[270] In a second retrospective investigation, 65 dogs treated with amputation and carboplatin at a dosage of 300 mg/m^2 every 21 days for four to six treatment cycles had a median DFI and ST of 137 and 277 days, respectively.[271]

Single-Agent Doxorubicin Chemotherapy

DOX is considered effective for delaying the development and progression of metastatic disease in dogs with OSA. The antimetastatic effects of DOX are more definitively substantiated when administered every 2 weeks rather than every 3 weeks. In one study, DOX was administered at a dose of 30 mg/m^2 every 2 weeks for five treatments to 35 dogs with appendicular OSA in a neoadjuvant setting. Dogs were treated with two or three doses of DOX before amputation and continued to receive DOX postoperatively for a total of five treatments.[272] The 1- and 2-year survival rates were 50.5% and 9.7%, respectively. In a second study evaluating the activity of a matrix metalloproteinase inhibitor (BAY 12-9566), 303 dogs were treated with amputation and DOX (30 mg/m^2 every 2 weeks for a total of five treatments), and then randomized to receive a daily oral placebo or BAY 12-9566.[180] No difference in ST was identified between dogs receiving placebo or BAY 12-9566, and the overall MST was 8 months.

Doxorubicin-Carboplatin Combined Chemotherapy

Given the modest to severe toxicity associated with DOX-cisplatin combination therapy,[273,274] one study investigated if combination tolerability could be improved by replacing cisplatin with carboplatin. The rationale to use carboplatin was based upon its comparable anticancer activities and improved side effect profile relative to cisplatin, which removes the need for saline diuresis and minimizes the likelihood of severe emesis. Twenty-four dogs were treated with definitive surgery

TABLE 25.2 **Abbreviated Summary of Historic and Adjuvant Chemotherapy Protocols Derived From Studies With a Minimum of 20 Dogs**

Drug	Dose Regime and Number of Dogs	Disease-Free Interval	Survival Outcomes	Comments
Cisplatin[17] Single agent	70 mg/m^2 IV for two treatments, every 21 days $n = 36$	Median 177–226 days	Median 262–282 days 1-year survival rate 38%–43% 2-year survival rate 16%–18%	No significant difference in survival data for dogs given cisplatin before or after amputation
Cisplatin[201] (some dogs treated with limb salvage surgery) Single agent	60 mg/m^2 IV for one to six treatments, every 21 days $n = 22$	-	Median 325 days 1-year survival rate 45.5% 2-year survival rate 20.9%	Apparent increase in treatment failures due to bone metastasis
SPI-77[269] liposome encapsulated cisplatin Single agent	350 mg/m^2 IV for four treatments, every 21 days $n = 20$	Median 156 days	Median 333 days	Dramatic increase in cumulative cisplatin dose without the need for diuresis
Lobaplatin[407] Single agent	35 mg/m^2 IV for four treatments, every 21 days		1-year overall survival rate 31.8% 1-year disease-free survival rate 21.8%	No need for diuresis with this platinum analog
Doxorubicin and cisplatin[408] Concurrent combination	Doxorubicin at 12.5–25 mg/m^2 IV followed in 2 hours by cisplatin at 60 mg/m^2 IV or three treatments $n = 102$	-	Median 345 days 1-year survival rate 48% 2-year survival rate 28%	Unacceptable toxicity with doxorubicin at 25 mg/m^2
Doxorubicin and cisplatin[273] Concurrent combination	Cisplatin at 50 mg/m^2 IV on day 1 and doxorubicin at 15 mg/m^2 IV on day 2 for four treatments $n = 35$	Median 240 days	Median 300 days	Much better tolerated protocol compared with concurrent cisplatin-doxorubicin[408]
Doxorubicin and cisplatin[409] Alternating combination	Doxorubicin at 30 mg/m^2 IV followed by cisplatin at 60 mg/m^2 IV 21 days later for two treatments, every 21 days $n = 38$		Median 300 days	Alternating combination well tolerated with no grade III or IV dose-limiting toxicities
Carboplatin and gemcitabine[410] Concurrent combination	Carboplatin at 300 mg/m^2 IV then gemcitabine 2 mg/kg IV as a 20-minute infusion 4 hours postcarboplatin for four treatments, every 21 days $n = 50$	Median 203 days	Median 279 days 1-year survival rate 29.5% 2-year survival rate 11.3%	Well-tolerated protocol with low incidence of grade III or IV hematologic toxicities

followed by combination chemotherapy consisting of carboplatin (175 mg/m^2) administered on day 1, followed by DOX (15 mg/m^2) on day 2.[275] Combination DOX-carboplatin was administered every 21 days for a maximum of four treatment cycles. Nineteen dogs completed four treatment cycles. The tolerability of the combination was good with mild GI toxicity reported in approximately 50% of dogs; grade III hematologic toxicity or greater was rare. The median DFI and MST were 195 and 235 days, respectively, and not considered superior to historical single-agent studies.

Doxorubicin-Carboplatin Alternating Chemotherapy

The tolerability and activity of full-dose, alternating combinations with DOX and carboplatin have been investigated. In one study, 32 dogs were treated with amputation or LSS and then with adjuvant carboplatin (300 mg/m^2 or 10 mg/kg if <15 kg) followed 21 days later with DOX (30 mg/m^2 or 1.0 mg/kg if <15 kg).[276] Dogs were treated with up to three treatment cycles (three carboplatin and three DOX). Alternating carboplatin and

DOX therapy was well tolerated; only one grade III neutropenia, one grade III thrombocytopenia, and one grade III vomiting were recorded from a total of 88 doses of carboplatin and 82 doses of DOX administered. The median DFI and MST were 227 and 320 days, respectively, with 1- and 2-year survival rates of 48% and 18%, respectively.

In a second study, 50 dogs were treated with amputation and, 10 to 14 days postoperatively, alternating combination chemotherapy with carboplatin (300 mg/m^2) and DOX (30 mg/m^2) every 21 days for three cycles (three carboplatin and three DOX).[277] Adverse events, including grade III or IV hematologic toxicity, were reported in 18% of dogs and grade III or IV GI toxicity was recorded in 12% of dogs. The median DFI and MST were 202 and 258, respectively.

Doxorubicin-Carboplatin Modified Combination Sequencing or Dose Interval

Combination sequencing or dose interval alterations with carboplatin and DOX have been investigated to assess whether this may improve the outcome in dogs with OSA. In one study, the safety and efficacy of adjuvant chemotherapy, consisting of two doses of DOX (30 mg/m^2 or 1 mg/kg in dogs <15 kg) given 2 weeks apart, followed by four consecutive doses of carboplatin (300 mg/m^2) every 3 weeks, was evaluated retrospectively in 33 dogs after amputation. Tolerability to this protocol was reasonable with the greatest hematologic toxicity occurring post-DOX administration; approximately 10% of dogs experienced grade III or IV neutropenia. Similarly, 16% of dogs experienced grade III to IV GI toxicity. The drug combination also exerted anticancer activities with dogs achieving median DFI and overall MST of 232 and 247 days, respectively.[278]

In another study, 38 dogs were treated with amputation and a combination of three doses of DOX (30 mg/m^2 or 1 mg/kg in dogs <15 kg) every 14 days, followed by three consecutive doses of carboplatin (300 mg/m^2 for dogs ≥15 kg or 250 mg/m^2 for dogs <15 kg) every 21 days. This combinatorial strategy was tolerable with 5.2% of dogs requiring hospitalization for complications associated with toxicity. Additionally, anticancer activity were comparable to most treatment protocols with dogs achieving a MST of 317 days and 1- and 2-year survival rates of 43.2% and 13.9%, respectively.[279]

Head-to-Head Comparison Studies

Despite multiple published studies evaluating the anticancer activities of carboplatin, DOX, or the combination in dogs with OSA, few investigations can offer prescriptive recommendations on the best adjuvant treatment options, either due to insufficient power as a consequence of small study populations or limited study design being either retrospective in nature or the absence of relevant contemporaneous comparator arms. To address some of these limitations, two recent studies have been published. The first investigation, although retrospective in nature, included a large number of dogs with OSA treated at a single institution and compared carboplatin and DOX-based chemotherapy protocols in 470 dogs after amputation. Five different chemotherapy protocols were compared for tolerability and anticancer effects: carboplatin 300 mg/m^2 IV every 21 days for four or six cycles; DOX 30 mg/m^2 IV every 14 or 21 days for five cycles; and alternating carboplatin 300 mg/m^2 IV and DOX 30 mg/m^2 IV every 21 days for three cycles. Overall, the median DFI and MST were 291 and 284 days, respectively. Although no chemotherapy protocol proved superior, a lower proportion of dogs treated with six cycles of carboplatin experienced adverse effects, necessitating treatment delay, dose reduction, or hospitalization.[208]

In a second study, carboplatin and alternating carboplatin and DOX were evaluated in a randomized, open-label trial study. Dogs were treated with either six doses of carboplatin (300 mg/m^2 IV) every 3 weeks or three cycles of alternating carboplatin (300 mg/m^2 IV) and DOX (30 mg/m^2 IV) every 3 weeks. Of the 50 dogs recruited at a 1:1 ratio for either carboplatin alone or alternating carboplatin and DOX, 32 dogs completed their planned chemotherapy protocols and the remaining 18 dogs developed metastatic disease before completion of their targeted chemotherapy course. Toxicity was similar in both treatment arms. Dogs treated with carboplatin alone had a significantly longer DFI (425 days) than dogs treated with the alternating protocol (135 days).[280]

Conventional Chemotherapy Combined with Metronomic Therapies

Several studies have investigated the combination of systemic chemotherapy with concurrent and/or maintenance metronomic

chemotherapy. In one retrospective study of 30 dogs treated with amputation, dogs received one of two chemotherapy protocols (carboplatin alone [300 mg/m^2 IV every 21 days for six cycles] or alternating carboplatin [300 mg/m^2 IV] and DOX [30 mg/m^2 IV] every 21 days for a total of five treatments [three carboplatin and two DOX]) and concurrent daily piroxicam (0.3 mg/kg PO) and cyclophosphamide (10–12 mg/m^2 PO). The initiation of combinatorial systemic therapies was started 2 days postamputation and metronomic chemotherapy continued indefinitely after the completion of systemic chemotherapy. Although adverse side effects were tolerable for both combinatorial protocols, grade III to IV toxicities were more commonly observed in dogs treated with carboplatin alone plus piroxicam/cyclophosphamide therapy. No significant difference in DFI was identified between the protocols.[281]

In a second study, the potential benefit of metronomic cyclophosphamide and meloxicam administered as a maintenance therapy after amputation and carboplatin was evaluated retrospectively in 39 dogs. Carboplatin therapy (300 mg/m^2 IV every 21 days for four to six cycles) was started 10 to 14 days postamputation. Of the 39 dogs evaluated and treated with carboplatin, 19 dogs were treated with maintenance metronomic cyclophosphamide (15 mg/m^2 PO daily) and meloxicam (0.1 mg/kg PO daily), and the remaining 20 dogs were not treated with maintenance metronomic chemotherapy. Sterile hemorrhagic cystitis was reported in 58% of dogs treated with metronomic chemotherapy. The median progression-free (PFS) and MST were 402 and 464 days, respectively. Though dogs receiving maintenance metronomic chemotherapy did achieve longer median PFS (480 days) and MST (480 days) than dogs treated with carboplatin alone (244 days and 458 days, respectively), the differences were not statistically significant.[282]

Chemoimmunotherapy

Harnessing and directing the immune system is a highly desirable anticancer strategy. Despite the various forms of immunotherapies, such as monoclonal antibodies and dendritic cell vaccines, currently used for the treatment of metastatic tumors in people, only a few canine immunotherapy studies have been conducted as randomized, double-blind trials. The best documented and clinically effective immunotherapy trials for dogs with OSA have evaluated the anticancer immune effects of liposome-encapsulated muramyl tripeptide-phosphatidylethanolamine (L-MTP-PE). Being a lipophilic derivative of muramyl dipeptide, a synthetic analog of a Mycobacterium cell wall component, L-MTP-PE has been demonstrated to augment canine alveolar macrophage tumoricidal properties with enhanced cytotoxicity against OSA cells in vitro.[283]

In an initial clinical study of 27 dogs, the single-agent activity of IV L-MTP-PE was assessed immediately after amputation. Dogs were treated twice weekly with either L-MTP-PE or empty liposomes for 8 weeks. Dogs treated with L-MTP-PE had a significantly longer median DFI (168 days) than dogs treated with empty liposomes (58 days). Similarly, the MST was significantly longer for dogs treated with L-MTP-PE (222 days) than for dogs treated with empty liposomes (77 days).[284] Based upon these findings, it was concluded that L-MTP-PE induced beneficial immunobiologic effects capable of delaying the development of pulmonary metastasis.

After establishing the anticancer activity of single-agent L-MTP-PE when used in the adjuvant setting, two subsequent randomized, double-blind studies were conducted to determine the effectiveness of combining L-MTP-PE with cisplatin.[285] In one study, dogs were treated with limb amputation and cisplatin every 4 weeks for four treatments. Upon completion of cisplatin therapy, 25 dogs without overt evidence of pulmonary metastasis were randomized to receive either L-MTP-PE or empty liposomes twice a week for 8 weeks. Dogs treated with L-MTP-PE had a significantly longer MST (14.4 months) than dogs treated with empty liposomes (9.8 months).

Unlike the first study in which cisplatin and L-MTP-PE was administered serially, the second study investigated the anticancer activities of concurrently administered cisplatin and L-MTP-PE in 64 dogs. All dogs were treated with limb amputation and cisplatin every 3 weeks for four treatments. Within 24 hours after the first cisplatin treatment, dogs were randomized to concurrently receive either L-MTP-PE twice weekly, L-MTP-PE once weekly, or empty liposomes once weekly for 8 weeks. Dogs treated with concurrent L-MTP-PE (once or twice weekly) and cisplatin did not have an improvement in median DFI or MST compared with dogs treated with concurrent empty liposomes and cisplatin. The MSTs for the twice weekly, once weekly L-MTP-PE, and empty liposome groups were 10.3, 10.5, and 7.6 months, respectively.

These studies suggest that innate immune activation may be a strategy for improving outcomes in dogs with OSA. This priming of the innate immune system has been leveraged through different strategies. The potential to create localized inflammation, apoptosis, and necrosis within the immediate tumor microenvironment with subsequent adaptive immune cell priming was evaluated in dogs with OSA receiving an intratumoral adenoviral vector for FasL (Ad-FasL). Through an open-label clinical trial, 52 dogs with OSA were treated with intratumoral Ad-FasL and subsequent limb amputation 10 days post-Ad-FasL administration and carboplatin chemotherapy. After amputation, histologic examination of the primary tumor was performed to characterize degree of inflammation, apoptosis, necrosis, and lymphocyte infiltration. Dogs with greater inflammation and lymphocyte infiltration scores had improved median DFIs and MSTs. When inflammation induced by Ad-FasL was categorized into low (score 1) versus high (score 2 or 3), the MSTs were 198 versus 359 days, respectively. Collectively, these studies support the notion that creating a robust innate immune response within the immediate primary tumor microenvironment has the capacity to induce sufficient immunogenic abscopal effects to delay the onset of metastatic disease.[286]

In addition to innate immune activation strategies, a vaccine approach to specifically induce tumor-specific T-cell responses against the dominant immune epitopes of HER2/neu expressed by canine OSA cells has been reported. Through the generation and IV administration of a highly attenuated, recombinant *Listeria monocytogenes* expressing a chimeric human HER2/neu+ fusion protein (ADXS31-164), the capacity to elicit a HER2-specific immune response was evaluated in 18 dogs with OSA treated with three consecutive dosages of ADXS31-164 every 3 weeks after the completion of conventional therapy (amputation or LSS and four doses of carboplatin chemotherapy). In 15 dogs, HER2-specific responses could be serially assessed through the quantification of antigen-induced T-cell interferon-gamma (IFNγ) secretion, and this served as an immune biomarker to measure the immune reaction elicited by vaccination with ADXS31-164. Although T-cell IFNγ secretion profiles did not correlate with long-term survival outcomes, the magnitude of white blood cell, neutrophil, and monocyte elevations 24 hours after ADXS31-164 administration were significantly greater in dogs with STs exceeding 18 months. These collective findings would suggest that innate immune responses are contributing to the anticancer immune effects exerted by ADXS31-164. Overall, the adjuvant use of ADXS31-164 after standard-of-care therapy was well tolerated, and treated dogs achieved prolonged disease control with a median DFI and MST of 615 and 956 days, respectively.[287]

Molecular Targeted Therapies for Dogs with Osteosarcoma

The GH and IGF-1 growth factor signaling cascade has been thoroughly investigated in OSA. The putative roles of GH and IGF-1 in OSA pathogenesis are supported by several clinical observations in both humans and dogs. Given the central roles of GH and IGF-1 in skeletal growth and homeostasis, as well as their role in cell survival, it has been hypothesized that aberrant or excessive GH and IGF-1 signaling is likely involved in OSA pathogenesis.[288] To investigate the biologic consequences of attenuating GH and IGF-1 autocrine and/or paracrine signaling in OSA, a randomized clinical trial of 44 dogs with OSA was conducted in which circulating IGF-1 concentrations were suppressed with the administration of a long-acting somatostatin analog (OncoLAR).[268] All dogs were treated with amputation and carboplatin in combination with either OncoLAR or control vehicle. The administration of OncoLAR resulted in a 43% reduction in circulating IGF-1 concentrations in comparison to baseline values; however, incomplete suppression in IGF-1 did not result in improved DFIs or overall MSTs in comparison to dogs treated with carboplatin and the vehicle.

Molecular therapies with the capacity to delay or inhibit the development of pulmonary metastases would dramatically improve current treatment outcomes. As such, novel anticancer agents have been designed to selectively inhibit obligate steps necessary for successful tumor cell invasion and metastasis. One specific strategy has been the inhibition of matrix metalloproteinases (MMPs), which are proteolytic enzymes involved in local tissue invasion and metastases. Based upon documented gelatinolytic activities of MMP-2 and MMP-9 in canine cell lines and OSA samples,[91,93] it has been rationalized that specific inhibitors of MMP activity may have the potential to increase the metastasis-free period after amputation and systemic chemotherapy. A prospective, double-blind, randomized, placebo-controlled clinical trial evaluating the adjuvant activity of a MMP-2 and -9 inhibitor (BAY 12-9566) was conducted in 223 dogs with nonmetastatic OSA.[180] After amputation and DOX therapy, dogs were randomized and treated with either BAY 12-9566 (10 mg/kg) or placebo control daily until clinical failure. The addition of BAY 12-9566 did not improve DFI or MST in comparison to placebo control. Correlating with the absence of biologic effect, serum MMP-2 and -9 activities were not different between dogs receiving BAY 12-9566 or placebo.

With the approval of toceranib phosphate (TOC) in veterinary medicine, this small molecule inhibitor of multiple kinase signaling pathways (KIT, VEGF receptor 2 [VEGFR2], platelet-derived growth factor receptor [PDGFR]) has generated scientific interest for its inclusion as an adjuvant treatment for dogs with appendicular OSA. In a randomized, prospective clinical trial, 126 dogs with OSA were treated with amputation and four doses of carboplatin and, if there was no evidence of metastatic disease, this was followed by either oral metronomic therapy (cyclophosphamide and piroxicam) alone or oral metronomic therapy and TOC. Although the inclusion of toceranib phosphate was tolerable, there was no statistical difference in the median DFI for dogs treated with the control protocol (215 days) or TOC (233 days).

Similarly, the MSTs were not different between control (242 days) and TOC (318 days) groups.[289]

Increasing the sensitivity of OSA cells to conventional cytotoxic therapies has the potential to delay the development of metastatic disease. Suramin, a polysulfonated napthylurea, has shown promise to increase tumor sensitivity to chemotherapy and has been evaluated in combination with DOX in 47 dogs with OSA. Suramin was administered at a dose of 6.75 mg/kg IV, and this was followed 4 hours later with 30 mg/m^2 IV DOX every 14 days for a total of five treatments. The combination of suramin and DOX was well tolerated; the median DFI and overall MST were 203 and 369 days, respectively. Although principally a feasibility study, the single-arm design precluded any definitive conclusions to be drawn regarding the ability of adjuvant suramin to augment the anticancer activities of DOX.[290]

Treating Gross Metastatic Disease

Surgery for Gross Metastatic Disease

Resection of pulmonary metastasis from OSA or other solid tumors has been reported in dogs and people.[207,291] In one study of 36 dogs with metastatic OSA to the lungs, metastasectomy was performed by either local resection or partial or total lung lobectomy. Chemotherapy was not administered after pulmonary metastasectomy. Although the initial treatments varied among dogs, the overall MST was 487 days. The MST after pulmonary metastasectomy was 176 days. The criteria established for case selection for pulmonary metastasectomy to maximize the probability of long survival periods were: (1) primary tumor in complete remission, preferably for >300 days; (2) one or two nodules visible on survey thoracic radiographs; (3) metastasis confined to the lungs (negative bone scan); and perhaps (4) long doubling time (>30 days) with no new visible lesions within this time. In a small series, pulmonary metastasectomy was also effective in ameliorating the clinical effects of hypertrophic osteopathy in four dogs with metastatic appendicular OSA.[292]

Chemotherapy and Receptor Tyrosine Kinase Inhibitors for Gross Osteosarcoma

The treatment of gross measurable OSA with conventional cytotoxic agents or receptor tyrosine kinase inhibitors remains unsatisfactory. In part, the ineffectiveness of systemic therapies to cytoreduce gross measurable OSA lesions is likely secondary to drug-resistant clones in conjunction with unfavorable and altered drug biodistribution within large tumor microenvironments. Because formidable biologic barriers exist within macroscopic tumors that favor cancer cell survival, the majority of studies demonstrate only marginal effectiveness of conventional cytotoxic agents or receptor tyrosine kinase inhibitors for the management of gross, measurable OSA.

In one study, 45 dogs that had either developed gross metastatic OSA after standard-of-care therapy (amputation and systemic chemotherapy) or diagnosed at presentation with metastatic OSA were treated with single-agent chemotherapies including cisplatin, DOX, or mitoxantrone.[293] Only one dog achieved a short-lived (21 days) partial response. These findings suggest that conventional cytotoxic agents, which are effective in the adjuvant setting, are not efficacious for managing macroscopic metastatic OSA. In a second study evaluating the tolerability and anticancer activities of paclitaxel in dogs with measurable tumor burdens, two of nine dogs with macroscopic pulmonary metastatic OSA achieved a partial response, suggesting that inhibitors of microtubule depolymerization might have modest activity for the management of gross measurable OSA lesions.[294]

In addition to cytotoxic agents, TOC has recently evaluated for anticancer activity across a broad range of tumor histologies, including metastatic pulmonary OSA.[295] Based on the ability of TOC to inhibit multiple signaling pathways, its potential activity was evaluated retrospectively in 23 dogs with measurable pulmonary OSA metastases.[296] TOC was orally administered at a median dose 2.7 mg/kg (every other day or Monday-Wednesday-Friday). A partial response was noted in one dog (4.3%) and stable disease in 10 dogs (43.5%). Given the initial potential activity of TOC phosphate in dogs with macroscopic pulmonary metastatic disease, its activity was further evaluated in two subsequent follow-up studies. In one prospective study, 22 dogs with measurable pulmonary metastases were treated with TOC at a target dosage of 2.75 mg/kg PO on Monday-Wednesday-Friday schedule. Dogs were reevaluated at weeks 2, 3, 4, and 8 week to assess for biochemical tolerability, and at 8 weeks for radiographic response. In addition to radiographic response, changes in circulating VEGF and Tregs associated with TOC therapy were quantified. Nine dogs were withdrawn from study before radiographic assessment due to reduced quality of life and/or disease progression. Stable and progressive disease was documented in 17.6% and 83.4% of the remaining dogs, respectively. The median PFS and overall MSTs were 57 and 89 days, respectively. Circulating VEGF increased with TOC treatment, but there was no effect on Tregs.[297] A second retrospective study in 20 dogs confirmed the overall low efficacy of TOC in the treatment of dogs with pulmonary metastases. In this second study, TOC was administered at a median dose of 2.52 mg/kg. A partial response and stable disease was documented in one dog each for an overall 10% clinical benefit rate. The median PFS and overall MST were 36 and 90 days, respectively.[298] Based upon these two studies, the anticancer activities of TOC as a single agent managing macroscopic OSA metastases is relatively low.

Strategies to enhance the susceptibility of metastatic cancers to conventional chemotherapeutic agents have also been investigated. By virtue of their chromatin remodeling effects, histone deacetylase inhibitors (HDACi) used in combination with cytotoxic agents may enhance the nuclear accumulation of cytotoxic agents and improve therapeutic outcomes. Based on this premise and a systems biology approach to identifying molecular pathways altered by HDAC inhibition in OSA,[299] a phase I dose-escalation study combining valproic acid and DOX was conducted in dogs with various spontaneous tumors to determine the tolerability and activity of this HDACi-chemotherapy combination.[300] Three dogs with macroscopic OSA pulmonary metastases were treated with valproic acid and DOX, and one dog achieved durable stable disease.

Investigational Therapies for Gross Metastatic Disease

Aerosol Drug Delivery

Two studies have been conducted to evaluate the feasibility, tolerability, and anticancer activities of aerosolized cytotoxic therapies in dogs diagnosed with pulmonary OSA metastases.[301,302] In one study, six dogs with pulmonary OSA metastasis were treated with inhaled DOX, paclitaxel, or both every 14 days for a total of six treatments.[301] Aerosolization therapy was well tolerated with no dose-limiting hematologic or biochemical toxicity; however, in dogs treated with aerosolized DOX, pulmonary histologic changes were identified at necropsy in some patients, consisting of toxin-induced pneumonitis, multifocal interstitial fibrosis, alveolar histiocytosis, and type II pneumocyte proliferation. A partial response was documented in two dogs treated with inhaled DOX and a complete response in one dog treated with inhaled paclitaxel. In the one dog with a complete response, the response was durable and persisted for more than 325 days.

In addition to DOX and paclitaxel, aerosolized gemcitabine has been evaluated in dogs with metastatic OSA. Gemcitabine, a pyrimidine antimetabolite belonging to the nucleoside analog family, has anticancer activity when administered through an aerosolized route in mouse OSA xenograft models; these are mediated though the upregulation of Fas receptor expression on the surface of pulmonary metastatic OSA cells.[303] Because lung epithelium basally expresses Fas ligand, the restoration of Fas receptor expression by OSA cells would consequently render them susceptible to Fas receptor/Fas ligand-mediated apoptosis. Based on this preclinical information, a comparative study with aerosolized gemcitabine was conducted in 20 dogs with pulmonary OSA metastasis.[302] Dogs were treated twice weekly with inhalation gemcitabine and monitored for toxicity and anticancer activity. Aerosolized gemcitabine was well tolerated with no dose-limiting hematologic or biochemical toxicity reported and minimal histologic lung pathology after inhalation therapy. Mechanistic anticancer activities of aerosolized gemcitabine were supported by the identification of increases in percent necrosis, Fas receptor expression, and TUNEL positivity in macroscopic pulmonary OSA metastatic lesions; however, clinically relevant responses were not documented.

Augmentation of Antitumor Immunity

Cytokines are cellular peptides that actively aid or stimulate the immune system to recognize and attack cancer cells. Although numerous cytokines participate in shaping the strength, specificity, and longevity of antitumor immune responses, interleukin-2 (IL-2) is a critical cytokine necessary for stimulating the growth, differentiation, and survival of antigen-specific cytotoxic T cells. Additional immune effects orchestrated by IL-2 include the facilitation of immunoglobulin production by B cells and the differentiation and proliferation of natural killer cells. Despite the pleiotropic and desirable antitumor immune activities of IL-2, its systemic administration has been clinically limited due to severe toxicities. As such, alternative delivery strategies have been investigated to attenuate IL-2 associated toxicities yet maximize its potent immunomodulatory effects.

For the treatment of pulmonary metastasis, the localized deposition of IL-2 or the preferential gene expression of IL-2 within the lung parenchyma has been investigated as a novel treatment option in dogs with metastatic OSA. Initial studies evaluated the antitumor activities of inhaled liposomal IL-2.[304] Dogs were nebulized with liposomal IL-2 daily for 30 days. The immunomodulatory effects of IL-2 were confirmed by increases in bronchoalveolar lavage effector cell numbers and lytic activities with resultant complete regression of macroscopic pulmonary OSA metastasis in two of four dogs. The duration of this response was between 12 and 20 months. IV gene therapy as liposome-DNA complexes encoding IL-2 has also been investigated as an alternative to inhaled liposomal IL-2 delivery strategies.[305] Based on its preferential accumulation and subsequent transgene expression within the lung parenchyma, the tolerability, immunomodulatory effects, and antitumor activity of IV liposome DNA complexes encoding IL-2 were evaluated in 20 dogs with chemotherapy-resistant OSA metastasis. After administration, the immunomodulatory effects

of liposome DNA complexes were substantiated by the induction of fever, leukogram changes, monocyte activation, and increased natural killer cell activities. After completion of 12 consecutive weekly IV treatments with liposome DNA complexes, measurable responses were achieved in three dogs with one complete response and two partial responses.

Other investigations have evaluated alternative strategies for activating the immune system, including IV administration of a genetically modified and attenuated bacterial species, *Salmonella typhimurium* (VNP20009).[306] Based on the premise that anaerobic bacteria have potential as novel immunomodulatory cancer therapeutics, a phase I dose escalation study was conducted with VNP20009 in 41 dogs with spontaneous cancers. Dose-limiting toxicity included fever and vomiting; both were attributed to systemic immune activation. Importantly, preferential tumor tissue tropism of VNP20009 was confirmed by gene transcription and bacterial culture techniques in a substantial proportion of tumor samples. In a subset of four dogs with OSA pulmonary metastasis, one dog had a partial response for a duration of 68 days.

Palliative Treatment: Primary and Metastatic Bone Cancer Pain

Palliative Radiation Therapy

RT is considered the most effective treatment modality for the management of osteolytic bone pain in human cancer patients and, likewise, has been investigated and extensively applied for alleviating bone cancer pain in dogs with primary bone tumors. Mechanistically, the analgesic effects of ionizing radiation can be partially attributed to the induction of cell death in both malignant osteoblasts and resorbing osteoclasts,[307] and this has been documented in dogs by an assessment of percentage TN.[205,239,308] As such, ionizing radiation may reduce overall tumor burden and attenuate the degree of osteoclast resorption. The rapid onset of analgesia that occurs before a change in tumor volume suggests other, as yet unknown, mechanisms are involved in the analgesic effects of RT. Other proposed mechanisms of radiation-induced analgesia include depletion of local inflammatory cells and inhibition of osteoclast precursor recruitment.[309]

Multiple palliative RT protocols have been evaluated and reported in the veterinary literature with the majority of dosing schemes using two to four fractions of 6 to 10 Gy. Although variable and subjectively reported in these studies, the alleviation of bone cancer pain was achieved in 74% to 93% of dogs. Although the majority of dogs symptomatically improved after palliative RT, the median time interval of subjective pain alleviation was not durable and ranged from 53 to 130 days.[234,310–314] Given that most conventional palliative RT protocols only include two to four fractions, the total cumulative radiation dose administered is relatively low (<32 Gy). As a result, acute and late radiation toxicities are not a limiting factor for the majority of patients treated. Although megavoltage palliative RT appears effective when used as a single-agent treatment option for short-term pain management, some investigations suggest that the concurrent administration of IV systemic chemotherapy along with palliative RT may enhance analgesic response rates, durations of responses, and overall STs.[313,315]

Radiopharmaceuticals

^{153}Sm is a radioisotope that undergoes gamma (103 keV) and beta decay (max 810 keV), allowing for concurrent biodistribution tracking studies as well as therapeutic ionizing radiation delivery within a 2 to 3 mm deposition radius. When ^{153}Sm is conjugated to EDTMP, which is a bisphosphonate, the resultant ^{153}Sm-EDTMP compound preferentially concentrates in areas of increased osteoblastic activity and binds to exposed hydroxyapatite crystals.[316] By virtue of its osteotropism and defined radius of ionizing radiation deposition, ^{153}Sm-EDTMP is currently used as a radiopharmaceutical for the palliative treatment of multifocal skeletal metastases in people with breast or prostate carcinoma.[317]

Similar to people diagnosed with skeletal malignant osteolysis, the use of ^{153}Sm-EDTMP has been investigated for alleviating bone cancer pain in dogs with appendicular and axial OSA.[318–322] In dogs treated with ^{153}Sm-EDTMP, the predicted radiation dose equivalent achieved within the immediate bone tumor microenvironment has been estimated to approximate 20 Gy,[318] although its intratumoral biodistribution is expected to be nonhomogenous based upon regional differences in reparative osteoblastic activities. After IV ^{153}Sm-EDTMP administration, the 63% to 83% of dogs with OSA demonstrate improved lameness scores and activity levels, suggesting palliation of pain.[318–321] In axial skeletal lesions, four dogs were documented to have an improvement at 21 days posttreatment based on reduced tumor size or improved clinical signs, whereas 13 dogs had progressive disease based on worsening of clinical signs or tumor growth.[322]

^{177}Lutetium (^{177}Lu) is an isotope that emits gamma photons (208 keV) and beta particles (max 497 keV). ^{177}Lu has been investigated when complexed with EDTMP or DOTMP, a macrocyclic analog of EDMTP.[266] ^{177}Lu is proposed to offer greater bone marrow sparing effects in comparison to ^{153}Sm-EDTMP due to a lower soft tissue penetration of 670 μm. The toxicity profile of ^{177}Lu-DOTMP has been evaluated in normal dogs and no significant changes in platelet or white cell counts were observed, but mild changes in red cell counts were noted on day 84.[323] A pilot study was performed in four dogs with primary or metastatic skeletal lesions, and analgesic effect was demonstrated in three dogs.[324] In human patients, ^{177}Lu-EDTMP appears equally effective at inducing analgesia compared with ^{153}Sm-EDTMP with a similar toxicity profile.[325]

Aminobisphosphonates

Aminobisphosphonates (NBPs) are synthetic analogs of inorganic pyrophosphate that were initially utilized for diagnostic purposes in bone scanning based on their ability to preferentially adsorb to sites of active bone mineral remodeling. The pharmaceutical use of NBPs has gained wide acceptance in the therapy of human nonneoplastic bone resorptive disorders such as osteoporosis and Paget's disease.[326] In addition to the management of these metabolic disorders, NBPs are considered first-line options for the treatment of malignant skeletal osteolytic conditions, including paraneoplastic hypercalcemia, multiple myeloma, and metastatic bone diseases in human cancer patients.[327,328]

The effective treatment of bone disorders by NBPs is attributed to their differential effect on bone resorption and bone mineralization. At concentrations safely achievable in vivo, NBPs inhibit bone resorption without inhibiting bone mineralization. Mechanistically, the bone protective effects exerted by NBPs are through the induction of osteoclast apoptosis, which results in the net attenuation of pathologic bone resorption.[329,330] Specifically, NBPs interfere with posttranslational prenylation of small GTP-binding proteins, including Ras, Rho, and Rac.[331] The disruption of these small GTP-binding protein results in the failure of normal intracellular signaling and interaction with the extracellular matrix, thereby triggering osteoclast apoptosis.

Given that OSA is characterized by focal and aggressive malignant osteolysis, the investigation of NBPs has been a focus of clinical interest. The first reported description in the veterinary literature was the use of oral alendronate for the palliative management of two dogs with OSA.[332] Based upon the unexpectedly long STs reported in this anecdotal study, the authors suggested that NBPs therapy may have a role in managing dogs malignant bone diseases. Given that IV NBPs have been historically used for the management of malignant osteolysis in people, a prospective study principally evaluating the safety of IV pamidronate (PAM) was conducted in 33 dogs diagnosed with primary and secondary skeletal tumors.[333] IV PAM (1.0 mg/kg diluted with 0.9% sodium chloride to a total volume of 250 mL) as a 2-hour constant rate infusion (CRI) every 28 days was well-tolerated and, in a subset of dogs, the bone biologic and clinically relevant therapeutic effects of IV PAM were documented with significant reductions in urine N-telopeptide (NTx) concentrations, increases in relative primary tumor bone mineral density (rBMD) as assessed by dual-energy x-ray absorptiometry (DEXA), and subjective pain alleviation.

After the established safety of IV PAM in dogs with skeletal tumors, a second study of 43 dogs treated with IV PAM (1.0 mg/kg versus 2.0 mg/kg) was conducted to further characterize the biologic activity of PAM specifically for the management of appendicular OSA associated bone pain and pathologic bone resorption.[334] Overall, 28% of 43 OSA-bearing dogs achieved pain alleviation for more than 4 months. In addition to the subjective analgesic effects of PAM reported by pet owners, changes in urine NTx concentrations and DEXA-assessed rBMD correlated with therapeutic response.

Although original studies have focused on the palliative effects of PAM when used as a single-agent, a recent study documented the synergistic activity of PAM when coupled with palliative RT in dogs with appendicular OSA.[335] In a prospective, double-blind, randomized, placebo controlled clinical trial, 17 dogs with appendicular OSA were treated with palliative RT (8 Gy on days 1 and 2) and either 0.9% saline infusion or PAM once every 4 weeks for three treatments. Before initial palliative RT and after each IV treatment with either 0.9% saline or PAM, all dogs were evaluated by force plate gait analysis, urine NTx concentrations, numerical lameness evaluation, and owner quality of life (QOL) questionnaires. The saline placebo group dogs experienced a significant increase in numerical lameness score between weeks 0 and 12, and PAM significantly lowered the lameness scores on week 12 compared with saline. In addition, dogs receiving PAM had a significantly greater vertical impulse and total stance time from week 4 to week 12. Based on these findings, the addition of PAM to palliative RT appeared to improved limb function compared with palliative RT alone.

In a double-blind, placebo-controlled study, 50 dogs with OSA were treated with palliative RT, DOX, and either a saline placebo or PAM.[336] The median pain-free intervals for dogs treated adjuvant PAM or saline was 76 days and 75 days, respectively. Despite the apparent lack of pet owner-perceived analgesia, dogs treated with adjuvant PAM had better QOL scores and, more importantly, decreased malignant bone resorption in the primary tumor. Collectively, these findings suggest that adjuvant PAM may not subjectively improve analgesia when dogs are already receiving treatment with megavoltage RT and DOX, but PAM still exerts beneficial bone biologic effects within the bone tumor microenvironment in dogs with OSA.

Although most palliative studies have documented the effects of PAM, other more potent IV NBPs for managing malignant

TABLE 25.3	A Comparison of Canine and Human Osteosarcoma Characteristics	
Variable	**Dog**	**Human**
Incidence in United States	>8000/year	1000/year
Mean age	7 years	14 years
Race/breed	Large or giant purebreds	None
Body weight	90% >20 kg	Heavy
Site	77% long bones Metaphyseal Distal radius > proximal humerus Distal femur > tibia	90% long bones Metaphyseal Proximal humerus Distal femur > proximal tibia
Etiology	Generally unknown	Generally unknown
Percentage clinically confined to the limb at presentation	80%–90%	80%–90%
Percentage histologically high grade	95%	85%–90%
DNA index	75% aneuploid	75% aneuploid
Genetic and molecular alterations	See Etiology Section	See Etiology Section
Prognostic indicators[178,179]	Alkaline phosphatase	Alkaline phosphatase
Metastatic rate without chemotherapy	90% before 1 year	80% before 2 years
Metastatic sites	Lung > bone > soft tissue	Lung > bone > soft tissue
Improved survival with chemotherapy	Yes	Yes
Regional lymph node metastasis	<5%, negative prognostically	Poor prognosis

Modified with permission from Withrow SJ, Powers BE, Straw RC, et al. *Clin Orthop Relat Res.* 1991; 270:159–167.[7]

bone pain have been evaluated in dogs with skeletal tumors. Zoledronate (ZOL) has a 100-fold greater antiresorptive potency than PAM and has the advantage of being safely administered over a shorter period of time than other NBPs. In one case report, IV ZOL administered every 28 days was effective for the long-term pain management of a dog with a distal radial OSA.[337] The bone biologic effects of IV ZOL were evaluated in 10 dogs with primary and secondary skeletal tumors.[338] ZOL was administered at a dose of 0.25 mg/kg as a 15-minute CRI every 28 days. This was well tolerated with no overt biochemical evidence of renal toxicity in patients receiving multiple monthly infusions. Pain was alleviated in 50% of the 10 dogs with appendicular OSA for more than 4 months. These dogs demonstrated significant increases in rBMD, which suggests that ZOL inhibits local malignant osteolysis and the generation of pain within the immediate bone tumor microenvironment. Although studies evaluating the safety of long-term PAM or ZOL in dogs with primary and secondary bone tumors have not been thoroughly evaluated, infrequent and severe bone metabolic changes, such as osteonecrosis of the jaw, have been reported in one dog treated with monthly ZOL (0.1 mg/kg IV, 15-minute CRI) for 43 consecutive months.[339]

Comparative Aspects

Animal models for the study of human diseases are important to better understand the mechanisms and etiology of diseases and to develop and refine therapeutic strategies. Spontaneously developing diseases in animal populations are particularly useful for translational purposes.[340–342] Canine OSA has many similarities to human OSA in terms of genetic similarities, clinical presentation,

biologic behavior, and metastatic progression and has been shown through many studies to be a valuable comparative model for study (Table 25.3).[7,341] OSA is more common in dogs than in humans, and therefore case accrual is more rapid. Because disease progression is more rapid in dogs than in humans, results of novel treatment protocols can be reported earlier than in similar trials in humans. Research costs for clinical trials in dogs are less compared with those in human clinical trials, and, from an animal welfare standpoint, no disease is induced and dogs with cancer can potentially be helped through the course of the research.

OSA is an uncommon cancer in humans, affecting mainly adolescents in their second decade of life, and it remains a very serious, aggressive tumor. Fortunately, there has been an improvement in survival rates with the use of established multidrug adjuvant protocols incorporating high-dose methotrexate, DOX, and cisplatin. The long-term survival rate for human OSA is presently 60% to 70% at 5 years, which contrasts with the 20% 5-year survival rate of the early 1980s. A recent retrospective study of 251 patients showed that the 5-year survival rate increased from 36% in the 1980s to 67% in the early 2000s. During the same period, LSS for local disease control increased from 53% to 97%, and the need for amputation due to failure of the LSSs concurrently decreased, indicating that the increased adoption of LSSs did not negatively affect outcome.[343]

Poor prognostic factors include older age, advanced local or systemic stage, axial location, larger size, and percentage TN.[344] Tumor necrosis of more than 90% after neoadjuvant chemotherapy is highly prognostic for improved patient outcome with 5-year survival rates of 75% to 80% compared with 45% to 50% for those with less than 90% necrosis. A recent phase III

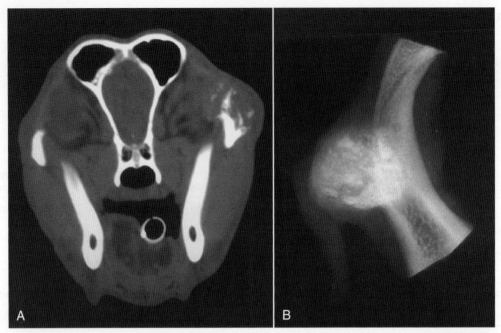

• **Fig. 25.12** (A) Computed tomography scan of a low-grade parosteal osteosarcoma of the zygomatic arch in a dog. Low-grade primary bone tumors are often more radiodense and well circumscribed. (B) Specimen radiograph after zygomatic arch resection.

trial randomly assigned 618 patients with less than 90% tumor necrosis after neoadjuvant chemotherapy to a protocol that incorporated ifosphamide and etoposide in addition to the standard-of-care drugs methotrexate, DOX, and cisplatin. This study failed to show any prolongation in PFS after administration of the additional chemotherapy agents and resulted in more frequent grade IV hematologic toxicity.[345]

Bone Surface Osteosarcoma

OSA usually originates from elements within the medullary canal of bones (intraosseous OSA); however, there are forms of this cancer that originate from the outer surface of bones. Periosteal OSA is a high-grade form of surface OSA and seems to arise from the periosteal surface but has invasive characteristics that can be seen radiographically.[346] There is cortical lysis with extension of the tumor into the bone and surrounding soft tissues. These tumors are histologically similar to intraosseous OSA and have a similar aggressive biological behavior.

In contrast, parosteal or juxtacortical OSA arises from the periosteal surface of bones but is less aggressive than periosteal OSA both radiographically and biologically. Parosteal OSAs are uncommon and have a moderately well-circumscribed radiographic appearance. These tumors grow out from the periosteal side of a cortex, and cortical lysis is usually very mild on radiographs. Histologically, these tumors look more benign compared with intraosseous or periosteal OSA. These tumors contain well-differentiated cartilage, fibrous tissue, and bone with sparse regions of sarcoma cells adjacent to tumor osteoid. Histologic specimens must be evaluated carefully because it is often easy to miss the areas of tumor cells and misdiagnose the lesion as an osteoma, chondroma, or reactive bone. They generally do not invade the medullary canal and tend to grow out from the bone on broad pedicles. Diagnosis is based on typical histologic and radiographic findings.

Parosteal OSA is usually slow growing, but can induce pain at the local site. Metastasis can occur, but the prognosis for long-term survival is much better than for intraosseous OSA.[347,348] Control of parosteal OSA can be achieved by en bloc resection of the tumor with the adjacent cortical bone, as has been reported for tumors of the zygomatic arch (Fig. 25.12).[348] If full thickness cortex needs to be removed for tumors in the long bones, reconstruction may be performed using autogenous corticocancellous bone such as a rib, ileal crest, or allogeneic cortical bone.

Other Primary Bone Tumors of Dogs

Primary bone tumors other than OSA account for 2% to 15% of bone malignancies in dogs. These tumors include CSAs, FSAs, HSAs, lymphomas, and plasma cell tumors.

It can be difficult to distinguish chondroblastic OSA from CSA, fibroblastic OSA from FSA, and telangiectatic OSA from HSA when only small amounts of tissue are evaluated.[140] This makes interpretation of older reports difficult in terms of trying to establish the true incidence of the different types of primary bone tumors; however, more recent studies have identified IHC markers which may aid in bone sarcoma differentiation.[349–351]

Chondrosarcoma

CSA is the second most common primary tumor of bone in humans and dogs and accounts for approximately 5% to 10% of all canine primary bone tumors.[2–5,352] CSAs are characterized histologically by anaplastic cartilage cells that elaborate a cartilaginous matrix. There is a spectrum of degree of differentiation and maturation of the cells within and between each tumor. Histologic grading systems have been described. The etiology is generally unknown, although CSA can arise in dogs with preexisting multiple cartilaginous exostosis.[353,354] In a clinicopathologic study of 97 dogs with CSA, the mean age was 8.7 years, and Golden

Retrievers were at a higher risk of developing CSA than any other breed.[355] There was no sex predilection, and 61% of the tumors occurred on flat bones. CSA can originate in the nasal cavity, ribs, long bones, pelvis, extraskeletal sites (such as the mammary gland, heart valves, aorta, larynx, trachea, lung, and omentum), vertebrae, facial bones, digits, and os penis.[29,355–362] The nasal cavity is the most common site for canine CSA.[355]

CSA is generally considered to have a lower metastatic rate than OSA; however, a more aggressive variant, dedifferentiated CSA, has been described in seven dogs and one cat, and the metastatic rate in these animals was 63%.[363] Tumor location rather than histologic grade was prognostic in one study,[344] but histologic grade was prognostic in two other studies.[364,365] The MST for dogs with nasal CSA ranges from 210 days to 580 days with various treatments (RT, rhinotomy and RT, and rhinotomy alone).[355,366] Metastatic disease is rare in dogs with nasal CSA. The MST for dogs with CSA of ribs varies widely.[20,171,367] Reports before 1992 contained few cases that were treated with intent to cure, but MSTs in more contemporary reports range from 1080 days to more than 3820 days.[172,181,364,365] The overall MST for 25 dogs with appendicular CSA treated with limb amputation alone was 979 days, but outcomes were dependent on histologic grade. The metastatic rates and MSTs for grade I, II, and III appendicular CSAs were 0% and 6.0 years, 31% and 2.7 years, and 50% and 0.9 years, respectively. A reliable adjuvant chemotherapeutic agent is not known for canine CSA.

Hemangiosarcoma

Primary HSA of bone is rare and accounts for less than 5% of all bone tumors. This disease generally affects middle-aged to older dogs and can occur in dogs of any size. This is a highly metastatic tumor, and most dogs affected will develop metastatic disease within 6 months of diagnosis. Metastases can be widely spread throughout various organs such as lungs, liver, spleen, heart, skeletal muscles, kidney, brain, and bones. Dogs can present with multiple lesions making it difficult to determine the site of primary disease. Histologically, HSA is composed of highly anaplastic mesenchymal cells, which are precursors to vascular endothelium. The cells are arranged in chords separated by a collagenous background and may appear to be forming vascular channels or sinuses. Cellular pleomorphism and numerous mitotic figures are features of this highly malignant disease. There is profound bone lysis, and the malignant cells aggressively invade adjacent normal structures. Appendicular HSA may be confused with telangiectatic OSA, especially if the diagnosis is based on small tissue samples.[349] The dominant radiographic feature is often lysis; however, HSA does not have an unequivocally unique radiographic appearance, and diagnosis is based on histology.

If HSA is diagnosed, the dog must be thoroughly staged with thoracic and abdominal films, bone survey radiographs or bone scintigraphy, and ultrasonographic evaluation, particularly of the heart and abdominal organs. Right atrial HSA may be present without clinical or radiographic signs of pericardial effusion. Cyclophosphamide, vincristine, and DOX have been used in combination as an adjuvant protocol, and the reported MST for dogs with nonskeletal HSA is 172 days.[368] In a recent study of 41 dogs with primary appendicular HSA, a predilection for the pelvic limb was noted, especially the tibia. The overall MST was 299 days after treatment with limb amputation and chemotherapy.[350]

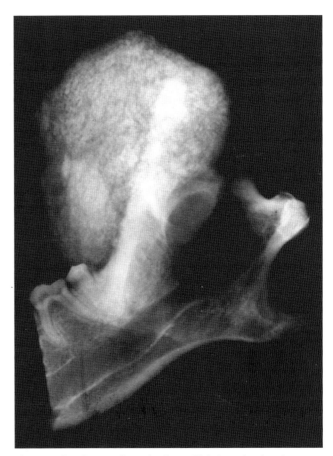

• **Fig. 25.13** Specimen radiograph of a multilobular osteochondrosarcoma arising from the vertical ramus of the mandible in a dog. These tumors have a granular radiographic appearance often referred to as "popcorn ball."

Fibrosarcoma

Primary FSA is also a rare tumor of dogs and accounts for less than 5% of all primary bone tumors.[4] Unfortunately, the difficulty in distinguishing FSA from fibroblastic OSA histologically renders study of this tumor difficult. In one report, 11 dogs thought to have appendicular FSA were reevaluated after complete resection and the histologic diagnosis was changed to OSA in six dogs.[369] Histologic characteristics of FSA include interwoven bundles of fibroblasts within a collagen matrix of permeating cancellous and cortical bone that is not associated with osteoid produced by the tumor cells. Limb amputation or LSS may be curative, although metastatic potential may be considerable. There is no good evidence that adjuvant chemotherapy is beneficial in preventing metastatic disease. It has been postulated that primary FSA of bone has a propensity to metastasize to such sites as heart, pericardium, skin, and bones rather than lung.[369]

Multilobular Osteochondrosarcoma

Multilobular osteochondrosarcoma (MLO) is an uncommon tumor that generally arises from the skull of dogs.[162,370–372] Many names have been used to describe this disease, including chondroma rodens, multilobular osteoma, and multilobular tumor of bone. These tumors have a characteristic appearance on radiographs, CT, and MRI; the borders of the tumor are sharply demarcated with limited lysis of adjacent bone, and there is a coarse granular mineral density throughout (Fig. 25.13).[373,374]

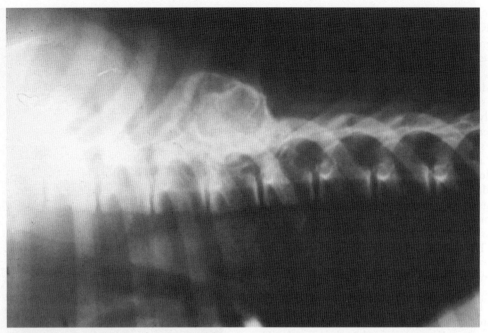

• **Fig. 25.14** Lateral radiograph of a multiple cartilaginous exostosis lesion of the dorsal spinous process in a dog.

There is one report of an MLO of the vertebra that did not have radiographic abnormalities.[375] Histologically, these tumors are composed of multiple lobules, each centered on a core of cartilaginous or bony matrix that is surrounded by a thin layer of spindle cells. A histologic grading system has been described.[162,371] In one report of 39 dogs with MLOs, the median age was 8 years, the median weight was 29 kg, and there was no breed or sex predilection.[373] Local tumor recurrence was reported in 47% of dogs after a median time of 797 days.[373] Metastasis was reported in 56% of dogs; however, time to metastasis was prolonged with a median of 542 days. The MST was 800 days. Local tumor recurrence and metastasis after treatment were predicted by histologic grade and the ability to obtain histologically complete resection.[373] Local tumor excision with histologically complete surgical margins appears to offer a good opportunity for long-term tumor control, especially for low-grade lesions. When metastatic lesions are identified by thoracic radiography, dogs may remain asymptomatic for their lung disease for 1 year or more. The role of chemotherapy and RT in the management of MLO is not well defined.

Metastatic Tumors of Bone

Almost any malignant tumor can metastasize to bone via the hematogenous route. The lumbar vertebrae, femur, humerus, rib, and pelvis are common sites for metastasis, possibly because these are predilection sites for bone metastasis from urinogenital malignancies such as prostate, bladder, urethral, and mammary cancer.[376] Metastatic lesions in long bones frequently affect the diaphysis, likely because of the proximity to a nutrient foramen. Nuclear scintigraphy is a sensitive technique to detect bone metastasis. A whole-body bone scan or PET/CT imaging is recommended when metastatic bone cancer is suspected because it is common for multiple sites of metastasis to be present, even if the patient is symptomatic for only one bone.

Benign Tumors of Bone

Osteomas

Osteomas are benign tumors of bone.[377] Radiographically, these are well circumscribed, dense bony projections that are usually not painful on palpation. Histologically, they are composed of tissue nearly indistinguishable from reactive bone. The diagnosis is made after considering the history and physical examination as well as the radiographic and histologic findings. The most important differential diagnosis is MLO when the lesion occurs on the skull. Treatment for osteoma is simple surgical excision and this is usually curative.

Multiple Cartilaginous Exostosis

Multiple cartilaginous exostosis (MCE) is a developmental condition of growing dogs. There is evidence that the etiology of this condition may have a heritable component.[354,378] The actual incidence of MCE is difficult to determine because affected dogs may show no clinical signs and the diagnosis is often incidental. Endochondral ossification is responsible for formation of these lesions with new bone being formed from a cartilage cap analogous to a physis. Lesions are located on bones that form from endochondral ossification, and lesions stop growing at skeletal maturity. Malignant transformation of MCE lesions has been reported, but generally they remain as unchanged, mature, bony projections from the surface of the bone from which they arose.[353]

Dogs typically present because of a nonpainful or moderately painful palpable mass on the surface of a bone or bones. The pain and lameness is thought to be due to mechanical interference of the mass with overlying soft tissue structures. In the case of MCE of vertebral bodies, animals can present with clinical signs associated with spinal cord impingement. Radiographically, there is a bony mass on the surface of the affected bone that has a benign appearance and a fine trabecular pattern in the body of the mass (Fig. 25.14). To obtain a histologic diagnosis, biopsy material must be collected so that sections include the cartilaginous cap and the underlying stalk of bone. Histologically, this cartilaginous cap gives rise to an orderly array of maturing bone according to the sequence of endochondral ossification. The cortical bone surfaces of the mass and the adjacent bone are confluent.[353] A strong presumptive diagnosis is made by evaluation of the history, physical examination findings, and radiographic features.

Treatment involves conservative surgical excision, but this is only necessary if clinical signs do not abate after the dog reaches skeletal maturity. Because of the likelihood of a heritable etiology, affected dogs should be neutered. Owners should also be advised of the possibility of late malignant transformation. Dogs with a previous history of MCE should be carefully evaluated for bone malignancy if clinical signs return later in life.

Bone Cysts

Cysts are rare, benign lesions of bone. The majority of the veterinary literature pertaining to bone cysts centers on several small series of cases or single case reports.[379–381] Affected animals are often young and present because of mild or moderate lameness; however, pathologic fracture can occur through cystic areas of long bones leading to severe lameness. There appears to be a familial tendency in Doberman Pinschers and Old English Sheepdogs. These lesions are usually in metaphyseal regions of long bones, and they can cross an open growth plate; however, unicameral bone cysts can sometimes be diaphyseal or epiphyseal. The etiology and pathogenesis are unknown, but it is speculated that the lesions may be the result of trauma to the growth plate interfering with proper endochondral ossification. Others have theorized that with the rapid resorption and deposition of bone occurring in the metaphysis of a young animal, a cyst might develop if resorption is so rapid that a focus of loose fibrous tissue forms. The focus of fibrous tissue may then obstruct the thin-walled sinusoids causing interstitial fluid to build up and form a cyst. Cysts have been described in bone immediately below articular cartilage (subchondral bone cysts or juxtacortical bone cysts).[376,379,381] In these, it is possible to demonstrate a direct communication with the articular synovial membrane. Radiographically, bone cysts are either single or, more commonly, multilocular, sharply defined, centrally located, radiolucent defects in the medullary canal of long bones. Variable degrees of thinning of the cortex with symmetric bone "expansion" are often a radiographic feature. Diagnosis of bone cyst relies on the histologic finding of a thin, fibrous wall lined by flat to slightly plump layers of mesothelial or endothelial cells. Treatment consists of meticulous curettage and packing the space with autogenous bone graft.

Aneurysmal bone cysts (ABCs) are spongy, multiloculated masses filled with free-flowing blood. The walls of an ABC are rarely lined by epithelium, and the lesion possibly represents an arteriovenous malformation. A proposed pathogenesis of ABCs is that a primary event, such as trauma or a benign bone tumor, occurs within the bone or periosteum. This event disrupts the vasculature, resulting in a rapidly enlarging lesion with anomalous blood flow that damages the bone mesenchyme. The bone reacts by proliferating. As the vascular anomaly becomes stabilized, the reactive bone becomes more consolidated and matures. The age of affected dogs ranges from 2 to 14 years, but it has been reported in a 6-month-old dog.[380] Treatment options include en bloc resection and reconstruction or extensive curettage with packing of the defect with autogenous bone graft.

Periarticular Tumors

Periarticular tumors in dogs include histiocytic sarcoma (HS), synovial myxoma/myxoma sarcoma, malignant fibrous histiocytoma, and synovial cell sarcoma (SCS). Typical presenting clinical signs include lameness and a firm mass or swelling near the joint. These tumors typically occur in the large joints (particularly the stifle) of the extremities and occur most commonly in large breed, middle-aged dogs. Radiographs show lytic and/or proliferative changes in the bones surrounding the involved joint. The involvement of more than one bone near an affected joint distinguishes the radiographic appearance of a periarticular tumor from a primary bone tumor. The gold standard for the diagnosis of periarticular tumors is biopsy with IHC staining to differentiate the various tumor types. Classic IHC markers include cytokeratin, CD18, vimentin, and smooth muscle actin. The distinction between SCS and periarticular HS is important as these two tumors have differing biologic behaviors and recommended treatments. SCS is typically vimentin positive, cytokeratin positive, and CD18 negative, whereas HS is typically vimentin positive, CD18 positive, and cytokeratin negative. Thus to avoid confusion, some authors suggest that SCS should be replaced with cytokeratin-positive joint associated sarcoma because this better describes the distinction between HS and the classical SCS.[382] Canine SCS can be further subclassified into monophasic or biphasic depending on the presence or absence of an epithelioid component (biphasic) in addition to the spindle cells typically noted with SCS. Amputation is recommended as more conservative resections result in a significantly worse outcome. The overall MST for dogs with SCS is 455 to 967 days, but STs are also dependent on histologic grade. The MSTs for dogs with grade I, II, and III SCSs are 365 to 1460 days, 156 to 1095 days, and 183 days, respectively. The metastatic rate for dogs with SCS is 8% to 32%[383] but up to 91% for dogs with periarticular HS. Treatment for dogs with periarticular HS should include amputation and adjuvant CCNU as MSTs are superior with this multimodality therapy (568 days) than amputation alone (161 days).[382,384,385]

Myxoma sarcomas have a similar radiographic appearance to SCS but, on histology, typically contain multiple myxomatous islands containing widely spaced stellate cells. On gross inspection, these tumors are composed of gelatinous nodules that fill the joint cavity and exude viscous fluid when incised. They occur in the stifle and digits most commonly. They are distinguishable from SCS and HS because they stain positive for vimentin and HSP, variably positive for CD18 (20%–40%), and negative for cytokeratin. Myxomas of the joint are treated with either amputation or local resection (synovectomy) and can have long STs (>2 years) even with incomplete excision.[384]

Primary Bone Tumors of Cats

Incidence and Risk

Primary tumors involving the bones of cats are rare. An estimate of the incidence of all bone tumors in cats is 4.9 per 100,000.[386] Between 67% and 90% of bone tumors in cats are histologically malignant. OSAs are the most common primary bone tumor in cats and account for 70% to 80% of all primary malignant bone cancers of cats. Feline OSA occurs in appendicular and axial skeletal sites and extraskeletal sites. OSA occurs in the appendicular skeleton approximately twice as often as in axial sites;[387,388] however, in one study, 55% of 90 skeletal OSA cases were appendicular and 44% occurred in the axial skeleton.[389] Axial OSA originates most commonly in the skull (especially oral cavity) and pelvis but has also been reported in the ribs and vertebrae. The disease in cats differs from that in dogs in that the primary lesions occur more often in pelvic limbs in cats (distal femur and proximal tibia) and it is less metastatic than in dogs.[390] In a series of 146 cats with OSA, 56 cats had extraskeletal OSA; these were most commonly associated with common injection sites, but other locations included ocular/orbital, oral, intestinal, and mammary sites.[389] There is no difference in histopathologic findings for extraskeletal, axial, or appendicular sites.[388] There are also reports of feline extraskeletal OSA in the flank, liver, spleen, kidney, stomach, duodenum, mammary gland, and subcutaneous tissues.[388,391–394]

OSA generally affects older cats with mean ages of 8.5 to 10.7 years,[387,388,390] but OSA has been reported in cats as young as 5 months and as old as 20 years.[394] The age at presentation for axial OSA is greater than appendicular OSA.[389] Conflicting reports on gender predisposition exist with either no difference between sexes or a slight male predisposition.[387–390] OSA has been reported to arise after fracture repair in two cats and after RT in another cat.[34,395] OSA has also been diagnosed at a site of prior surgical resection of a unicameral bone cyst.[396]

Osteochondroma and the multicentric form (osteochondromatosis or MCE) have both been reported in the cat.[397–399] Osteochondromas are solitary lesions composed of hard, irregular exostoses having a fibrous and cartilaginous cap.[400] Endochondral ossification occurs from the cartilage cap and extends to a variable thickness. This cap tends to blend with adjacent tissue, making surgical removal difficult. The lesions in cats differ from dogs because they continue to develop after skeletal maturity and in sites not associated with endochondral ossification, such as the skull. Osteochondromas in cats have a potential for malignant transformation and metastasis.

MCE or osteochondromatosis also occurs after skeletal maturity in cats. In contrast to dogs, the lesions seldom affect long bones, are rarely symmetric, and are probably of viral rather than familial origin. There does not appear to be any breed or sex predisposition, although early reports of this condition were in Siamese cats.[401] Affected cats range in age from 1.3 to 8 years (mean 3.2 years). Virtually all cats with MCE are FeLV positive. This disease has an aggressive natural behavior.

Pathology and Natural Behavior

The histologic characteristics of feline OSA are like canine OSA. OSA of cats is composed of mesenchymal cells embedded in malignant osteoid. There may be a considerable amount of cartilage present, and osteoid may be scant. A feature of some feline OSA cases is the presence of multinucleate giant cells, which may be numerous. Reactive host bone and remnants of host bone are often present in specimens. Tumors are seen to be invasive; however, some surrounding soft tissue may be compressed rather than infiltrated. There is often variation of the histologic appearance within the tumor with some portions having a more fibrosarcomatous appearance and others more cartilaginous. Feline skeletal OSA appears similar with respect to grade and histology to canine OSA; however, mitoses are seen almost half as frequently.[388] Some authors have described subtypes that resemble those seen in dogs: chondroblastic, fibroblastic, and telangiectatic, as well as the giant cell variant. These histologic subtypes, however, do not appear to confer any prognostic predictive value.[402,403] OSAs in cats are locally aggressive but have a low metastatic rate compared with canine OSA.

More recently, several studies have compared cellular protein expression in canine and feline OSA to investigate their behavioral disparity. The expression of the cytoskeletal linker proteins ezrin and moesin were found to differ between dogs and cats; however, the implication of these differences is unclear. Cats more commonly expressed the phosphorylated (active) form of ezrin, but dogs more commonly expressed it in a membranous location suggesting greater biologic activity.[404] KIT IHC expression was present in 79% of canine OSA but absent in all feline cases. Canine KIT mRNA expression was also higher when assessed with RT-PCR.[405] MMP-9 and -2 have also been shown to be expressed at higher levels in canine OSA compared with feline OSA, and this may be associated with greater invasive and metastatic behaviors.[406]

History and Clinical Signs

The most common clinical signs associated with appendicular OSA in cats are lameness, swelling, and deformity, depending on the location of the lesion. Radiographically, feline OSA appears similar to OSA in dogs with mixed osteoblastic and osteolytic changes and an ill-defined zone of transition between normal and neoplastic bone; however, juxtacortical OSA has also been reported in cats.[387] Tumors can reach a large size without evidence of severe clinical signs. It is rare for cats to have metastasis at presentation.

Cats with virally associated MCE have rapidly progressing, conspicuous, hard swellings over affected sites causing pain and loss of function. Common sites for MCE include the scapula, vertebrae, and mandible; however, any bone can be affected. Radiographically, the lesions are either sessile or pedunculated protuberances from bone surfaces, and the borders between the mass and normal bone are indistinct. There may be a loss of smooth contour with evidence of lysis, particularly if there is malignant transformation.

Diagnostic Workup

Both OSA and MCE may be suspected based on the radiographic appearance of the lesions and the FeLV status of the cat. Definitive diagnosis is made by histopathologic evaluation of properly collected biopsy tissue. Although metastatic rates for cats with primary bone tumors are low compared with dogs (5%–10% compared with >90%), three-view thoracic radiographs are recommended as part of the clinical staging process. Presurgical evaluation with a complete blood count, serum biochemistry profile, and urinalysis are recommended to rule out concurrent disease.

Therapy and Prognosis

Amputation is the recommended treatment for nonmetastatic appendicular OSA. Complete surgical excision of the primary tumor is prognostic for increased ST, DFI, and PFS.[388] Due to the low metastatic rate and prolonged MSTs of 24 to 44 months with limb amputation alone,[366,368] adjuvant chemotherapy is not indicated or recommended in cats. The MST for cats with axial OSA (6.7 months) is lower than either appendicular or extraskeletal OSA.[389] This most likely reflects the difficulty of achieving complete resection and local tumor control in axial sites rather than a difference in their biologic behavior. A combination of surgical resection and RT may be appropriate in these cases. SRT has been used in several cats with appendicular and axial OSA for local tumor control.

Histologic grade, using a grading scheme that evaluates tumor vascular invasion, pleomorphism, mitotic index, and tumor matrix and cell necrosis, is prognostic for survival.[388] The overall metastatic rate is 5% to 10%, and reported anatomic sites include lung, kidney, liver, brain, and spleen. Cats with MCE have a guarded prognosis. Lesions may be removed surgically for palliation; however, local recurrences and/or the development of new lesions are common. An effective treatment protocol is not known for MCE in cats.

Fibrosarcoma, Chondrosarcoma, and Hemangiosarcoma

Non-OSA primary bone tumors in cats are rare. FSA is the second most common primary bone tumor of cats,[402] followed by CSA and then rarely HSA.[390] Little is known about the biologic behavior of these rare bone tumors in cats. Aggressive surgical resection is the preferred treatment for these tumors. The metastatic rate is low; however, metastasis have been reported in cats with primary bone CSA and HSA.[390,403]

References

1. Brodey RS, Mc GJ, Reynolds H: A clinical and radiological study of canine bone neoplasms. I, *J Am Vet Med Assoc* 134:53–71, 1959.
2. Brodey RS, Riser WH: Canine osteosarcoma. A clinicopathologic study of 194 cases, *Clin Orthop Relat Res* 62:54–64, 1969.
3. Brodey RS, Sauer RM, Medway W: Canine bone neoplasms, *J Am Vet Med Assoc* 143:471–495, 1963.
4. Dorfman SK, Hurvitz AI, Patnaik AK: Primary and secondary bone tumours in the dog, *J Small Anim Pract* 18:313–326, 1977.
5. Ling GV, Morgan JP, Pool RR: Primary bone tumors in the dog; a combined clinical, radiographic, and histologic approach to early diagnosis, *J Am Vet Med Assoc* 165:55–67, 1974.
6. Priester WA, McKay FW: The occurrence of tumors in domestic animals, *Natl Cancer Inst Monogr* 1–210, 1980.
7. Withrow SJ, Powers BE, Straw RC, et al.: Comparative aspects of osteosarcoma. Dog versus man, *Clin Orthop Relat Res* 159–168, 1991.
8. Alexander JW, Patton CS: Primary tumors of the skeletal system, *Vet Clin North Am Small Anim Pract* 13:181–195, 1983.
9. Brodey RS, Abt DA: Results of surgical treatment in 65 dogs with osteosarcoma, *J Am Vet Med Assoc* 168:1032–1035, 1976.
10. Jongeward SJ: Primary bone tumors, *Vet Clin North Am Small Anim Pract* 15:609–641, 1985.
11. Knecht CD, Priester WA: Musculoskeletal tumors in dogs, *J Am Vet Med Assoc* 172:72–74, 1978.
12. Misdorp W: Skeletal osteosarcoma. Animal model; canine osteosarcoma, *Am J Pathol* 98:285–288, 1980.
13. Misdorp W, Hart AA: Some prognostic and epidemiologic factors in canine osteosarcoma, *J Natl Cancer Inst* 62:537–545, 1979.
14. Nielsen SW, Schroder JD, Smith DL: The pathology of osteogenic sarcoma in dogs, *J Am Vet Med Assoc* 124:28–35, 1954.
15. Smith RL, Sutton RH: Osteosarcoma in dogs in the Brisbane area, *Aust Vet Pract* 18:97–100, 1988.
16. Spodnick GJ, Berg J, Rand WM, et al.: Prognosis for dogs with appendicular osteosarcoma treated by amputation alone;162 cases (1978-1988), *J Am Vet Med Assoc* 200:995–999, 1992.
17. Straw RC, Withrow SJ, Richter SL, et al.: Amputation and cisplatin for treatment of canine osteosarcoma, *J Vet Intern Med* 5:205–210, 1991.
18. Tjalma RA: Canine bone sarcoma; estimation of relative risk as a function of body size, *J Natl Cancer Inst* 36:1137–1150, 1966.
19. Wolke RE, Nielsen SW: Site incidence of canine osteosarcoma, *J Small Anim Pract* 7:489–492, 1966.
20. Feeney DA, Johnston GR, Grindem CB, et al.: Malignant neoplasia of canine ribs; clinical, radiographic, and pathologic findings, *J Am Vet Med Assoc* 180:927–933, 1982.
21. Heyman SJ, Diefenderfer DL, Goldschmidt MH, et al.: Canine axial skeletal osteosarcoma. A retrospective study of 116 cases (1986 to 1989), *Vet Surg* 21:304–310, 1992.
22. Ru G, Terracini B, Glickman LT: Host related risk factors for canine osteosarcoma, *Vet J* 156:31–39, 1998.
23. Cooley DM, Beranek BC, Schlittler DL, et al.: Endogenous gonadal hormone exposure and bone sarcoma risk, *Cancer Epidemiol Biomarkers Prev* 11:1434–1440, 2002.
24. Gamblin RM, Straw RC, Powers BE, et al.: Primary osteosarcoma distal to the antebrachiocarpal and tarsocrural joints in nine dogs (1980-1992), *J Am Anim Hosp Assoc* 31:86–91, 1995.
25. LaRue SM, Withrow SJ, Wrigley RH: Radiographic bone surveys in the evaluation of primary bone tumors in dogs, *J Am Vet Med Assoc* 188:514–516, 1986.
26. Bech-Nielsen S, Haskins ME, Reif JS, et al.: Frequency of osteosarcoma among first-degree relatives of St. Bernard dogs, *J Natl Cancer Inst* 60:349–353, 1978.
27. Kuntz CA, Dernell WS, Powers BE, et al.: Extraskeletal osteosarcomas in dogs;14 cases, *J Am Anim Hosp Assoc* 34:26–30, 1998.
28. Langenbach A, Anderson MA, Dambach DM, et al.: Extraskeletal osteosarcomas in dogs; a retrospective study of 169 cases (1986-1996), *J Am Anim Hosp Assoc* 34:113–120, 1998.
29. Patnaik AK: Canine extraskeletal osteosarcoma and chondrosarcoma; a clinicopathologic study of 14 cases, *Vet Pathol* 27:46–55, 1990.
30. Ringenberg MA, Neitzel LE, Zachary JF: Meningeal osteosarcoma in a dog, *Vet Pathol* 37:653–655, 2000.
31. Thamm DH, Mauldin EA, Edinger DT, et al.: Primary osteosarcoma of the synovium in a dog, *J Am Anim Hosp Assoc* 36:326–331, 2000.
32. Owen LN: Transplantation of canine osteosarcoma, *Eur J Cancer* 5:615–620, 1969.
33. Gellasch KL, Kalscheur VL, Clayton MK, et al.: Fatigue microdamage in the radial predilection site for osteosarcoma in dogs, *Am J Vet Res* 63:896–899, 2002.
34. Bennett D, Campbell JR, Brown P: Osteosarcoma associated with healed fractures, *J Small Anim Pract* 20:13–18, 1979.
35. Knecht CD, Priester WA: Osteosarcoma in dogs - study of previous trauma, fracture, and fracture fixation, *J Am An Hosp Assoc* 14:82–84, 1978.
36. Sinibaldi K, Rosen H, Liu SK, et al.: Tumors associated with metallic implants in animals, *Clin Orthop Relat Res* 257–266, 1976.
37. Stevenson S, Hohn RB, Pohler OE, et al.: Fracture-associated sarcoma in the dog, *J Am Vet Med Assoc* 180:1189–1196, 1982.
38. Vasseur PB, Stevenson S: Osteosarcoma at the site of a cortical bone allograft in a dog, *Vet Surg* 16:70–74, 1987.
39. Gillette SM, Gillette EL, Powers BE, et al.: Radiation-induced osteosarcoma in dogs after external beam or intraoperative radiation therapy, *Cancer Res* 50:54–57, 1990.
40. Lloyd RD, Taylor GN, Angus W, et al.: Distribution of skeletal malignancies in beagles injected with 239Pu citrate, *Health Phys* 66:407–413, 1994.
41. McEntee MC, Page RL, Theon A, et al.: Malignant tumor formation in dogs previously irradiated for acanthomatous epulis, *Vet Radiol Ultrasound* 45:357–361, 2004.
42. Miller SC, Lloyd RD, Bruenger FW, et al.: Comparisons of the skeletal locations of putative plutonium-induced osteosarcomas in humans with those in beagle dogs and with naturally occurring tumors in both species, *Radiat Res* 160:517–523, 2003.
43. Powers BE, Gillette EL, McChesney SL, et al.: Bone necrosis and tumor induction following experimental intraoperative irradiation, *Int J Radiat Oncol Biol Phys* 17:559–567, 1989.
44. Robinson E, Neugut AI, Wylie P: Clinical aspects of postirradiation sarcomas, *J Natl Cancer Inst* 80:233–240, 1988.
45. Tillotson C, Rosenberg A, Gebhardt M, et al.: Postradiation multicentric osteosarcoma, *Cancer* 62:67–71, 1988.

46. White RG, Raabe OG, Culbertson MR, et al.: Bone sarcoma characteristics and distribution in beagles fed strontium-90, *Radiat Res* 136:178–189, 1993.

47. White RG, Raabe OG, Culbertson MR, et al.: Bone sarcoma characteristics and distribution in beagles injected with radium-226, *Radiat Res* 137:361–370, 1994.

48. Johnson AS, Couto CG, Weghorst CM: Mutation of the p53 tumor suppressor gene in spontaneously occurring osteosarcomas of the dog, *Carcinogenesis* 19:213–217, 1998.

49. Kirpensteijn J, Kik M, Teske E, et al.: TP53 gene mutations in canine osteosarcoma, *Vet Surg* 37:454–460, 2008.

50. Levine RA, Fleischli MA: Inactivation of p53 and retinoblastoma family pathways in canine osteosarcoma cell lines, *Vet Pathol* 37:54–61, 2000.

51. Loukopoulos P, Thornton TR, Robinson WF: Clinical and pathologic relevance of p53 index in canine osseous tumors, *Vet Pathol* 40:237–248, 2003.

52. Mendoza S, Konishi T, Dernell WS, et al.: Status of the p53, Rb and MDM2 genes in canine osteosarcoma, *Anticancer Res* 18:4449–4453, 1998.

53. Sagartz JE, Bodley WL, Gamblin RM, et al.: p53 tumor suppressor protein overexpression in osteogenic tumors of dogs, *Vet Pathol* 33:213–221, 1996.

54. Setoguchi A, Sakai T, Okuda M, et al.: Aberrations of the p53 tumor suppressor gene in various tumors in dogs, *Am J Vet Res* 62:433–439, 2001.

55. vanLeeuwen IS, Comelisse CJ, Misdorp W, et al.: p53 gene mutations in osteosarcomas in the dog, *Cancer Lett* 111:173–178, 1997.

56. Thomas R, Wang HXJ, Tsai PC, et al.: Influence of genetic background on tumor karyotypes; evidence for breed-associated cytogenetic aberrations in canine appendicular osteosarcoma, *Chromosome Res* 17:365–377, 2009.

57. Levine AJ, Chang AW, Dittmer D, et al.: The P53 tumor-suppressor gene, *J Lab Clin Med* 123:817–823, 1994.

58. Cam M, Gardner HL, Roberts RD, et al.: DeltaNp63 mediates cellular survival and metastasis in canine osteosarcoma, *Oncotarget* 7:48533–48546, 2016.

59. Wadayama B, Toguchida J, Shimizu T, et al.: Mutation spectrum of the retinoblastoma gene in osteosarcomas, *Cancer Res* 54:3042–3048, 1994.

60. Scott MC, Sarver AL, Tomiyasu H, et al.: Aberrant retinoblastoma (RB)-E2F transcriptional regulation defines molecular phenotypes of osteosarcoma, *J Biol Chem* 290:28070–28083, 2015.

61. Levine RA, Forest T, Smith C: Tumor suppressor PTEN is mutated in canine osteosarcoma cell lines and tumors, *Vet Pathol* 39:372–378, 2002.

62. Angstadt AY, Motsinger-Reif A, Thomas R, et al.: Characterization of canine osteosarcoma by array comparative genomic hybridization and RT-qPCR; signatures of genomic imbalance in canine osteosarcoma parallel the human counterpart, *Genes Chromosomes Cancer* 50:859–874, 2011.

63. Angstadt AY, Thayanithy V, Subramanian S, et al.: A genome-wide approach to comparative oncology; high-resolution oligonucleotide a CGH of canine and human osteosarcoma pinpoints shared microaberrations, *Cancer Genet* 205:572–587, 2012.

64. Cooley DM, Waters DJ: Skeletal neoplasms of small dogs;a retrospective study and literature review, *J Am Anim Hosp Assoc* 33:11–23, 1997.

65. Phillips J, Lembcke L, Chamberlin T: Genetics of osteosarcoma in the scottish deerhound, *J Vet Intern Med* 24:675–675, 2010.

66. Phillips JC, Lembcke L, Chamberlin T: A novel locus for canine osteosarcoma (OSA1) maps to CFA34, the canine orthologue of human 3q26, *Genomics* 96:220–227, 2010.

67. Phillips JC, Stephenson B, Hauck M, et al.: Heritability and segregation analysis of osteosarcoma in the Scottish deerhound, *Genomics* 90:354–363, 2007.

68. Rosenberger JA, Pablo NV, Crawford PC: Prevalence of and intrinsic risk factors for appendicular osteosarcorna in dogs; 179 cases (1996-2005), *J Am Vet Med Assoc* 231:1076–1080, 2007.

69. Urfer SR, Gaillard C, Steiger A: Lifespan and disease predispositions in the Irish Wolfhound; a review, *Vet Q* 29:157–157, 2017.

70. Karlsson EK, Sigurdsson S, Ivansson E, et al.: Genome-wide analyses implicate 33 loci in heritable dog osteosarcoma, including regulatory variants near CDKN2A/B, *Genome Biol* 14:R132, 2013.

71. Dillberger JE, McAtee SA: Osteosarcoma inheritance in two families of Scottish deerhounds, *Canine Genet Epidemiol* 4(3), 2017.

72. Sarver AL, Thayanithy V, Scott MC, et al.: MicroRNAs at the human 14q32 locus have prognostic significance in osteosarcoma, *Orphanet J Rare Dis* 8(7), 2013.

73. Fenger JM, Roberts RD, Iwenofu OH, et al.: MiR-9 is overexpressed in spontaneous canine osteosarcoma and promotes a metastatic phenotype including invasion and migration in osteoblasts and osteosarcoma cell lines, *BMC Cancer* 16:784, 2016.

74. Lopez CM, Yu PY, Zhang X, et al.: MiR-34a regulates the invasive capacity of canine osteosarcoma cell lines, *PLoS One* 13:e0190086, 2018.

75. Fox MH, Armstrong LW, Withrow SJ, et al.: Comparison of DNA aneuploidy of primary and metastatic spontaneous canine osteosarcomas, *Cancer Res* 50:6176–6178, 1990.

76. Liao AT, McCleese J, Kamerling S, et al.: A novel small molecule Met inhibitor, PF2362376, exhibits biological activity against osteosarcoma, *Vet Comp Oncol* 5:177–196, 2007.

77. Liao AT, McMahon M, London C: Characterization, expression and function of c-Met in canine spontaneous cancers, *Vet Comp Oncol* 3:61–72, 2005.

78. MacEwen EG, Kutzke J, Carew J, et al.: c-Met tyrosine kinase receptor expression and function in human and canine osteosarcoma cells, *Clin Exp Metastasis* 20:421–430, 2003.

79. Ferracini R, Angelini P, Cagliero E, et al.: MET oncogene aberrant expression in canine osteosarcoma, *J Orthop Res* 18:253–256, 2000.

80. Liao AT, McMahon M, London CA: Identification of a novel germline MET mutation in dogs, *Anim Genet* 37:248–252, 2006.

81. Fieten H, Spee B, Ijzer J, et al.: Expression of hepatocyte growth factor and the proto-oncogenic receptor c-Met in canine osteosarcoma, *Vet Pathol* 46:869–877, 2009.

82. MacEwen EG, Pastor J, Kutzke J, et al.: IGF-1 receptor contributes to the malignant phenotype in human and canine osteosarcoma, *J Cell Biochem* 92:77–91, 2004.

83. Maniscalco L, Iussich S, Morello E, et al.: Increased expression of insulin-like growth factor-1 receptor is correlated with worse survival in canine appendicular osteosarcoma, *Vet J* 205:272–280, 2015.

84. Gorlick R, Huvos AG, Heller G, et al.: Expression of HER2/erbB-2 correlates with survival in osteosarcoma, *J Clin Oncol* 17:2781–2788, 1999.

85. Scotlandi K, Manara MC, Hattinger CM, et al.: Prognostic and therapeutic relevance of HER2 expression in osteosarcoma and Ewing's sarcoma, *Eur J Cancer* 41:1349–1361, 2005.

86. Flint AF, U'Ren L, Legare ME, et al.: Overexpression of the erbB-2 proto-oncogene in canine osteosarcoma cell lines and tumors, *Vet Pathol* 41:291–296, 2004.

87. Gordon IK, Ye F, Kent MS: Evaluation of the mammalian target of rapamycin pathway and the effect of rapamycin on target expression and cellular proliferation in osteosarcoma cells from dogs, *Am J Vet Res* 69:1079–1084, 2008.

88. Paoloni MC, Mazcko C, Fox E, et al.: Rapamycin pharmacokinetic and pharmacodynamic relationships in osteosarcoma; a comparative oncology study in dogs, *PLoS One* 5:e11013, 2010.

89. Shahi MH, Holt R, Rebhun RB: Blocking signaling at the level of GLI regulates downstream gene expression and inhibits proliferation of canine osteosarcoma cells, *PLoS One* 9:e96593, 2014.

90. Dailey DD, Anfinsen KP, Pfaff LE, et al.: HES1, a target of Notch signaling, is elevated in canine osteosarcoma, but reduced in the most aggressive tumors, *BMC Vet Res* 9:130, 2013.

91. Loukopoulos P, O'Brien T, Ghoddusi M, et al.: Characterisation of three novel canine osteosarcoma cell lines producing high levels of matrix metalloproteinases, *Res Vet Sci* 77:131–141, 2004.

92. Barger AM, Fan TM, de Lorimier LP, et al.: Expression of receptor activator of nuclear factor kappa-B ligand (RANKL) in neoplasms of dogs and cats, *J Vet Intern Med* 21:133–140, 2007.

93. Lana SE, Ogilvie GK, Hansen RA, et al.: Identification of matrix metalloproteinases in canine neoplastic tissue, *Am J Vet Res* 61:111–114, 2000.

94. Schmit JM, Pondenis HC, Barger AM, et al.: Cathepsin K expression and activity in canine osteosarcoma, *J Vet Intern Med* 26:126–134, 2012.

95. Marley K, Bracha S, Seguin B: Osteoprotegerin activates osteosarcoma cells that co-express RANK and RANKL, *Exp Cell Res* 338:32–38, 2015.

96. Neumann ZL, Pondenis HC, Masyr A, et al.: The association of endothelin-1 signaling with bone alkaline phosphatase expression and protumorigenic activities in canine osteosarcoma, *J Vet Intern Med* 29:1584–1594, 2015.

97. Shor S, Fadl-Alla BA, Pondenis HC, et al.: Expression of nociceptive ligands in canine osteosarcoma, *J Vet Intern Med* 29:268–275, 2015.

98. Khanna C, Wan X, Bose S, et al.: The membrane-cytoskeleton linker ezrin is necessary for osteosarcoma metastasis, *Nat Med* 10:182–186, 2004.

99. Fan TM, Barger AM, Fredrickson RL, et al.: Investigating CXCR4 expression in canine appendicular osteosarcoma, *J Vet Intern Med* 22:602–608, 2008.

100. Byrum ML, Pondenis HC, Fredrickson RL, et al.: Downregulation of CXCR4 expression and functionality after zoledronate exposure in canine osteosarcoma, *J Vet Intern Med* 30:1187–1196, 2016.

101. Barger A, Graca R, Bailey K, et al.: Use of alkaline phosphatase staining to differentiate canine osteosarcoma from other vimentin-positive tumors, *Vet Pathol* 42:161–165, 2005.

102. Neihaus SA, Locke JE, Barger AM, et al.: A novel method of core aspirate cytology compared to fine-needle aspiration for diagnosing canine osteosarcoma, *J Am Anim Hosp Assoc* 47:317–323, 2011.

103. Britt T, Clifford C, Barger A, et al.: Diagnosing appendicular osteosarcoma with ultrasound-guided fine-needle aspiration; 36 cases, *J Small Anim Pract* 48:145–150, 2007.

104. Kirpensteijn J, Kik M, Rutteman GR, et al.: Prognostic significance of a new histologic grading system for canine osteosarcoma, *Vet Pathol* 39:240–246, 2002.

105. Schott CR, Tatiersky LJ, Foster RA, et al.: Histologic grade does not predict outcome in dogs with appendicular osteosarcoma receiving the standard of care, *Vet Pathol* 55:202–211, 2018.

106. O'Donoghue LE, Ptitsyn AA, Kamstock DA, et al.: Expression profiling in canine osteosarcoma; identification of biomarkers and pathways associated with outcome, *BMC Cancer* 10:506, 2010.

107. Bhandal J, Boston SE: Pathologic fracture in dogs with suspected or confirmed osteosarcoma, *Vet Surg* 40:423–430, 2011.

108. Kim MS, Lee SY, Lee TR, et al.: Prognostic effect of pathologic fracture in localized osteosarcoma; a cohort/case controlled study at a single institute, *J Surg Oncol* 100:233–239, 2009.

109. Ebeid W, Amin S, Abdelmegid A: Limb salvage management of pathologic fractures of primary malignant bone tumors, *Cancer Control* 12:57–61, 2005.

110. Bacci G, Ferrari S, Longhi A, et al.: Nonmetastatic osteosarcoma of the extremity with pathologic fracture at presentation;local and systemic control by amputation or limb salvage after preoperative chemotherapy, *Acta Orthop Scand* 74:449–454, 2003.

111. Boston SE, Vinayak A, Lu X, et al.: Outcome and complications in dogs with appendicular primary bone tumors treated with stereotactic radiotherapy and concurrent surgical stabilization, *Vet Surg* 46:829–837, 2017.

112. Covey JL, Farese JP, Bacon NJ, et al.: Stereotactic radiosurgery and fracture fixation in 6 dogs with appendicular osteosarcoma, *Vet Surg* 43:174–181, 2014.

113. Hillers KR, Dernell WS, Lafferty MH, et al.: Incidence and prognostic importance of lymph node metastases in dogs with appendicular osteosarcoma; 228 cases (1986-2003), *J Am Vet Med Assoc* 226:1364–1367, 2005.

114. Boston SE, Ehrhart NP, Dernell WS, et al.: Evaluation of survival time in dogs with stage III osteosarcoma that undergo treatment;90 cases (1985-2004), *J Am Vet Med Assoc* 228:1905–1908, 2006.

115. Giuliano AE, Feig S, Eilber FR: Changing metastatic patterns of osteosarcoma, *Cancer* 54:2160–2164, 1984.

116. Bacci G, Avella M, Picci P, et al.: Metastatic patterns in osteosarcoma, *Tumori* 74:421–427, 1988.

117. Moore GE, Mathey WS, Eggers JS, et al.: Osteosarcoma in adjacent lumbar vertebrae in a dog, *J Am Vet Med Assoc* 217(1008):1038–1040, 2000.

118. Talbott JL, Boston SE, Milner RJ, et al.: Retrospective evaluation of whole body computed tomography for tumor staging in dogs with primary appendicular osteosarcoma, *Vet Surg* 46:75–80, 2017.

119. Oblak ML, Boston SE, Woods JP, et al.: Comparison of concurrent imaging modalities for staging of dogs with appendicular primary bone tumours, *Vet Comp Oncol* 13:28–39, 2015.

120. Sivacolundhu RK, Runge JJ, Donovan TA, et al.: Ulnar osteosarcoma in dogs;30 cases (1992-2008), *J Am Vet Med Assoc* 243:96–101, 2013.

121. Montinaro V, Boston SE, Buracco P, et al.: Clinical outcome of 42 dogs with scapular tumors treated by scapulectomy;a Veterinary Society of Surgical Oncology (VSSO) retrospective study (1995-2010), *Vet Surg* 42:943–950, 2013.

122. Straw RC, Powers BE, Klausner J, et al.: Canine mandibular osteosarcoma; 51 cases (1980-1992), *J Am Anim Hosp Assoc* 32:257–262, 1996.

123. Dickerson ME, Page RL, LaDue TA, et al.: Retrospective analysis of axial skeleton osteosarcoma in 22 large-breed dogs, *J Vet Intern Med* 15:120–124, 2001.

124. Selmic LE, Lafferty MH, Kamstock DA, et al.: Outcome and prognostic factors for osteosarcoma of the maxilla, mandible, or calvarium in dogs; 183 cases (1986-2012), *J Am Vet Med Assoc* 245:930–938, 2014.

125. Coyle VJ, Rassnick KM, Borst LB, et al.: Biological behaviour of canine mandibular osteosarcoma. A retrospective study of 50 cases (1999-2007), *Vet Comp Oncol* 13:89–97, 2015.

126. Amsellem PM, Selmic LE, Wypij JM, et al.: Appendicular osteosarcoma in small-breed dogs; 51 cases (1986-2011), *J Am Vet Med Assoc* 245:203–210, 2014.

127. Boulay JP, Wallace LJ, Lipowitz AJ: Pathological fracture of long bones in the dog, *J Am An Hosp Assoc* 23:297–303, 1987.

128. Mazzaferro EM, Hackett TB, Stein TP, et al.: Metabolic alterations in dogs with osteosarcoma, *Am J Vet Res* 62:1234–1239, 2001.

129. Story AL, Boston SE, Kilkenny JJ, et al.: Evaluation of weight change during carboplatin therapy in dogs with appendicular osteosarcoma, *J Vet Intern Med* 31:1159–1162, 2017.

130. Kazmierski KJ, Ogilvie GK, Fettman MJ, et al.: Serum zinc, chromium, and iron concentrations in dogs with lymphoma and osteosarcoma, *J Vet Intern Med* 15:585–588, 2001.

131. Wrigley RH: Malignant versus nonmalignant bone disease, *Vet Clin North Am Small Anim Pract* 30:315–347, 2000. vi-vii.

132. Charney VA, Miller MA, Heng HG, et al.: Skeletal metastasis of canine urothelial carcinoma; pathologic and computed tomographic features, *Vet Pathol* 54:380–386, 2017.

133. Reinhardt S, Stockhaus C, Teske E, et al.: Assessment of cytological criteria for diagnosing osteosarcoma in dogs, *J Small Anim Pract* 46:65–70, 2005.

134. Samii VF, Nyland TG, Werner LL, et al.: Ultrasound-guided fine-needle aspiration biopsy of bone lesions; a preliminary report, *Vet Radiol Ultrasound* 40:82–86, 1999.

135. Ehrhart N: Principles of tumor biopsy, *Clin Tech Small Anim Pract* 13:10–16, 1998.

136. Mankin HJ, Lange TA, Spanier SS: The hazards of biopsy in patients with malignant primary bone and soft-tissue tumors, *J Bone Joint Surg Am* 64:1121–1127, 1982.

137. de Santos LA, Murray JA, Ayala AG: The value of percutaneous needle biopsy in the management of primary bone tumors, *Cancer* 43:735–744, 1979.

138. Simon MA: Biopsy of musculoskeletal tumors, *J Bone Joint Surg Am* 64:1253–1257, 1982.

139. Wykes PM, Withrow SJ, Powers BE, et al.: Closed biopsy for diagnosis of long-bone tumors - accuracy and results, *J Am Anim Hosp Assoc* 21:489–494, 1985.

140. Powers BE, LaRue SM, Withrow SJ, et al.: Jamshidi needle biopsy for diagnosis of bone lesions in small animals, *J Am Vet Med Assoc* 193:205–210, 1988.

141. Vignoli M, Ohlerth S, Rossi F, et al.: Computed tomography-guided fine-needle aspiration and tissue-core biopsy of bone lesions in small animals, *Vet Radiol Ultrasound* 45:125–130, 2004.

142. Barthez PY, Hornof WJ, Theon AP, et al.: Receiver operating characteristic curve analysis of the performance of various radiographic protocols when screening dogs for pulmonary metastases, *J Am Vet Med Assoc* 204:237–240, 1994.

143. Picci P, Vanel D, Briccoli A, et al.: Computed tomography of pulmonary metastases from osteosarcoma; the less poor technique. A study of 51 patients with histological correlation, *Ann Oncol* 12:1601–1604, 2001.

144. Waters DJ, Coakley FV, Cohen MD, et al.: The detection of pulmonary metastases by helical CT; a clinicopathologic study in dogs, *J Comput Assist Tomogr* 22:235–240, 1998.

145. Karnik KS, Samii VF, Weisbrode SE, et al.: Accuracy of computed tomography in determining lesion size in canine appendicular osteosarcoma, *Vet Radiol Ultrasound* 53:273–279, 2012.

146. Armbrust LJ, Biller DS, Bamford A, et al.: Comparison of three-view thoracic radiography and computed tomography for detection of pulmonary nodules in dogs with neoplasia, *J Am Vet Med Assoc* 240:1088–1094, 2012.

147. Eberle N, Fork M, von Babo V, et al.: Comparison of examination of thoracic radiographs and thoracic computed tomography in dogs with appendicular osteosarcoma, *Vet Comp Oncol* 9:131–140, 2011.

148. Berg J, Lamb CR, O'Callaghan MW: Bone scintigraphy in the initial evaluation of dogs with primary bone tumors, *J Am Vet Med Assoc* 196:917–920, 1990.

149. Hahn KA, Hurd C, Cantwell HD: Single-phase methylene diphosphate bone scintigraphy in the diagnostic evaluation of dogs with osteosarcoma, *J Am Vet Med Assoc* 196:1483–1486, 1990.

150. Jankowski MK, Steyn PF, Lana SE, et al.: Nuclear scanning with 99mTc-HDP for the initial evaluation of osseous metastasis in canine osteosarcoma, *Vet Comp Oncol* 1:152–158, 2003.

151. Lamb CR: Bone scintigraphy in small animals, *J Am Vet Med Assoc* 191:1616–1622, 1987.

152. Parchman MB, Flanders JA, Erb HN, et al.: Nuclear medical bone imaging and targeted radiography for evaluation of skeletal neoplasms in 23 dogs, *Vet Surg* 18:454–458, 1989.

153. Sacornrattana O, Dervisis NG, McNiel EA: Abdominal ultrasonographic findings at diagnosis of osteosarcoma in dogs and association with treatment outcome, *Vet Comp Oncol* 11:199–207, 2013.

154. Wallace M, Selmic L, Withrow SJ: Diagnostic utility of abdominal ultrasonography for routine staging at diagnosis of skeletal OSA in dogs, *J Am Anim Hosp Assoc* 49:243–245, 2013.

155. Enneking WF, Spanier SS, Goodman MA: A system for the surgical staging of musculoskeletal sarcoma, *Clin Orthop Relat Res* 106–120, 1980.

156. Lamb CR, Berg J, Bengtson AE: Preoperative measurement of canine primary bone tumors, using radiography and bone scintigraphy, *J Am Vet Med Assoc* 196:1474–1478, 1990.

157. Leibman NF, Kuntz CA, Steyn PF, et al.: Accuracy of radiography, nuclear scintigraphy, and histopathology for determining the proximal extent of distal radius osteosarcoma in dogs, *Vet Surg* 30:240–245, 2001.

158. Davis GJ, Kapatkin AS, Craig LE, et al.: Comparison of radiography, computed tomography, and magnetic resonance imaging for evaluation of appendicular osteosarcoma in dogs, *J Am Vet Med Assoc* 220:1171–1176, 2002.

159. Schmidt AF, Nielen M, Klungel OH, et al.: Prognostic factors of early metastasis and mortality in dogs with appendicular osteosarcoma after receiving surgery; an individual patient data meta-analysis, *Prev Vet Med* 112:414–422, 2013.

160. Bergman PJ, MacEwen EG, Kurzman ID, et al.: Amputation and carboplatin for treatment of dogs with osteosarcoma; 48 cases (1991 to 1993), *J Vet Intern Med* 10:76–81, 1996.

161. Cho WH, Song WS, Jeon DG, et al.: Differential presentations, clinical courses, and survivals of osteosarcomas of the proximal humerus over other extremity locations, *Ann Surg Oncol* 17:702–708, 2010.

162. Kuntz CA, Asselin TL, Dernell WS, et al.: Limb salvage surgery for osteosarcoma of the proximal humerus; outcome in 17 dogs, *Vet Surg* 27:417–422, 1998.

163. Sottnik JL, Rao S, Lafferty MH, et al.: Association of blood monocyte and lymphocyte count and disease-free interval in dogs with osteosarcoma, *J Vet Intern Med* 24:1439–1444, 2010.

164. Boerman I, Selvarajah GT, Nielen M, et al.: Prognostic factors in canine appendicular osteosarcoma - a meta-analysis, *BMC Vet Res* 8:56, 2012.

165. Hammer AS, Weeren FR, Weisbrode SE, et al.: Prognostic factors in dogs with osteosarcomas of the flat or irregular bones, *J Am Anim Hosp Assoc* 31:321–326, 1995.

166. Kosovsky JK, Matthiesen DT, Marretta SM, et al.: Results of partial mandibulectomy for the treatment of oral tumors in 142 dogs, *Vet Surg* 20:397–401, 1991.

167. Schwarz PD, Withrow SJ, Curtis CR, et al.: Partial maxillary resection as a treatment for oral-cancer in 61 dogs, *J Am Anim Hosp Asoc* 27:617–624, 1991.

168. Wallace J, Matthiesen DT, Patnaik AK: Hemimaxillectomy for the treatment of oral tumors in 69 dogs, *Vet Surg* 21:337–341, 1992.

169. Baines SJ, Lewis S, White RAS: Primary thoracic wall tumours of mesenchymal origin in dogs; a retrospective study of 46 cases, *Vet Rec* 150:335–339, 2002.

170. Matthiesen DT, Clark GN, Orsher RJ, et al.: En-bloc resection of primary rib tumors in 40 dogs, *Vet Surg* 21:201–204, 1992.

171. Montgomery RD, Henderson RA, Powers RD, et al.: Retrospective study of 26 primary tumors of the osseous thoracic wall in dogs, *J Am Anim Hosp Assoc* 29:68–72, 1993.

172. Pirkeyehrhart N, Withrow SJ, Straw RC, et al.: Primary rib tumors in 54 dogs, *J Am Anim Hosp Assoc* 31:65–69, 1995.

173. Trout NJ, Pavletic MM, Kraus KH: Partial scapulectomy for management of sarcomas in 3 dogs and 2 cats, *J Am Vet Med Assoc* 207:585–587, 1995.

174. Norton C, Drenen CM, Emms SG: Subtotal scapulectomy as the treatment for scapular tumour in the dog; a report of six cases, *Aust Vet J* 84:364–366, 2006.

175. Dernell WS, Van Vechten BJ, Straw RC, et al.: Outcome following treatment of vertebral tumors in 20 dogs (1986-1995), *J Am Anim Hosp Assoc* 36:245–251.

176. Bray JP, Worley DR, Henderson RA, et al.: Hemipelvectomy; outcome in 84 dogs and 16 cats. A Veterinary Society of Surgical Oncology Retrospective Study, *Vet Surg* 43:27–37, 2014.

177. Turner H, Seguin B, Worley DR, et al.: Prognosis for dogs with stage III osteosarcoma following treatment with amputation and chemotherapy with and without metastasectomy, *J Am Vet Med Assoc* 251:1293–1305, 2017.

178. Garzotto CK, Berg J, Hoffmann WE, et al.: Prognostic significance of serum alkaline phosphatase activity in canine appendicular osteosarcoma, *J Vet Intern Med* 14:587–592, 2000.

179. Ehrhart N, Dernell WS, Hoffmann WE, et al.: Prognostic importance of alkaline phosphatase activity in serum from dogs with appendicular osteosarcoma; 75 cases (1990-1996), *J Am Vet Med Assoc* 213:1002–1006, 1998.

180. Moore AS, Dernell WS, Ogilvie GK, et al.: Doxorubicin and BAY 12-9566 for the treatment of osteosarcoma in dogs; a randomized, double-blind, placebo-controlled study, *J Vet Intern Med* 21:783–790, 2007.

181. Liptak JM, Kamstock DA, Dernell WS, et al.: Oncologic outcome after curative-intent treatment in 39 dogs with primary chest wall tumors (1992-2005), *Vet Surg* 37:488–496, 2008.

182. Sternberg RA, Pondenis HC, Yang X, et al.: Association between absolute tumor burden and serum bone-specific alkaline phosphatase in canine appendicular osteosarcoma, *J Vet Intern Med* 27:955–963, 2013.

183. Holmes KE, Thompson V, Piskun CM, et al.: Canine osteosarcoma cell lines from patients with differing serum alkaline phosphatase concentrations display no behavioural differences in vitro, *Vet Comp Oncol* 13:166–175, 2015.

184. McCleese JK, Bear MD, Kulp SK, et al.: Met interacts with EGFR and Ron in canine osteosarcoma, *Vet Comp Oncol* 11:124–139, 2013.

185. Mullins MN, Lana SE, Dernell WS, et al.: Cyclooxygenase-2 expression in canine appendicular osteosarcomas, *J Vet Intern Med* 18:859–865, 2004.

186. Shoeneman JK, Ehrhart 3rd EJ, Eickhoff JC, et al.: Expression and function of survivin in canine osteosarcoma, *Cancer Res* 72:249–259, 2012.

187. Thamm DH, O'Brien MG, Vail DM: Serum vascular endothelial growth factor concentrations and postsurgical outcome in dogs with osteosarcoma, *Vet Comp Oncol* 6:126–132, 2008.

188. Selvarajah GT, Bonestroo FA, Kirpensteijn J, et al.: Heat shock protein expression analysis in canine osteosarcoma reveals HSP60 as a potentially relevant therapeutic target, *Cell Stress Chaperones* 18:607–622, 2013.

189. Millanta F, Asproni P, Cancedda S, et al.: Immunohistochemical expression of COX-2, mPGES and EP2 receptor in normal and reactive canine bone and in canine osteosarcoma, *J Comp Pathol* 147:153–160, 2012.

190. Pang LY, Gatenby EL, Kamida A, et al.: Global gene expression analysis of canine osteosarcoma stem cells reveals a novel role for COX-2 in tumour initiation, *PLoS One* 9:e83144, 2014.

191. Selvarajah GT, Kirpensteijn J, van Wolferen ME, et al.: Gene expression profiling of canine osteosarcoma reveals genes associated with short and long survival times, *Mol Cancer* 8:72, 2009.

192. Scott MC, Sarver AL, Gavin KJ, et al.: Molecular subtypes of osteosarcoma identified by reducing tumor heterogeneity through an interspecies comparative approach, *Bone* 49:356–367, 2011.

193. Biller BJ, Elmslie RE, Burnett RC, et al.: Use of FoxP3 expression to identify regulatory T cells in healthy dogs and dogs with cancer, *Vet Immunol Immunopathol* 116:69–78, 2007.

194. O'Neill K, Guth A, Biller B, et al.: Changes in regulatory T cells in dogs with cancer and associations with tumor type, *J Vet Intern Med* 23:875–881, 2009.

195. Rissetto KC, Rindt H, Selting KA, et al.: Cloning and expression of canine CD25 for validation of an anti-human CD25 antibody to compare T regulatory lymphocytes in healthy dogs and dogs with osteosarcoma, *Vet Immunol Immunopathol* 135:137–145, 2010.

196. Biller BJ, Guth A, Burton JH, et al.: Decreased ratio of CD8+ T cells to regulatory T cells associated with decreased survival in dogs with osteosarcoma, *J Vet Intern Med* 24:1118–1123, 2010.

197. Tuohy JL, Lascelles BD, Griffith EH, et al.: Association of canine osteosarcoma and monocyte phenotype and chemotactic function, *J Vet Intern Med* 30:1167–1178, 2016.

198. Withers SS, Skorupski KA, York D, et al.: Association of macrophage and lymphocyte infiltration with outcome in canine osteosarcoma, *Vet Comp Oncol*, 2018. epub ahead of print.

199. Withrow SJ, Hirsch VM: Owner response to amputation of a pet's leg, *Vet Med Small Anim Clin* 74(332):334, 1979.

200. Carberry CA, Harvey HJ: Owner satisfaction with limb amputation in dogs and cats, *J Am Anim Hosp Assoc* 23:227–232, 1987.

201. Berg J, Weinstein MJ, Schelling SH, et al.: Treatment of dogs with osteosarcoma by administration of cisplatin after amputation or limb-sparing surgery; 22 cases (1987-1990), *J Am Vet Med Assoc* 200:2005–2008, 1992.

202. LaRue SM, Withrow SJ, Powers BE, et al.: Limb-sparing treatment for osteosarcoma in dogs, *J Am Vet Med Assoc* 195:1734–1744, 1989.

203. Thrall DE, Withrow SJ, Powers BE, et al.: Radiotherapy prior to cortical allograft limb sparing in dogs with osteosarcoma; a dose response assay, *Int J Radiat Oncol Biol Phys* 18:1351–1357, 1990.

204. Vasseur P: Limb preservation in dogs with primary bone tumors, *Vet Clin North Am Small Anim Pract* 17:889–903, 1987.

205. Withrow SJ, Thrall DE, Straw RC, et al.: Intra-arterial cisplatin with or without radiation in limb-sparing for canine osteosarcoma, *Cancer* 71:2484–2490, 1993.

206. Straw RC, Withrow SJ: Limb-sparing surgery versus amputation for dogs with bone tumors, *Vet Clin North Am Small Anim Pract* 26:135–143, 1996.

207. O'Brien MG, Straw RC, Withrow SJ, et al.: Resection of pulmonary metastases in canine osteosarcoma; 36 cases (1983-1992), *Vet Surg* 22:105–109, 1993.

208. Selmic LE, Burton JH, Thamm DH, et al.: Comparison of carboplatin and doxorubicin-based chemotherapy protocols in 470 dogs after amputation for treatment of appendicular osteosarcoma, *J Vet Intern Med* 28:554–563, 2014.

209. Liptak JM, Dernell WS, Straw RC, et al.: Intercalary bone grafts for joint and limb preservation in 17 dogs with high-grade malignant tumors of the diaphysis, *Vet Surg* 33:457–467, 2004.

210. Morello E, Buracco P, Martano M, et al.: Bone allografts and adjuvant cisplatin for the treatment of canine appendicular osteosarcoma in 18 dogs, *J Small Anim Pract* 42:61–66, 2001.

211. Tomford WW, Doppelt SH, Mankin HJ, et al.: 1983 bone bank procedures, *Clin Orthop Relat R*15–21, 1983.

212. Straw RC, Powers BE, Withrow SJ, et al.: The effect of intramedullary polymethylmethacrylate on healing of intercalary cortical allografts in a canine model, *J Orthopaed Res* 10:434–439, 1992.

213. Kirpensteijn J, Steinheimer D, Park RD, et al.: Comparison of cemented and non-cemented allografts in dogs with osteosarcoma, *Vet Comp Orthopaed* 11:178–184, 1998.

214. Liptak JM, Dernell WS, Ehrhart N, et al.: Cortical allograft and endoprosthesis for limb-sparing surgery in dogs with distal radial osteosarcoma; a prospective clinical comparison of two different limb-sparing techniques, *Vet Surg* 35:518–533, 2006.

215. Mitchell KE, Boston SE, Kung M, et al.: Outcomes of limb-sparing surgery using two generations of metal endoprosthesis in 45 dogs with distal radial osteosarcoma. A Veterinary Society of Surgical Oncology retrospective study, *Vet Surg* 45:36–43, 2016.

216. Bray JP, Kersley A, Downing W, et al.: Clinical outcomes of patient-specific porous titanium endoprostheses in dogs with tumors of the mandible, radius, or tibia; 12 cases (2013-2016), *J Am Vet Med Assoc* 251:566–579, 2017.

217. Fitzpatrick N, Guthrie JW: Hemipelvic and proximal femoral limb salvage endoprosthesis with tendon ongrowth in a dog, *Vet Surg* 47:963–969, 2018.

218. Degna MT, Ehrhart N, Feretti A, et al.: Bone transport osteogenesis for limb salvage - Following resection of primary bone tumors; experience with six cases (1991-1996), *Vet Comp Orthopaed* 13:18–22, 2000.

219. Ehrhart N: Longitudinal bone transport for treatment of primary bone tumors in dogs; technique description and outcome in 9 dogs, *Vet Surg* 34:24–34, 2005.

220. Jehn CT, Lewis DD, Farese JP, et al.: Transverse ulnar bone transport osteogenesis;a new technique for limb salvage for the treatment of distal radial osteosarcoma in dogs, *Vet Surg* 36:324–334, 2007.

221. Ehrhart N, Eurell JA, Tommasini M, et al.: Effect of cisplatin on bone transport osteogenesis in dogs, *Am J Vet Res* 63:703–711, 2002.

222. Rovesti GL, Bascucci M, Schmidt K, et al.: Limb sparing using a double bone-transport technique for treatment of a distal tibial osteosarcoma in a dog, *Vet Surg* 31:70–77, 2002.

223. Pooya HA, Seguin B, Mason DR, et al.: Biomechanical comparison of cortical radial graft versus ulnar transposition graft limb-sparing techniques for the distal radial site in dogs, *Vet Surg* 33:301–308, 2004.
224. Seguin B, Walsh PJ, Mason DR, et al.: Use of an ipsilateral vascularized ulnar transposition autograft for limb-sparing surgery of the distal radius in dogs; an anatomic and clinical study, *Vet Surg* 32:69–79, 2003.
225. Liptak JM, Dernell WS, Lascelles BD, et al.: Intraoperative extracorporeal irradiation for limb sparing in 13 dogs, *Vet Surg* 33:446–456, 2004.
226. Boston SE, Duerr F, Bacon N, et al.: Intraoperative radiation for limb sparing of the distal aspect of the radius without transcarpal plating in five dogs, *Vet Surg* 36:314–323, 2007.
227. Oya N, Kokubo M, Mizowaki T, et al.: Definitive intraoperative very high-dose radiotherapy for localized osteosarcoma in the extremities, *Int J Radiat Oncol* 51:87–93, 2001.
228. Sakayama K, Kidani T, Fujibuchi T, et al.: Definitive intraoperative radiotherapy for musculoskeletal sarcomas and malignant lymphoma in combination with surgical excision, *Int J Clin Oncol* 8:174–179, 2003.
229. Tsuboyama T, Toguchida J, Kotoura Y, et al.: Intra-operative radiation therapy for osteosarcoma in the extremities, *Int Orthop* 24:202–207, 2000.
230. Farese JP, Milner R, Thompson MS, et al.: Stereotactic radiosurgery for treatment of osteosarcomas involving the distal portions of the limbs in dogs, *J Am Vet Med Assoc* 225:1567–1572, 2004.
231. Kubicek L, Vanderhart D, Wirth K, et al.: Association between computed tomography characteristics and fractures following stereotactic radiosurgery in dogs with appendicular osteosarcoma, *Vet Radiol Ultrasound* 57:321–330, 2016.
232. Curtis RC, Custis JT, Ehrhart NP, et al.: Combination therapy with zoledronic acid and parathyroid hormone improves bone architecture and strength following a clinically-relevant dose of stereotactic radiation therapy for the local treatment of canine osteosarcoma in athymic rats, *PLoS One* 11:e0158005, 2016.
233. Powers BE, Withrow SJ, Thrall DE, et al.: Percent tumor necrosis as a predictor of treatment response in canine osteosarcoma, *Cancer* 67:126–134, 1991.
234. Pagano C, Boudreaux B, Shiomitsu K: Safety and toxicity of an accelerated coarsely fractionated radiation protocol for treatment of appendicular osteosarcoma in 14 dogs; 10 Gy x 2 fractions, *Vet Radiol Ultrasound* 57:551–556, 2016.
235. Van Ginkel RJ, Hoekstra HJ, Meutstege FJ, et al.: Hyperthermic isolated regional perfusion with cisplatin in the local treatment of spontaneous canine osteosarcoma; assessment of short-term effects, *J Surg Oncol* 59:169–176, 1995.
236. Rossi CR, Pasquali S, Mocellin S, et al.: Long-term results of melphalan-based isolated limb perfusion with or without low-dose tnf for in-transit melanoma metastases, *Ann Surg Oncol* 17:3000–3007, 2010.
237. Deroose JP, Van Geel AN, Burger JWA, et al.: Isolated limb perfusion with TNF-alpha and melphalan for distal parts of the limb in soft tissue sarcoma patients, *J Surg Oncol* 105:563–569, 2012.
238. Zachos TA, Aiken SW, DiResta GR, et al.: Interstitial fluid pressure and blood flow in canine osteosarcoma and other tumors, *Clin Orthop Relat Res* 230–236, 2001.
239. Powers BE, Withrow SJ, Thrall DE, et al.: Percent tumor necrosis as a predictor of treatment response in canine osteosarcoma, *Cancer* 67:126–134, 1991.
240. Withrow SJ, Liptak JM, Straw RC, et al.: Biodegradable cisplatin polymer in limb-sparing surgery for canine osteosarcoma, *Ann Surg Oncol* 11:705–713, 2004.
241. Lascelles BDX, Dernell WS, Correa MT, et al.: Improved survival associated with postoperative wound infection in dogs treated with limb-salvage surgery for osteosarcoma, *Ann Surg Oncol* 12:1073–1083, 2005.
242. Culp WT, Olea-Popelka F, Sefton J, et al.: Evaluation of outcome and prognostic factors for dogs living greater than one year after diagnosis of osteosarcoma; 90 cases (1997-2008), *J Am Vet Med Assoc* 245:1141–1146, 2014.
243. Jeys LM, Grimer RJ, Carter SR, et al.: Post operative infection and increased survival in osteosarcoma patients; are they associated? *Ann Surg Oncol* 14:2887–2895, 2007.
244. Sottnik JL, U'Ren LW, Thamm DH, et al.: Chronic bacterial osteomyelitis suppression of tumor growth requires innate immune responses, *Cancer Immunol Immunother* 59:367–378, 2010.
245. Kramer A, Walsh PJ, Seguin B: Hemipelvectomy in dogs and cats; technique overview, variations, and description, *Vet Surg* 37:413–419, 2008.
246. Straw RC, Withrow SJ, Powers BE: Partial or total hemipelvectomy in the management of sarcomas in nine dogs and two cats, *Vet Surg* 21:183–188, 1992.
247. Bray JP: Hemipelvectomy; modified surgical technique and clinical experiences from a retrospective study, *Vet Surg* 43:19–26, 2014.
248. Chauvet AE, Hogge GS, Sandin JA, et al.: Vertebrectomy, bone allograft fusion, and antitumor vaccination for the treatment of vertebral fibrosarcoma in a dog, *Vet Surg* 28:480–488, 1999.
249. Nakata K, Miura H, Sakai H, et al.: Vertebral replacement for the treatment of vertebral osteosarcoma in a cat, *J Vet Med Sci* 79:999–1002, 2017.
250. Liptak JM, Dernell WS, Rizzo SA, et al.: Partial foot amputation in 11 dogs, *J Am Anim Hosp Assoc* 41:47–55, 2005.
251. Fitzpatrick N, Smith TJ, Pendegrass CJ, et al.: Intraosseous transcutaneous amputation prosthesis (ITAP) for limb salvage in 4 dogs, *Vet Surg* 40:909–925, 2011.
252. Drygas KA, Taylor R, Sidebotham CG, et al.: Transcutaneous tibial implants; a surgical procedure for restoring ambulation after amputation of the distal aspect of the tibia in a dog, *Vet Surg* 37:322–327, 2008.
253. Kirpensteijn J, Straw RC, Pardo AD, et al.: Partial and total scapulectomy in the dog, *J Am Anim Hosp Assoc* 30:313–319, 1994.
254. Montinaro V, Boston SE, Buracco P, et al.: Clinical outcome of 42 dogs with scapular tumors treated by scapulectomy; a Veterinary Society of Surgical Oncology (VSSO) retrospective study (1995–2010), *Vet Surg* 42:943–950, 2013.
255. Straw RC, Withrow SJ, Powers BE: Primary osteosarcoma of the ulna in 12 dogs, *J Am Anim Hosp Assoc* 27:323–326, 1991.
256. Duncan B, Lascelles X, Thomson MJ, et al.: Combined dorsolateral and intraoral approach for the resection of tumors of the maxilla in the dog, *J Am Anim Hosp Assoc* 39:294–305, 2003.
257. Fox LE, Geoghegan SL, Davis LH, et al.: Owner satisfaction with partial mandibulectomy or maxillectomy for treatment of oral tumors in 27 dogs, *J Am Anim Hosp Assoc* 33:25–31, 1997.
258. White RAS: Mandibulectomy and maxillectomy in the dog - long-term survival in 100 cases, *J Sm Anim Pract* 32:69–74, 1991.
259. Withrow SJ, Holmberg DL: Mandibulectomy in the treatment of oral cancer, *J Am Anim Hosp Assoc* 19:273–286, 1983.
260. OBrien MG, Withrow SJ, Straw RC, et al.: Total and partial orbitectomy for the treatment of periorbital tumors in 24 dogs and 6 cats; a retrospective study, *Vet Surg* 25:471–479, 1996.
261. Liptak JM, Dernell WS, Rizzo SA, et al.: Reconstruction of chest wall defects after rib tumor resection; a comparison of autogenous, prosthetic, and composite techniques in 44 dogs, *Vet Surg* 37:479–487, 2008.
262. Caceres E, Zaharia M, Valdivia S, et al.: Local control of osteogenic-sarcoma by radiation and chemotherapy, *Int J Radiat Oncol* 10:35–39, 1984.
263. Gaitanyanguas M: A Study of the response of osteogenic-sarcoma and adjacent normal-tissues to radiation, *Int J Radiat Oncol* 7:593–595, 1981.
264. Machak GN, Tkachev SI, Solovyev YN, et al.: Neoadjuvant chemotherapy and local radiotherapy for high-grade osteosarcoma of the extremities, *Mayo Clin Proc* 78:147–155, 2003.

265. Walter CU, Dernell WS, LaRue SM, et al.: Curative-intent radiation therapy as a treatment modality for appendicular and axial osteosarcoma; a preliminary retrospective evaluation of 14 dogs with the disease, *Vet Comp Oncol* 3:1–7, 2005.

266. Chakraborty S, Das T, Sarma HD, et al.: Comparative studies of 177Lu-EDTMP and 177Lu-DOTMP as potential agents for palliative radiotherapy of bone metastasis, *Appl Radiat Isot* 66:1196–1205, 2008.

267. Zhou JJ, Gonzalez A, Lenox MW, et al.: Dosimetry of a (90) Y-hydroxide liquid brachytherapy treatment approach to canine osteosarcoma using PET/CT, *Appl Radiat Isot* 97:193–200, 2015.

268. Khanna C, Prehn J, Hayden D, et al.: A randomized controlled trial of octreotide pamoate long-acting release and carboplatin versus carboplatin alone in dogs with naturally occurring osteosarcoma; evaluation of insulin-like growth factor suppression and chemotherapy, *Clin Cancer Res* 8:2406–2412, 2002.

269. Vail DM, Kurzman ID, Glawe PC, et al.: STEALTH liposome-encapsulated cisplatin (SPI-77) versus carboplatin as adjuvant therapy for spontaneously arising osteosarcoma (OSA) in the dog; a randomized multicenter clinical trial, *Cancer Chemoth Pharmacol* 50:131–136, 2002.

270. Philips B, Powers BE, Dernell WS, et al.: Use of single-agent carboplatin as adjuvant or neoadjuvant therapy in conjunction with amputation for appendicular osteosarcoma in dogs, *J Am Anim Hosp Assoc* 45:33–38, 2009.

271. Saam DE, Liptak JM, Stalker MJ, et al.: Predictors of outcome in dogs treated with adjuvant carboplatin for appendicular osteosarcoma; 65 cases (1996-2006), *J Am Vet Med Assoc* 238:195–206, 2011.

272. Berg J, Weinstein MJ, Springfield DS, et al.: Results of surgery and doxorubicin chemotherapy in dogs with osteosarcoma, *J Am Vet Med Assoc* 206:1555–1560, 1995.

273. Chun R, Garrett LD, Henry C, et al.: Toxicity and efficacy of cisplatin and doxorubicin combination chemotherapy for the treatment of canine osteosarcoma, *J Am Anim Hosp Assoc* 41:382–387, 2005.

274. Chun R, Kurzman ID, Couto CG, et al.: Cisplatin and doxorubicin combination chemotherapy for the treatment of canine osteosarcoma; a pilot study, *J Vet Intern Med* 14:495–498, 2000.

275. Bailey D, Erb H, Williams L, et al.: Carboplatin and doxorubicin combination chemotherapy for the treatment of appendicular osteosarcoma in the dog, *J Vet Intern Med* 17:199–205, 2003.

276. Kent MS, Strom A, London CA, et al.: Alternating carboplatin and doxorubicin as adjunctive chemotherapy to amputation or limb-sparing surgery in the treatment of appendicular osteosarcoma in dogs, *J Vet Intern Med* 18:540–544, 2004.

277. Bacon NJ, Ehrhart NP, Dernell WS, et al.: Use of alternating administration of carboplatin and doxorubicin in dogs with microscopic metastases after amputation for appendicular osteosarcoma; 50 cases (1999-2006), *J Am Vet Med Assoc* 232:1504–1510, 2008.

278. Lane A, Black M, Wyatt K: Toxicity and efficacy of a novel doxorubicin and carboplatin chemotherapy protocol for the treatment of canine appendicular osteosarcoma following limb amputation, *Aust Vet J* 90:69–74, 2012.

279. Frimberger AE, Chan CM, Moore AS: Canine osteosarcoma treated by post-amputation sequential accelerated doxorubicin and carboplatin chemotherapy; 38 cases, *J Am Anim Hosp Assoc* 52:149–156, 2016.

280. Skorupski KA, Uhl JM, Szivek A, et al.: Carboplatin versus alternating carboplatin and doxorubicin for the adjuvant treatment of canine appendicular osteosarcoma; a randomized, phase III trial, *Vet Comp Oncol* 14:81–87, 2016.

281. Bracha S, Walshaw R, Danton T, et al.: Evaluation of toxicities from combined metronomic and maximal-tolerated dose chemotherapy in dogs with osteosarcoma, *J Small Anim Pract* 55:369–374, 2014.

282. Matsuyama A, Schott CR, Wood GA, et al.: Evaluation of metronomic cyclophosphamide chemotherapy as maintenance treatment for dogs with appendicular osteosarcoma following limb amputation and carboplatin chemotherapy, *J Am Vet Med Assoc* 252:1377–1383, 2018.

283. Kurzman ID, Shi F, Vail DM, et al.: In vitro and in vivo enhancement of canine pulmonary alveolar macrophage cytotoxic activity against canine osteosarcoma cells, *Cancer Biother Radiopharm* 14:121–128, 1999.

284. MacEwen EG, Kurzman ID, Rosenthal RC, et al.: Therapy for osteosarcoma in dogs with intravenous injection of liposome–encapsulated muramyl tripeptide, *J Natl Cancer Inst* 81:935–938, 1989.

285. Kurzman ID, MacEwen EG, Rosenthal RC, et al.: Adjuvant therapy for osteosarcoma in dogs; results of randomized clinical trials using combined liposome-encapsulated muramyl tripeptide and cisplatin, *Clin Cancer Res* 1:1595–1601, 1995.

286. Modiano JF, Bellgrau D, Cutter GR, et al.: Inflammation, apoptosis, and necrosis induced by neoadjuvant fas ligand gene therapy improves survival of dogs with spontaneous bone cancer, *Mol Ther* 20:2234–2243, 2012.

287. Mason NJ, Gnanandarajah JS, Engiles JB, et al.: Immunotherapy with a HER2-targeting listeria induces HER2-specific immunity and demonstrates potential therapeutic effects in a phase I trial in canine osteosarcoma, *Clin Cancer Res* 22:4380–4390, 2016.

288. Polednak AP: Human biology and epidemiology of childhood bone cancers; a review, *Hum Biol* 57:1–26, 1985.

289. London CA, Gardner HL, Mathie T, et al.: Impact of toceranib/piroxicam/cyclophosphamide maintenance therapy on outcome of dogs with appendicular osteosarcoma following amputation and carboplatin chemotherapy; a multi-institutional study, *PLoS One* 10:e0124889, 2015.

290. Alvarez FJ, Kisseberth W, Hosoya K, et al.: Postoperative adjuvant combination therapy with doxorubicin and noncytotoxic suramin in dogs with appendicular osteosarcoma, *J Am Anim Hosp Assoc* 50:12–18, 2014.

291. Downey RJ: Surgical treatment of pulmonary metastases, *Surg Oncol Clin North Amer* 8:341, 1999.

292. Liptak JM, Monnet E, Dernell WS, et al.: Pulmonary metastatectomy in the management of four dogs with hypertrophic osteopathy, *Vet Comp Oncol* 2:1–12, 2004.

293. Ogilvie GK, Straw RC, Jameson VJ, et al.: Evaluation of single-agent chemotherapy for treatment of clinically evident osteosarcoma metastases in dogs; 45 cases (1987-1991uo), *J Am Vet Med Assoc* 202:304–306, 1993.

294. Poirier VJ, Hershey AE, Burgess KE, et al.: Efficacy and toxicity of paclitaxel (Taxol) for the treatment of canine malignant tumors, *J Vet Intern Med* 18:219–222, 2004.

295. London CA, Hannah AL, Zadovoskaya R, et al.: Phase I dose-escalating study of SU11654, a small molecule receptor tyrosine kinase inhibitor, in dogs with spontaneous malignancies, *Clin Cancer Res* 9:2755–2768, 2003.

296. London C, Mathie T, Stingle N, et al.: Preliminary evidence for biologic activity of toceranib phosphate (Palladia((R))) in solid tumours, *Vet Comp Oncol* 10:194–205, 2012.

297. Laver T, London CA, Vail DM, et al.: Prospective evaluation of toceranib phosphate in metastatic canine osteosarcoma, *Vet Comp Oncol* 16:E23–E29, 2018.

298. Kim C, Matsuyama A, Mutsaers AJ, et al.: Retrospective evaluation of toceranib (Palladia) treatment for canine metastatic appendicular osteosarcoma, *Can Vet J* 58:1059–1064, 2017.

299. Wittenburg LA, Ptitsyn AA, Thamm DH: A systems biology approach to identify molecular pathways altered by HDAC inhibition in osteosarcoma, *J Cell Biochem* 113:773–783, 2012.

300. Wittenburg LA, Gustafson DL, Thamm DH: Phase I pharmacokinetic and pharmacodynamic evaluation of combined valproic acid/doxorubicin treatment in dogs with spontaneous cancer, *Clin Cancer Res* 16:4832–4842, 2010.

301. Hershey AE, Kurzman ID, Forrest LJ, et al.: Inhalation chemotherapy for macroscopic primary or metastatic lung tumors; proof of principle using dogs with spontaneously occurring tumors as a model, *Clin Cancer Res* 5:2653–2659, 1999.

302. Rodriguez CO, Crabbs TA, Wilson DW, et al.: Aerosol gemcitabine; preclinical safety and in vivo antitumor activity in osteosarcoma-bearing dogs, *J Aerosol Med Pulm D* 23:197–206, 2010.

303. Koshkina NV, Kleinerman ES: Aerosol gemcitabine inhibits the growth of primary osteosarcoma and osteosarcoma lung metastases, *Int J Cancer* 116:458–463, 2005.
304. Khanna C, Anderson PM, Hasz DE, et al.: Interleukin-2 liposome inhalation therapy is safe and effective for dogs with spontaneous pulmonary metastases, *Cancer* 79:1409–1421, 1997.
305. Dow S, Elmslie R, Kurzman I, et al.: Phase I study of liposome-DNA complexes encoding the interleukin-2 gene in dogs with osteosarcoma lung metastases, *Hum Gene Ther* 16:937–946, 2005.
306. Thamm DH, Kurzman ID, King I, et al.: Systemic administration of an attenuated, tumor-targeting Salmonella typhimurium to dogs with spontaneous neoplasia; phase I evaluation, *Clin Cancer Res* 11:4827–4834, 2005.
307. Goblirsch M, Mathews W, Lynch C, et al.: Radiation treatment decreases bone cancer pain, osteolysis and tumor size, *Radiat Res* 161:228–234, 2004.
308. Withrow SJ, Powers BE, Straw RC, et al.: Tumor necrosis following radiation therapy and/or chemotherapy for canine osteosarcoma, *Chir Organi Mov* 75:29–31, 1990.
309. Vakaet LA, Boterberg T: Pain control by ionizing radiation of bone metastasis, *Int J Dev Biol* 48:599–606, 2004.
310. Green EM, Adams WM, Forrest LJ: Four fraction palliative radiotherapy for osteosarcoma in 24 dogs, *J Am Anim Hosp Assoc* 38:445–451, 2002.
311. Knapp-Hoch HM, Fidel JL, Sellon RK, et al.: An expedited palliative radiation protocol for lytic or proliferative lesions of appendicular bone in dogs, *J Am Anim Hosp Assoc* 45:24–32, 2009.
312. Mueller F, Poirier V, Melzer K, et al.: Palliative radiotherapy with electrons of appendicular osteosarcoma in 54 dogs, *Vivo* 19:713–716, 2005.
313. Ramirez 3rd O, Dodge RK, Page RL, et al.: Palliative radiotherapy of appendicular osteosarcoma in 95 dogs, *Vet Radiol Ultrasound* 40:517–522, 1999.
314. Mcentee MC, Page RL, Novotney CA, et al.: Palliative radiotherapy for canine appendicular osteosarcoma, *Vet Radiol Ultrasound* 34:367–370, 1993.
315. Oblak ML, Boston SE, Higginson G, et al.: The impact of pamidronate and chemotherapy on survival times in dogs with appendicular primary bone tumors treated with palliative radiation therapy, *Vet Surg* 41:430–435, 2012.
316. Holmes RA: [153Sm]EDTMP; a potential therapy for bone cancer pain, *Semin Nucl Med* 22:41–45, 1992.
317. Serafini AN: Samarium Sm-153 lexidronam for the palliation of bone pain associated with metastases, *Cancer* 88:2934–2939, 2000.
318. Aas M, Moe L, Gamlem H, et al.: Internal radionuclide therapy of primary osteosarcoma in dogs, using 153Sm-ethylene-diamino-tetramethylene-phosphonate (EDTMP), *Clin Cancer Res* 5:3148s–3152s, 1999.
319. Barnard SM, Zuber RM, Moore AS: Samarium Sm 153 lexidronam for the palliative treatment of dogs with primary bone tumors; 35 cases (1999-2005), *J Am Vet Med Assoc* 230:1877–1881, 2007.
320. Lattimer JC, Corwin Jr LA, Stapleton J, et al.: Clinical and clinicopathologic response of canine bone tumor patients to treatment with samarium-153-EDTMP, *J Nucl Med* 31:1316–1325, 1990.
321. Milner RJ, Dormehl I, Louw WK, et al.: Targeted radiotherapy with Sm-153-EDTMP in nine cases of canine primary bone tumours, *J S Afr Vet Assoc* 69:12–17, 1998.
322. Vancil JM, Henry CJ, Milner RJ, et al.: Use of samarium Sm 153 lexidronam for the treatment of dogs with primary tumors of the skull; 20 cases (1986-2006), *J Am Vet Med Assoc* 240:1310–1315, 2012.
323. Bryan JN, Bommarito D, Kim DY, et al.: Comparison of systemic toxicities of 177Lu-DOTMP and 153Sm-EDTMP administered intravenously at equivalent skeletal doses to normal dogs, *J Nucl Med Technol* 37:45–52, 2009.
324. Chakraborty S, Balogh L, Das T, et al.: Evaluation of (1)(7)(7)Lu-EDTMP in dogs with spontaneous tumor involving bone; pharmacokinetics, dosimetry and therapeutic efficacy, *Curr Radiopharm* 9:64–70, 2016.
325. Thapa P, Nikam D, Das T, et al.: Clinical efficacy and safety comparison of 177Lu-EDTMP with 153Sm-EDTMP on an equidose basis in patients with painful skeletal metastases, *J Nucl Med* 56:1513–1519, 2015.
326. Lipton A: New therapeutic agents for the treatment of bone diseases, *Expert Opin Biol Ther* 5:817–832, 2005.
327. Coleman RE: Therapeutic use of bisphosphonates in oncology, *Brit Med J* 309, 1994. 1233–1233.
328. Coleman RE, McCloskey EV: Bisphosphonates in oncology, *Bone* 49:71–76, 2011.
329. Carano A, Teitelbaum SL, Konsek JD, et al.: Bisphosphonates directly inhibit the bone resorption activity of isolated avian osteoclasts in vitro, *J Clin Invest* 85:456–461, 1990.
330. Hughes DE, Wright KR, Uy HL, et al.: Bisphosphonates promote apoptosis in murine osteoclasts in vitro and in vivo, *J Bone Miner Res* 10:1478–1487, 1995.
331. Luckman SP, Hughes DE, Coxon FP, et al.: Nitrogen-containing bisphosphonates inhibit the mevalonate pathway and prevent post-translational prenylation of GTP-binding proteins, including Ras, *J Bone Miner Res* 13:581–589, 1998.
332. Tomlin JL, Sturgeon C, Pead MJ, et al.: Use of the bisphosphonate drug alendronate for palliative management of osteosarcoma in two dogs, *Vet Rec* 147:129–132, 2000.
333. Fan TM, de Lorimier LP, Charney SC, et al.: Evaluation of intravenous pamidronate administration in 33 cancer-bearing dogs with primary or secondary bone involvement, *J Vet Intern Med* 19:74–80, 2005.
334. Fan TM, de Lorimier LP, O'Dell-Anderson K, et al.: Single-agent pamidronate for palliative therapy of canine appendicular osteosarcoma bone pain, *J Vet Intern Med* 21:431–439, 2007.
335. Tuohy J, Haussler K, Adrian C, et al.: Interim analysis of randomized placebo-controlled clinical trial of radiation therapy +/- pamidronate for palliative treatment of canine appendicular osteosarcoma, *Vete Comp Oncol* 9:e1–e49, 2011.
336. Fan TM, Charney SC, de Lorimier LP, et al.: Double-blind placebo-controlled trial of adjuvant pamidronate with palliative radiotherapy and intravenous doxorubicin for canine appendicular osteosarcoma bone pain, *J Vet Intern Med* 23:152–160, 2009.
337. Spugnini EP, Vincenzi B, Caruso G, et al.: Zoledronic acid for the treatment of appendicular osteosarcoma in a dog, *J Small Anim Pract* 50:44–46, 2009.
338. Fan TM, de Lorimier LP, Garrett LD, et al.: The bone biologic effects of zoledronate in healthy dogs and dogs with malignant osteolysis, *J Vet Intern Med* 22:380–387, 2008.
339. Lundberg AP, Roady PJ, Somrak AJ, et al.: Zoledronate-associated osteonecrosis of the jaw in a dog with appendicular osteosarcoma, *J Vet Intern Med* 30:1235–1240, 2016.
340. Vail DM, MacEwen EG: Spontaneously occurring tumors of companion animals as models for human cancer, *Cancer Invest* 18:781–792, 2000.
341. Withrow SJ, Wilkins RM: Cross talk from pets to people; translational osteosarcoma treatments, *ILAR J* 51:208–213, 2010.
342. Rowell JL, McCarthy DO, Alvarez CE: Dog models of naturally occurring cancer, *Trends Mol Med* 17:380–388, 2011.
343. Ayerza MA, Farfalli GL, Aponte-Tinao L, et al.: Does increased rate of limb-sparing surgery affect survival in osteosarcoma? *Clin Orthop Relat Res* 468:2854–2859, 2010.
344. Mankin HJ, Hornicek FI, Rosenberg AE, et al.: Survival data for 648 patients with osteosarcoma treated at one institution, *Clin Orthop Relat Res* 286–291, 2004.
345. Marina NM, Smeland S, Bielack SS, et al.: Comparison of MAPIE versus MAP in patients with a poor response to preoperative chemotherapy for newly diagnosed high-grade osteosarcoma (EURAMOS-1); an open-label, international, randomised controlled trial, *Lancet Oncol* 17:1396–1408, 2016.
346. Okada K, Unni KK, Swee RG, et al.: High grade surface osteosarcoma - a clinicopathologic study of 46 cases, *Cancer* 85:1044–1054, 1999.

347. Banks WC: Parosteal osteosarcoma in a dog and a cat, *J Am Vet Med Assoc* 158:1412,1971.
348. Withrow SJ, Doige CE: En bloc resection of a juxtacortical and 3 intra-osseous osteosarcomas of the zygomatic arch in dogs, *J Am Anim Hosp Assoc* 16:867–872, 1980.
349. Giuffrida MA, Bacon NJ, Kamstock DA: Use of routine histopathology and factor VIII-related antigen/von Willebrand factor immunohistochemistry to differentiate primary hemangiosarcoma of bone from telangiectatic osteosarcoma in 54 dogs, *Vet Comp Oncol* 15:1232–1239, 2017.
350. Giuffrida MA, Kamstock DA, Selmic LE, et al.: Primary appendicular hemangiosarcoma and telangiectatic osteosarcoma in 70 dogs; a Veterinary Society of Surgical Oncology retrospective study, *Vet Surg* 47:774–783, 2018.
351. Wehrle-Martinez AS, Dittmer KE, Aberdein D, et al.: Osteocalcin and osteonectin expression in canine osteosarcoma, *Vet Pathol* 53:781–787, 2016.
352. Brodey RS, Riser WH, Ro Vanderhe: Canine skeletal chondrosarcoma - clinicopathologic study of 35 cases, *J Am Vet Med Assoc* 165:68–78, 1974.
353. Doige CE, Pharr JW, Withrow SJ: Chondrosarcoma arising in multiple cartilaginous exostoses in a dog, *J Am Anim Hosp Assoc* 14:605–611, 1978.
354. Gee BR, Doige CE: Multiple cartilaginous exostoses in a litter of dogs, *J Am Vet Med Assoc* 156:53,1970.
355. Popovitch CA, Weinstein MJ, Goldschmidt MH, et al.: Chondrosarcoma - a retrospective study of 97 dogs (1987-1990), *J Am Anim Hosp Assoc* 30:81–85, 1994.
356. Anderson WI, Carberry CA, King JM, et al.: Primary aortic chondrosarcoma in a dog, *Vet Pathol* 25:180–181, 1988.
357. Aron DN, Devries R, Short CE: Primary tracheal chondrosarcoma in a dog - case-report with description of surgical and anesthetic techniques, *J Am Anim Hosp Assoc* 16:31–37, 1980.
358. Flanders JA, Castleman W, Carberry CA, et al.: Laryngeal chondrosarcoma in a dog, *J Am Vet Med Assoc* 190:68–70, 1987.
359. Greenlee PG, Liu SK: Chondrosarcoma of the mitral leaflet in a dog, *Vet Pathol* 21:540–542, 1984.
360. Patnaik AK, Matthiesen DT, Zawie DA: 2 cases of canine penile neoplasm - squamous-cell carcinoma and mesenchymal chondrosarcoma, *J Am Anim Hosp Assoc* 24:403–406, 1988.
361. Southerland EM, Miller RT, Jones CL: Primary right atrial chondrosarcoma in a dog, *J Am Vet Med Assoc* 203:1697–1698, 1993.
362. Weller RE, Dagle GE, Perry RL, et al.: Primary pulmonary chondrosarcoma in a dog, *Cornell Vet* 82:447–452, 1992.
363. Vinayak A, Worley DR, Withrow SJ, et al.: Dedifferentiated chondrosarcoma in the dog and cat; a case series and review of the literature, *J Am Anim Hosp Assoc* 54:50–59, 2018.
364. Farese JP, Kirpensteijn J, Kik M, et al.: Biologic behavior and clinical outcome of 25 dogs with canine appendicular chondrosarcoma treated by amputation; a veterinary society of surgical oncology retrospective study, *Vet Surg* 38:914–919, 2009.
365. Waltman SS, Seguin B, Cooper BJ, et al.: Clinical outcome of nonnasal chondrosarcoma in dogs; thirty-one cases (1986-2003), *Vet Surg* 36:266–271, 2007.
366. Lana SE, Dernell WS, LaRue SM, et al.: Slow release cisplatin combined with radiation for the treatment of canine nasal tumors, *Vet Radiol Ultrasound* 38:474–478, 1997.
367. Yamaguchi T, Toguchida J, Yamamuro T, et al.: Allelotype analysis in osteosarcomas - frequent allele loss on 3q, 13q, 17p, and 18q, *Cancer Res* 52:2419–2423, 1992.
368. Hammer AS, Couto CG, Filppi J, et al.: Efficacy and toxicity of VAC chemotherapy (vincristine, doxorubicin, and cyclophosphamide) in dogs with hemangiosarcoma, *J Vet Intern Med* 5:160–166, 1991.
369. Ablin LW, Berg J, Schelling SH: Fibrosarcoma of the canine appendicular skeleton, *J Am Anim Hosp Assoc* 27:303–309, 1991.
370. Banks TA, Straw RC: Multilobular osteochondrosarcoma of the hard palate in a dog, *Aust Vet J* 82:409–412, 2004.
371. Straw RC, Lecouteur RA, Powers BE, et al.: Multilobular osteochondrosarcoma of the canine skull - 16 cases (1978-1988), *J Am Vet Med Assoc* 195:1764–1769, 1989.
372. Dernell WS, Straw RC, Cooper MF, et al.: Multilobular osteochondrosarcoma in 39 dogs; 1979-1993, *J Am Anim Hosp Assoc* 34:11–18, 1998.
373. Hathcock JT, Newton JC: Computed tomographic characteristics of multilobular tumor of bone involving the cranium in 7 dogs and zygomatic arch in 2 dogs, *Vet Radiol Ultrasound* 41:214–217, 2000.
374. Lipsitz D, Levitski RE, Berry WL: Magnetic resonance imaging features of multilobular osteochondrosarcoma in 3 dogs, *Vet Radiol Ultrasound* 42:14–19, 2001.
375. Stoll MR, Roush JK, Moisan PG: Multilobular tumour of bone with no abnormalities on plain radiography in a dog, *J Small Anim Pract* 42:453–455, 2001.
376. Grabias S, Mankin HJ: Chondrosarcoma arising in histologically proved unicameral bone-cyst - case report, *J Bone Joint Surg A* 56:1501–1509, 1974.
377. Johnson KA, Cooley AJ, Darien DL: Zygomatic osteoma with atypical heterogeneity in a dog, *J Comp Pathol* 114:199–203, 1996.
378. Chester DK: Multiple cartilaginous exostoses in two generations of dogs, *J Am Vet Med Assoc* 159:895–897, 1971.
379. Basher AWP, Doige CE, Presnell KR: Subchondral bone cysts in a dog with osteochondrosis, *J Am Anim Hosp Assoc* 24:321–326, 1988.
380. Pernell RT, Dunstan RW, DeCamp CE: Aneurysmal bone cyst in a six-month-old dog, *J Am Vet Med Assoc* 201:1897–1899, 1992.
381. Schrader SC, Burk RL, Liu SK: Bone cysts in two dogs and a review of similar cystic bone lesions in the dog, *J Am Vet Med Assoc* 182:490–495, 1983.
382. Monti P, Barnes D, Adrian AM, et al.: Synovial cell sarcoma in a dog; a misnomer-cytologic and histologic findings and review of the literature, *Vet Clin Pathol* 47:181–185, 2018.
383. Vail DM, Powers BE, Getzy DM, et al.: Evaluation of prognostic factors for dogs with synovial sarcoma - 36 cases (1986-1991), *J Am Vet Med Assoc* 205:1300–1307, 1994.
384. Craig LE, Krimer PM, Cooley AJ: Canine synovial myxoma; 39 cases, *Vet Pathol* 47:931–936, 2010.
385. Craig LE, Julian ME, Ferracone JD: The diagnosis and prognosis of synovial tumors in dogs; 35 cases, *Vet Pathol* 39:66–73, 2002.
386. Dorn CR, Taylor DO, Schneider R, et al.: Survey of animal neoplasms in Alameda and Contra Costa Counties, California. II. Cancer morbidity in dogs and cats from Alameda County, *J Natl Cancer Inst* 40:307–318, 1968.
387. Bitetto WV, Patnaik AK, Schrader SC, et al.: Osteosarcoma in cats; 22 cases (1974-1984), *J Am Vet Med Assoc* 190:91–93, 1987.
388. Dimopoulou M, Kirpensteijn J, Moens H, et al.: Histologic prognosticators in feline osteosarcoma; a comparison with phenotypically similar canine osteosarcoma, *Vet Surg* 37:466–471, 2008.
389. Heldmann E, Anderson MA, Wagner-Mann C: Feline osteosarcoma;145 cases (1990-1995), *J Am Anim Hosp Assoc* 36:518–521, 2000.
390. Turrel JM, Pool RR: Primary bone tumors in the cat - a retrospective study of 15 cats and a literature-review, *Vet Radiol* 23:152–166, 1982.
391. Spugnini EP, Ruslander D, Bartolazzi A: Extraskeletal osteosarcoma in a cat, *J Am Vet Med Asoc* 219:60–62, 2001.
392. Stimson EL, Cook WT, Smith MM, et al.: Extraskeletal osteosarcoma in the duodenum of a cat, *J Am Anim Hosp Assoc* 36:332–336, 2000.
393. Dhaliwal RS, Johnson TO, Kitchell BE: Primary extraskeletal hepatic osteosarcoma in a cat, *J Am Vet Med Assoc* 222:340–342, 2003.
394. Simerdova V, Vavra M, Skoric M, et al.: What is your diagnosis? Multilobate nasal mass in a 5-month-old Sphynx cat, *Vet Clin Pathol* 46:369–370, 2017.

395. Sonnenschein B, Dickomeit MJ, Bali MS: Late-onset fracture-associated osteosarcoma in a cat, *Vet Comp Orthop Traumatol* 25:418–420, 2012.

396. Berger B, Bruhschwein A, Eddicks L, et al.: Malignant transformation of a unicameral bone cyst in a cat, *Can Vet J* 57:377–381, 2016.

397. Rosa C, Kirberger RM: Extraskeletal osteochondroma on a cat's elbow, *J S Afr Vet Assoc* 83;104, 2012.

398. Ickes JC, Moore KW, Morales SC: What is your diagnosis? Osteochondroma, *J Am Vet Med Assoc* 241:1155–1156, 2012.

399. Tan C, Allan GS, Barfield D, et al.: Synovial osteochondroma involving the elbow of a cat, *J Feline Med Surg* 12:412–417, 2010.

400. Riddle WE, Leighton RL: Osteochondromatosis in a cat, *J Am Vet Med Assoc* 156;1428, 1970.

401. Pool RR, Carrig CB: Multiple cartilaginous exostoses in a cat, *Vet Pathol* 9:350–359, 1972.

402. Liu SK, Dorfman HD, Patnaik AK: Primary and secondary bone tumours in the cat, *J Small Anim Pract* 15:141–156, 1974.

403. Quigley PJ, Leedale AH: Tumors involving bone in the domestic cat - a review of 58 cases, *Vet Pathol* 20:670–686, 1983.

404. Hlavaty J, Wolfesberger B, Hauck M, et al.: Ezrin and moesin expression in canine and feline osteosarcoma, *Histol Histopathol* 32:805–816, 2017.

405. Wolfesberger B, Fuchs-Baumgartinger A, Hlavaty J, et al.: Stem cell growth factor receptor in canine vs. feline osteosarcomas, *Oncol Lett* 12:2485–2492, 2016.

406. Gebhard C, Fuchs-Baumgartinger A, Razzazi-Fazeli E, et al.: Distribution and activity levels of matrix metalloproteinase 2 and 9 in canine and feline osteosarcoma, *Can J Vet Res* 80:66–73, 2016.

407. Kirpensteijn J, Teske E, Kik M, et al.: Lobaplatin as an adjuvant chemotherapy to surgery in canine appendicular osteosarcoma;a phase II evaluation, *Anticancer Res* 22:2765–2770, 2002.

408. Berg J, Gebhardt MC, Rand WM: Effect of timing of postoperative chemotherapy on survival of dogs with osteosarcoma, *Cancer* 79:1343–1350, 1997.

409. Mauldin GN, Matus RE, Withrow SJ, et al.: Canine osteosarcoma - treatment by amputation versus amputation and adjuvant chemotherapy using doxorubicin and cisplatin, *J Vet Intern Med* 2:177–180, 1988.

410. McMahon M, Mathie T, Stingle N, et al.: Adjuvant carboplatin and gemcitabine combination chemotherapy postamputation in canine appendicular osteosarcoma, *J Vet Intern Med* 25:511–517, 2011.

26

Tumors of the Endocrine System

KATHARINE F. LUNN AND SARAH E. BOSTON

Pituitary Tumors

Primary tumors of the pituitary gland can arise from several different cell types, including corticotrophs, somatotrophs, thyrotrophs, gonadotrophs, and lactotrophs. The clinical signs associated with these tumors depend on the tumor's size and secretory properties. In a recent study of pituitary glands collected from 136 dogs and 65 cats during routine necropsy, pituitary neoplasia was detected in 14% of the middle-aged and old dogs; however, in most cases the lesions were considered to be incidental.[1] Pituitary tumors also may be detected incidentally when brain imaging is performed for unrelated reasons.[2] The most clinically important pituitary tumor in the dog is the corticotroph adenoma. This tumor produces chronically excessive amounts of adrenocorticotrophic hormone (ACTH) and is associated with clinical signs of hypercortisolism. In the cat, the most clinically significant pituitary tumor is the growth hormone (GH)–secreting somatotroph adenoma, which causes hypersomatotropism and acromegaly.

Nonfunctional pituitary tumors become clinically significant when they are large enough to cause neurologic signs, including obtundation, stupor, behavioral changes, decreased appetite, gait abnormalities, seizures, blindness, narcolepsy-cataplexy, and other cranial nerve abnormalities.[3–7] The pituitary gland may also be affected by secondary tumors, either through direct extension or by metastatic spread from a distant site.[1] Locally invasive or compressive primary or secondary pituitary tumors also have the potential to cause loss of pituitary function, resulting in hypothyroidism, hypocortisolism, gonadal atrophy, or central diabetes insipidus.[8]

Pituitary Corticotroph Tumors: Hyperadrenocorticism

Pathogenesis

Hyperadrenocorticism (HAC), also termed *hypercortisolism* or *Cushing's syndrome*, is a common endocrine disease of middle-aged and older dogs.[9] It is uncommon in cats. This clinical syndrome results from chronic exposure to excessive blood levels of glucocorticoids. Naturally occurring canine and feline HAC is usually either pituitary dependent or a result of excessive glucocorticoid secretion from an adrenocortical tumor.

Pituitary-dependent hypercortisolism (PDH) is the most common form of spontaneous HAC in dogs and cats, accounting for 80% to 85% of cases in these species. This disorder is a consequence of autonomous synthesis and secretion of ACTH from a pituitary tumor. The secretion of ACTH from the pituitary tumor is chronically excessive, leading to bilateral adrenal cortical hyperplasia and hypercortisolemia. The pituitary tumor is relatively insensitive to negative feedback by cortisol, and a loss of hypothalamic control over ACTH release occurs because corticotropin-releasing hormone (CRH) secretion is suppressed by the chronic hypercortisolemia.[10]

Pituitary tumors that secrete ACTH are derived from pituitary corticotroph cells; approximately 70% to 80% arise from the pars distalis of the pituitary gland, which is mainly under the control of CRH. The remainder of these tumors arise from the pars intermedia, which is predominantly under dopaminergic and serotoninergic control, with less regulation by CRH. This distinction between pars intermedia and pars distalis tumors typically is not made clinically or from the results of diagnostic testing, but it does potentially help explain why some pituitary-directed medical therapies are not efficacious in all dogs with PDH. The specific molecular defects that lead to the development of canine corticotroph tumors continue to be investigated, and it generally is believed that these tumors result from somatic mutations that occur within the corticotroph cells, rather than from chronic stimulation of the corticotrophs by hypothalamic factors in combination with decreased dopaminergic tone.[10] There is only one clearly documented report of ectopic ACTH secretion in the dog,[11] which may reflect the fact that it is very difficult to prove this diagnosis.

Pituitary tumors may be described as macrotumors or microtumors. The latter distinction is derived from human medicine: microtumors are less than 1 cm in diameter, and macrotumors are 1 cm or larger in diameter. The use of this size-based classification is controversial in veterinary medicine, at least partly because of variability in patient size and conformation.[4] Pituitary tumors may also be classified as noninvasive adenomas, invasive adenomas, or adenocarcinomas. The latter term is reserved for tumors in which there is demonstrated evidence of metastatic disease. Canine pituitary adenocarcinomas are uncommon. In a study of 33 dogs with pituitary tumors that underwent necropsy evaluation after brain imaging, 61% had a pituitary adenoma, 33% had an invasive adenoma, and 6% had an adenocarcinoma.[3]

Adrenal-dependent hypercortisolism (ADH) refers to disease of the adrenal cortex, including neoplasia, dysplasia, or hyperplasia, and is discussed in the section on adrenal gland tumors.

Clinical Findings and Diagnostic Evaluation in Dogs

Most dogs with PDH are older than 9 years of age, and female dogs are slightly overrepresented. Breed predispositions have been noted in dachshunds, terrier breeds, German shepherd dogs, and poodle breeds. The onset of canine Cushing's syndrome is often slow, and the signs can progress slowly. Affected dogs are often not considered by their owners to be sick; they have a good appetite and do not show signs such as vomiting, diarrhea, coughing, or weight loss. Because spontaneous HAC typically affects elderly dogs, the signs initially may be attributed to normal aging. The progress of the disorder is generally insidious, but eventually the owners of affected dogs seek veterinary care because of frustration with signs such as polyuria, polydipsia, panting, and exercise intolerance.

The clinical signs in dogs with HAC are the result of the gluconeogenic, catabolic, immunosuppressive, and anti inflammatory effects of excessive circulating glucocorticoids. These signs include polyuria, polydipsia, polyphagia, abdominal enlargement, lethargy, panting, exercise intolerance, muscle weakness, alopecia, calcinosis cutis, thinning of the skin, poor wound healing, muscle wasting, decreased bone density, and reproductive abnormalities. Dogs with HAC are also predisposed to diabetes mellitus and are more susceptible to infection, particularly urinary tract infections. More serious disorders associated with canine HAC include hypertension and proteinuria. Although uncommon, pulmonary thromboembolism is another potentially life-threatening complication of HAC.

The most commonly used screening tests for HAC are the low-dose dexamethasone suppression test (LDDST) and the ACTH stimulation test. For patients with typical clinical signs of HAC and positive results on a screening test, further testing is often necessary to differentiate between pituitary- and adrenal-dependent disease. Differentiation tests that are commonly used include the high-dose dexamethasone suppression test (HDDST) and the measurement of endogenous ACTH levels. The interested reader should consult the many excellent resources that provide further detail on the clinical and clinicopathologic findings in dogs with HAC, in addition to extensive discussion of the pros and cons of the different screening and differentiation tests.[9,10,12]

The results of imaging studies, including ultrasonography, computed tomography (CT), or magnetic resonance imaging (MRI), may assist in distinguishing between PDH and ADH. Abdominal ultrasonography should not be used as a screening test for HAC, and it should also not be used as the sole mechanism for discriminating between PDH and ADH; however, it can provide useful information.[13–17] The adrenals of patients with PDH are often bilaterally enlarged with increased thickness; they typically maintain a normal shape and are homogeneous in echogenicity.[14] However, there can be overlap between adrenal gland measurements in normal dogs, dogs with nonadrenal disease, and dogs with HAC. Adrenal gland asymmetry may also be detected in dogs with PDH because of nodular hyperplasia. In some cases this appearance can be confused with adrenal neoplasia. To further complicate the diagnostic accuracy of abdominal ultrasonography, a small percentage of patients with HAC may have concurrent PDH and ADH.[18] Bilateral adrenal tumors may also occur,

including both functional or nonfunctional adrenocortical tumors and pheochromocytomas.[16,19–23] Thus ultrasound findings must always be interpreted concurrently with clinical findings and endocrine test results. Abdominal CT is used less commonly than ultrasonography to evaluate the adrenals, but CT findings may also assist in the discrimination between PDH and ADH.[24,25] This technique also demonstrates overlap between adrenal volume in dogs with PDH and dogs with nonadrenal disease and also confirms that dogs with PDH can have nodular adrenal lesions.[25]

Although 80% to 85% of dogs with spontaneous HAC have PDH and the great majority of cases of PDH are the result of the presence of a pituitary tumor, canine patients do not often show clinical signs directly referable to the local effects of the tumor. Most patients initially are presented for veterinary care because of the typical clinical signs of HAC, particularly once they affect the quality of life of the patient or the owner. Pituitary tumors may be detected by CT,[4,6] dynamic CT,[26,27] MRI,[4,6,28–32] or dynamic MRI[33]; however, these techniques are not routinely performed in all dogs diagnosed with PDH. In most cases the diagnosis is based on the presence of typical clinical signs and clinicopathologic changes of hypercortisolemia, together with the results of endocrine testing.

As noted previously, brain imaging is not performed in most dogs with PDH, and most receive treatment to address adrenal hyperfunction rather than the pituitary tumor itself. This is most likely because brain imaging and pituitary surgery or radiation therapy (RT) is not affordable or accessible to many clients. Although medical therapy for PDH has a long history of successful use, it is important to note that the pituitary lesion in dogs with PDH will progress over time. In a study of 13 dogs that underwent MRI evaluation of the brain at the time of diagnosis of PDH and before medical therapy was instituted, eight of the dogs had a visible pituitary mass and none of the dogs had clinical signs of neurologic disease.[31] Four of the dogs showed enlargement of the pituitary tumor on MRI 1 year later, and a pituitary tumor also was detected in two dogs that did not have a visible mass on the initial MRI. Two of the 13 dogs had developed neurologic signs at the time of the 1-year follow-up MRI. In a study evaluating diagnostic imaging findings in 157 dogs with PDH with and without neurologic signs, central nervous system (CNS)–specific signs such as circling, seizures, and ataxia were neither sensitive nor specific for predicting the presence of a pituitary macrotumor.[6] However, signs such as lethargy, mental dullness, and decreased appetite were highly specific for detection of a pituitary macrotumor but not highly sensitive. Other studies also have documented that mentation and appetite changes are the most common signs associated with pituitary tumors.[5,34]

When considering brain imaging in dogs with PDH, several factors should be taken into account: 40% to 50% of dogs with PDH have tumors that are not visible on CT or MRI, and these dogs are unlikely to develop neurologic signs associated with the tumor; 15% to 25% of dogs with PDH are at risk for the development of neurologic signs as the result o the presence of an enlarging tumor, and these signs typically develop within 6 to 18 months of the diagnosis of PDH; brain imaging may be helpful in predicting dogs likely to develop neurologic signs in patients with PDH that initially have no signs directly attributable to the tumor[35]; and if RT is being considered, early treatment will likely improve the prognosis.[5,36] One approach that has been suggested is that CT or MRI should be considered at the time of diagnosis of PDH, with medical therapy alone recommended if no mass is seen. If a pituitary mass is detected but is less than 8 mm in diameter, medical therapy and repeat imaging in 12–18 months should be recommended. For masses greater than 8 mm in diameter, RT should be recommended.[9] Unfortunately this approach is not available or feasible for many clients, and medical therapy alone is often the mainstay of treatment. Theoretically, measurement of plasma ACTH precursor concentrations could help in the selection of patients for brain imaging because it has been shown that pro-opiomelanocortin/pro-ACTH levels in plasma are correlated with pituitary tumor size in dogs with PDH. However these tests are not commercially available.[37,38] Unfortunately, plasma cortisol concentrations at baseline and 4 or 8 hours after administration of a low dose of dexamethasone do not appear to correlate with the development of neurologic signs.[6] Consequently, there is no readily available, inexpensive, simple diagnostic test that can predict pituitary tumor size in dogs with PDH.

Treatment of Canine Pituitary-Dependent Hypercortisolism

Medical Therapy

Although PDH is a disease of the pituitary gland, most dogs with this disorder are treated with medical therapies that address adrenocortical hyperplasia and hyperfunction. The most commonly used medications are trilostane and mitotane. Mitotane (o,p'-DDD, Lysodren) is a potent adrenocorticolytic agent that is cytotoxic to the adrenal cortex, particularly the zona fasciculata and zona reticularis. Trilostane (Vetoryl) is an orally active synthetic corticosteroid analog that competitively inhibits 3-β-hydroxysteroid dehydrogenase.[39] This enzyme is essential for synthesis of cortisol and other steroids, such as corticosterone, androstenedione, and aldosterone. Both mitotane and trilostane are widely and successfully used in the management of PDH, and each has its own advantages and disadvantages.[40–43] A detailed discussion of these treatment modalities for PDH is beyond the scope of this chapter, and readers are strongly encouraged to consult any of several excellent reviews of this subject before initiating medical therapy in any patient.[9,10]

As noted previously, the two medications most commonly used to treat PDH in dogs are trilostane and mitotane. But several other medications also have been used in dogs with PDH, some of which are targeted against the pituitary lesion in these patients. When canine pituitary corticotroph adenomas were evaluated for expression of receptors that are potential therapeutic targets for human Cushing's disease, it was found that canine tumors removed after transsphenoidal surgery expressed a predominance of somatostatin receptor subtype 2 (SST2), in contrast to human tumors, which express predominantly subtype 5 (SST5). Canine tumors express much lower levels of SST5 and express the dopamine receptor D2 at levels that were described as moderate and comparatively less than expressed in tumors from humans.[44] Pasireotide is a somatostatin receptor analog that binds to receptors of the subtypes SST1, SST2, SS, and SST5. In a small study of 20 dogs with PDH, pasireotide therapy produced improvements in plasma ACTH concentrations, urine cortisol:creatinine ratios, tumor size, and clinical signs in most dogs, although three dogs developed diabetes mellitus.[45] In a more recent study, pasireotide therapy was combined with trilostane therapy (eight dogs) or mitotane therapy (one dog) in nine dogs with PDH resulting from a macroadenoma. No adverse effects were noted, and tumor volume decreased in six of the nine dogs, but it increased in three of the nine.[46] Unfortunately pasireotide is extremely expensive,

which may limit its current use in many patients. Selegiline (L-deprenyl, Anipryl) acts by inhibiting degradation of dopamine, thereby potentially inhibiting ACTH secretion from the intermediate lobe of the pituitary gland; unfortunately only 20% of canine PDH cases arise from disease in this area. Additional disadvantages are documented poor efficacy,[47] expense, and inability to monitor response with ACTH stimulation testing. Cabergoline is a dopamine D2 receptor agonist that also acts to reduce pituitary ACTH secretion by increasing dopaminergic tone. In the only published study of cabergoline use in dogs with PDH, 17 of 40 dogs showed a favorable clinical response. Decreases in ACTH concentrations, urine cortisol:creatinine ratios, and pituitary tumor size also were reported.[48] Further studies are needed before this is likely to become a widely adopted treatment for canine PDH. Bromocriptine is a dopamine agonist and also acts to reduce plasma ACTH concentrations. Because of adverse effects and lack of demonstrated efficacy, it is not recommended for treatment of canine PDH.[49] Use of the antiserotoninergic medication cyproheptadine arose from the hypothesis that excessive ACTH secretion could result from excessive serotoninergic stimulation of the pituitary gland. This drug has been shown to be ineffective in clinical cases.[50] Retinoic acid also has been used in the management of canine PDH. This medication may inhibit pituitary tumor development, reduce ACTH production, and inhibit cell proliferation. One study showed promise in terms of a decrease in the size of pituitary tumors and subjective improvement in clinical signs.[51] Unfortunately experience with this medication is very limited, particularly when contrasted with proven therapies such as trilostane and mitotane. Availability and cost of the appropriate formulation of retinoic acid are also significant concerns.

Surgery

Hypophysectomy is the treatment of choice for PDH in humans and can be successful in dogs.[2,52–55] Once PDH is diagnosed, if surgical management is an option, advanced imaging is required. Both CT and MRI have been used to evaluate the pituitary gland before surgery.[53,56–58] The relative size of the pituitary gland is assessed by evaluating the pituitary height:brain area (P:B) ratio; a P:B ratio >0.31 is consistent with pituitary enlargement.[56,59]

Transsphenoidal hypophysectomy first was reported in a large cohort of dogs in 1998.[53] In that study the 1- and 2-year estimated survival rates were 84% and 80%, respectively. Forty-three dogs went into remission, and recurrence of HAC was reported in five dogs.[53] The same group since has published the largest cohort of dogs with PDH treated with transsphenoidal hypophysectomy to date, reporting the outcomes in 306 dogs.[56] In that study 91% of the dogs survived the 4-week perioperative period. The median survival time (MST) was 781 days, and the median disease-free interval (DFI) was 951 days. The recurrence rate was 27%, and recurrence of HAC was diagnosed a median of 555 days from surgery. When the pituitary gland size was evaluated using the P:B ratio, dogs with larger tumors had a shorter survival time (ST) and an increased risk of recurrence.[56] Postoperative ACTH and cortisol concentrations may give some indication of the risk of residual disease. However, this should be evaluated in light of the tumor size, baseline ACTH levels, and individual patient hormone profiles.[60] Postoperative management includes lifelong administration of thyroid hormone and glucocorticoids, and either short- or long-term administration of desmospressin.[53,56]

In a prospective study of 150 dogs treated with transsphenoidal hypophysectomy for PDH, the 1-, 2-, 3-, and 4-year estimated survival rates were 84%, 76%, 72%, and 68%, respectively. Twelve dogs died postoperatively, and 127 went into remission, of which 32 later experienced a recurrence of disease. Complications included central diabetes insipidus in 53% of dogs undergoing remission and incomplete hypophysectomy in nine dogs. The overall success rate of transsphenoidal hypophysectomy was determined to be 65% in this study.[54] Reported complications of transsphenoidal hypophysectomy include hemorrhage, electrolyte imbalance, postoperative neurologic deficits, decreased tear production, thromboembolic disease, recurrence of PDH, and perioperative death.[54,56] However, the overall outcome of this procedure is favorable, resulting in rapid resolution of disease and a long period of remission or complete resolution in patients that survive the perioperative period.[53,56]

Although most of the publications on the surgical management of canine pituitary tumors originated in Europe, this technique is becoming more widely available in the United States. A recent publication documented the outcome of transsphenoidal surgery using a high-definition video telescope, and this approach is now available at Washington State University Veterinary Teaching Hospital. In this case series of 26 dogs with PDH, the overall mortality associated with the surgery was 19%; however, the five deaths occurred in the first 10 dogs treated, with no mortality in the subsequent 16 dogs.[55] This serves as a reminder that transsphenoidal hypophysectomy is a specialized procedure with a steep learning curve. A successful outcome is most likely with careful patient selection and a coordinated approach from a team of specialists in surgery, medicine, neurology, and critical care.[2]

Radiation Therapy

Several reports have been published on the successful use of radiation in the treatment of canine PDH.[5,36,61–65] Dow and colleagues treated six dogs with functional pituitary macrotumors; the dogs were given 40 Gy in 10 equal fractions. The MST was 743 days; neurologic signs resolved in all the dogs; and ACTH levels remained high for at least 1 year after therapy.[61] Cobalt 60 RT was used to treat six dogs with PDH caused by a pituitary tumor that was detectable on MRI; tumor size was significantly reduced in all cases, but clinical signs of PDH were adequately controlled only in one dog.[62] The effects of megavoltage irradiation on pituitary tumors was evaluated in 24 dogs with neurologic signs; 10 dogs experienced complete remission of neurologic signs, and another 10 achieved partial remission; 4 dogs died, either during radiation therapy or shortly thereafter.[36] As in previous studies a correlation was noted between relative tumor size and the severity of neurologic signs in dogs with pituitary tumors. A correlation between tumor size and remission of neurologic signs also was noted after pituitary irradiation, which suggests that early treatment of these tumors should improve the prognosis, although control of ACTH secretion was unlikely.[36] A retrospective study of RT for the treatment of pituitary masses demonstrated significantly improved STs and control of neurologic signs in 19 dogs that received RT compared to 27 untreated control dogs with pituitary masses.[5] The mean ST in the treated group was 1405 days, compared to 551 days in the nonirradiated group. The 1-, 2-, and 3-year estimated survival rates were 93%, 87%, and 55% for the irradiated dogs and 45%, 32%, and 25% for the nonirradiated dogs, respectively.

Treated dogs with smaller tumors lived longer than those with larger tumors; again, this suggests that early diagnosis and treatment of pituitary tumors are beneficial. Five of 14 dogs with PDH in this study were reported to show resolution of clinical signs of HAC, together with at least one normal ACTH stimulation test result after completion of RT.[5] A recent nonrandomized observational study compared two coarse fractionated radiation protocols for canine pituitary macrotumors and found that dogs treated with 10 fractions of 3.8 Gy/fraction on a Monday/Wednesday/Friday protocol had a longer ST than dogs treated once weekly to a total dose of 38 Gy.[64]

Most of the reports that document the use of RT for the treatment of pituitary tumors in dogs provide little detailed information about the progress of the clinical syndrome of HAC in these patients. Therefore, although RT appears effective in controlling neurologic signs and increasing survival,[5] it is difficult to predict the endocrinologic outcome of RT for dogs with PDH. Current and future developments in the use of RT for the management of canine PDH likely will include the more widespread use of stereotactic RT (SRT; see Chapter 13).

Feline Pituitary-Dependent Hyperadrenocorticism

As noted previously, approximately 80% to 85% of cases of HAC in the cat are the result of pituitary disease.[66–68] Most of these cats will have a pituitary adenoma that secretes excessive ACTH; however, pituitary carcinoma has been reported,[69] and cases have been described of cats with pituitary tumors that secrete other hormones in addition to ACTH.[70–72] Cushing's syndrome is considerably less common in cats than in dogs, and in general affected cats are much more "sick" than their canine counterparts. The mean age of cats with PDH is approximately 10 years. Feline HAC is commonly associated with insulin-resistant diabetes mellitus, with signs of polyuria, polydipsia, polyphagia, and weight loss. Cats with HAC often have a potbellied appearance as a result of hepatomegaly and muscle weakness, and they frequently have thin, fragile skin that tears and bruises easily. The clinician should keep this in mind when examining these cats and performing diagnostic tests, because it is easy to cause significant, debilitating skin damage. Additional clinical signs include lethargy, generalized muscle atrophy, weakness, alopecia, and an unkempt hair coat (Fig. 26.1).

On routine laboratory testing, increased alkaline phosphatase activity is much less frequently detected in cats with HAC compared to dogs. Cats may have increased alanine aminotransferase activity, hypercholesterolemia, azotemia, and a minimally concentrated urine. Hyperglycemia and glycosuria are expected in cats with concurrent diabetes mellitus. No consistent complete blood count (CBC) changes have been reported in cats with HAC. Tests used to screen for spontaneous HAC in cats include the urine cortisol:creatinine ratio, ACTH stimulation test, and LDDST. It is important to note that the details of these protocols differ between dogs and cats; readers are directed to more complete references for further information.[66–68] The HDDST, endogenous ACTH concentrations, and abdominal ultrasound examination may be used to assist in differentiation of PDH from ADH in the cat.[73]

Because PDH is relatively uncommon in the cat, there have historically been few case series and case reports on which to base treatment recommendations. However, recent years have yielded some additional information about the management of this condition. Direct treatment of the pituitary tumor has been reported with either surgical hypophysectomy or RT.[52,66,70,74–76]

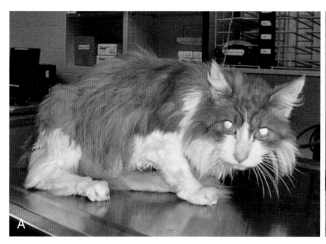
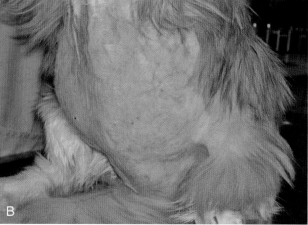

• **Fig. 26.1** A 14-year-old male neutered domestic long-hair cat with pituitary-dependent hypercortisolism. (A) The patient appears weak with muscle atrophy and has an unkempt hair coat. (B) The abdomen has a potbellied appearance with thinning of the skin.

Transsphenoidal hypophysectomy was described in seven cats with PDH.[74] Two of the cats died within 4 weeks of surgery from unrelated causes, and the remaining five cats experienced remission of their disease. Two additional cats died several months after surgery, and one cat experienced a relapse of PDH 19 months after treatment, likely associated with pituitary remnants after surgery.[74] Potential complications of this surgery include transient or long-term hypopituitarism, electrolyte disturbances, soft palate dehiscence, and reduced tear production. Relatively few reports have been published on the outcome of RT for cats with PDH, and it is still unclear if this modality leads to robust management of endocrine disease.[66,67] SRT is an appealing option for these cats because it requires significantly fewer anesthetic events in patients that often are clinically fragile. Surgical bilateral adrenalectomy also has been described in cats with PDH and historically was considered the treatment of choice.[77] However, these cats are often poor surgical candidates, they have diminished healing ability, and complications are common. Laparoscopic adrenalectomy potentially is a better option for these patients because the incisions are much smaller; however, this has not yet been reported in cats with PDH. Trilostane currently appears to be the most reasonable medical therapy for cats with PDH.[66,73,78–80] Clinicians intending to pursue this therapy are encouraged to become familiar with resources that provide detailed protocols for the use of trilostane in cats.[66,67]

Pituitary Somatotroph Tumors (Feline Acromegaly)

Feline acromegaly is a disease of older cats that results from chronic excessive GH secretion, usually from a functional somatotroph adenoma of the pars distalis of the pituitary gland.[81–83] The genetic cause of feline acromegaly is unknown; however, the arylhydrocarbon-receptor interacting protein gene has been the subject of preliminary investigations because it is known to play a role in the development of human familial acromegaly.[84] The term *hypersomatotropism* refers to a condition of excessive growth hormone, whereas *acromegaly* refers to the constellation of associated clinical signs.[85]

Feline acromegaly historically was regarded as a rare condition; however, more recent findings indicate that it may be underdiagnosed. In an early study of 184 diabetic cats, 59 had markedly increased serum insulin–like growth factor-1 (IGF-1) concentrations, and acromegaly was confirmed in 17 of 18 cats that were examined by CT, MRI, or necropsy.[86] The same group subsequently published the results of screening for acromegaly in a much larger group of 1221 diabetic cats. They found that 319 (26.1%) of the cats had serum insulin-like growth factor 1 (IGF-1) concentrations consistent with acromegaly; 63 of these cats underwent pituitary imaging, and the presence of a pituitary lesion was confirmed in 94% of this group.[87] A study of diabetic cats in Europe recently found that 36 of 202 (17.8%) cats evaluated had serum IGF-1 concentrations consistent with acromegaly.[88] Clearly the prevalence of acromegaly differs between these studies, and selection bias may play in role in some of the data. For example, in an initial study of 184 cats, the IGF-1 assays were performed on blood samples submitted to a laboratory at a referral institution for measurement of serum fructosamine,[86] which is a test that may be more likely to be performed in cats with diabetes that is difficult to regulate. The prevalence of acromegaly in the average or typical diabetic cat is likely in the range of 10% to 15%, but the prevalence in cats that are difficult to regulate is probably closer to 30%.[83] Regardless of the exact numbers or differences between studies, considerable evidence now suggests that acromegaly is neither rare nor uncommon. Most veterinary endocrinologists agree that a cat with any of the clinical features of acromegaly, including insulin resistance, should be screened for this disorder.[89]

Acromegaly is more common in male cats, with no apparent breed predilection, and most affected cats are middle-aged or older. The typical history is one of insulin-resistant diabetes mellitus, with affected cats requiring 10 to 20 units of insulin per dose or more, often with inadequate control of the diabetes. This insulin resistance is due to a GH-induced postreceptor defect in the action of insulin on target cells. Affected cats remain polyuric, polydipsic, and polyphagic and continue to gain weight. Most cats with poorly regulated diabetes mellitus lose weight; therefore weight gain in this situation may be suggestive of feline acromegaly.

The physical changes of acromegaly develop slowly and often are not noted by the owner until they are advanced. These changes may include enlarged feet, broadening of the face, protrusion of the mandible (Fig. 26.2), increased spacing between the teeth, and

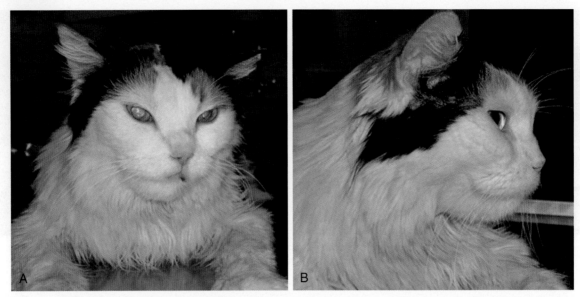

• **Fig. 26.2** (A) and (B) A 12-year-old female spayed domestic long-hair cat with acromegaly caused by a pituitary tumor. Note the broad forehead and large mandible.

abdominal enlargement. Owners of affected cats also frequently note noisy or stertorous breathing or respiratory stridor.[86,87,90,91] A physical examination may reveal additional abnormalities, such as enlarged abdominal organs and cardiac murmurs, arrhythmias, or a gallop rhythm.[81,86,92] However, it also is likely that acromegalic cats with few physical features of the disease will be increasingly recognized as awareness of the disorder increases and patients are diagnosed at an earlier stage. In addition, more cats may be diagnosed with acromegaly in the absence of diabetes, as has been reported in a small number of cases[93]; however, the prevalence of acromegaly in the nondiabetic cat population is unknown.

Neurologic signs associated with the pituitary tumor generally appear to be uncommon but may be underrecognized or underreported. Lethargy, mental dullness, or impaired vision may occur but often can be subtle. Affected cats also may demonstrate signs of diabetic neuropathy or lameness, possibly because of acromegaly-associated arthropathy.[81,86] An additional significant complication of acromegaly is the development of structural and functional cardiac disease, including increased thickness of the left ventricular wall, increased left atrial diameter, and evidence of abnormal diastolic function.[94,95] Some evidence indicates that many of these changes are reversible if the acromegaly is treated successfully.[95]

Acromegaly is the result of excessive GH secretion from a pituitary gland tumor, and increased serum GH concentrations have been reported in several cats with acromegaly. Unfortunately, a feline GH assay currently is not reliably available in the United States. The physical changes in patients with acromegaly are due to the anabolic effects of GH, which are mediated by peripherally synthesized IGF-1.[83] This hormone is produced in the liver and other tissues, and serum concentrations of IGF-1 increase in the presence of chronically increased GH production. Because GH secretion may be pulsatile, even in some acromegalics, and because it has a short half-life, an increased serum IGF-1 level has been suggested to be a more sensitive test for acromegaly because it may reflect GH levels over the preceding 24 hours.[83] Serum IGF-1 values are widely reported in acromegalic cats. One study confirmed that IGF-1 measurement is a useful screening test for feline acromegaly, with a sensitivity and specificity of 84% and 92%, respectively.[90] No difference in serum IGF-1 concentrations

was seen among well-controlled diabetic cats, poorly controlled diabetic cats, and healthy cats.[90] The highest IGF-1 noted in a diabetic cat was 153 nM, with a normal reference range of 12 to 92 nM; thus some overlap exists between the IGF-1 values found in acromegalic cats and those found in poorly regulated diabetic cats. However, this author's experience (KL) is that IGF-1 levels in cats with acromegaly usually are at least twice the value of the high end of this reference range, at least by the time the cats are investigated for causes of insulin resistance. In Europe, the serum IGF-1 concentration typically is expressed in ng/mL, with a positive predictive value of 95% for an IGF-1 >1000 ng/mL.[87] Feline IGF-1 measurement is readily available to veterinarians in the United States, and this test should be considered for cats with diabetes mellitus that appear to be insulin resistant or that have any physical features consistent with acromegaly.[89]

The presence of a pituitary tumor can be demonstrated either by CT or by MRI in cats with acromegaly, and both techniques have been reported in the literature.[86,96–99] MRI likely is more sensitive than CT,[99] but both imaging modalities may reveal a normal pituitary in a cat with acromegaly if the size of the mass is below the limit of detection. Brain imaging may also reveal bone or soft tissue changes that support a diagnosis of acromegaly.[98] In a case-control study of CT findings, 68 acromegalic diabetic cats were compared to 36 control cats. Cats with acromegaly had significantly thicker bones, skin, and subcutaneous tissues, and narrower nasopharynges compared to the control cats.[99] Additional imaging findings supportive of acromegaly include echocardiographic changes as noted previously, enlarged kidneys and adrenal glands, and evidence of pancreatic changes on abdominal ultrasound examination.[100]

Treatment options for acromegaly in human medicine include surgery, conventional external-beam RT, SRT, and medical therapy. Many of these therapies also have been evaluated in cats. In humans, transsphenoidal surgery to remove the pituitary tumor generally is regarded as the treatment of choice; however, currently only rare published reports are available on the use of surgery for the treatment of feline acromegaly.[70,101,102] The largest reported case series of cats undergoing hypophysectomy focused on anesthetic management and complications in 37 cats with acromegaly[103]; the same group reported the outcome of surgical hypophysectomy in 21 diabetic cats in abstract form.[104] These two publications provide relatively little detail but in summary: 3 of 21 cats died postoperatively; all 18 surviving cats experienced a reduction in serum IGF-1 concentrations; and 14 of these cats achieved diabetic remission.[104] As was noted previously transsphenoidal hypophysectomy is technically challenging, and it requires an experienced surgeon and coordinated team of specialists.

RT rarely is used as a first-line therapy in human medicine.[105] In contrast, RT is the treatment for feline acromegaly that has been most widely reported in the veterinary literature.[a] Conventional fractionated RT protocols range from five fractions given weekly to as many as 20 fractions given over a period of 4 weeks. Improved diabetic control is one potential outcome of RT therapy, although IGF-1 concentrations do not appear to correlate with this improved control.[76,109] Few reports are available on the long-term follow-up of acromegalic cats receiving conventional RT; therefore it is difficult to assess the risk of complications of this modality in this species. However, published case reports and case series of cats receiving conventional RT suggest that short- and long-term adverse effects are relatively uncommon.

Disadvantages of RT as a treatment for feline acromegaly include cost, availability, and the necessity for repeated anesthetic events. The latter disadvantage can be lessened by the use of SRT, which is widely used in the treatment of pituitary tumors in human patients. In an early case series in veterinary medicine, cats with pituitary tumors received treatment with a linear accelerator-based modified radiosurgical approach.[76] Cats received a single large dose of radiation, but it was delivered in a nonconformal fashion. The technique was reported to be safe and effective. A recent study documented the outcome of SRT, delivered in 3 or 4 doses, for the treatment of acromegaly in 53 cats.[110] The overall MST was 1072 days, with no association noted between tumor size or serum IGF-1 concentration and survival. Causes of death included neurologic disease, heart disease, kidney disease, and unrelated diseases. Ten cats experienced acute radiation effects, all of which responded to prednisolone therapy. Seven of 50 cats in which serum T_4 concentrations were monitored developed hypothyroidism months to years after SRT. Diabetic regulation was followed in 41 of the 53 cats, and 39 experienced a reduction in insulin dose, with 13 (32%) cats going into diabetic remission.[110] SRT, therefore, appears to be a safe and effective therapy for feline acromegaly. This therapy is becoming more widely available, at least compared to hypophysectomy, and compared to conventional RT, it offers considerable advantages in terms of owner time commitment and the risks of anesthesia and hospitalization in elderly diabetic cats.

Medical therapy for acromegaly commonly is used in humans either as a first-line treatment or as an adjunct to surgery or RT. The classes of drugs used are somatostatin analogs, GH-receptor antagonists, and dopamine agonists. GH-receptor antagonists have not been evaluated in cats, and dopamine agonists do not appear to be useful in this species.[111]

Somatostatin analogs, also termed *somatostatin receptor ligands* (SRLs), bind to somatostatin receptors, suppressing the release of GH from the pituitary gland. These medications are available as long- or short-acting preparations, and the response to SRLs is assessed by measurement of IGF-1 and GH levels and tumor size, and evaluation of clinical signs. Octreotide has been evaluated in a small number of cats with acromegaly. In five cats short-acting octreotide was used

for up to 4 weeks with no apparent improvement in GH levels.[81,112] However, another study showed that GH levels were significantly reduced for up to 120 minutes postinjection in five cats with acromegaly that received a single dose of octreotide.[113] These studies used the short-acting form of octreotide and were performed over a very short time without assessment of the clinical response. Both short- and long-acting pasireotide have been studied in acromegalic cats, with encouraging results.[114,115] Treated cats experienced improved insulin sensitivity, and serum IGF-1 concentrations were reduced. Diarrhea was a common side effect, and the expense of this medication is a significant impediment for most cat owners.

For many cats with acromegaly, insulin therapy is the only treatment available or acceptable to the owner. In general these patients should receive the amount of insulin necessary to control their diabetes, although adequate blood glucose regulation can be difficult to achieve in many cases. In-home blood glucose monitoring, with close cooperation between the owner and the veterinarian, is strongly recommended. Feeding a low-carbohydrate diet also may be beneficial. These patients should be expected to receive insulin doses in the range of 10 to 20 units per dose or more. Concurrent illnesses and complications of acromegaly and diabetes mellitus also should be addressed. The short-term prognosis for cats diagnosed with acromegaly generally is fair to good, but the long-term prognosis is poor without specific therapy.[83] Patients may succumb to cardiac or renal failure, neurologic disease, or complications of poorly regulated diabetes mellitus. In one early case series the MST was 20.5 months.[81]

Adrenal Gland Neoplasia

The prevalence of primary adrenal gland tumors in the dog and cat is difficult to discern from the literature. For dogs and cats undergoing necropsy or adrenal surgery, tumors of the adrenal cortex appear to be more common than those of the medulla. A number of case series over the past 15 years have documented the outcome of adrenal surgery in dogs.[20,22,116–120] When the data from these cases was combined, a histopathologic diagnosis was reported for a total of 304 adrenal tumors, with 227 (75%) arising from the adrenal cortex and 72 (23%) from the medulla. The remaining tumors included two myelolipomas and one each of fibrosarcoma, lymphoma, and leiomyosarcoma. For the adrenocortical tumors that were further classified, 114 of 199 (57%) were carcinomas, 77 of 199 (39%) were adenomas, and 8 of 199 (4%) were described as hyperplastic lesions. It is important to note the bias inherent in this data because only dogs that underwent surgery were included. Functional cortisol-secreting tumors of the adrenal cortex are responsible for 15% to 20% of canine and feline cases of naturally occurring HAC, with PDH accounting for 80% to 85%. Functional adrenocortical tumors in dogs and cats also can secrete one or more sex hormones, including androstenedione, progesterone, 17-hydroxyprogesterone, testosterone, and estradiol. These tumors may or may not secrete glucocorticoids, and some patients show signs of HAC in the absence of elevated cortisol levels on typical screening tests. Signs of sex hormone excess with sex hormone–secreting adrenal tumors appear to be more common in cats than dogs.

Imaging techniques such as ultrasonography, CT, and MRI have greatly enhanced the ability to identify both clinical and subclinical adrenal abnormalities; it appears that the adrenal gland is affected with neoplasia more commonly than previously suspected. The ability to detect these adrenal lesions also leads to diagnostic dilemmas as the clinician attempts to elucidate

---

[a] References 62, 75, 76, 81, and 106–109.

whether the lesions arise from the cortex or medulla, whether they are functional or nonfunctional, and whether they are benign or malignant. Functional adrenal tumors may secrete cortisol, catecholamines, aldosterone, sex hormones, or steroid hormone precursors, and these may be associated with specific clinical and laboratory findings. Hormonal testing and imaging techniques are central to the diagnostic evaluation of these patients, helping ensure that the most appropriate course of therapy can be pursued. Large adrenal masses may be detected on abdominal radiographs.[121–123] The presence of mineralization suggests an adrenal tumor, but this finding is not highly specific, and it cannot be used to differentiate between benign and malignant masses. The normal ultrasonographic appearance of canine adrenal glands has been described,[124,125] and many reports of the ultrasonographic appearance of adrenal lesions in dogs are available, although no particular ultrasound findings are pathognomonic for a specific diagnosis.[126] Abdominal ultrasound examination frequently is used to detect metastatic disease and to determine the local invasiveness of adrenal tumors. Ultrasonography has been reported to be 80% to 100% sensitive and approximately 90% specific for the detection of adrenal tumor invasion into the caudal vena cava.[20,22,127] Contrast-enhanced ultrasonography may provide additional information about tumor type and malignancy.[128,129]

The CT appearance of both normal and abnormal canine adrenal glands has been described.[24,123,130–134] Contrast-enhanced CT has been shown to provide accurate preoperative evaluation of canine adrenal masses with 92% sensitivity and 100% specificity for the detection of vascular invasion by adrenal tumors.[135,136] The MRI appearance of presumed normal canine adrenal glands also has been described,[137] but as yet, few reports document the systematic use of MRI for evaluation of adrenal lesions in dogs and cats.

Canine Adrenocortical Tumors

A review of case reports of functional adrenocortical tumors in dogs suggests that carcinomas are slightly more common than adenomas, although this could reflect the fact that tumors with features of malignancy are more likely to be removed surgically. Adenomas typically are smaller; tumors larger than 2 cm are more likely to be carcinomas.[138] On histopathologic examination, adenocarcinomas appear more likely to exhibit a trabecular growth pattern, peripheral fibrosis, capsular invasion, necrosis, and/or hemorrhage.[138] They are less likely to exhibit cytoplasmic vacuolization, extramedullary hematopoiesis, or fibrin thrombi.

Approximately 20% of adrenocortical carcinomas invade into the phrenicoabdominal vein with extension into the renal vein and/or caudal vena cava.[19,139] Intravascular invasion has the potential to cause severe and life-threatening intraabdominal or retroperitoneal hemorrhage.[22,140] Metastasis was identified in approximately 50% of dogs with adrenocortical carcinomas.[138,139] Although involvement of the liver and lungs is most common, metastasis to the kidney, ovary, mesenteric lymph nodes, peritoneal cavity, and thyroid gland also has been reported. In the absence of evidence of tumor invasion or metastasis, no consistent clinical, biochemical, or imaging findings reliably distinguish between functional adrenocortical adenomas and carcinomas.

Dogs with PDH and dogs with ADH are similar in age, but almost 50% of dogs with ADH weigh more than 20 kg compared to approximately 25% of dogs with PDH.[121] The historic features, physical changes, clinical signs, and basic laboratory findings in canine Cushing's syndrome essentially are the same in dogs with

PDH and ADH (these are described in detail elsewhere).[9,10] Similar screening tests are used to confirm the diagnosis of HAC; however, the sensitivity of the ACTH stimulation test for the diagnosis of ADH is only approximately 60%.[141] Therefore the LDDST is a better screening test when ADH is suspected. Dogs with ADH fail to show suppression on LDDST or HDDST, and differentiation from PDH generally is determined by imaging studies, particularly abdominal ultrasound examination, and measurement of endogenous ACTH levels. Excessive secretion of glucocorticoids by a functional adrenocortical adenoma or adenocarcinoma occurs independently of pituitary control, with secondary atrophy of the normal adrenocortical cells in both the affected and contralateral adrenal glands. Unfortunately, the functional atrophy of the contralateral adrenal gland is not always easily detected on abdominal ultrasonography.[16] This finding, termed equivocal adrenal asymmetry, is also observed in some dogs with PDH and is associated with asymmetric hyperplasia of the glands.[14] An ultrasound study of dogs with equivocal adrenal asymmetry suggested that a maximal dorsoventral thickness of the smaller gland of less than 5.00 mm was consistent with a diagnosis of ADH.[17]

Surgical adrenalectomy is the treatment of choice for dogs with ADH. In one series of 144 dogs undergoing surgical removal of a functional adrenocortical tumor, the prognosis was described as excellent for patients that survived 4 weeks postoperatively, and the average life expectancy was 3 years. Nine of 144 dogs were euthanized at the time of surgery, and 29 dogs died during surgery or immediately postoperatively.[35] MSTs of 230 to 778 days have been reported for dogs undergoing adrenalectomy for adrenal carcinomas,[19,116,117] compared to an MST of 688 days for dogs with adenomas.[116]

SRT has been reported in a small number of dogs with adrenocortical tumors with vascular invasion. In the nine dogs evaluated, of which six dogs had nonsecretory tumors, the MST was 1030 days, tumor size was reduced, and no dogs experienced severe radiotoxicity.[142] However, more studies involving larger numbers are necessary to further evaluate this mode of therapy.

Mitotane or trilostane therapy for ADH should be used when surgery is not a good option for the patient or client, or they may be used before adrenalectomy in patients that are significantly debilitated by HAC. Treatment with mitotane as an alternative to surgical adrenalectomy uses the drug as a true cytotoxic agent. Detailed protocols are readily available[9,143]; clinicians should be aware that this approach typically requires higher doses of mitotane than those used in PDH,[144] and relapses are common. However, this treatment can be effective; a mean ST of 16.4 months was reported in a series of 32 dogs, and dogs without evidence of metastatic disease appeared to have a better response to mitotane therapy.[145] Trilostane is not a cytotoxic drug, but it has been used successfully to manage patients with ADH,[42,146,147] including a small number of dogs with metastatic disease.[148] In a retrospective study comparing trilostane and mitotane in dogs with ADH, the MSTs for dogs treated with trilostane and mitotane were 353 days and 102 days, respectively. These STs were not significantly different; however, this study did further confirm that STs are significantly reduced with metastatic disease.[149] The MSTs in a more recent study were 15.6 months and 14 months for dogs with ADH treated with mitotane or trilostane, respectively[150]; thus either medication is a reasonable option for ADH if surgery is not feasible.

Aldosterone-secreting adrenocortical tumors have rarely been reported in dogs.[151–155] Clinical findings include lethargy, anorexia, polyuria/polydipsia, hypokalemia, metabolic alkalosis, and hypertension. The diagnosis is confirmed by ruling out other causes of hypokalemia, together with finding a markedly increased plasma aldosterone concentration.[156]

Feline Adrenocortical Tumors

Hyperadrenocorticism in cats is rare, and only 15% to 20% of cases are due to a functional adrenocortical tumor. A recent case series documented the clinical findings in 33 cats with adrenal neoplasia that had a histopathologic diagnosis.[157] Thirty of the 33 cats were diagnosed with a cortical tumor, and only three had a pheochromocytoma. Of the 25 cats that underwent adrenal function tests, 19 cats were diagnosed with a functional tumor, and of these 16 cats had hyperaldosteronism, one had hypercortisolemia, one had high estradiol, and one had hypersecretion of multiple hormones. Increasing evidence indicates that primary hyperaldosteronism (also termed *primary aldosteronism* or *Conn's syndrome*) has been an underrecognized condition in cats. In fact, it has been suggested to be the most common adrenocortical disorder in this species.[158] Affected cats are middle-aged or older, and the most common clinical sign is muscle weakness resulting from hypokalemia. Arterial hypertension frequently is detected in these patients and may be associated with ocular changes. Routine laboratory testing often reveals hypokalemia and sometimes metabolic alkalosis, but hypernatremia is uncommon, presumably because of intact water balance mechanisms in these patients. Some cats also may have evidence of concurrent renal disease.

Plasma aldosterone can be measured in cats, and normal or increased plasma concentrations in the face of hypokalemia would be regarded as inappropriate. However, definitive diagnosis using aldosterone levels is difficult without measurement of the plasma renin activity and calculation of an aldosterone:renin ratio.[159] Unfortunately, a plasma renin activity assay is not readily available. The oral fludrocortisone suppression test had been shown to be useful in the diagnosis of feline hyperaldosteronism.[160–163] Imaging of the adrenal glands often is performed in the evaluation of these patients,[164,165] and this may distinguish between unilateral and bilateral lesions and also reveal vascular invasion or metastatic disease. Most cats with hyperaldosteronism have an adrenal adenoma or carcinoma.[157,166,167] Bilateral adenomas have been reported,[166] and some cats have adrenal hyperplasia.[159]

Adrenalectomy is the treatment of choice for cats with unilateral disease, and good outcomes have been reported both for adenomas and for carcinomas, in addition to tumors associated with vena cava thrombosis.[157,166–170] Medical management with potassium supplementation, antihypertensive drugs, and the aldosterone antagonist spironolactone can give reasonable STs in patients that are not surgical candidates.[156]

Adrenal Medullary Tumors

Chromaffin cells are part of the sympathetic nervous system and are present in the adrenal medulla and other locations throughout the body. Neoplastic chromaffin cells in the adrenal medulla give rise to pheochromocytomas, which are tumors that predominantly secrete catecholamines. Chromaffin cell tumors (termed *paragangliomas* or *extraadrenal pheochromocytomas*) can arise in other parts of the body, but these are rare in veterinary medicine.

Pheochromocytomas are uncommon in dogs and rare in cats.[171,172] In past decades the diagnosis of pheochromocytoma most often was made incidentally at necropsy, but these tumors are now likely to be detected antemortem because abdominal imaging techniques are used routinely in small animal patients. Pheochromocytomas generally are considered malignant tumors in dogs.[173] Metastasis is reported in up to 40% of affected dogs; sites include liver, spleen, lung, regional lymph nodes, bone, and CNS.[171,172,174] Vascular invasion by the tumor has been reported in as many as 82% of cases.[20,22,175] This finding is not specific for pheochromocytoma because vascular invasion can also occur with adrenocortical tumors.

Pheochromocytoma usually is diagnosed in older dogs, and no clear breed predilection has been found. Catecholamine release by pheochromocytomas typically is episodic, therefore clinical signs may be intermittent and often are absent at the time of physical examination. Signs can include weakness, episodic collapse, panting, anxiety, restlessness, exercise intolerance, decreased appetite, weight loss, polyuria, and polydipsia. Physical examination findings may be normal because of the episodic nature of catecholamine release or may reveal tachypnea, panting, tachycardia, weakness, pallor, cardiac arrhythmias, or hypertension. Some dogs have signs referable to an abdominal mass, and acute collapse may occur secondary to tumor rupture with abdominal or retroperitoneal bleeding.[140] No consistent abnormalities are seen on the CBC, serum biochemistry profile, or urinalysis in dogs with pheochromocytomas.[83]

Diagnostic imaging is central to the evaluation of patients with pheochromocytoma. In many dogs evaluation for pheochromocytoma occurs after an adrenal mass is found when abdominal ultrasonography is performed for other reasons. In addition to revealing the presence of an adrenal tumor, abdominal ultrasonography may reveal metastatic disease, and it is sensitive and specific for detecting vascular invasion by adrenal tumors.[20,22] CT and MRI are the imaging modalities of choice for humans with pheochromocytomas, and experience with these techniques in canine patients has been encouraging.[134,176] Unfortunately no ultrasound or CT findings can distinguish definitively between pheochromocytoma and other adrenal tumors. Thoracic radiographs or CT scans are recommended to evaluate the cardiovascular system and for detection of pulmonary metastases in any patient with a suspected adrenal tumor. Abdominal radiographs sometimes may reveal the presence of a large adrenal mass, but they generally are less informative than ultrasonography or CT. Rare reports exist of positron emission tomography (PET) or nuclear scintigraphy imaging in dogs with pheochromocytomas.[177,178] Immunohistochemical staining for chromogranin-A can distinguish pheochromocytomas from adrenocortical tumors on tissue obtained at surgery or necropsy.[179]

Plasma and urinary concentrations of catecholamines and their metabolites are measured routinely in humans for the diagnosis of pheochromocytoma, and these have also been evaluated in dogs and cats.[180–188] The best differentiation between pheochromocytoma and other diseases appears to be provided by measurement of normetanephrine, either in urine or plasma.[174,187,188]

Surgery is the only definitive treatment for pheochromocytoma. Chemotherapy and RT have not been evaluated in dogs with pheochromocytoma. Radiotherapy using ^{131}I-metaiodobenzylguanidine was reported in one dog.[189] The prognosis for dogs with pheochromocytoma depends on tumor size, the presence of metastases, and local invasion. An MST of 374 days has been reported after surgical treatment of pheochromocytoma.[116] Dogs without metastatic disease that survive the perioperative period appear to have a good prognosis. A pheochromocytoma-associated cardiomyopathy recently was described in dogs, and further studies are needed to determine if management of this condition affects morbidity or mortality in dogs with pheochromocytoma.[190]

Surgical Management of Adrenal Tumors

Before adrenalectomy every attempt should be made to determine whether an adrenal tumor is functional, whether evidence of metastatic disease exists, and whether vascular invasion has occurred. Patients with ADH also may be medically managed with trilostane or mitotane before surgery to mitigate metabolic derangements and potentially reduce the risk of thromboembolic disease that can result from their prothrombotic state.[9] Important components of the presurgical workup for a patient with an adrenal tumor include blood pressure measurement, an ACTH stimulation test as a preoperative baseline, CBC, serum biochemistry, and blood typing, with or without cross-matching, in preparation for potential blood transfusion. Pretreatment with α-blockade has been recommended before surgery, because phenoxybenzamine was shown in one study to improve the ST significantly in dogs undergoing adrenalectomy.[175] However, the exact dosage and number of days that dogs should be on this medication, and even the decision to pretreat, are somewhat controversial. This recommendation likely deserves re-examination, particularly because this also is an area of controversy in human medicine,[191] and the recommendation is not necessarily supported by findings in other veterinary studies.[118]

Abdominal CT is a precise method for planning a resection and for evaluating the extent of an adrenal mass and the presence of caval tumor thrombus.[134,135] CT also allows for further staging of the lungs and the rest of the abdomen and will allow for assessment of kidney and/or renal vein involvement, so that the surgeon and owner can be prepared for possible nephrectomy. A recent study indicated that triple-phase contrast CT may aid in preoperative diagnosis of the tumor type.[136]

Blood loss from adrenalectomy can be significant and even fatal, particularly in patients that have extensive invasion of the surrounding tissues or caudal vena cava. The patient should be cross-matched and blood typed, and blood should be available for transfusion intraoperatively and postoperatively. Dogs with HAC have a higher risk of being hypercoagulable.[192–194] Perioperative management of this potential complication is somewhat controversial and will vary among clinicians. When available, thromboelastography (TEG) may be useful as a preoperative baseline and postoperatively to monitor for evidence of hypercoagulability, to allow directed anticoagulant therapy when indicated.

The technical difficulty of adrenalectomy depends on the size and invasiveness of the tumor. For small tumors with no invasion, a ventral midline, flank, intercostal, or minimally invasive approach can be considered.[195–198] The approach used generally is based on the surgeon's preference and experience. For large right-sided tumors, the right lateral abdomen also should be aseptically prepared in case the standard ventral midline approach needs to be extended to include a paracostal approach. A vessel sealing device facilitates adrenalectomy. Hemaclips or ligaclips also should be available to assist with hemostasis.

When caval invasion exists, the surgery requires a focused team. Blunt dissection, electrosurgery, and the vessel sealing device are used to dissect the adrenal tumor from surrounding tissues. Considerable neovascularization, and possibly invasion into the vasculature of the surrounding tissues, often is seen. Caval thrombus is more common in cases of pheochromocytoma but can occur with

adrenal cortical tumors.[116–118] The adrenal gland is freed from all surrounding tissues except for the phrenicoabdominal vein as it enters the vena cava. The dorsolateral aspect of the phrenicoabdominal vein should be isolated and ligated. For a thrombus that does not extend beyond the hepatic hilus, Rummel tourniquets are placed around the vena cava cranial and caudal to the tumor thrombus and on the contralateral renal vein. The Rummel tourniquets are tightened, and a cavotomy is made at the level of the phrenicoabdominal vein as it enters the vena cava. The length of the venotomy should be limited to the diameter of the tumor thrombus, or just slightly longer than this. The tumor thrombus is removed by gently sliding it out of the vena cava. The Satinsky clamps are placed tangentially across the cavotomy in a manner that allows partial flow through the vena cava. Preplacement of a small-gauge, nonabsorbable suture may facilitate placement of the Satinsky clamp and management of the venotomy. If stay sutures of 5-0 polypropylene suture material are used at the cranial and caudal extent of the proposed venotomy, the suture can be used to close the venotomy site. The Rummel tourniquets are released, and the venotomy site is sutured in a simple continuous pattern. If further bleeding is noted, the Rummel tourniquets can be re-engaged and the repair can be augmented with additional suture as required. A recent publication reported phrenicoabdominal venotomy, rather than caval venotomy, for removal of adrenal tumors with caval invasion.[120] This technique can be used for a relatively small caval thrombus, and it offers the advantage that a cavotomy is not necessary. The tumor thrombus can be milked into the phrenicoabdominal vein, and a Satinsky clamp can be placed between the thrombus and the vena cava. Rummel tourniquets still should be placed as a precaution, but engagement of the Rummel tourniquets is not needed.

Bilateral adrenalectomy first was reported in 1972 for the surgical management of canine Cushing's disease.[199] Medical management of Cushing's disease has replaced surgical therapy in cases of PDH. However, the surgical management of bilateral adrenal tumors is possible and is no more challenging technically than managing a unilateral tumor. The preoperative management is the same as for a unilateral adrenal tumor, with the exception that a single patient may have both a pheochromocytoma and HAC, so this should be considered. The postoperative management is slightly more challenging in cases of bilateral adrenalectomy because the patient becomes acutely Addisonian. However, this can be managed with an appropriate dose of desoxycorticosterone pivalate (DOCP) and a supraphysiologic dose of dexamethasone intraoperatively. In the short-term these patients need to be monitored for signs of Addisonian crisis during recovery, and careful attention should be paid to their fluid requirements, urine production, and electrolytes. In the long-term these dogs essentially are treated as Addisonian patients and should be managed with DOCP injections approximately monthly and daily physiologic doses of prednisone. As with any Addisonian patient, the frequency of DOCP injections and the dose of prednisone should be tailored to the patient. Similarly, the dose of prednisone should be increased during times of stress. The reported success rate in a recent retrospective study of bilateral adrenalectomy was similar to that reported with unilateral adrenalectomy when the acute Addison's disease was managed preemptively and appropriately.[119]

The perioperative mortality rate for adrenalectomy ranges from 15% to 37%.[116–118] Perioperative morbidity for adrenalectomy also is high, with reported complications including gastrointestinal (GI) problems, pancreatitis, hemorrhage, hypotension, electrolyte imbalances, renal failure, disseminated intravascular coagulation (DIC), pulmonary thromboembolism, and death.[116–118] Prognostic factors include the presence and size of a tumor thrombus, whether nephrectomy is performed, whether a transfusion is performed, the tumor type (pheochromocytoma), and the tumor's size (>5 cm).[116–118]

Dogs with preoperative HAC require a postoperative ACTH stimulation test, and it could be argued that this test should be performed after adrenalectomy in all cases because some tumors can secrete more than one hormone and the tumor type is not always clearly defined before surgery. Dogs undergoing adrenalectomy for ADH need a supraphysiologic dose of corticosteroids postoperatively that can be weaned down over several weeks. ACTH stimulation tests can be used to monitor recovery of function in the remaining adrenal gland. Even in cases with a presumptive pheochromocytoma, if a patient is not recovering as well as expected postoperatively, an ACTH stimulation test should be considered to rule out a relative insufficiency of cortisol. TEG should be performed postoperatively and the result compared to the preoperative status. Long-term survival is reported if the patient survives the perioperative period.[116–118]

Compared with dogs, significantly fewer accounts are available of adrenalectomy in cats. In one series of 33 cats with adrenal neoplasia, 26 cats underwent adrenalectomy and 20 (77%) survived for at least 2 weeks postoperatively.[157] Causes of death included euthanasia, hemorrhage and refractory hypotension, and acute kidney injury. The MST for cats undergoing surgery was 50 weeks. Complications included pancreatitis, lethargy and anorexia, and significant hemorrhage. Three of the cats developed postoperative hypoadrenocorticism. In a series of 10 cats undergoing unilateral adrenalectomy for management of aldosterone-secreting tumors, eight cats survived to discharge and the overall MST was 1297 days, with none of the cats requiring further medical therapy.[167] Laparoscopic adrenalectomy for unilateral adrenal tumors also has been described in cats, but 4 of the 11 reported cases required conversion to laparotomy. Ten of the 11 cats survived to discharge, and the MST was 803 days.[200]

Incidental Adrenal Masses

Advances in abdominal imaging have led to the diagnostic dilemma of the incidental adrenal mass ("incidentaloma") in both human and veterinary medicine. In a published study of dogs undergoing abdominal ultrasound examination, 4% were found to have an incidental adrenal gland lesion, with affected dogs being older than a control population with no adrenal lesions.[201] Twenty of these dogs underwent surgery or necropsy; six were determined to have malignant tumors, all of which had a maximum dimension greater than 20 mm. In another study of 20 dogs with non–cortisol-secreting adrenal tumors that did not undergo surgery, the MST was 17.8 months[202]; however, not all the tumors in those cases were truly incidental findings. Adrenal masses may also be incidentally found on abdominal CT studies. In a series of 270 dogs undergoing abdominal CT for reasons unrelated to adrenal disease, 25 (9.3%) had adrenal gland masses; as with the ultrasound findings, these incidental masses were more likely in older dogs.[203]

When an incidental adrenal mass is identified in a dog or cat, a thorough history and physical examination, including blood pressure measurement and fundic examination, are indicated. Endocrine testing should be pursued to rule out a functional tumor. Given the high incidence of metastasis to the adrenal glands in cats and dogs, imaging of the thorax and abdomen should be performed to rule out another primary tumor. Aspiration cytology and ultrasound- or CT-guided biopsies are not routinely recommended for incidentalomas because of the high risk of complications and the inability to reliably differentiate benign and malignant lesions[15,204]; however, a recent study suggested that cytology can be valuable in distinguishing between cortical and medullary tumors.[205]

Adrenalectomy should be considered for masses that are functional, locally invasive, or larger than 2.5 cm in maximum dimension. Masses smaller than 2 cm with no evidence of hormonal activity should be monitored with regular imaging. A suggested protocol is to repeat the sonogram monthly for 3 months after the initial study and then less frequently if no significant change is noted, with further intervals determined by the appearance of the mass and the clinical status of the patient. However, the growth of these masses is not necessarily predictable or uniform over time.[9,156]

Thyroid Gland Neoplasia in Dogs

Thyroid carcinoma is a tumor of middle-aged to older, medium to large breed dogs.[206] Siberian huskies, golden retrievers, and beagles are overrepresented. The median age is 10 to 15 years, with no gender predilection.[206] Carcinomas or adenocarcinomas were diagnosed in 90% of thyroid tumors.[206] Thyroid adenomas that cause clinical signs are very rare in dogs.[207] Carcinomas can be further divided into follicular and medullary carcinomas with immunohistochemistry; follicular tumors are more common.[208] It has been suggested that medullary carcinomas may have a less aggressive behavior,[208,209] although this distinction rarely is used clinically. This tumor often is detected as an incidental finding by the owner or primary care veterinarian, which highlights the importance of careful neck palpation on every physical examination. It should be noted that palpation of the mass is not sensitive or specific for determining histopathologic invasion[210,211]; therefore incidentally detected cervical masses always should be investigated further. With the increasing adoption of advanced imaging techniques, incidental thyroid masses also have been identified on CT scans[212] and cervical ultrasound studies.[213] In one study of dogs that had a cervical CT scan for an unrelated reason, the overall incidence of a thyroid mass identified as an incidental finding was 0.76%.[212] If dogs present with clinical signs, these generally are due either to a mass effect or to invasion of the thyroid tumor into adjacent tissue; such signs include dysphagia, voice change, laryngeal paralysis, Horner's syndrome, and dyspnea.[214–216]

Potential causes of thyroid carcinoma in humans include exposure to radiation, persistently elevated thyroid-stimulating hormone (TSH), and dietary and genetic factors.[207] In dogs, breed predisposition suggests a genetic factor. Persistently elevated TSH also has been suggested as a potential risk factor.[207,217] Most dogs with thyroid carcinoma are euthyroid, with some hypothyroid and some hyperthyroid dogs.[207,218] The serum concentrations of thyroid hormone and TSH should be assessed preoperatively because some patients require postoperative monitoring and treatment. The term "functional thyroid carcinoma" in dogs generally refers to the production of thyroid hormone and a hyperthyroid patient. Functional thyroid carcinoma in human patients generally refers to the ability of thyroid carcinoma cells to trap and organify iodine. This is more clinically important in human patients because radioactive iodine therapy is a routine part of treatment.

The workup of a suspect thyroid tumor involves confirmation of the tumor type and clinical staging. Ultrasound examination of the neck is useful as a screening tool for a mass suspicious for thyroid carcinoma. However, ultrasound was not found to be as sensitive or specific as MRI or CT for determining the degree of invasiveness and for confirming thyroid origin.[210] The decision to aspirate a mass in the region of the thyroid gland under ultrasound guidance is clinician dependent. Because a mass definitively arising from the thyroid gland has a very high likelihood of being a thyroid carcinoma and the mass ultimately will be removed and submitted for histopathology, some clinicians do not perform aspiration of the mass if imaging is to be performed. Ultrasound is not as sensitive or specific as a CT scan in determining that a mass is originating from the thyroid gland,[210] so in the absence of advanced imaging, cytology may be warranted. Fine-needle aspiration should be done under ultrasound guidance to avoid hemorrhage; also, because this procedure is painful, the patient should be sedated before thyroid mass aspiration. Thyroid carcinomas are extremely vascular; therefore needle core biopsy and incisional biopsy should *never* be performed, because they carry a high risk of severe hemorrhage in a noncompressible area. Aspiration or biopsy also could lead to the formation of a large hematoma and the spread of tumor cells within this area.

Thyroid carcinoma tends to metastasize to the draining lymph nodes and lungs, but metastasis to abdominal organs also has been reported.[219] The local lymph nodes (mandibular) should be palpated and aspirated. Three-view thoracic radiographs also are recommended before therapy. Preoperatively a CT scan is very useful for determining the origin and invasiveness of the tumor and for staging the disease. CT has been shown to be more sensitive for assessing the invasiveness of thyroid carcinomas than palpation or neck ultrasound.[210,211] Masses that have invaded dorsal to the trachea are difficult to assess ultrasonographically because of the presence of air in the trachea. Furthermore, because of the high iodine content of precontrast and postcontrast thyroid tissue, CT has been shown to be useful in diagnosing nonthyroid cervical masses, such as carotid body tumors, because the normal thyroid tissue is more easily identifiable using a contrast-enhanced CT scan compared with ultrasound or MRI.[210] CT also is very useful for assessing the lungs for evidence of metastatic disease.

Thyroid tumors are categorized as invasive or noninvasive. The invasiveness of a thyroid mass can be determined by a combination of palpation characteristics and advanced imaging. In general, a noninvasive mass is round to ovoid and mobile. Size alone is not a predictor of whether a thyroid mass is resectable. On imaging, evaluation of whether the thyroid mass remains encapsulated or invades adjacent structures is important for determining whether the mass can be removed.

The thyroid gland is composed of two lobes that lie adjacent to the left and right sides of the trachea from the fifth to eighth rings.[220,221] The recurrent laryngeal nerves run dorsal to the thyroid gland, and the carotid sheaths are lateral to the gland. Evaluation of laryngeal function before surgery is recommended as a baseline for potential damage to the recurrent laryngeal nerve, as a result either of tumor invasion or of iatrogenic damage at the time of surgery. The external and internal parathyroid glands are intimately associated with the thyroid gland[221] and often are obscured completely in cases of thyroid carcinoma. This is of little consequence for unilateral tumors. The primary blood supply and drainage are the cranial thyroid artery and vein. The caudal thyroid artery and vein also are significant, and the cranial and caudal thyroid arteries anastomose across the surface of the gland.[221] This can be quite apparent in cases of thyroid carcinoma with significant hypertrophy and neovascularization of the blood supply as

common features noted at surgery.[220] The lymphatic drainage of the thyroid gland is to the cranial deep cervical lymph node (cranial portion) and the caudal deep cervical lymph node (caudal portion).[221] The lymph nodes are extremely small and are not present or identifiable in most dogs.[221] Because of this, elective lymph node dissection is not routinely performed in dogs with thyroid carcinoma.

Surgical removal of a thyroid carcinoma includes a routine ventral approach to the neck and trachea between the paired sternohyoideus muscles.[220] The thyroid glands should be evaluated bilaterally. The thyroid mass is identified and removed by blunt dissection, taking care to preserve the recurrent laryngeal nerve and with careful attention to hemostasis using hemoclips, electrocautery, or a vessel sealing device. In the author's (SB) experience, gently retracting the thyroid mass ventrally and working outside of the neck can help protect the critical structures that lie adjacent to the thyroid gland. Potential complications of surgery include hemorrhage and laryngeal paralysis arising from iatrogenic damage to the recurrent laryngeal nerve. Postoperative care for these patients should involve multimodal analgesia, intravenous fluids, and monitoring for dyspnea and hemorrhage. Most patients can be discharged from the hospital within 24 hours.

Bilateral thyroid carcinomas have been reported. Two recent reports of bilateral, noninvasive thyroid carcinoma treated with surgery alone demonstrated STs comparable to those for unilateral thyroid carcinoma.[222,223] One additional potential complication of total thyroidectomy is transient or permanent postoperative hypocalcemia.[222] In one study of 15 dogs treated with total thyroidectomy because of bilateral disease, parathyroid tissue was preserved in two dogs, reimplanted in four dogs, and removed completely in nine dogs. In that study postoperative hypocalcemia occurred in 11 dogs, with only seven dogs requiring long-term management of hypocalcemia.[222] Another study reported the intentional preservation of at least one external parathyroid gland in six cases of total thyroidectomy for thyroid carcinoma. The blood supply was preserved in five dogs, and the parathyroid gland was reimplanted in one dog. The MST was not reached, and the mean ST was 920 days, with no evidence of recurrence.[223] Attempts should be made to preserve parathyroid tissue in cases of total thyroidectomy in dogs.

Ectopic thyroid carcinoma has been reported in dogs at the base of tongue, involving the hyoid apparatus, cranial mediastinum, and the right heart base.[224–228] The treatment approach to these tumors is similar to that for eutopic thyroid carcinomas, with long-term survival reported with surgery alone or with radioactive iodine.[224]

Invasive thyroid carcinomas generally are not amenable to surgery because of invasion of critical structures in the neck, such as the trachea, esophagus, carotid artery, and recurrent laryngeal nerve. Treatment options for invasive thyroid carcinoma include external beam RT and radioactive iodine. External beam RT generally is more available at most facilities. Two reports exist on the use of external beam RT to treat thyroid carcinoma in dogs. A hypofractionated protocol reported in 13 dogs resulted in an MST of 96 weeks.[229] Interestingly, evidence of pulmonary metastasis at the time of diagnosis was not prognostic.[229] Definitive fractionated RT was reported in eight dogs with invasive thyroid carcinoma, with a similar MST of 24.5 months.[230] A more recent study reported an MST of only 170 days for 20 dogs treated with palliative radiation for advanced thyroid carcinoma.[231] In that study, achieving a partial or complete response was the only variable that was prognostic.[231] Hypothyroidism has been reported as a consequence of RT for thyroid carcinoma,[232] therefore monitoring of the patient's thyroid status after RT or surgery is recommended.

Radioactive iodine (^{131}I) is not readily available for dogs because of the facilities required for isolation after high-dose ^{131}I therapy. Two reports of ^{131}I therapy for invasive thyroid carcinoma indicate relatively long STs.[233,234] One study reported 43 dogs treated with ^{131}I, either as sole therapy or in combination with surgery. The first 24 dogs were treated with a dose that was calculated by means of scintigraphy, with a dose range of 555 to 1850 MBq; the remaining 19 dogs were treated with a dose of 1600 MBq without dose calculation or taking body weight into account.[233] The MSTs for ^{131}I used alone and in combination with surgery were 30 months and 34 months, respectively, and no adverse events were noted.[233] A similar study reported ^{131}I therapy as primary therapy in 39 dogs with nonresectable thyroid carcinoma.[234] The MSTs for dogs without metastatic disease and those with metastatic disease were 839 and 366 days, respectively. The dose of ^{131}I was calculated using scintigraphy and body weight. The mean and median doses were 3.60 GBq and 3.70 GBq, respectively. Three dogs in this study developed fatal bone marrow suppression.[234] It is notable that the dose used in this study was more than twice that used in the previous study. The advantage of external beam RT is that the radiation dose can be evenly distributed throughout the tumor. The advantage of ^{131}I is that metastatic lesions also can be treated with this therapy. RT should be considered in cases of invasive thyroid carcinoma because prolonged STs may be possible.

The prognosis for dogs with unilateral mobile thyroid carcinoma is excellent with surgery alone, with a reported MST of 36 months and a 70% 2-year survival rate.[214] Tumor diameter, tumor volume, and bilateral location have been associated with metastatic disease, and gross and histologic evidence of vascular invasion were associated with a reduced disease-free survival.[208] The role of chemotherapy is not well defined with this disease. In general, large tumors with evidence of vascular invasion or metastasis are treated with systemic chemotherapy. Carboplatin most commonly is used. However, no definitive evidence exists that chemotherapy improves STs in dogs with thyroid carcinoma. One study showed no benefit to the addition of chemotherapy for dogs that had been treated surgically for thyroid carcinoma.[216] A recent study showed that dogs with thyroid carcinoma treated with isotretinoin 9-cis postoperatively had an increased survival rate compared to dogs treated with surgery alone or surgery with adjuvant doxorubicin.[235] The response to toceranib has been reported in dogs with metastatic thyroid carcinoma in a phase I study of this therapy for solid tumors in dogs. A clinical benefit was noted in 12 of 15 dogs with thyroid carcinoma, with four dogs having a partial response and eight dogs having stable disease.[219] This has not been reported as first-line therapy but may be considered in cases of metastatic disease. For dogs with functional thyroid tumors, if surgery, RT or ^{131}I therapy is not feasible, treatment with methimazole or an iodine-restricted diet could be considered.[236–238]

Thyroid Gland Neoplasia in Cats

Hyperthyroidism (thyrotoxicosis) is the most common endocrine disorder in cats.[239,240] The closest human counterpart to this disease is toxic nodular goiter.[241] Feline hyperthyroidism is most often caused by a primary thyroid abnormality that results in the production and secretion of excessive thyroxine (T_4) and triiodothyronine (T_3). Multinodular adenomatous hyperplasia is identified histologically in most thyrotoxic cats.[239,240,242] Both thyroid lobes are affected in 70% to 90% of cases,[240,242,243] although they may be asymmetrically enlarged at the time of diagnosis. Ectopic hyperplastic functional thyroid tissue also is found in a proportion of hyperthyroid cats.[242,244,245] Malignant carcinomas are the least common cause of hyperthyroidism, occurring in only 1% to 3% of thyrotoxic cats[239,240,242,245]; however, one group recently proposed that the prevalence of malignant disease increases with disease duration.[246] Feline thyroid carcinomas are more locally invasive than their benign counterparts, and their metastatic rate can be as high as 70%, with regional lymph nodes and lungs affected most commonly.[245,247,248] Unfortunately, no noninvasive tests are available that can reliably distinguish between benign and malignant thyroid disease in hyperthyroid cats, although clinicians may be more suspicious of thyroid carcinoma if thyroid palpation or the appearance at surgery is atypical or if the patient does not respond as expected to medical therapy.[249] Nonfunctional thyroid carcinomas are uncommon.[249,250] Thyroid cysts also have been reported in hyperthyroid and euthyroid cats in association with both benign and malignant tumors.[251]

Hyperthyroidism was not recognized as a clinical disorder in cats until 1979, and evidence indicates that the prevalence has increased since that time.[252] The prevalence has been reported to be as high as 10% in older cats in the United States[253] and as high as 12.3% in parts of Europe.[254] These high prevalence rates may reflect a true increase in incidence over time, heightened awareness and testing by veterinarians, or both. If the incidence truly has increased, environmental factors may have contributed.[239] Environmental factors (e.g., the availability of commercially prepared cat food) may also help explain why prevalence rates vary between geographic regions.[239] Several risk factors have been variably associated with hyperthyroidism, including the consumption of commercially prepared canned cat food, the iodine content of cat food, indoor residence, use of cat litter, exposure to brominated flame retardants, and use of flea-control products.[252,255–258] None of these has been definitively shown to be a primary inciting cause, and the evidence for the role of some of these risk factors remains contradictory. The cause of feline hyperthyroidism may well be multifactorial; however, many authors consider that the consumption of canned food likely plays a significant role.[239,254,259–263] The molecular events underlying the development of feline hyperthyroidism have been investigated,[264–270] but currently no single unifying hypothesis explains the development and increasing prevalence of this disease in cats.

The following discussion reviews the clinical features, diagnosis, and treatment of feline hyperthyroidism, highlighting new information and including information pertaining to the malignant form of the disease. Many excellent and detailed reviews are available for the reader who wishes to read in more depth about this common feline endocrinopathy.[239,240,253]

Hyperthyroidism is a disease of older cats with mean and median ages in the range of 12 to 15 years. It is rarely diagnosed in cats younger than 8 years of age.[239] There is no sex predilection, but several breeds of cat appear to be at decreased risk compared to domestic short-hair and long-hair, nonpurebred cats appear to be at increased risk.[259,271] The classic clinical signs of feline hyperthyroidism are well described and readily recognized by most clinicians. The "typical" hyperthyroid cat would be expected to be losing weight despite polyphagia, hyperactive, and possibly have GI signs such as vomiting and/or diarrhea, in addition to polyuria and polydipsia. Physical examination in affected cats may reveal a palpable thyroid nodule (goiter), tachycardia, cardiac arrhythmia, heart murmur, gallop rhythm, premature beats, and poor hair coat. However, because measurement of serum thyroxine (T_4) is a common component of wellness laboratory testing in cats and because awareness of the condition is high, this "typical" presentation of feline hyperthyroidism likely is becoming less common, with an increasing proportion of cats being diagnosed with mild signs, no signs, or atypical signs.[239,272] In a recent study of more than 400 hyperthyroid cats, most had lost body weight, but this was associated with muscle wasting, and most cats had an ideal or overweight body condition score at diagnosis, with only approximately one third determined to be underweight.[273] No historical or physical examination findings can distinguish definitively between benign and malignant thyroid disease in cats.

The serum total T_4 concentration is highly sensitive and specific for the diagnosis of feline hyperthyroidism,[239,274] but false positive or false negative results are possible.[275] Approximately 10% of hyperthyroid cats have a total serum T_4 concentration within the reference range.[275] This may be due to the presence of early disease, normal fluctuations in serum thyroid hormone concentrations, and/or the presence of concurrent nonthyroidal illness.[274,276] Thus the clinician always must consider test results in light of the clinical signs in the patient. If hyperthyroidism is suspected in a cat with a normal total T_4 concentration, the total T_4 should be measured again in 1 to 2 weeks, particularly if the total T_4 is in the upper half of the reference range. Free T_4 measurement also may aid in the diagnosis of hyperthyroidism when the total T_4 is within the reference range. However, this test should be used only in cats with clinical signs of hyperthyroidism in which the total T_4 is in the high normal range. Free T_4 concentrations can be high in cats with nonthyroidal illness,[274,277,278] and these patients would be expected to have low serum total T_4 concentrations. Thus free T_4 should never be used as a screening test for hyperthyroidism. For patients in which hyperthyroidism is suspected but not confirmed by measurement of the total or free T_4, additional tests have been used to confirm the diagnosis. These include thyroid scintigraphy, the TSH stimulation test, the thyrotropin-releasing hormone (TRH) stimulation test, and the triiodothyronine suppression test. Both the TSH and TRH stimulation tests are of limited utility,[279,280] and the triiodothyronine suppression test can provide useful information but relies on significant owner and patient compliance.[281,282] Measurement of the serum TSH concentration is very sensitive but poorly specific for the diagnosis of feline hyperthyroidism,[283] and the results of this assay should be interpreted in conjunction with clinical signs and the serum total and free T_4 concentrations. Thyroid function tests cannot be used to differentiate benign and malignant tumors.

The diagnostic workup for cats with hyperthyroidism minimally should include a baseline CBC, serum biochemistry profile, urinalysis, and blood pressure measurement.[284] These tests may reveal abnormalities caused by hyperthyroidism (e.g., increased liver enzyme activity) and also provide evidence of concurrent disease. Additional diagnostic tests that may be recommended include thoracic radiography, electrocardiography, and echocardiography.[243,285,286] An abdominal ultrasound examination typically is performed only if the clinician suspects concurrent illness because this test rarely provides evidence against recommending definitive treatment for hyperthyroidism.[287] If performed, an abdominal ultrasound examination may reveal bilateral moderate adrenomegaly in hyperthyroid cats.[288] Thyroid scintigraphy (most commonly using ^{99m}Tc-pertechnetate) is valuable for determining the anatomic extent of functional thyroid tissue and for planning therapy, in addition to confirming the diagnosis of

hyperthyroidism.[244,245,289] Unilateral uptake occurs in cats with a solitary adenoma and atrophy of the normal contralateral gland. Bilateral uptake, even if asymmetric, is indicative of adenomatous hyperplasia. Thyroid scintigraphy is particularly useful for revealing the presence of ectopic thyroid tissue or multiple areas of hyperfunctioning thyroid tissue. Metastatic disease caused by thyroid carcinoma may be detected by scintigraphy, and the pattern of uptake of radionuclide may be suggestive of the presence of malignant disease[245,289]; however, other studies have demonstrated that no scintigraphic findings can distinguish definitively between benign and malignant thyroid disease in all hyperthyroid cats.[239,244,249]

Treatment options for feline hyperthyroidism include antithyroid drugs, dietary management, surgical thyroidectomy, and radioactive iodine therapy.[239,253] Homeopathic therapy is ineffective.[290] Methimazole is the most widely used antithyroid drug in North America.[291] Carbimazole is used more widely in Europe.[253,292] These are thioureylene drugs that inhibit thyroid hormone synthesis by interfering with the oxidation of iodide, iodination of tyrosyl residues in thyroglobulin, and the coupling of iodotyrosines to iodothyronines.[239] Methimazole and carbimazole are both highly effective in lowering serum thyroid hormone concentrations and controlling hyperthyroidism. Carbimazole is converted to methimazole in the body, and a dose of 5 mg of carbimazole is considered to be equivalent to 3 mg of methimazole.[239] Methimazole is usually administered at a starting dose of 2.5 mg orally twice daily for 2 weeks.[240,293] Based on clinical signs and serum T_4 levels, the dosage can be adjusted incrementally with monitoring of serum T_4 concentrations. Once daily administration of methimazole has been reported to be less effective,[294] but this approach can be successful in some cats, particularly those that need very low doses to control their disease. Carbimazole usually is administered 2 or 3 times daily, but a controlled-release formulation has been shown to be effective when administered once daily.[295] For cats that are difficult to medicate orally or that have GI side effects, methimazole compounded in pluronic lecithin organogel (PLO)[296-298] or in a lipophilic formulation[299] can be applied topically to the ear pinna. Transdermal carbimazole also has been shown to be effective.[300] Although transdermal application of antithyroid medications appears to be safe and effective and often is more convenient for cat owners, dose adjustments, particularly dose increases, often are necessary for long-term control.[301] Approximately 10% to 25% of patients treated with methimazole develop adverse effects, including lethargy, anorexia, vomiting, facial excoriations, hepatotoxicity, bleeding diatheses, and blood dyscrasias.[239,291,293,302] GI side effects are often self-limiting or can be avoided by transdermal drug delivery. Blood dyscrasias are rare but most likely to occur within the first 3 months of treatment; therefore CBCs should be monitored most closely during this time. Medication should be discontinued in patients that experience facial excoriations, blood dyscrasias, or hepatotoxicity. Carbimazole or transdermal methimazole are likely to have the same effects and therefore should not be used in patients experiencing these adverse effects with oral methimazole. These drugs often are used for assessing the effect of resolution of hyperthyroidism on renal function and preparing a cat for anesthesia and thyroidectomy. They also frequently are used as a long-term treatment modality, but it is important to note that they have no antitumor activity and no cytotoxic effect on thyroid follicular cells. A recent study demonstrated that the duration of disease, despite antithyroid drug therapy, is correlated positively with the development of more severe hyperthyroid disease, characterized by increasing size, volume, and number of thyroid nodules, in addition to suspected increasing prevalence of thyroid carcinoma.[246] In other words, the longer a patient is managed with these drugs, the more likely it is to develop disease that may be less responsive to definitive therapy with [131]I. Other medical therapies that have been used to treat feline hyperthyroidism include ipodate and iopanoic acid[303,304]; however, these are unlikely to be effective for long-term control and rarely are used.

A more recent development in the management of feline hyperthyroidism is the use of an iodine-restricted diet to control the disease. Hill's Prescription Diet y/d Feline is a commercially available diet that is extremely restricted in iodine, containing only 0.2 ppm, compared to the recommended minimum of 0.46 ppm for adult cats.[253] Dietary management appears to be effective in most cats[305]; however, up to 25% of cats continue to have increased serum total T_4 concentrations after several weeks on the diet, and not all clinical signs of hyperthyroidism appear to resolve.[306,307] A significant disadvantage of this approach is that the cat must be fed the prescription diet exclusively. Feeding of other diets (even in very small amounts), treats, flavored medications, or hunting negates the effects of the highly iodine-restricted diet. Therefore compliance can be poor, particularly in multicat households. Furthermore, as with antithyroid medications, dietary therapy does not inhibit the growth and progression of the primary thyroid lesion in these cats, perhaps leading to an increased risk of the development of malignant disease over time. However, this is only a theoretical concern, because no studies have been published evaluating the long-term risks of dietary management of feline hyperthyroidism. An additional consideration is that scintigraphy studies showed that cats that consume the iodine-restricted diet for at least 6 months had a greater percentage uptake of ^{123}I by the thyroid gland 8 hours after isotope administration compared to baseline values.[305] Further studies are needed to determine if consumption of this diet affects the response to ^{131}I therapy in hyperthyroid cats. Whenever possible, definitive therapy is recommended for cats with hyperthyroidism; however, dietary management may be a valuable option for cats with concurrent illnesses and for owners who cannot medicate their cats or are unable to pursue definitive therapy.

Definitive therapy for feline hyperthyroidism currently consists of surgical thyroidectomy or radioactive iodine. Surgical excision of the affected thyroid lobe(s) is an effective treatment,[239,242,308,309] although it is less commonly performed as access to radioactive iodine therapy expands.[239] Although most cats have bilateral disease, this may be asymmetric and not apparent on palpation or surgical exploration. Thus thyroid scintigraphy is recommended before surgery to determine whether unilateral or bilateral thyroidectomy is necessary.[242] Intracapsular and extracapsular thyroidectomy techniques have been described.[239,308,310] When bilateral thyroidectomy is indicated, preservation of one of the parathyroid glands is important to maintain calcium homeostasis. Extracapsular thyroidectomy is most commonly performed.[220,309] This involves removal of the thyroid gland and its capsule, using gentle dissection and meticulous hemostasis, from caudal to cranial. At the cranial extent of the thyroid, the external parathyroid gland must be identified and its blood supply preserved.[220,309] The intracapsular technique involves dissection of the thyroid gland within its capsule in an effort to preserve the external parathyroid gland.[220,309] Unfortunately, this technique can lead to recurrence of hyperthyroidism as the result of remnants of thyroid tissue that are left with the capsule.[220,309] Hyperthyroid cats often are poor anesthetic candidates, and preoperative stabilization with oral antithyroid medications or β-adrenergic blockers should be considered. The most significant intraoperative complication of thyroidectomy in hyperthyroid cats may be cardiac dysrhythmias.[309] Otherwise, the surgery is not technically demanding.[242,309] Hypocalcemia resulting from transient or permanent hypoparathyroidism is the most commonly reported postoperative complication, with rates ranging from 6% to 15%.[242,309] Other potential complications include hypothyroidism and, in rare cases, Horner's syndrome or laryngeal paralysis. All surgically excised tissue should be submitted for histopathology to rule out the presence of a thyroid carcinoma. Cats with thyroid carcinoma that undergo thyroidectomy usually experience improvement in their clinical signs, but most remain hyperthyroid or develop recurrent hyperthyroidism within a few months of surgery.[247,250] Cats with ectopic hyperplastic thyroid tissue also are at risk for postoperative recurrence of hyperthyroidism.[242] Radioactive iodine therapy is recommended for patients with thyroid carcinoma or ectopic hyperplastic thyroid tissue.

Radioactive iodine, or ^{131}I therapy, generally is regarded as the treatment of choice for cats with hyperthyroidism, particularly those with bilateral thyroid hyperplasia, ectopic thyroid tissue, or thyroid carcinoma.[a] [131]I has a half-life of 8 days and emits both beta and gamma radiation. Beta particles, which account for 80% of the tissue damage, travel a maximum of 2 mm in tissue and have an average path length of 400 μm. They therefore cause local destruction while sparing adjacent hypoplastic thyroid tissue, parathyroid glands, and other cervical structures. The dose of ^{131}I can be calculated from tracer kinetic studies,[312,313] but these are rarely performed. The administration of a fixed dose of ^{131}I is reported by some authors,[314-317] whereas others use doses that take into account variables such as the number or size of thyroid nodules, the patient's body weight, the severity of the clinical signs, or the magnitude of elevation in the serum total T_4.[239,311,318,319] [131]I usually is administered by the subcutaneous route because it is effective, less stressful for the patient, and safer for personnel.[318] For cats with benign thyroid disease, reported ^{131}I doses typically range from 2 to 6 mCi. Regardless of the wide variety of dosing strategies used, overall less than 5% of cats remain hyperthyroid or experience relapse of clinical signs after ^{131}I therapy. When treatment failure occurs, a second treatment often is curative. One recent study compared the efficacy of a 2 mCi dose of ^{131}I to a "standard" dose of 4 mCi for cats with serum T_4 concentrations in the range of 4 to 10.3 μg/dL.[316] No significant difference was seen in the prevalence of persistent hyperthyroidism between the two groups; the lower dose resulted in euthyroidism in greater than 95% of cats by 6 months after treatment. The use of a lower dose is appealing because it reduces radiation exposure, shortens quarantine times, and reduces costs. The proportion of cats that develop persistent hypothyroidism after ^{131}I therapy varies among studies, and the risk of this has been suggested to be higher in cats with scintigraphic evidence of bilateral disease.[320] In the recent study comparing a 2 mCi dose to a 4 mCi dose, overt or subclinical hypothyroidism was more likely in the group that received 4 mCi.[316] Minimizing the risk of iatrogenic hypothyroidism after ^{131}I therapy is important because cats with iatrogenic hypothyroidism that become azotemic after treatment have shorter STs than cats that remain nonazotemic.[321] In one large study of hyperthyroid cats treated with ^{131}I, the MST was 2 years, with survival rates at 1, 2, and 3 years of 89%, 72%, and 52%, respectively.[311] The most common causes of death or euthanasia were cancer or

---

[a] References 239, 247, 249, 250, and 311.

renal disease, which is perhaps not surprising in this population of older cats. The MST was 4 years in another study of cats treated with ^{131}I compared to 2 years for cats treated with methimazole.[322] Relatively few publications address the management of cats with hyperthyroidism caused by malignant thyroid disease. Cats with thyroid carcinomas usually have larger tumor burdens, and malignant cells trap and retain iodine less efficiently.[250,318] These cats therefore are treated with higher ablative doses of ^{131}I, in the range of 20 to 30 mCi.[249,250] Another approach to the treatment of thyroid carcinoma is to combine surgery and ^{131}I therapy.[239,247,250] Thyroid cysts occasionally are detected in both euthyroid and hyperthyroid cats and may be associated with either benign or malignant disease. Thyroid cysts may persist after ^{131}I therapy in hyperthyroid cats, therefore a surgical approach also may be needed in these cases.[251]

Ultrasound-guided percutaneous ethanol injection has been evaluated as a treatment for feline hyperthyroidism. Cats with solitary adenomas have a good response, with resolution of clinical signs persisting for longer than 12 months.[323] This technique is not recommended for bilateral hyperplasia.[324] Ultrasound-guided percutaneous radiofrequency heat ablation has been shown to be ineffective for long-term control of hyperthyroidism.[325] Given the ready availability of permanent effective treatments for unilateral or bilateral disease, these alternative treatments are unlikely to be used widely.

Chronic kidney disease (CKD) is a relatively common problem in older cats, and concurrent CKD and hyperthyroidism frequently occur in this population.[326] The hyperthyroid state increases the glomerular filtration rate (GFR),[327,328] thereby reducing serum creatinine values. The implications of this are that hyperthyroid cats with normal serum creatinine values actually may have concurrent masked CKD and that decline in renal function is a risk of all effective treatments for feline hyperthyroidism, with some nonazotemic cats becoming azotemic, or the potential for worsening of preexisting azotemia.[319,327,329,330] This decline in renal function occurs within 1 month after treatment and appears to remain stable thereafter.[319,331] Measurement of the pretreatment GFR may help predict which cats will become azotemic after resolution of the hyperthyroidism[319,330]; however, this is impractical for most patients. A recent study found that a high serum symmetric dimethylarginine (SDMA) concentration in a hyperthyroid cat can help predict the development of azotemia after treatment, but this has poor sensitivity.[332] Unfortunately, no readily available clinical data can predict the effects of therapy on renal function in an individual cat.[326,333] For this reason, many clinicians recommend a therapeutic trial with methimazole before definitive therapy for feline hyperthyroidism.[333] This may have value in providing owners with information about the likely consequence of therapy for these cats, but regardless of the detected change in renal function, effective therapy for hyperthyroidism still is required in these patients. One study showed that the development of azotemia was not significantly associated with the survival of cats treated for hyperthyroidism,[334] but the same group also demonstrated a significantly shorter ST in cats with iatrogenic hypothyroidism that became azotemic after treatment compared with those that remained nonazotemic.[321]

Parathyroid Tumors

Parathyroid tumors are uncommon in dogs and rare in cats. These tumors arise from the chief cells and autonomously secrete parathyroid hormone (PTH), leading to hypercalcemia as a result of primary hyperparathyroidism. Hypercalcemia is the result of direct effects of PTH on bone and the kidneys and indirect effects on the intestine, mediated by vitamin D. Approximately 90% of dogs and cats with primary hyperparathyroidism have a single parathyroid mass.[335–341] Adenomas are most commonly diagnosed; cystadenoma, carcinoma, and hyperplasia are diagnosed less frequently; and metastatic disease is extremely rare.[335–337,339–347] Two or more parathyroid masses may be found in some canine and feline patients, and they may not necessarily all be of the same histologic type. The presence of four hyperplastic parathyroid masses should prompt careful evaluation for causes of secondary hyperparathyroidism.

Primary hyperparathyroidism is most common in older dogs and cats, with reported mean ages of approximately 11 years in dogs[337,339] and 13 years in cats.[335] A breed predisposition has been reported in keeshond dogs, in which the disease appears to follow an autosomal dominant mode of inheritance, although the affected gene has not yet been identified in this breed.[337,341,343,348] It is not clear whether a breed predilection exists in cats.

The clinical signs of hyperparathyroidism result from hypercalcemia; they include polyuria/polydipsia, weakness, lethargy, decreased appetite, weight loss, muscle wasting, vomiting, and trembling. It is not uncommon for owners to detect no clinical signs in affected dogs or cats, and the hypercalcemia is diagnosed when blood is drawn for a routine health check or for investigation of an unrelated problem. However, signs can be subtle and may be recognized only in retrospect, after the hyperparathyroidism has been treated and the hypercalcemia has resolved. In a large case series, the most common clinical problems reported in dogs with hyperparathyroidism were related to the lower urinary tract, usually associated with urolithiasis or urinary tract infection.[337] Specific physical examination abnormalities are rare in dogs and cats. A palpable parathyroid mass has been reported in some cats with hyperparathyroidism, but this is an extremely rare finding in dogs.[336,337,347]

Hyperparathyroidism usually is diagnosed after hypercalcemia is found on a serum biochemistry profile, either as an incidental finding or when a problem such as calcium oxalate urolithiasis, polyuria/polydipsia, or weakness is investigated. The presence of hypercalcemia should be verified by measuring the serum ionized calcium, with appropriate careful sample handling.[349,350] Hypercalcemia has many causes in dogs and cats,[351,352] and diagnostic tests may be performed to investigate several possible causes simultaneously. (The reader is directed to Chapter 5 for a further discussion of the causes of hypercalcemia in dogs and cats.) Hypercalcemia resulting from primary hyperparathyroidism often is accompanied by hypophosphatemia, or a serum inorganic phosphorus level at the low end of the reference range. This finding is not pathognomonic for hyperparathyroidism and can be associated with humoral hypercalcemia of malignancy, but it can assist in ranking the differential diagnoses because vitamin D toxicosis and renal failure both would be expected to cause hyperphosphatemia. The diagnosis of hyperparathyroidism is confirmed by documenting an inappropriately high serum PTH level in the presence of ionized hypercalcemia. It is important to note that PTH frequently is within the reference range in patients with hyperparathyroidism, with 73% of cases reported to have a normal PTH in one large series.[337] A normal PTH in the face of hypercalcemia is an abnormal finding because PTH should be suppressed as serum calcium increases. The lack of suppression of PTH indicates loss of the normal negative feedback effects of calcium due to autonomous hormone secretion by hyperplastic or neoplastic parathyroid tissue. Ultrasound examination of the neck commonly is used in the diagnosis of hyperparathyroidism in dogs and cats and is particularly useful for localizing parathyroid mass(es) before surgery or other ablative procedures.[a] The normal sonographic appearance of canine parathyroid glands has been described,[355] and parathyroid masses as small as 3 mm in greatest diameter have been identified ultrasonographically.[337] Parathyroid scintigraphy and selective venous sampling to assess local PTH concentrations do not appear to be helpful in localizing hyperplastic or neoplastic parathyroid tissue.[353,356,357]

The management of hypercalcemia is further addressed in Chapter 5. Primary hyperparathyroidism in dogs and cats usually is associated with slowly progressing hypercalcemia, and the increased calcium itself rarely requires emergency treatment. Hypercalcemia is a risk factor for acute kidney injury (AKI); the mechanisms include altered glomerular capillary permeability, reduced renal blood flow, and mineralization of the kidneys. The risk of mineralization is increased when the calcium × phosphorus product exceeds 70. As noted previously, patients with hyperparathyroidism often have a decreased or low normal phosphorus level, which reduces the risk of renal mineralization. In fact, AKI appears to be rare in dogs with primary hyperparathyroidism. In a large canine case series, the mean blood urea nitrogen (BUN) and serum creatinine both were significantly lower in 210 dogs with primary hyperparathyroidism compared with 200 control dogs.[337] In addition, 95% of the hyperparathyroid dogs had BUN and serum creatinine values within or below the reference range. This partly may be a result of the secondary nephrogenic diabetes insipidus that causes polyuria/polydipsia in these patients.

Definitive therapy for primary hyperparathyroidism requires removal of the hyperfunctioning gland(s). This is most commonly achieved by surgery in both dogs and cats; however, percutaneous ultrasound-guided ablation techniques also have been described in the dog. There are four parathyroid glands, and two are closely associated with each thyroid lobe. The external parathyroid glands are outside the thyroid lobe but within the capsule and generally associated with the cranial pole.[221] The internal parathyroid glands are within the thyroid capsule and lobe and can vary in location, but they generally are located in the caudal portion of the lobe.[221] Normal parathyroid glands in the dog are small (2–5 mm × 0.5–1 mm), disk shaped, and tan in color. They are distinct from thyroid tissue.[221] Parathyroid adenomas are larger than normal parathyroid glands, round, and firm in texture. Once a diagnosis of primary hyperparathyroidism has been made, a preoperative ultrasound examination of the neck may be useful to establish the side and site of the parathyroid nodule. This can be an important tool to confirm the presence of a nodule and the surgical site of interest. However, it is important to note that false positive and negative results are possible with ultrasound; for example, thyroid nodules may be incidentally found in hypercalcemic dogs undergoing cervical ultrasound studies.[213] In addition, patients with primary hyperparathyroidism may have disease in more than one parathyroid gland and/or ectopic parathyroid tissue. Up to three of the four parathyroid glands can be removed without risk of permanent hypoparathyroidism. Patients with involvement of all four glands present a dilemma, and it is important to ensure that hyperplasia in these cases is not secondary.

A routine ventral midline approach to the thyroid glands is made. The area is explored bilaterally, even if the location of the parathyroid nodule is known preoperatively, to evaluate for additional sites of disease. The nodule can be identified with a combination of visualization and digital palpation. Once a nodule has been identified, it is bluntly dissected from the thyroid gland and hemostasis is achieved with bipolar electrocautery.

The postoperative care generally is more involved than the surgery itself. Patients must be monitored closely for hypocalcemia, which occurs as a result of downregulation of normal parathyroid tissue with prolonged hypercalcemia. Serum ionized calcium concentrations should be monitored at least twice daily for as long as 5 to 7 days after surgery or other ablative procedures. Hypocalcemia should be treated if the ionized calcium falls below 0.8 to 0.9 mmol/L; the total calcium is less than 8 to 9 mg/dL; or the patient has signs of tetany. Intravenous (IV) calcium salts are used for acute therapy for hypocalcemia; subcutaneous (SQ) administration should be avoided. Vitamin D and oral calcium are used for subacute and chronic therapy.

Several excellent references are available on the treatment of hypoparathyroidism.[340,358] In summary, 1,25-dihydroxyvitamin D_3 (calcitriol) is recommended for vitamin D supplementation because it has a rapid onset of action and a short half-life. This facilitates dose adjustments and reduces the risk of hypercalcemia. Oral calcium supplementation alone is not sufficient to treat hypoparathyroidism, and in fact this therapy can be withdrawn gradually once the calcium is stable because most maintenance diets contain an adequate amount of calcium. The approach to these patients postoperatively remains somewhat controversial; some clinicians treat with calcitriol and oral calcium immediately postoperatively, whereas others monitor the ionized calcium carefully for the development of hypocalcemia. In the author's (SB) opinion, careful monitoring without administering oral calcium or calcitriol is preferred because not all patients will develop hypocalcemia, and it is more straightforward in those patients to allow them to regulate their own calcium. Furthermore, in one study prophylactic calcitriol administration was not shown to have a protective effect for preventing hypocalcemia in patients after parathyroidectomy.[359] Several studies have attempted to correlate the preoperative ionized calcium concentrations with the risk of hypocalcemia postoperatively, with varying results. One study found a moderate correlation with a high preoperative ionized calcium and postoperative hypocalcemia,[360] whereas other studies have failed to show a correlation between preoperative ionized calcium[361,362] and PTH[362] and postoperative serum calcium concentrations. A small number of patients may be resistant to the postoperative management of hypocalcemia,[363] and this may be the result of "hungry bone syndrome," marked by aggressive, unregulated uptake of calcium by the bones.[364] In human medicine this syndrome has been managed with preoperative bisphosphonate administration[365] or the use of recombinant PTH.[366] Neither of these approaches has been used in veterinary medicine, and most patients eventually respond to high doses of calcitriol and calcium supplementation.

Ideally the calcium will decline into the normal range and then plateau. Once a plateau has been documented, the patient can be discharged from the hospital. Some patients become hypocalcemic and require administration of both calcitriol and calcium. Once their serum calcium concentrations stabilize, they can be discharged, but they must have careful and regular follow-up. When adjusting the dose of calcitriol, the goal is to maintain calcium

---

[a]References 337, 338, 347, 353, and 354.

concentrations barely below, rather than within, the normal reference range. This reduces the risk of hypercalcemia and provides the stimulus for recovery of function of the remaining normal parathyroid glands. Once the serum calcium has been stable for at least 1 to 2 weeks in an outpatient, the dose of calcitriol can be reduced gradually, with careful monitoring. The time for return of normal parathyroid function is unpredictable, therefore clients should expect frequent rechecks of calcium levels for several weeks to months after treatment of hyperparathyroidism.

A small percentage of patients have persistent hypercalcemia after parathyroidectomy. This likely is due to a nodule of another parathyroid gland that was not discovered at the time of surgery, or to hyperplasia or neoplasia in ectopic parathyroid tissue. Ectopic parathyroid tissue is a frustrating clinical problem. Anecdotally the author (SB) has found a parathyroid adenoma under the tongue in one patient. A rapid parathyroid assay now is available for intraoperative measurement of PTH.[357] This may be helpful for confirming that the offending parathyroid tissue has been removed successfully intraoperatively.[367] When ectopic parathyroid tissue cannot be located easily, MRI or CT can be attempted. However, the nodules typically are small and may be difficult to diagnose.

Ultrasound-guided ablative techniques also have been reported to treat primary hyperparathyroidism. Ultrasound-guided radiofrequency ablation (RFA) was first reported in 2001 in 11 dogs. One treatment was required in six dogs, two treatments in two dogs, and the treatment was unsuccessful in three dogs.[368] In another study persistent or recurrent disease was reported in 31% of 32 dogs; larger nodules and/or concurrent hypothyroidism were associated with treatment failure.[369] Ultrasound-guided ethanol ablation also has been reported as a minimally invasive method to treat primary hyperparathyroidism. This technique first was reported in eight dogs, with seven dogs requiring one treatment and one dog requiring two treatments. Hypercalcemia resolved in all cases, but one dog developed recurrent hypercalcemia 1 month later and was treated with surgical removal of the mass.[370] Another larger study reported ethanol ablation of parathyroid nodules in 27 dogs; hypercalcemia resolved in 85% of the cases, but three dogs required a second treatment.[371] A direct comparison of the three techniques for the treatment of primary hyperparathyroidism was reported retrospectively. That study found that control of hypercalcemia was achieved in 94%, 72%, and 90% of cases treated with parathyroidectomy, ethanol ablation, and RFA, respectively.[339]

The long-term prognosis after surgical or ablative treatment for hyperparathyroidism is very good both for control of hypercalcemia and for the tumor itself. Metastatic disease is extremely rare, and the complication of hypocalcemia generally is amenable to medical therapy. Histopathology most commonly reveals a parathyroid adenoma or hyperplastic nodule, although histologic classification is not straightforward.[340] In rare cases a parathyroid adenocarcinoma has been diagnosed. These are functional parathyroid nodules, and in a report of 19 dogs with parathyroid adenocarcinoma, no features of the disease differed from those of a benign functional adenoma except for the finding of carcinoma on histopathology. The prognosis in these cases was excellent both for tumor control and for resolution of hyperparathyroidism.[344] Approximately 10% of dogs treated for hyperparathyroidism experience a recurrence of the disease.[340] If this occurs, a second surgery or ablative procedure should be performed. The short-term prognosis for dogs and cats that do not undergo definitive surgical or ablative therapy for hyperparathyroidism still may be favorable because the disease tends to be slowly progressive, clinical signs may be mild, and renal failure may be a less common outcome than previously suspected.[337]

Pancreatic Beta-Cell Tumors (Insulinomas)

Pancreatic beta-cell tumors are rare in humans and cats and uncommon in dogs.[372–375] These tumors often are functional, but the neoplastic beta cells fail to inhibit insulin secretion appropriately at low blood glucose concentrations. Thus the hallmark of insulinoma is a normal or increased blood insulin concentration in the presence of low blood glucose levels. Molecular studies of a feline insulinoma revealed abnormal glucokinase and hexokinase expression, suggesting that these changes may contribute to enhanced glucose sensitivity and an abnormal insulin secretory response in insulinoma cells.[374] Although the clinical signs of insulinoma result from hypoglycemia associated with unregulated insulin secretion, immunocytochemical analysis reveals that these tumors often produce many additional hormones, including glucagon, somatostatin, pancreatic polypeptide, GH, IGF-1, and gastrin.[374,376–380] A more recent study demonstrated that some canine insulinomas express genes more typically associated with the exocrine pancreas; the study also revealed that these tumors contain small subpopulations of cells with mixed endocrine-exocrine features, termed *amphicrine cells*.[381]

In humans 90% of insulinomas are solitary and benign, and 5% to 10% are associated with multiple endocrine neoplasia type 1 (MEN1). Insulinomas in dogs are much more likely to be malignant, although morphologic classification into adenoma or adenocarcinoma does not consistently reflect the biologic behavior of these tumors.[375,378,382] Metastatic lesions are detected in approximately 50% of canine insulinomas, with the regional lymph nodes and liver most commonly affected. Pulmonary metastases are rare in dogs.[379,383–387] The World Health Organization (WHO) recommendations have been used to stage canine pancreatic tumors.[384] Stage I tumors involve only the pancreas, with no evidence of local or distant lymph node involvement and no distant metastasis (T1N0M0); stage II tumors have lymph node involvement (T1N1M0); and stage III tumors have distant metastasis (T1N1M1 or T1N0M1).

Beta-Cell Tumors in Dogs

The cellular and molecular events causing beta-cell tumors in dogs are unknown; however, studies of these tumors have provided insights into tumor biology and molecular genetics. Canine insulinomas have been shown to express somatostatin receptors, which may have implications for both diagnosis and therapy.[388] Local production of GH and IGF-1 also have been demonstrated in canine insulinomas, with a higher level of expression of GH and IGF-1 mRNA in metastases compared to primary tumors.[380,389] It has been suggested that the locally produced hormones may have autocrine or paracrine effects on cell proliferation, and tumor growth and progression. Furthermore, it is speculated that locally produced somatostatin has inhibitory effects on insulinomas within the pancreas, but that these effects are decreased in metastases leading to increased GH production.[389] Gene expression profiling of canine insulinomas and their metastases have demonstrated differential expression of genes between low-metastatic and high-metastatic subsets of insulinomas with genes for acinar enzymes being more substantially down-regulated in the more malignant subset of tumors. In addition, pathways involved in

DNA repair and cell cycle regulation were also down-regulated in the high-metastatic canine insulinomas.[381,390] In studies of potential prognostic biomarkers for canine insulinoma, tumor size, TNM stage, Ki67 index (a marker of proliferation), presence of necrosis, nuclear atypia, and stromal fibrosis have all been identified as being predictive for DFI and/or ST, depending on the model used in analysis.[382,391]

Canine insulinomas are most commonly reported in medium and large breed dogs, particularly Labrador retrievers, golden retrievers, German shepherd dogs, German short-haired pointers, Irish setters, boxers, and mixed breed dogs. Small breed dogs also can be affected; West Highland white terriers are overrepresented in some reports.[379,385] Depending on the case series, the median reported age is 9 to 10 years, with a range of 3 to 15 years, and no sex predilection.[379,383–385,389,392]

The clinical signs of insulinoma result from the effects of hypoglycemia on the nervous system, which is termed *neuroglycopenia*; these signs include weakness, ataxia, collapse, disorientation, behavioral changes, and seizures. Catecholamine release stimulated by low blood glucose levels also may cause muscle tremors, shaking, anxiety, and hunger. Clinical signs can be present for days to months and often are intermittent, episodic, or precipitated by fasting, exercise, excitement, or eating. Signs may be less pronounced with more chronic hypoglycemia, and patients can be clinically normal, with significantly low blood glucose levels. Physical examination findings otherwise are unremarkable in most patients. A paraneoplastic peripheral neuropathy has been described in dogs with insulinoma. This is rare, although subclinical neuropathies may be present and undetected.[393–397] Brain lesions associated with hypoglycemia also have been reported in rare cases.[398,399]

The diagnosis of insulinoma is confirmed by documenting hypoglycemia (blood glucose <60 mg/dL) with a concurrent normal or increased serum insulin concentration. In some cases it may be necessary to fast the patient, with careful monitoring, and repeat blood glucose measurements every 30 to 60 minutes. Once the blood glucose is less than 60 mg/dL, a serum sample should be submitted for concurrent insulin measurement. The presence of a normal or high serum insulin concentration in the face of hypoglycemia is inappropriate and generally sufficient to confirm the diagnosis of insulinoma. This insulin-glucose pair should be performed more than once if the initial sample provides equivocal results.[400] The use of insulin:glucose or glucose:insulin ratios is not recommended because these do not improve diagnostic accuracy.[401] Provocative testing is rarely used in veterinary medicine because of risks, expense, and poor sensitivity.[385,401] Serum fructosamine and glycosylated hemoglobin concentrations also can be measured in dogs to support a suspicion of insulinoma.[402–405] Concentrations of these glycosylated proteins would be expected to be lower than normal in dogs with chronic hypoglycemia, although this is not necessarily pathognomonic for insulinoma.

Imaging studies often are used in the evaluation of insulinoma patients, either to investigate other differential diagnoses for hypoglycemia or for local and distant staging in preparation for surgical management. Thoracic and abdominal radiographs usually are unremarkable,[401] and abdominal ultrasonography, although commonly performed, cannot be used to rule in or rule out a diagnosis of insulinoma. This technique has been reported to clearly identify and localize a pancreatic mass in less than 50% of patients with insulinoma,[387,392,406,407] and it has low sensitivity and specificity for the detection of metastatic lesions. In human medicine, endoscopic and intraoperative ultrasonography are used to identify small pancreatic tumors, but these approaches have yet to be significantly used in canine patients.[408–410] Contrast-enhanced ultrasound techniques are widely used in human medicine and are may be of value for the detection of pancreatic tumors in dogs. In this procedure, gas-filled microbubbles are injected into the circulation and ultimately reach the vascular supply to the organ of interest, where they are detected on ultrasound examination.[128] Because the microbubbles remain in the vasculature, this technique is particularly valuable for assessing tissue blood supply and perfusion. Contrast-enhanced ultrasonography has been described for the normal canine pancreas,[411–414] patients with pancreatitis,[415,416] and a small number of dogs with pancreatic tumors,[417,418] and the apparent safety and relative accessibility of this technique indicate that its use very likely will increase.[128] CT findings have been reported in a small number of dogs with insulinoma.[407,419,420] In a study comparing ultrasound, CT, and single-photon emission CT (SPECT), CT was found to be the most sensitive technique, identifying 10 of 14 confirmed primary insulinomas. However, CT also identified a significant number of false positive metastatic lesions.[407] The results of SPECT with ^{111}In-DTPA-D-Phe[1]-octreotide have been reported in a total of 19 dogs with insulinoma, with an overall sensitivity of 50% for detection and correct localization of the primary tumor.[388,407] Enhanced CT techniques, such as dynamic CT or dual-phase CT angiography, hold promise for greater sensitivity of detection of insulinomas in dogs, but large-scale studies have yet to be reported in the veterinary literature.[419–421] Somatostatin receptor scintigraphy (SRS) is an important imaging modality in humans with pancreatic endocrine tumors, including insulinomas. Indium In-111 pentetreotide SRS has been reported in a total of six dogs with insulinoma; positive results were reported in five cases, although an accurate anatomic localization was obtained only in one dog.[422,423] PET has been used in human patients to localize insulinomas when CT, MRI, and ultrasound are negative.[424] This modality has yet to be explored in canine insulinoma patients.

Therapy for canine insulinoma involves acute and chronic treatment of hypoglycemia and long-term management of the tumor. Acute treatment of hypoglycemia is accomplished through administration of intravenous dextrose, often as a slow bolus, followed by continuous rate infusion (CRI). This should be given with caution because this treatment can stimulate further unregulated insulin secretion and worsened hypoglycemia. Glucagon infusion also has been safely and effectively used in the management of hyperinsulinemic-hypoglycemic crises in a small number of dogs.[425,426]

Surgery is the recommended treatment for insulinoma in dogs and is indicated in patients with hypoglycemia and inappropriately increased serum insulin concentrations, regardless of the results of abdominal imaging studies.[383–385,387,392] Ultimately, an exploratory laparotomy is necessary to evaluate the pancreas for the primary tumor and the remainder of the abdomen for metastatic disease. Most canine insulinomas are visible or palpable at surgery, and tumors are identified in both lobes of the pancreas with equal frequency.[375] Treatment before surgery with corticosteroids may help improve blood glucose levels.[401] The patient should not have a long period of fasting, and some cases may require intravenous dextrose.[401] Conventionally the abdomen is explored via a ventral midline approach, although laparoscopic evaluation and partial pancreatectomy has been reported.[427] A partial pancreatectomy of the affected portion of the pancreas and a margin of normal tissue is performed. This can be performed by intracapsular dissection and ligation or with a vessel sealing device.[428] If evidence of metastatic disease is seen, especially to the liver, then as much metastatic disease as possible should be removed. Potential postoperative complications include persistent hypoglycemia, pancreatitis, and hyperglycemia.[375,429] In general, hyperglycemia will be transient if it occurs, but a small percentage of cases require insulin therapy.[375,429] Postoperatively patients should be managed with intravenous fluid therapy, multimodal analgesia, and antinausea medications, and with careful monitoring of the blood glucose level and for signs of pancreatitis. Any tissue removed or biopsied at surgery should be submitted for histopathologic examination to confirm the diagnosis.[401] Limited reports exist on the use of cytology, typically performed during preoperative patient evaluation, to support the diagnosis of insulinoma. [401,430,431]

Medical treatment of insulinoma is used to stabilize patients preoperatively, as an alternate therapy if surgery is not possible, and in conjunction with surgical management. Medical therapies primarily are used to control hypoglycemia, but cytotoxic agents also have been used to destroy pancreatic beta cells. Streptozocin (streptozotocin) is the chemotherapeutic drug that has been used most often, albeit infrequently, in dogs. Its use in dogs historically was limited by its nephrotoxicity,[375] but more recent reports suggest that the risk of nephrotoxicity is reduced significantly if streptozocin is administered in combination with intensive saline diuresis.[432–434] Other side effects include vomiting during administration, diabetes mellitus, hypoglycemia, increased liver enzyme activity, and mild hematologic changes.[432–434] The administration of streptozocin does not significantly increase the duration of normoglycemia in dogs with insulinoma compared with control dogs treated medically or surgically.[432] Although individual dogs have demonstrated reductions in tumor size or resolution of paraneoplastic neuropathy with streptozocin, it still is unclear whether the risks of therapy outweigh the benefits of this treatment for dogs with insulinoma.[375,434]

Strategies used to control hypoglycemia consist of dietary modification and medical therapy with prednisone, diazoxide, or octreotide. Excitement should be avoided in these patients and exercise limited. Diets high in fat, protein, and complex carbohydrates should be fed in small, frequent meals, and simple sugars should be avoided.[375] Prednisone is used for its insulin-antagonizing, gluconeogenic, and glycogenolytic effects.[375] A starting dose of 0.25 mg/kg by mouth (PO) twice daily is recommended, with gradual dose increases as needed to control hypoglycemia.[375,401] Typical glucocorticoid side effects should be anticipated. Diazoxide is a nondiuretic benzothiadiazine that suppresses insulin release from beta cells. It also stimulates hepatic gluconeogenesis and glycogenolysis and inhibits cellular uptake of glucose. Diazoxide is not cytotoxic and does not inhibit insulin synthesis. A starting dose of 5 mg/kg PO twice daily is recommended, and the dose can be increased gradually to 30 mg/kg daily dose ose can be ates hepatic glucon.[375,401] Approximately 70% of canine insulinoma patients respond to diazoxide therapy.[375,383] Adverse effects are uncommon but may include ptyalism, vomiting, anorexia, and diarrhea.[375,401,435] The use of diazoxide is limited by its cost and inconsistent availability.[401] Octreotide is a somatostatin receptor ligand that inhibits synthesis and secretion of insulin by pancreatic beta cells. It has been reported to alleviate hypoglycemia in up to 50% of dogs with insulinoma, although some may become refractory to treatment.[375,388] The suggested dose is 10 to 50 µg SQ 2 or 3 times daily, and side effects appear to be rare. In a more recent study a single 50 µg dose of octreotide was administered to 12 dogs with insulinoma. Plasma insulin concentrations decreased significantly after administration of octreotide in dogs with insulinoma, but GH, ACTH, cortisol, and glucagon levels did not change, and glucose levels increased.[436] These findings suggest that the use of octreotide warrants further investigation in canine patients with insulinoma, although the cost of the medication may be a significant impediment.

The prognosis for dogs with insulinomas is good in the short term but guarded to poor in the long term. Patients that undergo surgery and then medical management are more likely to become euglycemic, remain euglycemic for longer periods, and have longer STs compared to patients that receive only medical therapy.[387,392] MSTs after partial pancreatectomy range from 12 to 14 months.[435] The prognosis after surgery depends on the clinical stage of the disease.[375] Dogs with stage I disease have a longer DFI compared to dogs with stages II and III disease; 50% of dogs with stage I disease are free of hypoglycemia 14 months after surgery, whereas less than 20% of dogs in stage II and III disease are free of hypoglycemia at this time.[384] Dogs with stage III disease have a significantly shorter ST than dogs with stage I and II disease – approximately 50% of dogs with metastasis are dead by 6 months.[384] A more recent retrospective study showed an improved ST in dogs with insulinoma compared to earlier reports with a median DFI and MST of 496 days and 785 days, respectively, for 19 dogs undergoing partial pancreatectomy.[392] A subset of nine dogs treated with partial pancreatectomy and postoperative prednisolone had an MST of 1316 days. For eight dogs that received medical therapy alone, the MST was 196 days. When all the dogs that received medical therapy were considered as a group, the MST after institution of the medical treatment was 452 days.[392] These results lend strong support to the use of medical therapy in canine patients with insulinoma, particularly when clinical signs recur after surgery.

Beta-Cell Tumors in Cats

Compared to dogs, significantly fewer reports of insulinomas exist for cats.[373,437–441] History, clinical signs, and biologic behavior in this species appear to be similar to those in the dog, and concurrent measurements of blood glucose and serum insulin concentrations are used to confirm the diagnosis; however, it is important to use an insulin assay that has been validated in cats.[375] Surgical management has been reported in cats, with STs ranging from 1 to 32 months. Conservative therapy with dietary management and prednisolone also has been used in cats. Octreotide may be considered, although little evidence supports its use, and no evidence supports the use of diazoxide or streptozotocin in this species.[375]

Gastrointestinal Endocrine Tumors

Gastrinoma

Gastrinomas are neuroendocrine tumors that secrete excessive amounts of gastrin. Zollinger-Ellison syndrome refers to the triad of a non–beta-cell neuroendocrine tumor in the pancreas, hypergastrinemia, and GI ulceration. Gastrinomas are rare in dogs and very rare in cats.[442,443] Almost all reported gastrinomas in these species were identified in the pancreas, although one report exists of a duodenal gastrinoma in a dog.[444] Gastrinomas are highly metastatic, with involvement of the liver, regional lymph nodes, spleen, peritoneum, small intestine, omentum, or mesentery identified in 85% of dogs and cats at the time of initial diagnosis.[442,443,445–447]

Gastrinomas typically are reported in middle-aged dogs and older cats.[442,443] No obvious breed or sex predilections have been identified. Clinical signs result from gastric acid hypersecretion and gastric mucosal hyperplasia. The most common signs are vomiting and weight loss. Melena, abdominal pain, anorexia, regurgitation, hematemesis, hematochezia, and diarrhea also may occur.[441–443,445,447–454] Physical examination findings range from unremarkable to a patient in hypovolemic shock because of perforation of an ulcer. A serum biochemistry profile, CBC, and urinalysis may demonstrate changes associated with protein loss and bleeding resulting from GI ulceration or may reflect the consequences of severe or persistent vomiting or the presence of hepatic metastases. One case of common bile duct obstruction caused by a duodenal gastrinoma has been reported in a dog.[444] Abdominal radiographs often are unremarkable unless GI perforation has occurred. Contrast radiographs and abdominal ultrasound examination may show evidence of GI ulceration and a thickened pyloric antrum and gastric wall. Ultrasound examination also may reveal metastatic lesions in the liver or regional lymph nodes; however, the primary tumor in the pancreas usually is too small to be detected with this modality.[447] The results of techniques such as CT and MRI have not been widely reported in dogs and cats with gastrinomas. Endoscopy may reveal esophagitis, with ulceration, gastric and duodenal ulceration, thickened gastric rugae, and hypertrophy of the pyloric antrum. The diagnosis may be supported by measuring basal serum gastrin levels or levels after provocative testing or by scintigraphy using radiolabeled pentetreotide.[455] Basal gastrin levels have been significantly increased in dogs and cats with gastrinoma; however, gastrin levels also can be increased in renal or gastric disease, and no specific cutoff values for diagnosis have been determined.[443,456] Although it has been suggested that treatment with medications such as proton pump inhibitors and H$_2$-antihistamines can lead to increased serum gastrin concentrations, recent studies indicate that these effects are mild and short-lived and may not in fact inhibit the diagnosis of gastrinoma.[457–460] Provocative testing to diagnose gastrinoma rarely has been reported in veterinary medicine.[442,443,461]

Exploratory laparotomy is recommended for dogs and cats with a suspected gastrinoma. Even though most dogs and cats have visible metastasis at the time of initial diagnosis, surgical debulking reduces the gastrin secretory capacity and enhances the efficacy of medical therapy.[462] In addition, deep or perforated GI ulcers can be identified and excised. Long-term medical management includes the use of proton pump inhibitors, H$_2$-antihistamines, and sucralfate.[448,452] Octreotide has been used in three dogs with success.[455,463,464] STs for dogs and cats with gastrinoma range from 1 week to 26 months.[442,462,465]

Glucagonoma

Glucagonomas are rare in dogs, and currently only a single published case report exists in a cat.[443,466] These tumors are associated with a crusting dermatologic condition termed *necrolytic migratory erythema* (NME). Other associated problems include hyperglycemia or overt diabetes mellitus, hypoaminoacidemia, and increased liver enzyme activity. Skin lesions associated with NME include hyperkeratosis, crusting, and ulceration and erosions of the footpads, mucocutaneous junctions, external genitalia, distal extremities, pressure points, and ventral abdomen.[461,466–471] Glucagonomas usually arise from alpha cells in the pancreas; however, extrapancreatic glucagon-secreting tumors also have

been reported.[466,470] The tumors sometimes can be detected on abdominal ultrasound examination or CT.[443,466,469,471] Plasma glucagon concentrations have been measured in some cases, and amino acid concentrations also have been evaluated in a small number of patients,[468–470,472] but the sensitivity and specificity of these diagnostic tests have not been evaluated. Surgical resection or debulking is the treatment of choice for canine glucagonoma. Rare reports exist of the use of somatostatin analogs.[470,471] The dermatologic lesions of NME may improve after surgery or medical therapy,[471,472] but metastasis is common at the time of diagnosis and the prognosis is generally poor.[461,469] When NME is suspected, it is important to rule out liver disease, a more common cause of this dermatologic condition in dogs.

Intestinal Carcinoid

Intestinal carcinoid tumors are rare in dogs and cats. They arise from neuroendocrine cells that are found in a variety of locations, including the GI tract, liver, gallbladder, and pancreas.[443,473–478] Clinical signs generally are associated with the anatomic location of the tumor, although the physiologic effects of vasoactive substances released from the tumor were suspected to be the cause of clinical signs in one dog with an intestinal carcinoid.[477] In general, the prognosis for these tumors is guarded because metastasis is common at the time of diagnosis.[443] Surgical removal is recommended; a single case report has described adjuvant chemotherapy in a dog.[479]

References

1. Polledo L, Grinwis GCM, Graham P, et al.: Pathological findings in the pituitary glands of dogs and cats, *Vet Pathol* 55:880–888, 2018.
2. Owen TJ, Martin LG, Chen AV: Transsphenoidal surgery for pituitary tumors and other sellar masses, *Vet Clin North Am Small Anim Pract* 48:129–151, 2018.
3. Pollard RE, Reilly CM, Uerling MR, et al.: Cross-sectional imaging characteristics of pituitary adenomas, invasive adenomas and adenocarcinomas in dogs: 33 cases (1988-2006), *J Vet Intern Med* 24:160–165, 2010.
4. Moore SA, O'Brien DP: Canine pituitary macrotumors, *Compend Contin Educ Vet* 30:33–41, 2008.
5. Kent MS, Bommarito D, Feldman E, et al.: Survival, neurologic response, and prognostic factors in dogs with pituitary masses treated with radiation therapy and untreated dogs, *J Vet Intern Med* 21:1027–1033, 2007.
6. Wood FD, Pollard RE, Uerling MR, et al.: Diagnostic imaging findings and endocrine test results in dogs with pituitary-dependent hyperadrenocorticism that did or did not have neurologic abnormalities: 157 cases (1989-2005), *J Am Vet Med Assoc* 231:1081–1085, 2007.
7. Schmid S, Hodshon A, Olin S, et al.: Pituitary macrotumor causing narcolepsy-cataplexy in a Dachshund, *J Vet Intern Med* 31:545–549, 2017.
8. Goossens MM, Rijnberk A, Mol JA, et al.: Central diabetes insipidus in a dog with a pro-opiomelanocortin-producing pituitary tumor not causing hyperadrenocorticism, *J Vet Intern Med* 9:361–365, 1995.
9. Behrend EN: Canine hyperadrenocorticism. In Feldman EC, Nelson RW, Reusch CE, et al. editors: *Canine and feline endocrinology*, ed 4., St. Louis, 2015, Elsevier, pp 377–451.
10. Perez-Alenza D, Melian C: Hyperadrenocorticism in dogs. In Ettinger SJ, Feldman EC, Cote E, editors: *Textbook of veterinary internal medicine*, ed 8, St. Louis, 2017, Elsevier, pp 1795–1811.

11. Galac S, Kooistra HS, Voorhout G, et al.: Hyperadrenocorticism in a dog due to ectopic secretion of adrenocorticotropic hormone, *Domest Anim Endocrinol* 28:338–348, 2005.

12. Behrend EN, Kooistra HS, Nelson R, et al.: Diagnosis of spontaneous canine hyperadrenocorticism: 2012 ACVIM consensus statement (small animal), *J Vet Intern Med* 27:1292–1304, 2013.

13. Gould SM, Baines EA, Mannion PA, et al.: Use of endogenous ACTH concentration and adrenal ultrasonography to distinguish the cause of canine hyperadrenocorticism, *J Small Anim Pract* 42:113–121, 2001.

14. Grooters AM, Biller DS, Theisen SK, et al.: Ultrasonographic characteristics of the adrenal glands in dogs with pituitary-dependent hyperadrenocorticism: comparison with normal dogs, *J Vet Intern Med* 10:110–115, 1996.

15. Besso JG, Penninck DG, Gliatto JM: Retrospective ultrasonographic evaluation of adrenal lesions in 26 dogs, *Vet Radiol Ultrasound* 38:448–455, 1997.

16. Hoerauf A, Reusch C: Ultrasonographic characteristics of both adrenal glands in 15 dogs with functional adrenocortical tumors, *J Am Anim Hosp Assoc* 35:193–199, 1999.

17. Benchekroun G, de Fornel-Thibaud P, Pineiro MIR, et al.: Ultrasonography criteria for differentiating ACTH dependency from ACTH independency in 47 dogs with hyperadrenocorticism and equivocal adrenal asymmetry, *J Vet Intern Med* 24:1077–1085, 2010.

18. Greco DS, Peterson ME, Davidson AP, et al.: Concurrent pituitary and adrenal tumors in dogs with hyperadrenocorticism: 17 cases (1978-1995), *J Am Vet Med Assoc* 214:1349–1353, 1999.

19. Anderson CR, Birchard SJ, Powers BE, et al.: Surgical treatment of adrenocortical tumors: 21 cases (1990-1996), *J Am Anim Hosp Assoc* 37:93–97, 2001.

20. Kyles AE, Feldman EC, De Cock HE, et al.: Surgical management of adrenal gland tumors with and without associated tumor thrombi in dogs: 40 cases (1994-2001), *J Am Vet Med Assoc* 223:654–662, 2003.

21. Morandi F, Mays JL, Newman SJ, et al.: Imaging diagnosis-bilateral adrenal adenomas and myelolipomas in a dog, *Vet Radiol Ultrasound* 48:246–249, 2007.

22. Lang JM, Schertel E, Kennedy S, et al.: Elective and emergency surgical management of adrenal gland tumors: 60 cases (1999-2006), *J Am Anim Hosp Assoc* 47:428–435, 2011.

23. Nabeta R, Osada H, Ogawa M, et al.: Clinical and pathological features and outcome of bilateral incidental adrenocortical carcinomas in a dog, *J Vet Med Sci* 79:1489–1493, 2017.

24. Voorhout G, Stolp R, Lubberink AA, et al.: Computed tomography in the diagnosis of canine hyperadrenocorticism not suppressible by dexamethasone, *J Am Vet Med Assoc* 192:641–646, 1988.

25. Bertolini G, Furlanello T, Drigo M, et al.: Computed tomographic adrenal gland quantification in canine adrenocorticotroph hormone-dependent hyperadrenocorticism, *Vet Radiol Ultrasound* 49:449–453, 2008.

26. van der Vlugt-Meijer RH, Meij BP, van den Ingh TS, et al.: Dynamic computed tomography of the pituitary gland in dogs with pituitary-dependent hyperadrenocorticism, *J Vet Intern Med* 17:773–780, 2003.

27. van der Vlugt-Meijer RH, Meij BP, Voorhout G: Dynamic helical computed tomography of the pituitary gland in healthy dogs, *Vet Radiol Ultrasound* 48:118–124, 2007.

28. Auriemma E, Barthez PY, van der Vlugt-Meijer RH, et al.: Computed tomography and low-field magnetic resonance imaging of the pituitary gland in dogs with pituitary-dependent hyperadrenocorticism: 11 cases (2001-2003), *J Am Vet Med Assoc* 235:409–414, 2009.

29. Bertoy EH, Feldman EC, Nelson RW, et al.: Magnetic resonance imaging of the brain in dogs with recently diagnosed but untreated pituitary-dependent hyperadrenocorticism, *J Am Vet Med Assoc* 206:651–656, 1995.

30. Duesberg CA, Feldman EC, Nelson RW, et al.: Magnetic resonance imaging for diagnosis of pituitary macrotumors in dogs, *J Am Vet Med Assoc* 206:657–662, 1995.

31. Bertoy EH, Feldman EC, Nelson RW, et al.: One-year follow-up evaluation of magnetic resonance imaging of the brain in dogs with pituitary-dependent hyperadrenocorticism, *J Am Vet Med Assoc* 208:1268–1273, 1996.

32. Taoda T, Hara Y, Masuda H, et al.: Magnetic resonance imaging assessment of pituitary posterior lobe displacement in dogs with pituitary-dependent hyperadrenocorticism, *J Vet Med Sci* 73:725–731, 2011.

33. Zhao Q, Lee S, Kent M, et al.: Dynamic contrast-enhanced magnetic resonance imaging of canine brain tumors, *Vet Radiol Ultrasound* 51:122–129, 2010.

34. Nelson RW, Ihle SL, Feldman EC: Pituitary macroadenomas and macroadenocarcinomas in dogs treated with mitotane for pituitary-dependent hyperadrenocorticism - 13 Cases (1981-1986), *J Am Vet Med Assoc* 194:1612–1617, 1989.

35. Feldman EC, Nelson RW: Canine hyperadrenocorticism (Cushing's syndrome). In Feldman EC, Nelson RW, editors: *Canine and feline endocrinology and reproduction*, ed 3, St. Louis, 2004, Saunders, pp 252–357.

36. Theon AP, Feldman EC: Megavoltage irradiation of pituitary macrotumors in dogs with neurologic signs, *J Am Vet Med Assoc* 213:225–231, 1998.

37. Bosje JT, Rijnberk A, Mol JA, et al.: Plasma concentrations of ACTH precursors correlate with pituitary size and resistance to dexamethasone in dogs with pituitary-dependent hyperadrenocorticism, *Domest Anim Endocrinol* 22:201–210, 2002.

38. Granger N, de Fornel P, Devauchelle P, et al.: Plasma pro-opiomelanocortin, pro-adrenocorticotropin hormone, and pituitary adenoma size in dogs with Cushing's disease, *J Vet Intern Med* 19:23–28, 2005.

39. Ramsey IK: Trilostane in dogs, *Vet Clin North Am Small Anim Pract* 40:269–283, 2010.

40. Kintzer PP, Peterson ME: Mitotane (o,p'-DDD) treatment of 200 dogs with pituitary-dependent hyperadrenocorticism, *J Vet Intern Med* 5:182–190, 1991.

41. Neiger R, Ramsey I, O'Connor J, et al.: Trilostane treatment of 78 dogs with pituitary-dependent hyperadrenocorticism, *Vet Rec* 150:799–804, 2002.

42. Vaughan MA, Feldman EC, Hoar BR, et al.: Evaluation of twice-daily, low-dose trilostane treatment administered orally in dogs with naturally occurring hyperadrenocorticism, *J Am Vet Med Assoc* 232:1321–1328, 2008.

43. Barker EN, Campbell S, Tebb AJ, et al.: A comparison of the survival times of dogs treated with mitotane or trilostane for pituitary-dependent hyperadrenocorticism, *J Vet Intern Med* 19:810–815, 2005.

44. de Bruin C, Hanson JM, Meij BP, et al.: Expression and functional analysis of dopamine receptor subtype 2 and somatostatin receptor subtypes in canine cushing's disease, *Endocrinology* 149:4357–4366, 2008.

45. Castillo V, Theodoropoulou M, Stalla J, et al.: Effect of SOM230 (pasireotide) on corticotropic cells: action in dogs with Cushing's disease, *Neuroendocrinology* 94:124–136, 2011.

46. Lottati M, Bruyette DS: Outcomes of the addition of pasireotide to traditional adrenal-directed treatment for dogs with pituitary-dependent hyperadrenocorticism secondary to macroadenoma: 9 cases (2013-2015), *J Am Vet Med Assoc* 252:1403–1408, 2018.

47. Braddock JA, Church DB, Robertson ID, et al.: Inefficacy of selegiline in treatment of canine pituitary-dependent hyperadrenocorticism, *Aust Vet J* 82:272–277, 2004.

48. Castillo VA, Gomez NV, Lalia JC, et al.: Cushing's disease in dogs: cabergoline treatment, *Res Vet Sci* 85:26–34, 2008.

49. Rijnberk A, Mol JA, Kwant MM, et al.: Effects of bromocriptine on corticotrophin, melanotrophin and corticosteroid secretion in dogs with pituitary-dependent hyperadrenocorticism, *J Endocrinol* 118:271–277, 1988.

50. Stolp R, Croughs RJ, Rijnberk A: Results of cyproheptadine treatment in dogs with pituitary-dependent hyperadrenocorticism, *J Endocrinol* 101:311–314, 1984.

51. Castillo V, Giacomini D, Paez-Pereda M, et al.: Retinoic acid as a novel medical therapy for Cushing's disease in dogs, *Endocrinology* 147:4438–4444, 2006.

52. Meij B, Voorhout G, Rijnberk A: Progress in transsphenoidal hypophysectomy for treatment of pituitary-dependent hyperadrenocorticism in dogs and cats, *Mol Cell Endocrinol* 197:89–96, 2002.

53. Meij BP, Voorhout G, van den Ingh TS, et al.: Results of transsphenoidal hypophysectomy in 52 dogs with pituitary-dependent hyperadrenocorticism, *Vet Surg* 27:246–261, 1998.

54. Hanson JM, van 't HM, Voorhout G, et al.: Efficacy of transsphenoidal hypophysectomy in treatment of dogs with pituitary-dependent hyperadrenocorticism, *J Vet Intern Med* 19:687–694, 2005.

55. Mamelak AN, Owen TJ, Bruyette D: Transsphenoidal surgery using a high definition video telescope for pituitary adenomas in dogs with pituitary dependent hypercortisolism: methods and results, *Vet Surg* 43:369–379, 2014.

56. van Rijn SJ, Galac S, Tryfonidou MA, et al.: The influence of pituitary size on outcome after transsphenoidal hypophysectomy in a large cohort of dogs with pituitary-dependent hypercortisolism, *J Vet Intern Med* 30:989–995, 2016.

57. Del Magno S, Grinwis GCM, Voorhout G, et al.: Dynamic computed tomography of the pituitary gland using a single slice scanner in dogs with pituitary-dependent hypercortisolism, *Res Vet Sci* 107:42–49, 2016.

58. Sato A, Teshima T, Ishino H, et al.: A magnetic resonance imaging-based classification system for indication of trans-sphenoidal hypophysectomy in canine pituitary-dependent hypercortisolism, *J Small Anim Pract* 57:240–246, 2016.

59. Kooistra HS, Voorhout G, Mol JA, et al.: Correlation between impairment of glucocorticoid feedback and the size of the pituitary gland in dogs with pituitary-dependent hyperadrenocorticism, *J Endocrinol* 152:387–394, 1997.

60. van Rijn SJ, Hanson JM, Zierikzee D, et al.: The prognostic value of perioperative profiles of ACTH and cortisol for recurrence after transsphenoidal hypophysectomy in dogs with corticotroph adenomas, *J Vet Intern Med* 29:869–876, 2015.

61. Dow SW, Lecouteur RA, Rosychuk RAW, et al.: Response of dogs with functional pituitary macroadenomas and macrocarcinomas to radiation, *J Small Anim Pract* 31:287–294, 1990.

62. Goossens MM, Feldman EC, Nelson RW, et al.: Cobalt 60 irradiation of pituitary gland tumors in three cats with acromegaly, *J Am Vet Med Assoc* 213:374–376, 1998.

63. De Fornel P, Delisle F, Devauchelle P, et al.: Effects of radiotherapy on pituitary corticotroph macrotumors in dogs: a retrospective study of 12 cases, *Can Vet J* 48:481–486, 2007.

64. Marcinowska A, Warland J, Brearley M, et al.: Comparison of two coarse fractionated radiation protocols for the management of canine pituitary macrotumor: an observational study of 24 dogs, *Vet Radiol Ultrasound* 56:554–562, 2015.

65. Sawada H, Mori A, Lee P, et al.: Pituitary size alteration and adverse effects of radiation therapy performed in 9 dogs with pituitary-dependent hypercortisolism, *Res Vet Sci* 118:19–26, 2018.

66. Feldman EC: Hyperadrenocorticism in cats. In Feldman EC, Nelson RW, Reusch CE, et al.: *Canine and feline endocrinology*, ed 4, St. Louis, 2015, Elsevier, pp 452–484.

67. Ramsey IK, Herrtage ME: Feline hyperadrenocorticism. In Ettinger SJ, Feldman EC, Cote E, editors: *Textbook of veterinary internal medicine*, ed 8, St. Louis, 2017, Elsevier, pp 1811–1818.

68. Boland LA, Barrs VR: Peculiarities of feline hyperadrenocorticism: update on diagnosis and treatment, *J Feline Med Surg* 19:933–947, 2017.

69. Kimitsuki K, Boonsriroj H, Kojima D, et al.: A case report of feline pituitary carcinoma with hypercortisolism, *J Vet Med Sci* 76:133–138, 2014.

70. Meij BP, van der Vlugt-Meijer RH, van den Ingh TS, et al.: Somatotroph and corticotroph pituitary adenoma (double adenoma) in a cat with diabetes mellitus and hyperadrenocorticism, *J Comp Pathol* 130:209–215, 2004.

71. Cross E, Moreland R, Wallack S: Feline pituitary-dependent hyperadrenocorticism and insulin resistance due to a plurihormonal adenoma, *Top Companion Anim Med* 27:8–20, 2012.

72. Sharman M, FitzGerald L, Kiupel M: Concurrent somatotroph and plurihormonal pituitary adenomas in a cat, *J Feline Med Surg* 15:945–952, 2013.

73. Valentin SY, Cortright CC, Nelson RW, et al.: Clinical findings, diagnostic test results, and treatment outcome in cats with spontaneous hyperadrenocorticism: 30 cases, *J Vet Intern Med* 28:481–487, 2014.

74. Meij BP, Voorhout G, Van Den Ingh TS, et al.: Transsphenoidal hypophysectomy for treatment of pituitary-dependent hyperadrenocorticism in 7 cats, *Vet Surg* 30:72–86, 2001.

75. Mayer MN, Greco DS, LaRue SM: Outcomes of pituitary tumor irradiation in cats, *J Vet Intern Med* 20:1151–1154, 2006.

76. Sellon RK, Fidel J, Houston R, et al.: Linear-accelerator-based modified radiosurgical treatment of pituitary tumors in cats: 11 cases (1997-2008), *J Vet Intern Med* 23:1038–1044, 2009.

77. Duesberg CA, Nelson RW, Feldman EC, et al.: Adrenalectomy for treatment of hyperadrenocorticism in cats: 10 cases (1988-1992), *J Am Vet Med Assoc* 207:1066–1070, 1995.

78. Skelly BJ, Petrus D, Nicholls PK: Use of trilostane for the treatment of pituitary-dependent hyperadrenocorticism in a cat, *J Small Anim Pract* 44:269–272, 2003.

79. Neiger R, Witt AL, Noble A, et al.: Trilostane therapy for treatment of pituitary-dependent hyperadrenocorticism in 5 cats, *J Vet Intern Med* 18:160–164, 2004.

80. Mellett Keith AM, Bruyette D, Stanley S: Trilostane therapy for treatment of spontaneous hyperadrenocorticism in cats: 15 cases (2004-2012), *J Vet Intern Med* 27:1471–1477, 2013.

81. Peterson ME, Taylor RS, Greco DS, et al.: Acromegaly in 14 cats, *J Vet Intern Med* 4:192–201, 1990.

82. Hurty CA, Flatland B: Feline acromegaly: a review of the syndrome, *J Am Anim Hosp Assoc* 41:292–297, 2005.

83. Reusch CE: Disorders of Growth Hormone. In Feldman EC, Nelson RW, Reusch CE, et al.: *Canine and feline endocrinology*, ed 4, St. Louis, 2015, Elsevier, pp 37–76.

84. Scudder CJ, Niessen SJ, Catchpole B, et al.: Feline hypersomatotropism and acromegaly tumorigenesis: a potential role for the AIP gene, *Domest Anim Endocrinol* 59:134–139, 2017.

85. Niessen SJ, Church DB, Forcada Y: Hypersomatotropism, acromegaly, and hyperadrenocorticism and feline diabetes mellitus, *Vet Clin North Am Small Anim Pract* 43:319–350, 2013.

86. Niessen SJ, Petrie G, Gaudiano F, et al.: Feline acromegaly: an underdiagnosed endocrinopathy? *J Vet Intern Med* 21:899–905, 2007.

87. Niessen SJ, Forcada Y, Mantis P, et al.: Studying cat (Felis catus) diabetes: beware of the acromegalic imposter, *PloS one* 10:e0127794, 2015.

88. Schaefer S, Kooistra HS, Riond B, et al.: Evaluation of insulin-like growth factor-1, total thyroxine, feline pancreas-specific lipase and urinary corticoid-to-creatinine ratio in cats with diabetes mellitus in Switzerland and the Netherlands, *J Feline Med Surg* 19:888–896, 2017.

89. Peterson ME: Acromegaly in cats: are we only diagnosing the tip of the iceberg? *J Vet Intern Med* 21:889–891, 2007.

90. Berg RI, Nelson RW, Feldman EC, et al.: Serum insulin-like growth factor-1 concentration in cats with diabetes mellitus and acromegaly, *J Vet Intern Med* 21:892–898, 2007.

91. Norman EJ, Mooney CT: Diagnosis and management of diabetes mellitus in five cats with somatotrophic abnormalities, *J Feline Med Surg* 2:183–190, 2000.

92. Niessen SJ: Feline acromegaly: an essential differential diagnosis for the difficult diabetic, *J Feline Med Surg* 12:15–23, 2010.

93. Fletcher JM, Scudder CJ, Kiupel M, et al.: Hypersomatotropism in 3 cats without concurrent diabetes mellitus, *J Vet Intern Med* 30:1216–1221, 2016.

94. Myers JA, Lunn KF, Bright JM: Echocardiographic findings in 11 cats with acromegaly, *J Vet Intern Med* 28:1235–1238, 2014.

95. Borgeat K, Niessen SJM, Wilkie L, et al.: Time spent with cats is never wasted: lessons learned from feline acromegalic cardiomyopathy, a naturally occurring animal model of the human disease, *PloS one* 13:e0194342, 2018.

96. Elliott DA, Feldman EC, Koblik PD, et al.: Prevalence of pituitary tumors among diabetic cats with insulin resistance, *J Am Vet Med Assoc* 216:1765–1768, 2000.

97. Posch B, Dobson J, Herrtage M: Magnetic resonance imaging findings in 15 acromegalic cats, *Vet Radiol Ultrasound* 52:422–427, 2011.

98. Fischetti AJ, Gisselman K, Peterson ME: CT and MRI evaluation of skull bones and soft tissues in six cats with presumed acromegaly versus 12 unaffected cats, *Vet Radiol Ultrasound* 53:535–539, 2012.

99. Lamb CR, Ciasca TC, Mantis P, et al.: Computed tomographic signs of acromegaly in 68 diabetic cats with hypersomatotropism, *J Feline Med Surg* 16:99–108, 2014.

100. Lourenco BN, Randall E, Seiler G, et al.: Abdominal ultrasonographic findings in acromegalic cats, *J Feline Med Surg* 17:698–703, 2015.

101. Meij BP, Auriemma E, Grinwis G, et al.: Successful treatment of acromegaly in a diabetic cat with transsphenoidal hypophysectomy, *J Feline Med Surg* 12:406–410, 2010.

102. Blois SL, Holmberg DL: Cryohypophysectomy used in the treatment of a case of feline acromegaly, *J Small Anim Pract* 49:596–600, 2008.

103. Neilson DM, Viscasillas J, Alibhai H, et al.: Anaesthetic management and complications during hypophysectomy in 37 cats with acromegaly, *J Feline Med Surg*, 2018. 1098612x18778697.

104. Kenny P, Scudder C, Keyte S, et al.: Treatment of feline hypersomatotropism - efficacy, morbidity and mortality of hypophysectomy, *J Vet Intern Med* 29:1271, 2015.

105. Melmed S, Colao A, Barkan A, et al.: Guidelines for acromegaly management: an update, *J Clin Endocrinol Metab* 94:1509–1517, 2009.

106. Littler RM, Polton GA, Brearley MJ: Resolution of diabetes mellitus but not acromegaly in a cat with a pituitary macroadenoma treated with hypofractionated radiation, *J Small Anim Pract* 47:392–395, 2006.

107. Kaser-Hotz B, Rohrer CR, Stankeova S, et al.: Radiotherapy of pituitary tumours in five cats, *J Small Anim Pract* 43:303–307, 2002.

108. Brearley MJ, Polton GA, Littler RM, et al.: Coarse fractionated radiation therapy for pituitary tumours in cats: a retrospective study of 12 cases, *Vet Comp Oncol* 4:209–217, 2006.

109. Dunning MD, Lowrie CS, Bexfield NH, et al.: Exogenous insulin treatment after hypofractionated radiotherapy in cats with diabetes mellitus and acromegaly, *J Vet Intern Med* 23:243–249, 2009.

110. Wormhoudt TL, Boss MK, Lunn K, et al.: Stereotactic radiation therapy for the treatment of functional pituitary adenomas associated with feline acromegaly, *J Vet Intern Med* 32:1383–1391, 2018.

111. Abraham LA, Helmond SE, Mitten RW, et al.: Treatment of an acromegalic cat with the dopamine agonist L-deprenyl, *Aust Vet J* 80:479–483, 2002.

112. Morrison SA, Randolph J, Lothrop Jr CD: Hypersomatotropism and insulin-resistant diabetes mellitus in a cat, *J Am Vet Med Assoc* 194:91–94, 1989.

113. Slingerland LI, Voorhout G, Rijnberk A, et al.: Growth hormone excess and the effect of octreotide in cats with diabetes mellitus, *Domest Anim Endocrinol* 35:352–361, 2008.

114. Scudder CJ, Gostelow R, Forcada Y, et al.: Pasireotide for the medical management of feline hypersomatotropism, *J Vet Intern Med* 29:1074–1080, 2015.

115. Gostelow R, Scudder C, Keyte S, et al.: Pasireotide long-acting release treatment for diabetic cats with underlying hypersomatotropism, *J Vet Intern Med* 31:355–364, 2017.

116. Schwartz P, Kovak JR, Koprowski A, et al.: Evaluation of prognostic factors in the surgical treatment of adrenal gland tumors in dogs: 41 cases (1999-2005), *J Am Vet Med Assoc* 232:77–84, 2008.

117. Massari F, Nicoli S, Romanelli G, et al.: Adrenalectomy in dogs with adrenal gland tumors: 52 cases (2002-2008), *J Am Vet Med Assoc* 239:216–221, 2011.

118. Barrera JS, Bernard F, Ehrhart EJ, et al.: Evaluation of risk factors for outcome associated with adrenal gland tumors with or without invasion of the caudal vena cava and treated via adrenalectomy in dogs: 86 cases (1993-2009), *J Am Vet Med Assoc* 242:1715–1721, 2013.

119. Oblak ML, Bacon NJ, Covey JL: Perioperative management and outcome of bilateral adrenalectomy in 9 dogs, *Vet Surg* 45:790–797, 2016.

120. Mayhew PD, Culp WTN, Balsa IM, et al.: Phrenicoabdominal venotomy for tumor thrombectomy in dogs with adrenal neoplasia and suspected vena caval invasion, *Vet Surg* 47:227–235, 2018.

121. Reusch CE, Feldman EC: Canine hyperadrenocorticism due to adrenocortical neoplasia. Pretreatment evaluation of 41 dogs, *J Vet Intern Med* 5:3–10, 1991.

122. Penninck DG, Feldman EC, Nyland TG: Radiographic features of canine hyperadrenocorticism caused by autonomously functioning adrenocortical tumors: 23 cases (1978-1986), *J Am Vet Med Assoc* 192:1604–1608, 1988.

123. Voorhout G, Stolp R, Rijnberk A, et al.: Assessment of survey radiography and comparison with X-ray computed-tomography for detection of hyperfunctioning adrenocortical tumors in dogs, *J Am Vet Med Assoc* 196:1799–1803, 1990.

124. Widmer WR, Guptill L: Imaging techniques for facilitating diagnosis of hyperadrenocorticism in dogs and cats, *J Am Vet Med Assoc* 206:1857–1864, 1995.

125. Douglass JP, Berry CR, James S: Ultrasonographic adrenal gland measurements in dogs without evidence of adrenal disease, *Vet Radiol Ultrasound* 38:124–130, 1997.

126. Pagani E, Tursi M, Lorenzi C, et al.: Ultrasonographic features of adrenal gland lesions in dogs can aid in diagnosis, *BMC Vet Res* 12:267, 2016.

127. Davis MK, Schochet RA, Wrigley R: Ultrasonographic identification of vascular invasion by adrenal tumors in dogs, *Vet Radiol Ultrasound* 53:442–445, 2012.

128. Seiler GS, Brown JC, Reetz JA, et al.: Safety of contrast-enhanced ultrasonography in dogs and cats: 488 cases (2002-2011), *J Am Vet Med Assoc* 242:1255–1259, 2013.

129. Pey P, Rossi F, Vignoli M, et al.: Use of contrast-enhanced ultrasonography to characterize adrenal gland tumors in dogs, *Am J Vet Res* 75:886–892, 2014.

130. Voorhout G: X-ray-computed tomography, nephrotomography, and ultrasonography of the adrenal glands of healthy dogs, *Am J Vet Res* 51:625–631, 1990.

131. Voorhout G, Rijnberk A, Sjollema BE, et al.: Nephrotomography and ultrasonography for the localization of hyperfunctioning adrenocortical tumors in dogs, *Am J Vet Res* 51:1280–1285, 1990.

132. Emms SG, Wortman JA, Johnston DE, et al.: Evaluation of canine hyperadrenocorticism, using computed tomography, *J Am Vet Med Assoc* 189:432–439, 1986.

133. Bertolini G, Furlanello T, De Lorenzi D, et al.: Computed tomographic quantification of canine adrenal gland volume and attenuation, *Vet Radiol Ultrasound* 47:444–448, 2006.

134. Gregori T, Mantis P, Benigni L, et al.: Comparison of computed tomographic and pathologic findings in 17 dogs with primary adrenal neoplasia, *Vet Radiol Ultrasound* 56:153–159, 2015.

135. Schultz RM, Wisner ER, Johnson EG, et al.: Contrast-enhanced computed tomography as a preoperative indicator of vascular invasion from adrenal masses in dogs, *Vet Radiol Ultrasound* 50:625–629, 2009.

136. Yoshida O, Kutara K, Seki M, et al.: Preoperative differential diagnosis of canine adrenal tumors using triple-phase helical computed tomography, *Vet Surg* 45:427–435, 2016.

137. Llabres-Diaz FJ, Dennis R: Magnetic resonance imaging of the presumed normal canine adrenal glands, *Vet Radiol Ultrasound* 44:5–19, 2003.

138. Labelle P, Kyles AE, Farver TB, et al.: Indicators of malignancy of canine adrenocortical tumors: histopathology and proliferation index, *Vet Pathol* 41:490–497, 2004.

139. Scavelli TD, Peterson ME, Matthiesen DT: Results of surgical treatment for hyperadrenocorticism caused by adrenocortical neoplasia in the dog: 25 cases (1980-1984), *J Am Vet Med Assoc* 189:1360–1364, 1986.

140. Whittemore JC, Preston CA, Kyles AE, et al.: Nontraumatic rupture of an adrenal gland tumor causing intra-abdominal or retroperitoneal hemorrhage in four dogs, *J Am Vet Med Assoc* 219:329–333, 2001.

141. Behrend EN, Kemppainen RJ: Diagnosis of canine hyperadrenocorticism, *Vet Clin North Am Small Anim Pract* 31:985–1001, 2001.

142. Dolera M, Malfassi L, Pavesi S, et al.: Volumetric-modulated arc stereotactic radiotherapy for canine adrenocortical tumours with vascular invasion, *J Small Anim Pract* 57:710–717, 2016.

143. Kintzer PP, Peterson ME: Diagnosis and management of canine cortisol-secreting adrenal tumors, *Vet Clin North Am Small Anim Pract* 27:299–307, 1997.

144. Feldman EC, Nelson RW, Feldman MS, et al.: Comparison of mitotane treatment for adrenal tumor versus pituitary-dependent hyperadrenocorticism in dogs, *J Am Vet Med Assoc* 200:1642–1647, 1992.

145. Kintzer PP, Peterson ME: Mitotane treatment of 32 dogs with cortisol-secreting adrenocortical neoplasms, *J Am Vet Med Assoc* 205:54–61, 1994.

146. Feldman EC: Evaluation of twice-daily lower-dose trilostane treatment administered orally in dogs with naturally occurring hyperadrenocorticism, *J Am Vet Med Assoc* 238:1441–1451, 2011.

147. Eastwood JM, Elwood CM, Hurley KJ: Trilostane treatment of a dog with functional adrenocortical neoplasia, *J Small Anim Pract* 44:126–131, 2003.

148. Benchekroun G, de Fornel-Thibaud P, Lafarge S, et al.: Trilostane therapy for hyperadrenocorticism in three dogs with adrenocortical metastasis, *Vet Rec* 163:190–192, 2008.

149. Helm JR, McLauchlan G, Boden LA, et al.: A comparison of factors that influence survival in dogs with adrenal-dependent hyperadrenocorticism treated with mitotane or trilostane, *J Vet Intern Med* 25:251–260, 2011.

150. Arenas C, Melian C, Perez-Alenza MD: Long-term survival of dogs with adrenal-dependent hyperadrenocorticism: a comparison between mitotane and twice daily trilostane treatment, *J Vet Intern Med* 28:473–480, 2014.

151. Rijnberk A, Kooistra HS, van Vonderen IK, et al.: Aldosteronoma in a dog with polyuria as the leading symptom, *Domest Anim Endocrinol* 20:227–240, 2001.

152. Behrend EN, Weigand CM, Whitley EM, et al.: Corticosterone- and aldosterone-secreting adrenocortical tumor in a dog, *J Am Vet Med Assoc* 226:1662–1666, 2005.

153. Machida T, Uchida E, Matsuda K, et al.: Aldosterone-, corticosterone- and cortisol-secreting adrenocortical carcinoma in a dog: case report, *J Vet Med Sci* 70:317–320, 2008.

154. Gojska-Zygner O, Lechowski R, Zygner W: Functioning unilateral adrenocortical carcinoma in a dog, *Can Vet J* 53:623–625, 2012.

155. Frankot JL, Behrend EN, Sebestyen P, et al.: Adrenocortical carcinoma in a dog with incomplete excision managed long-term with metastasectomy alone, *J Am Anim Hosp Assoc* 48:417–423, 2012.

156. Behrend EN: Non-cortisol-secreting adrenocortical tumors and incidentalomas. In Ettinger SJ, Feldman EC, Cote E, editors: *Textbook of veterinary internal medicine*, ed 8, St. Louis, 2017, Elsevier, pp 1819–1825.

157. Daniel G, Mahony OM, Markovich JE, et al.: Clinical findings, diagnostics and outcome in 33 cats with adrenal neoplasia (2002-2013), *J Feline Med Surg* 18:77–84, 2016.

158. Djajadiningrat-Laanen S, Galac S, Kooistra H: Primary hyperaldosteronism: expanding the diagnostic net, *J Feline Med Surg* 13:641–650, 2011.

159. Javadi S, Djajadiningrat-Laanen SC, Kooistra HS, et al.: Primary hyperaldosteronism, a mediator of progressive renal disease in cats, *Domest Anim Endocrinol* 28:85–104, 2005.

160. Djajadiningrat-Laanen SC, Galac S, Cammelbeeck SE, et al.: Urinary aldosterone to creatinine ratio in cats before and after suppression with salt or fludrocortisone acetate, *J Vet Intern Med* 22:1283–1288, 2008.

161. Djajadiningrat-Laanen SC, Galac S, Boeve MH, et al.: Evaluation of the oral fludrocortisone suppression test for diagnosing primary hyperaldosteronism in cats, *J Vet Intern Med* 27:1493–1499, 2013.

162. Matsuda M, Behrend EN, Kemppainen R, et al.: Serum aldosterone and cortisol concentrations before and after suppression with fludrocortisone in cats: a pilot study, *J Vet Diagn Invest* 27:361–368, 2015.

163. Koutinas CK, Soubasis NC, Djajadiningrat-Laanen SC, et al.: Urinary aldosterone/creatinine ratio after fludrocortisone suppression consistent with PHA in a cat, *J Am Anim Hosp Assoc* 51:338–341, 2015.

164. Moore LE, Biller DS, Smith TA: Use of abdominal ultrasonography in the diagnosis of primary hyperaldosteronism in a cat, *J Am Vet Med Assoc* 217:213–215, 2000.

165. Schulman RL: Feline primary hyperaldosteronism, *Vet Clin North Am Small Anim Pract* 40:353–359, 2010.

166. Ash RA, Harvey AM, Tasker S: Primary hyperaldosteronism in the cat: a series of 13 cases, *J Feline Med Surg* 7:173–182, 2005.

167. Lo AJ, Holt DE, Brown DC, et al.: Treatment of aldosterone-secreting adrenocortical tumors in cats by unilateral adrenalectomy: 10 cases (2002-2012), *J Vet Intern Med* 28:137–143, 2014.

168. Flood SM, Randolph JF, Gelzer AR, et al.: Primary hyperaldosteronism in two cats, *J Am Anim Hosp Assoc* 35:411–416, 1999.

169. MacKay AD, Holt PE, Sparkes AH: Successful surgical treatment of a cat with primary aldosteronism, *J Feline Med Surg* 1:117–122, 1999.

170. Rose SA, Kyles AE, Labelle P, et al.: Adrenalectomy and caval thrombectomy in a cat with primary hyperaldosteronism, *J Am Anim Hosp Assoc* 43:209–214, 2007.

171. Gilson SD, Withrow SJ, Wheeler SL, et al.: Pheochromocytoma in 50 dogs, *J Vet Intern Med* 8:228–232, 1994.

172. Barthez PY, Marks SL, Woo J, et al.: Pheochromocytoma in dogs: 61 cases (1984-1995), *J Vet Intern Med* 11:272–278, 1997.

173. Galac S: Pheochromocytoma. In Ettinger SJ, Feldman EC, Cote E, editors: *Textbook of veterinary internal medicine*, ed 8, St. Louis, 2017, Elsevier, pp 1838–1843.

174. Reusch CE: Pheochromocytoma and multiple endocrine neoplasia. In Feldman EC, Nelson RW, Reusch CE, et al.: *Canine and feline endocrinology*, ed 4, St. Louis, 2015, Elsevier, pp 521–554.

175. Herrera MA, Mehl ML, Kass PH, et al.: Predictive factors and the effect of phenoxybenzamine on outcome in dogs undergoing adrenalectomy for pheochromocytoma, *J Vet Intern Med* 22:1333–1339, 2008.

176. Rosenstein DS: Diagnostic imaging in canine pheochromocytoma, *Vet Radiol Ultrasound* 41:499–506, 2000.

177. Berry CR, DeGrado TR, Nutter F, et al.: Imaging of pheochromocytoma in 2 dogs using p-[18F] fluorobenzylguanidine, *Vet Radiol Ultrasound* 43:183–186, 2002.

178. Head LL, Daniel GB: Scintigraphic diagnosis-an unusual presentation of metastatic pheochromocytoma in a dog, *Vet Radiol Ultrasound* 45:574–576, 2004.

179. Doss JC, Grone A, Capen CC, et al.: Immunohistochemical localization of chromogranin A in endocrine tissues and endocrine tumors of dogs, *Vet Pathol* 35:312–315, 1998.

180. Kook PH, Boretti FS, Hersberger M, et al.: Urinary catecholamine and metanephrine to creatinine ratios in healthy dogs at home and in a hospital environment and in 2 dogs with pheochromocytoma, *J Vet Intern Med* 21:388–393, 2007.

181. Kook PH, Grest P, Quante S, et al.: Urinary catecholamine and metadrenaline to creatinine ratios in dogs with a phaeochromocytoma, *Vet Rec* 166:169–174, 2010.

182. Wimpole JA, Adagra CF, Billson MF, et al.: Plasma free metanephrines in healthy cats, cats with non-adrenal disease and a cat with suspected phaeochromocytoma, *J Feline Med Surg* 12:435–440, 2010.

183. Quante S, Boretti FS, Kook PH, et al.: Urinary catecholamine and metanephrine to creatinine ratios in dogs with hyperadrenocorticism or pheochromocytoma, and in healthy dogs, *J Vet Intern Med* 24:1093–1097, 2010.

184. Green BA, Frank EL: Comparison of plasma free metanephrines between healthy dogs and 3 dogs with pheochromocytoma, *Vet Clin Pathol* 42:499–503, 2013.

185. Gostelow R, Syme H: Plasma metadrenalines in canine phaeochromocytoma, *Vet Rec* 166:538, 2010.

186. Gostelow R, Syme HM: Plasma free metanephrine and normetanephrine concentrations are elevated in dogs with pheochromocytoma, *J Vet Intern Med* 25:680–681, 2011.

187. Gostelow R, Bridger N, Syme HM: Plasma-free metanephrine and free normetanephrine measurement for the diagnosis of pheochromocytoma in dogs, *J Vet Intern Med* 27:83–90, 2013.

188. Salesov E, Boretti FS, Sieber-Ruckstuhl NS, et al.: Urinary and plasma catecholamines and metanephrines in dogs with pheochromocytoma, hypercortisolism, nonadrenal disease and in healthy dogs, *J Vet Intern Med* 29:597–602, 2015.

189. Bommarito DA, Lattimer JC, Selting KA, et al.: Treatment of a malignant pheochromocytoma in a dog using 131I metaiodobenzylguanidine, *J Am Anim Hosp Assoc* 47:e188–194, 2011.

190. Edmondson EF, Bright JM, Halsey CH, et al.: Pathologic and cardiovascular characterization of pheochromocytoma-associated cardiomyopathy in dogs, *Vet Pathol* 52:338–343, 2015.

191. Lentschener C, Gaujoux S, Tesniere A, et al.: Point of controversy: perioperative care of patients undergoing pheochromocytoma removal-time for a reappraisal? *Eur J Endocrinol* 165:365–373, 2011.

192. Rose L, Dunn ME, Bedard C: Effect of canine hyperadrenocorticism on coagulation parameters, *J Vet Intern Med* 27:207–211, 2013.

193. Kol A, Nelson RW, Gosselin RC, et al.: Characterization of thrombelastography over time in dogs with hyperadrenocorticism, *Vet J* 197:675–681, 2013.

194. Pace SL, Creevy KE, Krimer PM, et al.: Assessment of coagulation and potential biochemical markers for hypercoagulability in canine hyperadrenocorticism, *J Vet Intern Med* 27:1113–1120, 2013.

195. Andrade N, Rivas LR, Milovancev M, et al.: Intercostal approach for right adrenalectomy in dogs, *Vet Surg* 43:99–104, 2014.

196. Mayhew PD, Culp WT, Hunt GB, et al.: Comparison of perioperative morbidity and mortality rates in dogs with noninvasive adrenocortical masses undergoing laparoscopic versus open adrenalectomy, *J Am Vet Med Assoc* 245:1028–1035, 2014.

197. Pitt KA, Mayhew PD, Steffey MA, et al.: Laparoscopic adrenalectomy for removal of unilateral noninvasive pheochromocytomas in 10 Dogs, *Vet Surg* 45:O70–O76, 2016.

198. van Sluijs FJ, Sjollema BE, Voorhout G, et al.: Results of adrenalectomy in 36 dogs with hyperadrenocorticism caused by adrenocortical tumour, *Vet Q* 17:113–116, 1995.

199. Walker RG, Halliwell RE, Hall LW: The surgical treatment of Cushing's disease in a dog, *Vet Rec* 90:723–726, 1972.

200. Mitchell JW, Mayhew PD, Culp WTN, et al.: Outcome of laparoscopic adrenalectomy for resection of unilateral noninvasive adrenocortical tumors in 11 cats, *Vet Surg* 46:714–721, 2017.

201. Cook AK, Spaulding KA, Edwards JF: Clinical findings in dogs with incidental adrenal gland lesions determined by ultrasonography: 151 cases (2007-2010), *J Am Vet Med Assoc* 244:1181–1185, 2014.

202. Arenas C, Perez-Alenza D, Melian C: Clinical features, outcome and prognostic factors in dogs diagnosed with non-cortisol-secreting adrenal tumours without adrenalectomy: 20 cases (1994-2009), *Vet Rec* 173:501, 2013.

203. Baum JI, Boston SE, Case JB: Prevalence of adrenal gland masses as incidental findings during abdominal computed tomography in dogs: 270 cases (2013-2014), *J Am Vet Med Assoc* 249:1165–1169, 2016.

204. Myers 3rd NC, incidentalomas Adrenal: Diagnostic workup of the incidentally discovered adrenal mass, *Vet Clin North Am Small Anim Pract* 27:381–399, 1997.

205. Bertazzolo W, Didier M, Gelain ME, et al.: Accuracy of cytology in distinguishing adrenocortical tumors from pheochromocytoma in companion animals, *Vet Clin Pathol* 43:453–459, 2014.

206. Wucherer KL, Wilke V: Thyroid cancer in dogs: an update based on 638 cases (1995-2005), *J Am Anim Hosp Assoc* 46:249–254, 2010.

207. Barber LG: Thyroid tumors in dogs and cats, *Vet Clin North Am Small Anim Pract* 37:755–773, 2007.

208. Campos M, Ducatelle R, Rutteman G, et al.: Clinical, pathologic, and immunohistochemical prognostic factors in dogs with thyroid carcinoma, *J Vet Intern Med* 28:1805–1813, 2014.

209. Carver JR, Kapatkin A, Patnaik AK: A comparison of medullary thyroid carcinoma and thyroid adenocarcinoma in dogs: a retrospective study of 38 cases, *Vet Surg* 24:315–319, 1995.

210. Taeymans O, Penninck DG, Peters RM: Comparison between clinical, ultrasound, CT, MRI, and pathology findings in dogs presented for suspected thyroid carcinoma, *Vet Radiol Ultrasound* 54:61–70, 2013.

211. Deitz K, Gilmour L, Wilke V, et al.: Computed tomographic appearance of canine thyroid tumours, *J Small Anim Pract* 55:323–329, 2014.

212. Bertolini G, Drigo M, Angeloni L, et al.: Incidental and nonincidental canine thyroid tumors assessed by multidetector row computed tomography: a single-centre cross sectional study in 4520 dogs, *Vet Radiol Ultrasound* 58:304–314, 2017.

213. Pollard RE, Bohannon LK, Feldman EC: Prevalence of incidental thyroid nodules in ultrasound studies of dogs with hypercalcemia (2008-2013), *Vet Radiol Ultrasound* 56:63–67, 2015.

214. Klein MK, Powers BE, Withrow SJ, et al.: Treatment of thyroid carcinoma in dogs by surgical resection alone: 20 cases (1981-1989), *J Am Vet Med Assoc* 206:1007–1009, 1995.

215. Liptak JM: Canine thyroid carcinoma, *Clin Tech Small Anim Pract* 22:75–81, 2007.

216. Nadeau ME, Kitchell BE: Evaluation of the use of chemotherapy and other prognostic variables for surgically excised canine thyroid carcinoma with and without metastasis, *Can Vet J* 52:994–998, 2011.

217. Haley PJ, Hahn FF, Muggenburg BA, et al.: Thyroid neoplasms in a colony of beagle dogs, *Vet Pathol* 26:438–441, 1989.

218. Harari J, Patterson JS, Rosenthal RC: Clinical and pathologic features of thyroid tumors in 26 dogs, *J Am Vet Med Assoc* 188:1160–1164, 1986.

219. London C, Mathie T, Stingle N, et al.: Preliminary evidence for biologic activity of toceranib phosphate (Palladia)in solid tumours, *Vet Comp Oncol* 10:194–205, 2012.

220. Radlinsky MG: Thyroid surgery in dogs and cats, *Vet Clin North Am Small Anim Pract* 37:789–798, 2007.

221. Hullinger RL: The endocrine Ssstem. In Evans HE, de Lahunta A, editors: *Miller's anatomy of the dog*, ed 4, St. Louis, 2013, Elsevier, pp 406–427.

222. Tuohy JL, Worley DR, Withrow SJ: Outcome following simultaneous bilateral thyroid lobectomy for treatment of thyroid carcinoma in dogs: 15 cases (1994-2010), *J Am Vet Med Assoc* 241:95–103, 2012.

223. Fukui S, Endo Y, Hirayama K, et al.: Identification and preservation of the parathyroid gland during total thyroidectomy in dogs with bilateral thyroid carcinoma: a report of six cases, *J Vet Med Sci* 77:747–751, 2015.

224. Broome MR, Peterson ME, Walker JR: Clinical features and treatment outcomes of 41 dogs with sublingual ectopic thyroid neoplasia, *J Vet Intern Med* 28:1560–1568, 2014.

225. Milovancev M, Wilson DM, Monnet E, et al.: Partial resection of the hyoid apparatus during surgical treatment of ectopic thyroid carcinomas in dogs: 5 cases (2011-2013), *J Am Vet Med Assoc* 244:1319–1324, 2014.

226. Kang MH, Kim DY, Park HM: Ectopic thyroid carcinoma infiltrating the right atrium of the heart in a dog, *Can Vet J* 53:177–181, 2012.

227. Lantz GC, Salisbury SK: Surgical excision of ectopic thyroid carcinoma involving the base of the tongue in dogs: three cases (1980-1987), *J Am Vet Med Assoc* 195:1606–1608, 1989.

228. Liptak JM, Kamstock DA, Dernell WS, et al.: Cranial mediastinal carcinomas in nine dogs, *Vet Comp Oncol* 6:19–30, 2008.

229. Brearley MJ, Hayes AM, Murphy S: Hypofractionated radiation therapy for invasive thyroid carcinoma in dogs: a retrospective analysis of survival, *J Small Anim Pract* 40:206–210, 1999.

230. Pack L, Roberts RE, Dawson SD, et al.: Definitive radiation therapy for infiltrative thyroid carcinoma in dogs, *Vet Radiol Ultrasound* 42:471–474, 2001.

231. Tsimbas K, Turek M, Christensen N, et al.: Short survival time following palliative-intent hypofractionated radiotherapy for nonresectable canine thyroid carcinoma: a retrospective analysis of 20 dogs, *Vet Radiol Ultrasound*, 2018. https://doi.org/10.1111/vru.12680.

232. Amores-Fuster I, Cripps P, Blackwood L: Post-radiotherapy hypothyroidism in dogs treated for thyroid carcinomas, *Vet Comp Oncol* 15:247–251, 2017.

233. Worth AJ, Zuber RM, Hocking M: Radioiodide (131I) therapy for the treatment of canine thyroid carcinoma, *Aust Vet J* 83:208–214, 2005.

234. Turrel JM, McEntee MC, Burke BP, et al.: Sodium iodide i 131 treatment of dogs with nonresectable thyroid tumors: 39 cases (1990-2003), *J Am Vet Med Assoc* 229:542–548, 2006.

235. Castillo V, Pessina P, Hall P, et al.: Post-surgical treatment of thyroid carcinoma in dogs with retinoic acid 9 cis improves patient outcome, *Open Vet J* 6:6–14, 2016.

236. Scott-Moncrieff JCR: Canine thyroid tumors and hyperthyroidism. In Feldman EC, Nelson RW, Reusch CE, et al.: *Canine and feline endocrinology*, ed 4, St. Louis, 2015, Elsevier, pp 196–212.

237. Ward CW: Canine hyperthyroidism. In Ettinger SJ, Feldman EC, Cote E, editors: *Textbook of veterinary internal medicine*, ed 8, St. Louis, 2017, Elsevier, pp 1757–1761.

238. Looney A, Wakshlag J: Dietary management of hyperthyroidism in a dog, *J Am Anim Hosp Assoc* 53:111–118, 2017.

239. Scott-Moncrieff JCR: Feline hyperthyroidism. In Feldman EC, Nelson RW, Reusch CE, et al.: *Canine and feline endocrinology*, ed 4, St. Louis, 2015, Elsevier, pp 136–195.

240. Graves TK: Feline hyperthyroidism. In Ettinger SJ, Feldman EC, Cote E, editors: *Textbook of veterinary internal medicine*, ed 8, St. Louis, 2017, Elsevier, pp 1747–1757.

241. Peterson ME: Animal models of disease: feline hyperthyroidism: an animal model for toxic nodular goiter, *J Endocrinol* 223:T97–114, 2014.

242. Naan EC, Kirpensteijn J, Kooistra HS, et al.: Results of thyroidectomy in 101 cats with hyperthyroidism, *Vet Surg* 35:287–293, 2006.

243. Peterson ME, Kintzer PP, Cavanagh PG, et al.: Feline hyperthyroidism: pretreatment clinical and laboratory evaluation of 131 cases, *J Am Vet Med Assoc* 183:103–110, 1983.

244. Harvey AM, Hibbert A, Barrett EL, et al.: Scintigraphic findings in 120 hyperthyroid cats, *J Feline Med Surg* 11:96–106, 2009.

245. Peterson ME, Broome MR: Thyroid scintigraphy findings in 2096 cats with hyperthyroidism, *Vet Radiol Ultrasound* 56:84–95, 2015.

246. Peterson ME, Broome MR, Rishniw M: Prevalence and degree of thyroid pathology in hyperthyroid cats increases with disease duration: a cross-sectional analysis of 2096 cats referred for radioiodine therapy, *J Feline Med Surg* 18:92–103, 2016.

247. Turrel JM, Feldman EC, Nelson RW, et al.: Thyroid carcinoma causing hyperthyroidism in cats: 14 cases (1981-1986), *J Am Vet Med Assoc* 193:359–364, 1988.

248. Cook SM, Daniel GB, Walker MA, et al.: Radiographic and scintigraphic evidence of focal pulmonary neoplasia in three cats with hyperthyroidism: diagnostic and therapeutic considerations, *J Vet Intern Med* 7:303–308, 1993.

249. Hibbert A, Gruffydd-Jones T, Barrett EL, et al.: Feline thyroid carcinoma: diagnosis and response to high-dose radioactive iodine treatment, *J Feline Med Surg* 11:116–124, 2009.

250. Guptill L, Scott-Moncrieff CR, Janovitz EB, et al.: Response to high-dose radioactive iodine administration in cats with thyroid carcinoma that had previously undergone surgery, *J Am Vet Med Assoc* 207:1055–1058, 1995.

251. Miller ML, Peterson ME, Randolph JF, et al.: Thyroid Cysts in Cats: A Retrospective Study of 40 Cases, *J Vet Intern Med* 31:723–729, 2017.

252. Peterson M: Hyperthyroidism in cats: what's causing this epidemic of thyroid disease and can we prevent it? *J Feline Med Surg* 14:804–818, 2012.

253. Carney HC, Ward CR, Bailey SJ, et al.: 2016 AAFP guidelines for the management of feline hyperthyroidism, *J Feline Med Surg* 18:400–416, 2016.

254. Kohler I, Ballhausen BD, Stockhaus C, et al.: Prevalence of and risk factors for feline hyperthyroidism among a clinic population in Southern Germany, *Tierarztl Prax Ausg K Kleintiere Heimtiere* 44:149–157, 2016.

255. Wakeling J, Everard A, Brodbelt D, et al.: Risk factors for feline hyperthyroidism in the UK, *J Small Anim Pract* 50:406–414, 2009.

256. Edinboro CH, Scott-Moncrieff JC, Glickman LT: Feline hyperthyroidism: potential relationship with iodine supplement requirements of commercial cat foods, *J Feline Med Surg* 12:672–679, 2010.

257. van Hoek I, Hesta M, Biourge V: A critical review of food-associated factors proposed in the etiology of feline hyperthyroidism, *J Feline Med Surg* 17:837–847, 2015.

258. Walter KM, Lin YP, Kass PH, et al.: Association of polybrominated diphenyl ethers (PBDEs) and polychlorinated biphenyls (PCBs) with hyperthyroidism in domestic felines, sentinels for thyroid hormone disruption, *BMC Vet Res* 13:120, 2017.

259. Kass PH, Peterson ME, Levy J, et al.: Evaluation of environmental, nutritional, and host factors in cats with hyperthyroidism, *J Vet Intern Med* 13:323–329, 1999.

260. Martin KM, Rossing MA, Ryland LM, et al.: Evaluation of dietary and environmental risk factors for hyperthyroidism in cats, *J Am Vet Med Assoc* 217:853–856, 2000.

261. Edinboro CH, Scott-Moncrieff JC, Janovitz E, et al.: Epidemiologic study of relationships between consumption of commercial canned food and risk of hyperthyroidism in cats, *J Am Vet Med Assoc* 224:879–886, 2004.

262. McLean JL, Lobetti RG, Schoeman JP: Worldwide prevalence and risk factors for feline hyperthyroidism: a review, *J S Afr Vet Assoc* 85:1097, 2014.

263. McLean JL, Lobetti RG, Mooney CT, et al.: Prevalence of and risk factors for feline hyperthyroidism in South Africa, *J Feline Med Surg* 19:1103–1109, 2017.

264. Hammer KB, Holt DE, Ward CR: Altered expression of G proteins in thyroid gland adenomas obtained from hyperthyroid cats, *Am J Vet Res* 61:874–879, 2000.

265. Ward CR, Achenbach SE, Peterson ME, et al.: Expression of inhibitory G proteins in adenomatous thyroid glands obtained from hyperthyroid cats, *Am J Vet Res* 66:1478–1482, 2005.

266. Peeters ME, Timmermans-Sprang EP, Mol JA: Feline thyroid adenomas are in part associated with mutations in the G(s alpha) gene and not with polymorphisms found in the thyrotropin receptor, *Thyroid* 12:571–575, 2002.

267. Ward CR, Windham WR, Dise D: Evaluation of activation of G proteins in response to thyroid stimulating hormone in thyroid gland cells from euthyroid and hyperthyroid cats, *Am J Vet Res* 71:643–648, 2010.

268. Pearce SH, Foster DJ, Imrie H, et al.: Mutational analysis of the thyrotropin receptor gene in sporadic and familial feline thyrotoxicosis, *Thyroid* 7:923–927, 1997.

269. Watson SG, Radford AD, Kipar A, et al.: Somatic mutations of the thyroid-stimulating hormone receptor gene in feline hyperthyroidism: parallels with human hyperthyroidism, *J Endocrinol* 186:523–537, 2005.

270. Merryman JI, Buckles EL, Bowers G, et al.: Overexpression of c-Ras in hyperplasia and adenomas of the feline thyroid gland: an immunohistochemical analysis of 34 cases, *Vet Pathol* 36:117–124, 1999.

271. Crossley VJ, Debnath A, Chang YM, et al.: Breed, coat color, and hair length as risk factors for hyperthyroidism in cats, *J Vet Intern Med* 31:1028–1034, 2017.

272. Watson N, Murray JK, Fonfara S, et al.: Clinicopathological features and comorbidities of cats with mild, moderate or severe hyperthyroidism: a radioiodine referral population, *J Feline Med Surg*, 2018.

273. Peterson ME, Castellano CA, Rishniw M: Evaluation of body weight, body condition, and muscle condition in cats with hyperthyroidism, *J Vet Intern Med* 30:1780–1789, 2016.

274. Peterson ME, Melian C, Nichols R: Measurement of serum concentrations of free thyroxine, total thyroxine, and total triiodothyronine in cats with hyperthyroidism and cats with nonthyroidal disease, *J Am Vet Med Assoc* 218:529–536, 2001.

275. Peterson ME: More than just T(4): diagnostic testing for hyperthyroidism in cats, *J Feline Med Surg* 15:765–777, 2013.

276. Peterson ME, Graves TK, Cavanagh I: Serum thyroid hormone concentrations fluctuate in cats with hyperthyroidism, *J Vet Intern Med* 1:142–146, 1987.

277. Mooney CT, Little CJ, Macrae AW: Effect of illness not associated with the thyroid gland on serum total and free thyroxine concentrations in cats, *J Am Vet Med Assoc* 208:2004–2008, 1996.

278. Wakeling J, Moore K, Elliott J, et al.: Diagnosis of hyperthyroidism in cats with mild chronic kidney disease, *J Small Anim Pract* 49:287–294, 2008.

279. Mooney CT, Thoday KL, Doxey DL: Serum thyroxine and triiodothyronine responses of hyperthyroid cats to thyrotropin, *Am J Vet Res* 57:987–991, 1996.

280. Tomsa K, Glaus TM, Kacl GM, et al.: Thyrotropin-releasing hormone stimulation test to assess thyroid function in severely sick cats, *J Vet Intern Med* 15:89–93, 2001.

281. Peterson ME, Graves TK, Gamble DA: Triiodothyronine (T3) suppression test. An aid in the diagnosis of mild hyperthyroidism in cats, *J Vet Intern Med* 4:233–238, 1990.

282. Refsal KR, Nachreiner RF, Stein BE, et al.: Use of the triiodothyronine suppression test for diagnosis of hyperthyroidism in ill cats that have serum concentration of iodothyronines within normal range, *J Am Vet Med Assoc* 199:1594–1601, 1991.

283. Peterson ME, Guterl JN, Nichols R, et al.: Evaluation of serum thyroid-stimulating hormone concentration as a diagnostic test for hyperthyroidism in cats, *J Vet Intern Med* 29:1327–1334, 2015.

284. Taylor SS, Sparkes AH, Briscoe K, et al.: ISFM Consensus guidelines on the diagnosis and management of hypertension in cats, *J Feline Med Surg* 19:288–303, 2017.

285. Bond BR, Fox PR, Peterson ME, et al.: Echocardiographic findings in 103 cats with hyperthyroidism, *J Am Vet Med Assoc* 192:1546–1549, 1988.

286. Fox PR, Peterson ME, Broussard JD: Electrocardiographic and radiographic changes in cats with hyperthyroidism: comparison of populations evaluated during 1992-1993 vs. 1979-1982, *J Am Anim Hosp Assoc* 35:27–31, 1999.

287. Nussbaum LK, Scavelli TD, Scavelli DM, et al.: Abdominal ultrasound examination findings in 534 hyperthyroid cats referred for radioiodine treatment between 2007-2010, *J Vet Intern Med* 29:1069–1073, 2015.

288. Combes A, Vandermeulen E, Duchateau L, et al.: Ultrasonographic measurements of adrenal glands in cats with hyperthyroidism, *Vet Radiol Ultrasound* 53:210–216, 2012.

289. Daniel GB, Neelis DA: Thyroid scintigraphy in veterinary medicine, *Semin Nucl Med* 44:24–34, 2014.

290. Bodey AL, Almond CJ, Holmes MA: Double-blinded randomised placebo-controlled clinical trial of individualised homeopathic treatment of hyperthyroid cats, *Vet Rec* 180:377, 2017.

291. Peterson ME, Kintzer PP, Hurvitz AI: Methimazole treatment of 262 cats with hyperthyroidism, *J Vet Intern Med* 2:150–157, 1988.

292. Mooney CT, Thoday KL, Doxey DL: Carbimazole therapy of feline hyperthyroidism, *J Small Anim Pract* 33:228–235, 1992.

293. Daminet S, Kooistra HS, Fracassi F, et al.: Best practice for the pharmacological management of hyperthyroid cats with antithyroid drugs, *J Small Anim Pract* 55:4–13, 2014.

294. Trepanier LA, Hoffman SB, Kroll M, et al.: Efficacy and safety of once versus twice daily administration of methimazole in cats with hyperthyroidism, *J Am Vet Med Assoc* 222:954–958, 2003.

295. Frenais R, Rosenberg D, Burgaud S, et al.: Clinical efficacy and safety of a once-daily formulation of carbimazole in cats with hyperthyroidism, *J Small Anim Pract* 50:510–515, 2009.

296. Hoffman SB, Yoder AR, Trepanier LA: Bioavailability of transdermal methimazole in a pluronic lecithin organogel (PLO) in healthy cats, *J Vet Pharmacol Ther* 25:189–193, 2002.

297. Hoffmann G, Marks SL, Taboada J, et al.: Transdermal methimazole treatment in cats with hyperthyroidism, *J Feline Med Surg* 5:77–82, 2003.

298. Sartor LL, Trepanier LA, Kroll MM, et al.: Efficacy and safety of transdermal methimazole in the treatment of cats with hyperthyroidism, *J Vet Intern Med* 18:651–655, 2004.

299. Hill KE, Gieseg MA, Kingsbury D, et al.: The efficacy and safety of a novel lipophilic formulation of methimazole for the once daily transdermal treatment of cats with hyperthyroidism, *J Vet Intern Med* 25:1357–1365, 2011.

300. Buijtels JJ, Kurvers IA, Galac S, et al.: Transdermal carbimazole for the treatment of feline hyperthyroidism, *Tijdschr Diergeneeskd* 131:478–482, 2006.

301. Boretti FS, Sieber-Ruckstuhl NS, Schafer S, et al.: Transdermal application of methimazole in hyperthyroid cats: a long-term follow-up study, *J Feline Med Surg* 16:453–459, 2014.

302. Trepanier LA: Pharmacologic management of feline hyperthyroidism, *Vet Clin North Am Small Anim Pract* 37:775–788, 2007.

303. Murray LA, Peterson ME: Ipodate treatment of hyperthyroidism in cats, *J Am Vet Med Assoc* 211:63–67, 1997.

304. Gallagher AE, Panciera DL: Efficacy of iopanoic acid for treatment of spontaneous hyperthyroidism in cats, *J Feline Med Surg* 13:441–447, 2011.

305. Scott-Moncrieff JC, Heng HG, Weng HY, et al.: Effect of a limited iodine diet on iodine uptake by thyroid glands in hyperthyroid cats, *J Vet Intern Med* 29:1322–1326, 2015.

306. van der Kooij M, Becvarova I, Meyer HP, et al.: Effects of an iodine-restricted food on client-owned cats with hyperthyroidism, *J Feline Med Surg* 16:491–498, 2014.

307. Hui TY, Bruyette DS, Moore GE, et al.: Effect of feeding an iodine-restricted diet in cats with spontaneous hyperthyroidism, *J Vet Intern Med* 29:1063–1068, 2015.

308. Flanders JA: Surgical options for the treatment of hyperthyroidism in the cat, *J Feline Med Surg* 1:127–134, 1999.

309. Birchard SJ: Thyroidectomy in the cat, *Clin Tech Small Anim Pract* 21:29–33, 2006.

310. Padgett S: Feline thyroid surgery, *Vet Clin North Am Small Anim Pract* 32:851–859, 2002.

311. Peterson ME, Becker DV: Radioiodine treatment of 524 cats with hyperthyroidism, *J Am Vet Med Assoc* 207:1422–1428, 1995.

312. Turrel JM, Feldman EC, Hays M, et al.: Radioactive iodine therapy in cats with hyperthyroidism, *J Am Vet Med Assoc* 184:554–559, 1984.

313. Meric SM, Hawkins EC, Washabau RJ, et al.: Serum thyroxine concentrations after radioactive iodine therapy in cats with hyperthyroidism, *J Am Vet Med Assoc* 188:1038–1040, 1986.

314. Chun R, Garrett LD, Sargeant J, et al.: Predictors of response to radioiodine therapy in hyperthyroid cats, *Vet Radiol Ultrasound* 43:587–591, 2002.

315. Meric SM, Rubin SI: Serum thyroxine concentrations following fixed-dose radioactive iodine treatment in hyperthyroid cats: 62 cases (1986-1989), *J Am Vet Med Assoc* 197:621–623, 1990.

316. Lucy JM, Peterson ME, Randolph JF, et al.: Efficacy of low-dose (2 millicurie) versus standard-dose (4 millicurie) radioiodine treatment for cats with mild-to-moderate hyperthyroidism, *J Vet Intern Med* 31:326–334, 2017.

317. Vagney M, Desquilbet L, Reyes-Gomez E, et al.: Survival times for cats with hyperthyroidism treated with a 3.35 mCi iodine-131 dose: a retrospective study of 96 cases, *J Feline Med Surg* 20:528–534, 2018.

318. Peterson ME: Radioiodine treatment of hyperthyroidism, *Clin Tech Small Anim Pract* 21:34–39, 2006.

319. Boag AK, Neiger R, Slater L, et al.: Changes in the glomerular filtration rate of 27 cats with hyperthyroidism after treatment with radioactive iodine, *Vet Rec* 161:711–715, 2007.

320. Nykamp SG, Dykes NL, Zarfoss MK, et al.: Association of the risk of development of hypothyroidism after iodine 131 treatment with the pretreatment pattern of sodium pertechnetate Tc 99m uptake in the thyroid gland in cats with hyperthyroidism: 165 cases (1990-2002), *J Am Vet Med Assoc* 226:1671–1675, 2005.

321. Williams TL, Elliott J, Syme HM: Association of iatrogenic hypothyroidism with azotemia and reduced survival time in cats treated for hyperthyroidism, *J Vet Intern Med* 24:1086–1092, 2010.

322. Milner RJ, Channell CD, Levy JK, et al.: Survival times for cats with hyperthyroidism treated with iodine 131, methimazole, or both: 167 cases (1996-2003), *J Am Vet Med Assoc* 228:559–563, 2006.

323. Goldstein RE, Long C, Swift NC, et al.: Percutaneous ethanol injection for treatment of unilateral hyperplastic thyroid nodules in cats, *J Am Vet Med Assoc* 218:1298–1302, 2001.

324. Wells AL, Long CD, Hornof WJ, et al.: Use of percutaneous ethanol injection for treatment of bilateral hyperplastic thyroid nodules in cats, *J Am Vet Med Assoc* 218:1293–1297, 2001.

325. Mallery KF, Pollard RE, Nelson RW, et al.: Percutaneous ultrasound-guided radiofrequency heat ablation for treatment of hyperthyroidism in cats, *J Am Vet Med Assoc* 223:1602–1607, 2003.

326. Vaske HH, Schermerhorn T, Grauer GF: Effects of feline hyperthyroidism on kidney function: a review, *J Feline Med Surg* 18:55–59, 2016.

327. Graves TK, Olivier NB, Nachreiner RF, et al.: Changes in renal function associated with treatment of hyperthyroidism in cats, *Am J Vet Res* 55:1745–1749, 1994.

328. Becker TJ, Graves TK, Kruger JM, et al.: Effects of methimazole on renal function in cats with hyperthyroidism, *J Am Anim Hosp Assoc* 36:215–223, 2000.

329. DiBartola SP, Broome MR, Stein BS, et al.: Effect of treatment of hyperthyroidism on renal function in cats, *J Am Vet Med Assoc* 208:875–878, 1996.

330. Adams WH, Daniel GB, Legendre AM, et al.: Changes in renal function in cats following treatment of hyperthyroidism using 131I, *Vet Radiol Ultrasound* 38:231–238, 1997.

331. van Hoek I, Lefebvre HP, Peremans K, et al.: Short- and long-term follow-up of glomerular and tubular renal markers of kidney function in hyperthyroid cats after treatment with radioiodine, *Domest Anim Endocrinol* 36:45–56, 2009.

332. Peterson ME, Varela FV, Rishniw M, et al.: Evaluation of serum symmetric dimethylarginine concentration as a marker for masked chronic kidney disease in cats with hyperthyroidism, *J Vet Intern Med* 32:295–304, 2018.

333. Riensche MR, Graves TK, Schaeffer DJ: An investigation of predictors of renal insufficiency following treatment of hyperthyroidism in cats, *J Feline Med Surg* 10:160–166, 2008.

334. Williams TL, Peak KJ, Brodbelt D, et al.: Survival and the development of azotemia after treatment of hyperthyroid cats, *J Vet Intern Med* 24:863–869, 2010.

335. Kallet AJ, Richter KP, Feldman EC, et al.: Primary hyperparathyroidism in cats: seven cases (1984-1989), *J Am Vet Med Assoc* 199:1767–1771, 1991.

336. Barber PJ: Disorders of the parathyroid glands, *J Feline Med Surg* 6:259–269, 2004.

337. Feldman EC, Hoar B, Pollard R, et al.: Pretreatment clinical and laboratory findings in dogs with primary hyperparathyroidism: 210 cases (1987-2004), *J Am Vet Med Assoc* 227:756–761, 2005.

338. Gear RN, Neiger R, Skelly BJ, et al.: Primary hyperparathyroidism in 29 dogs: diagnosis, treatment, outcome and associated renal failure, *J Small Anim Pract* 46:10–16, 2005.

339. Rasor L, Pollard R, Feldman EC: Retrospective evaluation of three treatment methods for primary hyperparathyroidism in dogs, *J Am Anim Hosp Assoc* 43:70–77, 2007.

340. Feldman EC: Hypercalcemia and primary hyperparathyroidism. In Feldman EC, Nelson RW, Reusch CE, et al.: *Canine and feline endocrinology*, ed 4, St. Louis, 2015, Elsevier, pp 579–624.

341. Skelly BJ: Primary hyperparathyroidism. In Ettinger SJ, Feldman EC, Cote E, editors: *Textbook of veterinary internal medicine*, ed 8, St. Louis, 2017, Elsevier, pp 1715–1727.

342. Cavana P, Vittone V, Capucchio MT, et al.: Parathyroid adenocarcinoma in a nephropathic Persian cat, *J Feline Med Surg* 8:340–344, 2006.

343. Skelly BJ, Franklin RJ: Mutations in genes causing human familial isolated hyperparathyroidism do not account for hyperparathyroidism in Keeshond dogs, *Vet J* 174:652–654, 2007.

344. Sawyer ES, Northrup NC, Schmiedt CW, et al.: Outcome of 19 dogs with parathyroid carcinoma after surgical excision, *Vet Comp Oncol* 10:57–64, 2012.

345. Faucher MR, Freiche V, Bongrand Y, et al.: Primary hyperparathyroidism caused by a parathyroid carcinoma in a 16-year-old male neutered cat with concurrent chronic kidney disease, *Vet Q* 34:37–40, 2014.

346. Kishi EN, Holmes SP, Abbott JR, et al.: Functional metastatic parathyroid adenocarcinoma in a dog, *Can Vet J* 55:383–388, 2014.

347. Parker VJ, Gilor C, Chew DJ: Feline hyperparathyroidism: pathophysiology, diagnosis and treatment of primary and secondary disease, *J Feline Med Surg* 17:427–439, 2015.

348. Goldstein RE, Atwater DZ, Cazolli DM, et al.: Inheritance, mode of inheritance, and candidate genes for primary hyperparathyroidism in Keeshonden, *J Vet Intern Med* 21:199–203, 2007.

349. Schenck PA, Chew DJ: Prediction of serum ionized calcium concentration by use of serum total calcium concentration in dogs, *Am J Vet Res* 66:1330–1336, 2005.

350. Schenck PA, Chew DJ: Prediction of serum ionized calcium concentration by serum total calcium measurement in cats, *Can J Vet Res* 74:209–213, 2010.

351. Savary KC, Price GS, Vaden SL: Hypercalcemia in cats: a retrospective study of 71 cases (1991-1997), *J Vet Intern Med* 14:184–189, 2000.

352. Messinger JS, Windham WR, Ward CR: Ionized hypercalcemia in dogs: a retrospective study of 109 cases (1998-2003), *J Vet Intern Med* 23:514–519, 2009.

353. Feldman EC, Wisner ER, Nelson RW, et al.: Comparison of results of hormonal analysis of samples obtained from selected venous sites versus cervical ultrasonography for localizing parathyroid masses in dogs, *J Am Vet Med Assoc* 211:54–56, 1997.

354. Sueda MT, Stefanacci JD: Ultrasound evaluation of the parathyroid glands in two hypercalcemic cats, *Vet Radiol Ultrasound* 41:448–451, 2000.

355. Liles SR, Linder KE, Cain B, et al.: Ultrasonography of histologically normal parathyroid glands and thyroid lobules in normocalcemic dogs, *Vet Radiol Ultrasound* 51:447–452, 2010.

356. Matwichuk CL, Taylor SM, Daniel GB, et al.: Double-phase parathyroid scintigraphy in dogs using technetium-99M-sestamibi, *Vet Radiol Ultrasound* 41:461–469, 2000.

357. Ham K, Greenfield CL, Barger A, et al.: Validation of a rapid parathyroid hormone assay and intraoperative measurement of parathyroid hormone in dogs with benign naturally occurring primary hyperparathyroidism, *Vet Surg* 38:122–132, 2009.

358. Chew DJ, Nagode LA, Schenck PA: Treatment of hypoparathyroidism. In Bonagura JD, Twedt DC, editors: *Kirk's current veterinary therapy XIV*, St. Louis, 2009, Saunders Elsevier, pp 241–247.

359. Armstrong AJ, Hauptman JG, Stanley BJ, et al.: Effect of prophylactic calcitriol administration on serum ionized calcium concentrations after parathyroidectomy: 78 cases (2005-2015), *J Vet Intern Med* 32:99–106, 2018.

360. Dear JD, Kass PH, Della Maggiore AM, et al.: Association of hypercalcemia before treatment with hypocalcemia after treatment in dogs with primary hyperparathyroidism, *J Vet Intern Med* 31:349–354, 2017.

361. Milovancev M, Schmiedt CW: Preoperative factors associated with postoperative hypocalcemia in dogs with primary hyperparathyroidism that underwent parathyroidectomy: 62 cases (2004-2009), *J Am Vet Med Assoc* 507–515, 2013.

362. Arbaugh M, Smeak D, Monnet E: Evaluation of preoperative serum concentrations of ionized calcium and parathyroid hormone as predictors of hypocalcemia following parathyroidectomy in dogs with primary hyperparathyroidism: 17 cases (2001-2009), *J Am Vet Med Assoc* 241:233–236, 2012.

363. Reinhart JM, Nuth EK, Byers CG, et al.: Pre-operative fibrous osteodystrophy and severe, refractory, post-operative hypocalcemia following parathyroidectomy in a dog, *Can Vet J* 56:867–871, 2015.

364. Witteveen JE, van Thiel S, Romijn JA, et al.: Hungry bone syndrome: still a challenge in the post-operative management of primary hyperparathyroidism: a systematic review of the literature, *Eur J Endocrinol* 168:R45–53, 2013.

365. Lee IT, Sheu WH, Tu ST, et al.: Bisphosphonate pretreatment attenuates hungry bone syndrome postoperatively in subjects with primary hyperparathyroidism, *J Bone Miner Metab* 24:255–258, 2006.

366. Mahajan A, Narayanan M, Jaffers G, et al.: Hypoparathyroidism associated with severe mineral bone disease postrenal transplantation, treated successfully with recombinant PTH, *Hemodial Int* 13:547–550, 2009.

367. Graham KJ, Wilkinson M, Culvenor J, et al.: Intraoperative parathyroid hormone concentration to confirm removal of hypersecretory parathyroid tissue and time to postoperative normocalcaemia in nine dogs with primary hyperparathyroidism, *Aust Vet J* 90:203–209, 2012.

368. Pollard RE, Long CD, Nelson RW, et al.: Percutaneous ultrasonographically guided radiofrequency heat ablation for treatment of primary hyperparathyroidism in dogs, *J Am Vet Med Assoc* 218:1106–1110, 2001.

369. Bucy D, Pollard R, Nelson R: Analysis of factors affecting outcome of ultrasound-guided radiofrequency heat ablation for treatment of primary hyperparathyroidism in dogs, *Vet Radiol Ultrasound* 58:83–89, 2017.

370. Long CD, Goldstein RE, Hornof WJ, et al.: Percutaneous ultrasound-guided chemical parathyroid ablation for treatment of primary hyperparathyroidism in dogs, *J Am Vet Med Assoc* 215:217–221, 1999.

371. Guttin T, Knox VWt, Diroff JS: Outcomes for dogs with primary hyperparathyroidism following treatment with percutaneous ultrasound-guided ethanol ablation of presumed functional parathyroid nodules: 27 cases (2008-2011), *J Am Vet Med Assoc* 247:771–777, 2015.

372. Batcher E, Madaj P, Gianoukakis AG: Pancreatic neuroendocrine tumors, *Endocr Res* 36:35–43, 2011.

373. Schaub S, Wigger A: Ultrasound-aided diagnosis of an insulinoma in a cat, *Tierarztl Prax Ausg K Kleintiere Heimtiere* 41:338–342, 2013.

374. Jackson TC, Debey B, Lindbloom-Hawley S, et al.: Cellular and molecular characterization of a feline insulinoma, *J Vet Intern Med* 23:383–387, 2009.

375. Nelson RW: Beta-cell neoplasia: insulinoma. In Feldman EC, Nelson RW, Reusch CE, et al.: *Canine and feline endocrinology*, ed 4, St. Louis, 2015, Elsevier, pp 348–375.

376. Hawkins KL, Summers BA, Kuhajda FP, et al.: Immunocytochemistry of normal pancreatic islets and spontaneous islet cell tumors in dogs, *Vet Pathol* 24:170–179, 1987.

377. Myers 3rd NC, Andrews GA, Chard-Bergstrom C: Chromogranin A plasma concentration and expression in pancreatic islet cell tumors of dogs and cats, *Am J Vet Res* 58:615–620, 1997.

378. Minkus G, Jutting U, Aubele M, et al.: Canine neuroendocrine tumors of the pancreas: a study using image analysis techniques for the discrimination of metastatic versus nonmetastatic tumors, *Vet Pathol* 34:138–145, 1997.

379. Madarame H, Kayanuma H, Shida T, et al.: Retrospective study of canine insulinomas: eight cases (2005-2008), *J Vet Med Sci* 71:905–911, 2009.

380. Buishand FO, van Erp MG, Groenveld HA, et al.: Expression of insulin-like growth factor-1 by canine insulinomas and their metastases, *Vet J*, 2011.

381. Buishand FO, Kirpensteijn J, Jaarsma AA, et al.: Gene expression profiling of primary canine insulinomas and their metastases, *Vet J* 197:192–197, 2013.

382. Buishand FO, Kik M, Kirpensteijn J: Evaluation of clinico-pathological criteria and the Ki67 index as prognostic indicators in canine insulinoma, *Vet J* 185:62–67, 2010.

383. Leifer CE, Peterson ME, Matus RE: Insulin-secreting tumor: diagnosis and medical and surgical management in 55 dogs, *J Am Vet Med Assoc* 188:60–64, 1986.

384. Caywood DD, Klausner JS, O'Leary TP, et al.: Pancreatic insulin-secreting neoplasms: clinical, diagnostic, and prognostic features in 73 dogs, *J Am Anim Hosp Assoc* 24:577–584, 1988.

385. Steiner JM, Bruyette DS: Canine insulinoma, *Compend Contin Educ Vet* 18:13–25, 1996.

386. Trifonidou MA, Kirpensteijn J, Robben JH: A retrospective evaluation of 51 dogs with insulinoma, *Vet Q* 20(Suppl 1):S114–115, 1998.

387. Tobin RL, Nelson RW, Lucroy MD, et al.: Outcome of surgical versus medical treatment of dogs with beta cell neoplasia: 39 cases (1990-1997), *J Am Vet Med Assoc* 215:226–230, 1999.

388. Robben JH, Visser-Wisselaar HA, Rutteman GR, et al.: In vitro and in vivo detection of functional somatostatin receptors in canine insulinomas, *J Nucl Med* 38:1036–1042, 1997.

389. Robben JH, Van Garderen E, Mol JA, et al.: Locally produced growth hormone in canine insulinomas, *Mol Cell Endocrinol* 197:187–195, 2002.

390. Schermerhorn T: Canine insulinoma as a model for studying molecular genetics of tumorigenesis and metastasis, *Vet J* 197:126–127, 2013.

391. Buishand FO, Visser J, Kik M, et al.: Evaluation of prognostic indicators using validated canine insulinoma tissue microarrays, *Vet J* 201:57–63, 2014.

392. Polton GA, White RN, Brearley MJ, et al.: Improved survival in a retrospective cohort of 28 dogs with insulinoma, *J Small Anim Pract* 48:151–156, 2007.

393. Shahar R, Rousseaux C, Steiss J: Peripheral polyneuropathy in a dog with functional islet B-cell tumor and widespread metastasis, *J Am Vet Med Assoc* 187:175–177, 1985.

394. Braund KG, McGuire JA, Amling KA, et al.: Peripheral neuropathy associated with malignant neoplasms in dogs, *Vet Pathol* 24:16–21, 1987.

395. Braund KG, Steiss JE, Amling KA, et al.: Insulinoma and subclinical peripheral neuropathy in two dogs, *J Vet Intern Med* 1:86–90, 1987.

396. Schrauwen E: Clinical peripheral polyneuropathy associated with canine insulinoma, *Vet Rec* 128:211–212, 1991.

397. Van Ham L, Braund KG, Roels S, et al.: Treatment of a dog with an insulinoma-related peripheral polyneuropathy with corticosteroids, *Vet Rec* 141:98–100, 1997.

398. Shimada A, Morita T, Ikeda N, et al.: Hypoglycaemic brain lesions in a dog with insulinoma, *J Comp Pathol* 122:67–71, 2000.

399. Fukazawa K, Kayanuma H, Kanai E, et al.: Insulinoma with basal ganglion involvement detected by magnetic resonance imaging in a dog, *J Vet Med Sci* 71:689–692, 2009.

400. Siliart B, Stambouli F: Laboratory diagnosis of insulinoma in the dog: a retrospective study and a new diagnostic procedure, *J Small Anim Pract* 37:367–370, 1996.

401. Goutal CM, Brugmann BL, Ryan KA: Insulinoma in dogs: a review, *J Am Anim Hosp Assoc* 48:151–163, 2012.

402. Thoresen SI, Aleksandersen M, Lonaas L, et al.: Pancreatic insulin-secreting carcinoma in a dog: fructosamine for determining persistent hypoglycaemia, *J Small Anim Pract* 36:282–286, 1995.

403. Elliott DA, Nelson RW, Feldman EC, et al.: Glycosylated hemoglobin concentrations in the blood of healthy dogs and dogs with naturally developing diabetes mellitus, pancreatic beta-cell neoplasia, hyperadrenocorticism, and anemia, *J Am Vet Med Assoc* 211:723–727, 1997.

404. Loste A, Marca MC, Perez M, et al.: Clinical value of fructosamine measurements in non-healthy dogs, *Vet Res Commun* 25(109–115), 2001.

405. Mellanby RJ, Herrtage ME: Insulinoma in a normoglycaemic dog with low serum fructosamine, *J Small Anim Pract* 43:506–508, 2002.

406. Lamb CR, Simpson KW, Boswood A, et al.: Ultrasonography of pancreatic neoplasia in the dog: a retrospective review of 16 cases, *Vet Rec* 137:65–68, 1995.

407. Robben JH, Pollak YW, Kirpensteijn J, et al.: Comparison of ultrasonography, computed tomography, and single-photon emission computed tomography for the detection and localization of canine insulinoma, *J Vet Intern Med* 19:15–22, 2005.

408. Ekeblad S: Islet cell tumours, *Adv Exp Med Biol* 654:771–789, 2010.

409. Gaschen L, Kircher P, Lang J: Endoscopic ultrasound instrumentation, applications in humans, and potential veterinary applications, *Vet Radiol Ultrasound* 44:665–680, 2003.

410. Gaschen L, Kircher P, Wolfram K: Endoscopic ultrasound of the canine abdomen, *Vet Radiol Ultrasound* 48:338–349, 2007.

411. Haers H, Saunders JH: Review of clinical characteristics and applications of contrast-enhanced ultrasonography in dogs, *J Am Vet Med Assoc* 234:460–470, 2009. 430.

412. Johnson-Neitman JL, O'Brien RT, Wallace JD: Quantitative perfusion analysis of the pancreas and duodenum in healthy dogs by use of contrast-enhanced ultrasonography, *Am J Vet Res* 73:385–392, 2012.

413. Lim SY, Nakamura K, Morishita K, et al.: Qualitative and quantitative contrast enhanced ultrasonography of the pancreas using bolus injection and continuous infusion methods in normal dogs, *J Vet Med Sci* 75:1601–1607, 2013.

414. Rademacher N, Schur D, Gaschen F, et al.: Contrast-enhanced ultrasonography of the pancreas in healthy dogs and in dogs with acute pancreatitis, *Vet Radiol Ultrasound* 57:58–64, 2016.

415. Lim SY, Nakamura K, Morishita K, et al.: Qualitative and quantitative contrast-enhanced ultrasonographic assessment of cerulein-induced acute pancreatitis in dogs, *J Vet Intern Med* 28:496–503, 2014.

416. Lim SY, Nakamura K, Morishita K, et al.: Quantitative contrast-enhanced ultrasonographic assessment of naturally occurring pancreatitis in dogs, *J Vet Intern Med* 29:71–78, 2015.

417. Vanderperren K, Haers H, Van der Vekens E, et al.: Description of the use of contrast-enhanced ultrasonography in four dogs with pancreatic tumours, *J Small Anim Pract* 55:164–169, 2014.

418. Nakamura K, Lim SY, Ochiai K, et al.: Contrast-enhanced ultrasonographic findings in three dogs with pancreatic insulinoma, *Vet Radiol Ultrasound* 56:55–62, 2015.

419. Iseri T, Yamada K, Chijiwa K, et al.: Dynamic computed tomography of the pancreas in normal dogs and in a dog with pancreatic insulinoma, *Vet Radiol Ultrasound* 48:328–331, 2007.

420. Mai W, Caceres AV: Dual-phase computed tomographic angiography in three dogs with pancreatic insulinoma, *Vet Radiol Ultrasound* 49:141–148, 2008.

421. Fukushima K, Fujiwara R, Yamamoto K, et al.: Characterization of triple-phase computed tomography in dogs with pancreatic insulinoma, *J Vet Med Sci* 77:1549–1553, 2016.

422. Lester NV, Newell SM, Hill RC, et al.: Scintigraphic diagnosis of insulinoma in a dog, *Vet Radiol Ultrasound* 40:174–178, 1999.

423. Garden OA, Reubi JC, Dykes NL, et al.: Somatostatin receptor imaging in vivo by planar scintigraphy facilitates the diagnosis of canine insulinomas, *J Vet Intern Med* 19:168–176, 2005.

424. Sundin A, Garske U, Orlefors H: Nuclear imaging of neuroendocrine tumours, *Best Pract Res Clin Endocrinol Metab* 21:69–85, 2007.

425. Fischer JR, Smith SA, Harkin KR: Glucagon constant-rate infusion: a novel strategy for the management of hyperinsulinemic-hypoglycemic crisis in the dog, *J Am Anim Hosp Assoc* 36:27–32, 2000.

426. Datte K, Guillaumin J, Barrett S, et al.: Retrospective evaluation of the use of glucagon infusion as adjunctive therapy for hypoglycemia in dogs: 9 cases (2005-2014), *J Vet Emerg Crit Care* 26:775–781, 2016.

427. McClaran JK, Pavia P, Fischetti AJ, et al.: Laparoscopic resection of a pancreatic beta cell tumor in a dog, *J Am Anim Hosp Assoc* 53:338–345, 2017.

428. Wouters EG, Buishand FO, Kik M, et al.: Use of a bipolar vessel-sealing device in resection of canine insulinoma, *J Small Anim Pract* 52:139–145, 2011.

429. de Brito Galvao JF, Chew DJ: Metabolic complications of endocrine surgery in companion animals, *Vet Clin North Am Small Anim Pract* 41:847–868, 2011.

430. Cordner AP, Sharkey LC, Armstrong PJ, et al.: Cytologic findings and diagnostic yield in 92 dogs undergoing fine-needle aspiration of the pancreas, *J Vet Diagn Invest* 27:236–240, 2015.

431. Moore AR, Chu C, Singh K, et al.: What is your diagnosis? Liver aspirate from a hypoglycemic dog, *Vet Clin Pathol* 44:463–464, 2015.

432. Moore AS, Nelson RW, Henry CJ, et al.: Streptozocin for treatment of pancreatic islet cell tumors in dogs: 17 cases (1989-1999), *J Am Vet Med Assoc* 221:811–818, 2002.

433. Bell R, Mooney CT, Mansfield CS, et al.: Treatment of insulinoma in a springer spaniel with streptozotocin, *J Small Anim Pract* 46:247–250, 2005.

434. Northrup NC, Rassnick KM, Gieger TL, et al.: Prospective evaluation of biweekly streptozotocin in 19 dogs with insulinoma, *J Vet Intern Med* 27:483–490, 2013.

435. Schoeman JP: Insulin-secreting tumors. In Ettinger SJ, Feldman EC, Cote E, editors: *Textbook of veterinary internal medicine*, ed 8, St. Louis, 2017, Elsevier, pp 1762–1767.

436. Robben JH, van den Brom WE, Mol JA, et al.: Effect of octreotide on plasma concentrations of glucose, insulin, glucagon, growth hormone, and cortisol in healthy dogs and dogs with insulinoma, *Res Vet Sci* 80:25–32, 2006.

437. McMillan FD, Barr B, Feldman EC: Functional pancreatic islet cell tumor in a cat, *J Am Anim Hosp Assoc* 21:741–746, 1985.

438. O'Brien TD, Norton F, Turner TM, et al.: Pancreatic endocrine tumor in a cat: clinical, pathological, and immunohistochemical evaluation, *J Am Anim Hosp Assoc* 26:453–457, 1990.

439. Hawks D, Peterson ME, Hawkins KL, et al.: Insulin-secreting pancreatic (islet cell) carcinoma in a cat, *J Vet Intern Med* 6:193–196, 1992.

440. Kraje AC: Hypoglycemia and irreversible neurologic complications in a cat with insulinoma, *J Am Vet Med Assoc* 223:812–814, 2003.

441. Greene SN, Bright RM: Insulinoma in a cat, *J Small Anim Pract* 49:38–40, 2008.

442. Feldman EC, Nelson RW: Gastrinoma, glucagonoma, and other APUDomas. In Feldman EC, Nelson RW, editors: *Canine and feline endocrinology and reproduction*, ed 3, St. Louis, 2004, Saunders, pp 645–658.

443. Schermerhorn T: Gastrointestinal endocrinology. In Ettinger SJ, Feldman EC, Cote E, editors: *Textbook of veterinary internal medicine*, ed 8, St. Louis, 2017, Elsevier, pp 1833–1838.

444. Vergine M, Pozzo S, Pogliani E, et al.: Common bile duct obstruction due to a duodenal gastrinoma in a dog, *Vet J* 170:141–143, 2005.

445. Shaw DH: Gastrinoma (Zollinger-Ellison syndrome) in the dog and cat, *Can Vet J* 29:448–452, 1988.

446. Green RA, Gartrell CL: Gastrinoma: a retrospective study of four cases (1985-1995), *J Am Anim Hosp Assoc* 33:524–527, 1997.

447. Simpson KW, Dykes NL: Diagnosis and treatment of gastrinoma, *Semin Vet Med Surg (Small Anim)* 12:274–281, 1997.

448. Brooks D, Watson GL: Omeprazole in a dog with gastrinoma, *J Vet Intern Med* 11:379–381, 1997.

449. Liptak JM, Hunt GB, Barrs VR, et al.: Gastroduodenal ulceration in cats: eight cases and a review of the literature, *J Feline Med Surg* 4:27–42, 2002.

450. Fukushima R, Ichikawa K, Hirabayashi M, et al.: A case of canine gastrinoma, *J Vet Med Sci* 66:993–995, 2004.

451. Fukushima U, Sato M, Okano S, et al.: A case of gastrinoma in a Shih-Tzu dog, *J Vet Med Sci* 66:311–313, 2004.

452. Hughes SM: Canine gastrinoma: a case study and literature review of therapeutic options, *N Z Vet J* 54:242–247, 2006.

453. Diroff JS, Sanders NA, McDonough SP, et al.: Gastrin-secreting neoplasia in a cat, *J Vet Intern Med* 20:1245–1247, 2006.

454. Gal A, Ridgway MD, Fredrickson RL: An unusual clinical presentation of a dog with gastrinoma, *Can Vet J* 52:641–644, 2011.

455. Altschul M, Simpson KW, Dykes NL, et al.: Evaluation of somatostatin analogues for the detection and treatment of gastrinoma in a dog, *J Small Anim Pract* 38:286–291, 1997.

456. McLeland SM, Lunn KF, Duncan CG, et al.: Relationship among serum creatinine, serum gastrin, calcium-phosphorus product, and uremic gastropathy in cats with chronic kidney disease, *J Vet Intern Med* 28:827–837, 2014.

457. Mordecai A, Sellon RK, Mealey KL: Normal dogs treated with famotidine for 14 days have only transient increases in serum gastrin concentrations, *J Vet Intern Med* 25:1248–1252, 2011.

458. Parente NL, Bari Olivier N, Refsal KR, et al.: Serum concentrations of gastrin after famotidine and omeprazole administration to dogs, *J Vet Intern Med* 28:1465–1470, 2014.

459. Tolbert MK, Graham A, Odunayo A, et al.: Repeated famotidine administration results in a diminished effect on intragastric pH in dogs, *J Vet Intern Med* 31:117–123, 2017.

460. Heilmann RM, Berghoff N, Grutzner N, et al.: Effect of gastric acid-suppressive therapy and biological variation of serum gastrin concentrations in dogs with chronic enteropathies, *BMC Vet Res* 13:321, 2017.

461. Lurye JC, Behrend EN: Endocrine tumors, *Vet Clin North Am Small Anim Pract* 31:1083–1110, 2001.

462. Ward CR: Gastrointestinal endocrine disease. In Ettinger SJ, Feldman EC, editors: *Textbook of veterinary internal medicine*, ed 7, St. Louis, 2010, Saunders Elsevier, pp 1857–1865.

463. Lothrop CD: Medical treatment of neuroendocrine tumors of the gastroenteropancreatic system with somatostatin. In Kirk RW, editor: *Current veterinary therapy X*, Philadelphia, 1989, W. B. Saunders, pp 1020–1024.

464. Kim S, Hosoya K, Takagi S, et al.: Treatment of gastrin-secreting tumor with sustained-release octreotide acetate in a dog, *J Am Anim Hosp Assoc* 51:407–412, 2015.

465. Hughes AM, Bannasch DL, Kellett K, et al.: Examination of candidate genes for hypoadrenocorticism in Nova Scotia Duck Tolling Retrievers, *Vet J* 187:212–216, 2011.

466. Asakawa MG, Cullen JM, Linder KE: Necrolytic migratory erythema associated with a glucagon-producing primary hepatic neuroendocrine carcinoma in a cat, *Vet Dermatol* 24:466–469, 2013.

467. Gross TL, O'Brien TD, Davies AP, et al.: Glucagon-producing pancreatic endocrine tumors in two dogs with superficial necrolytic dermatitis, *J Am Vet Med Assoc* 197:1619–1622, 1990.

468. Allenspach K, Arnold P, Glaus T, et al.: Glucagon-producing neuroendocrine tumour associated with hypoaminoacidaemia and skin lesions, *J Small Anim Pract* 41:402–406, 2000.

469. Langer NB, Jergens AE, Miles KG: Canine glucagonoma, *Compend Contin Educ Vet* 25:56–63, 2003.

470. Mizuno T, Hiraoka H, Yoshioka C, et al.: Superficial necrolytic dermatitis associated with extrapancreatic glucagonoma in a dog, *Vet Dermatol* 20:72–79, 2009.

471. Oberkirchner U, Linder KE, Zadrozny L, et al.: Successful treatment of canine necrolytic migratory erythema (superficial necrolytic dermatitis) due to metastatic glucagonoma with octreotide, *Vet Dermatol* 21:510–516, 2010.

472. Torres SM, Caywood DD, O'Brien TD, et al.: Resolution of superficial necrolytic dermatitis following excision of a glucagon-secreting pancreatic neoplasm in a dog, *J Am Anim Hosp Assoc* 33:313–319, 1997.

473. Rossmeisl Jr JH, Forrester SD, Robertson JL, et al.: Chronic vomiting associated with a gastric carcinoid in a cat, *J Am Anim Hosp Assoc* 38:61–66, 2002.

474. Morrell CN, Volk MV, Mankowski JL: A carcinoid tumor in the gallbladder of a dog, *Vet Pathol* 39:756–758, 2002.

475. Sako T, Uchida E, Okamoto M, et al.: Immunohistochemical evaluation of a malignant intestinal carcinoid in a dog, *Vet Pathol* 40:212–215, 2003.

476. Lippo NJ, Williams JE, Brawer RS, et al.: Acute hemobilia and hemocholecyst in 2 dogs with gallbladder carcinoid, *J Vet Intern Med* 22:1249–1252, 2008.

477. Tappin S, Brown P, Ferasin L: An intestinal neuroendocrine tumour associated with paroxysmal ventricular tachycardia and melaena in a 10-year-old boxer, *J Small Anim Pract* 49:33–37, 2008.

478. Baker SG, Mayhew PD, Mehler SJ: Choledochotomy and primary repair of extrahepatic biliary duct rupture in seven dogs and two cats, *J Small Anim Pract* 52:32–37, 2011.

479. Spugnini EP, Gargiulo M, Assin R, et al.: Adjuvant carboplatin for the treatment of intestinal carcinoid in a dog, *Vivo* 22:759–761, 2008.

27

Tumors of the Female Reproductive System

COREY F. SABA AND JESSICA A. LAWRENCE

Ovarian Tumors

Incidence

Ovarian tumors are uncommon in dogs and cats, resulting in part from the routine practice of ovariohysterectomy (OHE) in many areas of the world. The overall reported prevalence in dogs is 0.5% to 1.2%,[1–3] with an estimated prevalence of 6.25% in intact females.[4] Ovarian tumors are equally rare in cats, with a reported prevalence of 0.7% to 3.6% in intact females.[5,6] These numbers are derived primarily from pathology surveys and likely overestimate the true incidence in the pet population. Breed predilections are also difficult to discern; however, German shepherd dogs, boxers, Yorkshire terriers, poodles, and Boston terriers appear to be most commonly affected.[2,7,8] Aside from germ cell tumors and specifically teratomas, most ovarian tumors develop in older dogs (approximately 6 years of age and older).[2,7–9] Teratomas are often found in younger dogs (≤6 years of age).[7,8,10,11] Ovarian tumors have been reported in cats ranging from less than 1 year to 20 years (mean age: 6.7 years).[12–15]

Pathology and Natural Behavior

Canine Ovarian Tumors

Owing to the complexity of the canine ovary, a variety of histologic tumor types may occur. Historically, canine ovarian tumors have been classified based on the World Health Organization (WHO) classification scheme for human ovarian tumors, with primary tumor types including epithelial tumors, germ cell tumors, sex cord stromal (gonadostromal) tumors, and mesenchymal tumors.[2,8,16,17] Later, the human WHO classification system was revised to subdivide each of the aforementioned categories into histologic types based on morphologic similarities; the use of immunohistochemistry has aided in further differentiating ovarian tumors.[18] Attempts to recapitulate such classification schemes in dogs have been reported, but are not routinely employed.[19,20]

Epithelial Tumors

Epithelial tumors arise from the outer surface of the ovary[9,21] and according to several reports are most common.[2,8,16] Malignant tumors outnumber benign tumors,[7,8,16] and larger size is suggestive of malignancy.[8,16] Malignant histologies include papillary

adenocarcinomas, tubular adenocarcinomas, and undifferentiated carcinomas; benign tumors such as rete adenomas, papillary adenomas, and cystadenomas also occur.[2,8,16] Reportedly, 48% of adenocarcinomas will metastasize, generally within the peritoneal cavity to the intraabdominal lymph nodes, omentum, and liver.[8] Direct tumor cell implantation and subsequent malignant effusion may also occur.[3,8] Although most are unilateral, bilateral epithelial ovarian tumors have been described.[8] Cysts in the contralateral ovary and cystic endometrial hyperplasia may also be found.

Epithelial ovarian tumors routinely express cytokeratin AE1/AE3 (CK AE1/AE3), vimentin, and desmin.[19,20] Although papillary adenocarcinomas also demonstrate placental alkaline phosphatase (PLAP) and cytokeratin 7 (CK7) immunoreactivity, positive immunoreactivity appears to be less frequent in tubular adenocarcinomas.[19] Alpha-fetoprotein (AFP),[19] S-100,[19] and endothelin-A (ET-A)[22] are variably expressed. Faint to strong intracytoplasmic cyclooxygenase-2 (COX-2)[23] and endothelin-1 (ET-1)[22] immunoreactivity has been reported in 81% and 83% of canine ovarian carcinomas, respectively. Inhibin-alpha (INH-α), a glycopeptide synthesized in gonadal cells of the ovaries, inhibits pituitary secretion of follicle-stimulating hormone (FSH), and it has been described as a sensitive and specific marker for granulosa-theca cell tumor (GTCT).[24] Therefore epithelial tumor cells should not express INH-α, and demonstration of INH-α expression has resulted in reclassification of epithelial tumors as GTCT.[20] The immunohistochemical marker HBME-1 (Hector Battifora mesothelial epitope) has been used in human medicine to aid in the diagnosis of epithelial ovarian tumors. Results from a study in canine ovaries and ovarian tumors suggest that HBME-1 may be of similar value in dogs.[25]

Sex Cord Stromal Tumors

Sex cord stromal tumors, specifically GTCT, are likely second in occurrence to epithelial tumors. Less common histologies include Sertoli–Leydig tumors, thecomas, and luteomas. These tumors arise from the specialized estrogen- and progesterone-producing gonadal stroma of the ovary and therefore have the potential to secrete these steroid hormones if functional.[3,4,8,16] The metastatic rate of GTCT is low, occurring in approximately 20% of cases.[3,8,9,16] Metastatic sites include sublumbar lymph nodes, pancreas, and lungs, with peritoneal carcinomatosis noted in some

597

cases.[1,3,8,16] Although rare, thecomas and luteomas are for the most part considered benign.[8,16]

Although most sex cord stromal tumors are unilateral, bilateral tumors are possible, especially among Sertoli–Leydig tumors.[8] Concomitant cystic endometrial hyperplasia and cysts in the contralateral ovary appear common within this group.[8]

Solid, nest, cord, palisade, cystic, and spindle are the histologic patterns described for GTCT, and a mixture of these may exist within a single tumor.[8,19] GTCTs are generally vimentin,[19] S-100,[19] and INH-α[20] positive, although one study has reported INH-α–negative GTCT.[19] Variable expression of CK AE1/AE3,[20] CK 7,[20] and ET-A[22] has been described. Moderate-to-strong intracytoplasmic ET-1 immunoreactivity has been detected in 88% of canine GTCT, [22] whereas GTCT should be HBME-1 negative.[25]

Germ Cell Tumors

Germ cell tumors, including dysgerminomas, teratomas, and malignant teratomas (teratocarcinomas), arise from primordial germ cells of the ovary.[8,16,26] Concurrent cysts in the contralateral ovary and uterine abnormalities such as pyometra and cystic endometrial hyperplasia are common.[26]

Dysgerminomas, also known as *ovarian seminomas*, are most common in this group and arise from undifferentiated germ cells. Histologically, these tumors consist of a uniform population of cells resembling ovarian primordial germ cells.[3,8,16] Bilateral dysgerminomas have been reported; however, most are unilateral.[8,16,26] The reported metastatic rate is low (10%–30%), with sites of metastasis including lymph nodes, liver, kidney, omentum, pancreas, and adrenal glands.[3,8,9,26–28]

Teratomas are composed of germ cells that undergo differentiation into at least two germinal cell layers and any combination of tissues can be seen. These tissues are usually well differentiated, and tissues from virtually any organ (excluding ovary or testis) may be present. Malignant teratomas are composed of predominantly immature, undifferentiated tissues resembling those of the embryo.[26] Metastasis has been noted in up to 50%. Although distant visceral metastasis can occur, peritoneal metastasis with carcinomatosis is most common.[8,9,26]

Germ cell tumors, specifically dysgerminomas, are vimentin positive and PLAP, CK7, desmin, S-100, CK AE1/AE3, and INH-α negative.[19]

Mesenchymal Tumors

Mesenchymal ovarian tumors are rare. Reported tumor types include hemangiosarcoma,[2,16] hemangioma,[16] and leiomyoma.[2,16] Behavior of this group is difficult to predict because information in the literature is sparse.

Miscellaneous

In addition to the various primary ovarian tumors, other differential diagnoses should be considered. These include ovarian cysts, paraovarian cysts, cystic rete tubules, vascular hamartomas, and adenomatous hyperplasia of the rete ovarii. Although rare, metastasis to the ovary has been reported in cases of mammary (especially inflammatory carcinoma),[29] intestinal and pancreatic carcinoma, and lymphoma.[16]

Feline Ovarian Tumors

Reported feline ovarian tumor classifications include epithelial, germ cell, and sex cord stromal tumors. Although mesenchymal ovarian tumors have not been reported in cats, it seems plausible that they may occur. Ovarian involvement with lymphoma has been documented.[15]

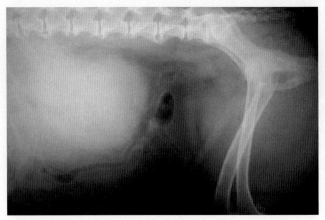

• **Fig. 27.1** Right lateral caudal abdominal radiograph of a dog with an ovarian tumor. (Courtesy Dr. T. Schwarz, University of Edinburgh.)

Sex cord stromal tumors are most common in cats, accounting for at least half of reported cases. They are often unilateral. Of these, GTCTs are most common and approximately 50% are malignant. Metastatic sites include the peritoneum, regional lymph nodes, omentum, diaphragm, kidney, spleen, liver, and lungs.[15] Luteomas, thecomas, and Sertoli–Leydig cell tumors are rare and typically benign.

Germ cell tumors are also rare in cats. Of these, dysgerminomas are most common.[15] They are generally considered benign, yet metastasis has been reported in 20% to 33% of cases.[15] Teratomas have been rarely documented.[15,30] A malignant estrogen-producing teratoma has been reported in a cat.[31]

Epithelial tumors are perhaps the least common ovarian tumor in the cat. Cystadenomas and adenocarcinomas have been described. Metastasis to the lungs, liver, and abdominal peritoneum was seen in one case of ovarian adenocarcinoma.[15]

History and Clinical Signs

Canine Ovarian Tumors

History and clinical signs associated with canine ovarian tumors vary, depending on the tissue of origin. Although initially insidious, ovarian tumors grow to the point of being palpable and clinical signs are typically referable to a space-occupying abdominal mass (Fig. 27.1).[9,32–34] Functional sex cord stromal tumors may produce one or multiple hormones, or they may be nonfunctional.[8,16,35] Sex cord stromal tumors that produce steroid hormones, such as estrogen, may cause vulvar enlargement, sanguineous vulvar discharge, persistent estrus, alopecia, and aplastic pancytopenia; whereas excessive progesterone production may cause cystic endometrial hyperplasia and pyometra.[3,8,9,16,33] Hyperadrenocorticism was reported in a dog with an ovarian-steroid tumor resembling a luteoma, and the associated clinical signs resolved after OHE.[36] Germ cell tumors have been associated with evidence of hormonal dysfunction, although they are most often associated with clinical signs referable to a space-occupying abdominal mass.[26]

Feline Ovarian Tumors

Ovarian tumors in cats also have an insidious onset and eventually grow to the point of being detectable by abdominal palpation. Signs referable to a space-occupying abdominal mass such as weight loss, lethargy, vomiting, ascites, and abdominal distension are often noted. GTCTs are most common, and they are generally functional, producing estrogen, progesterone, or testosterone. Clinical signs of hyperestrogenism, including persistent estrus,

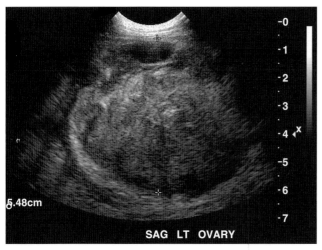

• **Fig. 27.2** A large, irregularly shaped mixed echogenic left ovarian mass identified on abdominal ultrasound. The mass was histologically consistent with a granulosa cell tumor. (Courtesy Dr. D. Jimenez, University of Georgia.)

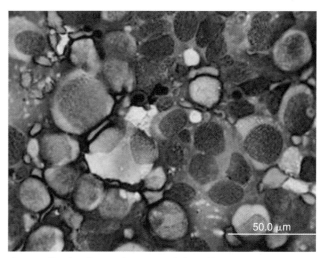

• **Fig. 27.3** Ovarian dysgerminoma population of highly pleomorphic round cells. These cells have a scant amount of lightly basophilic cytoplasm and round to irregularly shaped nuclei with a coarsely granular to smudged chromatin pattern with occasional indistinct nucleoli. Binucleated and multinucleated cells are seen and occasional micronuclei are observed. There is moderate-to-marked anisocytosis and anisokaryosis. (Courtesy Dr. M. Camus, University of Georgia.)

alopecia, and endometrial hyperplasia, have been reported.[15] Virilizing behavior secondary to a testosterone-producing thecoma of the ovarian stump was reported in a 6-year-old domestic shorthair cat.[37]

Diagnostic Techniques and Workup

Laboratory abnormalities attributable to ovarian tumors are generally not noted. However, hypercalcemia secondary to tumor production of parathyroid hormone–related peptide (PTH-rP) has been reported in a dog with ovarian adenocarcinoma.[34] Thoracic radiographs should be evaluated for evidence of metastatic disease. Abdominal imaging, specifically ultrasound, is useful in identifying ovarian masses and associated abdominal metastasis or uterine abnormalities (Fig. 27.2). Ultrasonographic patterns include solid, solid with cystic component, and cystic[38]. Malignant tumors are typically solid, whereas benign tumors are generally cystic with smooth borders.[38] Concurrent uterine abnormalities such as pyometra and cystic endometrial hyperplasia may be detectable via ultrasound in up to 50% of dogs.[38] Because the risk of tumor seeding is high, transabdominal needle biopsies of ovarian tumors are not recommended. If present, abdominal fluid may be safely collected, and cytologic evaluation of fluid often is suggestive of malignant effusions. In a series of 19 cases with a variety of ovarian tumors, cytologic diagnosis was consistent with histopathology in 94.7% of cases (Fig. 27.3).[2] Finally, if a functional tumor is suspected, evaluation of vaginal cytology for evidence of estrogen-induced cornification is also indicated.

Therapy

Complete OHE is the treatment of choice for most localized ovarian tumors. Standard oncologic surgical principles must be practiced to minimize tumor seeding of the abdominal cavity. A thorough exploration of the abdominal cavity with biopsy of any abnormalities is recommended for definitive diagnosis and to rule out metastatic lesions.[9]

Use of chemotherapy and/or radiation therapy in the treatment of ovarian tumors has not been widely investigated in veterinary medicine; therefore recommendations are difficult to make. Palliation of malignant effusions with intracavitary instillation of

chemotherapeutics, such as the platinum agents, may be considered.[39,40] It is important to remember that the use of cisplatin is considered unsafe in cats.[41]

Prognosis

Prognosis for both dogs and cats with ovarian tumors is difficult to predict because of lack of evidence in the literature. Intuitively, it seems the prognosis is good with complete excision of benign or localized malignant tumors, but poor with detection of metastatic disease.

Comparative Aspects

As in dogs, ovarian cancer in women includes tumors of epithelial, germ cell, or sex cord stromal origin. Epithelial tumors are most common and generally occur in postmenopausal women (median age: 60 years), whereas germ cell tumors are often diagnosed in younger women. An increased incidence of epithelial tumors has been noted in Caucasian women compared with African American women, and ovarian cancer risk (specifically epithelial tumors) appears lower in women who have had children, who have breastfed, or who have taken oral contraceptives. Although uncommon, germline mutations in the *BRCA1* or *BRCA2* genes have been identified in women with familial ovarian cancer. Such mutations also convey an increased risk of other cancers, specifically breast cancer.[42]

Epithelial ovarian tumors in women also resemble the canine counterpart in terms of biologic behavior. They typically metastasize locoregionally within the abdomen; however, distant metastasis may also occur. Patients are often asymptomatic until the disease spreads to the upper abdomen, and presenting symptoms, including abdominal discomfort, bloating, and ascites, are nonspecific. Approximately 70% of women present with advanced disease; as a result, epithelial ovarian cancer is the leading cause of gynecologic cancer mortality.[42]

Cytoreductive surgery and chemotherapy are preferred treatments in epithelial ovarian cancer patients. Even in cases with advanced disease, cytoreductive surgery appears beneficial. Removal of large, necrotic tumors with poor blood supply theoretically improves chemotherapy delivery. Platinum agents (primarily cisplatin) and taxanes are commonly used chemotherapeutic agents. Radiation therapy has fallen out of use in high-risk early stage patients because it has proven less effective and more toxic than platinum-containing chemotherapy regimens.[42]

Stage is the most important predictor of prognosis. The 5-year survival rate in patients with stage III, optimally debulked, gross residual disease is 20% to 30%.[42]

Uterine Tumors

Incidence

Uterine tumors are rare, accounting for 0.3% to 0.4%[6] and 0.29%[43] of all canine and feline tumors, respectively. Middle-aged to older animals are most commonly affected, although uterine carcinoma has been reported in dogs and cats <1 year of age.[44,45] No specific breed predilections have been reported.

Pathology and Natural Behavior

Benign mesenchymal tumors (leiomyomas) are most common in the canine uterus.[9,46–48] Other reported but rare uterine tumors include leiomyosarcoma, fibroma, fibrosarcoma, hemangiosarcoma, angiolipoleiomyoma, lymphoma, and lipoma.[47,49] Epithelial tumors are rarely reported but may occur in dogs.[48] Most epithelial tumors are malignant,[50] but benign histologies have been reported.[51]

Leiomyomas generally are slow growing, noninvasive, and do not metastasize.[9] Grossly, they are difficult to distinguish from their malignant counterparts.[47] A syndrome characterized by multiple uterine leiomyomas, bilateral renal cystadenomas, and nodular dermatofibrosis has been characterized in German shepherd dogs.[52,53] This syndrome has been noted to have a hereditary component associated with a mutation in the canine Birt–Hogg–Dube (*BHD*) gene.[54]

A majority of studies suggest that adenocarcinoma is the most common tumor in the feline uterus.[15,43,55,56] Less common histologies include Müllerian tumor (adenosarcoma), leiomyoma, leiomyosarcoma, fibrosarcoma, lymphoma, fibroma, hemangioma, lipoma, and squamous cell carcinoma.[15,43,57–63] Metastasis to the cerebrum, eyes, ovaries, adrenal glands, lungs, liver, kidneys, bladder, colon, diaphragm, and regional lymph nodes has been reported.[15,43,55,64,65] One study evaluating immunohistochemical reactivity of six feline endometrial adenocarcinomas suggests these tumors routinely express CK AE1/AE3, COX-2, E-cadherin, and β-catenin. Five of six tumors demonstrated expression of progesterone receptors, but infrequent vimentin and estrogen receptor staining was seen.[56] Another study demonstrated a significant loss of expression of ER-α and a significant increase in Ki-67 immunoreactivity compared with normal feline endometrium.[66]

History and Clinical Signs

Although it seems logical that uterine tumors occur in intact animals, it is important to note that these may arise from uterine stumps after incomplete OHE (Fig. 27.4).[49] Clinical signs associated with uterine tumors are not commonly reported, and most are incidental findings.[9] However, in some cases, they grow large enough to produce

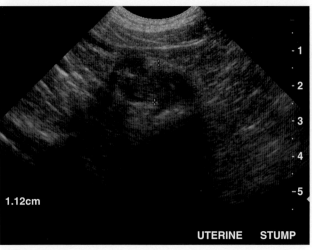

• **Fig. 27.4** Irregular, hypoechoic mass at the uterine stump in a dog after ovariohysterectomy. (Courtesy Dr. D. Jimenez, University of Georgia.)

abdominal distension and signs referable to a space-occupying abdominal mass. Abnormal estrus cycles, vaginal discharge, stranguria, constipation, pyometra, polyuria, polydipsia, vomiting, abdominal distension, and weight loss may also occur.[9,15,33,43,49,50,55,62]

Diagnostic Therapeutics and Workup

Although abdominal imaging helps confirm the presence of an abdominal or uterine mass, histologic evaluation via complete surgical excision is required for definitive diagnosis.[67] As a result, complete staging, including thoracic radiographs and abdominal ultrasound, should be considered before surgery to rule out the possibility of locoregional and distant metastasis. Advanced imaging, such as CT scan, may also be of diagnostic value (Fig. 27.5A).

Therapy

Complete OHE is the treatment of choice for uterine tumors. At the time of surgery, thorough examination of the abdominal cavity must be performed with biopsy of any suspected metastatic foci. Little is known about the role of chemotherapy.

Prognosis

As most uterine tumors in dogs are benign, surgery is often curative. The prognosis is also potentially good for completely excised, localized malignant tumors. However, the presence of metastatic disease warrants a grave prognosis. Feline uterine adenocarcinomas have well-documented metastatic potential[43,55]; therefore the prognosis must be considered guarded. A favorable outcome, with a survival of 19 months, has been reported in a cat with a focal uterine T-cell lymphoma treated with hysterectomy alone.[62]

Vaginal and Vulvar Tumors

Incidence

Vaginal and vulvar tumors account for 2.4% to 3%[46,68] of all canine tumors. Excluding skin tumors arising on the labia of the vulva, most are benign smooth muscle tumors (leiomyomas). These generally occur in middle-aged to older intact female dogs.

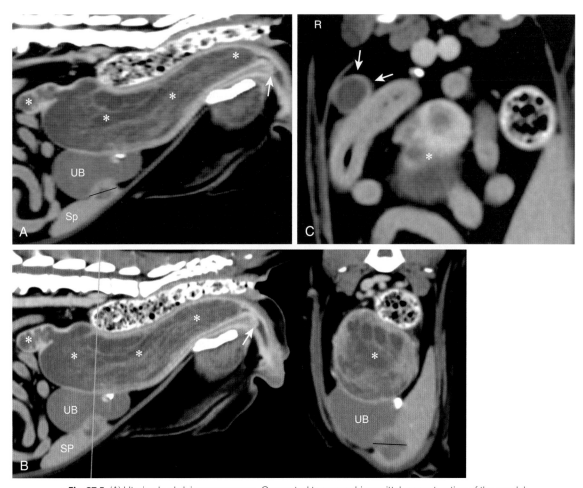

• **Fig. 27.5** (A) Uterine body leiomyosarcoma. Computed tomographic sagittal reconstruction of the caudal abdomen, postcontrast in delayed phase and displayed in soft tissue window. A uterine body mass (*) extends 1 cm proximal to the external urethral orifice (*white arrow*). The mass is irregularly, mildly contrast enhancing. (B) Uterine body leiomyosarcoma. Computed tomographic sagittal reconstruction (*left*) and transverse plane (*right*) of the caudal abdomen, post-contrast in delayed phase and displayed in soft tissue window. A uterine body mass (*) extends 1 cm proximal to the external urethral orifice (*white arrow*). The mass is irregularly, mildly enhancing, a behavior consistent with the cystic spaces and dense cellular arrangement observed on pathologic examination. The nodule on the splenic tail (calipers) was confirmed to be lymphoid hyperplasia. SP: spleen, UB: urinary bladder. (C) Computed tomographic transverse reconstruction of the caudal abdomen at the level of L4/5, postcontrast in delayed phase, soft tissue window. In the region of the right ovary, a nodule (*arrows*) has a thin enhancing rim around a fluid dense center. These findings correlate with histopathologic findings of a fluid to mucus-filled cyst partially lined by cells and ovarian tissue, diagnosed as an interstitial cell tumor of an ovarian remnant. Cranial aspect of the uterine body mass (*). (B Courtesy Dr. K. Gendron, University of Georgia.)

Lipomas often occur in younger dogs ranging in age from 1 to 8 years (mean age: 6.3 years).[46,68]

Malignant vaginal and vulvar tumors have been reported; however, these appear to be more common in spayed female dogs. Primary clitoral carcinomas have been reported in a small number of dogs, all of whom were spayed.[69]

Incidence rates are not available for the cat. Leiomyomas are reported most commonly, occurring in older intact queens.[15,70]

Pathology and Natural Behavior

Benign smooth muscle tumors, including leiomyoma, fibroleiomyoma, fibroma, and polyps, comprise approximately 83% of reported vaginal tumors.[9,68] The most common malignant tumor is leiomyosarcoma, and associated distant metastasis has been reported.[46,68] Other less common tumor types include lipoma, fibrous histiocytoma, benign melanoma, myxoma, myxofibroma, adenocarcinoma, hemangiosarcoma, osteosarcoma, epidermoid carcinoma, and, in endemic areas, transmissible venereal tumor (TVT).[68,71] Carcinomas arising from the bladder or urethra may manifest as vaginal masses near the urethral papilla, and any skin tumor (e.g., mast cell tumors) may develop on the labia of the vulva.[68]

Macroscopically, tumors of the vestibule or vagina are described as extraluminal or intraluminal.[9] Extraluminal tumors appear as slowly growing, well-encapsulated, perineal masses. Intraluminal tumors are attached to the vestibular or vaginal wall by a pedicle, and multiple tumors may occur.[9] In one study, all pedunculated or polypoid tumors were benign; however, it is important to note that definitive diagnosis requires histopathology.[68]

It has been suggested that vaginal leiomyomas may be hormone dependent, as most dogs with these tumors are intact at diagnosis.[9,46,68] Furthermore, one study reported a recurrence rate of 0% in dogs undergoing OHE at the time of tumor removal, whereas 15% of dogs that were left intact experienced local recurrence.[9,68]

Information from the few reported cases of canine clitoral carcinoma (CCC) suggests that the cytologic, histologic, and clinical features appear to mimic those of apocrine gland anal sac adenocarcinoma (AGASA). Cytologically, cells from CCC are arranged in cohesive clusters, with what appear to be "bare" nuclei floating in a background of cytoplasm. Histologically, CCC is described as a partially encapsulated epithelial neoplasm displaying three distinct patterns (tubular, solid, and rosette type). CCC cells consistently express CK AE1/AE3, but expression of neuroendocrine markers is more variable.[69] In a study by Verin et al, neuron-specific enolase (NSE) was expressed in 6 of 6 CCC, whereas chromogranin A (CGA) and synaptophysin (SYN) were mildly expressed in two of six tumors. S-100 expression was not detected in any of the tumors.[69] Like AGASA, hypercalcemia of malignancy has been reported, and locoregional nodal metastasis is a common finding at the time of diagnosis.[69]

History and Clinical Signs

Presence of a mass protruding from the vulva is the most common clinical sign, although vaginal bleeding or discharge is often noted. Other clinical signs may include dysuria, hematuria, tenesmus, constipation, excessive vulvar licking, and dystocia.[9,68]

Lipomas are generally slow growing but eventually impinge on adjacent structures. These tumors can arise from the perivascular and perivaginal fat and lie within the pelvic canal and may attach to the tuber ischium. All lipomas are reported to be well circumscribed and relatively avascular.[68]

Concurrent cystic ovaries and mammary adenocarcinoma have also been reported in a cat with vaginal leiomyoma.[68]

Diagnostic Techniques and Workup

A presumptive diagnosis may be made based on patient signalment and tumor location, although definitive diagnosis requires histopathology. Vaginal and rectal palpation, vaginoscopic examination, and vaginal cytology are often the first steps performed in evaluation of vaginal and vulvar tumors. Retrograde vaginography or urethrocystography may also be used to help delineate the extent of the mass. For some tumor types (e.g., TVT), aspiration cytology of the tumor may be diagnostic; alternatively, incisional biopsy may be performed. Although most vaginal and vulvar tumors are benign, complete staging, including thoracic radiographs and thorough abdominal ultrasound, should be considered in cases in which malignancy is suspected (e.g., rapidly growing, nonpedunculated tumors) or confirmed.

Therapy

Surgical excision combined with OHE is the treatment of choice for most vaginal and vulvar tumors. For benign tumors, this is likely curative, and wide resections are not necessary, especially if OHE is performed. Intraluminal tumors can be removed easily by transecting the pedicle. A dorsal episiotomy may be performed if needed for adequate visualization and exposure.[9,68]

Surgical removal of extraluminal tumors also can be accomplished through a dorsal episiotomy. Because these tumors are often well encapsulated and poorly vascularized, blunt dissection generally removes them entirely. On rare occasions, a perineal approach or pelvic split may be required. Urethral catheterization prevents accidental damage to the urethra during tumor excision. Malignant, infiltrative vaginal neoplasms can be addressed with complete vulvovaginectomy and perineal urethrostomy in carefully selected cases. OHE is indicated in cases with multifocal disease because stable disease or regression may be obtained with hormone ablation.

Prognosis

For benign tumors, surgical excision and OHE are nearly always curative. The prognosis for malignant tumors must be considered guarded because of high rates of local recurrence and metastasis.[68] Surgery with OHE was curative in the one feline leiomyoma reported.

References

1. Hayes A, Harvey HJ: Treatment of metastatic granulosa cell tumor in a dog, *J Am Vet Med Assoc* 174:1304–1306, 1979.
2. Sforna M, Brachelente C, Lepri E, et al.: Canine ovarian tumours: a retrospective study of 49 cases, *Vet Res Commun* 27(Suppl 1):359–361, 2003.
3. Cotchin E: Canine ovarian neoplasms, *Res Vet Sci* 2:133–142, 1961.
4. Dow C: Ovarian abnormalities in the bitch, *J Comp Pathol* 70:59–69, 1960.
5. Cotchin E: Some tumours of dogs and cats of comparative veterinary and human interest, *Vet Rec* 71:1040–1054, 1959.
6. Brodey RS: Canine and feline neoplasia, *Adv Vet Sci Comp Med* 14:309–354, 1970.
7. Bertazzolo W, Dell'Orco M, Bonfanti U, et al.: Cytological features of canine ovarian tumours: a retrospective study of 19 cases, *J Small Anim Pract* 45:539–545, 2004.
8. Patnaik AK, Greenlee PG: Canine ovarian neoplasms: a clinicopathologic study of 71 cases, including histology of 12 granulosa cell tumors, *Vet Pathol* 24:509–514, 1987.
9. Herron MA: Tumors of the canine genital system, *J Am Anim Hosp Assoc* 19:981–994, 1983.
10. Jergens AE, Knapp DW, Shaw DP: Ovarian teratoma in a bitch, *J Am Vet Med Assoc* 191:81–83, 1987.
11. Elena Gorman M, Bildfell R, Seguin B. What is your diagnosis? Peritoneal fluid from a 1-year-old female German Shepherd dog. Malignant teratoma. *Vet Clin Pathol* 39: 393–394.
12. Gruys E, van Dijk JE: Four canine ovarian teratomas and a nonovarian feline teratoma, *Vet Pathol* 13:455–459, 1976.
13. Gelberg HB, McEntee K: Feline ovarian neoplasms, *Vet Pathol* 22:572–576, 1985.
14. Basaraba RJ, Kraft SL, Andrews GA, et al.: An ovarian teratoma in a cat, *Vet Pathol* 35:141–144, 1998.
15. Stein BS: Tumors of the feline genital tract, *J Am Anim Hosp Assoc* 17:1022–1025, 1981.
16. Nielsen SW, Misdorp W, McEntee K: Tumours of the ovary, *Bull World Health Organ* 53:203–215, 1976.
17. Kennedy PC, Cullen JM, Edwards JF, et al.: *Tumors of the Ovary In: WHO. Histological Classification of Tumors of the Genital System of Domestic Animals*, Washington, DC, 1998, AFIP.
18. McCluggage WG: Recent advances in immunohistochemistry in the diagnosis of ovarian neoplasms, *J Clin Pathol* 53:327–334, 2000.
19. Akihara Y, Shimoyama Y, Kawasako K, et al.: Immunohistochemical evaluation of canine ovarian tumors, *J Vet Med Sci* 69:703–708, 2007.
20. Riccardi E, Grieco V, Verganti S, et al.: Immunohistochemical diagnosis of canine ovarian epithelial and granulosa cell tumors, *J Vet Diagn Invest* 19:431–435, 2007.

21. Agnew D, MacLachlan N: *Tumors of the gential systems. Tumors in domestic animals*, 5th ed., Ames, IA, 2017, John Wiley & Sons, pp 699–706.

22. Borzacchiello G, Mogavero S, Tortorella G, et al. Expression of endothelin-1 and endothelin receptor a in canine ovarian tumours. *Reprod Domest Anim* 45:e465–468.

23. Borzacchiello G, Russo V, Russo M: Immunohistochemical expression of cyclooxygenase-2 in canine ovarian carcinomas, *J Vet Med A Physiol Pathol Clin Med* 54:247–249, 2007.

24. Pelkey TJ, Frierson Jr HF, Mills SE, et al.: The diagnostic utility of inhibin staining in ovarian neoplasms, *Int J Gynecol Pathol* 17:97–105, 1998.

25. Banco B, Antuofermo E, Borzacchiello G, et al.: Canine ovarian tumors: an immunohistochemical study with HBME-1 antibody, *J Vet Diagn Invest* 23:977–981, 2011.

26. Greenlee PG, Patnaik AK: Canine ovarian tumors of germ cell origin, *Vet Pathol* 22:117–122, 1985.

27. Andrews EJ, Stookey JL, Helland DR, et al.: A histopathological study of canine and feline ovarian dysgerminomas, *Can J Comp Med* 38:85–89, 1974.

28. Dehner LP, Norris HJ, Garner FM, et al.: Comparative pathology of ovarian neoplasms. Germ cell tumours of canine, bovine, feline, rodent and human species, *J Comp Pathol* 80:299–306, 1970.

29. Clemente M, Perez-Alenza MD, Pena L. Metastasis of canine inflammatory versus non-inflammatory mammary tumours. *J Comp Pathol* 143: 157–163.

30. Sato T, Hontake S, Shibuya H, et al.: A solid mature teratoma of a feline ovary, *J Feline Med Surg* 5:349–351, 2003.

31. Machida Y, Michishita M, Wada M, et al.: Malignant oestrogen-producing teratoma in a cat, *J Comp Pathol* 156:178–182, 2017.

32. Olsen J, Komtebedde J, Lackner A, et al.: Cytoreductive treatment of ovarian carcinoma in a dog, *J Vet Intern Med* 8:133–135, 1994.

33. McEntee MC: Reproductive oncology, *Clin Tech Small Anim Pract* 17:133–149, 2002.

34. Hori Y, Uechi M, Kanakubo K, et al.: Canine ovarian serous papillary adenocarcinoma with neoplastic hypercalcemia, *J Vet Med Sci* 68:979–982, 2006.

35. McCandlish IA, Munro CD, Breeze RG, et al.: Hormone producing ovarian tumours in the dog, *Vet Rec* 105:9–11, 1979.

36. Yamini B, VanDenBrink PL, Refsal KR: Ovarian steroid cell tumor resembling luteoma associated with hyperadrenocorticism (Cushing's disease) in a dog, *Vet Pathol* 34:57–60, 1997.

37. Cellio LM, Degner DA: Testosterone-producing thecoma in a female cat, *J Am Anim Hosp Assoc* 36:323–325, 2000.

38. Diez-Bru N, Garcia-Real I, Martinez EM, et al.: Ultrasonographic appearance of ovarian tumors in 10 dogs, *Vet Radiol Ultrasound* 39:226–233, 1998.

39. Moore AS, Kirk C, Cardona A: Intracavitary cisplatin chemotherapy experience with six dogs, *J Vet Intern Med* 5:227–231, 1991.

40. Best MP, Frimberger AE: Ovarian carcinomatosis in a dog managed with surgery and intraperitoneal, systemic, and intrapleural chemotherapy utilizing indwelling pleural access ports, *Can Vet J* 58:493–497, 2017.

41. Knapp DW, Richardson RC, DeNicola DB, et al.: Cisplatin toxicity in cats, *J Vet Intern Med* 1:29–35, 1987.

42. Cannistra SA, Gershenson DM, Recht A: Ovarian Cancer, Fallopian Tube Carcinoma, and Peritoneal Carcinoma. In DeVita VT, Lawrence TS, Rosenberg SA, editors: *Cancer principles & practice of oncology*, 8th ed., Philadelphia, PA, 2008, Lippincott Williams & Wilkins, pp 1568–1594.

43. Miller MA, Ramos-Vara JA, Dickerson MF, et al.: Uterine neoplasia in 13 cats, *J Vet Diagn Invest* 15:515–522, 2003.

44. Cave TA, Hine R, Howie F, et al.: Uterine carcinoma in a 10-month-old golden retriever, *J Small Anim Pract* 43:133–135, 2002.

45. Payan-Carreira R, Saraiva AL, Santos T, et al.: Feline endometrial adenocarcinoma in females <1 year old: a description of four cases, *Reprod Domest Anim* 48:e70–e77, 2013.

46. Brodey RS, Roszel JF: Neoplasms of the canine uterus, vagina, and vulva: a clinicopathologic survey of 90 cases, *J Am Vet Med Assoc* 151:1294–1307, 1967.

47. McEntee K, Nielsen SW: Tumours of the female genital tract, *Bull World Health Organ* 53:217–226, 1976.

48. Cotchin E: Spontaneous Uterine Cancer in Animals, *Br J Cancer* 18:209–227, 1964.

49. Wenzlow N, Tivers MS, Selmic LE, et al.: Haemangiosarcoma in the uterine remnant of a spayed female dog, *J Small Anim Pract* 50:488–491, 2009.

50. Murphy ST, Kruger JM, Watson GL: Uterine adenocarcinoma in the dog: a case report and review, *J Am Anim Hosp Assoc* 30:440–444, 1994.

51. Marino G, Quartuccio M, Cristarella S, et al.: Adenoma of the uterine tube in the bitch: two case reports, *Vet Res Commun* 31(Suppl 1):173–175, 2007.

52. Lium B, Moe L: Hereditary multifocal renal cystadenocarcinomas and nodular dermatofibrosis in the German shepherd dog: macroscopic and histopathologic changes, *Vet Pathol* 22:447–455, 2007.

53. Moe L, Lium B: Hereditary multifocal renal cystadenocarcinomas and nodular dermatofibrosis in 51 German shepherd dogs, *J Small Anim Pract* 38:498–505, 1997.

54. Lingaas F, Comstock KE, Kirkness EF, et al.: A mutation in the canine BHD gene is associated with hereditary multifocal renal cystadenocarcinoma and nodular dermatofibrosis in the German Shepherd dog, *Hum Mol Genet* 12:3043–3053, 2003.

55. Anderson C, Pratschke K. Uterine adenocarcinoma with abdominal metastases in an ovariohysterectomised cat. *J Feline Med Surg* 13: 44–47.

56. Gil da Costa RM, Santos M, Amorim I, et al.: An immunohistochemical study of feline endometrial adenocarcinoma, *J Comp Pathol* 140:254–259, 2009.

57. Fukui K, Matsuda H: Uterine haemangioma in a cat, *Vet Rec* 113:375, 1983.

58. Cooper TK, Ronnett BM, Ruben DS, et al.: Uterine myxoid leiomyosarcoma with widespread metastases in a cat, *Vet Pathol* 43:552–556, 2006.

59. Nicotina PA, Zanghi A, Catone G: Uterine malignant mixed Mullerian tumor (Metaplasic carcinoma) in the cat: clinicopathologic features and proliferation indices, *Vet Pathol* 39:158–160, 2002.

60. Papparella S, Roperto F: Spontaneous uterine tumors in three cats, *Vet Pathol* 21:257–258, 1984.

61. Gilmore CE: Tumors of the female reproductive tract, *Calif Vet* 19:12–15, 1965.

62. Conversy B, Freulon AL, Graille M: Focal uterine T-cell lymphoma in an ovariectomized cat, *J Am Vet Med Assoc* 251:1059–1063, 2017.

63. Hayashi A, Tanaka H, Tajima T, et al.: A spayed female cat with squamous cell carcinoma in the uterine remnant, *J Vet Med Sci* 75:391–393, 2013.

64. O'Rourke MD, Geib LW: Endometrial adenocarcinoma in a cat, *Cornell Vet* 60:598–604, 1970.

65. Schmidt RE, Langham RF: A survey of feline neoplasms, *J Am Vet Med Assoc* 151:1325–1328, 1967.

66. Saraiva AL, Payan-Carreira R, Gartner F, et al.: An immunohistochemical study on the expression of sex steroid receptors, Ki-67 and cytokeratins 7 and 20 in feline endometrial adenocarcinomas, *BMC Vet Res* 11:204, 2015.

67. Patsikas M, Papazoglou LG, Jakovljevic S, et al.: Radiographic and ultrasonographic findings of uterine neoplasms in nine dogs, *J Am Anim Hosp Assoc* 50:330–337, 2014.

68. Thacher C, Bradley RL: Vulvar and vaginal tumors in the dog: a retrospective study, *J Am Vet Med Assoc* 183:690–692, 1983.

69. Verin R, Cian F, Stewart J, et al.: Canine clitoral carcinoma: a clinical, cytologic, histopathological, immunohistochemical, and ultrastructural study, *Vet Pathol* 300985818759772, 2018.

70. Wolke RE: Vaginal leiomyoma as a cause of chronic constipation in the cat, *J Am Vet Med Assoc* 143:1103–1105, 1963.

71. Hill TP, Lobetti RG, Schulman ML: Vulvovaginectomy and neourethrostomy for treatment of haemangiosarcoma of the vulva and vagina, *J S Afr Vet Assoc* 71:256–259, 2000.

28
Tumors of the Mammary Gland

KARIN U. SORENMO, DEANNA R. WORLEY, AND VALENTINA ZAPPULLI

Mammary Gland Tumors in Dogs

Epidemiology and Risk Factors

Epidemiology

Mammary gland (MG) tumors (MGTs) are common in dogs and represent the most common neoplasms in sexually intact female dogs.[1-8] The incidence rates reported vary depending on the origin of the studies and characteristics of the source population. The current incidence of MGTs in the United States is lower than in many other countries owing to the common practice of performing ovariohysterectomy (OHE) at a young age. Data from several European national or regional canine cancer registries, including from Norway,[2] Denmark,[5] and Italy,[6,7] as well as Mexican[8] registries, provide information regarding MGT incidence in general, in addition to details regarding the relative frequency of various tumors according to site, age, and breed. These registries consist of a population of predominantly sexually intact dogs and thus provide insight into the natural or true MGT risk in unaltered dogs. Results from these registries show that MGTs are the most common tumors in female dogs and represent 50% to 70% of all tumors in this subset of the population.[2,6] Interestingly, results from the two most recent studies suggest that the ratio of malignant versus benign MGTs has shifted toward an increase in malignant tumors in dogs, similar to the epidemiologic trends in women.[7,8]

In general, open population-based and insurance-based studies may underestimate the true incidence of disease, especially if the diagnosis and subsequent registration require a surgical biopsy. Furthermore, the insured dog population may be skewed toward younger animals because of age restriction and may be void after the tenth year of age, which coincides with the peak incidence age of MGT diagnosis.[3,4] Early data from the surveys of Alameda and Contra Costa counties reported an estimated annual incidence rate of 257.7 malignant MGTs per 100,000 in intact female dogs.[1] A later large Swedish study based on 80,000 insured female dogs, most of which were sexually intact, reported a rate of 111 MGTs (including both benign and malignant) per 10,000 dog-years at risk.[3] This study also reported an increasing risk for tumors with advancing age; 6% of all 8-year-old dogs and 13% of all 10-year-old dogs were diagnosed with at least one MGT. Another large insurance-based study from the United Kingdom reported an annual incidence rate of 205 MGTs per 100,000 dogs. This study included all MGTs regardless of histology.[4]

In addition to these open and more heterogeneous population-based studies, closed population studies provide another source of incidence and natural progression data. Longitudinal studies may provide a more accurate estimate of the total lifetime risk of MGTs because dogs are monitored closely and all tumors are noted, biopsied, and reported. In a large beagle colony morbidity and mortality study, 71% of female dogs developed at least one MGT in their lifetime[9]; however, this may not accurately represent the incidence in other breeds. Many of the various tumor registries have reported significant breed variations in MGT incidence, suggesting that, in addition to age and hormonal factors, hereditary breed-associated genetic susceptibility may also contribute to MGT risk.

Risk Factors

As noted, the incidence of MGTs varies depending on where the studies are performed and the specific characteristics of the population in terms of OHE status, age, and breed distribution. Thus in addition to providing data regarding incidence, epidemiologic studies also help identify risk factors for MGTs. Three main factors have been identified that play important roles in MGT risk: age, hormonal exposure, and breed. To a lesser degree, diet and body weight or obesity may also contribute to risk.

Age

MGTs affect middle-aged and older dogs.[1,10-13] MGTs, especially malignant tumors, are extremely rare in dogs younger than 5 years old.[1,10,14] The tumor risk increases with age and becomes clinically significant when dogs turn 7 or 8 years old, and continues to increase until the age of 11 to 13 years.[10,14] Dogs with malignant tumors are significantly older than dogs with benign tumors: the mean age of dogs with malignant tumors is 9 to 11 years versus 7 to 9 years with benign tumors.[15,16] The peak incidence age also depends on the lifespan of various breeds. In general, larger breeds have a naturally shorter lifespan and therefore tend to be younger than smaller breeds when they are diagnosed. These differences may be further exaggerated in high-risk breeds such as English springer spaniels.[3,17]

Hormonal Exposure

Many MGTs in dogs are preventable. Dogs spayed before their first estrus have only a 0.5% risk of developing MGTs in their lifetime.[18] The protective effect of OHE decreases over the first few estrus cycles and most of the earlier studies have not found significant benefit after 4 years of age. According to Schneider's original study, the risk increases and the benefit diminishes with each estrus cycle, as illustrated by an increasing risk of 8% and 26% depending on whether the OHE was performed before the second or third heat cycle.[18] No significant risk reduction was seen in dogs spayed after 2.5 years of age, although other researchers have found some modest benefit in dogs spayed later. These studies were all retrospective case-control studies.[14,19,20] A recent prospective randomized study, however, documented significant decreased risk for new tumor development by performing OHE concurrent with tumor removal in dogs with benign MGTs.[21] Notably, these dogs were older, with a mean age of 9 years, confirming that hormonal deprivation via OHE later in life significantly decreases the risk for new tumor development. Nevertheless, the greatest benefit on MGT prevention is seen if the dog is not allowed to go through any heat cycles, suggesting that some of the initial effects of ovarian hormones on the MGs in terms of cancer risk occur early in life, likely during puberty when the MG develops and matures. Other factors resulting in physiologic variation in hormonal influence on the mammary tissues, such as pseudopregnancy, pregnancy, or parity, which typically occur after a few estrus cycles, have not been found to significantly influence the tumor risk, but none of these studies were controlled or randomized.[14,18,22] Exposure to exogenous or pharmacologic doses of hormones (both progestins and estrogens) has been found to increase the risk for developing MGTs in dogs. Dogs treated with progestins are more likely to develop tumors and at a younger age.[20] According to the Norwegian Canine Cancer Registry, dogs treated with progestins to prevent estrus had a 2.3-fold higher risk for MGTs compared with dogs not receiving such treatment.[23] Similarly, a Dutch study found that privately owned dogs with MGTs were significantly more likely to have received progestins.[20] Numerous studies have investigated the effect of dose, duration, and type of hormones (progestins, estrogens, or a combination of both) on MGT development in laboratory dogs. Although some discordance exists, most conclude that low-dose progestins alone increase the risk for predominantly benign tumors, whereas a combination of estrogens and progestins tends to induce malignant tumors.[24–28]

Breeds and Genetic Susceptibility

In general, MGTs tend to be more common in the smaller breeds. Purebred dogs are more commonly affected[1]; poodles, Chihuahuas, dachshunds, Yorkshire terriers, Maltese, and cocker spaniels are frequently listed as high-risk breeds in the small-breed category.[1,2,16,29] However, some of the larger breeds are also at increased risk, including the English springer spaniel, English setters, Brittany spaniels, German shepherds, pointers, Doberman pinschers, and boxers.[1–3,16,29] Some noteworthy discrepancies exist, specifically between the US and European reports. Boxers are noted to have a decreased risk for MGTs according to data from the University of Pennsylvania, whereas Scandinavian studies reflect an increased risk in boxers.[2,3,16] A closed population beagle study showed that two different lines or families of beagles have very different MGT risks.[30] These results collectively support a genetic influence on MGT development. Familial or inherited germline mutations in BRCA1 and BRCA2 account for 5% to 10% of all human breast cancers (BCs) and are associated with an 85% cumulative lifetime risk of BC in affected individuals.[31–34] Studies of BRCA mutations in canine MGTs have so far been limited to tumor gene expression studies and the results have varied;

some found underexpression of BRCA1 in malignant tumors and others have documented overexpression of BRCA2 in metastatic tumors.[35,36] Germline polymorphisms in both BRCA1 and BRCA2 were associated with significantly increased risk in English springer spaniels in a large Swedish study.[3,17]

Other Risk Factors

Body weight, specifically during puberty (9–12 months), is found to have a significant effect on later MGT risk; being underweight during this time period provides significant protection against later tumor development.[19] This study did not find an increased risk for tumors in dogs fed a high-fat diet or dogs that were obese around the time of tumor detection; however, a subsequent case-control study did document an association between diet and mammary cancer in which obesity early in life and a diet high in red meat were found to increase risk.[37] Obesity has also been recognized as a risk factor for developing postmenopausal BC in women.[38,39] One of the proposed mechanisms by which diet/obesity may be linked to breast carcinogenesis is via its effect on serum estrogen levels. Obesity is associated with decreased concentration of sex hormone–binding globulin and thus results in elevated serum free estrogen levels.[40–44] In addition, adipose tissues may be a source of increased estrogen production via aromatase-mediated conversion of androgens. Interestingly, the mammary cancer–sparing influence of being underweight is most significant during the first year of life, when the effects of the endogenous hormones are the greatest.

Tumor Biology: Development, Hormones, Growth Factors, and Clinical Implications

Based on the previous discussion of risk factors, it is clear that exposure to ovarian hormones is important in the development of MGTs in dogs. Both estrogens and progesterone are necessary for normal MG development and maturation. The MGs undergo distinct clinical and histopathologic changes as hormone levels fluctuate according to the phases of the estrus cycle.[45,46] Estrogens and progesterone are mitogens of breast epithelium and induce proliferation of intralobular ductal epithelium and development of ducts and lobules, resulting in expansion of the MGs. Historically, the tumorigenic effects of estrogen in human BC were thought to be mediated via their receptor binding and enhanced production of growth factors resulting in increased cellular proliferation[47]; however, more recent research shows that estrogen and its metabolites also have direct genotoxic effects by increasing mutations and induction of aneuploidy independent of the estrogen receptors.[48–50] The tumorigenic effects of progesterone are in part thought to be mediated via a progesterone-induced increased MG production of growth hormone (GH) and GH receptors.[51–53] GH has direct stimulatory effects on mammary tissues and indirect effects via increasing insulin-like growth factor-1 (IGF-1).[54] The GH/IGF-1 axis has been implicated in human breast carcinogenesis. IGF-1 is both a proproliferative and a survival factor for breast epithelial cells and regulates the expression of numerous genes involved in BC development.[55–60] The complex dysregulation of growth factors and hormones that precedes, initiates, and potentially drives canine mammary tumorigenesis is far from understood; evidence exists indicating that both growth factors and steroid hormones are intrinsically implicated and contribute in an autocrine/paracrine manner. Malignant tumors have significantly higher tissue concentrations of GH, IGF-1, progesterone, and 17β-estradiol than benign tumors; moreover, levels correspond with important clinicopathologic parameters such as growth rate, size, and histotype.[61,62] A complete review of the biologic and molecular aspects of MGT carcinogenesis is beyond the scope of this chapter, but recent reviews provide more complete information.[63,64]

The entire mammary chain is exposed to growth factors and sex hormones, resulting in a field carcinogenesis effect. Consequently, most dogs develop tumors in multiple glands.[9,14,15,65–67] Histologic progression with increasing tumor size is often noted in dogs with multiple tumors and areas of transitions such as carcinoma in situ (CIS) can be seen in benign tumors.[15,65] This provides direct evidence that benign and malignant MGTs are not separate entities; instead, they are part of a biologic and histopathologic continuum in which the malignant invasive carcinomas are the end stage of the process. Earlier publications support this hypothesis and document associations between tumors of benign and malignant histology. For instance, dogs with carcinomas often had concurrent benign tumors of the same cell type and dogs with benign MGTs were at increased risk for developing subsequent malignant tumors.[66] Furthermore, risk was even higher in dogs diagnosed with CIS or carcinomas.[15,65,67] Evidence of histologic progression has also been reported in which a high incidence of CIS and intraepithelial lesions with atypia was noted adjacent to invasive carcinomas.[65,68] There are likely regional variations in terms of exposure resulting in a range of histopathologic and clinical changes. Some tumors may never change and remain small and benign whereas others progress and become malignant and many develop new tumors in other glands. This suggests that canine MGTs provide unique comparative opportunities to study mammary carcinogenesis and progression with direct applications to human BC research.

Tumor Hormone Receptors/Molecular-Based Classification: Prognostic, Clinical, and Therapeutic Implications

Hormonal exposure plays an important role in MGT development and many tumors, specifically tumors of epithelial origin, express hormone receptors (HRs), suggesting continued hormonal influence and dependence. Benign tumors are more likely than malignant tumors to retain HRs, both estrogen receptors (ERs) and progesterone receptors (PRs).[69–73] The HR status is also influenced by age and hormonal status: dogs that are intact, younger, and in estrus are more likely to have receptor-positive tumors than dogs that are spayed, older, and anestrous.[73–75] Furthermore, the HR expression is inversely correlated with tumor size and histopathologic differentiation; larger tumors and undifferentiated or anaplastic tumors are less likely to express receptors than tumors with more differentiated histology, reflecting a biologic drift toward hormone independence and corresponding with aggressive histology and clinical behavior.[74,76,77] HR expression analysis is most commonly performed by immunohistochemistry (IHC). Results from various studies are quite disparate, especially in terms of ER-alpha positivity in malignant tumors, and range from 10% to 92%.[69–74,76–79] These variations may in part be due to differences between study populations (tumor size, OHE status, tumor types) and the fact that IHC methods vary and, up until recently, have not been validated or tested for their ability to predict response to hormonal therapy.[79] A prospective randomized trial on the effect of OHE in dogs with mammary carcinoma determined the threshold positive immunostaining of both ERs and PRs to be an Allred score

of greater than 3.[79] Despite these discrepancies, several studies have documented that tumor expression of ER and PR is associated with a more favorable outcome.[74,76,77] Endocrine therapy is recommended to all women with ER-positive tumors, regardless of intensity of staining, and results in significant improvement in survival when used in the adjuvant setting.[80–85] In addition to the presence of HRs, the overexpression of human epidermal growth factor receptor-2 (HER-2/erb-2), a member of the epidermal growth factor receptor family involved in signal transduction pathways that regulate cell growth and differentiation, may also provide clinical and prognostic insight and therapeutic opportunities in MGTs. Overexpression or amplification of HER-2 is found in 20% to 25% of all human BC patients and is associated with aggressive behavior, resistance to hormonal therapy, and a poor prognosis.[86–88] HER-2 overexpression has also been documented in canine MGTs using the same HercepTest scoring systems used in human BC; positive staining has ranged from 17% to 48% in malignant tumors.[89–94] HER-2 staining was associated with negative histologic features and short survival times (STs) according to one of these studies[89] but, contrary to the human studies, HER-2 expression was associated with improved survival in two other independent studies.[90,91] Discrepancies can be related to IHC protocols and scoring systems, which are still controversial in human BC. Recently preanalytical, analytical, and postanalytical guidelines have been suggested to test HER-2 expression in canine MGTs.[95] They suggest 6- to 48-hour formalin fixation, evaluation of the invasive portions of the tumor, and threshold positive immunostaining to be greater than 30% of cells with complete membrane staining.[95]

Information about HR and HER-2, added to data on the expression of luminal versus basal cell differentiation markers and Ki67, allows for the molecular classification of human BC. More precisely, IHC-based surrogates of gene expression–based molecular subtypes are routinely applied. In human BC, the IHC subtypes include *luminal A* (high HR, HER-2–, low Ki67, luminal markers +, basal markers +/–), *luminal B* (low HR, HER-2+/–, any/high Ki67, luminal markers +, basal markers +/–), *HER-2-overexpressing* (HR–, HER-2+, any Ki67, luminal markers +/–, basal markers +/–), and *triple-negative* (HR–, HER-2–, any Ki67, luminal markers +/–, basal markers +/–). The latter includes the molecular *basal-like* tumors which are triple-negative for receptors (ER, PR, HER-2) and express basal markers (CK5, CK6, CK14, CK17, SMA, calponin, vimentin, and p63) and not luminal markers; the *normal-like* subtype, which is negative to all markers and shows a adipose tissue signature; and the *claudin-low* subtype, which is also triple-negative (ER, PR, HER-2) and, regardless of basal markers, expresses low claudin and high vimentin.[96–100]

In women, these subtypes are associated with different clinical outcomes, ranging from the best prognosis for *luminal A* tumors to the worst prognosis for two of the *triple-negative* subtypes (*basal-like* and *claudin-low*).[100] In women with BC, treatment is determined using these molecular signatures, histopathologic subtype, histologic grading, and clinical staging.[99]

Recently a few studies have attempted a molecular classification of canine MGTs by applying the same human BC IHC panels.[91,92,94] In one study,[91] this classification was prognostic with the *basal-like* phenotype significantly associated with shorter disease-free interval (DFI) and overall survival time (OST); however, the results differ between studies and highlight the need for continued investigations and standardizing the IHC protocols. This represents the first and crucial step toward using results from molecular classification to inform precise and patient-specific treatment recommendations in canine MGTs, similar to the approach in human BC therapy.

History and Clinical Presentation

MGTs are usually easy to detect through routine physical examinations; however, high-risk dogs, specifically older intact female dogs, should undergo a thorough examination of the MGs. MGTs typically affect the two caudal glands where the MGs or tissues are naturally larger; thus careful palpation may be necessary to detect small tumors.[9,14,66,67] The MGs should be palpated again under general anesthesia to ensure that all tumors are found and included in the surgical planning, and both chains should be carefully evaluated. A recent study documented that 70% of intact females had more than one MGT at diagnosis.[15] The size of the tumor(s), stage of disease, and presence of systemic signs of illness vary widely. Inflammatory mammary carcinomas represent a rare but clinically important subset of MGTs in dogs. Affected dogs may easily be misdiagnosed as having mastitis or severe dermatitis because, rather than presenting with discrete well-circumscribed tumors, the entire mammary chain may appear edematous, swollen, warm, and painful (Fig. 28.1).[101,102] In addition to the extensive locoregional involvement, most dogs with inflammatory carcinomas have distant metastatic disease and signs of systemic illness.[101,102] These dogs are therefore poor surgical candidates. The majority of dogs with MGTs are systemically healthy and the tumors are confined to the MGs when they are diagnosed.

Clinical Assessment, Diagnosis, Workup, and Staging

Because of the risk of metastasis associated with MGTs, staging before initiating therapy is strongly recommended, especially if benign disease cannot be histologically confirmed. Minimal diagnostic workup and staging can include complete blood count (CBC), serum biochemistry, three-view thoracic radiographs, and fine-needle aspiration (FNA) of regional lymph nodes (LNs) or more accurately, sentinel LN mapping and biopsy (see Chapter 9).[103,104] In women, the use of sentinel LN mapping has dramatically altered the surgical treatment of BC. As canine mammary carcinoma has been demonstrated as a relevant model for human disease,[105,106] incorporation of human LN staging techniques should be reconsidered for the dog.[107] Sentinel LN mapping is a means of detecting which LNs are receiving draining tumor lymph and thus most at risk for metastasis. Some techniques described for sentinel LN mapping in the dog include lymphoscintigraphy using technetium, contrast-enhanced ultrasonography, autogenous hemosiderin, computed tomographic indirect lymphography, and intraoperative dyes (Fig. 28.2).[103,104,107–111] Clinically normal LNs can be difficult to identify in dogs with MGTs, as the axillary LNs are often not palpable and the superficial inguinal LNs reside deep to the fifth MG in the inguinal fat pad. Furthermore, many dogs have more than one tumor; thus multiple LNs may represent draining LNs. Lymphatic drainage of normal MGs is in addition very complex with documented drainage occurring to multiple ipsilateral LNs and even to contralateral LNs.[104,112,113] The amount of variation in lymphatic drainage increases in the neoplastic MG.[112] Tumor-induced lymphangiogenesis, well documented in human BC, may be responsible for the unpredictable and erratic location of susceptible or "at-risk" LNs in dogs having malignant MGTs.[114] Thus exclusive anatomic sampling of nearby LNs may not be sufficient for accurate LN staging and may miss the presence of locoregional disease.[107]

The first description of sentinel LN mapping in any animal was done in cats almost 30 years ago.[115] Benefits in human medicine include greater ease in identifying the at-risk LNs intraoperatively with minimal surgical incisions and with efficiency, especially for the rarely assessed axillary nodes. The prognostic value of sentinel LN mapping is currently unknown for the dog,[116] although a study of computed tomographic indirect lymphography found imaging characteristics of sentinel LNs positive for histologic mammary tumor metastasis having decreased or heterogeneous LN contrast enhancement compared with the homogeneous contrast enhancement pattern of sentinel LNs negative for histologic metastasis.[103]

Abdominal ultrasound may be indicated in dogs with suspected regional LN involvement or changes on preoperative blood work suggesting tumor-related or non–tumor-related serum biochemistry changes. Even though osseous metaplasia occurs occasionally with mammary adenocarcinoma and the MGs are a common site for extraskeletal osteosarcoma (OSA), there has been no prognostic value found for serum alkaline phosphatase activity.[117,118] There may be value in performing MGT cytology to help rule out nonmammary dermal

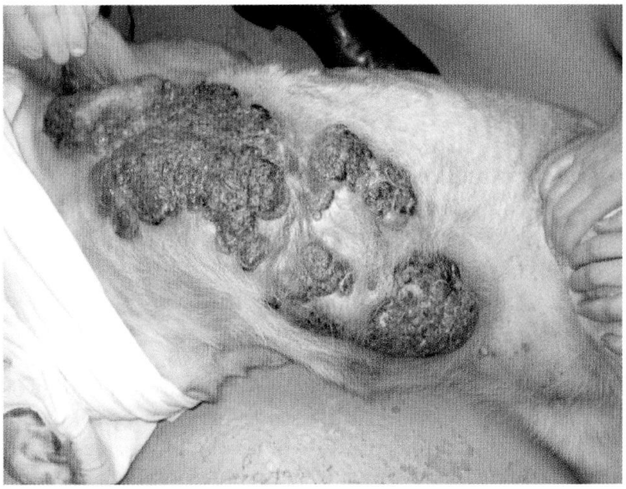

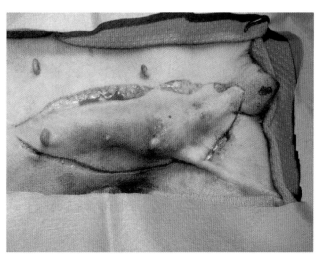

• **Fig. 28.1** Inflammatory mammary carcinoma in a dog. (Courtesy Dr. Nicholas Bacon, Fitzpatrick Referrals, Guildford, United Kingdom.)

• **Fig. 28.2** Regional mastectomy in a dog. (Courtesy Dr. Julius Liptak, VCA Canada—Alta Vista Animal Hospital, Ottawa, Canada.)

		Lymph Node	
Stage	Tumor Size	Status	Metastasis
Stage I	T1 <3 cm	N_0	M_0
Stage II	T2 3–5 cm	N_0	M_0
Stage III	T3 >5 cm	N_0	M_0
Stage IV	Any	N_1 (positive)	M_0
Stage V	Any	Any	M_1 (metastasis)

TABLE 28.1 Staging of Canine Mammary Tumors[15,125]

and subcutaneous tumors (e.g., mast cell tumors, lipomas). In addition, correlations between cytopathology and ex vivo histopathology have been reported to be between 68% and 93%,[119,120] and the reported cytologic sensitivity and specificity for a malignant MGT diagnosis were 88% and 96%, respectively.[121] Computed tomography (CT) imaging of the thoracic cavity provides more sensitive detection of pulmonary nodules than does thoracic radiography, but this may not be applicable for every patient because of increased expense and limited availability.[121,122] Distant metastatic sites can include LNs, liver, lungs, and bone.[123]

Staging System

MGTs are staged according to the T (tumor), N (lymph node), and M (metastasis) system. A modified version of the original staging system published by Owen[124] is currently used by most oncologists: stage advances from I to II to III as the size of the primary tumor increases from smaller than 3 cm, to between 3 and 5 cm, to larger than 5 cm.[125] These size categories capture important changes in prognosis and outcome. LN metastasis represents stage IV disease, regardless of tumor size, and distant metastasis constitutes stage V disease. This staging system should be used for dogs with epithelial tumors (noninflammatory) but not sarcomas (Table 28.1).

Histopathologic Classification Systems

The normal MG is a complex branching structure and the histologic and IHC characteristics are equally complex; the interested reader is referred to a thorough review on the subject.[126]

Two early classifications of canine and feline MGTs were published in 1974 and 1999,[127,128] and a revised system for the dog was published in 2011.[129] In dogs, although there may be histopathologic evidence of malignancy, only a small percentage of cases will have lymphatic and vascular invasion and metastatic disease, whereas in cats the majority are malignant and metastasis to local LNs is more common. The classification used in this text is based on both morphology[129] and prognosis.[130,131] When discussing the classification of MGTs, the terms *simple* and *complex* are commonly used. Simple denotes that the neoplasm is composed of one cell type resembling either luminal epithelial cells or myoepithelial cells, whereas complex neoplasms are composed of two cell types, both luminal and myoepithelial cells, in which the myoepithelial cells extend into the interstitium, show a typical spindle to stellate morphology, and are embedded in a myxoid matrix.[129]

When distinguishing between benign and malignant tumors, criteria of malignancy have been listed in the 2011 classification

for canine MGTs[129]; however, particularly when applied to low-grade or borderline lesions, some variability can be due to subjective interpretation and experience of the pathologist. This may lead to overreporting of malignant over benign tumors affecting epidemiologic data.

Canine Mammary Hyperplasia and Dysplasia

Several hyperplastic and dysplastic lesions are diagnosed in the canine MG and, in some cases, they can be considered precursor lesions to the development of MGTs.[129] These include duct ectasia, lobular hyperplasia (regular, with secretory [lactational] activity, with fibrosis [interlobular fibrous connective tissue], and with atypia), epitheliosis, papillomatosis, and fibroadenomatous change (fibroepithelial hyperplasia, fibroepithelial hypertrophy, mammary hypertrophy). The latter is frequent in the cat, but has not been clearly described in the canine MG; nodular lesions with fibroadenomatous morphology in the dog should be more correctly classified as fibroadenomas.

Benign Mammary Neoplasms

Several types of benign MGTs exist in the dog and include adenoma, intraductal papillary adenoma (duct papilloma), ductal adenoma, fibroadenoma, myoepithelioma, complex adenoma (adenomyoepithelioma), and benign mixed tumors. A histologic description of these various entities is beyond the scope of this chapter and interested readers are directed to a more thorough review.[129]

Malignant Canine Mammary Neoplasms

Malignant Epithelial Tumors

Several types of malignant epithelial tumors (Table 28.2) exist, including a variety of simple and complex carcinomas. CIS is described in the human breast as a well-demarcated, noninfiltrative nodule(s) that has not extended through the basement membrane; it is rarely diagnosed in dogs because early lesions are less frequently detected than in women and criteria to differentiate CIS from lobular hyperplasia with atypia and atypical epitheliosis in the canine MG are still under discussion. In addition, several less common subtypes of malignant epithelial neoplasm in the dog include squamous cell carcinomas, adenosquamous carcinomas, mucinous carcinomas, lipid-rich carcinomas, and spindle cell carcinomas.[129] The predominant morphologic pattern in each nodule is used to classify each nodule separately.

Malignant Mesenchymal Neoplasms: Sarcomas

Malignant mesenchymal neoplasms of the MG most commonly include OSA, chondrosarcoma, fibrosarcoma, and hemangiosarcoma.[129]

OSA is the most common mesenchymal neoplasm of the canine MG and there is often a history of recent rapid growth of a mammary mass that might have been present for some time. A proliferation of cells varies from fusiform to stellate to ovoid, and there is an association with islands of tumor osteoid and/or bone formation. Cartilage can also be present in variable amounts. Mitoses are frequently found. Metastasis occurs via the hematogenous route, mainly to the lungs.

TABLE 28.2	Classification of Malignant Epithelial Mammary Tumors
Classification	**Histologic Characteristics**
Carcinoma in situ	Well-demarcated, noninfiltrative nodule(s) (noninvading basement membrane and myoepithelial layer) of closely packed cells arranged in irregular tubules or nests that have not extended through the basement membrane. • Loss of normal architecture, cell and nuclear polarity with anisocytosis, anisokaryosis, and increased numbers of mitotic figures. • Difficult to differentiate from hyperplastic/dysplastic lesions with atypia.

Carcinomas: Simple	• Tubular carcinoma
	   • Cells arranged in a predominant tubular pattern associated with variable fibrovascular stroma.
	 • Cribriform
	   • Proliferation of neoplastic cells forming a sieve-like arrangement (very small undetectable tubules).
	 • Tubulopapillary
	   • Papillae extend into tubular lumina and this is the main pattern. They are supported by a fine fibrovascular stroma.
	 • Cystic-papillary
	   • Papillae extending into cystic lumina.

Carcinoma: Micropapillary invasive	• Neoplastic cells form small irregular aggregates and small papillae that do not have a supporting fibrovascular stalk and that are surrounded by empty lacunar spaces. • There is often infiltration of neoplastic cells into the peripheral tissue.
Carcinoma: Solid	• Closely packed cells arranged in nests and cords form dense, irregularly sized lobules surrounded by fine fibrovascular stroma.
Comedocarcinoma	• Multinodular appearance with well-demarcated necrosis within the center of the nodular areas surrounded by neoplastic cells. • Necrotic areas characterized by abundant amorphous eosinophilic material admixed with cell debris.
Carcinoma: Anaplastic	• Most malignant of the carcinomas. • Neoplastic cells individualized or in small nests. • Invading cells often evoke a desmoplastic host response. • Anaplastic histology can be characterized by extensive histologic lymphovascular invasion with neoplastic emboli in the overlying dermal lymphatic vessels. This can appear as inflammatory carcinoma, which is a clinical diagnosis. Inflammatory carcinoma can also be associated with other histologic subtype.
Carcinoma arising in a complex adenoma/ mixed tumor	• Benign counterpart detectable with areas of more pleomorphic epithelial cells showing increased number of mitoses and higher pleomorphism compared with the preexisting benign epithelial component.
Carcinomas: Complex	• Malignant epithelial component, but myoepithelium is nonmalignant. The myoepithelium as a typical spindle to stellate morphology admixed with variable amount of myxoid matrix. • Only the epithelial cells exhibit considerable anisokaryosis and anisocytosis.
Ductal carcinoma	• Cells arranged in cords and tubules that surround slit-like lumina lined by a double layer of epithelial cells (luminal and basal/myoepithelial cells). • Exhibit anisokaryosis, anisocytosis, and increased mitotic figures. • Basal/myoepithelial cells can extend into the interstitium but retain a basal morphology.
Intraductal papillary carcinoma	• Proliferation of multilayered epithelial cells forming intraductal papillae. • Fibrous connective tissue and normal myoepithelial cells are retained as the supporting stroma for the papillae.

Carcinosarcoma (Malignant Mixed Mammary Tumor)

Carcinosarcoma (malignant mixed mammary tumor) is composed partly of cells morphologically resembling the epithelial component and partly of cells morphologically resembling mesenchymal tissue elements, both types of which are malignant. It is an uncommon mammary neoplasm, but it most often presents as a carcinoma and OSA. The mesenchymal component can less commonly be represented by fibrous connective tissue alone or in combination with malignant bone/cartilage tissue. Myoepithelial cells (benign or malignant) can occasionally be present. The epithelial component metastasizes via lymphatic vessels to regional LNs and the lungs, and the mesenchymal component metastasizes via the hematogenous route to the lungs.

Hyperplasia/Dysplasia/Neoplasia of the Nipple

Ductal adenoma and carcinoma are rare and involve only the nipple (ducts) with no neoplastic tissue in the underlying MG.

The nipple is enlarged and firm. The histopathology mimics that of ductal adenomas and carcinomas of the underlying gland.[129] Carcinoma with epidermal infiltration (Paget-like disease) is a neoplasm occasionally seen in the dog that mimics Paget's disease of the nipple in women. In this lesion, the carcinoma is present within the MG and carcinoma cells, either as individual cells or small aggregates, are present within the epidermis of the nipple.

Histopathologic Prognostic Factors and Grading

The epithelial tumors are graded according to specific histopathologic criteria. Several systems for both canine and feline tumors exist, most of which are based on the Elston and Ellis grading system,[132] which incorporates information regarding (1) tubule formation, (2) nuclear pleomorphism, and (3) mitoses per 10 high-power fields (HPFs) (Table 28.3).[133–135] Based on the total score derived from this system, the grade of the tumor will be determined: grade I (low score) is a well-differentiated tumor, grade II (intermediate score) is moderately differentiated, and grade III (high total score)

TABLE 28.3 Criteria Used for Histologic Grading of Malignancy in Feline and Canine Mammary Carcinomas

Tubule Formation[a]	Nuclear Pleomorphism[a]	MITOSES/10 HPFS[b]	
		Canine	Feline
Tubule formation >75% of the specimen: **1 point**	Uniform or regular small nucleus and occasional nucleoli: **1 point**	0–9: **1 point**	0–8: **1 point**
Moderate formation of tubular arrangements (10%–75% of the specimen) admixed with areas of solid tumor growth: **2 points**	Moderate degree of variation in nuclear size and shape, hyperchromatic nucleus, and presence of nucleoli (some of which can be prominent): **2 points**	10–19: **2 points**	9–17: **2 points**
Minimal or no tubule formation (<10%): **3 points**	Marked variation in nuclear size and hyperchromatic nucleus, often with one or more prominent nucleoli: **3 points**	>19: **3 points**	>17: **3 points**

[a]In complex and mixed tumors, the percentage of tubular formation and the nuclear pleomorphism are evaluated only in the malignant component. In malignant myoepithelioma tubular formation is 2
[b]HPF, High-power field. The fields are selected at the periphery or the most mitotically active parts of the sample (including also myeopithelial cells if part of the tumor). Diameter of the field of view = 0.55 mm; area = 0.237 mm[2]; 10 HPFs = 2.37 mm[2]. The mitotic count has to be proportional to the field diameter.

TABLE 28.4A Tumor Grade Based on Histologic Score from Table 28.3 in Cats and Dogs[133,134,136,137,210]

Total Score	Grade of Malignancy
3–5	I (low) Well differentiated
6–7	II (intermediate) Moderately differentiated
8–9	III (high) Poorly differentiated

TABLE 28.4B Newly Proposed Histologic Grading System for Invasive Mammary Carcinoma in Cats

Lymphovascular Invasion	Points
Present	1
Absent	0
Nuclear Form[a]	**Points**
≤5% Abnormal	0
>5% Abnormal	1
Mitotic Count (mitoses per 10 HPFs)[b]	**Points**
≤62	0
>62	1
Histologic Grade	**Sum of Points**
Grade I (low, well differentiated)	0
Grade II (intermediate, moderately differentiated)	1
Grade III (high, poorly differentiated)	2–3

[a]Abnormal nuclear form includes any deviation from smooth nuclear contour or round/oval nuclear shape such as clefting, angularity, corrugation, or ameboid morphology assessed at high power (40–60× objective) in the least differentiated and/or most invasive portions of the tumor. The number of nuclei exhibiting the abnormal nuclear form is estimated and expressed as a percentage of the total number of nuclei within any given field.
[b]Cumulative number of mitoses in 10 consecutive high-power fields (HPFs) in the most mitotically active area with a microscope field diameter of 0.53 mm (40× objective).[218]

is poorly differentiated (Table 28.4a,b). Tumor grade has been found to provide consistent and reliable prognostic information in both cats and dogs.[82,129,130,132–135] More recently, details on how to perform grading, particularly in MGTs with myoepithelial or mesenchymal components[136] and on how to standardize the mitotic count,[137] have been published. In addition to the grading system, information regarding vascular/lymphatic invasion, surrounding stromal invasion, LN involvement, and tumor type may also predict behavior.[13,29,65,130,131,135,138,139] Specifically for histotypes,[131] dogs carrying adenosquamous (median survival time [MST] of 18 months), comedo- (MST of 14 months), solid (MST of 8 months), and anaplastic (MST of 3 months) carcinomas experienced the worst prognosis. Prolonged survival was observed for complex carcinoma and simple tubular carcinoma, whereas a more than 10-fold higher risk of tumor-related death was associated with certain other types such as simple tubulopapillary carcinoma, intraductal papillary carcinoma, and carcinoma and malignant myoepithelioma. Carcinosarcomas and sarcomas are typically not graded via this system, but the majority tend to be biologically aggressive tumors and associated with a very poor long-term survival.[135,138]

MGTs in dogs represent a wide histologic spectrum with both benign and malignant lesions originating from different tissue types or a combination of tissues. Many dogs present with several different tumors and tumors of different types and can as such represent a rather daunting histopathologic picture; prognosis is determined by the most aggressive tumor and decisions regarding adjuvant treatments should be based on the largest or the most aggressive histology. In many cases, the most aggressive tumor is the largest.[15]

Clinical Prognostic Factors

The three prognostic factors that are most consistently reported to be associated with prognosis include tumor size, LN involvement, and World Health Organization (WHO) stage (modified and original). These are the only factors that will be discussed here.

Tumor Size

According to MacEwen et al, dogs with tumor volume larger than 40 cc (approximately 3.4 cm in diameter) have a statistically significant worse outcome than smaller tumors, both in terms of remission and survival.[140] Other investigators have classified tumors as stage I, smaller than 3 cm; stage II, between 3 cm and 5 cm; and stage III, larger than 5 cm.[124,140] Dogs with stage I tumors have a significantly longer survival.[13,74,141] Others, however, have found that a change in prognosis only becomes significant when tumors are larger than 5 cm.[29,142] The change in prognosis is likely gradual as tumors increase in size. The modified WHO staging system has incorporated these three size categories representing stage I, stage II, and stage III disease, respectively.[125] Importantly, however, the size of the tumor becomes irrelevant if the local LN is involved.[13] A positive LN constitutes stage IV disease according to the revised WHO system, attributing a worse prognosis to LN involvement rather than tumor size.

Lymph Node Status

A large retrospective study, including only dogs with carcinomas, all of which had the local or draining LN removed and biopsied, found that the status of the local LNs was highly prognostic.[13] Others have confirmed these findings.[29,74,77,135,138,143] Therefore information regarding the status of the local LN is extremely important when considering the need for adjuvant or systemic therapy in dogs with MGTs. Earlier publications did not quantify the extent of LN involvement or did not use IHC to facilitate identification of microscopic clusters or isolated tumor cells, potentially including only dogs with macrometastasis in their analysis. More recent publications, however, have investigated the significance of microscopic LN metastasis. Micrometastasis, defined as clusters of cells ranging from 0.2 to 2.0 mm in diameter,[116,144] did not predict a significantly worse outcome compared with dogs with no evidence of metastasis. Interestingly, dogs with isolated metastatic tumor cells (not in clusters) had a worse outcome according to one of these studies.[144]

WHO Staging System

Both the original and the revised WHO staging system provide prognostic information. When performing a side-by-side comparison of the two systems, the revised system appears to better reflect the stronger effect of LN status on prognosis.[126] Nevertheless, the original staging system also provides useful prognostic information as illustrated in two larger separate retrospective studies in which dogs with higher WHO stage disease had a significantly worse prognosis than dogs with lower stage disease.[29,143]

Therapy

Surgical Treatment

The challenge in preparing surgical recommendations is the lack of uniform, robust prospective clinical trials that clarify the extent or "dose" of surgical excision: simple lumpectomy, local mastectomy, regional mastectomy, chain mastectomy, or bilateral mastectomies. The goal of the surgery must be defined through staging and counseling with the owner. Is the goal to remove the current tumor(s) with clean margins or remove the current tumor(s) with clean margins *and* prevent new tumors in the remaining glands? The latter option as elaborated in the next paragraph would require prophylactic mastectomies of clinically normal glands in addition to affected glands.

Several studies have evaluated the effect of surgical dose in canine mammary tumors. A prospective randomized trial of 144 dogs with naïve malignant tumors comparing the DFI and OST benefit relative to either chain mastectomy or simple mastectomy found no differences.[140] Similarly, a retrospective case series of 79

dogs treated at a single institution found no difference in DFI or OST compared with the type of surgical procedure performed, whether lumpectomy, local mastectomy, regional mastectomy with en bloc LN excision, or chain mastectomy with en bloc LN excision.[143] However, the relative hazard for death within the first 2 years after surgery was slightly higher for dogs receiving a regional mastectomy over a chain mastectomy.[143] Interestingly, in one study, the hazard curves for DFI and survival were quite similar, suggesting that most dogs that experienced recurrence developed metastasis and not new tumors; however, the rate of new tumors was not reported in this study.[140] A different study indicated that surgical "dose" is important. In this case series of 99 dogs, all intact female dogs underwent either a regional or chain mastectomy for a single MGT with unknown histology.[145] Of these, 58% of dogs developed a new tumor in the remaining ipsilateral MG tissue after a regional mastectomy and those whose initial tumor was subsequently determined to be malignant were more likely to develop an ipsilateral tumor. The authors advocated for an initial unilateral chain mastectomy for female intact dogs with a single MGT, although, in their population, 42% of dogs did not develop a subsequent tumor and would have experienced a larger surgical dose than needed.[145] Although a more aggressive surgical approach does not affect MGT development in the contralateral mammary chain or improve STs, it does decrease the need for further surgery for the management of subsequent MGTs in the ipsilateral mammary chain in approximately 60% of dogs. It is worth noting, however, the significant incidence of postoperative complications (77%) in dogs undergoing radical mastectomies when making such recommendations[146] Other large useful studies investigating the association between OHE and survival did not report on the completeness or extent of MGT removal.[20,147,148] Development of second MGTs is well documented and has been reported in more than 70% of dogs with malignant MGTs after lumpectomy, although the effect of second MGT development on survival is not well delineated.[18,140,145] It is clear from a prospective randomized study trial for intact dogs having benign MGTs that concurrent OHE significantly reduces the risk of future MGT development by almost 50% and reduces the risk for additional life-threatening uterine and ovarian diseases.[21] A related prospective randomized clinical trial of 60 intact dogs having malignant MGTs demonstrated that a small subset of dogs benefited from concurrent OHE, specifically those dogs with grade II ER+ tumors or dogs with increased peri-surgical serum E_2 concentration.[79] A single standardized guideline for surgical treatment omits consideration of factors such as the age, tumor size, tumor number, previous MGTs, and clinical stage, and may not provide the optimal outcome. Future carefully constructed clinical trials may offer more tailored recommendations based on the individual patient's risk.

Current recommendations based on available data suggest that for dogs with a single MGT of known or unknown histotype, surgical excision wide enough to completely remove the tumor is adequate.[149] Incomplete excision or cytoreductive procedures are not recommended.[123] Tumors that are fixed or have skin ulceration and are less than 1 cm in diameter may be sufficiently managed with a local mastectomy (Fig. 28.3).[123] Wide excision has not been well defined, but for larger tumors, this may be generalized to a 2-cm lateral margin and modified according to the size of the patient and tumor.[123] The deep margin may need to include the abdominal muscular fascia and/or portions of the abdominal wall to be excised en bloc with the

MGT, depending on size and fixation.[123] If abdominal surgery is to be performed simultaneously for OHE, accidental penetration of the tumor capsule before abdominal entry is to be avoided to prevent direct spread of tumor cells; rather, tumor removal should follow abdominal closure. For animals with multiple MGTs, more extensive resections such as a regional mastectomy, unilateral chain mastectomy, or bilateral mastectomy may be pursued. As with other tumor resections, surgical margin

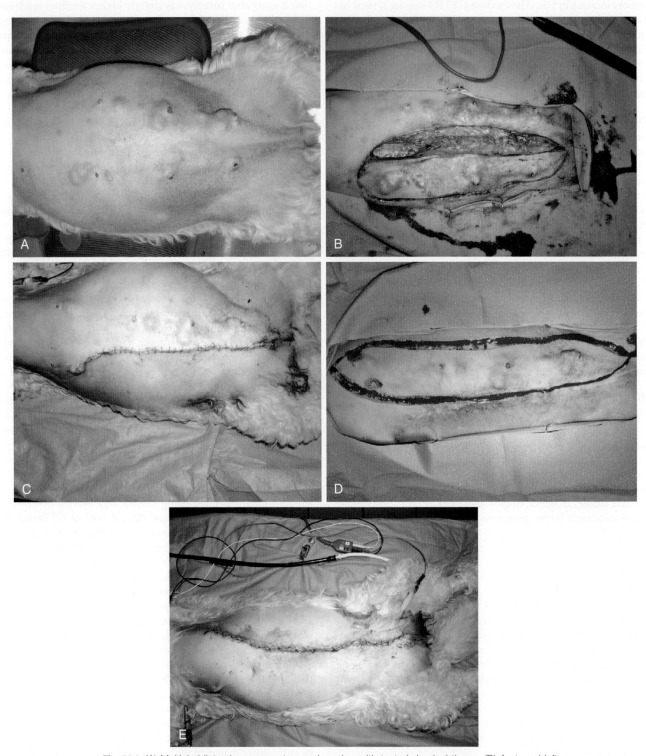

• **Fig. 28.3** (A) Multiple bilateral mammary tumors in a dog with taut abdominal tissue. (B) A staged left chain mastectomy was performed initially of the side with the larger tumors. (C) Immediate postsurgical appearance after the staged unilateral chain mastectomy without undue tension. (D) The staged right chain mastectomy was performed 6 weeks later. (E) Immediate postsurgical appearance after completed resection of all mammary tumors in this dog. (Courtesy Dr. Julius Liptak, VCA Canada—Alta Vista Animal Hospital, Ottawa, Canada.)

assessment is critical for malignant MGTs, and additional surgery should be pursued if incompletely excised. In one retrospective study, the MST was 15.5 months for dogs with incomplete histologic excision of their MGT versus 22.8 months for dogs with complete histologic excision, and 70 days versus 872 days, respectively, in another retrospective study.[150,75] Elective unilateral or bilateral chain mastectomies may be reasonable for young intact bitches with multiple MGTs because there is the possibility of development of additional tumors (Fig. 28.4).[123]

Surgical excision is questionable as a treatment for dogs presenting with inflammatory carcinoma because of the profound diffuse microscopic extent of cutaneous disease, the significant metastatic rate, and the local tissue coagulopathy that may be present. In 43 dogs with inflammatory carcinoma, only three dogs were considered suitable for unilateral chain mastectomy based on physical examination, yet all three had residual neoplastic cells at the surgical margins.[102] Interestingly, two of the dogs also received adjuvant chemotherapy and were among the longest survivors in that study.[102] Radiation therapy can be considered for palliation of dogs having clinical signs associated with presence of an inflammatory carcinoma.[151]

Systemic Treatment

Few clinical studies have investigated systemic therapy for MGTs, and efficacy has not been evaluated and confirmed according to the highest evidence-based standards. Despite this uncertainty, chemotherapy is routinely recommended and administered in dogs with "high-risk" tumors. This practice is based on the recognition that dogs with large tumors, positive LNs, and aggressive histology are not treated effectively

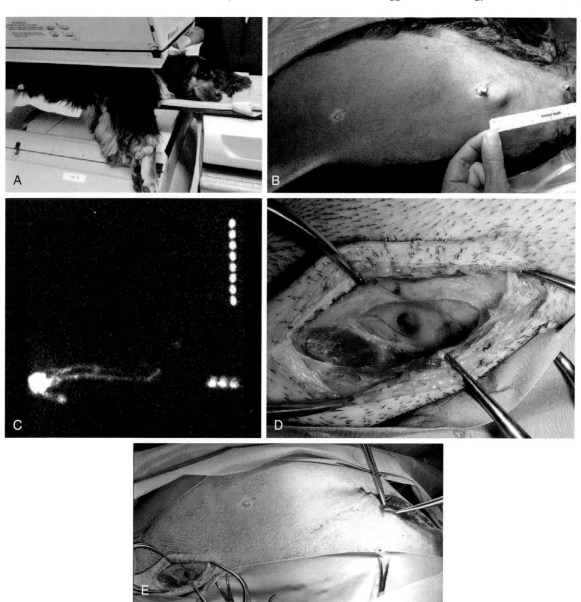

• **Fig. 28.4** (A) Regional lymphoscintigraphy being performed in a dog with a single mammary carcinoma. Technetium was injected in four quadrants around the primary tumor in the cranial abdominal mammary gland. (B) Gross image of the same tumor in vivo. (C) Regional lymphoscintigram of the patient highlighting radiopharmaceutical uptake in the mammary tumor and in the sentinel ipsilateral axillary lymph nodes. (D) Close-up surgical appearance of a "hot" and "blue" sentinel accessory axillary lymph node visualized on the lymphoscintigram enhanced with intraoperative methylene blue dye mapping. (E) Surgical field highlighting the distance between the mammary tumor and the same sentinel lymph node.

TABLE 28.5	Prognostic Factors and Indication for Adjuvant Chemotherapy with Supporting Level of Evidence in Dogs with Malignant Mammary Tumors			
Tumor Size	Lymph Node Involvement	Histopathologic Type	Indication for Chemotherapy (No or Yes)	Evidence Level 1–5[a]
<3 cm/40 cc	Negative	Carcinoma	No[b]	1[140]
>3 cm/40 cc	Negative	Carcinoma	Yes[c]	1,[140] 2,[226] 4,[227] 5[80]
Any	Positive	Carcinoma	Yes	3,[13,29,74,77,135,138,143] 2,[226] 5[80]
Any	Any	Osteosarcoma	Yes	3[138,164]
Any	Any	Inflammatory carcinoma	Yes	3[101,102,162]

[a]Evidence level 1: Prospective randomized trial; level 2: Prospective, nonrandomized trial; level 3: Retrospective; level 4: Case report(s); level 5: Extrapolation from human breast cancer studies.
[b]Chemotherapy may be considered if unfavorable histology (vascular invasion or high grade).[134,135,138,139]
[c]Dogs with stage III disease according to the original WHO staging system were included.[226] Stage III disease includes dogs with tumors >5 cm with or without lymph node metastasis.[124]

with surgery alone. The use of hormonal therapy in canine MGTs is based on tumor hormone dependence (tumor risk and HRs) and the potential to significantly reduce recurrence and prolong survival in HR-positive cancers similar to human hormonal therapy. This can be achieved by surgical means (ovariectomy [OVE] or OHE) or medical means, including specific ER modulators and suppression of estrogen synthesis by aromatase inhibitors or luteinizing hormone–releasing hormone agonists. Tamoxifen, an ER antagonist commonly used in women with ER-positive breast cancer, has been evaluated in dogs both with and without MGTs. Because of the side effects, mostly from proestrogenic signs, this strategy may not be tolerable or feasible in dogs.[152,153] Surgical ovarian ablation, specifically OVE/OHE, is a more practical solution in the dog. This will also eliminate the ovarian production of progesterone, the other main player in canine mammary tumorigenesis. Alternatively, specific drugs targeting the progesterone receptor may be considered. A recent randomized study documented improvements in DFI in specific subset of dogs randomized to receive a progesterone receptor antagonist (aglepristone) (see Table 28.6).[154] There are numerous publications on the topic of OHE in canine MGTs. The results are in discordance; most of the earlier studies did not report benefit in ovariohysterectomized dogs compared with intact dogs.[18,140,141,152,155] A few of these earlier studies, however, did report benefit; one study found that the benefit of OHE was only significant in dogs with complex carcinomas.[143] Another study found that the timing of OHE in relation to tumor surgery was important; only dogs with OHE performed within 2 years before or concurrently with tumor removal benefited.[148] None of these studies were randomized and the results were not analyzed in the context of tumor HRs, thus the results must be interpreted with caution. A recently published prospective randomized study may provide new insight regarding OHE in dogs with mammary carcinoma.[79] As to be expected, no benefit was noted when all dogs were included in the analysis; however, when the effect of OHE was stratified based on HR positivity, a modest improvement was noted in dogs that underwent OHE. This difference did not reach significance, likely due to lack of power. Interestingly, OHE conferred a significant improvement in survival in dogs with grade II tumors and dogs that had higher than median peri-surgical serum estradiol, regardless of ER expression.[79] These results reflect the diversity in the biology and behavior in canine mammary carcinoma and

therefore the need for more individualized recommendations regarding adjuvant care, including whether to perform OHE (one size does not fit all).

Chemotherapy is often administered to dogs with MGTs considered to be at risk for metastasis or recurrence. Most of the evidence regarding the efficacy of adjuvant chemotherapy is weak, but some studies have reported improved outcomes in dogs treated with chemotherapy, alone or in combination with nonsteroidal antiinflammatory drugs (NSAIDs) (see Table 28.6). Anthracycline or taxane combinations are considered part of first-line protocols in human BC in women requiring adjuvant therapy[80,156–158]; however, only inadequately powered nonrandomized studies on the efficacy of doxorubicin (DOX), docetaxel, gemcitabine, mitoxantrone, and carboplatin in dogs with high risk or advanced MGTs have been performed and none clearly establish benefit.[150,159–161] Interestingly, NSAIDs, with or without chemotherapy, were found to be effective in prolonging survival in dogs with high risk (grade III and/or advanced clinical stage) or inflammatory carcinomas according to several retrospective and prospective studies (see Table 28.6).[102,160,162,163] Chemotherapy may also have a role in the treatment of primary MG OSA. The MG is one of the most common sites for extraskeletal OSA and, according to one small retrospective case series (including primary MG OSA and other extraskeletal sites), dogs treated with adjuvant chemotherapy were significantly less likely to die of tumor-related causes than dogs treated with surgery alone.[164]

Lastly, a prospective randomized trial documented significant improvement in survival in dogs with histologic grade II or III carcinoma treated with perioperative desmopressin.[165] The antimetastatic properties of desmopressin are not fully understood, but it is hypothesized that they in part are mediated through improving hemostasis and preventing cancer cells from gaining access to the vasculature during surgical manipulation.[166,167] The results are intriguing, however, further confirmatory studies are warranted in light of the fact that only two dogs with grade III tumors were randomized to the placebo arm in this particular study and both dogs died shortly after surgery (MST 35 days). This unusually short survival may contribute to the apparent improvement in survival in the desmopressin arm. As illustrated earlier, there is currently a paucity of high-quality trial evidence from which to draw information and guidance for treating dogs with malignant high-risk MGTs. Table 28.5 provides general guidance and treatment consideration/options and the level of supporting evidence. Table 28.6 summarizes trials reporting benefit from systemic therapy in dogs with MGTs.

TABLE 28.6	Summary of Published Studies Reporting Benefit from Systemic Therapy in Dogs with Malignant Mammary Tumors			
Tumor Stage	**Grade/Histopathology**	**Treatment**	**Comments and Effect**	**Reference**
Stage III–IV	Any grade Various carcinomas	Cyclophosphamide, 5-fluorouracil vs none	Evidence level 2[a] DFS: $p < 0.01$	226
Stage I–IV	Grade 3 Various carcinomas	NSAID: firocoxib vs none	Evidence level 2 DFS: $p = 0.015$	160
Stage IV–V	Grade: NA	Carboplatin +/– NSAIDs vs none	Evidence level 2 OS: $p = 0.07$[b]	163
Advanced	Inflammatory carcinomas	NSAIDs +/– chemotherapy vs None	Evidence level 3 Palliative intent OS: $p = 0.01$	102
Advanced	Inflammatory carcinomas	NSAID (piroxicam) vs doxorubicin	Evidence level 3 Palliative intent PFS: $p < 0.01$	162
Stage I	Grades 1, 2 Complex and mixed carcinomas, PR+	Hormonal Tx Antiprogestin (aglepristone) vs none	Evidence level 1 $p = 0.002–0.02$	154
Stage I–IV	Grade 2	Hormonal Tx OHE vs intact	Evidence level 1 $p = 0.03$	79
Stage III–IV	Grades 2, 3 Various carcinomas	DDAVP (desmopressin) vs none	Evidence level 1 DSF: $p = 0.001$	165
NA	Extraskeletal Osteosarcoma, including mammary	Doxorubicin or cisplatin vs none	Evidence level 3 Mixed primary sites OS: $p = 0.02$	164

[a]Evidence level 1: Prospective randomized trial; level 2: Prospective, nonrandomized trial; level 3: Retrospective; level 4: Case report(s); level 5: Extrapolation from human breast cancer studies.
[b]Significance set at $p = 0.1$.
NSAID, Nonsteroidal antiinflammatory drug; *OST*, overall survival time; *PFS*, progression-free survival; *PR*, progesterone receptor.

Mammary Tumors in Cats

Epidemiology and Risk Factors

Epidemiology

There are fewer epidemiologic studies regarding the incidence of mammary neoplasia in cats compared with dogs. Furthermore, because of differences in veterinary care for cats, the available data likely underestimate the true incidence of disease. According to data from one of the largest Swedish insurance companies, approximately 40% to 50 % of all dogs had insurance to cover veterinary expenses, whereas only 20% of cats had such coverage.[168,169] Another study from the United States also reported that a significantly lower percentage of cats receives regular veterinary care compared with dogs.[170]

The overall MGT incidence is lower in cats than in dogs. According to the California Animal Neoplasia Registry (CANR), MGTs represent the third most common tumor in female cats (after skin tumors and lymphoma) with an annual incidence rate of 25.4/100,000 and 12% of tumors in cats regardless of sex.[1] Data from an animal tumor registry from two provinces in northern Italy reported that MGTs represented 16% of all tumors in cats and 25% in female cats.[171] Data from a Swedish insurance company indicate that MGTs were the most common cancer representing 40% of all tumor-related claims in cats.[168] It is unclear whether the higher relative incidence of MGTs in the latter studies is due to differences in neutering practices or use of progestins

in the source population because no information regarding OHE status was provided.

Risk Factors

Three main risk factors in cats have been identified: age, breed, and hormonal influence.

Age

As in the dog, mammary neoplasia is a disease seen predominantly in middle-aged to older cats. The mean age of diagnosis is between 10 and 12 years of age.[1,172–175] Risk increases incrementally with age but does not become significant until 7 to 9 years, according to the age-specific incidence curves from the CANR, and continues to increase up until 12 to 14 years.[1]

Breed

Siamese cats are significantly younger when diagnosed with MGTs and risk plateaus at 9 years of age.[176] In general, genetic predisposition for a disease is often associated with a younger age of diagnosis. Siamese cats appear overrepresented compared with other breeds.[176,177] However, Siamese cats have an increased risk for many tumor types and not only MGTs.[178–182] It is therefore possible that the increased incidence in Siamese cats is due to breed-associated germline alterations in common tumor susceptibility genes or defective tumor suppressor gene function that confers increased risk for many different malignancies.

Hormonal Association

Exposure to ovarian hormones is also strongly implicated in mammary tumorigenesis in the cat. Sexually intact cats have a 7-fold higher risk than spayed cats.[1] The increased risk in intact cats has been confirmed by others.[173,176,183] Similar to findings in dogs, exposure from ovarian hormones in cats at an early age appears crucial. The protective effect of OHE diminishes quickly over the first few years; risk reductions of 91%, 86%, and 11% are seen in cats that are ovariohysterectomized before 6 months, between 7 and 12 months, and between 13 and 24 months, respectively. No benefit was found after 24 months.[183] According to the same study, parity did not influence risk for MGTs.

In addition to endogenous ovarian hormonal influence, exposure to exogenous progestins also increases risk. Cats treated with progestins have an overall relative risk of 3.4 compared with those not receiving such treatments, although benign tumors arise more commonly than malignant tumors (relative risk 5.3 vs 2.8).[173] Unlike dogs, progestin-treated cats were not younger than non-treated cats when they developed tumors.[173] The tumorigenic effects of oral progestins in cats are supported by reports of male cats with MGTs. MGTs are rare in males, but in a report of 22 cases, eight (36%) had a history of progestin use.[184] In a recent case series of three male cats with MGTs, all had received multiple injections of a long-lasting progestin over 5 to 6 years before tumor development. All had malignant tumors and all developed subsequent malignant tumors in other glands after initial surgery.[185] Shorter duration of treatment or inconsistent administration is less likely to result in malignant tumors, but nevertheless induce changes in the MGs.[186] Fibroepithelial hyperplasia (fibroadenomatous change, fibroepithelial hypertrophy, mammary hypertrophy) is the most common histopathologic change in cats treated for shorter periods of time and can occur relatively quickly, even after one injection; however, studies show that regular and prolonged administration is needed for malignant tumors to develop.[173]

Tumor Biology: Development, Hormones, Growth Factors, and Prognostic Implications

The risk for MGT development in cats is determined by exposure to ovarian hormones early in life, but the latency period appears long because most cats are older when diagnosed. In many species, ovarian hormones are necessary for normal MG development and maturation, but few studies have examined hormonal effects on mammary tumorigenesis in cats. The complex interactions between sex hormones, GH, and IGF-1 have been discussed in more detail in the section on canine MGTs, but progestin-induced mammary production of GH has been documented in the cat.[187,188] It is, however, biologically plausible that the tumorigenic effects on mammary tissues are similar across species and that the same general mechanisms are involved, specifically sex hormones and GH. Despite ER and PR expression being implicated in the initial stages of MGT development, many investigators have reported that most feline mammary carcinomas are ER and PR negative, although slightly more than one-third are PR positive.[72,189–192] The percentage of ER/PR expression varies between studies and is likely the result of differences in case selection, methods, and interpretation of the results. The biochemical method, the dextran-coated charcoal (DCC) method, may be more sensitive than IHC when

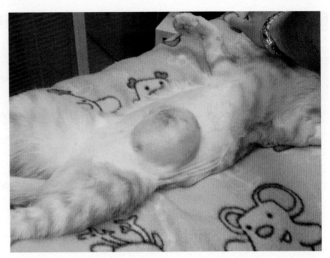

• **Fig. 28.5** Fibroepithelial hyperplasia in a cat. (Courtesy Dr. Lisa Mestrinho, Faculdade de Medicina Veterinária, Universidade Lusofona de Humanidades e Tecnologias, Lisboa, Portugal.)

analyzing ER in cats.[191] Standardized IHC methods have high concordance with DCC methods; 38.5% of the malignant tumors and 66.7% of the benign lesions expressed PR according to IHC.[191] In this particular study, sexually intact cats were more likely to have PR-positive tumors. Lower concordance was found between ER analysis by DCC and IHC with IHC being less sensitive than DCC; only 20% of the malignant tumors expressed ER according to IHC compared with 44% according to the DCC assay.[191] These results are consistent with other publications showing a relatively low ER expression in feline MGTs when using IHC.

The low HR positivity in the tumors is consistent with the higher rate of malignancy and a more aggressive clinical behavior in feline MGTs. In contrast to malignant tumors, normal mammary tissue and dysplastic lesions in the MG express both ER and PR[72,189,190]; however, this hormone dependence appears to wane with histologic progression from benign to malignant. None of the intermediate- or high-grade ductal CIS (nomenclature referring to breast intraepithelial lesions in women) were ER or PR positive,[189] whereas the normal and hyperplastic adjacent mammary tissue expressed HRs.[72,189,190] Fibroepithelial hyperplasia, a progesterone-induced change, has been reported to have high PR expression[186] and can be effectively treated by OHE or antiprogestins (Fig. 28.5).[193]

In human BC, an inverse relationship between the HR status and HER-2 expression is documented. HER-2 expression tends to be higher in cats than in dogs and humans; however, a wide range (6%–90%) of HER-2–positive tumors is reported.[194–197]

History and Clinical Presentation

Cats with MGTs are often older and may be sexually intact or spayed after they were 2 years old. Tumors are easy to detect on physical examination and appear as firm discrete mass(es) in the MG(s). One study reported that all glands are equally susceptible to tumor development, but a later study showed that the cranial glands were less commonly affected.[198,199] Multiple tumors are common; 60% of cats had more than one tumor at diagnosis in one report.[174] Careful examination of the remaining MGs is important when evaluating a cat with a prior history of MGTs, especially if treated with local mastectomy, because new primary tumors are common. Tumor(s) size at diagnosis depends on how early it is detected and how aggressive the tumor behaves. Larger tumors may become ulcerated, inflamed, and infected. Local LNs may or may not appear enlarged. Inflammatory mammary carcinomas are rare in cats and the clinical picture and outcome are similar to those described in the dog.[200]

Clinical Assessment, Diagnosis, Workup, and Clinical Staging

Cats with mammary masses tend to be older and their tumors are commonly malignant; therefore a thorough workup is recommended to ascertain any comorbidity and advanced disease. This may include CBC, serum biochemistry, serum T_4 concentration, three-view thoracic radiographs, abdominal ultrasound, and urinalysis, in addition to FNA of any mammary masses and any palpable (including normal-sized) regional LNs.

Staging System

Feline MGTs are staged similar to canine tumors using a modification of the original system published by Owen.[124,201] In the modified system, stage advances from I to II to III as the size increases from smaller than 2 cm, to between 2 and 3 cm, to larger than 3 cm.[125] Unlike the canine system, stage III disease also includes T1 or T2 tumors with concurrent LN metastasis and LN metastasis does not need to be present with T3 tumors. Stage IV disease is any tumor with any LN metastasis and distant metastasis.[201] This staging system should not be used with MG sarcomas (see Table 28.6).

Histopathology

The vast majority of feline MGTs are malignant (85%–95%) with an aggressive biologic behavior, and lymphatic invasion and LN metastasis are more common at the time of initial diagnosis than in dogs. Early classifications of feline MGTs were simpler than that used for canine tumors.[128] Complex and mixed tumors showing the same features of the canine counterparts have not been diagnosed in the feline MG; however, new and previously unclassified subtypes have been reported.[202] Morphologic features of each subtype are identical to the canine counterparts and, as per dogs, the predominant morphologic pattern is used to classify the tumor.

Similar to dogs, a molecular approach to MGT classification has been attempted in cats.[203–208] Despite lack of standardized methods and variability of results, mammary carcinomas in cats were associated with the highest percentage of triple-negative (HR– and HER-2–) MGTs, associated with frequent expression of both basal cytokeratins and vimentin, and had the worst prognosis. This seems to suggest that the cat may be a suitable model for some subtypes of human BC, such as the HR-independent basal-like cancers.

Hyperplasia and Dysplasia

The various hyperplastic and dysplastic lesions seen in cats include duct ectasia, lobular hyperplasia (regular, with secretory [lactational] activity, with fibrosis [interlobular fibrous connective tissue], and with atypia), epitheliosis, papillomatosis, and

TABLE 28.7 Staging of Feline Mammary Tumors[201]

Stage	Tumor Size	Lymph Node Status	Metastasis
Stage I	T_1 <2 cm	N_0	M_0
Stage II	T_2 2–3 cm	N_0	M_0
Stage III	T_1 or T_2	N_1 (positive)	M_0
	T_3 >3 cm	N_0 or N_1	M_0
Stage IV	Any	Any	M_1

From McNeill CJ, Sorenmo KU, Shofer FS, et al.: Evaluation of adjuvant doxorubicin-based chemotherapy for the treatment of feline mammary carcinoma, *J Vet Intern Med* 23:123–129, 2009.

fibroadenomatous change.[209] Fibroadenomatous change (fibroepithelial hyperplasia, fibroepithelial hypertrophy, mammary hypertrophy) is common in the cat, usually affects several glands, and is characterized by the proliferation of interlobular ducts, tubules, and periductal stromal cells. The stroma is often edematous or myxomatous, and both the epithelial and stromal cell nuclei exhibit some pleomorphism with mitoses. This lesion is hormonally induced and occurs in progestin-treated female and male cats, as well as being associated with pregnancy. Most cases regress at the end of pregnancy or cessation of progestin treatment.[128,202]

Benign Feline Mammary Neoplasms

Benign tumors in cats are uncommon and include simple adenoma, ductal adenoma, fibroadenoma, and intraductal papillary adenoma (duct papilloma).[128,202]

Malignant Mammary Neoplasms

The predominant malignant tumor types in cats are simple and epithelial in origin and as such represent carcinomas of various types. Tubular carcinomas, tubulopapillary carcinomas, and solid carcinomas are most common. Other variants include cystic-papillary carcinoma, cribriform carcinoma (when tubules are nearly undetectable), micropapillary invasive carcinoma, comedocarcinoma, anaplastic carcinoma, intraductal papillary carcinoma, ductal carcinoma, and, less commonly, squamous cell carcinoma, mucinous carcinoma, lipid-rich carcinoma, adenosquamous carcinoma, and spindle cell carcinoma.[128,197,200,202,209–216]

Histopathologic Prognostic Factors and Grading

Grading was initially thought not to be prognostic in cats; therefore the classification of mammary tumors was based on morphologic criteria only. More recently, histologic grading using a system similar to that in dogs (see Tables 28.3 and 28.4a) has been shown to be prognostic in cats.[210,217] In addition to histologic grade, lymphovascular invasion and LN metastasis are independent prognostic factors.[210,217] Thus the histopathologic criteria used in dogs (i.e., grade, vascular invasion, LN status) can be used in cats when assessing risk for metastasis and prognosis, and should be incorporated into decisions regarding the need for systemic treatment in cats with MGTs (Table 28.7).

Recently a novel grading system for feline MGTs has been proposed which includes lymphovascular invasion (see Table 28.4b).[218] A limitation of this system is that when evaluating histologic section(s) of a tumor, lymphovascular invasion might not be present in the selected section(s). Standardization of this method would be improved by additional information, such as number of sections, and trimming procedure. Pathologists might then consider including both systems in their report to allow a comparison and a more robust assessment of its prognostic value. Using this grading system, the median OST of cats with grade I tumors was 31 months (36 months with the Elston and Ellis–based scoring system), grade II tumors was 14 months (18 months with the Elston and Ellis–based scoring system), and grade III tumors was 8 months (6 months with the Elston and Ellis–based scoring system).[218]

Clinical Prognostic Factors

Few studies reporting prognostic factors in cats with MGTs are prospective, only one is randomized, and most are underpowered or not stratified according to treatment. Therefore the results vary and may be significantly affected by bias. Tumor size has, however, consistently been reported to have prognostic significance, including the results of two large prospective studies.

Tumor Size

Three size categories have shown prognostic significance: (1) smaller than 8 cm³ or smaller than 2 cm diameter; (2) 8 to 27 cm³ or 2 to 3 cm diameter; and (3) larger than 27 cm³ or larger than 3 cm diameter. Cats with small (<2 cm) tumors can be effectively treated with surgery alone, specifically radical mastectomy, with a MST of more than 3 years, whereas cats with tumors larger than 3 cm have a MST of only 6 months according to a large retrospective study.[219] Cats with 2- to 3-cm diameter tumors survived an average of 2 years. Several other publications have confirmed this association between survival and tumor size.[175,177,199,220,221]

Lymph Node Status

Surprisingly few studies have evaluated LN status and its prognostic significance in cats with MGTs. In a large prospective study of 202 cats, those with LN metastasis had significantly shorter STs than cats with negative LNs.[199] A retrospective study with 92 cats supported these findings; all cats with LN metastasis died within the first 9 months of diagnosis.[217] A retrospective study of 107 cats treated with either unilateral mastectomy or bilateral mastectomy for mammary adenocarcinomas revealed that LN metastasis at the time of mastectomy had a significant negative association with progression-free ST and an increased risk of death, but a third of cats having histologic evidence of LN metastasis did not progress to additional metastasis.[222]

Breed

Domestic shorthair cats had significantly better outcomes than purebred cats in a prospective randomized trial of cats with mammary carcinomas.[220] Another study reported that Siamese cats had a worse prognosis than domestic shorthairs.[223] These studies may in fact complement each other; however, the first study did not provide information regarding how many Siamese cats were included in the purebred group. Several other studies have not found breed to be prognostic when adjusted for other factors.

Age

The results regarding age and prognosis are conflicting. Several studies report that older cats have a worse prognosis; however, bias due to differences in treatments or differences in tumor size and clinical stage may exist. Importantly, a prospective randomized trial found no difference according to age when comparing cats that were younger or older than 10 years.[220]

Therapy

Surgical Treatment

The surgical dose recommended for treating feline MGTs is much clearer than in the dog. A chain mastectomy (unilateral for cats possessing a single tumor or a staged bilateral chain mastectomy for cats with bilateral tumors) resulted in a statistically significant improvement in DFI and ST, as opposed to cats receiving conservative tumor excision in a series of 100 cats.[219] In a retrospective case series of 53 cats, although no significant difference was found between the type of surgical procedure performed, cats experienced longer DFIs after either unilateral or bilateral chain mastectomies compared with partial mastectomy.[177] Recently, a multiinstitutional retrospective case series of 107 cats having either unilateral mastectomy or bilateral mastectomy for mammary adenocarcinoma found a longer median progression-free ST of 542 days for cats treated with bilateral mastectomies versus 289 days for cats treated with unilateral mastectomy.[222] In the multivariable analysis, disease-specific death was greater for those cats treated with a unilateral mastectomy and those that developed metastasis.[222] In addition, the disease-specific ST was statistically improved for cats treated with both mastectomy and adjuvant chemotherapy.[222] In a multiinstitutional retrospective case series comparing patients treated with surgery versus surgery and adjuvant DOX-based chemotherapy, the subset of cats having unilateral mastectomies followed with chemotherapy had significantly longer MSTs than cats having unilateral mastectomies without chemotherapy (1998 vs 414 days).[201] In that series, local recurrence developed in 50% of cats and, although not statistically significant, also appears to support the use of bilateral mastectomies for feline mammary carcinomas.[201] In a report of male cats diagnosed with mammary carcinomas, a trend toward more frequent local recurrence correlated with more conservative resections.[184] Thus, for cats, a unilateral or staged bilateral chain mastectomy is recommended for curative-intent treatment of mammary carcinoma. For some cats with excessively loose mammary tissue, a bilateral chain mastectomy can be performed during a single surgical session if minimal postsurgical tension can be achieved, but these cats can have a more difficult recovery with increased complication rates (Fig. 28.6).[222] For tumors that are fixed, muscular fascia or portions of the body wall should be included with en bloc resections. In a retrospective case series, bilateral mastectomy in cats with LN metastasis was found to be protective against disease progression on multivariable study analysis.[222] Thus bilateral mastectomy is recommended for MGTs in cats.

The high malignancy rate of mammary carcinoma and the poor prognosis associated with LN metastasis supports aggressive LN assessment. This could include ultrasound-guided FNA of difficult to palpate LNs and inguinal lymphadenectomy concurrent with chain mastectomy. Sentinel LN mapping has been described in the cat and was the original model for the procedure, which is common for human breast cancer patients.[111,115] Published techniques in the cat include CT evaluation after

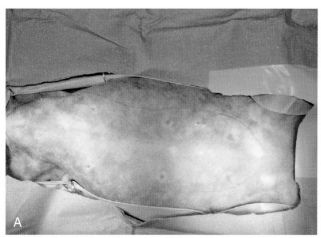
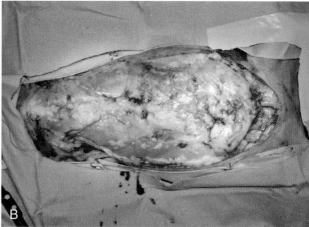
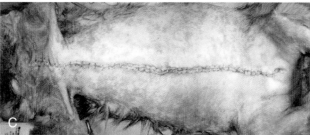

• **Fig. 28.6** (A) Cat having mammary adenocarcinoma prepared for bilateral simultaneous chain mastectomies. (B) Intraoperative view after excision of all mammary tissue. (C) Immediate postsurgical appearance after the bilateral chain mastectomies. (Courtesy Dr. Julius Liptak, VCA Canada—Alta Vista Animal Hospital, Ottawa, Canada.)

intramammary injection of iopamidol and radiographic imaging after intramammary ethiodized oil injections.[111] There are no clinical reports utilizing nuclear lymphoscintigraphy in the cat. Use of blue dyes for node visualization is recommended with caution because their use may cause Heinz body anemia and methemoglobinemia in this species. LNs extirpated during mastectomy surgery frequently yield metastasis, as found in 48 of 51,[204] 41 of 93,[222] and 17 of 66[218] cats having surgical resection of malignant MGTs.

Fibroepithelial hyperplasia has a classic appearance that is very difficult to mistake for malignant MGTs. This condition is typically treated with either OHE or medical hormone therapy management. Inflammatory mammary carcinoma has very rarely been reported in cats; in a sole case series of three cats, the disease was described as occurring secondary to postsurgical mastectomy with nonhealing incisions, edema, and suture rejections.[200]

Systemic Treatment

Early detection and aggressive surgery (including prophylactic chain mastectomy) can result in long-term survival in cats with early stage MGTs; however, cats with delayed diagnosis, large primary tumors, or metastatic local LNs are not treated effectively with surgery alone. The incidence of distant metastasis, primarily to the lungs and pleura, is high, although other organs are also frequently involved.[199] Despite the high rate of metastasis after surgery, relatively few advances have been made in identifying effective adjuvant systemic treatments.

Owing to low HR expression in feline mammary carcinoma, hormonal therapy is not likely to be effective; however, randomized trials have not been performed to confirm this.

Several studies, all retrospective, have evaluated the use of chemotherapy in cats with mammary cancer. Two case series of cats with macroscopic primary and/or metastatic tumors documented objective responses in 40% to 50% of the cats treated with a combination of DOX and cyclophosphamide.[224,225] The relatively high response rate in the macroscopic setting suggests that this may be an effective protocol in patients with microscopic minimal residual disease (i.e., after surgical cytoreduction). Results from adjuvant studies are, however, mixed, but two more recent studies suggest a benefit from chemotherapy in cats undergoing radical mastectomy (chain or bilateral). The chemotherapy varied in these studied, but DOX-based protocols were used most commonly in both of these studies: cats treated with chain mastectomy and adjuvant chemotherapy survived significantly longer than cats treated with chain mastectomy alone (1998 days vs 414 days).[202] Similar findings were also demonstrated in a separate multiinstitutional study whereby the disease-specific survival was significantly improved for 53 cats receiving adjuvant chemotherapy in 105 cats being followed after mastectomy.[222] These results support the use of adjuvant chemotherapy in this setting. It is interesting that none of these retrospective studies reported STs as long as earlier studies using surgery alone, especially in the subset of cats with small tumors. This further illustrates the difficulty in comparing outcomes between retrospective studies, especially noncontemporaneous ones. Ultimately, prospective, randomized trials will be necessary to determine the appropriate use of chemotherapy in cats with MGTs. Despite the lack of quality evidence in the literature to support it, veterinary oncologists continue to recommend the use of chemotherapy in some cats with MGTs. Table 28.8 summarizes the most important prognostic factors, general guidelines for systemic treatments, and the strength of supporting evidence.

TABLE 28.8   Prognostic Factors and Indications for Adjuvant Chemotherapy with Level of Supporting Evidence in Cats with Malignant Mammary Tumors

Tumor Size	Lymph Node Involvement	Histopathologic Parameters	Indication for Chemotherapy No or Yes	Evidence Level[a]
<2 cm /8 cm³	Negative	Carcinoma	No Yes[b]	1[220] 3[210,217,221]
2–3 cm/8–27 cm³	Negative	Carcinoma	No Yes[b]	3[219,222] 3[210,217,221]
>3 cm/ 27 cm³	Negative	Carcinoma	Yes	1,[220]2,[199] 3[219,222]
Any	Positive	Carcinoma	Yes	2,[199]3,[217] 5[80]

[a]Evidence level 1: Prospective randomized trial; level 2: Prospective, nonrandomized trial; level 3: Retrospective; level 5: Extrapolation from human breast cancer studies.
[b]Vascular invasion and high grade were found to be independent negative prognostic factors in multivariate analysis.

References

1. Dorn CR, Taylor DO, Schneider R, et al.: Survey of animal neoplasms in Alameda and Contra Costa Counties, California. II. Cancer morbidity in dogs and cats from Alameda County, *J Natl Cancer Inst* 40:307–318, 1968.
2. Moe L: Population-based incidence of mammary tumours in some dog breeds, *J Reprod Fertil Suppl* 57:439–443, 2001.
3. Egenvall A, Bonnett BN, Ohagen P, et al.: Incidence of and survival after mammary tumors in a population of over 80,000 insured female dogs in sweden from 1995 to 2002, *Prev Vet Med* 69:109–127, 2005.
4. Dobson JM, Samuel S, Milstein H, et al.: Canine neoplasia in the UK: estimates of incidence rates from a population of insured dogs, *J Small Anim Pract* 43:240–246, 2002.
5. Bronden LB, Nielsen SS, Toft N, et al.: Data from the danish veterinary cancer registry on the occurrence and distribution of neoplasms in dogs in Denmark, *Vet Rec* 166:586–590, 2010.
6. Merlo DF, Rossi L, Pellegrino C, et al.: Cancer incidence in pet dogs: findings of the animal tumor registry of genoa, Italy, *J Vet Intern Med* 22:976–984, 2008.
7. Vascellari M, Capello K, Carminato A, et al.: Incidence of mammary tumors in the canine population living in the veneto region (northeastern Italy): risk factors and similarities to human breast cancer, *Prev Vet Med* 126:183–189, 2016.
8. Salas Y, Marquez A, Diaz D, et al: Epidemiological study of mammary tumors in female dogs diagnosed during the period 2002–2012: a growing animal health problem, *PLoS One* 10:e0127381.
9. Benjamin SA, Lee AC, Saunders WJ: Classification and behavior of canine mammary epithelial neoplasms based on life-span observations in beagles, *Vet Pathol* 36:423–436, 1999.
10. Schneider R: Comparison of age, sex, and incidence rates in human and canine breast cancer, *Cancer* 26:419–426, 1970.
11. Priester WA, Mantel N: Occurrence of tumors in domestic animals. Data from 12 United States and Canadian colleges of veterinary medicine, *J Natl Cancer Inst* 47:1333–1344, 1971.
12. Brodey RS, Goldschmidt MH, Roszel JR: Canine mammary gland neoplasms, *J Am Anim Hosp Assoc* 19:61–90, 1983.
13. Kurzman ID, Gilbertson SR: Prognostic factors in canine mammary tumors, *Semin Vet Med Surg (Small Anim)* 1:25–32, 1986.
14. Taylor GN, Shabestari L, Williams J, et al.: Mammary neoplasia in a closed beagle colony, *Cancer Res* 36:2740–2743, 1976.
15. Sorenmo KU, Kristiansen VM, Cofone MA, et al.: Canine mammary gland tumours; a histological continuum from benign to malignant; clinical and histopathological evidence, *Vet Comp Oncol* 7:162–172, 2009.
16. Goldschmidt M, Shofer FS, Smelstoys JA: Neoplastic lesions of the mammary gland. In Mohr U, Carlton WW, Dungworth DL, et al.: *Pathobiology of the aging dog.* Ames, Iowa State University Press, 2001, pp 168–178.
17. Rivera P, Melin M, Biagi T, et al.: Mammary tumor development in dogs is associated with BRCA1 and BRCA2, *Cancer Res* 69:8770–8774, 2009.
18. Schneider R, Dorn CR, Taylor DO: Factors influencing canine mammary cancer development and postsurgical survival, *J Natl Cancer Inst* 43:1249–1261, 1969.
19. Sonnenschein EG, Glickman LT, Goldschmidt MH, et al.: Body conformation, diet, and risk of breast cancer in pet dogs: a case-control study, *Am J Epidemiol* 133:694–703, 1991.
20. Misdorp W: Canine mammary tumours: protective effect of late ovariectomy and stimulating effect of progestins, *Vet Q* 10:26–33, 1988.
21. Kristiansen VM, Nodtvedt A, Breen AM, et al.: Effect of ovariohysterectomy at the time of tumor removal in dogs with benign mammary tumors and hyperplastic lesions: a randomized controlled clinical trial, *J Vet Intern Med* 27:935–942, 2013.
22. Brodey RS, Fidler IJ, Howson AE: The relationship of estrous irregularity, pseudopregnancy, and pregnancy to the development of canine mammary neoplasms, *J Am Vet Med Assoc* 149:1047–1049, 1966.
23. Stovring M, Moe L, Glattre E: A population-based case-control study of canine mammary tumours and clinical use of medroxyprogesterone acetate, *APMIS* 105:590–596, 1997.
24. Concannon PW, Spraker TR, Casey HW, et al.: Gross and histopathologic effects of medroxyprogesterone acetate and progesterone on the mammary glands of adult beagle bitches, *Fertil Steril* 36:373–387, 1981.
25. Giles RC, Kwapien RP, Geil RG, et al.: Mammary nodules in beagle dogs administered investigational oral contraceptive steroids, *J Natl Cancer Inst* 60:1351–1364, 1978.
26. Kwapien RP, Giles RC, Geil RG, et al.: Malignant mammary tumors in beagle dogs dosed with investigational oral contraceptive steroids, *J Natl Cancer Inst* 65:137–144, 1980.
27. Selman PJ, van Garderen E, Mol JA, et al.: Comparison of the histological changes in the dog after treatment with the progestins medroxyprogesterone acetate and proligestone, *Vet Q* 17:128–133, 1995.
28. Geil RG, Lamar JK: Fda studies of estrogen, progestogens, and estrogen/progestogen combinations in the dog and monkey, *J Toxicol Environ Health* 3:179–193.
29. Yamagami T, Kobayashi T, Takahashi K, et al.: Prognosis for canine malignant mammary tumors based on tnm and histologic classification, *J Vet Med Sci* 58:1079–1083, 1996.

30. Schafer KA, Kelly G, Schrader R, et al.: A canine model of familial mammary gland neoplasia, *Vet Pathol* 35:168–177, 1998.

31. Ford D, Easton DF, Stratton M, et al.: Genetic heterogeneity and penetrance analysis of the *BRCA1* and *BRCA2* genes in breast cancer families. The breast cancer linkage consortium, *Am J Hum Genet* 62:676–689, 1998.

32. King MC, Marks JH, Mandell JB: Breast and ovarian cancer risks due to inherited mutations in *BRCA1* and *BRCA2*, *Science* 302:643–646, 2003.

33. Easton DF, Ford D, Bishop DT: Breast and ovarian cancer incidence in *BRCA1*–mutation carriers. Breast cancer linkage consortium, *Am J Hum Genet* 56:265–271, 1995.

34. Fackenthal JD, Olopade OI: Breast cancer risk associated with *BRCA1* and *BRCA2* in diverse populations, *Nat Rev Cancer* 7:937–948, 2007.

35. Klopfleisch R, Gruber AD: Increased expression of *BRCA2* and *Rad51* in lymph node metastases of canine mammary adenocarcinomas, *Vet Pathol* 46:416–422, 2009.

36. Nieto A, Perez-Alenza MD, Del Castillo N, et al.: BRCA1 expression in canine mammary dysplasias and tumours: relationship with prognostic variables, *J Comp Pathol* 128:260–268, 2003.

37. Perez Alenza D, Rutteman GR, Pena L, et al.: Relation between habitual diet and canine mammary tumors in a case-control study, *J Vet Intern Med* 12:132–139, 1998.

38. Calle EE, Kaaks R: Overweight, obesity and cancer: epidemiological evidence and proposed mechanisms, *Nat Rev Cancer* 4:579–591, 2004.

39. Carmichael AR, Bates T: Obesity and breast cancer: a review of the literature, *Breast* 13:85–92, 2004.

40. Tymchuk CN, Tessler SB, Barnard RJ: Changes in sex hormone-binding globulin, insulin, and serum lipids in postmenopausal women on a low-fat, high-fiber diet combined with exercise, *Nutr Cancer* 38:158–162, 2000.

41. Wu AH, Pike MC, Stram DO: Meta-analysis: dietary fat intake, serum estrogen levels, and the risk of breast cancer, *J Natl Cancer Inst* 91:529–534, 1999.

42. Hankinson SE, Willett WC, Manson JE, et al.: Plasma sex steroid hormone levels and risk of breast cancer in postmenopausal women, *J Natl Cancer Inst* 90:1292–1299, 1998.

43. Cleary MP, Grossmann ME: Minireview: obesity and breast cancer: the estrogen connection, *Endocrinology* 150:2537–2542, 2009.

44. Cleary MP, Grossmann ME, Ray A: Effect of obesity on breast cancer development, *Vet Pathol* 47:202–213, 2010.

45. Rehm S, Stanislaus DJ, Williams AM: Estrous cycle-dependent histology and review of sex steroid expression in dog reproductive tissues and mammary gland and associated hormone levels, *Birth Defects Res B Dev Reprod Toxicol* 80:233–245, 2007.

46. Santos M, Marcos R, Faustino AM: Histological study of canine mammary gland during the oestrous cycle, *Reprod Domest Anim* 45:e146–154, 2010.

47. Pike MC, Spicer DV, Dahmoush L, et al.: Estrogens, progestogens, normal breast cell proliferation, and breast cancer risk, *Epidemiol Rev* 15:17–35, 1993.

48. Russo J, Russo IH: The role of estrogen in the initiation of breast cancer, *J Steroid Biochem Mol Biol* 102:89–96, 2006.

49. Okoh V, Deoraj A, Roy D: Estrogen-induced reactive oxygen species-mediated signalings contribute to breast cancer, *Biochim Biophys Acta* 1815:115–133, 2011.

50. Dickson RB, Lippman ME, Slamon D: UCLA colloquium. New insights into breast cancer: the molecular biochemical and cellular biology of breast cancer, *Cancer Res* 50:4446–4447, 1990.

51. Mol JA, Lantinga-van Leeuwen IS, van Garderen E, et al.: Mammary growth hormone and tumorigenesis—lessons from the dog, *Vet Q* 21:111–115, 1999.

52. Selman PJ, Mol JA, Rutteman GR, et al.: Progestin-induced growth hormone excess in the dog originates in the mammary gland, *Endocrinology* 134:287–292, 1994.

53. van Garderen E, Schalken JA: Morphogenic and tumorigenic potentials of the mammary growth hormone/growth hormone receptor system, *Mol Cell Endocrinol* 197:153–165, 2002.

54. Mol JA, Selman PJ, Sprang EP, et al.: The role of progestins, insulin-like growth factor (IGF) and IGF-binding proteins in the normal and neoplastic mammary gland of the bitch: a review, *J Reprod Fertil Suppl* 51:339–344, 1997.

55. Hamelers IH, van Schaik RF, van Teeffelen HA, et al.: Synergistic proliferative action of insulin-like growth factor 1 and 17 beta-estradiol in MCF-7s breast tumor cells, *Exp Cell Res* 273:107–117, 2002.

56. Thorne C, Lee AV: Cross talk between estrogen receptor and IGF signaling in normal mammary gland development and breast cancer, *Breast Dis* 17:105–114, 2003.

57. Laban C, Bustin SA, Jenkins PJ: The GH-IGF-i axis and breast cancer, *Trends Endocrinol Metab* 14:28–34, 2003.

58. van der Burg B, Rutteman GR, Blankenstein MA, et al.: Mitogenic stimulation of human breast cancer cells in a growth factor-defined medium: synergistic action of insulin and estrogen, *J Cell Physiol* 134:101–108, 1988.

59. Osborne CK, Clemmons DR, Arteaga CL: Regulation of breast cancer growth by insulin-like growth factors, *J Steroid Biochem Mol Biol* 37:805–809, 1990.

60. Dupont J, Le Roith D: Insulin-like growth factor 1 and oestradiol promote cell proliferation of MCF-7 breast cancer cells: new insights into their synergistic effects, *Mol Pathol* 54:149–154, 2001.

61. Queiroga FL, Perez-Alenza D, Silvan G, et al.: Serum and intratumoural GH and IGF-i concentrations: prognostic factors in the outcome of canine mammary cancer, *Res Vet Sci* 89:396–403, 2010.

62. Queiroga FL, Perez-Alenza MD, Silvan G, et al.: Crosstalk between GH/IGF-1 axis and steroid hormones (progesterone, 17beta-estradiol) in canine mammary tumours, *J Steroid Biochem Mol Biol* 110:76–82, 2008.

63. Klopfleisch R, von Euler H, Sarli G, et al.: Molecular carcinogenesis of canine mammary tumors: news from an old disease, *Vet Pathol* 48:98–116, 2011.

64. Rivera P, von Euler H: Molecular biological aspects on canine and human mammary tumors, *Vet Pathol* 48:132–146, 2011.

65. Gilbertson SR, Kurzman ID, Zachrau RE, et al.: Canine mammary epithelial neoplasms: biologic implications of morphologic characteristics assessed in 232 dogs, *Vet Pathol* 20:127–142, 1983.

66. Moulton JE, Rosenblatt LS, Goldman M: Mammary tumors in a colony of beagle dogs, *Vet Pathol* 23:741–749, 1986.

67. Bender AP, Dorn CR, Schneider R: An epidemiologic study of canine multiple primary neoplasma involving the female and male reproductive systems, *Prev Vet Med* 2:715–731, 1984.

68. Antuofermo E, Miller MA, Pirino S, et al.: Spontaneous mammary intraepithelial lesions in dogs—a model of breast cancer, *Cancer Epidemiol Biomarkers Prev* 16:2247–2256, 2007.

69. MacEwen EG, Patnaik AK, Harvey HJ, et al.: Estrogen receptors in canine mammary tumors, *Cancer Res* 42:2255–2259, 1982.

70. Rutteman GR, Misdorp W, Blankenstein MA, et al.: OEstrogen (ER) and progestin receptors (PR) in mammary tissue of the female dog: different receptor profile in non-malignant and malignant states, *Br J Cancer* 58:594–599, 1988.

71. Illera JC, Perez-Alenza MD, Nieto A, et al.: Steroids and receptors in canine mammary cancer, *Steroids* 71:541–548, 2006.

72. Millanta F, Calandrella M, Bari G, et al.: Comparison of steroid receptor expression in normal, dysplastic, and neoplastic canine and feline mammary tissues, *Res Vet Sci* 79:225–232, 2005.

73. Donnay I, Rauis J, Devleeschouwer N, et al.: Comparison of estrogen and progesterone receptor expression in normal and tumor mammary tissues from dogs, *Am J Vet Res* 56:1188–1194, 1995.

74. de Las Mulas JM, Millan Y, Dios R: A prospective analysis of immunohistochemically determined estrogen receptor alpha and progesterone receptor expression and host and tumor factors as predictors of disease-free period in mammary tumors of the dog, *Vet Pathol* 42:200–212, 2005.

75. Mainenti M, Rasotto R, Carnier P, et al.: OEstrogen and progesterone receptor expression in subtypes of canine mammary tumours in intact and ovariectomised dogs, *Vet J* 202:62–68, 2014.

76. Chang CC, Tsai MH, Liao JW, et al.: Evaluation of hormone receptor expression for use in predicting survival of female dogs with malignant mammary gland tumors, *J Am Vet Med Assoc* 235:391–396, 2009.

77. Nieto A, Pena L, Perez-Alenza MD, et al.: Immunohistologic detection of estrogen receptor alpha in canine mammary tumors: clinical and pathologic associations and prognostic significance, *Vet Pathol* 37:239–247, 2000.

78. Geraldes M, Gartner F, Schmitt F: Immunohistochemical study of hormonal receptors and cell proliferation in normal canine mammary glands and spontaneous mammary tumours, *Vet Rec* 146:403–406, 2000.

79. Kristiansen VM, Pena L, Diez Cordova L, et al.: Effect of ovariohysterectomy at the time of tumor removal in dogs with mammary carcinomas: a randomized controlled trial, *J Vet Intern Med* 30:230–241, 2016.

80. Effects of chemotherapy and hormonal therapy for early breast cancer on recurrence and 15–year survival: an overview of the randomised trials, *Lancet* 365:1687–1717, 2005.

81. Winer EP, Hudis C, Burstein HJ, et al.: American Society of Clinical Oncology technology assessment on the use of aromatase inhibitors as adjuvant therapy for postmenopausal women with hormone receptor-positive breast cancer: status report 2004, *J Clin Oncol* 23:619–629, 2005.

82. Network NCC: *Clinical practice guidelines in oncology - version 2.2006*, National Comprehensive Cancer Network, Inc., 2005.

83. Tamoxifen for early breast cancer: An overview of the randomised trials. Early breast cancer trialists' collaborative group, *Lancet* 351:1451–1467, 1998.

84. Thuerlimann B, Koeberle D, Senn HJ: Guidelines for the adjuvant treatment of postmenopausal women with endocrine-responsive breast cancer: past, present and future recommendations, *Eur J Cancer* 43:46–52, 2007.

85. Fisher B, Costantino JP, Wickerham DL, et al.: Tamoxifen for prevention of breast cancer: report of the National Surgical Adjuvant Breast and Bowel Project P-1 study, *J Natl Cancer Inst* 90:1371–1388, 1998.

86. Sjogren S, Inganas M, Lindgren A, et al.: Prognostic and predictive value of c-*erbb-2* overexpression in primary breast cancer, alone and in combination with other prognostic markers, *J Clin Oncol* 16:462–469, 1998.

87. Slamon DJ, Clark GM, Wong SG, et al.: Human breast cancer: correlation of relapse and survival with amplification of the *HER-2/neu* oncogene, *Science* 235:177–182, 1987.

88. Slamon DJ, Leyland-Jones B, Shak S, et al.: Use of chemotherapy plus a monoclonal antibody against her2 for metastatic breast cancer that overexpresses *HER2*, *N Engl J Med* 344:783–792, 2001.

89. Martin de las Mulas J, Ordas J, Millan Y, et al.: Oncogene *HER-2* in canine mammary gland carcinomas: an immunohistochemical and chromogenic in situ hybridization study, *Breast Cancer Res Treat* 80:363–367, 2003.

90. Hsu WL, Huang HM, Liao JW, et al.: Increased survival in dogs with malignant mammary tumours overexpressing HER-2 protein and detection of a silent single nucleotide polymorphism in the canine *her-2* gene, *Vet J* 180:116–123, 2009.

91. Gama A, Alves A, Schmitt F: Identification of molecular phenotypes in canine mammary carcinomas with clinical implications: application of the human classification, *Virchows Arch* 453:123–132, 2008.

92. Im KS, Kim IH, Kim NH, et al.: Breed-related differences in altered *BRCA1* expression, phenotype and subtype in malignant canine mammary tumors, *Vet J* 195:366–372, 2013.

93. Rungsipipat A, Tateyama S, Yamaguchi R, et al.: Immunohistochemical analysis of c-*yes* and c-*erbb-2* oncogene products and p53 tumor suppressor protein in canine mammary tumors, *J Vet Med Sci* 61:27–32, 1999.

94. Sassi F, Benazzi C, Castellani G, et al.: Molecular-based tumour subtypes of canine mammary carcinomas assessed by immunohistochemistry, *BMC Vet Res* 6(5), 2010.

95. Pena L, Gama A, Goldschmidt MH, et al.: Canine mammary tumors: a review and consensus of standard guidelines on epithelial and myoepithelial phenotype markers, HER2, and hormone receptor assessment using immunohistochemistry, *Vet Pathol* 51:127–145, 2014.

96. The Cancer Genome Atlas Network: Comprehensive molecular portraits of human breast tumours, *Nature* 490:61–70, 2012.

97. Sørlie T, Perou CM, Tibshirani R, et al.: Gene expression patterns of breast carcinomas distinguish tumor subclasses with clinical implications, *Proc Natl Acad Sci USA* 98:10869–10874, 2001.

98. Malhotra GK, Zhao X, Band H, et al.: Histological, molecular and functional subtypes of breast cancers, *Cancer Biol Ther* 10:955–960, 2010.

99. Coleman WB, Anders CK: Discerning clinical responses in breast cancer based on molecular signatures, *Am J Pathol* 187:2199–2207, 2017.

100. Yam C, Mani SA, Moulder SL: Targeting the molecular subtypes of triple negative breast cancer: understanding the diversity to progress the field, *Oncologist* 22:1086–1093, 2017.

101. Perez Alenza MD, Tabanera E, Pena L: Inflammatory mammary carcinoma in dogs: 33 cases (1995–1999), *J Am Vet Med Assoc* 219:1110–1114, 2001.

102. Marconato L, Romanelli G, Stefanello D, et al.: Prognostic factors for dogs with mammary inflammatory carcinoma: 43 cases (2003–2008), *J Am Vet Med Assoc* 235:967–972, 2009.

103. Soultani C, Patsikas MN, Karayannopoulou M, et al.: Assessment of sentinel lymph node metastasis in canine mammary gland tumors using computed tomographic indirect lymphography, *Vet Radiol Ultrasound* 58:186–196, 2017.

104. Pereira CT, Luiz Navarro Marques F, Williams J, et al.: ^{99}MTC-labeled dextran for mammary lymphoscintigraphy in dogs, *Vet Radiol Ultrasound* 49:487–491, 2008.

105. MacEwen EG: Spontaneous tumors in dogs and cats: models for the study of cancer biology and treatment, *Cancer Metastasis Rev* 9:125–136, 1990.

106. Vail DM, MacEwen EG: Spontaneously occurring tumors of companion animals as models for human cancer, *Cancer Invest* 18:781–792, 2000.

107. Tuohy JL, Milgram J, Worley DR, et al.: A review of sentinel lymph node evaluation and the need for its incorporation into veterinary oncology, *Vet Comp Oncol* 7:81–91, 2009.

108. Gelb HR, Freeman LJ, Rohleder JJ, et al.: Feasibility of contrast-enhanced ultrasound-guided biopsy of sentinel lymph nodes in dogs, *Vet Radiol Ultrasound* 51:628–633, 2010.

109. Pinheiro LG, Oliveira Filho RS, Vasques PH, et al.: Hemosiderin: a new marker for sentinel lymph node identification, *Acta Cir Bras* 24:432–436, 2009.

110. Balogh L, Thuroczy J, Andocs G, et al.: Sentinel lymph node detection in canine oncological patients, *Nucl Med Rev Cent East Eur* 5:139–144, 2002.

111. Patsikas MN, Papadopoulou PL, Charitanti A, et al.: Computed tomography and radiographic indirect lymphography for visualization of mammary lymphatic vessels and the sentinel lymph node in normal cats, *Vet Radiol Ultrasound* 51:299–304, 2010.

112. Pereira CT, Rahal SC, de Carvalho Balieiro JC, et al.: Lymphatic drainage on healthy and neoplasic mammary glands in female dogs: can it really be altered? *Anat Histol Embryol* 32:282–290, 2003.

113. Patsikas MN, Dessiris A: The lymph drainage of the mammary glands in the bitch: a lymphographic study. Part II: the 3rd mammary gland, *Anat Histol Embryol* 25:139–143, 1996.

114. Ran S, Volk L, Hall K, et al.: Lymphangiogenesis and lymphatic metastasis in breast cancer, *Pathophysiology* 17:229–251, 2010.

115. Wong JH, Cagle LA, Morton DL: Lymphatic drainage of skin to a sentinel lymph node in a feline model, *Ann Surg* 214:637–641, 1991.

116. Szczubial M, Lopuszynski W: Prognostic value of regional lymph node status in canine mammary carcinomas, *Vet Comp Oncol* 9:296–303, 2011.

117. Karayannopoulou M, Koutinas AF, Polizopoulou ZS, et al.: Total serum alkaline phosphatase activity in dogs with mammary neoplasms: a prospective study on 79 natural cases, *J Vet Med A Physiol Pathol Clin Med* 50:501–505, 2003.

118. Karayannopoulou M, Polizopoulou ZS, Koutinas AF, et al.: Serum alkaline phosphatase isoenzyme activities in canine malignant mammary neoplasms with and without osseous transformation, *Vet Clin Pathol* 35:287–290, 2006.

119. Cassali GD, Gobbi H, Malm C, et al.: Evaluation of accuracy of fine needle aspiration cytology for diagnosis of canine mammary tumours: comparative features with human tumours, *Cytopathology* 18:191–196, 2007.

120. Simon D, Schoenrock D, Nolte I, et al.: Cytologic examination of fine-needle aspirates from mammary gland tumors in the dog: diagnostic accuracy with comparison to histopathology and association with postoperative outcome, *Vet Clin Pathol* 38:521–528, 2009.

121. Eberle N, Fork M, von Babo V, et al.: Comparison of examination of thoracic radiographs and thoracic computed tomography in dogs with appendicular osteosarcoma, *Vet Comp Oncol* 9:131–140, 2011.

122. Otoni CC, Rahal SC, Vulcano LC, et al.: Survey radiography and computerized tomography imaging of the thorax in female dogs with mammary tumors, *Acta Vet Scand* 52:20, 2010.

123. Lana SE, Rutteman GR, Withrow SJ: Tumors of the mammary gland. In Withrow SJ, Vail DM, editors: *Withrow & MacEwen's small animal clinical oncology*, ed 4, St. Louis, 2007, Saunders Elsevier.

124. Owens L: *Classification of tumors in domestic animals*, ed 1, Geneva, 1980, World Health Organization.

125. Rutteman G, Withrow SJ, MacEwen EG: Tumors of the mammary gland. In Withrow SJ, MacEwen EG, editors: *Small animal clinical oncology*, ed 3, Philadelphia, 2001, WB Saunders.

126. Sorenmo KU, Rasotto R, Zappulli V, et al.: Development, anatomy, histology, lymphatic drainage, clinical features, and cell differentiation markers of canine mammary gland neoplasms, *Vet Pathol* 48:85–97, 2011.

127. Hampe JF, Misdorp W: Tumours and dysplasias of the mammary gland, *Bull World Health Organ* 50:111–133, 1974.

128. Misdorp W, Else R, Hellmen E, et al.: *Histological classification of mammary tumors of the dog and the cat*, ed 2, Washington, DC, 1999, Armed Forces Institute of Pathology, pp 3–29.

129. Goldschmidt M, Pena L, Rasotto R, et al.: Classification and grading of canine mammary tumors, *Vet Pathol* 48:117–131, 2011.

130. Rasotto R, Zappulli V, Castagnaro M, et al.: A retrospective study of those histopathologic parameters predictive of invasion of the lymphatic system by canine mammary carcinomas, *Vet Pathol* 49:330–340, 2011.

131. Rasotto R, Berlato D, Goldschmidt MH, et al.: Prognostic significance of canine mammary tumor histologic subtypes: an observational cohort study of 229 cases, *Vet Pathol* 54:571–578, 2017.

132. Elston CW, Ellis IO: Pathological prognostic factors in breast cancer. I. The value of histological grade in breast cancer: experience from a large study with long-term follow-up, *Histopathology* 19:403–410, 1991.

133. Misdorp W: Tumors of the mammary gland. In Meuten DJ, editor: *Tumors in domestic animals*, ed 4, Ames, Iowa, 2002, Iowa State Press, pp 575–606, 764.

134. Clemente M, Perez-Alenza MD, Illera JC, et al.: Histological, immunohistological, and ultrastructural description of vasculogenic mimicry in canine mammary cancer, *Vet Pathol* 47:265–274, 2010.

135. Karayannopoulou M, Kaldrymidou E, Constantinidis TC, et al.: Histological grading and prognosis in dogs with mammary carcinomas: application of a human grading method, *J Comp Pathol* 133:246–252, 2005.

136. Pena L, De Andres PJ, Clemente M, et al.: Prognostic value of histological grading in noninflammatory canine mammary carcinomas in a prospective study with two-year follow-up: relationship with clinical and histological characteristics, *Vet Pathol* 50:94–105, 2013.

137. Meuten DJ, Moore FM, George JW: Mitotic count and the field of view area: time to standardize, *Vet Pathol* 53:7–9, 2016.

138. Hellmen E, Bergstrom R, Holmberg L, et al.: Prognostic factors in canine mammary tumors: a multivariate study of 202 consecutive cases, *Vet Pathol* 30:20–27, 1993.

139. Perez Alenza MD, Pena L, Nieto AI, et al.: Clinical and pathological prognostic factors in canine mammary tumors, *Ann Ist Super Sanita* 33:581–585, 1997.

140. MacEwen EG, Harvey HJ, Patnaik AK, et al.: Evaluation of effects of levamisole and surgery on canine mammary cancer, *J Biol Response Mod* 4:418–426, 1985.

141. Philibert JC, Snyder PW, Glickman N, et al.: Influence of host factors on survival in dogs with malignant mammary gland tumors, *J Vet Intern Med* 17:102–106, 2003.

142. Morris JS, Dobson JM, Bostock DE: Use of tamoxifen in the control of canine mammary neoplasia, *Vet Rec* 133:539–542, 1993.

143. Chang SC, Chang CC, Chang TJ, et al.: Prognostic factors associated with survival two years after surgery in dogs with malignant mammary tumors: 79 cases (1998–2002), *J Am Vet Med Assoc* 227:1625–1629, 2005.

144. de Araujo MR, Campos LC, Ferreira E, et al.: Quantitation of the regional lymph node metastatic burden and prognosis in malignant mammary tumors of dogs, *J Vet Intern Med* 29:1360–1367, 2015.

145. Stratmann N, Failing K, Richter A, et al.: Mammary tumor recurrence in bitches after regional mastectomy, *Vet Surg* 37:82–86, 2008.

146. Horta RS, Figueiredo MS, Lavalle GE, et al.: Surgical stress and postoperative complications related to regional and radical mastectomy in dogs, *Acta Vet Scand* 57:34, 2015.

147. Morris JS, Dobson JM, Bostock DE, et al.: Effect of ovariohysterectomy in bitches with mammary neoplasms, *Vet Rec* 142:656–658, 1998.

148. Sorenmo KU, Shofer FS, Goldschmidt MH: Effect of spaying and timing of spaying on survival of dogs with mammary carcinoma, *J Vet Intern Med* 14:266–270, 2000.

149. Hermo GA, Torres P, Ripoll GV, et al.: Perioperative desmopressin prolongs survival in surgically treated bitches with mammary gland tumours: a pilot study, *Vet J* 178:103–108, 2008.

150. Tran CM, Moore AS, Frimberger AE: Surgical treatment of mammary carcinomas in dogs with or without postoperative chemotherapy, *Vet Comp Oncol* 14:252–262, 2016.

151. Rossi F, Sabattini S, Vascellari M, et al.: The impact of toceranib, piroxicam and thalidomide with or without hypofractionated radiation therapy on clinical outcome in dogs with inflammatory mammary carcinoma, *Vet Comp Oncol*, 2018. https://doi.org/10.1111/vco.12407. Epub ahead of print.

152. Allen S, Mahaffey E: Canine mammary neoplasia: prognostic indicators and response to surgical therapy, *J Am Anim Hosp Assoc* 25:504–546, 1989.

153. Tavares WL, Lavalle GE, Figueiredo MS, et al.: Evaluation of adverse effects in tamoxifen exposed healthy female dogs, *Acta Vet Scand* 52:67, 2010.

154. Guil-Luna S, Millan Y, De Andres J, et al.: Prognostic impact of neoadjuvant aglepristone treatment in clinicopathological parameters of progesterone receptor-positive canine mammary carcinomas, *Vet Comp Oncol* 15:391–399, 2017.

155. Yamagami T, Kobayashi T, Takahashi K, et al.: Influence of ovariectomy at the time of mastectomy on the prognosis for canine malignant mammary tumours, *J Small Anim Pract* 37:462–464, 1996.

156. Nabholtz JM, Senn HJ, Bezwoda WR, et al.: Prospective randomized trial of docetaxel versus mitomycin plus vinblastine in patients with metastatic breast cancer progressing despite previous anthracycline-containing chemotherapy. 304 study group, *J Clin Oncol* 17:1413–1424, 1999.

157. Sjostrom J, Blomqvist C, Mouridsen H, et al.: Docetaxel compared with sequential methotrexate and 5–fluorouracil in patients with advanced breast cancer after anthracycline failure: a randomised phase III study with crossover on progression by the Scandinavian Breast Group, *Eur J Cancer* 35:1194–1201, 1999.

158. Morabito A, Piccirillo MC, Monaco K, et al.: First-line chemotherapy for HER-2 negative metastatic breast cancer patients who received anthracyclines as adjuvant treatment, *Oncologist* 12:1288–1298, 2007.

159. Simon D, Schoenrock D, Baumgartner W, et al.: Postoperative adjuvant treatment of invasive malignant mammary gland tumors in dogs with doxorubicin and docetaxel, *J Vet Intern Med* 20:1184–1190, 2006.

160. Arenas C, Pena L, Granados-Soler JL, et al.: Adjuvant therapy for highly malignant canine mammary tumours: COX-2 inhibitor versus chemotherapy: a case-control prospective study, *Vet Rec* 179:125, 2016.

161. Marconato L, Lorenzo RM, Abramo F, et al.: Adjuvant gemcitabine after surgical removal of aggressive malignant mammary tumours in dogs, *Vet Comp Oncol* 6:90–101, 2008.

162. de Mello Souza CH, Toledo-Piza E, Amorin R, et al.: Inflammatory mammary carcinoma in 12 dogs: clinical features, cyclooxygenase-2 expression, and response to piroxicam treatment, *Can Vet J* 50:506–510, 2009.

163. Lavalle GE, De Campos CB, Bertagnolli AC, et al.: Canine malignant mammary gland neoplasms with advanced clinical staging treated with carboplatin and cyclooxygenase inhibitors, *Vivo* 26:375–379, 2012.

164. Kuntz CA, Dernell WS, Powers BE, et al.: Extraskeletal osteosarcomas in dogs: 14 cases, *J Am Anim Hosp Assoc* 34:26–30, 1998.

165. Hermo GA, Turic E, Angelico D, et al.: Effect of adjuvant perioperative desmopressin in locally advanced canine mammary carcinoma and its relation to histologic grade, *J Am Anim Hosp Assoc* 47:21–27, 2011.

166. Terraube V, Marx I, Denis CV: Role of Von Willebrand factor in tumor metastasis, *Thromb Res* 120(suppl 2):S64–70, 2007.

167. Ripoll GV, Giron S, Krzymuski MJ, et al.: Antitumor effects of desmopressin in combination with chemotherapeutic agents in a mouse model of breast cancer, *Anticancer Res* 28:2607–2611, 2008.

168. Egenvall A, Bonnett BN, Haggstrom J, et al.: Morbidity of insured Swedish cats during 1999–2006 by age, breed, sex, and diagnosis, *J Feline Med Surg* 12:948–959, 2010.

169. Bonnett BN, Egenvall A: Age patterns of disease and death in insured Swedish dogs, cats and horses, *J Comp Pathol* 142(suppl 1):S33–38, 2010.

170. Teclaw R, Mendlein J, Garbe P, et al.: Characteristics of pet populations and households in the Purdue Comparative Oncology Program catchment area, 1988, *J Am Vet Med Assoc* 201:1725–1729, 1992.

171. Vascellari M, Baioni E, Ru G, et al.: Animal tumour registry of two provinces in northern Italy: incidence of spontaneous tumours in dogs and cats, *BMC Vet Res* 5(39), 2009.

172. Hayden DW, Nielsen SW: Feline mammary tumours, *J Small Anim Pract* 12:687–698, 1971.

173. Misdorp W, Romijn A, Hart AA: Feline mammary tumors: a case-control study of hormonal factors, *Anticancer Res* 11:1793–1797, 1991.

174. Hayes AA, Mooney S: Feline mammary tumors, *Vet Clin North Am Small Anim Pract* 15:513–520, 1985.

175. Weijer K, Head KW, Misdorp W, et al.: Feline malignant mammary tumors. I. Morphology and biology: some comparisons with human and canine mammary carcinomas, *J Natl Cancer Inst* 49:1697–1704, 1972.

176. Hayes Jr HM, Milne KL, Mandell CP: Epidemiological features of feline mammary carcinoma, *Vet Rec* 108:476–479, 1981.

177. Ito T, Kadosawa T, Mochizuki M, et al.: Prognosis of malignant mammary tumor in 53 cats, *J Vet Med Sci* 58:723–726, 1996.

178. Patnaik AK, Liu SK, Hurvitz AI, et al.: Nonhematopoietic neoplasms in cats, *J Natl Cancer Inst* 54:855–860, 1975.

179. Rissetto K, Villamil JA, Selting KA, et al.: Recent trends in feline intestinal neoplasia: an epidemiologic study of 1,129 cases in the Veterinary Medical Database from 1964 to 2004, *J Am Anim Hosp Assoc* 47:28–36, 2011.

180. Louwerens M, London CA, Pedersen NC, et al.: Feline lymphoma in the post-feline leukemia virus era, *J Vet Intern Med* 19:329–335, 2005.

181. Gabor LJ, Malik R, Canfield PJ: Clinical and anatomical features of lymphosarcoma in 118 cats, *Aust Vet J* 76:725–732, 1998.

182. Miller MA, Nelson SL, Turk JR, et al.: Cutaneous neoplasia in 340 cats, *Vet Pathol* 28:389–395, 1991.

183. Overley B, Shofer FS, Goldschmidt MH, et al.: Association between ovariohysterectomy and feline mammary carcinoma, *J Vet Intern Med* 19:560–563, 2005.

184. Skorupski KA, Overley B, Shofer FS, et al.: Clinical characteristics of mammary carcinoma in male cats, *J Vet Intern Med* 19:52–55, 2005.

185. Jacobs TM, Hoppe BR, Poehlmann CE, et al.: Mammary adenocarcinomas in three male cats exposed to medroxyprogesterone acetate (1990–2006), *J Feline Med Surg* 12:169–174, 2010.

186. Loretti AP, Ilha MR, Ordas J, et al.: Clinical, pathological and immunohistochemical study of feline mammary fibroepithelial hyperplasia following a single injection of depot medroxyprogesterone acetate, *J Feline Med Surg* 7:43–52, 2005.

187. Mol JA, van Garderen E, Rutteman GR, et al.: New insights in the molecular mechanism of progestin-induced proliferation of mammary epithelium:induction of the local biosynthesis of growth hormone (GH) in the mammary glands of dogs, cats and humans, *J Steroid Biochem Mol Biol* 57:67–71, 1996.

188. Mol JA, van Garderen E, Selman PJ, et al.: Growth hormone mRNA in mammary gland tumors of dogs and cats, *J Clin Invest* 95:2028–2034, 1995.

189. Burrai GP, Mohammed SI, Miller MA, et al.: Spontaneous feline mammary intraepithelial lesions as a model for human estrogen receptor- and progesterone receptor-negative breast lesions, *BMC Cancer* 10(156), 2010.

190. Millanta F, Calandrella M, Vannozzi I, et al.: Steroid hormone receptors in normal, dysplastic and neoplastic feline mammary tissues and their prognostic significance, *Vet Rec* 158:821–824, 2006.

191. de las Mulas JM, van Niel M, Millan Y, et al.: Immunohistochemical analysis of estrogen receptors in feline mammary gland benign and malignant lesions: comparison with biochemical assay, *Domest Anim Endocrinol* 18:111–125, 2000.

192. Martin de las Mulas J, Van Niel M, Millan Y, et al.: Progesterone receptors in normal, dysplastic and tumourous feline mammary glands. Comparison with oestrogen receptors status, *Res Vet Sci* 72:153–161, 2002.

193. Meisl D, Hubler M, Arnold S: Treatment of fibroepithelial hyperplasia (FEH) of the mammary gland in the cat with the progesterone antagonist aglepristone (alizine), *Schweiz Arch Tierheilkd* 145:130–136, 2003.

194. Ordas J, Millan Y, Dios R, et al.: Proto-oncogene *HER-2* in normal, dysplastic and tumorous feline mammary glands: an immunohistochemical and chromogenic in situ hybridization study, *BMC Cancer* 7:179, 2007.

195. Millanta F, Calandrella M, Citi S, et al.: Overexpression of *HER-2* in feline invasive mammary carcinomas: an immunohistochemical survey and evaluation of its prognostic potential, *Vet Pathol* 42:30–34, 2005.

196. Winston J, Craft DM, Scase TJ, et al.: Immunohistochemical detection of *HER-2/neu* expression in spontaneous feline mammary tumours, *Vet Comp Oncol* 3:8–15, 2005.

197. Rasotto R, Caliari D, Castagnaro M, et al.: An immunohistochemical study of *HER-2* expression in feline mammary tumours, *J Comp Pathol* 144:170–179, 2011.

198. Brodey RS: Canine and feline neoplasms, *Adv Vet Sci* 24:434, 1957.

199. Weijer K, Hart AA: Prognostic factors in feline mammary carcinoma, *J Natl Cancer Inst* 70:709–716, 1983.

200. Perez-Alenza MD, Jimenez A, Nieto AI, et al.: First description of feline inflammatory mammary carcinoma: clinicopathological and immunohistochemical characteristics of three cases, *Breast Cancer Res* 6:R300–307, 2004.

201. McNeill CJ, Sorenmo KU, Shofer FS, et al.: Evaluation of adjuvant doxorubicin-based chemotherapy for the treatment of feline mammary carcinoma, *J Vet Intern Med* 23:123–129, 2009.

202. Goldschmidt MH, Pena L, Zappulli V: Tumors of the mammary gland. In Meuten DJ, editor: *Tumors in domestic animals*, ed 5, Oxford, UK, 2017, John Wiley and Sons.

203. Soares M, Madeira S, Correia J, et al.: Molecular based subtyping of feline mammary carcinomas and clinicopathological characterization, *Breast* 27:44–51, 2016.

204. Soares M, Correia J, Peleteiro MC, et al.: St Gallen molecular subtypes in feline mammary carcinoma and paired metastases-disease progression and clinical implications from a 3-year follow-up study, *Tumour Biol* 37:4053–4064, 2016.

205. Caliari D, Zappulli V, Rasotto R, et al.: Triple-negative vimentin-positive heterogeneous feline mammary carcinomas as a potential comparative model for breast cancer, *BMC Vet Res* 10(185), 2014.

206. Beha G, Muscatello LV, Brunetti B, et al.: Molecular phenotype of primary mammary tumours and distant metastases in female dogs and cats, *J Comp Pathol* 150:194–197, 2014.

207. Wiese DA, Thaiwong T, Yuzbasiyan-Gurkan V, et al.: Feline mammary basal-like adenocarcinomas: a potential model for human triple-negative breast cancer (TNBC) with basal-like subtype, *BMC Cancer* 13:403, 2013.

208. Brunetti B, Asproni P, Beha G, et al.: Molecular phenotype in mammary tumours of queens: correlation between primary tumour and lymph node metastasis, *J Comp Pathol* 148:206–213, 2013.

209. Hayden DW, Barnes DM, Johnson KH: Morphologic changes in the mammary gland of megestrol acetate-treated and untreated cats: a retrospective study, *Vet Pathol* 26:104–113, 1989.

210. Castagnaro M, Casalone C, Bozzetta E, et al.: Tumour grading and the one-year post-surgical prognosis in feline mammary carcinomas, *J Comp Pathol* 119:263–275, 1998.

211. Seixas F, Palmeira C, Pires MA, et al.: Mammary invasive micropapillary carcinoma in cats: clinicopathologic features and nuclear DNA content, *Vet Pathol* 44:842–848, 2007.

212. Seixas F, Pires MA, Lopes CA: Complex carcinomas of the mammary gland in cats: pathological and immunohistochemical features, *Vet J* 176:210–215, 2008.

213. Sarli G, Brunetti B, Benazzi C: Mammary mucinous carcinoma in the cat, *Vet Pathol* 43:667–673, 2006.

214. Kamstock DA, Fredrickson R, Ehrhart EJ: Lipid-rich carcinoma of the mammary gland in a cat, *Vet Pathol* 42:360–362, 2005.

215. Matsuda K, Kobayashi S, Yamashita M, et al.: Tubulopapillary carcinoma with spindle cell metaplasia of the mammary gland in a cat, *J Vet Med Sci* 70:479–481, 2008.

216. Zappulli V, Caliari D, Rasotto R, et al.: Proposed classification of the feline "complex" mammary tumors as ductal and intraductal papillary mammary tumors, *Vet Pathol* 50:1070–1077, 2013.

217. Seixas F, Palmeira C, Pires MA, et al.: Grade is an independent prognostic factor for feline mammary carcinomas: a clinicopathological and survival analysis, *Vet J* 187:65–71, 2011.

218. Mills SW, Musil KM, Davies JL, et al.: Prognostic value of histologic grading for feline mammary carcinoma: a retrospective survival analysis, *Vet Pathol* 52:238–249, 2015.

219. MacEwen EG, Hayes AA, Harvey HJ, et al.: Prognostic factors for feline mammary tumors, *J Am Vet Med Assoc* 185:201–204, 1984.

220. MacEwen EG, Hayes AA, Mooney S, et al.: Evaluation of effect of levamisole on feline mammary cancer, *J Biol Response Mod* 3:541–546, 1984.

221. Viste JR, Myers SL, Singh B, et al.: Feline mammary adenocarcinoma: tumor size as a prognostic indicator, *Can Vet J* 43:33–37, 2002.

222. Gemignani F, Mayhew PD, Giuffrida MA, et al.: Association of surgical approach with complication rate, progression-free survival time, and disease-specific survival time in cats with mammary adenocarcinoma: 107 cases (1991–2014), *J Am Vet Med Assoc* 252:1393–1402, 2018.

223. Borrego JF, Cartagena JC, Engel J: Treatment of feline mammary tumours using chemotherapy, surgery and a COX-2 inhibitor drug (meloxicam): a retrospective study of 23 cases (2002–2007), *Vet Comp Oncol* 7:213–221, 2009.

224. Jeglum KA, deGuzman E, Young KM: Chemotherapy of advanced mammary adenocarcinoma in 14 cats, *J Am Vet Med Assoc* 187:157–160, 1985.

225. Mauldin GN, Matus RE, Patnaik AK, et al.: Efficacy and toxicity of doxorubicin and cyclophosphamide used in the treatment of selected malignant tumors in 23 cats, *J Vet Intern Med* 2:60–65, 1988.

226. Karayannopoulou M, Kaldrymidou E, Constantinidis TC, et al.: Adjuvant post-operative chemotherapy in bitches with mammary cancer, *J Vet Med A Physiol Pathol Clin Med* 48:85–96, 2001.

227. Hahn K, Richardson R, Knapp D: Canine malignant mammary neoplasia: biological behavior, diagnosis, and treatment alternatives, *J Am Anim Hosp Assoc* 28:251–256, 1992.

29

Tumors of the Male Reproductive System

JESSICA A. LAWRENCE AND COREY F. SABA

Canine Testicular Tumors

Prevalence/Incidence

Testicular tumors are the most common tumors of the canine male genitalia and account for approximately 90% of all cancers in the male reproductive tract.[1-4] In the intact male dog, the testis is the second most common anatomic site for tumor development, with an overall prevalence ranging between 6% and 27%.[1,3-7] Many of these reports are case series and involve dogs submitted for routine necropsy and/or castration for cryptorchidism, making comparisons between study prevalence data difficult. However, a recent population-based study conducted in Norway, where elective castration is rare, reported a similar prevalence of 7% for testicular tumors.[8]

The rate of development of testicular cancer in humans has increased in some populations over time and across successive birth cohorts, and a similar phenomenon has been suggested in dogs.[7,9-13] One relatively recent population-based study published in 2011 did not find increased rates of testicular tumors among dogs; however, only an 8-year period was evaluated.[8] Testicular tumors are most often diagnosed in geriatric male dogs with a median age of approximately 10 years.[1,3,4,14,15]

The three most common testicular tumors arise from distinct testicular subsets: sustentacular cells of Sertoli, the spermatic germinal epithelium, and the interstitial cells of Leydig, giving rise to Sertoli cell tumors, seminomas, and interstitial cell tumors, respectively (Table 29.1).[2] The World Health Organization (WHO) classification of tumors of domestic animals differentiates the major types of testicular tumors in dogs as sex-cord stromal tumors (Sertoli cell tumors, interstitial cell tumors), germ cell tumors (seminoma, teratoma), and mixed germ cell–sex-cord stromal tumors.[16] Sertoli cell tumors, interstitial cell tumors, and seminomas have historically developed with equal frequency, although recent studies have suggested that the prevalence of Sertoli cell tumors is lower, at 8% to 16%.[1,3,4,7,17,18] Seminoma occurred most frequently in a study of lifetime occurrence of neoplasia in German shepherd dogs and Belgian Malinois.[17] Human testicular tumors are often divided into seminoma and nonseminoma, and seminomas are further differentiated as classical (SE), atypical, and spermatocytic seminoma (SS) according to the WHO, and some effort has been made to apply this to canine tumors.[9,13,19-23] Sertoli cell tumors and seminomas occur with higher frequency in cryptorchid testes.[3,24,25]

Rarely, other cell lineages can give rise to testicular tumors such as hemangiomas, granulosa cell tumors, teratomas, sarcomas, embryonal carcinomas, gonadoblastomas, lymphomas, schwannoma, mesothelioma, and rete testis mucinous adenocarcinomas.[26-30] Many dogs diagnosed with testicular cancer have more than one primary tumor.[3,6,18,31] In three separate studies evaluating a relatively large numbers of dogs with testicular tumors, between 4% and 20% of dogs had more than one type of testicular tumor.[3,8,32]

Risk Factors

Several factors may influence the development of testicular tumors in the dog, including cryptorchidism, age, breed, and carcinogen exposure. There is a significant association between cryptorchidism and the development of Sertoli cell tumors and seminomas, but not interstitial cell tumors.[4,15,25,33] An early prospective epidemiologic study compared the incidence of testicular tumors in cryptorchid dogs to age- and breed-matched control dogs.[15] None of the control dogs developed testicular tumors during the study, in which the average duration of monitoring was 2 years. The incidence of testicular neoplasia in the cryptorchid dogs was 12.7 per 1000 dog-years at risk, whereas for cryptorchid dogs older than 6 years the incidence increased to 68.1 per 1000 dog-years at risk.[15] Inguinal cryptorchidism may further increase the risk of testicular tumor development compared with abdominal cryptorchidism (Fig. 29.1).[4,15,25] In cryptorchid dogs, tumors more frequently develop in the right testicle, potentially because the right testicle is more likely to be retained.[4,15,32] Chronologic age is a risk factor for development of a primary testicular tumor; in one study, dogs older than 10 years were more likely to develop tumors than dogs younger than 6 years.[15] Another study indicated that the detection rate of testicular tumors in dogs younger than 10 years was significantly associated with cryptorchidism, with more than 60% of cryptorchid testicular tumors identified in middle-aged dogs (6–10 years).[4]

Several breeds have been reported to have increased risk of developing primary testicular tumors, including the boxer,

TABLE 29.1	Characteristics of the Three Most Common Testicular Tumors in the Dog					
Tumor Type	Incidence (% of all testicular tumors)	Origin	Hormone Production	Clinical Findings	Gross Appearance	Biologic Behavior and Potential for Metastasis
Sertoli Cell Tumor	8%–33%	Sustentacular cells of seminiferous tubules	≥50% Estrogen	Feminization syndrome Pancytopenia	Firm Lobulated White-gray "Greasy"	<15% regional or distant metastasis
Interstitial Cell Tumor (Leydig Cell Tumor)	33%–50%	Leydig cells between seminiferous tubules	Rarely estrogen Testosterone	Often incidental finding Perianal gland hyperplasia/ adenomas	Soft Expansive Yellow-orange Often cystic	Rarely metastasize
Seminomas	33%–52%	Germinal epithelium of seminiferous tubules	Rarely estrogen	Often incidental finding Metastasis may cause lethargy	Soft Homogeneous May be lobulated Ivory	<15% regional or distant metastasis

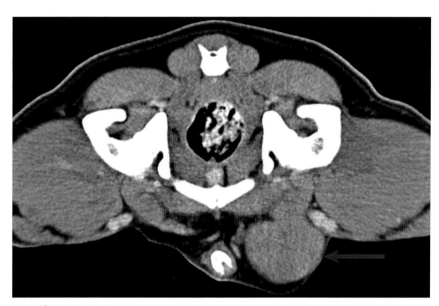

• **Fig. 29.1** Cross-sectional computed tomography image demonstrating an enlarged, minimally rim-enhancing Sertoli cell tumor (*blue arrow*) in a dog with inguinal cryptorchidism. (Image courtesy Dr. T. Schwarz, University of Edinburgh.)

German shepherd dog, Afghan hound, Weimaraner, Shetland sheepdog, collie, and Maltese.[3,8,14,25,32,34,35] Flat-coated retrievers, Rottweilers, Bouvier de Flandres, and Leonbergers may have a reduced risk of developing testicular tumors, although low numbers of the latter two breeds were evaluated.[8]

Two studies evaluating military working dogs suggested evidence of environmental carcinogen exposure during the Vietnam War as a contributor to testicular tumor development.[36,37] Pathologic changes in the testicles were noted, such as hemorrhage, epididymitis, orchitis, sperm granuloma, testicular degeneration, and seminoma, although the causative factor of these lesions could not be definitively determined. These epidemiologic studies postulated that exposure to phenoxy herbicide, dioxin, or tetracycline may have promoted the development of testicular tumors.[36,37]

Pathology and Pathogenesis

Sertoli cell tumors arise from the sustentacular cells of seminiferous tubules and seminomas arise from the germinal epithelium of seminiferous tubules. Interstitial cell tumors arise from Leydig cells located between seminiferous tubules. All three tumors have relatively distinct appearances grossly, but require histopathology for definitive diagnosis. Sertoli cell tumors are firm, lobulated, white-to-gray in appearance, and often characterized as "greasy" on palpation.[38] Seminomas tend to be homogeneous, soft, and occasionally lobulated with an ivory appearance when sectioned (Fig. 29.2).[38] Interstitial cell tumors are soft, expansive, and yellow-to-orange in color when sectioned and often contain cysts with serous or serosanguineous fluid.[38]

The molecular and cellular biology of primary testicular tumors has been investigated in recent years. Proliferation markers

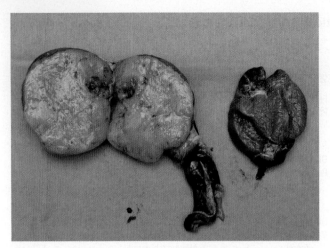

• **Fig. 29.2** Sectioned seminoma in a dog, demonstrating its ivory, homogeneous appearance in comparison to a mildly atrophied contralateral testicle.

(proliferating cell nuclear antigen [PCNA], Ki67, and argyrophilic nucleolar organizer regions [AgNORs]) and TERT expression (the catalytic reverse transcriptase subunit of telomerase) have been interrogated as indicators of degree of malignancy, local progression, and metastasis with discordant results.[39–44] Investigators sought to relate TERT to proliferation indices and p53 expression; however, because PCNA and TERT were expressed in all testicular tumors, their prognostic potential is limited.[41] Aggressive testicular tumors did express high levels TERT, p53, PCNA, and Ki67, suggesting these may provide some indication of biologic behavior.[41] Proliferative activity using AgNORs was assessed in canine seminomas, in which mean AgNOR scores were higher in invasive or diffuse tumors compared with well-differentiated intraductal seminomas.[43] Results suggest that testicular tumors develop a proliferative advantage as they become less differentiated, although larger studies should be performed before proliferative indices can be definitively relied on for prognostication in canine testicular tumors. Cyclins, which are intracellular proteins that form complexes with cyclin-dependent kinases to regulate cell-cycle checkpoints, have also been evaluated in normal and neoplastic testes; however, their significance is yet to be determined.[45]

The neoplastic cellular environment plays an important role in tumor invasion and progression, and a few studies have attempted to investigate changes in canine testicular tumors. Laminin is an extracellular matrix protein involved that plays a role in anchoring cells to the basement membrane. As tumors became more invasive, laminin expression became fragmented or lost in Sertoli cell tumors and seminomas, and this correlated with increasing proliferative activity as assessed by PCNA scoring, Ki67 index, and mitotic index.[39] Connexin 43 is the predominant gap junction protein of the testis and plays a role in phenotypic differentiation, cell pattern formation, and morphogenesis; and altered expression patterns may contribute to tumorigenesis and progression.[46–50] Similar to other work, differential alterations in connexin 34 expression occur in canine testicular tumors, and its expression may aid in differentiating neoplastic Sertoli cells from seminomas.[51]

Mutations of the *p53* tumor suppressor gene are common in both human and canine tmalignancies, and increased *p53* expression has been associated with tumor progression.[52–56] Nuclear *p53* immunoreactivity was detected in 15 of 20 seminomas, 6 of

12 Sertoli cell tumors, and all three interstitial cell tumors evaluated.[41] Interestingly, staining intensity was stronger in diffuse type Sertoli cell tumors and seminomas, similar to findings in another study.[41,55] Results suggest that *p53* expression may be an indicator of tumor aggression; however, further studies should be done to corroborate this.[41,55]

Similar to *p53* and proliferation indices, angiogenesis plays an important role in cancer progression and metastasis. Vascular endothelial growth factor (VEGF) and microvessel density (MVD) have been investigated as indicators of the degree of angiogenesis in multiple human and canine tumor types. VEGF expression and MVD were higher in seminomas compared with normal testes in one study.[57] In addition, both VEGF and MVD were higher in diffuse seminomas compared with more well-differentiated intratubular seminomas, potentially providing a histologic indicator of malignant behavior.[57]

The KIT protein or CD117 is a transmembrane protein for a tyrosine kinase receptor encoded by the proto-oncogene c-*kit*, which, when bound to its ligand stem cell factor (SCF), is essential to the development, proliferation, and maturation of several cell types, including germ cells.[58–60] Primordial germinal cells express KIT and migrate to interact with Sertoli cells that express SCF to guide the differentiation of the primordial cells into gonocytes.[61] Interstitial cells of Leydig also express KIT and, when stimulated by SCF, produce testosterone subsequent to Sertoli cell stimulation.[58,61,62] The expression of KIT is maintained by spermatogonia until differentiation into spermatocytes, making it a useful marker to define primordial germinal cells and early germinal cells.[61,63] In human seminomas, immunohistochemical (IHC) labeling for KIT and placental alkaline phosphatase (PLAP) is used to distinguish SE and SS, because SE expresses both KIT and PLAP whereas SS is negative for both.[64,65] Results in dogs with seminomas have suggested that, like in humans, canine seminomas may be differentiated into SE and SS using KIT and PLAP, although the frequency of each subset may affect how relevant the dog is as a model for human seminoma.[21,22,63,66,67] Recent histopathologic and IHC studies have suggested that SE may be rare in dogs, whereas canine SS may be a good model for humans, despite the rarity of SS in men.[66,67] In addition, intratubular germ cell neoplasia of undifferentiated origin and carcinoma in situ are frequent precursor lesions of SS in men, but these are infrequently identified in dogs.[22,33]

Natural Behavior

Most primary testicular tumors in the dog are characterized by local invasion and rarely metastasize. Regional or distant metastasis occurs in fewer than 15% of dogs diagnosed with Sertoli cell tumors or seminomas.[6,32,33,68–74] Interstitial cell tumors very rarely metastasize.[6] Sites of metastasis may include regional lymph nodes (LNs), eyes, brain, lungs, kidney, spleen, liver, adrenal glands, pancreas, skin, and peritoneum.[6,32,68–74]

Primary testicular tumors can also cause imbalances in sex hormone levels, regardless of the degree of local invasion and presence or absence of metastasis. Sertoli cell tumors can cause signs of feminization and more than 50% of affected dogs display signs of estrogen overproduction.[14,25,32,69] Seminomas and interstitial cell tumors are rarely associated with feminization.[75–77] Excess estrogen can cause signs such as bilateral symmetric alopecia, cutaneous hyperpigmentation, epidermal thinning, squamous metaplasia of the prostatic epithelium, gynecomastia, galactorrhea, attraction of other males, preputial atrophy, atrophy of the nonneoplastic testicle, and bone marrow suppression.[32] Sertoli cell tumors that develop in retained testicles are more likely to produce signs of hyperestrogenism; however, 17% of dogs with scrotal Sertoli cell tumors developed feminization.[14,25,32,69] Plasma sex hormone concentrations from dogs with primary testicular tumors have been investigated to better understand their contribution to tumor type and clinical signs.[77–80] Estradiol-17β concentrations were higher in dogs with Sertoli cell tumors compared with normal dogs, and were significantly higher in dogs with associated feminization syndrome.[77] Testosterone and testosterone/estradiol ratios are lower in dogs with Sertoli cell tumors compared with healthy control dogs.[76] Plasma estradiol concentrations have been variable, with one study suggesting they were lower in dogs with seminomas compared with normal dogs, but concentrations were not different in another study.[76,77] Clinical signs of feminization due to Sertoli cell tumors may best correlate to testosterone/estradiol ratio reductions rather than absolute increases in estradiol, accounting for this difference in reporting.[76] Because of variation in hormone levels, other biomarkers have been evaluated, including anti-Müllerian hormone (AMH), inhibins (inhibins α, β, βα), 3β-hydroxysteroid dehydrogenases, and insulin-like growth factors (IGF-1 and IGF-2).[77–81] AMH, alternatively termed Müllerian inhibiting substance (MIS), is a glycoprotein in the transforming growth factor-beta (TGF-β) family that is produced by Sertoli cells to stimulate regression of the Müllerian ducts in males.[82] Serum AMH may have promise as a biomarker for Sertoli cell tumors in dogs; significantly higher serum AMH has been found in a small number of dogs with Sertoli cell tumors compared with healthy adult dogs.[81]

History and Clinical Signs

Most dogs with testicular tumors are asymptomatic and a testicular mass is discovered as an incidental finding; however, clinical signs may be attributable to the primary tumor, to the presence of metastasis, or to paraneoplastic syndromes such as hyperestrogenism. In addition, breeding dogs may present with fertility problems. Diagnosis is usually made via palpation of an enlarged testicle or a testicular mass during routine physical examination, abdominal ultrasound, or necropsy. Atrophy of the remaining normal testicle is common (Fig. 29.3). Tumors in cryptorchid

dogs may cause a regional mass effect within the caudal abdominal cavity or inguinal region (Fig. 29.4).

Excess estrogen may cause signs of feminization and is the most common paraneoplastic syndrome associated with canine testicular tumors. As stated previously, seminomas and interstitial cell tumors are rarely associated with feminization whereas 50% of dogs with Sertoli cell tumors can show signs of hyperestrogenism.[14,32,69,75–77] Common clinical signs include bilateral symmetric alopecia and hyperpigmentation, pendulous prepuce, gynecomastia, galactorrhea, atrophy of the penis, and squamous metaplasia of the prostate.[32] The most deleterious effect of hyperestrogenism is bone marrow suppression, which may be irreversible and life threatening. Early effects of estrogen on the bone marrow include a transient increase in granulopoiesis with peripheral neutrophilia followed by progressive neutropenia, thrombocytopenia, and nonregenerative anemia.[75,83] Severe pancytopenia from bone marrow hypoplasia and blood dyscrasias can be fatal, and clinical signs can range from hemorrhage secondary to thrombocytopenia, anemia, and febrile neutropenia.[75,83] Less common signs associated with testicular neoplasia include lethargy (Sertoli cell tumors), presence of concurrent prostatic cyst or abscess, hematuria, hemoperitoneum, spermatic cord torsion, hypertrophic osteopathy, and perianal gland hyperplasia/adenomas (interstitial cell tumors).[3,32,69,84–87] Sertoli cell tumors have also been reported in cryptorchid male pseudohermaphrodites, which may disproportionately affect miniature Schnauzers.[88–92]

Diagnosis and Staging

Physical examination of intact male dogs, and particularly older dogs, should always include palpation of the testicles for masses and/or asymmetry. A thorough rectal examination should be performed to evaluate the prostate gland, regional LNs, and perianal region. In dogs with clinical signs of hormone imbalance (excess estrogen or testosterone), serum testosterone and estradiol-17β can be measured along with testosterone/estradiol ratio.[76,77] It is important to note that not all dogs with signs of feminization have absolute increases in estradiol-17β and clinical signs may be more closely linked to altered androgen/estrogen ratios.[76]

Definitive diagnosis is achieved by histopathologic evaluation, although the presence of a testicular mass and cytology may be supportive of testicular neoplasia. Because most dogs with testicular tumors are older and therefore have a high risk of another

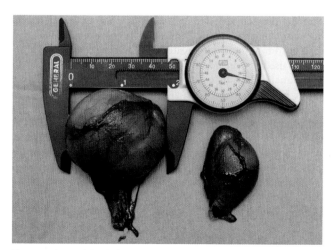

• **Fig. 29.3** Large left seminoma with mild atrophy of the right normal testicle identified as an incidental finding on physical examination.

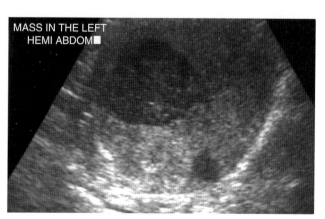

• **Fig. 29.4** Large mixed echogenic and cavitated testicle within the left midabdomen on abdominal ultrasound in a cryptorchid dog. (Image courtesy Dr. T. Schwarz, University of Edinburgh.)

primary tumor (up to 50%) or concurrent diseases, complete staging before surgery is generally recommended. Preoperative staging typically includes a complete blood count (CBC) to evaluate for hematologic abnormalities, chemistry profile, urinalysis, abdominal ultrasound, and three-view thoracic radiographs. A coagulation profile may be warranted in dogs with anemia and signs of hemorrhage. Abdominal ultrasound may serve multiple purposes: it can aid in identification of undescended testicles in the abdominal cavity or inguinal canal, assessment of regional LNs, assessment of prostatic changes, and evaluation of common sites of metastasis, such as the spleen and liver (Fig. 29.5). Testicular ultrasonography may aid in differentiating neoplastic processes from orchitis, testicular torsion, and epididymitis; however, changes are not specific enough to identify tumor type.[93–95] Ultrasound-guided fine needle-aspiration (FNA) may support a

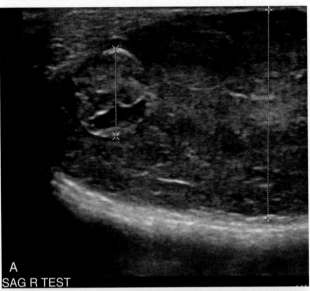

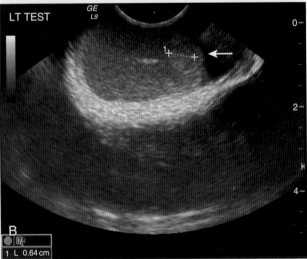

• **Fig. 29.5** (A) Sagittal ultrasound image of the testicle of a dog demonstrating a mixed echogenic neoplastic nodule (*blue arrow*). (B) Sagittal ultrasound image demonstrating an incidental, nonspecific, hyperechoic nodule (*purple arrow*) within the left testicle that was detected during routine abdominal ultrasound in a dog that presented with hematuria and benign prostatic hyperplasia. ((A) Image courtesy Dr. D. Jimenez, University of Georgia. (B) Image courtesy Dr. K. Anderson, University of Minnesota.)

suspicion of neoplasia before orchiectomy, particularly in breeding animals.[93,96] For owners with financial constraints, minimum staging should consist of CBC, chemistry profile, and urinalysis. Castration may be performed before full staging for some cases, with the decision to do full workup after histopathologic evaluation, because it is appropriate therapy for most testicular tumors. Histopathologic diagnosis is generally straightforward; however, IHC staining for vimentin, cytokeratin, desmin, c-kit, PLAP, and inhibin may be indicated to identify the underlying cell of origin.[26,33,78,97–100]

Treatment and Prognosis

As most primary canine testicular tumors are characterized by local infiltration with low potential for metastasis, orchiectomy with scrotal ablation is the treatment of choice and is often curative. Bilateral orchiectomy is the treatment of choice for testicular tumors, given that up to 50% of dogs in one report had bilateral tumors with only 12% being clinically detected in the opposite testicle.[15] In valuable breeding dogs, unilateral orchiectomy can be considered with continued monitoring afterward.[101,102] Exploratory laparotomy is indicated in cryptorchid dogs so the regional LNs can be visually assessed and biopsied if indicated. In dogs with signs of hyperestrogenism secondary to the primary tumor, clinical signs typically resolve within 1 to 3 months after castration, unless metastatic lesions provide persistent estrogen release.[68,69,74] Recurrence of feminization after castration may be associated with the development of metastasis.[69] Serum sex hormone levels may be monitored as well after castration and may correlate with resolution of clinical signs.[76,103] Dogs with bone marrow hypoplasia secondary to estrogen toxicity require close monitoring perioperatively and postoperatively for complications requiring medical intervention with blood products and/or antibiotics. These dogs carry a guarded prognosis owing to the high morbidity and mortality associated with neutropenia and hemorrhage.[75,83] Dogs with aplastic anemia likely warrant a poor prognosis.[75]

Primary testicular tumors occasionally metastasize to regional LNs and distant sites, and therapy other than surgery may be warranted in these dogs. Optimal management employing chemotherapy, radiation therapy (RT), and novel targeted therapies is not currently known. Cisplatin, actinomycin-D, chlorambucil, mithramycin, and bleomycin have been used; however, too few dogs have been treated and evaluated to formulate any conclusions regarding efficacy.[70,71,73,104] Cisplatin was evaluated in three dogs with aggressive testicular tumors with survival times (STs) ranging from 5 months to greater than 31 months.[70] RT was successfully used in four dogs with metastatic seminoma confined to the regional LNs using total doses ranging from 17 to 40 Gy with cesium-137 teletherapy.[105] In all four cases, tumors regressed and STs ranged from 6 to 37 months; importantly, none of the dogs died of seminoma. One dog that died 6 months after RT had no evidence of seminoma at necropsy.[105] Even though this was a small report, further studies are warranted to evaluate the role of external beam RT in managing metastatic seminomas because of its inherent high radiosensitivity.[106]

Feline Testicular Tumors

Feline testicular tumors are rare, although Sertoli cell tumor, seminoma, interstitial cell tumor, and teratoma have been reported.[35,107–113] The biologic behavior of testicular neoplasia in the cat is unclear because of the sparse literature available. Metastasis of a Sertoli cell tumor to the liver and spleen, and a teratoma to the omentum have been reported; therefore staging is recommended.[110,113] Optimal therapy other than orchiectomy is not known.

Comparative Aspects

In the United States testicular cancer is the most common cancer in men 15 to 44 years old, but is one of the most curable cancers with early diagnosis.[107–109] Studies have shown an increase in testicular cancer over the past half-century, with significant shifts in the age at presentation over time.[107,108,110] Causal factors such as genetic predisposition, maternal estrogen exposure, occupational hazards, dietary factors, smoking habits, and birthplace have been evaluated but, to date, the most established risk factor remains cryptorchidism.[23,107,111–120] Most cancers in men are germ cell tumors and are broadly divided into pure seminomas and nonseminomas, with seminomas comprising 50% of tumors in this group.[13,20,109] Seminomas are further classified into SE, atypical, or SS subtypes; however, diagnostic and therapeutic management does not vary considerably between tumor types.[20,109] Pure seminomas are more likely to behave in a clinically aggressive fashion; therefore when both seminoma and nonseminoma features are present, therapeutic management follows the guidelines for nonseminoma.[109] Standard staging in human seminomas consists of physical examination, radiographic studies, determination of serum markers, including alpha-fetoprotein, human chorionic gonadotropin, and lactate dehydrogenase, and histopathologic assessment. SS is a rare variant of germ cell neoplasia that is most commonly seen in older men and carries a low risk of metastasis, suggesting similar behavior to most canine seminomas.[21,23] Treatment generally includes surgery for stage I seminomas, and/or RT and chemotherapy for individuals with higher stage disease.[106,121–123] Cisplatin-based chemotherapy protocols are generally employed for patients with greater than stage I disease, with cure rates in the range of 70% to 80% despite high tumor burdens.[23,106,109,124] The dog has been proposed as a model for studies of the male reproductive system, and in particular for studies evaluating the development of testicular tumors.[18,21,22,33] Further work on the molecular pathogenesis, classification system, and behavior of canine tumors may yield more support for use of spontaneously occurring testicular tumors as good comparative models for human disease.

Canine Prostate Tumors

Incidence/Prevalence

Prostatic tumors are relatively uncommon in dogs and have a low prevalence at less than 1% (0.2%–0.6%).[132–136] In a collection of more than 17,000 confirmed neoplasms of the dog collected from veterinary schools in North America, only 11 prostate carcinomas (PCAs) were identified (0.06%).[34] A study evaluating lifetime occurrence of neoplasia in predominantly intact German shepherd dogs and Belgian Malinois working dogs showed that more than 30% developed at least one cancer; however only 2 of the 104 primary tumors were PCAs.[17] Despite this low incidence, the dog is one of the few domestic species to develop spontaneous prostate cancer, thus sparking interest in the dog as a model for prostate cancer in men.[135,137–143] In three retrospective reviews of dogs with prostatic disease, between 7%

and 16% were diagnosed with PCA.[144–146] One study of 177 dogs found that PCA was the most common disease in neutered dogs whereas bacterial prostatitis and prostatic cysts were more common in intact male dogs.[145] Elderly dogs are more commonly diagnosed with PCA, with a median age at diagnosis of 10 years.[135,146–148] The underlying etiology of canine prostatic cancer is unknown; however, high-grade prostatic intraepithelial neoplasia (PIN or HGPIN), which is believed to be a precursor of human prostate carcinoma, has been detected in both dogs without evidence of prostatic disease and in those with existing PCA.[149–152] The occurrence of PIN in dogs with concurrent carcinoma varies from 7% to 72%, although in two large studies of dogs without histologic evidence of PCA, the occurrence was low at 0% to 3%.[134,149–152]

Most tumors of the canine prostate are carcinomas, with most being transitional cell carcinoma (TCC) or adenocarcinoma in origin.[153–156] Prostate tumors in the dog likely have a urothelial or ductular origin rather than acinar because most canine tumors are androgen independent.[153,154,157–160] Other types of carcinomas include mixed carcinomas and squamous cell carcinomas (SCCs). Classifying carcinomas on the basis of subtype is somewhat subjective and there is not currently a standard for definitive diagnosis of canine prostate tumors as there is with humans.[151,152,161–165] Fibrosarcoma, leiomyosarcoma, osteosarcoma, lymphoma, and hemangiosarcoma have also been reported to affect the prostate.[134,166–171] Benign tumors of the prostate are rare.[172] TCC of the prostatic urethra will frequently invade the prostate, and it may be difficult to distinguish primary PCA from secondary invasion of a urethral tumor.

Risk Factors

Both intact and castrated dogs develop PCAs, although multiple studies have suggested there is an increased risk of PCA in castrated male dogs compared with intact male dogs, with an odds ratio of approximately 2.3 to 4.3.[132,146,147,153,157] More aggressive tumors may develop in castrated males with a higher risk of metastasis.[147] The reason for this difference is unclear, although it is possible that castrated dogs live longer than intact dogs and are thus predisposed to developing age-related cancers.[146,153] It is also possible that androgens provide a protective effect on prostatic tissue, or that, after castration, the relative estrogen effect aids in neoplastic transformation.[153,173–175] The lowest relative risk of neutered males in a recent study was for PCA, which may occur relatively more frequently in intact male dogs.[134,151,153] Although several studies have suggested that androgens may not be required for initiation or progression of adenocarcinoma of the canine prostate, further controlled studies should be done to definitively determine the role of androgens or the effect of early or late castration.[153,154,157,159,160,176]

Breeds that may be at increased risk of developing PCA include the Bouvier des Flandres, Doberman pinscher, Shetland sheepdog, Scottish terrier, beagle, miniature poodle, German shorthaired pointer, Airedale terrier, and Norwegian elkhound.[146,153] The Shetland sheepdog and Scottish terrier remained at increased risk even when TCC was excluded in one study.[153] Mixed-breed dogs have also been reported as at increased risk for PCA, regardless of neutering status, suggesting that environmental influences may play a significant role in tumor development.[153] The American cocker spaniel, miniature poodle, and dachshund may be at decreased risk for developing PCA.[153]

Natural Behavior

At the time of diagnosis, most canine prostatic tumors are characterized by local invasion with a high propensity for regional and distant metastasis. In one postmortem study of 76 dogs, 80% of dogs with PCA had evidence of measurable metastatic disease, with lung and LNs being the most common sites of spread.[134] Importantly, similar to high-grade PCA in men, canine PCA has a tendency to metastasize to bone: 22% to 42% of dogs develop skeletal metastasis, predominantly to the lumbar vertebrae and pelvis.[134,159,177,178] Younger dogs diagnosed with PCA may be at increased risk for metastasis than older dogs, although the role of castration status in these two groups is unclear.[134,179] As long-term studies in dogs with evidence of PIN but without PCA are not available, it is unclear if PCA in dogs can behave in a slowly progressive fashion in its early phase of development. It is presumed that most dogs are diagnosed at an advanced stage of disease because of the high metastatic rate; however, the true behavior from time of onset is not definitively known and PCA may behave differently in intact and castrated dogs.[146,147]

Pathogenesis

The underlying cause of prostate tumors is unknown, and it is possible that both genetic and environmental factors contribute to tumor development. HGPIN is considered a precursor of human PCA and occurs under the influence of androgenic stimulation in those patients at risk for carcinoma.[180] Although PIN has been detected in dogs with existing PCA, it has also been detected in dogs without evidence of prostatic disease, making its role in the dog less clear.[149–151] HGPIN as a predictor of carcinoma occurrence may not be as reliable in the dog as it is in men.[150,173] It is not known with certainty if low- and intermediate-grade PIN occurs in dogs, although one IHC study suggested the presence of low-grade PIN.[181] Investigators evaluated five prostates from middle-aged to older intact dogs containing lesions of PIN and compared nuclear protein p63 (marker of prostatic basal cells), androgen receptor expression, and PCNA to normal prostatic tissue also obtained from intact dogs. PIN foci had higher p63 expression, higher PCNA index, and heterogeneous androgen receptor (AR) expression, suggesting similarities to human low-grade PIN.[181] Prostatic inflammatory atrophy has also been identified in dogs and humans, which may be a precursor of PIN lesions or PCA.[143,152,182–185] Several studies have attempted to elucidate key changes in gene and protein expression in prostate carcinogenesis to develop and investigate targeted approaches that interrupt carcinogenesis and progression.[143,163,182,183,186–188]

The role of hormones in prostate development and tumor progression is unclear in the dog. Castration does not provide a protective effect and, in fact, may contribute to tumor development and/or progression, although PCA may behave differently in the intact male compared with the neutered male.[146,147] Normal prostate development and regulation in humans and dogs is androgen dependent; however, neoplastic human prostate most commonly remains androgen dependent as opposed to the dog. AR expression within the nuclei can be identified in 90% to 95% of normal (intact) prostatic secretory epithelial cells and in the majority of acinar basal cells.[159,160,189,190] In neutered dogs and in dogs with PCA, nuclear AR expression decreases and is usually lost.[159,160] The role of estrogen and progesterone has yet to be fully defined, although nuclear estrogen receptor expression appears to be decreased in PCA tissue compared with normal and hyperplastic prostate tissue.[158,190]

Because of its aggressive behavior at the time of diagnosis, some investigators have considered mechanisms that may contribute to PCA progression and metastasis. Activating mutations in the *BRAF* gene, which lead to constitutive MAPK signaling, were found in the majority of PCA in dogs. Moreover, the mutation frequency was similar between PCA and urothelial (bladder) TCC.[191,192] This is uncommon in nonmetastatic human prostate cancer, but may support the current hypothesis that most canine PCAs arise from the prostatic ducts or prostatic urethra.[134,154,157,193–196]

Cyclooxgyenase-2 (COX-2) expression may play a role in carcinogenesis and progression in PCA. Expression of COX-2 was noted in 75% of PCAs in one study, whereas none of the normal prostate tissue stained positively.[197] Two other studies have supported the notion that COX-2 and downstream prostaglandin E_2 production may play a role in PCA development.[198,199] Indeed, a clinical study identified COX-2 protein expression in 88% of 16 PCAs examined and was further able to show a survival benefit in dogs treated with either piroxicam or carprofen.[200]

PCA has a predilection for bone, which may be mediated in part by TGF-β, parathyroid hormone–related protein (PTHrp), and endothelin.[201–203] PTHrp mediates pathologic bone resorption in many different tumors, including PCA, which may encourage release of TGF-β into the microenvironment. In a positive feedback loop, canine PCA cells can increase gene transcription for PTHrp in response to exogenous TGF-β.[202] Although PTHrp and TGF-β may be important in establishing skeletal metastases, it is interesting to note that PCA metastases are more commonly osteoblastic in nature.[173,204,205] In a rat model, osteoblast activation was increased after incubation with normal canine prostate protein homogenates through an endothelin-dependent pathway, suggesting a possible contribution to bone metastasis formation.[203] Recent gene expression profiling work in human castration-resistant prostate cancer (CRPC) has shown high AR expression is correlated to genes controlling osteoblast/osteoclast activity, cellular metabolism (i.e., cholesterol synthesis, fatty acid oxidation, pyrimidine synthesis), and immune cell infiltration, all of which may influence therapeutic regimens.[206,207]

History and Clinical Signs

Clinical signs in dogs with PCA are variable and may be reflective of local and/or metastatic disease. Common historical findings and clinical examination signs include hematuria, dysuria, stranguria, dyschezia, tenesmus, bacteriuria, and altered stool shape (flattened or ribbonlike stools).[134,147,155,178,208] With complete obstruction of urinary outflow due to prostatic compression or direct tumor extension into the urethra, hydroureter, hyrdronephrosis, and renal failure may occur. Local invasion into the lumbar vertebrae or nerve roots may cause signs of pain, gait abnormalities, lameness, and/or constipation. Nonspecific systemic illness, typically associated with advanced disease, include lethargy, exercise intolerance, tachypnea or dyspnea, hyporexia, and weight loss. Dogs with skeletal metastasis may present with signs of severe bone pain, pathologic fracture, or rarely with a palpable mass.[134,178,209] Dogs may present with a history of clinical signs that partially improved with empiric therapy for prostatitis.

Diagnosis and Staging

Dogs that present with suspected PCA should be fully staged to determine extent of disease and to rule out other causes of prostatic disease such as benign prostatic hypertrophy (BPH), prostatitis, and prostatic cysts or abscesses.[155,210,211] Physical examination, including a thorough rectal examination, should be performed on every patient. Rectal palpation often reveals a large, firm, and asymmetric or irregular prostate that may be painful. Sublumbar lymphadenomegaly may be detected on rectal or abdominal palpation. A normal-sized prostate on rectal examination in a castrated dog is considered abnormal, even if symmetric and nonpainful. CBC and serum chemistry profile may demonstrate anemia, leukocytosis, hypocalcemia, elevated bone alkaline phosphatase activity, or signs of concurrent disease.[147,148,212] Urinalysis and culture may show pyuria, bacteriuria, dysplastic urinary epithelial cells, and secondary urinary bacterial infection.[134,145,147,173,212,213] Three-view thoracic radiographs may show evidence of pulmonary metastatic disease, sternal lymphadenomegaly, or rarely metastasis to the extrathoracic skeletal structures (ribs, scapula).[178] Abdominal radiographs may show evidence of an enlarged prostate, with or without evidence of mineralization; periosteal reactions on the vertebrae, femur, or pelvic bones; and/or sublumbar or retroperitoneal lymphadenomegaly (Fig. 29.6A, B).[147,178,214,215] It is important to note that the presence of mineralization, particularly in intact dogs, is not pathognomonic for neoplasia and can occur in dogs with prostatitis, BPH, or prostatic cysts[215–217]; however, neutered dogs with prostatic mineralization are highly likely to have prostatic neoplasia and should undergo further diagnostics.[215] If a clinical suspicion of skeletal metastasis exists, survey radiographs or bone scintigraphy may be useful for localization.[209] PCA metastases to bone most commonly have an osteoproductive component, but may be osteolytic, osteoproductive, or mixed. Contrast studies such as retrograde urethrography may be useful to evaluate irregularities in the prostatic urethra or reflux of contrast into a prostatic mass; however, they are not specific enough to differentiate neoplasia from inflammatory or infectious processes.[214,218] Abdominal ultrasound can be useful to further evaluate the prostate, urethra, bladder, regional LNs, and cranial abdominal organs. Lymphadenomegaly, echogenicity changes, and mineralization may be visualized on ultrasound in dogs with prostatic neoplasia, although they can also be features of nonneoplastic diseases (see Fig. 29.6C).[214,215]

Obtaining tissue samples is considered the gold standard of diagnosis of canine prostatic neoplasia. One retrospective histopathologic study highlighted several different histologic patterns that may be important to providing an accurate diagnosis of PCA.[152] More recently, proposals for a Gleason-type grading system have been made to provide some level of prognostication in dogs and to better correlate findings to prostate cancer in men.[163–165] In human PCA, the Gleason grading system assesses the architecture of biopsy sections and is used to assign a Gleason score based on the sum of the Gleason pattern identified in the largest area (the primary grade) and the highest grade (secondary grade).[219,220] The Gleason score has been modified over time but has maintained its reliable and robust prognostic significance; thus there is interest in adapting this type of system to dogs.[220]

A definitive diagnosis of prostatic neoplasia may be garnered from cytology samples as well.[155,213] A number of methods may provide adequate samples for diagnosis, including ejaculation, traumatic catheterization, prostatic massage, prostatic wash, ultrasound-guided FNA cytology, impression smears during surgery,

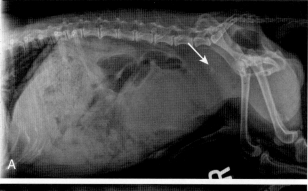
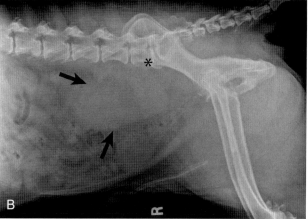
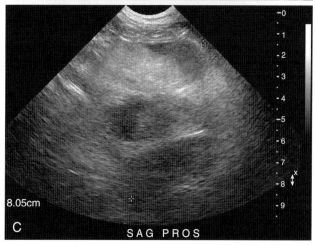

• **Fig. 29.6** (A) Right lateral abdominal radiograph demonstrating prostatic mineralization (*white arrow*), which may be a feature of benign and malignant disease in intact dogs. (B) Right lateral abdominal radiograph of a dog with prostatic carcinoma with metastasis to the sublumbar lymph nodes (*black arrows*) and local invasion along the sacrum and ventral aspect of the seventh lumbar vertebral body (*star*). (C) Ultrasound image of a symmetric, yet severely enlarged prostate of heterogeneous echogenicity in a dog diagnosed with Rocky Mountain spotted fever and bacterial prostatitis. ((A and B) Images courtesy of Dr. S. Holmes, AXIS - Animal Cross-Sectional Imaging Specialists. (C) Image courtesy Dr. D. Jimenez, University of Georgia.)

or biopsy via percutaneous, perineal transrectal, or surgical routes. Risks of percutaneous biopsies, ultrasound-guided aspirates or biopsies, and transrectal aspirates include hemorrhage, urethral trauma, and tumor seeding[210,221–224] Cytology or histology of suspected metastatic lesions (e.g., LN) may also aid with diagnosis and offer a simpler method of diagnosis (Fig. 29.7). Histologic grading of PCA is not routinely performed because there is no

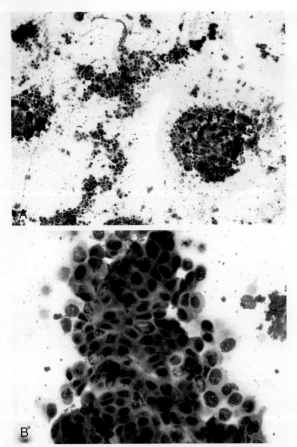

• **Fig. 29.7** (A) Cytology from a prostatic carcinoma (4×) demonstrating clusters of variably sized polygonal epithelial cells with a moderate amount of basophilic cytoplasm, which often contains clear, nonstaining vacuoles. (B) Cytology from a prostatic carcinoma (20×) showing cellular detail and moderate anisocytosis and anisokaryosis. Cells have round to ovoid nuclei with a coarsely granular chromatin pattern and distinct nucleoli. (Images courtesy Dr. D. Seelig and Dr. D. Heinrich, University of Minnesota.)

support for its effect on prognostication.[134,225] Cytologic evaluation of samples collected via traumatic catheterization or prostatic wash may prove challenging, as it can be difficult to differentiate dysplastic epithelial cells from neoplasia.[213,226] In one study, discordant results between cytology and histology in prostatic disorders occurred in 20% of cases, but were not considered a flaw of aspiration techniques but rather of the pathologic process.[213] Multiple techniques were employed, including ultrasound-guided FNA, prostatic massage and wash, and impression smears of biopsies. Other factors, such as serum and seminal plasma concentrations of acid phosphatase (AP), prostate-specific antigen (PSA), and canine prostate-specific esterase, have not been useful in the definitive diagnosis of PCA in the dog.[133,227] Although significantly higher serum total AP, prostatic AP, and nonprostatic AP concentrations were noted in dogs with PCA compared with healthy dogs or dogs with BPH, they were neither sufficiently sensitive nor specific for definitive diagnosis.[227]

Treatment and Prognosis

Because PCA in dogs is characterized by insidious local progression and a high rate of metastasis, most dogs are diagnosed with advanced disease and the overall prognosis is poor. Median survival times (MSTs) for dogs without therapy are often less than 30 days and, in one report of 76 dogs, most dogs were euthanized at the time of diagnosis.[134,200] If therapy is attempted, effort is generally made to control local disease in addition to locoregional and distant metastases, although therapy is considered largely palliative. There is currently no standard-of-care consensus therapy for canine prostate tumors, although use of nonsteroidal antiinflammatory drugs (NSAIDs) is recommended as minimal therapy.

Therapeutic options for managing local disease include partial or total prostatectomy, electrosurgical transurethral resection (TUR), photodynamic therapy (PDT), RT, laser therapy, and medical management. Prostatectomy is generally recommended for dogs with early stage, intracapsular disease, but case selection is likely important for good outcome. Total prostatectomy is associated with a moderate to high rate of postoperative morbidity and a survival benefit over medical management has not been investigated.[148,228–233] The entire prostate gland and associated urethra are removed with total prostatectomy, thus requiring reconstruction for urinary drainage. The most common complication is urinary incontinence, occurring in 33% to 35% of dogs.[148,231,232] A recent multiinstitutional retrospective study described total prostatectomy in 25 dogs that included 9 dogs with extracapsular extension of tumor and 11 dogs with intracapsular tumors. All dogs survived prostatectomy and 21 received variable adjunctive therapy, most commonly mitoxantrone and NSAIDs (*n* = 14).[148] The MST for all dogs was 231 days and dogs with intracapsular tumors had a significantly longer MST than those with extracapsular tumors (248 days vs 138 days).[148] Local recurrence and/or distant metastasis were suspected in over 30% of dogs, thus justifying the prospective exploration of surgery and additional local and systemic therapy for some dogs.[148] Subtotal intracapsular prostatectomy may be a useful alternative in some dogs. In one study that compared 10 dogs that underwent total prostatectomy to 11 dogs that underwent subtotal intracapsular prostatectomy, the latter procedure was associated with longer mean STs (112 days vs 20 days) and a decreased rate of postoperative complications.[230] Importantly, 7 of the 10 dogs that underwent total prostatectomy were euthanized within 2 weeks of surgery compared with only two dogs in the subtotal intracapsular prostatectomy group.[230] The high acute (within 2 weeks) postoperative mortality rate in dogs that underwent total prostatectomy in this randomized study may be reflective of less stringent case selection given the results of the more recent report of total prostatectomy in dogs.[148,230] As urinary incontinence is common after prostatectomy, attempts have been made to reduce trauma to the prostatic urethra, including use of a neodymium:yttrium–aluminum–garnet (Nd:YAG) laser; however, there is still a risk of significant postoperative complications.[229,232,233] Rapid palliation of dysuria was reported after TUR using an electrocautery cutting loop with or without intraoperative RT in three dogs with prostatic TCC or undifferentiated carcinoma.[212] Complications occurred in all dogs and included urinary tract infection, tumor seeding, and urethral perforation, and STs were relatively short.[212]

In dogs with urethral obstruction due to a prostatic tumor, palliative measures may be attempted to alleviate the obstruction. Placement of a cystostomy tube permits urinary diversion and bladder emptying, but owners should be aware that it generally does not resolve incontinence or stranguria and secondary urinary tract infections are common.[234–236] Palliative stenting of the urethra in the obstructed area is a reasonable alternative to cystostomy tubes and is the authors' preferred option. The extent and location of the obstruction is determined using fluoroscopy or digital radiography and stents are typically selected to extend approximately 1 cm proximal and distal to the obstruction.[166,237–239] The use of digital radiography to guide stent placement is relatively new and may require more cautious placement.[237] Stents can be ordered in various diameters and are recommended to be 10% greater than the diameter of healthy-appearing urethra. The procedure is considered palliative and complications include incontinence (which may be severe in 25% of cases), stranguria, reobstruction, and stent migration.[166,237–239] Although the literature reporting outcome for dogs treated with stenting and chemotherapy is still maturing, studies suggest that the addition of NSAIDs with or without chemotherapy may be beneficial.[238]

PDT may be a viable option for some dogs with minimally invasive PCA, although its availability is not widespread.[240] PDT remains predominantly investigational at this time, although several reports have suggested that the dog provides a good model to support clinical applications for novel treatments for PCA.[241–246] Challenges in delivering homogeneous doses may limit the utility of PDT in advanced tumors.

RT may be useful in the palliation of clinical signs related to local PCA and to painful skeletal metastases, although optimal dose and fractionation are unknown. In an older study, 10 dogs with PCA were treated with intraoperative orthovoltage therapy.[247] Nine of the dogs were prescribed 20 Gy to 30 Gy to the prostate with an MST of 114 days, although the range extended to 750 days.[247] It is probable that with advances in RT planning and delivery involving the routine use of 3D conformal RT (CRT) or intensity-modulated RT (IMRT) with image-guided RT (IGRT) to confirm target positioning, local disease may be better targeted and controlled (Fig. 29.8). A recent retrospective study described definitive-intent IMRT/IGRT in 21 dogs with genitourinary carcinomas that were prescribed 54 to 58 Gy in 20 fractions to the primary target volume.[248] Ten dogs had prostatic carcinomas completed treatment and had an event-free survival time of 317 days; the overall event free survival time and overall survival time reported for all 21 dogs was 317 days and 654 days, respectively.[248] Although multimodality therapy and NSAIDs were not standardized, results support further prospective evaluation of RT for long-term control. Given the potential for durable tumor control after RT, it will be important to monitor for late radiation toxicity, as approximately 20% of dogs developed manageable grade 3 late toxicity (including urethral, ureteral, and rectal stricture), despite the small fraction size.[248] It is unclear if improving local control with RT will alter the time or pattern of metastasis but prospective efforts to elucidate the role of RT are warranted.

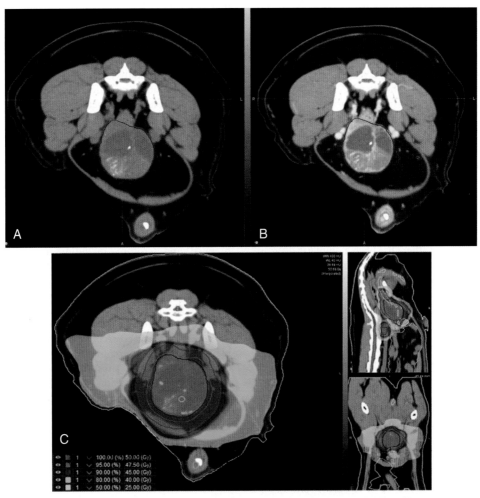

• **Fig. 29.8** Precontrast (A) and postcontrast (B) films of a dog with a large, mineralized, and heterogeneous prostatic carcinoma causing dorsal deviation and compression of the colon. The *blue outline* represents the gross tumor volume. (C) Radiation dose distribution illustrated with colored isodose lines around the prostate on an axial CT image.

The benefit of systemic therapy to manage canine prostatic tumors is also unclear, although a study demonstrated a clear survival benefit in dogs with PCAs treated with piroxicam or carprofen compared with those dogs that were untreated (MSTs of 6.9 months vs 0.7 months, respectively).[200] The role of chemotherapy is less clear.

For dogs with skeletal metastasis, palliative options include systemic analgesics, RT, bisphosphonates, and samarium-153–ethylenediamine–tetramethylene–phosphonic acid ([153]SM-EDTMP).[249,251] Standardized protocols have not yet been determined, although RT and bisphosphonates are widely available and relatively easy to administer.[249,251–253]

Feline Prostate Tumors

Prostate tumors in the cat are rare and reports in the veterinary literature are sparse.[254–259] Of the few case reports, most tumors appear to be adenocarcinomas and affect older castrated cats. Definitive risk factors have not been identified because of the lack of frequent cases and epidemiologic data. Clinical signs often include lower urinary tract signs and obstipation or constipation, tenesmus, and dyschezia. Rectal palpation can reveal the presence of a mass, which may be further characterized with abdominal ultrasound. There is no standard-of-care therapy in cats and given the paucity of reports in the literature, it is difficult to state overall prognosis. Metastasis appears common and sites of spread can include pancreas, lung, and LNs; most cats died within 3 months of diagnosis.[254–258] Prostatectomy for a low-grade prostatic sarcomatoid carcinoma in one cat provided long-term control with no evidence of local or metastatic disease at 2 years.[259] Prostatectomy followed by doxorubicin and cyclophosphamide was reported to yield a survival duration of 10 months in another cat.[255] Until more cats with PCA prostatic carcinoma are evaluated, therapy and prognosis are unclear.

Comparative Aspects

The recommendations for diagnosis and treatment of PCA in men have changed markedly in the past decade, particularly in the United States, where the value of PSA as a reliable biomarker has been debated.[219,260] Where much emphasis is placed on early detection in most tumor types, there has been a dramatic decrease in the screening for PCA owing to the increased treatment of clinically insignificant tumors, which increase morbidity and mortality compared with that associated with natural cancer progression.[219,261] Active surveillance is now implemented for many men with low-risk PCA and screening recommendations have recently been updated to align with other countries.[260–264] After modifications to the US Preventative Services Task Force (USPSTF) draft guidelines, the USPSTF, American Cancer Society, American Urological Association, the American Society of Clinical Oncology, the American College of Physicians, and the National Comprehensive Cancer Network all advocate for patient education and "shared decision making" when considering screening high-risk groups, men with a family history, or when other factors may influence the likelihood of nonindolent PCA.[260,261,263] Newer PCA biomarker panels may outperform PSA alone as useful screening tools, especially in high-risk disease.[260,265–267]

Well-established and consistent risk factors for PCA in men are race/ethnicity, family history, and age, although other factors such as diet and lifestyle may contribute as well.[219,268] Despite the lack of clear evidence for a direct causal role in the development of PCA, preventative measures have focused on low-fat diets, regular exercise, and maintenance of a normal body mass index.[219] Like in dogs, most prostatic tumors in men are carcinomas; however, the incidence of disease is considerably higher in men. Because the dog is one of the few domestic species to develop spontaneous PCA, there is indeed considerable interest in the dog as a model for PCA in men.[135,137–143] Challenges that exist when considering the dog as a model include the lack of canine PSA that is similar to human PSA, and the most tumors in dogs are likely androgen independent.[133,219,269] PCA in men typically initiates as PIN, which is often seen as multifocal premalignant lesions that progress to neoplasia; the role of PIN in the development of canine prostatic diseases in either the intact or castrated dog is unclear. High-grade PCA in men behaves similarly to the disease in dogs, with significant local invasion and a propensity for skeletal metastasis. Although less common in man, the dog may serve as a good model for interventional strategies for androgen-independent, aggressive PCA. Therapy in humans is highly dependent on the stage at presentation and partially dependent on a summary of risks versus benefit of intervention.[219,270–272] Newer robotic surgery approaches are currently being evaluated in an attempt to improve perioperative and postoperative outcome after prostatectomy, which has traditionally been performed as an open or laparoscopic surgery.[272–274] Advances in RT technology have also led to the safe delivery of higher doses of radiation to prostate tumors, which has improved disease control while maintaining quality-of-life measures.[219,264,270,275,276] Although there are many nuances to treatment beyond the scope of this chapter, androgen deprivation therapy generally forms the basis for therapy for hormone-sensitive prostate cancer; for CRPC, improvements in outcome may be possible with docetaxel with or without novel targeted drugs such as abiraterone, a cytochrome P450 (17) inhibitor, and enzalutamide, an antiandrogen.[219,277–279] The approaches to screening and treatment are changing rapidly and warrant attention as novel drugs are developed, as many of these drugs that have efficacy against CRPC may be applicable to canine PCA.

Canine Penile, Preputial, and Scrotal Tumors

Multiple tumor types can affect the soft tissues of the canine penis, prepuce, and scrotum, including transmissible venereal tumor (TVT), SCC, sebaceous gland adenoma, mesothelioma, papilloma, lymphoma, plasma cell tumor, mast cell tumor, hemangioma, melanoma, and fibrosarcoma.[38,280–287] Overall, TVT and SCC are the most common neoplasms of the canine penis. Ossifying fibroma, benign mesenchymoma, multilobular osteochondrosarcoma and osteosarcoma can arise from the penile bone (os penis).[288–293] Osteosarcoma of the os penis may behave similarly to other axial skeleton sites with a potential to develop local recurrence after narrow excision and distant metastasis.[288,290]

Clinical signs are often associated with local disease and many dogs present with hematuria, stranguria, or dysuria. Occasionally, dogs may present with a visible mass and the absence of urinary signs; this is likely more common in scrotal tumors compared with other tumor sites. It is also possible for clinical signs to be secondary to locoregional or distant metastasis, as the biologic behavior for most tumors is poorly defined. Full workup and clinical staging, including CBC, serum chemistry, urinalysis, and thoracic and abdominal imaging, is recommended in dogs with penile tumors before definitive therapy. Surgical excision is generally recommended and often involves partial or complete penile amputation and perineal urethrostomy. TVT is an exception, because it is a chemoresponsive and radioresponsive tumor, although surgery may be used for refractory cases.[294,295] For dogs with scrotal tumors, castration (if intact) with scrotal ablation is recommended. Depending on the underlying tumor type, adjuvant therapy such as RT or chemotherapy may be indicated. Prognosis is heavily dependent on underlying histology and the ability to obtain adequate local control.

Feline Penile, Preputial, and Scrotal Tumors

Little information exists on tumors that affect the feline penis, prepuce, and scrotum. There is a report of fibroma affecting the scrotum of a cat; however, it is probable that clinical signs would be similar to those in dogs.[296]

Comparative Aspects

Penile tumors in the United States are rare, although they remain a problem in a number of countries in Asia, Africa, and South America, where up to 10% of cancers may arise in the penis.[297] The incidence of penile cancer has been declining in part as a result of increased personal hygiene and circumcision.[298–300] Indeed, neonatal circumcision virtually eliminates penile carcinoma from the population.[299] Poor local hygiene, phimosis, tobacco, chronic inflammation, lack of circumcision, infection with human papilloma virus, and having multiple sexual partners are associated with the development of malignant penile lesions.[299,301–303] Most penile tumors are carcinomas and more than 95% of carcinomas are SCC.[304] Clinical signs in men are varied and range from a subtle erythematous local lesion to an ulcerated, infected mass lesion. Full staging is important in men who present with penile cancer because nodal status is one of the most significant prognostic variables for survival.[305] The prognosis is generally excellent for patients with early-stage disease and treatment typically consists of surgery. Occasionally, RT is used for primary treatment of early-stage disease, but local recurrence rates are higher than with surgery.[306–309] In advanced cases, aggressive surgery may include emasculation procedures or hemipelvectomy followed by RT. Although surgery is the mainstay of treatment, multimodal treatment with radical surgery and adjuvant chemotherapy is important for outcome when lymphatic spread is present.[297,305] Of note, because penile carcinoma is rare in developed countries, it is recommended that patients seek care with experienced multidisciplinary specialty teams, as this approach is associated with improved outcomes.[305,310–312]

References

1. Cotchin E: Testicular neoplasms in dogs, *J Comp Pathol* 70:232–248, 1960.
2. von-Bomhard D, Pukkavesa C, Haenichen T: The ultrastructure of testicular tumours in the dog. I. Germinal cells and seminomas, *J Comp Pathol* 88:49–57, 1978.
3. Hayes HM, Pendergrass TW: Canine testicular tumors: epidemiologic features of 410 dogs, *Int J Cancer* 18:482–487, 1976.
4. Liao AT, Chu PY, Yeh LS, et al.: A 12-year retrospective study of canine testicular tumors, *Theriogenology* 71:919–923, 2009.
5. Cohen D, Reif J, Brodey R, et al.: Epidemiologic analysis of the most prevalent sites and types of canine neoplasia observed in a veterinary hospital, *Cancer Res* 34:2859–2868, 1974.
6. Dow C: Testicular tumours in the dog, *J Comp Pathol* 72:247–265, 1962.
7. Grieco V, Riccardi E, Greppi GF, et al.: Canine testicular tumours: a study on 232 dogs, *J Comp Pathol* 138:86–89, 2008.
8. Nodtvedt A, Gamlem H, Gunnes G, et al.: Breed differences in the proportional morbidity of testicular tumours and distribution of histopathologic types in a population-based canine cancer registry, *Vet Comp Oncol* 9:45–54, 2011.
9. Bray F, Ferlay J, Devesa SS, et al.: Interpreting the international trends in testicular seminoma and nonseminoma incidence, *Nat Clin Pract Urol* 3:532–543, 2006.
10. Chia VM, Quraishi SM, Devesa SS, et al.: International trends in the incidence of testicular cancer, 1973-2002 *Cancer Epidemiol Biomarkers Prev* 19:1151–1159, 2010.
11. Shah MN, Devesa SS, McGlynn KA: Trends in testicular germ cell tumours by ethnic group in the United States, *Int J Androl* 30:206–213, 2007.
12. Townsend JS, Richardson LC, German RR: Incidence of testicular cancer in the United States, 1999-2004, *Am J Mens Health* 4:353–360, 2010.
13. Bray F, Richiardi L, Ekbom A, et al.: Do testicular seminoma and nonseminoma share the same etiology? Evidence from an age-period-cohort analysis of incidence trends in eight European countries, *Cancer Epidemiol Biomarkers Prev* 15:652–658, 2006.
14. Weaver AD: Survey with follow-up of 67 dogs with testicular sertoli cell tumours, *Vet Rec* 113:105–107, 1983.
15. Reif JS, Maguire TG, Kenney RM, et al.: A cohort study of canine testicular neoplasia, *J Am Vet Med Assoc* 175:719–723, 1979.
16. Kennedy PC, Cullen JM, Edwards JF, et al.: *Histological classifications of tumors of the genital system of domestic animals*, Washington, D.C, 1998, American Registry of Pathology.
17. Peterson JR, Frommelt RA, Dunn DG: A study of the lifetime occurrence of neoplasia and breed differences in a cohort of German shepherd dogs and Belgian Malinois military working dogs that died in 1992, *J Vet Intern Med* 14:140–145, 2000.
18. Peters MA, DeRooij DG, Teerds KJ, et al.: Spermatogenesis and testicular tumours in ageing dogs, *J Reprod Fertil* 120:443–452, 2000.
19. Maiolino P, Restucci B, Papparella S, et al.: Correlation of nuclear morphometric features with animal and human World Health Organization international histological classifications of canine spontaneous seminomas, *Vet Pathol* 41:608–611, 2004.
20. Mostofi FK, Sesterhenn IA: *Histologic typing of testis tumors*, ed 2, Geneva, 1998, Springer.
21. Kim JH, Yu CH, Yhee JY, et al.: Canine classical seminoma: a specific malignant type with human classifications is highly correlated with tumor angiogenesis, *BMC Cancer* 10:243–251, 2010.
22. Grieco V, Riccardi E, Rondena M, et al.: Classical and spermatocytic seminoma in the dog: histochemical and immunohistochemical findings, *J Comp Pathol* 137:41–46, 2007.
23. Pagliaro LC, Logothetis CJ: Cancer of the testis. In DeVita Jr VT, Lawrence TS, Stevens GH, editors: *Cancer: principles and practice of oncology*, ed 10, Philadelphia, 2006, Wolters Kluwer Health / Lippincott Wiliams & Wilkins, pp 988–1004.
24. Ortega-Pacheco A, Rodriguez-Buenfil JC, Segura-Correa JC, et al.: Pathological conditions of the reproductive organs of male stray dogs in the tropics: prevalence, risk factors, morphological findings and testosterone concentrations, *Reprod Domest Anim* 41:429–437, 2006.
25. Reif JS, Brodey RS: The relationship between cryptorchidism and canine testicular neoplasia, *J Am Vet Med Assoc 1969* 155:2005–2010, 2005.
26. Patnaik AK, Mostofi FK: A clinicopathologic, histologic, and immunohistochemical study of mixed germ cell-stromal tumors of the testis in 16 dogs, *Vet Pathol* 30:287–295, 1993.
27. Radi ZA, Miller DL, Hines ME: Rete testis mucinous adenocarcinoma in a dog, *Vet Pathol* 41:75–78, 2004.
28. Turk JR, Turk MA, Gallina AM: A canine testicular tumor resembling gonadoblastoma, *Vet Pathol* 18:201–207, 1981.
29. Rothwell TLW, Papdimitriou JM, Zu FN, et al.: Schwannoma in the testis of a dog, *Vet Pathol* 23:629–631, 1986.

30. Vascellari M, Carminato A, Camall G, et al.: Malignant mesothelioma of the tunica vaginalis testis in a dog: histological and immunohistochemical characterization, *J Vet Diagn Invest* 23:135–139, 2011.

31. Scully RE, Coffin DL: Canine testicular tumors with special reference to their histogenesis, comparative morphology, and endocrinology, *Cancer Epidemiol Biomarkers Prev* 5:592–605, 1952.

32. Lipowitz AJ, Schwartz A, Wilson GP, et al.: Testicular neoplasms and concomitant clinical changes in the dog, *J Am Vet Med Assoc* 163:1364–1368, 1973.

33. Hohsteter M, Artukovic B, Severin K, et al.: Canine testicular tumors: two types of seminomas can be differentiated by immunohistochemistry, *BMC Vet Res* 10(169), 2014.

34. Priester WA, McKay FW: The occurrence of tumors in domestic animals, *Natl Cancer Inst Monogr* 54:1–210, 1980.

35. Sapierzynski R, Malicka E, Bielecki W, et al.: Tumors of the urogenital system in dogs and cats. Retrospective review of 138 cases, *Pol J Vet Sci* 10:97–103, 2007.

36. Hayes HM, Tarone RE, Casey HW: A cohort study of the effects of Vitenam service on testicular pathology of US military working dogs, *Mil Med* 160:248–255, 1995.

37. Hayes HM, Tarone RE, Casey HW, et al.: Excess of seminomas observed in Vietnam service U.S. military working dogs, *J Natl Cancer Inst* 82:1042–1046, 1990.

38. McEntee MC: Reproductive oncology, *Clin Tech Sm Anim Pract* 17:133–149, 2002.

39. Benazzi C, Sarli G, Preziosi R, et al.: Laminin expression in testicular tumours of the dog, *J Comp Pathol* 112:141–150, 1995.

40. Sarli G, Benazzi C, Preziosi R, et al.: Proliferative activity assessed by anti-PCNA and Ki67 Mabs in canine testicular tumours, *J Comp Pathol* 110:357–368, 1994.

41. Papaioannou N, Psalla D, Zavlaris M, et al.: Immunohistochemical expression of dogTERT in canine testicular tumours in relation to PCNA, ki67 and p53 expression, *Vet Res Commun* 33:905–919, 2009.

42. Nasir L: Telomeres and telomerase: biological and clinical importance in dogs, *Vet J* 175:155–163, 2008.

43. DeVico G, Papparella S, DiGuardo G: Number and size of sliver-stained nucleoli (Ag-NOR clusters) in canine seminomas: correlation with histological features and tumour behaviour, *J Comp Pathol* 110:267–273, 1994.

44. Nasir L, Devlin P, McKevitt T, et al.: Telomere lengths and telomerase activity in dog tissues: a potential model system to study human telomere and telomerase biology, *Neoplasia* 3:351–359, 2001.

45. Murakami Y, Tateyama S, Uchida K, et al.: Immunohistochemical analysis of cyclins in canine normal testes and testicular tumors, *J Vet Med Sci* 63:909–912, 2001.

46. Brehm R, Ruttinger C, Fischer P, et al.: Transition from preinvasive carcinoma in situ to seminoma is accompanied by a reduction of connexin 43 expression in Sertoli cells and germ cells, *Neoplasia* 8:499–509, 2006.

47. Lin JH, Takano T, Cotrina ML, et al.: Connexin 43 enhances the adhesivity and mediates the invasion of malignant glioma cells, *J Neurosci* 22:4302–4311, 2002.

48. Risley MS, Tan IP, Roy C, et al.: Cell-, age-, and stage-dependent distribution of connexin43 gap junctions in testes, *J Cell Sci* 103:81–96, 1992.

49. Steger K, Tetens F, Bergmann M: Expression of connexin43 in human testis, *Histochem Cell Biol* 112:215–220, 1999.

50. Zhang W, Nwagwu C, Le DM, et al.: Increased invasive capacity of connexin43-overexpressing malignant glioma cells, *J Neurosci* 99:1039–1046, 2003.

51. Ruttinger C, Bergmann M, Fink L, et al.: Expression of connexin 43 in normal canine testes and canine testicular tumors, *Histochem Cell Biol* 130:537–548, 2008.

52. Lee CH, Kim WH, Lim JH, et al.: Mutation and overexpression of p53 as a prognostic factor in canine mammary tumors, *J Vet Sci* 5:63–69, 2004.

53. Lee CH, Kweon OK: Mutations of p53 tumor suppressor gene in spontaneous canine mammary tumors, *J Vet Sci* 3:321–325, 2002.

54. Queiroga FL, Raposo T, Carvalho MI, et al.: Canine mammary tumours as a model to study human breast cancer: most recent findings, *In Vivo* 25:455–465, 2011.

55. Inoue M, Wada N: Immunohistochemical detection of p53 and p21 proteins in canine testicular tumours, *Vet Rec* 146:370–372, 2000.

56. Vitellozzi G, Mariotti F, Ricci G: Immunohistochemical expression of the p53 protein in testicular tumours in the dog, *Eur J Vet Pathol* 4:61–65, 1998.

57. Restucci B, Maiolino P, Paciello O, et al.: Evaluation of angiogenesis in canine seminomas by quantitative immunohistochemistry, *J Comp Pathol* 128:252–259, 2003.

58. Yoshinaga K, Nishikawa S, Ogawa M, et al.: Role of c-kit in mouse spermatogenesis: identification of spermatogonia as a specific site of c-kit expression and function, *Development* 113:689–699, 1991.

59. Sattler M, Salgia R: Targeting c-kit mutation: basic science to novel therapies, *Leuk Res* 28S1:S11–S20, 2004.

60. Goddard NC, McIntyre A, Summersgill B, et al.: KIT and RAS signalling pathways in testicular germ cell tumours: new data and a review of the literature, *Int J Androl* 30:337–348, 2007.

61. Mauduit C, Hamamah S, Benahmed M: Stem cell factor/c-kit system in spermatogenesis, *Hum Reprod Update* 5:535–545, 1999.

62. Rothschild G, Sottas CM, Kissel H, et al.: A role for kit receptor signaling in Leydig cell steroidogenesis, *Biol Reprod* 69:925–932, 2003.

63. Grieco V, Banco B, Giudice C, et al.: Immunohistochemical expression of the KIT protein (CD117) in normal and neoplastic canine testes, *J Comp Pathol* 142:213–217, 2010.

64. Stoop H, Honecker F, vandeGeijn GJ, et al.: Stem cell factor as a novel diagnostic marker for early malignant germ cells, *J Pathol* 216:43–54, 2008.

65. Cummings OW, Ulbright TM, Eble JN, et al.: Spermatocytic seminoma: an immunohistochemical study, *Hum Pathol* 25:54–59, 1994.

66. Bush JM, Gardiner DW, Palmer JS, et al.: Testicular germ cell tumours in dogs are predominantly of spermatocytic seminoma type and are frequently associated with somatic cell tumours, *Int J Androl* 34:e288–e295, 2011.

67. Thorvaldsen TE, Nodtvedt A, Grotmol T, et al.: Morphological and immunohistochemical characterisation of seminomas in Norwegian dogs, *Acta Vet Scand* 54:52, 2012.

68. Hogenesch H, Whitely HE, Vicini DS, et al.: Seminoma with metastases in the eyes and the brain in a dog, *Vet Pathol* 24:278–280, 1987.

69. Brodey RS, Martin JE: Sertoli cell neoplasms in the dog: the clinicopathological and endocrinological findings in thirty-seven dogs, *J Am Vet Med Assoc* 133:249–257, 1958.

70. Dhaliwal RS, Kitchell BE, Knight BL, et al.: Treatment of aggressive testicular tumors in four dogs, *J Am An Hosp Assoc* 35:311–318, 1999.

71. Spugnini EP, Bartolazzi A, Ruslander D: Seminoma with cutaneous metastases in a dog, *J Am An Hosp Assoc* 36:253–256, 2000.

72. Takiguchi M, Iida T, Kudo T, et al.: Malignant seminoma with systemic metastases in a dog, *J Sm An Pract* 42:360–362, 2001.

73. Weller RE, Palmer B: Metastatic seminoma in a dog, *Mod Vet Pract* 64:275–278, 1983.

74. Gopinath D, Draffan D, Philbey AW, et al.: Use of intralesional oestradiol concentration to identify a functional pulmonary metastasis of canine sertoli cell tumor, *J Sm An Pract* 50:198–200, 2009.

75. Morgan RV: Blood dyscrasias associated with testicular tumors in the dog, *J Am An Hosp Assoc* 18:970–975, 1982.

76. Mischke R, Meurer D, Hoppen HO, et al.: Blood plasma concentrations of oestradiol-17B, testosterone and testosterone/oestradiol ratio in dogs with neoplastic and degenerative testicular diseases, *Res Vet Sci* 73:267–272, 2002.

77. Peters MAJ, Jong FS, Teerds KJ, et al.: Ageing, testicular tumours and the pituitary-testis axis in dogs, *J Endocrinol* 166: 153–161, 2000.

78. Taniyama H, Hirayama K, Nakada K, et al.: Immunohistochemical detection of inhibin-alpha, -betaB, and -betaA chains and 3beta-hydroxysteroid dehydrogenase in canine testicular tumors and normal testes, *Vet Pathol* 38:661–666, 2001.

79. Grootenhuis AJ, vanSluijs FJ, Klaij IA, et al.: Inhibin, gonadotrophins and sex steroids in dogs with Sertoli cell tumours, *J Endocrinol* 127:235–242, 1990.

80. Peters MA, Mol JA, vanWolferen Me, et al.: Expression of the insulin-like growth factor (IGF) system and steroidogenic enzymes in canine testis tumors, *Reprod Biol Endocrinol* 14: 22–29, 2003.

81. Holst BS, Dreimanis U: Anti-Mullerian hormone: a potentially useful biomarker for the diagnosis of canine Sertoli cell tumours, *BMC Vet Res* 11:166, 2015.

82. Roly ZY, Backhouse B, Cutting A, et al.: The cell biology and molecular genetics of Mullerian duct development, *Wiley Interdiscip Rev Dev Biol* 7:e310, 2018.

83. Sherding RG, Wilson GP, Kociba GJ: Bone marrow hypoplasia in eight dogs with Sertoli cell tumor, *J Am Vet Med Assoc* 178:497–501, 1981.

84. Scott DW, Reimers TJ: Tail gland and perianal gland hyperplasia associated with testicular neoplasia and hypertestosteronemia in a dog, *Canine Pract* 13:15–17, 1986.

85. Laing EJ, Harari J, Smith CW: Spermatic cord torsion and Sertoli cell tumor in a dog, *J Am Vet Med Assoc* 183:879–881, 1983.

86. Spackman CJ, Roth L: Prostatic cyst and concurrent Sertoli cell tumor in a dog, *J Am Vet Med Assoc* 192:1096–1098, 1988.

87. Barrand KR, Scudamore CL: Canine hypertrophic osteoarthropathy associated with a malignant Sertoli cell tumour, *J Sm Anim Pract* 42:143–145, 2001.

88. Brown TT, Burek JD, McEntee K: Male pseudohermaphroditism, cryptorchism, and Sertoli cell neoplasia in three miniature Schnauzers, *J Am Vet Med Assoc* 169:821–825, 1976.

89. Norrdin RW, Baum AC: A male pseudohermaphrodite dog with a Sertoli's cell tumor, mucometra, and vaginal glands, *J Am Vet Med Assoc* 156:204–207, 1970.

90. Frey DC, Tyler DE, Ramsey FK: Pyometra associated with bilateral cryptorchidism and Sertoli's cell tumor in a male pseudohermaphroditic dog, *J Am Vet Med Assoc* 146:723–727, 1965.

91. Park EJ, Lee SH, Jo YK, et al.: Coincidence of Persistent Mullerian duct syndrome and testicular tumors in dogs, *BMC Vet Res* 13:156, 2017.

92. Bigliardi E, Parma P, Peressotti P, et al.: Clinical, genetic, and pathological features of male pseudohermaphrodism in dog, *Reprod Biol Endocrinol* 9:12–18, 2011.

93. Johnston GR, Feeney DA, Johnston SD, et al.: Ultrasonographic features of testicular neoplasia in dogs: 16 cases (1980-1988), *J Am Vet Med Assoc* 198:1779–1784, 1991.

94. Pugh CR, Konde LJ: Sonographic evaluation of canine testicular and scrotal abnormalities: a review of 26 case histories, *Vet Radiol* 32:243–250, 1991.

95. Eilts BE, Pechman RD, Hedlund CS, et al.: Use of ultrasonography to diagnose Sertoli cell neoplasia and cryptorchidism in a dog, *J Am Vet Med Assoc* 192:533–534, 1988.

96. Masserdotti C, DeLorenzi D, Gasparotto L: Cytologic detection of Call-Exner bodies in Sertoli cell tumors from 2 dogs, *Vet Clin Pathol* 37:112–114, 2008.

97. Banco B, Giudice C, Veronesi MC, et al.: An immunohistochemical study of normal and neoplastic canine sertoli cells, *J Comp Pathol* 143:239–247, 2010.

98. Peters MA, Teerds KJ, vanderGaag I, et al.: Use of antibodies against LH receptor, 3beta-hydroxysteroid dehydrogenase and vimentin to characterize different types of testicular tumour in dogs, *Reproduction* 121:287–296, 2001.

99. Yu CH, Hwang DN, Kim JH, et al.: Comparative immunohistochemical characterization of canine seminomas and Sertoli cell tumors, *J Vet Sci* 10:1–7, 2009.

100. Doxsee AL, Yager JA, Best SJ, et al.: Extratesticular interstitial and Sertoli cell tumors in previously neutered dogs and cats: a report of 17 cases, *Can Vet J* 47:763–766, 2006.

101. Archbald LI, Waldow D, Gelatt K: Interstitial cell tumor, *J Am Vet Med Assoc* 210:1423–1424, 1997.

102. England GC: Ultrasonographic diagnosis of non-palpable Sertoli cell tumours in infertile dogs, *J Sm An Pract* 36:476–480, 1995.

103. Metzger FL, Hattel AL: Hematuria, hyperestrogenemia, and hyperprogesteronemia due to a sertoli-cell tumor in a bilaterally cryptorchid dog, *Canine Pract* 18:32–35, 1993.

104. Madewell BR, Theilen GH: Tumors of the genital tract. In Theilen GH, Madewell BR, editors: *Veterinary cancer medicine*, ed 2, Philadelphia, 1987, Lea & Febiger, pp 583–600.

105. McDonald RK, Walker M, Legendre A, et al.: Radiotherapy of metastatic seminoma in the dog. Case reports, *J Vet Intern Med* 2:103–107, 1988.

106. Albers P, Albrecht W, Algaba F, et al.: EAU guidelines on testicular cancer: 2011 update, *Eur Uol* 60:304–319, 2011.

107. Rosen DK, Carpenter JL: Functional ectopic interstitial cell tumor in a castrated male cat, *J Am Vet Med Assoc* 202:1865–1866, 1993.

108. Cotchin E: Neoplasia. In Wilkinson GT, editor: *Diseases of the cat and their management*, Oxford, 1984, Blackwell, pp 366–387.

109. Miller MA, Hartnett SE, Ramos-Vara JA: Interstitial cell tumor and Sertoli cell tumor in the testis of a cat, *Vet Pathol* 44:394–397, 2007.

110. Miyoshi N, Yasuda N, Kamimura Y, et al.: Teratoma in a feline unilateral cryptorchid testis, *Vet Pathol* 38:729–730, 2001.

111. Ferreira-da-Silva J: Teratoma in a feline unilateral cryptorchid testis (letter to the editor), *Vet Pathol* 39:516, 2002.

112. Benazzi C, Sarli G, Brunetti B: Sertoli cell tumour in a cat, *J Vet Med A Physiol Pathol Clin Med* 51:124–126, 2004.

113. Meier H: Sertoli-cell tumor in the cat. Report of two cases, *North Am Vet* 37:979–981, 1956.

114. Rosen A, Jayram G, Drazer M, et al.: Global trends in testicular cancer incidence and mortality, *Eur Urol* 60: 374–379, 2011.

115. Ruf CG, Isbarn H, Wagner W, et al.: Changes in epidemiologic features of testicular germ cell cancer: age at diagnosis and relative frequency of seminoma are constantly and significantly increasing, *Urol Oncol* 32(33):e31–e36, 2014.

116. Motzer RJ, Jonasch E, Agarwal N, et al.: Testicular cancer, version 2.2015, *J Natl Compr Canc Netw* 13:772–799, 2015.

117. Jacobsen R, Moller H, Thoresen S, et al.: Trends in testicular cancer incidence in the Nordic countries, focusing on the recent decrease in Denmark, *Int J Androl* 29:199–204, 2006.

118. Myrup C, Wohlfahrt J, Oudin A, et al.: Risk of testicular cancer according to brithplace and birth cohort in Denmark, *Int J Cancer* 126:217–223, 2010.

119. Henderson BE, Benton B, Jing J, et al.: Risk factors for cancer of the testis in young men, *Int J Cancer* 23:598–602, 1979.

120. Weir HK, Marrett LD, Kreiger N, Darlington GA: Pre-natal and peri-natal exposures and risk of testicular germ-cell cancer, *Int J Cancer* 87:438–443, 2000.

121. Garner MJ, Birkett NJ, Johnson KC, et al.: Dietary risk factors for testicular carcinoma, *Int J Cancer* 106:934–941, 2003.

122. Hu J, LaVecchia C, Morrison H, et al.: Salt, processed meta and the risk of cancer, *Eur J Cancer Prev* 20:132–139, 2011.

123. Kratz CP, Mai PL, Greene MH: Familial testicular germ cell tumours, *Best Pract Res Clin Endocrinol Metab* 24: 503–513, 2010.

124. VandenEeden SK, Weiss NS, Strader CH, et al.: Occupation and the occurrence of testicular cancer, *Am J Ind Med* 19: 327–337, 1991.

125. Garner MJ, Turner MC, Ghadirian P, et al.: Epidemiology of testicular cancer: an overview, *Int J Cancer* 116:331–339, 2005.

126. Pinczowski D, McLaughlin JK, Lackgren G, et al.: Occurrence of testicular cancer in patients operated on for cryptorchidism and inguinal hernia, *J Urol* 146:1291–1294, 1991.

127. Looijenga LH, Van Agthoven T, Biermann K: Development of malignant germ cells - the genvironmental hypothesis, *Int J Dev Biol* 57:241–253, 2013.

128. Tandstad T, Smaaland R, Solberg A, et al.: Management of seminomatous testicular cancer: a binational prospective population-based study from the Swedish Norwegian testicular cancer study group, *J Clin Oncol* 29:719–725, 2011.

129. Aparicio J, delMuro G, Maroto P, et al.: Multicenter study evaluating a dual policy of postorchiectomy surveillance and selective adjuvant single-agent carboplatin for patients with clinical stage I seminoma, *Ann Oncol* 14:867–872, 2003.

130. Oliver RT, mead GM, Rustin GJ, et al.: Randomized trial of carboplatin versus radiotherapy for stage I seminoma: mature results on relapse and contralateral testis cancer rates in MRC TE19/EORTC 30982 study (ISRCTN27163214), *J Clin Oncol* 29:957–962, 2011.

131. Motzer RJ, Nichols CJ, Margolin KA, et al.: Phase III randomized trial of conventional-dose chemotherapy with or without high-dose chemotherapy and autologous hematopoietic stem-cell rescue as first-line treatment for patients with poor-prognosis metastatic germ cell tumors, *J Clin Oncol* 25:247–256, 2007.

132. Obradovich J, Walshaw R, Goullaud E: The influence of castration on the development of prostatic carcinoma in the dog: 43 cases, *J Vet Intern Med* 1:183–187, 1987.

133. Bell FW, Klausner JS, Hayden DW, et al.: Evaluation of serum and seminal plasma markers in the diagnosis of canine prostatic disorders, *J Vet Intern Med* 9:149–153, 1995.

134. Cornell KK, Bostwick DG, Cooley DM, et al.: Clinical and pathological aspects of spontaneous canine prostate carcinoma: a retrospective analysis of 76 cases, *Prostate* 45:173–183, 2000.

135. Waters DJ, Sakr WA, Hayden DW, et al.: Workgroup 5: spontaneous prostate cancer in dogs and non-human primates, *Prostate* 36:64–67, 1998.

136. Weaver AD: Fifteen cases of prostatic carcinoma in the dog, *Vet Rec* 109:71–75, 1981.

137. Waters DJ, Shen S, Glickman LT, et al.: Prostate cancer risk and DNA damage: translational significance of selenium supplementation in a canine model, *Carcinogenesis* 26:1256–1262, 2005.

138. Maini A, Archer C, Wang CY, et al.: Comparative pathology of benign prostatic hyperplasia and prostate cancer, *Vivo* 11:293–300, 1997.

139. Usui T, Sakurai M, Nishikawa S, et al.: Establishment of a dog primary prostate cancer organoid using the urine cancer stem cells, *Cancer Sci* 108:2383–2392, 2017.

140. Keller JM, Schade GR, Ives K, et al.: A novel canine model for prostate cancer, *Prostate* 73:952–959, 2013.

141. Elshafae SM, Kohart NA, Altstadt LA, et al.: The effect of a histone deacetylase inhibitor (AR-42) on canine prostate cancer growth and metastasis, *Prostate* 77:776–793, 2017.

142. Kato Y, Ochiai K, Kawakami S, et al.: Canine REIC/Dkk-3 interacts with SGTA and restores androgen receptor signalling in androgen-independent prostate cancer cell lines, *BMC Vet Res* 13:170, 2017.

143. Rivera-Calderon LG, Fonseca-Alves CE, Kobayashi PE, et al.: Alterations in PTEN, MDM2, TP53 and AR protein and gene expression are associated with canine prostate carcinogenesis, *Res Vet Sci* 106:56–61, 2016.

144. Hornbuckle WE, MacCoy DM, Allan GS, et al.: Prostatic disease in the dog, *Cornell Vet* 68:284–305, 1978.

145. Krawiec DR, Heflin D: Study of prostatic disease in dogs: 177 cases (1981-1986), *J Am Vet Med Assoc* 200:1119–1122, 1992.

146. Teske E, Naan EC, vanDijk EM, et al.: Canine prostate carcinoma: epidemiological evidence of an increased risk in castrated dogs, *Mol Cell Endocrinol* 197:251–255, 2002.

147. Bell FW, Klausner JS, Hayden DW, et al.: Clinical and pathologic features of prostatic adenocarcinoma in sexually intact and castrated dogs: 31 cases (1970-1987), *J Am Vet Med Assoc* 199:623–630, 1991.

148. Bennett TC, Matz BM, Henderson RA, et al.: Total prostatectomy as a treatment for prostatic carcinoma in 25 dogs, *Vet Surg* 47:367–377, 2018.

149. Waters DJ, Bostwick DG: Prostatic intraepithelial neoplasia occurs spontaneously in the canine prostate, *J Urol* 157, 1997.

150. Madewell BR, Gandour-Edwards R, DeVere-White RW: Canine prostatic intraepithelial neoplasia: is the comparative model relevant? *Prostate* 58:314–317, 2004.

151. Aquilina JW, McKinney L, Pacelli A, et al.: High grade prostatic intraepithelial neoplasia in military working dogs with and without prostate cancer, *Prostate* 36:189–193, 1998.

152. Palmieri C, Lean FZ, Akter SH, et al.: A retrospective analysis of 111 canine prostatic samples: histopathological findings and classification, *Res Vet Sci* 97:568–573, 2014.

153. Bryan JN, Keeler MR, Henry CJ, et al.: A population study of neutering status as a risk factor for canine prostate cancer, *Prostate* 67:1174–1181, 2007.

154. LeRoy BE, Nadella MV, Toribio RE, et al.: Canine prostate carcinomas express markers of urothelial and prostatic differentiation, *Vet Pathol* 41:131–140, 2004.

155. Smith J: Canine prostatic disease: a review of anatomy, pathology, diagnosis, and treatment, *Theriogenology* 70:375–383, 2008.

156. Mochizuki H, Shapiro SG, Breen M: Detection of BRAF mutation in urine DNA as a molecular diagnostic for canine urothelial and prostatic carcinoma, *PloS One* 10:e0144170, 2015.

157. Sorenmo KU, Goldschmidt M, Shofer F, et al.: Immunohistochemical characterization of canine prostatic carcinoma and correlation with castration status and castration time, *Vet Comp Oncol* 1:48–56, 2003.

158. Grieco V, Riccardi E, Rondena M, et al.: The distribution of oestrogen receptors in normal, hyperplastic and neoplastic canine prostate, as demonstrated immunohistochemically, *J Comp Pathol* 135:11–16, 2006.

159. Leav I, Schelling KH, Adams JY, et al.: Role of canine basal cells in postnatal prostatic development, induction of hyperplasia, and sex hormone-stimulated growth; and the ductal origin of carcinoma, *Prostate* 48:210–224, 2001.

160. Lai CL, vandenHam R, Mol J, et al.: Immunostaining of the androgen receptor and sequence analysis of its DNA-binding domain in canine prostate cancer, *Vet J* 181:256–260, 2009.

161. Humphrey PA: Gleason grading and prognostic factors in carcinoma of the prostate, *Mod Pathol* 17:292–306, 2004.

162. Young RH, Srigley JR, Amin MB, et al.: *Tumors of the prostate gland, seminal vesicles, male urethra, and penis. Atlas of tumor pathology: third series, Fascicle 28*, Washington D.C, 2000, Armed Forces Institute of Pathology.

163. Di Donato G, Laufer-Amorim R, Palmieri C: Nuclear morphometry in histological specimens of canine prostate cancer: correlation with histological subtypes, Gleason score, methods of collection and survival time, *Res Vet Sci* 114:212–217, 2017.

164. Palmieri C, Grieco V: Proposal of Gleason-like grading system of canine prostate carcinoma in veterinary pathology practice, *Res Vet Sci* 103:11–15, 2015.

165. Lin HY, Palmieri C: Is STAT3 and PTEN expression altered in canine prostate cancer? *J Comp Pathol* 155:185–189, 2016.

166. Weisse C, Berent A, Todd K, et al.: Evaluation of palliative stenting for management of malignant urethral obstructions in dogs, *J Am Vet Med Assoc* 229:226–234, 2006.

167. Mainwaring CJ: Primary lymphoma of the prostate in a dog, *J Sm Anim Pract* 31:617–619, 1990.

168. Winter MD, Locke JE, Penninck DG: Imaging diagnosis - urinary obstruction secondary to prostatic lymphoma in a young dog, *Vet Radiol Ultrasound* 47:597–601, 2006.

169. Hayden DW, Klausner JS, Waters DJ: Prostatic leiomyosarcoma in a dog, *J Vet Diagn Invest* 11:283–286, 1999.
170. Bacci B, Vignoli M, Rossi F, et al.: Primary prostatic leiomyosarcoma with pulmonary metastases in a dog, *J Am An Hosp Assoc* 46:103–106, 2010.
171. Hayden DW, Bartges JW, Bell FW, et al.: Prostatic hemangiosarcoma in a dog: clinical and pathologic findings, *J Vet Diagn Invest* 4:2009–2011, 1992.
172. Gilson SD, Miller RT, Hardie EM, et al.: Unusual prostatic mass in a dog, *J Am Vet Med Assoc* 200:702–704, 1992.
173. LeRoy BE, Northrup N: Prostate cancer in dogs: comparative and clinical aspects, *Vet J* 180:149–162, 2009.
174. Dore M, Chevalier S, Sirois J: Estrogen-dependent induction of cyclooxygenase-2 in the canine prostate in vivo, *Vet Pathol* 42:100–103, 2005.
175. Shidaifat F, Daradka M, Al-Omari R: Effect of androgen ablation on prostatic cell differentiation in dogs, *Endocr Res* 30:327–334, 2004.
176. Grieco V, Patton V, Romussi S, et al.: Cytokeratin and vimentin expression in normal and neoplastic canine prostate, *J Comp Pathol* 129:78–84, 2003.
177. Cooley DM, Waters DJ: Skeletal metastasis as the initial clinical manifestation of metastatic carcinoma in 19 dogs, *J Vet Intern Med* 12:288–293, 1998.
178. Durham SK, Dietze AE: Prostatic adenocarcinoma with and without metastasis to bone in dogs, *J Am Vet Med Assoc* 188:1432–1436, 1986.
179. Waters DJ, Cooley DM, Allen DK, et al.: Host age influences the biological behavior of cancer: studies in pet dogs with naturally occurring malignancies, *Gerontologist* 38(110), 1998.
180. Ross RK, Pike MC, Coetzee GA, et al.: Androgen metabolism and prostate cancer: establishing a model of genetic susceptibility, *Cancer Res* 58:4497–4504, 1998.
181. Matsuzaki P, Cogliati B, Sanches DS, et al.: Immunohistochemical characterization of canine prostatic intraepithelial neoplasia, *J Comp Pathol* 142:84–88, 2010.
182. Fonseca-Alves CE, Kobayashi PE, Palmieri C, et al.: Investigation of c-KIT and Ki67 expression in normal, preneoplastic and neoplastic canine prostate, *BMC Vet Res* 13:380, 2017.
183. Kobayashi PE, Fonseca-Alves CE, Rivera-Calderon LG, et al.: Deregulation of E-cadherin, beta-catenin, APC and caveolin-1 expression occurs in canine prostate cancer and metastatic processes, *Res Vet Sci* 118:254–261, 2018.
184. Servian P, Celma A, Planas J, et al.: Clinical significance of proliferative inflammatory atrophy finding in prostatic biopsies, *Prostate* 75:1669–1675, 2015.
185. Servian P, Celma A, Planas J, et al.: Clinical significance of proliferative inflammatory atrophy in negative prostatic biopsies, *Prostate* 76:1501–1506, 2016.
186. Fonseca-Alves CE, Kobayashi PE, Rivera-Calderon LG, et al.: Evidence of epithelial-mesenchymal transition in canine prostate cancer metastasis, *Res Vet Sci* 100:176–181, 2015.
187. Fonseca-Alves CE, Kobayashi PE, Laufer-Amorim R: Evaluation of NKX3.1 and C-MYC expression in canine prostatic cancer, *Res Vet Sci* 118:365–370, 2018.
188. Palmieri C, Mancini M, Benazzi C, et al.: Heat shock protein 90 is associated with hyperplasia and neoplastic transformation of canine prostatic epithelial cells, *J Comp Pathol* 150:393–398, 2014.
189. Gallardo F, Lloreta J, Garcia F, et al.: Immunolocalization of androgen receptors, estrogen alpha receptors, and estrogen beta receptors in experimentally induced canine prostatic hyperplasia, *J Androl* 30:240–247, 2009.
190. Gallardo F, Mogas T, Baro T, et al.: Expression of androgen, oestrogen alpha and beta, and progesterone receptors in the canine prostate: differences between normal, inflamed, hyperplastic and neoplastic glands, *J Comp Pathol* 136:1–8, 2007.
191. Mochizuki H, Kennedy K, Shapiro SG, et al.: BRAF mutations in canine cancers, *PloS One* 10:e0129534, 2015.

192. Mochizuki H, Breen M: Sequence analysis of RAS and RAF mutation hot spots in canine carcinoma, *Vet Comp Oncol* 15:1598–1605, 2017.
193. Kollermann J, Albrecht H, Schlomm T, et al.: Activating BRAF gene mutations are uncommon in hormone refractory prostate cancer in Caucasian patients, *Oncol Lett* 1:729–732, 2010.
194. Mochizuki H, Breen M: Comparative aspects of BRAF mutations in canine cancers, *Vet Sci* 2:231–245, 2015.
195. Taylor BS, Schultz N, Hieronymus H, et al.: Integrative genomic profiling of human prostate cancer, *Cancer Cell* 18:11–22, 2010.
196. Salmaninejad A, Ghadami S, Dizaji MZ, et al.: Molecular characterization of KRAS, BRAF, and EGFR genes in cases with prostatic adenocarcinoma; reporting bioinformatics description and recurrent mutations, *Clin Lab* 61:749–759, 2015.
197. Tremblay C, Dore M, Bochsler PN, et al.: Induction of prostaglandin G/H synthase-2 in a canine model of spontaneous prostatic adenocarcinoma, *J Natl Cancer Inst* 91:1398–1403, 1999.
198. Mohammed SI, Coffman K, Glickman NW, et al.: Prostaglandin E2 concentrations in naturally occurring canine cancer, *Prostaglandins Leukot Essent Fatty Acids* 64:1–4, 2001.
199. Mohammed SI, Khan KN, Sellers RS, et al.: Expression of cyclooxygenase-1 and 2 in naturally-occurring canine cancer, *Prostaglandins Leukot Essent Fatty Acids* 70:479–483, 2004.
200. Sorenmo KU, Goldschmidt MH, Shofer FS, et al.: Evaluation of cyclooxygenase-1 and cyclooxygenase-2 expression and the effect of cyclooxygenase inhibitors in canine prostatic carcinoma, *Vet Comp Oncol* 2:13–23, 2004.
201. Keller ET, Zhang J, Cooper CR, et al.: Prostate carcinoma skeletal metastases: cross-talk between tumor and bone, *Cancer Metastasis Rev* 20:333–349, 2001.
202. Sellers RS, LeRoy BE, Blomme EA, et al.: Effects of transforming growth factor-beta1 on parathyroid hormone-related protein mRNA expression and protein secretion in canine prostate epithelial, stromal, and carcinoma cells, *Prostate* 58:366–373, 2004.
203. LeRoy BE, Sellers RS, Rosol TJ: Canine prostate stimulates osteoblast function using the endothelin receptors, *Prostate* 59:148–156, 2004.
204. Simmons JK, Hildreth 3rd BE, Supsavhad W, et al.: Animal models of bone metastasis, *Vet Pathol* 52:827–841, 2015.
205. Hibberd C, Cossigny DA, Quan GM: Animal cancer models of skeletal metastasis, *Cancer Growth Metastasis* 6:23–34, 2013.
206. Ylitalo EB, Thysell E, Jernberg E, et al.: Subgroups of castration-resistant prostate cancer bone metastases defined through an inverse relationship between androgen receptor activity and immune response, *Eur Urol* 71:776–787, 2017.
207. Nordstrand A, Bovinder Ylitalo E, Thysell E, et al.: Bone cell activity in clinical prostate cancer bone metastasis and its inverse relation to tumor cell androgen receptor activity, *Int J Mol Sci* 19, 2018.
208. Leav I, Ling GV: Adenocarcinoma of the canine prostate, *Cancer* 22:1329–1345, 1968.
209. Lee-Parritz DE, Lamb CR: Prostatic adenocarcinoma with osseous metastases in a dog, *J Am Vet Med Assoc* 192:1569–1572, 1988.
210. Barsanti JA, Finco DR: Canine prostatic disease, *Vet Clin North Am* 16:587–599, 1986.
211. Johnston SD, Kamolpatana K, Root-Kustritz MV, et al.: Prostatic disorders in the dog, *Anim Reprod Sci* 61:405–415, 2000.
212. Liptak JM, Brutscher SP, Monnet E, et al.: Transurethral resection in the management of urethral and prostatic neoplasia in 6 dogs, *Vet Surg* 33:505–516, 2004.
213. Powe JR, Canfield PJ, Martin PA: Evaluation of the cytologic diagnosis of canine prostatic disorders, *Vet Clin Pathol* 33:150–154, 2004.
214. Feeney DA, Johnston GR, Klausner JS, et al.: Canine prostatic disease—comparison of radiographic appearance with morphologic and microbiologic findings: 30 cases (1981-1985), *J Am Vet Med Assoc* 190:1018–1026, 1987.

215. Bradbury CA, Westropp JL, Pollard RE: Relationship between prostatomegaly, prostatic mineralization, and cytologic diagnosis, *Vet Radiol Ultrasound* 50:167–171, 2009.

216. Head LL, Francis DA: Mineralized paraprostatic cyst as a potential contributing factor in the development of perineal hernias in a dog, *J Am Vet Med Assoc* 221:533–535, 2002.

217. Zekas LJ, Forrest LJ, Swainson S, et al.: Radiographic diagnosis: mineralized paraprostatic cyst in a dog, *Vet Radiol Ultrasound* 45:310–311, 2004.

218. Ackerman N: Prostatic reflux during positive contrast retrograde urethrography in the dog, *Vet Radiol* 24, 1983.

219. Scher HI, Scardino PT, Zelefsky MJ: Cancer of the Prostate. In DeVita VT, Lawrence TS, Rosenberg SA, editors: *Cancer: principles & practice of oncology*, ed 10, Philadelphia, 2015, Wolters Kluwer, pp 932–980.

220. Epstein JI, Egevad L, Amin MB, et al.: The 2014 International Society of Urological Pathology (ISUP) consensus conference on gleason grading of prostatic carcinoma: definition of grading patterns and proposal for a new grading system, *Am J Surg Pathol* 40:244–252, 2016.

221. Barsanti JA, Shotts EB, Prasse K, et al.: Evaluation of diagnostic techniques for canine prostatic diseases, *J Am Vet Med Assoc* 177:160–163, 1980.

222. Barsanti JA, Finco DR: Evaluation of techniques for diagnosis of canine prostatic diseases, *J Am Vet Med Assoc* 185:198–200, 1984.

223. Leeds EB, Leav I: Perineal punch biopsy of the canine prostate gland, *J Am Vet Med Assoc* 154:925–934, 1969.

224. Nyland TG, Wallack ST, Wisner ER: Needle-tract implantation following us-guided fine-needle aspiration biopsy of transitional cell carcinoma of the bladder, urethra, and prostate, *Vet Radiol Ultrasound* 43:50–53, 2002.

225. MacLachan NJ, Kennedy PC: Tumors of the genital systems. In Meuten DJ, editor: *Tumors in domestic animals*, Ames, IA, 2002, Iowa State University Press, pp 568–570.

226. Thrall MA, Olsen PN, Freemyer FG: Cytologic diagnosis of canine prostatic disease, *J Am An Hosp Assoc* 21:95–102, 1985.

227. Corazza M, Guidi G, Romagnoli S, et al.: Serum total prostatic and non-prostatic acid phosphatases in healthy dogs and in dogs with prostatic diseases, *J Sm Anim Pract* 35:307–310, 1994.

228. Hardie EM, Barsanti JA, Rawlings CA: Complications of prostatic surgery, *J Am An Hosp Assoc* 20:50–56, 1984.

229. Hardie EM, Stone EA, Spaulding KA, et al.: Subtotal canine prostatectomy with the neodymium:yttrium-aluminum-garnet laser, *Vet Surg* 19:348–355, 1990.

230. Vlasin M, Rauser P, Fichtel T, et al.: Subtotal intracapsular prostatectomy as a useful treatment for advanced-stage prostatic malignancies, *J Sm Anim Pract* 47:512–516, 2006.

231. Basinger RR, Rawlings CA, Barsanti JA, et al.: Urodynamic alterations associated with clinical prostatic diseases and prostate surgery in 23 dogs, *J Am An Hosp Assoc* 25:385–392, 1989.

232. Goldsmid SE, Bellenger CR: Urinary incontinence after prostatectomy in dogs, *Vet Surg* 20:253–256, 1991.

233. L'Epplattenier HF, Klem B, Teske E, et al.: Partial prostatectomy using Nd:YAG laser for management of canine prostate carcinoma, *Vet Surg* 35:406–411, 2006.

234. Williams JM, White RAS: Tube cystostomy in the dog and cat, *J Sm Anim Pract* 32:598–602, 2007.

235. Smith JD, Stone EA, Gilson SD: Placement of a permanent cystostomy catheter to relieve urine outflow obstruction in dogs with transitional cell carcinoma, *J Am Vet Med Assoc* 206:496–499, 1995.

236. Mann FA, Barrett RJ, Henderson RA: Use of a retained urethral catheter in three dogs with prosatatic neoplasia, *Vet Surg* 21:342–347, 1992.

237. Radhakrishnan A: Urethral stenting for obstructive uropathy utilizing digital radiography for guidance: feasibility and clinical outcome in 26 Dogs, *J Vet Intern Med* 31:427–433, 2017.

238. Blackburn AL, Berent AC, Weisse CW, et al.: Evaluation of outcome following urethral stent placement for the treatment of obstructive carcinoma of the urethra in dogs: 42 cases (2004-2008), *J Am Vet Med Assoc* 242:59–68, 2013.

239. McMillan SK, Knapp DW, Ramos-Vara JA, et al.: Outcome of urethral stent placement for management of urethral obstruction secondary to transitional cell carcinoma in dogs: 19 cases (2007-2010), *J Am Vet Med Assoc* 241:1627–1632, 2012.

240. Lucroy MD, Bowles MH, Higbee RG, et al.: Photodynamic therapy for prostatic carcinoma in a dog, *J Vet Intern Med* 19:235–237, 2003.

241. Chevalier S, Anidjar M, Scarlata E, et al.: Preclinical study of the novel vascular occluding agent, WST11, for photodynamic therapy of the canine prostate, *J Urol* 186:302–309, 2011.

242. Xiao Z, Owen RJ, Liu W, et al.: Lipophilic photosensitizer administration via the prostate arteries for photodynamic therapy of the canine prostate, *Photodiagnosis Photodyn Ther* 7:106–114, 2010.

243. Du KL, Mick R, Busch TM, et al.: Preliminary results of interstitial motexafin lutetium-mediated PDT for prostate cancer, *Lasers Surg Med* 38:427–434, 2006.

244. Huang Z, Chen Q, Luck D, et al.: Studies of a vascular-acting photosensitizer, Pd-bacteriopheophorbide (Tookad), in normal canine prostate and spontaneous canine prostate cancer, *Lasers Surg Med* 36:390–397, 2005.

245. Swartling J, Hoglund OV, Hansson K, et al.: Online dosimetry for temoporfin-mediated interstitial photodynamic therapy using the canine prostate as model, *J Biomed Opt* 21:28002, 2016.

246. Hsi RA, Kapatkin A, Strandberg J, et al.: Photodynamic therapy in the canine prostate using motexafin lutetium, *Clin Cancer Res* 7:651–660, 2001.

247. Turrel JM: Intraoperative radiotherapy of carcinoma of the prostate gland in ten dogs, *J Am Vet Med Assoc* 190:48–52, 1987.

248. Nolan MW, Kogan L, Griffin LR, et al.: Intensity-modulated and image-guided radiation therapy for treatment of genitourinary carcinomas in dogs, *J Vet Intern Med* 26:987–995, 2012.

249. Fan TM, deLorimier LP, Charney SC, et al.: Evaluation of intravenous pamidronate administration in 33 cancer-bearing dogs with primary or secondary bone involvement, *J Vet Intern Med* 19:74–80, 2005.

250. Lattimer Jr JC: LAC, Stapleton J, et al. Clinical and clinicopathologic response of canine bone tumor patients to treatment with samarium-153-EDTMP, *J Nucl Med* 31:1316–1325, 1990.

251. Fan TM, de Lorimier LP, Garrett LD, et al.: The bone biologic effects of zoledronate in healthy dogs and dogs with malignant osteolysis, *J Vet Intern Med* 22:380–387, 2008.

252. Fan TM, Charney SC, deLorimier LP, et al.: Double-blind placebo-controlled trial of adjuvant pamidronate with palliative radiotherapy and intravenous doxorubicin for canine appendicular osteosarcoma bone pain, *J Vet Intern Med* 23:152–160, 2009.

253. Klausner JS, Johnston SD, Bell FW: Canine prostatic diseases. In Kirk RW, editor: *Current veterinary therapy XII*, Philadelphia, 1995, WB Saunders, pp 1103–1108.

254. Hawe JS: What is your diagnosis? Prostatic adenocarcinoma in a cat, *J Am Vet Med Assoc* 182:1257–1258, 1983.

255. Hubbard BS, Vulgamott JC, Liska WD: Prostatic adenocarcinoma in a cat, *J Am Vet Med Assoc* 197:1493–1494, 1990.

256. Caney SM, Hold PE, Day MJ, et al.: Prostatic carcinoma in two cats, *J Sm Anim Pract* 39:140–143, 1998.

257. LeRoy BE, Lech ME: Prostatic carcinoma causing urethral obstruction and obstipation in a cat, *J Fel Med Surg* 6:397–400, 2004.

258. Tursi M, Costa T, Valenza F, et al.: Adenocarcinoma of the disseminated prostate in a cat, *J Fel Med Surg* 10:600–602, 2008.

259. Zambelli D, Cunto M, Raccagni R, et al.: Successful surgical treatment of a prostatic biphasic tumour (sarcomatoid carcinoma) in a cat, *J Fel Med Surg* 12:161–165, 2010.

260. Printz C: Evolving detection and treatment methods change approaches to prostate cancer: US preventive services task force draft recommendations now align more closely with others, *Cancer* 124:11–12, 2018.

261. Mottet N, Bellmunt J, Bolla M, et al.: EAU-ESTRO-SIOG guidelines on prostate cancer. part 1: screening, diagnosis, and local treatment with curative intent, *Eur Urol* 71:618–629, 2017.

262. Jeldres C, Cullen J, Hurwitz LM, et al.: Prospective quality-of-life outcomes for low-risk prostate cancer: active surveillance versus radical prostatectomy, *Cancer* 121:2465–2473, 2015.

263. Punnen S, Cowan JE, Chan JM, et al.: Long-term health-related quality of life after primary treatment for localized prostate cancer: results from the CaPSURE registry, *Eur Urol* 68:600–608, 2015.

264. Banerji JS, Hurwitz LM, Cullen J, et al.: A prospective study of health-related quality-of-life outcomes for patients with low-risk prostate cancer managed by active surveillance or radiation therapy, *Urol Oncol* 35:234–242, 2017.

265. Chistiakov DA, Myasoedova VA, Grechko AV, et al.: New biomarkers for diagnosis and prognosis of localized prostate cancer, *Semin Cancer Biol*, 2018, epub ahead of print. https://doi.org/10.1013/j.semcancer.2018.2018.01.012.

266. Friedl A, Stangl K, Bauer W, et al.: Prostate-specific antigen parameters and prostate health index enhance prostate cancer prediction with the in-bore 3-T magnetic resonance imaging-guided transrectal targeted prostate biopsy after negative 12-core biopsy, *Urology* 110:148–153, 2017.

267. Druskin SC, Tosoian JJ, Young A, et al.: Combining prostate health index density, magnetic resonance imaging and prior negative biopsy status to improve the detection of clinically significant prostate cancer, *BJU Int* 121:619–626, 2018.

268. Campi R, Brookman-May SD, Subiela Henriquez JD, et al.: Impact of metabolic diseases, drugs, and dietary factors on prostate cancer risk, recurrence, and survival: a systematic review by the european association of urology section of oncological urology, *Eur Urol Focus*, 2018, epub ahead of print. https://doi.org/10.1016/j.euf.2018.04.001.

269. Anidjar M, Villette JM, Devauchelle P, et al.: In vivo model mimicking natural history of dog prostate cancer using DPC-1, a new canine prostate carcinoma cell line, *Prostate* 46:2–10, 2001.

270. Kishan AU, Shaikh T, Wang PC, et al.: Clinical outcomes for patients with Gleason score 9-10 prostate adenocarcinoma treated with radiotherapy or radical prostatectomy: a multi-institutional comparative analysis, *Eur Urol* 71:766–773, 2017.

271. Kishan AU, Cook RR, Ciezki JP, et al.: Radical prostatectomy, external beam radiotherapy, or external beam radiotherapy with brachytherapy boost and disease progression and mortality in patients with Gleason score 9-10 prostate cancer, *J Am Med Assoc* 319:896–905, 2018.

272. Ploussard G: Robotic surgery in urology: facts and reality. What are the real advantages of robotic approaches for prostate cancer patients? *Curr Opin Urol* 28:153–158, 2018.

273. Ilic D, Evans SM, Allan CA, et al.: Laparoscopic and robotic-assisted versus open radical prostatectomy for the treatment of localised prostate cancer, *Cochrane Database Syst Rev* 9:CD009625, 2017.

274. Huang X, Wang L, Zheng X, et al.: Comparison of perioperative, functional, and oncologic outcomes between standard laparoscopic and robotic-assisted radical prostatectomy: a systemic review and meta-analysis, *Surg Endosc* 31:1045–1060, 2017.

275. Phak JH, Kim HJ, Kim WC: Prostate-specific antigen kinetics following hypofractionated stereotactic body radiotherapy boost as post-external beam radiotherapy versus conventionally fractionated external beam radiotherapy for localized prostate cancer, *Prostate Int* 4:25–29, 2016.

276. Anwar M, Weinberg V, Chang AJ, et al.: Hypofractionated SBRT versus conventionally fractionated EBRT for prostate cancer: comparison of PSA slope and nadir, *Radiat Oncol* 9:42, 2014.

277. Gordon JA, Buonerba C, Pond G, et al.: Statin use and survival in patients with metastatic castration-resistant prostate cancer treated with abiraterone or enzalutamide after docetaxel failure: the international retrospective observational STABEN study, *Oncotarget* 9:19861–19873, 2018.

278. James ND, de Bono JS, Spears MR, et al.: Abiraterone for prostate cancer not previously treated with hormone therapy, *N Eng J Med* 377:338–351, 2017.

279. Cornford P, Bellmunt J, Bolla M, et al.: EAU-ESTRO-SIOG Guidelines on prostate cancer. Part II: treatment of relapsing, metastatic, and castration-resistant prostate cancer, *Eur Urol* 71:630–642, 2017.

280. Michels GM, Knapp DW, David M, et al.: Penile prolapse and urethral obstruction secondary to lymphosarcoma of the penis in a dog, *J Am An Hosp Assoc* 37:474–477, 2001.

281. Cornegliani L, Vercelli A, Abramo F: Idiopathic mucosal penile squamous papillomas in dogs, *Vet Dermatol* 18:439–443, 2007.

282. Ndiritu CG: Lesions of the canine penis and prepuce, *Mod Vet Pract* 60:712–715, 1979.

283. Patnaik AK, Matthiesen DT, Zawie DA: Two cases of canine penile neoplasm: squamous cell carcinoma and mesenchymal chondrosarcoma, *J Am An Hosp Assoc* 24:403–406, 1988.

284. Hall WC, Nielsen SW, McEntee K: Tumours of the prostate and penis, *Bull World Health Organ* 53:247–256, 1976.

285. Bloom F: *Pathology of the dog and cat: the genitourinary system with clinical considerations*, Evanston, 1954, American Veterinary Publications.

286. Vascellari M, Carminato A, Camali G, et al.: Malignant mesothelioma of the tunica vaginalis testis in a dog: histological and immunohistochemical characterization, *J Vet Diagn Invest* 23:135–139, 2011.

287. Cihak RW, Roen DR, Klaassen J: Malignant mesothelioma of the tunica vaginalis in a dog, *J Comp Pathol* 96:459–462, 1986.

288. Peppler C, Weissert D, Kappe E, et al.: Osteosarcoma of the penile bone (os penis) in a dog, *Aust Vet J* 87:52–55, 2009.

289. Webb JA, Liptak JM, Hewitt SA, et al.: Multilobular osteochondrosarcoma of the os penis in a dog, *Can Vet J* 50:81–84, 2009.

290. Bleier T, Lewitschek HP, Reinacher M: Canine osteosarcoma of the penile bone, *J Vet Med A Physiol Pathol Clin Med* 50:397–398, 2003.

291. Mirkovic TK, Shmon CL, Allen AL: Urinary obstruction secondary to an ossifying fibroma of the os penis in a dog, *J Am An Hosp Assoc* 40:152–156, 2004.

292. Root-Kustritz MV, Fick JL, Theriogenologists ACo: Theriogenology question of the month. Neoplasia of the os penis in a dog, *J Am Vet Med Assoc* 230:197–198, 2007.

293. Patnaik AK: Canine extraskeletal osteosarcoma and chondrosarcoma: a clinicopathologic study of 14 cases, *Vet Pathol* 27:46–55, 1990.

294. Rogers KS, Walker MA, Dillon HB: Transmissible venereal tumor: a retrospective study of 29 cases, *J Am An Hosp Assoc* 34:463–470, 1998.

295. Thrall DE: Orthovoltage radiotherapy of canine transmissible venereal tumors, *Vet Radiol* 23:217–219, 1982.

296. Milks HJ: Some diseases of the genito-urinary system, *Cornell Vet* 29:105–114, 1939.

297. Trabulsi EJ, Gomella LG: Cancer of the urethra and penis. In DeVita VT, Lawrence TS, Rosenberg SA, editors: *Cancer: principles & practice of oncology*, ed 10, Philadelphia, 2015, Wolters Kluwer.

298. Yeole BB, Jussawalla DJ: Descriptive epidemiology of the cancers of male genital organs in greater Bombay, *Indian J Cancer* 34:30–39, 1997.

299. Maden C, Sherman KJ, Beckman AM, et al.: History of circumcision, medical conditions, and sexual activity and risk of penile cancer, *J Natl Cancer Inst* 85:19–24, 1993.

300. Hanash KA, Furlow WL, Utz DC, et al.: Carcinoma of the penis: a clinicopathologic study, *J Urol* 104:291–297, 1970.

301. Shabbir M, Minhas S, Muneer A: Diagnosis and management of premalignant penile lesions, *Ther Adv Urol* 3:151–158, 2011.

302. Harish K, Ravi R: The role of tobacco in penile carcinoma, *Br J Urol* 75:375–377, 1995.

303. Backes DM, Kurman RJ, Pimenta JM, et al.: Systematic review of human papillomavirus prevalence in invasive penile cancer, *Cancer Causes Control* 20:449–557, 2009.

304. Nicolai N, Biasoni D, Catanzaro MA, et al.: Testicular germ-cell tumours and penile squamous cell carcinoma: appropriate management makes the difference, *Eur J Surg Oncol*, 2018.

305. Hakenberg OW, Comperat EM, Minhas S, et al.: EAU guidelines on penile cancer: 2014 update, *Eur Urol* 67: 142–150, 2015.

306. Trabulsi EJ, Gomella LG: Cancer of the urethra and penis. In Devita VT, Lawrence TS, Rosenberg SA, editors: *Cancer principles and practice of oncology*, Philadelphia, 2008, Lippincott Williams and Wilkins, pp 1452–1462.

307. Shapiro D, Shasha D, Tareen M, et al.: Contemporary management of localized penile cancer, *Expert Rev Anticancer Ther* 11: 29–36, 2011.

308. Stancik I, Holtl W: Penile cancer: review of the recent literature, *Curr Opin Urol* 13:467–472, 2003.

309. Lawindy SM, Rodriguez AR, Horenblas S, et al.: Current and future strategies in the diagnosis and management of penile cancer, *Adv Urol* 1–9, 2011 May 30.

310. Kumar P, Singh S, Goddard JC, et al.: The development of a supra-regional network for the management of penile cancer, *Ann R Coll Surg Engl* 94:204–209, 2012.

311. Davis NF, Fitzgerald M, Burke JP, et al.: Is there a role for the development of a supra-regional network for the management of penile cancer in the Republic of Ireland? *Surgeon* 14:82–86, 2016.

312. Breen KJ, O'Connor KM, Power DG, et al.: Penile cancer— Guideline adherence produces optimum results, *Surgeon* 13: 200–206, 2015.

30

Tumors of the Urinary System

CHRISTOPHER M. FULKERSON AND DEBORAH W. KNAPP

Canine Urinary Bladder Tumors

Urinary bladder cancer accounts for approximately 2% of all reported malignancies in the dog.[1-3] With more than 65 million dogs in the United States, and the estimated 6 million new canine cancer cases in the United States each year, even less frequent forms of cancer, such as bladder cancer, affect tens of thousands of dogs each year.[2,3] Invasive urothelial carcinoma (iUC), also referred to as invasive transitional cell carcinoma, is the most common form of canine urinary bladder cancer.[1-3] Most iUCs are intermediate- to high-grade papillary infiltrative tumors.[1-3] A series of 232 iUCs included 70% grade 3 (high grade) tumors, 29% grade 2 (intermediate grade) tumors, and 1% grade 1 (low grade) tumors.[3] Other types of bladder tumors reported less frequently include squamous cell carcinoma, adenocarcinoma, undifferentiated carcinoma, rhabdomyosarcoma, lymphoma, hemangiosarcoma, fibroma, and other mesenchymal tumors.[1-8]

iUC is most often located in the trigone region of the bladder. Papillary lesions and a thickened bladder wall (Fig. 30.1) are common features, and can lead to partial or complete urinary tract obstruction. In a series of 102 dogs with iUC of the bladder, the cancer also involved the urethra in 56% of dogs and the prostate in 29% of male dogs.[1] Nodal and distant metastases were present in 16% and 14% of dogs, respectively, at diagnosis.[1] Following World Health Organization (WHO) criteria for staging canine bladder tumors (Box 30.1),[9] 78% of dogs had T_2 tumors and 20% had T_3 tumors.[1] In a necropsy study of 137 dogs with iUC, 58% of dogs had distant metastases and 42% had nodal metastases (including 33% of dogs with both nodal and distant metastases).[3] The lung was the most common site of distant metastases (50% of dogs), with other sites including liver, kidney, adrenal gland, spleen, bone, skin, heart, brain, and gastrointestinal (GI) tract.[3] At necropsy, second primary tumors were noted in 13% of dogs, including hemangiosarcoma, lymphoma, thyroid carcinoma, and others.[3] Bone metastases were reported in 17 (9%) of 188 canine iUC cases reviewed retrospectively, and in 3 (14%) of 21 dogs prospectively undergoing total body computed tomography (CT) at euthanasia followed by a standardized pathologic examination.[10] In a series of 12 dogs with cutaneous iUC metastases, gross lesions consisted of plaques, papules, and nodules.[11] iUC can occur in the abdominal wall, either through seeding from instruments and needles used in surgical and nonsurgical procedures, or through natural spread of transmural lesions along bladder ligaments.[12] iUC in the abdominal wall is typically aggressive and poorly responsive to medical therapy.[12]

Etiology and Prevention

The etiology of canine bladder cancer is multifactorial. Risk factors include exposure to older generation flea control products and lawn chemicals, obesity, possibly cyclophosphamide exposure, female gender, and a very strong breed-associated risk (Table 30.1).[1-3,13-15] The female-to-male ratio of dogs with TCC has been reported to range from 1.71:1 to 1.95:1, although the sex predilection is less pronounced in high-risk breeds.[3] TCC risk is higher in neutered dogs than intact dogs of both genders, although the reason for this has not been determined.[1-3,13]

In a case control study of 166 Scottish terriers (STs), TCC risk was significantly higher in STs that had been exposed to lawn herbicides and insecticides than in dogs not exposed, and the risk was significantly lower in dogs that ate vegetables at least three times per week in addition to their dog food.[14,16] The specific vegetable with the most benefit could not be determined, but carrots, given as treats, were the most frequently fed vegetable. In contrast to older types of flea dips, exposure to spot-on products containing fipronil was not associated with an increased TCC risk.[15] It would appear appropriate to inform owners of dogs in high-risk breeds

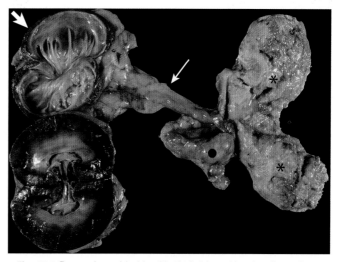

• **Fig. 30.1** Dog, urinary bladder. Urothelial (transitional cell) carcinoma. Transmural neoplastic growth involving the entire bladder (*asterisk*). One of the iliac lymph nodes (*black circle*) is also infiltrated by this neoplasm. One of the ureters is dilated (hydroureter, *thin arrow*) and the corresponding kidney (opened, *thick arrow*) has hydronephrosis as a result of blockage of the ureter at the trigone. (Courtesy J. A. Ramos-Vara, Purdue University.)

of the risk, to limit exposure to lawn chemicals and older types of flea control products, and to feed vegetables at least three times per week, especially in dogs in breeds at high risk for iUC.

Urinary tract ultrasonography and urinalysis with sediment examination at 6-month intervals, plus cystoscopy and biopsy of suspicious lesions, has allowed detection of iUC in STs before the onset of clinical signs, and treatment response has been better than in more advanced iUC (D. Knapp, personal communication). Other screening tests for iUC are emerging. A $BRAF^{V595E}$ mutation has been detected in more than 80% of canine iUC cases with urine detection closely correlating to tumor tissue genotype.[17,18] In one study, the $BRAF^{V595E}$ mutation was detected in 19 of 23 dogs presenting with iUC and in 0 of 37 dogs that were either normal or had cystitis.[18] Copy number aberrations in urine DNA from dogs with iUC have also been reported.[19] Screening strategies including these tests could help identify dogs for further evaluation for potential iUC.

• BOX 30.1 TNM Clinical Staging System for Canine Bladder Cancer

T—Primary Tumor

T_{is}	Carcinoma in situ
T_0	No evidence of a primary tumor
T_1	Superficial papillary tumor
T_2	Tumor invading the bladder wall, with induration
T_3	Tumor invading neighboring organs (prostate, uterus, vagina, and pelvic canal)

N—Regional Lymph Node (Internal and External Iliac Lymph Node)

N_0	No regional lymph node involvement
N_1	Regional lymph node involved
N_2	Regional lymph node and juxtaregional lymph node involved

M—Distant Metastases

M_0	No evidence of metastasis
M_1	Distant metastasis present

Modified from Owen LN: TNM classification of tumors in domestic animals, Geneva, 1980, World Health Organization.[9]

Presentation, Diagnosis and Differential Diagnoses, and Clinical Staging

Common clinical signs in dogs with iUC include hematuria, dysuria, pollakiuria, and less commonly lameness caused by bone metastasis or hypertrophic osteopathy.[1] Urinary tract signs mimic those of dogs with urinary tract infections (UTIs) and may resolve temporarily with antibiotic therapy if a concurrent UTI is present. Concern for iUC or other urinary tract abnormalities, such as calculi, arise when clinical signs do not resolve with antibiotics or recur soon after a course of antibiotics is completed. In dogs with iUC, a physical examination, which includes a rectal examination, may reveal thickening of the urethra and trigone region of the bladder, enlargement of lymph nodes, prostatomegaly in male dogs, and sometimes a mass in the bladder or a distended bladder. However, a normal physical examination does not rule out iUC.

Many conditions mimic iUC in regard to clinical signs, presence of abnormal epithelial cells in urine, and mass lesions within the urinary tract (Fig. 30.2 and 30.3). Differential diagnoses include other neoplasia, chronic bacterial cystitis, polypoid cystitis, fibroepithelial polyp, granulomatous cystitis/urethritis, gossypiboma, calculi, and inflammatory pseudotumor.[4–8,20–22] It is important to differentiate non-iUC conditions from iUC because the treatments and prognosis differ considerably and are dependent on the condition present.

A definitive diagnosis of iUC is made through histopathologic examination of tissues. Immunohistochemistry for uroplakin III and potentially GATA-3 can be used to determine urothelial origin of the cancer in difficult cases.[3] Methods for obtaining tissue for histopathologic diagnosis include cystotomy, cystoscopy (Fig. 30.2), and traumatic catheterization.[1,23] Cystoscopy provides the opportunity to visually inspect the urethra and bladder and to obtain biopsies via a noninvasive method. With the small size of cystoscopic biopsies, the operator must be diligent to collect sufficient tissue for diagnosis. Placing tissue samples in a histology cassette before processing helps prevent loss of small samples (Fig. 30.2F). The use of a wire basket designed to capture stones during cystoscopy (Fig. 30.2D, E) allows collection of larger samples. Traumatic catheterization to collect tissues for diagnosis can also be performed, although samples are usually small and the diagnostic quality is variable. Percutaneous biopsy methods can lead to tumor seeding and should be avoided.[24]

TABLE 30.1 Breed and Risk of Invasive Urothelial Carcinoma (iUC) in Pet Dogs[3]

Breed	Number of Dogs in That Breed in Database	TCC Cases in That Breed in Database	OR compared with mixed breed	95% confidence intervals
Mixed breed dog (Reference Category)	42,777	269	1.0	NA
Scottish terrier	670	79	21.12	16.23–27.49
Eskimo dog	225	9	6.58	3.34–12.96
Shetland sheepdog	2521	93	6.05	4.76–7.69
West Highland white terrier	1234	44	5.84	4.23–8.08
Keeshond	381	10	4.26	2.25–8.07
Samoyed	471	10	3.43	1.81–6.49
Beagle	3236	62	3.09	2.34–4.08
Dalmatian	1253	19	2.43	1.52–3.89

The odds ratios (ORs) of TCC risk compared with the risk in mixed breed dogs are included for breeds with an OR > 2.0 and at least 9 cases of iUC in the breed.

In dogs with confirmed or suspected iUC, evaluation should include an assessment of overall health (complete blood count, serum biochemistry profile, urinalysis, ± urine culture) and staging of the cancer (three-view thoracic radiograps, abdominal ultrasonography or computed tomography [CT], and urinary tract imaging). To avoid the risk of seeding iUC through cystocentesis, urine may be collected by free catch or catheterization. Catheterization must be performed carefully to avoid penetrating the diseased bladder or urethral wall. Urinary tract imaging is used to assess the tumor location for potential surgical intervention

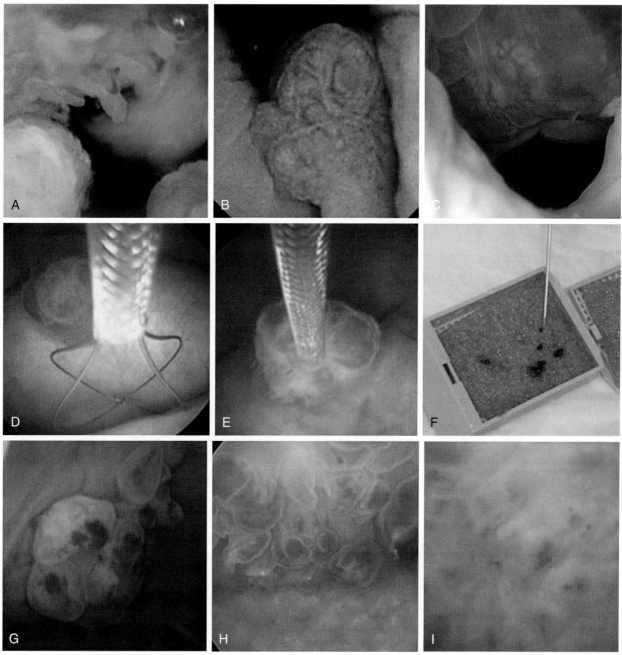

• **Fig. 30.2** Images from cystoscopy of dogs with invasive urothelial carcinoma (iUC, A–E) and biopsy material obtained (F), and images of dogs with polypoid cystitis (G–I). TCC can appear as a ruffled frond-like mass, a solid smooth mass, or as polyp-like lesions. High-quality images can be obtained with rigid cystoscopes typically used in female dogs (A, C–E) and in digital flexible scopes used in male dogs (B, image from a male Scottish terrier). The use of a cystoscopic wire stone basket (D, E) allows collection of larger biopsies. Regardless of the biopsy instrument used, however, cystoscopic biopsies are relatively small, and placing the samples in a tissue cassette (F) may facilitate processing. Polypoid cystitis (G–I) appears very similar to TCC, but it is treated differently and has a better prognosis than TCC. Images (H) and (I) are from a dog with polypoid cystitis before (H) and after (I) a month of clavamox treatment alone with no other therapy. The polpys had regressed by more than 80% (I) at the time of rescoping. Cases such as this one emphasize the importance of histopathology in the diagnosis of urinary tract masses, especially when selecting therapy, and even more so when dogs are participating in clinical trials. (Courtesy L. G. Adams and D. W. Knapp, Purdue University.)

and to map and measure iUC masses to subsequently determine response to therapy. Cystosonography, cystography, or CT may be employed.[25–28] To accurately track response to therapy, regardless of the imaging approach, it is essential to follow a consistent protocol from visit to visit for imaging modality, bladder distention, patient positioning, and images acquired. When using cystosonography to monitor response, it is critical to have the same operator perform examinations over multiple visits.

Treatment

Localized Therapy

Surgery

Surgery may be indicated to (1) obtain tissue for a definitive diagnosis, (2) eradicate lesions amenable to wide excision (e.g., tumors distant from the trigone), and (3) relieve urinary tract obstruction. Local recurrence after partial cystectomy and the presence of multifocal lesions within the bladder in many dogs with iUC support the notion of the field effect or malignant transformation of the entire urothelium in response to carcinogen exposure.[29] Surgical removal of iUC is typically followed by systemic therapy, usually with a cyclooxygenase (COX) inhibitor, to reduce

risk of recurrence.[1,29] When considering surgery, patient selection and owner counseling regarding risks (procedural risk, risk of recurrence) are essential. The risk of tumor seeding at the time of surgery is well documented and careful surgical technique is critical.[12,29,30]

Full-thickness removal of part of the bladder may be considered in dogs with discrete iUC lesions away from the trigone. In a retrospective study of 37 dogs with iUC treated with partial cystectomy (all gross tumor removal in 92% of dogs) plus COX inhibitors, with or without chemotherapy, the median progression-free interval (PFI) was 235 days, and the median survival time (MST) was 348 days.[29] In a subset of 22 dogs treated with surgery and daily piroxicam (with or without other systemic therapy), the MST was 722 days.[29] This result is similar to results in a series of nine dogs that had surgical resection of iUC (three dogs with tumor-free margins and six dogs with residual microscopic disease) followed by single-agent deracoxib, in which the MST was 749 days.[1] More complex surgical approaches in dogs with iUC have also been reported including total cystectomy plus various urinary diversion strategies, but serious complications limit the success of these approaches.[31–34] Prepubic cystostomy catheters or low-profile cystostomy tubes can be placed to bypass urethral

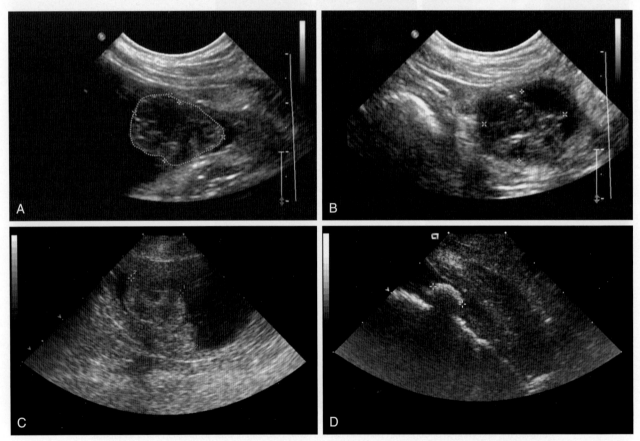

• **Fig. 30.3** Cystosonography images from dogs with bladder masses. Images made in the sagittal (A) and transverse (B) planes (5 mL/kg fluid distention of the bladder) of an 11-year-old neutered male Shih Tzu with invasive urothelial carcinoma. To measure bladder masses over multiple time points, it is important to follow a consistent protocol in regard to level of bladder distention, and patient and probe positioning; and to have the same operator perform the ultrasonography on each visit. Polypoid cystitis (C, D), which can appear very similar to iUC, can occur in any part of the bladder including the mid/apex (C) and trigone (D). The dog imaged in (D) was a 13-year-old spayed female Bichon Frise with history of previous urinary tract infection, current hematuria, stranguria, atypical epithelial cells in urine, and masses in the mid and trigone areas of the bladder. Surgical biopsies of the masses confirmed they were polyps. (Courtesy J. F. Naughton, Purdue University.)

obstruction in a palliative setting or to maintain urine flow while other therapies are instituted.[35–37] Complications can include urine leakage and tumor seeding, infection, tube displacement, and tube damage if the dog is allowed to chew on the tube.

Urethral and Ureteral Stent Placement and Laser Ablation

In recent years, the use of interventional radiology approaches has gained favor over tube cystostomy and other surgical procedures for palliative management of obstruction secondary to iUC.[30,38–41] Most urethral stents and some ureteral stents can be placed with minimally invasive approaches, and stents do not require pet owners to manipulate a urine collection system. Survival after urethral and ureteral stent placement is variable and largely dependent on the extent of tumor lesions. In three reports, MSTs have ranged from 20 to 78 days (range, 2–536 days) after urethral stent placement for iUC or prostatic adenocarcinoma.[39–41] After urethral stent placement, lower urinary tract signs, including stranguria, can persist. Incontinence has been reported in 25% to 39% of dogs.[39–41] Urethral stents are typically placed using fluoroscopic guidance, but the use of digital radiography to guide stent placement has also been reported.[42] Ureteral stents can be placed surgically, and in some cases, nonsurgically in dogs with iUC. The MST after ureteral stent placement was 57 days (range, 7–337 days) in one study.[43] Nephrectomy can be considered for severe unilateral hydronephrosis if persistent renal pain or infection is present.

Transurethral carbon dioxide (CO_2) and near-infrared diode laser ablation of iUC (performed in combination with cytotoxic chemotherapy and COX inhibitors) has been reported, with its main application being in dogs with discrete tumor masses causing urinary tract obstruction.[44,45] Complications include perforation with iUC spread, transient postprocedural worsening of stranguria and hematuria, urethral stenosis, and infection.[44,45] In a small series, the outcome of dogs treated with laser ablation and medical therapy was not better than medical therapy alone.[44]

Radiation Therapy

Although iUC cells are generally thought to be sensitive to radiation therapy (RT), an in vitro study of three canine iUC cell lines revealed a low α/β ratio, suggesting moderate radioresistance and supporting treatment protocols using higher doses and less fractionation.[46] The early use of large doses and less fractionation, however, was associated with chronic colitis, cystitis, and urethral strictures, and little improvement in MST compared with medical therapy alone.[47,48]

With new advanced image-guided targeting technology and increasing availability of RT, there is renewed interest in RT to treat iUC.[49–53] A retrospective report of intensity-modulated and image-guided radiation therapy revealed lower complication rates compared with earlier studies in the dog.[49] In a series of 21 dogs, acute side effects were mild and self-limiting and included colitis (38%), erythema or hyperpigmentation (19%), and stranguria (5%).[49] Late complications included urethral stricture (9%), ureteral stricture (5%), or rectal stricture (5%). The median event-free survival was 317 days and the overall MST was 654 days.[49] In a report of 13 dogs with urogenital carcinomas treated with a low dose palliative RT (10 daily fractions of 2.7 Gy with CT planning) plus antineoplastic drugs, acute side effects were mild including colitis, cystitis, vaginitis, and dermatitis, and no late complications were noted.[50] Complete remission (CR) or partial remission (PR) was reported in 61% of dogs and stable disease (SD) in 38% of dogs.[50]

Medical Therapy

Systemic Medical Therapy

Systemic medical therapy is the mainstay of iUC treatment in dogs, and usually consists of chemotherapy, COX inhibitors (nonselective and COX-2 selective inhibitors), and combinations thereof (Table 30.2).[1–3,27,54–62] Although medical therapy is not usually curative, several different drugs lead to remission or SD of iUC, and most therapies are well tolerated. Resistance to one drug does not imply resistance to other drugs. Some of the best results are seen in dogs

TABLE 30.2	Study Results Reported for the Medical Therapy of Invasive Urothelial Carcinoma (iUC) in Dogs								
Drug(s)	Number of Dogs: Total/Evaluable for Tumor Response	N_1 or N_2/M_1/Any Metastasis, (% of Total Dogs)	CR (%)	PR (%)	SD (%)	PD (%)	PFI (d)	Median Survival From Start of That Drug(s)	Refs.
Randomized Trials									
Vinblastine (2.5 mg/m²)[a]	27/26	4/7/11	0	22	70	4	143	531[b]	59
Vinblastine (2.5 mg/m²)/piroxicam[a]	24/24	0/4/4	0	58	33	8	199	299	59
Cisplatin (60 mg/m²)[a]	8/8	12/12/12	0	0	50	50	84	300[c]	1–3
Cisplatin (60 mg/m²)/piroxicam[a,d]	14/14	28/14/43	14	57	28	0	124	246	1–3
Cisplatin (60 mg/m²)[a]	15/14	20/20/33	0	13	53	27	87	338[e]	62
Firocoxib (5 mg/kg)[a]	15/12	33/27/53	0	20	33	27	105	152	62
Cisplatin (60 mg/m²/firocoxib (5 mg/kg)[a]	14/11	21/14/29	0	57	21	0	186	179	62
Mitoxantrone/piroxicam[f]	26/NA	8/NA/8	0	8	69	23	106	247	56
Carobplatin/piroxicam[f]	24/NA	29/NA/29	0	13	54	33	73	263	56

Continued

TABLE 30.2   Study Results Reported for the Medical Therapy of Invasive Urothelial Carcinoma (iUC) in Dogs—cont'd

Drug(s)	Number of Dogs: Total/Evaluable for Tumor Response	N₁ or N₂/M₁/Any Metastasis, (% of Total Dogs)	CR (%)	PR (%)	SD (%)	PD (%)	PFI (d)	Median Survival From Start of That Drug(s)	Refs.
Single-Arm Trials									
Piroxicam[a]	94/76	9/11/16	3	18	59	20	120	244	3
Deracoxib[a]	26/24	4/11/15	0	17	71	12	133	323	54
Vinblastine[a,g,h]	28/28	11/21/28	0	36	50	14	122	147	58
Vinblastine–folate conjugate[a]	10/9	10/40/40	0	56	44	0	58	115	66
Vinblastine/toceranib/COX inhibitor[f]	10/9	20/0/20	0	33–55[i]	NA	NA	NA	NA	27
Mitoxantrone/piroxicam[f]	55/48	NA/NA/11	2	33	46	19	194	291	1
Carboplatin[a]	14/12	21/14/28	0	0	8	92	41	132	1
Carboplatin/piroxicam[a]	31/29	13/13/19	0	38	45	17	NA	161	1
Doxorubicin/piroxicam[f]	34/23	NA/NA/NA	0	9	60	30	103	168	55
Gemcitabine/piroxicam[f]	38/37	11/3/11	5	22	51	22	NA	230	57
Cisplatin (60 mg/m²)[a]	18/16	NA/28/33	0	19	25	56	75	130	1–3
Cisplatin (40–50 mg/m²)[a]	14/14	7/7/7	0	7	36	57	78	307	1–3
Cisplatin (60 mg/m²)/piroxicam[a]	14/12	14/14/28	0	50	17	33	NA	329	1–3
Cisplatin (60 mg/m²/piroxicam/tavocept[f]	14/11	NA/NA/NA	0	27	73	0	NA	253	60
Chlorambucil (4 mg/m² daily)[a]	30/30	10/30/33	0	3	67	30	119	221	61
5-Azacitidine[a]	19/18	5/15/15	0	22	50	22	NA	203	67
Mitomycin C—intravesical[a]	13/12	0/0/0	0	42	58	0	120	223	69

[a]Diagnosis based on histopathology.

[b]When dogs receiving vinblastine alone failed, there was then the option for the dogs to receive piroxicam alone or other drugs. Twenty dogs received piroxicam alone after failing vinblastine alone. The responses to piroxicam were 3 (15%) PR, 9 (45%) SD, 5 (25%) PD, and 3 (15%) NA. Twelve of these dogs received additional therapy after failing piroxicam. In the combined therapy arm, 15 dogs received additional therapy after failing vinblastine/piroxicam.

[c]Dogs that initially received cisplatin alone and had tumor progression were then treated with piroxicam alone; two dogs had PR and five dogs had SD with piroxicam treatment. This could have contributed to the favorable survival in that treatment arm.

[d]Despite favorable tumor response, the combination of cisplatin and piroxicam is not recommended for routine use because of frequent renal toxicity.

[e]After failing cisplatin alone, options were given for the dogs to receive firocoxib alone or other drugs. Thirteen dogs received firocoxib alone after failing cisplatin alone, and tumor responses included 2 PR, 4 SD, and 7 PD. This (and other drugs) could have contributed to the longer survival time.

[f]Study included dogs with cytologic evidence of TCC and dogs with biopsy-proven TCC.

[h]The majority of dogs had failed prior therapy before receiving vinblastine. The dosage of vinblastine used in this trial was 3 mg/m² every 2 weeks. In most dogs in the trial, however, subsequent dose reduction was necessary because of myelosuppression. The currently recommended starting dosage of vinblastine for dogs with iUC is 2.5 mg/m² every 2 weeks for medium to large dogs and 2.0 mg/m² every 2 weeks for small dogs with subsequent dose escalation in the absence of toxicity.

[i]Seventeen of the dogs had failed a COX inhibitor before enrolling in the trial and continued to receive the COX inhibitor during the vinblastine treatment.

[j]In the study, the tumor masses were measured by ultrasound and by computed tomography. At 8 weeks, two different ultrasound operators reported tumor responses of 33% and 55% respectively.

More advanced TNM stage is associated with a poorer prognosis; the percentages of dogs with metastasis for each study are included.

CR, Complete remission; *NA,* information not available; *PD,* progressive disease; *PFI,* progression-free interval; *PR,* partial remission; *SD,* stable disease.

that sequentially receive multiple different treatment protocols over the course of their disease. Baseline measurements of the iUC masses are obtained, an initial treatment protocol is instituted, and the iUC masses remeasured at 4- to 8-week intervals. The initial treatment is continued as long as the iUC is controlled (PR, SD), side effects are acceptable, and quality of life is good. Clinical signs do not consistently follow changes in tumor size with therapy; thus remeasuring the tumor is essential. If cancer progression or unacceptable toxicity occurs, then a different treatment is instituted.

Subsequent treatment changes are based on change in tumor size and treatment tolerability. With this approach, iUC growth can be controlled in approximately 75% to 80% of dogs, quality of life is usually very good, and MSTs have extended well beyond a year.[1–3] Simultaneously combining multiple chemotherapy agents in dogs with iUC is not currently recommended because the benefit has not been determined, toxicity is likely to increase, and the potential development of resistance to multiple drugs at the same time could limit the options for subsequent therapy.

The optimal length of chemotherapy for iUC has not been defined. Although the authors continue a chemotherapy protocol as long as the cancer is controlled, quality of life is good, and no serious adverse events are noted, other oncologists cap the number of chemotherapy doses because of concerns of chronic toxicity. The effects of discontinuing chemotherapy in dogs with PR or SD, or administering COX inhibitors or metronomic chemotherapy as "maintenance therapy," have not been determined. It is certainly expected that residual iUC will progress if drugs controlling it are withdrawn. Anecdotally, the authors have administered vinblastine or mitoxantrone for well beyond a year without ill effects (D. Knapp, personal communication), but further study is needed.

Systemic chemotherapy agents investigated in dogs with iUC are summarized in Table 30.2.[1-3,48,55-62] Although cisplatin appears to be one of the more active agents, it is seldom used because of renal, GI, and bone marrow toxicities.[1-3,60,62] In a recent report, the administration of cisplatin and piroxicam concurrently with a chemoprotectant agent (Tavocept) was associated with less renal toxicity than a historic control group receiving similar doses of cisplatin and piroxicam, but the response rate was inferior in the dogs that received Tavocept.[60]

In recent years, vinblastine has emerged as a preferred chemotherapy agent in dogs with iUC because of very good antitumor activity and a good safety profile.[58,59] After promising results in a single arm trial in dogs with advanced resistant iUC, a follow-up trial was performed in which dogs with histologically diagnosed iUC were randomly assigned to receive vinblastine (2.5 mg/m^2 intravenously every 2 weeks) plus piroxicam (0.3 mg/kg daily PO) or vinblastine alone (same dose).[59] Remission was more frequent with vinblastine–piroxicam (58%) than with vinblastine alone (22%). The median PFI was 143 days with vinblastine alone and 199 days with the combination. Interestingly, the MST was significantly longer in dogs receiving vinblastine alone followed by piroxicam alone (531 days) than in dogs receiving the two drugs given concurrently (299 days). The longer survival was possibly due to the dogs not developing resistance to both drugs simultaneously. The treatment was well tolerated in both arms. Therefore vinblastine combined with piroxicam (or another COX inhibitor) has become the preferred chemotherapy protocol at the authors' institution.

Another commonly used chemotherapy protocol, mitoxantrone combined with piroxicam, induced remission in 35% of dogs with iUC with a MST was 291 days.[1] Carboplatin combined with piroxicam induced remission in 38% of dogs, but is usually reserved for later use because of more frequent side effects.[1] Other chemotherapy studies are summarized in Table 30.2.

Low-dose frequent (metronomic) chemotherapy has also been used in dogs with iUC.[61] A clinical trial of metronomic oral chlorambucil (4 mg/m^2 daily) was performed in 31 dogs with iUC, 29 of which had failed prior therapy.[61] Tumor responses included PR in one dog (3%) and SD in 20 dogs (67%). The median PFI and MST from the start of chlorambucil was 119 days and 221 days, respectively. The quality of life was excellent. Although toxicity was minimal in this study, with increased use of chlorambucil, especially for several months in dogs, chronic myelosuppression persisting for weeks to months has emerged as a concern. The chlorambucil dose used in the iUC trial (4 mg/m^2 daily) was selected because it was more effective than lower or less frequent doses in early work.[63] In a recent study, three different doses of chlorambucil (4 mg/m^2, 6 mg/m^2, or 8 mg/m^2) were given to 78 dogs with a variety of cancer types.[64] Doses greater than 4 mg/m^2 were associated with more GI and bone marrow toxicity, but no improvement in antitumor effects. Of 34 dogs receiving 4 mg/m^2,

bone marrow suppression was noted in 10% of dogs at 90 days and in 80% of dogs at 1 year. Most toxicity was grade 1 or 2, but this justifies the need for careful monitoring.

A more conservative treatment for iUC is a single-agent COX inhibitor, including the nonselective COX inhibitor piroxicam or COX-2 selective inhibitors such as deracoxib and firocoxib.[1,3,54,62] All three of these agents have induced remission (with most being PRs) in 15 to 20% of dogs with iUC, and have resulted in SD in up to 55% of dogs. Information on 94 dogs with iUC treated with piroxicam (0.3 mg/kg daily) has been published.[3] Tumor responses were known in 76 dogs and included 3% CR, 18% PR, 59% SD, and 20% PD. The median PFI was 120 days, and MST was 244 days.[3] The MST compared favorably to that of 55 dogs in the Purdue Comparative Oncology Program Tumor Registry that were treated with cytoreductive surgery alone (median survival 109 days).[3] GI adverse events (due to piroxicam or comorbid conditions) were noted in 31% of dogs.[3] Although most were grade 1 or 2, piroxicam can cause GI ulceration. It is critical for pet owners to observe their dog, stop piroxicam, and contact their veterinarian if anorexia, vomiting, or melena occurs. If the clinical signs are thought to be piroxicam related, it is safest to give a drug holiday and then switch to a COX-2 inhibitor. Interestingly, in an expanded series of dogs with multiple types of cancer receiving piroxicam, the use of GI-protectant drugs was associated with greater GI toxicity, but the reasons for this require further study.[65] Although piroxicam can cause toxicity, the majority of dogs have notably improved quality of life on the drug.[3]

COX-2 selective inhibitors are also used in dogs with iUC. In a randomized trial, firocoxib (Previcox, Merial) had antitumor activity as a single agent (20% PR and 33% SD) and greatly enhanced the activity of cisplatin.[62] Firocoxib did not worsen the renal toxicity of cisplatin (as piroxicam does), but other toxicities inherent to cisplatin still limit its use. In a clinical trial of single-agent deracoxib (Deramaxx, Novartis, 3 mg/kg PO daily) in 26 dogs with iUC, tumor responses included 17% PR, 71% SD, and 12% PD.[54] The MST after deracoxib and subsequent therapies was 323 days. Mild GI toxicity occurred in 20% of dogs.

Targeted therapies are also receiving considerable interest in treating TCC and other cancers in dogs. Folate-targeted vinblastine (EC0905, Endocyte) and the BRAF targeted drug vemurafenib have shown good promise in iUC (D. Knapp, personal communication).[66] Toceranib combined with vinblastine and COX inhibitor has been studied, although responses did not appear better than for other vinblastine protocols.[27] The injectable demethylating agent 5-azacitidine resulted in PR in 22% and SD in 50% of treated dogs.[67] The pharmacokinetics, toxicity, and dosing of the oral demethylating agent zebularine in dogs with iUC have been reported, and a phase II trial is in progress (C. Fulkerson, personal communication).[68]

Localized Drug Delivery

The use of localized drug delivery in dogs with iUC has been limited, but has included intravesical mitomycin C and photodynamic therapy (PDT).[69,70] Both have shown promise, but neither is used to any extent owing to the risk for systemic toxicity (when drugs instilled enter the circulation via vascularized tumors), local irritation to the bladder, and initial inflammation and tissue swelling after PDT.[69,70]

Urinary Tract Infections

The risk of urinary tract infections (UTIs) is high in dogs with iUC, especially in female dogs with urethral disease.[71,72] This is due at least in part to urine retention, acquired structural defects in the bladder and urethra, damaged urothelium, and, in some cases, potentially compromised immune function.[71,72] UTIs are problematic because they can result in worsening clinical signs, the false impression of cancer progression, and further malignant transformation, invasion, and metastasis secondary to inflammation.[73–75] Antibiotic use can negatively affect the immune response through changes in the microbiome and other mechanisms.[73] Another major problem with UTIs is the increasing resistance to antibiotics.[71,76–79] For example, between January 2013 and February 2015, 168 resistant bacterial isolates from urine were reported at the Purdue University Veterinary Teaching Hospital, and 60% of the resistant isolates were from dogs with TCC (Fulkerson, unpublished data). In a 1-year period, 7 of 57 dogs with iUC developed infections that were sensitive only to nephrotoxic antibiotics, very expensive antibiotics, or were not sensitive to any antibiotics tested.[1] These issues point out the need to appropriately treat UTIs, but to also refrain from prescribing antibiotics when not indicated, as this can promote antibiotic resistance. A positive urine culture, especially with a low colony count in the absence of worsening clinical signs and supporting findings on urinalysis, is not an indication to treat with antibiotics.

If a dog with iUC develops new or progressive lower urinary tract signs, a urinalysis with sediment evaluation should be performed. If the urinalysis reveals pyuria or the presence of intracellular bacteria, a urine culture is recommended. Because of the risk of tumor seeding, urine samples for culture are collected via midstream voiding or through a urinary catheter. While waiting on culture results, an initial antimicrobial choice should target *Escherichia coli* and *Staphylococcus* spp., which are among the most common uropathogens in non–tumor-bearing and tumor-bearing dogs with UTIs.[72] The authors typically prescribe amoxicillin–clavulanate or trimethoprim–sulfa pending culture results. Amoxicillin, doxycycline, and enrofloxacin (but not amoxicillin-clavulanate or cephalexin) have been associated with resistance patterns in cultures performed within 30 days after use.[80] The benefits and risk of other approaches to treat or control UTIs, such as methenamine maleate or bacterial transfer, have not yet been determined.[81,82]

Prognosis

Although iUC is not usually curable in dogs, it is considered very treatable because of the 75% chance of cancer control or remission with treatment. The quality of life in most dogs is excellent. Survival has been strongly associated with the TNM stage at the time of diagnosis.[1,3] Factors associated with a more advanced TNM stage at diagnosis include younger age (increased risk of nodal metastasis), prostate involvement (increased risk of distant metastasis), and higher T stage (increased risk of nodal and distant metastasis).[1,3]

Feline Urinary Bladder Tumors

Bladder cancer is rarely reported in cats. iUC is the most frequently reported form of feline bladder cancer, with mesenchymal tumors, lymphoma, and other tumors being less common.[83–89] Clinical signs of iUC in the cat are similar to those in the dog.[84] In contrast to dogs, more than half of iUCs in a series of 20 cats were away from the trigone.[84] Cats in this series were treated with surgery, cytotoxic chemotherapy, COX inhibitors, or combinations thereof, and the MST was 261 days.[84] As in canine and human iUC, most feline iUCs express COX-1 and COX-2.[89] The MST of 11 cats treated with meloxicam was 311 days.[89] The optimal drugs

for feline iUC and possible role of RT requires more study. Surgical approaches and the placement of stents and cystostomy tubes to improve urine flow have been reported in cats with iUC.[35,90–92]

Canine Urethral Tumors

Most urethral tumors in dogs are malignant epithelial tumors including iUC and squamous cell carcinoma, with other cancers being less common.[93] Staging procedures and treatment recommendations for urethral iUC are generally the same as for iUC located in the bladder. It is important to note that granulomatous/chronic active urethritis comprised 24% of urethral lesions in a series of 41 dogs, and the clinical signs and lesions associated with granulomatous urethritis can mimic iUC.[93] Complete urethral obstruction has been reported with granulomatous urethritis. Histopathology is particularly important for urethral masses to rule out granulomatous urethritis, as treatment and prognosis differ from those of iUC.[93]

Canine Renal Tumors

Canine renal cancer includes renal cell carcinoma (RCC), adenocarcinomas, iUC, papillary cystadenocarcinomas, and less commonly, sarcomas.[94–97] Nodular dermatofibrosis in association with renal cystadenocarcinoma and uterine tumors has been reported, mostly in German shepherd dogs.[98,99] This condition arises as a result of a dominantly inherited missense mutation in *FLCN*, a tumor suppressor gene coding for the protein folliculin, and is similar to Birt–Hogg–Dubé syndrome in people.[98,99]

Epithelial renal tumors and sarcomas tend to occur in older dogs.[94] Nephroblastoma has been reported in young dogs (including a 3-month-old dog), middle-aged, and older dogs.[94–96] A male predisposition has been reported.[97] Clinical signs, when present, include hematuria, pain in the area of the kidneys, a palpable abdominal mass, bone pain secondary to hypertrophic osteopathy, or other nonspecific signs such as GI upset or behavior changes.[94–96,100]

Laboratory findings can include mild to moderate anemia, neutrophilia, azotemia, elevated alkaline phosphatase, hypoalbuminemia, hypercalcemia, and paraneoplastic polycythemia secondary to erythropoietin production.[94,101–104] In a case report of a dog with renal carcinoma and suspected paraneoplastic leukocytosis, immunohistochemistry revealed expression of granulocyte-macrophage colony-stimulating factor by the tumor.[103]

Clinical staging should include thoracic and abdominal imaging. Tumor extension into the caudal vena cava is possible; thus CT may be useful for surgical planning. Evaluation of glomerular filtration rate via scintigraphy can also be useful. Histopathology is required for a definitive diagnosis and can be obtained by ultrasound-guided percutaneous biopsy or at the time of nephrectomy. Immunohistochemistry can help differentiate subtypes of RCC.[105]

Nephrectomy remains the treatment of choice for dogs with unilateral renal tumors with no evidence of metastasis and normal renal function. Even in dogs with metastasis, surgery can be palliative. Renal lymphoma is typically treated with chemotherapy (see Chapter 33), but effective chemotherapy protocols have yet to be described for most primary renal tumors.

In one study, the MSTs were 16 months for 49 dogs with renal carcinomas, 9 months for 28 dogs with renal sarcomas, and 6 months for 5 dogs with nephroblastomas.[94] Higher mitotic index, increased COX-2 expression, specific histologic subtypes, and Fuhrman nuclear grade have reported negative prognostic value for RCCs.[106,107] The MSTs for dogs with a mitotic index of <10, 10 to 30, and >30 were 1184 days, 452 days, and 187 days, respectively.[106] The MST appears shorter for clear cell (87 days) versus chromophobe, papillary, and multilocular cystic RCCs.[106] Fuhrman nuclear grade, a human RCC histologic grading scheme based on morphologic features of nuclei and nucleoli, was prognostic in one study of 70 dogs with RCC with MSTs not reached, 1065 days, 379 days, and 87 days in dogs with grade 1, 2, 3, and 4 RCCs, respectively.[106] Radiographic evidence of metastasis is present in 16% to 34% of dogs with primary renal tumors.[94,97] Metastasis at death was reported in 88% of dogs with sarcomas, 75% with nephroblastomas, and 69% with carcinomas.[94]

Feline Renal Tumors

Primary renal tumors are rare in the cat. Excluding lymphoma, reported feline primary renal tumors include tubular RCC, tubulopapillary RCC, sarcomatoid RCC, adenocarcinoma, adenoma, iUC, squamous cell carcinoma, leiomyosarcoma, nephroblastoma, and hemangiosarcoma.[108–115] The tubular and tubulopapillary RCC were most common in a series of 19 cats.[108] The most common presenting complaint was weight loss. Metastasis was frequently detected at the time of diagnosis.[108]

Polycythemia has been reported in cats with primary renal tumors.[108,115] In two cats with renal adenocarcinoma, polycythemia resolved after nephrectomy.[115] Hypertrophic osteopathy has been reported in a cat with renal adenoma.[110] In contrast to canine and human RCC, immunohistochemistry did not correlate with RCC subtype in a small series of cats.[114] Nephrectomy could be considered in unilateral cancer. The role of chemotherapy is undefined. Limited information on survival is present, but most reports are associated with short survival times.

Comparative Aspects

Invasive Urothelial Carcinoma

There are more than 65,000 new cases and more than 16,000 deaths from urinary bladder cancer in the United States each year, with most deaths from iUC.[116] Cigarette smoking is by far the most common cause of human bladder cancer.[116] In humans, more than two-thirds of bladder tumors are superficial low-grade non–muscle-invasive tumors.[116] These tumors generally respond well to transurethral resection and intravesical therapy, although recurrence is common and progression to iUC is a risk. Approximately 20% of human bladder cancers are higher grade muscle-invasive urothelial carcinoma at the time of diagnosis. Metastasis to the regional lymph nodes, lungs, and other organs occurs in approximately 50% of human iUC cases.[116] iUC in dogs is very similar to iUC in humans in histopathologic characteristics, cellular features, biologic behavior including metastasis, and response to therapy.[2,3,116–125] Canine iUC has emerged as a highly relevant naturally occurring model for human invasive bladder cancer.[2,3] Successful therapies in dogs have been translated into human clinical trials, and similar effects observed between the two species.[2,3,126]

Molecular analyses have further strengthened the role of canine TCC as a model for human iUC.[127–134] In microarray and RNA-seq analyses, hundreds of genes that are differentially expressed between normal bladder tissues and iUC have been found that are shared between dogs and humans.[127,128] Altered expression of genes shared between canine and human iUC includes *COX-2*, *EGFR*, *HER2*, *p53* family genes, *DNMT1*, and *VIM*.[121–125,129–133] The *BRAF*[V595E] mutation, which is present in 80% of canine iUC, leads to continuous activation of the MAPK pathway.[17] This mutation is the canine homolog

of the *BRAF*[V600E] mutation that drives 8% of all human cancer. Although *BRAF* mutations are rare in human iUC, other molecular variants are present that turn on the MAPK pathway in approximately 30% of human iUC cases.[133] Mutations in several other genes implicated in the development and progression of iUC and other cancers in humans have been identified in canine iUC including *EGFR*, *CDKN2B*, *PIK3CA*, *BRCA2*, *NFκB*, *ARHGEF4*, *XPA*, *NCOA4*, *MDC1*, *UBR5*, *RB1CC1*, *RPS6*, *CIITA*, *MITF*, and *WT1*.[17,128,133] Another intriguing finding in canine iUC is the presence of molecular subtypes defined by gene signatures including luminal and basal subtypes initially observed in human breast cancer and then found in human iUC.[127,134] This is important because cancer behavior, treatment response, and prognosis differ between subtypes in humans.[134]

Renal Cancer

Major types of renal cancer in humans include RCC, urothelial carcinoma of the renal pelvis, and Wilms' tumor (nephroblastoma), which is most commonly diagnosed in children.[135] Renal cancer is newly diagnosed in 64,000 people and results in 15,000 deaths each year in the United States. RCC accounts for 90% of adult renal carcinomas.[135] Risk factors for RCC include cigarette smoking, obesity, and hypertension.[136] Multiple subtypes of RCC exist including clear cell, papillary types I and II, and chromophobe types. The clear cell type can be sporadic or associated with von Hippel–Lindau disease in which mutations occur in the *VHL* gene. With recent progress in targeted and immunotherapies, the outlook for human RCC has improved substantially in recent years.

References

1. Fulkerson CM, Knapp DW: Management of transitional cell carcinoma of the urinary bladder in dogs: a review, *Vet J* 205:217–225, 2015.
2. Fulkerson CM, Dhawan D, Ratliff TL, et al.: Naturally occurring canine invasive urinary bladder cancer: a complementary animal model to improve the success rate in human clinical trials of new cancer drugs, *Int J Genomics* 2017:1–9, 2017.
3. Knapp DW, Ramos-Vara JA, Moore GE, et al.: Urinary bladder cancer in dogs, a naturally occurring model for cancer biology and drug development, *ILAR J* 55:100–118, 2014.
4. Shrader S, Lauridson J, King Z, et al.: Urachal adenocarcinoma in a dog, *J Comp Pathol* 154:304–308, 2016.
5. Gelberg HB: Urinary bladder mass in a dog, *Vet Pathol* 47:181–184, 2010.
6. Kessler M, Kandel-Tschiederer B, Pfleghaar S, et al.: Primary malignant lymphoma of the urinary bladder in a dog: longterm remission following treatment with radiation and chemotherapy, *Schweiz Arch Tierheilkd* 150:565–569, 2008.
7. Bae I-H, Kim Y, Pakhrin B, et al.: Genitourinary rhabdomyosarcoma with systemic metastasis in a young dog, *Vet Pathol* 44:518–520, 2007.
8. Mineshige T, Kawarai S, Yauchi T, et al.: Cutaneous epitheliotropic T-cell lymphoma with systemic dissemination in a dog, *J Vet Diagn Invest* 28:327–331, 2016.
9. Owen LN: *TNM classification of tumours in domestic animals*, Geneva, 1980, World Health Organization.
10. Charney VA, Miller MA, Heng HG, et al.: Skeletal metastasis of canine urothelial carcinoma: pathologic and computed tomographic features, *Vet Pathol* 54:380–386, 2017.
11. Reed LT, Knapp DW, Miller MA: Cutaneous metastasis of transitional cell carcinoma in 12 dogs, *Vet Pathol* 50:676–681, 2013.

12. Higuchi T, Burcham GN, Childress MO, et al.: Characterization and treatment of transitional cell carcinoma of the abdominal wall in dogs: 24 cases (1985-2010), *J Am Vet Med Assoc* 242:499–506, 2013.

13. Bryan JN, Keeler MR, Henry CJ, et al.: A population study of neutering status as a risk factor for canine prostate cancer, *Prostate* 67:1174–1181, 2007.

14. Glickman LT, Raghavan M, Knapp DW, et al.: Herbicide exposure and the risk of transitional cell carcinoma of the urinary bladder in Scottish Terriers, *J Am Vet Med Assoc* 224:1290–1297, 2004.

15. Raghavan M, Knapp DW, Dawson MH, et al.: Topical flea and tick pesticides and the risk of transitional cell carcinoma of the urinary bladder in Scottish Terriers, *J Am Vet Med Assoc* 225:389–394, 2004.

16. Raghavan M, Knapp DW, Bonney PL, et al.: Evaluation of the effect of dietary vegetable consumption on reducing risk of transitional cell carcinoma of the urinary bladder in Scottish Terriers, *J Am Vet Med Assoc* 227:94–100, 2005.

17. Decker B, Parker HG, Dhawan D, et al.: Homologous mutation to human BRAF V600E is common in naturally occurring canine bladder cancer, evidence for a relevant model system and urine-based diagnostic test, *Mol Cancer Res* 13:993–1002, 2015.

18. Mochizuki H, Shapiro SG, Breen M: Detection of BRAF mutation in urine DNA as a molecular diagnostic for canine urothelial and prostatic carcinoma, Scarpa A, ed *PLoS One* 10:e0144170, 2015.

19. Mochizuki H, Shapiro SG, Breen M: Detection of copy number imbalance in canine urothelial carcinoma with droplet digital polymerase chain reaction, *Vet Pathol* 53:764–772, 2016.

20. Deschamps J-Y, Roux FA: Extravesical textiloma (gossypiboma) mimicking a bladder tumor in a dog, *J Am Anim Hosp Assoc* 45:89–92, 2009.

21. Böhme B, Ngendahayo P, Hamaide A, et al.: Inflammatory pseudotumours of the urinary bladder in dogs resembling human myofibroblastic tumours: a report of eight cases and comparative pathology, *Vet J* 183:89–94, 2010.

22. Martinez I, Mattoon JS, Eaton KA, et al.: Polypoid cystitis in 17 dogs (1978-2001), *J Vet Intern Med* 17:499–509, 2003.

23. Childress MO, Adams LG, Ramos-Vara J, et al.: Comparison of cystoscopy vs surgery in obtaining diagnostic biopsy specimens from dogs with transitional cell carcinoma of the urinary bladder and urethra, *J Am Vet Med Assoc* 239:350–356, 2011.

24. Vignoli M, Rossi F, Chierici C, et al.: Needle tract implantation after fine needle aspiration biopsy (FNAB) of transitional cell carcinoma of the urinary bladder and adenocarcinoma of the lung, *Schweiz Arch Tierheilkd* 149:314–318, 2007.

25. Hume C, Seiler G, Porat-Mosenco Y, et al.: Cystosonographic measurements of canine bladder tumours, *Vet Comp Oncol* 8:122–126, 2010.

26. Honkisz SI, Naughton JF, Weng HY: Evaluation of two-dimensional ultrasonography and computed tomography in the mapping and measuring of canine urinary bladder tumors, *Vet J* 232:23–26, 2018.

27. Rippy SB, Gardner HL, Nguyen SM, et al.: A pilot study of toceranib/vinblastine therapy for canine transitional cell carcinoma, *BMC Vet Res* 257(12), 2016.

28. Naughton JF, Widmer WR, Constable PD, et al.: Accuracy of three-dimensional and two-dimensional ultrasonography for measurement of tumor volume in dogs with transitional cell carcinoma of the urinary bladder, *Am J Vet Res* 73:1919–1924, 2012.

29. Marvel SJ, Seguin B, Dailey DD, Thamm DH: Clinical outcome of partial cystectomy for transitional cell carcinoma of the canine bladder, *Vet Comp Oncol* 15:1417–1427, 2017.

30. Hosoya K, Takagi S, Okumura M: Iatrogenic tumor seeding after ureteral stenting in a dog with urothelial carcinoma, *J Am Anim Hosp Assoc* 49:262–266, 2013.

31. Saeki K, Fujita A, Fujita N, et al.: Total cystectomy and subsequent urinary diversion to the prepuce or vagina in dogs with transitional cell carcinoma of the trigone area: a report of 10 cases (2005-2011), *Can Vet J* 56:73–80, 2015.

32. Ricardo Huppes R, Crivellenti LZ, Barboza De Nardi A, et al.: Radical cystectomy and cutaneous ureterostomy in 4 dogs with trigonal transitional cell carcinoma: description of technique and case series, *Vet Surg* 46:111–119, 2017.

33. Boston S, Singh A: Total cystectomy for treatment of transitional cell carcinoma of the urethra and bladder trigone in a dog, *Vet Surg* 43:294–300, 2014.

34. Wongsetthachai P, Pramatwinai C, Banlunara W, et al.: Urinary bladder wall substitution using autologous tunica vaginalis in male dogs, *Res Vet Sci* 90:156–159, 2011.

35. Beck AL, Grierson JM, Ogden DM, et al.: Outcome of and complications associated with tube cystostomy in dogs and cats: 76 cases (1995-2006), *J Am Vet Med Assoc* 230:1184–1189, 2007.

36. Bray JP, Doyle RS, Burton CA: Minimally invasive inguinal approach for tube cystostomy, *Vet Surg* 38:411–416, 2009.

37. Zhang J-T, Wang H-B, Shi J, et al.: Laparoscopy for percutaneous tube cystostomy in dogs, *J Am Vet Med Assoc* 236:975–977, 2010.

38. Berent AC: Ureteral obstructions in dogs and cats: a review of traditional and new interventional diagnostic and therapeutic options, *J Vet Emerg Crit Care (San Antonio)* 21:86–103, 2011.

39. Weisse C, Berent A, Todd K, et al.: Evaluation of palliative stenting for management of malignant urethral obstructions in dogs, *J Am Vet Med Assoc* 229:226–234, 2006.

40. Blackburn AL, Berent AC, Weisse CW, et al.: Evaluation of outcome following urethral stent placement for the treatment of obstructive carcinoma of the urethra in dogs: 42 cases (2004-2008), *J Am Vet Med Assoc* 242:59–68, 2013.

41. McMillan SK, Knapp DW, Ramos-Vara JA, et al.: Outcome of urethral stent placement for management of urethral obstruction secondary to transitional cell carcinoma in dogs: 19 cases (2007-2010), *J Am Vet Med Assoc* 241:1627–1632, 2012.

42. Radhakrishnan A: Urethral stenting for obstructive uropathy utilizing digital radiography for guidance: feasibility and clinical outcome in 26 dogs, *J Vet Intern Med* 31:427–433, 2017.

43. Berent AC, Weisse C, Beal MW, et al.: Use of indwelling, double-pigtail stents for treatment of malignant ureteral obstruction in dogs: 12 cases (2006-2009), *J Am Vet Med Assoc* 238:1017–1025, 2011.

44. Upton ML, Tangner CH, Payton ME: Evaluation of carbon dioxide laser ablation combined with mitoxantrone and piroxicam treatment in dogs with transitional cell carcinoma, *J Am Vet Med Assoc* 228:549–552, 2006.

45. Cerf DJ, Lindquist EC: Palliative ultrasound-guided endoscopic diode laser ablation of transitional cell carcinomas of the lower urinary tract in dogs, *J Am Vet Med Assoc* 240:51–60, 2012.

46. Parfitt SL, Milner RJ, Salute ME, et al.: Radiosensitivity and capacity for radiation-induced sublethal damage repair of canine transitional cell carcinoma (TCC) cell lines, *Vet Comp Oncol* 9:232–240, 2011.

47. Arthur JJ, Kleiter MM, Thrall DE, et al.: Characterization of normal tissue complications in 51 dogs undergoing definitive pelvic region irradiation, *Vet Radiol Ultrasound* 49:85–89, 2008.

48. Poirier VJ, Forrest LJ, Adams WM, et al.: Piroxicam, mitoxantrone, and coarse fraction radiotherapy for the treatment of transitional cell carcinoma of the bladder in 10 dogs: a pilot study, *J Am Anim Hosp Assoc* 40:131–136, 2004.

49. Nolan MW, Kogan L, Griffin LR, et al.: Intensity-modulated and image-guided radiation therapy for treatment of genitourinary carcinomas in dogs, *J Vet Intern Med* 26:987–995, 2012.

50. Choy K, Fidel J: Tolerability and tumor response of a novel low-dose palliative radiation therapy protocol in dogs with transitional cell carcinoma of the bladder and urethra, *Vet Radiol Ultrasound* 57:341–351, 2016.

51. Yoshikawa H, Nolan MW, Lewis DW, et al.: Retrospective evaluation of interfraction ureteral movement in dogs undergoing radiation therapy to eluicidate appropriate setup margins, *Vet Radiol Ultrasound* 57:170–179, 2016.

52. Nieset JR, Harmon JF, Johnson TE, et al.: Comparison of adaptive radiotherapy techniques for external radiation therapy of canine bladder cancer, *Vet Radiol Ultrasound* 55:644–650, 2014.

53. Nieset JR, Harmon JF, Larue SM: Use of cone-beam computed tomography to characterize daily urinary bladder variations during fractionated radiotherapy for canine bladder cancer, *Vet Radiol Ultrasound* 52:580–588, 2011.

54. McMillan SK, Boria P, Moore GE, et al.: Antitumor effects of deracoxib treatment in 26 dogs with transitional cell carcinoma of the urinary bladder, *J Am Vet Med Assoc* 239:1084–1089, 2011.

55. Robat C, Burton J, Thamm D, et al.: Retrospective evaluation of doxorubicin-piroxicam combination for the treatment of transitional cell carcinoma in dogs, *J Small Anim Pract* 54:67–74, 2013.

56. Allstadt SD, Rodriguez Jr CO, Boostrom B, et al.: Randomized phase III trial of piroxicam in combination with mitoxantrone or carboplatin for first-line treatment of urogenital tract transitional cell carcinoma in dogs, *J Vet Intern Med* 29:261–267, 2015.

57. Marconato L, Zini E, Lindner D, et al.: Toxic effects and antitumor response of gemcitabine in combination with piroxicam treatment in dogs with transitional cell carcinoma of the urinary bladder, *J Am Vet Med Assoc* 238:1004–1010, 2011.

58. Arnold EJ, Childress MO, Fourez LM, et al.: Clinical trial of vinblastine in dogs with transitional cell carcinoma of the urinary bladder, *J Vet Intern Med* 25:1385–1390, 2011.

59. Knapp DW, Ruple-Czerniak A, Ramos-Vara JA, et al.: A nonselective cyclooxygenase inhibitor enhances the activity of vinblastine in a naturally-occurring canine model of invasive urothelial carcinoma, *Bladder Cancer* 2:241–250, 2016.

60. Henry CJ, Flesner BK, Bechtel SA, et al.: Clinical evaluation of tavocept to decrease diuresis time and volume in dogs with bladder cancer receiving cisplatin, *J Vet Intern Med*, 2017. https://doi.org/10.1111/jvim.14848. Epub ahead of print.

61. Schrempp DR, Childress MO, Stewart JC, et al.: Metronomic administration of chlorambucil for treatment of dogs with urinary bladder transitional cell carcinoma, *J Am Vet Med Assoc* 242:1534–1538, 2013.

62. Knapp DW, Henry CJ, Widmer WR, et al.: Randomized trial of cisplatin versus firocoxib versus cisplatin/firocoxib in dogs with transitional cell carcinoma of the urinary bladder, *J Vet Intern Med* 27:126–133, 2013.

63. Leach TN, Childress MO, Greene SN, et al.: Prospective trial of metronomic chlorambucil chemotherapy in dogs with naturally occurring cancer, *Vet Comp Oncol* 10:102–120, 2012.

64. Custead MR, Weng HY, Childress MO: Retrospective comparison of three doses of metronomic chlorambucil for tolerability and efficacy in dogs with spontaneous cancer, *Vet Comp Oncol* 15:808–819, 2017.

65. Eichstadt LR, Moore GE, Childress MO: Risk factors for treatment-related adverse events in cancer-bearing dogs receiving piroxicam, *Vet Comp Oncol* 15:1346–1353, 2017.

66. Dhawan D, Ramos-Vara JA, Naughton JF, et al.: Targeting folate receptors to treat invasive urinary bladder cancer, *Cancer Res* 73:875–884, 2013.

67. Hahn NM, Bonney PL, Dhawan D, et al.: Subcutaneous 5-azacitidine treatment of naturally occurring canine urothelial carcinoma: a novel epigenetic approach to human urothelial carcinoma drug development, *J Urol* 187:302–309, 2012.

68. Fulkerson CM, Dhawan D, Jones DR, et al.: Pharmacokinetics and toxicity of the novel oral demethylating agent zebularine in laboratory and tumor bearing dogs, *Vet Comp Oncol* 15:226–236, 2017.

69. Abbo AH, Jones DR, Masters AR, et al.: Phase I clinical trial and pharmacokinetics of intravesical mitomycin C in dogs with localized transitional cell carcinoma of the urinary bladder, *J Vet Intern Med* 24:1124–1130, 2010.

70. Lucroy MD, Ridgway TD, Peavy GM, et al.: Preclinical evaluation of 5-aminolevulinic acid-based photodynamic therapy for canine transitional cell carcinoma, *Vet Comp Oncol* 1:76–85, 2003.

71. Thompson MF, Litster AL, Platell JL, et al.: Canine bacterial urinary tract infections: new developments in old pathogens, *Vet J* 190:22–27, 2011.

72. Budreckis DM, Byrne BA, Pollard RE, et al.: Bacterial urinary tract infections associated with transitional cell carcinoma in dogs, *J Vet Intern Med* 29:828–833, 2015.

73. Iida N, Dzutsev A, Stewart CA, et al.: Commensal bacteria control cancer response to therapy by modulating the tumor microenvironment, *Science* 342:967–970, 2013.

74. Ohnishi S, Ma N, Thanan R, et al.: DNA damage in inflammation-related carcinogenesis and cancer stem cells, *Oxid Med Cell Longev* 2013387014, 2013.

75. Chung S-D, Tsai M-C, Lin C-C, et al.: A case-control study on the association between bladder cancer and prior bladder calculus, *BMC Cancer* 13:117, 2013.

76. Hall JL, Holmes MA, Baines SJ: Prevalence and antimicrobial resistance of canine urinary tract pathogens, *Vet Rec* 173:549, 2013.

77. Boothe D, Smaha T, Carpenter DM, et al.: Antimicrobial resistance and pharmacodynamics of canine and feline pathogenic *E. coli* in the United States, *J Am Anim Hosp Assoc* 48:379–389, 2012.

78. Wagner S, Gally DL, Argyle SA: Multidrug-resistant *Escherichia coli* from canine urinary tract infections tend to have commensal phylotypes, lower prevalence of virulence determinants and ampC-replicons, *Vet Microbiol* 169:171–178, 2014.

79. Nam E-H, Ko S, Chae J-S, et al.: Characterization and zoonotic potential of uropathogenic *Escherichia coli* isolated from dogs, *J Microbiol Biotechnol* 23:422–429, 2013.

80. Wong C, Epstein SE, Westropp JL: Antimicrobial susceptibility patterns in urinary tract infections in dogs (2010-2013), *J Vet Intern Med* 29:1045–1052, 2015.

81. Lee BSB, Bhuta T, Simpson JM, et al.: Methenamine hippurate for preventing urinary tract infections, *Cochrane database Syst Rev* 10:CD003265, 2012.

82. Tariq R, Pardi DS, Tosh PK, et al.: Fecal microbiota transplantation for recurrent *clostridium difficile* infection reduces recurrent urinary tract infection frequency, *Clin Infect Dis* 65:1745–1747, 2017.

83. Schwarz PD, Greene RW, Patnaik AK: Urinary bladder tumors in the cat: a review of 27 cases, *J Am Anim Hosp Assoc* 21:237–245, 1985.

84. Wilson HM, Chun R, Larson VS, et al.: Clinical signs, treatments, and outcome in cats with transitional cell carcinoma of the urinary bladder: 20 cases (1990-2004), *J Am Vet Med Assoc* 231:101–106, 2007.

85. Sapierzyński R, Malicka E, Bielecki W, et al.: Tumors of the urogenital system in dogs and cats. retrospective review of 138 cases, *Pol J Vet Sci* 10:97–103, 2007.

86. Geigy CA, Dandrieux J, Miclard J, et al.: Extranodal B-cell lymphoma in the urinary bladder with cytological evidence of concurrent involvement of the gall bladder in a cat, *J Small Anim Pract* 51:280–287, 2010.

87. Pavia PR, Havig ME, Donovan TA, et al.: Malignant peripheral nerve sheath tumour of the urinary bladder in a cat, *J Small Anim Pract* 53:245–248, 2012.

88. Khodakaram-Tafti A, Shirian S, Vesal N, et al.: Lipoma of the urinary bladder in a cat, *J Comp Pathol* 144:212–213, 2011.

89. Bommer NX, Hayes AM, Scase TJ, et al.: Clinical features, survival times and COX-1 and COX-2 expression in cats with transitional cell carcinoma of the urinary bladder treated with meloxicam, *J Feline Med Surg* 14:527–533, 2012.

90. Brace MA, Weisse C, Berent A: Preliminary experience with stenting for management of non-urolith urethral obstruction in eight cats, *Vet Surg* 43:199–208, 2014.

91. Christensen NI, Culvenor J, Langova V: Fluoroscopic stent placement for the relief of malignant urethral obstruction in a cat, *Aust Vet J* 88:478–482, 2010.

92. Newman RG, Mehler SJ, Kitchell BE, et al.: Use of a balloon-expandable metallic stent to relieve malignant urethral obstruction in a cat, *J Am Vet Med Assoc* 234:236–239, 2009.

93. Moroff SD, Brown BA, Matthiesen DT, et al.: Infiltrative urethral disease in female dogs: 41 cases (1980-1987), *J Am Vet Med Assoc* 199:247–251, 1991.

94. Bryan JN, Henry CJ, Turnquist SE, et al.: Primary renal neoplasia of dogs, *J Vet Intern Med* 20:1155–1160, 2006.

95. Michael HT, Sharkey LC, Kovi RC, et al.: Pathology in practice. renal nephroblastoma in a young dog, *J Am Vet Med Assoc* 242:471–473, 2013.

96. Montinaro V, Boston SE, Stevens B: Renal nephroblastoma in a 3-month-old golden retriever, *Can Vet J* 54:683–686, 2013.

97. Klein MK, Campbell GC, Harris CK, et al.: Canine primary renal neoplasms: a retrospective review of 54 cases, *J Am Anim Hosp Assoc* 24:443–452, 1987.

98. Lingaas F, Comstock KE, Kirkness EF, et al.: A mutation in the canine BHD gene is associated with hereditary multifocal renal cystadenocarcinoma and nodular dermatofibrosis in the German Shepherd dog, *Hum Mol Genet* 12:3043–3053, 2003.

99. Bønsdorff TB, Jansen JH, Thomassen RF, et al.: Loss of heterozygosity at the FLCN locus in early renal cystic lesions in dogs with renal cystadenocarcinoma and nodular dermatofibrosis, *Mamm Genome* 20:315–320, 2009.

100. Grillo TP, Brandão CVS, Mamprim MJ, et al.: Hypertrophic osteopathy associated with renal pelvis transitional cell carcinoma in a dog, *Can Vet J* 48:745–747, 2007.

101. Froment R, Gara-Boivin C: Bilateral renal T-cell lymphoma with hepatic infiltration and secondary polycythemia in a dog: utility of cytology slides, *Can Vet J* 56:1287–1291, 2015.

102. Durno AS, Webb JA, Gauthier MJ, et al.: Polycythemia and inappropriate erythropoietin concentrations in two dogs with renal T-cell lymphoma, *J Am Anim Hosp Assoc* 47:122–128, 2011.

103. Petterino C, Luzio E, Baracchini L, et al.: Paraneoplastic leukocytosis in a dog with a renal carcinoma, *Vet Clin Pathol* 40:89–94, 2011.

104. Merrick CH, Schleis SE, Smith AN, et al.: Hypercalcemia of malignancy associated with renal cell carcinoma in a dog, *J Am Anim Hosp Assoc* 49:385–388, 2013.

105. Gil da Costa RM, Oliveira JP, Saraiva AL, et al.: Immunohistochemical characterization of 13 canine renal cell carcinomas, *Vet Pathol* 48:427–432, 2011.

106. Edmondson EF, Hess AM, Powers BE: Prognostic significance of histologic features in canine renal cell carcinomas: 70 nephrectomies, *Vet Pathol* 52:260–268, 2015.

107. Carvalho S, Stoll AL, Priestnall SL, et al.: Retrospective evaluation of COX-2 expression, histological and clinical factors as prognostic indicators in dogs with renal cell carcinomas undergoing nephrectomy, *Vet Comp Oncol* 15:1280–1294, 2017.

108. Henry CJ, Turnquist SE, Smith A, et al.: Primary renal tumours in cats: 19 cases (1992-1998), *J Feline Med Surg* 1:165–170, 1999.

109. Gulbahar MY, Arslan HH, Gacar A, et al.: Sarcomatoid renal cell carcinoma with scant epithelial components in an Angora cat, *N Z Vet J* 61:362–366, 2013.

110. Johnson RL, Lenz SD: Hypertrophic osteopathy associated with a renal adenoma in a cat, *J Vet Diagn Invest* 23:171–175, 2011.

111. Gómez Selgas A, Scase TJ, Foale RD: Unilateral squamous cell carcinoma of the renal pelvis with hydronephrosis in a cat, *J Feline Med Surg* 16:183–188, 2014.

112. Hanzlicek AS, Ganta C, Myers CB, et al.: Renal transitional-cell carcinoma in two cats with chronic kidney disease, *J Feline Med Surg* 14:280–284, 2012.

113. Evans D, Fowlkes N: Renal leiomyosarcoma in a cat, *J Vet Diagn Invest* 28:315–318, 2016.

114. Bonsembiante F, Benali SL, Trez D, et al.: Histological and immunohistochemical characterization of feline renal cell carcinoma: a case series, *J Vet Med Sci* 78:1039–1043, 2016.

115. Klainbart S, Segev G, Loeb E, et al.: Resolution of renal adenocarcinoma-induced secondary inappropriate polycythaemia after nephrectomy in two cats, *J Feline Med Surg* 10:264–268, 2008.

116. Czerniak B, Dinney C, McConkey D: Origins of bladder cancer, *Annu Rev Pathol* 11:149–174, 2016.

117. McCleary-Wheeler AL, Williams LE, Hess PR, et al.: Evaluation of an in vitro telomeric repeat amplification protocol assay to detect telomerase activity in canine urine, *Am J Vet Res* 71:1468–1474, 2010.

118. Rankin WV, Henry CJ, Turnquist SE, et al.: Identification of survivin, an inhibitor of apoptosis, in canine urinary bladder transitional cell carcinoma, *Vet Comp Oncol* 6:141–150, 2008.

119. Lee J-Y, Tanabe S, Shimohira H, et al.: Expression of cyclooxygenase-2, P-glycoprotein and multi-drug resistance-associated protein in canine transitional cell carcinoma, *Res Vet Sci* 83:210–216, 2007.

120. Dill AL, Ifa DR, Manicke NE, et al.: Lipid profiles of canine invasive transitional cell carcinoma of the urinary bladder and adjacent normal tissue by desorption electrospray ionization imaging mass spectrometry, *Anal Chem* 81:8758–8764, 2009.

121. Hanazono K, Fukumoto S, Kawamura Y, et al.: Epidermal growth factor receptor expression in canine transitional cell carcinoma, *J Vet Med Sci* 77:1–6, 2015.

122. Hanazono K, Nishimori T, Fukumoto S, et al.: Immunohistochemical expression of p63, Ki67 and β-catenin in canine transitional cell carcinoma and polypoid cystitis of the urinary bladder, *Vet Comp Oncol* 14:263–269, 2016.

123. Suárez-Bonnet A, Herráez P, Aguirre M, et al.: Expression of cell cycle regulators, 14-3-3σ and p53 proteins, and vimentin in canine transitional cell carcinoma of the urinary bladder, *Urol Oncol* 33(7):332.e1–332.e7, 2015.

124. Dhawan D, Ramos-Vara JA, Stewart JC, et al.: Canine invasive transitional cell carcinoma cell lines: in vitro tools to complement a relevant animal model of invasive urinary bladder cancer, *Urol Oncol* 27:284–292, 2009.

125. Dhawan D, Ramos-Vara JA, Hahn NM, et al.: DNMT1: an emerging target in the treatment of invasive urinary bladder cancer, *Urol Oncol* 31:1761–1769, 2013.

126. Dhawan D, Craig BA, Cheng L, et al.: Effects of short-term celecoxib treatment in patients with invasive transitional cell carcinoma of the urinary bladder, *Mol Cancer Ther* 9:1371–1377, 2010.

127. Dhawan D, Paoloni M, Shukradas S, et al.: Comparative gene expression analyses identify luminal and basal subtypes of canine invasive urothelial carcinoma that mimic patterns in human invasive bladder cancer. St-Pierre Y, *PLoS One* 10:e0136688, 2015.

128. Ramsey SA, Xu T, Goodall C, et al.: Cross-species analysis of the canine and human bladder cancer transcriptome and exome, *Genes Chromosomes Cancer* 56:328–343, 2017.

129. Khan KN, Knapp DW, Denicola DB, et al.: Expression of cyclooxygenase-2 in transitional cell carcinoma of the urinary bladder in dogs, *Am J Vet Res* 61:478–481, 2000.

130. Cekanova M, Uddin MJ, Bartges JW, et al.: Molecular imaging of cyclooxygenase-2 in canine transitional cell carcinomas in vitro and in vivo, *Cancer Prev Res (Phila)* 6:466–476, 2013.

131. Sledge DG, Patrick DJ, Fitzgerald SD, et al.: Differences in expression of uroplakin III, cytokeratin 7, and cyclooxygenase-2 in canine proliferative urothelial lesions of the urinary bladder, *Vet Pathol* 52:74–82, 2015.

132. Millanta F, Impellizeri J, McSherry L, et al.: Overexpression of HER-2 via immunohistochemistry in canine urinary bladder transitional cell carcinoma - a marker of malignancy and possible therapeutic target, *Vet Comp Oncol*, 2017. https://doi.org/10.1111/vco.12345. Epub ahead of print.

133. Cancer Genome Atlas Research Network JN, Akbani R, Broom BM, et al.: Comprehensive molecular characterization of urothelial bladder carcinoma, *Nature* 507:315–322, 2014.

134. Choi W, Ochoa A, McConkey DJ, et al.: Genetic alterations in the molecular subtypes of bladder cancer: illustration in The Cancer Genome Atlas Dataset, *Eur Urol* 72:354–365, 2017.

135. Sánchez-Gastaldo A, Kempf E, González Del Alba A, et al.: Systemic treatment of renal cell cancer: a comprehensive review, *Cancer Treat Rev* 60:77–89, 2017.

136. Chow W-H, Dong LM, Devesa SS: Epidemiology and risk factors for kidney cancer, *Nat Rev Urol* 7:245–257, 2010.

31

Tumors of the Nervous System

JOHN H. ROSSMEISL, JR AND THERESA E. PANCOTTO

Nervous System Tumor Classification and Grading

Tumors of the nervous system can be broadly categorized into primary and secondary varieties.[1–4] Primary brain (PBT) or spinal cord (SC) tumors arise from the constitutive tissues of the brain or SC, such as neurons, glia, and the meninges. Secondary brain (SBT) or SC tumors represent those cancers that metastasize to the brain or SC from a distant site or affect nervous tissue by direct extension from an adjacent tissue (e.g., pituitary, nasal, or calvarial tumors).[4]

In recent years, efforts have been made to model classification of domestic animal nervous system neoplasms after the 2007 World Health Organization (WHO) criteria applied to human tumors.[5] This has been motivated principally by the remarkable clinical, diagnostic imaging, phenotypic, molecular, and genomic similarities observed between many canine and human PBTs,[6–10] as well as attempts to address limitations in the previous system used to describe nervous system tumors of animals.[11] The 2007 WHO criteria are grounded in traditional principles of histogenesis where light microscopic phenotypic similarities define the various tumor types, each type putatively originating from different cellular lineages (Table 31.1). The benefits of using this WHO system include the availability of a more comprehensive descriptive library of histologic tumor subtypes and the inclusion of a tumor grading scheme applicable across tumor types.

The tumor grades represent the range of potential biologic behaviors displayed by tumors. Grades are assigned based on the presence and degree of classic cytoarchitectural features of malignancy, such as cellular atypia, nuclear pleomorphism, mitotic rate, microvascular proliferation, and necrosis.[5] For example, in humans, grade I tumors are well differentiated with low proliferative potential that may often be cured by surgical excision, whereas grade IV tumors are cytologically malignant, mitotically active tumors that are refractory to therapy. Thus in humans, the tumor grade represents one piece of a composite system that uses patient clinicopathologic data to guide therapeutic decision making and predict long-term prognosis.[5] Within the closed confines of the calvarium or vertebral column, even slow-growing grade I tumors will cause progressive morbidity and eventual death of the patient in the absence of therapy regardless of presence of benign versus malignant characteristics. By prospectively applying WHO criteria in animal populations with nervous system tumors, efforts

are ongoing to assess if this type of methodological approach can provide clinically useful correlations between tumor histology, biologic behavior, and therapeutic outcomes in a manner similar to those that exist for other veterinary neoplasms, such as mast cell tumors.[12]

Since the late 1990s, key discoveries have been made regarding the fundamental genetic aberrations that drive tumorigenesis in many types of human nervous system tumors. These studies have revealed that considerable molecular and genotypic heterogeneity exists between tumor types, even among of tumors of the same histology, and these features can have important prognostic implications that transcend phenotype.[13] This has resulted in a departure of the most recent human WHO classification of nervous system tumors from a histology-based platform to an integrated system that incorporates tumor genotypic, molecular, and classic phenotypic information into the definition of neoplastic entities.[13] As the genetic characterization of canine and feline nervous system tumors continues to advance, it is likely that this approach to classification will also become relevant in veterinary medicine.[7–10]

Intracranial Tumors

Epidemiology

Besides humans, dogs and cats are the only mammalian species in which spontaneous brain tumors are encountered frequently.[1–4,14–19] The overall estimated incidences of canine and feline nervous system tumors have been reported as 14.5 cases per 100,000 and 3.5 per 100,000 at risk, respectively.[14,18] Other studies indicate that intracranial neoplasms are observed in 2.0% to 4.5% of dogs and 2% of cats at necropsy.[1,17–19]

Dogs

In dogs, approximately 90% of PBTs (see Table 31.1) are represented by meningiomas (45%), gliomas (40%), and choroid plexus tumors (CPTs; 5%), although the distribution of specific PBTs in individual studies varies substantially.[1,2,17–19] Less commonly reported PBTs in dogs include ependymomas, primary central nervous system (CNS) lymphoma, primitive neuroectodermal tumors (PNETs), gliomatosis cerebri, and primary CNS histiocytic sarcoma (HS) (see Table 31.1); numerous other rare PBT have been described[1,2,14–19] SBTs comprise one-half of all

TABLE 31.1	World Health Organization Classification and Frequency of Primary Brain Tumors in Dogs and Cats		
Tissue of Origin	Tumor Types/Grades	Frequency of Tumor Diagnosis[a]	
		Canine[1,2,5–7,20,21,24,25]	Feline[3,5,6,21–23]
Meninges	Meningioma • Grade I • Grade II (atypical) • Grade III (malignant)	42%–52%	40%–59%
Neuroepithelium	Astrocytic tumors • Grade I (pilocytic) • Grade II (diffuse) • Grade III (anaplastic) • Grade IV (glioblastoma)	13%–60%	<1%–3%
	Oligodendroglial tumors • Grade II (oligodendroglioma) • Grade III (anaplastic)	1%–23%	<1%–3%
	Oligoastrocytic tumors • Grade II (oligoastrocytoma) • Grade III (anaplastic)	<5%	NA
	Choroid plexus tumors • Grade I (papilloma) • Grade II (atypical papilloma) • Grade III (carcinoma)	5%–8%	<1%
	Embryonal tumors • Primitive neuroectodermal tumor (Grade IV)	<0.5%	<1%
	Ependymoma • Grade II (ependymoma) • Grade III (anaplastic)	0.2%–6%	3%

[a]Frequency of diagnosis among all primary brain tumors.

NA, data not available.

canine intracranial tumors, with hemangiosarcoma (HSA, 29%–35%), pituitary tumors (11%–25%), lymphoma (12%–20%), and metastatic carcinomas (11%–20%) accounting for 77% to 86% of all SBTs.[1,4]

Brain tumors in dogs may occur at any age and in any breed with no reported sex predispositions. Most PBTs and SBTs occur in middle-aged to older dogs, with the majority of cases described being greater than 5 years of age. Pooled data from the most current retrospective studies indicate that the median ages at diagnosis for dogs with meningiomas, gliomas, and CPTs were 10.5 years, 8.0 years, and 5.5 years, respectively.[1,2,20,21] There is a propensity for PBTs in juvenile animals to be neuroepithelial tumors of glial, neuronal, or embryonal origin.[1,22] One study identified a significant linear relationship between age and body weight and the occurrence of PBTs; large-breed dogs were at significantly increased risk for developing meningiomas and CPTs.[1] Golden retrievers, boxers, miniature schnauzers, and rat terriers have been identified as breeds in which intracranial meningiomas are overrepresented.[1,2,19,20]

Although CPTs were overrepresented in golden retrievers in one report,[21] this breed predisposition was not corroborated in a subsequent investigation.[1] Gliomas (astrocytomas and oligodendrogliomas) are highly overrepresented in brachycephalic breeds including boxers, Boston terrier, bullmastiffs, and English and French bulldogs.[1,2] A recent study has also identified a locus on canine chromosome (CFA) 26 that is strongly associated with glioma across multiple dog breeds, with subsequent mapping of

the region revealing single nucleotide variants in three neighboring genes *DENR*, *CAMKK2*, and *P2RX7* that are highly associated with glioma susceptibility.[23] The *CAMKK2* and *P2RX7* genes have been previously recognized as relevant to the development or progression of human cancers.[23]

Cats

Intracranial tumors are less common in cats compared with dogs. Approximately 70% of all feline intracranial tumors are PBTs and more than 50% of PBTs in cats are meningiomas.[3,6,15] Other types of PBTs, such as ependymomas, gliomas, and choroid plexus tumors, are infrequently reported (see Table 31.1).[3,6,15] The most common SBTs in cats are lymphoma and pituitary tumors, which accounted for nearly 50% and 30%, respectively, of all feline SBTs in one study.[3] The median age at diagnosis of cats with meningioma is 11 years, whereas neuroepithelial tumors and lymphoma are typically seen in cats in the 7- to 8-year age range.[3,24] There are no known breed or sex predilections for cats to develop brain tumors.

Pathophysiology, History, and Clinical Signs

PBTs and SBTs are space-occupying intracranial lesions that cause clinical signs of brain dysfunction by directly compressing or invading brain tissue and indirectly through secondary effects, such as induction of peritumoral edema, neuroinflammation, obstructive

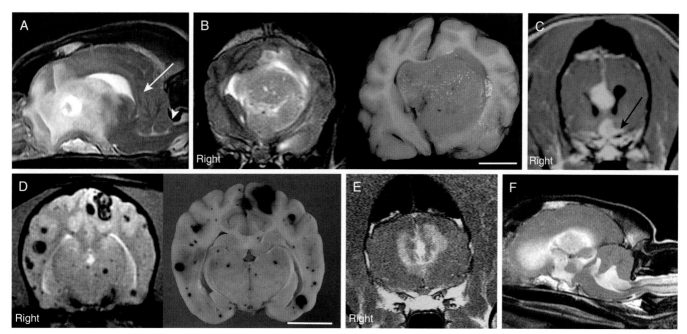

• **Fig. 31.1** MRI and pathologic phenotypes of canine brain tumors causing multifocal intracranial clinical signs. (A) MRI of a cerebral meningioma with marked perilesional edema and transtentorial (*arrow*) and foramen magnum herniations (*arrowhead*). (B) MRI (*left*) and gross specimen (*right*) of primitive neuroectodermal tumor causing mass effect in both cerebral hemispheres and obliterating the lateral and third ventricles. (C) MRI of multiple meningiomas. A dural tail sign (*arrow*) can be seen associated with parasellar mass. (D) MRI (*left*) and gross specimen (*right*) of multifocal metastatic hemangiosarcoma. (E) MRI of butterfly glioblastoma demonstrating bilaterally symmetric wing-like tumor extensions into both cerebral hemispheres. (F) MRI of a choroid plexus carcinoma resulting in obstructive hydrocephalus, fourth ventricular dilatation, and syringohydromyelia.

hydrocephalus, and intracranial hemorrhage.[25] In early stages of tumor growth, compensatory autoregulatory mechanisms, such as decreased cerebrospinal fluid (CSF) production and shifting of CSF into the spinal subarachnoid space, are effective at maintaining the intracranial pressure within physiologic ranges. For some slow-growing tumor types, such as meningiomas, intracranial pressure–volume homeostatic regulatory mechanisms can remain surprisingly intact despite large tumor volumes associated with significant mass effect; however, with progressive increases in tumor volume, autoregulatory mechanisms become overwhelmed and intracranial hypertension (ICH) develops. ICH, and the resulting detrimental decrease in cerebral perfusion pressure, is the common pathophysiologic denominator underlying many of the primary and secondary mechanisms of tumor-associated brain injury. Acute clinical deterioration observed in animals with brain tumors and ICH is often the result of vasogenic or interstitial (i.e., obstructive hydrocephalus) brain edema, abnormalities of cerebral blood flow (ischemia or hemorrhage), brain herniations, or combinations of these mechanisms (Figs. 31.1A, B).[25]

A brain tumor should be considered as a differential diagnosis in any middle-aged or older animal with a clinical history consistent with peracute, acute, or chronic brain dysfunction, especially if clinical signs are progressive. In dogs, seizures are the most common clinical manifestation of intracranial neoplasia and occur in approximately 50% of dogs with forebrain tumors.[2,26–28] The index of suspicion for a brain tumor should increase in dogs that experience a new onset of seizure activity after 5 years of age, especially in at-risk breeds.[26] Significant risk factors for tumor-associated structural epilepsy based on magnetic resonance imaging (MRI) diagnosis include the presence

of tumor involving the frontal lobe, falcine or subtentorial brain herniations, and marked contrast enhancement of the tumor.[28] In cats, the overall incidence of tumor-associated epilepsy is lower than dogs, with approximately 25% of cats with brain tumors experiencing seizures.[3,24,29] In one study, seizures were more common in cats with glioma (27%) and lymphoma (26%) than meningioma (15%).[24] Behavioral changes are the most frequently reported clinical sign associated with feline brain tumors, being observed in 16% to 67% of cats.[3,29] Central vestibular dysfunction is the most common clinical manifestation of brain tumors affecting the brainstem.[26,30] Nonspecific complaints (e.g., lethargy, inappetance) were identified in more than 20% of cats with brain tumors and are frequently reported in dogs with pituitary tumors.[3,31]

Tumors involving forebrain structures are more common than those in the brainstem.[1–3,30] In many cases with solitary masses, observed neurologic deficits are reflective of the focal neuroanatomic area involved. However, dogs and cats may present with neurologic deficits indicative of multifocal intracranial disease (see Fig. 31.1).

In 50% of dogs with solitary PBTs, multifocal signs result from the tumor or its secondary effects involving multiple region of the brains.[2] The phenotype of some PBTs, such as butterfly glioblastomas, by definition requires tumor invasion of both cerebral hemispheres.[32] Multiple tumors may also be present, which occurs occasionally in canine meningiomas, but is seen in approximately 20% of cats with meningiomas.[3,33,34] Canine oligodendrogliomas can manifest with multifocal or diffuse leptomeningeal involvement.[35] Rare case reports describing synchronous PBTs of different histologies and synchronous PBTs and SBTs also exist.[36]

Choroid plexus carcinomas may metastasize within the CNS by a unique mechanism termed *drop metastases* in which cancer cells are exfoliated into the subarachnoid space or ventricular system with eventual distant implantation of tumor foci.[37] Finally, SBTs that spread hematogenously often result in multiple metastases within the brain (see Fig. 31.1).[4]

Diagnosis of Intracranial Tumors

The index of suspicion for a brain tumor as a potential etiology for the observed clinical signs is based upon signalment, history, and neurologic examination findings. In addition to brain tumors, differential diagnoses in dogs and cats with focal intracranial disease include anomalies/malformations, infectious or immune-mediated meningoencephalitis, traumatic brain injury, and stroke. For those animals with a multifocal or diffuse localization, metabolic disorders, neurodegenerative diseases, and meningoencephalitides should be considered. A logical and prioritized diagnostic approach to patients with suspected brain tumors is indicated.

Minimum Database

Laboratory evaluation of health status (complete blood count, serum biochemistry, urinalysis) is important, as anesthesia is recommended for diagnosis of structural brain disease. The at-risk population of middle-aged to older animals with brain tumors may also have significant concurrent disease that affects management.[2,38]

Thoracic radiographs and an abdominal ultrasound (AUS) should be considered in an attempt to identify concurrent unrelated neoplasia or other significant comorbidities. Studies have reported contemporaneous and unrelated neoplasms in 3% to 23% of dogs with PBTs, the majority of which involved the thoracic or abdominal cavities.[2,39] Recent studies have shown that although abnormalities are frequently identified on thoracic radiographs and AUS in dogs with PBT, the results of these procedures uncommonly (1.3%) negatively affected the decision to pursue advanced neurodiagnostics indicated for the neurologic condition of the patient, and significantly altered therapeutic recommendations for the brain tumor in 8.0% of cases.[38,39] For clinically stable patients with a suspected brain tumor and unremarkable general physical examination, the authors do not routinely perform screening radiographs or AUS before MRI, but do recommend these procedures before brain tumor treatment.

Diagnostic Imaging

Computed tomography (CT) and MRI have revolutionized the antemortem clinical diagnosis and management of brain tumors in veterinary medicine.[40–43] MRI is the preferred modality for the evaluation of intracranial disease. Information obtained from imaging such as tumor number, origin within the neuraxis (extraaxial, intraaxia, or intraventricular) and intrinsic signal appearances, often collectively provides characteristic patterns that allow for the presumptive diagnosis of the most frequently encountered PBTs and SBTs. In one investigation, the accuracy of predicting the type of PBT based on MR images of was 70%.[40]

Meningiomas (Fig. 31.2 and see Figs. 31.1A, C) are the most common extraaxial origin tumors in dogs and cats.[3,33–34] Meningiomas typically have a broad-based skull attachment, have distinct tumor margins, and demonstrate marked and often uniform contrast enhancement (see Fig. 31.2). Some meningiomas will also display intratumoral fluid (see Fig. 31.2A), large cystic regions, intratumoral mineralization, calvarial hyperostosis, or a dural tail sign (see Fig. 31.2). Calvarial hyperostosis can result from tumor-induced reactive osseous changes or tumor invasion into bone.[3,44] The dural tail sign is a contrast-enhancing, linear thickening of the dura mater extending from an adjacent extraaxial mass and is not specific for meningioma (see Fig. 31.2) or for neoplastic diseases in general.[45,46] Peritumoral edema is observed in more than 90% of canine meningiomas (see Fig. 31.1A).[20,40,41] In canine studies, reported sensitivities of MRI to correctly identify intracranial meningiomas range between 60% and 100%,[20,40,47] but specific grades and subtypes cannot be distinguished.[20] The MRI sensitivity for meningiomas has been estimated to be 96% in cats.[48] The imaging features of HS, granular cell tumors, and hemangioblastomas share similarities with those of meningiomas (see Fig. 31.2).[41,42,49]

As gliomas originate within and may infiltrate and displace the neuropil, they often appear poorly marginated and may or may not demonstrate contrast enhancement.[40–42,50] Among contrast-enhancing gliomas, the patterns and degree of enhancement seen can be highly variable. A "ring enhancing" pattern, in which a circular ring of contrast enhancement surrounds nonenhancing abnormal tissue, is often associated with gliomas (Fig. 31.3). However, ring enhancement is a nonspecific finding that has been associated with neoplastic, vascular, and inflammatory brain diseases.[51] Currently, using conventional CT or MRI sequences, it is not possible to reliably differentiate types of gliomas (astrocytomas from oligodendrogliomas) or accurately predict the grade of gliomas.[40,50] The considerable overlap that exists in the imaging

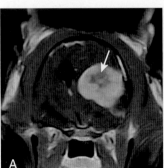 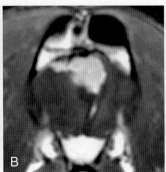 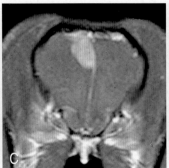 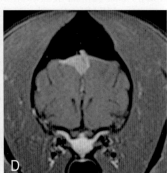

• **Fig. 31.2** Postcontrast magnetic resonance image features of intracranial meningioma and its imaging mimics. (A) Feline meningioma, with intratumoral fluid (*arrow*). (B) Canine histiocytic sarcoma. (C) Canine granular cell tumor. (D) Canine parasagittal meningioma. Each of the canine tumors features a dural tail sign.

features of gliomas, cerebrovascular accidents, and inflammatory lesions results in frequent misdiagnosis of these categories of intraaxial lesions.[52,53] The addition of diffusion-weighted, spectroscopic, and perfusion-weighted imaging sequences (see Fig. 31.3) to conventional MRI sequences has shown promise in improving the ability of MRI to discriminate between neoplastic and non-neoplastic lesions, and differentiation of tumor grades.[54,55]

Choroid plexus tumors (see Fig. 31.1F) and ependymomas are the most common tumors found in an intraventricular location, and both of these tumors types often uniformly contrast enhance.[21,56] Other intraventricular tumors that are occasionally or rarely seen include meningiomas arising from the tela choroidea of the third ventricle, oligodendroglioma, PNET, and central neurocytoma.[2,3] The identification of intraventricular or subarachnoid metastatic tumor implants on MRI studies is a reliable means to clinically discriminate grade III choroid plexus carcinomas (CPC) from grade I papillomas (CPP).

Finally, although MRI is sensitive for the detection of intracranial neoplasms, a normal MRI does not rule out a brain tumor. Lymphomatosis and gliomatosis cerebri are notable for their propensity to be occult on imaging studies of the brain.

Tumor Biopsy and Pathology

In practice, it is common to make clinical decisions in patients with presumptively diagnosed tumors based on imaging derived data. However, it is important to recognize the potential consequences that the previously described limitations of imaging can have on individual patients. Histopathologic examination of representative tissue is required for the definitive diagnosis and grading of nervous system tumors. Excisional biopsy performed during curative-intent surgery remains the most frequently employed biopsy technique for PBTs, but these procedures have been historically limited to patients with superficially located, extraaxial forebrain or cerebellar tumors. In cases in which surgical resection

may not be a possible or optimal, minimally invasive brain biopsy (MIBB) techniques are a viable alternative.

Several MIBB techniques have been used in dogs and cats with brain tumors including endoscopic-assisted, free-hand, and image-guided procedures.[56–58] When MIBB is performed in animals with brain tumors by operators experienced with contemporary CT and MRI stereotactic systems, diagnostic yields approach 95%, and serious adverse events occur in approximately 5% of cases.[8,58] The histologic classification and grading of anaplastic CNS tumors can be challenging when evaluating the limited sample sizes associated with MIBB, but often can be facilitated with additional immunohistochemical evaluation of tumors.[59,60]

Not surprisingly, as intracranial tumors are more common in dogs, a wider variety of histologic types and subtypes have been described in dogs compared with cats. There are multiple histologic subtypes of grade I meningiomas including angiomatous, meningothelial, transitional, fibroblastic, psammomatous, microcystic, and papillary variants. Meningothelial, transitional, and psammomatous subtypes of meningiomas are the most common in both species.[20,29] The majority of feline meningiomas are grade I tumors.[29] Atypical (grade II) meningiomas account for a significantly higher proportion (40%) of meningiomas in dogs.[20] In addition, all grades of canine meningiomas can display invasion into the neural parenchyma, a mechanism that may contribute to therapeutic failure.[20] Anaplastic (grade III) meningiomas are rare in humans, dogs and cats, and account for about 1% of all canine and feline meningiomas.[20]

The histopathologic features of canine gliomas are remarkably similar to what is seen in humans.[60–64] Their propensity to locally or distantly infiltrate brain tissue contributes to their malignant clinical behavior.[32,60–64] A diverse spectrum of types and grades of astrocytomas, oligodendrogliomas, and oligoastrocytomas that occur in people have been documented in dogs. However, the frequency of glioma types encountered in dogs differs from

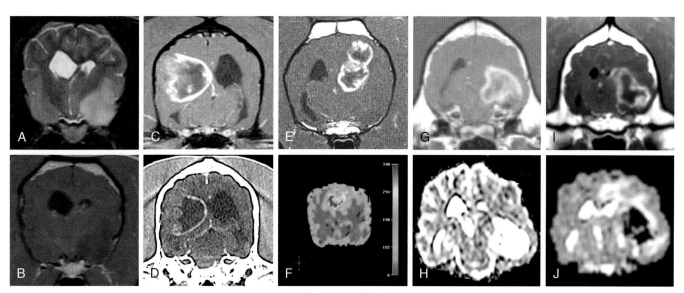

• **Fig. 31.3** Comparative magnetic resonance image (MRI) features of canine gliomas and other ring enhancing lesions. Top panels are all transverse, T1-weighted postcontrast images. (A, B) Nonenhancing grade II astrocytoma in the left piriform lobe. MRI (C, E) and CT (D) images of ring-enhancing grade III oligodendrogliomas causing marked attenuation of the lateral ventricles. (E) Ring-enhancing glioblastoma (F) Dynamic contrast MRI perfusion map of the tumor depicted in panel ((G, H) and hemorrhagic infarction with peripheral revascularization (I, J) in the left occipital lobes of two dogs. The glioblastoma (G) appears hyperintense on the apparent diffusion coefficient map (ADC; H) generated from DWI sequences, whereas restricted diffusion in the infarction (J) appears as a hypointense region on the ADC map.

that seen in humans, with oligodendrogliomas accounting for a significantly higher proportion of all canine gliomas.[1,2,64] Insufficient data currently exist in veterinary medicine to evaluate the effect of glioma grade on clinical outcome.[5] Intracranial gliomas are rare in cats, and oligodendrogliomas are the most common type observed.[3,65,66]

In the dog, approximately 40% of CPTs are grade I CPP, 60% are grade III CPC, and nearly 50% of CPTs occur in the fourth ventricular region.[21] Atypical (grade II) choroid plexus papillomas have not yet been recognized in veterinary medicine.[5,21] The morphology of CPTs usually allows for rapid and accurate cytologic diagnosis of tumor type when performed on surgical or MIBB specimens.[21] In dogs and humans, CPCs frequently demonstrate local invasion and commonly metastasize via the ventricular system.[21]

Although the genetic and epigenetic studies performed to date in canine brain tumors have identified similarities in molecular signatures, differentially expressed genes, and methylation profiles in developmentally regulated genes between human and canine tumors, these studies were performed with fairly limited microarray platforms.[8,10,67-74] It is likely that additional common denominators are shared among canine and human tumors and will be discovered with the use of more robust whole exome sequencing and single nucleotide polymorphism analytical systems.[23] It is also probable that aberrations in key pathways unique to the dog will continue to be revealed.[10]

Cerebrospinal Fluid Analysis

CSF analysis provides data that are complementary to clinical examination and diagnostic imaging results, and helps the clinician refine the list of differential diagnosis. Obtaining CSF when ICH is present carries a risk of causing clinical deterioration. Although this risk is low, it should be critically assessed in each patient and evaluated in context of the likelihood of obtaining a nonspecific test result. Advanced imaging of the brain should always precede CSF collection to best evaluate patient risk.

Although CSF is a sensitive indicator of intracranial disease and is frequently abnormal in patients with brain tumors, white blood cell (WBC) counts, WBC differentials, and total protein concentrations are highly variable and are often nonspecific for neoplasia.[75,76] In one study of CPTs, CSF analysis was helpful for the differentiation of CPCs from CPPs, as observation of a CSF total protein concentration greater than 80 mg/dL was exclusively associated with a diagnosis of CPC.[21] Exfoliated neoplastic cells may be observed in the CSF cytology of patients with any type of brain tumor, but choroid plexus tumors, lymphoma, HS, and cats with caudal brainstem oligodendrogliomas have been the most frequently reported.[2,21,65,77]

Treatment and Prognosis of Intracranial Tumors

Many veterinary studies regarding the treatment of brain tumors are limited by the inclusion of presumptively diagnosed cases, variable survival definitions and end-points, lack of inclusion or reporting of objective imaging-based criteria of therapeutic response or other unbiased quantitative follow-up metrics, retrospective study designs, and small case numbers[7,9,78] Thus there currently exists a significant void in the literature with respect to meaningful data regarding tumor type-specific therapeutic outcomes for many PBTs, as well as a lack of large and rigorously designed trials comparing treatment modalities.

Palliative Care

The primary palliative therapies administered to brain tumor patients are anticonvulsant drugs (ACD) for tumor-associated structural epilepsy, corticosteroids targeting peritumoral vasogenic edema, and analgesics for signs consistent with somatic, visceral, or neuropathic cancer pain.[7,9,30] Although seizures are one of the most common clinical signs associated with brain tumors, ideal ACD protocols for the treatment of tumor-associated epilepsy are currently unknown.[2,24,27,28] Phenobarbital, levetiracetam, and zonisamide are popular clinical ACD monotherapy choices.[24,28,30] Multidrug ACD protocols are frequently needed to control refractory seizures in brain tumor patients, and the aggressiveness and diligence of the approach to seizure management is often as important to the therapeutic outcome as the tumor response to other treatment modalities.[30]

Animals that have peritumoral vasogenic edema on MRI are more likely to respond favorably to corticosteroid treatment (Figs. 31.4A, B and see Fig. 31.1A) however, animals without significant vasogenic edema may benefit also from the antiinflammatory and euphoric effects of corticosteroids; corticosteroid therapy alone may also transiently reduce the tumor burden in some cases (see Figs. 31.4A, B) or provide modest benefit to animals with tumors causing secondary obstructive hydrocephalus.[7] Polyuria, polydipsia, polyphagia, and sedation are commonly anticipated and reported adverse effects of palliative treatment, but palliative therapies are rarely associated with significant treatment-associated morbidity that necessitates discontinuation of therapy.[9,30,78]

Pain associated with nervous system tumors can arise from compression or stretching of the meninges, nerve roots, or vasculature, tumor-associated meningitis, neuritis, or radiculitis, and tumor infiltration of the periosteum or musculature.[44] Hyperesthesia of the head or neck is frequently observed in dogs with brain tumors, being reported in 12% of dogs with PBTs in one study.[2] Clinical signs consistent with pain often respond to corticosteroid treatment, and additional opioid or neuropathic pain agents can be added if necessary.

Studies published to date indicate that 6% and up to 19% of canine and feline meningiomas, respectively, are identified incidentally.[2,3] Given the increasing clinical usage of serial cross-sectional imaging techniques to manage numerous diseases in veterinary medicine, it is likely that the frequency of identification of incidental brain tumors will increase. Thus objective observation (e.g., watchful monitoring) also represents a reasonable approach to the management of some small and asymptomatic brain tumors (see Figs. 31.4C–E). Further elucidation of the natural disease history for specific brain tumors will be paramount to identifying optimal indications for watchful monitoring, as well as recommended observation intervals and protocols.

Currently, there is no robust information regarding survival associated with palliative care of specific PBT types or grades. Pooled data indicates a median survival time (MST) after palliative care of PBT of approximately 9 weeks, with a range of 1 to 13 weeks.[3,7,9,30,79] Dogs with supratentorial tumors treated palliatively have a better prognosis (MST 25 weeks) than those with infratentorial tumors (MST 4 weeks).[30] The prognosis associated with palliative care of pituitary tumors is more favorable than PBTs, with a MST of 51 weeks reported in one study.[80]

Chemotherapy

Data evaluating the efficacy of chemotherapy for the management of brain tumors is limited by the lack of histologic tumor diagnoses in the vast majority of reported cases, and the preponderance

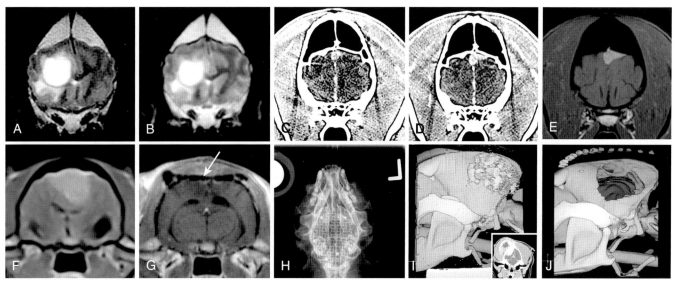

• **Fig. 31.4** Serial imaging of brain tumors treated with different approaches. (A, B) Grade III oligodendroglioma in the right frontal lobe associated with perilesional vasogenic edema. Compared with the pretreatment (A) image there is improvement in the edema and a decrease in the size of the mass after 3 days of dexamethasone therapy (B). Sequential CT (C, D) and magnetic resonance imaging (E) examinations of an incidental meningioma managed with annual watchful monitoring. There is minimal enlargement of the mass over the depicted 3-year period. Feline parasagittal meningioma with calvarial hyperostosis (F) treated via bilateral radical rostrotentorial craniectomy and reconstructive titanium mesh cranioplasty (G, *arrow*; H). Pre- (I) and immediate postresection (J) computed tomography reconstructions of a dog with a multilobular osteochondroma compressing the cerebrum (I, *inset*).

of case reports or small case series examining specific drugs. The most commonly used chemotherapeutics for brain tumors are the alkylating agents lomustine (CCNU), carmustine (BCNU), and temozolomide (TMZ), or the antimetabolite hydroxyurea, all of which penetrate the blood–brain barrier (BBB).[79–81] A small number of case reports have reported objective tumor responses or survival benefits associated with chemotherapy.[82,83] In general, however, chemotherapy appears to have very limited objective efficacy for the treatment of brain tumors, especially when used as a monotherapy in the setting of gross disease. One retrospective study in 71 dogs with presumptively diagnosed brain tumors reported that CCNU-treated dogs (MST 93 days) experienced no survival benefit compared with dogs receiving palliative therapy (MST 60 days).[79] No difference in survival was reported between groups of dogs with predominantly presumptively diagnosed gliomas treated with stereotactic volume modulated arc radiotherapy (VMAT) with (MST 420 days) or without (MST 383 days) TMZ.[81] At the dose intensities reported in the literature, toxicities associated with CCNU, TMZ, and hydroxyurea appear to be uncommon and rarely life-threatening in companion animals with brain tumors.[79,81]

In vitro studies have demonstrated that therapeutic responses to chemotherapeutic agents (such as bleomycin, carboplatin, CCNU, irinotecan, and TMZ), as well as mechanisms of chemoresistance observed in canine glioma cell lines, parallel those seen in human glioma cell lines.[70] Thus it is reasonable to expect that the inclusion of adjuvant chemotherapy in multimodality companion animal brain tumor treatment protocols could result in modest clinical benefits, as is generally seen in humans. Metronomic chemotherapy with chlorambucil in conjunction with surgical resection is currently being evaluated in an early phase trial in dogs with gliomas.[84] The creation of animal patient-derived tumor cell lines will be paramount to efforts necessary to develop and evaluate brain tumor-specific drug protocols, such as high-throughput drug library screening and the identification of biomarkers that predict chemoresponsiveness.

Surgery

Advantages associated with surgical resection of brain tumors include the rapid reduction or elimination of the tumor burden, the secondary beneficial effect this has on reducing intracranial pressure, and definitive histopathologic diagnosis of the tumor. Several variables complicate critical comparisons of studies evaluating the efficacy surgical treatment of specific tumor types including the experience of the surgeon, availability or standardized protocols for usage of a growing number of operating room technologies, and a nearly universal lack of inclusion of quantifiable surrogates of surgical success, such as the extent of resection (EOR) in PBT studies. Given that attainment of wide excision margins of brain tumors is generally not possible, objective evaluation of EOR is currently dependent on MRI-based assessments, which are associated with practical limitations, including expense and difficulties distinguishing residual tumor from surgically induced reactive changes in the acute postoperative period.[85,86]

Cytoreductive surgery is currently the preferred primary mode of therapy for feline supratentorial meningiomas.[3,29,87,88] Feline supratentoral meningiomas are often located over the cerebral convexities, visibly well demarcated, and are not usually infiltrative into the underlying brain parenchyma. These characteristics make them amenable to gross total resection (see Figs. 31.4F, G) with low procedural mortality, even in instances of large tumor burdens, multiple tumor foci, or recurrent tumor.[34] Reconstruction of extensive cranial surgical defects necessary to remove large tumors can be performed using MRI-compatible materials, including fascial or calvarial autografts, or polymethylmethacrylate or titanium mesh cranioplasties (see Figs. 31.4G, H).[89]

Cats with cerebral meningiomas treated surgically often survive in excess of 2 years, with reported MSTs ranging from 23 to 37 months.[3,29,87,88] Approximately 25% of feline meningiomas will recur after surgery, with highly variable times to recurrence ranging from 3 to 69 months.[87,88]

Outcomes associated with surgical management of canine meningiomas are more variable than those of feline meningiomas, reflective of the previously identified operator and technical factors, in addition to the propensity for all grades of canine meningiomas to locally invade brain tissue.[20] Most surgical studies of canine meningiomas have included superficially located cerebral or cerebellar convexity, falcine, parasagittal, or olfactory tumors.[90–94] Surgical treatment of basilar, cerebellopontomedullary angle, foramen magnum, parasellar, and tentorial meningiomas is technically challenging and has not been frequently reported.[90] When standard cytoreductive surgical techniques are used, the MST for canine meningiomas is approximately 7 months.[91–93] Studies describing the use of techniques or technologies that facilitate removal of infiltrative tumor or intraoperative visualization such as cortical resection, extirpation with an ultrasonic aspirator, or endoscopic assisted resection in canine meningiomas report superior MSTs (16–70 months) compared with conventional surgical methods.[90,94] Dogs with meningiomas treated surgically also benefit from the addition of adjunctive radiation therapy (RT), as MSTs associated with multimodal surgery and RT protocols range from 16 to 30 months.[92,95,96]

There is a paucity of data regarding the potential efficacy of surgery as a primary treatment of other PBTs, such as ependymomas, gliomas, and choroid plexus tumors, although a few individual animals with these tumor types experienced prolonged survival times (STs) after surgery or multimodal investigational therapies.[7,21,84,97] Surgical removal of these tumors is seldom attempted because approaching and removing them is technically demanding due to their intraaxial or intraventricular locations. In addition, as high-grade variants of these tumors are poorly delineated and locally invasive, it is inherently more difficult to discriminate the margins of tumor from the neighboring neuropil. Clinician attitudes and abilities with respect to the resection of these tumors types are evolving in parallel with improvements in brain imaging techniques, intraoperative stereotactic and neuronavigational systems, minimally invasive automated tissue resection devices, and "tumor painting" with fluorophores to assist with delineation of tumors from the surrounding brain.[7,84,97,98] The literature also suggests that the prognosis for some tumor types, such as HS, is poor, irrespective of the types of treatment administered.[99]

Surgery also has utility in the management of some SBTs. Transsphenoidal hypophysectomy is an effective technique for the treatment canine and feline pituitary-dependent hyperadrenocorticism (PDH) and feline acromegaly, producing durable endocrinologic and clinical remissions.[100–102] However, microsurgical hypophysectomy has limited value in cases with pituitary macrotumors, is associated with a steep operator learning curve, and is currently only offered at a few centers worldwide.[101,102] Some calvarial SBTs, such as multilobular osteochondrosarcoma can also be managed surgically with good long-term outcomes depending on histologic grade and completeness of excision (see Figs. 31.4I, J).[103]

The frequency of significant adverse events associated surgical treatment of PBTs varies widely between individual studies, ranging from 6% to 100%.[29,78,84,87,88,90–92,98,104,105] If the outlier study with 100% perioperative mortality is excluded from analysis, the average rate of surgical adverse events is approximately 11%.[104] Common causes of morbidity and early perioperative mortality include aspiration pneumonia, intracranial hemorrhage or infarction, pneumocephalus, medically refractory provoked seizures, transient or permanent neurologic disability, electrolyte and osmotic disturbances, and thermoregulatory dysfunction.[78]

Radiation Therapy

RT is beneficial for the treatment of PBTs and SBTs when used as a sole or adjunctive therapeutic modality. As with other treatments, extrapolating meaningful data from the veterinary brain tumor RT literature with respect to the outcomes associated with specific tumor types in confounded by a general lack of histologically diagnosed tumors included in RT studies, grouping of heterogeneous intracranial masses in data analyses, and considerable variability in the RT types and dose prescriptions used. RT equipment and techniques have advanced to current predominantly linear accelerator-based options, including intensity-modulated RT (IMRT) capabilities such as VMAT and tomotherapy, as well as stereotactic RT (SRT).[81] The advantages of IMRT, VMAT, and SRT are improved target volume conformity, particularly in volumes with complex shapes, and improved sparing of normal tissues resulting in reduced risk for toxicities.[81] SRT broadly encompasses treatments that involve the precision delivery of high doses of ionizing radiation to a stereotactically defined anatomic target in a limited number (1–5) of fractions, compared with the 16 to 20 fractions for standard RT protocols.[9]

Studies of cohorts of dogs treated with RT as a sole treatment modality for brain tumors report MSTs ranging from 7 to 23 months when all treated intracranial masses are included.[81,96,106–111] MSTs associated with RT treatment of extraaxial masses, the majority of which were presumptively diagnosed meningiomas, range from 9 to 19 months; and MSTs reported for intraaxial masses ranges from 9 to 13 months.[78,81,96,106–111] Some RT studies report that extraaxial tumors have a more favorable prognosis than intraaxial tumors.[110] Given the variable outcomes associated with both RT and surgery, there is currently no clearly superior choice between these two modalities when either is used a sole treatment for canine meningiomas.[78]

RT is also useful for the adjunctive therapy of canine meningiomas, with combined surgical and RT therapy producing MSTs of 16 to 30 months.[92,95,96] Selected biomarkers have been shown to have prognostic value in dogs with meningiomas treated with surgery and RT. In one study of 17 dogs treated with surgery and adjunctive hypofractionated RT, survival was negatively correlated with VEGF expression.[8] The MST was 25 months for dogs with tumors with 75% or fewer cells demonstrating immunoreactivity to VEGF compared with 15 months for dogs with tumors with greater than 75% of cell staining for VEGF, and dogs with tumors demonstrating more intense VEGF immunoreactivity also had a significantly shorter MST.[112] Progesterone receptor expression has also been shown to be inversely related to the tumor proliferative index (PF_{PCNA} index), which was predictive of survival in dogs with meningiomas after surgery and postoperative RT. The 2-year progression-free survival rate was 42% for tumors with a PF_{PCNA} index 24% or greater and 91% for tumors with a PF_{PCNA} index less than 24%.[95]

Compared with palliative therapy, RT is effective at reducing tumor size, improving neurologic signs, and providing a survival benefit in dogs and cats with pituitary tumors.[80,108,113–117] RT is the preferred therapeutic modality for pituitary macrotumors.[80,115] In cases of PDH treated with RT, the reported rates of endocrinologic remission are variable, with some studies reporting persistent hypercortisolinemia for up to a year after RT.[80,113,116] Thus continued medical management and serial endocrinologic evaluations are necessary after RT of PDH. Negative prognostic indicators associated with RT for pituitary masses include severe neurologic dysfunction at presentation and large relative tumor size.[80,115]

SRT is actively being investigated for the treatment of multiple types of brain tumors. SRT offers the distinct advantage of a reduced number of anesthetic episodes required for treatment. However, SRT is associated with limitations as to the size of masses that can be treated (likely several centimeters) and it is not suitable for treating residual microscopic disease after surgery.[9] Preliminary data suggest that SRT results in tumor control that is comparable to standard fractionated RT protocols with potentially fewer short-term adverse effects and, in the case of pituitary tumors, provide results that are similar to those of hypophysectomy.[111,115–117]

Approximately 10% of brain tumor cases treated with RT will experience treatment-related mortality or adverse effects.[78] Frequently reported adverse effects include aspiration pneumonia, pulmonary thromboembolism, acute CNS toxicity which often manifests as a decreased level of consciousness, damage to organs in the treatment field including deafness, cataract formation, and keratitis, and late-onset radiation necrosis.[78] Important radiobiologic considerations when treating brain tumors include the radiation dose per fraction, total radiation dose, and the volume of the brain irradiated. In one study of hypofractionated RT, delivery of a high dose per fraction resulted in the death of nearly of 15% of treated dogs because of suspected delayed radiation side effects.[110] Although significant adverse events associated with SRT have been uncommonly reported in animals to date, the more frequent use of high-dose per fraction prescriptions may eventually influence the incidence of observed toxicity.

Novel Therapeutics

The identification and use of novel animal models that allow for the study of fundamental cancer drug and device development questions would meet a critical and shared need among stakeholders in the cancer research and global healthcare communities. A growing body of evidence indicates that canine brain tumors are clinically, phenotypically, and molecularly similar to their human analogs, thus providing unique avenues for preclinical discovery.[7,9,10,118] Translational studies of investigational agents in tumor-bearing dogs can provide a variety of pharmacokinetic, mechanistic, toxicity, and antitumor activity data in an immunocompetent host, and thus offer numerous opportunities to guide the therapeutic development process to mutually improve the lives of dogs and humans with brain tumors.[118]

The repertoire of agents and techniques that are being investigated in canine brain tumors is rapidly expanding. General areas that capture the efforts of active veterinary neuro-oncology research programs can be summarized into (1) macroscopic tumor targeting or CNS delivery techniques, (2) novel molecular therapeutics targeting tumor-specific markers or aberrant cellular pathways, (3) immunotherapy, and (4) modifications of the dosing or chemistry of existing therapeutics based on new mechanistic discoveries. Reviews of early-phase trials evaluating these approaches in dogs with brain tumors are available.[7,9,119]

The objectives of macroscopic tumor targeting techniques are to facilitate the gross surgical resection of tumors or to overcome therapeutic drug delivery limitations imposed by the BBB. The use of intraoperative microsurgical or stereotactic equipment and

neuronavigational systems with various tissue resection devices and techniques are being actively investigated for the surgical biopsy and treatment of canine brain tumors.[7,9,58,84] The safety and feasibility of brain tumor ablation techniques using lasers and pulsed electrical fields have also been demonstrated in canine gliomas.[119] Technologies capable of focally disrupting the BBB to allow for CNS drug delivery, such as transcranial focused ultrasound and irreversible electroporation, are also being used to treat canine brain tumors.[119]

Approaches that bypass the BBB and allow for direct intratumoral delivery of therapeutically relevant concentrations of macromolecular drugs, such as convection-enhanced delivery (CED) of chemotherapeutics and implantation of various biodegradable nanomaterial drug carriers, have also been investigated in dogs. CED of nonselective chemotherapy drugs, such as liposomal CPT-11, and novel agents targeting the overexpression of cell surface EGFR (EGFRvIII-antibody bioconjugated nanoparticles), EphA2, and IL-13RA2 (recombinant bacterial cytotoxins) receptors that occur in canine and human gliomas, have been performed in dogs with glioma.[7,9,67,119–121] These studies have illustrated the safety of the CED procedure and have provided preliminary evidence of efficacy of these investigational agents.

There is a considerable library of targeted agents being develop for and tested in canine brain tumors, and these agents encompass a wide variety of mechanistic approaches including protease-conjugated oncolytic viruses, immunomodulatory microRNAs or small interfering RNAs, immune-checkpoint inhibitors, apoptosis promoters, radiosensitizing agents, and nanoparticular cytotoxic drugs. These compounds have shown promising antitumor effects in vitro or in vivo against non-CNS tumors, the ability to penetrate the BBB when administered systemically, or favorable safety and pharmacokinetic profiles in healthy dogs, and are currently in early phase trials in dogs with tumors.[7,9,122,123] In a proof-of-concept trial, bacterially derived minicells were packaged with doxorubicin, targeted to EGFR using bispecific antibodies to EFGR, and administered intravenously to dogs with brain tumors. Durable and objective tumor responses were seen in 24% of dogs and no significant toxicities were observed.[123]

There has been a paradigm shift away from the brain being considered an immune-privileged organ unfavorable to immunotherapeutic (IT) interventions toward an elucidation and exploitation of the unique mechanisms that characterize immunocompetency and tumor–host interactions within the brain. A diverse array of IT strategies, whose unifying goal is to introduce, stimulate, or otherwise augment the patient's T-cell–mediated immune response against cancer cells, are being explored for use in the treatment of companion animal brain tumors.[7,9,] IT approaches that involve tumor vaccinations with stimulated patient-derived dendritic cells and autologous tumor lysates combined with toll-like receptor ligands have demonstrated the safety, feasibility, and potential efficacy of IT for use in canine glioma and meningioma.[7,9,93,97]

Recent studies have provided data that indicates that novel repurposing approaches using existing drugs are capable of achieving intratumoral drug concentrations that may result in favorable therapeutic and adverse effects profiles compared with traditionally administered doses or other chemotherapy agents with the same mechanism of action.[84] An in vitro study of benzimidazole anthelmintics in canine glioma cell line demonstrated that drug treatment increased depolymerization of tubulin and increased tumor cell apoptosis compared with the controls.[124]

Tumors of the Spinal Cord

Classification and Epidemiology

As with brain tumors, SC neoplasms are classified as primary or secondary according to their tissue of origin. However, a classification scheme based on the tumor location relative to the neuraxis (Table 31.2) is the most commonly used method of clinical classification of tumors affecting the SC in veterinary medicine. The overall incidence in dogs and cats is unknown, but SC tumors appear to be less common than intracranial neoplasms.

Extradural tumors account for approximately 50% of all tumors affecting the SC and frequently arise from the vertebrae. Vertebral tumors such as osteosarcoma (OSA), chondrosarcoma (CSA), plasma cell tumors, fibrosarcoma (FSA), and HSA are commonly encountered extradural tumors (Fig. 31.5; see Table 31.2)[125–133] Intradural-extramedullary (ID-EM) tumors account for 35% of all tumors, and meningiomas are the most common ID-EM tumor (Fig. 31.6) and also the most common primary

spinal cord tumor diagnosed in dogs and cats.[125,126,131] Approximately 15% of spinal cord neoplasms are intramedullary (IM), although up to one-third of tumors may involve multiple compartments.[125–127,134,135] In dogs, ependymomas and gliomas are the most frequently diagnosed primary IM tumors, and HSA and transitional cell carcinoma are the most common secondary IM tumors.[135]

In dogs and cats, CNS lymphoma may affect any or all compartments of the SC and may occur as a primary or secondary tumor.[77,136–139] Lymphoma is the second most prevalent SC disease of cats and the most common feline SC tumor, although 85% of cases of SC lymphoma in cats are secondary and part of a multicentric process.[137–139] Older studies report that 80% to 90% of cats with CNS lymphoma were seropositive for FeLV p27 antigen; a more recent reported indicated that only 56% of cats with CNS lymphoma were infected with FeLV.[138,140] This may reflect the decreasing overall prevalence of feline retroviral infections attributable to vaccination and improved management practices, or infer the importance of other factors that contribute to development of CNS lymphomas.[141] Cats with lymphoma are typically younger (median 4 years) at diagnosis than cats with other tumor types affecting the SC (median 9 years).[138]

Large-breed, older dogs are predisposed to the development of vertebral tumors.[129,130] SC tumors such as ependymomas and nephroblastomas are more commonly seen in dogs less than 6 years old.[142,143] Young German shepherd dogs and golden retrievers (<3 years of age) are predisposed to nephroblastoma.[142,143] Boxer dogs were overrepresented in one study of intraspinal meningiomas, and both boxers and other brachycephalic breeds are predisposed to tumors of glial origin.[131,134]

Pathophysiology, History, and Clinical Signs

Dogs and cats with SC tumors commonly present for progressive myelopathic signs reflecting the neuroanatomic location of the tumor with or without evidence of pain. Tumors in ED or ID-EM locations cause clinical signs of neurologic dysfunction, mainly by compression of the spinal cord or nerve roots by the neoplasm (see Fig. 31.6). IM tumors may cause signs of spinal cord disease by compression, invasion, or destruction of the SC parenchyma, as well as by obstructing CSF flow and inducing

TABLE 31.2	Clinical Classification and Examples of Tumors Affecting the Spinal Cord	
Anatomic Location Relative to Spinal Cord		
Extradural	*Intradural-Extramedullary*	*Intramedullary*
Osteosarcoma	Meningioma	Astrocytoma
Chondrosarcoma	Peripheral nerve sheath tumor	Ependymoma
Fibrosarcoma	Nephroblastoma	Oligodendroglioma
Plasmacytoma	Histiocytic sarcoma	Gliomatosis cerebri
Multiple myeloma	Lymphoma	Hemangiosarcoma
Lymphoma		Transitional cell carcinoma
Hemangiosarcoma		Lymphmoma
Various carcinomas		

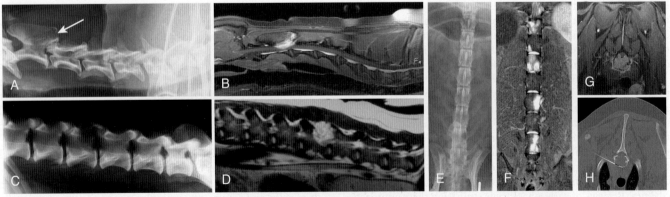

• **Fig. 31.5** Imaging features of extradural vertebral tumors. Lytic and sclerotic lesion in the C2 spinous process (A, *arrow*) and corresponding postcontrast MRI (B) illustrating spinal cord compression from a plasmacytoma. Radiographic lysis in the L4 lamina and pedicle (C), and corresponding sagittal MRI (D) demonstrating chondrosarcoma. Normal lumbar spinal radiograph (E) in dog with multifocal hyperintense foci of lymphoma in the vertebral bodies on MRI (F). MRI (G) and CT-guided needle biopsy (H) of T3 osteosarcoma.

syringomyelic syndrome (see Fig. 31.6).[135] All types of SC tumors can cause numerous secondary changes within the SC including edema, inflammation, gliosis, and hemorrhage. Signs of paraspinal hyperesthesia arise from compression, stretching, inflammation, or invasion of the meninges, nerve roots, periosteum, or paraspinal musculature. Early reports have described IM tumors as non-painful because of lack of nociceptors in the parenchyma[126,144]; however, in one study that specifically reported on the prevalence of paraspinal hyperpathia, 68% of all dogs with IM tumors displayed paraspinal hyperpathia.[135] Development of hyperpathia in association with IM tumors may be a result of altered neurotransmitter modulation association with destruction of the dorsal horn of the gray matter known as syringomyelic syndrome (see Fig. 31.6D–F).[135] Another theory postulates that intramedullary mass expansion may lead to stretching of meninges and stimulation of nociceptive pathways.

Primary IM tumors have a protracted clinical course compared with metastatic IM neoplasms.[135] Acute decompensation can occur because of pathologic fracture of neoplastic vertebra, hemorrhage in or around the tumor or SC, or necrosis of the tumor itself. Clinical signs of SC disease, rather than primary organ dysfunction, is a frequent chief complaint for animals with secondary SC tumors, occurring in up to 44% of dogs with metastatic tumors.[135,140]

Diagnosis of Spinal Cord Tumors

The minimum database for a patient with a suspected SC neoplasm is identical to that for a brain tumor patient. Although these laboratory tests will seldom provide a definitive answer regarding the etiology of SC neoplasia, they can provide valuable information with respect to hematologic abnormalities, paraneoplastic syndromes, and primary organ dysfunction that is often detected in patients with metastatic cancers such as lymphoma and multiple myeloma.[132,145]

Diagnostic Imaging

Survey radiographs may identify primary vertebral body tumors (see Fig. 31.5A, E), pathologic fractures, osseous metastases, as well as evidence of concurrent malignancy or disease, but are frequently normal (see Fig. 31.5C).[135,145] In cats, radiographically apparent lytic lesions are seen more commonly in nonlymphoid neoplasms.[133,138]

As with brain tumors, MRI is the modality of choice for the evaluation of SC tumors.[130–131,135,146,147] However, CT myelography can be helpful for determination of the longitudinal and axial location of many neoplastic lesions.[147] Irrespective of the imaging modality used, in some cases it can be difficult to distinguish ID-EM from IM origin masses.[146] Similar to what is observed with

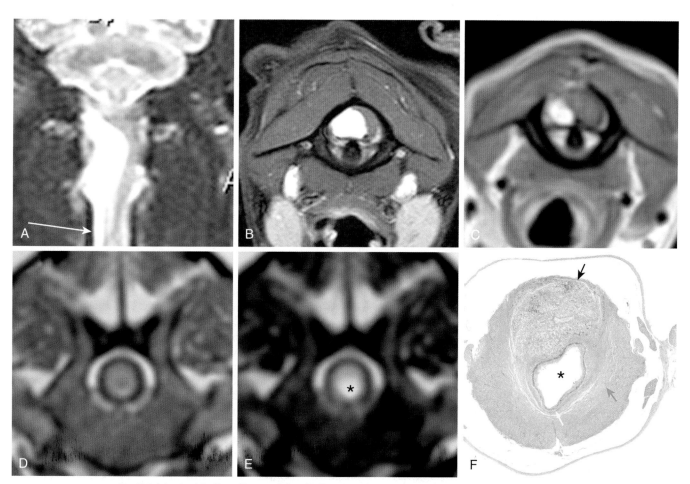

• **Fig. 31.6** Intradural (A–C) and intramedullary (D–F) canine spinal cord tumors. Dorsal STIR (A) and postcontrast magnetic resonance image (MRI) (B, C) images of C1 meningioma causing marked spinal cord compression dural tail (A, *arrow*). Recurrent tumor is visible 9 months after surgery (C). MRI of heterogeneously contrast enhancing (D) and T2 hyperintense (E) grade III oligodendroglioma that effaces the spinal cord architecture at T10. Necropsy specimen demonstrating intramedullary tumor (F, *arrow*) and syringomyelic cavity (*).

intracranial tumors, the commonly encountered vertebral and SC tumors often display characteristic MRI features that allow for presumptive diagnosis, but definitive diagnosis can only be obtained with histopathology, as there exists considerable overlap in the MRI features of specific tumor types with other neoplasms and non-neoplastic lesions.[130,131,135,146,147] Meningiomas usually appear as focal ID-EM masses, often strongly enhancing on postcontrast MRI sequences, and frequently demonstrate a dural tail (see Figs. 31.6A, B).[131] Although spinal lymphoma is commonly described as an extradural mass lesion, especially in cats, it is very often a mixed compartment neoplasm in dogs and involves extraneural tissues in both species.[77,136–139] Plasma cell tumors and lymphoma both cause osteolysis, though the latter typically spares the cortex.[148] Short tau inversion recovery (STIR) MR sequences have been reported to have the most utility for the detection of vertebral (see Figs. 31.5D, 31.6A) or SC tumors involving multiple compartments.[148]

Tumor Biopsy and Pathologys

Biopsy of tumors affecting the vertebrae or SC is required for definitive diagnosis. Biopsy is often achieved at the time of surgical excision, but needle biopsy can be performed using percutaneous, surgical free-hand and image-guided techniques, including ultrasonography and CT (see Fig. 31.5H).[149]

Among ED tumors arising from the vertebra, OSA is the most common followed by CSA and FSA.[125,130,133] A variety of ED (often epidural) tumors that often do not involve the vertebra but arise from adipose tissue have also been reported, including lipomas, infiltrative lipomas, liposarcomas, and myelolipomas. Solitary plasma cell tumors affecting the vertebra are classified as plasmacytomas (see Figs. 31.5A, B) and may precede multiple myeloma.[132] Meningiomas and nerve sheath tumors are the two most common ID-EM neoplasms, with meningiomas predominating. Nephroblastomas also are predominantly ID-EM tumors, and almost always are found between T9 and L2 spinal cord segments because of the embryologic origin of the metanephric blastema from which they arise.[142,143] Approximately 80% of canine nephroblastomas will demonstrate immunoreactivity to WT-1, a human nephroblastoma gene product.[142]

When lymphoma involves the neuraxis in dogs and cats, it is most often a manifestation of multicentric disease.[136,138,139] In cats with SC lymphoma, more than 80% had extraneural organ involvement that commonly included the bone marrow, kidneys, liver, spleen, lymph nodes, and 43% had concurrent brain involvement.[138] Immunophenotypic characterizations of the vast majority of canine and feline cases of nervous system lymphomas have not been performed, but both B- and T-cell lymphomas have been reported.[136,139] In a recent report of canine lymphoma, the only case of primary CNS lymphoma identified in the patient cohort was restricted to the SC, and was a diffuse large B-cell lymphoma characterized by CD79a staining.[136] Among the 36 cases of metastatic canine CNS lymphomas in this series, 55% were B-cell lymphomas and 45% were of T-cell lineage.[136]

Cerebrospinal Fluid Analysis

CSF analysis is frequently done in combination with cross-sectional imaging and is a sensitive but nonspecific test that does not usually provide a diagnosis, with the exception of lymphoma. In 68% of dogs with CNS lymphoma in one series, a diagnosis was made using CSF analysis, and a diagnostic CSF was more likely when infiltrative meningeal lesions were seen on MRI.[136]

Treatment and Prognosis for Tumors Affecting the Spinal Cord

There is limited information on the results of treatment of vertebral or SC tumors in veterinary medicine; however, treatment options parallel those available for brain tumor management. The principles and outcomes associated with palliative treatment of SC tumors are also generally similar those of brain tumors, with the major exception of the more intensive and multimodal pain and urinary bladder management plans that are often required in animals with SC tumors. Palliative treatment of vertebral and SC tumors rarely results in prolonged STs or satisfactory functional outcomes, with MST ranging from 0 to 105 days.[128,129,134,135] In general, despite the type of treatments currently administered, many dogs and cats with vertebral and SC tumors die or are euthanized because of tumor-related causes, which often present as a recurrence or progression of neurologic signs.[126,128,130,131] Thus presumed and confirmed local treatment failures remain a significant source of morbidity and mortality in animals with vertebral and SC tumors (see Figs. 31.6A–C).

Chemotherapy

Chemotherapy may be used as an effective primary treatment modality in cases of vertebral plasma cell tumors, multiple myeloma, or lymphoma.[132,138,140] Dogs with vertebral plasmacytomas and multiple myeloma may have favorable and durable responses to melphalan and prednisone chemotherapy, even in the face of multiple or diffuse vertebral lesions and signs of moderate SC dysfunction.[132] Although there exist numerous reports on SC lymphoma in dogs in cats, there is limited information on specific chemotherapy protocols used and the results of treatment, specifically with respect to survival and neurologic functional endpoints.[138,140] Six cats with lymphoma treated with a combination of vincristine, cyclophosphamide, and prednisone had a complete remission rate of 50% and the median duration of remission was 14 weeks.[150] Platinum-based chemotherapeutic agents are often use as adjunctive treatment in cases of vertebral OSA.[129]

Surgery and Radiation Therapy

In addition to providing a histopathologic diagnosis, cytoreductive surgery often results in a significant acute clinical benefit from SC decompression.[128,129,131,133] Depending on the tumor type, surgery alone may convey sustained improvement in neurologic function.

Meningiomas can be treated effectively with surgery, with or without postoperative RT.[131,133] The MSTs for dogs with intraspinal meningioma treated with surgery alone vary widely and range from 6 to 47 months.[129,131,151,152] Serious surgical adverse events are more common with treatment of cranial cervical meningiomas because of compromise of critical respiratory or vascular structures.[131] The addition of postoperative RT in dogs with meningiomas increased the MST to approximately 45 months; dogs receiving RT took significantly longer to neurologically decline than dogs that did not, thus delaying the period to clinical deterioration because of local treatment failure.[131] In cats with spinal meningiomas treated surgically, reported MSTs are 6 to 17 months.[133,144]

Vertebral tumors in dogs and cats are frequently treated with multimodal therapy consisting of surgery, RT, and/or chemotherapy. The long-term prognosis associated with vertebral tumors is guarded, with one study reporting an overall MST of 4.5 months in dogs with a variety of vertebral tumors.[129] In this study, the posttreatment neurologic status was the only significant prognostic factor where a nonambulatory status was significantly associated with shorter STs.[129] Two dogs with CSAs treated with surgery alone both had a recurrence of clinical signs because of imaging confirmed tumor recurrence within 5 months of surgery.[130]

Cats with malignant vertebral tumors also have a guarded to poor long-term prognosis with surgical treatment, with a reported MST of 3.7 months in one study.[133] The literature indicates that common contemporary veterinary neurosurgical techniques are generally insufficient to attain the goal of en bloc surgical excision of vertebral tumors, which is critical to the therapeutic outcome in humans.[129,130,133] Thus, although currently largely unexplored in veterinary medicine, aggressive surgical techniques, including vertebrectomy with vertebral stabilization, will likely become an important component of advancing the surgical treatment of vertebral and SC tumors.[153]

Currently, there is insufficient information to clearly identify the superior method of treatment of solitary vertebral plasma cell tumors in dogs and cats. Solitary plasmacytomas have been treated successfully with surgery, RT, and various combinations of these modalities.[132,154]

Dogs with nephroblastomas treated with surgery and RT may also experience improved functional outcomes and STs compared with those not treated surgically, although reported MSTs vary widely.[142,143] In one study, MST for dogs that were not treated surgically was 1 day compared with 71 days for dogs that underwent cytoreductive surgery.[142] Another investigation reported that dogs with nephroblastoma treated with cytoreductive surgery or RT survived longer (MST 374 days) than dogs treated palliatively (MST 55 days).[143] Tumors confined to an ID-EM location were associated with superior STs (MST 380 days) than tumors with IM involvement (MST 140 days).[143] As nephroblastoma affects young dogs, the literature suggests that the majority of dogs will experience life-limiting local tumor recurrence or treatment complications regardless of treatment type.[142,143]

The outcomes associated with other specific types of SC tumors are unknown owing to very limited numbers of reported cases that received treatment, and in some instances, cases received RT treatment without histologic confirmation of the type of lesion being treated.[155] A few case reports suggest that primary IM neuroepithelial neoplasms may be resected if well-demarcated and that long-term successful outcomes are possible with combinations of surgery, with and without RT.[156] However, most animals with IM tumors are euthanized at or near the time of diagnosis because of poor prognosis or failure to respond to palliative therapy.[134,135]

Tumors of Cranial, Paraspinal, and Peripheral Nerves

Classification, Epidemiology, and Comparative Pathology

Peripheral nerve tumors (often collectively called *peripheral nerve sheath tumors* [PNSTs]) are uncommon in dogs and rare in cats. PNSTs may arise from Schwann cells, perineurial cells, or intraneural fibroblasts. Descriptive terminology that reflects the cellular origin of these tumors (schwannoma, neurofibroma, neurofibrosarcoma) is not routinely used because of the inherent level of difficulty in determining the tissue of origin of these tumors in veterinary medicine. Instead, PNSTs are divided into benign peripheral nerve sheath tumors (BPNSTs) or malignant peripheral nerve sheath tumors (MPNSTs) based on microscopic evidence of malignancy.[157–159] This latter classification scheme is more useful from a clinical standpoint, as the majority of reported PNSTs in dogs are histologically and biologically aggressive tumors. Cats have a higher proportion of BPNSTs compared with dogs.[158]

PNSTs may arise in any cranial nerve, spinal nerve root, or somatic or autonomic peripheral nerve.[157–160] PNSTs occur most commonly in middle-aged to older dogs of medium and large breeds. No breed or sex predilection has been noted. The most frequently affected cranial nerve is the trigeminal nerve, and the most common spinal nerve roots affected are in the caudal cervical region (C6–T2) followed by nerves of the lumbar intumescence (Fig. 31.7).[157–160] Metastasis is rare. Secondary tumors, such as lymphoma, malignant sarcomas, HS, and hamartomas, can occasionally involve peripheral nerves.[136,138,139] In cats, diffuse infiltrative peripheral nerve lymphoma (neurolymphomatosis) is usually B-cell origin, but one case of peripheral T-cell lymphoma in an FeLV-positive cat has been reported.[161,162] In dogs, peripheral nerve lymphoma is typically of T-cell origin.[136]

Pathophysiology, History, and Clinical Signs

As with brain and spinal tumors, the clinical signs of PNSTs reflect the location of the tumor. As the majority of reported canine PNSTs involve the nerve roots and/or nerves of the brachial and

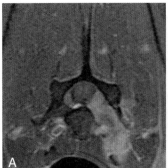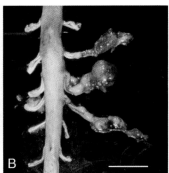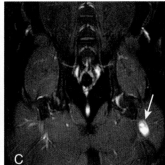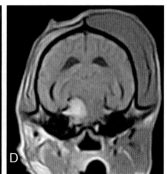

• **Fig. 31.7** MRI and pathologic features of PNST. (A) Postcontrast MRI of C7 MPNST manifesting as thickening and contrast enhancement of the affected nerve, as well as intradural invasion. (B) At necropsy, a MPNST appears as nodular masses on the C7, C8, and T1 nerves. Bar = 1.5 cm. (C) Dorsal MRI image of a sciatic PNST causing enlargement of hyperintensity of the affected nerve (*arrow*). (D) MRI of a trigeminal PNST with compression of the midbrain and atrophy of the muscles of mastication ipsilateral to the tumor.

lumbar plexi, the classic clinical scenario is one of chronic lameness without identifiable orthopedic abnormalities.[163,164] The etiology of the observed clinical signs may remain elusive for months and may not be appreciated until signs progress to monoparesis with neurogenic atrophy or signs of spinal cord disease appear. Signs of myelopathy are often asymmetric and occur when the mass invades the vertebral canal and compresses or invades the SC. Clinical signs of pain on palpation or paresthesia are also common.

Trigeminal PNSTs cause signs of severe, unilateral masticatory muscular atrophy, diminished jaw tone, decreased facial sensation, and Horner's syndrome.[160] Brainstem involvement may result in other regional cranial nerve deficits and long tract signs depending on size and invasiveness of the mass (see Fig. 31.7D). Peripheral nerve lymphoma may present with a clinical history similar to PNST or with neurolymphomatosis. In the latter scenario, flaccid tetraparesis and hyporeflexia can reflect the diffuse neoplastic infiltrative neuropathy.[161]

Diagnosis of PNSTs

Approximately 33% of cases with PNST affecting the brachial plexus will have a palpable mass on physical examination.[157,163,165] Ultrasound of the axillary region appears to be more sensitive for the detection of mass lesions than palpation, but not as useful as MRI.[166]

PNST can be challenging to diagnose, and exploratory surgery and biopsy is sometimes required. The most useful imaging tool for diagnosing PNST and discriminating other etiologies of the observed clinical signs is MRI, whether the lesion involves a plexus, the SC, or a cranial nerve, although CT-myelography is described.[160,166] To facilitate the diagnosis of PNST, cross-sectional imaging should include sequences with a wide field of view to incorporate the plexi and limb structures (see Fig. 31.7C). On MRI examinations of PNST cases, up to 50% of patients display only nerve thickening rather than a discrete mass (see Fig. 31.7A).[160,166,167] Postcontrast sequences are particularly helpful in the identification of subtle tumors. Idiopathic neuritis, hypertrophic ganglioneuritis, and peripheral nerve lymphomas may have an identical appearance on MRI to PNST.[166,168]

Treatment and Prognosis of PNSTs

Surgery is the preferred treatment of PNSTs in dogs and cats.[157,158] The prognosis for paraspinal or plexus PNSTs depends in part on tumor location and whether or not the tumor is amenable to complete resection using amputation, compartmental resection with limb sparing, laminectomy, or combinations of techniques.[157,158,169] Proximity to and invasion into the vertebral canal, which occurs in 45% of dogs, and the presence of tumor infiltrated margins after compartmental resection are negative prognostic indicators.[157,169] In dogs, the overall prognosis historically is considered guarded to poor, with MSTs of approximately 6 months for dogs with paraspinal and plexus PNST, reflecting the more malignant biologic behavior of canine PNST. Long-term survival is possible after complete resection of tumors,[163] including the use of limb sparing techniques (MST 1303 days).[169] Recently, a study investigating VMAT radiotherapy for the treatment of canine PNST reported outcomes that were superior to earlier reports of surgically treated dogs with evidence of nerve root and vertebral canal invasion, with a mean progression-free

ST of 8 months.[170] The prognosis for cats is more favorable. In one study of 45 surgically treated cats, 31% (5/16) of MPNST recurred compared with 14% (4/43) of BPNST.[158] Treatment failures typically manifest as neurologic signs attributed to local recurrence.

Canine trigeminal PNST may have an insidious clinical course, with some untreated dogs experiencing STs in excess of 18 months without significant clinical progression.[160,167,171] Trigeminal PNSTs may be surgically removed or irradiated and successful outcomes have been reported for both treatment modalities.[160,167,171] The MSTs for dogs with trigeminal PNST treated with SRS or SRT is reported as 745 days[167] and 441 days.[171] RT may be superior to palliative and surgical treatment, particularly with respect to resolving neurologic signs in cases with clinical and imaging evidence of brainstem involvement.[111,167,171] Peripheral nerve lymphomas, which may be indistinguishable from PNST, may respond to radiation or chemotherapy, although no current literature provides specific treatment recommendations or outcomes of dogs or cats with peripheral nerve lymphoma or neurolymphomatosis.

References

1. Song RB, Vite CH, Bradley CE, et al.: Postmortem evaluation of 435 cases of intracranial neoplasia in dogs and relationship of neoplasm with breed, age, and body weight, *J Vet Intern Med* 27:1143–1152, 2013.
2. Snyder JM, Shofer FS, Van Winkle TJ, et al.: Primary intracranial neoplasia in dogs: 173 cases (1986–2003), *J Vet Intern Med* 20:669–675, 2006.
3. Troxel MT, Vite CH, Van Winkle TJ, et al.: Feline intracranial neoplasia: retrospective review of 160 cases (1985–2001), *J Vet Intern Med* 17:850–859, 2003.
4. Snyder JM, Lipitz L, Skorupski KA, et al.: Secondary intracranial neoplasia in the dog: 177 cases (1986-2003), *J Vet Intern Med* 22:172–177, 2008.
5. Louis DN, Ohgaki K, Wiestler OD, et al.: The 2007 WHO classification of tumours of the central nervous system, *Acta Neuropathol* 114:97–109, 2007.
6. Solleveld HA, Bigner DD, Averill DR, et al.: Brain tumors in man and animals: report of a workshop, *Environ Health Perspect* 68:155–173, 1986.
7. Dickinson PJ: Advances in diagnostic and treatment modalities for intracranial tumors, *J Vet Intern Med* 28:1165–1185, 2014.
8. Dickinson PJ, York D, Higgins RJ, et al.: Chromosomal aberrations in canine gliomas define candidate genes and common pathways in dogs and humans, *J Neuropathol Exp Neurol* 75:700–710, 2016.
9. Rossmeisl JH: New treatment modalities for brain tumors in dogs and cats, *Vet Clin North Am Sm Anim Pract* 44:1013–1038, 2014.
10. Connolly NP, Shetty AC, Stokum JA, et al.: Cross-species transcriptional analysis reveals conserved and host-specific neoplastic processes in mammalian glioma, *Sci Rep* 8:1180, 2018.
11. Koestner A, Bilzer T, Fatzer R, et al.: *Histological classification of tumors of the nervous system of domestic animals*, vol. 5. Washington, DC, 1999, Armed Forces Institute of Pathology.
12. Patnaik AK, Ehler WJ, MacEwen EG: Canine cutaneous mast cell tumor: morphologic grading and survival time in 83 dogs, *Vet Pathol* 21:469–474, 1984.
13. Louis DN, Perry A, Reifenberger G, et al.: The 2016 World Health Organization classification of tumors of the central nervous system: a summary, *Acta Neuropathol* 131:803–820, 2016.
14. Vandevelde M: Brain tumors in domestic animals: an overview, *Proceedings of the Conference on Brain Tumors in Man and Animals* NC, 1984, Research Triangle Park. September 5-6.

15. Hayes HM, Priester Jr WA, Pendergrass TW: Occurrence of nervous-tissue tumors in cattle, horses, cats and dogs, *Int J Cancer* 15:39–47, 1975.
16. Priester WA, Mantel N: Occurrence of tumors in domestic animals. Data from 12 United States and Canadian colleges of veterinary medicine, *J Natl Cancer Inst* 47:1333–1344, 1971.
17. Zaki FA, Hurvita AI: Spontaneous neoplasms of the central nervous system of the cat, *J Sm Anim Pract* 17:733–782, 1976.
18. Dorn CR, Taylor DO, Frye FL, et al.: Survey of animal neoplasms in Alameda and Contra Costa Counties, California. I. Methodology and description of cases, *J Natl Cancer Inst* 40:295–305, 1968.
19. McGrath JT: Intracranial pathology of the dog, *Acta Neuropathol (Berl)* (Suppl I):3–4, 1962.
20. Sturges BK, Dickinson PJ, Bollen AW, et al.: Magnetic resonance imaging and histological classification of intracranial meningiomas in 112 dogs, *J Vet Intern Med* 22, 2008. 586–585.
21. Westworth DR, Dickinson PJ, Vernau W, et al.: Choroid plexus tumors in 56 dogs (1985-2007), *J Vet Intern Med* 22:1157–1165, 2008.
22. Kube SA, Bruyette DS, Hanson SM: Astrocytomas in young dogs, *J Am Anim Hosp Assoc* 39:288–293, 2003.
23. Truvé K, Dickinson P, Xiong A, York Daniel, et al.: Utilizing the dog genome in the search for novel candidate genes involved in glioma development—Genome Wide Association Mapping followed by targeted massive parallel sequencing identifies a strongly associated locus, *PLOS Genetics* 12:e1006000, 2016.
24. Tomek A, Cizinauskas S, Doherr M, et al.: Intracranial neoplasia in 61 cats: localization, tumour types and seizure patterns, *J Feline Med Surg* 8:243–253, 2006.
25. Rossmeisl JH, Pancotto TE: Intracranial neoplasia and secondary pathological effects. In Platt S, Garosi L, editors: *Small animal neurological emergencies*, ed 1, London, 2012, Manson Publishing, pp 461–478.
26. Bagley RS, Gavin PR, Moore MP, et al.: Clinical signs associated with brain tumors in dogs: 97 cases (1992–1997), *J Am Vet Med Assoc* 215:818–819, 1999.
27. Bagley RS, Gavin PR: Seizures as a complication of brain tumors in dogs, *Clin Tech Sm Anim Pract* 13:179–184, 1998.
28. Schwartz M, Lamb CR, Brodbelt DC, et al.: Canine intracranial neoplasia: clinical risk factors for the development of epileptic seizures, *J Sm Anim Pract* 52:632–637, 2011.
29. Cameron S, Rishiniw M, Miller AD, et al.: Characteristics and survival of 121 cats undergoing excision of intracranial meningiomas (1994-2011), *Vet Surg* 44:772–776, 2015.
30. Rossmeisl JH, Jones JC, Zimmerman KL, et al.: Survival time following hospital discharge in dogs with palliatively treated brain tumors, *J Am Vet Med Assoc* 242:193–198, 2013.
31. Wood FD, Pollard RE, Uerling MR, et al.: Diagnostic imaging findings and endocrine test results in dogs with pituitary-dependent hyperadrenocorticism that did or did not have neuro-logic abnormalities: 157 cases (1989–2005), *J Am Vet Med Assoc* 231:1081–1085, 2007.
32. Rossmeisl JH, Clapp K, Pancotto TE, et al.: Canine butterfly glioblastomas: A neuroradiological review, *Front Vet Sci* 3:40, 2016.
33. McDonnell JJ, Kalbko K, Keating JH, et al.: Multiple meningiomas in three dogs, *J Am Anim Hosp Assoc* 43:201–208, 2007.
34. Forterre F, Tomek A, Konar M, et al.: Multiple meningiomas: clinical, radiological, surgical and pathological findings with outcome in four cats, *J Feline Med Surg* 9:36–43, 2007.
35. Koch MW, Sánchez MD, Long S: Multifocal oligodendroglioma in three dogs, *J Am Anim Hosp Assoc* 47:77–85, 2011.
36. Alves A, Prada J, Almeida JM, et al.: Primary and secondary tumours occurring simultaneously in the brain of a dog, *J Small Anim Pract* 47:607–610, 2006.
37. Patnaik AK, Erlandson RA, Lieberman PH, et al.: Choroid plexus carcinoma with meningeal carcinomatosis in a dog, *Vet Pathol* 17:381–385, 1980.
38. Tong MN, Zwingenberger AL, Blair WH, et al.: Effect of screening abdominal ultrasound examination on the decision to pursue advanced diagnostic tests and treatment in dogs with neurologic disease, *J Vet Intern Med* 29:893–899, 2015.
39. Bigio Marcello A, Gieger TL, Jimenez DA, et al.: Detection of comorbidities and synchronous primary tumours via thoracic radiography and abdominal ultrasonography and their influence on treatment outcome in dogs with soft tissue sarcomas, primary brain tumours and intranasal tumours, *Vet Comp Oncol* 13:433–442, 2013.
40. Rodenas S, Pumarola M, Gaitero L, et al.: Magnetic resonance imaging findings in 40 dogs with histologically confirmed intracranial tumours, *Vet J* 187:85–91, 2011.
41. Wisner ER, Dickinson PJ, Higgins RJ: Magnetic resonance imaging features of canine intracranial neoplasia, *Vet Radiol Ultrasound* 52:S52–S61, 2011.
42. Bentley RT: Magnetic resonance imaging diagnosis of brain tumors in dogs, *Vet J* 205:204–216, 2015.
43. Stadler K, Ruth JD, Pancotto TE, et al.: Computed tomography and magnetic resonance imaging are equivalent in mensuration and similarly inaccurate in type and grade predictability of canine intracranial gliomas, *Front Vet Sci* 4:157, 2017.
44. Rossmeisl JH, Kopf K, Ruth J: Magnetic resonance imaging of meningiomas associated with transcalvarial extension through osteolytic skull defects in a cat and two dogs, *J Vet Med Res* 2:1025, 2015.
45. Graham JP, Newell SM, Voges AK, et al.: The dural tail sign in the diagnosis of meningiomas, *Vet Rad Ultrasound* 39:297–302, 1998.
46. Cherubini GB, Mantis P, Martinez TA, et al.: Utility of magnetic resonance imaging for distinguishing neoplastic from non-neoplastic brain lesions in dogs and cats, *Vet Radiol Ultrasound* 46:384–387, 2005.
47. Wolff CA, Holmes BD, Young BD, et al.: Magnetic resonance imaging for the differentiation of neoplastic, inflammatory, and cerebrovascular brain disease in dogs, *J Vet Intern Med* 26:589–597, 2012.
48. Troxel MT, Vite CH, Massicotte C, et al.: Magnetic resonance imaging features of feline intracranial neoplasia: retrospective analysis of 46 cats, *J Vet Intern Med* 18:176–189, 2004.
49. Mariani CL, Jennings MK, Olby NJ, et al.: Histiocytic sarcoma with central nervous system involvement in dogs; 19 cases (2006-2012), *J Vet Intern Med* 29:607–613, 2015.
50. Young BD, Levine JM, Porter BF, et al.: Magnetic resonance imaging features of intracranial astrocytomas and oligodendrogliomas in dogs, *Vet Radiol Ultrasound* 52:132–141, 2011.
51. Vite CH, Cross JR: Correlating magnetic resonance finding with neuropathology and clinical signs in dogs and cats, *Vet Radiol Ultrasound* 52:S23–S31, 2011.
52. Cervera V, Mai W, Vite CH, et al.: Comparative magnetic resonance imaging findings between gliomas and presumed cerebrovascular accidents in dogs, *Vet Radiol Ultrasound* 52:33–40, 2011.
53. Young BD, Fosgate GT, Holmes SP, et al.: Evaluation of standard magnetic resonance characteristics used to differentiate neoplastic, inflammatory, and vascular brain lesions in dogs, *Vet Radiol Ultrasound* 55:399–406, 2014.
53. Sutherland-Smith J, King R, Faissler D, et al.: Magnetic resonance imaging apparent diffusion coefficients for histologically confirmed intracranial lesions in dogs, *Vet Radiol Ultra-sound* 52:142–148, 2011.
54. Zhao Q, Lee S, Kent M, et al.: Dynamic contrast-enhanced magnetic resonance imaging of canine brain tumors, *Vet Radiol Ultrasound* 51:122–129, 2010.
55. DeJesus A, Cohen EB, Galban E, et al.: Magnetic resonance imaging features of intraventricular ependymomas in five cats, *Vet Radiol Ultrasound* 58:326–333, 2017.

56. Koblik PD, LeCouteur RA, Higgins RJ, et al.: CT-guided brain biopsy using a modified Pelorus Mark III stereotactic system: experience with 50 dogs, *Vet Radiol Ultrasound* 40:434–440, 1999.

57. Moissonnier P, Blot S, Devauchelle P, et al.: Stereotactic CT-guided brain biopsy in the dog, *J Small Anim Pract* 43:115–123, 2002.

58. Rossmeisl JH, Andriani RA, Cecere TE, et al.: Frame-based stereotactic biopsy of canine brain masses: technique and clinical results in 26 cases, *Front Vet Sci* 2:20, 2015.

59. Barnhart KF, Wojcieszyn J, Storts RW: Immunohistochemical staining patterns of canine meningiomas and correlation with published immunophenotypes, *Vet Pathol* 39:311–321, 2002.

60. Ide T, Uchida K, Kikuta F, et al.: Immunohistochemical characterization of canine neuroepithelial tumors, *Vet Pathol* 47:741–750, 2010.

61. Lipsitz D, Higgins RJ, Kortz GD, et al.: Glioblastoma multiforme: clinical findings, magnetic resonance imaging, and pathology in five dogs, *Vet Pathol* 40:659–669, 2003.

62. Stoica G, Kim HT, Hall DG, et al.: Morphology, immunohistochemistry, and genetic alterations in dog astrocytomas, *Vet Pathol* 41:10–19, 2004.

63. Stoica G, Levine J, Wolff J, Murphy K: Canine astrocytic tumors: a comparative review, *Vet Pathol* 48:266–275, 2011.

64. Sloma EA, Creneti CT, Erb HN, et al.: Characterization of inflammatory changes associated with canine oligodendroglioma, *J Comp Pathol* 153:92–100, 2015.

65. Dicksinson PJ, Keel MK, Higgins RJ, et al.: Clinical and pathological features of oligodendrogliomas in two cats, *Vet Pathol* 37:16–167, 2000.

66. Rissi DR, Miller AD: Feline glioma: A retrospective study and review of the literature, *J Fel Med Surg* 19:1307–1314, 2017.

67. Debinski W, Dickinson P, Rossmeisl JH, et al.: New agents for targeting of IL-13RA2 expressed in primary human and canine brain tumors, *PLoS One* 8:e77719, 2013.

68. Courtay-Cahen C, Platt SR, De Risio L, et al.: Preliminary analysis of genomic abnormalities in canine meningiomas, *Vet Comp Oncol* 6:182–192, 2008.

69. Thomas R, Duke SE, Wang HJ, et al.: 'Putting our heads together': insights into genomic conservation between human and canine intracranial tumors, *J Neurooncol* 94:333–349, 2009.

70. Boudreau CE, York D, Higgins RJ, et al.: Molecular signaling pathways in canine gliomas, *Vet Comp Oncol* e15:133–150, 2017.

71. York D, Higgins RJ, LeCouteur RA, et al.: TP53 mutations in canine brain tumors, *Vet Pathol* 49:796–801, 2012.

72. Ancona D, York D, Higgins RJ, et al.: Comparative cytogenetic analysis of dog and human choroid plexus tumors defines sytenic regions of genomic loss, *J Neuropathol Exp Neurol* 77:413–419, 2018.

73. Thomson SA, Kennerly E, Olby N, et al.: Microarray analysis of differentially expressed genes of primary tumors in the canine central nervous system, *Vet Pathol* 42:550–558, 2005.

74. Dickinson PJ, Surace EI, Cambell M, et al.: Expression of the tumor suppressor genes NF2, 4.1B, and TSLC1 in canine meningiomas, *Vet Pathol* 46:884–892, 2009.

75. Bailey CS, Higgins RJ: Characteristics of cisternal cerebrospinal fluid associated with primary brain tumors in the dog: a retrospective study, *J Am Vet Med Assoc* 188:414–417, 1986.

76. Dickinson PJ, Sturges BK, Kass PH, et al.: Characteristics of cisternal cerebrospinal fluid associated with intracranial meningiomas in dogs: 56 cases (1985-2004), *J Am Med Vet Assoc* 15:564–567, 2006.

77. Palus V, Volk HA, Lamb CR, et al.: MRI features of CNS lymphoma in dogs and cats, *Vet Radiol Ultrasound* 53:44–49, 2012.

78. Hu H, Barker A, Harcourt-Brown T, et al.: Systematic review of brain tumor treatment in dogs, *J Vet Intern Med* 29:1456–1463, 2015.

79. Van Meervenne S, Verhoeven PS, de Vos J, et al.: Comparison between symptomatic treatment and lomustine supplementation in 71 dogs with intracranial, space-occupying lesions, *Vet Comp Oncol* 12:67–77, 2014.

80. Kent MS, Bommarito D, Feldman E, et al.: Survival, neurologic response, and prognostic factors in dogs with pituitary masses treated with radiation therapy and untreated dogs, *J Vet Intern Med* 21:1027–1033, 2007.

81. Dolera M, Malfassi, Bianchi C, et al.: Frameless stereotactic radiotherapy alone and combined with temozolamide for presumed canine gliomas, *Vet Comp Oncol* 16:90–101, 2018.

82. Jeffrey N, Brearley MJ: Brain tumors in the dog: Treatment of 10 cases and review of recent literature, *J Small Anim Pract* 34:367–372, 1993.

83. Jung DI, Kim HJ, Park C, et al.: Long-term chemotherapy with lomustine of intracranial meningioma occurring in a miniature schnauzer, *J Vet Med Sci* 68:383–386, 2006.

84. Bentley RT, Thomovsky SA, Miller MA, et al. Canine (pet dog) tumor microsurgery and intratumoral concentration and safety of metronomic chlorambucil for spontaneous glioma: a phase I clinical trial. *World Neurosurg* e-pub ahead of print 5/19/18; https://doi:10.1016/j.wneu.2018.05.027 2018.

85. Rossmeisl Jr JH, Garcia PA, Daniel GB, et al.: Invited review-neuroimaging response assessment criteria for brain tumors in veterinary patients, *Vet Radiol Ultrasound* 55:115–132, 2014.

86. Chow KE, Tyrell D, Long SN: Early post-operative magnetic resonance imaging findings in five dogs with confirmed and suspected brain tumors, *Vet Radiol Ultrasound* 56:531–539, 2015.

87. Gordon LE, Thacher C, Matthiesen DT, et al.: Results of craniotomy for the treatment of cerebral meningioma in 42 cats, *Vet Surg* 23:94–100, 1994.

88. Gallagher JG, Berg J, Knowles KE, et al.: Prognosis after surgical excision of cerebral meningiomas in cats: 17 cases (1986–1992), *J Am Vet Med Assoc* 203:1437–1440, 1993.

89. Bryant KJ, Steinberg H, McAnulty JF: Cranioplasty by means of molded polymethylmethacrylate prosthetic reconstruction after radical excision of neoplasms of the skull in two dogs, *J Am Vet Med Assoc* 223:67–72, 2003.

90. Klopp LS, Rao S: Endoscopic-assisted intracranial tumor removal in dogs and cats: long-term outcome of 39 cases, *J Vet Intern Med* 23:108–115, 2009.

91. Kostolich M, Dulisch ML: A surgical approach to the canine olfactory bulb for meningioma removal, *Vet Surg* 16:273277, 1987.

92. Axlund TW, McGlasson ML, Smith AN: Surgery alone or in combination with radiation therapy for treatment of intra-cranial meningiomas in dogs: 31 cases (1989–2002), *J Am Vet Med Assoc* 221:1597–1600, 2002.

93. Andersen BM, Pluhar E, Seiler C, et al.: Vaccination for invasive canine meningioma induces in situ production of antibodies capable of antibody dependent cell-mediated cytotoxicity, *Cancer Res* 73:2987–2997, 2013.

94. Greco JJ, Aiken SA, Berg JM, et al.: Evaluation of intracranial meningioma resection with a surgical aspirator in dogs: 17 cases (1996–2004), *J Am Vet Med Assoc* 229:394–400, 2006.

95. Theon AP, Lecouteur RA, Carr EA, et al.: Influence of tumor cell proliferation and sex-hormone receptors on effectiveness of radiation therapy for dogs with incompletely resected meningiomas, *J Am Vet Med Assoc* 216:701–707, 2000.

96. Keyerleber MA, McEntee MC, Farrely J, et al.: Three-dimensional conformal radiation therapy alone or in combination with surgery for treatment of canine intracranial meningiomas, *Vet Comp Oncol* 13:385–397, 2015.

97. Maclellan JD, Arnold SA, Dave AC, et al.: Association of magnetic resonance imaging-based preoperative tumor volume with postsurgical survival time in dogs with primary intracranial glioma, *J Am Vet Med Assoc* 252:98–102, 2018.

98. Nakano Y, Nakata K, Shibata S, et al.: Fluorescein sodium-guided resection of intracranial lesions in 22 dogs, *Vet Surg* 47:302–309, 2018.

99. Mariani CL, Jennings MK, Olby NJ, et al.: Histiocytic sarcoma with central nervous system involvement in dogs; 19 cases (2006-2012), *J Vet Intern Med* 29:607–613, 2015.

100. Meij B, Voorhout G, Rijnberk A: Progress in transsphenoidal hypophysectomy for treatment of pituitary-dependent hyperadrenocorticism in dogs and cats, *Mol Cell Endocrinol* 197:89–96, 2002.

101. Meij BP, Auriemma E, Grinwis G, et al.: Successful treatment of acromegaly in a diabetic cat with transsphenoidal hypophysectomy, *J Feline Med Surg* 12:406–410, 2010.

102. Mamelak AN, Owe TN, Bruyette D: Transsphenoidal surgery using a high-definition video telescope for pituitary adenomas in dogs with pituitary dependent hypercortisolism: methods and results, *Vet Surg* 43:369–379, 2014.

103. Dernell WS, Straw RC, Cooper MF, et al.: Multilobular osteochondrosarcoma in 39 dogs: 1979-1993, *J Am Anim Hosp Assoc* 34:11–18, 1998.

104. Marino DJ, Dewey CW, Loughin CA, et al.: Severe hyperthermia, hypernatremia, and early postoperative death after transethmoidal cavitron ultrasonic surgical aspirator (CUSA)-assisted diencephalic mass removal in 4 dogs and 2 cats, *Vet Surg* 43:888–894, 2014.

105. Forward AK, Volk HA, De Decker S: Postoperative survival and early complications after intracranial surgery in dogs, *Vet Surg* 47:549–554, 2018.

106. Evans SM, Dayrell-Hart B, Powlis W, et al.: Radiation therapy of canine brain masses, *J Vet Intern Med* 7:216–219, 1993.

107. Lester NV, Hopkins AL, Bova FJ, et al.: Radiosurgery using a stereotactic headframe system for irradiation of brain tumors in dogs, *J Am Vet Med Assoc* 219:1562–1567, 2001.

108. Bley CR, Sumova A, Roos M, et al.: Irradiation of brain tumors in dogs with neurologic disease, *J Vet Intern Med* 19:849–854, 2005.

109. Spugnini EP, Thrall DE, Price GS, et al.: Primary irradiation of canine intracranial masses, *Vet Radiol Ultrasound* 41:377–380, 2000.

110. Brearley MJ, Jeffery ND, Phillips SM, et al.: Hypofractionated radiation therapy of brain masses in dogs: a retrospective analysis of survival of 83 cases (1991–1996), *J Vet Intern Med* 13:408–412, 1999.

111. Mariani CL, Schubert TA, House RA, et al.: Frameless stereotactic radiosurgery for the treatment of primary intracranial tumours in dogs, *Vet Comp Oncol* 13:409–423, 2015.

112. Platt SR, Scase TJ, Adams V, et al.: Vascular endothelial growth factor expression in canine intracranial meningiomas and association with patient survival, *J Vet Intern Med* 20:663–668, 2006.

113. Dow SW, Lecouteur RA, Rosychuk RA, et al.: Response of dogs with functional pituitary macroadenomas and macrocarcinomas to radiation, *J Small Anim Pract* 31:287–294, 1990.

114. Mayer MN, Greco DS, LaRue SM: Outcomes of pituitary tumor irradiation in cats, *J Vet Intern Med* 20:1151–1154, 2006.

115. Theon AP, Feldman EC: Megavoltage irradiation of pituitary macrotumors in dogs with neurologic signs, *J Am Vet Med Assoc* 213:225–231, 1998.

116. Goossens MM, Feldman EC, Theon AP, et al.: Efficacy of cobalt 60 radiotherapy in dogs with pituitary-dependent hyperadrenocorticism, *J Am Vet Med Assoc* 212:374–376, 1998.

117. Marcinowska A, Warland J, Brearley M, et al.: Comparison of two course fractionated radiation protocols for the management of canine pituitary macrotumor: an observational study of 24 dogs, *Vet Radiol Ultrasound* 56:554–562, 2015.

118. LeBlanc AK, Mazcko C, Brown DE, et al.: Creation of an NCI comparative brain tumor consortium: informing the translation of new knowledge from canine to human brain tumor patients, *Neuro Oncol* 18:1209–1218, 2016.

119. Rossmeisl JH: Maximizing local access to therapeutic deliveries in glioblastoma. Part V: Clinically relevant model for testing new therapeutic approaches. In De Vleeschouwer S, editor: *Glioblastoma*. Brisbane, Codon Publications, 2017, pp 405–425.

120. Dickinson PJ, LeCouteur RA, Higgins RJ, et al.: Canine spontaneous glioma: a translational model system for convection-enhanced delivery, *Neuro Oncol* 12:928–940, 2010.

121. Platt SR, Nduom E, Kent M, et al.: Canine model of convection-enhanced delivery of cetuximab-conjugated iron-oxide nanoparticles monitored with magnetic resonance imaging, *Clin Neurosurg* 59:107–113, 2012.

122. Joshi AD, Botham RC, Roth HS, et al.: An oral procaspase activating drug, PAC-1, shows preclinical promise for glioblastoma therapy, *Cancer Res* 75:S3620, 2015.

123. MacDiarmid JA, Langova V, Bailey D, et al.: Targeted doxorubicin delivery to brain tumors via minicells: proof of principle using dogs with spontaneously occurring tumors as a model, *PLoS One* 11:e0151832, 2016.

124. Lai S, Koehler J: In vitro anti-tubulin effects of benzimidazole anthelmintics mebendazole and fenbendazole on canine glioblastoma cells, *J Vet Intern Med* 30:1434–1435, 2016.

125. Johnson KB, Manhart K, Vite C, et al.: 399 spinal tumors in dogs, *J Vet Intern Med* 21:639–640, 2007.

126. Luttgen PJ, Braund KG, Brawner Jr WR, et al.: A retrospective study of 29 spinal tumors in the dog and cat, *J Sm Anim Pract* 21:213–216, 1980.

127. Wright JA: The pathological features associated with spinal tumours in 29 dogs, *J Comp Pathol* 95:549–557, 1985.

128. Levy MS, Kapatkin AS, Patnaik AK, et al.: Spinal tumors in 37 dogs: clinical outcome and long-term survival (1987-1994), *J Am Anim Hosp Assoc* 33:307–312, 1997.

129. Dernell WS, Van Vechten BJ, Straw R, et al.: Outcome following treatment of vertebral tumors in 20 dogs (1986-1995), *J Am Anim Hosp Assoc* 36:245–251, 2000.

130. Roynard PFP, Bilderback A, Falzone C, et al.: Magnetic resonance imaging, treatment, and outcome of canine vertebral chondrosarcomas. Six cases, *J Sm Anim Pract* 57:610–616, 2016.

131. Petersen SA, Sturges BK, Dickinson PJ, et al.: Canine intraspinal meningiomas: imaging features, histopathologic classification, and long-term outcome in 34 dogs, *J Vet Intern Med* 22:946–953, 2008.

132. Rusbridge C, Wheeler SJ, Lamb CR, et al.: Vertebral plasma cell tumors in 8 dogs, *J Vet Intern Med* 13:126–133, 1999.

133. Rossmeisl JH, Lanz OI, Waldron DR, et al.: Surgical cytoreduction for the treatment of non-lymphoid vertebral and spinal cord neoplasms in cats: retrospective evaluation of 26 cases (1990-2005), *Vet Comp Oncol* 4:411–450, 2006.

134. Rissi DR, Barber R, Burnum A, et al.: Canine spinal cord glioma: a case series and review of the literature, *J Vet Diag Invest* 29:126–132, 2017.

135. Pancotto TE, Rossmeisl JH, Zimmerman K, et al.: Intramedullary spinal cord neoplasia in 53 dogs (1990-2010): distribution, clinicopathologic characteristics, and clinical behavior, *J Vet Intern Med* 3:1500–1508, 2013.

136. Siso S, Marco-Salazar P, Moore PF, et al.: Canine nervous system lymphoma subtypes display characteristic neuroanatomical patterns, *Vet Pathol* 54:53–60, 2017.

137. Marioni-Henry K, Vite CH, Newton AL, et al.: Prevalence of disease of the spinal cord of cats, *J Vet Intern Med* 18:851–858, 2004.

138. Marioni-Henry K, Van Winkle TJ, Smith SH, et al.: Tumors affecting the spinal cord of cats: 85 (1980-2005), *J Am Vet Med Assoc* 232:237–243, 2008.

139. Mandara MT, Motta L, Calo P: Distribution of feline lymphoma in the central and peripheral nervous systems, *Vet J* 216:109–116, 2016.

140. Lane SB, Kornegay JN, Duncan JR, et al.: Feline spinal lymphosarcoma: a retrospective evaluation of 23 cats, *J Vet Intern Med* 8:99–104, 1994.

141. Meichner K, Kruse DB, Hirschberger J, et al.: Changes in the prevalence of progressive feline leukaemia virus infection in cats with lymphoma in Germany, *Vet Rec* 171:348, 2012.

142. Brewer DM, Cerda-Gonzalez S, Dewey CW, et al.: Spinal cord nephroblastoma in dogs: 11 cases (1985-2007), *J Am Vet Med Assoc* 238:618–624, 2011.

143. Liebel FX, Rossmeisl JH, Lanz OI, et al.: Canine spinal nephroblastoma: long-term outcomes associated with treatment of 10 cases (1996-2009), *Vet Surg* 40:244–252, 2011.

144. Levy MS, Mauldin G, Kapatkin AS, et al.: Nonlymphoid vertebral canal tumors in cats: 11 cases (1987-1995), *J Am Vet Med Assoc* 210:663–664, 1997.

145. Mellor PJ, Haugland S, Murphy S, et al.: Myeloma-related disorders in cats commonly present as extramedullary neoplasms in contrast to myeloma in human patients: 24 cases with clinical follow-up, *J Vet Intern Med* 20:1376–1383, 2006.

146. Kippenes H, Gavin PR, Bagley RS, et al.: Magnetic resonance imaging features of tumors of the spine and spinal cord in dogs, *Vet Radiol Ultrasound* 40:627–633, 1999.

147. Drost WT, Love NE, Berry CR: Comparison of radiography, myelography, and computed tomography for the evaluation of canine vertebral and spinal cord tumors in sixteen dogs, *Vet Radiol Ultrasound* 37:28–33, 1996.

148. Allett B, Hecht S: Magnetic resonance imaging findings in the spine of six dogs diagnosed with lymphoma, *Vet Radiol Ultrasound* 57:154–161, 2016.

149. Nanai B, Lyman R, Bichsel PS: Use of intraoperative ultrasonography in canine spinal cord lesions, *Vet Radiol Ultrasound* 48:254–261, 2007.

150. Spodnick GJ, Berg J, Moore FM, et al.: Spinal lymphoma in cats: 21 cases (1976-1989), *J Am Vet Med Assoc* 200:373–376, 1992.

151. Fingeroth JM, Prata RG, Patnaik AK: Spinal meningiomas in dogs: 13 cases (1972-1987), *J Am Vet Med Assoc* 191:720–726, 1987.

152. Forterre F, Kaiser S, Matiasek K, et al.: Spinal cord canal tumor in dogs: 33 cases (retrospective study), *Kleintierpraxis* 47:357–364, 2002.

153. Chauvet AE, Hogge GS, Sandin JA, et al.: Vertebrectomy, bone allograft fusion, and antitumor vaccination for the treatment of vertebral fibrosarcoma in a dog, *Vet Surg* 28:480–488, 1999.

154. Clark GN, Berg J, Engler SJ, et al.: Extramedullary plasmacytomas in dogs: results of surgical excision in 131 cases, *J Am Anim Hosp Assoc* 28:105–111, 1992.

155. Moore TW, Bentley T, Moore SA, et al.: Spinal mast cell tumors in dogs: imaging features and clinical outcome of four cases, *Vet Radiol Ultrasound* 58:44–52, 2017.

156. Tamura S, Hori Y, Tamura Y, et al.: Long-term follow-up of surgical treatment of spinal anaplastic astrocytoma in a cat, *J Feline Med Surg* 15:921–926, 2013.

157. Brehm DM, Vite CH, Steinberg HS, et al.: A retrospective evaluation of 51 cases of peripheral nerve sheath tumors in the dog, *J Am Anim Hosp Assoc* 31:349–359, 1995.

158. Schulman FY, Johnson TO, Facemire PR, et al.: Feline peripheral nerve sheath tumors: histologic, immunohistochemical, and clinicopathologic correlation (59 tumors in 53 cats), *Vet Pathol* 46:1166–1180, 2009.

159. Chijiwa K, Uchida K, Tateyama S: Immunohistochemical evaluation of canine peripheral nerve sheath tumors and other soft tissue sarcomas, *Vet Pathol* 41:307–318, 2004.

160. Bagley RS, Wheeler SJ, Klopp L, et al.: Clinical features of trigeminal nerve-sheath tumor in 10 dogs, *J Am Anim Hosp Assoc* 34:19–25, 1998.

161. Higgins MA, Rossmeisl Jr JH, Saunders GK, et al.: B-cell lymphoma in the peripheral nerves of a cat, *Vet Pathol* 45:54–57, 2008.

162. Mandrioli I, Morini M, Biserni R, et al.: A case of feline neurolymphomatosis: pathological and molecular investigations, *J Vet Diag Invest* 24:1083–1086, 2012.

163. Bradley RL, Withrow SJ, Snyder SP: Nerve sheath tumors in the dog, *J Am Anim Hosp Assoc* 18:915–921, 1992.

164. le Chevoir M, Thibaud TL, Labruyere J, et al.: Electrophysiological features in dogs with peripheral nerve sheath tumors: 51 cases (11993-2010), *J Am Vet Med Assoc* 241:1194–1201, 2012.

165. daCosta RC, Parent JM, Dobson H, et al.: Ultrasound-guided fine needle aspiration in the diagnosis of peripheral nerve sheath tumors in 4 dogs, *Can Vet J* 49:77–81, 2007.

166. Kraft S, Ehrhart EJ, Gall D, et al.: Magnetic resonance imaging characteristics of peripheral nerve sheath tumors of the canine brachial plexus in 18 dogs, *Vet Rad Ultrasound* 48:1–7, 2007.

167. Hansen KS, Zwingenberger AL, Theon AP, et al.: Treatment of MRI-diagnosed trigeminal peripheral nerve sheath tumors by stereotactic radiotherapy in dogs, *J Vet Intern Med* 30:1112–1120, 2016.

168. Joslyn S, Driver C, McConell F, et al.: Magnetic resonance imaging of suspected idiopathic bilateral C2 hypertrophic ganglioneuritis in dogs, *J Sm Anim Pract* 56:184–189, 2015.

169. van Stee L, Boston S, Teske E, et al.: Compartmental resection of peripheral nerve tumours with limb preservation in 16 dogs (1995-2011), *Vet J* 226:40–45, 2017.

170. Dolera M, Malfassi L, Bianchi C, et al.: Frameless stereotactic volumetric modulated arc radiotherapy of brachial plexus tumours in dogs: 10 cases, *Br J Radiol* 90:1069, 2017.

171. Swift KE, McGrath S, Nolan MW, et al.: Clinical and imaging findings, treatments, and outcomes in 27 dogs with imaging diagnosed trigeminal nerve sheath tumor: a multi-center study, *Vet Radiol Ultrasound* 58:679–689, 2017.

32

Ocular Tumors

PAUL E. MILLER AND LEANDRO B.C. TEIXEIRA

Tumors of the eye, orbit, or adnexa can have devastating consequences for an animal's vision, appearance, and comfort and may be harbingers of potentially life-threatening disease elsewhere in the body. By virtue of their location, even benign ocular tumors may cause blindness and loss of the eye. Although these tumors reportedly affected only 0.87% of all dogs and 0.34% of all cats recorded in the Veterinary Medical Database (VMDB) over a 10-year period, their actual frequency is undoubtedly greater because many presumably benign ocular tumors are not histologically examined. Additional insights into the relative frequency of ocular tumors can also be gained by reviewing submissions over several decades to the large ophthalmic pathology database compiled by the Comparative Ocular Pathology Laboratory of Wisconsin (COPLOW) (Fig. 32.1). This chapter describes the more common ocular tumors in small animals and also uses the database of the COPLOW laboratory to estimate the relative frequency of various ocular tumors.

Tumors of the Eyelids, Third Eyelid, Conjunctiva, and Ocular Surface

Incidence and Risk Factors

Benign adenomas and melanomas of the haired skin or eyelid margin make up 76% of canine eyelid tumors in the COPLOW database and tend to affect old dogs. One study suggests Boxers, collies, Weimaraners, cocker spaniels, and springer spaniels are at greater risk for eyelid neoplasia than the general hospital population,[1] and another study suggests that beagles, Siberian huskies, and English setters are at greater risk than mixed-breed dogs.[2] Canine juvenile histiocytomas affect the eyelid skin of young to middle-aged dogs[1,2] but are relatively uncommon, comprising only 3% of eyelid biopsy samples submitted to COPLOW. Squamous cell carcinoma (SCC) comprises up to two-thirds of feline eyelid and third eyelid tumors and has a predilection for the lower eyelid and medial canthus of white cats.[3] Ocular SCC is less frequent in dogs, but in both cats and dogs increased exposure to solar radiation, lack of adnexal pigmentation, and possibly chronic ocular surface irritation are believed to be predisposing factors (Fig. 32.2).[1,4,5]

Vascular endothelial cell tumors of the lateral limbus or the leading edge of the third eyelid constitute 25% of conjunctival tumors in dogs and tend to occur in the nonpigmented conjunctiva in Bassett hounds, springer spaniels, and beagles (Fig. 32.3).

Melanomas often occur in dogs with a pigmented conjunctiva and are the most common malignant tumor of the canine conjunctiva, making up 16% of conjunctival tumor biopsies. Older (mean = 11 years), female, Weimaraner, and possibly German shepherd/large-breed dogs may be predisposed to conjunctival melanomas.[6] Melanomas also have a propensity for the nictitating membrane and superior palpebral conjunctiva.[6,7] Ocular viral papillomas compose about 3% of conjunctival tumors and tend to occur in young dogs and are believed to have a papillomavirus etiology (perhaps canine oral papillomavirus).[8] However, one study failed to identify papillomaviral genetic material in older dogs with smaller solitary lesions, suggesting that the cause of ocular surface papillomas in dogs may be heterogeneous.[9] Canine squamous papilloma is a benign papillary tumor of unknown etiology and makes up 9% of conjunctival tumor biopsies. Reactive papilloma is seen secondary to other conditions such as meibomian tumors, but they make up 18% of conjunctival tumor biopsies. Corneal tumors have a predilection for the limbus.

Pathology and Natural Behavior

Sebaceous or meibomian gland adenomas and epitheliomas, papillomas, and melanomas comprise more than 80% of canine eyelid and conjunctival neoplasms, and a substantial majority of these tumors are histologically benign.[1,2] Even histologically malignant eyelid tumors in dogs rarely metastasize, although they are more likely to be locally invasive and recur after surgery.[1,2] In contrast, most feline eyelid and ocular surface tumors such as SCC are malignant.[3]

Viral papillomas tend to be well demarcated and superficial, minimally altering deeper tissues. Surgical manipulation has occasionally been associated with dispersal of papillomas throughout the ocular surface.[10,11] Papillomas, like histiocytomas, often spontaneously regress in young dogs, although they may persist in the older dog where they may not be of viral origin. SCC may also develop superficially, but after malignant transformation the preinvasive actinic plaque can invade deeper tissues. SCC may spread to regional lymph nodes late in the course of the disease and uncommonly distantly metastasize. SCC of the third eyelid may more readily invade the orbit than corneal or eyelid SCC. Primary corneal SCC is more common in brachycephalic dogs and has been reported to be associated with chronic keratitis and topical immunosuppressive therapy.[12]

Adenocarcinomas of the gland of the third eyelid constitute 12% of conjunctival tumors in dogs and approximately 85% of all third eyelid tumors in dogs and cats.[13] They are variable in morphology and often show moderate infiltrative growth.[13] They may mimic prolapse of the gland of the nictitans ("cherry eye") by appearing as localized, firm, smooth, pink swellings on the posterior surface of the nictitans, but a key differentiating feature is their occurrence in much older dogs (10–16 years). Although excision of the grossly visible tumor may initially appear adequate, recurrence is common if the entire gland is not removed, and metastasis, especially to the regional lymph nodes and orbit, is

possible.[13–15] Adenomas of the gland of the third eyelid are less frequently reported in dogs (approximately 14% of all third eyelid tumors) as are SCC (approximately 1% of all canine and 16% of all feline third eyelid tumors).[13]

The natural behavior of conjunctival vascular, melanocytic, and mast cell tumors (MCTs) is poorly understood, in part because they are uncommon. Conjunctival hemangiomas and hemangiosarcomas tend to remain relatively superficial but may recur after simple excision.[15–19] Hemangiosarcomas may exhibit a more aggressive course and a primary ocular hemangiosarcoma must be differentiated from a metastatic lesion. However, metastasis of primary conjunctival vascular tumors, even when classified as hemangiosarcomas, appears to be rare.[15–19]

Feline conjunctival melanomas originate on the bulbar conjunctiva and invade the eyelid.[20,21] Melanoma of the conjunctiva in dogs is most often morphologically malignant, but metastatic disease is not common. As in cats, canine conjunctival melanomas have been reported to recur locally after surgical excision in 55% of cases, and at least 17% of the dogs experienced orbital invasion or spread to the regional lymph nodes or lungs.[6] Melanomas originating from the palpebral conjunctiva may have greater metastatic potential.[6] Mitotic index, cell type, and degree of pigmentation are not useful predictors of malignancy for canine conjunctival melanomas.[6] Conjunctival (subconjunctival) MCTs make up 4% of conjunctival tumors, but their natural history is poorly understood in part because they are uncommon. Nevertheless, they have been suggested to have a relatively benign course in dogs, even with incomplete excision and if the tumors present more malignant histologic features.[22,23] Conjunctival MCTs are not typically graded as the grading system was developed for cutaneous tumors and the criteria are not applicable to conjunctival tissues. In the largest review to date, local recurrence was observed in only 2 of 32 dogs, even though residual tumor was histologically present in 25 dogs.[23] In addition, none of the 32 dogs died of conjunctival MCT-related disease.[23]

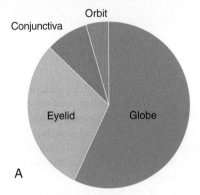

Anatomic Distribution of Canine Primary Ocular Neoplasms (*n* = 11091)

A

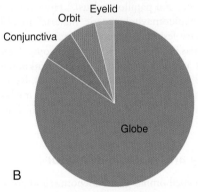

Anatomic Distribution of Feline Primary Ocular Neoplasms (*n* = 4631)

B

• **Fig. 32.1** The distribution of canine (A) and feline (B) ocular tumors submitted to the Comparative Ocular Pathology Laboratory of Wisconsin.

History and Clinical Signs

Vascular tumors are often focal, raised, soft, red masses with visible feeder vessels arising from the surface of the conjunctiva or third eyelid.[15–19] SCC of the eyelid, third eyelid, or ocular surface

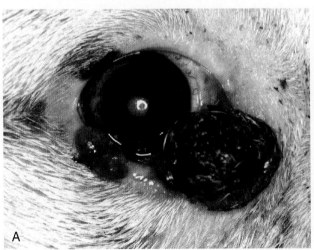

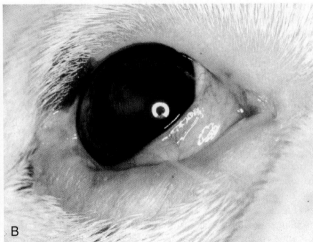

• **Fig. 32.2** (A) Squamous cell carcinoma affecting the lower eyelids of a boxer. (B) Same dog after cryosurgical ablation of the tumor. Lid function is spared.

may appear as a focally thickened, roughened, and usually pink-to-red lesion in older animals or, more commonly, as an ulcerated lesion with a protracted course.[3–5] In contrast, papillomas in young dogs appear verrucous and usually progress rapidly over weeks to a few months whereas they tend to be solitary and slowly progressive in older dogs. Conjunctival MCTs often have smooth surfaces and appear tan or red in color. Nonneoplastic conditions such as nodular granulomatous episcleritis, which is an inflammatory disorder, can be mistaken for neoplasia.

In addition to a mass lesion, other clinical signs of eyelid or ocular surface tumors may include epiphora, conjunctival vascular injection, mucopurulent ocular discharge, protrusion of the third eyelid, conjunctival/corneal roughening or ulceration, and corneal neovascularization or pigmentation. Occasionally, palpebral conjunctival masses protrude only when their bulk no longer can be accommodated by the space between the eyelid and globe, and very advanced tumors may create exophthalmia or enophthalmia if the orbit is invaded. Large tumors and sebaceous adenomas often have a substantial inflammatory component and may be secondarily infected. Mesenchymal hamartoma appears to have a predisposition for the skin of lateral canthus of dogs.[24]

Diagnostic Techniques and Workup

In addition to fluorescein staining and examination of the ocular surface with a cobalt filter or black light, the extent of involvement of the bulbar and palpebral conjunctiva should be determined by everting the eyelid (and third eyelid if affected). Careful palpation of the lesion by inserting a lubricated finger in the conjunctival cul-de-sac can be invaluable for determining the full extent of the tumor and whether bony involvement has occurred. Nasolacrimal lavage and possibly positive contrast dacryocystorhinography may help characterize medial canthal masses. In general, small eyelid and ocular surface tumors are best diagnosed and treated by excisional biopsy. Fine-needle aspiration (FNA) or incisional biopsies

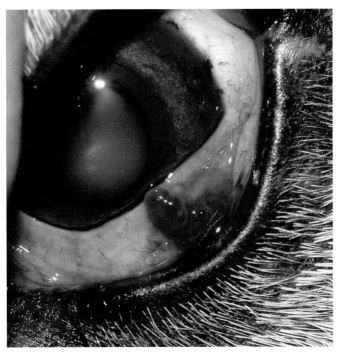

• **Fig. 32.3** Hemangiosarcoma of the third eyelid in a dog.

of larger tumors aid in determining prognosis and planning definitive therapy. Occasionally, orbital ultrasound, skull radiographs, computed tomography (CT), magnetic resonance imaging (MRI), regional lymph node cytology, and thoracic radiographs are required to localize or clinically stage potentially malignant tumors such as SCC, MCTs, adenocarcinomas of the third eyelid, and conjunctival melanomas.

Therapy

Specific therapy varies with the type of tumor; its location, size, and extent; whether the eye still has useful vision; the animal's expected lifespan; the degree of discomfort the mass is creating; and the owner's financial limitations. All eyelid tumors, whether benign or malignant, have the potential to affect vision or ocular comfort. Indications for tumor removal include any eyelid tumor in a cat, rapid growth, ocular surface irritation, impaired eyelid function, owner concern, or an unappealing appearance. In young dogs, observation of nonirritating papillomas or histiocytomas, even if quite large, may be appropriate as spontaneous regression is common.

Tumors involving less than one-fourth to one-third of the length of the eyelid are best treated by a V-plasty (wedge) or four-sided excision.[25] The latter technique affords superior apposition of the eyelid margins and wound stability, especially in tumors approaching the one-fourth to one-third limit, because the initial incision is made perpendicular to the eyelid margin rather than obliquely. In general, only one-third to one-fourth of the eyelid in dogs and one-fourth of the eyelid in cats can be removed with these techniques. Antibiotic or antiinflammatory therapy may reduce the size of large tumors that are infected or inflamed so that a wedge or four-sided excision becomes possible. Electrosurgical excision should be avoided because it may result in substantial scarring of the eyelids. Carbon dioxide (CO_2) laser ablation may be appropriate for some tumors.[26]

Tumors greater than one-fourth to one-third of the eyelid typically require more advanced reconstructive blepharoplasty or use of other therapeutic modalities. Some tumors may be responsive to systemic chemotherapy (e.g., lymphoma, MCTs), local infiltration with chemotherapeutic agents such as cisplatin (e.g., SCC),[27] and/or local radiation therapy (RT; e.g., SCC). In some cases, these modalities will completely eliminate the tumor or shrink it to the point in which a less extensive surgical procedure can be performed. Reconstructive blepharoplasty, however, is the procedure of choice if surgical cure is a possibility and these other modalities have failed or are unlikely to substantially affect the tumor or if the nature of the tumor indicates extensive margins are required.

Cryosurgery is an attractive alternative to extensive blepharoplasty and has been reported to be effective in several canine eyelid tumor types (see Fig. 32.2; see also Chapter 10).[2,28] It is quick, less technically demanding than reconstructive blepharoplasty, and usually permits preservation of the nasolacrimal puncta and canaliculus. In many old or debilitated patients, cryosurgery can be accomplished with only sedation or local/topical anesthesia. After pretreatment with dexamethasone (0.1 mg/kg intravenous [IV]), the mass is isolated with a chalazion forceps (if possible) and debulked flush with the lid margin. Using liquid nitrogen and a closed probe that approximates the diameter of the mass as much as possible, a double freeze-thaw is performed so that the ice ball extends 3 to 5 mm beyond the visible margins of the mass. Ice balls should overlap in large tumors. Freezing may be repeated a second or third time if complete regression is not achieved after the first session. Substantial postoperative swelling and usually transient depigmentation of the frozen tissue are to be expected.

Tumors involving the conjunctiva and third eyelid (especially conjunctival hemangiosarcomas, melanomas, and nictitans adenocarcinomas) are most effectively treated by surgical excision, occasionally to the point of exenterating the orbit. If the globe is to be spared, however, excision of the entire nictitans should not be taken lightly because undesirable sequelae such as ocular drying and chronic keratitis frequently result. Bulbar conjunctival tumors move freely and, if small, are generally amenable to excision under only topical anesthesia and perhaps sedation. Cryosurgery may permit the nictitans to be spared in the cases of papillomas and early SCC, or it can be used as an adjunct to excision in advanced canine conjunctival melanomas and SCC.[6,28]

Superficial keratectomy/sclerectomy is preferred for many corneal and scleral tumors, although some tumors require a full-thickness resection of the cornea or sclera. In the latter case, corneal or scleral allografts or autologous tissue grafts should be used to maintain ocular structural integrity. Limbal SCC and epibulbar melanoma may also be amenable to cryosurgery, although the ice ball should be carefully monitored to avoid unnecessary freezing of intraocular structures.

Prognosis

The prognosis for most canine primary eyelid tumors is excellent, whether treated by excision or cryosurgery. Metastasis is rare, even in histologically malignant primary lid tumors, and recurrence rates are low (approximately 10%–15%).[2] New primary eyelid tumors are not uncommon and must be distinguished from recurrence. Because most eyelid tumors in cats are malignant, the prognosis is not as good as that for dogs, but it is unclear how prognosis correlates with the histologic features. Conjunctival melanomas and nictitans adenocarcinomas frequently recur after partial excision of the nictitans, even if all the clinically visible tumor has been removed.[6] Conjunctival hemangiosarcomas appear to have a good prognosis because total excision may be curative, although recurrence and loss of the eye is still possible.[15–19] Conjunctival MCTs also appear to have a good prognosis.[23]

Limbal (Epibulbar) Melanomas

Limbal melanomas are typically benign, slightly raised, heavily pigmented masses originating from melanocytes in the sclera or subconjunctival connective tissue (Fig. 32.4).[29–35] They comprise 3.5% of all canine ocular tumors and 1% of feline ocular tumor submissions to COPLOW. The majority of these slow-growing tumors originate in the superior limbal region, suggesting exposure to solar radiation may be a risk factor.[15] Affected dogs average age 5 to 6 years old (cats 8+ years), and a female sex and German shepherd, golden retriever and Labrador retriever breed predilection has been inconsistently reported.[29–35] Confirmed metastasis has not been reported in dogs or cats and mitotic figures are rarely encountered; although in one study, two of four cats also had feline leukemia virus (FeLV)-associated lymphoma or leukemia, and a third cat had a second intraocular pigmented mass unassociated with the limbal tumor.[34] Lightly pigmented spindle cells capable of division are seen histologically, but the dominant cell is presumably a hypermature spindle cell that is large, round, pigment laden, and benign.[30] These masses are often only incidentally noted and the clinical signs are typically minimal, although

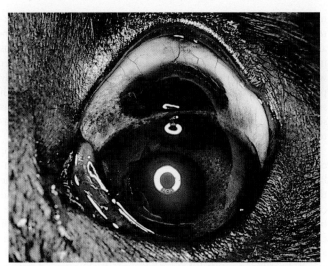

• **Fig. 32.4** Epibulbar melanomas typically originate from the superior limbal region of the globe. (Image courtesy Dr. Elizabeth Adkins.)

local corneal invasion, epiphora, and mild conjunctival irritation may be seen.[32,33] Differential diagnoses include conjunctival melanoma, invasive uveal melanoma, metastatic melanoma, and staphyloma or coloboma. Gonioscopy aids in differentiating invasive intraocular tumors from limbal melanomas.

Therapy should be considered if the tumor has invaded the eye or if growth is rapid. Given its benign nature and usually slow growth rate (imperceptible growth over 18 months has been described), observation alone may be appropriate in older dogs. If intervention is required, lamellar keratectomy/sclerectomy with graft placement is often curative.[36–38] Beta-irradiation and cryosurgery have been used as adjuncts to surgery.[36,39] Cryosurgery alone or laser photocoagulation[35] has also been described as effective means of treatment. Regrowth after local surgical excision occurs in approximately 30% of patients, but 2 to 3 years may pass before the anterior chamber is invaded and enucleation is required.[30,32,33] The addition of adjunctive therapy such as cryotherapy or beta-irradiation substantially reduces the risk of recurrence after local excision.[36,39] Enucleation is curative and indicated if painful intraocular disease is present.[30]

Primary Ocular Tumors

Canine Anterior Uveal Melanomas
Incidence and Risk Factors

In one review of data from the Armed Forces Institute of Pathology, intraocular melanomas, other primary intraocular tumors, and metastatic intraocular neoplasms constituted 12%, 14%, and 9%, respectively, of canine ophthalmic/orbital/adnexal tumors.[40] In the COPLOW archive, uveal melanocytic tumors make up 25% of all ocular tumor submissions. Any age is at risk, but most affected dogs are older than 7 years of age, and breed or sex predilections are inconsistent.[30]

Pathology and Natural Behavior

Approximately 75% of canine intraocular melanomas are benign, and 95% arise from the iris or ciliary body (Fig. 32.5).[30,32,41] The most clinically useful classification scheme classifies these tumors simply as melanocytoma (benign) and melanoma (potentially malignant) based on nuclear features of the tumor cells, with

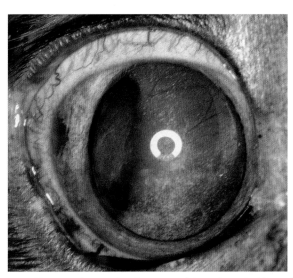

• **Fig. 32.5** Most anterior uveal melanomas originate from the iris or ciliary body and are benign.

mitotic rate being the most important.[30,31] Benign tumors have fewer than two to four mitotic figures/10 HPFs (mitotic index), and malignant tumors demonstrate nuclear pleomorphism and a mitotic index of at least four and often more than 30. Destruction of the eye is not by itself sufficient for a diagnosis of malignancy.[30] The overall rate of metastasis of intraocular melanomas is approximately 4%[41] and usually occurs via the hematogenous route. Local spread along ocular vessels and nerves or via direct penetration of the sclera or cornea also occurs. Benign tumors tend to be smaller, more darkly pigmented and have a lower mitotic index than malignant tumors.[30,31]

Circumscribed, nevus-like pigmented iridal growths have been described in young dogs (7 months to 2 years old).[32] The natural history of these lesions is variable because enlargement may not occur over several years.[32,40] Some, however, are capable of rapid growth, but to date all are clinically and histologically benign.

Ocular melanosis of Cairn terriers resembles feline diffuse iris melanoma in some respects.[42] This disorder is probably an autosomal-dominant condition with a variable age of onset and rate of progression. It results in a thickening and pigmentation of the iris, release of pigment into the aqueous, pigment deposition in the sclera/episclera, and to a lesser extent posterior segment pigment deposition. Secondary glaucoma is common, and overt uveal melanocytic neoplasia occurs in a small percentage of dogs.[42]

History and Clinical Signs

Common presentations of intraocular tumors include a visible intraocular or scleral mass, glaucoma, hyphema, anterior uveitis, or extrabulbar spread, or they can be an incidental finding during an ophthalmic examination.[30,41] Because glaucoma or hyphema are often the only overtly visible clinical signs,[30,41] intraocular neoplasia should always be considered in animals with hyphema, glaucoma, or both when there is no history of trauma or coagulopathy. Small masses frequently create few symptoms other than pupillary distortion. Pigmentation is variable and not a reliable indicator of tumor type.

Diagnostic Techniques and Workup

Usually, the clinical or ultrasonographic appearance (if the media are opaque) is strongly suggestive of intraocular neoplasia, although

it may be difficult to arrive at a definitive diagnosis without invading the eye or removing it because organizing blood clots are not always distinguishable from neoplastic mass lesions. Because most anterior uveal brown or black masses are cystic and not neoplastic, transillumination should be attempted before more invasive procedures. Uveal cysts typically permit bright light to pass through them, are roughly spherical, and may be attached to the ciliary body or free-floating in the anterior chamber. Once suspected, most primary canine intraocular tumors are observed for progression, although occasionally FNA (with its risks of inflammation, infection, and hemorrhage) or attempts at intraocular resection or enucleation are used for diagnostic purposes. The possibility of metastasis from another primary site (i.e., oral cavity or nail bed) to the eye or from the eye to other organs should be eliminated.

Therapy

Canine primary intraocular tumors are often carefully observed, although surgical intervention (sector iridectomy/cyclectomy, laser ablation, enucleation) should also be considered. Digital photographs are a valuable aid in assessing progression. Enucleation is advised if there is concern about malignancy or if complications such as intractable uveitis, chronic hyphema or secondary glaucoma occur.[43] In the COPLOW collection, 14% of canine globes with glaucoma that are removed also had melanoma. The low risk of metastasis and unproved efficacy of enucleation at preventing metastasis in the few malignant tumors that have been reported make it difficult to automatically advise enucleation of normotensive, noninflamed, visual eyes.[30] Isolated primary masses involving only the iris or a portion of the ciliary body may be amenable to local resection by sector iridectomy/cyclectomy to preserve the eye and vision.[32,40] These intraocular procedures, however, require an accomplished ophthalmic surgeon and often have unsatisfactory long-term results. Transscleral and transcorneal Nd:YAG or diode laser therapy has induced remission in some small- to moderate-sized primary intraocular tumors.[43,44] Specialized goniolenses may also allow laser treatment of masses that have invaded into the iridocorneal angle. Although the results were variable, perhaps because these tumors varied histologically in nature, laser therapy holds promise for the palliation or potential cure of a number of intraocular tumor types while also preserving vision. Metastasis was not observed after this procedure, although this obviously remains a risk when the tumor is malignant.[43]

Prognosis

Although the data in most studies are heavily "censored," the prognosis for histologically benign melanomas appears to be excellent. Enucleation is curative, but attempts at local excision or laser photoablation may be only palliative, especially if the ciliary body or trabecular meshwork is involved. The presence of black, nonsolid material within the orbit after the enucleation of benign melanomas with scleral invasion apparently does not affect prognosis because these cells appear incapable of continued growth.[32] In one study, approximately 25% of histologically malignant melanomas demonstrated metastasis, typically within 3 months of enucleation, and most dogs with metastasis were euthanatized within 6 months of enucleation.[30] This surprisingly poor prognosis has not been the experience of cases followed recently in the COPLOW data set, and in a larger study, dogs with tumors classified as malignant were reported to have only a somewhat decreased survival time compared with dogs with melanocytoma and dogs from a control population.[45]

Choroidal Melanomas

Choroidal melanomas are rare intraocular melanocytic tumors, comprising only 4% to 7% of canine uveal melanomas, with no clear breed or sex predisposition.[46] Middle-aged (6–7 years), medium- to large-breed dogs predominate.[46] Generally, these tumors are well-delineated, raised subretinal pigmented masses with tapering margins, bulging centers, and a propensity for the peripapillary region and optic nerve.[46,47] In some cases, the tumor may remain virtually static for many years, whereas others exhibit infiltration into the overlying retina, through the sclera, up the optic nerve, and into the orbit.[46] Nuclear anaplasia is minimal and generally mitotic figures are absent.[47] Despite these benign cytologic features, metastasis has been described in one dog 21 months after exenteration, and follow-up in most studies is incomplete.[48] In general, however, these tumors appear to be benign in the vast majority of dogs. Most dogs with tumors involving a limited portion of the choroid are asymptomatic, and the mass is noted incidentally on ophthalmoscopy. Larger tumors frequently present with chronic uveitis, secondary glaucoma, retinal detachment, intraocular hemorrhage, or blindness.[46,47] Extension into the orbit can occur, and documentation of this is important in planning for enucleation surgery. Ocular ultrasonography may demonstrate mass lesions if anterior segment changes or retinal detachment obscures an underlying mass. Therapy usually consists of enucleation once progression has been documented or if the eye is painful. Diode laser ablation may offer an alternative to enucleation if the lesion is small and does not involve the optic nerve. Optic nerve or scleral invasion may warrant a more cautious prognosis.

Feline Primary Intraocular Melanomas (Feline Diffuse Iris Melanoma)

Incidence and Risk Factors

Anterior uveal melanomas are the most common primary intraocular tumor in cats (Fig. 32.6).[49] They account for 55% of all neoplastic submissions to the COPLOW in cats. There appears to be no breed or sex predisposition, and most cats are more than 9 years of age at the time of diagnosis,[49,50] although the prodromal period for many of these tumors may be quite long.

Pathology and Natural Behavior

In the malignant form of uveal melanoma, the rate of metastasis (frequently to the liver and lungs) has been reported to vary from 55% to 66% or higher.[49–52] Iridal hyperpigmentation, however, frequently takes months to years to progress to the extent to which the eye must be enucleated, and an additional 1 to 3 years after enucleation are required before metastatic disease may become evident.[49,50,52,53] No single morphologic feature is predictive of outcome, but in some studies metastasis has been linked to a greater mitotic index, larger tumors, and extension through the iris into the ciliary body stroma and involvement of the scleral venous plexus.[49,50] In a recent study,[54] an increased risk for metastasis was found if there was extrascleral extension, necrosis within the neoplasm, a mitotic index of more than seven mitoses in 10 high-power (×400) fields, choroidal invasion, increased labeling for E-cadherin (a transmembrane protein responsible for cell adhesion) or melan-A (an antigen expressed by melanocytes) label intensity. PNL2 label homogeneity was associated with a decreased rate of metastasis.[54] PNL2 is an antibody directed against an unidentified antigen expressed by normal and neoplastic melanocytes.

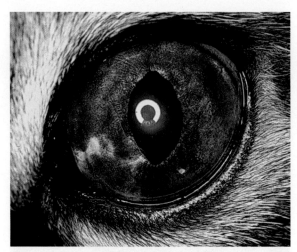

• **Fig. 32.6** Diffuse iris melanomas may first appear as multifocal to diffuse pigmentary changes, as seen in the coalescing darker regions of the iris in this cat.

Most ophthalmologists have noted unilateral or occasionally bilateral slowly progressive iridal pigmentary changes (especially in older orange cats) over many years to a decade or more that apparently do not lead to disease beyond the pigmentation, although eventual removal of these eyes can show melanoma. It is possible in some cats that these initially benign-appearing accumulations of small, angular pigmented cells on the anterior iridal surface undergo transformation to the larger, rounded cells typical of the potentially malignant diffuse iris melanoma. Of concern to the clinician waiting to document progression before advising treatment, however, is that malignant transformation is not readily observable clinically and that these cells, once transformed, appear to be capable of quickly dropping off into the anterior chamber and entering the drainage apparatus and vasculature.[50]

History, Clinical Signs, Diagnostic Techniques, and Workup

Slowly progressive, diffuse iridal hyperpigmentation is the most common clinical sign, although occasionally a pigmented iridal nodule or amelanotic mass is seen. Secondary glaucoma will eventually occur, and the diffuse form may be mistaken for chronic anterior uveitis with iridal hyperpigmentation.

The diagnosis of melanoma, generally made clinically, requires demonstration of progression and iridal thickening or irregularity of the iris surface or pupil. The prognostic and diagnostic value of FNAs of the iridal surface or iridal biopsies is unclear and worthy of further study. A recent report described multiple cases of darkly pigmented iridociliary cysts in cats that were erroneously diagnosed as iris melanomas.[55] These cases presented single to multiple cysts that failed to transilluminate and caused distortion and discoloration of the iris, leading to enucleation of the globe. The presence of bilateral masses protruding through the pupil may help distinguish iridociliary cysts from melanomas and should prompt the clinician to pursue additional diagnostic imaging, such as high-resolution ultrasound.

Therapy

The treatment of feline uveal melanomas is controversial. Ideally, enucleation would be delayed until just *before* malignant transformation, invasion into other ocular structures, secondary glaucoma, or metastasis. Such precise timing, however, is seldom attainable in a clinical setting, and enucleation is commonly performed if iridal pigment changes have been demonstrated to progressively increase to the point that virtually the entire iridal surface is involved, pigmented cells are present in the trabecular meshwork, the pupil is distorted (indicating iridal invasion), ciliary body or scleral invasion is threatened, uveitis is present, or glaucoma is impending. Although it would seem logical that early enucleation would optimize survival, this is unproved. In one study, enucleation has been shown to markedly enhance the rate of metastasis in cats with feline sarcoma virus–induced uveal melanomas.[56] The applicability of this experimental model to spontaneous disease, however, is unclear and neither feline sarcoma virus nor FeLV were found in a study of 10 eyes with spontaneous diffuse iris melanoma.[57] Some ophthalmologists have attempted to ablate small, focal, hyperpigmented foci on the iris of cats with a diode laser, thereby preserving vision and the eye. The long-term success rate and side effects of this procedure, however, are not known. Finally, most slowly progressing lesions are simply monitored, ideally by comparison to baseline photographs. This option is particularly suitable for older cats with other diseases that limit their expected lifespan. In many cats, progression may be so slow as to permit the patient to be followed for many years to a decade or more without apparent metastasis.

Prognosis

The metastatic potential of feline uveal melanomas has been correlated with the extent of ocular involvement seen histologically.[50,54] Because the tumor is relatively slow-growing, however, the period until metastatic disease becomes apparent may be measured in years, and even then, substantial additional time may elapse before the metastasis is life threatening. Cats with tumors confined to iris stroma and trabecular meshwork at the time of enucleation have survival times comparable to those of age-matched controls. Enucleation after the tumor has invaded into the ciliary body but not the sclera warrants a poorer prognosis, but the median survival time (MST) is still approximately 5 years.[50] Enucleation after the tumor has invaded into the ciliary body and the sclera merits an even poorer prognosis, with an MST of approximately 1.5 years.[50] The MST is also reduced if secondary glaucoma has occurred.[50] In one study of 47 cats enucleated for diffuse iris melanoma, confirmed or suspected metastasis occurred in nine cases.[54] However, cats being enucleated for diffuse iris melanoma most likely reflect the more extensive form of the disease and the rate of metastasis in cats with all forms of diffuse iris melanoma is likely substantially lower.

Feline Ocular Posttraumatic Sarcoma

Sarcomas after ocular trauma, although uncommon, are second only to melanomas in frequency as a primary ocular tumor of cats (Fig. 32.7).[58–61] In the COPLOW collection, 8% of feline ocular tumors are posttraumatic sarcoma. These tumors are subdivided into three morphologic subtypes: spindle cell sarcoma (the most common), round cell sarcoma (posttraumatic lymphoma), and osteosarcoma/chondrosarcoma. All three have similar histories leading up to tumor presentation. Cats that are 7 to 15 years of age are most commonly affected, the latency period after trauma averages 5 years,[59] and 67% of affected cats are males or neutered males. Damage to the lens and chronic uveitis may be risk factors.[58–60] Ciliary body ablation with gentamicin for glaucoma may also be a risk factor.[62]

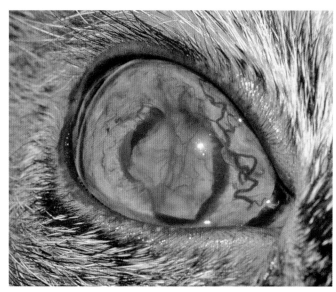

• **Fig. 32.7** Posttraumatic sarcoma in a cat. (Image courtesy Dr. Elizabeth Adkins.)

Because of the risk of posttraumatic sarcoma, many clinicians are cautious about cataract surgery, intravitreous injections of gentamicin for the treatment of glaucoma or the use of an intrascleral prosthesis in cats. The cell of origin varies and is not definitively known for all three subtypes. There is good evidence that the spindle cell variant originates from the lens epithelial cell, and that the initial pathogenesis of the tumor is related to lens capsule rupture, release, and proliferation of the lens epithelial cells and epithelial-to-mesenchymal transition, leading to the sarcoma phenotype of the tumor.[63,64] Neoplastic cells of the round cell variant are positive on immunohistochemistry for CD79a (a B-lymphocyte marker) and this variant likely represents a form of anaplastic, primary ocular, B-cell lymphoma.[65] Chronic inflammation may support neoplastic transformation of a pluripotent cell.[58–60] These tumors, often within the same eye, exhibit a spectrum of changes ranging from granulation tissue to fibrosarcoma, osteosarcoma, and anaplastic spindle cell sarcoma.[59,60] All of these tumors tend to circumferentially line the choroid and quickly infiltrate the retina and optic nerve.[59,60] The round cell variant tends to infiltrate the retina early.[65,66] White or pinkish discoloration of the affected eye or change in the shape or consistency of the globe are the most common presenting signs. Skull radiographs may demonstrate bone involvement or metallic foreign bodies.[61]

Because this tumor is uncommon, many ophthalmologists will not remove a comfortable phthisical feline eye unless it changes appearance. The advanced stage at which many of these tumors are first identified, however, and the propensity for early optic nerve involvement indicate that enucleation at this point may be only palliative and not prolong life. This has led some authors to advocate prophylactic enucleation of phthisical feline eyes or of feline eyes that are blind and have been severely traumatized or are chronically inflamed.[58,61] Further support for this approach comes from the observation that approximately 7.5% of globes removed prophylactically in the COPLOW collection already have tumors. Extension beyond the sclera or into the optic nerve may occur and are poor prognostic indicators, further supporting the concept of early enucleation. As much of the optic nerve as possible should be removed during enucleation for confirmed or suspected ocular sarcoma so that the extent of infiltrative disease and prognosis may be accurately determined. There is reason to believe that the prognosis is considerably better if enucleation is performed before the tumor invades the optic nerve or extends beyond the sclera.[67] To date, there have been no reports of treatment by RT or chemotherapy.

Extraocular extension is common, as is recurrence after orbital exenteration.[58,61] Continued growth up the remainder of the optic nerve into the chiasm and brain, with vision loss or other neurologic signs, involvement of regional lymph nodes, and distant metastasis, has been reported.[47,59] The vast majority of animals die of local invasion and recurrence, typically within several months of enucleation.[58,61]

Spindle Cell Tumors (Uveal Schwannoma) of Blue-Eyed Dogs

Dogs with a blue, or partially blue, iris appear to be at risk of developing a spindle cell sarcoma in the uvea.[68,69] These tumors usually involve the iris but can originate or extend into the ciliary body, choroid, and even the vitreous. Breeds that commonly have blue irides are more likely to develop an iridal spindle cell sarcoma, but any dog with any blue in its iris appears to be at risk. The origin of these tumors is thought to be Schwann cells of nonmyelinated peripheral nerves and the term "uveal Schwannoma of blue-eyed dogs" has been proposed.[69,70] The cells stain positive with glial fibrillary acidic protein (GFAP), as do the Schwann cells of nonmyelinating nerves. In a case series involving 11 dogs, more than half of the tumors were not clinically recognized and the diagnosis of neoplasia was not made until histopathology was performed. Metastatic disease appears uncommon, although one case has been reported and local recurrence within the scleral shell was seen in another dog that had been treated by evisceration and placement of an intrascleral prosthesis.[68,70]

Iridociliary Epithelial Tumors

Primary iridociliary epithelial tumors (ciliary body adenomas, adenocarcinomas, pleomorphic adenocarcinoma, and less commonly, medulloepitheliomas and other primitive neuroectodermal tumors [PNETs]) are the second most common primary intraocular tumors in dogs after melanocytic neoplasms and the third most common in cats.[71,72] They account for 12% of all canine and 3.5% of all feline tumors in the COPLOW database. The two main histologic forms of iridociliary adenomas/carcinomas that have been described are papillary (57% of cases in one study) and solid tumors (43%).[71] In the authors' experience, these tumors often appear nonpigmented clinically, but histologically at least some pigmented cells are present in approximately one-half of cases. Pigmented tumors of the ciliary body may be grossly indistinguishable from anterior uveal melanomas. Middle-aged to older dogs are the most commonly affected and golden and Labrador retrievers may be predisposed, for they comprised 27% of dogs with iridociliary epithelial tumors in one survey.[71] Most of these tumors appear to be benign, fairly well-delineated, sometimes pedunculated, slow-growing masses that originate in the pars plicata of the ciliary body or the iris epithelium.[71-73] Although approximately 60% invade the uveal tract, only 21% invade the sclera.[71] Tumors that invade the sclera are typically classified as adenocarcinomas and have anaplastic features, but metastasis is uncommon and occurs late in the course of the disease, if at all.[71-75] A small series of truly malignant pleomorphic adenocarcinomas

with potentially fatal metastasis has been described in dogs.[76,77] These tumors are rare (0.2% of COPLOW's canine tumors) and affected dogs usually have long-standing disease thought to be inflammatory or traumatic. One retrospective study reported that 13% of cases had a history of known or suspected ocular trauma and 33% received an intravitreous gentamicin injection for the treatment of glaucoma.[77]

Clinical signs include a retroiridal mass that may displace the iris or lens by expansive growth, and if the tumor is large, secondary glaucoma, ocular pain, and intraocular hemorrhage may be noted.[74] The diagnostic workup and differential diagnosis are similar to that of anterior uveal melanomas. Given the high frequency of ciliary body cysts in some predisposed breeds (especially the golden retriever), it is essential to differentiate ciliary body tumors from a benign cystic lesion before enucleation. Cystic lesions, which rarely require any intervention, are usually seen as lightly pigmented, ovoid, retroiridal masses that can be shown to be hollow by transillumination or hypoechoic by ultrasonography. Early enucleation of ciliary body tumors has been recommended, although benign adenomas may remain static for years, making enucleation controversial for small tumors unassociated with secondary ocular disease. Local intraocular resection or laser photoablation may permit vision and ocular comfort to be maintained for at least some period of time.[43] However, in one study,[72] the vast majority of local excisional biopsies for iridociliary epithelial tumors had "dirty" margins and of the 19 dogs with follow-up only four did not have recurrence (which occurred an average of 23 months postbiopsy). In that study, adenomas were indistinguishable from adenocarcinomas on the basis of biopsy alone, although adenocarcinomas seldom metastasize. Complications of excisional biopsy include tumor recurrence, intraocular hemorrhage, chronic uveitis, cataract, glaucoma, lens displacement and retinal detachment. Systemic administration of 5-fluorouracil (5-FU) has been described as an adjunct to local resection of ciliary body tumors, but the efficacy of this therapy is unknown.[75]

Secondary Uveal Neoplasms

Numerous malignant tumors, especially adenocarcinomas, have been reported to metastasize to the highly vascular uveal tract. Metastatic tumors to the eye in dogs account for approximately 5% of all tumor submissions in the COPLOW database. Of those, the most common tumors in descending order are lymphomas, histiocytic sarcomas, hemangiosarcomas, respiratory (nasal and pulmonary) carcinomas, digital and oral melanomas, osteosarcomas and SCC.[78] In cats, the most common metastatic tumors to the eye are lymphomas, respiratory (nasal and pulmonary) carcinomas and SCC.

Lymphoma is the most common secondary intraocular tumor in the dog and cat, and ocular lesions are present in approximately one-third of dogs with the disease.[74,79–81] Ocular lymphomas are typically thought to be associated with systemic disease; however, a recent study found that, 60% of dogs with ocular lymphomas are free of systemic disease at the time of enucleation and hence were classified as presumed solitary ocular lymphoma (PSOL).[82] In this study, dogs with PSOL experienced a longer median survival time (MST, 769 days) than dogs with known systemic involvement (MST of 103 days). Histiocytic sarcomas account for 1.5% of all canine tumor submissions in the COPLOW database. In dogs, the diagnosis of ocular histiocytic sarcomas carries a poor prognosis with rapid progression of systemic disease and clinical decline. Unpublished data from the COPLOW laboratory indicates that dogs diagnosed with histiocytic sarcoma in the eye have an average survival time of 3 months. Common presentations include severe uveitis, glaucoma, retinal hemorrhages, hyphema, conjunctivitis, and keratitis characterized by corneal infiltrates, edema, vascularization, and intrastromal hemorrhage.[74,79–81] Exophthalmia resulting from orbital invasion by the tumor and vision loss due to optic nerve or central nervous system (CNS) disease may also be present. Posterior segment lesions may include retinal vascular tortuosity, papilledema, multiple intraretinal hemorrhages, and retinal detachment. In one study, the lifespan of dogs with intraocular lymphoma was only 60% to 70% as long as dogs without ocular involvement when treated with cyclophosphamide, vincristine, and prednisolone (COP), or with doxorubicin.[80] Topical or systemic corticosteroid therapy or enucleation is palliative. (See Chapter 33 for the definitive therapy of lymphoma.) Ophthalmic disease, especially intraocular or retinal hemorrhage, may also be the presenting complaint in animals with multiple myeloma.[83]

Tumors of the Orbit and Optic Nerve

Incidence and Risk Factors

Risk factors other than middle to old age, possibly large-breed dogs,[84] and possibly sex (female dogs, male cats) have not been described.[84–92] Tumors involving the optic nerve are rare, although secondary invasion occurs in feline posttraumatic sarcomas, feline SCC, and canine choroidal melanomas. Canine orbital meningioma is the most common tumor of the optic nerve but comprises only 3% of all meningiomas in dogs.[88,90] Orbital rhabdomyosarcoma is a relatively rare but highly malignant neoplasm in juvenile dogs that accounts for 0.2% of all canine tumor submissions in the COPLOW database.[93] Lobular adenomas of unspecified glandular origin have been recently reported to involve the anterior orbit in dogs.[89]

Pathology and Natural Behavior

Orbital neoplasia may be primary (most common in dogs), secondary to extension of adjacent tumors into the orbit (most common in cats), or the result of distant metastasis. In cats and dogs, more than 90% of orbital tumors are malignant, and regional infiltration (including into the CNS) or distant metastasis is common.[84–87] At least 26 types of orbital tumors, roughly equally divided among connective tissue, bone, epithelial, and hemolymphatic origins, have been reported in dogs.[87] Osteosarcomas, MCTs, histiocytic sarcomas, fibrosarcomas, and neurofibrosarcomas are the most common canine primary orbital tumors.[87] More than two-thirds of feline orbital tumors are epithelial in origin, with SCC being the most common,[86] but at least 15 other tumor types have been described in cats.

Canine orbital meningiomas exhibit predictable biologic behavior. They are slowly progressive and rarely metastasize; they may be osteolytic and invade surrounding tissues, including the CNS via the optic foramen.[87,89,90] Primary optic nerve tumors in dogs include glioma and meningioma.[87,88,90,91] Retinal and optic nerve gliomas may be considered as differential diagnoses of intraocular and orbital masses. The metastatic potential of gliomas appears to be low, but ascending invasion into the ventral aspect of the brain is possible.[92]

Canine orbital rhabdomyosarcomas (COR) are embryonal tumors that usually exhibit an aggressive biologic behavior. A recent case series reported that the age of the patient had a direct effect on the prognosis of the disease.[93] Dogs younger than 4 years old diagnosed with COR had high rates of recurrence and/ or metastasis and were euthanized within 6 months (median 2.5 months). On the other hand, COR in dogs 6 years of age or older had a less aggressive biologic behavior with no clinical signs of recurrence or metastasis 8 to 13 months postdiagnosis.

Lobular orbital adenomas are made up of multiple soft friable lobules in the anterior orbit, making complete surgical excision difficult.[89] We have noted that for this tumor, excision of the multiple soft masses is possible with a large diameter surgical suction tip or a Sims Connector. This increases the ability to completely remove the tumor and limits the surgical exposure required.

History and Clinical Signs

Slowly progressive exophthalmia, absent to minimal pain on opening the mouth, difficulty in retropulsing the eye, and deviation of the globe typify orbital neoplasia. Sudden erosion of nasal or sinus tumors into the orbit occasionally results in acute exophthalmia and substantial orbital pain. Enophthalmia may occur if the mass is anterior to the equator of the globe. Lobular adenomas may present as soft, raised, subconjunctival masses and create either enophthalmia or exophthalmia. Chronic epiphora secondary to obstruction of the nasolacrimal duct, exposure keratoconjunctivitis, palpable orbital masses after enucleation, or unexplained orbital pain also suggests orbital neoplasia.[84–87] Measurement of corneal diameters and intraocular pressure (IOP) aids in differentiating glaucomatous ocular enlargement (large corneal diameter, high IOP) from exophthalmia (normal corneal diameter and IOP).

Optic nerve lesions may result in unilateral or bilateral blindness (the latter if the optic chiasm is affected), optic nerve head pallor, papilledema, or marked protrusion and congestion of the optic disc on ophthalmoscopy. A relatively mild degree of exophthalmia with vision loss suggests optic nerve neoplasia because tumors of other orbital tissues typically cause profound exophthalmos before visual loss. Tumors affecting the retrobulbar, intracanalicular, or chiasmal portions of the optic nerve may not result in exophthalmia or a visible change in the optic nerve head.

Diagnostic Techniques and Workup

It is essential to differentiate nonneoplastic orbital inflammatory diseases (granulomas, cellulitis, abscesses, myositis of the extraocular and masticatory muscles) from neoplasia. Animals with inflammatory disease typically exhibit significant pain on opening the mouth. The location of an orbital mass can usually be determined by careful physical examination, including retropulsion of the globe, oral examination caudal to the last molar, and determination of the direction of malposition of the eye.

In addition to physical examination, cytology of regional lymph nodes, orbital ultrasound, orbital and thoracic radiographs and orbital CT/MRI imaging should be considered. In one study of cats with orbital neoplasia, 59% had radiographic signs of orbital bone lesions and 15% had evidence of metastasis on thoracic radiographs.[86] CT or MRI offer superior depictions of the orbit and facilitate planning of either radiation or surgical therapy (Fig. 32.8). Histologic characterization by FNA or needle core biopsies (performed via the mouth or through the orbital skin), with ultrasound or CT guidance if necessary, are helpful in arriving at a definitive diagnosis. The globe, major orbital blood vessels, and optic nerve should be avoided. Because 50% of orbital tumors

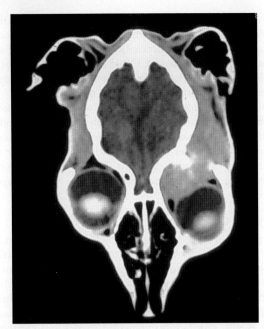

• **Fig. 32.8** CT (dorsal view) provides detailed information about the location and extent of orbital tumors, as in this 17-year-old cat with orbital osteosarcoma.

may have a nondiagnostic FNA, especially in cases of SCC,[86] exploratory orbitotomy via a number of approaches[94–99] or exenteration may be required to characterize the mass and resect it if possible. Cerebrospinal fluid taps may aid in distinguishing optic nerve neoplasia from optic neuritis.

Therapy

Primary orbital and optic nerve tumors that lack metastasis or regional lymph node involvement may be amenable to surgical excision. If bony involvement is not present, orbital exenteration by widely dissecting around the mass (stripping periorbita if necessary) is usually the preferred procedure, as the advanced stage of the tumor at the time of diagnosis typically makes it impossible to excise the mass completely and preserve a functional or comfortable eye. If periorbital bones are involved, radical "orbitectomy," which resects the affected orbital tissues and surrounding bones, should be considered.[96] When treating optic nerve tumors, as much of the ipsilateral optic nerve as possible should be removed in an attempt to obtain complete excision.[87]

If preservation of a comfortable eye and vision appears possible, a variety of orbitotomy/partial orbitectomy techniques, ranging from small incisions through the eyelid or mouth to reflection of the zygomatic arch, temporalis muscle elevation, zygomatic process osteotomy and ostectomy of a variety of orbital bony structures have been described.[94–99] Recently orbital reconstruction techniques have also been described which improve the tectonic, cosmetic and functional results of the procedure.[99] Postoperative complications are common and may include secondary enophthalmia with entropion and possibly diplopia (double vision). Surgical debulking as an alternative to "radical orbitectomy" can be palliative, and some dogs may survive a year or more with minimal therapy.

The role of chemotherapy and RT, either alone or as an adjunct to surgery, is yet to be defined in the treatment of orbital tumors, although chemotherapy for orbital lymphoma may be effective. Systemic corticosteroids may permit some patients with optic nerve meningioma to maintain vision for several weeks to months. RT may be helpful in the case of nasal tumors with orbital extension, in subtotally excised or recurrent meningiomas, and in other select cases.

Prognosis

With conservative treatment, the prognosis for most tumors involving the orbit and optic nerve is poor,[86,87] especially if there is bony involvement on skull radiographs. Recurrence at the primary site and involvement of adjacent or distant sites are common, often occurring within weeks to a few months. Even benign-appearing tumors such as lobular orbital adenomas and orbital meningiomas may be locally invasive and have a propensity for recurrence after wide excison.[84–90,96] In one study, however, radical orbitectomy (with or without chemotherapy or RT) provided a local disease-free interval of more than 1 year in more than 50% of patients and a 70% survival rate for the first year.[96] In another study, the mean survival time for cats with orbital tumors treated by RT, chemotherapy, or surgery that included resection of affected orbital bones was only 4.3 months.[86] In a study of 23 dogs with orbital tumors, most of which were treated by exenteration with or without adjunct therapy, only three survived 3 years or longer.[87] The majority of these animals died as a direct result of the tumor or were euthanatized at the time of diagnosis.[84–87]

Ocular Effects of Cancer Therapeutic Modalities

The ocular effect of external-beam RT for nasal and periocular tumors can have a substantial effect on an animal's quality of life. Common complications include chronic keratoconjunctivitis, corneal ulceration, "dry eye," enophthalmia, entropion, cataracts, retinal hemorrhages, retinal detachments, and blindness.[100–103] Many of these conditions respond poorly to treatment, and vigorous attempts at prevention should be made to avoid chronic ocular pain and blindness. Recently intensity-modulated RT (IMRT), which uses conformal avoidance, has been shown to significantly decrease the ocular toxicity seen in dogs treated by RT for spontaneous sinonasal tumors.[102,103]

In humans, blurred vision, partial visual field defects, loss of color vision, and diplopia have been associated with several antineoplastic drugs.[104–107] Similar effects probably occur in animals but would be difficult to detect. In addition, in humans, the bacillus Calmette-Guérin (BCG) has been associated with uveitis; cyclophosphamide has been associated with dry eye; cisplatin has been associated with neuroretinal toxicity; doxorubicin has been associated with excessive lacrimation and conjunctivitis; 5-FU has been associated with blurred vision, excessive lacrimation, blepharitis, conjunctivitis, and keratitis; and vincristine has been associated with cranial nerve palsies, optic neuropathy, and cortical and night blindness.[104] Monoclonal antibodies directed at the vasculature supporting the tumor also have been associated with uveitis.[105] Antibody–drug conjugates have been associated with blurred vision, dry eye, and corneal abnormalities including microcystic corneal disease.[106]

Comparative Aspects

Malignant melanoma of the choroid is the most common primary ocular malignancy in adult humans. Initially, it was believed that enucleation of these patients may enhance the risk of metastasis;

thus a large randomized clinical trial (the Collaborative Ocular Melanoma Study) was conducted comparing enucleation with iodine-125 brachytherapy, which left the globe intact.[108,109] Both treatment modalities yielded similar results, although many patients still died from metastatic melanoma, and it appears that significant improvement in survival rates will depend on developing effective systemic therapeutic modalities for melanoma.[108,109]

Retinoblastoma is the most common malignant intraocular tumor of children and has a genetic basis. No cases of retinoblastoma have been described in nonhuman primates, and only one case of retinoblastoma has been described in a dog.[110] With therapy, long-term survival in children is over 85%, but many patients develop second tumors, especially osteosarcoma.[111] Cancer-associated retinopathy is an uncommon, immune-mediated paraneoplastic phenomenon in humans in which antibodies are directed against specific retinal autoantigens, such as recoverin.[112–114] In this condition, patients with small-cell lung carcinoma and other tumors may develop blurred vision, impaired color vision, substantial visual field defects, or complete blindness as tumor antigens cross-react with specific retinal components.[112–114] Treatment with IV immunoglobulin has been reported to return vision to some patients.[112] Although cancer-associated retinopathy has been suggested to occur in dogs, especially those with sudden acquired retinal degeneration syndrome (SARDS), definitive proof is lacking and one study did not identify antibody activity against retinal proteins or evidence of neoplasia in dogs with SARDS.[115]

Acknowledgments

The authors wish to thank Dr. Richard R. Dubielzig for his invaluable contributions to earlier editions of this chapter.

References

1. Krehbiel JD, Langham RF: Eyelid neoplasms in dogs, *Am J Vet Res* 36:115–119, 1975.
2. Roberts SM, Severin GA, Lavach JD: Prevalence and treatment of palpebral neoplasms in the dog: 200 cases (1975-1983), *J Am Vet Med Assoc* 189:1355–1359, 1986.
3. McLaughlin SA, Whitley RD, Gilger BC, et al.: Eyelid neoplasms in cats: A review of demographic data (1979 to 1989), *J Am Anim Hosp Assoc* 29:63–67, 1983.
4. Barrie KP, Gelatt KN, Parshall CP: Eyelid squamous cell carcinoma in four dogs, *J Am Anim Hosp Assoc* 18:123–127, 1982.
5. Bernays ME, Flemming D, Peiffer RL: Primary corneal papilloma and squamous cell carcinoma associated with pigmentary keratitis in four dogs, *J Am Vet Med Assoc* 214:215–217, 1999.
6. Collins BK, Collier LL, Miller MA, et al.: Biologic behavior and histologic characteristics of canine conjunctival melanoma, *Prog Vet Comp Ophthalmol* 3:135–140, 1993.
7. Roels S, Ducatelle R: Malignant melanoma of the nictitating membrane in a cat (Felix vulgaris), *J Comp Pathol* 119:189–193, 1998.
8. Brandes K, Fritsche J, Mueller N, et al.: Detection of canine oral papillomavirus DNA in conjunctival epithelial hyperplastic lesions of three dogs, *Vet Pathol* 46:34–38, 2009.
9. Beckwith-Cohen B, Teixeira LB, Ramos-Vara JA, et al.: Squamous papillomas of the conjunctiva in dogs: a condition not associated with papillomavirus infection, *Vet Pathol* 52:676–680, 2015.
10. Bonney CH, Koch SA, Dice PF, et al.: Papillomatosis of conjunctiva and adnexa in dogs, *J Am Vet Med Assoc* 176:48–51, 1980.
11. Collier LL, Collins BK: Excision and cryosurgical ablation of severe periocular papillomatosis in a dog, *J Am Vet Med Assoc* 204:881–885, 1994.
12. Dreyfus J, Schobert CS, Dubielzig RR: Superficial corneal squamous cell carcinoma occurring in dogs with chronic keratitis, *Vet Ophthalmol* 14:161–168, 2011.
13. Dees DD, Schobert CS, Dubielzig RR, et al.: Third eyelid gland neoplasms of dogs and cats: a retrospective histopathologic study of 145 cases, *Vet Ophthalmol* 19:138–143, 2016.
14. Schäffer EH, Pfleghaar S, Gordon S, et al.: Malignant nictitating membrane tumors in dogs and cats, *Tierarztliche Praxis* 22:382–389, 1994.
15. Hargis AM, Lee AC, Thomassen RW: Tumor and tumor-like lesions of perilimbal conjunctiva in laboratory dogs, *J Am Vet Med Assoc* 173:1185–1190, 1978.
16. Mughannam AJ, Hacker DV, Spangler WL: Conjunctival vascular tumors in six dogs, *Vet Comp Ophthalmol* 7:56–59, 1997.
17. Multari D, Vascellari M, Mutinelli F: Hemangiosarcoma of the third eyelid in a cat, *Vet Ophthalmol* 5:273–276, 2002.
18. Pirie CG, Knollinger AM, Thomas CB, et al.: Canine conjunctival hemangioma and hemangiosarcoma: a retrospective evaluation of 108 cases (1989-2004), *Vet Ophthalmol* 9:215–226, 2006.
19. Pirie CG, Dubielzig RR: Feline conjunctival hemangioma and hemangiosarcoma: a retrospective evaluation of eight cases (1993-2004), *Vet Ophthalmol* 9:227–231, 2006.
20. Patnaik AK, Mooney S: Feline melanoma: a comparative study of ocular, oral and dermal neoplasms, *Vet Pathol* 25:105–112, 1988.
21. Schobert CS, Labelle P, Dubielzig RR: Feline conjunctival melanoma: histopathological characteristics and clinical outcomes, *Vet Ophthalmol* 13:43–46, 2010.
22. Johnson BW, Brightman, Whiteley HE: Conjunctival mast cell tumor in two dogs, *J Am Anim Hosp Assoc* 24:439–442, 1988.
23. Fife M, Blocker T, Fife T, et al.: Canine conjunctival mast cell tumors: a retrospective study, *Vet Ophthalmol* 14:153–160, 2011.
24. Kafarnik C, Calvarese S, Dubielzig RR: Canine mesenchymal hamartoma of the eyelid, *Vet Ophthalmol* 13:94–98, 2010.
25. Bettenay S, Mueller RS, Maggs DJ: Diseases of the Eyelids. In Maggs DJ, Miller PE, Ofri R, editors: *Slatter's fundamentals of veterinary ophthalmology*, 6th ed., St. Louis, 2018, Elsevier.
26. Dees DD, Knollinger AM, MacLaren NE: Carbon dioxide (CO_2) laser third eyelid excision: surgical description and report of 7 cases, *Vet Ophthalmol* 18:381–384, 2015.
27. Guiliano EA: Diseases of the adnexal and nasolacrimal system. In Gilger BC, editor: *Equine ophthalmology*, ed 3, St. Louis, 2017, Elsevier, pp 197–251.
28. Holmberg DL, Withrow SJ: Cryosurgical treatment of palpebral neoplasms: clinical and experimental results, *Vet Surg* 8:68–73, 1979.
29. Donaldson D, Sansom J, Scase T, et al.: Canine limbal melanoma: 30 cases (1992-2004). Part 1. Signalment, clinical and histological features and pedigree analysis, *Vet Ophthalmol* 9:115–119, 2006.
30. Wilcock BP, Peiffer RL: Morphology and behavior of primary ocular melanomas in 91 dogs, *Vet Pathol* 23:418–424, 1986.
31. Zoroquiain P, Mayo-Goldberg E, Alghamdi S, et al.: Melanocytoma-like melanoma may be the missing link between benign and malignant uveal melanocytic lesions in humans and dogs: a comparative study, *Melanoma Res* 26:565–571, 2016.
32. Diters RW, Dubielzig RR, Aquirre GD, et al.: Primary ocular melanoma in dogs, *Vet Pathol* 20:379–395, 1983.
33. Diters RW, Ryan AM: Canine limbal melanoma, *Vet Med Small Anim Clin* 78:1529–1534, 1983.
34. Harling DE, Peiffer RL, Cook CS, et al.: Feline limbal melanoma: four cases, *J Am Anim Hosp Assoc* 22:795–802, 1986.
35. Sullivan TC, Nasisse MP, Davidson MG, et al.: Photocoagulation of limbal melanoma in dogs and cats: 15 cases (1989-1993), *J Am Vet Med Assoc* 208:891–894, 1996.
36. Featherstone HJ, Renwick P, Heinrich CL, et al.: Efficacy of lamellar resection, cryotherapy, and adjunctive grafting for the treatment of canine limbal melanoma, *Vet Ophthalmol* 12(Suppl 1):65–72, 2009.

37. Mathes RL, Moore PA, Ellis AE: Penetrating sclerokeratoplasty and autologous pinnal cartilage and conjunctival grafting to treat a large limbal melanoma in a dog, *Vet Ophthalmol* 18:152–159, 2015.

38. Maggio F, Pizzirani S, Peña T, et al.: Surgical treatment of epibulbar melanocytomas by complete excision and homologous corneoscleral grafting in dogs: 11 cases, *Vet Ophthalmol* 16:56–64, 2013.

39. Donaldson D, Sansom J, Scase T, et al.: Canine limbal melanoma: 30 cases (1992-2004). Part 2. Treatment with lamellar resection and adjunctive strontium-90 beta plesiotherapy—efficacy and morbidity, *Vet Ophthalmol* 9:179–185, 2006.

40. Gelatt KN, Johnson KA, Peiffer RL: Primary iridal pigmented masses in three dogs, *J Am Anim Hosp Assoc* 15:339–344, 1979.

41. Bussanich NM, Dolman PJ, Rootman J, et al.: Canine uveal melanomas: series and literature review, *J Am Anim Hosp Assoc* 23:415–422, 1987.

42. Petersen-Jones SM, Forcier J, Mentzer AL: Ocular melanosis in the Cairn Terrier: clinical description and investigation of mode of inheritance, *Vet Ophthalmol* 10(Suppl 1):63–69, 2007.

43. Nasisse MP, Davidson MG, Olivero DK, et al.: Neodymium:YAG laser treatment of primary canine intraocular tumors, *Prog Vet Comp Ophthalmol* 3:152–157, 1993.

44. Cook CS, Wilkie DA: Treatment of presumed iris melanoma in dogs by diode laser photocoagulation: 23 cases, *Vet Ophthalmol* 2:217–225, 1999.

45. Giuliano EA, Chappell R, Fischer B, et al.: A matched observational study of canine survival with primary melanocytic neoplasia, *Vet Ophthalmol* 2:185–190, 1999.

46. Collinson PN, Peiffer RL: Clinical presentation, morphology, and behavior of primary choroidal melanomas in eight dogs, *Prog Vet Comp Ophthalmol* 3:158–164, 1993.

47. Dubielzig RR, Aquirre GD, Gross SL, et al.: Choroidal melanomas in dogs, *Vet Pathol* 22:582–585, 1985.

48. Hyman JA, Koch SA, Wilcock BP: Canine choroidal melanoma with metastases, *Vet Ophthalmol* 5:113–117, 2002.

49. Duncan DE, Peiffer RL: Morphology and prognostic indicators of anterior uveal melanomas in cats, *Prog Vet Comp Ophthalmol* 1:25–32, 1991.

50. Kalishman JB, Chappell R, Flood LA, et al.: A matched observational study of survival in cats with enucleation due to diffuse iris melanoma, *Vet Ophthalmol* 1:21–24, 1998.

51. Bellhorn RW, Henkind P: Intraocular malignant melanomas in domestic cats, *J Small Anim Pract* 10:631–637, 1970.

52. Patnaik AK, Mooney S: Feline melanoma: a comparative study of ocular, oral and dermal neoplasms, *Vet Pathol* 25:105–112, 1988.

53. Acland GM, McLean IW, Aquirre GD, et al.: Diffuse iris melanoma in cats, *J Am Vet Med Assoc* 176:52–56, 1980.

54. Wiggans KT, Reilly CM, Kass PH, et al.: Histologic and immunohistologic predictors for clinical behavior for feline diffuse iris melanoma, *Vet Ophthalmol* 19:44–55, 2016.

55. Fragola J, Dubielzig RR, Bentley E, et al.: Iridociliary cysts masquerading as neoplasia in cats: a morphologic review of 14 cases, *Veterinary Ophthalmol Epub ahead of print*, 2017.

56. Niederkorn JY, Shadduck JA, Albert DM: Enucleation and the appearance of second primary tumors in cats bearing virally induced intraocular tumors, *Invest Ophthalmol Vis Sci* 23:719–725, 1982.

57. Cullen CL, Haines DM, Jackson ML, et al.: Lack of detection of feline leukemia and feline sarcoma viruses in diffuse iris melanomas of cats by immunohistochemistry and polymerase chain reaction, *J Vet Diagn Invest* 14:340–343, 2002.

58. Peiffer RL, Monticello T, Bouldin TW: Primary ocular sarcomas in the cat, *J Small Anim Pract* 29:105–116, 1988.

59. Dubielzig RR, Everitt J, Shadduck JA, et al.: Clinical and morphologic features of post-traumatic ocular sarcomas in cats, *Vet Pathol* 27:62–65, 1990.

60. Dubielzig RR, Hawkins KL, Toy KA, et al.: Morphologic features of feline ocular sarcomas in 10 cats: light microscopy, ultrastructure, and immunohistochemistry, *Vet Comp Ophthalmol* 4:7–12, 1994.

61. Håkansson N, Shively JN, Reed RE, et al.: Intraocular spindle cell sarcoma following ocular trauma in a cat: case report and literature review, *J Am Anim Hosp Assoc* 26:63–66, 1990.

62. Duke FD, Strong TD, Bentley E, et al.: Feline ocular tumors following ciliary body ablation with intravitreal gentamicin, *Vet Ophthalmol* 16:188–190, 2013.

63. Albert DM, Phelps PO, Surapaneni KR, et al.: The significance of the discordant occurrence of lens tumors in humans versus other species, *Ophthalmol* 122:1765–1770, 2015.

64. Takahashi H, Ueda S, Matsubayashi J, et al.: An immunohistochemical study for the tumorigenesis of feline ocular post-traumatic sarcoma, *Invest Ophthalmol Vis Sci (Abstract)* 56:3413, 2015.

65. Naranjo C, Schobert CS, Dubielzig RR: Round cell variant of feline ocular posttraumatic sarcoma: a retrospective study, *Vet Ophthalmol (Abstract)* 10:399, 2007.

66. Dubielzig RR, Zeiss C: Feline post-traumatic ocular sarcoma: Three morphologic variants and evidence that some are derived from lens epithelial cells, *Invest Ophthalmol Vis Sci* 45:3562, 2004.

67. Dubielzig RR: Feline post-traumatic ocular sarcoma: a review of 110 cases, *Proc Am Coll Vet Pathol, New Orleans, Vet Pathol* 39:619, 2002.

68. Klauss G, Dubielzig RR: Characteristics of primary spindle cell neoplasm of the anterior uveal tract: 11 dogs. *Proc Am Coll Vet Pathol, Salt Lake City, Vet Pathol* 38:574, 2001.

69. Zarfoss MK, Klauss G, Newkirk K, et al.: Uveal spindle cell tumor of blue-eyed dogs: an immunohistochemical study, *Vet Pathol* 44:276–284, 2007.

70. Duke FD, Brudenall DK, Scott EM, et al.: Metastatic uveal schwannoma of blue-eyed dogs, *Vet Ophthalmol* 16:141–144, 2013.

71. Dubielzig RR, Steinberg H, Garvin H, et al.: Iridociliary epithelial tumors in 100 dogs and 17 cats: a morphological study, *Vet Ophthalmol* 1:223–231, 1998.

72. Beckwith-Cohen B, Bentley E, Dubielzig RR: Outcome of iridociliary epithelial tumour biopsies in dogs: a retrospective study, *Vet Record* 176:147–151, 2015.

73. Peiffer RL: Ciliary body epithelial tumors in the dog and cat: a report of thirteen cases, *J Small Anim Pract* 24:347–370, 1983.

74. Gwin RM, Gelatt KN, Williams LW: Ophthalmic neoplasms in the dog, *J Am Anim Hosp Assoc* 18:853–866, 1982.

75. Clerc B: Surgery and chemotherapy for the treatment of adenocarcinoma of the iris and ciliary body in five dogs, *Vet Comp Ophthalmol* 6:265–270, 1996.

76. Bell CM, Dubielzig RR: Canine iridociliary epithelial tumors: a morphologic review of 702 cases, *Vet Pathol (Abstract)* 46:1064, 2009.

77. Shaw G, Dubielzig RR, Teixeira LBC: A case series of canine pleomorphic iridociliary adenocarcinomas, *Invest Ophthalmol Vis Sci (Abstract)* 56:3414, 2015.

78. Teixeira LBC, Dubielzig RR: Ocular metastasis in dogs: a retrospective study of 320 cases, *Invest Ophthalmol Vis Sci (Abstract)* 579(7):4114, 2016.

79. Williams LW, Gelatt KN, Gwin RM: Ophthalmic neoplasms in the cat, *J Am Anim Hosp Assoc* 17:999–1008, 1981.

80. Krohne SG, Henderson NM, Richardson RC, et al.: Prevalence of ocular involvement in dogs with multicentric lymphoma: prospective evaluation of 94 cases, *Vet Comp Ophthalmol* 4:127–135, 1994.

81. Corcoran KA, Peiffer RL, Koch SA: Histopathologic features of feline ocular lymphosarcoma: 49 cases (1978-1992), *Vet Comp Ophthalmol* 5:35–41, 1995.

82. Lanza MR, Musciano AR, Dubielzig RD, et al.: Clinical and pathological classification of canine intraocular lymphoma, *Vet Ophthalmol* Epub ahead of print, 2017.

83. Hendrix DV, Gelatt KN, Smith PJ, et al.: Ophthalmic disease as the presenting complaint in five dogs with multiple myeloma, *J Am Anim Hosp Assoc* 34:121–128, 1998.

84. Attali-Soussay K, Jegou JP, Clerc B: Retrobulbar tumors in dogs and cats: 25 cases, *Vet Ophthalmol* 4:19–27, 2001.

85. Mauldin EA, Deehr AJ, Hertzke D, et al.: Canine orbital meningiomas: a review of 22 cases, *Vet Ophthalmol* 3:11–16, 2000.

86. Gilger BC, McLaughlin SA, Whitley RD, et al.: Orbital neoplasms in cats: 21 cases (1974-1990), *J Am Vet Med Assoc* 201:1083–1086, 1992.

87. Kern TJ: Orbital neoplasia in 23 dogs, *J Am Vet Med Assoc* 186:489–491, 1985.

88. Braund KG, Ribas JL: Central nervous system meningiomas, *Compend Contin Educ Pract Vet* 8:241–248, 1986.

89. Headrick JK, Bentley E, Dubielzig RR: Canine lobular orbital adenoma: a report of 15 cases with distinctive features, *Vet Ophthalmol* 7:47–51, 2004.

90. Dugan SJ, Schwarz PD, Roberts SM, et al.: Primary optic nerve meningioma and pulmonary metastasis in a dog, *J Am Anim Hosp Assoc* 29:11–16, 1993.

91. Spiess BM, Wilcock BP: Glioma of the optic nerve with intraocular and intracranial involvement in a dog, *J Comp Pathol* 97:79–84, 1987.

92. Naranjo C, Schobert C, Dubielzig RR: Canine ocular gliomas: a retrospective study, *Vet Ophthalmol* 11:356–362, 2008.

93. Scott EM, Teixeira LBC, Flanders DJ, et al.: Canine orbital rhabdomyosarcoma: a report of 18 cases, *Vet Ophthalmol* 19:130–137, 2016.

94. Slatter DH, Abdelbaki Y: Lateral orbitotomy by zygomatic arch resection in the dog, *J Am Vet Med Assoc* 175:1179–1182, 1979.

95. Gilger BC, Whitely RD, McLaughlin SA: Modified lateral orbitotomy for removal of orbital neoplasms in two dogs, *Vet Surg* 23:53–58, 1994.

96. O'Brien MG, Withrow SJ, Straw RC, et al.: Total and partial orbitectomy for the treatment of periorbital tumors in 24 dogs and 6 cats: a retrospective study, *Vet Surg* 25:471–479, 1996.

97. Håkansson NW, Håkansson BW: Transfrontal orbitotomy in the dog: an adaptable three-step approach to the orbit, *Vet Ophthalmol* 13:377–383, 2010.

98. Bartoe JT, Brightman AH, Davidson HJ: Modified lateral orbitotomy for vision-sparing excision of a zygomatic mucocele in a dog, *Vet Ophthalmol* 10:127–131, 2007.

99. Wallin-Håkansson N, Berggren K: Orbital reconstruction in the dog, cat and horse, *Vet Ophthalmol* 20:316–328, 2017.

100. Adams WM, Miller PE, Vail DM, et al.: An accelerated technique for irradiation of malignant canine nasal and paranasal sinus tumors, *Vet Radiol Ultrasound* 5:475–481, 1998.

101. Roberts SM, Lavach JD, Severin GA, et al.: Ophthalmic complications following megavoltage irradiation of the nasal and paranasal cavities in dogs, *J Am Vet Med Assoc* 190:43–47, 1987.

102. Miller PE, Turek MM, Forrest LJ, et al.: Ocular sparing using intensity modulated radiation therapy (IMRT) in a canine model of spontaneous sinonasal cancer: proof of principle of conformal avoidance, *Invest Ophthalmol Vis Sci* 46:5408, 2005.

103. Lawrence JA, Forrest LJ, Turek MM: Proof of principle of ocular sparing in dogs with sinonasal tumors treated with intensity-modulated radiation therapy, *Vet Radiol Ultrasound* 51:561–570, 2010.

104. Imperia PS, Lazarus HM, Lass JH: Ocular complications of systemic cancer chemotherapy, *Surg Ophthalmol* 34:209–230, 1989.

105. Martin PL, Miller PE, Mata M, et al.: Ocular inflammation in cynomolgus macaques following intravenous administration of a human monoclonal antibody, *J Toxicol* 28:5–16, 2009.

106. Eaton JS, Miller PE, Mannis MJ, et al.: Ocular adverse events associated with antibody drug conjugates in human clinical trials, *J Ocular Pharm Ther* 31:589–604, 2015.

107. Kheir WJ, Sniegowski MC, El-Sawy T, et al.: Ophthalmic complications of targeted cancer therapy and recently recognized ophthalmic complications of traditional chemotherapy, *Surv Ophthalmol* 59:493–502, 2014.

108. Chattopahdyay C, Kim DW, Gombos D, et al.: Uveal melanoma: from diagnosis to treatment and the science in between, *Cancer* 122:2299–2312, 2016.

109. Diener-West M, Earle JD, Fine SL, et al.: The COMS randomized trial of iodine 125 brachytherapy for choroidal melanoma, III: Initial mortality findings, COMS Report No. 18, *Arch Ophthalmol* 119:969–982, 2001.

110. Syed NA, Nork TM, Poulsen GL, et al.: Retinoblastoma in a dog, *Arch Ophthalmol* 115:758–763, 1997.

111. Shields CL, Meadows AT, Leahey AM, et al.: Continuing challenges in the management of retinoblastoma with chemotherapy, *Retina* 24:849–862, 2004.

112. Guy J, Aptiauri N: Treatment of paraneoplastic visual loss with intravenous immunoglobulin: report of 3 cases, *Arch Ophthalmol* 117:471–477, 1999.

113. Subramanian L, Polan AS: Cancer-related diseases of the eye: the role of calcium-binding proteins, *Biochem Biophys Res Commun* 322:1153–1165, 2004.

114. Ohgura H, Yokoi Y, Ohguro I, et al.: Clinical and immunologic aspects of cancer-associated retinopathy, *Am J Ophthalmol* 137:1117–1119, 2004.

115. Gilmour MA, Cardenas MR, Blaik MA, et al.: Evaluation of a comparative pathogenesis between cancer-associated retinopathy in humans and sudden acquired retinal degeneration syndrome in dogs via diagnostic imaging and western blot analysis, *Am J Vet Res* 67:877–881, 2006.

33

Hematopoietic Tumors

**DAVID M. VAIL, MARIE PINKERTON, AND
KAREN M. YOUNG**

Lymphoma

Lymphoma (malignant lymphoma or lymphosarcoma) comprises a diverse group of neoplasms that have in common their origin from lymphocytes. The neoplasms usually arise in lymphoid tissues such as lymph nodes (LNs), spleen, and bone marrow; however, they may arise in almost any tissue in the body. Although the annual incidence of lymphoma is difficult to predict in the absence of a national canine tumor registry, it is clear that it represents one of the most common neoplasms seen in the dog. The annual incidence has been estimated to range between 13 and 114 per 100,000 dogs at risk. The rates at specific ages are estimated to be 1.5 per 100,000 for dogs less than 1 year of age and 84 per 100,000 for dogs 10 to 11 years old.[1–4] Lymphoma comprises approximately 7% to 24% of all canine neoplasias and 83% of all canine hematopoietic malignancies.[5,6] In a review of the Veterinary Medical Database Program (VMDP) at Purdue University from 1987 to 1997, the frequency of dogs presented with lymphoma to 20 veterinary institutions increased from 0.75% to 2.0% of total case load, and it appears the frequency is continuing to increase. A similar trend is present in physician-based oncology; non-Hodgkin's lymphoma (NHL) represents 5% of all new cancer cases, the fifth leading cause of cancer death, and the second fastest growing cancer in terms of mortality in humans.[7] Middle-aged to older (median age of 6–9 years) dogs are primarily affected, although dogs with T-cell lymphoma tend to be younger.[8] A decreased risk for lymphoma is reported for intact females.[9] Breeds reported to have a higher incidence include boxers, bullmastiffs, basset hounds, St. Bernards, Scottish terriers, Airedales, pitbulls, Briards, Irish setters, Rottweilers, and bulldogs; breeds at lower risk include dachshunds and Pomeranians.[8,10,11] See Box 33.1.

Etiology

The etiology of canine lymphoma is likely multifactorial and largely unknown; however, investigations are currently shedding significant light on the subject.

Genetic and Molecular Factors

Advances in molecular cytogenetics (see Chapter 1, Section A), including array-comparative genomic hybridization and chromosome painting, have been and are currently being applied to investigations of chromosomal aberrations in dogs with lymphoma.[12–18] Publication of the canine genome and commercial availability of canine gene microarrays (GeneChip Canine Genome 2.0 Array, Affymetrix, Inc.) have led to advances in our understanding of deregulations of gene expression occurring in lymphoma.[19] Gains of canine chromosomes 13 and 31 and loss of chromosome 14 have been documented as the most common aberrations in a group of 25 cases analyzed.[17] Chromosomal aberrations have also been associated with prognosis in dogs with lymphoma. A study of 61 dogs with lymphoma demonstrated a prognostic advantage in dogs with trisomy of chromosome 13 (25% of the dogs studied), as evidenced by increase in duration of first remission and overall survival time (ST).[20] Germline and somatic genetic mutations and altered oncogene/tumor suppressor gene expression, epigenetic changes (e.g., DNA hypomethylation), signal transduction, and death-pathway alterations (e.g., Bcl-2 family) are common in human lymphomas and have been reported in the dog as well (see Chapter 1, Section A, and Chapter 15, Section B).[21–25] These include N-ras, p53, Rb, p16 cyclin-dependent kinase, telomerase, and NF-κB among others.[22,26–31] Somatic mutations, as determined by exome sequencing, have shown much overlap in canine breeds with respect to B-cell lymphoma, specifically mutations in TRAF3-MAP3K14, FBXW7, and POT1, but little overlap in somatic mutations among breeds with T-cell lymphoma.[21] In addition, differences in the prevalence of immunophenotypic subtypes of lymphoma among different breeds indicate heritable risks.[32] Telomerase activity (see Chapter 2) has also been documented in canine lymphoma tissues.[33–35] As somatic mutations are often implicated, it is not surprising that alterations or deficiencies in DNA repair mechanisms would also be implicated, as has been demonstrated in golden retrievers with lymphoma.[36]

Infectious Factors

The hypothesis that a retrovirus may be involved in the pathogenesis of canine lymphoma has not been confirmed. Epstein–Barr virus, a gammaherpesvirus linked to some forms of lymphoma in humans, has also been investigated in canine lymphoma; however, there was no association between serologic or molecular detection of gammaherpesvirus and development of lymphoma.[37,38]

In humans, a direct association between *Helicobacter* sp. infections and development of gastric lymphoma has been made.[39] Although this has not been definitively shown in dogs, there is

Key Clinical Summary Points: Canine Lymphoma

- Lymphoma is a catch-all term for approximately two dozen lymphocyte cancer subtypes (Table 33.1).
- Most are intermediate or high grade, but indolent forms exist.
- Dogs with lymphoma most commonly have peripheral lymphadenopathy, although varied anatomic locations can be affected (Box 33.2).
- For nodal disease, needle aspirate cytology is a good first screening step; ancillary diagnostics are required to subtype for prognosis or to confirm diagnosis in equivocal cases (Figs. 33.3, 33.8).
- Many treatment protocols exist, but most involve CHOP-based combination chemotherapy (Table 33.4).
- Initially gratifying to treat, as response rates are high and often durable (>6 months); however, cures are rare (<10%) and it is ultimately a uniformly fatal disease.
- Dogs with indolent subtypes may live years, often without therapeutic intervention.
- A veterinary oncology specialist should be consulted on individual cases, as the clinical, diagnostic, and therapeutic landscape changes rapidly.

evidence of *Helicobacter* sp. infection in laboratory beagle dogs resulting in gastric lymphoid follicle formation that is considered a precursor of mucosa-associated lymphoid tissue (MALT) lymphoma in humans.[40]

Alterations in the gut microbiome have been implicated as playing a role in susceptibility to certain tumors. Fecal microbiota of dogs with lymphoma have been shown to be significantly different than control dogs, although a cause–effect relationship is unclear.[41]

Environmental Factors

In humans, evidence has accumulated implicating phenoxyacetic acid herbicides, in particular 2,4-dichlorophenoxyacetic acid (2, 4-D), in the development of NHL. Some epidemiologic evidence also implicates lawn herbicide use and occurrence of lymphoma incidence in dogs.[42–45] In one case-control study, the risk of canine lymphoma was reported to rise two-fold (odds ratio [OR] = 1.3) with four or more yearly owner applications of 2,4-D. The results of this study have come under criticism, and three additional follow-up investigations have not validated this increased risk.[46–48] In another study, dogs exposed to lawn treatment within 7 days of application were greater than 50 times more likely to have 2,4-D urinary levels of 50 μg/L or higher.[45] In an environmental case-control study performed in Europe, two variables, residency in industrial areas and use of chemicals (defined as paints or solvents) by owners, modestly increased the risk of developing lymphoma; however, no link was found with pesticide use.[49] A more recent epidemiologic study investigating multiple environmental factors showed increased risk of canine lymphoma with use of lawn care products, in particular professionally applied pesticides.[43] This study did not find an association with flea and tick control products.

A weak association between lymphoma in dogs and exposure to strong magnetic fields was observed in a preliminary epidemiologic study.[50] In this hospital-based case-control study, the risk of developing lymphoma with high or very high exposure was increased (OR = 1.8). More thorough studies are necessary to evaluate this association further. Proximity to environmental waste was implicated in two European studies; however, it was felt to be a risk indicator rather than a risk factor and would require further case-control investigations.[51,52] Exposure to tobacco smoke was also implicated in one study.[53]

Immunologic Factors

Impaired immune function has also been implicated in dogs with lymphoma. Immune system alterations, such as immune-mediated thrombocytopenia, independent of age and sex, have been associated with a higher risk of subsequently developing lymphoma compared with the normal population.[54,55] Additional evidence comes from observations in human and feline transplantation patients.[56–58] In a case-control study of cats undergoing renal transplant, 24% of cases developed cancer (36% of those were lymphoma) while on cyclosporine immunosuppressive therapy compared with 5.1% of control cats, none of which developed lymphoma (OR, 6.1; *p* = 0.001).[58] A case of lymphoma developing in a dog after treatment with cyclosporine also exists.[57] One report suggests an association between the immunodysregulation observed in dogs with atopic dermatitis and the risk of developing epitheliotropic T-cell lymphoma; whether lymphoma is associated with the primary disease or the immunomodulatory treatments commonly applied is unknown.[59]

Classification and Pathology

Classification of malignant lymphoma in dogs is based on anatomic location, histologic criteria, and immunophenotypic characteristics. The most common anatomic forms of lymphoma, in order of decreasing prevalence, are multicentric, gastrointestinal (GI), mediastinal, and cutaneous forms.[60] Primary extranodal forms, which can occur in any location outside the lymphatic system, include the eyes, skin, central nervous system (CNS), bone marrow, bladder, heart, and nasal cavity. The pathologic characteristics of the various anatomic classifications will be discussed in this section and clinical characteristics will be described in subsequent sections.

More than 80% of dogs with lymphoma are presented with the multicentric form, which is usually characterized by the presence of peripheral lymphadenopathy (Fig. 33.1).[60] The alimentary form of lymphoma is much less common, accounting for 5% to 7% of all canine lymphomas. Primary GI lymphoma in dogs may occur focally, but more often affects multiple segments with thickening of the wall, narrowing of the lumen, and frequently mucosal ulceration.[61,62] Histologically, there is infiltration of neoplastic lymphocytes throughout the mucosa and submucosa with occasional transmural infiltration. Liver and local LNs are often secondarily involved. Lymphocytic-plasmacytic inflammatory bowel disease (LP-IBD) can be seen adjacent to or distant from the primary tumor. Pathologically, some of these neoplasms may resemble plasma cell tumors and aberrant production of immunoglobulins may occur. Histologically, distinguishing between GI lymphoma and LP-IBD can be difficult. Some have suggested that LP-IBD may be a prelymphomatous change in the GI tract. A syndrome of immunoproliferative intestinal disease characterized by LP-IBD has been described in Basenjis, which subsequently develop GI lymphoma.[63] In addition, plasma cell–rich areas with heterogeneous lymphomatous infiltration may resemble lesions of LP-IBD. Only a few reports specifically identify the immunophenotype of the lymphocyte subpopulations in GI lymphoma in dogs. Historically, it was presumed that they most likely originate from B cells; however, recent evidence suggests that most GI lymphomas in dogs arise from T cells and often exhibit epitheliotropism.[62,64,65] The boxer and Shar-pei breeds may be overrepresented in cases of alimentary lymphoma.[65,66]

The mediastinal form of the disease occurs in approximately 5% of cases.[60] This form is characterized by enlargement of the cranial mediastinal LNs, thymus, or both (Fig. 33.2). Hypercalcemia is reported to occur in 10% to 40% of dogs with lymphoma and is most common with the mediastinal form. In a study of 37 dogs with lymphoma and hypercalcemia, 16 (43%) had mediastinal lymphoma.[67] The mediastinal form in dogs is most commonly associated with a T-cell phenotype.[68,69] A single case of mediastinal γδT-cell lymphoma with large granular lymphocyte morphology has been reported.[70]

Cutaneous lymphoma can be solitary or more generalized and is usually classified as epitheliotropic (mycosis fungoides) or nonepitheliotropic.[71,72] Canine epitheliotropic cutaneous lymphoma

originates from T cells,[73–77] similar to the case in humans. In dogs, these more commonly represent CD8+ cells, whereas in humans they are typically CD4+ cells.[76] A rare form of cutaneous T-cell lymphoma, characterized by skin involvement with evidence of peripherally circulating large (15–20 μm in diameter) malignant T cells with folded, grooved nuclei, has been described. In humans, this is referred to as Sézary syndrome and has been reported in both dogs and cats.[78–80] Nonepitheliotropic cutaneous lymphomas form single or multiple dermal or subcutaneous nodules or plaques; histologically, they spare the epidermis and papillary dermis and affect the middle and deep portions of the dermis and subcutis.[72] An inflamed form of nonepitheliotropic cutaneous T-cell lymphoma (NE-CTCL) is more pleocellular and can be difficult to differentiate from reactive histiocytosis.[71]

Atypical Anatomic Forms of Lymphoma

Hepatosplenic lymphoma is a relatively uncommon, distinct presentation in the dog marked by a lack of significant peripheral lymphadenopathy in the face of hepatic, splenic, and bone marrow infiltration with malignant lymphocytes, usually of T-cell origin.[81–83] Biologically, this form of lymphoma is extremely aggressive and poorly responsive to therapy. In humans and dogs, the tumor usually is composed of γδT cells (i.e., T cells that express the γδT-cell receptor).[81,82]

Intravascular (angiotropic, angioendotheliomatosis) lymphoma is a distinct form of lymphoma defined as proliferations of neoplastic lymphocytes within the lumen and wall of blood vessels in the absence of a primary extravascular mass or leukemia. It has been reported several times in the veterinary literature and often involves the CNS and peripheral nervous system (PNS), including the eye.[84–89] The B-cell immunophenotype is most common in humans; however, in most reported cases in dogs, the origin is either T cell or null cell (neither B nor T cell), although one case of a B-cell phenotype has been reported.

Pulmonary lymphomatoid granulomatosis (PLG), also termed angiocentric B-cell lymphoma, is a rare neoplasm of the lung and

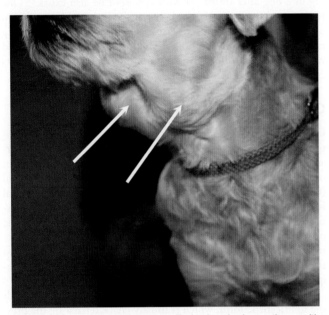

• **Fig. 33.1** A dog with obvious mandibular lymphadenopathy resulting from multicentric lymphoma.

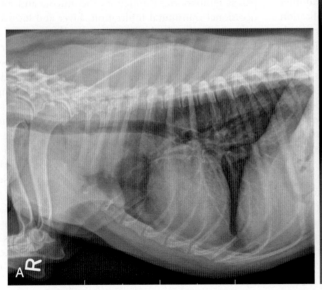
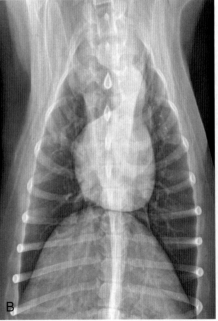

• **Fig. 33.2** (A) Lateral radiographic projection of a dog with mediastinal lymphoma. (B) Ventrodorsal projection of the same dog.

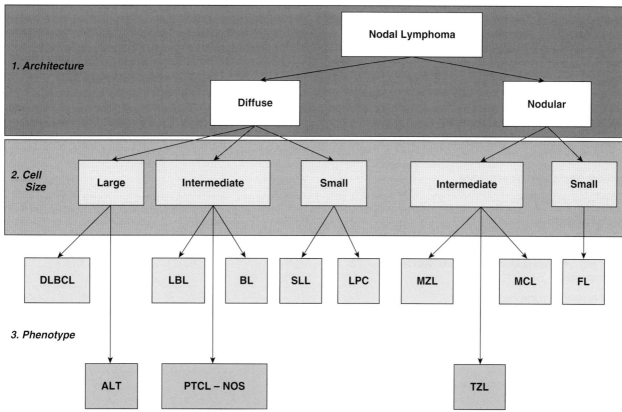

• **Fig. 33.3** The histologic approach toward the classification of canine nodal lymphoma. Using excisional lymph node sections, lymphoma is initially divided into diffuse (effacing) or nodular (noneffacing) forms of the disease. Next, using a red blood cell or a small lymphocyte as a guideline, the neoplastic population is divided into large, small, and intermediate forms of the disease. Finally, using knowledge of additional cellular and nuclear features, including mitotic rate and immunophenotype (B cell, blue boxes; T cell, red boxes), a final diagnosis is established. *ALT*, Anaplastic large cell T-cell lymphoma; *BL*, Burkitt lymphoma; *DLBCL*, diffuse large B-cell lymphoma; *FL*, follicular lymphoma; *LBL*, lymphoblastic lymphoma; *LPC*, lymphoplasmacytoid lymphoma; *MCL*, mantle cell lymphoma; *MZL*, marginal zone lymphoma; *PTCL, NOS*, peripheral T-cell lymphoma, not otherwise specified; *SLL*, small lymphocytic lymphoma; *TZL*, T-zone lymphoma. (Reproduced and modified with permission from Seelig DM, Avery AC, Ehrhart EJ, Linden MA. The comparative diagnostic features of canine and human lymphoma. *Vet Sci.* 2016;3(2). Epub 2017/04/25. https://doi.org/10.3390/vetsci3020011. PubMed PMID: 28435836; PubMed Central PMCID: PMCPMC5397114.)

occasionally other tissues, characterized by a heterogeneous accumulation of lymphocytes (both B and T cell), neutrophils, plasma cells, and macrophages, often arranged angiocentrically.[90–94] Clinical signs are related to respiratory compromise, and various chemotherapeutic protocols have been used with reported results varying from rapid progression to long-term clinical remissions.

Histologic Classification Systems

Lymphomas arise from clonal expansion of lymphocytes with distinctive morphologic and immunophenotypic features. Many histologic systems have been used to classify NHL in humans, and some of these have been applied to lymphoma in the dog and other species. Histologic classification of lymphoma currently follows the Revised European American Lymphoma/World Health Organization (REAL/WHO) system, which incorporates anatomic, morphologic (cytology and histology), and immunophenotypic criteria (B- and T-cell immunophenotype), with the goal of enabling accurate and reproducible diagnosis of specific neoplastic entities.[90,95,96] Fig. 33.3 represents an overall histologic approach to the classification of various subtypes in the dog as reviewed by Seelig et al.[96,97] This theoretically should assist in better tailoring

of treatment protocols, better correlation of prognosis with subtype, and better comparative capabilities once larger data sets with correlate outcomes are generated. Table 33.1 shows some of the WHO categories in three different surveys, including a 2-year survey (2008–2009) of canine necropsy and biopsy cases at the University of Wisconsin–Madison Veterinary Care Hospital[29,95,96,98]; some of the less common categories in the REAL/WHO system were not represented and are not listed. Most canine lymphomas fall into the following categories, in decreasing frequency: diffuse large B-cell lymphoma (DLBCL), peripheral T-cell lymphoma not otherwise specified (PTCL-NOS), T-zone lymphoma (TZL), T-lymphoblastic lymphoma (also called "precursor T-cell neoplasia"), and marginal zone lymphoma (MZL).[90] The REAL/WHO system provides accurate and consistent reproducible diagnostic results similar to the system used in human pathology; agreement among a group of pathologists examining 300 cases was 83%, and accuracy in evaluating the six most common diagnoses (80% of the cases) was 87%.[99] It is clear that lymphoma is not a single disease, and classification by subtype will become increasingly important as clinical studies are performed to correlate the various categories of disease with biologic behavior, response to treatment, and

TABLE 33.1	World Health Organization Classification System for Canine Lymphoma		
		PERCENTAGE	
Category	Seelig et al[96] (n = 3 data sets)	Vezzali et al[98] (n = 123)	University of Wisconsin (n = 122)
B-Cell Neoplasms	69	78.9	59.0
Precursor B lymphoblastic leukemia/lymphoma[a]	—	2.4	8.2
B-cell chronic lymphocytic leukemia/small lymphocytic lymphoma	—	2.4	0.8
Lymphocytic lymphoma—intermediate type	—	0.8	—
Lymphoplasmacytic lymphoma	—	3.3	0.8
Mantle cell lymphoma	2	1.6	—
Follicular center cell lymphomas	—	2.4	—
Marginal zone lymphoma (splenic, nodal, mucosa-associated lymphoid tissue)	8	3.3	2.5
Plasma cell myeloma/plasmacytoma	—	16.3	9.8
Diffuse large cell lymphoma	52	33.3	24.6
T-cell–rich, B-cell lymphoma	—	0.8	—
Large cell immunoblastic lymphoma	—	10.6	10.7
Mediastinal (thymic) large B-cell lymphoma	—	0.8	—
Burkitt's lymphoma/leukemia	—	0.8	1.6
Other B cell	8[d]	—	—
T-Cell and Natural Killer (NK[b]) Cell Lymphomas	31	21.1	41.0
Precursor T lymphoblastic lymphoma/leukemia[a]	3	6.5	9.8
T-cell chronic lymphocytic leukemia (CLL)	—	3.3	0.8
Intestinal T-cell lymphoma	—	4.1	4.1
Mycosis fungoides/Sézary syndrome	—	1.6	11.5
Cutaneous nonepitheliotropic lymphoma	—	3.3	—
Anaplastic large cell lymphoma	—	—	0.8
Peripheral T-cell lymphoma-not otherwise specified	15	2.4	13.1[c]
T-zone lymphoma	4		
Other T cell	7[d]	—	—
Other	3[d]		

[a]Acute leukemias and lymphoblastic lymphomas of both B and T derivation are also classified as lymphoid "precursor neoplasms."

[b]Non-B, non-T lymphomas.

[c]Includes T-zone lymphoma in this data set.

[d]Other in Seelig include those not otherwise subclassified.

prognosis. Preliminary results indicate that dogs with indolent lymphoma (e.g., MZL, follicular lymphoma, B- or T-cell small cell lymphoma, T-cell–rich B-cell lymphoma, and TZL) maintain normal activity and appetite levels even during advanced stages of disease and experience long-term survival even with limited or no therapy.[90,99–102]

Other classification systems that have been used include the National Cancer Institute Working Formulation (WF)[103] and the updated Kiel system.[104] The WF was developed to allow investigators to "translate" among the numerous classification systems so that clinical trials could be compared in humans. Most of the larger compilations agree that most canine lymphomas are intermediate or high grade. The WF categorizes tumors according to pattern (diffuse or follicular) and cell type (e.g., small cleaved cell, large cell, immunoblastic), but it does not include information about the immunophenotype of the tumor.[103] The WF subtypes are related to the biology of the tumor and patient survival. The updated Kiel classification includes the architectural pattern, morphology (centroblastic, centrocytic, or immunoblastic), and immunophenotype (B or T cell) of the tumor cells.[104] In both systems, the tumors can then be categorized as low-grade, intermediate-grade, or high-grade malignancies. Low-grade lymphomas composed of small cells with a low mitotic rate typically progress slowly and are associated with long STs, but are ultimately incurable. High-grade lymphomas with a high mitotic rate progress rapidly, but are more likely to respond initially to chemotherapy and, in humans, are potentially curable. In the REAL/WHO system, each subtype of lymphoma is classified as a distinct disease based on characteristics that include biologic behavior (indolent versus aggressive, response to treatment).[90]

Several features of canine lymphomas become apparent when these classification systems are applied. The most striking difference between canine and human lymphomas is the scarcity of follicular lymphomas in the dog. The most common form of canine lymphoma is DLBCL, a high-grade tumor.[90,98,99,105] A small percentage of canine lymphomas (5.3%–29%) are considered low-grade.

A documented difference exists in the prevalence of the various immunophenotypes based on breed.[32,106,107] For example, cocker spaniels and Doberman pinschers are more likely to develop B-cell lymphoma, boxers are more likely to have T-cell lymphoma, and golden retrievers appear to have an equal likelihood of B- and T-cell tumors.

To be clinically useful, these classification systems in the end must yield information about response to therapy, maintenance of remission, and survival. In most studies, high-grade lymphomas achieve a complete response (CR) to chemotherapy significantly more often than low-grade tumors. However, dogs with low-grade tumors may live years without aggressive chemotherapy.[100–102,108–111] Dogs with T-cell lymphomas have shown a lower rate of CR to chemotherapy and shorter remission and STs than dogs with B-cell tumors (with the exception of low-grade T-cell subtypes).[68,69,112,113] Furthermore, T-cell lymphomas are more commonly associated with hypercalcemia.[8,114,115]

In the veterinary literature, 60% to 80% of canine lymphomas are of B-cell origin; T-cell lymphomas account for 10% to 38%; mixed B- and T-cell lymphomas account for as many as 22%; and null-cell tumors represent fewer than 5%.[8,68,69,116–118] The development of monoclonal antibodies to detect specific markers on canine lymphocytes has made immunophenotyping of tumors in dogs routinely available in many commercial laboratories. Such techniques can be performed on paraffin-embedded samples, from tissue microarrays, on cytologic specimens obtained by fine-needle aspiration (FNA) of lesions, or by flow cytometric analysis of cellular fluid samples (e.g., peripheral blood, effusions) and lesion aspirates.

One criticism of the Kiel and WF classification systems is that they fail to include extranodal lymphomas as a separate category. The REAL/WHO system does include anatomic location as a factor in determining certain categories. Although differences between nodal and extranodal tumors in biologic behavior and prognosis are well recognized, comparative information about the histogenesis of these tumors is lacking. For example, in humans, small-cell lymphomas arising from MALT are composed of cells with a different immunophenotype than that of other small-cell lymphomas (i.e., MALT lymphomas typically are negative for both CD5 and CD10). With the exception of cutaneous lymphoid neoplasms, detailed characterization of extranodal lymphomas in dogs has not been done. Although cutaneous lymphoma is a heterogeneous group of neoplasms that includes an epitheliotropic form resembling mycosis fungoides and a nonepitheliotropic form, most cutaneous lymphomas have a T-cell phenotype.[119]

To summarize, it is important to determine the histologic grade of canine lymphomas as low (small lymphocytic or centrocytic lymphomas), intermediate, or high (diffuse large cell, centroblastic, and immunoblastic lymphomas), and the architecture as diffuse or nodular/follicular. Furthermore, determining the immunophenotype of the tumor provides useful information and is essential to accurately subtype lymphoma. Response rates to chemotherapy are, in general, better in animals with B-cell tumors and intermediate- to high-grade lymphomas. Dogs with low-grade indolent lymphomas can have long STs without aggressive therapy.

History and Clinical Signs

The clinical signs associated with canine lymphoma are variable and depend on the extent and location of the tumor. Multicentric lymphoma, the most common form, is usually distinguished by the presence of generalized peripheral lymphadenopathy (see Fig. 33.1). Enlarged LNs are usually painless, rubbery, and discrete. In addition, hepatosplenomegaly and bone marrow involvement can be associated with generalized lymphadenopathy. Most dogs with multicentric lymphoma are presented without dramatic signs of systemic illness (WHO substage a) (Box 33.2); however, a diversity of nonspecific signs such as anorexia, weight loss, vomiting, diarrhea, emaciation, ascites, dyspnea, polydipsia, polyuria, and fever can occur (WHO substage b). Dogs with T-cell lymphoma are more likely to have constitutional (i.e., substage b) signs. Most veterinary oncologists consider mild-moderate severity of clinical signs sufficient for a substage b designation.[120] Polydipsia and polyuria are often evident in dogs with hypercalcemia of malignancy. Dogs may also be presented with clinical signs related to blood dyscrasias secondary to marked tumor infiltration of bone marrow (myelophthisis) or paraneoplastic anemia, thrombocytopenia, or neutropenia. These could include fever, sepsis, anemia, and hemorrhage. Diffuse pulmonary infiltration, as detected by radiographic changes, is seen in 27% to 34% of dogs with the multicentric form (Fig. 33.4).[121,122] Based on bronchoalveolar lavage, the actual incidence of lung involvement may be higher.[123,124]

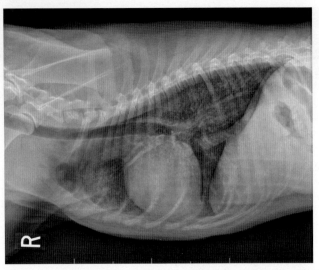

• **Fig. 33.4** Lateral projection of a thoracic radiograph of a dog with diffuse interstitial infiltration with lymphoma secondary to multicentric lymphoma.

Dogs with GI lymphoma usually present with nonspecific GI signs, such as vomiting, diarrhea, weight loss, and malabsorption.[61,64,125–128] Mesenteric LNs, spleen, and liver may be involved.

The mediastinal form of lymphoma is characterized by enlargement of the cranial mediastinal structures and/or thymus (see Fig. 33.2), and clinical signs are associated with the extent of disease with resulting respiratory compromise or polydipsia/polyuria from hypercalcemia. In advanced cases, dogs present with respiratory distress caused by a space-occupying mass and pleural effusion, exercise intolerance, and possibly regurgitation. In addition, dogs with mediastinal lymphoma may have precaval syndrome, characterized by pitting edema of the head, neck, and forelimbs secondary to tumor compression or invasion of the cranial vena cava (Fig. 33.5).

Clinical signs in dogs with extranodal lymphoma depend on the specific organ involved. Cutaneous lymphoma can be mucocutaneous, cutaneous, or both. Lesions can be solitary, generalized, or multifocal.[71,74–76,129–132] Tumors occur as nodules, plaques, ulcers, and erythemic or exfoliative dermatitis with focal

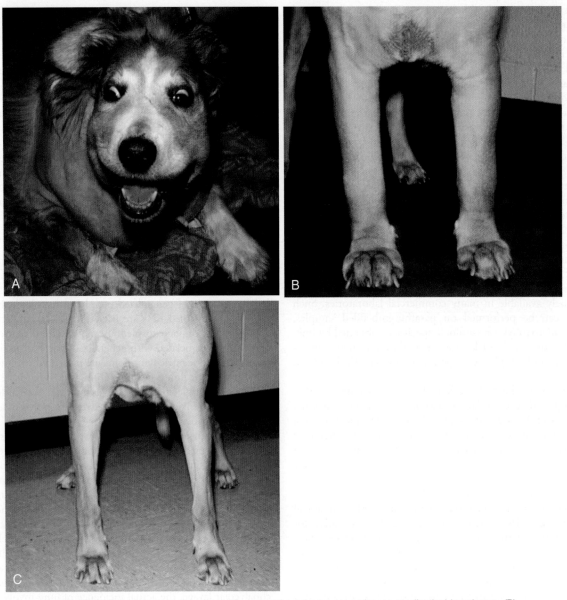

• **Fig. 33.5** (A) Facial edema in a dog with precaval syndrome secondary to mediastinal lymphoma. (B) Forelimb edema in a dog with precaval syndrome secondary to mediastinal lymphoma. (C) The dog in (B) 24 hours after radiation therapy to the cranial mediastinal mass, showing resolution of pitting edema.

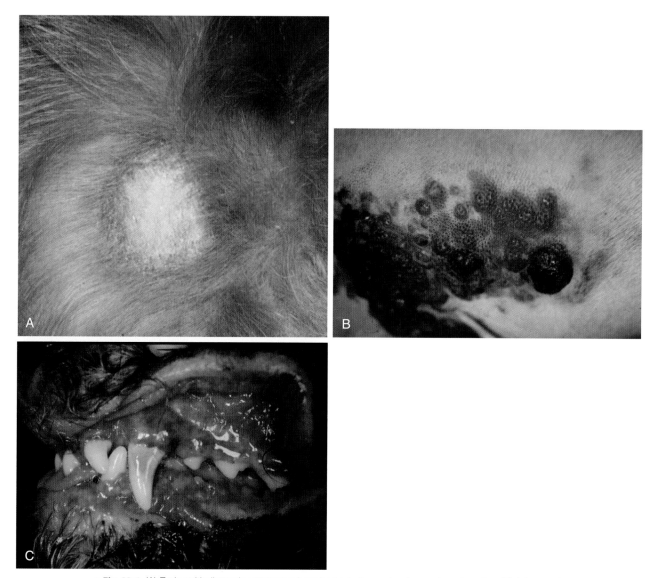

• **Fig. 33.6** (A) Early epitheliotropic cutaneous lymphoma in the scaly, plaque stage in a dog. (B) Advanced epitheliotropic cutaneous lymphoma in the nodular stage in a dog. (C) Oral mucosal epitheliotropic cutaneous lymphoma in a dog.

hypopigmentation and alopecia. Epitheliotropic T-cell lymphoma (e.g., mycosis fungoides) typically has a clinical course with three apparent clinical stages. Initially, there will be scaling, alopecia, and pruritus (Fig. 33.6A), which can mimic a variety of other skin conditions. As the disease progresses, the skin becomes more erythematous, thickened, ulcerated, and exudative. The final stage is characterized by proliferative plaques and nodules with progressive ulceration (Fig. 33.6B). Oral mucocutaneous involvement may also occur and this can appear as multicentric erythematous plaque-like hypopigmented lesions or nodules associated with the gum and lips (Fig. 33.6C). Extracutaneous involvement can also occur, most often in the LNs, spleen, liver, and bone marrow/peripheral blood. Nonepitheliotropic cutaneous lymphomas are also quite variable in appearance and can form single or multiple dermal or subcutaneous nodules or plaques that may be nonpuritic, ulcerated, or alopecic with crusts.[71] The face (lips, nasal planum, eyelids), lower extremities (paws, interdigital folds), neck, and trunk are often affected.

Dogs with CNS lymphoma may be presented with either multifocal or solitary involvement.[133–135] The majority of cases involve secondary extension into the CNS. Most have a B-cell immunophenotype and have meningeal, perivascular, and periventricular locations, whereas T-cell varieties are more likely to involve the peripheral nerves.[136] Seizures, paralysis, and paresis may be noted.

Ocular lymphoma is characterized by infiltration and thickening of the iris, uveitis, hypopyon, hyphema, posterior synechia, and glaucoma, and is discussed in more detail in Chapter 32.[137–139] Although it is often secondary to multicentric systemic lymphoma, in a compilation of 100 cases, 61% were presumed solitary ocular lymphoma (PSOL) without systemic involvement at diagnosis and no progression postenucleation.[137] Peripheral T-cell lymphoma and DLBCL are the most common subtypes. Importantly, dogs with PSOL had median survival times (MSTs) of 769 days versus 103 days for dogs having systemic involvement at diagnosis. In one study of 94 cases of canine multicentric lymphoma, 37% had ocular changes consistent with lymphoma; and, in a series of 102 cases of uveitis in dogs, 17% were secondary to lymphoma.[139] Anterior uveitis was most commonly seen in the advanced stage of disease (stage V).

Dogs with intravascular lymphoma usually present with signs related to CNS, PNS, or ocular involvement,[84–88] including paraparesis, ataxia, hyperesthesia, seizures, blindness, lethargy, anorexia, weight loss, diarrhea, polyuria, polydipsia, and intermittent fever. Finally, dogs with pure hepatosplenic lymphoma usually present with nonspecific signs of lethargy, inappetence and weakness, and often are icteric.[81–83]

Canine lymphoma also may be associated with paraneoplastic syndromes (see Chapter 5). Anemia is the most common lymphoma-related paraneoplastic syndrome.[140] Paraneoplastic hypercalcemia is also common and is characterized clinically by anorexia, weight loss, muscle weakness, lethargy, polyuria, polydipsia, and, rarely, CNS depression and coma. Lymphoma-induced hypercalcemia in most cases results from parathyroid hormone–related peptide (PTHrP), elaborated by neoplastic cells; however, it can also be related to the production of several other humoral factors, including interleukin-1 (IL-1), tumor necrosis factor-alpha (TNF-α), transforming growth factor-beta (TGF-β), and vitamin D analogs (e.g., 1,25-dihydroxyvitamin D).[114,115,141–143] As previously discussed, hypercalcemia is most commonly associated with the T-cell immunophenotype. Other paraneoplastic syndromes that may be encountered include monoclonal gammopathies, neuropathies, and cancer cachexia.

Diagnostics

For dogs with suspected lymphoma, the diagnostic evaluation should include a thorough physical examination; complete blood count (CBC), including differential leukocyte and platelet counts; a serum biochemical profile; and urinalysis. Optimally, plasma ionized calcium concentration should be measured. Ultimately, obtaining tissue or cytologic specimens (or both) for a definitive diagnosis is essential. The differential diagnosis of lymphadenopathy depends on the travel history of the dog (i.e., relative to infectious disease) and the size, consistency, and location of affected LNs. Other causes of lymphadenopathy include infections caused by bacteria, viruses, protozoa (*Toxoplasma* sp., *Leishmania* sp.), rickettsial organisms (salmon poisoning, *Ehrlichia* sp.), and fungal agents (*Blastomyces* and *Histoplasma* sp.). The potential for hypercalcemia to accompany systemic fungal diseases may further complicate differentiation from lymphoma. Discrete, hard, asymmetric LNs, particularly if they are fixed to underlying tissues, may indicate metastatic tumors such as mast cell tumor or carcinoma. Immune-mediated diseases (e.g., pemphigus, systemic lupus erythematosus, and immune-mediated polyarthropathy) also may result in mildly to moderately enlarged LNs. The various differential diseases or conditions that can resemble canine lymphoma are listed in Table 33.2.

Physical Examination

A thorough physical examination should include palpation of all assessable LNs and rectal examination, as in the authors' experience, a significant proportion of dogs will have rectal polyps consisting of aggregates of neoplastic lymphocytes. Inspection of mucous membranes for pallor, icterus, petechiae, and ulceration should be undertaken as these signs may indicate anemia or thrombocytopenia secondary to myelophthisis or immune-mediated disease or may be evidence of major organ failure or uremia. Abdominal palpation may reveal organomegaly, intestinal wall thickening (if marked), or mesenteric lymphadenopathy. The presence of a mediastinal mass and/or pleural effusion can be suspected after thoracic auscultation. Ocular examination, including

TABLE 33.2	Differential Diseases or Conditions That Can Resemble Canine Lymphoma
Form of Lymphoma	**Other Disorders**
Multicentric	Disseminated infections: bacterial, viral, rickettsial, parasitic, fungal Immune-mediated disorders: dermatopathies, vasculitis, polyarthritis, lupus erythrematosus Tumors metastatic to nodes Other hematopoietic tumors: leukemia, multiple myeloma, malignant or systemic histiocytosis
Mediastinal	Other tumors: thymoma, chemodectoma, ultimobranchial cyst, ectopic thyroid carcinoma, pleural carcinomatosis, pulmonary lymphomatoid granulomatosis[a] Infectious disease: granulomatous disease, pyothorax Miscellaneous: congestive heart failure, chylothorax, hemothorax
Alimentary	Other gastrointestinal tumors, foreign body, lymphangiectasia, lymphocytic-plasmacytic enteritis, systemic mycosis, gastroduodenal ulceration
Cutaneous	Infectious dermatitis: advanced pyoderma Immune-mediated dermatitis: pemphigus Other cutaneous neoplasms (in particular histiocytic disorders)
Extranodal	Variable, depending on organ/system involved

[a]The existence of this disease is controversial; in most cases the disease has been reclassified as a lymphoid neoplasm.

funduscopic assessment, may reveal abnormalities (e.g., uveitis, retinal hemorrhage, ocular infiltration, glaucoma) in approximately one-third to one-half of dogs with lymphoma.[139,144]

Complete Blood Count, Biochemical Profile, and Urinalysis

Anemia, the most common lymphoma-related hematologic abnormality, is usually normochromic and normocytic (nonregenerative), consistent with anemia of chronic disease[140]; however, hemorrhagic and hemolytic anemias may also occur, and regenerative anemias may reflect concomitant blood loss or hemolysis. In addition, if significant myelophthisis is present, anemia may be accompanied by thrombocytopenia and leukopenia.[145,146] In animals with anemia or evidence of bleeding, in addition to a platelet count, a reticulocyte count and coagulation testing may be indicated. Thrombocytopenia occurs in 30% to 50% of cases, but bleeding is seldom a clinical problem. Neutrophilia occurs in 25% to 40% of dogs and lymphocytosis occurs in approximately 20% of affected dogs. Circulating atypical lymphocytes may be indicative of bone marrow involvement and leukemia. It is important to differentiate multicentric lymphoma with bone marrow involvement (i.e., stage V disease) from primary lymphocytic leukemia because the prognosis for each may be different. Hypoproteinemia is observed more frequently in animals with alimentary lymphoma. In dogs with a high total protein concentration or evidence of an increased globulin fraction on a biochemical profile, serum proteins may be evaluated by serum protein electrophoresis. Monoclonal gammopathies have been reported to occur in approximately 6% of dogs with lymphoma.[147]

Serum biochemical abnormalities often reflect the anatomic site involved as well as paraneoplastic syndromes, such as hypercalcemia. In dogs with lymphoma, ionized calcium concentrations should be obtained, as they may be increased even if the total calcium concentration is within the reference interval. In cases of hypercalcemia of unknown origin, lymphoma should always be considered high on the differential disease list and diagnostic testing directed at this possibility should be undertaken (see Chapter 5). In addition, the presence of hypercalcemia can serve as a biomarker for response to therapy and relapse. Increased urea nitrogen and creatinine concentrations can occur secondary to renal infiltration with tumor, hypercalcemic nephrosis, or prerenal azotemia from dehydration. Increases in liver-specific enzyme activities or bilirubin concentrations may result from hepatic parenchymal infiltration. Increased serum globulin concentrations, usually monoclonal, occur infrequently with B-cell lymphoma.

Urinalysis is part of the minimum database used to assess renal function and the urinary tract. For example, isosthenuria and proteinuria in the absence of an active sediment may indicate renal disease, and hematuria may result from a hemostatic abnormality. It is important to note that isosthenuria in hypercalcemic dogs is not necessarily indicative of renal disease, as high calcium concentrations interfere with tubular concentrating capabilities through impairment of response to antidiuretic hormone; however, clinicians should be aware that there is a risk of renal calcification and subsequent failure with sustained high calcium concentrations.

Histologic and Cytologic Evaluation of Lymph Nodes

Morphologic and phenotypic examination of the tissue and cells that constitute the tumor is essential to the diagnosis and subtyping of lymphoma. In humans, a combination of histologic, immunophenotypic, clinical, and genetic features are used in the diagnosis and subtyping of NHL. An excellent review of the morphologic and immunophenotypic diagnostic features of canine lymphoma has recently been published.[96] In veterinary medicine, care should be taken to avoid sampling LNs from reactive areas (e.g., mandibular LNs), unless those nodes are the only ones enlarged; the prescapular or popliteal LNs are preferable if also involved. Also, lymphocytes are fragile, and in preparing smears of aspirated material only gentle pressure should be applied in spreading material on the slides. As the majority of dogs with nodal lymphomas are presented with multicentric effacement of peripheral LNs by intermediate or large lymphocytes, cytologic examination of FNAs of affected LNs or other tissues is a highly sensitive and specific first-line or screening diagnostic step.[96] Typically, most of the cells are large lymphocytes (>2 times the diameter of a red blood cell or larger than a neutrophil), and they may have visible nucleoli and basophilic cytoplasm with or without paranuclear clear zones (Fig. 33.7A) or fine chromatin with indistinct nucleoli. Because tissue architecture is not maintained in cytologic specimens, effacement of the node or capsular disruption cannot be detected. Therefore marked reactive hyperplasia characterized by increased numbers of large lymphocytes may be difficult to distinguish from lymphoma. In some forms of lymphoma, intermediate lymphocytes that are similar in diameter to neutrophils predominate; these specimens can be more challenging for novice cytopathologists. Small-cell lymphomas may have few cytologic clues that point to

malignancy. Therefore classification of lymphoma into subtypes that make up the low-, intermediate-, and high-grade forms can be attempted using cytologic appearance and immunophenotypic analysis of cytologic specimens (Fig. 33.7B),[96,148–150] but is performed most accurately on histologic sections. Although cytologic findings identified by an experienced cytopathologist may suggest a particular subtype of lymphoma, subsequent analysis that may include flow cytometry, immunocytochemistry, biopsy for histologic examination, clonality assays, and cytogenetic analysis are required to further subtype the lymphoma or to confirm or establish a diagnosis in equivocal cases. Fig. 33.8 presents a diagnostic algorithm for assessing peripheral lymphadenopathy in dogs applying these techniques, beginning with initial screening by cytologic examination.

For accurate histopathologic evaluation, an entire LN, including the capsule, should be removed, placed in buffered formalin, and submitted to a pathologist. Needle-core biopsies are generally inadequate to evaluate nodal morphology. Effacement of normal nodal architecture by neoplastic lymphocytes and capsular disruption are characteristic findings (Fig. 33.7C, D).

Histologic and Cytologic Evaluation of Extranodal Sites

Diagnostic ultrasonography and ultrasound-guided FNA or needle biopsy have been useful for evaluation of involvement of the liver, spleen, or abdominal LNs.[151–153] Aspiration of ultrasonographically normal splenic tissue is rarely contributory to a diagnosis. If possible, the diagnosis should be made by sampling peripheral nodes, avoiding percutaneous biopsies of the liver and spleen. However, if there is no peripheral node involvement, it is appropriate to biopsy affected tissues in the abdominal cavity.

When GI lymphoma is suspected, an open surgical wedge biopsy of the intestine is preferred in most cases to differentiate lymphoma from lymphocytic enteritis. If associated abdominal LNs also appear involved, image-guided biopsies may be obtained with less morbidity than intestinal biopsies. Multiple samples may be necessary to accurately diagnose segmental disease. Endoscopic biopsies may be inadequate as only a superficial specimen is obtained; however, more aggressive endoscopic biopsy techniques combined with more accurate histopathologic, immunophenotypic, and molecular assessments are improving the diagnostic yield of these less invasive techniques.[125,126,154–162] In many dogs with primary GI lymphoma, an inflammatory nonneoplastic infiltrate (i.e., LP-IBD) may be misdiagnosed on biopsy specimens that are too superficial. The application of assays for clonal expansion (e.g., receptor gene rearrangement [PARR]) does not appear as yet to be as accurate for endoscopically derived intestinal biopsies as it is for other solid lymphoid tumors in dogs.

Cytologic examination of cerebrospinal fluid (CSF), thoracic fluid, or mass aspirates is indicated in animals with CNS disease, pleural effusion, or an intrathoracic mass, respectively. In two studies, CSF analysis was diagnostic of lymphoma in 74% of 27 samples.[133,136] Characteristics of the CSF in one study included an increased nucleated cell count in seven dogs with 95% to 100% of the cells comprising atypical lymphocytes.[133] CSF protein concentration was increased in five of the dogs, ranging from 34 to 310 mg/dL (reference interval <25 mg/dL). Flow cytometric and molecular diagnostic procedures may also be applied to CSF samples,[136] although cell counts may be a limiting factor as some of these assays require at least 10,000 cells.

For cutaneous lymphoma, dermal punch biopsies (4–8 mm) should be taken from the most representative and infiltrative, but not secondarily infected, skin lesions. Application of

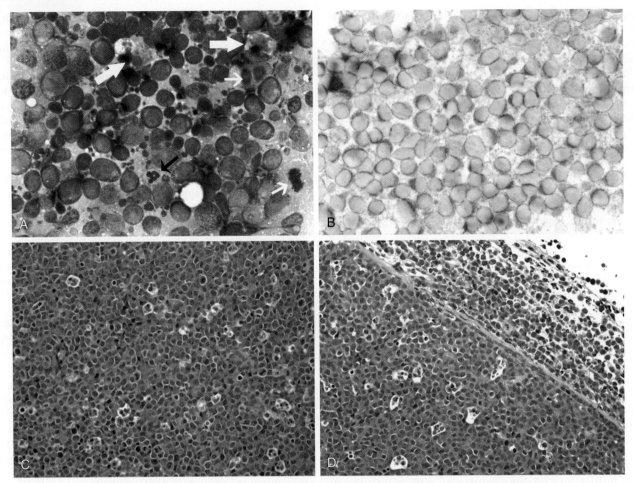

• **Fig. 33.7** Lymph nodes from dogs with lymphoma. (A) Fine-needle aspirate. Note the homogeneous population of large lymphoid cells with prominent nucleoli and basophilic cytoplasm. These cells are larger than the neutrophil *(black arrow)* in the field. Mitotic figures *(thin white arrows)* and tingible-body macrophages *(thick white arrows)* also are present. (Wright's stain, ×60 objective.) (B) Fine-needle aspirate stained for immunoreactivity for CD79a. Note that nearly all of the lymphocytes express CD79a. The diagnosis was B-cell lymphoma. (Alkaline phosphatase/Fast Red, ×60 objective.) (C) Histologic section. Note effacement of normal architecture. The white spaces are macrophages, giving a "starry sky" appearance to the lymph node. (H&E, ×20 objective.) (D) Histologic section. Note the presence of tumor cells outside the capsule of the lymph node. (H&E, ×20 objective.)

immunophenotypic and clonality assessments of cutaneous biopsies can aid in differentiating lymphoma from benign lymphocytic lesions.[71,75,77,163]

Molecular Diagnostic Techniques

Molecular techniques can be used to establish a diagnosis of lymphoma, but are best used to further characterize the tumor after the initial diagnosis is made. Indeed, in people, genetic characterization of NHL are often used in diagnosis and subtyping.[96] Tissues and cells from peripheral blood, LNs, nonlymphoid sites, and effusions can be analyzed by various molecular and cytogenetic means to aid in categorization of subtypes and in cases that represent a more difficult diagnostic challenge, particularly in cases where reactive lymphocytosis and lymphoma are both possible based on standard histologic or cytologic assessment. These include histochemical and cytochemical, immunohistochemical (IHC) and immunocytochemical, flow cytometric, polymerase chain reaction (PCR), and cytogenetic techniques. For example, the immunophenotype (B vs T cell),[118,164–171] proliferation rate (e.g., expression of Ki67, proliferating cell nuclear

antigen expression, argyrophilic nucleolar organizer regions [AgNOR]),[68,74,101,154,171–177] and clonality (PCR for antigen PARR)[81,160,178–187] of the tumor can be determined. Genetic characterizations of canine lymphoma samples have been investigated and are showing potential for both diagnostic and prognostic utility, but are not widely applied and clinical correlates are currently preliminary.[21,22,24,178,179,188,189] The availability of molecular and genetic analyses is increasing in veterinary oncology; however, at present, only immunophenotype and PARR clonality assays are routinely used in dogs to inform clinical decision making.

Immunophenotyping

Immunophenotyping is used to determine the type of cells that comprise the tumor, but this technique also can be helpful for making the initial diagnosis and predicting outcome.[96,164,166–171,190,191] When a heterogeneous population of lymphocytes is expected in a tissue, documentation of a homogeneous population of the same immunophenotype is supportive of a neoplastic process. The immunophenotype of a lymphocyte

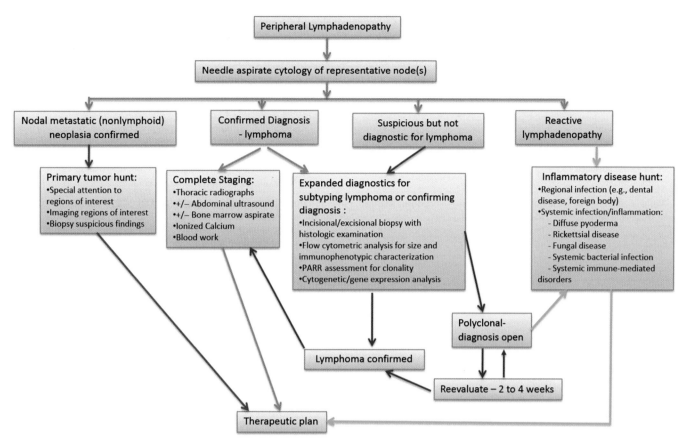

• **Fig. 33.8** Diagnostic algorithm for peripheral lymphadenopathy in dogs. *PARR*, polymerase chain reaction for receptor gene rearrangement.

is identified by determining the expression of molecules specific for B cells (e.g., CD79a, CD20) and T cells (e.g., CD3), and have been recently reviewed.[96] Although tumor cells sometimes have morphologic characteristics that typify a particular immunophenotype, exceptions occur and morphologic appearance cannot be used as the sole determinant of immunophenotype. For example, in a series of nine high-grade T-cell lymphomas and leukemias in dogs, the cells had a plasmacytoid appearance typically associated with B-cell lymphoma.[123,192] Similarly, anatomic location does not always predict the immunophenotype.

For accurate determination of immunophenotype, antibodies against lymphocyte markers are applied to tissue sections (IHC), cytologic specimens (immunocytochemistry), or individual cells in a fluid medium (flow cytometry). Flow cytometric evaluation of cells obtained by needle aspiration is also feasible. For T cells, markers include CD3 (pan T), CD4 (helper T), and CD8 (cytotoxic T); for B cells, the markers are CD79a (see Fig. 33.7B), CD20, and CD21, although dogs with indolent TZL can express CD21.[178] Increasingly, aberrant expression of CD molecules has been reported in canine lymphoma. In a study of 59 dogs with lymphoma, tumor cells from six dogs were positive for both T- and B-cell markers; however, a clonality assay revealed clonality either of the T-cell or the immunoglobulin receptor, but not both. This indicates that, in some cases, the malignant cells may coexpress B- and T-cell markers.[118] Antibodies against these molecules are used to determine the immunophenotype; however, they also have potential utility as a therapeutic modality if tumor cells could be targeted using these antibodies. Table 33.3 presents the histologic and immunophenotypic characteristics of the more common lymphoma subtypes in dogs.

Clonality Assays

Information about the clinical presentation and morphologic and immunophenotypic characteristics of the lymphocytes, obtained by IHC or flow cytometric analysis, must be integrated to select appropriate targets for clonality testing and to interpret results accurately.[193] Occasionally, diagnosis of lymphoma and differentiation of malignant versus benign proliferation of lymphocytes are not possible based on standard histologic and cytologic criteria. In these cases, advanced molecular analyses may be helpful to confirm a diagnosis. Clonality is the hallmark of malignancy; that is, the malignant cell population theoretically should be derived from expansion of a single malignant clone characterized by a particular DNA region unique to that tumor. For example, in a dog with T-cell lymphoma, all the malignant cells theoretically should have the same DNA sequence for the variable region of the T-cell receptor gene. Likewise, in a dog with B-cell lymphoma, the tumor cells should have identical DNA sequences in the variable region of the immunoglobulin (Ig) receptor gene. Conversely, in reactive lymphocytosis, the cells are polyclonal for their antigen receptors. Using this knowledge, investigators have used PCR technology to amplify the variable regions of the T-cell and immunoglobulin receptor genes to detect the presence of clonal lymphocyte populations in dogs (see Fig. 8.3 of Chapter 8). These techniques are reviewed in Chapter 8 and elsewhere.[158,180,193–195] In physician-based medicine, such assays of clonality are approximately 70% to 90% sensitive and have a false-positive rate of approximately 5%, and recent studies report similar rates in dogs. False-negative and false-positive

TABLE 33.3	Histologic and Immunophenotypic Characteristics of Common Canine Non-Hodgkin's Lymphomas in Relative Order of Frequency				
Subtype	Typical Location	Histologic Architecture	Cellular Features	Immunophenotype
Diffuse large B-cell (DLBCL)	Usually multicentric lymphadenopathy	Diffuse	Large cells; round nuclei; one (central) or multiple nucleoli; high mitotic rate; "starry sky" appearance	CD1+, CD20+, CD21+, CD45+, CD79a+, Pax5+, MHCII+, CD18^{low}
Peripheral T-cell lymphoma-not otherwise specified (PTCL-NOS)	Usually multicentric lymphadenopathy	Diffuse	Variable size (small to large); irregular nuclei, variable chromatin, prominent nucleoli; varied mitotic activity	CD3+, CD79a−, CD21−, CD45+, CD5+, CD4+/−, CD8+/−, CD18^{high}, TCRαβ
Marginal zone lymphoma (MZL)	Nodal (nMZL) or splenic (sMZL) or extranodal mucosal	Nodular/ follicular	Mostly intermediate- sized cells-abundant pale cytoplasm; irregular nuclei with peripheralized chromatin and a single central nucleolus; rare mitotic figures (except nMZL)	CD1+, CD20+, CD21+, CD45+, CD79a+, MHCII+, CD18^{intermediate}
T-zone lymphoma (TZL)	Usually multicentric Lymphadenopathy	Nodular, paracortical, progressing to diffuse	Small to intermediate- sized cells; moderate amount of pale cytoplasm; oval to elliptical nuclei with sharp, shallow indentations; nucleoli and mitotic figures are sparse	CD45−, CD3+, CD5+, CD21+, CD4+/−, CD8+/−
Precursor lymphoma[a]	Multicentric and/or leukemia	Diffuse and/or leukemia	Intermediate-sized cells; round nuclei; scant Cytoplasm; high mitotic rate	**If T-cell:** CD45+, CD34+/−, CD5+/−, CD3+/−, CD4+/−, CD8− **If B-cell:** CD45+, CD18+, CD34+/−, CD79a+, CD21+/−, CD20+/−
Mantle cell lymphoma (MCL)	Splenic white pulp	Nodular/ follicular	Small to intermediate- sized cells; scant cytoplasm; round nuclei with dense chromatin, inconspicuous nucleoli; varied mitotic rate	CD20+, CD21+, CD45+, CD79a+, MHCII+
Follicular lymphoma	Lymphadenopathy, solitary or multiple	Nodular/ follicular	Mixed—mostly small cells with clear cytoplasm, pale chromatin, and inconspicuous nucleoli (centrocytes) with fewer large cells with dark blue cytoplasm, vesicular nuclei, and 1–3 nucleoli (centroblasts)	CD20+, CD21+, CD45+, CD79a+, MHCII+

[a]Precursor lymphoma includes lymphoblastic B- or T-cell lymphomas and B- or T-cell acute leukemias.

Adapted with permission from Seelig DM, Avery AC, Ehrhart EJ, Linden MA. The comparative diagnostic features of canine and human lymphoma. *Vet Sci*. 2016;3: Epub ahead of print. https://doi.org/10.3390/vetsci3020011; and Burkhard MJ, Bienzle D. Making sense of lymphoma diagnostics in small animal patients. *Vet Clin North Am Small Anim Pract*. 2013;43:1331-1347.

results can occur with clonality assays. For example, cells from a dog with lymphoma may be negative for clonality if the clonal segment of DNA is not detected with the PCR primers used, mutation of the primer site has occurred, there are background nonneoplastic lymphocytes (noise) within the tumor, the malignant cells are natural killer (NK) cells (rare), or the malignant cells are present in too low a frequency to be detected. False positives occur rarely in some infectious diseases (e.g., ehrlichiosis and leishmaniasis). In these cases, a diagnosis should be made only after considering the results of all the diagnostic tests, including histologic/cytologic evaluation, immunophenotyping, and clonality studies in conjunction with signalment and physical examination findings. These

molecular techniques, although helpful for diagnosis, could also have utility in detecting relapse and in determining more accurate clinical stage and so-called "molecular remission rates" because they are more sensitive than standard cytologic assessment of peripheral blood, bone marrow, or LNs.

Other Immunohistochemical and Immunocytochemical Assessments

Assessments of several markers of multidrug resistance and apoptotic pathways (e.g., P-glycoprotein, p53, Bcl-2 proteins) have been evaluated in dogs with lymphoma[29,30,174,196,197]; however, their clinical significance and utility have not been established.

Proteomics and Serum Biomarkers

Proteomics comprises, simplistically, methodologies that analyze the entire protein component or protein signature of cells (the proteome). Protein components of a cell (normal or malignant) change over time with upregulation and downregulation of gene expression in response to varied stimuli (e.g., growth factors, environmental cues). It may therefore be possible to use the field of proteomics to identify serum biomarkers of malignancy (i.e., cancer-specific protein markers) and to further analyze response to therapy or even to predict which therapies are appropriate for an individual patient's tumor. Although in its infancy in veterinary oncology, preliminary investigations of the proteome of dogs with lymphoma have been reported[198–201]; however, they have yet to reach the level of sophistication in which useful output would have a significant effect on clinical decision making.

Several analytes in serum have been explored as biomarkers of lymphoma in the dog and have been reviewed.[202] These include tumor and metabolic products, cytokines, cellular leakage enzymes, and serum proteins. Examples include thymidine kinase 1, C-reactive protein, alpha-fetoprotein, alpha-1 glycoprotein levels, zinc, chromium, iron, endostatin, vascular endothelial growth factor (VEGF), lactate dehydrogenase, haptoglobin, and antioxidants/oxidative stress markers.[203–214] Although some have been grouped and commercialized (e.g., TK Canine Cancer Panel [VDI Labs, Simi Valley, CA, USA], Canine Lymphoma Blood Test [cLBT; Avacta Animal Health, Whetherby, UK]), the clinical, biologic, and prognostic significance of these assays has yet to be definitively characterized. Intuitively, use of biomarkers to detect early relapse would have clinical utility if meaningful therapeutic decisions and options were identified that would result in enhancement of quantity and quality of life. Currently, the lead-time provided over standard clinical diagnosis of relapse is relatively short, limiting their routine utility; definitive studies to support their application in larger and more varied general populations of dogs with lymphoma are currently lacking.

Clinical Staging

After a diagnosis has been established, the extent of disease should be determined and categorized by clinical staging. The WHO staging system routinely used to stage dogs with lymphoma is presented in Box 33.2. Most dogs (>80%) are presented in advanced stages (III–IV). Diagnostic imaging and assessment of bone marrow involvement may be indicated for staging. The degree to which thorough staging is implemented depends on whether the result will alter the treatment plan, whether relevant prognostic information is gleaned, and whether the clients need to know the stage before initiating (or declining) a treatment plan. In addition, when comparing different treatment protocols with respect to efficacy, consistent and similar staging diagnostics should be used to avoid so-called "stage migration," which results when one staging methodology is more accurate than another.[215] The effect of stage migration on prognosis should be considered when comparing different published outcomes.

Bone Marrow Evaluation

A bone marrow aspirate or core biopsy (from the proximal humerus or iliac crest) is recommended for complete staging and prognostication and may be indicated in dogs with anemia,

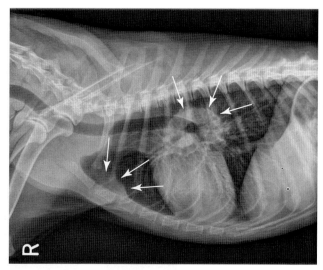

• **Fig. 33.9** Lateral radiographic projection of a dog with sternal and hylar lymphadenopathy due to lymphoma.

lymphocytosis, circulating atypical lymphocytes, or other peripheral cytopenias. In one study of 53 dogs with lymphoma, 28% had circulating malignant cells and were considered leukemic, whereas bone marrow examination indicated involvement in 57% of the dogs.[216] The presence of a few prolymphocytes and large lymphocytes with nucleoli in the circulation of dogs with lymphoma may indicate bone marrow involvement. It is important to remember these cells also can be seen with immune-mediated and inflammatory/infectious diseases. As discussed previously, tumor cells within the peripheral and bone marrow compartments can also be identified using clonality assays (PARR) that are more sensitive than routine microscopic examination in detecting malignant cells; however, the prognostic significance of the knowledge gained with more sensitive staging methodologies has yet to be determined.[216–218] Although bone marrow evaluation may offer prognostically valuable information, it is not necessary to perform the procedure if the client is committed to treat regardless of stage.

Imaging

Evaluation of thoracic and abdominal radiographs may be important in determining the extent of internal involvement (Fig. 33.9).[121,219] Approximately 60% to 75% of dogs with multicentric lymphoma have abnormalities on thoracic radiographs, with one-third having evidence of pulmonary infiltrates (see Fig. 33.4) and two-thirds having thoracic lymphadenopathy (sternal and tracheobronchial LNs [see Fig. 33.9]) and widening of the cranial mediastinum (see Fig. 33.2).[121,122] Pulmonary infiltrates usually are represented by an interstitial and/or alveolar pattern; however, nodules (rarely) and bronchial infiltrates can also occur.[220] Pleural effusion may be present. Cranial mediastinal lymphadenopathy is detected in 20% of dogs with lymphoma.[122,220] Abdominal radiographs reveal evidence of involvement of medial iliac (sublumbar) and/or mesenteric LNs, spleen, or liver in approximately 50% of cases. In the authors' practice, for the typical cases of canine multicentric lymphoma, imaging is limited to thoracic radiographs as there is no prognostic difference between dogs with stage III and IV disease (i.e., liver/spleen involvement); however, cranial mediastinal lymphadenopathy is of prognostic significance. If there are

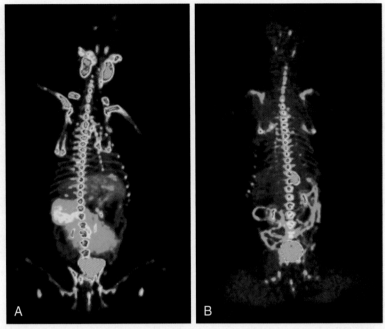

• **Fig. 33.10** (A) FLT-PET/CT image of a 3-year-old MN Hound cross illustrating FLT uptake in the peripheral nodes, bone marrow, kidneys bladder and spleen. (B) FLT-PET/CT image of the same dog 3 weeks after his final dose of chemotherapy. The lymph nodes were small on CT with minimal FLT uptake on PET images. Note the persistent uptake in the bone marrow, kidneys, and bladder. (Reprinted with permission from Lawrence J, Vanderhoek M, Barbee D, et al Use of 3'-deoxy-3'-[18F]fluorothymidine PET/CT for evaluating response to cytotoxic chemotherapy in dogs with non-Hodgkin's lymphoma. *Vet Radiol Ultrasound.* 2009;50:660–668.)

clinical signs attributable to abdominal disease, if complete staging is necessary (e.g., for clinical trial inclusion), or if peripheral lymphadenopathy is not part of the presentation, further imaging of the abdomen is warranted. Abdominal ultrasonography can be important for obtaining ultrasound-guided intraabdominal samples for diagnosis if more peripheral lesions are not evident (e.g., GI, abdominal nodal, and hepatosplenic lymphoma) or if complete clinical staging is required.[152] Ultrasonographic (including Doppler ultrasound) assessment of peripheral LNs has also been explored[153]; however, its clinical applicability is questionable because cytologic assessment of peripheral nodes is easy, inexpensive, and of higher diagnostic utility.

Advanced imaging modalities, including computed tomography (CT), magnetic resonance imaging (MRI), positron emission tomography (PET), or PET/CT and PET/MR imaging, are becoming more commonplace in veterinary practice and their utility is only now being determined.[221–226] PET/CT imaging is the current standard of care for following and predicting durability of treatment response in human patients with lymphoma, and both [18F]fluorothymidine (18FLT) PET/CT and [18F]fluoro-D-glucose (18FDG) PET imaging have been reported in dogs with lymphoma.[224–226] 18FLT-PET/CT functional and anatomic imaging shows promise for the evaluation of response to cytotoxic chemotherapy in dogs with lymphoma and for predicting relapse before standard clinical and clinicopathologic confirmation (Fig. 33.10).

Treatment of Multicentric Lymphoma

The therapeutic approach to a particular patient with lymphoma is determined by the subtype, stage, and substage of disease, the presence or absence of paraneoplastic disease, the overall physiologic status of the patient, financial and time commitment of the clients, and their level of comfort with respect to likelihood of treatment-related success and/or side effects. Without treatment, most dogs with intermediate- or high-grade lymphoma will die of their disease within 4 to 6 weeks of diagnosis, although significant variability exists.[147] With few exceptions, canine lymphoma is considered a systemic disease and therefore requires systemic therapy to achieve remission and prolong survival. The majority of canine multicentric lymphomas are intermediate- to high-grade, and, currently, histologic and immunophenotypic characterization does not play a significant role in determining the initial treatment protocol unless a diagnosis of indolent or low-grade lymphoma is confirmed. It is hoped that in the near future, as more clinically correlative information on the significance of the various subclassifications of lymphoma in dogs is acquired, more tailored therapeutic approaches may become available.

Systemic multiagent chemotherapy continues to be the therapy of choice for canine intermediate- and high-grade lymphoma. In general, combination chemotherapy protocols are superior in efficacy to single-agent protocols. In rare cases in which lymphoma is limited to one site (especially an extranodal site), the animal can be treated with a local modality such as surgery or radiation therapy (RT) as long as the client and clinician are committed to diligent reevaluation (active surveillance) to document subsequent progression to systemic involvement, should it occur.

Multidrug Combination Protocols

Many chemotherapeutic protocols for dogs with lymphoma have been developed over the past 30 years (Table 33.4).[116,227–251] Significant limitations arise when comparing efficacy studies in the veterinary literature for the various published protocols. Few of

TABLE 33.4 Summary of First Remission Outcomes of Combination or Single-Agent Doxorubicin Lymphoma Chemotherapy Protocols[a]

PRIVATE Protocol	No. of Dogs	Remission Rate (%)	Median Remission Duration (Months)	% 1-Year Survival	References
COP	77	75	6.0	19	248
A	37	59	4.4	NR	250
A[b]	121	85	4.3	NR	246
A	42	74	4.9	NR	239
A + piroxicam	33	79	4.3	NR	239
VMC-L	59	90	4.4	25	236
VMC-L	147	77	4.7	25	237
VCA-L	112	73	7.9	50	116
L-COPA	41	76	11.0[c]	48	251
L-COPA(II)	68	75	9.0[c]	27 (13 at 2 yr)	240
COPLA/LVP	75	92 (80[c])	5.8	17	415
VELCAP-SC	94	70	5.6	44	238
VLCAP-Long	98	69	12.5[c]	NR	247
L-VCAMP (UW-Madison CHOP)	55	84	8.4	50 (24 at 2 yr)	235
L-VCAMP (continuous maintenance CHOP)	96 86	79 (CR) 90	9 6.8[c]	NR 35[c]	234 243
L-VCAMP (+/− intensification CHOP)	130	94.6	7.3[d]	NR	245
L-VCAP (25-week CHOP)	51	94	9.1	NR	232
L-VCAP-Mx	65	94	10	NR	231
L-VCAP	71	88	9.7[c]	32 (13 at 2 yr)	241
L-VCAP (12-week CHOP)	77	89	8.1[c]	28[c]	244
VCAP (15-week CHOP)	31 134	100 (84 CR) 98 (78 CR)	4.7[d] 5.9[d]	NR NR	227 228
L-VCAP/CCNU/MOPrP	66	94	10.6[c]	46 (35 at 2 yr)	241
COArP	71	92	3	NR	233
L-VCADP	39	100	11[d]	NR	242
L-VCEP	97	100 (96 CR)	7.2	NR	229
RA	54	98 (68 CR)	6.5[d]	NR	230

[a]Minimum of 30 cases required for inclusion. Few of these protocols include sufficient numbers for adequate statistical power and fewer compare treatment protocols in a randomized prospective fashion. In addition, staging, inclusion, and response criteria vary considerably between protocols presented. Therefore evaluations of efficacy between the various protocols are subject to bias, making direct comparisons difficult and indeed precarious.

[b]With COP rescue.

[c]Only durations of cases achieving CR reported.

[d]Time to progression.

[e]Questionable (only one-third reportedly finished).

A, Adriamycin (doxorubicin); *Ar*, cytosine arabinoside; *C*, cyclophosphamide; *CR*, complete response; *D*, dactinomycin; *E*, epirubicin; *L*, ʟ-asparaginase; *M*, methotrexate; *Mx*, mitoxantrone; *NR*, not reported; *O*, Oncovin (vincristine); *P*, prednisone; *Pr*, procarbazine; *R*, rabacfosadine; *V*, vincristine.

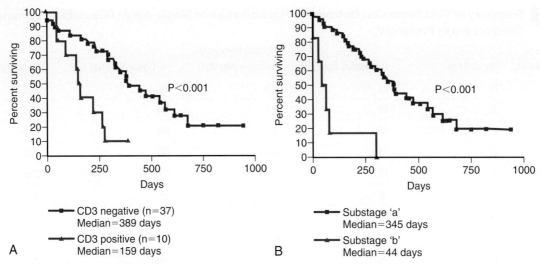

• **Fig. 33.11** (A) Kaplan–Meier survival duration estimates for a group of 55 dogs with lymphoma treated with an identical CHOP-based combination chemotherapy protocol. Dogs with CD3 immunoreactive (T-cell) lymphoma had significantly shorter survival durations. (B) Kaplan–Meier survival duration estimates for a group of 55 dogs with lymphoma treated with an identical CHOP based combination chemotherapy protocol at the University of Wisconsin. Dogs with substage *b* disease (i.e., clinically ill) had significantly shorter survival durations. (From Vail DM. Hematopoietic tumors. In Ettinger SJ, Feldman EC, eds. *Textbook of Veterinary Internal Medicine*. 6th ed. St. Louis: Elsevier; 2005.)

these studies include sufficient numbers of dogs for adequate statistical power and even fewer compare treatment protocols in a randomized prospective fashion. In addition, staging, inclusion, and response criteria vary considerably among reports. Therefore evaluations of efficacy among various protocols are subject to substantial bias, making direct comparisons difficult and indeed precarious. A recurring theme in the concluding statement in most of these published protocols is some variation of "prospective randomized trials will be required to confirm these suggestive findings." Despite the plethora of available combination protocols, most are modifications of CHOP protocols initially designed for human oncologic use, and currently randomized prospective evidence does not exist in dogs to clearly recommend one over the other as long as the basic CHOP components are present. CHOP represents combinations of cyclophosphamide (C), doxorubicin (H, hydroxydaunorubicin), vincristine (O, Oncovin), and prednisone (P). In the 1980s and early 1990s, physicians treating human patients with advanced, intermediate- or high-grade lymphoma faced a similar dilemma in that many different variations of CHOP existed and no randomized data were available to determine which protocols were superior. Eventually, a national randomized trial involving more than 1000 people with intermediate/high grade NHL was conducted comparing the plethora of protocols available, and the results indicated that CHOP was as effective as any of the more complicated protocols and had the safest adverse event profile.[252] CHOP subsequently became (and remains, with the addition of monoclonal antibody therapy) the standard of care for people with intermediate-/high-grade NHL.

Conventional CHOP-based chemotherapy induces remission in approximately 80% to 95% of dogs, with overall MSTs of 10 to 12 months. Approximately 20% to 25% of treated dogs will be alive 2 years after initiation of these protocols (Fig. 33.11). Response rates and durations of response vary according to the presence or absence of prognostic factors discussed in the text that follows. The relative cost of the various protocols to the client depends on the drug(s) selected, the size of the animal, the

frequency of administration, and the laboratory tests required to monitor adverse events and response.

In an attempt to better standardize response criteria and outcome reporting of future trials, the Veterinary Cooperative Oncology Group (VCOG) published response evaluation criteria (v1.0)[253] that can be applied in the routine practice setting. The greatest obstacle to performance of prospective randomized comparative lymphoma trials in veterinary oncology is financial; that is, clinical trials are inherently costly, and because most of the known effective drugs are unregistered off-label human generic (i.e., off-patent) drugs, the incentive for pharmaceutical-funded, sufficiently powered, randomized field trials is low, resulting in a general lack of comparative data.

Dogs responding to chemotherapy and undergoing complete "clinical" remission are usually free of clinical signs associated with lymphoma and subsequently return to a very good quality of life, making the treatment of dogs with lymphoma initially gratifying. Most dogs tolerate chemotherapy well, and although dose reductions and treatment breaks ("treatment holidays") are sometimes required in individual cases, only a minority of dogs develop significant adverse events requiring hospitalization.[254,255] Studies assessing client perceptions of medical treatment for cancer in general and lymphoma in particular report a positive experience; most owners feel treatment was worthwhile, that it resulted in improvement in the well-being of their pet, and that quality of life during treatment was good.[256,257] Very few clients express regret about treating lymphoma using a multidrug protocol.

Importantly, it must be realized that cures are rare, and though complete clinical remissions are the norm, complete molecular remissions (iCR), which can be documented only with molecular techniques, are rarely achieved in dogs; thus the utility of documenting iCR, in the absence of meaningful therapeutic options, is limited to investigative trials striving to achieve them.

With lymphoma, the fundamental goals of chemotherapy are to induce a complete durable (>6 months) first remission (termed *induction*), to reinduce a remission when the tumor recrudesces (the patient relapses) after achievement of a remission (termed *reinduction*), and, finally, to induce remissions when the cancer fails to respond to induction or reinduction using drugs not present in the initial protocols (termed *rescue*).

An unanswered question in the treatment of lymphoma has been whether long-term maintenance chemotherapy is useful after an initial course of aggressive induction chemotherapy lasting 6 months or less. Long-term maintenance chemotherapy has not been shown to be of significant value in humans with most aggressive forms of NHL; however, in humans, the initial induction course of chemotherapy is much more aggressive than that used in veterinary patients. Although no randomized prospective studies have been performed to address the therapeutic benefit of long-term maintenance chemotherapy in dogs, most comparisons of dogs treated with CHOP-based protocols do not show any clear advantage for a maintenance or consolidation phase after induction therapy.[229,231,232,234,240,242–245,247,258–262] Indeed, in most reports, dogs receiving shorter, less costly protocols that do not include a prolonged maintenance phase have comparable remission and progression-free survival (PFS) durations and appear to more readily achieve second remissions when they relapse after completion of chemotherapy than their counterparts receiving long-term maintenance. These data, taken together, suggest that maintenance therapy is not beneficial for most dogs with lymphoma. Until well-designed randomized prospective trials indicate otherwise, the author (DMV) prefers protocols that utilize an aggressive induction without maintenance.

Single-Agent Chemotherapy with Known Activity for Dogs with Lymphoma

The most effective currently available chemotherapeutic agents for canine lymphoma include doxorubicin (DOX), L-asparaginase, vincristine, cyclophosphamide, and prednisone, most of which are represented to one degree or another in most first-line multiagent chemotherapy protocols. Other drugs that have documented activity are often considered second-line agents and include rabacfosadine (Tanovea-CA1), lomustine, vinblastine, actinomycin-D, mitoxantrone, mustargen, chlorambucil, methotrexate, dacarbazine (DTIC), 9-aminocamptothecin, ifosfamide, cytosine arabinoside, procarbazine, bleomycin, and gemcitabine. Of these, cytosine arabinoside,[263] ifosfamide,[264] bleomycin,[265] and gemcitabine[266] appear to have minimal activity. With the exception of DOX, single-agent induction therapy does not typically result in durable remission durations compared with standard combination protocols. Incorporation of other standard cytotoxic drugs with single-agent activity into standard CHOP-based protocols has not resulted in significant gains or has not been adequately evaluated, and most are reserved for subsequent rescue settings.

The use of rabacfosadine (Tanovea-CA1) warrants a brief discussion as it is the only chemotherapy agent currently approved, albeit conditionally, by the US Food and Drug Administration (FDA) for the treatment of dogs with lymphoma (see Chapter 12 for a specific discussion of rabacfosadine). Rabacfosadine has been evaluated in hundreds of dogs with lymphoma and activity has been documented as a single-agent for treatment of cutaneous lymphoma, multiple myeloma, and naïve and relapsed multicentric lymphoma, as well as in combination with DOX for lymphoma.[226,230,267–270] Currently, rabacfosadine is most commonly used as a rescue agent at relapse or as a first-line treatment in combination with DOX owing to a less intense treatment protocol while maintaining similar remission durations compared with CHOP in a nonrandomized fashion.[230]

• BOX 33.3 **Current Canine Lymphoma Protocol (UW-Madison-19)**

Week 1: Vincristine, 0.7 mg/m² IV
Prednisone, 2 mg/kg, PO, daily
Week 2: Cyclophosphamide,ᵃ 250 mg/m² IV or PO
Prednisone, 1.5 mg/kg, PO, daily
Week 3: Vincristine, 0.7 mg/m² IV
Prednisone, 1.0 mg/kg, PO, daily
Week 4: Doxorubicin,ᵇ 30 mg/m² IV
Prednisone, 0.5 mg/kg, PO, daily
Week 6: Vincristine, 0.7 mg/m² IV
Week 7: Cyclophosphamide,ᵃ 250 mg/m² IV or PO
Week 8: Vincristine, 0.7 mg/m² IV
Week 9: Doxorubicin,ᵇ 30 mg/m² IV
Week 11: Vincristine, 0.7 mg/m² IV
Week 12: Cyclophosphamide,ᵃ 250 mg/m² IV or PO
Week 13: Vincristine, 0.7 mg/m² IV
Week 14: Doxorubicin,ᵇ 30 mg/m² IV
Week 16: Vincristine, 0.7 mg/m² IV
Week 17: Cyclophosphamide,ᵃ 250 mg/m² IV or PO
Week 18: Vincristine, 0.7 mg/m² IV
Week 19: Doxorubicin,ᵇ 30 mg/m² IV

1. All treatments are discontinued after week 19 if in complete remission.
2. A complete blood count (CBC) should be performed before each chemotherapy. If neutrophil count is <1500 wait 5 to 7 days and repeat CBC.
3. If sterile hemorrhagic cystitis occurs on cyclophosphamide, discontinue and substitute chlorambucil (1.4 mg/kg PO) for subsequently scheduled cyclophosphamide treatments.
4. For acute lymphocytic leukemia (ALL)–administer L-asparaginase 400 IU/kg SQ with each vincristine injection, until a complete response is achieved.

ᵃFurosemide (1–2 mg/kg) is given IV or PO, concurrent with cyclophosphamide to lessen the incidence of sterile hemorrhagic cystitis.
ᵇIn dogs less than 15 kg in body weight, a doxorubicin dose of 1 mg/kg is substituted for 30 mg/m²

Overall Chemotherapy Recommendations for Multicentric Lymphoma (Author [DMV] Preference)

Several factors should be considered and discussed with caregivers on a case-by-case basis when choosing the treatment protocol. These factors include cost, time commitment involved, efficacy, adverse event profiles, and experience of the clinician with the protocols under consideration.

Induction in Treatment-Naïve Patients

It is now clearly established that "standard-of-care" combination protocols used in dogs with intermediate- and high-grade lymphoma are essentially variations of CHOP protocols (see Table 33.4). Specific details regarding dose and timing of the CHOP protocol currently preferred by the author (DMV) are outlined in Box 33.3. This protocol does not have a maintenance component and all treatments cease at 19 weeks, provided the animal is in complete clinical remission. Although several other CHOP-based protocols include L-asparaginase either at initiation or at varying times throughout the protocol, several studies suggest this does not result in clinically relevant increases in remission rate, speed of attaining remission, or first-remission duration, and therefore the author reserves its use for rescue situations.[246,260,271,272]

If client or other considerations preclude a CHOP-based protocol, single-agent DOX (30 mg/m², intravenous [IV], every 3 weeks for five total treatments) is offered along with a 4-week tapering oral prednisone regimen (same prednisone regimen in Box 33.3) as a less aggressive, less time-consuming, and less costly approach. The expected CR rate for the single-agent DOX protocol will range from 50% to 75%, with an anticipated MST of 6 to 8 months.[246,250,273,274] The addition of oral cyclophosphamide (50 mg/m² daily for 3 days starting on the same day as DOX) to single-agent DOX resulted in a numerically, but not statistically, improved outcome in a randomized trial comparing DOX/prednisone with DOX/cyclophosphamide/prednisone (PFS of 5.6 months vs 8.2 months, respectively).[274] This trial was powered only to detect a three-fold difference in PFS; therefore larger trials should be undertaken to confirm any benefit. Alternatively, a less time-intense protocol with treatments every 3 weeks involves the previously mentioned rabacfosadine/DOX protocol.[230]

If clients are reticent to include IV medications, the author often recommends a protocol of either oral lomustine (CCNU; 70 mg/m² by mouth [PO] every 3 weeks for five treatments) and prednisone or oral cyclophosphamide (250 mg/m² [PO] every 2–3 weeks) with prednisone. The CCNU protocol has been associated with short median remissions (40 days) in one small case series[275]; however, in the author's experience, a subset of dogs have remained in remission for several months on this protocol when clients decline IV medication.

If financial or other client concerns preclude the use of systemic chemotherapy, prednisone alone (2 mg/kg PO, daily) will often result in short-lived remissions of approximately 1 to 2 months; however, an occasional durable remission will result. In these cases, it is important to educate clients that, should they decide to pursue more aggressive therapy at a later date, dogs receiving single-agent prednisone therapy are more likely to develop multidrug resistance (MDR) and experience shorter remission and survival durations with subsequent combination protocols.[258,276–278] This is especially true after long-term prednisone use or in dogs that have experienced a relapse while receiving prednisone. Therefore the earlier that clients opt for more aggressive therapy, the more likely a durable response will result.

A CBC should be performed before each chemotherapy treatment. Dogs should have a minimum of 1500 neutrophils/μL (some oncologists use a cut-off of 2000 neutrophils/μL) and 50,000 platelets/μL before the administration of myelosuppressive chemotherapy.[279] If the neutrophil count is lower than 1500/μL, it is recommended to wait 5 to 7 days and repeat the CBC; if the neutrophil count has increased to more than 1500 cells/μL, the drug can be safely administered. A caveat to these restrictions is that for dogs presenting before initiation of chemotherapy with low neutrophil and platelet counts due to bone marrow effacement (myelophthisis), myelosuppressive chemotherapy is instituted in the face of cytopenias to clear the bone marrow of neoplastic cells and allow hematopoiesis to normalize.

In those breeds likely to have homozygous *MDR1* gene mutations (e.g., collies; see Chapter 12), and therefore to be at risk for serious chemotherapy toxicity,[280] the author [DMV] will initiate a CHOP protocol out of sequence, beginning with non-MDR1–substrate drugs, such as cyclophosphamide. This ensures treatment of the lymphoma while allowing sufficient time for analysis of *MDR1* gene mutations before initiating MDR1 substrate drugs. No specific protocols have been scrutinized for treating dogs that are double-mutant for *MDR1*; however, if using *MDR1*-substrate drugs, the author initiates treatment using a 40% to 50% dose reduction. Subsequent dose modifications (increased or decreased dosage) can be implemented, depending on the level of adverse events observed, particularly low neutrophil counts at nadir. The author does not dose-modify for heterozygous *MDR1* gene mutations as little documented clinically significant chemosensitivity exists in these animals.

The Case for Treating T-Cell Lymphoma Differently

With some exceptions (e.g., TZL), multicentric T-cell lymphoma, compared with multicentric B-cell lymphoma, is associated with similar initial response rates, but significantly lower response durations (e.g., PFS) after chemotherapy (including CHOP-based protocols).[68,112,113,116,123,226,242,244,277,281–283] In addition, the effectiveness of a single treatment of DOX in the treatment of naïve lymphoma in one retrospective case series suggested a lower initial response rate for T-cell, compared with B-cell, immunophenotypes; however, this study performed only a single day 7 evaluation.[281] Many question whether dogs diagnosed with T-cell lymphoma should be treated with standard CHOP-based protocols or with alternative protocols. This is a valid question; however, the answer remains elusive because adequately powered randomized controlled trials do not currently exist to demonstrate if an alternate protocol is better for this immunophenotype. Several alternative protocols (MOPP, LOPP, VELCAP-TSC) have been reported and reviewed for induction therapy in dogs with multicentric T-cell lymphoma.[110,284–286] These alternative protocols tend to add or substitute alkylating agents (e.g., nitrogen mustard, lomustine, procarbazine) for DOX. Although reports have suggested improvements in remission durations in dogs with either confirmed T-cell lymphoma or lymphoma with hypercalcemia and no immunophenotypic classification, the confidence intervals of the medians all overlap with data from CHOP-based protocols, and differences in determining PFS, response evaluation, and study population (in particular, some do not adequately distinguish indolent multicentric lymphoma) in these reports preclude confident comparisons. As yet, no controlled, randomized trials have documented improvement with this approach. Ultimately, the development of better protocols for treating T-cell lymphoma awaits careful, randomized, prospective trial assessment. Until such time, the author prefers to initiate CHOP-based induction and switch to lomustine-based rescue at the first sign of progression or to enter dogs into clinical trials with novel agents. Although species differences may exist, in people with aggressive T-cell NHL, alternative protocols rich in alkylating agents have not shown superiority over CHOP-based protocols, and the National Comprehensive Cancer Network recommend human patient participation in clinical trials as the "gold standard" for aggressive nonindolent T-cell lymphomas.

Evaluation of Treatment Response

VCOG has published criteria for evaluation of treatment response (v1.0) to standardize reporting of outcome results and comparisons among protocols for peripheral nodal disease using criteria readily available in the practice setting.[253] The most important of these outcome measures and the preferred temporal outcome criterion for assessing protocol activity is now considered to be PFS, which is defined as being the time from treatment initiation to tumor progression or death from any cause. This brings veterinary outcome reporting more in line with human standards. Because the majority of dogs with lymphoma eventually experience relapse after chemotherapy-induced remissions and because methodology for differentiating complete and partial responses is analysis dependent on how responses are determined, PFS removes many sources of bias. Further, overall survival in published reports invariably includes patients who go on to receive varied rescue protocols that bias the overall result, making it a less comparable outcome. Widespread application of these standardized criteria should permit more suitable comparisons in the future. True iCR rarely occur in dogs with lymphoma; documenting iCRs is limited to investigative trials striving to achieve them because we lack meaningful therapeutic options.

Improved methods of detecting minimal residual disease (MRD) or early recurrence have been investigated in dogs with lymphoma and include advanced imaging and detection of molecular and biologic markers of MRD. Advanced functional and anatomic imaging techniques (i.e., PET/CT) are the current standard for assessing treatment response and early relapse of lymphoma in humans and have also been investigated in dogs (see Fig. 33.10).[221,223–226] As these techniques become available to a broader veterinary population, their clinical application will surely increase. Molecular detection of MRD applies clonality and PCR techniques. Beyond diagnostic applications, these techniques have been applied to determine cytoreductive efficacy of various chemotherapeutic drugs and to document and predict early relapse in patients before more conventional methods.[123,217,246,287–293] Regarding biomarkers of MRD, preliminary investigations have suggested serum lactate dehydrogenase activity, thymidine kinase 1 activity, haptoglobin, and serum C-reactive protein may be candidates in the dog.[202–206,294]

As we become more proficient at defining MRD, the pressing clinical question becomes how we use this information. Theoretically, such information could suggest when more aggressive therapy or alternative therapy should be instituted in patients who have not achieved a "molecular remission" or who are undergoing early relapse; however, until we determine what these interventions should be based on prospective trial assessment, the clinical utility of MRD analytics remain theoretical.

Reinduction and Rescue Chemotherapy

Eventually, the vast majority of dogs that achieve a remission will relapse or experience recrudescence of lymphoma. This usually represents the emergence of tumor clones or tumor stem cells (see Chapter 2) that are inherently more resistant to chemotherapy than the original tumor, the so-called MDR clones that either were initially drug resistant or became so after exposure to selected chemotherapy agents.[295] Evidence suggests that in dogs with relapsed lymphoma, tumor cells are more likely to express genes (e.g., *MDR1*) that encode ABC-transporter protein transmembrane drug pumps often associated with MDR.[196,197,296–299] *MDR1* represents only one of the plethora of mechanisms that lead to drug-resistant disease (see Chapter 12). Other causes of

relapse after chemotherapy include inadequate dosing and/or frequency of administration of chemotherapy, failure to achieve high concentrations of chemotherapeutic drugs in certain sites such as the CNS, and initial treatment with prednisone alone.

At the first recurrence of lymphoma, it is recommended that reinduction be attempted first by reintroducing the induction protocol that was initially successful, provided the recurrence occurred temporally far enough from the conclusion of the initial protocol (e.g., ≥2 months) to make reinduction likely. The cumulative dose of DOX that will result from reinduction, baseline cardiac assessment, the use of cardioprotectants, alternative drug choices, and client education should all be considered. In general, the duration of reinduction remission will be half that encountered in the initial therapy; however, a subset of animals will enjoy long-term reinductions, especially if the dog completed the initial induction treatment protocol and was currently not receiving chemotherapy for several months when relapse occurred. Reinduction rates of nearly 80% to 90% can be expected in dogs that have completed CHOP-based protocols and then relapse while not receiving therapy.[232,300] The duration of a second CHOP-based remission in one report was predicted by the duration of the interval between protocols and the duration of the first remission.[123,300]

If reinduction fails or the dog does not respond to the initial induction, the use of so-called "rescue" agents or "rescue" protocols may be attempted. These are single drugs or drug combinations that are typically not found in standard CHOP protocols and are withheld for use in the drug-resistant setting. The most common rescue protocols used in dogs include single-agent use or a combination of rabacfosadine, actinomycin D, mitoxantrone, DOX (if DOX was not part of the original induction protocol), dacarbazine (DTIC), temozolomide, lomustine (CCNU), L-asparaginase, mechlorethamine, vincristine, vinblastine, procarbazine, prednisone, and etoposide. Some rescue protocols are relatively simple and convenient single-agent treatments, whereas others are more complicated (and expensive) multiagent protocols, such as MOPP. Overall rescue response rates of 40% to 90% are reported; however, responses are usually not durable with median response durations of 1.5 to 2.5 months being typical regardless of the complexity of the protocol. A small (<20%) subset of animals will enjoy longer rescue durations. Table 33.5 provides a summary of canine rescue protocols and published results.[270,301–320] Current published data from rescue protocols do not include sufficient numbers for adequate statistical power, nor do they compare protocols in a controlled, randomized prospective fashion. Therefore comparative evaluations of efficacy among various protocols are subject to substantial bias, making direct comparisons difficult. Choice

TABLE 33.5	Summary of Response for Rescue Protocols[a]					
PRIVATE Protocol	Number of Animals	Overall Response (%)	Complete Response (%)	Median Response Duration[c]	Median Duration of Complete Response	References
Actinomycin-D	25	0	0	0 days	0 days	316
Actinomycin-D	49[b]	41	41	129 days	129 days	310
Dacarbazine	40	35	3	43 days	144 days	313
Dacarbazine or temozolomide-anthracycline	63	71	55	45 days	NR	311

Continued

TABLE 33.5	Summary of Response for Rescue Protocols[a]—cont'd					
PRIVATE Protocol	Number of Animals	Overall Response (%)	Complete Response (%)	Median Response Duration[c]	Median Duration of Complete Response	References
DMAC (dexamethasone, melphalan, actinomycin-D, cytosine arabinoside)	54 86	72 43	44 16	61 days 24 days	112 days NR	309 306
Lomustine (CCNU)	43	27	7	86 days	110 days	314
Lomustine, L-asparaginase, prednisone	48	77	65	70 days	90 days	319
Lomustine, L-asparaginase, prednisone	31	87	52	63 days	111 days	320
Lomustine, DTIC	57	35	23	62 days	83 days	312
Mitoxantrone	44	41	30	NR	127 days	315
MOPP (mechlorethamine, vincristine, procarbazine, prednisone)	117	65	31	61 days	63 days	318
MPP (mechlorethamine, procarbazine, prednisone)	41	34	17	56 days	238 days	317
MOMP (mechlorethamine, vincristine, melphalan, prednisone)	88	51	12	56 days	81 days	301
LOPP (lomustine, vincristine, procarbazine, prednisone)	33	61	36	84 days	NR	302
Vinblastine (second rescue)	39	25.6	7.7	30 days	NR	304
Rabacfosadine (B cell only)	50	74	45	108 days	203 days	270
LPP (lomustine, procarbazine, prednisone)	41	61	29	34 days	84 days	307
Temozolomide	26	32	13	15 days	NR	308

[a]Minimum of 25 cases. Few of these protocols include sufficient numbers for adequate statistical power and fewer compare treatment protocols in a randomized prospective fashion. In addition, staging, inclusion, and response criteria vary considerably between protocols presented. Therefore evaluations of efficacy between the various protocols are subject to bias making direct comparisons difficult and indeed precarious.

[b]Prednisone often used concurrently.

[c]Various temporal response end-points were used including disease-free interval, time to progression, progression-free survival, time to discontinuation, and remission duration.

TABLE 33.6 First-Line Rescue Protocol[a]

Cycle 1

Week 1	**Baseline ALT _____ Units/L** L-Asparaginase, 400 Units/kg SC CCNU[b] 70 mg/m² PO Prednisone, 2 mg/kg PO, once daily
Week 2	Prednisone, 1.5 mg/kg PO, once daily
Week 3	Prednisone, 1.0 mg/kg PO, once daily

Cycle 2

Week 1	**Optional ALT _____ Units/L** L-Asparaginase, 400 U/kg SC CCNU 70 mg/m² PO Prednisone, 1.0 mg/kg PO, EOD
Week 2	Prednisone, 1.0 mg/kg PO, EOD
Week 3	Prednisone, 1.0 mg/kg PO, EOD

Cycle 3–5

Week 1	**Mandatory ALT _____ Units/L** CCNU 70 mg/m² PO Prednisone, 1.0 mg/kg PO, EOD
Week 2	Prednisone, 1.0 mg/kg PO, EOD
Week 3	Prednisone, 1.0 mg/kg PO, EOD

[a]Treatment discontinuation criteria: (1) After completion of protocol, two treatments beyond complete response (CR); (2) progressive disease; (3) increase in ALT activity >2× upper limit of normal (or 2× baseline if higher than baseline at initiation)—institute drug discontinuation and reinstitution/dose reduction dependent on normalization of ALT.

[b]Prophylactic liver protectants recommended (e.g., Denamarin).

ALT, Alanine aminotransferase.

of a particular rescue protocol should depend on several factors, including cost, time commitment required, efficacy, adverse event profile, and experience of the clinician with the protocols in question. As the complexity of rescue protocols does not yet appear to be associated with significant gains in rescue durability, the author (DMV) tends to choose simpler and less costly protocols (e.g., CCNU/L-asparaginase/prednisone) (Table 33.6); however, the use of multiple varied rescue protocols, switching as needed based on response, continues as long as clients are comfortable with their dog's quality of life. This sequential application of several different rescue protocols can result in several months of extended survival with acceptable quality of life.

Strategies to Enhance Effectiveness of Therapy in Lymphoma

Despite the plethora of published chemotherapeutic protocols for dogs with lymphoma, it appears we have achieved as much as we can from currently available cytotoxic chemotherapeutics in standard settings. The 12-month median survival "wall" and the 20% to 25% 2-year survival rates have not improved dramatically. Further advances in remission and survival durations await the development of new methods of delivering or targeting traditional chemotherapeutic drugs, new generations of chemotherapeutic drugs, or novel nonchemotherapeutic treatment modalities; in particular, the development of targeted immunotherapies, which is the standard of care in physician-based oncology. Mechanisms of avoiding or abrogating MDR, enhancing tumor apoptosis

(programmed cell death), tumor ablation, and immune-system reconstitution, as well as novel immunomodulatory therapies for lymphoma, are all active areas of investigation in both human and veterinary medicine.

Treatment Approaches Using Immunologic or Biologic Agents

Monoclonal Antibody Approaches

Enhanced durability of first remissions in humans with B-cell NHL has been achieved primarily through the institution of monoclonal antibody (mAb)-based therapies (so-called R-CHOP protocols that are the current "standard-of-care" in people). The "R" refers to rituximab (Rituxan), a recombinant chimeric murine/human antibody directed against the CD20 antigen, a hydrophobic transmembrane protein located on normal pre-B and mature B lymphocytes. After binding, rituximab triggers a host cytotoxic immune response against CD20-positive cells. Unfortunately, rituximab does not have therapeutic activity in dogs because of a lack of external recognition of a similar antigen on canine lymphoma cells and the inherent antigenicity of human-derived antibodies in dogs.[321,322] Recently, caninized mAb designed to target either B-cell (blontuvetmab; Blontress) or T-cell (tamtuvetmab; Tactress) lymphomas were conditionally approved by the USDA for use in dogs with lymphoma; however, after being assessed in prospective clinical trials involving a large number of dogs, their target specificity was found to be inadequate to effect clinical efficacy, and they are no longer available and are not currently recommended for use. Several laboratories throughout the world are working to characterize and develop more specific and effective mAb therapies for use in canine lymphoma,[323–326] and practitioners await their development.

Antitumor Vaccine Approaches

Several antitumor vaccine approaches have been investigated in dogs with lymphoma, including tumor vaccine extract using killed lymphoma cells combined with Freund's adjuvant[327,328] and autologous killed and/or gene engineered lymphoma tumor cell vaccines[329,330]; however, no significant gains in remission times or overall survival have been documented. Exploratory vaccines targeting telomerase[331,332] (see Chapter 15, Section D), heat shock proteins,[333,334] and RNA-loaded CD40-activated B cells[335,336] in dogs with lymphoma have also been conducted. These studies involved small numbers of nonrandomized patients and lacked controlled populations for comparison. A xenogeneic DNA vaccine designed to target canine CD20 is currently undergoing clinical trials in the United States. Although preliminary activity is suggested in many of these reports and they are serving to enhance our basic understanding of immunotherapeutic methodologies, their development is still early; complete safety and efficacy trials have not been completed to date.

Adaptive Immunotherapy Approaches

Much excitement has been generated in physician-based medicine about adaptive immunotherapy approaches, in particular the application of chimeric antigen receptor T cells (CAR-T; see Chapter 14). These approaches are currently the subject of several proof-of-concept trials in dogs with NHL.[337,338]

Surgery

Most dogs with lymphoma have multicentric disease and therefore require systemic chemotherapy to effectively treat their disease.

However, surgery has been used to treat solitary lymphoma (stage I) or solitary extranodal disease. Careful staging is necessary in such cases to rule out multicentric involvement before treating local disease. Surgery has also occasionally been applied for palliative removal of nodes that are mechanical obstructions in drug resistant settings.

The benefit of surgical removal of the spleen in dogs with massive splenomegaly remains unclear; however, for indolent lymphomas confined to the spleen, long-term survival after splenectomy is the norm.[100,102,339,340] In an older report, 16 dogs with lymphoma underwent splenectomy to remove a massively enlarged spleen and were subsequently treated with chemotherapy.[340] Within 6 weeks of splenectomy, five of the 16 dogs died of disseminated intravascular coagulation (DIC) and sepsis. The remaining 11 dogs (66%) had a CR, and seven dogs had a MST of 14 months. No staging or histologic information was provided, so the information appears of limited usefulness, although those with follow-up lived approximately 1 year. In two reports of indolent nodular lymphoma of the spleen (MZL and mantle cell lymphoma [MCL]), outcome was available on seven MZL cases, including three cases that did not receive adjuvant chemotherapy after surgery,[100,102] and only one died of lymphoma after splenectomy. In a recent report of indolent lymphomas, four splenic lymphomas (three MZL and one MCL) underwent splenectomy alone and all survived more than 1 year, with none dying of their primary disease.[101] In another report of 41 dogs undergoing splenectomy for lymphoma, those dogs with indolent forms enjoyed long-term survival.[339] Splenectomy should be considered if the lymphoma is not documented in other sites after thorough staging, if lymphoma is an indolent form, or if splenic rupture has occurred. Of note, no control population consisting of dogs that did not undergo splenectomy exists, so the natural history of indolent splenic lymphoma remains uncertain.

Radiation Therapy

Radiation therapy, although of limited routine use in the treatment of lymphoma, may be indicated in selected cases.[341-351] Potential indications are as follows:

1. Curative intent therapy for stage I LN and solitary extranodal disease (i.e., nasal, cutaneous, spinal lymphoma)
2. Palliation for local disease (e.g., mandibular lymphadenopathy, rectal lymphoma, mediastinal lymphoma where precaval syndrome is present, localized bone involvement)
3. Total body radiation combined with bone marrow or stem cell reconstitution
4. Whole or staged half-body RT after chemotherapy-induced remissions

In the latter case, staged half-body irradiation sandwiched between chemotherapy cycles or after attainment of remission by induction chemotherapy has been preliminarily investigated as a form of consolidation or maintenance.[261,344,345,349,352-354] RT is delivered to either the cranial or caudal half of the body in 4 to 8 Gy fractions and, after a 2- or 4-week rest, the other half of the body is irradiated in a similar fashion. Although these preliminary investigations were not randomized, they suggest that RT applied when dogs are in either complete or partial remission is safe and warrants further investigation to determine whether significant therapeutic gain can be realized. A pilot study of low-dose (1 Gy) single-fraction total body irradiation in seven dogs with relapsed drug-resistant lymphoma, although safely applied, resulted in only partial nondurable (1–4 week) remissions.[341]

Total body irradiation (and/or ablative chemotherapy) for complete or partial bone marrow ablation followed by reconstitution

with bone marrow or stem-cell transplant in dogs, although a recognized model in comparative research settings,[355] is still in its early phases of development and application in clinical veterinary practice.[356-359] Because of the high cost, limited accessibility to relatively sophisticated equipment, and management requirements, these types of procedures are limited to preliminary investigations at a few centers. Currently, long-term results documenting significantly enhanced efficacy in sufficient numbers of treated cases have yet to be presented.

Treatment of Extranodal Lymphoma

In general, the veterinary literature contains little information on treating various extranodal forms of lymphoma in dogs, and our ability to predict outcome is thus limited. In general, it is recommended that, after extensive staging, in those cases where disease is shown to be localized to a solitary site, local therapies (e.g., surgery, local RT) can be used while withholding systemic therapies (i.e., chemotherapy) until systemic progression or recurrence is documented. In contrast, if multiple extranodal sites are involved or they are part of a more generalized process, systemic chemotherapy should be chosen.

Alimentary Lymphoma

Most dogs with alimentary lymphoma are presented with diffuse involvement of the intestinal tract, and involvement of local LNs and liver is common. Chemotherapy in dogs with diffuse intermediate- or high-grade disease has been reported to be unrewarding for the most part[61,126,360,361] with MSTs of only a few months after CHOP-based chemotherapy; however, durable remissions in a small subset of cases have been reported. A small-cell T-cell intestinal lymphoma has been reported in dogs that appears to have a more indolent course similar to small-cell T-cell intestinal lymphoma in cats.[64,125] In reports of 17 and 20 dogs, MSTs after receiving conservative treatment (prednisone and chlorambucil most commonly) were 1.5 to 2.0 years.[64,125] Solitary alimentary lymphoma is rare in the dog; however, if the tumor is localized and can be surgically removed, results (with or without follow-up chemotherapy) can be encouraging. Colorectal lymphoma, generally a high-grade B-cell phenotype, is also associated with an indolent outcome with median progression-free and overall survival times greater than 3 years after initiation of chemotherapy.[362,363]

Primary Central Nervous System Lymphoma

CNS lymphoma in dogs usually results from extension of multicentric lymphoma; however, primary CNS lymphoma has been reported.[87,133,135,136,364] If tumors are localized (rare), local RT should be considered. Few studies have reported the use of chemotherapy. In one study, cytosine arabinoside (Ara-C) at a dosage of 20 mg/m^2 was given intrathecally; this treatment was combined with systemic chemotherapy and CNS RT.[133] Overall, the response rates are low and of short duration (several weeks to months), although occasional durable responses are encountered.

Cutaneous Lymphoma

The cutaneous lymphomas represent an assorted group of clinical entities that vary considerably in presentation and outcome.[71,74,77,119,129,130,365,366] Epitheliotropic cutaneous lymphoma is most common and has been categorized into two clinically separate entities (mucocutaneous and cutaneous) based on outcome differences, with the mucocutaneous form appearing to have better overall outcomes.[129] Treatment of cutaneous and mucocutaneous lymphoma depends on the extent of disease. Solitary lesions have a better prognosis and may be treated with surgical excision or RT, although thorough staging for systemic disease should be undertaken before local therapy and active surveillance for subsequent development of recurrent or systemic involvement should be implemented. Fractionated RT has been associated with long-term control.[366,367] Diffuse cutaneous lymphoma is best managed with systemic therapy, although the rate and durability of response is generally less than in multicentric lymphoma. The most widely used protocols for epitheliotropic and nonepitheliotropic cutaneous T-cell lymphoma (CTCL) include CCNU (with or without L-asparaginase [see Table 33.6]) along with prednisone, pegylated L-asparaginase (very costly), and oral retinoic acid analogs (limited availability; acitretin, etretinate, isotretinoin).[269,366,368–372] Multiagent protocols (generally CHOP-based) may also be used, but have generally been instituted after single-agent therapies have failed. Although reported response rates can range from 40% to 80%, median remission durations are generally short (approximately 3–6 months); occasionally, durable remissions are encountered. Sporadic reports of other therapies for cutaneous lymphoma in small numbers of cases include the use of COAP (cyclophosphamide, vincristine [Oncovin], Ara-C, and prednisone), topical mechlorethamine (Mustargen), rabacfosadine, recombinant human interferon-alpha, and masitinib.[132,269,368,373] All these reports involved small numbers of cases and resulted in relatively short response durations. Whole-body surface RT has also been explored for the treatment of diffuse cutaneous lymphoma in preliminary trials.[348,374]

A form of cutaneous lymphocytic infiltration has been characterized as an indolent T-cell lymphoma based on clonality.[77] It is associated with slow progression and long-term survival after corticosteroid management; however, it does have the potential to progress to high-grade lymphoma.

Prognosis

The prognosis for dogs with lymphoma is highly variable and depends on a wide variety of factors that are documented or presumed to affect response to therapy. Although rarely curable (<10% of cases), CRs and a good quality of life during extended remissions and survival are typical. Factors that have been shown to influence treatment response and survival for peripheral nodal lymphoma are summarized in Tables 33.7 and 33.8.[a] The prognostic factors most consistently identified for peripheral nodal lymphoma are immunophenotype, WHO substage (see Fig. 33.11B), and an indolent subclassification (Fig. 33.12). Many reports have confirmed that dogs with nonindolent intermediate- and high-grade T-cell lymphomas have significantly shorter remissions and survival durations than dogs with intermediate or high-grade B-cell disease.[68,69,112,113,116,277,391] This holds true primarily for dogs with multicentric lymphoma because the immunophenotype of solitary or extranodal forms of lymphoma has not been thoroughly investigated with respect to prognosis. In addition, it has been shown that dogs with B-cell lymphomas that express lower than normal levels of B5 antigen (expressed in 95% of nonneoplastic lymphocytes) or low levels of class II MHC expression experience shorter remissions and survival durations.[69,391] Dogs presented with WHO substage *b* disease (i.e., clinically ill) also do poorly compared with dogs with substage *a* disease.[68,112,116,235,387] Dogs with stage I and II disease have a better prognosis than those dogs in more advanced stages (stage III, IV, and V).

Proliferative assays such as analysis of bromodeoxyuridine (BrdU) uptake, Ki67 antibody reactivity, and AgNOR indices to measure proliferative activity of tumor cells have been shown to provide prognostic information in dogs treated with combination chemotherapy; however, different studies are contradictory and the information is rarely helpful clinically. In addition, in one report, the proportion of tumor cells undergoing apoptosis was modestly predictive of remission duration.[123,174]

The anatomic site of disease is also of considerable prognostic importance. Primary diffuse cutaneous, diffuse GI, hepatosplenic, and primary CNS lymphomas tend to be associated with a poor prognosis. Dogs with indolent cutaneous T-cell lymphocytic infiltration experience long-term survivals.[77] Sex has been shown to influence prognosis in some studies.[235,237] Neutered females tend to have a better prognosis; male dogs may have a higher incidence of the T-cell phenotype, which may account for the poorer prognosis.

Reported biomarkers of prognosis, summarized in Table 33.8, include increased circulating levels of glutathione-S-transferase, thymidine kinase, lactate dehydrogenase, C-reactive proteins, and VEGF. Finally, one report suggests that a history of chronic inflammatory disease of several types predicts likelihood of early relapse.[202,398] These putative prognostic indicators require further confirmation in larger trials.

Of particular interest is the capacity of gene expression analysis to predict and indeed subcategorize the lymphomas into prognostic categories.[14,20,178,179,384] Although these types of analysis are not currently widely available in the veterinary clinical setting, they are routinely used for prognostication and therapeutic decision making in people and are likely to become more readily available to veterinary clinicians in the next decade. The potential of genetic molecular profiling in veterinary oncology is illustrated by Frant et al[178]: they were able to subcategorize dogs with peripheral nodal lymphoma into three prognostic categories based on a benchtop quantitative real-time (qRT)-PCR diagnostic analysis of expression of only four genes.[178]

The Indolent Lymphomas

Histologic grade (subtype) greatly influences prognosis. Dogs with lymphoma classified as intermediate or high grade tend to respond to chemotherapy, but can relapse early. Dogs with low-grade indolent lymphomas have a poorer response to chemotherapy, yet have a survival advantage over dogs with intermediate- and high-grade lymphomas (see Fig. 33.12). Several case compilations have documented that dogs with indolent lymphoma (e.g., MZL, MCL, TZL) experience prolonged STs, often in the absence of any or aggressive chemotherapy; that is, they often enjoy prolonged survival despite intervention rather than because of intervention.[100–102] One caveat is that canine nodal marginal zone lymphoma, which is designated as an indolent disorder, is generally more aggressive with median progression-free intervals of 5 months and overall STs of only 8.5 months; this is substantially less than splenic MZL, which is associated with long-term survival or cure after splenectomy.[108] Many dogs with indolent lymphoma will live near normal life-spans and ultimately die of non–lymphoma-related disorders. Generally, with the indolent lymphomas, unless the presence of disease is having an effect on the quality of life or results in clinically significant cytopenias (myelophthisis), active surveillance in the absence of treatment is recommended. If treatment is deemed necessary, more conservative protocols (e.g., chlorambucil/prednisone or cyclophosphamide/prednisone) are initiated. The goal of therapy is to control the disease (stable disease or partial response) as CRs are unusual with the indolent lymphomas.

---

[a]108, 111, 123, 139, 177–179, 207, 210, 213, 235, 237, 273, 276–278, 287, 290, 293, 294, 299, 328, 365, 375–397.

TABLE 33.7   Prognostic Factors for Peripheral Nodal Lymphoma in Dogs

Factor	Strong Association	Modest Association Requiring Further Investigation	Comments	References
Histopathology/Subclassification	X		High/intermediate-grade: unfavorable Indolent/low-grade: favorable	29,90,96,98–102,107–113,116–119
Immunophenotype	X		T cell phenotype: unfavorable (except TZL) Low MHC II expression: unfavorable	68,69,112,113,116,277,365,379,391
WHO clinical stage		X	Stage I/II: favorable Stage V with significant bone marrow involvement: unfavorable	248,273,379,387
WHO clinical substage	X		Substage *b* (clinically ill): unfavorable	68,112,116,235,379,387
Sex		X	Females/neutered females: unfavorable	235,237
Genetic/gene expression analysis	X		Some signatures highly predictive of outcome	14,20,29,378,384,385
Anatomic location	X		Leukemia, diffuse cutaneous and alimentary, hepatosplenic forms: unfavorable	See text for extra nodal sites
Peripheral blood counts at presentation Anemia Neutrophilia Neutrophil/lymphocyte ratio Thrombocytopenia Lymphocyte/monocyte ratio	X	X X X X	Unfavorable Unfavorable Low: unfavorable Unfavorable Low: unfavorable	277,375,376,379,386,390 376 379 375 382
Molecular assessment of minimal residual disease (e.g., PCR, flow)		X	Likely to become more important when "curative" therapeutic approaches are developed and instituted	123,217,287–290,293,393,416
Measures of proliferation		X	Contradictory reports exist	123,177,380,388,389
Steroid pretreatment	X		Prolonged steroid pretreatment: unfavorable	276,278
Cranial mediastinal lymphadenopathy	X		Present: unfavorable	122
Chemotherapy-induced hematologic toxicity		X	Grade III or IV chemotherapy-induced neutropenias: favorable	381,392
Geographic location		X	Mixed	383

Lymphocytic Leukemia

Lymphocytic leukemia is typically defined as proliferation of neoplastic lymphocytes in bone marrow. Neoplastic cells usually originate in the bone marrow, but occasionally in the spleen, and may or may not be circulating in the peripheral blood. Our ability to diagnose lymphocytic leukemias using morphologic, flow cytometric, immunophenotypic, and cytochemical techniques has increased significantly in the past decade. Although little information on treatment and prognosis is available for acute lymphocytic leukemias (ALL), clinically relevant information on

chronic lymphocytic leukemias (CLL), their prognosis, and treatment have recently come to light. Differentiating between true leukemia and stage V lymphoma can be difficult and arbitrary, and is often based on lack of significant lymphadenopathy, degree of blood and bone marrow involvement, and immunophenotypic characteristics.

Incidence, Risk Factors, and Etiology

Lymphocytic leukemia is more common than acute myeloid leukemia and myeloproliferative disorders, but the true incidence

TABLE 33.8	Circulating (Serum/Plasma) Biomarkers as Prognostic Indices in Dogs with Lymphoma	
Biomarker	**Comments**	**References**
Lactate dehydrogenase activity	Increased: unfavorable	202,210
Thymidine kinase activity	Increased: unfavorable	202,205,206,396,397
Haptoglobin	Increased: unfavorable	202–204
Serum VEGF	Increased: unfavorable	213,417
Glutathione-*S*-transferase	Increased: unfavorable	418
Hypercalcemia	Unfavorable	116,395,419,420
Serum cobalamin	Decreased: unfavorable	395
Serum albumin	Decreased: unfavorable	375,377
Serum C-reactive protein	Although it may be used to characterize remission status, variable levels preclude utility.	202–205,294

VEGF, Vascular endothelial growth factor.

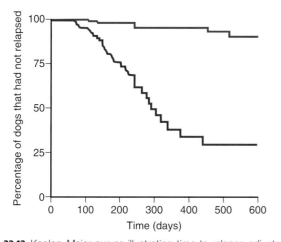

• **Fig. 33.12** Kaplan–Meier curves illustrating time to relapse adjusted for clinical stage and immunophenotype among dogs treated for low-grade (*n* = 17) (*blue line*) or high-grade (*n* = 51) (*red line*) Kiel classification lymphoma. (From Teske E, van Heerde P, Rutteman GR, et al. Prognostic factors for treatment of malignant lymphoma in dogs. *J Am Vet Med Assoc.* 1994;205:1722-1728.)

is unknown. Overall, CLL is much more common than ALL. Smaller reports state that German shepherd dogs and golden retrievers may be overrepresented.[170,399] Based on a recent compilations of more than 400 dogs with B-cell CLL (B-CLL), small-breed dogs are much more likely to be affected.[106] Lymphocytic leukemia can occur in dogs of any age, but typically occurs in middle-aged to older dogs (mean of 7–10 years of age); CLL usually occurs in older dogs (mean of 10–11 years of age),[106,170,394,399,400] although a distinct form of B-CLL in English bulldogs occurs in younger dogs (mean, 6 years of age).[106] A significant sex predilection is not reported. As with lymphoma, the etiology of lymphocytic leukemia is for the most part unknown. Genetic factors likely play a role and have been compared between dogs and humans.[12]

Pathology and Classification

Lymphocytic leukemias can be subdivided based on cell size, maturity, genetic aberrations, microRNA expression, and immunophenotype.[12,170,180,394,399–402] The simplest classification divides leukemia into two groups: chronic (small cells with a mature cytologic phenotype) and acute (large cells with an immature cytologic phenotype). Immunophenotypic assessment using flow cytometric and molecular assays can further characterize these two major subtypes.

Of the CLLs, approximately two-thirds are T cell (T-CLL) and one-third are B-CLL. Three primary subtypes of CLL, based primarily on immunophenotyping, have been reported[106,164,170,394,400]: (1) T-CLL, which is the most common form, with cells in the majority of cases being CD3⁺/CD8⁺ granular lymphocytes; (2) B-CLL (CD21⁺), which is the next most common subtype; and (3) atypical CLL, which represents a combination of immunophenotypes (CD3⁻, CD8⁺; CD3⁺, CD4⁻, CD8⁻; CD3⁺, CD4⁺, CD8⁺, and CD3⁺ + CD21⁺). This is in contrast to CLL in humans, which is primarily a disease of B cells. In CLL, lymphocytes often are indistinguishable morphologically from normal small lymphocytes (Fig. 33.13) and have a low rate of proliferation; accumulation of lymphocytes likely results from their prolonged lifespan.

ALL has also been classified as a lymphoid precursor neoplasm and can be derived from either B cells (B-ALL) or T cells (T-ALL). The majority are B-ALL (CD21⁺, CD3⁻, CD4⁻, CD8⁻), although a smaller percentage (<10%) are T-ALL (CD3⁺, CD4⁻, CD8⁻, CD21⁻).[170] In general, these cells tend to be intermediate or large cells with moderate amounts of basophilic cytoplasm. Perhaps the most distinguishing feature of the large lymphocytes is the nuclear chromatin pattern, which typically is less condensed than the chromatin in small lymphocytes but more condensed than the chromatin in myeloblasts. Large lymphocytes are larger than neutrophils, have a high nuclear-to-cytoplasmic ratio, and contain basophilic cytoplasm (see Fig. 33.13). Nucleoli, although present, are less prominent in large lymphocytes than in myeloblasts. Nevertheless, these cells cannot be distinguished easily from immature cells of other hematopoietic lineages, and identification of lineage-specific markers by immunocytochemical, flow cytometric, or molecular/genetic analysis is required to ascertain their lineage.[401,403,404] If the cells express CD34, a stem-cell marker, an acute phenotype is implied[170,394,399]; however, both myeloid and lymphoid lineages express CD34 and our ability to differentiate ALL from acute myeloid leukemia relies on detection of other markers, including T- and B-cell markers and myeloperoxidase, a myeloid marker. Furthermore, some T-ALLs do not express CD34.[404]

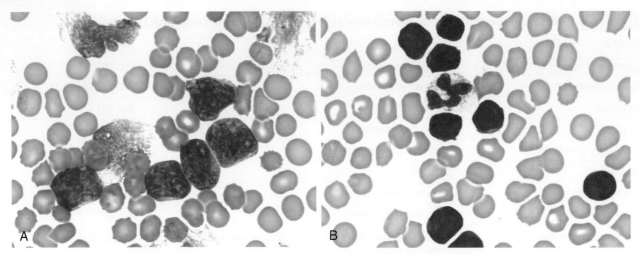

• **Fig. 33.13** (A) Peripheral blood from a dog with acute lymphocytic leukemia (ALL). Note the large lymphoid cells with visible nucleoli. Chromatin from disintegrated cells also is visible. (Wright's stain, ×60 objective.) (B) Peripheral blood from a dog with chronic lymphocytic leukemia (CLL). Note the small lymphocytes of normal mature morphology (smaller than the neutrophil). (Wright's stain, ×60 objective.)

History and Clinical Signs

Dogs with CLL are often asymptomatic and a diagnosis is pursued based on an incidental finding of increased circulating mature lymphocytes on routine CBCs. In more advanced disease, some owners report lethargy and decreased appetite. Mild lymphadenopathy and splenomegaly may be present, although late in the disease splenomegaly may be marked.[405] In a compilation of nearly 500 dogs with B-CLL, 50% had some degree of peripheral lymphadenopathy, 50% had splenomegaly, 30% had hepatomegaly, 23% had visceral lymphadenopathy, and 3% had a mediastinal mass.[106] The white blood cell (WBC) count is usually >30,000 cells/μL but can vary from normal to more than 100,000 cells/μL because of an increase in circulating mature lymphocytes. Lymphocytosis is persistent, and granulocytes are usually present in normal numbers. Other than lymphocytosis, hemograms of dogs with CLL tend to have few abnormalities when lymphocytes are less than 30,000/μL.[170,394,400] Mild anemia, neutropenia, and thrombocytopenia are common, but may become marked as the disease progresses and lymphocyte counts increase above 30,000/μL. In B-CLL, the median lymphocyte count was 24,600/μL and neutropenia and thrombocytopenia were uncommon (1% and 7%, respectively).[106] Despite the well-differentiated appearance of the lymphocytes in CLL, these cells may function abnormally. Paraneoplastic syndromes include monoclonal gammopathies, immune-mediated hemolytic anemia, pure red cell aplasia, and, rarely, hypercalcemia; 80% of dogs with B-CLL were reported to be hyperglobulinemic and 13% were hypercalcemic.[106,406,407] In 22 dogs with CLL, 68% had monoclonal gammopathies (usually IgM or IgA).[407] The immunophenotypes were not reported in this latter report, but a monoclonal gammopathy would be more likely to occur in B-CLL.

Dogs with ALL usually present with clinical signs of anorexia, weight loss, and lethargy. Splenomegaly is typical and other physical abnormalities may include hemorrhage, lymphadenopathy, and hepatomegaly.[408] Infiltration of bone marrow by neoplastic lymphocytes may be extensive, resulting in significant depression of normal hematopoietic elements or myelophthisis.[170,394,399,404,408,409] Anemia, neutropenia, and thrombocytopenia are typically much more severe than with CLL and may become life threatening. Infiltration of extramedullary sites, such as the CNS, bone, and GI tract, may also occur and can result in neuropathies, bone pain, and GI signs, respectively.

Diagnostics and Clinical Staging

Consideration of signalment, history, physical findings, and morphologic appearance and immunophenotype of cells is essential in making an accurate diagnosis. It is helpful to know the profile of lymphocyte subsets in the peripheral blood of normal dogs to determine whether a particular subset has expanded. Approximately 80% of circulating lymphocytes in normal dogs are T cells and about 15% are B cells. NK cells and double-negative (CD4-, CD8-) T cells constitute the remaining fraction. In the T-cell fraction, helper T cells (CD4+) outnumber cytotoxic T cells (CD8+).[407] Lymphocytic leukemia should be a consideration if atypical lymphocytes are in circulation, the immunophenotype of the lymphocytes in circulation is homogeneous as determined by flow cytometric analysis, a phenotype typically present in low frequency has increased, or if clonality is documented (e.g., by PARR analysis). Other differential diagnoses for lymphocytosis include infectious diseases, such as chronic ehrlichiosis, postvaccinal responses in young dogs, IL-2 administration, and transient physiologic or epinephrine-induced lymphocytosis. In some cases, reactive and neoplastic lymphocytoses are difficult to distinguish.

Expansion of neoplastic lymphocytes in bone marrow is the hallmark of ALL and, in most cases, CLL. Careful examination of peripheral blood and bone marrow by an experienced cytopathologist is important in establishing a diagnosis of lymphocytic leukemia; in cases of marked lymphocytosis with atypia, peripheral blood can be used for analysis of immunophenotype and clonality, and examination of bone marrow is not essential. If diagnostic bone marrow cannot be adequately obtained by aspiration, bone marrow core biopsy should be performed. In ALL, large lymphocytes predominate in the bone marrow and are also present in peripheral blood, and other lineages are decreased. In B- and T-cell CLL, lymphocytes are small mature cells that occur in excessive numbers in bone marrow (≥30% of all nucleated cells) early in the disease.[405] In T-CLL, lymphocytes may contain pink granules. Infiltration becomes more extensive as the disease slowly progresses, and eventually the neoplastic cells replace normal marrow.

A separate clinical staging system has not been developed for lymphocytic leukemias. Currently, all dogs with leukemia are classified as stage V based on the WHO Staging System for lymphoma as presented in Box 33.2.

Treatment of Chronic Lymphocytic Leukemia

Because of the indolent and often asymptomatic nature of CLL, the decision to treat is often based on the clinical and laboratory findings in the individual dog. Most oncologists recommend active surveillance (monthly or bimonthly physical examination and CBC) over active therapy when CLL is identified incidentally, there are no accompanying clinical signs, and other significant hematologic abnormalities are not identified. If the dog is significantly anemic or thrombocytopenic or is showing evidence of significant lymphadenopathy or hepatosplenomegaly, therapy should be considered. There is no consensus on what degree of lymphocytosis is used to initiate therapy; the definition of "excessively high" varies among oncologists, and a standard has not been established in veterinary medicine. The author (DMV) prefers to base treatment decisions on the presence of significant constitutional signs and peripheral cytopenias rather than an absolute lymphocyte count. Currently, the most effective drug available for treatment of CLL, once therapy is deemed necessary, is chlorambucil.[400,405] Chlorambucil is given orally at a dose of 0.2 mg/kg or 6 mg/m^2 PO once daily for 7 to 14 days; the dose can then be reduced to 0.1 mg/kg or 3 mg/m^2 PO daily. For long-term maintenance, a dose of 2.0 mg/m^2 every other day can be used. The dose is adjusted based on clinical response and bone marrow tolerance. Pulse-dose chlorambucil (20–30 mg/m^2 q 2 weeks) has been anecdotally used for CLL in some cases; however, no compilations of cases have been reported to assess effectiveness of this protocol. Oral prednisone is used concurrently with chlorambucil at doses of 1 mg/kg daily for 1 to 2 weeks, then 0.5 mg/kg every other day thereafter. The addition of vincristine or the substitution of cyclophosphamide for chlorambucil has been advocated in animals that do not respond to chlorambucil.

Treatment of CLL, once initiated, is primarily palliative with rare complete remissions and a uniformly fatal course. Owing to the indolent nature of this disease, however, STs have been in the range of 1 to 3 years with a good quality of life.[400,405,410] The phenotype of CLL is usually stable over months to years; however, the disease may evolve into an acute phase, and some dogs will develop a form of lymphoma that is rapidly progressive and characterized by the presence of pleomorphic large lymphocytes[411,412]; in humans, this is termed *Richter's syndrome*.[413] Based on a data set of 153 cases, 2% of T-CLLs and 10% of B-CLLs progressed to a Richter-like acute disease often characterized by lymphadenopathy, coughing, vomiting, weight loss, and neurologic signs.[412] In these eight dogs, the progression to acute disease occurred 2 to 16 months after initial diagnosis of their CLL and MST after this progression was only 41 days despite aggressive (CHOP-based) chemotherapy in half of the cases.[412]

Treatment of Acute Lymphocytic Leukemia

Much of the morbidity in dogs with ALL results from effacement of bone marrow (myelophthisis) and subsequent life-threatening peripheral cytopenias. Neutropenia, thrombocytopenia, and anemia may be severe. Dogs often require supportive therapy, such as fresh whole-blood transfusions, broad-spectrum antibiotics, fluid therapy, and nutritional support. Careful monitoring for sepsis, hemorrhage, and DIC is important. Specific treatment of ALL would require aggressive chemotherapy; however, consistently efficacious protocols have not been developed in veterinary medicine, and there are few published reports. CHOP-based protocols, similar to those used for lymphoma (see Table 33.4), have

been used by the author (DMV) and others for dogs with ALL; however, responses and durability of response are generally disappointing. The standard of care in humans with acute leukemia generally involves bone marrow ablative treatments with stem cell or marrow replacement, technology that is not widely available or often pursued in veterinary oncology.

Prognosis

In general, CLL is an indolent disease (with the aforementioned exception of atypical CLL), and many dogs will not require therapy for some time after diagnosis; several dogs have been reported to survive a year or more without treatment.[400,414] For those dogs that are treated, normalization of lymphocyte counts can be expected in 70% of cases. In one report of 17 dogs treated with vincristine, chlorambucil, and prednisone, MST was approximately 12 months with an expected 30% survival at 2 years.[405] In larger compilations of cases that include immunophenotypic analysis, treatment protocols were poorly documented, although most received chlorambucil and prednisone. The immunophenotype of CLL has been shown to be prognostic; in a report of 43 cases, MSTs of 930 days, 480 days, and 22 days were reported for T-CLL, B-CLL, and atypical CLL, respectively.[400] In this group of dogs, young age and anemia were also associated with a poor prognosis. In another series with limited treatment information, dogs with CLL of a CD8$^+$ immunophenotype that presented with less than 30,000 lymphocytes/μL or greater than 30,000 lymphocytes/μL had MSTs of 1098 and 131 days, respectively.[400]

Prognosis for dogs with ALL is generally very poor. In a study of 21 dogs treated with vincristine and prednisone, dogs achieving complete or partial remission (29%) had an MST of 120 days, and few dogs survived longer than 8 months.[408] In one report of 46 cases of ALL with a CD34$^+$ phenotype, dogs had a MST of 16 days (range, 3–128 days), even though the majority received a CHOP-based treatment protocol.[394] In addition, dogs with B-cell ALL (CD21$^+$) in which the lymphocytes were large cells (forward scatter lymphocyte/forward scatter neutrophil ratio of greater than 0.58 by flow cytometric analysis) had a MST of only 129 days, independent of treatment protocol.[394]

SECTION B: FELINE LYMPHOMA AND LEUKEMIA

DAVID M. VAIL AND MARIE PINKERTON

Lymphoma

Lymphoma (malignant lymphoma or lymphosarcoma) comprises a diverse group of neoplasms that have in common their origin from lymphocytes. The neoplasms usually arise in lymphoid tissues such as lymph nodes, spleen, and bone marrow; however, they may arise in almost any tissue in the body. Lymphoma is one of the most common neoplasms seen in the cat. See Box 33.4.

Incidence

Epidemiologic reports before 1990 suggested that lymphoma accounted for 50% to 90% of all hematopoietic tumors in the cat,[421,422] and because hematopoietic tumors (lymphoid and

- A varied group of lymphoid cancers discussed in three major groups based on varied presentation, diagnosis, management, and outcome (Table 33.9): Alimentary/Gastrointestinal, Peripheral Nodal, and Extranodal.
- Feline leukemia virus (FeLV) infection, a major etiologic agent of the disease, is no longer relevant in the majority of cases because of viral elimination and vaccination programs instituted in the 1980s.
- The alimentary/gastrointestinal forms predominate, and distinct subtypes exist representing both indolent (majority) and aggressive (intermediate-/high-grade) lymphomas (Table 33.10).
- Indolent (low-grade) subtypes in any anatomic site are managed with conservative chemotherapy (chlorambucil and prednisolone), with high response rates and durable survival durations (≥1.5–3 years) expected.
- Intermediate- or high-grade subtypes of any anatomic site are managed with more aggressive CHOP- or COP-based chemotherapy protocols (Tables 33.11, 33.12), with moderate response rates (50%–65%) and less durable (<1 year) survival durations expected.
- Cats with intermediate- or high-grade lymphoma that achieve a complete response with chemotherapy (approximately 35% of cases) often enjoy more durable (>1 year) survival durations.
- Solitary forms of lymphoma may be managed with local therapies (i.e., surgery, radiation therapy) provided thorough staging has ruled out systemic spread and active surveillance for identifying recurrence is instituted.

myeloid) represent approximately one-third of all feline tumors, it was estimated that lymphoid neoplasia accounted for an incidence of 200 per 100,000 cats at risk.[423] In one series of 400 cats with hematopoietic tumors, 61% had lymphoma and 39% had leukemias and myeloproliferative diseases (MPDs), of which 21% were categorized as undifferentiated leukemias, most likely myeloid in origin.[424] However, a significant change in the epidemiology and characteristics of lymphoma in cats coincided with the widespread integration of feline leukemia virus (FeLV) diagnostic assays and affected animal elimination regimens of the late 1970s and 1980s, and was further enhanced by the commercially available FeLV vaccines appearing in the late 1980s. The decline in FeLV-associated lymphoma is mirrored by a global decline in the overall prevalence per year of FeLV positivity in cats tested.[425–429] Importantly, many of these studies reveal that despite a sharp drop in FeLV-associated lymphoma, the overall prevalence of lymphoma in cats is increasing. The increased prevalence appears because of an increase in the number and relative frequency of the alimentary (and, in particular, the intestinal) and extranodal anatomic forms of lymphoma.[426,430–433] This is supported by an epidemiologic survey of several hundred cases of feline intestinal lymphoma; 534 (86%) were from the 20 years after 1985 and only 14% were from cases diagnosed in the 20 years before 1985.[432] This change in incidence has also been observed in Europe.[426,431]

The true annual incidence rate for lymphoma in cats is currently unknown. With respect to feline pediatric (<1 year of age) tumors, a study in the United Kingdom (n = 233 pathology specimens) found that 73 (31%) represented hematopoietic tumors, of which 51 (70%) were lymphoma; note that FeLV status was unavailable for this compilation of cases.[433]

The typical signalment for cats with lymphoma cannot be uniformly stated as it varies widely based on anatomic site and FeLV status, and therefore will be discussed individually under site-specific discussions. In general, based on two large compilations (n = 850) of cases in North America and Europe,[427,428] domestic

shorthair (DSH) cats are most commonly affected and Siamese cats appear overrepresented in some reports. A 1.5:1 male-to-female ratio was observed in two studies, with no association with gender or neutering status observed in one.[427,428] In a large compilation of Australian cases, male cats and the Siamese/oriental breeds were overrepresented,[434] and similar breed findings have been observed in North America, although similar gender predilections have not been found. Within the Siamese/oriental breeds, there appears to be a predisposition for a mediastinal form that is not FeLV-associated and represents a younger population (median of 2 years).

Etiology

Viral Factors

FeLV was the most common cause of hematopoietic tumors in the cat in the so-called "FeLV era" of the 1960s through the 1980s, when approximately two-thirds of lymphoma cases were associated with FeLV antigenemia. Several studies have documented the potential molecular means by which FeLV can result in lymphoid neoplasia (see Chapter 1, Section C). As one would predict, along with a shift away from FeLV-associated tumors came a shift away from traditional signalment and relative frequency of anatomic sites. This is also supported outside of North America by similar signalment and anatomic frequency data observed in Australia, where FeLV infection is less common, and in Europe, where FeLV incidence has declined and signalment and anatomic site prevalence has shifted accordingly.[426,431,434,435] The median age of approximately 11 to 12 years now reported in North America and Europe is considerably higher than the median ages of 3 to 5 years reported in the FeLV era.[421,422,426–429,431] The median age of cats within various anatomic tumor groupings has not changed, and anatomic forms traditionally associated with FeLV, such as the mediastinal form, may still occur in younger, FeLV antigenemic cats. Similarly, the alimentary form and extranodal forms occur most often in older, FeLV-negative cats.[436–441] Table 33.9 presents an overview of the characteristics of the various anatomic sites of lymphoma in cats. As our ability to interrogate FeLV associations on a molecular basis has improved (e.g., PCR amplification and fluorescent in situ hybridization), several reports exist defining the role or potential role of FeLV in cats with and without FeLV antigenemia.[442–447] Collectively, these studies indicate FeLV proviral insertion exists in a proportion of feline lymphoma tissues and is more common in those of T-cell origin, particularly the thymic and peripheral lymph node anatomic forms. They also suggest that several common FeLV integration sites exist.

There is also evidence that feline immunodeficiency virus (FIV) infection can increase the incidence of lymphoma in cats.[425,448–456] In contrast to the direct role of FeLV in tumorigenesis, most evidence suggests an indirect role for FIV secondary to the immunosuppressive effects of the virus. Shelton et al determined that FIV infection alone in cats was associated with a five-fold increased risk for development of lymphoma.[454] Coinfection with FeLV further potentiates the development of lymphoproliferative disorders. Experimentally, cats infected with FIV have developed lymphoma in the kidney, alimentary tract, liver, and multicentric sites. FIV-associated lymphoma is more likely to be of B-cell immunophenotype, as opposed to the T-cell predominance associated with FeLV. It has been suggested that FIV infection may be associated more commonly with alimentary lymphoma of B-cell origin,[449,457] and this may be related to chronic dysregulation of the immune system or the activation of oncogenic pathways; however,

TABLE 33.9 General Characteristics of the Most Commonly Encountered Anatomic Forms of Lymphoma in Cats

Anatomic Form	Relative Frequency	Median Age (yr)	Immuno-Phenotype (Generally)	FeLV Antigenicity	Local versus Diffuse/ Multicentric	Biologic Behavior	General Prognosis
Alimentary/ Gastroin-testinal							
LGAL	Common	10–13	T-cell, small	Rare	Diffuse	Indolent	Good
I/HGAL	Uncommon	12	B-cell, large	Rare	Generally Diffuse	Aggressive	Poor–Fair
LGL	Uncommon	9	T-cell, large	Rare	Generally Diffuse	Aggressive	Poor
Nasal	Uncommon	9–10	B cell (75%)	Rare	Local common	More indolent	Good–Fair
Mediastinal	Uncommon	2–4	T-cell, large	More common	Local common	Indolent or aggressive forms	Fair–Poor
Peripheral nodal							
Non-Hodg-kin's	Uncommon	3–4	B-cell (75%), large	More common	Multicentric	Aggressive	Fair–Poor
Hodgkin's-like	Rare	11	T-cell rich B-cell, large	Rare	Local initially	Indolent	Good–Fair
Laryngeal/ Tracheal	Rare	9	ID	Rare	Local common	ID	Fair–Good
Renal	Uncommon	9	B-cell	Rare	Multicentric	Aggressive	Poor–Fair
CNS	Rare	4–10	ID	Rare	Multicentric	Aggressive	Poor
Cutaneous	Rare	10–13	T-cell	Rare	Local initially	Indolent to aggressive	Fair
Subcutane-ous	Rare	10–13	B-cell, large	Rare	Local initially	Aggressive	Fair
Ocular (PSOL)	Rare	10–11	B-cell	Rare	Local	Often indolent	Good–Fair

Common = >50% of clinical presentations; Moderate = 20%–50% of clinical presentations;
Uncommon = 5%–20% of clinical presentation; Rare = <5% of clinical presentations.

ID, Insufficient data; *I/HGAL*, intermediate-/high-grade alimentary lymphoma; *LGAL*, low-grade alimentary lymphoma; *LGL*, = large granular lymphoma; *PSOL*, presumed solitary ocular lymphoma.

FIV antigenemia was only rarely associated with alimentary lymphoma in other large compilations of cases.[428,458–461]

Interrogations of gammaherpesvirus 1(FcGHV1) in cats with lymphoma did not show an association; however, FcGHV1 antigenemia was associated with an overall poorer prognosis for cats with lymphoma, the causality of which is speculative.[462]

Genetic and Molecular Factors

As discussed in Section A of this chapter (canine lymphoma), recent advances in molecular cytogenetics (see also Chapter 1, Section A, and Chapter 8), including gene microarray techniques, have and are currently being applied to investigations of chromosomal aberrations and gene expression changes in veterinary species with lymphoma. Indeed, a predisposition of the oriental cat breeds to develop lymphoma suggests a genetic predisposition and indicates heritable risk.[427,435,436] Altered oncogene/tumor suppressor gene expression, epigenetic changes, signal transduction, and cell death-pathway alterations are common in lymphomas of humans and are likely also involved in the cat. Several genetic factors have already been discussed as they relate to FeLV associations. In addition, N-*ras* aberrations have been implicated, although they are rare in cats.[463] Furthermore, telomerase activity

(see Chapter 2) has been documented in feline lymphoma tissues.[464,465] Alterations in cellular proliferation and in cell-cycle and death (apoptosis) pathways, in particular the cyclin-dependent kinase cell-cycle regulators and the Bcl-2 family of proapoptotic and antiapoptotic governing molecules, have also been implicated in feline lymphoma.[466–468]

Environmental Factors

Evidence for exposure to environmental tobacco smoke (ETS) as a risk factor for lymphoma in humans has prompted investigations in cats. In one report, the relative risk of developing lymphoma in cats with any exposure to ETS and with 5 or more years of exposure to ETS was 2.4 and 3.2, respectively.[469] A large European study documenting an association between proximity of waste management and cancer in dogs failed to show increased risk in cats.[470]

Immunosuppression

Immune system alterations in the cat, such as those accompanying FIV infection, has been implicated in the development of lymphoma.[450,452,454,471] As is the case in immunosuppressed human organ transplantation patients, reports of immunosuppressed feline renal transplant recipients document increased risk of lymphoma after transplant and associated immunosuppressive therapy.[472–474] In these studies, approximately 10% of transplanted cats developed de novo malignant lymphoma and, in one report, all cats had intermediate- or high-grade multicentric B cell lymphoma.

Chronic Inflammation

Although definitive proof is lacking, there is a growing body of indirect evidence to suggest that lymphoma can be associated with the presence of chronic inflammation, which theoretically could be the case with intestinal and nasal lymphoma. In particular, an association has been suggested between intestinal lymphoma and inflammatory bowel disease[427,475]; however, others have not found support for this concept.[476] In addition, an association between gastric *Helicobacter* infection and gastric mucosa-associated lymphoid tissue (MALT) lymphoma in cats is suggested in one study, and it warrants further investigation because this is a recognized syndrome in humans.[477,478] In a case-control study investigating mucosa-invading and intravascular bacteria in feline intestinal lymphomas, statistically significant differences were found in prevalence of mucosa-invading bacteria, which were identified in 82%, 18% and 3% of large cell lymphoma, small cell lymphoma and lymphocytic-plasmacytic enteritis biopsy samples, respectively.[477] Furthermore, intravascular bacteria were only present in cases of large cell intestinal lymphoma (29% of cases). The etiologic significance of this has not been explored, but is also warranted. Finally, a suggestion that chronic inflammation from injection sites may be involved in the risk of developing subcutaneous lymphoma in cats,[431] similar to its documented association with subcutaneous soft tissue sarcomas.

Diet and Intestinal Lymphoma

Although no direct evidence exists, a link between diet and the development of intestinal lymphoma in cats has been suggested.[427] Support is offered by the relative and absolute increase in the alimentary form of lymphoma in the past 20 years and the fact that several dietary modifications in cat food have occurred in a similar timeframe in response to diseases, such as urinary tract disease. Further investigation is warranted to prove or disprove such assertions.

Pathology and Natural Behavior

Lymphoma can be classified based on anatomic location and histologic and immunophenotypic (flow cytometric or immunohistochemical) criteria; often, the two are intimately associated because certain histologic and immunophenotypic types are commonly associated with specific anatomic locations (see Table 33.9). The interrogation of lymphoma subtypes by flow cytometric analysis, PARR clonality analysis and genetic characterization, as is the standard of practice for human lymphoma and becoming so in canine lymphoma, is less well described and applied in the feline lymphomas, partly due to the prevalence of intrabdominal anatomic forms making sampling more difficult and partly due to variable PCR primer availability and sensitivity.[479,480] The largest compilation of feline cases subjected to rigorous histologic classification was reported by Valli and others using the NCI Working Formulation.[481] The WHO has also published a histologic classification system that uses the REAL system as a basis for defining histologic categories of hematopoietic tumors in domestic animals.[482,483] This system incorporates both histologic criteria and immunohistologic criteria (e.g., B- and T-cell immunophenotype) and was discussed in length in Section A of this chapter. The updated Kiel classification system has also been used to classify feline lymphoma.[484,485] Regarding anatomic location, a profound change in presentation,

signalment, FeLV antigenemia, immunophenotype, and frequency of anatomic sites has occurred in cats with lymphoma in the "post-FeLV" era (see Table 33.9). Because of this shift, characteristics of feline lymphoma discussed in this chapter will be primarily limited to reports collected from cases presenting after 1995.

Several anatomic classifications exist for lymphoma in the cat, and some categorize the disease as mediastinal, alimentary, multicentric, nodal, leukemic, and individual extranodal forms. Others have combined various nodal and extranodal forms into categories of atypical, unclassified, and mixed, and others have combined intestinal, splenic, hepatic, and mesenteric nodal forms into one category termed *intraabdominal*. Some discrepancies in the discussion of frequency will inevitably result from the variations in classification used in the literature. The relative frequency of anatomic forms and their associated immunophenotype may also vary with geographic distribution and may be related to genetic and FeLV strain differences, as well as prevalence of FeLV vaccine use. For the purposes of this chapter, the feline lymphomas will be discussed in three separate sections: alimentary/gastrointestinal, peripheral nodal, and extranodal. Signalment, clinical presentation, diagnosis, treatment, and prognosis will be discussed individually under each of these three sections.

Alimentary/Gastrointestinal Lymphoma

Lymphoma is the most common tumor type found in the GI tract of cats, representing 55% of cases in an epidemiologic survey of 1129 intestinal tumors in the species.[432] The Siamese breed is reported at increased risk; however, the majority of cases occur in DSH cats.[427,432,436,441] Although lymphoma may occur in cats of any age, it is primarily a disease of aged cats with a mean of 10 to 13 years for T-cell alimentary lymphoma and 12 years for B-cell lymphoma.[427,432,441,486,487] Alimentary/GI lymphoma can be confined to intestinal/gastric infiltration or a combination of intestinal, mesenteric lymph node, and hepatosplenic involvement. Uncommonly, cats may be presented with extraabdominal coinvolvement. The tumors can be solitary, but more commonly are diffuse throughout the intestines. No consistent sex bias is noted. Anatomically, alimentary lymphoma is nearly four times more likely to occur in the small intestine than the large intestine.[486] In a series of colonic neoplasia in cats, lymphoma was the second most common malignancy (41%), second only to adenocarcinoma.[459] Most feline GI lymphomas can be categorized into one of three types based on histopathology and immunohistopathology: (1) low-grade alimentary lymphoma (LGAL), (2) intermediate- or high-grade alimentary lymphoma (I/HGAL), and (3) large granular lymphoma (LGL). Salient, generalizable characteristics of each are presented in Table 33.10.

Pathology and Natural Behavior

Low-Grade Alimentary Lymphoma

It is now clear that the vast majority of LGALs represent mucosal, epitheliotropic, small T-cell immunophenotypes that arise primarily from MALT.[436,441,487–492] Thus the major differential for LGAL is benign lymphocytic-plasmacytic enteritis (LPE; commonly referred to as inflammatory bowel disease [IBD]), which is also most commonly characterized by a small, T-cell, epitheliotropic infiltration. The largest compilation of LGAL (*n* = 120) classified GI lymphoma based on immunophenotype, then as either mucosal (infiltrate confined to mucosa and lamina propria with minimal submucosal extension) or transmural (significant extension into submucosa and muscularis propria).[487] They then compared

TABLE 33.10 Characteristics of the Three Most Common Forms of Alimentary/Gastrointestinal Lymphoma in Cats

Characteristic	Low-Grade Alimentary Lymphoma (LGAL)	Intermediate-/High-Grade Alimentary Lymphoma (I/HGAL)	Large Granular Lymphoma (LGL)
Incidence	50%–80% of cases	≈20% of cases	≈10% of cases
Clinical presentation	Nonspecific gastrointestinal signs (anorexia, weight loss, diarrhea, inappetence)	Nonspecific gastrointestinal signs; vomiting common if gastric; hematochezia more common if large bowel	Nonspecific gastrointestinal signs; vomiting more common
Clinical course	Indolent clinical progression	Acute clinical progression	Acute clinical progression
Abdominal palpation	Generally normal, modest intestinal thickening and abdominal lymphadenopathy possible	More common to palpate gastric/intestinal mass, mesenteric lymphadenopathy, organomegaly	More common to palpate gastric/intestinal mass, mesenteric lymphadenopathy
Abdominal ultrasound findings	Often unremarkable; diffuse intestinal wall thickening if present is limited to muscularis propria /submucosa; normal intestinal wall layering; mild lymphadenopathy/organomegaly possible	More commonly thickened transmural intestinal wall; loss of normal intestinal wall layering; mass effect more likely; mesenteric lymphadenopathy more likely	More commonly thickened transmural intestinal wall; loss of normal intestinal wall layering; mass effect more likely; mesenteric lymphadenopathy more likely; effusion uncommon but more likely
Topography[a]			
General diagnostics	Cytology generally not helpful; biopsy (full thickness preferred, but endoscopic helpful) with histopathology, immunophenotype, and clonality analysis often helpful to differentiate from LPE	Cytology (mass/lymph node) often diagnostic; biopsy with histopathology, immunophenotype, and clonality analysis less commonly required.	Cytology (mass/lymph node) often diagnostic; biopsy with histopathology, immunophenotype, and clonality analysis less commonly required.
Cell size	>80% small, <20% large	>90% intermediate/large	Intermediate/large
Immunophenotype	>80% T-cell (CD3+)	≈100% B-cell (CD79a+)	Cytotoxic T-cell (CD3+/CD8+/CD79a−), or NK cell (CD3−/CD79a−); often CD103+ and granzyme B+
Clonality	>90% clonal or oligoclonal	>70% clonal or oligoclonal	>90% clonal or oligoclonal
WHO EATCL classification	90% type II (mucosal) 10% type I (transmural)	90% type I (transmural) 10% type II (mucosal)	≥90% type I (transmural)
Epitheliotropism	Common	Rare	Common
Recommended treatment	Chlorambucil/prednisolone	CHOP- or COP-based chemotherapy; surgery considered if large discreet lesion prechemo; surgery performed if obstruction/perforation	CHOP- or COP-based chemotherapy; surgery considered if large discreet lesion prechemo; surgery performed if obstruction/perforation
Chemotherapy response and outcome	>80% response; median survival 1.5–3 years	≈50%–60% response (30% CR); median survival 3–10 months; more durable if CR	≈30% response; median survival 45–90 days; occasionally more durable

[a]Numbers indicate number of cases having lymphoma at that location. Areas in red indicate most commonly affected regions of the intestine.

CR, Complete response; *LPE*, lymphocytic-plasmacytic enteritis; *WHO EATCL*, World Health Organization enteropathy-associated T-cell lymphoma.

Topography diagrams used with permission from: Moore PF, Rodriguez-Bertos A, Kass PH. Feline gastrointestinal lymphoma: mucosal architecture, immunophenotype, and molecular clonality. *Vet Pathol.* 2012;49:658-668.

infiltration patterns with the WHO classification scheme[493] as well as documenting anatomic location, cell size, presence of epitheliotropism, clonality, and outcome data. This information is summarized in Table 33.10. Of the 120 cases, none tested serologically positive for FeLV and only three cats tested positive for FIV. Four cats had large B-cell lymphoma (gastric, cecal, or colonic) concurrent with small T-cell lymphoma of the small intestine. Topographically, T-cell variants are much more likely to occur in the small intestine (94%) and rarely in the stomach or large intestine. The majority of T-cell variants are mucosal (equivalent to WHO enteropathy-associated T-cell lymphoma [WHO EATCL] type II), and the majority of B-cell tumors are transmural (equivalent to WHO EATCL type I classification). Regarding cell size, nearly all mucosal T-cell tumors were composed of small lymphocytes, and slightly more than half of transmural T-cell and all B-cell variants were composed of larger cells. Epitheliotropism is common with LGAL T-cell tumors, but is rare in B-cell tumors. Other abdominal organ involvement is common, and in one report of 29 cases of low-grade T-cell intestinal lymphoma, liver and mesenteric node involvement was documented in 53% and 33% of cases, respectively.[494] Hepatic lymphoma can occur concurrently with GI lymphoma or be confined solely to the liver.[486,495] Most are T-cell and clonal or oligoclonal based on PCR analysis.

Intermediate- or High-Grade Alimentary Lymphoma

Unlike LGAL, the majority of I/HGALs are large or intermediate sized B-cell lymphomas. They arise from organized lymphoid tissues; MALT in the stomach and Peyer's patches and mucosal lymphoid nodules concentrated in the distal small intestine, cecum, and colon.[436,487,488,496,497] Therefore I/HGAL is more common in the stomach, distal small intestine, cecum, and colon (see Table 33.10). These B-cell variants can be solitary or at multiple sites that occur simultaneously within the stomach, small intestine, and ileocecocolic junction. The majority are transmural (equivalent to WHO EATCL type I classification) and epitheliotropism is rarely observed.

Large Granular Lymphoma

LGL represents a less common, distinct form of alimentary lymphoma occurring in older (median age 9–10 years) cats.[436,438,487,497–501] These granulated round cell tumors have also been termed *globule leukocyte tumors,* although they are likely variations of the same disease. LGL is characterized by lymphocytes described as 12 to 20 μm in diameter with a round, clefted, or cerebriform nucleus, variably distinct nucleoli, finely granular to lacey chromatin, and a moderate amount of basophilic granular cytoplasm that is occasionally vacuolated.[500] Prominent magenta or azurophilic granules are characteristic (Fig. 7.34, Chapter 7). They are usually granzyme B positive by immunohistochemistry.[487] This population of cells includes cytotoxic T cells and occasionally NK cells: most are CD3+, CD8+, and CD20- and have T-cell receptor gene rearrangements.[487,501] In one report, nearly 60% expressed CD103 (integrin alpha E).[501,502] LGL was confined to the intestines in 93% of cases in a large compilation,[438] but can occur extraabdominally (e.g., nasal).[438,498] Approximately 10% express neither B- or T-cell markers and are thus classified as NK cells. These NK tumors commonly originate in the small intestine, especially the jejunum, are transmural, often exhibit epitheliotropism, and at least two-thirds present with other organs involved; most with mesenteric lymph node involvement and many with liver, spleen, kidney, peritoneal malignant effusions, and bone marrow infiltration. Also, thoracic involvement may

occur with malignant pleural effusion and a mediastinal mass present. Peripheral blood involvement was present in 10% to 15% in some reports[438,500] and as often as 86% in another report.[501] Affected cats are generally FeLV/FIV negative.

History, Clinical Signs, and Physical Examination Findings

Low-Grade Alimentary Lymphoma

LGAL is most commonly associated with nonspecific signs associated with the GI tract; most cats present with weight loss (>80%), vomiting and/or diarrhea (70%–90%), and hyporexia (70%–90%), whereas icterus is uncommon (7%).[436,486,503,504] Abdominal palpation is often unremarkable, but intestinal thickening, mesenteric lymphadenopathy, and organomegaly can occasionally be appreciated. Clinical signs are usually present for several months before diagnosis (median, 6 months).[504]

Intermediate- or High-Grade Alimentary Lymphoma

I/HGAL tends to cause similar clinical signs as LGAL; however, they tend to progress more acutely and are more likely to present with a palpable abdominal mass originating from the GI tract, enlarged mesenteric lymph nodes, or liver.[436,439,461,496,503,505] Icterus is also more common in large cell forms. Hematochezia and tenesmus may also be present if the colon is involved.[459] Rarely, cats may present with signs consistent with an acute abdomen due to intestinal obstruction or perforation and concurrent peritonitis.

Large Granular Lymphoma

Cats with intestinal LGL have typical GI clinical signs, but are also more likely to be acutely presented.[438,498,500,501] A palpable abdominal mass is present in approximately half of cases, and hepatomegaly, splenomegaly, and renomegaly are common. Abdominal and pleural effusions, and icterus are observed in nearly 10% of cases.

Diagnosis and Clinical Staging

For most cats with suspect alimentary/GI lymphoma, the diagnostic evaluation should include a baseline assessment consisting of a CBC with differential cell and platelet count, serum biochemistry profile, urinalysis, and retroviral (FeLV/FIV) screen. Anemia and neutrophilia are common findings in all forms of alimentary lymphoma; however, they tend to be more profound in I/HGAL and LGL.[436,438,488,498] Circulating neoplastic lymphocytes are rare with LGAL, but may be observed in up to 15% of I/HGAL and LGL. Serum biochemistry profiles can help establish the overall health of the animal and suggest extra-GI involvement (e.g., liver enzymes elevations/icterus may indicate hepatic infiltration; azotemia may indicate renal involvement). For cats with alimentary lymphoma, hypoproteinemia and anemia are reported to occur in up to 23% and 76% of cases, respectively.[461,486,506] Hypercalcemia is rarely seen in cats, but has been reported in cats with lymphoma at various anatomic sites. Hypoglycemia, hypoalbuminemia, hyperglobulinemia, abnormal serum folate (high or low), elevated lactate dehydrogenase (LDH), and hypocobalaminemia are often reported.[436,438,506,507]

Low-Grade Alimentary Lymphoma

LGAL must be differentiated from LPE, which have similar clinical presentations and histologic cell populations.[441,487–491,508] LGAL is more commonly associated with modest (or palpably absent) intestinal thickening without mass effect similar if not identical in presentation to LPE. The key elements necessary for the diagnosis of LGAL (and differentiation from IBD) include procurement of tissue for histopathology, and if necessary, assessment of immunophenotype and clonality.

Abdominal ultrasound is by no means pathognomonic as both LGAL and LPE can have normal ultrasound appearance or reveal modest intestinal wall thickening with preservation of wall layering.[436,461,486,488,508–510] Changes, if present, predominantly involves the muscularis propria and submucosal layers, although mucosal thickening can also occur. Focal mural masses are uncommon. Mesenteric lymphadenopathy is also common and reported in 45% to 80% of affected cats. LGAL generally involves the small intestine and, less commonly, the stomach and large intestine. Cats with LGAL will uncommonly have ultrasonographic abnormalities in other abdominal organs such as the stomach, liver, spleen, colon, and pancreas, and occasionally, mild effusions are observed.

Cytologic evaluation of thickened bowel or associated mesenteric lymphadenopathy alone is generally not sufficient for differentiating LGAL from LPE.[486,488,502] Therefore tissue procurement is required for diagnosis (and differentiation from LPE). The debate still exists as to whether endoscopically obtained tissue is sufficient for diagnosis or if full-thickness tissue procured during laparotomy or laparoscopy is necessary in light of similarities with LPE.[436,487,491,509,511,512] Although histologic morphology and intestinal infiltrative patterns (e.g., villous nests or plaques) can be highly suggestive of lymphoma, they may not provide a definitive diagnosis. Most agree that although full thickness biopsies are preferred, less invasive endoscopic biopsies, with ancillary immunophenotypic and molecular (i.e., PARR; see Chapter 8) assessments, are sufficient in the majority of cases (see Table 33.10). If the differentiation of lymphoma and LPE is equivocal after standard histopathologic assessment, the addition of immunophenotypic and clonality analysis in a stepwise fashion, as proposed by several reports, enhances specificity and sensitivity and usually provides a definitive diagnosis.[436,441,479,480,487,489,491,513,514] As LGAL most commonly involves the jejunum and ilium, endoscopic biopsy by both gastroduodenoscopy and ileocolonoscopy may be necessary to procure representative samples.

Intermediate- or High-Grade Alimentary Lymphoma and Large Granular Lymphoma

The diagnosis of I/HGAL and LGL is generally less complicated than for LGAL.[436,438,488,498] The former are often diagnosed with physical examination, abdominal imaging (e.g., ultrasound), and cytologic or histologic assessment of needle aspirate or needle biopsy samples from intestinal masses, enlarged mesenteric lymph nodes, or liver because mass lesions and gross lymphadenopathy are more commonly present. Ultrasonographically, I/HGAL is more likely to involve the stomach and colon than LGAL. In a series of 16 cats with I/HGAL of the stomach, all had either ultrasonic evidence of wall thickening or the presence of a mass, and 20% had abdominal lymphadenopathy.[439] Less commonly, abdominal exploration is necessary if lesions are subtle or not amenable to transabdominal sampling. Further staging via thoracic imaging, peripheral lymph node aspiration, and bone marrow assessment may be performed, but rarely contributes prognostic information or alters treatment decisions because the disease is already widespread and systemic therapy is required.

Treatment and Prognosis

In general, cats tolerate chemotherapy for lymphoma quite well, most clients are happy with their choice to initiate treatment, and quality of life generally improves after commencement of therapy.[515,516]

Low-Grade Alimentary Lymphoma

LGAL is a gratifying disease to treat as durable remissions are generally achieved with well-tolerated, conservative treatment protocols (e.g., oral chlorambucil and prednisolone).[486–488,504,517,518] Chlorambucil (20 mg/m^2 PO every 2 weeks [preferred by the author] or 2 mg PO every other day) and prednisolone (initially 1–2 mg/kg PO daily, reduced to 0.5–1.0 mg/kg every other day over several weeks) results in response rates (i.e., resolution of clinical signs) of greater than 80% and MSTs of approximately 1.5 to 3.0 years.[486,488,491,504,517,518] Most clinical oncologists continue these conservative protocols for 2 years or longer; however, one report discontinued chlorambucil/prednisolone therapy at 1 year.[517] Cats that relapse while receiving this protocol often will subsequently respond to alternative alkylating agents, such as cyclophosphamide (200–250 mg/m^2, PO, q2–3 weeks) or lomustine, or to reintroduction of chlorambucil if this had been discontinued.[505,517–519] Rescue protocols have reported MSTs ranging from 9 to 29 months. Anecdotally, many will also respond to vinblastine chemotherapy if they no longer are responsive to alkylating agents. Ultimately, more aggressive CHOP- or MOPP-based protocols may be utilized when more conservative protocols are no longer effective.

Prognostic factors for cats with LGAL are not well-defined owing to the indolent nature of the disease and typical long-term survival. Only lack of response to initial induction chemotherapy is consistently observed as a negative factor, although transmural extension may also be associated with shorter STs.[487]

Intermediate- or High-Grade Alimentary Lymphoma

More aggressive multiagent combination chemotherapy is recommended for I/HGAL and LGL subtypes of lymphoma. The agents used most commonly to treat intermediate- or high-grade lymphoma in cats are similar to those used for dogs with lymphoma (see Section A in this chapter), and induction protocols currently employed in cats are modifications of CHOP protocols initially designed for humans.[428,438–440,488,496,498,515,520–528] CHOP represents combinations of cyclophosphamide (C), doxorubicin (H, hydroxydaunorubicin), vincristine (O, Oncovin) and prednisone (P). In general, CHOP-based protocols are appropriate for cats with intermediate- and high-grade lymphoma involving any anatomic site (e.g., peripheral nodal, mediastinal, and extranodal forms), but should not be first-line therapy for low-grade variants such as LGAL. As in the dog, a plethora of CHOP-based protocols have been reported for use in cats, although virtually no high-quality comparative data exist to compare outcomes. As such, the protocol used should be based on cost, ease, client/veterinarian preference, and level of comfort. One report found that cats may better tolerate CHOP protocols that substitute vinblastine for vincristine; GI adverse events were less frequent and of lesser grade in cats receiving vinblastine.[529] The current CHOP-based protocol in use by the author for cats is presented in Table 33.11. This protocol has been used in many cats with various forms of intermediate- and high-grade lymphoma and is generally well tolerated. At present, most canine lymphoma protocols involve a 12- to 25-week induction phase whereupon chemotherapy is discontinued and no

TABLE 33.11	The CHOP-Based Chemotherapy Protocol for Cats with Intermediate/High-grade Lymphoma Employed by the Author
Treatment Week	**Drug, Dosage, and Route**
1	Vincristine, 0.5–0.7 mg/m², IV L-Asparaginase, 400 Units/kg, SC Prednisolone, 2.0 mg/kg, PO
2	Cyclophosphamide 200 mg/m², PO Prednisolone, 2.0 mg/kg, PO
3	Vincristine, 0.5–0.7 mg/m², IV Prednisolone, 1.0 mg/kg, PO
4	Doxorubicin, 25 mg/m², IV Prednisolone, 1.0 mg/kg, PO[a]
6	Vincristine, 0.5–0.7 mg/m², IV
7	Cyclophosphamide 200 mg/m², PO
8	Vincristine, 0.5–0.7 mg/m², IV
9[b]	Doxorubicin, 25 mg/m², IV
11	Vincristine, 0.5–0.7 mg/m², IV
13	Cyclophosphamide 200 mg/m², PO
15	Vincristine, 0.5–0.7 mg/m², IV
17	Doxorubicin, 25 mg/m², IV
19	Vincristine, 0.5–0.7 mg/m², IV
21	Cyclophosphamide 200 mg/m², PO
23	Vincristine, 0.5–0.7 mg/m², IV
25[c]	Doxorubicin, 25 mg/m², IV

CHOP, Combinations of cyclophosphamide (C), doxorubicin (H, hydroxydaunorubicin), vincristine (O, Oncovin), and prednisolone (P); *IV*, intravenous; *PO*, by mouth; *SQ*, subcutaneous.

[a]Prednisolone is continued (1 mg/kg, PO) every other day from this point on.

[b]If in complete remission at week 9, continue to week 11.

[c]If in complete remission at week 25, therapy is discontinued after this doxorubicin, and cat is rechecked monthly for recurrence.

Note: A complete blood count (CBC) should be performed before each chemotherapy. If neutrophils are <1500 cells/μL, wait 5–7 days, repeat CBC, then administer the drug if neutrophils have risen above the 1500 cell/μL cutoff.

TABLE 33.12	COP Protocol for Lymphoma in Cats
Drug	**Frequency of Drug Delivery**
Cyclophosphamide: 250–300 mg/m², PO[a]	Given every 3 weeks on the day after vincristine
Vincristine: 0.7 mg/m², IV	Given weekly on weeks 1, 2, 3, and 4, then given every 3 weeks thereafter on the days before cyclophosphamide. Discontinue if in remission at 1 year.
Prednisolone: 1–2 mg/kg, PO	Given daily for 1 year.

[a]Some divide the cyclophosphamide over 3 consecutive days.

Note: A complete blood count (CBC) should be performed before each chemotherapy. If neutrophils are <1500 cells/μL, wait 5–7 days, repeat CBC, then administer the drug if neutrophils have risen above the 1500 cell/μL cutoff.

predicting more durable responses.[488,527,534] The use of intraperitoneal-delivered COP in a small number of cats (*n* = 26) was reported; three-quarters achieved a CR with a MST of 1 year.[535] This study included only three GI cases and did not histologically or immunophenotypically subtype cases beyond saying all were "large cell"; therefore larger, more controlled studies would be necessary to establish/confirm efficacy of this protocol.

Response rates and durability of response for cats with I/HGAL treated with combination protocols are generally not as good as in dogs with intermediate- or high-grade peripheral nodal lymphoma. Remission rates of 50% to 65% can be expected with approximately one-third achieving CR. Remission and survival are only durable in cases achieving a CR; MSTs for cats in CR are approximately 7 to 10 months with a subset living to 1 year or longer.[439,440,488,496,520–522,529,428,515,523–528] Rescue protocols involving alternate drugs (e.g., melphalan, lomustine, mechlorethamine, actinomycin-D, cytarabine) or reinduction with CHOP generally do not result in durable subsequent remissions.[519,536,537]

Several prognostic factors have been reported for cats with I/HGAL; however, by far the most predictive is whether a CR is achieved.[439,440,487,488,491,496,520–522,529] Negative prognostic factors identified for I/HGAL include transmural extension, FeLV antigenemia, weight loss, elevated LDH, hypoalbuminemia, hypocobalaminemia, and bicavitary involvement, while stage I disease (rare) is associated with a more favorable prognosis. Factors not found to be prognostic were immunophenotype and various proliferation indices (e.g., PCNA, AgNOR, Ki67).

Large Granular Lymphoma

Cats with LGL typically have the lowest reported response rates and shortest response durations of any of the GI lymphomas. Approximately one-third of cases will experience a response and MSTs in larger reports of cases were only 21 days; cats receiving CHOP-based or CCNU-based protocols experienced MSTs of 45 to 90 days.[438,488,500] That being said, a small subset (7% in this report) enjoyed more durable (>6 month survivals) responses and, in one small study (*n* = 6), a MST of 9 months was reported after a variety of interventions.[498]

The Role of Surgery in Cats with Gastrointestinal Lymphoma

Surgery is primarily reserved for I/HGAL that have discrete lesions and in cats that are presented with intestinal perforation

maintenance chemotherapy is used. Although data exist in dogs for a maintenance-free approach, similar comparative data do not currently exist in the cat. DOX alone (25 mg/m² every 3 weeks for five total treatments), CCNU (lomustine; 40–50 mg/m² PO q 3 weeks),[440] or palliative prednisone therapy is offered if clients decline more aggressive CHOP-based therapy.[440,530,531] Cats are generally less tolerant of DOX than are dogs; therefore a lower dosage (25 mg/m² or 1 mg/kg IV) is used (see Chapter 12). Cardiac toxicity does not appear to be a clinically significant problem in cats, although renal toxicity is more commonly encountered,[532] and renal function should be monitored (i.e., serial blood urea nitrogen [BUN], creatinine, and urine specific gravity) closely before and during therapy. The use of COP (i.e., CHOP without the addition of DOX) is often used in cats in Europe, and one compilation reported similar results to CHOP.[533] A COP (cyclophosphamide, vincristine, and prednisolone) protocol commonly employed in cats is presented in Table 33.12; however, several studies have reported that the inclusion of DOX is important for and obstructive lesions.[439,488,496] Of current debate is whether surgery should be performed on discrete lesions that are not perforated or obstructed before initiating systemic chemotherapy. This question is currently unanswered as comparative trials have not clearly established a benefit or detriment to this approach. The motivation behind performing surgery before chemotherapy often lies with concern for GI perforation resulting from robust chemotherapy response in cases with full-thickness involvement with lymphoma. Crouse reported on 23 cats with discrete I/HGAL undergoing chemotherapy without surgery. Although four cats (17%) experienced perforation, these events occurred 2 to 87 days after initiation of chemotherapy rather than in the acute postchemotherapy period, they were not associated with size or degree of hypoalbuminemia, and progressive disease was documented in three cats and only a partial response in the other cat at the time of perforation.[437] Taken together, this implies that perforations were likely due to progressive disease rather than robust response to chemotherapy. An additional motivation for surgical intervention is the theoretical advantage of immediate creation of a "minimal residual disease" state if staging does not reveal disease distant from a large GI primary tumor; chemotherapy is generally thought to result in more favorable outcomes in the minimal disease state, rather than in the macroscopic disease state. The author generally recommends surgery, albeit in the absence of convincing support in the literature, if lesions are large, discrete, and no (or minimal) involvement is documented outside the primary mass after complete staging. Multiagent chemotherapy is then initiated at suture removal owing to the high-grade nature and overall short STs associated with I/HGAL.

The Role of Radiation Therapy in Cats with Gastrointestinal Lymphoma

Radiation therapy (RT) for GI lymphoma in cats has not been thoroughly explored and is generally reserved for consolidation therapy (during or after chemotherapy) or as a rescue modality.[538,539] In one report, 11 cats (six small cell, four large cell, and one LGL) that progressed after chemotherapy received abdominal radiation (8 Gy in two fractions over 2 days) and experienced a MST of 7 months, although numbers were small and 40% were lost to follow-up.[538] In a second report, eight cats (seven with I/HGAL) underwent 6 weeks of CHOP-based combination chemotherapy followed 2 weeks later by whole abdomen radiation consisting of 10 daily 1.5 Gy fractions.[539,540] Although three cats died within 3 weeks of RT, five experienced durable remissions. These preliminary results warrant further investigation before RT can be recommended as standard care.

Supportive Care for Cats with Gastrointestinal Lymphoma

Intuitively, GI disease may compromise the nutritional status of affected cats. As such, careful and repeated assessments of nutritional state, caloric intake, and body weight should be undertaken. Nutritional support (see Chapter 16, Section B) should be instituted sooner rather than later in affected cats. A good plan of nutrition should help maintain or improve quality of life, immunologic status, and tolerance of chemotherapy. Cobalamin supplementation should be instituted in those cats with documented hypocobalaminemia.

Peripheral Nodal Lymphoma in Cats

Involvement limited to peripheral lymph nodes is unusual in cats with lymphoma, representing approximately 4% to 10% of cases.[427,428]

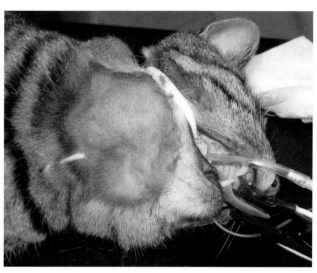

• **Fig. 33.14** A cat presented with mandibular lymphadenopathy that was confirmed to be Hodgkin's-like lymphoma after histologic assessment.

In contrast, approximately one-quarter of all other anatomic forms of lymphoma have some component of lymph node involvement. One-third of cats with nodal lymphoma are T-cell immunophenotype and FeLV antigenemic; however, complete categorizations have not occurred in the post-FeLV era and this may no longer be true.[427,428,435,492] Peripheral nodal lymphoma was the most common anatomic form of lymphoma reported in a compilation of cases in cats under the age of 1 year, representing one-third of cases in this age group.[433] As lymphoma progresses, bone marrow and hepatic infiltration may develop. Clinical staging and diagnostic approach for peripheral lymphadenopathy and peripheral nodal lymphoma is similar to the dog (see Section A of this chapter).

Cats with the nodal form of lymphoma present with variable clinical signs depending on the extent of disease; however, they are often depressed and lethargic. Peripheral lymphadenopathy, as the only physical finding, is an uncommon presentation.

An uncommon and distinct form of nodal lymphoma in cats referred to as "Hodgkin's-like" lymphoma has been reported.[541,542] This form typically involves solitary or regional lymph nodes of the head and neck (Fig. 33.14) and histologically resembles Hodgkin's lymphoma in humans. Affected cats generally present with enlargement of one or two mandibular or cervical nodes initially, and tumors are immunophenotypically classified as T-cell–rich, B-cell lymphoma. Histologically, lymph nodes can be effaced by either nodular or diffuse small to large lymphocytes with characteristic bizarre or multinucleated cells (Reed–Sternberg-like cells) (Fig. 33.15). No association with FeLV or FIV has been documented. Cats with Hodgkin's-like nodal lymphoma usually present without overt clinical signs.[541,542] Inguinal node, multicentric nodal, subcutaneous, and conjunctival involvement have been reported.[542–545] Interestingly, in both reports of subcutaneous Hodgkin's lymphoma in cats, spontaneous remissions were observed suggesting these may not have been be true lymphoid neoplasia.[543,544] The clinical course of Hodgkin's-like lymphoma is generally more indolent than for peripheral nodal non-Hodgkin's lymphoma in the cat.

The treatment choice for peripheral nodal lymphoma in cats depends on whether the individual case represents a low-grade (e.g., indolent [rare]) versus an intermediate- or high-grade (e.g., intermediate/large cell) lymphoma; the latter are

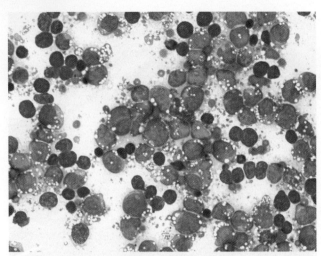

• **Fig. 33.15** Fine-needle aspirate cytology of a lymph node in a cat with Hodgkin's-like lymphoma. The large lymphocytes have prominent nucleoli and smooth basophilic cytoplasm. Several binucleate lymphocytes are present.

best treated with CHOP- or COP-based protocols (discussed under I/HGAL earlier) and carry a less favorable prognosis, whereas the former generally respond to less aggressive chlorambucil/corticosteroid protocols and enjoy durable responses. Less is known regarding the treatment of Hodgkin's-like lymphoma involving solitary or regional nodes of the head and neck.[541,542] Clinical outcome after surgical extirpation of or RT to the affected node (or nodes if a reasonable number) is often associated with long-term disease control and MSTs of approximately 1 year, suggesting that it is a more indolent form of lymphoma. Eventual recurrence in distal nodes after surgical excision or RT is common, and the author currently offers clients the option of adjuvant chlorambucil/corticosteroids after surgery. This theoretically may have benefit; however, insufficient data currently exist to document a survival advantage with this approach.

Mediastinal Lymphoma

The mediastinal form can involve the thymus and mediastinal and sternal lymph nodes. Pleural effusion is common. In two large compilations, 63% of cats with thymic disease and 17% of cats with pleural effusion were documented as having lymphoma.[546,547] Hypercalcemia occurs frequently with mediastinal lymphoma in dogs, but is rare in cats. The majority of cats with mediastinal lymphoma in older reports were young (median age, 2–4 years), FeLV positive, and had T-cell immunophenotype tumor; however, many reports did not report immunophenotypic data.[427,428,433–435,548] The disease is confined to the mediastinum in most cases. A form of mediastinal lymphoma also occurs primarily in young, FeLV-negative Siamese cats that appears to be less biologically aggressive and more responsive to chemotherapy than FeLV-associated forms.[533] In a more recent report of 55 cats with mediastinal lymphoma from the United Kingdom, the majority were antigenically FeLV/FIV negative, young (median age, 3 years), male (3.2:1 male-to-female ratio), and nearly one-third were Siamese.[548] In this large cohort, immunophenotype was not reported.

The clinical signs associated with mediastinal lymphoma include dyspnea (80%), tachypnea, and a noncompressible cranial thorax with dull heart and lung sounds.[549] Rarely, a Horner's

syndrome and precaval syndrome may be observed. Pleural effusion is observed in 50% of cases and characterized by serohemorrhagic to chylous effusion and, in most cases, neoplastic cells (lymphoblasts) are identified.[546,548,550] Diagnostic suspicion may begin with a noncompressible cranial thorax on physical examination and confirmation of a mediastinal mass/pleural effusion on thoracic radiographs. Fine-needle aspirate (FNA) cytology of the mass or cytologic evaluation of pleural fluid may be sufficient to establish a diagnosis. In most cats, the finding of a monotonous population of intermediate or large lymphoid cells will establish a diagnosis; however, definitive diagnosis of lymphoma in cats with a mediastinal mass and concurrent chylothorax can be challenging. CT appearance may be helpful, but generally does not contribute to a definitive diagnosis. If large lymphocytes are not identified in the pleural chylous effusion, then cholesterol and triglyceride concentrations can be measured.[551] In chylous effusions, the pleural fluid triglyceride concentration will be greater than in the serum; however, anorectic cats may have lower triglyceride levels in the pleural fluid. A major differential for mediastinal lymphoma is thymoma. The cytologic features of thymoma can be distinct from lymphoma in many cases, but the diagnosis can be challenging because of a preponderance of small lymphocytes in thymoma. Mast cells can also be seen in up to 50% of aspirations from thymomas. The addition of immunophenotypic and clonality assessment may be helpful in equivocal cases.

In the largest report, cats with mediastinal lymphoma treated with either COP- or CHOP-based protocols experienced an overall response rate of 95% with a MST of 373 days (980 days if CR was achieved).[548] In contrast, mediastinal lymphoma in young FeLV-positive cats is generally associated with a poor prognosis and MSTs of approximately 2 to 3 months are expected after treatment with CHOP- or COP-based protocols.[428,524]

Extranodal Lymphoma

Collectively, extranodal lymphoma represents the second most common site of lymphoma after GI lymphoma in cats.[431] The most common extranodal sites for lymphoma in cats include nasal (including nasopharyngeal and sinonasal), kidney, CNS, laryngeal and tracheal, cutaneous, subcutaneous, and ocular.

The clinical signs associated with feline extranodal lymphoma are variable and depend on anatomic location and extent of disease. Many, if confined to the primary site (stage I), will appear clinically healthy. However, cats with lymphoma, regardless of site, may present with nonspecific constitutional signs including anorexia, weight loss, lethargy, or depression. Secondary bone marrow infiltration, although uncommon, may lead to anemia. Signs related to paraneoplastic hypercalcemia (polyuria/polydipsia [PU/PD]) can occur in cats, however, much less commonly than in the dog. In one survey of hypercalcemia in cats, approximately 10% were diagnosed with lymphoma of various anatomic types.[552]

For most cats with suspected extranodal lymphoma, the diagnostic evaluation should include a baseline assessment consisting of a CBC with differential cell count, platelet count, serum chemistry profile, urinalysis, and retroviral (FeLV/FIV) screen. Serum biochemistry profiles can help establish the overall health of the animal, as well as, in some cases, suggest site-specific tumor involvement. For example, increased liver enzymes levels may indicate hepatic infiltration and increased BUN and creatinine may indicate renal lymphoma. Hypoglycemia was reported in approximately one-third of cats with lymphoma in one Australian study.[506] In a series of cats with various anatomic forms of lymphoma, serum albumin concentrations were significantly lower and β-globulin concentrations (as measured by protein electrophoresis) were significantly higher than a healthy control population.[507]

The use of various imaging modalities in cats with lymphoma depends on the anatomic site and will be discussed in site-specific discussions to follow.

Cytopathologic or histopathologic evaluation of involved lymph node(s) or involved organ tissue, procured via FNA cytology (see Chapter 7) or surgical, endoscopic, or needle-core biopsy (see Chapter 9), is required for a definitive diagnosis. Cytology alone may not be sufficient in some cases, owing to difficulties encountered in distinguishing lymphoma from benign hyperplastic or reactive lymphoid conditions. In such cases, incisional or excisional biopsy is preferred as orientation and information regarding invasiveness and architectural abnormalities may be necessary for diagnosis. In addition, involved tissue, needle aspirate, and fluid samples can be further interrogated by various histochemical, immunohistochemical, flow cytometric analysis (e.g., size and immunophenotypic assessment), and molecular techniques (e.g., PARR to assess clonality) to further characterize the disease process and refine the diagnosis in equivocal cases. The reader is referred to Chapter 8 for a general discussion of flow cytometric analysis and molecular diagnostic techniques, as well as Section A of this chapter for specific applications to lymphoma. PARR in cats is approximately 80% sensitive for the diagnosis of lymphoma[553]; however, assessment of specificity has not been clearly established. Clonality assessment tools (e.g., primers) for both Ig and T-cell receptor variable region genes have been developed in cats.[479,480,554–557]

Assessment of tumor proliferation rates (e.g., Ki67, PCNA, AgNOR), telomerase activity, and serum protein electrophoresis can also be performed on involved tissues in cats; however, consistent prognostic value across the anatomic, histopathologic, and immunophenotypic variants of lymphoma in cats is not well characterized.

Thorough staging, including a bone marrow aspiration or biopsy, peripheral lymph node assessment (clinically normal or abnormal nodes), and thoracic and/or abdominal imaging, is indicated when (1) solitary site disease is suspected (stage I) and a decision between locoregional therapy (i.e., surgery and/or RT) versus systemic therapy (i.e., chemotherapy) is being considered; (2) it provides prognostic information that will help a caregiver make treatment decisions; and (3) complete staging of the extent of disease is required as part of a clinical trial. Bone marrow evaluation may be of particular interest if anemia, cellular atypia, and/or leukopenia are present. A WHO staging system exists for the cat that is similar to that used in the dog (see Box 33.2); however, because of the high incidence of visceral/extranodal involvement in cats, a separate staging system has been evaluated and is often used (Box 33.5).[558] Because lymphoma in cats is more varied with respect to anatomic locations, staging systems are generally less helpful for predicting response.

Our knowledge base for treating cats with extranodal lymphoma is not well established, and outcomes are less predictable than that in dogs, primarily due to the greater variation in histologic type and anatomic location observed in cats. This is further complicated by the plethora of papers that include very small numbers of cases representing multiple anatomic/immunophenotypic and histologic subtypes (e.g., small cell vs large cell variants) together when reporting survival analysis after chemotherapy.

• BOX 33.5 Clinical Staging System for Feline Lymphoma[558]

Stage 1
- A single tumor (extranodal) or single anatomic area (nodal)
- Includes primary intrathoracic tumors

Stage 2
- A single tumor (extranodal) with regional lymph node involvement
- Two or more nodal areas on the same side of the diaphragm
- Two single (extranodal) tumors with or without regional lymph node involvement on the same side of the diaphragm
- A resectable primary gastrointestinal tract tumor, usually in the ileocecal area, with or without involvement of associated mesenteric nodes only

Stage 3
- Two single tumors (extranodal) on opposite sides of the diaphragm
- Two or more nodal areas above and below the diaphragm
- All extensive primary unresectable intraabdominal disease
- All paraspinal or epidural tumors, regardless of other tumor site or sites

Stage 4
- Stages 1–3 with liver and/or spleen involvement

Stage 5
- Stages 1–4 with initial involvement of CNS or bone marrow or both

---

This provides only general observations rather than specific outcome information (i.e., response rate and durability of response) that can vary significantly with respect to anatomic and histologic subtype. Most treatment decisions should be based on assessment of whether the individual case represents a low-grade (e.g., indolent) versus an intermediate- or high-grade (e.g., large cell) lymphoma and whether the disease is limited to the local extranodal site. Chemotherapy protocols for the cat have been previously discussed under sections in GI lymphoma; low-grade tumors are generally treated with chlorambucil/prednisolone protocols and intermediate- or high-grade tumors with CHOP- or COP-based protocols. Finally, much of the early work on chemotherapy protocol development for cats with lymphoma occurred during the FeLV era and care should be exercised when applying this information in the post-FeLV era.

Nasal Lymphoma

Nasal lymphoma is the most common extranodal lymphoma in cats.[559] It is usually a localized disease; however, 20% have local extension or distant metastasis at necropsy.[560] The majority of nonviral nasal/paranasal diseases in cats are neoplasia, and lymphoma represents one-third to one-half of these cases.[561–564] It occurs primarily in older (median age, 9–10 years; range, 3–17 years), FeLV/FIV antigenemic negative cats, and at least three-quarters are B-cell in origin, although T-cell and mixed B-cell/T-cell immunophenotypes are reported in 10% to 15% of cases.[428,559–561,565] An Italian report documented FeLV antigen (p27 or gp70) expression in nasal lymphoma tissues by immunohistochemistry (IHC); however, FeLV antigenemia was not reported in this cohort.[561] Siamese cats appear overrepresented and a 2:1 male-to-female ratio has also been observed.[561,565] Most are of intermediate- or high-grade histology; however, small-cell low-grade variants have been reported in up to 25% of some cohorts.[560,561,565] Epitheliotropism is common if the epithelium is present in the biopsy.

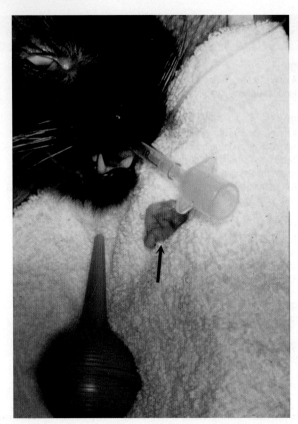

• **Fig. 33.16** Flush biopsy of nasal lymphoma. Note the large sample *(arrow)* procured by retrograde flushing of saline through on nares while occluding the contralateral nares. The sample is flushed through the pharynx and out the mouth.

Cats with nasal lymphoma present with nasal discharge (60%–85%), sneezing (20%–70%), upper respiratory noise (stridor, stertor, wheezing; 20%–60%), facial deformity (0%–20%), hyporexia (10%–60%), epiphora (10%–30%), and occasionally increased respiratory effort and coughing.[559–561,565] The nasal discharge is usually mucopurulent, although epistaxis is present in up to one-third of cases. Regional lymphadenopathy can also occur. The median duration of clinical signs before diagnosis is 2 months (range, 1–1800 days).

If nasal lymphoma is suspected, advanced imaging (CT, MRI), rhinoscopy, and biopsy are usually necessary for diagnosis (see Chapter 24, Section B). CT or MRI is useful to determine the extent of involvement and to help plan biopsy procurement and RT if that treatment option is pursued. CT characteristics include the presence of a unilateral or bilateral nasal/sinus mass or fluid, bulla effusion, and lysis of associated bony structures.[561,566–568] A biopsy can be procured either by intranasal procurement (with or without rhinoscopy) or by flushing one hemicavity with a bulb syringe and saline while occluding the contralateral cavity and collecting samples flushed out of the nasopharynx (Fig. 33.16). Thorough staging (i.e., regional node assessment, thoracic and abdominal staging, and bone marrow assessment) to ensure the disease is confined to the nasal passages is recommended if local RT without systemic chemotherapy is being considered. IHC may be necessary to differentiate nasal carcinoma from nasal lymphoma in a subset of cases; approximately 7% of samples required IHC to differentiate carcinoma from lymphoma in one large cohort of cases.[569]

In one report, 38 cats with nasal lymphoma that were not treated had MSTs of only 53 days.[561] However, in cats that are treated, durable remissions and lengthy MSTs can be expected in the majority of cases.[428,502,559,565,570–574] If disease is documented to be confined to the nasal cavity (i.e., stage I) after thorough staging, then RT is the treatment of choice. CR rates of 75% to 95% are reported with MSTs after RT of 1.5 to 3.0 years.[565,573] Cats that do not achieve a CR with RT have an MST of approximately 4.5 months. Total radiation dosage does affect STs, and a total dose greater than 32 Gy is recommended. The addition of chemotherapy to RT has not been definitively shown to enhance STs for cats with locally confined disease; combinations of RT and chemotherapy result in similar response rates and STs.[565,570,571,573,574] Chemotherapy (COP- or CHOP-based protocols) is a reasonable alternative to RT, with CR rates of approximately 75% and MSTs of approximately 2 years for cats achieving CR.[559] The author's preference is to initiate systemic chemotherapy only for cases that have confirmed disease beyond the nasal passage, cases that relapse after RT, or cases in which RT is unavailable or declined.

Renal Lymphoma

Renal lymphoma is the second most common form of extranodal lymphoma, occurring in approximately one-third of cases.[559,572] Although it can present as confined to the kidneys (<25%), it more commonly presents as concurrent with alimentary or multicentric lymphoma. The median age at presentation is 9 years, although 6% occur in cats under 1 year of age.[559,575] The majority of cases are not associated with FeLV and, although most are not associated with FIV, approximately one-half of cats reported in an Australian study were FIV positive. Little contemporary information exists on the immunohistologic classification of renal lymphoma; however, the majority are of high-grade B-cell immunophenotype.[428,435] Extension to the CNS was frequent in one report, but not similarly reported elsewhere.[575]

Cats with renal lymphoma present with signs consistent with renal insufficiency: hyporexia, weight loss, and polyuria/polydipsia.[559,575] On physical examination, marked renomegaly (bilateral, lumpy, and irregular; although a smooth variant has been observed) is palpated in the majority of cases (Fig. 33.17). Radiographic appearance is smooth-to-irregular renomegaly (Fig. 33.17A). Ultrasonographic imaging usually reveals bilateral (>80%), irregular renomegaly with hypoechoic subcapsular thickening.[156] Approximately one-third of cases will have ultrasonographic evidence of other abdominal organ involvement. The disease is usually diffuse throughout the renal cortex (Fig. 33.17B) and transabdominal FNA cytology or core biopsy is diagnostic in most cases.[576]

Treatment and outcome appears similar to other high-grade lymphomas in the cat; approximately two-thirds will experience clinical benefit with COP- or CHOP-based protocols with MSTs reported from 4 to 7 months. Owing to an inability to differentiate how much of the renal insufficiency at presentation is lymphoma-related versus due to underlying renal disease of older cats, most oncologists will start COP-based protocols and only add in DOX if renal values normalize during remission because of the potential for renal toxicity with DOX in cats.

CNS Lymphoma

CNS lymphoma can be intracranial, extracranial (i.e., spinal), or both.[157] CNS lymphoma accounted for 14% of 110 reported cases of extranodal lymphoma,[559] 15% to 31% of intracranial tumors,[158,577] and 39% of spinal cord tumors,[578] making it one of

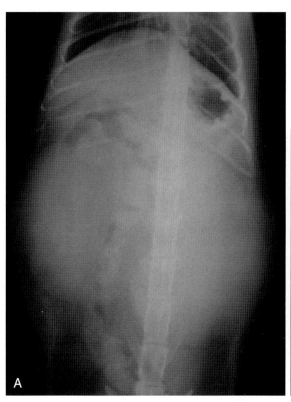
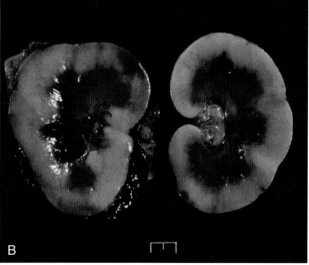

• **Fig. 33.17** (A) Ventrodorsal projection of a cat with real lymphoma. Massive bilateral renomegaly is observed. (B) Necropsy specimen of a cat with bilateral renal lymphoma illustrating the diffuse cortical nature of the disease that is most common.

the most common malignancies encoutered in the CNS in cats.[579] Although some discordance exists in the literature, cats with CNS lymphoma are younger (median age, 4.0–10.5 years) and 17%[580] to 50% of cases are FeLV antigenemic.[577,578,581] As most reports are older, these data may no longer hold true in the current era. Approximately two-thirds of intracranial cases also have multicentric and extracranial disease; and approximately 40% of spinal lymphoma cases occur in multiple spinal cord sites with one-third also involving intracranial locations.[559,577–579,581] In a compilation of 160 cases of intracranial tumors in cats, diffuse cerebral and brainstem involvement was most common for lymphoid malignancies.[577] Spinal lesions are usually both extradural and intradural, although they can be limited to one or the other compartment.[578] Feline CNS lymphoma may be primary, but more commonly (approximately 80%) represents a multicentric process (especially with renal or bone marrow involvement).[577,581–583] A paucity of information exists on the immunophenotype of CNS lymphoma.

Cats with CNS lymphoma can present with constitutional signs (hyporexia, lethargy) and signs referring to intracranial lesions, spinal lesions, or both.[577–580,582,583] Intracranial signs may include ataxia, altered consciousness, aggression, central blindness, and vestibular abnormalities. In a study of cats with seizures, of those diagnosed with intracranial lesions, 8% were due to lymphoma.[580] Clinical signs referring to spinal cord involvement may include paresis or paraplegia (>80% with tetraparesis in 20%), ataxia, pain, constipation, and nonspecific constitutional signs (e.g., hyporexia, lethargy, weight loss).[578,582] Neurologic examination may further reveal lower or upper motor neuron bladder, tail flaccidity, and absent deep pain; approximately one-third of cats will be asymmetric and most refer to thoracolumbar involvement. The neurologic dysfunction may be insidious or progress rapidly.

In cats with suspected spinal lymphoma, survey radiographs of the spine will rarely reveal osseous lesions. CT or MRI are preferred and, in approximately 75% of the cases, an extradural or intradural mass will be detected.[577,579,580,582–584] Most lesions occur at a thoracolumbar or lumbosacral location and are often multifocal. Image-guided FNA of epidural lesions may yield a cytologic diagnosis. CT or MRI also reveals multifocal disease in the majority of cats with intracranial lymphoma.[577,580] CSF analysis may be helpful and could provide a definitive diagnosis in some cases. One of 11 cats with confirmed spinal lymphoma in one study[578] and six of 17 with confirmed intracranial lymphoma in another study[577] had evidence of neoplastic lymphocytes in the CNS, and an increased protein content was commonly found. Bone marrow and renal involvement are often present, and cytologic assessment of these or other more accessible involved organs is generally more easily attainable than from spinal sites.

Few cases report chemotherapy treatment and outcome for CNS lymphoma, and although an occasional case has experienced durable response to systemic chemotherapy, generally fewer than 50% will respond and MSTs of 1 to 4 months can be expected.[528,559,572,577,578] RT may be used and generally brisk responses would be expected owing to the inherent radiosensitivity of lymphocytes. Adjuvant chemotherapy should be considered, as many cases with CNS lymphoma have documented bone marrow or renal involvement.[582,583]

Cutaneous Lymphoma

Cutaneous lymphoma is a rarely encountered anatomic form in the cat. It is usually seen in older cats (median age, 10.0–13.5 years) with no sex or breed predominance, and is not associated with FeLV/FIV.[585,586] Cutaneous lymphoma may be solitary or diffuse with a varied presentation.[585,587] In decreasing order of likelihood, lesions may include erythematous patches, alopecia, scaling, dermal nodules, or ulcerative plaques. Nasal hypopigmentation, miliary dermatitis, and mucosal lesions are rarely observed. Peripheral lymphadenopathy may also be present. In most cats, the duration of signs will be prolonged, lasting several months.

Cutaneous lymphoma often affects the head and face and is generally an indolent disease. Two forms have been distinguished histologically and immunohistochemically. Most reports in the cat are epitheliotropic and consist of T cells, although, unlike in dogs, adnexal structures are often spared. A report of nonepitheliotropic cutaneous lymphoma in cats also found 5 of 6 cases to be of T-cell derivation.[588] "Cutaneous lymphocytosis," an uncommon disease histologically resembling well-differentiated lymphoma, was characterized in 23 cats.[502] Solitary lesions were most common. All were composed primarily of T cells, with two-thirds having some B-cell aggregates. Cutaneous lymphocytosis was characterized as a slowly progressive disorder; however, a few cases went on to develop internal organ infiltration. Two case reports exist of cats with cutaneous T-cell lymphoma and circulating atypical lymphocytes.[589,590] The circulating cells were lymphocytes with large, hyperchromatic, grooved nuclei, and one case was immunophenotyped as a CD3/CD8 population. In humans, cutaneous T-cell lymphoma with circulating malignant cells is termed *Sézary syndrome*.

For cats suspected of cutaneous lymphoma, dermal punch biopsies (4–8 mm) should be taken from the most representative and infiltrative sites, while avoiding overtly infected skin lesions. Immunophenotypic and PARR analysis are often helpful in definitive diagnosis. Complete staging to rule out systemic disease is also recommended for cats with cutaneous lymphoma, as local therapy may be applied in cases of solitary disease.

Very little has been published regarding the treatment of cutaneous lymphoma in cats[585]; however, a report of a CR to lomustine exists.[591] Cats with a solitary disease could theoretically be treated with surgical excision or RT, although clinical staging is necessary to rule out possible further systemic involvement. For multiple sites, combination chemotherapy should be considered.

Subcutaneous Lymphoma

Recently several retrospective compilations of a subcutaneous form of lymphoma (SC-L) have been reported.[431,592,593] Although these have been referred to as "cutaneous" lymphoma in some reports, their clinical and histologic characteristics imply a SC localization. Most affected cats are older DSH cats, and males may be overrepresented. Overall, this appears to be an uncommon presentation, representing 0.4% of all cutaneous/SC masses submitted in a report of 97 cases.[431] Retroviral (FeLV/FIV) antigenemia is rare, although in one report of 17 cats, FeLV gp70 and/or p27 protein was expressed in the majority of tumor tissues.[593]

Cats with SC-L are presented with firm, painless SC nodules with a predilection for lateral thoracic, lateral abdominal wall, intrascapular, and tarsal locations (Fig. 33.18). Histologically, they are characterized by deep SC invasion with a monomorphic round cell population, extension into underlying tissues and overlying superficial tissue (but not epitheliotropic), and with extensive central necrosis and peripheral inflammation ("collaring"). Angiocentricity and angioinvasion are often observed. Mitotic index ranges from 3 to more than 25/10 HPF. The round cell population has been characterized as a large high-grade B cell in approximately two-thirds of cases and high-grade T cell in one-third, with an occasional NK immunophenotype reported.[431,592,593]

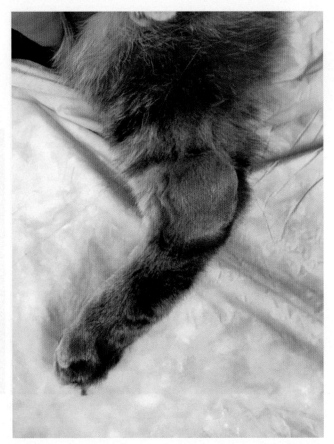

• **Fig. 33.18** Subcutaneous lymphoma of the tarsus in a cat. (Image courtesy Dr. Samuel Hocker.)

Most animals are otherwise healthy (substage *a*) and the disease is generally confined to the local site at presentation (stage I), although in one report the tarsal location was associated with regional popliteal lymph node involvement in nearly 20% of cases.[592] In two cases, concurrent feline injection-site sarcoma (FISS) was found at other sites. SC-L has several similarities to FISS, including clinical presentation, site of occurrence, poor demarcation, central necrosis and peripheral inflammation, although macrophages with phagocytized vaccine-like product has not been observed within the inflammatory component.[431] These similarities suggest the possibility that injection-site inflammation may play a role in the disease etiology; however, this has not been confirmed. Regardless, SC-L should remain an important differential in consideration of FISS.

The treatment of SC-L in the literature is varied and, as such, a standard of care is not currently established.[431,592,593] Although the disease is initially confined to the local primary site in most cases, recurrence after local therapy, whether surgical excision, RT, or both, occurs in nearly half of cases and eventual distant metastasis occurs in one-third of cases. Approximately 75% of affected cats go on to die of their lymphoma; therefore SC-L should be considered to have an aggressive biologic behavior. In the largest report, median progression-free and overall STs after primary site surgical removal were 101 days and 148 days respectively.[431] In the case of tarsal SC-L, even with hindlimb amputation in three cats, regional nodal or distant involvement was documented in all cases (at 56, 350, and 525 days), albeit durable disease-free intervals were observed in two cats. In a limited number of cats treated with RT, responses were brisk, but some progressed beyond the radiation field. The efficacy of chemotherapy is currently not well known; in a small number of cases receiving a variety of

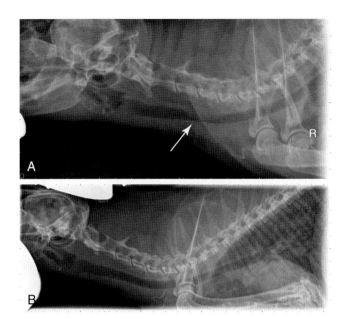

• **Fig. 33.19** (A) Lateral radiographic projection of a cat with tracheal lymphoma before treatment. (B) The same cat 6 weeks after initiation of CHOP-based chemotherapy protocol.

chemotherapy protocols, although many responded or stabilized, durability was poor and MSTs were approximately 6 months.[592] Seven cases of tarsal SC-L received chemotherapy and RT with an MST of 216 days. Because the disease has a high recurrence and metastatic behavior, it is likely that a multimodality approach involving local therapy (surgery and/or RT) and systemic chemotherapy would intuitively provide the best outcomes.

Laryngeal/Pharyngeal/Tracheal Lymphoma

Laryngeal lymphoma comprised 10% of 110 cases of extranodal forms in one report and represented 11% of all laryngeal disease in the species.[559,572,594] It occurs in older cats (median age, 9 years), is not associated with FeLV, and may be a solitary lesion or occur in the presence of other multicentric sites. No information on immunophenotype is currently available. Signs associated with this location in affected cats include dyspnea, dysphonia, stridor, gagging or retching, and rarely, coughing.[559,594] Although it is generally localized to the primary site (stage I), approximately 25% had regional nodal involvement in one report. The vast majority of cats with laryngeal or tracheal lymphoma respond to either RT (if localized) or systemic chemotherapy (90% CR to COP- or CHOP-based protocols) (Fig. 33.19).[528,559] Whereas the author's experience is that most have durable responses and STs typically approach or exceed 1 year, published reported MSTs range from 5.5 to 9.0 months after achievement of a CR.[561]

Ocular Lymphoma

In a compilation of 75 cases of intraocular tumors of cats, 15 (20%) were lymphoma (seven B-cell, four T-cell and four not evaluated).[506] It was presumed, but not proved, that the majority of these were part of a systemic multicentric process. Indeed, lymphoma was the most common metastatic cancer in the feline eye. In 26 cats surveyed with systemic lymphoma, nearly half had some ocular changes with uveitis being most common, followed by exophthalmos, corneal ulceration, and chemosis.[595] In a

histologic characterization of uveitis in cats, lymphoma was diagnosed in approximately one-third of cases; however, whether these were part of a systemic process or limited to the eye was unclear.[596] Nearly half of these cases were documented before 1988 and because nearly half were FeLV antigenemic cats, these data likely have little bearing on modern incidence of the disease.

Presumed solitary ocular lymphoma (PSOL) is rare in cats and was identified in 5 of 110 cases of extranodal lymphoma in one report.[559] Cats with ocular lymphoma are presented with uveitis or iridial masses, as well as signs related to systemic involvement of disease.

Only sporadic reports appear in the literature with the majority (approximately 75%) being B-cell immunophenotyped. One case of LGL PSOL is documented.[559] Intraocular, retinal, and conjunctival locations are reported.[597–600] Outcomes are poorly defined in reports; those cases that underwent enucleation often experienced long-term outcomes with STs of 6 months to 4 years reported.

General Summary of Prognosis for Cats with Lymphoma

As previously discussed, the prediction of outcome in cats with lymphoma is not generalizable because of the wide spectrum of histologic and anatomic subtypes encountered. Much has been mentioned in the previous treatment sections, and Tables 33.9 and 33.10 summarize prognostic parameters for lymphoma in cats.

Feline Leukemias, Myeloproliferative Disorders, and Myelodysplasia

For a complete discussion of leukemias and MPDs, including a general discussion of hematopoiesis, etiologies, lineage classification and descriptions, see Section C of this chapter. The classification of leukemias in cats is difficult because of the similarity of clinical and pathologic features and the transition, overlap, or mixture of cell types involved.[601–605] Most cases are from the FeLV era and generally only single case reports exist from the more contemporary post-FeLV era, which further confuses our understanding of their biology and outcome. For this reason, only a simplistic discussion, primarily relating to the lymphoid leukemias will be presented here and the interested reader is again referred to Section C of this chapter for a general discussion of nonlymphoid leukemia.

For cats with suspected leukemia, peripheral blood assessment (e.g., CBC with differential, flow cytometric analysis for size and immunophenotype, and PARR [for lymphoid leukemias]), and bone marrow aspiration or biopsy may contribute to a diagnosis. Cats with acute leukemia are likely to have malignant cellular infiltrates in organs other than bone marrow.[603] A bone marrow aspirate with greater than 30% abnormal blast cells is sufficient to make a diagnosis of an acute leukemia. In cats with suspected CLL, infiltration of the bone marrow with more than 15% mature lymphocytes helps support the diagnosis.[606] All cats with leukemia should be tested for FeLV/FIV. Determining the lineage of some leukemias can be challenging; most can be distinguished by histologic appearance, histochemical stains, or immunohistochemical or flow cytometric analysis of the leukemic cells for cellular antigens that identify their lineage (see Chapter 8 and Section C of this chapter).[601,605,607] In addition, examination of blast cells by electron microscopy may reveal characteristic ultrastructural features. The French–American–British (FAB) classification system is considered useful in cats with myelodysplastic syndromes and almost all reported cases have been FeLV antigenemic.[607,608]

Lymphoid Leukemia

ALL was the most commonly encountered type of leukemia in cats in the FeLV era; however, it is much less common today. ALL is characterized by poorly differentiated lymphoblasts and prolymphocytes in blood and bone marrow. Approximately 60% to 80% of cats with ALL are FeLV positive, and most malignant cells have T-cell immunophenotypes[609]; however, little information is available in the contemporary literature.

CLL is rarely reported in cats and is characterized by well-differentiated, small, mature lymphocytes in peripheral blood and bone marrow.[606,607,610,611] In the largest compilation, most cats were older, half were presented incidentally, and half with nonspecific constitutional signs (weight loss, hyporexia).[606] No specific serum biochemical abnormalities were noted; however, 50% were anemic, 10% thrombocytopenic, and all had peripheral lymphocyte counts of greater than 9000/μL (although this was the cutoff required for diagnosis). All cats tested (*n* = 13) were negative for FeLV/FIV. Median peripheral lymphocyte counts were 34,200/μL (range, 9 to >300,000/μL). Whereas most are of the T-cell lineage, B-cell CLL has also been reported in cats.[606,607,610,611] In one report of 18 cases of CLL in cats, most were found to be T-helper cells (CD3+/CD4+/CD8−).[611]

Treatment of Leukemias

The use of chemotherapy to treat ALL has been disappointing. Using COP-based protocols, a 27% CR rate has been reported.[612]

CLL can be treated with chlorambucil (0.2 mg/kg PO or 2 mg/cat qod; alternatively, 20 mg/m² q2 weeks) and prednisolone (1 mg/kg PO daily). In 16 cats treated with chlorambucil and prednisolone, approximately 90% responded with a median remission duration of 6 months; however, half achieved CR with a median remission duration of 14 months.[606] Several of these cats were rescued with various protocols after recurrence, many with prolonged second remissions. As in humans and dogs, if significant clinical signs or profound cytopenias are not present, treatment can be withheld; one cat with CLL remained stable without chemotherapy for over a year.[610]

The prognoses for feline ALLs are generally very poor, although some exceptions exist in case report form in the historic literature.

SECTION C: CANINE ACUTE MYELOID LEUKEMIA, MYELOPROLIFERATIVE NEOPLASMS, AND MYELODYSPLASIA

DAVID M. VAIL AND KAREN M. YOUNG

Myeloproliferative disorders (MPDs) are a group of neoplastic diseases of bone marrow in which there are clonal disorders of hematopoietic stem cells.[613] Aberrant proliferation of cells with defective maturation and function leads to reduction of normal hematopoiesis and invasion of other tissues. These disorders have been classified based on biologic behavior, degree of cellular differentiation, and lineage of the neoplastic cells (granulocytic,

---

> **• BOX 33.6** Key Clinical Summary Points: Myeloid Leukemia, Myeloproliferative Neoplasms, and Myelodysplasia
>
> - Myeloid leukemias and myeloproliferative disorders are rare neoplastic diseases of bone marrow in which there are clonal disorders of hematopoietic stem cells (Table 33.13).
> - Clonal disorders of bone marrow include *myeloaplasia* (usually referred to as *aplastic anemia*), *myelodysplasia*, and *myeloproliferation*.
> - The terms *acute* and *chronic* refer to the degree of cellular differentiation of the leukemic cells, but these terms also correlate with the biologic behavior of the neoplasm.
> - The *acute myeloid leukemias* (AMLs) are aggressive leukemias that progress rapidly, are poorly responsive to treatment, and are associated with short survival times (typically <2 months).
> - In AML, determination of the leukemic lineage (i.e., neutrophilic, monocytic, erythroid, or megakaryocytic origin) requires advanced diagnostic testing (cytochemical staining, flow cytometric analysis, clonality testing, or genetic analysis).
> - *Myeloproliferative neoplasms* (MPNs), previously termed chronic myeloproliferative disorders, are characterized by excessive production of differentiated bone marrow cells, resulting in the accumulation of erythrocytes (*polycythemia vera*), granulocytes and/or monocytes (*chronic myelogenous leukemia* and its variants), or platelets (*essential thrombocythemia*).
> - Because of the degree of differentiation of cells in MPNs, these disorders must be distinguished from nonneoplastic causes of increases in these cell types.
> - Compared with AMLs, MPNs and myelodysplasias have a more chronic course and may have better responses to therapy, although most will progress and ultimately result in mortality.

monocytic, erythroid, megakaryocytic, or mixed). Newer classification systems in humans have incorporated genetics and molecular genetic analysis; these are currently areas of active investigation in the study of animal MPDs.[614] In 1991, the Animal Leukemia Study Group made recommendations for classifying nonlymphoid leukemias in dogs and cats.[615] More recently, the Oncology Committee of the American College of Veterinary Pathologists (ACVP) has been reexamining criteria for a classification system and spearheading large multiinstitutional studies to validate the criteria. Long-term objectives of these studies are to define molecular lesions, establish prognostic markers, and identify effective therapeutic approaches.[616] See Box 33.6.

Incidence and Risk Factors

Myeloid neoplasms are uncommon or rare in the dog and occur 10 times less frequently than lymphoproliferative disorders.[617] Accurate information about incidence and other epidemiologic information has been generally lacking owing to a lack of a consistent use of a uniform classification system; however, several larger compilations have been published recently.[618–622] There is no consistent breed predilection; most are large-breed dogs with a median age of 7 to 8 years, although acute myeloid leukemia (AML) can occur in dogs as young as 7 months of age. AML occurred more frequently in males than females (2:1 ratio) in two large compilations.[618,621] In dogs, the etiology of spontaneously occurring leukemia is unknown. It is likely that genetic and environmental factors (including exposure to radiation, drugs, or toxic chemicals) play a role. In humans, acquired chromosomal derangements lead to clonal overgrowth with arrested development.[623] Chromosomal

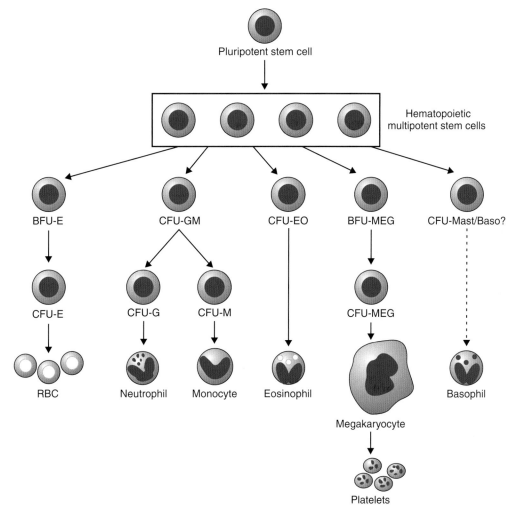

• **Fig. 33.20** A simplified scheme of hematopoiesis. *BFU*, Blast-forming units; *CFU*, colony-forming units; *E*, erythroid; *EO*, eosinophil; *GM*, granulocytic-monocytic; *MEG*, megakaryocyte.

abnormalities have been reported in dogs with AML, chronic myelogenous leukemia (CML), and lymphoid leukemia.[624–627] However, because karyotyping is difficult to perform in dogs because of the large number and morphologic similarity of their chromosomes and their resistance to banding, defining genetic factors in canine myeloid neoplasms has awaited application of molecular technologies and use of the canine genome mapping.[614,626,628–630] Certain forms of leukemia in dogs have been produced experimentally after irradiation.[631–633] In contrast to MPDs in cats, no causative viral agent has been demonstrated in dogs, although retrovirus-like budding particles were observed in the neoplastic cells of a dog with granulocytic leukemia.[634]

Pathology and Natural Behavior

A review of normal hematopoiesis will aid in understanding the various manifestations of MPDs. Hematopoiesis is the process of proliferation, differentiation, and maturation of stem cells into terminally differentiated blood cells. A simplified scheme is presented in Fig. 33.20. Pluripotent stem cells differentiate into either lymphopoietic or hematopoietic multipotent stem cells.[635] Under the influence of specific regulatory and microenvironmental factors, multipotent stem cells in bone marrow differentiate into progenitor cells committed to a specific hematopoietic cell

line, for example, erythroid, granulocytic-monocytic, or megakaryocytic. Maturation results in the production of terminally differentiated blood cells (erythrocytes, granulocytes, monocytes, and platelets) that are delivered to the circulation. In some cases, as in the maturation of reticulocytes to erythrocytes, final development may occur in the spleen.

The proliferation and differentiation of hematopoietic cells are controlled by a group of regulatory growth factors.[635,636] Of these, erythropoietin is the best characterized; it regulates erythroid proliferation and differentiation and is produced in the kidney, where changes in oxygen tension are detected. The myeloid compartment depends on a group of factors, collectively referred to as *colony-stimulating factors* (CSFs). These factors act at the level of the committed progenitor cells, but also influence the functional capabilities of mature cells. Some of these factors have a broad spectrum of activity; others are more restricted in their target cells and actions. CSFs are produced in vitro by a multitude of cell types, including monocytes, macrophages, lymphocytes, and endothelial cells, and these cells likely play a role in the production and regulation of these factors in vivo. The gene for thrombopoietin also has been cloned, and it appears that this hormone alone can induce differentiation of megakaryocytes and platelet production.[637] Recombinant forms of many of these growth factors are increasingly available.

Clonal disorders of bone marrow include myeloaplasia (usually referred to as *aplastic anemia*), myelodysplasia, and myeloproliferation. A preleukemic syndrome, characterized by peripheral pancytopenia and bone marrow hyperplasia with maturation arrest, is more correctly termed *myelodysplasia* because the syndrome does not always progress to overt leukemia. This syndrome has been described in cats, usually in association with FeLV infection, but is rarely recognized in dogs.[638–641] These clonal disorders may be manifested by abnormalities in any or all lineages because hematopoietic cells share a common stem cell. In addition, transformation from one form to another may occur.[642]

Myeloid neoplasms are classified in several ways. The terms *acute* and *chronic* refer to the degree of cellular differentiation of the leukemic cells, but these terms also correlate with the biologic behavior of the neoplasm.[643] Disorders resulting from uncontrolled proliferation or decreased apoptosis of cells incapable of maturation lead to the accumulation of poorly differentiated or "blast" cells. These disorders are included under the umbrella term of AML. Disorders resulting from unregulated proliferation of cells that exhibit progressive, albeit incomplete and defective, maturation lead to the accumulation of differentiated cells and thus are called chronic disorders. These disorders are termed *myeloproliferative neoplasms* (MPN) and include polycythemia vera, CML and its variants, essential thrombocythemia, and possibly primary myelofibrosis. Myeloid neoplasms are further classified by the lineage of the dominant cell type(s), defined by Romanowsky stains, special cytochemical stains, ultrastructural features, flow cytometric analysis, molecular genetic analysis, and immunologic cell markers, and they have been classified into subtypes.

AML has a more sudden onset and is more clinically aggressive. In both acute and chronic disorders, however, abnormalities in proliferation, maturation, and functional characteristics can occur in any hematopoietic cell line.[613] In addition, normal hematopoiesis is adversely affected. Animals with acute leukemias usually have decreased numbers of circulating normal cells. The pathogenesis of cytopenias is complex and may result in part from production of inhibitory factors. Eventually, neoplastic cells displace normal hematopoietic cells, termed *myelophthisis*. Anemia and thrombocytopenia are particularly common. Neutropenia and thrombocytopenia result in infection and hemorrhage, respectively, which may be more deleterious to the animal than the primary disease process.

Acute Myeloid Leukemia

AML is rare and is characterized by aberrant proliferation and/or decreased apoptosis of a clone of cells without maturation. This results in accumulation of immature blast cells in bone marrow and peripheral blood (Fig. 33.21). The white blood cell (WBC) count is variable and ranges from leukopenia to counts greater than 250,000/μL. Spleen, liver, and lymph nodes are frequently involved, and other tissues, including tonsils, kidney, heart, and the CNS, may be infiltrated as well.[621] The median age is approximately 7 to 8 years; however, young dogs may be affected.[618–621,644] The clinical course of these disorders tends to be rapid. Production of normal peripheral blood cells is usually diminished or absent, and anemia, neutropenia, and thrombocytopenia are common with infection and hemorrhage occurring as frequent sequelae. Occasionally, neoplastic blasts are present in bone marrow, but not in peripheral blood. This is termed *aleukemic* leukemia, whereas *subleukemic* suggests a normal or decreased WBC count with some neoplastic cells in circulation.

In 1985, the Animal Leukemia Study Group was formed under the auspices of the American Society for Veterinary Clinical Pathology to develop specific morphologic and cytochemical criteria for classifying acute nonlymphocytic leukemias. Recognition of specific subtypes of leukemia is required to compile accurate and useful information about prognosis and response to treatment, as well as to compare studies from different sites. In 1991 this group proposed a classification system following adaptation of the FAB system and criteria established by the NCI Workshop.[615] Group members examined blood and bone marrow from 49 dogs and cats with myeloid neoplasms. Romanowsky-stained specimens were examined first to identify blast cells and their percentages. Lineage specificity was then determined using cytochemical markers. The percentage of blasts and the information about lineage specificity were used in combination to classify disorders as acute undifferentiated leukemia (AUL), AML (subtypes M1–M5 and M7), and erythroleukemia with or without erythroid predominance (M6 and M6Er). A description of these subtypes is presented in Table 33.13.

Because the modified FAB system has been adopted only recently, the names given to these disorders in the literature vary considerably. In addition, in the absence of cytochemical staining, immunophenotyping, or electron microscopic evaluation, the specific subtype of leukemia has often been uncertain, making retrospective analysis of epidemiologic information, prognosis, and response to therapy confusing at best. Although defining specific subtypes may seem to be an academic exercise owing to the uniformly poor prognosis of acute leukemias, this information is critical to improving their management. Because of the low incidence of AML, national and international cooperative efforts will be required to accumulate information on the pathogenesis and response to different treatment modalities of specific subtypes. Utilization of a uniform classification system is an essential first step. Different forms of AML are demonstrated in Fig. 33.21. With the exception of acute promyelocytic leukemia or M3, all AML subtypes have been described in dogs. Combining three recent compilations of 85 dogs with AML, the relative frequency of subtypes in decreasing order were: 42% monocytic leukemia (M5a, M5b), 33% myelomonocytic leukemia (M4), 13% myeloblastic leukemia without differentiation (M1), 5% megakaryoblastic leukemia (M7), and one each of myeloblastic leukemia with some differentiation (M2) and erythroleukemia (M6).[619–621] AML of mixed lineages comprised 5% of cases. Many single case or small case series reports also exist describing various subtypes in dogs.[617,632–637,639–671] Monocytic leukemias have likely included those with and without monocytic differentiation (M5a and M5b),[672,673] but in some cases the diagnosis may have been chronic myelomonocytic or chronic monocytic leukemia. There are few reports in dogs of spontaneously occurring erythroleukemia (M6) in which the leukemic cells include myeloblasts, monoblasts, and erythroid elements.[674–676] AULs have uncertain lineages because they are negative for all cytochemical markers. These leukemias should be distinguished from lymphoid leukemias by flow cytometric analysis of the leukemic cells for cellular antigens that identify their lineage.[620,677] In addition, examination of blast cells by electron microscopy may reveal characteristic ultrastructural features.

Canine karyotyping is difficult, but with advancements in molecular cytogenetic analysis, chromosome painting, and genomic hybridization, AML in dogs can now be analyzed at the base-pair level,[626,628,629] and missense mutations in *flt3*, *c-kit*, and *ras* sequences have been identified in dogs with AML, similar to

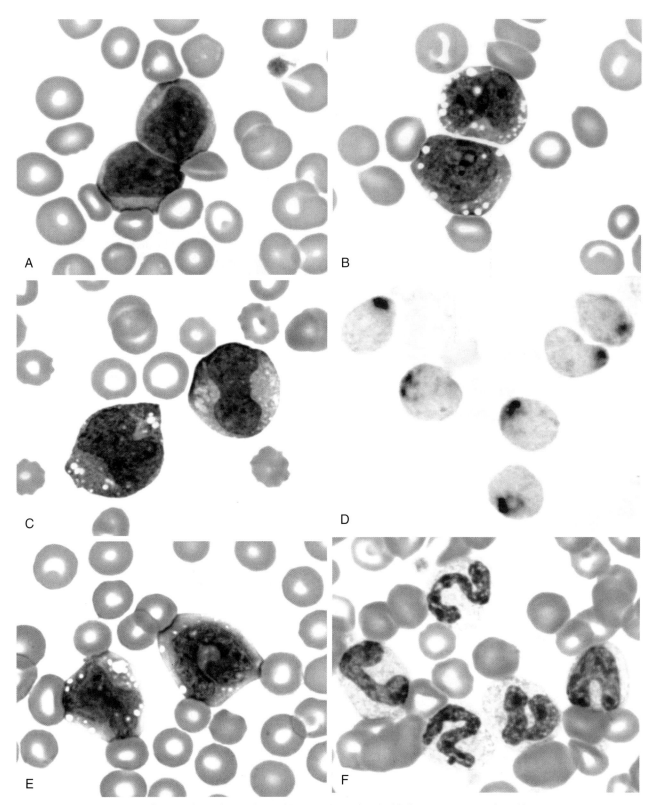

• **Fig. 33.21** Peripheral blood from dogs with myeloid neoplasms. All diagnoses were confirmed by cytochemical staining. Note how similar the blast cells appear in A–C. (A) Acute myeloblastic leukemia (M1). Wright's stain, ×100 objective. (B) Acute myelomonocytic leukemia (M4). Wright's stain, ×100 objective. (C) Acute monocytic leukemia (M5a). Wright's stain. (D) Acute monocytic leukemia (M5a). Cytochemical stain: α-naphthyl butyrate esterase (nonspecific esterase) with red reaction product. (E) Acute monocytic leukemia with some differentiation (M5b). Wright's stain, ×100 objective. (F) Chronic myelogenous leukemia (CML). Wright's stain, ×100 objective.

TABLE 33.13	Subtypes of Leukemias and Dysplasias Adapting the FAB System
Subtype	Description
Acute Leukemias	
AUL	Acute undifferentiated leukemia (formerly called reticuloendotheliosis)
M1	Myeloblastic leukemia, without differentiation
M2	Myeloblastic leukemia, with some neutrophilic differentiation
M3	Promyelocytic leukemia (not recognized in animals)
M4	Myelomonocytic leukemia
M5a	Monocytic leukemia, without differentiation
M5b	Monocytic leukemia, with some monocytic differentiation
M6	Erythroleukemia
M6Er	Variant of M6 with erythroblasts comprising erythroid component
M7	Megakaryoblastic leukemia
Chronic Myeloid Leukemias	
CML	Chronic myelogenous leukemia
CMML	Chronic myelomonocytic leukemia
CMoL	Chronic monocytic leukemia
Hematopoietic Dysplasia	
MDS	Myelodysplastic syndrome
MDS-Er	Myelodysplastic syndrome with erythroid predominance

what has been found for human AML.[678] BCR–ABL translocation is also reported in dogs with acute myeloblastic leukemia.[679] Recurrent DNA copy number abnormalities (CNA) have been interrogated in 24 dogs with AML and there is potential for CNA clustering to be used in diagnostic models.[626] In addition to serving as diagnostic and prognostic markers, cytogenetic lesions may be therapeutic targets. As cytogenetic abnormalities continue to be identified, this information will need to be incorporated into classification schemes.

Myeloproliferative Neoplasms

Myeloproliferative neoplasms (MPNs), previously termed *chronic myeloproliferative disorders,* are characterized by excessive production of differentiated bone marrow cells, resulting in the accumulation of erythrocytes (polycythemia vera), granulocytes and/or monocytes (CML and its variants), or platelets (essential thrombocythemia). Primary myelofibrosis, a clonal disorder of bone marrow stromal cells characterized by proliferation of megakaryocytes and granulocytic precursors with accumulation of collagen in bone marrow, has been recognized only rarely in animals. Phenotypic-driver mutations in

the *JAK2, CALR,* and *MPL* genes have been identified in people with polycythemia vera (PV), essential thrombocythemia (ET), and primary myelofibrosis.[680] Only *JAK2* mutations have been investigated in dogs with PV, and an identical mutation to that in people was found in 1 of 5 cases in dogs.[681] Myelofibrosis is considered a response to injury and may occur secondary to other neoplasms, systemic inflammation, drug exposure, or FeLV infection in cats.

Polycythemia Vera

Polycythemia vera (PV) is a clonal disorder of stem cells, although whether the defect is in the pluripotent stem cell or the hematopoietic multipotent stem cell is still not clear. The disease is rare and must be distinguished from more common causes of polycythemia. In PV, there is neoplastic proliferation of the erythroid series with terminal differentiation to RBCs. The disease has been reported in dogs that tend to be middle-aged with no breed or sex predilection[682–692] and is characterized by an increased RBC mass evidenced by an increased packed cell volume (PCV), RBC count, and hemoglobin concentration. The PCV is typically in the range of 65% to 85%. The bone marrow is hyperplastic, although the myeloid-to-erythroid (M:E) ratio tends to be normal. In contrast to the disease in humans, other cell lines do not appear to be involved and transformation to other MPNs has not been reported. The disease in dogs may be more appropriately termed *primary erythrocytosis.* In humans, progenitor cells have an increased sensitivity to insulin-like growth factor 1, which stimulates hematopoiesis.[691] It is not known whether this hypersensitivity is the primary defect or is secondary to another gene mutation. In any case, the result is overproduction of red blood cells (RBCs). Acquired *JAK2* gene mutations are identified in 90% of humans with PV, and an identical mutation in the *JAK2* gene of 1 of 5 dogs with PV was reported.[681]

Chronic Myelogenous Leukemia

In dogs, CML is more similar to chronic neutrophilic leukemia, a rare form of MPN in humans, than to CML in humans because it is a neoplastic proliferation of the neutrophil series, although concurrent eosinophilic and basophilic differentiation can occur. CML can occur in dogs of any age.[693–698] Neutrophils and neutrophilic precursors accumulate in bone marrow and peripheral blood as well as in other organs. The peripheral WBC count is usually, but not always, greater than 100,000/μL. Both immature and mature neutrophils are present (see Fig. 33.21F). Mature forms are usually more numerous, but sometimes an "uneven" left shift is present. Signs of dysplasia may be evident, including hypersegmentation, ringed nuclei, and giant forms. Eosinophils and basophils may also be increased. The bone marrow is characterized by granulocytic hyperplasia and morphologic abnormalities may not be present. Erythroid and megakaryocytic lines may be affected, resulting in anemia, thrombocytopenia, or less commonly, thrombocytosis. This disorder must be distinguished from severe or extreme neutrophilic leukocytosis ("leukemoid reactions") caused by inflammation or immune-mediated diseases. Extreme neutrophilia can also occur as a paraneoplastic syndrome. In humans with CML, characteristic cytogenetic abnormalities are present in all bone marrow cells, signifying a lesion at the level of an early multipotent stem cell. Typically, these individuals have a chromosomal translocation, resulting in the Philadelphia chromosome or BCR–ABL translocation between chromosomes 9 and 22.[699] The analogous chromosomes in dogs are chromosomes 9 and 26, and BCR–ABL translocation, termed the "Raleigh chromosome," has been reported in several cases of CML in dogs.[614,627,700,701] Variants of CML are chronic myelomonocytic leukemia and chronic monocytic leukemia (CMoL).[702–704] CMoL has also been associated with BCR–ABL translocation in the dog.[702] These diagnoses are made based on the percentage of monocytes in the leukemic cell population. An infrequent myeloproliferative neoplasm, atypical chronic myeloid leukemia, has been reported in a dog and had features of both myelodysplastic syndrome and chronic leukemia.[700] In this dog, BCR–ABL translocation was present in fewer than 10% of cells, considered a negative finding.

In addition to accumulating in bone marrow and peripheral blood, leukemic cells also are found in the red pulp of the spleen, the periportal and sinusoidal areas of the liver, and sometimes lymph nodes. Other organs, such as the kidney, heart, and lung, are less commonly affected. In addition, extramedullary hematopoiesis may be present in the liver and spleen. Death is usually due to complications of infection or hemorrhage secondary to neutrophil dysfunction and thrombocytopenia, respectively. In some cases, CML may terminate in "blast crisis," in which there is a transformation from a predominance of well-differentiated granulocytes to excessive numbers of poorly differentiated blast cells in peripheral blood and bone marrow. This phenomenon is well documented in the dog.[693,696,698]

Basophilic and Eosinophilic Leukemia

Basophilic leukemia, although rare, has been reported in dogs and is characterized by an increased WBC count with a high proportion of basophils in peripheral blood and bone marrow.[705–707] Hepatosplenomegaly, lymphadenopathy, and thrombocytosis may be present. All the dogs have been anemic. Basophilic leukemia should be distinguished from mast cell leukemia (mastocytosis). Whether dogs develop eosinophilic leukemia remains in question. Reported cases have had high blood eosinophil counts and eosinophilic infiltrates in organs.[708,709] One dog responded well to treatment with corticosteroids. The distinction between neoplastic proliferation of eosinophils and idiopathic hypereosinophilic syndrome remains elusive. Nonmyeloproliferative disorders associated with eosinophilia such as parasitism, skin diseases, or diseases of the respiratory and GI tracts should be considered first in an animal with eosinophilia. One distinguishing feature should be clonality, with reactive eosinophilia comprising polyclonal cells and the neoplastic condition arising from a single clone. As clonality assays become more available, this discrepancy may be resolved.

Essential Thrombocythemia

In humans, ET, or primary thrombocytosis, is characterized by platelet counts that are persistently greater than 600,000/μL. There are no blast cells in circulation and marked megakaryocytic hyperplasia of the bone marrow without myelofibrosis is present. Thrombosis and bleeding are the most common sequelae, and most patients have splenomegaly. Other MPDs, especially

PV, should be ruled out, and importantly, there should be no primary disorders associated with reactive thrombocytosis,[710] including inflammation, hemolytic anemia, iron deficiency anemia, malignancies, recovery from severe hemorrhage, rebound from immune-mediated thrombocytopenia, and splenectomy. In addition, certain drugs such as vincristine can induce thrombocytosis. ET has been recognized in dogs.[642,711–714] In one dog, the platelet count exceeded 4 million/μL and bizarre giant forms with abnormal granulation were present. The bone marrow contained increased numbers of megakaryocytes and megakaryoblasts, but circulating blast cells were not seen. Other findings included splenomegaly, GI bleeding, and increased numbers of circulating basophils. Causes of secondary or reactive thrombocytosis were ruled out.[713] Basophilia was also reported in a more recent case.[711] In another dog, ET was diagnosed and then progressed to CML.[642] In some cases reported in the literature as ET, the dogs had microcytic hypochromic anemias. Because iron deficiency anemia is associated with reactive or secondary thrombocytosis, care must be taken to rule out this disorder. However, spurious microcytosis may be reported if a dog has many giant platelets that are counted by some analyzers as small RBCs.[712] Microscopic review of the blood film may be helpful in these cases.

Other Bone Marrow Disorders

Myelofibrosis

Primary myelofibrosis has been reported only rarely in dogs, and myelofibrosis is more typically a secondary, or reactive, process.[715,716] In humans, myelofibrosis is characterized by collagen deposition in bone marrow and increased numbers of megakaryocytes and granulocytic precursors, many of which exhibit morphologic abnormalities. In fact, breakdown of intramedullary megakaryocytes and subsequent release of factors that promote fibroblast proliferation or inhibit collagen breakdown may be the underlying pathogenesis of the fibrosis.[717] Focal osteosclerosis is sometimes present. Anemia, thrombocytopenia, splenomegaly, and myeloid metaplasia (production of hematopoietic cells outside the bone marrow) are consistent features.

In dogs, myelofibrosis occurs secondary to MPDs, radiation damage, and congenital hemolytic anemias.[718–721] In some cases, the inciting cause is unknown (idiopathic myelofibrosis). There may be concurrent marrow necrosis in cases of ehrlichiosis, septicemia, or drug toxicity (estrogens, cephalosporins), and there is speculation that fibroblasts proliferate in response to release of inflammatory mediators associated with the necrosis.[715] Myeloid metaplasia has been reported to occur in the liver, spleen, and lung.[721] Extramedullary hematopoiesis is ineffective in preventing or correcting the pancytopenia that eventually develops.

Myelodysplastic Syndrome

Dysfunction of the hematopoietic system can be manifested by a variety of abnormalities that constitute myelodysplastic syndrome (MDS). In dogs, in which the syndrome is rare, there usually are cytopenias in two or three lines in the peripheral blood (anemia, neutropenia, and/or thrombocytopenia). Other blood abnormalities can include macrocytic erythrocytes and metarubricytosis. The bone marrow is typically normocellular or hypercellular, and dysplastic changes are evident in several cell lines. If blast cells are present, they make up fewer than 30% of all nucleated cells,[614] although this threshold is being changed to less than 20%.[616,722] Myelodysplasia is sometimes referred to as *preleukemia* because, in some cases, it may progress to acute leukemia.[639–641] Based on reported cases, poor prognostic factors include increased percentage of blast cells, cytopenias involving more than one lineage, and cellular atypia.[616] Primary MDSs are clonal disorders and are considered neoplastic. Complex classification schemes for human MDS, based on percentages of blasts in bone marrow, cytogenetic analysis, cytopenias, need for transfusions, and other variables, comprise at least nine subtypes; their applicability to veterinary medicine is unknown.[617] Three subtypes are proposed for dogs and cats and include MDS with excessive blasts (MDS-EB), in which blast percentages are greater than 5% and less than 20%, and progression to AML may occur; MDS with refractory cytopenia (MDS-RC) with blast percentages less than 5% and cytopenias in one or more lineages; and MDS with erythroid predominance (MDS-ER) in which the M : E ratio is less than one and prognosis is poor.[616] Larger studies are needed to determine the utility of this classification scheme and other potential prognostic factors, such as sex and age and, in cats, FeLV positivity. In addition to accumulating enough cases, another confounding factor to studying and classifying MDS is the presence of reversible MDSs that occur secondary to immune-mediated, infectious, and other diseases in both dogs and cats.

History and Clinical Signs

Dogs with myeloid neoplasms have similar presentations regardless of the specific disease entity, although animals with AML have a more acute onset of illness and a more rapid clinical course. A history of constitutional signs (e.g., lethargy, hyporexia, and weight loss) is common.[618–621] Clinical signs include emaciation, persistent fever, pallor, and petechiation. Peripheral lymphadenopathy is reported in 40% to 75% of cases and hepatosplenomegaly in approximately 40% of cases. Shifting leg lameness, ocular lesions, and recurrent infections are also seen. Vomiting, diarrhea, dyspnea, and neurologic signs are variable features. Serum biochemical analytes may be within reference intervals, but can change if significant organ infiltration occurs. Animals with MDS may be lethargic and anorectic and have pallor, fever, and hepatosplenomegaly. In PV, dogs often have erythema of mucous membranes owing to the increase in RBC mass. Some dogs are polydipsic. In addition, neurologic signs such as disorientation, ataxia, or seizures may be present and are thought to be the result of hyperviscosity or hypervolemia.[690] Hepatosplenomegaly is usually absent.

Peripheral blood abnormalities are consistently found in more than 90% of cases.[615,618–621] In addition to the presence of neoplastic cells, other abnormalities, including bi- and pancytopenia, may be present. Low numbers of nucleated RBCs are present in the blood of about half the dogs with acute nonlymphocytic leukemia. Nonregenerative anemia and thrombocytopenia are present in most cases. Anemia is usually normocytic and normochromic, although macrocytic anemia is sometimes present. Pathogenic mechanisms include effects of inhibitory factors leading to ineffective hematopoiesis, myelophthisis, immune-mediated anemia secondary to neoplasia, and hemorrhage secondary to thrombocytopenia, platelet dysfunction, or disseminated intravascular coagulation. Anemia is most severe in AML, although both anemia and thrombocytopenia may be milder in animals with the M5 subtype (acute monocytic leukemia). In myelofibrosis, anemia is characterized by anisocytosis and poikilocytosis. In addition, pancytopenia and leukoerythroblastosis, in which immature erythroid and myeloid cells are in circulation, may be present. These phenomena probably result from replacement of marrow by fibrous tissue with resultant shearing of red cells and escape of immature cells normally confined to bone marrow. In PV, the PCV is increased, usually in the range of 65% to 85%. The bone marrow is hyperplastic and the M : E ratio is usually in the normal range.

Neoplastic cells are often defective functionally. Platelet dysfunction has been reported in a dog with acute megakaryoblastic leukemia (M7)[658]; and, in CML, neutrophils have decreased phagocytic capacity and other abnormalities. One exception to this was a report of CML in a dog in which the neutrophils had enhanced phagocytic capacity and superoxide production.[723] The authors hypothesized that increased synthesis of granulocyte-macrophage (GM)-CSF resulted from a lactoferrin deficiency in the neoplastic neutrophils and mediated the enhanced function of these cells.

Diagnostic Techniques and Workup

In all cases of myeloid neoplasms, diagnosis depends on examination of peripheral blood and bone marrow. AML is diagnosed on the basis of finding blast cells with clearly visible nucleoli in blood and bone marrow. Most dogs with acute leukemia have circulating blasts. These cells may be present in low numbers in peripheral blood, and careful examination of the smear, especially at the feathered edge, should be made. Even if blasts are not detected in circulation, indications of bone marrow disease such as nonregenerative anemia or thrombocytopenia are usually present. Occasionally, neoplastic cells can be found in CSF in animals with invasion of the CNS. Smears of aspirates from tissues such as the lymph nodes, spleen, or liver may contain blasts but usually contribute little to the diagnostic workup.

Examination of blasts stained with standard Romanowsky stains may give clues as to the lineage of the cells (see Fig. 33.21A–C, and E). In myelomonocytic leukemia, the nuclei of the blasts are usually pleomorphic, with round to lobulated forms. In some cells, the cytoplasm may contain large azurophilic granules or vacuoles. Blasts in megakaryocytic leukemia may contain vacuoles and have cytoplasmic blebs. In addition, bizarre macroplatelets may be present. Although these distinguishing morphologic features may suggest a definitive diagnosis, cytochemical staining, immunophenotyping, flow cytometric analysis, clonality testing, and genetic analysis are usually required to definitively define the lineage of the blasts; the reader is referred to several large compilations for which these methodologies have been discussed and applied in dogs.[618–621,626,671,724–726] Several investigators have reported modification of diagnoses after cytochemical staining. It is especially important to distinguish AML from lymphocytic leukemia to provide accurate prognostic information to the owner and institute appropriate therapy.

The Animal Leukemia Group has recommended the following diagnostic criteria, summarized in Fig. 33.22.[615] Using well-prepared Romanowsky-stained blood and bone marrow films, a minimum of 200 cells are counted to determine the leukocyte differential in blood and the percentage of blast cells in bone marrow and/or blood. In bone marrow, blast cells are calculated both as a percentage of all nucleated cells (ANC) and nonerythroid cells, and are further characterized using cytochemical markers.[724,725,727] Neutrophil differentiation is identified by positive staining of blasts for peroxidase, Sudan Black B, and chloracetate esterase. Nonspecific esterases (α-naphthyl acetate esterase or α-naphthyl butyrate esterase), especially if they are inhibited by

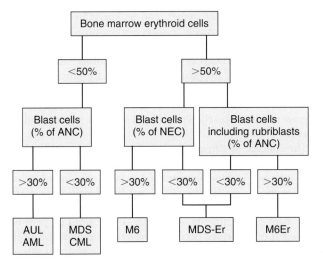

• **Fig. 33.22** A scheme to classify myeloid neoplasms and myelodysplastic syndromes in dogs and cats. *AML,* Acute myeloid leukemias M1–M5 and M7; *ANC,* all nucleated cells in bone marrow, including lymphocytes, plasma cells, macrophages, and mast cells; *AUL,* acute undifferentiated leukemia; *Blast cells,* myeloblasts, monoblasts, and megakaryoblasts; *CML,* chronic myeloid leukemias, including chronic myelogenous, chronic myelomonocytic, and chronic monocytic leukemias; *M6,* erythroleukemia; *M6Er,* erythroleukemia with erythroid predominance; *MDS,* myelodysplastic syndrome; *MDS-Er,* myelodysplastic syndrome with erythroid predominance; *NEC,* nonerythroid cells in bone marrow. (Reprinted with permission from Jain NC, Blue JT, Grindem CB, et al. Proposed criteria for classification of acute myeloid leukemia in dogs and cats. *Vet Clin Pathol.* 1991;20(3):63-82.)

sodium fluoride, mark monocytes. Canine monocytes may also contain a few peroxidase-positive granules. Acetylcholinesterase is a marker for megakaryocytes in dogs and cats. In addition, positive immunostaining for von Willebrand's factor (factor VIII–related antigen) and platelet glycoproteins on the surface of blasts identifies them as megakaryocyte precursors.[648,658,659,661,665,667] Alkaline phosphatase (ALP) only rarely marks normal cells in dogs and cats, but is present in blasts cells in acute myeloblastic and myelomonocytic leukemias. However, owing to reports of ALP activity in lymphoid leukemias in dogs, its specificity as a marker for myeloid cells is not certain. A recent study indicated that ALP was a useful marker for the diagnosis of AML if neoplastic cells express only CD34.[728] Omega exonuclease is a specific marker for basophils, which are also positive for chloracetate esterase activity.[707]

Blood and bone marrow differential counts and cytochemical staining should be performed and interpreted by experienced veterinary cytopathologists. If erythroid cells are less than 50% of ANC and the blast cells are greater than 20%, a diagnosis of AML or AUL is made. If erythroid cells are greater than 50% of ANC and the blast cells are greater than 20%, a diagnosis of erythroleukemia (M6) is made. If rubriblasts are a significant proportion of the blast cells, a diagnosis of M6Er, or erythroleukemia with erythroid predominance, can be made. It should be noted that in the human AML classification system, the blast threshold has been lowered from 30% to 20%, and similar recommendations are now made for AML in dogs and cats.

In some cases, electron microscopy is required to identify the lineage of the blast cells. For example, megakaryocyte precursors are positive for platelet peroxidase activity and contain demarcation membranes and alpha granules.[648,665] Both of these features are detected at the ultrastructural level. Increasingly, cytogenetic

abnormalities are being identified in animal leukemias; cytogenetic analysis may yield important diagnostic and prognostic information and become a valuable tool for identifying targeted therapeutic approaches.

Although morphologic and cytochemical analyses have formed the mainstay of cell identification, newer technologies now are routinely used to classify leukemias by using monoclonal antibodies to detect antigens associated with certain cell types. Cells can be immunophenotyped using flow cytometric analysis or immunocytochemistry.[618–621,671,677,722,729–732] Cells from both acute lymphoid leukemia and AML are positive for CD34. Many lymphocyte markers, including CD3, CD4, CD8, CD21, CD79, and IgG, are available for dogs and can be used to rule out lymphoblastic leukemia in dogs with acute leukemias. Other markers include myeloperoxidase (MPO) and CD11b for myeloid cells and CD41 for megakaryoblasts. There is some overlap in expression of these cellular antigens. For example, canine (but not human) granulocytes express CD4. It is highly recommended to use a panel of antibodies (similar to using a battery of cytochemical stains) because antigens are often expressed on multiple lineages, and lineage infidelity can occur. These tests have become more valuable with the availability of canine reagents. Currently, the ACVP Oncology Committee recommends that the following immunophenotyping panel be done on bone marrow and/or blood smears to characterize animal leukemias: for B lymphocytes, CD79a; for T lymphocytes, CD3; for myeloid cells, MPO and CD11b; for megakaryoblasts, CD41; for dendritic cells, CD1c; and for acute leukemias, CD34.[632] In 2 large reports of 60 cases of AML in dogs, most were CD45/CD18/CD34 positive and, in one report, 64% had clonal or biclonal rearrangements of either the T- or B-cell receptor.[619,621]

Because of the degree of differentiation of cells in MPN, these disorders must be distinguished from nonneoplastic causes of increases in these cell types. To make a diagnosis of PV, it must first be established that the polycythemia is absolute rather than relative. In relative polycythemias, plasma volume is decreased from hemoconcentration, dehydration, or hypovolemia, and the absolute RBC mass is not increased. Splenic contraction can also result in relative polycythemia. Absolute polycythemia, in which RBC mass is increased, is usually secondary to tissue hypoxia, causing appropriately increased production of erythropoietin. Rarely, erythropoietin may be produced inappropriately by a tumor (e.g., renal cell carcinoma) or in renal disease (pyelonephritis) or localized renal hypoxia.[733–735] These causes of polycythemia should be eliminated by appropriate laboratory work, thoracic radiographs, arterial blood gas analysis, and renal ultrasonography. In humans with PV, plasma erythropoietin (EPO) concentrations are low. EPO concentrations in dogs with PV tend to be low or low-normal, whereas in animals with secondary absolute polycythemia, the levels are high.[736,737] Samples for determination of EPO concentrations should be taken before therapeutic phlebotomy used to treat hyperviscosity and, owing to fluctuations in EPO concentrations, should be repeated if results are incongruous with other information.

There are no pathognomonic features of CML in dogs, and other common causes for marked leukocytosis with a left shift (extreme neutrophilia) and granulocytic hyperplasia of bone marrow must be eliminated. These include infections, especially pyogenic infections; immune-mediated diseases; and some neoplasms that cause neutrophilia by elaborating CSFs. In CML, maturation sometimes appears disorderly, and there may be variation in the size and shape of neutrophils at the same level of maturation. In addition, neoplastic leukocytes may disintegrate more rapidly and appear vacuolated.[697] Because of the invasive nature of CML, biopsy of liver or spleen may also help distinguish true leukemia from a leukemoid reaction, assuming the animal can tolerate the procedure. Fluorescent in situ hybridization analysis is available to identify chromosomal rearrangements, including translocations (e.g., Raleigh chromosome), inversions, and deletions, in dogs; some of these aberrations are associated with certain forms of leukemia, and continued investigations will likely yield a larger database of cytogenetic abnormalities and their links to hematologic malignancies.[614,624–630,678,679,681,699–702]

Basophilic leukemia is diagnosed by finding excessive numbers of basophils in circulation and in bone marrow. Basophilic leukemia must be differentiated from mastocytosis based on the morphology of the cell type present. Basophils have a segmented "ribbon-like" nucleus and variably sized granules, whereas mast cells have a round-to-oval nucleus that may be partially or totally obscured by small, round, metachromatic-staining granules. This distinction is usually easy to make; however, in basophilic leukemia, changes in the morphology of the nucleus and granules make the distinction less clear.[706]

ET has been diagnosed based on finding persistent and excessive thrombocytosis (>600,000/μL) without circulating blast cells and in the absence of another MPD (e.g., PV), myelofibrosis, or disorders known to cause secondary thrombocytosis,[710] including iron deficiency anemia, chronic inflammatory diseases, recovery from severe hemorrhage, rebound from immune-mediated thrombocytopenia, and absence of a spleen. Thrombocytosis is transient in these disorders or abates with resolution of the primary disease. In ET, platelet morphology may be abnormal with bizarre giant forms and abnormal granulation.[713] In the bone marrow, megakaryocytic hyperplasia is a consistent feature and dysplastic changes may be evident in megakaryocytes.[712] Spurious hyperkalemia may be present in serum samples from dogs with thrombocytosis from any cause due to the release of potassium from platelets during clot formation.[738] Measuring potassium in plasma is recommended in these cases and usually demonstrates a potassium concentration within reference interval. Platelet aggregability has been variably reported as impaired[713] or enhanced.[712] In the one dog in which it was measured, plasma thrombopoietin (TPO) concentration was normal.[711] It is unclear whether TPO plays a role in ET or is suppressed by the high platelet mass.

In MDS, abnormalities in two or three cell lines are usually manifested in peripheral blood as neutropenia with or without a left shift, nonregenerative anemia, or thrombocytopenia. Other changes include macrocytosis and metarubricytosis. The bone marrow is typically normocellular or hypercellular with an increased M:E ratio, and blasts cells, although increased, constitute less than 20% of nucleated cells; in a report of 13 dogs with primary or secondary MDS, in all but one dog the blast cell percentage was less than 20%.[739] Dysplastic changes can be detected in any cell line. Dyserythropoiesis is characterized by asynchronous maturation of erythroid cells typified by large hemoglobinized cells with immature nuclei (megaloblastic change). If the erythroid component is dominant, the MDS is called *MDS-Er* (see Table 33.13).[615,638] In dysgranulopoiesis, giant neutrophil precursors and abnormalities in nuclear segmentation and cytoplasmic granulation can be seen. Finally, dysthrombopoiesis is characterized by giant platelets and micromegakaryocytes.

Myelofibrosis should be suspected in animals with nonregenerative anemia or pancytopenia, abnormalities in erythrocyte morphology (especially shape), and leukoerythroblastosis. Bone marrow aspiration is usually unsuccessful, resulting in a "dry tap." This necessitates a bone marrow biopsy obtained with a Jamshidi needle.[740] The specimen is processed for routine histopathologic examination and, if necessary, special stains for fibrous tissue can be used. Because myelofibrosis occurs secondary to other diseases of bone marrow, such as chronic hemolytic anemia or bone marrow necrosis, the clinician should look for a primary disease process.

The concept of clinical staging of patients with AML, MPD, and MDS is obviously much different than that of patients with solid tumors. As these hematologic tumors are "liquid," that is they involve primarily the peripheral blood and bone marrow compartments, clinical staging is generally not performed beyond these two compartments. Certainly, infiltration of peripheral nodes and other organs occurs; however, documentation of their involvement with advanced imaging or tissue aspirates does not alter treatment or prognosis in any significant way. Two studies have documented the proof-of-concept use of 3-T body MRI to distinguish diffuse versus focal bone marrow and/or parenchymal involvement of hematopoetic neoplasia; however, the clinical utility of this methodology is currently unknown.[741,742]

Treatment

Acute Myeloid Leukemia

Treatment of acute nonlymphocytic leukemias has been unrewarding to date. There is limited information on the response of specific subtypes of leukemia to uniform chemotherapeutic protocols, in part owing to the rarity of these diseases and the paucity of cases in the literature. Veterinarians are advised to contact a veterinary oncologist for discussion of new protocols and appropriate management of these cases, as novel agents are currently in development and may become available in the future.

The overriding therapeutic goal is to eradicate leukemic cells and reestablish normal hematopoiesis. Currently, this is best accomplished by cytoreductive chemotherapy and the agents most commonly utilized include combinations of anthracyclines, such as doxorubicin, cyclophosphamide, vincristine, 6-thioguanine, and prednisone.[618–620,640,644,646,707,743–746] In dogs, cytosine arabinoside (Ara-C), 100 to 200 mg/m², given by slow infusion (12–24 hours) daily for 3 days and repeated weekly, has been used, as well as several other variations using subcutaneous injections of Ara-C (see Chapter 12). Several variations of CHOP- or COP-based protocols (see Section A of this chapter), with or without Ara-C, have been used as well. The overall prognosis with currently available treatment is poor. Although response rates to multiagent protocols are relatively high (50%–70%), responses are not durable and MSTs, despite aggressive protocols, are generally 0.5 to 2.0 months.[618–620] Obviously, effective therapies for AML in dogs await further investigation.

Regardless of the chemotherapy protocol used, significant cytopenias either persist or are sequela to chemotherapy, and intensive supportive care will be necessary. Transfusions of whole blood or platelet-rich plasma may be required to treat anemia and thrombocytopenia, and infection should be managed with aggressive antibiotic therapy. Because of the generally poor response, many clients will choose palliative supportive care; however, the acute progression of disease does not allow for prolonged palliation in most cases and MSTs with supportive care are generally only 1 to 2 weeks.

Polycythemia Vera

In treating PV, therapy is directed at reducing RBC mass. The PCV should be reduced to 50% to 60% or by one-sixth of its starting value. Phlebotomies should be performed as needed, administering appropriate colloid and crystalloid solutions to replace lost electrolytes; 20 mL of whole blood/kg of body weight can be removed at regular intervals.[687] In humans, phlebotomy continues to be the therapeutic approach used most frequently.

The chemotherapeutic drug of choice is hydroxyurea, an inhibitor of DNA synthesis. This drug should be administered at an initial dose of 30 mg/kg for 10 days and then reduced to 15 mg/kg PO daily.[690] The major goal of treatment is to maintain the PCV as close to normal as possible. Radiophosphorus (^{32}P) has been shown to provide long-term control in people with PV and ET but has seen only limited use in veterinary medicine.[747,748] A *JAK2* inhibitor, ruxolitinib (Jakafi), has been approved for second-line use in people with PV.[680] A mutation in the *JAK2* gene that is identical to that observed in people was documented in one of five dogs with PV[681]; therefore one could speculate that oclacitinib (Apoquel), which has some *JAK2* inhibitory activity and is FDA-approved for use in dogs with atopy, could have therapeutic potential for PV in some dogs. This potential application for oclacitinib has not, as yet, been investigated.

Chronic Myelogenous Leukemia

It has now been documented that a subset of CML in dogs is associated with a BCR–ABL chromosomal abnormality ("Raleigh chromosome") similar to the "Philadelphia chromosome" translocation responsible for a large majority of CML in humans. Imatinib mesylate (Gleevec), a tyrosine kinase inhibitor, is known to be an effective therapy for CML in humans. For dogs with CML that have the Raleigh chromosomal abnormality, it is intuitive that these types of drugs may have activity, and indeed tyrosine kinase inhibitors have been investigated in dogs with BCR–ABL translocation CML.[701] One dog with chronic monocytic leukemia treated with toceranib (Palladia) and prednisone therapy achieved a clinical remission (before developing progressive disease) and a partial cytogenetic response. In addition, molecular techniques may be used to monitor cytogenetic aberrations, such as DNA copy number aberrations and BCR–ABL translocations, after treatment to gauge the cytogenetic response to therapy.[627,701] The author (DMV) and others have anecdotally used toceranib and/or imatinib in a handful of CML cases with responses that have lasted several months; the true activity and durability of response with these agents in dogs awaits further investigation.

CML has also been managed with chemotherapy to control the proliferation of the abnormal cell line and improve the quality of life. Hydroxyurea is the most effective agent for treating CML during the chronic phase.[627,696,749] The initial dosage is 20 to 25 mg/kg twice daily. Treatment with hydroxyurea should continue until the leukocyte count falls to 15,000 to 20,000 cells/μL.[694,696,705] Then the dosage of hydroxyurea can be reduced by 50% on a daily basis or to 50 mg/kg given biweekly or triweekly. In humans, the alkylating agent busulfan can be used as an alternative.[750] An effective dosage has not been established in the dog, but following human protocols, 0.1 mg/kg/day PO is given until the leukocyte count is reduced to 15,000 to 20,000 cells/μL. Vincristine and prednisone therapy resulted in a short remission in one dog with CML.[627]

Despite response to chemotherapy and control for many months, most dogs with CML will eventually enter a terminal phase of their disease. In one study of seven dogs with CML, 4 dogs underwent terminal phase blast crisis.[696] In humans, blast crisis may be lymphoid or myeloid.[751] Dogs with blast crisis have a poor prognosis, despite rescue with more aggressive multiagent chemotherapy.

Essential Thrombocythemia

Few cases have been reported, but one dog was treated successfully with a combination chemotherapy protocol that included vincristine, Ara-C, cyclophosphamide, and prednisone.[714] Treatment is controversial in humans because of the lack of evidence that asymptomatic patients benefit from chemotherapy. Patients with thrombosis or bleeding are given cytoreductive therapy. Hydroxyurea is the drug of choice for initially controlling the thrombocytosis.[710] *JAK2* small molecule inhibitors have been used in people with ET,[680] and although no studies have investigated *JAK2* mutations in dogs with ET, one could speculate on the use of oclacitinib (Apoquel) in dogs. Radiophosphorus treatment is also occasionally used in people with ET.[747]

Myelodysplastic Syndrome

There is no standard therapeutic regime for MDS. Often, humans receive no treatment if the cytopenias do not cause clinical signs. Transfusions are given when necessary, and patients with fever are evaluated aggressively to detect infections. Growth factors, such as EPO, GM-CSF, G-CSF, and IL-3, are sometimes used in patients who require frequent transfusions to increase their blood cell counts and enhance neutrophil function.[752,753] In one case report, human EPO was administered (100 U/kg SQ q48 hours) to a dog with MDS because of profound anemia. The rationale for use of EPO was to promote terminal differentiation of dysplastic erythrocytes. Human recombinant EPO should be used with caution in animals, as anti-EPO antibodies may be induced and target endogenous EPO. The PCV increased from 12% to 34% by day 19 of EPO treatment. This dog remained in remission for more than 30 months.[638] Other factors that induce differentiation of hematopoietic cells include retinoic acid analogs, 1,25 dihydroxyvitamin D3, interferon-α, and conventional chemotherapeutic agents, such as 6-thioguanine and Ara-C.[754-756] The propensity of these factors to enhance progression to leukemia is not known in many cases, but the potential risk exists.

Prognosis

In general, the prognosis for animals with MPN is better than for dogs with AML, in which it is grave. The prognosis for PV and CML is guarded, but significant remissions have been achieved with certain therapeutic regimes and careful monitoring. Animals commonly survive a year or more.[696,714]

SECTION D: MYELOMA-RELATED DISORDERS

DAVID M. VAIL

Myeloma-related disorders (MRDs) arise when a cell of the plasma cell or immunoglobulin-producing B-lymphocyte precursor lineage transforms and proliferates to form a clonal neoplastic population of similar cells. This population is believed in most instances to be monoclonal (i.e., derived from a single cell) because they typically produce homogeneous immunoglobulin, although some examples of biclonal and polyclonal MRD neoplasms exist. A wide variety of clinical syndromes are represented by MRDs, including multiple myeloma (MM), extramedullary plasmacytoma (EMP [both cutaneous and noncutaneous]), IgM

(Waldenström's) macroglobulinemia, solitary osseous plasmacytoma (SOP), and Ig-secreting lymphomas and leukemias (including plasma cell leukemia). MM is the most important MRD based on clinical incidence and severity. There appears to be some discordance and blurring of the distinction between MM and multicentric noncutaneous EMP in cats and these two MRDs will be discussed together in this species. See Box 33.7.

Multiple Myeloma

Incidence and Etiology

Although MM represents fewer than 1% of all malignant tumors in animals, it is responsible for approximately 8% of all hematopoietic tumors and 3.6% of all primary and secondary tumors affecting bone in dogs.[757,758] In a compilation of bone marrow disorders in dogs ($n = 717$), MM represented 4.4% and 19.8% of all abnormal samples and neoplastic processes, respectively.[759] Furthermore, in a compilation of serum protein electrophoretic samples ($n = 147$ dogs), MM accounted for 4.3% of abnormal and 28.5% of neoplastic processes encountered, respectively.[760] Several compilations have suggested a male predisposition,[761–763] whereas others have not observed this.[758,764] Older dogs are affected with an average age of between 9 and 10 years (range, 3–14 years).[758,761–764] In one large case series, German shepherd dogs were overrepresented based on the hospital population.[758] The true incidence of MM in the cat is unknown; however, it is a more rare diagnosis than in the dog, representing only 1 of 395 and 4 of 3248 tumors in two large compilations of feline malignancies, and 0.9% of all malignancies and 1.9% of hematologic malignancies in another report.[765–767] MM represented 1.4% and

14% of abnormal and malignant serum protein electrophoretic samples, respectively, in a compilation of 155 feline samples.[768] MM occurs in aged cats (median age 12–14 years), most commonly in domestic short hair cats, and no sex predilection has been consistently reported, although a male preponderance may exist.[764,767,769–771] MM has not been associated with coronavirus, FeLV, or FIV infections.

The etiology of MM is for the most part unknown. Genetic predispositions, molecular aberrations (e.g., c-kit), viral infections, chronic immune stimulation, and carcinogen exposure have all been suggested as contributing factors.[764,772–779] Suggestion of a familial association in cats follows cases reported among siblings.[770] Evidence exists that molecular mechanisms of cellular control, including overexpression of cell cycle control components like cyclin D1 (see Chapter 2), and receptor tyrosine kinase dysregulation may be involved in canine MM and plasma cell tumors.[774,776] In rodent models, chronic immune stimulation and exposure to implanted silicone gel have been associated with development of MM,[778,779] as have chronic infections and prolonged hyposensitization therapy in humans.[775] Viral Aleutian disease of mink results in monoclonal gammopathies in a small percentage of cases.[777] Exposure to the agricultural industry, petroleum products, and irradiation are known risk factors for development in humans.[780–782] In addition, progression of solitary plasma cell tumors to MM has been reported in both dogs and cats, and a single case of a B-cell lymphoma progressing to MM exists in the dog.[783–785]

Pathology and Natural Behavior

MM is a systemic proliferation of malignant plasma cells or their precursors arising as a clone of a single cell that usually involves multiple bone marrow sites in dogs. In cats, as previously stated, a blurring of the distinction of MM and multicentric noncutaneous EMP within the MRD occurs because widespread abdominal organ involvement without significant bone marrow infiltration has been described in a proportion of cases in European compilations.[771,786] Because both MM and multicentric noncutaneous EMP have a similar clinical course and widespread systemic involvement with hyperglobulinemia in cats, they will be discussed as MM in this chapter. Malignant plasma cells can have a varied appearance on histologic sections and cytologic preparations. The degree of differentiation ranges from those resembling normal plasma cells in late stages of differentiation (Fig. 33.23) to very large anaplastic round cells (often referred to as *plasmablasts*) with a high mitotic index representing early stages of differentiation.[763,764,767,786] Binucleate and multinucleate cells are often present (see Fig. 7.32, Chapter 7). In 16 cats with MM in one case series,[787] the majority (83%) of plasma cells were immature and had marked atypia, including increased size, multiple nuclei, clefted nuclei, anisocytosis, anisokaryosis, variable nuclear : cytoplasmic ratios, decreased chromatin density, and variable nucleoli; nearly one quarter had "flame cell" morphology characterized by peripheral eosinophilic cytoplasmic processes.[767] However, in a European compilation of feline multicentric noncutaneous MRD cases ($n = 17$), 78% had well-differentiated morphologies.[786] The authors of this latter case series developed a grading system dependent on the percentage of plasmablasts within the neoplastic cells in which well-differentiated, intermediate-grade, and poorly differentiated MMs have less than 15%, 15% to 49%, and 50% or more plasmablasts, respectively.[786] Malignant plasma cells typically produce an overabundance of a single type of or component of immunoglobulin, which is referred to as the *M component*

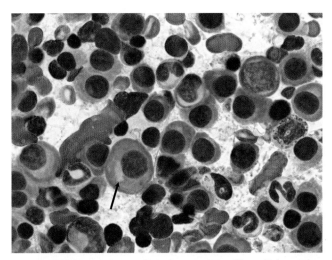

• **Fig. 33.23** Bone marrow aspirate from a dog with multiple myeloma showing an overabundance of large neoplastic plasma cells with characteristic paranuclear clear zone representing the Golgi apparatus *(arrow).* (Dif-quick stain, ×100 objective.)

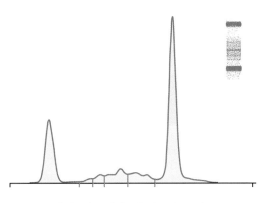

Animal protein electrophoresis

T.P.: 10.4 g/dL   A/G 0.32

Fractions	%	Conc.	Ref. Conc.
Albumin	24.4	2.54 L	2.60–4.00
Alpha 1	1.6	0.17	0.11–0.35
Alpha 2	3.0	0.31 L	0.92–1.66
Beta 1	8.7	0.90 H	0.22–0.61
Beta 2	7.8	0.81 H	0.08–0.50
Gamma	54.5	5.67 H	0.66–2.48

• **Fig. 33.24** Serum protein electrophoresis from a cat with multiple myeloma. Stained cellulose acetate electrophoretic strip *(upper right corner)* with accompanying densitogram. Note large M-component spike (representing an IgG monoclonal gammopathy) present in the gamma region. (Courtesy Dr. Frances Moore, Marshfield Laboratories, Marshfield, WI.)

(Fig. 33.24). The M component can be represented by any class of the entire immunoglobulin or only a portion of the molecule, such as the light chain (Bence Jones protein) or heavy chain (heavy chain disease) of the molecule. In the dog, the M component is usually represented by either IgA or IgG immunoglobulin types in nearly equal incidence, whereas the ratio of IgG to IgA in cats is approximately 5:1 in some reports and approximately 1:1 in others.[757,763–767,786,788] However, in two recent compilations of dogs with MM, including 27 dogs in which the immunoglobulin was typed, the vast majority (78%) were of the IgA type.[761,762] If the M component is the IgM type, the term *macroglobulinemia*

(Waldenström's) is often applied. Several cases of biclonal gammopathy in dogs and cats have been reported,[761,767,770,771,789–795] and several cases of nonsecretory MM have been reported in dogs.[762,796–798] Rarely, cryoglobulinemia occurs in dogs with MM and IgM macroglobulinemia, and this has also been reported in a cat with IgG myeloma.[764,799–801] Cryoglobulins are paraproteins that are insoluble at temperatures below 37°C and require blood collection and clotting to be performed at 37°C before serum separation. If whole blood is allowed to clot at temperatures below this, the protein precipitates in the clot and is lost. Pure light-chain M component is rare, but has been reported in both dogs and cats.[762,802,803]

The pathology associated with MM is a result of either high levels of circulating M component, organ or bone infiltration with neoplastic cells, or both. Associated pathologic conditions include bone disease, bleeding diathesis, hyperviscosity syndrome (HVS), renal disease, hypercalcemia, immunodeficiency (and subsequent susceptibility to infections), cytopenias secondary to myelophthisis, and cardiac failure.

Bone lesions can be isolated, discrete osteolytic lesions (including pathologic fractures) (Fig. 33.25A), diffuse osteopenias, or both (Fig. 33.26). Approximately one-quarter to two-thirds of dogs with MM have radiographic evidence of bony lysis or diffuse osteoporosis.[757,761,763,764] The incidence of radiographic skeletal lesions in cats varies tremendously within reports from as few as 8% in some case series to as high as 65% in others.[765,767,770,771,788] Those bones engaged in active hematopoiesis are more commonly affected and include the vertebrae, ribs, pelvis, skull, and the metaphyses of long bones. Skeletal lesions are rare with IgM (Waldenström's) macroglobulinemia, in which malignant cells often infiltrate the spleen, liver, and lymphoid tissue rather than bone.[764,804,805]

Bleeding diathesis can result from one or a combination of events. M components may interfere with coagulation by (1) inhibiting platelet aggregation and the release of platelet factor-3; (2) causing adsorption of minor clotting proteins; (3) generating abnormal fibrin polymerization; and (4) producing a functional decrease in calcium.[764,806,807] Approximately 10% to 30% of dogs and up to one-quarter of cats have clinical evidence of hemorrhage.[757,761,767,770,771] In dogs, nearly half have abnormal prothrombin (PT) and partial thromboplastin (PTT) times. Thrombocytopenia may also play a role if bone marrow infiltration is significant (i.e., myelophthisis).

HVS represents one of a constellation of clinicopathologic abnormalities resulting from greatly increased serum viscosity. The magnitude of viscosity changes is related to the type, size, shape, and concentration of the M component in the blood. HVS is more common with IgM macroglobulinemia because of the high molecular weight of this class of immunoglobulin. IgA-secreting myelomas (IgA is usually present as a dimer in the dog) may undergo polymerization resulting in increased serum viscosity.[757,764,808] IgG-associated HVS can also occur, albeit less frequently. High serum viscosity occurs in approximately 20% to 40% of dogs with MM and can result in bleeding diathesis, neurologic signs (e.g., dementia, depression, seizure activity, coma), ophthalmic abnormalities (e.g., dilated and tortuous retinal vessels, retinal hemorrhage [Fig. 33.27], retinal detachment), and increased cardiac workload with the potential for subsequent development of cardiomyopathy.[757,761,764,804,805,808–811] In a retrospective compilation of 83 dogs with retinal hemorrhage, 5% were due to MM.[812] These consequences of HVS are thought to be a result of sludging of blood in small vessels, ineffective delivery of oxygen and nutrients, and coagulation abnormalities. HVS

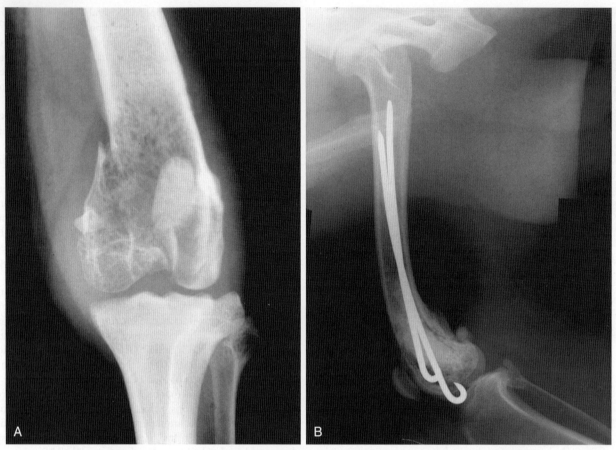

• **Fig. 33.25** (A) Radiograph of a distal femur in a dog demonstrating severe osteolysis and a pathologic fracture secondary to a plasma cell tumor. (B) Radiograph of the same pathologic fracture after surgical repair with Rush rods and bone cement. Local site was treated with adjuvant radiation. The dog was continued on chemotherapy for 2 more years and did well.

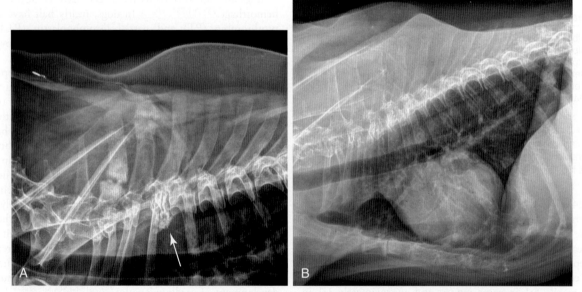

• **Fig. 33.26** (A) Lateral thoracic radiographs of a dog showing multiple expansile lytic lesions and pathologic fractures of the dorsal spinous processes and collapse fracture *(arrow)* of the third thoracic vertebral body. (B) Lateral thoracic radiographs of a dog with diffuse osteopenia secondary to multiple myeloma. Note the overall decreased opacity of the lumbar vertebrae and dorsal spinous processes secondary to diffuse marrow involvement causing loss of bone trabeculae and thinning of the cortices.

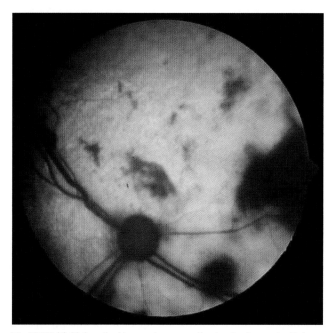

• **Fig. 33.27** Multiple retinal hemorrhages on the fundus in a cat with hyperviscosity syndrome secondary to multiple myeloma.

has been reported in cats with IgG-, IgA-, and IgM-secreting tumors.[764,765,813–818] In several of these cases, relative serum viscosity was increased above control ranges.

Renal disease is present in approximately one-quarter to one-half of dogs with MM, and azotemia is observed in 30% to 40% of cats.[757,761,763,767,769,771] The pathogenesis of renal failure is often multifactorial and can ensue as a result of Bence Jones (light-chain) proteinuria, tumor infiltration into renal tissue, hypercalcemia, amyloidosis, diminished perfusion secondary to HVS, dehydration, or ascending urinary tract infections.[757,764,806,807] Normally, heavy- and light-chain synthesis is well balanced in nonneoplastic immunoglobulin production. In the case of MM, an unbalanced excess of light-chain products may be produced. Light chains are of low molecular weight and are normally filtered by the renal glomerulus, and their presence in urine can result in protein precipitates and subsequent renal tubular injury. The presence of light chains in urine without a concomitant monoclonal spike in serum, although rare, is indicative of pure light-chain disease.[802] Tubules become obstructed by large laminated casts containing albumin, immunoglobulin, and light chains. Bence Jones proteinuria occurs in approximately 25% to 40% of dogs with MM.[757,763,764] Bence Jones proteinuria is reported to occur in approximately 40% of cats with MM/MRD.[767,768] Hypercalcemia is reported in 15% to 50% of dogs with MM and is thought to result primarily from the production of osteoclast-activating factor by neoplastic cells.[757,761,762,764,819] Other factors, including increased levels of various cytokines, TNF-α, IL-1, and IL-6, have been implicated in human MM. In two dogs with MM and hypercalcemia, serum elevations in circulating N-terminal parathyroid hormone-related peptide were noted.[820] Hypercalcemia may also be exacerbated by associated renal disease. Hypercalcemia, initially thought to be a rare event in cats with MM, occurred in 10% to 25% of recently reported cases.[767,769–771,821]

Susceptibility to infection and immunodeficiency have long been associated with MM and are often the ultimate cause of death in affected animals.[757,764,788] Infection rates in humans with MM are 15 times higher than normal and usually present as pneumonia or urinary tract infections.[822] Response to vaccination has also been shown to be suppressed in humans with MM.[822]

"Normal" immunoglobulin concentrations are often severely depressed in affected animals.[764] In addition, leukopenia may be present secondary to myelophthisis. Reports of multiple concurrent infections in both dogs and cats affected with MM exist and, in one dog with several concurrent infections, a polyclonal and a monoclonal gammopathy existed pretreatment, with the former persisting after successful treatment of the myeloma.[772,773]

Variable cytopenias may be observed in association with MM. A normocytic, normochromic, nonregenerative anemia is encountered in approximately one-half to two-thirds of dogs with MM.[757,761–764] This can result from marrow infiltration (myelophthisis), blood loss from coagulation disorders, anemia of chronic disease, or increased erythrocyte destruction secondary to high serum viscosity. Rare erythrophagocytic forms of MM have also been reported in both dogs and cats and may contribute to anemia.[823–825] Similar factors lead to thrombocytopenia and leukopenia in 30% and 80% of dogs with MM, respectively; and in cats, approximately two-thirds, one-half, and one-third will be anemic, thrombocytopenic, and neutropenic, respectively.[761,762,767,769–771]

Cardiac disease, if present, is usually a result of excessive cardiac workload and myocardial hypoxia secondary to hyperviscosity. Myocardial infiltration with amyloid and anemia may be complicating factors. Nearly one-half of cats with MM in two reports presented with a cardiac murmur, the etiology of which was not established.[767,769] Three cats with HVS presented with congestive heart failure, murmurs, and echocardiographic signs consistent with hypertrophic cardiomyopathy.[813]

History and Clinical Signs

Clinical signs of MM may be present up to a year before diagnosis with a median duration of 1 month reported in dogs.[757,764] In one cat, M-component elevations were detected 9 years before clinical presentation.[767] In this latter case, the M-component elevation was consistent with monoclonal gammopathy of unknown significance (MGUS). MGUS (i.e., benign, essential, or idiopathic monoclonal gammopathy) is a benign monoclonal gammopathy that is not associated with osteolysis, bone marrow infiltration, or Bence Jones proteinuria. MGUS has also been reported in dogs.[826,827] Signs of MM can be variable based on the wide range of pathologic effects possible. Tables 33.14 and 33.15 list the relative frequencies of clinical signs observed in the dog and cat, respectively, based on a compilation of several reports.[757,761,762,764,767,769–771,788] Bleeding diathesis is usually represented by epistaxis and gingival bleeding. Funduscopic abnormalities may include retinal hemorrhage (see Fig. 33.27), venous dilatation with sacculation and tortuosity, retinal detachment, and blindness.[757,761,6,764,769,771,808–812] CNS signs may include dementia, seizure activity, tremors, and deficiencies in midbrain or brainstem localizing reflexes secondary to HVS or extreme hypercalcemia. Signs reflective of transverse myelopathies secondary to vertebral column infiltration, pathologic fracture, or extradural mass compression can also occur.[757,764,799,828,829] One case of ataxia and seizure activity in a dog with EMP secondary to tumor-associated hypoglycemia has been reported.[830] In addition, paraneoplastic polyneuropathy has been reported in a dog with MM.[831] A history of chronic respiratory infections and persistent fever may also be present in cats. Hepatosplenomegaly and renomegaly can occur due to organ infiltration. Bleeding diathesis due to HVS is less common in the cat; however, epistaxis, pleural and peritoneal hemorrhagic effusions, retinal hemorrhage, and central neurologic signs have been reported in both dogs and cats.[761,764,765,769,813–818] Polydipsia and polyuria can occur

TABLE 33.14	Frequency of Clinical Signs Reported for Dogs with Multiple Myeloma (*n* = 112)[757,761,762]	
Clinical Sign	**Frequency Reported (%)**	
Lethargy and weakness	58	
Inappetence and weight loss	36	
Lameness	35	
Bleeding diathesis	28	
Funduscopic/ocular abnormalities	32	
Polyuria/polydipsia	30	
CNS deficits	8	

CNS, Central nervous system.

TABLE 33.15	Approximate Frequency of Clinical Signs Reported for Cats with Myeloma-Related Disorders (*n* = 68)[764,767,769–771,788]
Clinical Sign	**Frequency Range Reported (%)**
Lethargy and weakness	40–100
Anorexia	33–100
Pallor	30–100
Polyuria/polydipsia	13–40
Vomiting/diarrhea	10–30
Dehydration	20–33
Palpable organomegaly	20–25
Lameness	7–25
Heart murmur	0–45
Hind limb paresis/paralysis	0–45
Bleeding diathesis	0–40
CNS signs	13–30
Concurrent cutaneous plasma cell tumor	0–30
Fundic/ocular changes	13–33
Lymphadenopathy	0–10

CNS, Central nervous system.

secondary to renal disease or hypercalcemia, and dehydration may develop. Hindlimb paresis secondary to osteolysis and instability of lumbar vertebral bodies or extradural compression has been reported in cats.[770,832]

Diagnosis and Staging

The diagnosis of MM in dogs usually follows the demonstration of bone marrow plasmacytosis (see Fig. 33.23), the presence of osteolytic bone lesions (see Figs. 33.25 and 33.26), and the

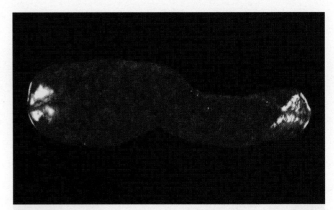

• **Fig. 33.28** Necropsy specimen of a spleen from a cat with multiple myeloma showing diffuse plasma cell infiltration.

demonstration of serum or urine myeloma proteins (M component) (see Fig. 33.24). In the absence of osteolytic bone lesions, a diagnosis can also be made if marrow plasmacytosis is associated with a progressive increase in the M-component or if plasma cell clonality (e.g., PARR) is documented. In the cat, because the degree of bone marrow infiltration may not be as marked, it has been suggested that consideration of plasma cell morphology and visceral organ infiltration (Fig. 33.28) be given in cases with demonstrable M-component disease in the absence of marked (<20%) marrow plasmacytosis.[767,771,786]

All animals suspected of plasma cell tumors should receive a minimal diagnostic evaluation including a CBC, platelet count, ionized calcium, serum biochemistry profile, and urinalysis. Particular attention should be paid to renal function and serum calcium levels. If clinical hemorrhage is present, a coagulation assessment (e.g., platelet count, PT, PTT) and serum viscosity measurements are indicated. All animals should undergo a careful funduscopic examination. Serum electrophoresis and immunoelectrophoresis are performed to determine the presence of a monoclonal M-component (see Fig. 33.24) and to categorize the immunoglobulin class involved. Heat precipitation and electrophoresis of urine may be performed to determine presence of Bence Jones proteinuria because commercial urine dipstick methods are not capable of this determination. Definitive diagnosis usually follows the performance of a bone marrow aspiration in the dog. A bone marrow core biopsy or multiple aspirations may be necessary because of the possibility of uneven clustering or infiltration of plasma cells in the bone marrow. Normal marrow contains less than 5% plasma cells, whereas myelomatous marrow often greatly exceeds this level. Current recommendations require more than 20% marrow plasmacytosis to be present, although a 10% cutoff in cats has been recently recommended with special attention to cellular atypia.[767] Even the 10% threshold may be problematic in cats, and cellular atypia and visceral organ involvement (assessed through needle aspiration cytology or tissue biopsy) should be considered equally important in this species.[767,771,786] Rarely, biopsy of osteolytic lesions (i.e., Jamshidi core biopsy; see Chapter 25) is necessary for diagnosis in the dog. In one case of MM in a dog, splenic aspirates were diagnostically helpful.[833] Overall frequencies of clinical diagnostic abnormalities for dogs and cats with MM are compiled from published series having at least five cases each and are listed in Table 33.16.

Immunohistochemical and Molecular Diagnostics

Histochemical and IHC analyses of cells or tissues suspected of MRD are more often applied in the case of solitary plasmacytomas

TABLE 33.16 Approximate Frequency of Clinical Diagnostic Abnormalities for Dogs and Cats with Multiple Myeloma (*n* = 68 cats, 134 dogs)[757,761,762,764,767,769–771,788]

Abnormality	FREQUENCY RANGE REPORTED (%)	
	Dogs	Cats
Increased M component	99	94–98
Monoclonal	95	77–100
Biclonal	5%[a]	16–23
IgG	40	84
IgA	60	16
Noncutaneous extramedullary extension	NR	65–100[b]
Marrow plasmacytosis (>10%)	100	50–100
Complete blood count (CBC) abnormalities		
Anemia (nonregenerative)	61	50–80
Thrombocytopenia	39	50
Neutropenia	26	37
Circulating plasma cells (leukemia)	7	5–25
Hypoalbuminemia	62	36–60
Hypocholesterolemia	NR	68
Proteinuria	45	71–91
Bence Jones proteinuria	38	40–59
Bone lysis	64	5–45
Serum hyperviscosity	35	35–44
Azotemia	29	22–40
Hypercalcemia	27	10–25
Increased activities of liver enzymes	NR	43–50

[a]Several single case reports exist for biclonal gammopathy in dogs with MM.

[b]11 of 11 in one report had evidence of infiltration in either spleen, lymph node, or liver.

NR, Not reported.

or where EMP is suspected in the absence of marrow involvement and will be discussed in subsequent sections; however, they have been occasionally useful in the diagnosis of MM. Molecular diagnostic techniques for MM have received limited use thus far in veterinary oncology; however, determining clonality of the immunoglobulin heavy chain variable region gene has been performed in feline and canine plasmacytoma and myeloma using PARR techniques (see Chapter 8),[762,834] and use of this technology in cases where diagnosis is not straightforward is expanding. The author has used PARR analysis both before treatment and after clinical remission in a small number of dogs with MM involved in clinical trials and documented its utility for (1) initial diagnosis and (2) to characterize molecular remission.[762]

Imaging

Routine thoracic and abdominal radiographs are recommended in suspected cases. Occasionally, bony lesions can be observed in skeletal areas on these standard films, and organomegaly (liver, spleen, kidney) is observed in the majority of cats.[767,769,771] Abdominal ultrasound is recommended in all cats suspected of

MM because this modality reveals involvement of one or more abdominal organs in the majority of cases. These include splenomegaly with or without nodules, diffuse hyperechoic hepatomegaly with or without nodules, renomegaly, and iliac lymph node enlargement. In one case series in cats with MM, 85% of organs with ultrasonographic abnormalities were subsequently confirmed to have plasma cell infiltration.[771] Skeletal survey radiographs are recommended to determine presence and extent of osteolytic lesions, which may have diagnostic, prognostic, and therapeutic implications. Although nuclear scintigraphy (bone scan) for clinical staging of dogs with MM has been performed, because of the predominant osteolytic activity with osteoblastic inactivity present, scans seldom give positive results and are therefore not useful for routine diagnosis.[835] In physician-based oncology, bone mineral density analysis (dual-energy x-ray absorptiometry [DEXA] scan) to document osteoporosis, MRI of bone marrow, and PET/CT are commonly used for staging; however, these modalities have not been applied consistently in the veterinary literature. A clinical staging system for canine MM has been suggested[757]; however, at present, no prognostic significance has been attributed to it.

Differential Diagnosis of MM

Disease syndromes other than plasma cell tumors can be associated with monoclonal gammopathies and should be considered in any list of differentials. These include other lymphoreticular tumors (B-cell lymphoma, extramedullary plasmacytoma, and chronic and acute B-lymphocytic leukemia), chronic infections (e.g., ehrlichiosis, leishmaniasis, feline infectious peritonitis), and MGUS.[763,767,826,71,836–839]

Treatment

Initial Therapy of Multiple Myeloma

Therapy for MM is directed at both the tumor cell mass and the secondary systemic effects they elicit. With the exception of treating life-threatening sequelae (e.g., marked hypercalcemia, infection, renal failure), all diagnostic procedures to confirm MM should be completed before initiating primary therapy to ensure a diagnosis is confirmed and baseline values are procured for monitoring response. Chemotherapy is effective at reducing malignant cell burden, relieving bone pain, allowing for skeletal healing, and reducing levels of serum immunoglobulins in the majority of dogs with MM, and will greatly extend both the quality and quantity of most patients' lives. MM in dogs is initially a gratifying disease to treat for both the clinician and the companion animal caregiver as durable remissions are the norm, although complete elimination of neoplastic myeloma cells is rarely achieved and eventual relapse is to be expected. Although most cats with MM will also initially respond to chemotherapy, overall response rates and durability of response and overall survival times are generally not as high nor as durable as in the dog; although a more recent compilation of 15 cats had a more favorable response to chemotherapy (see Prognosis section to follow).[769]

Melphalan, an alkylating agent, is the chemotherapeutic of choice for the treatment of multiple myeloma in the dog.[757,761,764] Two different melphalan protocols can be used. A continuous daily dosing regimen has been historically used in the dog with an initial starting dose of 0.1 mg/kg PO, once daily for 10 days, which is then reduced to 0.05 mg/kg PO, once daily continuously. The author prefers a pulse-dose protocol that was recently shown to result in statistically similar (albeit numerically superior) efficacy and with a similar adverse event profile.[761] The pulse-dosing regimen uses melphalan at 7 mg/m^2 PO, daily for 5 consecutive days every 3 weeks. This protocol also has the advantage of requiring the caregiver to administer fewer treatments with less overall exposure to chemotherapy during delivery and in body fluids. This protocol has been used successfully by the author in a small number of cases in which myelosuppression was limiting more traditional continuous low-dose therapy.

The addition of prednisone or prednisolone is thought to increase the efficacy of melphalan therapy. Prednisone is initiated at a dosage of 0.5 mg/kg PO, once daily for 10 days, then reduced to 0.5 mg/kg every other day before discontinuation after 60 days of therapy, although some continue every other day prednisone continuously. Melphalan is continued indefinitely until clinical relapse occurs or myelosuppression necessitates a dose reduction or discontinuation. The vast majority of dogs on melphalan and prednisone combination therapy tolerate the regimen well. The most clinically significant toxicity of melphalan is myelosuppression, in particular a delayed thrombocytopenia which can be slow to recover and in some cases irreversible. CBCs, including platelet counts, should be performed biweekly for 2 months of therapy and monthly thereafter in dogs on continuous protocols and just before pulse-dose when using the alternate protocol. If significant myelosuppression occurs (usually thrombocytopenia or neutropenia), a drug holiday is instituted with reintroduction at a lesser dose after marrow recovery. Alternatively, a different alkylating agent (e.g., cyclophosphamide, lomustine) may be substituted.

Although melphalan and prednisolone therapy can also be used in cats with multiple myeloma, it appears this protocol is more myelosuppressive than in the dog and many clinicians prefer to use a cyclophosphamide (250 mg/m^2 PO or IV every 2–3 weeks) and prednisolone (1 mg/kg PO daily for 2 weeks and then every other day) protocol or a COP protocol (see Section B of this chapter) in this species. Alternatively, some have used cyclophosphamide at a dose of 25 mg/cat twice weekly.[769,771] If using melphalan in the cat, a dosing schedule similar to the dog has been reported; 0.1 mg/kg once daily for 10 to 14 days, then every other day until clinical improvement or leukopenia develop. Long-term continuous maintenance (0.1 mg/kg, once every 7 days) has been advocated.[770] An alternative protocol advocated in the cat uses melphalan at 2 mg/m^2, once every 4 days continuously, and appears to be well tolerated.[771]

Cyclophosphamide has been used as an alternative alkylating agent or in combination with melphalan in dogs and cats with MM.[757,764,769,771] There is no evidence to suggest that it is superior to melphalan in the dog. In the author's practice, cyclophosphamide in dogs with MM is limited to those cases presenting with severe hypercalcemia or with widespread systemic involvement in which a faster acting alkylating agent may more quickly alleviate systemic effects of the disease. Cyclophosphamide is initiated at a dosage of 200 to 250 mg/m^2 IV or PO, once, at the same time oral melphalan is started. Because cyclophosphamide is less likely to affect platelets, it may be substituted in those patients in which thrombocytopenia has developed secondary to long-term melphalan use.

Chlorambucil, another alkylating agent, has been used successfully for the treatment of IgM macroglobulinemia in dogs at a dosage of 0.2 mg/kg PO, once daily.[764,804] Little or no clinical signs of toxicity result from this dosing schedule. Chlorambucil has also been used in cats with MRD.[771]

Lomustine (CCNU), yet another alkylating agent, has been used in a limited number of cats with MM and a partial response has been reported after dosing at 50 mg/m^2 PO, every 21 days.[840]

Evaluation of Response to Therapy

Evaluation of response to systemic therapy for MM is based on improvement in clinical signs, clinicopathologic parameters, radiographic improvement of skeletal lesions, ultrasonographic improvement of organ involvement, and, in some cases, bone marrow reassessment with molecular analysis of clonality.[757,761,762,764,771] Subjective improvement in clinical signs of bone pain, lameness, lethargy, and hyporexia should be evident within 3 to 4 weeks after initiation of therapy. Objective laboratory improvement, including reduction in serum total globulin, M component and calcium, along with normalization of the hemogram, is usually noted within 3 to 6 weeks (Fig. 33.29). Radiographic improvement in osteolytic bone lesions may take months and resolution may only be partial. Ophthalmic complications (including long-standing retinal detachments) and paraneoplastic neuropathies often resolve along with tumor mass.[810,831] In cats responding to chemotherapy, clinical improvement is noted in 2 to 4 weeks and serum protein and radiographic bone abnormalities were greatly improved by 8 weeks.[770,771]

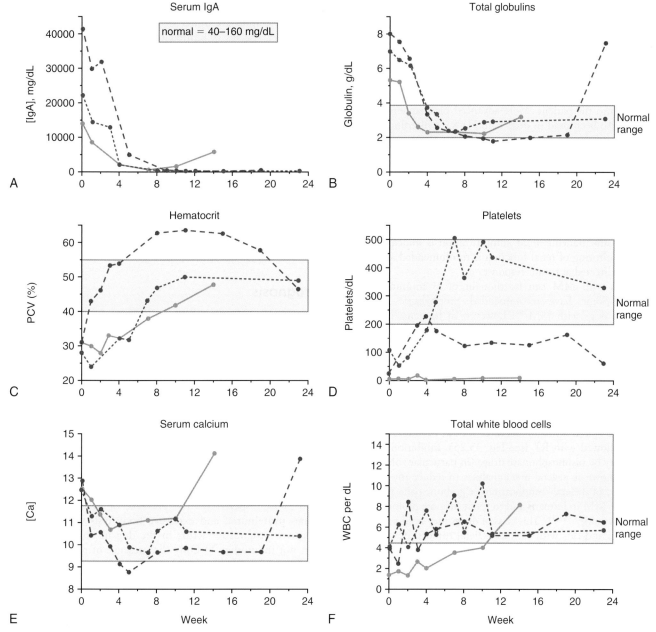

• **Fig. 33.29** Clinicopathologic data changes over time (weeks) after initiation of cytotoxic chemotherapy in three dogs with IgA multiple myeloma. *Light blue area,* Normal reference range. (A) Serum IgA (mg/dL); (B) Total globulins (g/dL). (C) Hematocrit (%). (D) Platelets/dL. (E) Serum calcium (mg/dL). (F) Total white blood cells/dL.

As previously discussed, complete resolution of MM does not generally occur and a good response is defined as a reduction in measured M-component (i.e., immunoglobulin or Bence Jones proteins) of at least 50% of pretreatment values.[764] Reduction in serum immunoglobulin levels may lag behind reductions in Bence Jones proteinuria because the half-lives are 15 to 20 days and 8 to 12 hours, respectively.[841] For routine follow-up, quantification of the increased serum globulin, immunoglobulin, or urine Bence Jones protein is performed monthly until a good response is noted and then every 2 to 3 months thereafter. Repeat bone marrow aspiration or imaging (in the case of visceral disease) for evaluation of plasma cell infiltration may be occasionally necessary. Bone marrow reevaluation is particularly prudent when cytopenias develop during chemotherapy, and drug-induced myelosuppression must be differentiated from myelophthisis due to neoplastic marrow recurrence.

Therapy Directed at Complications of Multiple Myeloma

The long-term control of complications, including hypercalcemia, HVS, bleeding diathesis, renal disease, immunosuppression with infection, ophthalmic complications, and pathologic skeletal fractures, depend on controlling the primary tumor mass. However, therapy directed more specifically at these complications may be indicated in the short term.

If hypercalcemia is marked and significant clinical signs exist, standard therapies, including fluid diuresis, with or without pharmacologic agents (e.g., zoledronate, calcitonin), may be indicated (see Chapter 5). Moderate hypercalcemia will typically begin to improve within 2 to 3 days after initiation of melphalan/prednisone chemotherapy without the addition of therapies directed at hypercalcemia specifically.

HVS is best treated in the short term by plasmapheresis.[764,808,813,838,844–846] Whole blood is collected from the patient and centrifuged to separate plasma from packed cells. Packed red cells are resuspended in normal saline or another crystalloid and reinfused into the patient. More advanced plasmapheresis methods have also been used in dogs with HVS.[842] Bleeding diathesis will usually resolve along with HVS; however, platelet-rich plasma transfusions may be necessary in the face of thrombocytopenia.

Renal impairment may necessitate aggressive fluid therapy in the short term and maintenance of adequate hydration in the long term. Careful attention to secondary urinary tract infections and appropriate antimicrobial therapy is indicated. Ensuring adequate water intake at home is important, and occasionally, educating owners in subcutaneous fluid administration is indicated. Continued monitoring of renal function is recommended along with follow-up directed at tumor response.

Patients with MM can be thought of as immunologically impaired. Some have recommended prophylactic antibiotic therapy in dogs with MM[764]; however, in humans, no benefit for this approach over diligent monitoring and aggressive antimicrobial management when indicated has been observed.[806] Cidal antimicrobials are preferred over static drugs, and avoidance of nephrotoxic antimicrobials is recommended.

Pathologic fractures of weight-bearing long bones and vertebrae resulting in spinal cord compression may require immediate surgical intervention in conjunction with systemic chemotherapy. Orthopedic stabilization of fractures should be undertaken and may be followed with RT (see Fig. 33.25). Inhibition of osteoclast activity by bisphosphonate drugs (in particular zoledronate), has been shown in several meta-analyses to reduce the incidence and severity of skeletal complications (e.g., bone pain, pathologic fracture) of MM in humans and to result in some prolongation of overall survival.[835,845,846] This class of drugs may hold promise for use in dogs and cats with various skeletal tumors; however, they have not been adequately evaluated for time-to-event efficacy in MRD in companion species.

Rescue Therapy

When MM eventually relapses in dogs and cats undergoing initial melphalan or alternative alkylator therapy or in the uncommon case that is initially resistant to alkylating agents, rescue therapy may be attempted. Switching to an alternate alkylating agent (e.g., cyclophosphamide, lomustine, chlorambucil) may be effective.[761,769] The author has also had limited success with VAD, which is a combination of doxorubicin (30 mg/m² IV, every 21 days), vincristine (0.7 mg/m² IV, days 8 and 15), and dexamethasone sodium phosphate (1.0 mg/kg IV, once a week on days 1, 8, and 15), given in 21-day cycles. Whereas most dogs initially respond to rescue protocols, the duration of response tends to be short, lasting only a few months. Liposomal doxorubicin has produced a long-term remission in a dog with MM previously resistant to native doxorubicin.[847]

Investigational Therapies

MM is ultimately a uniformly fatal disease in most species and thus significant effort is being placed on investigational therapies for this disease. Currently, bone marrow ablative therapy and marrow or stem cell rescue, thalidomide (and other antiangiogenic therapies), bortezomib (a proteasome inhibitor), arsenic trioxide, bisphosphonates, and several molecular targeting therapies are under investigation; however, their use in veterinary species is limited or completely absent at present. Bortezomib has been shown to have activity against canine melanoma in cell culture and mouse xenograft models.[848] A bortezomib protocol that is well-tolerated in dogs has been used successfully in the treatment of golden retriever muscular dystrophy but has not been, as yet, reported in dogs with MM.[849] One case report exists of a dog with MM that was resistant to melphalan, prednisone, and doxorubicin that subsequently achieved a partial response to tyrosine kinase inhibitor therapy (toceranib) that was maintained for 6 months.[776] Rabacfosadine (Tanovea-CA1) has been used investigationally in dogs with MM, either as induction therapy or for rescue in melphalan-resistant disease and significant efficacy, including durable molecular complete responses, was noted.[762] However, rabacfosadine is currently conditionally approved for use only in dogs with lymphoma.

Prognosis

The prognosis for dogs with MM is good for initial control of tumor and a return to good quality of life.[757,761,762] In a group of 60 dogs with MM, approximately 43% achieved complete remission (i.e., serum immunoglobulins normalized), 49% achieved a partial remission (i.e., immunoglobulins <50% pretreatment values), and only 8% did not respond to melphalan and prednisone chemotherapy.[757] Long-term survival is the norm, with a median survival time of 540 days reported (Fig. 33.30). More recently, in 38 dogs treated with melphalan/prednisone, 86% had objective responses (94% for pulse-dose protocol and 79% for continuous daily protocol) with a median progression-free and overall survival time (MST) of 601 and 930 days, respectively.[761] The 1-, 2-, and 3-year survival rates were 81%, 55%, and 30%, respectively. The presence of hypercalcemia, Bence Jones proteinuria, and extensive bony lysis were found to be negative prognostic factors in the dog in one large cohort,[757] but not in another.[761] Only the presence of renal disease and a high peripheral neutrophil:lymphocyte ratio at diagnosis were negative indices in the latter report.[761] Despite long-term durable responses in treated dogs, MM is generally a uniformly fatal disorder as drug-resistant recurrence of tumor mass and associated clinical signs is expected. Eventually, the tumor is no longer responsive to available chemotherapeutics and death follows from infection, renal failure, or euthanasia for intractable bone or spinal pain.[757,764]

The prognosis for MM in the cat is not as favorable as it is in the dog.[764,767,769–771,788] That being said, approximately 50% to 83% of cats with MM will respond to chemotherapy and although older compilations report MSTs of approximately 4 months, several long-term responses (i.e., >1 year) have been reported and a recent compilation documented MSTs of 8 to 13 months with treatment.[764,767,769–771,788,790,821] One investigator grouped MM in cats into two prognostic categories (Table 33.17) based on criteria known to predict behavior in dogs.[770] Although no rigorous statistical analysis was performed on this small group of nine cats, the MST for cats in "aggressive" and "nonaggressive" categories was 5 days and 387 days, respectively.

Experience in dogs with IgM macroglobulinemia is limited.[764,804–805] Response to chlorambucil is to be expected, and in nine treated dogs, 77% achieved remission with an MST of 11 months.[764]

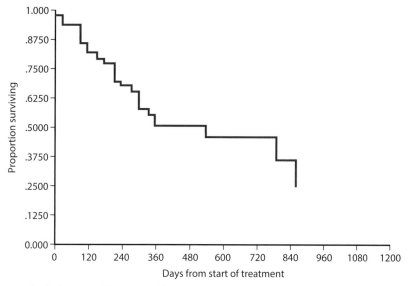

• **Fig. 33.30** Survival curve of 37 dogs with multiple myeloma treated with chemotherapy. The median survival time (MST) is 540 days. (From Matus RE, Leifer CE, MacEwen EG, et al. Prognostic factors for multiple myeloma in the dog. *J Am Vet Med Assoc.* 1986;188:1288-1292.)

TABLE 33.17	Classification of Multiple Myeloma in Cats Based on Clinical and Diagnostic Criteria Suspected of Predicting Prognosis[770]
Behavior Category	**Criteria**
Aggressive	Hypercalcemia, presence of bony lesions with pathologic fracture, low packed cell volume (PCV), presence of light-chain Bence Jones protein in urine, azotemia, hypercreatinemia, persistence of high serum protein level after 8 weeks of treatment, little or no clinical improvement
Less aggressive	Normal serum calcium, normal creatinine, blood urea nitrogen, PCV levels, presence of bony lesions without pathologic fractures, absence of light-chain Bence Jones protein, normalization of serum protein level after 8 weeks of treatment.

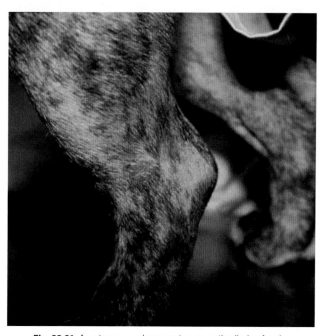

• **Fig. 33.31** A cutaneous plasmacytoma on the limb of a dog.

Solitary and Extramedullary Plasmacytic Tumors

Solitary collections of monoclonal plasmacytic tumors can originate in soft tissues or bone and are referred to as *extramedullary plasmacytoma* (EMP) and *solitary osseous plasmacytoma* (SOP), respectively. The systemic, multicentric, biologically aggressive EMP syndrome encountered in cats has been discussed in the MM section and will only receive limited discussion in this section.[771,786] A number of large case compilations of cutaneous plasmacytoma have been reported in the dog.[774,783,850–861] The most common locations for EMP in the dog are cutaneous (86%; Fig. 33.31), mucous membranes of the oral cavity and lips

(9%; Fig. 33.32), and the gastrointestinal tract (4%). The skin of the limbs and head (including the ears) are the most frequently reported cutaneous sites.[783] Oral plasmacytoma represents 5% of oral tumors, 2% of lingual tumors, and approximately 20% of all EMPs.[853] Other EMP sites uncommonly encountered include spleen, genitalia, eye, uterus, liver, larynx, trachea, third eyelid, sinonasal cavity (one case reported in the cat[862]), and intracranial sites.[863–871] The American cocker spaniel, English cocker spaniel, and West Highland white terrier (and perhaps Yorkshire terriers, boxers, German shepherds, and Airedale terriers) have been reported inconsistently to be at increased risk for developing plasmacytomas and the median age of affected dogs is 9 to 10 years of age.[783,853]

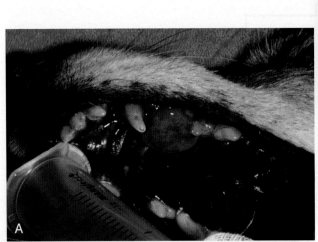
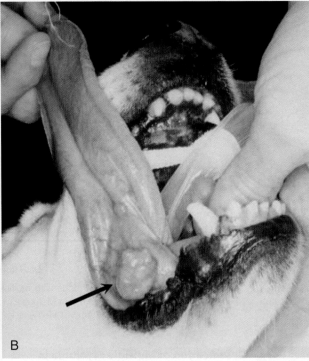

• **Fig. 33.32** Examples of oral solitary plasmacytoma in dogs; one involving the maxilla (A), the other involving the underside of the tongue (B). Both dogs were cured after surgical excision.

Pathology and Natural Behavior of Solitary and Extramedullary Plasmacytic Tumors

Cutaneous and oral EMP in dogs are typically benign tumors that are highly amenable to local therapy.[783,851,853,862,872] There exists, however, an uncommon form of multiple cutaneous plasmacytomas in the absence of MM referred to as *cutaneous plasmacytosis* in dogs that is a biologically aggressive disease with treatment and outcomes more like MM.[850,873,874] Three dogs with multiple oral plasmacytomas have been reported.[871] These were locally aggressive but did not metastasize and these dogs enjoyed long-term survival after surgical excision.

The natural behavior of noncutaneous/nonoral EMP appears to be somewhat more aggressive in the dog. Gastrointestinal EMP have been reported on a number of occasions in the veterinary literature, including the esophagus,[870] stomach,[874–877] and small[877] and large intestine.[876–880] Metastasis to associated lymph nodes is more common in these cases; however, bone marrow involvement and monoclonal gammopathies are less commonly encountered. Colorectal EMPs tend to be of low biologic aggressiveness, and most do not recur after surgical excision.[879] Conversely, the majority of SOPs eventually progress to systemic MM; however, the time course from local tumor development to systemic MM may be many months to years.[797,881] SOPs have been reported in the dog involving the appendicular skeleton, as well as the zygomatic arch, and ribs.[797]

SOPs are less common in cats, and fewer reports exist in the literature.[771,785,882–886] They occur in older cats (mean ages 9–14 years), with no significant sex predilection. The skin is the most common site; however, other sites include the oral cavity, eye, GI tract, liver, subcutaneous tissues, and brain. Reports exist of cutaneous EMP in cats that progressed to systemic MRD.[771,785,886]

History and Clinical Signs of Solitary and Extramedullary Plasmacytic Tumors

Clinical signs associated with EMPs and SOPs relate to the location of involvement, or in those rare cases with high levels of M component, HVS may occur. Most cutaneous plasmacytomas are solitary, smooth, raised pink, variably alopecic nodules from 1 to 2 cm in diameter (see Fig. 33.31), although tumors as large as 10 cm have been reported. Combining large series, greater than 95% occur as solitary masses and less than 1% occur as part of a systemic MM process.[774,98–861,873,874] Cutaneous and oral EMPs usually have a benign course with no related clinical signs.

Cutaneous plasmacytosis, however, is associated with multiple lesions, often with more than 10 and up to hundreds of lesions.[850] Some are ulcerated on presentation, but 81% were asymptomatic at presentation. Gastrointestinal EMPs typically have nonspecific signs which may suggest alimentary involvement. One dog with GI EMP was presented with intussusception.[878] Colorectal plasmacytomas often cause rectal bleeding, hematochezia, tenesmus, and rectal prolapse.[879] One case of ataxia and seizure activity in a dog with EMP secondary to tumor-associated hypoglycemia has been reported.[830] SOP is usually associated with pain and lameness if the appendicular skeleton is affected or neurologic signs if vertebral bodies are involved.

Diagnosis for Solitary and Extramedullary Plasmacytic Tumors

The diagnosis of SOP and EMP usually requires tissue biopsy or needle aspiration cytology for diagnosis. Cells making up solitary plasmacytic tumors in both cats and dogs have been histologically classified into mature, hyaline, cleaved, asynchronous, monomorphous blastic and polymorphous blastic cell types; however, no prognostic significance has been observed after classification, although it has been suggested that the polymorphous-blastic type may act more aggressively in the dog.[774,852,859,880] A divergent pseudoglandular histologic subtype has been reported in a small number of dogs that may be confused with epithelial neoplasia.[851] Intravascular tumor cells were observed in 16% of cutaneous plasmacytoma samples in one report, but this was not found to correlate with outcome and most were behaviorally benign.[783] A different classification was proposed for EMP in cats based on percentage of plasmablasts, and some prognostic importance has been documented.[786] In the case of poorly differentiated plasmacytic tumors, IHC studies, directed at detecting immunoglobulin, light and heavy chains, MM-1/interferon regulatory factor-4 (MUM1/IRF4), and thioflavin T, may be helpful in differentiation from other round cell tumors.[797,857,859,882,883,887–889] Of note, canine cutaneous histiocytoma (not histiocytic sarcoma) can be immunoreactive for MUM1 and therefore should be considered in any MUM1+ differential.[853] Immunoreactivity has been demonstrated for canine IgG F(ab)$_2$ and vimentin.[854] A variant characterized by an IgG-reactive amyloid interspersed with the neoplastic cells has also been described.[861] A panel of monoclonal antibodies (recognizing tryptase, chymase, serotonin, CD1a, CD3, CD79a, CD18, and MHC class II) in association with a histochemical stain (naphthol AS-D chloroacetate) has been advocated for use on formalin-fixed, paraffin-embedded sections of cutaneous round cell tumors to help classify poorly differentiated round cell tumors (mast cell tumors, histiocytomas, lymphomas, and plasmacytomas).[888] In addition, clonality of the immunoglobulin heavy chain variable region gene can be performed in plasmacytomas and myelomas using PCR technology, and this may have some diagnostic utility in difficult cases.[762]

It is important to thoroughly stage dogs and cats with plasmacytomas that are at higher risk for systemic spread if contemplating local or locoregional therapy without systemic therapy. This should include bone marrow aspiration cytology, serum electrophoresis, abdominal ultrasound, and skeletal survey radiographs to ensure the disease is confined to a local site before initiation of therapy. Several, albeit rare, instances of monoclonal gammopathy or plasma cell leukemia have been reported in dogs with cutaneous plasmacytoma, cutaneous plasmacytosis and gastrointestinal EMP.[850,874,890,891] Staging is likely most important in cases of cutaneous plasmacytosis, SOP, and GI EMP due to their relatively high metastatic rate, but is less important for cutaneous, oral, and colorectal plasmacytomas because of their more typical benign behavior. Cutaneous plasmacytosis was associated with lymph node or abdominal viscera involvement in approximately 30% of cases; however, no cases in a large compilation had positive bone marrow aspirates and only one dog had a monoclonal gammopathy.[850] For GI EMP (including colorectal EMP), endoscopic evaluation of the entire GI tract is recommended. A single case report of the use of PET/CT imaging for extramedullary splenic plasmacytoma in a dog exists; however, its utility remains unknown.[892]

Therapy for Solitary and Extramedullary Plasmacytic Tumors

Cutaneous and oral plasma cell tumors in the dog are almost always benign and carry an excellent prognosis after conservative surgical excision.[774,783,853,859,860,879,893] The exception is cutaneous plasmacytosis where excision is not possible due to the number of lesions and the fact that 30% of cases have documented

systemic disease.[850] Systemic chemotherapy is therefore indicated for dogs with cutaneous plasmacytosis; approximately three-quarters of 14 cases experienced objective responses to either melphalan or lomustine and median progression-free and overall STs were 153 and 542 days, respectively.[850] EMPs of the trachea, liver, and uterus have also been reported in dogs, and all had a benign course after local resection.[864–866] Successful therapy with melphalan and prednisone has been rarely applied for a local recurrence or incomplete margins in dogs and cats. RT has been used infrequently for cases that are not surgical candidates, including the application of strontium-90 plesiotherapy for lingual plasmacytoma in a dog.[894] Surgery is recommended, in combination with RT, for those cases of SOP in which the lesion results in an unstable, long bone fracture (see Fig. 33.25), or the patient is nonambulatory from neurologic compromise resulting from a vertebral body SOP. In the latter case, spinal cord decompression, mass excision, and possibly spinal stabilization may be necessary.[829] RT can be used alone (i.e., without surgery) in those cases where fractures are stable, as a palliative measure for bone pain, or in the case of vertebral SOP if the patient is ambulatory and stable. Good local control is usually achieved; however, most progress to systemic MM.[797,828,881] SOP of the axial skeleton can be managed by excision or RT alone. There is controversy as to whether systemic chemotherapy should be initiated at the time of local therapy for SOP when systemic involvement is not documented. Systemic spread may not occur for many months to even years beyond primary SOP diagnosis in humans and dogs, and studies in humans reveal no benefit to initiating systemic chemotherapy before progression to systemic disease.[807,828] Two cases of SOP in cats were recently reported; one was treated with external-beam RT and one managed with melphalan chemotherapy and both enjoyed durable remissions of greater than 4 years.[895] Similarly, EMP of the GI tract in humans are treated most commonly by surgical excision and thorough staging of disease. Systemic therapy is not initiated unless systemic involvement is documented. Systemic chemotherapy has been used after gastric EMP in a cat; however, the utility of adjuvant therapy in the species is unknown.[896]

Long-term follow-up of patients with SOP is indicated to recognize both recurrence of disease and systemic spread. Careful attention is given to serum globulin levels, bone pain, and radiographic appearance of bone healing in cases of SOP. Restaging of disease, including bone marrow evaluation, is indicated if systemic spread is suspected.

Prognosis for Solitary and Extramedullary Plasmacytic Tumors

Prognosis for solitary plasma cell tumors is generally good. Cutaneous and mucocutaneous plasmacytomas are usually cured after surgical excision.[774,859,893] In large compilations of cases in dogs, the local recurrence rate was approximately 5%, and nodal or distant metastasis occurred in only 7 of 349 cases (2%).[774,783,98,855,859,860] New cutaneous plasmacytomas at sites distant from the primary developed in fewer than 2% of cases. Neither tumor cell proliferation rate (as measured by Ki67 IHC), intravascular tumor infiltration/emboli in the dog, nor histopathologic grading in dogs and cats were prognostic in large compilations of cases, although it has been suggested that the polymorphous-blastic and plasmablastic type may act more aggressively in the dog and cat.[774,783,786,859] The presence of amyloid and overexpression of cyclin D1 (prognostic in human plasmacytomas) were not shown to be of prognostic value in dogs.[774] Dogs with EMP of the alimentary tract and other abdominal organs (e.g., liver, uterus) treated by surgical excision alone or in combination with systemic chemotherapy (if metastasis is present) can enjoy long-term survival in the majority of cases.[797,864–866,870,875–877,880] In a compilation of nine dogs with colorectal plasmacytoma, two dogs had local recurrence at 5 and 8 months after surgery, and the overall MST was 15 months after surgery alone.[879] DNA ploidy and Myc oncoprotein expression in biopsy samples were determined to be prognostic for EMPs in dogs; however, those that were malignant were all from noncutaneous sites (i.e., lymph node, colon, spleen). Therefore location appears to be as predictive.[897] As previously discussed, the majority of cases of SOP will eventually develop systemic disease; however, long disease-free periods usually precede the event.

The prognosis in cats is less well-defined because of the paucity of reported cases. If disease is confined to a local site and/or regional nodes, surgical excision and chemotherapy can result in long-term control; however, early, widespread metastasis and progression to MM is also reported in cats.[771,785,857,882,884,885,896]

References

1. Boerkamp KM, Teske E, Boon LR, et al.: Estimated incidence rate and distribution of tumours in 4,653 cases of archival submissions derived from the Dutch golden retriever population, *BMC Vet Res* 10(34), 2014.
2. Dorn CR, Taylor DO, Frye FL, et al.: Survey of animal neoplasms in Alameda and Contra Costa Counties, California. I. Methodology and description of cases, *J Natl Cancer Inst* 40:295–305, 1968.
3. Dorn CR, Taylor DO, Schneider R: The epidemiology of canine leukemia and lymphoma, *Bibl Haematol* 403–415, 1970.
4. Merlo DF, Rossi L, Pellegrino C, et al.: Cancer incidence in pet dogs: findings of the Animal Tumor Registry of Genoa, Italy, *J Vet Intern Med* 22:976–984, 2008.
5. Kaiser H: Animal neoplasia: a systemic review. In Kaiser H, editor: *neoplasms-comparative pathology in animals, plants and man*, Baltimore, 1981, Wiliams & Wilkins.
6. Moulton JE, Harvey HJ: Tumors of lymphoid and hematopoietic tissue. In Moulton JE, editor: *tumors of domestic animals*, ed 3, Berkley, CA, 1990, Univeristy of California Press.
7. Jemal A, Tiwari RC, Murray T, et al.: Cancer statistics, 2004, *CA Cancer J Clin* 54:8–29, 2004.
8. Ernst T, Kessler M, Lautscham E, et al.: Multicentric lymphoma in 411 dogs - an epidemiological study, *Tierarztl Prax Ausg K Kleintiere Heimtiere* 44:245–251, 2016.
9. Villamil JA, Henry CJ, Hahn AW, et al.: Hormonal and sex impact on the epidemiology of canine lymphoma, *J Cancer Epidemiol* 2009:591753, 2009.
10. Edwards DS, Henley WE, Harding EF, et al.: Breed incidence of lymphoma in a UK population of insured dogs, *Vet Comp Oncol* 1:200–206, 2003.
11. Priester WA, McKay FW: The occurrence of tumors in domestic animals, *Natl Cancer Inst Monogr* 1–210, 1980.
12. Breen M, Modiano JF: Evolutionarily conserved cytogenetic changes in hematological malignancies of dogs and humans—man and his best friend share more than companionship, *Chromosome Res* 16:145–154, 2008.
13. Devitt JJ, Maranon DG, Ehrhart EJ, et al.: Correlations between numerical chromosomal aberrations in the tumor and peripheral blood in canine lymphoma, *Cytogenet Genome Res* 124:12–18, 2009.
14. Thomas R, Fiegler H, Ostrander EA, et al.: A canine cancer-gene microarray for CGH analysis of tumors, *Cytogenet Genome Res* 102:254–260, 2003.
15. Thomas R, Seiser EL, Motsinger-Reif A, et al.: Refining tumor-associated aneuploidy through 'genomic recoding' of recurrent DNA copy number aberrations in 150 canine non-Hodgkin lymphomas, *Leuk Lymphoma* 52:1321–1335, 2011.
16. Thomas R, Smith KC, Gould R, et al.: Molecular cytogenetic analysis of a novel high-grade canine T-lymphoblastic lymphoma demonstrating co-expression of CD3 and CD79a cell markers, *Chromosome Res* 9:649–657, 2001.
17. Thomas R, Smith KC, Ostrander EA, et al.: Chromosome aberrations in canine multicentric lymphomas detected with comparative genomic hybridisation and a panel of single locus probes, *Br J Cancer* 89:1530–1537, 2003.
18. Starkey MP, Murphy S: Using lymph node fine needle aspirates for gene expression profiling of canine lymphoma, *Vet Comp Oncol* 2010(8):56–71, 2010.
19. Lindblad-Toh K, Wade CM, Mikkelsen TS, et al.: Genome sequence, comparative analysis and haplotype structure of the domestic dog, *Nature* 438:803–819, 2005.
20. Hahn KA, Richardson RC, Hahn EA, et al.: Diagnostic and prognostic importance of chromosomal aberrations identified in 61 dogs with lymphosarcoma, *Vet Pathol* 31:528–540, 1994.
21. Elvers I, Turner-Maier J, Swofford R, et al.: Exome sequencing of lymphomas from three dog breeds reveals somatic mutation patterns reflecting genetic background, *Genome Res* 25:1634–1645, 2015.
22. Mudaliar MA, Haggart RD, Miele G, et al.: Comparative gene expression profiling identifies common molecular signatures of NF-kappaB activation in canine and human diffuse large B cell lymphoma (DLBCL), *PLoS One* 8:e72591, 2013.
23. Thomas R, Demeter Z, Kennedy KA, et al.: Integrated immunohistochemical and DNA copy number profiling analysis provides insight into the molecular pathogenesis of canine follicular lymphoma, *Vet Comp Oncol* 15:852–867, 2017.
24. Tonomura N, Elvers I, Thomas R, et al.: Genome-wide association study identifies shared risk loci common to two malignancies in golden retrievers, *PLoS Genet* 11:e1004922, 2015.
25. Ulve R, Rault M, Bahin M, et al.: Discovery of human-similar gene fusions in canine cancers, *Cancer Res* 2017(77):5721–5727, 2017.
26. Nasir L, Argyle DJ: Mutational analysis of the tumour suppressor gene p53 in lymphosarcoma in two bull mastiffs, *Vet Rec* 145:23–24, 1999.
27. Pelham JT, Irwin PJ, Kay PH: Genomic hypomethylation in neoplastic cells from dogs with malignant lymphoproliferative disorders, *Res Vet Sci* 74:101–104, 2003.
28. Setoguchi A, Sakai T, Okuda M, et al.: Aberrations of the p53 tumor suppressor gene in various tumors in dogs, *Am J Vet Res* 62:433–439, 2001.
29. Sueiro FA, Alessi AC, Vassallo J: Canine lymphomas: a morphological and immunohistochemical study of 55 cases, with observations on p53 immunoexpression, *J Comp Pathol* 131:207–213, 2004.
30. Veldhoen N, Stewart J, Brown R, et al.: Mutations of the p53 gene in canine lymphoma and evidence for germ line p53 mutations in the dog, *Oncogene* 16:249–255, 1998.
31. Sokolowska J, Cywinska A, Malicka E: p53 expression in canine lymphoma, *J Vet Med A Physiol Pathol Clin Med* 52:172–175, 2005.
32. Modiano JF, Breen M, Burnett RC, et al.: Distinct B-cell and T-cell lymphoproliferative disease prevalence among dog breeds indicates heritable risk, *Cancer Res* 65:5654–5661, 2005.
33. Carioto LM, Kruth SA, Betts DH, et al.: Telomerase activity in clinically normal dogs and dogs with malignant lymphoma, *Am J Vet Res* 62:1442–1446, 2001.
34. Nasir L, Devlin P, McKevitt T, et al.: Telomere lengths and telomerase activity in dog tissues: a potential model system to study human telomere and telomerase biology, *Neoplasia* 3:351–359, 2001.
35. Yazawa M, Okuda M, Kanaya N, et al.: Molecular cloning of the canine telomerase reverse transcriptase gene and its expression in neoplastic and non-neoplastic cells, *Am J Vet Res* 64:1395–1400, 2003.
36. Thamm DH, Grunerud KK, Rose BJ, et al.: DNA repair deficiency as a susceptibility marker for spontaneous lymphoma in golden retriever dogs: a case-control study, *PLoS One* 8(e69192), 2013.

37. Waugh EM, Gallagher A, McAulay KA, et al.: Gammaherpesviruses and canine lymphoma: no evidence for direct involvement in commonly occurring lymphomas, *J Gen Virol* 96:1863–1872, 2015.

38. Milman G, Smith KC, Erles K: Serological detection of Epstein-Barr virus infection in dogs and cats, *Vet Microbiol* 150:15–20, 2011.

39. Farinha P, Gascoyne RD: Helicobacter pylori and MALT lymphoma, *Gastroenterology* 128:1579–1605, 2005.

40. Rossi G, Rossi M, Vitali CG, et al.: A conventional beagle dog model for acute and chronic infection with Helicobacter pylori, *Infect Immun* 67:3112–3120, 1999.

41. Gavazza A, Rossi G, Lubas G, et al.: Faecal microbiota in dogs with multicentric lymphoma, *Vet Comp Oncol*, 2017.

42. Ruple A, Avery AC, Morley PS: Differences in the geographic distribution of lymphoma subtypes in Golden retrievers in the USA, *Vet Comp Oncol* 15:1590–1597, 2017.

43. Takashima-Uebelhoer BB, Barber LG, Zagarins SE, et al.: Household chemical exposures and the risk of canine malignant lymphoma, a model for human non-Hodgkin's lymphoma, *Environ Res* 112:171–176, 2012.

44. Hayes HM, Tarone RE, Cantor KP, et al.: Case-control study of canine malignant lymphoma: positive association with dog owner's use of 2,4-dichlorophenoxyacetic acid herbicides, *J Natl Cancer Inst* 83:1226–1231, 1991.

45. Reynolds PM, Reif JS, Ramsdell HS, et al.: Canine exposure to herbicide-treated lawns and urinary excretion of 2,4-dichlorophenoxyacetic acid, *Cancer Epidemiol Biomarkers Prev* 3:233–237, 1994.

46. Carlo GL, Cole P, Miller AB, et al.: Review of a study reporting an association between 2,4-dichlorophenoxyacetic acid and canine malignant lymphoma: report of an expert panel, *Regul Toxicol Pharmacol* 16:245–252, 1992.

47. Garabrant DH, Philbert MA: Review of 2,4-dichlorophenoxyacetic acid (2,4-D) epidemiology and toxicology, *Crit Rev Toxicol* 32:233–257, 2002.

48. Kaneene JB, Miller R: Re-analysis of 2,4-D use and the occurrence of canine malignant lymphoma, *Vet Hum Toxicol* 41:164–170, 1999.

49. Gavazza A, Presciuttini S, Barale R, et al.: Association between canine malignant lymphoma, living in industrial areas, and use of chemicals by dog owners, *J Vet Intern Med* 15:190–195, 2001.

50. Reif JS, Lower KS, Ogilvie GK: Residential exposure to magnetic fields and risk of canine lymphoma, *Am J Epidemiol* 141:352–359, 1995.

51. Marconato L, Leo C, Girelli R, et al.: Association between waste management and cancer in companion animals, *J Vet Intern Med* 23:564–569, 2009.

52. Pastor M, Chalvet-Monfray K, Marchal T, et al.: Genetic and environmental risk indicators in canine non-Hodgkin's lymphomas: breed associations and geographic distribution of 608 cases diagnosed throughout France over 1 year, *J Vet Intern Med* 23:301–310, 2009.

53. Pinello KC, Santos M, Leite-Martins L, et al.: Immunocytochemical study of canine lymphomas and its correlation with exposure to tobacco smoke, *Vet World* 10:1307–1313, 2017.

54. Keller ET: Immune-mediated disease as a risk factor for canine lymphoma, *Cancer* 70:2334–2337, 1992.

55. Foster AP, Sturgess CP, Gould DJ, et al.: Pemphigus foliaceus in association with systemic lupus erythematosus, and subsequent lymphoma in a cocker spaniel, *J Small Anim Pract* 41:266–270, 2000.

56. Aronson LR: Update on the current status of kidney transplantation for chronic kidney disease in animals, *Vet Clin North Am Small Anim Pract* 46:1193–1218, 2016.

57. Blackwood L, German AJ, Stell AJ, et al.: Multicentric lymphoma in a dog after cyclosporine therapy, *J Small Anim Pract* 45:259–262, 2004.

58. Schmiedt CW, Grimes JA, Holzman G, et al.: Incidence and risk factors for development of malignant neoplasia after feline renal transplantation and cyclosporine-based immunosuppression, *Vet Comp Oncol* 7:45–53, 2009.

59. Santoro D, Marsella R, Hernandez J: Investigation on the association between atopic dermatitis and the development of mycosis fungoides in dogs: a retrospective case-control study, *Vet Dermatol* 18:101–106, 2007.

60. Madewell B: Hematopoietic neoplasms, sarcomas and related conditions. In Theilen GH, Madewell B, editors: *Veterinary Cancer Medicine*, ed 2, Philadelphia, 1987, Lea and Febiger.

61. Couto CG, Rutgers HC, Sherding RG, et al.: Gastrointestinal lymphoma in 20 dogs. A retrospective study, *J Vet Intern Med* 1989(3):73–78, 1989.

62. Ozaki K, Yamagami T, Nomura K, et al.: T-cell lymphoma with eosinophilic infiltration involving the intestinal tract in 11 dogs, *Vet Pathol* 43:339–344, 2006.

63. Breitschwerdt EB, Waltman C, Hagstad HV, et al.: Clinical and epidemiologic characterization of a diarrheal syndrome in Basenji dogs, *J Am Vet Med Assoc* 180:914–920, 1982.

64. Couto KM, Moore PF, Zwingenberger AL, et al.: Clinical characteristics and outcome in dogs with small cell T-cell intestinal lymphoma, *Vet Comp Oncol*, 2018. https://doi.org/10.1111/vco.12384. epub ahead of print.

65. Coyle KA, Steinberg H: Characterization of lymphocytes in canine gastrointestinal lymphoma, *Vet Pathol* 41:141–146, 2004.

66. Steinberg H, Dubielzig RR, Thomson J, et al.: Primary gastrointestinal lymphosarcoma with epitheliotropism in three Shar-pei and one boxer dog, *Vet Pathol* 32:423–426, 1995.

67. Rosenberg MP, Matus RE, Patnaik AK: Prognostic factors in dogs with lymphoma and associated hypercalcemia, *J Vet Intern Med* 5:268–271, 1991.

68. Vail DM, Kisseberth WC, Obradovich JE, et al.: Assessment of potential doubling time (Tpot), argyrophilic nucleolar organizer regions (AgNOR), and proliferating cell nuclear antigen (PCNA) as predictors of therapy response in canine non-Hodgkin's lymphoma, *Exp Hematol* 24:807–815, 1996.

69. Ruslander DA, Gebhard DH, Tompkins MB, et al.: Immunophenotypic characterization of canine lymphoproliferative disorders, *Vivo* 11:169–172, 1997.

70. Ortiz AL, Carvalho S, Leo C, et al.: Gamma delta T-cell large granular lymphocyte lymphoma in a dog, *Vet Clin Pathol* 44:442–447, 2015.

71. Moore PF, Affolter VK, Keller SM: Canine inflamed nonepitheliotropic cutaneous T-cell lymphoma: a diagnostic conundrum, *Vet Dermatol* 24:204–211, e244–205, 2013.

72. Gross T, Ihrke PJ, Walder EJ, et al.: Lymphocytic neoplasms. In Gross TL, Ihrke PJ, Walder EJ, et al.: *Skin diseases of the dog and cat*, ed 2, Oxford, 2005, Blackwell, pp 866–893.

73. Broder S, Muul L, Marshall S, et al.: Neoplasms of immunoregulatory T cells in clinical investigation, *J Invest Dermatol* 74:267–271, 1980.

74. Fontaine J, Heimann M, Day MJ: Canine cutaneous epitheliotropic T-cell lymphoma: a review of 30 cases, *Vet Dermatol* 21:267–275, 2010.

75. Moore PF, Affolter VK, Graham PS, et al.: Canine epitheliotropic cutaneous T-cell lymphoma: an investigation of T-cell receptor immunophenotype, lesion topography and molecular clonality, *Vet Dermatol* 20:569–576, 2009.

76. Moore PF, Olivry T, Naydan D: Canine cutaneous epitheliotropic lymphoma (mycosis fungoides) is a proliferative disorder of CD8+ T cells, *Am J Pathol* 144:421–429, 1994.

77. Affolter VK, Gross TL, Moore PF: Indolent cutaneous T-cell lymphoma presenting as cutaneous lymphocytosis in dogs, *Vet Dermatol* 20:577–585, 2009.

78. Foster AP, Evans E, Kerlin RL, et al.: Cutaneous T-cell lymphoma with Sezary syndrome in a dog, *Vet Clin Pathol* 26:188–192, 1997.

79. Schick RO, Murphy GF, Goldschmidt MH: Cutaneous lymphosarcoma and leukemia in a cat, *J Am Vet Med Assoc* 203:1155–1158, 1993.

80. Thrall MA, Macy DW, Snyder SP, et al.: Cutaneous lymphosarcoma and leukemia in a dog resembling Sezary syndrome in man, *Vet Pathol* 21:182–186, 1984.

81. Keller SM, Vernau W, Hodges J, et al.: Hepatosplenic and hepatocytotropic T-cell lymphoma: two distinct types of T-cell lymphoma in dogs, *Vet Pathol* 50:281–290, 2013.

82. Cienava EA, Barnhart KF, Brown R, et al.: Morphologic, immunohistochemical, and molecular characterization of hepatosplenic T-cell lymphoma in a dog, *Vet Clin Pathol* 33:105–110, 2004.

83. Fry MM, Vernau W, Pesavento PA, et al.: Hepatosplenic lymphoma in a dog, *Vet Pathol* 40:556–562, 2003.

84. Dargent FJ, Fox LE, Anderson WI: Neoplastic angioendotheliomatosis in a dog: an angiotropic lymphoma, *Cornell Vet* 78:253–262, 1988.

85. McDonough SP, Van Winkle TJ, Valentine BA, et al.: Clinicopathological and immunophenotypical features of canine intravascular lymphoma (malignant angioendotheliomatosis), *J Comp Pathol* 126:277–288, 2002.

86. Ridge L, Swinney G: Angiotrophic intravascular lymphosarcoma presenting as bi-cavity effusion in a dog, *Aust Vet J* 82:616–618, 2004.

87. Bush WW, Throop JL, McManus PM, et al.: Intravascular lymphoma involving the central and peripheral nervous systems in a dog, *J Am Anim Hosp Assoc* 39:90–96, 2003.

88. Cullen CL, Caswell JL, Grahn BH: Intravascular lymphoma presenting as bilateral panophthalmitis and retinal detachment in a dog, *J Am Anim Hosp Assoc* 36:337–342, 2000.

89. Summers BA, deLahunta A: Cerebral angioendotheliomatosis in a dog, *Acta Neuropathol* 68:10–14, 1985.

90. Valli VE, Kass PH, San Myint M, et al.: Canine lymphomas: association of classification type, disease stage, tumor subtype, mitotic rate, and treatment with survival, *Vet Pathol* 50:738–748, 2013.

91. Berry CR, Moore PF, Thomas WP, et al.: Pulmonary lymphomatoid granulomatosis in seven dogs (1976-1987), *J Vet Intern Med* 4:157–166, 1990.

92. Hatoya S, Kumagai D, Takeda S, et al.: Successful management with CHOP for pulmonary lymphomatoid granulomatosis in a dog, *J Vet Med Sci* 73:527–530, 2011.

93. Park HM, Hwang DN, Kang BT, et al.: Pulmonary lymphomatoid granulomatosis in a dog: evidence of immunophenotypic diversity and relationship to human pulmonary lymphomatoid granulomatosis and pulmonary Hodgkin's disease, *Vet Pathol* 44:921–923, 2007.

94. Fitzgerald SD, Wolf DC, Carlton WW: Eight cases of canine lymphomatoid granulomatosis, *Vet Pathol* 28:241–245, 1991.

95. Ponce F, Marchal T, Magnol JP, et al.: A morphological study of 608 cases of canine malignant lymphoma in France with a focus on comparative similarities between canine and human lymphoma morphology, *Vet Pathol* 47:414–433, 2010.

96. Seelig DM, Avery AC, Ehrhart EJ, et al.: The comparative diagnostic features of canine and human lymphoma, *Vet Sci* 3:11, 2016.

97. Burkhard MJ, Bienzle D: Making sense of lymphoma diagnostics in small animal patients, *Vet Clin North Am Small Anim Pract* 43:1331–1347, vii, 2013.

98. Vezzali E, Parodi AL, Marcato PS, et al.: Histopathologic classification of 171 cases of canine and feline non-Hodgkin lymphoma according to the WHO, *Vet Comp Oncol* 8:38–49, 2010.

99. Valli VE, San Myint M, Barthel A, et al.: Classification of canine malignant lymphomas according to the World Health Organization criteria, *Vet Pathol* 48:198–211, 2011.

100. Stefanello D, Valenti P, Zini E, et al.: Splenic marginal zone lymphoma in 5 dogs (2001-2008), *J Vet Intern Med* 25:90–93, 2011.

101. Flood-Knapik KE, Durham AC, Gregor TP, et al.: Clinical, histopathological and immunohistochemical characterization of canine indolent lymphoma, *Vet Comp Oncol* 11:272–286, 2013.

102. Valli VE, Vernau W, de Lorimier LP, et al.: Canine indolent nodular lymphoma, *Vet Pathol* 43:241–256, 2006.

103. National Cancer Institute sponsored study of classifications of non-Hodgkin's lymphomas: summary and description of a working formulation for clinical usage. The Non-Hodgkin's Lymphoma Pathologic Classification Project, *Cancer* 49:2112–2135, 1982.

104. Lennert KFA: *Histopathology of non-hodgkin's lymphomas (based on the updated kiel classification)*, ed 2, Berlin, 1990, Springer-Verlag.

105. Carter RF, Valli VE, Lumsden JH: The cytology, histology and prevalence of cell types in canine lymphoma classified according to the National Cancer Institute Working Formulation, *Can J Vet Res* 50:154–164, 1986.

106. Bromberek JL, Rout ED, Agnew MR, et al.: Breed distribution and clinical characteristics of b cell chronic lymphocytic leukemia in dogs, *J Vet Intern Med* 30:215–222, 2016.

107. Hughes KL, Labadie JD, Yoshimoto JA, et al.: Increased frequency of CD45 negative T cells (T zone cells) in older Golden retriever dogs, *Vet Comp Oncol* 16:E109–E116, 2018.

108. Cozzi M, Marconato L, Martini V, et al.: Canine nodal marginal zone lymphoma: descriptive insight into the biological behaviour, *Vet Comp Oncol* 16:246–252, 2018.

109. Mizutani N, Goto-Koshino Y, Takahashi M, et al.: Clinical and histopathological evaluation of 16 dogs with T-zone lymphoma, *J Vet Med Sci* 78:1237–1244, 2016.

110. Moore AS: Treatment of T cell lymphoma in dogs, *Vet Rec* 179:277, 2016.

111. Sayag D, Fournel-Fleury C, Ponce F: Prognostic significance of morphotypes in canine lymphomas: a systematic review of literature, *Vet Comp Oncol* 16:12–19, 2018.

112. Teske E, van Heerde P, Rutteman GR, et al.: Prognostic factors for treatment of malignant lymphoma in dogs, *J Am Vet Med Assoc* 205:1722–1728, 1994.

113. Appelbaum FR, Sale GE, Storb R, et al.: Phenotyping of canine lymphoma with monoclonal antibodies directed at cell surface antigens: classification, morphology, clinical presentation and response to chemotherapy, *Hematol Oncol* 2:151–168, 1984.

114. Rosol TJ, Capen CC: Mechanisms of cancer-induced hypercalcemia, *Lab Invest* 67:680–702, 1992.

115. Weir ECGP, Matus R, et al.: Hypercalcemia in canine lymphosarcoma is associated with the T cell subtype and with secretion of a PTH-like factor, *J Bone Miner Res* 3, 1988.

116. Greenlee PG, Filippa DA, Quimby FW, et al.: Lymphomas in dogs. A morphologic, immunologic, and clinical study, *Cancer* 66:480–490, 1990.

117. Fournel-Fleury C, Ponce F, Felman P, et al.: Canine T-cell lymphomas: a morphological, immunological, and clinical study of 46 new cases, *Vet Pathol* 39:92–109, 2002.

118. Wilkerson MJ, Dolce K, Koopman T, et al.: Lineage differentiation of canine lymphoma/leukemias and aberrant expression of CD molecules, *Vet Immunol Immunopathol* 106:179–196, 2005.

119. Day MJ: Immunophenotypic characterization of cutaneous lymphoid neoplasia in the dog and cat, *J Comp Pathol* 112:79–96, 1995.

120. Barber LG, Weishaar KM: Criteria for designation of clinical substage in canine lymphoma: a survey of veterinary oncologists, *Vet Comp Oncol* 14(Suppl 1):32–39, 2016.

121. Blackwood L, Sullivan M, Lawson H: Radiographic abnormalities in canine multicentric lymphoma: a review of 84 cases, *J Small Anim Pract* 38:62–69, 1997.

122. Starrak GS, Berry CR, Page RL, et al.: Correlation between thoracic radiographic changes and remission/survival duration in 270 dogs with lymphosarcoma, *Vet Radiol Ultrasound* 38:411–418, 1997.

123. Congress '99: what's new in the treatment of lymphoma? *J Small Anim Pract* 40:51, 1999.

124. Yohn SE, Hawkins EC, Morrison WB, et al.: Confirmation of a pulmonary component of multicentric lymphosarcoma with bronchoalveolar lavage in two dogs, *J Am Vet Med Assoc* 204:97–101, 1994.

125. Lane J, Price J, Moore A, et al.: Low-grade gastrointestinal lymphoma in dogs: 20 cases (2010 to 2016), *J Small Anim Pract* 59:147–153, 2018.
126. Sogame N, Risbon R, Burgess KE: Intestinal lymphoma in dogs: 84 cases (1997-2012), *J Am Vet Med Assoc* 252:440–447, 2018.
127. Gieger T: Alimentary lymphoma in cats and dogs, *Vet Clin North Am Small Anim Pract* 41:419–432, 2011.
128. Leib MS, et al.: Alimentary lymphosarcoma in a dog, *Compend Pract Vet Contin Educ* 9:809–815, 1987.
129. Chan CM, Frimberger AE, Moore AS: Clinical outcome and prognosis of dogs with histopathological features consistent with epitheliotropic lymphoma: a retrospective study of 148 cases (2003-2015), *Vet Dermatol* 29:154–159, 2018.
130. Fontaine J, Bovens C, Bettenay S, et al.: Canine cutaneous epitheliotropic T-cell lymphoma: a review, *Vet Comp Oncol* 7:1–14, 2009.
131. Fontaine J, Heimann M, Day MJ: Cutaneous epitheliotropic T-cell lymphoma in the cat: a review of the literature and five new cases, *Vet Dermatol* 22:454–461, 2011.
132. McKeever PJ, Grindem CB, Stevens JB, et al.: Canine cutaneous lymphoma, *J Am Vet Med Assoc* 180:531–536, 1982.
133. Couto CG, Cullen J, Pedroia V, et al.: Central nervous system lymphosarcoma in the dog, *J Am Vet Med Assoc* 184:809–813, 1984.
134. Dallman MJ, Saunders GK: Primary spinal cord lymphosarcoma in a dog, *J Am Vet Med Assoc* 189:1348–1349, 1986.
135. Rosin A: Neurologic diseases associated with lymphosarcoma in ten dogs, *J Am Vet Med Assoc* 181:50–53, 1982.
136. Siso S, Marco-Salazar P, Moore PF, et al.: Canine nervous system lymphoma subtypes display characteristic neuroanatomical patterns, *Vet Pathol* 54:53–60, 2017.
137. Lanza MR, Musciano AR, Dubielzig RD, et al.: Clinical and pathological classification of canine intraocular lymphoma, *Vet Ophthalmol* 21:167–173, 2018.
138. Swanson JF: Ocular manifestations of systemic disease in the dog and cat. Recent developments, *Vet Clin North Am Small Anim Pract* 20:849–867, 1990.
139. Krohne SDGVW, Richardson RC, et al.: Ocular involvement in canine lymphosarcoma: a retrospecive study of 94 cases, *Am College Vet Ophth Proc* 68–84, 1987.
140. Madewell BR, Feldman BF: Characterization of anemias associated with neoplasia in small animals, *J Am Vet Med Assoc* 176:419–425, 1980.
141. Kubota A, Kano R, Mizuno T, et al.: Parathyroid hormone-related protein (PTHrP) produced by dog lymphoma cells, *J Vet Med Sci* 64:835–837, 2002.
142. Rosol TJ, Nagode LA, Couto CG, et al.: Parathyroid hormone (PTH)-related protein, PTH, and 1,25-dihydroxyvitamin D in dogs with cancer-associated hypercalcemia, *Endocrinology* 131:1157–1164, 1992.
143. Gerber B, Hauser B, Reusch CE: Serum levels of 25-hydroxycholecalciferol and 1,25-dihydroxycholecalciferol in dogs with hypercalcaemia, *Vet Res Commun* 28:669–680, 2004.
144. Massa KL, Gilger BC, Miller TL, et al.: Causes of uveitis in dogs: 102 cases (1989-2000), *Vet Ophthalmol* 5:93–98, 2002.
145. Grindem CB, Breitschwerdt EB, Corbett WT, et al.: Thrombocytopenia associated with neoplasia in dogs, *J Vet Intern Med* 8:400–405, 1994.
146. BR m: Hematological and bone marrow cytological abnormalities in 75 dogs with malignant lymphoma, *J Am Anim Hosp Assoc* 22:235–240, 1986.
147. MacEwen EG, Hurvitz AI: Diagnosis and management of monoclonal gammopathies, *Vet Clin North Am* 7:119–132, 1977.
148. Ku CK, Kass PH, Christopher MM: Cytologic-histologic concordance in the diagnosis of neoplasia in canine and feline lymph nodes: a retrospective study of 367 cases, *Vet Comp Oncol* 2017(15):1206–1217, 2017.
149. Sapierzynski R, Kliczkowska-Klarowicz K, Jankowska U, et al.: Cytodiagnostics of canine lymphomas - possibilities and limitations, *Pol J Vet Sci* 19:433–439, 2016.
150. Sozmen M, Tasca S, Carli E, et al.: Use of fine needle aspirates and flow cytometry for the diagnosis, classification, and immunophenotyping of canine lymphomas, *J Vet Diagn Invest* 17:323–330, 2005.
151. Crabtree AC, Spangler E, Beard D, et al.: Diagnostic accuracy of gray-scale ultrasonography for the detection of hepatic and splenic lymphoma in dogs, *Vet Radiol Ultrasound* 51:661–664, 2010.
152. Kinns J, Mai W: Association between malignancy and sonographic heterogeneity in canine and feline abdominal lymph nodes, *Vet Radiol Ultrasound* 48:565–569, 2007.
153. Nyman HT, Lee MH, McEvoy FJ, et al.: Comparison of B-mode and Doppler ultrasonographic findings with histologic features of benign and malignant superficial lymph nodes in dogs, *Am J Vet Res* 67:978–984, 2006.
154. Carrasco V, Rodriguez-Bertos A, Rodriguez-Franco F, et al.: Distinguishing intestinal lymphoma from inflammatory bowel disease in canine duodenal endoscopic biopsy samples, *Vet Pathol* 52:668–675, 2015.
155. Maeda S, Tsuboi M, Sakai K, et al.: Endoscopic cytology for the diagnosis of chronic enteritis and intestinal lymphoma in dogs, *Vet Pathol* 54:595–604, 2017.
156. Ohmi A, Ohno K, Uchida K, et al.: Significance of clonal rearrangements of lymphocyte antigen receptor genes on the prognosis of chronic enteropathy in 22 Shiba dogs, *J Vet Med Sci* 79:1578–1584, 2017.
157. Ohmura S, Leipig M, Schopper I, et al.: Detection of monoclonality in intestinal lymphoma with polymerase chain reaction for antigen receptor gene rearrangement analysis to differentiate from enteritis in dogs, *Vet Comp Oncol* 15:194–207, 2017.
158. Takanosu M, Kagawa Y: Comparison of primer sets for T-cell clonality testing in canine intestinal lymphoma, *J Vet Diagn Invest* 27:645–650, 2015.
159. Fukushima K, Ohno K, Koshino-Goto Y, et al.: Sensitivity for the detection of a clonally rearranged antigen receptor gene in endoscopically obtained biopsy specimens from canine alimentary lymphoma, *J Vet Med Sci* 71:1673–1676, 2009.
160. Kaneko N, Yamamoto Y, Wada Y, et al.: Application of polymerase chain reaction to analysis of antigen receptor rearrangements to support endoscopic diagnosis of canine alimentary lymphoma, *J Vet Med Sci* 71:555–559, 2009.
161. Kleinschmidt S, Meneses F, Nolte I, et al.: Retrospective study on the diagnostic value of full-thickness biopsies from the stomach and intestines of dogs with chronic gastrointestinal disease symptoms, *Vet Pathol* 43:1000–1003, 2006.
162. Miura T, Maruyama H, Sakai M, et al.: Endoscopic findings on alimentary lymphoma in 7 dogs, *J Vet Med Sci* 66:577–580, 2004.
163. Chaubert P, Baur Chaubert AS, Sattler U, et al.: Improved polymerase chain reaction-based method to detect early-stage epitheliotropic T-cell lymphoma (mycosis fungoides) in formalin-fixed, paraffin-embedded skin biopsy specimens of the dog, *J Vet Diagn Invest* 22:20–29, 2010.
164. Comazzi S, Gelain ME: Use of flow cytometric immunophenotyping to refine the cytological diagnosis of canine lymphoma, *Vet J* 188:149–155, 2011.
165. Culmsee K, Simon D, Mischke R, et al.: Possibilities of flow cytometric analysis for immunophenotypic characterization of canine lymphoma, *J Vet Med A Physiol Pathol Clin Med* 48:199–206, 2001.
166. Fisher DJ, Naydan D, Werner LL, et al.: Immunophenotyping lymphomas in dogs: a comparison of results from fine needle aspirate and needle biopsy samples, *Vet Clin Pathol* 24:118–123, 1995.
167. Gelain ME, Mazzilli M, Riondato F, et al.: Aberrant phenotypes and quantitative antigen expression in different subtypes of canine lymphoma by flow cytometry, *Vet Immunol Immunopathol* 121:179–188, 2008.
168. Gibson D, Aubert I, Woods JP, et al.: Flow cytometric immunophenotype of canine lymph node aspirates, *J Vet Intern Med* 18:710–717, 2004.

169. Lana S, Plaza S, Hampe K, et al.: Diagnosis of mediastinal masses in dogs by flow cytometry, *J Vet Intern Med* 20:1161–1165, 2006.

170. Tasca S, Carli E, Caldin M, et al.: Hematologic abnormalities and flow cytometric immunophenotyping results in dogs with hematopoietic neoplasia: 210 cases (2002-2006), *Vet Clin Pathol* 38:2–12, 2009.

171. Vail DM, Kravis LD, Kisseberth WC, et al.: Application of rapid CD3 immunophenotype analysis and argyrophilic nucleolar organizer region (AgNOR) frequency to fine needle aspirate specimens from dogs with lymphoma, *Vet Clin Pathol* 26:66–69, 1997.

172. Bauer NB, Zervos D, Moritz A: Argyrophilic nucleolar organizing regions and Ki67 equally reflect proliferation in fine needle aspirates of normal, hyperplastic, inflamed, and neoplastic canine lymph nodes (n = 101), *J Vet Intern Med* 21:928–935, 2007.

173. Fournel-Fleury C, Magnol JP, Chabanne L, et al.: Growth fractions in canine non-Hodgkin's lymphomas as determined in situ by the expression of the Ki-67 antigen, *J Comp Pathol* 117:61–72, 1997.

174. Phillips BS, Kass PH, Naydan DK, et al.: Apoptotic and proliferation indexes in canine lymphoma, *J Vet Diagn Invest* 12:111–117, 2000.

175. Vajdovich P, Psader R, Toth ZA, et al.: Use of the argyrophilic nucleolar region method for cytologic and histologic examination of the lymph nodes in dogs, *Vet Pathol* 41:338–345, 2004.

176. Hung LC, Pong VF, Cheng CR, et al.: An improved system for quantifying AgNOR and PCNA in canine tumors, *Anticancer Res* 20:3273–3280, 2000.

177. Poggi A, Miniscalco B, Morello E, et al.: Prognostic significance of Ki67 evaluated by flow cytometry in dogs with high-grade B-cell lymphoma, *Vet Comp Oncol* 15:431–440, 2017.

178. Frantz AM, Sarver AL, Ito D, et al.: Molecular profiling reveals prognostically significant subtypes of canine lymphoma, *Vet Pathol* 50:693–703, 2013.

179. Su Y, Nielsen D, Zhu L, et al.: Gene selection and cancer type classification of diffuse large-B-cell lymphoma using a bivariate mixture model for two-species data, *Hum Genomics* 7(2), 2013.

180. Avery A: Molecular diagnostics of hematologic malignancies, *Top Companion Anim Med* 24:144–150, 2009.

181. Avery PR, Avery AC: Molecular methods to distinguish reactive and neoplastic lymphocyte expansions and their importance in transitional neoplastic states, *Vet Clin Pathol* 33:196–207, 2004.

182. Burnett RC, Vernau W, Modiano JF, et al.: Diagnosis of canine lymphoid neoplasia using clonal rearrangements of antigen receptor genes, *Vet Pathol* 40:32–41, 2003.

183. Dreitz MJ, Ogilvie G, Sim GK: Rearranged T lymphocyte antigen receptor genes as markers of malignant T cells, *Vet Immunol Immunopathol* 69:113–119, 1999.

184. Gentilini F, Calzolari C, Turba ME, et al.: GeneScanning analysis of Ig/TCR gene rearrangements to detect clonality in canine lymphomas, *Vet Immunol Immunopathol* 127:47–56, 2009.

185. Keller RL, Avery AC, Burnett RC, et al.: Detection of neoplastic lymphocytes in peripheral blood of dogs with lymphoma by polymerase chain reaction for antigen receptor gene rearrangement, *Vet Clin Pathol* 33:145–149, 2004.

186. Tamura K, Yagihara H, Isotani M, et al.: Development of the polymerase chain reaction assay based on the canine genome database for detection of monoclonality in B cell lymphoma, *Vet Immunol Immunopathol* 110:163–167, 2006.

187. Yagihara H, Tamura K, Isotani M, et al.: Genomic organization of the T-cell receptor gamma gene and PCR detection of its clonal rearrangement in canine T-cell lymphoma/leukemia, *Vet Immunol Immunopathol* 115:375–382, 2007.

188. Davis B, Schwartz M, Duchemin D, et al.: Validation of a multiplexed gene signature assay for diagnosis of canine cancers from formalin-fixed paraffin-embedded tissues, *J Vet Intern Med* 31:854–863, 2017.

189. Drazovska M, Sivikova K, Dianovsky J, et al.: Comparative genomic hybridization in detection of DNA changes in canine lymphomas, *An Sci J* 88:27–32, 2017.

190. Comazzi S, Avery PR, Garden OA, et al.: European canine lymphoma network consensus recommendations for reporting flow cytometry in canine hematopoietic neoplasms, *Cytometry Part B* 92:411–419, 2017.

191. Fournel-Fleury C, Magnol JP, Bricaire P, et al.: Cytohistological and immunological classification of canine malignant lymphomas: comparison with human non-Hodgkin's lymphomas, *J Comp Pathol* 117:35–59, 1997.

192. Ponce F, Magnol JP, Marchal T, et al.: High-grade canine T-cell lymphoma/leukemia with plasmacytoid morphology: a clinical pathological study of nine cases, *J Vet Diagn Invest* 15:330–337, 2003.

193. Keller SM, Vernau W, Moore PF: Clonality testing in veterinary medicine: a review with diagnostic guidelines, *Vet Pathol* 53:711–725, 2016.

194. Langner KF, Joetzke AE, Nerschbach V, et al.: Detection of clonal antigen receptor gene rearrangement in dogs with lymphoma by real-time polymerase chain reaction and melting curve analysis, *BMC Vet Res* 10(1), 2014.

195. Waugh EM, Gallagher A, Haining H, et al.: Optimisation and validation of a PCR for antigen receptor rearrangement (PARR) assay to detect clonality in canine lymphoid malignancies, *Vet Immunol Immunopathol* 182:115–124, 2016.

196. Bergman PJ, Ogilvie GK, Powers BE: Monoclonal antibody C219 immunohistochemistry against P-glycoprotein: sequential analysis and predictive ability in dogs with lymphoma, *J Vet Intern Med* 10:354–359, 1996.

197. Moore AS, Leveille CR, Reimann KA, et al.: The expression of P-glycoprotein in canine lymphoma and its association with multidrug resistance, *Cancer Invest* 13:475–479, 1995.

198. Gaines PJ, Powell TD, Walmsley SJ, et al.: Identification of serum biomarkers for canine B-cell lymphoma by use of surface-enhanced laser desorption-ionization time-of-flight mass spectrometry, *Am J Vet Res* 68:405–410, 2007.

199. McCaw DL, Chan AS, Stegner AL, et al.: Proteomics of canine lymphoma identifies potential cancer-specific protein markers, *Clin Cancer Res* 13:2496–2503, 2007.

200. Ratcliffe L, Mian S, Slater K, et al.: Proteomic identification and profiling of canine lymphoma patients, *Vet Comp Oncol* 7:92–105, 2009.

201. Wilson CR, Regnier FE, Knapp DW, et al.: Glycoproteomic profiling of serum peptides in canine lymphoma and transitional cell carcinoma, *Vet Comp Oncol* 6:171–181, 2008.

202. Bryan JN: The current state of clinical application of serum biomarkers for canine lymphoma, *Frontie Vet Sci* 3:87, 2016.

203. Alexandrakis I, Tuli R, Ractliffe SC, et al.: Utility of a multiple serum biomarker test to monitor remission status and relapse in dogs with lymphoma undergoing treatment with chemotherapy, *Vet Comp Oncol* 15:6–17, 2017.

204. Mirkes EM, Alexandrakis I, Slater K, et al.: Computational diagnosis and risk evaluation for canine lymphoma, *Comput Biol Med* 53:279–290, 2014.

205. Selting KA, Ringold R, Husbands B, et al.: Thymidine kinase type 1 and C-reactive protein concentrations in dogs with spontaneously occurring cancer, *J Vet Intern Med* 30:1159–1166, 2016.

206. Sharif H, von Euler H, Westberg S, et al.: A sensitive and kinetically defined radiochemical assay for canine and human serum thymidine kinase 1 (TK1) to monitor canine malignant lymphoma, *Vet J* 194:40–47, 2012.

207. Hahn KA, Freeman KP, Barnhill MA, et al.: Serum alpha 1-acid glycoprotein concentrations before and after relapse in dogs with lymphoma treated with doxorubicin, *J Am Vet Med Assoc* 214:1023–1025, 1999.

208. Kazmierski KJ, Ogilvie GK, Fettman MJ, et al.: Serum zinc, chromium, and iron concentrations in dogs with lymphoma and osteosarcoma, *J Vet Intern Med* 15:585–588, 2001.

209. Lechowski R, Jagielski D, Hoffmann-Jagielska M, et al.: Alpha-fetoprotein in canine multicentric lymphoma, *Vet Res Commun* 26:285–296, 2002.

210. Marconato L, Crispino G, Finotello R, et al.: Clinical relevance of serial determinations of lactate dehydrogenase activity used to predict recurrence in dogs with lymphoma, *J Am Vet Med Assoc* 236:969–974, 2010.

211. Mischke R, Waterston M, Eckersall PD: Changes in C-reactive protein and haptoglobin in dogs with lymphatic neoplasia, *Vet J* 174:188–192, 2007.

212. Winter JL, Barber LG, Freeman L, et al.: Antioxidant status and biomarkers of oxidative stress in dogs with lymphoma, *J Vet Intern Med* 23:311–316, 2009.

213. Zizzo N, Patruno R, Zito FA, et al.: Vascular endothelial growth factor concentrations from platelets correlate with tumor angiogenesis and grading in a spontaneous canine non-Hodgkin lymphoma model, *Leuk Lymphoma* 51:291–296, 2010.

214. Rossmeisl Jr JH, Bright P, Tamarkin L, et al.: Endostatin concentrations in healthy dogs and dogs with selected neoplasms, *J Vet Intern Med* 16:565–569, 2002.

215. Flory AB, Rassnick KM, Stokol T, et al.: Stage migration in dogs with lymphoma, *J Vet Intern Med* 21:1041–1047, 2007.

216. Raskin RE, Krehbiel JD: Prevalence of leukemic blood and bone marrow in dogs with multicentric lymphoma, *J Am Vet Med Assoc* 194:1427–1429, 1989.

217. Aresu L, Arico A, Ferraresso S, et al.: Minimal residual disease detection by flow cytometry and PARR in lymph node, peripheral blood and bone marrow, following treatment of dogs with diffuse large B-cell lymphoma, *Vet J* 200:318–324, 2014.

218. Weiss DJ: Evaluation of proliferative disorders in canine bone marrow by use of flow cytometric scatter plots and monoclonal antibodies, *Vet Pathol* 38:512–518, 2001.

219. Ackerman N, Madewell BR: Thoracic and abdominal radiographic abnormalities in the multicentric form of lymphosarcoma in dogs, *J Am Vet Med Assoc* 176:36–40, 1980.

220. Geyer NE, Reichle JK, Valdes-Martinez A, et al.: Radiographic appearance of confirmed pulmonary lymphoma in cats and dogs, *Vet Radiol Ultrasound* 51:386–390, 2010.

221. Jones ID, Daniels AD, Lara-Garcia A, et al.: Computed tomographic findings in 12 cases of canine multi-centric lymphoma with splenic and hepatic involvement, *J Small Anim Pract* 58:622–628, 2017.

222. Yoon J, Feeney DA, Cronk DE, et al.: Computed tomographic evaluation of canine and feline mediastinal masses in 14 patients, *Vet Radiol Ultrasound* 45:542–546, 2004.

223. Bassett CL, Daniel GB, Bochsler PN, et al.: Characterization of uptake of 2-deoxy-2-[18F]fluoro-D-glucose by fungal-associated inflammation: the differential uptake ratio for blastomyces-associated lesions is as high as for lymphoma and higher than for turpentine abscesses in experimentally induced lesions in rats, *Mol Imaging Biol* 4:193–200, 2002.

224. Lawrence J, Vanderhoek M, Barbee D, et al.: Use of 3'-deoxy-3'-[18F]fluorothymidine PET/CT for evaluating response to cytotoxic chemotherapy in dogs with non-Hodgkin's lymphoma, *Vet Radiol Ultrasound* 50:660–668, 2009.

225. LeBlanc AK, Jakoby BW, Townsend DW, et al.: 18FDG-PET imaging in canine lymphoma and cutaneous mast cell tumor, *Vet Radiol Ultrasound* 50:215–223, 2009.

226. Vail DM, Thamm DH, Reiser H, et al.: Assessment of GS-9219 in a pet dog model of non-Hodgkin's lymphoma, *Clin Cancer Res* 15:3503–3510, 2009.

227. Burton JH, Garrett-Mayer E, Thamm DH: Evaluation of a 15-week CHOP protocol for the treatment of canine multicentric lymphoma, *Vet Comp Oncol* 11:306–315, 2013.

228. Curran K, Thamm DH: Retrospective analysis for treatment of naive canine multicentric lymphoma with a 15-week, maintenance-free CHOP protocol, *Vet Comp Oncol* 14(Suppl 1):147–155, 2016.

229. Elliott JW, Cripps P, Marrington AM, et al.: Epirubicin as part of a multi-agent chemotherapy protocol for canine lymphoma, *Vet Comp Oncol* 11:185–198, 2013.

230. Thamm DH, Vail DM, Post GS, et al.: Alternating rabacfosadine/doxorubicin: efficacy and tolerability in naive canine multicentric lymphoma, *J Vet Intern Med* 31:872–878, 2017.

231. Daters AT, Mauldin GE, Mauldin GN, et al.: Evaluation of a multidrug chemotherapy protocol with mitoxantrone based maintenance (CHOP-MA) for the treatment of canine lymphoma, *Vet Comp Oncol* 8:11–22, 2010.

232. Garrett LD, Thamm DH, Chun R, et al.: Evaluation of a 6-month chemotherapy protocol with no maintenance therapy for dogs with lymphoma, *J Vet Intern Med* 16:704–709, 2002.

233. Hosoya K, Kisseberth WC, Lord LK, et al.: Comparison of COAP and UW-19 protocols for dogs with multicentric lymphoma, *J Vet Intern Med* 21:1355–1363, 2007.

234. Kaiser CI, Fidel JL, Roos M, et al.: Reevaluation of the University of Wisconsin 2-year protocol for treating canine lymphosarcoma, *J Am Anim Hosp Assoc* 43:85–92, 2007.

235. Keller ET, MacEwen EG, Rosenthal RC, et al.: Evaluation of prognostic factors and sequential combination chemotherapy with doxorubicin for canine lymphoma, *J Vet Intern Med* 7:289–295, 1993.

236. MacEwen EG, Brown NO, Patnaik AK, et al.: Cyclic combination chemotherapy of canine lymphosarcoma, *J Am Vet Med Assoc* 178:1178–1181, 1981.

237. MacEwen EG, Hayes AA, Matus RE, et al.: Evaluation of some prognostic factors for advanced multicentric lymphosarcoma in the dog: 147 cases (1978-1981), *J Am Vet Med Assoc* 190:564–568, 1987.

238. Morrison-Collister KE, Rassnick KM, Northrup NC, et al.: A combination chemotherapy protocol with MOPP and CCNU consolidation (Tufts VELCAP-SC) for the treatment of canine lymphoma, *Vet Comp Oncol* 1:180–190, 2003.

239. Mutsaers AJ, Glickman NW, DeNicola DB, et al.: Evaluation of treatment with doxorubicin and piroxicam or doxorubicin alone for multicentric lymphoma in dogs, *J Am Vet Med Assoc* 220:1813–1817, 2002.

240. Myers 3rd NC, Moore AS, Rand WM, et al.: Evaluation of a multi-drug chemotherapy protocol (ACOPA II) in dogs with lymphoma, *J Vet Intern Med* 11:333–339, 1997.

241. Rassnick KM, Bailey DB, Malone EK, et al.: Comparison between L-CHOP and an L-CHOP protocol with interposed treatments of CCNU and MOPP (L-CHOP-CCNU-MOPP) for lymphoma in dogs, *Vet Comp Oncol* 8:243–253, 2010.

242. Siedlecki CT, Kass PH, Jakubiak MJ, et al.: Evaluation of an actinomycin-D-containing combination chemotherapy protocol with extended maintenance therapy for canine lymphoma, *Can Vet J* 47:52–59, 2006.

243. Simon D, Moreno SN, Hirschberger J, et al.: Efficacy of a continuous, multiagent chemotherapeutic protocol versus a short-term single-agent protocol in dogs with lymphoma, *J Am Vet Med Assoc* 232:879–885, 2008.

244. Simon D, Nolte I, Eberle N, et al.: Treatment of dogs with lymphoma using a 12-week, maintenance-free combination chemotherapy protocol, *J Vet Intern Med* 20:948–954, 2006.

245. Sorenmo K, Overley B, Krick E, et al.: Outcome and toxicity associated with a dose-intensified, maintenance-free CHOP-based chemotherapy protocol in canine lymphoma: 130 cases, *Vet Comp Oncol* 8:196–208, 2010.

246. Valerius KD, Ogilvie GK, Mallinckrodt CH, et al.: Doxorubicin alone or in combination with asparaginase, followed by cyclophosphamide, vincristine, and prednisone for treatment of multicentric lymphoma in dogs: 121 cases (1987-1995), *J Am Vet Med Assoc* 210:512–516, 1997.

247. Zemann BI, Moore AS, Rand WM, et al.: A combination chemotherapy protocol (VELCAP-L) for dogs with lymphoma, *J Vet Intern Med* 12:465–470, 1998.

248. Cotter SMGM: Treatment of lymphoma and leukemia with cyclophosphamide, vincristine and prednisone: I. Treatment of dog, *J Am Anim Hosp Assoc* 19:159–165, 1983.

249. Boyce KLKB: Treatment of canine lymphoma with COPLA/LVP, *J Am Anim Hosp Assoc* 36:395–403, 2000.

250. Postorino NC, Susaneck SJ, Withrow SJ, et al.: Single agent therapy with adriamycin for canine lymphosarcoma, *J Am Anim Hosp Assoc* 25:221–225, 1989.

251. Stone MSGM, Cotter SM, et al.: Comparison of two protocols for induction of remission in dogs with lymphoma, *J Am Anim Hosp Assoc* 27:315–321, 1991.

252. Fisher RI, Gaynor ER, Dahlberg S, et al.: Comparison of a standard regimen (CHOP) with three intensive chemotherapy regimens for advanced non-Hodgkin's lymphoma, *N Engl J Med* 328:1002–1006, 1993.

253. Vail DM, Michels GM, Khanna C, et al.: Response evaluation criteria for peripheral nodal lymphoma in dogs (v1.0)—a Veterinary Cooperative Oncology Group (VCOG) consensus document, *Vet Comp Oncol* 8:28–37, 2010.

254. Tomiyasu H, Takahashi M, Fujino Y, et al.: Gastrointestinal and hematologic adverse events after administration of vincristine, cyclophosphamide, and doxorubicin in dogs with lymphoma that underwent a combination multidrug chemotherapy protocol, *J Vet Med Sci* 72:1391–1397, 2010.

255. Vail DM: Cytotoxic chemotherapy agents, *Clin Brief* 8:18–22, 2010.

256. Mellanby RJ, Herrtage ME, Dobson JM: Owners' assessments of their dog's quality of life during palliative chemotherapy for lymphoma, *J Small Anim Pract* 44:100–103, 2003.

257. Bronden LB, Rutteman GR, Flagstad A, et al.: Study of dog and cat owners' perceptions of medical treatment for cancer, *Vet Rec* 152:77–80, 2003.

258. Lautscham EM, Kessler M, Ernst T, et al.: Comparison of a CHOP-LAsp-based protocol with and without maintenance for canine multicentric lymphoma, *Vet Rec* 180:303, 2017.

259. Moore AS, Cotter SM, Rand WM, et al.: Evaluation of a discontinuous treatment protocol (VELCAP-S) for canine lymphoma, *J Vet Intern Med* 15:348–354, 2001.

260. Piek CJ, Rutteman GR, Teske E: Evaluation of the results of a L-asparaginase-based continuous chemotherapy protocol versus a short doxorubicin-based induction chemotherapy protocol in dogs with malignant lymphoma, *Vet Q* 21:44–49, 1999.

261. Rassnick KM, McEntee MC, Erb HN, et al.: Comparison of 3 protocols for treatment after induction of remission in dogs with lymphoma, *J Vet Intern Med* 21:1364–1373, 2007.

262. Zenker I, Meichner K, Steinle K, et al.: Thirteen-week dose-intensifying simultaneous combination chemotherapy protocol for malignant lymphoma in dogs, *Vet Rec* 167:744–748, 2010.

263. Ruslander D, Moore AS, Gliatto JM, et al.: Cytosine arabinoside as a single agent for the induction of remission in canine lymphoma, *J Vet Intern Med* 8:299–301, 1994.

264. Rassnick KM, Frimberger AE, Wood CA, et al.: Evaluation of ifosfamide for treatment of various canine neoplasms, *J Vet Intern Med* 14:271–276, 2000.

265. Smith AA, Lejeune A, Kow K, et al.: Clinical response and adverse event profile of bleomycin chemotherapy for canine multicentric lymphoma, *J Am Anim Hosp Assoc* 53:128–134, 2017.

266. Turner AI, Hahn KA, Rusk A, et al.: Single agent gemcitabine chemotherapy in dogs with spontaneously occurring lymphoma, *J Vet Intern Med* 20:1384–1388, 2006.

267. Reiser H, Wang J, Chong L, et al.: GS-9219—a novel acyclic nucleotide analogue with potent antineoplastic activity in dogs with spontaneous non-Hodgkin's lymphoma, *Clin Cancer Res* 14:2824–2832, 2008.

268. Thamm DH, Vail DM, Kurzman ID, et al.: GS-9219/VDC-1101—a prodrug of the acyclic nucleotide PMEG has antitumor activity in spontaneous canine multiple myeloma, *BMC Vet Res* 10(30), 2014.

269. Morges MA, Burton JH, Saba CF, et al.: Phase II evaluation of VDC-1101 in canine cutaneous T-cell lymphoma, *J Vet Intern Med* 28:1569–1574, 2014.

270. Saba CF, Vickery KR, Clifford CA, et al.: Rabacfosadine for relapsed canine B-cell lymphoma: Efficacy and adverse event profiles of 2 different doses, *Vet Comp Oncol* 16:E76–E82, 2018.

271. Jeffreys AB, Knapp DW, Carlton WW, et al.: Influence of asparaginase on a combination chemotherapy protocol for canine multicentric lymphoma, *J Am Anim Hosp Assoc* 41:221–226, 2005.

272. MacDonald VS, Thamm DH, Kurzman ID, et al.: Does L-asparaginase influence efficacy or toxicity when added to a standard CHOP protocol for dogs with lymphoma? *J Vet Intern Med* 19:732–736, 2005.

273. Carter RF, Harris CK, Withrow SJ, et al.: Chemotherapy of canine lymphoma with histopathologial correlation: doxorubicin alone compared to COP as first treatment regimen, *J Am Anim Hosp Assoc* 23:587–596, 1987.

274. Lori JC, Stein TJ, Thamm DH: Doxorubicin and cyclophosphamide for the treatment of canine lymphoma: a randomized, placebo-controlled study, *Vet Comp Oncol* 8:188–195, 2010.

275. Sauerbrey ML, Mullins MN, Bannink EO, et al.: Lomustine and prednisone as a first-line treatment for dogs with multicentric lymphoma: 17 cases (2004-2005), *J Am Vet Med Assoc* 230:1866–1869, 2007.

276. Khanna C, Lund EM, Redic KA, et al.: Randomized controlled trial of doxorubicin versus dactinomycin in a multiagent protocol for treatment of dogs with malignant lymphoma, *J Am Vet Med Assoc* 213:985–990, 1998.

277. Marconato L, Stefanello D, Valenti P, et al.: Predictors of long-term survival in dogs with high-grade multicentric lymphoma, *J Am Vet Med Assoc* 238:480–485, 2011.

278. Price GS, Page RL, Fischer BM, et al.: Efficacy and toxicity of doxorubicin/cyclophosphamide maintenance therapy in dogs with multicentric lymphosarcoma, *J Vet Intern Med* 5:259–262, 1991.

279. Fournier Q, Serra JC, Handel I, et al.: Impact of pretreatment neutrophil count on chemotherapy administration and toxicity in dogs with lymphoma treated with CHOP chemotherapy, *J Vet Intern Med* 32:384–393, 2018.

280. Mealey KL, Fidel J, Gay JM, et al.: ABCB1-1Delta polymorphism can predict hematologic toxicity in dogs treated with vincristine, *J Vet Intern Med* 22:996–1000, 2008.

281. Beaver LM, Strottner G, Klein MK: Response rate after administration of a single dose of doxorubicin in dogs with B-cell or T-cell lymphoma: 41 cases (2006-2008), *J Am Vet Med Assoc* 237:1052–1055, 2010.

282. Dobson JM, Blackwood LB, McInnes EF, et al.: Prognostic variables in canine multicentric lymphosarcoma, *J Small Anim Pract* 42:377–384, 2001.

283. Rebhun RB, Kent MS, Borrofka SA, et al.: CHOP chemotherapy for the treatment of canine multicentric T-cell lymphoma, *Vet Comp Oncol* 9:38–44, 2011.

284. Brown PM, Tzannes S, Nguyen S, et al.: LOPP chemotherapy as a first-line treatment for dogs with T-cell lymphoma, *Vet Comp Oncol* 16:108–113, 2018.

285. Goodman IH, Moore AS, Frimberger AE: Treatment of canine non-indolent T cell lymphoma using the VELCAP-TSC protocol: a retrospective evaluation of 70 dogs (2003-2013), *Vet J* 211:39–44, 2016.

286. Brodsky EM, Maudlin GN, Lachowicz JL, et al.: Asparaginase and MOPP treatment of dogs with lymphoma, *J Vet Intern Med* 23:578–584, 2009.

287. Gentilini F, Turba ME, Forni M: Retrospective monitoring of minimal residual disease using hairpin-shaped clone specific primers in B-cell lymphoma affected dogs, *Vet Immunol Immunopathol* 153:279–288, 2013.

288. Sato M, Yamazaki J, Goto-Koshino Y, et al.: Minimal residual disease in canine lymphoma: an objective marker to assess tumour cell burden in remission, *Vet J* 215:38–42, 2016.

289. Sato M, Yamzaki J, Goto-Koshino Y, et al.: The prognostic significance of minimal residual disease in the early phases of chemotherapy in dogs with high-grade B-cell lymphoma, *Vet J* 195:319–324, 2013.

290. Thilakaratne DN, Mayer MN, MacDonald VS, et al.: Clonality and phenotyping of canine lymphomas before chemotherapy and during remission using polymerase chain reaction (PCR) on lymph node cytologic smears and peripheral blood, *Can Vet J* 51:79–84, 2010.

291. Valerius KD, Ogilvie GK, Fettman MJ, et al.: Comparison of the effects of asparaginase administered subcutaneously versus intramuscularly for treatment of multicentric lymphoma in dogs receiving doxorubicin, *J Am Vet Med Assoc* 214:353–356, 1999.

292. Valli VE, Jacobs RM, Norris A, et al.: The histologic classification of 602 cases of feline lymphoproliferative disease using the National Cancer Institute working formulation, *J Vet Diagn Invest* 12:295–306, 2000.

293. Yamazaki J, Baba K, Goto-Koshino Y, et al.: Quantitative assessment of minimal residual disease (MRD) in canine lymphoma by using real-time polymerase chain reaction, *Vet Immunol Immunopathol* 126:321–331, 2008.

294. Nielsen L, Toft N, Eckersall PD, et al.: Serum C-reactive protein concentration as an indicator of remission status in dogs with multicentric lymphoma, *J Vet Intern Med* 21:1231–1236, 2007.

295. Ito D, Endicott MM, Jubala CM, et al.: A tumor-related lymphoid progenitor population supports hierarchical tumor organization in canine B-cell lymphoma, *J Vet Intern Med* 25:890–896, 2011.

296. Tomiyasu H, Tsujimoto H: Comparative aspects of molecular mechanisms of drug resistance through ABC transporters and other related molecules in canine lymphoma, *Vet Sci* 2:185–205, 2015.

297. Zandvliet M, Teske E: Mechanisms of drug resistance in veterinary oncology- a review with an emphasis on canine lymphoma, *Vet Sci* 2:150–184, 2015.

298. Zandvliet M, Teske E, Schrickx JA, et al.: A longitudinal study of ABC transporter expression in canine multicentric lymphoma, *Vet J* 205:263–271, 2015.

299. Lee JJ, Hughes CS, Fine RL, et al.: P-glycoprotein expression in canine lymphoma: a relevant, intermediate model of multidrug resistance, *Cancer* 77:1892–1898, 1996.

300. Flory AB, Rassnick KM, Erb HN, et al.: Evaluation of factors associated with second remission in dogs with lymphoma undergoing retreatment with a cyclophosphamide, doxorubicin, vincristine, and prednisone chemotherapy protocol: 95 cases (2000-2007), *J Am Vet Med Assoc* 238:501–506, 2011.

301. Back AR, Schleis SE, Smrkovski OA, et al.: Mechlorethamine, vincristine, melphalan and prednisone (MOMP) for the treatment of relapsed lymphoma in dogs, *Vet Comp Oncol* 13:398–408, 2015.

302. Fahey CE, Milner RJ, Barabas K, et al.: Evaluation of the University of Florida lomustine, vincristine, procarbazine, and prednisone chemotherapy protocol for the treatment of relapsed lymphoma in dogs: 33 cases (2003-2009), *J Am Vet Med Assoc* 239:209–215, 2011.

303. Gillem J, Giuffrida M, Krick E: Efficacy and toxicity of carboplatin and cytarabine chemotherapy for dogs with relapsed or refractory lymphoma (2000-2013), *Vet Comp Oncol* 15:400–410, 2017.

304. Lenz JA, Robat CS, Stein TJ: Vinblastine as a second rescue for the treatment of canine multicentric lymphoma in 39 cases (2005 to 2014), *J Small Anim Pract* 57:429–434, 2016.

305. Mastromauro ML, Suter SE, Hauck ML, et al.: Oral melphalan for the treatment of relapsed canine lymphoma, *Vet Comp Oncol* 16:E123–E129, 2018.

306. Parsons-Doherty M, Poirier VJ, Monteith G: The efficacy and adverse event profile of dexamethasone, melphalan, actinomycin D, and cytosine arabinoside (DMAC) chemotherapy in relapsed canine lymphoma, *Can Vet J* 55:175–180, 2014.

307. Tanis JB, Mason SL, Maddox TW, et al.: Evaluation of a multi-agent chemotherapy protocol combining lomustine, procarbazine and prednisolone (LPP) for the treatment of relapsed canine non-Hodgkin high-grade lymphomas, *Vet Comp Oncol*, 2018. https://doi.org/10.1111/vco.12387. epub ahead of print.

308. Treggiari E, Elliott JW, Baines SJ, et al.: Temozolomide alone or in combination with doxorubicin as a rescue agent in 37 cases of canine multicentric lymphoma, *Vet Comp Oncol* 16:194–201, 2018.

309. Alvarez FJ, Kisseberth WC, Gallant SL, et al.: Dexamethasone, melphalan, actinomycin D, cytosine arabinoside (DMAC) protocol for dogs with relapsed lymphoma, *J Vet Intern Med* 20:1178–1183, 2006.

310. Bannink EO, Sauerbrey ML, Mullins MN, et al.: Actinomycin D as rescue therapy in dogs with relapsed or resistant lymphoma: 49 cases (1999–2006), *J Am Vet Med Assoc* 233:446–451, 2008.

311. Dervisis NG, Dominguez PA, Sarbu L, et al.: Efficacy of temozolomide or dacarbazine in combination with an anthracycline for rescue chemotherapy in dogs with lymphoma, *J Am Vet Med Assoc* 231:563–569, 2007.

312. Flory AB, Rassnick KM, Al-Sarraf R, et al.: Combination of CCNU and DTIC chemotherapy for treatment of resistant lymphoma in dogs, *J Vet Intern Med* 22:164–171, 2008.

313. Griessmayr PC, Payne SE, Winter JE, et al.: Dacarbazine as single-agent therapy for relapsed lymphoma in dogs, *J Vet Intern Med* 23:1227–1231, 2009.

314. Moore AS, London CA, Wood CA, et al.: Lomustine (CCNU) for the treatment of resistant lymphoma in dogs, *J Vet Intern Med* 13:395–398, 1999.

315. Moore AS, Ogilvie GK, Ruslander D, et al.: Evaluation of mitoxantrone for the treatment of lymphoma in dogs, *J Am Vet Med Assoc* 204:1903–1905, 1994.

316. Moore AS, Ogilvie GK, Vail DM: Actinomycin D for reinduction of remission in dogs with resistant lymphoma, *J Vet Intern Med* 8:343–344, 1994.

317. Northrup NC, Gieger TL, Kosarek CE, et al.: Mechlorethamine, procarbazine and prednisone for the treatment of resistant lymphoma in dogs, *Vet Comp Oncol* 7:38–44, 2009.

318. Rassnick KM, Mauldin GE, Al-Sarraf R, et al.: MOPP chemotherapy for treatment of resistant lymphoma in dogs: a retrospective study of 117 cases (1989-2000), *J Vet Intern Med* 16:576–580, 2002.

319. Saba CF, Hafeman SD, Vail DM, et al.: Combination chemotherapy with continuous L-asparaginase, lomustine, and prednisone for relapsed canine lymphoma, *J Vet Intern Med* 23:1058–1063, 2009.

320. Saba CF, Thamm DH, Vail DM: Combination chemotherapy with L-asparaginase, lomustine, and prednisone for relapsed or refractory canine lymphoma, *J Vet Intern Med* 21:127–132, 2007.

321. Impellizeri JA, Howell K, McKeever KP, et al.: The role of rituximab in the treatment of canine lymphoma: an ex vivo evaluation, *Vet J* 171:556–558, 2006.

322. Jubala CM, Wojcieszyn JW, Valli VE, et al.: CD20 expression in normal canine B cells and in canine non-Hodgkin lymphoma, *Vet Pathol* 42:468–476, 2005.

323. Rue SM, Eckelman BP, Efe JA, et al.: Identification of a candidate therapeutic antibody for treatment of canine B-cell lymphoma, *Vet Immunol Immunopathol* 164:148–159, 2015.

324. Ito D, Brewer S, Modiano JF, et al.: Development of a novel anti-canine CD20 monoclonal antibody with diagnostic and therapeutic potential, *Leuk Lymphoma* 56:219–225, 2015.

325. Jain S, Aresu L, Comazzi S, et al.: The development of a recombinant scFv monoclonal antibody targeting canine CD20 for use in comparative medicine, *PLoS One* 11:e0148366, 2016.

326. Weiskopf K, Anderson KL, Ito D, et al.: Eradication of canine diffuse large B-Cell lymphoma in a murine xenograft model with CD47 blockade and anti-CD20, *Cancer Immunol Res* 4:1072–1087, 2016.

327. Crow SE, Theilen GH, Benjaminini E, et al.: Chemoimmunotherapy for canine lymphosarcoma, *Cancer* 40:2102–2108, 1977.

328. Weller RE, Theilen GH, Madewell BR, et al.: Chemoimmunotherapy for canine lymphosarcoma: a prospective evaluation of specific and nonspecific immunomodulation, *Am J Vet Res* 1980(41):516–521, 1980.

329. Jeglum KA, Young KM, Barnsley K, et al.: Chemotherapy versus chemotherapy with intralymphatic tumor cell vaccine in canine lymphoma, *Cancer* 61:2042–2050, 1988.

330. Turek MM, Thamm DH, Mitzey A, et al.: Human granulocyte-macrophage colony-stimulating factor DNA cationic-lipid complexed autologous tumour cell vaccination in the treatment of canine B-cell multicentric lymphoma, *Vet Comp Oncol* 5:219–231, 2007.

331. Gavazza A, Lubas G, Fridman A, et al.: Safety and efficacy of a genetic vaccine targeting telomerase plus chemotherapy for the therapy of canine B-cell lymphoma, *Hum Gene Ther* 24:728–738, 2013.

332. Peruzzi D, Gavazza A, Mesiti G, et al.: A vaccine targeting telomerase enhances survival of dogs affected by B-cell lymphoma, *Mol Ther* 18:1559–1567, 2010.

333. Marconato L, Frayssinet P, Rouquet N, et al.: Randomized, placebo-controlled, double-blinded chemoimmunotherapy clinical trial in a pet dog model of diffuse large B-cell lymphoma, *Clin Cancer Res* 20:668–677, 2014.

334. Marconato L, Stefanello D, Sabattini S, et al.: Enhanced therapeutic effect of APAVAC immunotherapy in combination with dose-intense chemotherapy in dogs with advanced indolent B-cell lymphoma, *Vaccine* 33:5080–5086, 2015.

335. Sorenmo KU, Krick E, Coughlin CM, et al.: CD40-activated B cell cancer vaccine improves second clinical remission and survival in privately owned dogs with non-Hodgkin's lymphoma, *PLoS One* 6:e24167, 2011.

336. Mason NJ, Coughlin CM, Overley B, et al.: RNA-loaded CD40-activated B cells stimulate antigen-specific T-cell responses in dogs with spontaneous lymphoma, *Gene Ther* 15:955–965, 2008.

337. O'Connor CM, Sheppard S, Hartline CA, et al.: Adoptive T-cell therapy improves treatment of canine non-Hodgkin lymphoma post chemotherapy, *Sci Rep* 2(249), 2012.

338. Panjwani MK, Smith JB, Schutsky K, et al.: Feasibility and safety of RNA-transfected CD20-specific chimeric antigen receptor t cells in dogs with spontaneous B cell lymphoma, *Mol Ther* 24:1602–1614, 2016.

339. van Stee LL, Boston SE, Singh A, et al.: Outcome and prognostic factors for canine splenic lymphoma treated by splenectomy (1995-2011), *Vet Surg* 44:976–982, 2015.

340. Brooks MB, Matus RE, Leifer CE, et al.: Use of splenectomy in the management of lymphoma in dogs: 16 cases (1976-1985), *J Am Vet Med Assoc* 191:1008–1010, 1987.

341. Brown EM, Ruslander DM, Azuma C, et al.: A feasibility study of low-dose total body irradiation for relapsed canine lymphoma, *Vet Comp Oncol* 4:75–83, 2006.

342. Deeg HJ, Appelbaum FR, Weiden PL, et al.: Autologous marrow transplantation as consolidation therapy for canine lymphoma: efficacy and toxicity of various regimens of total body irradiation, *Am J Vet Res* 46:2016–2018, 1985.

343. Gustafson NR, Lana SE, Mayer MN, et al.: A preliminary assessment of whole-body radiotherapy interposed within a chemotherapy protocol for canine lymphoma, *Vet Comp Oncol* 2:125–131, 2004.

344. Lurie DM, Gordon IK, Theon AP, et al.: Sequential low-dose rate half-body irradiation and chemotherapy for the treatment of canine multicentric lymphoma, *J Vet Intern Med* 23:1064–1070, 2009.

345. Lurie DM, Kent MS, Fry MM, et al.: A toxicity study of low-dose rate half-body irradiation and chemotherapy in dogs with lymphoma, *Vet Comp Oncol* 6:257–267, 2008.

346. Mayer MN, Larue SM: Radiation therapy in the treatment of canine lymphoma, *Can Vet J* 46:842–844, 2005.

347. Meleo KA: The role of radiotherapy in the treatment of lymphoma and thymoma, *Vet Clin North Am Small Anim Pract* 27:115–129, 1997.

348. Santoro D, Kubicek L, Lu B, et al.: Total skin electron therapy as treatment for epitheliotropic lymphoma in a dog, *Vet Dermatol* 28:246–e265, 2017.

349. Williams LE, Johnson JL, Hauck ML, et al.: Chemotherapy followed by half-body radiation therapy for canine lymphoma, *J Vet Intern Med* 18:703–709, 2004.

350. Williams LE, Pruitt AF, Thrall DE: Chemotherapy followed by abdominal cavity irradiation for feline lymphoblastic lymphoma, *Vet Radiol Ultrasound* 51:681–687, 2010.

351. George R, Smith A, Schleis S, et al.: Outcome of dogs with intranasal lymphoma treated with various radiation and chemotherapy protocols: 24 cases, *Vet Radiol Ultrasound* 57:306–312, 2016.

352. Axiak SM, Carreras JK, Hahn KA, et al.: Hematologic changes associated with half-body irradiation in dogs with lymphoma, *J Vet Intern Med* 20:1398–1401, 2006.

353. Dank G, Rassnick KM, Kristal O, et al.: Clinical characteristics, treatment, and outcome of dogs with presumed primary hepatic lymphoma: 18 cases (1992-2008), *J Am Vet Med Assoc* 239:966–971, 2011.

354. Gustafson NR, Lana SE, Mayer MN, et al.: A preliminary assessment of whole-body radiotherapy interposed within a chemotherapy protocol for canine lymphoma, *Vet Comp Oncol* 2:125–131, 2004.

355. Appelbaum FR, Deeg HJ, Storb R, et al.: Marrow transplant studies in dogs with malignant lymphoma, *Transplantation* 39:499–504, 1985.

356. Warry EE, Willcox JL, Suter SE: Autologous peripheral blood hematopoietic cell transplantation in dogs with T-cell lymphoma, *J Vet Intern Med* 28:529–537, 2014.

357. Willcox JL, Pruitt A, Suter SE: Autologous peripheral blood hematopoietic cell transplantation in dogs with B-cell lymphoma, *J Vet Intern Med* 26:1155–1163, 2012.

358. Escobar C, Grindem C, Neel JA, et al.: Hematologic changes after total body irradiation and autologous transplantation of hematopoietic peripheral blood progenitor cells in dogs with lymphoma, *Vet Pathol* 49:341–343, 2012.

359. Frimberger AE, Moore AS, Rassnick KM, et al.: A combination chemotherapy protocol with dose intensification and autologous bone marrow transplant (VELCAP-HDC) for canine lymphoma, *J Vet Intern Med* 20:355–364, 2006.

360. Rassnick KM, Moore AS, Collister KE, et al.: Efficacy of combination chemotherapy for treatment of gastrointestinal lymphoma in dogs, *J Vet Intern Med* 23:317–322, 2009.

361. Frank JDRS, Kass PH, et al.: Clinical outcomes of 30 cases (1997-2004) of canine gastrointestinal lymphoma, *J Am Anim Hosp Assoc* 43:313–321, 2007.

362. Desmas I, Burton JH, Post G, et al.: Clinical presentation, treatment and outcome in 31 dogs with presumed primary colorectal lymphoma (2001-2013), *Vet Comp Oncol* 15:504–517, 2017.

363. Van den Steen N, Berlato D, Polton G, et al.: Rectal lymphoma in 11 dogs: a retrospective study, *J Small Anim Pract* 53:586–591, 2012.

364. Long SN, Johnston PE, Anderson TJ: Primary T-cell lymphoma of the central nervous system in a dog, *J Am Vet Med Assoc* 218:719–722, 2001.

365. Deravi N, Berke O, Woods JP, et al.: Specific immunotypes of canine T cell lymphoma are associated with different outcomes, *Vet Immunol Immunopathol* 2017(191):5–13, 2017.

366. Risbon RE, de Lorimier LP, Skorupski K, et al.: Response of canine cutaneous epitheliotropic lymphoma to lomustine (CCNU): a retrospective study of 46 cases (1999-2004), *J Vet Intern Med* 20:1389–1397, 2006.

367. Berlato D, Schrempp D, Van Den Steen N, et al.: Radiotherapy in the management of localized mucocutaneous oral lymphoma in dogs: 14 cases, *Vet Comp Oncol* 10:16–23, 2012.

368. Holtermann N, Kiupel M, Kessler M, et al.: Masitinib monotherapy in canine epitheliotropic lymphoma, *Vet Comp Oncol* 14(suppl 1):127–135, 2016.

369. Laprais A, Olivry T: Is CCNU (lomustine) valuable for treatment of cutaneous epitheliotropic lymphoma in dogs? A critically appraised topic, *BMC Vet Res* 13:61, 2017.

370. Williams LE, Rassnick KM, Power HT, et al.: CCNU in the treatment of canine epitheliotropic lymphoma, *J Vet Intern Med* 20:136–143, 2006.

371. White SD, Rosychuk RA, Scott KV, et al.: Use of isotretinoin and etretinate for the treatment of benign cutaneous neoplasia and cutaneous lymphoma in dogs, *J Am Vet Med Assoc* 202:387–391, 1993.

372. Moriello KAME, Schultz KT: PEG-asparaginase in the treatment of canine epitheliotrophic lymphoma and histiocytic proliferative dermatitis. In Ihrke PJMI, White SD, editors: *Advances in Veterinary Dermatology*, New York, 1993, Perggamon Press.

373. Tzannes S, Ibarrola P, Batchelor DJ, et al.: Use of recombinant human interferon alpha-2a in the management of a dog with epitheliotropic lymphoma, *J Am Anim Hosp Assoc* 44:276–282, 2008.

374. Rechner KN, Weeks KJ, Pruitt AF: Total skin electron therapy technique for the canine patient, *Vet Radiol Ultrasound* 52:345–352, 2011.

375. Childress MO, Ramos-Vara JA, Ruple A: Retrospective analysis of factors affecting clinical outcome following CHOP-based chemotherapy in dogs with primary nodal diffuse large B-cell lymphoma, *Vet Comp Oncol* 16:E159–E168, 2018.

376. Davies O, Szladovits B, Polton G, et al.: Prognostic significance of clinical presentation, induction and rescue treatment in 42 cases of canine centroblastic diffuse large B-cell multicentric lymphoma in the United Kingdom, *Vet Comp Oncol* 16:276–287, 2018.

377. Fontaine SJ, McCulloch E, Eckersall PD, et al.: Evaluation of the modified Glasgow Prognostic Score to predict outcome in dogs with newly diagnosed lymphoma, *Vet Comp Oncol* 15:1513–1526, 2017.

378. Koshino A, Goto-Koshino Y, Setoguchi A, et al.: Mutation of p53 gene and its correlation with the clinical outcome in dogs with lymphoma, *J Vet Intern Med* 30:223–229, 2016.

379. Romano FR, Heinze CR, Barber LG, et al.: Association between body condition score and cancer prognosis in dogs with lymphoma and osteosarcoma, *J Vet Intern Med* 30:1179–1186, 2016.

380. Sierra Matiz OR, Santilli J, Anai LA, et al.: Prognostic significance of Ki67 and its correlation with mitotic index in dogs with diffuse large B-cell lymphoma treated with 19-week CHOP-based protocol, *J Vet Diagn Invest* 1040638717743280, 2017.

381. Wang SL, Lee JJ, Liao AT: Chemotherapy-induced neutropenia is associated with prolonged remission duration and survival time in canine lymphoma, *Vet J* 205:69–73, 2015.

382. Marconato L, Martini V, Stefanello D, et al.: Peripheral blood lymphocyte/monocyte ratio as a useful prognostic factor in dogs with diffuse large B-cell lymphoma receiving chemoimmunotherapy, *Vet J* 206:226–230, 2015.

383. Wilson-Robles H, Budke CM, Miller T, et al.: Geographical differences in survival of dogs with non-Hodgkin lymphoma treated with a CHOP based chemotherapy protocol, *Vet Comp Oncol* 15:1564–1571, 2017.

384. Zamani-Ahmadmahmudi M, Aghasharif S, Ilbeigi K: Prognostic efficacy of the human B-cell lymphoma prognostic genes in predicting disease-free survival (DFS) in the canine counterpart, *BMC Vet Res* 13:17, 2017.

385. Zamani-Ahmadmahmudi M, Najafi A, Nassiri SM: Detection of critical genes associated with overall survival (OS) and progression-free survival (PFS) in reconstructed canine B-cell lymphoma gene regulatory network (GRN), *Cancer Invest* 34:70–79, 2016.

386. Abbo AH, Lucroy MD: Assessment of anemia as an independent predictor of response to chemotherapy and survival in dogs with lymphoma: 96 cases (1993-2006), *J Am Vet Med Assoc* 231:1836–1842, 2007.

387. Jagielski D, Lechowski R, Hoffmann-Jagielska M, et al.: A retrospective study of the incidence and prognostic factors of multicentric lymphoma in dogs (1998-2000), *J Vet Med A Physiol Pathol Clin Med* 49:419–424, 2002.

388. Kiupel M, Bostock D, Bergmann V: The prognostic significance of AgNOR counts and PCNA-positive cell counts in canine malignant lymphomas, *J Comp Pathol* 119:407–418, 1998.

389. Larue SM, Fox MH, Ogilvie GK, et al.: Tumour cell kinetics as predictors of response in canine lymphoma treated with chemotherapy alone or combined with whole body hyperthermia, *Int J Hyperthermia* 15:475–486, 1999.

390. Miller AG, Morley PS, Rao S, et al.: Anemia is associated with decreased survival time in dogs with lymphoma, *J Vet Intern Med* 23:116–122, 2009.

391. Rao S, Lana S, Eickhoff J, et al.: Class II major histocompatibility complex expression and cell size independently predict survival in canine B-cell lymphoma, *J Vet Intern Med* 25:1097–1105, 2011.

392. Vaughan A, Johnson JL, Williams LE: Impact of chemotherapeutic dose intensity and hematologic toxicity on first remission duration in dogs with lymphoma treated with a chemoradiotherapy protocol, *J Vet Intern Med* 21:1332–1339, 2007.

393. Yamazaki J, Takahashi M, Setoguchi A, et al.: Monitoring of minimal residual disease (MRD) after multidrug chemotherapy and its correlation to outcome in dogs with lymphoma: a proof-of-concept pilot study, *J Vet Intern Med* 24:897–903, 2010.

394. Williams MJ, Avery AC, Lana SE, et al.: Canine lymphoproliferative disease characterized by lymphocytosis: immunophenotypic markers of prognosis, *J Vet Intern Med* 22:596–601, 2008.

395. Cook AK, Wright ZM, Suchodolski JS, et al.: Prevalence and prognostic impact of hypocobalaminemia in dogs with lymphoma, *J Am Vet Med Assoc* 235:1437–1441, 2009.

396. von Euler H, Einarsson R, Olsson U, et al.: Serum thymidine kinase activity in dogs with malignant lymphoma: a potent marker for prognosis and monitoring the disease, *J Vet Intern Med* 18:696–702, 2004.

397. Von Euler HP, Rivera P, Aronsson AC, et al.: Monitoring therapy in canine malignant lymphoma and leukemia with serum thymidine kinase 1 activity—evaluation of a new, fully automated non-radiometric assay, *Int J Oncol* 34:505–510, 2009.

398. Baskin CR, Couto CG, Wittum TE: Factors influencing first remission and survival in 145 dogs with lymphoma: a retrospective study, *J Am Anim Hosp Assoc* 36:404–409, 2000.

399. Adam F, Villiers E, Watson S, et al.: Clinical pathological and epidemiological assessment of morphologically and immunologically confirmed canine leukaemia, *Vet Comp Oncol* 7:181–195, 2009.

400. Comazzi S, Gelain ME, Martini V, et al.: Immunophenotype predicts survival time in dogs with chronic lymphocytic leukemia, *J Vet Intern Med* 25:100–106, 2011.

401. Roode SC, Rotroff D, Avery AC, et al.: Genome-wide assessment of recurrent genomic imbalances in canine leukemia identifies evolutionarily conserved regions for subtype differentiation, *Chromosome Res* 23:681–708, 2015.

402. Gioia G, Mortarino M, Gelain ME, et al.: Immunophenotype-related microRNA expression in canine chronic lymphocytic leukemia, *Vet Immunol Immunopathol* 142:228–235, 2011.

403. Stokol T, Schaefer DM, Shuman M, et al.: Alkaline phosphatase is a useful cytochemical marker for the diagnosis of acute myelomonocytic and monocytic leukemia in the dog, *Vet Clin Pathol* 44:79–93, 2015.

404. Bennett AL, Williams LE, Ferguson MW, et al.: Canine acute leukaemia: 50 cases (1989-2014), *Vet Comp Oncol* 15:1101–1114, 2017.

405. Leifer CE, Matus RE: Chronic lymphocytic leukemia in the dog: 22 cases (1974-1984), *J Am Vet Med Assoc* 189:214–217, 1986.

406. Kleiter M, Hirt R, Kirtz G, et al.: Hypercalcaemia associated with chronic lymphocytic leukaemia in a Giant Schnauzer, *Aust Vet J* 79:335–338, 2001.

407. Workman HC, Vernau W: Chronic lymphocytic leukemia in dogs and cats: the veterinary perspective, *Vet Clin North Am Small Anim Pract* 33:1379–1399, viii, 2003.

408. Matus RE, Leifer CE, MacEwen EG: Acute lymphoblastic leukemia in the dog: a review of 30 cases, *J Am Vet Med Assoc* 183:859–862, 1983.
409. Adams J, Mellanby RJ, Villiers E, et al.: Acute B cell lymphoblastic leukaemia in a 12-week-old greyhound, *J Small Anim Pract* 45:553–557, 2004.
410. Hodgkins EM, Zinkl JG, Madewell BR: Chronic lymphocytic leukemia in the dog, *J Am Vet Med Assoc* 177:704–707, 1980.
411. Comazzi S, Aresu L, Marconato L: Transformation of canine lymphoma/leukemia to more aggressive diseases: anecdotes or reality? *Front Vet Sci* 2(42), 2015.
412. Comazzi S, Martini V, Riondato F, et al.: Chronic lymphocytic leukemia transformation into high-grade lymphoma: a description of Richter's syndrome in eight dogs, *Vet Comp Oncol* 15:366–373, 2017.
413. Januszewicz E, Cooper IA, Pilkington G, et al.: Blastic transformation of chronic lymphocytic leukemia, *Am J Hematol* 15:399–402, 1983.
414. Harvey JW, Terrell TG, Hyde DM, et al.: Well-differentiated lymphocytic leukemia in a dog: long-term survival without therapy, *Vet Pathol* 18:37–47, 1981.
415. Boyce KL, Kitchell BE: Treatment of canine lymphoma with COPLA/LVP, *J Am Anim Hosp Assoc* 36:395–403, 2000.
416. Sato M, Yamazaki J, Goto-Koshino Y, et al.: Increase in minimal residual disease in peripheral blood before clinical relapse in dogs with lymphoma that achieved complete remission after chemotherapy, *J Vet Intern Med* 25:292–296, 2011.
417. Gentilini F, Calzolari C, Turba ME, et al.: Prognostic value of serum vascular endothelial growth factor (VEGF) and plasma activity of matrix metalloproteinase (MMP) 2 and 9 in lymphoma-affected dogs, *Leuk Res* 29:1263–1269, 2005.
418. Hahn KA, Barnhill MA, Freeman KP, et al.: Detection and clinical significance of plasma glutathione-S-transferases in dogs with lymphoma, *In Vivo* 13:173–175, 1999.
419. Heath 3rd H, Weller RE, Mundy GR: Canine lymphosarcoma: a model for study of the hypercalcemia of cancer, *Calcif Tissue Int* 30:127–133, 1980.
420. weller RHC, Theilen GH, et al.: Canine lymphosarcoma and hypercalcemia: clinical laboratory and pathologic evaluation of twenty-four cases, *J Small Anim Pract* 23:649–658, 1982.
421. Couto CG: Oncology. In R.G.S., editor: *The cat: diseases and clinical management*, New York, 1989, Churchill Livingstone.
422. Hardy WJ: Hematopoietic tumors of cats, *J Am Anim Hosp Assoc* 17:921–940, 1981.
423. Essex MFD: The risk to humans from malignant diseases of their pets: an unsettled issue, *J Am Anim Hosp Assoc* 12:386–390, 1976.
424. Theillen G, Madewell BR: Feline hematopoietic neoplasms. In Theilen GHMB, editor: *Veterinary cancer medicine*, ed 2, Philadelphia, 1987, Lea & Febiger.
425. Beatty J: Viral causes of feline lymphoma: retroviruses and beyond, *Vet J* 201:174–180, 2014.
426. Meichner K, Kruse DB, Hirschberger J, et al.: Changes in prevalence of progressive feline leukaemia virus infection in cats with lymphoma in Germany, *Vet Rec* 171:348, 2012.
427. Louwerens M, London CA, Pedersen NC, et al.: Feline lymphoma in the post-feline leukemia virus era, *J Vet Intern Med* 19:329–335, 2005.
428. Vail DM, Moore AS, Ogilvie GK, et al.: Feline lymphoma (145 cases): proliferation indices, cluster of differentiation 3 immunoreactivity, and their association with prognosis in 90 cats, *J Vet Intern Med* 12:349–354, 1998.
429. S.M.C.: Feline viral neoplasia. In Greene C, editor: *Infectious diseases of the dog and cat*, Philadelphia, 1998, WB Saunders.
430. Meichner K, Fogle JE, English L, et al.: Expression of apoptosis-regulating proteins Bcl-2 and Bax in lymph node aspirates from dogs with lymphoma, *J Vet Intern Med* 30:819–826, 2016.
431. Meichner K, von Bomhard W: Patient characteristics, histopathological findings and outcome in 97 cats with extranodal subcutaneous lymphoma (2007-2011), *Vet Comp Oncol* 14(Suppl 1):8–20, 2016.
432. Rissetto KVJ, Selting KA, et al.: Recent trends in feline intestinal neoplasia: an epidemiologic study of 1,129 cases in the veterinary medicanl database from 1964 to 2004, *J Am Anim Hosp Assoc* 47:28–36, 2011.
433. Schmidt JM, North SM, Freeman KP, et al.: Feline paediatric oncology: retrospective assessment of 233 tumours from cats up to one year (1993 to 2008), *J Small Anim Pract* 51:306–311, 2010.
434. Gabor LJ, Malik R, Canfield PJ: Clinical and anatomical features of lymphosarcoma in 118 cats, *Aust Vet J* 76:725–732, 1998.
435. Gabor LJ, Canfield PJ, Malik R: Immunophenotypic and histological characterisation of 109 cases of feline lymphosarcoma, *Aust Vet J* 77:436–441, 1999.
436. Barrs VR, Beatty JA: Feline alimentary lymphoma: 1. Classification, risk factors, clinical signs and non-invasive diagnostics, *J Feline Med Surg* 14:182–190, 2012.
437. Crouse Z, Phillips B, Flory A, et al.: Post-chemotherapy perforation in cats with discrete intermediate- or large-cell gastrointestinal lymphoma, *J Feline Med Surg*, 2017. https://doi.org/10.1177/1098612X17723773. epub ahead of print.
438. Finotello R, Vasconi ME, Sabattini S, et al.: Feline large granular lymphocyte lymphoma: an Italian Society of Veterinary Oncology (SIONCOV) retrospective study, *Vet Comp Oncol* 16:159–166, 2018.
439. Gustafson TL, Villamil A, Taylor BE, et al.: A retrospective study of feline gastric lymphoma in 16 chemotherapy-treated cats, *J Am Anim Hosp Assoc* 50:46–52, 2014.
440. Rau SE, Burgess KE: A retrospective evaluation of lomustine (CeeNU) in 32 treatment naive cats with intermediate to large cell gastrointestinal lymphoma (2006-2013), *Vet Comp Oncol* 15:1019–1028, 2017.
441. Sabattini S, Bottero E, Turba ME, et al.: Differentiating feline inflammatory bowel disease from alimentary lymphoma in duodenal endoscopic biopsies, *J Small Anim Pract* 57:396–401, 2016.
442. Ahmad S, Levy LS: The frequency of occurrence and nature of recombinant feline leukemia viruses in the induction of multicentric lymphoma by infection of the domestic cat with FeLV-945, *Virology* 403:103–110, 2010.
443. Fuhino YSH, Ohno K, et al.: Molecular cytogenetic analysis of feline leukemia virus insertions in cat lymphoid tumor cells, *J Virol Methods* 163:344–352, 2010.
444. Stutzer B, Simon K, Lutz H, et al.: Incidence of persistent viraemia and latent feline leukaemia virus infection in cats with lymphoma, *J Feline Med Surg* 13:81–87, 2011.
445. Fujino Y, Liao CP, Zhao YS, et al.: Identification of a novel common proviral integration site, flit-1, in feline leukemia virus induced thymic lymphoma, *Virology* 386:16–22, 2009.
446. Fujino Y, Ohno K, Tsujimoto H: Molecular pathogenesis of feline leukemia virus-induced malignancies: insertional mutagenesis, *Vet Immunol Immunopathol* 123:138–143, 2008.
447. Weiss AT, Klopfleisch R, Gruber AD: Prevalence of feline leukemia provirus DNA in feline lymphomas, *J Feline Med Surg* 12:929–935, 2010.
448. Beatty JA, Lawrence CE, Callanan JJ, et al.: Feline immunodeficiency virus (FIV)-associated lymphoma: a potential role for immune dysfunction in tumourigenesis, *Vet Immunol Immunopathol* 65:309–322, 1998.
449. Callanan JJ, McCandlish IA, O'Neil B, et al.: Lymphosarcoma in experimentally induced feline immunodeficiency virus infection, *Vet Rec* 130:293–295, 1992.
450. Endo Y, Cho KW, Nishigaki K, et al.: Molecular characteristics of malignant lymphomas in cats naturally infected with feline immunodeficiency virus, *Vet Immunol Immunopathol* 57:153–167, 1997.
451. Gabor LJ, Love DN, Malik R, et al.: Feline immunodeficiency virus status of Australian cats with lymphosarcoma, *Aust Vet J* 79:540–545, 2001.
452. Hutson CA, Rideout BA, Pedersen NC: Neoplasia associated with feline immunodeficiency virus infection in cats of southern California, *J Am Vet Med Assoc* 199:1357–1362, 1991.

453. Poli A, Abramo F, Baldinotti F, et al.: Malignant lymphoma associated with experimentally induced feline immunodeficiency virus infection, *J Comp Pathol* 110:319–328, 1994.

454. Shelton GH, Grant CK, Cotter SM, et al.: Feline immunodeficiency virus and feline leukemia virus infections and their relationships to lymphoid malignancies in cats: a retrospective study (1968-1988), *J Acquir Immune Defic Syndr* 3:623–630, 1990.

455. Terry A, Callanan JJ, Fulton R, et al.: Molecular analysis of tumours from feline immunodeficiency virus (FIV)-infected cats: an indirect role for FIV? *Int J Cancer* 61:227–232, 1995.

456. Wang J, Kyaw-Tanner M, Lee C, et al.: Characterisation of lymphosarcomas in Australian cats using polymerase chain reaction and immunohistochemical examination, *Aust Vet J* 79:41–46, 2001.

457. Rosenberg MPHA, Matus RE: Monoclonal gammopathy and lymphoma in a cat infected with feline immunodeficiency virus, *J Am Anim Hosp Assoc* 27:335–337, 1991.

458. Rassnick KM, Mauldin GN, Moroff SD, et al.: Prognostic value of argyrophilic nucleolar organizer region (AgNOR) staining in feline intestinal lymphoma, *J Vet Intern Med* 13:187–190, 1999.

459. Slawienski MJ, Mauldin GE, Mauldin GN, et al.: Malignant colonic neoplasia in cats: 46 cases (1990-1996), *J Am Vet Med Assoc* 211:878–881, 1997.

460. Zwahlen CH, Lucroy MD, Kraegel SA, et al.: Results of chemotherapy for cats with alimentary malignant lymphoma: 21 cases (1993-1997), *J Am Vet Med Assoc* 213:1144–1149, 1998.

461. Mahony OM, Moore AS, Cotter SM, et al.: Alimentary lymphoma in cats: 28 cases (1988-1993), *J Am Vet Med Assoc* 207:1593–1598, 1995.

462. McLuckie AJ, Barrs VR, Lindsay S, et al.: Molecular diagnosis of Felis catus gammaherpesvirus 1 (FcaGHV1) infection in cats of known retrovirus status with and without lymphoma, *Viruses* 10, 2018.

463. Mayr B, Winkler G, Schaffner G, et al.: N-ras mutation in a feline lymphoma. Low frequency of N-ras mutations in a series of feline, canine and bovine lymphomas, *Vet J* 163:326–328, 2002.

464. Cadile CD, Kitchell BE, Biller BJ, et al.: Telomerase activity as a marker for malignancy in feline tissues, *Am J Vet Res* 62:1578–1581, 2001.

465. Yazawa M, Okuda M, Uyama R, et al.: Molecular cloning of the feline telomerase reverse transcriptase (TERT) gene and its expression in cell lines and normal tissues, *J Vet Med Sci* 65:573–577, 2003.

466. Kano R, Sato E, Okamura T, et al.: Expression of Bcl-2 in feline lymphoma cell lines, *Vet Clin Pathol* 37:57–60, 2008.

467. Madewell B, Griffey S, Walls J, et al.: Reduced expression of cyclin-dependent kinase inhibitor p27Kip1 in feline lymphoma, *Vet Pathol* 38:698–702, 2001.

468. Dank G, Lucroy MD, Griffey SM, et al.: bcl-2 and MIB-1 labeling indexes in cats with lymphoma, *J Vet Intern Med* 16:720–725, 2002.

469. Bertone ER, Snyder LA, Moore AS: Environmental tobacco smoke and risk of malignant lymphoma in pet cats, *Am J Epidemiol* 156:268–273, 2002.

470. Marconato L, Leo C, Girelli R, et al.: Association between waste management and cancer in companion animals, *J Vet Intern Med* 23:564–569, 2009.

471. Beatty J, Terry A, MacDonald J, et al.: Feline immunodeficiency virus integration in B-cell lymphoma identifies a candidate tumor suppressor gene on human chromosome 15q15, *Cancer Res* 62:7175–7180, 2002.

472. Durham AC, Mariano AD, Holmes ES, et al.: Characterization of post transplantation lymphoma in feline renal transplant recipients, *J Comp Pathol* 150:162–168, 2014.

473. Schmiedt CW, Grimes JA, Holzman G, et al.: Incidence and risk factors for development of malignant neoplasia after feline renal transplantation and cyclosporine-based immunosuppression, *Vet Comp Oncol* 7:45–53, 2009.

474. Wooldridge JD, Gregory CR, Mathews KG, et al.: The prevalence of malignant neoplasia in feline renal-transplant recipients, *Vet Surg* 31:94–97, 2002.

475. Carreras JK, Goldschmidt M, Lamb M, et al.: Feline epitheliotropic intestinal malignant lymphoma: 10 cases (1997-2000), *J Vet Intern Med* 17:326–331, 2003.

476. Hart JFSE, Patnaik AK: Lymphocytic-plasmacytic enterocolitis in cats: 60 cases (1988-1990), *J Am Anim Hosp Assoc* 30:505–514, 1994.

477. Hoehne SN, McDonough SP, Rishniw M, et al.: Identification of mucosa-invading and intravascular bacteria in feline small intestinal lymphoma, *Vet Pathol* 54:23–241, 2017.

478. Bridgeford EC, Marini RP, Feng Y, et al.: Gastric Helicobacter species as a cause of feline gastric lymphoma: a viable hypothesis, *Vet Immunol Immunopathol* 123:106–113, 2008.

479. Martini V, Bernardi S, Marelli P, et al.: Flow cytometry for feline lymphoma: a retrospective study regarding pre-analytical factors possibly affecting the quality of samples, *J Feline Med Surg*, 1098612X17717175, 2017.

480. Hammer SE, Groiss S, Fuchs-Baumgartinger A, et al.: Characterization of a PCR-based lymphocyte clonality assay as a complementary tool for the diagnosis of feline lymphoma, *Vet Comp Oncol* 15:1354–1369, 2017.

481. Valli VE, Jacobs RM, Norris A, et al.: The histologic classification of 602 cases of feline lymphoproliferative disease using the National Cancer Institute working formulation, *J Vet Diagn Invest* 12:295–306, 2000.

482. Wolfesberger B, Skor O, Hammer SE, et al.: Does categorisation of lymphoma subtypes according to the World Health Organization classification predict clinical outcome in cats? *J Feline Med Surg* 19:897–906, 2017.

483. Valli VEJR, Parodi AL, et al.: *Histological classification of hematopoietic tumors of domestic animals*, Washington, DC, 2002, Armed Forces Institute of Pathology and The World health Organization.

484. Sato H, Fujino Y, Chino J, et al.: Prognostic analyses on anatomical and morphological classification of feline lymphoma, *J Vet Med Sci* 76:807–811, 2014.

485. Chino J, Fujino Y, Kobayashi T, et al.: Cytomorphological and immunological classification of feline lymphomas: clinicopathological features of 76 cases, *J Vet Med Sci* 75:701–707, 2013.

486. Lingard AE, Briscoe K, Beatty JA, et al.: Low-grade alimentary lymphoma: clinicopathological findings and response to treatment in 17 cases, *J Feline Med Surg* 11:692–700, 2009.

487. Moore PF, Rodriguez-Bertos A, Kass PH: Feline gastrointestinal lymphoma: mucosal architecture, immunophenotype, and molecular clonality, *Vet Pathol* 49:658–668, 2012.

488. Barrs VR, Beatty JA: Feline alimentary lymphoma: 2. Further diagnostics, therapy and prognosis, *J Feline Med Surg* 14:191–201, 2012.

489. Lalor S, Schwartz AM, Titmarsh H, et al.: Cats with inflammatory bowel disease and intestinal small cell lymphoma have low serum concentrations of 25-hydroxyvitamin D, *J Vet Intern Med* 28:351–355, 2014.

490. Russell KJ, Beatty JA, Dhand N, et al.: Feline low-grade alimentary lymphoma: how common is it? *J Feline Med Surg* 14:910–912, 2012.

491. Kiupel M, Smedley RC, Pfent C, et al.: Diagnostic algorithm to differentiate lymphoma from inflammation in feline small intestinal biopsy samples, *Vet Pathol* 48:212–222, 2011.

492. Vezzali E, Parodi AL, Marcato PS, et al.: Histopathologic classification of 171 cases of canine and feline non-Hodgkin lymphoma according to the WHO, *Vet Comp Oncol* 8:38–49, 2010.

493. Swerdlow SHCE, Harris NL, et al.: *WHO classification of tumor of the haematopoietic and lymphoid tissues*, France, 2008, International Agency for Research on Cancer.

494. Briscoe KA, Krockenberger M, Beatty JA, et al.: Histopathological and immunohistochemical evaluation of 53 cases of feline lymphoplasmacytic enteritis and low-grade alimentary lymphoma, *J Comp Pathol* 145:187–198, 2011.

495. Warren A, Center S, McDonough S, et al.: Histopathologic features, immunophenotyping, clonality, and eubacterial fluorescence in situ hybridization in cats with lymphocytic cholangitis/cholangiohepatitis, *Vet Pathol* 48:627–641, 2011.
496. Gouldin ED, Mullin C, Morges M, et al.: Feline discrete high-grade gastrointestinal lymphoma treated with surgical resection and adjuvant CHOP-based chemotherapy: retrospective study of 20 cases, *Vet Comp Oncol* 15:328–335, 2017.
497. Pohlman LM, Higginbotham ML, Welles EG, et al.: Immunophenotypic and histologic classification of 50 cases of feline gastrointestinal lymphoma, *Vet Pathol* 46:259–268, 2009.
498. Sapierzynski R, Jankowska U, Jagielski D, et al.: Large granular lymphoma in six cats, *Pol J Vet Sci* 18:163–169, 2015.
499. Ezura K, Ezura K, Nomura I, et al.: Natural killer-like T cell lymphoma in a cat, *Vet Rec* 154:268–270, 2004.
500. Krick EL, Little L, Patel R, et al.: Description of clinical and pathological findings, treatment and outcome of feline large granular lymphocyte lymphoma (1996-2004), *Vet Comp Oncol* 6:102–110, 2008.
501. Roccabianca P, Vernau W, Caniatti M, et al.: Feline large granular lymphocyte (LGL) lymphoma with secondary leukemia: primary intestinal origin with predominance of a CD3/CD8(alpha) phenotype, *Vet Pathol* 43:15–28, 2006.
502. Congress '99: what's new in the treatment of lymphoma? *J Small Anim Pract* 40:51, 1999.
503. Gieger T: Alimentary lymphoma in cats and dogs, *Vet Clin North Am Small Anim Pract* 41:419–432, 2011.
504. Kiselow MA, Rassnick KM, McDonough SP, et al.: Outcome of cats with low-grade lymphocytic lymphoma: 41 cases (1995-2005), *J Am Vet Med Assoc* 232:405–410, 2008.
505. Fondacaro JVRK, Carpenter JL, et al.: Feline gastrointestinal lymphoma: 67 cases, *Eur J Comp Gastroenterol* 4:199, 1999.
506. Gabor LJ, Canfield PJ, Malik R: Haematological and biochemical findings in cats in Australia with lymphosarcoma, *Aust Vet J* 78:456–461, 2000.
507. Gerou-Ferriani M, McBrearty AR, Burchmore RJ, et al.: Agarose gel serum protein electrophoresis in cats with and without lymphoma and preliminary results of tandem mass fingerprinting analysis, *Vet Clin Pathol* 40:159–173, 2011.
508. Daniaux LA, Laurenson MP, Marks SL, et al.: Ultrasonographic thickening of the muscularis propria in feline small intestinal small cell T-cell lymphoma and inflammatory bowel disease, *J Feline Med Surg* 16:89–98, 2014.
509. Evans SE, Bonczynski JJ, Broussard JD, et al.: Comparison of endoscopic and full-thickness biopsy specimens for diagnosis of inflammatory bowel disease and alimentary tract lymphoma in cats, *J Am Vet Med Assoc* 229:1447–1450, 2006.
510. Zwingenberger AL, Marks SL, Baker TW, et al.: Ultrasonographic evaluation of the muscularis propria in cats with diffuse small intestinal lymphoma or inflammatory bowel disease, *J Vet Intern Med* 24:289–292, 2010.
511. Jergens AE, Willard MD, Allenspach K: Maximizing the diagnostic utility of endoscopic biopsy in dogs and cats with gastrointestinal disease, *Vet J* 214:50–60, 2016.
512. Kleinschmidt S, Harder J, Nolte I, et al.: Chronic inflammatory and non-inflammatory diseases of the gastrointestinal tract in cats: diagnostic advantages of full-thickness intestinal and extraintestinal biopsies, *J Feline Med Surg* 12:97–103, 2010.
513. Awaysheh A, Wilcke J, Elvinger F, et al.: Evaluation of supervised machine-learning algorithms to distinguish between inflammatory bowel disease and alimentary lymphoma in cats, *J Vet Diagn Invest* 28:679–687, 2016.
514. Sawa M, Yabuki A, Setoguchi A, et al.: Development and application of multiple immunofluorescence staining for diagnostic cytology of canine and feline lymphoma, *Vet Clin Pathol* 44:580–585, 2015.
515. Malik R, Gabor LJ, Foster SF, et al.: Therapy for Australian cats with lymphosarcoma, *Aust Vet J* 79:808–817, 2001.
516. Tzannes S, Hammond MF, Murphy S, et al.: Owners 'perception of their cats' quality of life during COP chemotherapy for lymphoma, *J Feline Med Surg* 10:73–81, 2008.
517. Pope KV, Tun AE, McNeill CJ, et al.: Outcome and toxicity assessment of feline small cell lymphoma: 56 cases (2000-2010), *Vet Med Sci* 1:51–62, 2015.
518. Stein TJ, Pellin M, Steinberg H, et al.: Treatment of feline gastrointestinal small-cell lymphoma with chlorambucil and glucocorticoids, *J Am Anim Hosp Assoc* 46:413–417, 2010.
519. Dutelle AL, Bulman-Fleming JC, Lewis CA, et al.: Evaluation of lomustine as a rescue agent for cats with resistant lymphoma, *J Feline Med Surg* 14:694–700, 2012.
520. Collette SA, Allstadt SD, Chon EM, et al.: Treatment of feline intermediate- to high-grade lymphoma with a modified university of Wisconsin-Madison protocol: 119 cases (2004-2012), *Vet Comp Oncol* 14(Suppl 1):136–146, 2016.
521. Limmer S, Eberle N, Nerschbach V, et al.: Treatment of feline lymphoma using a 12-week, maintenance-free combination chemotherapy protocol in 26 cats, *Vet Comp Oncol* 14(Suppl 1):21–31, 2016.
522. Waite AH, Jackson K, Gregor TP, et al.: Lymphoma in cats treated with a weekly cyclophosphamide-, vincristine-, and prednisone-based protocol: 114 cases (1998-2008), *J Am Vet Med Assoc* 242:1104–1109, 2013.
523. Hadden AG, Cotter SM, Rand W, et al.: Efficacy and toxicosis of VELCAP-C treatment of lymphoma in cats, *J Vet Intern Med* 22:153–157, 2008.
524. Jeglum KA, Whereat A, Young K: Chemotherapy of lymphoma in 75 cats, *J Am Vet Med Assoc* 190:174–178, 1987.
525. Milner RJ, Peyton J, Cooke K, et al.: Response rates and survival times for cats with lymphoma treated with the University of Wisconsin-Madison chemotherapy protocol: 38 cases (1996-2003), *J Am Vet Med Assoc* 227:1118–1122, 2005.
526. Mooney SC, Hayes AA, MacEwen EG, et al.: Treatment and prognostic factors in lymphoma in cats: 103 cases (1977-1981), *J Am Vet Med Assoc* 194:696–702, 1989.
527. Moore AS, Cotter SM, Frimberger AE, et al.: A comparison of doxorubicin and COP for maintenance of remission in cats with lymphoma, *J Vet Intern Med* 10:372–375, 1996.
528. Simon D, Eberle N, Laacke-Singer L, et al.: Combination chemotherapy in feline lymphoma: treatment outcome, tolerability, and duration in 23 cats, *J Vet Intern Med* 22:394–400, 2008.
529. Krick EL, Cohen RB, Gregor TP, et al.: Prospective clinical trial to compare vincristine and vinblastine in a COP-based protocol for lymphoma in cats, *J Vet Intern Med* 27:134–140, 2013.
530. Kristal O, Lana SE, Ogilvie GK, et al.: Single agent chemotherapy with doxorubicin for feline lymphoma: a retrospective study of 19 cases (1994-1997), *J Vet Intern Med* 15:125–130, 2001.
531. Peaston AE, Maddison JE: Efficacy of doxorubicin as an induction agent for cats with lymphosarcoma, *Aust Vet J* 77:442–444, 1999.
532. Poirier VJ, Thamm DH, Kurzman ID, et al.: Liposome-encapsulated doxorubicin (Doxil) and doxorubicin in the treatment of vaccine-associated sarcoma in cats, *J Vet Intern Med* 16:726–731, 2002.
533. Teske E, van Straten G, van Noort R, et al.: Chemotherapy with cyclophosphamide, vincristine, and prednisolone (COP) in cats with malignant lymphoma: new results with an old protocol, *J Vet Intern Med* 16:179–186, 2002.
534. Vajdovich P, Psader R, Toth ZA, et al.: Use of the argyrophilic nucleolar region method for cytologic and histologic examination of the lymph nodes in dogs, *Vet Pathol* 41:338–345, 2004.
535. Teske E, van Lankveld AJ, Rutteman GR: Intraperitoneal antineoplastic drug delivery: experience with a cyclophosphamide, vincristine and prednisolone protocol in cats with malignant lymphoma, *Vet Comp Oncol* 12:37–46, 2014.
536. Elliott J, Finotello R: A dexamethasone, melphalan, actinomycin-D and cytarabine chemotherapy protocol as a rescue treatment for feline lymphoma, *Vet Comp Oncol* 16:E144–E151, 2018.

537. Martin OA, Price J: Mechlorethamine, vincristine, melphalan and prednisolone rescue chemotherapy protocol for resistant feline lymphoma, *J Feline Med Surg*, 2017. https://doi.org/10.1177/1098612X17735989. epub ahead of print.

538. Parshley DL, Larue SM, Kitchell B, et al.: Abdominal irradiation as a rescue therapy for feline gastrointestinal lymphoma: a retrospective study of 11 cats (2001-2008), *J Feline Med Surg* 13:63–68, 2011.

539. Williams LE, Pruitt AF, Thrall DE: Chemotherapy followed by abdominal cavity irradiation for feline lymphoblastic lymphoma, *Vet Radiol Ultrasound* 51:681–687, 2010.

540. Williams LE, Johnson JL, Hauck ML, et al.: Chemotherapy followed by half-body radiation therapy for canine lymphoma, *J Vet Intern Med* 18:703–709, 2004.

541. Day MJ, Kyaw-Tanner M, Silkstone MA, et al.: T-cell-rich B-cell lymphoma in the cat, *J Comp Pathol* 120:155–167, 1999.

542. Walton RM, Hendrick MJ: Feline Hodgkin's-like lymphoma: 20 cases (1992-1999), *Vet Pathol* 38:504–511, 2001.

543. Elliott J: Temporary spontaneous regression of feline non-Hodgkin's lymphoma, *Aust Vet J* 96:83–85, 2018.

544. Newton JA, de Vicente F, Haugland SP, et al.: Extra-nodal subcutaneous Hodgkin's-like lymphoma and subsequent regression in a cat, *J Feline Med Surg* 17:543–547, 2015.

545. Holt E, Goldschmidt MH, Skorupski K: Extranodal conjunctival Hodgkin's-like lymphoma in a cat, *Vet Ophthalmol* 9:141–144, 2006.

546. Davies C, Forrester SD: Pleural effusion in cats: 82 cases (1987 to 1995), *J Small Anim Pract* 37:217–224, 1996.

547. Day MJ: Review of thymic pathology in 30 cats and 36 dogs, *J Small Anim Pract* 38:393–403, 1997.

548. Fabrizio F, Calam AE, Dobson JM, et al.: Feline mediastinal lymphoma: a retrospective study of signalment, retroviral status, response to chemotherapy and prognostic indicators, *J Feline Med Surg* 16:637–644, 2014.

549. Court EA, Watson AD, Peaston AE: Retrospective study of 60 cases of feline lymphosarcoma, *Aust Vet J* 75:424–427, 1997.

550. Forrester SD, Fossum TW, Rogers KS: Diagnosis and treatment of chylothorax associated with lymphoblastic lymphosarcoma in four cats, *J Am Vet Med Assoc* 198:291–294, 1991.

551. Fossum TW, Jacobs RM, Birchard SJ: Evaluation of cholesterol and triglyceride concentrations in differentiating chylous and nonchylous pleural effusions in dogs and cats, *J Am Vet Med Assoc* 188:49–51, 1986.

552. Savary KC, Price GS, Vaden SL: Hypercalcemia in cats: a retrospective study of 71 cases (1991-1997), *J Vet Intern Med* 14:184–189, 2000.

553. Avery PR, Avery AC: Molecular methods to distinguish reactive and neoplastic lymphocyte expansions and their importance in transitional neoplastic states, *Vet Clin Pathol* 33:196–207, 2004.

554. Henrich M, Hecht W, Weiss AT, et al.: A new subgroup of immunoglobulin heavy chain variable region genes for the assessment of clonality in feline B-cell lymphomas, *Vet Immunol Immunopathol* 130:59–69, 2009.

555. Moore PF, Woo JC, Vernau W, et al.: Characterization of feline T cell receptor gamma (TCRG) variable region genes for the molecular diagnosis of feline intestinal T cell lymphoma, *Vet Immunol Immunopathol* 106:167–178, 2005.

556. Weiss AT, Klopfleisch R, Gruber AD: T-cell receptor gamma chain variable and joining region genes of subgroup 1 are clonally rearranged in feline B- and T-cell lymphoma, *J Comp Pathol* 144:123–134, 2011.

557. Werner JA, Woo JC, Vernau W, et al.: Characterization of feline immunoglobulin heavy chain variable region genes for the molecular diagnosis of B-cell neoplasia, *Vet Pathol* 42:596–607, 2005.

558. Mooney SC, Hayes AA: Lymphoma in the cat: an approach to diagnosis and management, *Semin Vet Med Surg (Small Anim)* 1:51–57, 1986.

559. Taylor SS, Goodfellow MR, Browne WJ, et al.: Feline extranodal lymphoma: response to chemotherapy and survival in 110 cats, *J Small Anim Pract* 50:584–592, 2009.

560. Little L, Patel R, Goldschmidt M: Nasal and nasopharyngeal lymphoma in cats: 50 cases (1989-2005), *Vet Pathol* 44:885–892, 2007.

561. Santagostino SF, Mortellaro CM, Boracchi P, et al.: Feline upper respiratory tract lymphoma: site, cyto-histology, phenotype, FeLV expression, and prognosis, *Vet Pathol* 52:250–259, 2015.

562. Demko JL, Cohn LA: Chronic nasal discharge in cats: 75 cases (1993-2004), *J Am Vet Med Assoc* 230:1032–1037, 2007.

563. Henderson SM, Bradley K, Day MJ, et al.: Investigation of nasal disease in the cat—a retrospective study of 77 cases, *J Feline Med Surg* 6:245–257, 2004.

564. Mukaratirwa S, van der Linde-Sipman JS, Gruys E: Feline nasal and paranasal sinus tumours: clinicopathological study, histomorphological description and diagnostic immunohistochemistry of 123 cases, *J Feline Med Surg* 3:235–245, 2001.

565. Haney SM, Beaver L, Turrel J, et al.: Survival analysis of 97 cats with nasal lymphoma: a multi-institutional retrospective study (1986-2006), *J Vet Intern Med* 23:287–294, 2009.

566. Nemanic S, Hollars K, Nelson NC, et al.: Combination of computed tomographic imaging characteristics of medial retropharyngeal lymph nodes and nasal passages aids discrimination between rhinitis and neoplasia in cats, *Vet Radiol Ultrasound* 56:617–627, 2015.

567. Detweiler DA, Johnson LR, Kass PH, et al.: Computed tomographic evidence of bulla effusion in cats with sinonasal disease: 2001-2004, *J Vet Intern Med* 20:1080–1084, 2006.

568. Tromblee TC, Jones JC, Etue AE, et al.: Association between clinical characteristics, computed tomography characteristics, and histologic diagnosis for cats with sinonasal disease, *Vet Radiol Ultrasound* 47:241–248, 2006.

569. Nagata K, Lamb M, Goldschmidt MH, et al.: The usefulness of immunohistochemistry to differentiate between nasal carcinoma and lymphoma in cats: 140 cases (1986-2000), *Vet Comp Oncol* 12:52–57, 2014.

570. Fu DR, Kato D, Endo Y, et al.: Apoptosis and Ki-67 as predictive factors for response to radiation therapy in feline nasal lymphomas, *J Vet Med Sci* 78:1161–1166, 2016.

571. Fujiwara-Igarashi A, Fujimori T, Oka M, et al.: Evaluation of outcomes and radiation complications in 65 cats with nasal tumours treated with palliative hypofractionated radiotherapy, *Vet J* 202:455–461, 2014.

572. Moore A: Extranodal lymphoma in the cat: prognostic factors and treatment options, *J Feline Med Surg* 15:379–390, 2013.

573. Elmslie RE Ogilvie GK, Gillette EL, et al.: Radiotherapy with and without chemotherapy for localized lymphoma in 10 cats, *Vet Radiol Ultrasound* 32:277–280, 1991.

574. Sfiligoi G, Theon AP, Kent MS: Response of nineteen cats with nasal lymphoma to radiation therapy and chemotherapy, *Vet Radiol Ultrasound* 48:388–393, 2007.

575. Mooney SC, Hayes AA, Matus RE, et al.: Renal lymphoma in cats: 28 cases (1977-1984), *J Am Vet Med Assoc* 191:1473–1477, 1987.

576. Valdes-Martinez A, Cianciolo R, Mai W: Association between renal hypoechoic subcapsular thickening and lymphosarcoma in cats, *Vet Radiol Ultrasound* 48:357–360, 2007.

577. Troxel MT, Vite CH, Van Winkle TJ, et al.: Feline intracranial neoplasia: retrospective review of 160 cases (1985-2001), *J Vet Intern Med* 17:850–859, 2003.

578. Marioni-Henry K, Van Winkle TJ, Smith SH, et al.: Tumors affecting the spinal cord of cats: 85 cases (1980-2005), *J Am Vet Med Assoc* 232:237–243, 2008.

579. Mandara MT, Motta L, Calo P: Distribution of feline lymphoma in the central and peripheral nervous systems, *Vet J* 216:109–116, 2016.

580. Tomek A, Cizinauskas S, Doherr M, et al.: Intracranial neoplasia in 61 cats: localisation, tumour types and seizure patterns, *J Feline Med Surg* 8:243–253, 2006.

581. Marioni-Henry K, Vite CH, Newton AL, et al.: Prevalence of diseases of the spinal cord of cats, *J Vet Intern Med* 18:851–858, 2004.

582. Lane SB, Kornegay JN, Duncan JR, et al.: Feline spinal lymphosarcoma: a retrospective evaluation of 23 cats, *J Vet Intern Med* 8:99–104, 1994.

583. Spodnick GJ, Berg J, Moore FM, et al.: Spinal lymphoma in cats: 21 cases (1976-1989), *J Am Vet Med Assoc* 200:373–376, 1992.

584. Palus V, Volk HA, Lamb CR, et al.: MRI features of CNS lymphoma in dogs and cats, *Vet Radiol Ultrasound* 53:44–49, 2012.

585. Fontaine J, Heimann M, Day MJ: Cutaneous epitheliotropic T-cell lymphoma in the cat: a review of the literature and five new cases, *Vet Dermatol* 22:454–461, 2011.

586. Caciolo PLNG, Patnaik AK, et al.: Cutaneous lymphosarcoma in the cat: a report of nine cases, *J Am Anim Hosp Assoc* 20:491–496, 1984.

587. Gilbert S, Affolter VK, Gross TL, et al.: Clinical, morphological and immunohistochemical characterization of cutaneous lymphocytosis in 23 cats, *Vet Dermatol* 15:3–12, 2004.

588. Day MJ: Immunophenotypic characterization of cutaneous lymphoid neoplasia in the dog and cat, *J Comp Pathol* 112:79–96, 1995.

589. Schick RO, Murphy GF, Goldschmidt MH: Cutaneous lymphosarcoma and leukemia in a cat, *J Am Vet Med Assoc* 203:1155–1158, 1993.

590. Wood C, Almes K, Bagladi-Swanson M, et al.: Sezary syndrome in a cat, *J Am Anim Hosp Assoc* 44:144–148, 2008.

591. Komori S, Nakamura S, Takahashi K, et al.: Use of lomustine to treat cutaneous nonepitheliotropic lymphoma in a cat, *J Am Vet Med Assoc* 226:237–239, 2005.

592. Burr HD, Keating JH, Clifford CA, et al.: Cutaneous lymphoma of the tarsus in cats: 23 cases (2000-2012), *J Am Vet Med Assoc* 244:1429–1434, 2014.

593. Roccabianca P, Avallone G, Rodriguez A, et al.: Cutaneous lymphoma at injection sites: pathological, immunophenotypical, and molecular characterization in 17 cats, *Vet Pathol* 53:823–832, 2016.

594. Taylor SS, Harvey AM, Barr FJ, et al.: Laryngeal disease in cats: a retrospective study of 35 cases, *J Feline Med Surg* 11:954–962, 2009.

595. Nerschbach V, Eule JC, Eberle N, et al.: Ocular manifestation of lymphoma in newly diagnosed cats, *Vet Comp Oncol* 2016(14):58–66, 2016.

596. Peiffer Jr RL: Wilcock BP: Histopathologic study of uveitis in cats: 139 cases (1978-1988), *J Am Vet Med Assoc* 198:135–138, 1991.

597. Malmberg JL, Garcia T, Dubielzig RR, et al.: Canine and feline retinal lymphoma: a retrospective review of 12 cases, *Vet Ophthalmol* 20:73–78, 2017.

598. McCowan C, Malcolm J, Hurn S, et al.: Conjunctival lymphoma: immunophenotype and outcome in five dogs and three cats, *Vet Ophthalmol* 17:351–357, 2014.

599. Ota-Kuroki J, Ragsdale JM, Bawa B, et al.: Intraocular and periocular lymphoma in dogs and cats: a retrospective review of 21 cases (2001-2012), *Vet Ophthalmol* 17:389–396, 2014.

600. Wiggans KT, Skorupski KA, Reilly CM, et al.: Presumed solitary intraocular or conjunctival lymphoma in dogs and cats: 9 cases (1985-2013), *J Am Vet Med Assoc* 244:460–470, 2014.

601. Grindem CB: Ultrastructural morphology of leukemic cells in the cat, *Vet Pathol* 22:147–155, 1985.

602. Gorman NT, Evans RJ: Myeloproliferative disease in the dog and cat: clinical presentations, diagnosis and treatment, *Vet Rec* 121:490–496, 1987.

603. Blue JT, French TW, Kranz JS: Non-lymphoid hematopoietic neoplasia in cats: a retrospective study of 60 cases, *Cornell Vet* 78:21–42, 1988.

604. Facklam NR, Kociba GJ: Cytochemical characterization of feline leukemic cells, *Vet Pathol* 23:155–161, 1986.

605. Grindem C: Morphological and clinical an pathological characteristics of spontaneous leukemia in 10 cats, *J Am Anim Hosp Assoc* 21:227, 1985.

606. Campbell MW, Hess PR, Williams LE: Chronic lymphocytic leukaemia in the cat: 18 cases (2000-2010), *Vet Comp Oncol* 11:256–264, 2013.

607. Weiss DJ: Differentiating benign and malignant causes of lymphocytosis in feline bone marrow, *J Vet Intern Med* 19:855–859, 2005.

608. Hisasue M, Okayama H, Okayama T, et al.: Hematologic abnormalities and outcome of 16 cats with myelodysplastic syndromes, *J Vet Intern Med* 15:471–477, 2001.

609. Essex ME: Feline leukemia: a naturally occurring cancer of infectious origin, *Epidemiol Rev* 4:189–203, 1982.

610. Tebb AJ, Cave T, Barron R, et al.: Diagnosis and management of B cell chronic lymphocytic leukaemia in a cat, *Vet Rec* 154:430–433, 2004.

611. Workman HC, Vernau W: Chronic lymphocytic leukemia in dogs and cats: the veterinary perspective, *Vet Clin North Am Small Anim Pract* 33:1379–1399, 2003.

612. Cotter SM: Treatment of lymphoma and leukemia with cyclophosphamide, vincristine and prednisone: I. Treatment of dogs, *J Am Anim Hosp Assoc* 19:159–165, 1983.

613. Lichtman MA: Classification and clinical manifestations of the clonal myeloid disorders. In Lichtman MA Kaushansky K, Seligsohn U, et al.: *Williams hematology*, ed 8, New York, 2011, McGraw-Hill.

614. Breen M, Modiano JF: Evolutionarily conserved cytogenetic changes in hematological malignancies of dogs and humans—man and his best friend share more than companionship, *Chromosome Res* 16:145–154, 2008.

615. Jain NC, Blue JT, Grindem CB, et al.: Proposed criteria for classification of acute myeloid leukemia in dogs and cats, *Vet Clin Pathol* 20:63–82, 1991.

616. Juopperi TA, Bienzle D, Bernreuter DC, et al.: Prognostic markers for myeloid neoplasms: a comparative review of the literature and goals for future investigation, *Vet Pathol* 48:182–197, 2011.

617. Nielson SW: myeloproliferative disorders in animals. In Clarke WJ Hacett EB, Hackett PL, editors: *Myeloproliferative disorders in animals and man*, Oak Ridge, Tenn, 1970, USAEC Division of Technical Information Extension.

618. Bennett AL, Williams LE, Ferguson MW, et al.: Canine acute leukaemia: 50 cases (1989-2014), *Vet Comp Oncol* 15:1101–1114, 2017.

619. Davis LL, Hume KR, Stokol T: A retrospective review of acute myeloid leukaemia in 35 dogs diagnosed by a combination of morphologic findings, flow cytometric immunophenotyping and cytochemical staining results (2007-2015), *Vet Comp Oncol* 16:268–275, 2018.

620. Novacco M, Comazzi S, Marconato L, et al.: Prognostic factors in canine acute leukaemias: a retrospective study, *Vet Comp Oncol* 14:409–416, 2016.

621. Stokol T, Nickerson GA, Shuman M, et al.: Dogs with acute myeloid leukemia have clonal rearrangements in T and B Cell receptors, *Front Vet Sci* 4:76, 2017.

622. Grindem CBSJ, Perman V: Morphologic classification and clinical and pathological charactersitics of spontaneous leukemia in 17 dogs, *J Am Anim Hosp Assoc* 21:219–226, 1985.

623. Jandl J: *Hematopoietic malignancies. blood: pathophysiology*, Boston, 1991, Blackwell Scientific.

624. Grindem CB, Buoen LC: Cytogenetic analysis of leukaemic cells in the dog. A report of 10 cases and a review of the literature, *J Comp Pathol* 96:623–635, 1986.

625. Reimann N, Bartnitzke S, Bullerdiek J, et al.: Trisomy 1 in a canine acute leukemia indicating the pathogenetic importance of polysomy 1 in leukemias of the dog, *Cancer Genet Cytogenet* 101:49–52, 1998.

626. Roode SC, Rotroff D, Avery AC, et al.: Genome-wide assessment of recurrent genomic imbalances in canine leukemia identifies evolutionarily conserved regions for subtype differentiation, *Chromosome Res* 23:681–708, 2015.

627. Culver S, Ito D, Borst L, et al.: Molecular characterization of canine BCR-ABL-positive chronic myelomonocytic leukemia before and after chemotherapy, *Vet Clin Pathol* 42:314–322, 2013.

628. Breen M: Canine cytogenetics—from band to basepair, *Cytogenet Genome Res* 120:50–60, 2008.

629. Breen M: Update on genomics in veterinary oncology, *Top Companion Anim Med* 24:113–121, 2009.

630. Reimann N, Bartnitzke S, Nolte I, et al.: Working with canine chromosomes: current recommendations for karyotype description, *J Hered* 90:31–34, 1999.

631. Andersen AC, Johnson RM: Erythroblastic malignancy in a beagle, *J Am Vet Med Assoc* 141:944–946, 1962.

632. Seed TM, Tolle DV, Fritz TE, et al.: Irradiation-induced erythroleukemia and myelogenous leukemia in the beagle dog: hematology and ultrastructure, *Blood* 50:1061–1079, 1977.

633. Tolle DV, Seed TM, Fritz TE, et al.: Acute monocytic leukemia in an irradiated Beagle, *Vet Pathol* 16:243–254, 1979.

634. Sykes GP, King JM, Cooper BC: Retrovirus-like particles associated with myeloproliferative disease in the dog, *J Comp Pathol* 95:559–564, 1985.

635. Quesenberry P: Hemopoietic stem cells, progenitor cells and cytokines. In Beutler ELM, Coller BS, et al.: *Williams hematology*, ed 5, New York, 1995, McGraw-Hill.

636. Metcalf D: *The hemopoietic colony stimulating factors*, New York, 1984, Elsevier.

637. Lok S, Kaushansky K, Holly RD, et al.: Cloning and expression of murine thrombopoietin cDNA and stimulation of platelet production in vivo, *Nature* 369:565–568, 1994.

638. Boone LI, Knauer KW, Rapp SW, et al.: Use of human recombinant erythropoietin and prednisone for treatment of myelodysplastic syndrome with erythroid predominance in a dog, *J Am Vet Med Assoc* 213:999–1001, 1998.

639. Couto CG: Clinicopathologic aspects of acute leukemias in the dog, *J Am Vet Med Assoc* 186:681–685, 1985.

640. Couto CG, Kallet AJ: Preleukemic syndrome in a dog, *J Am Vet Med Assoc* 184:1389–1392, 1984.

641. Weiss DJ, Raskin R, Zerbe C: Myelodysplastic syndrome in two dogs, *J Am Vet Med Assoc* 187:1038–1040, 1985.

642. Degen MA, Feldman BF, Turrel JM, et al.: Thrombocytosis associated with a myeloproliferative disorder in a dog, *J Am Vet Med Assoc* 194:1457–1459, 1989.

643. Evans RJ, Gorman NT: Myeloproliferative disease in the dog and cat: definition, aetiology and classification, *Vet Rec* 121:437–443, 1987.

644. Jain NC, Madewell BR, Weller RE, et al.: Clinical-pathological findings and cytochemical characterization of myelomonocytic leukaemia in 5 dogs, *J Comp Pathol* 91:17–31, 1981.

645. Clark P, Swenson CL, Drenen CM: A 6-year-old rottweiler with weight loss, *Aust Vet J* 75:709, 714–705, 1997.

646. Graves TK, Swenson CL, Scott MA: A potentially misleading presentation and course of acute myelomonocytic leukemia in a dog, *J Am Anim Hosp Assoc* 33:37–41, 1997.

647. Keller P, Sager P, Freudiger U, et al.: Acute myeloblastic leukaemia in a dog, *J Comp Pathol* 95:619–632, 1985.

648. Barthel CH: Acute myelomonocytic leukemia in a dog, *Vet Pathol* 11:79–86, 1974.

649. Bolon B, Buergelt CD, Harvey JW, et al.: Megakaryblastic leukemia in a dog, *Vet Clin Pathol* 18:69–74, 1989.

650. Green RABC: Acute myelomonocytic leukemia in a dog, *J Am Anim Hosp Assoc* 13:708–712, 1977.

651. Hayashi A, Tanaka H, Kitamura M, et al.: Acute myelomonocytic leukemia (AML-M4) in a dog with the extradural lesion, *J Vet Med Sci* 73:419–422, 2011.

652. Hisasue M, Nishimura T, Neo S, et al.: A dog with acute myelomonocytic leukemia, *J Vet Med Sci* 70:619–621, 2008.

653. Linnabary RDHM, Glick AD, et al.: Acute myelomonocytic leukemia in a dog, *J Am Anim Hosp Assoc* 14:71–75, 1978.

654. Madewell B: Unusual cytochemical reactivity in canine acute myeloblastic leukemia, *Comp Haematol Int* 1:117–120, 1991.

655. Moulton JEDD: Tumors of the lymphoid and hemopoietic tissues. In JE M, editor: *Tumors in domestic animals*, ed 2, Berkeley, 1978, University of California Press.

656. Ragan HA, Hackett PL, Dagle GE: Acute myelomonocytic leukemia manifested as myelophthisic anemia in a dog, *J Am Vet Med Assoc* 169:421–425, 1976.

657. Rohrig KE: Acute myelomonocytic leukemia in a dog, *J Am Vet Med Assoc* 182:137–141, 1983.

658. Cain GR, Feldman BF, Kawakami TG, et al.: Platelet dysplasia associated with megakaryoblastic leukemia in a dog, *J Am Vet Med Assoc* 188:529–530, 1986.

659. Cain GR, Kawakami TG, Jain NC: Radiation-induced megakaryoblastic leukemia in a dog, *Vet Pathol* 22:641–643, 1985.

660. Canfield PJCD, Russ IG: Myeloproliferative disorder involving the megakaryocytic line, *J Small Anim Pract* 34:296–301, 1993.

661. Colbatzky F, Hermanns W: Acute megakaryoblastic leukemia in one cat and two dogs, *Vet Pathol* 30:186–194, 1993.

662. Comazzi SGM, Belfanti U, et al.: Acute megakaryoblastic leukemia in a dog: a report of 3 cases and review of the literature, *J Am Anim Hosp Assoc* 46:327–335, 2010.

663. Ferreira HMT, Smith SH, Schwartz AM, et al.: Myeloperoxidase-positive acute megakaryoblastic leukemia in a dog, *Vet Clin Pathol* 40:530–537, 2011.

664. Holscher MA, Collins RD, Glick AD, et al.: Megakaryocytic leukemia in a dog, *Vet Pathol* 15:562–565, 1978.

665. Messick J, Carothers M, Wellman M: Identification and characterization of megakaryoblasts in acute megakaryoblastic leukemia in a dog, *Vet Pathol* 27:212–214, 1990.

666. Park HM, Doster AR, Tashbaeva RE, et al.: Clinical, histopathological and immunohistochemical findings in a case of megakaryoblastic leukemia in a dog, *J Vet Diagn Invest* 18:287–291, 2006.

667. Shull RM, DeNovo RC, McCracken MD: Megakaryoblastic leukemia in a dog, *Vet Pathol* 23:533–536, 1986.

668. Suter SE, Vernau W, Fry MM, et al.: CD34+, CD41+ acute megakaryoblastic leukemia in a dog, *Vet Clin Pathol* 36:288–292, 2007.

669. Willan MML, Schwendenwein I, et al.: Chemotherapy in canine acute megakaryoblastic leukemia: a case report and review of the literature, *Vivo* 23:911–918, 2009.

670. Mylonakis ME, Kritsepi-Konstantinou M, Vernau W, et al.: Presumptive pure erythroid leukemia in a dog, *J Vet Diagn Invest* 24:1004–1007, 2012.

671. Valentini F, Tasca S, Gavazza A, et al.: Use of CD9 and CD61 for the characterization of AML-M7 by flow cytometry in a dog, *Vet Comp Oncol* 10:312–318, 2012.

672. Latimer KS, Dykstra MJ: Acute monocytic leukemia in a dog, *J Am Vet Med Assoc* 184:852–854, 1984.

673. Mackey LJ: Monocytic leukaemia in the dog, *Vet Rec* 96:27–30, 1975.

674. Campbell MW, Hess PR, Williams LE: Chronic lymphocytic leukaemia in the cat: 18 cases (2000-2010), *Vet Comp Oncol* 11:256–264, 2013.

675. Tomiyasu H, Fujino Y, Takahashi M, et al.: Spontaneous acute erythroblastic leukaemia (AML-M6Er) in a dog, *J Small Anim Pract* 52:445–447, 2011.

676. Hejlasz Z: Three cases of erythroleukemia in a dog, *Medycyna Weterynaryjna* 42:346–349, 1986.

677. Grindem CB: Blood cell markers, *Vet Clin North Am Small Anim Pract* 26:1043–1064, 1996.

678. Usher SG, Radford AD, Villiers EJ, et al.: RAS, FLT3, and C-KIT mutations in immunophenotyped canine leukemias, *Exp Hematol* 37:65–77, 2009.

679. Figueiredo JF, Culver S, Behling-Kelly E, et al.: Acute myeloblastic leukemia with associated BCR-ABL translocation in a dog, *Vet Clin Pathol* 41:362–368, 2012.

680. Passamonti F, Maffioli M: The role of JAK2 inhibitors in MPNs 7 years after approval, *Blood* 131:2426–2435, 2018.

681. Beurlet S, Krief P, Sansonetti A, et al.: Identification of JAK2 mutations in canine primary polycythemia, *Exp Hematol* 39:542–545, 2011.

682. Prchal J: Primary polycythemias In JW A, editor, *Curr Opin Hematol* 2:146–152, 1995.

683. Bush BM, Fankhauser R: Polychthaemia vera in a bitch, *J Small Anim Pract* 13:75–89, 1972.

684. Carb AV: Polycythemia vera in a dog, *J Am Vet Med Assoc* 154:289–297, 1969.

685. Diogo CC, Fabretti AK, Camassa JA, et al.: Diagnosis and treatment of primary erythrocytosis in a dog: a case report, *Top Companion Anim Med* 30:65–67, 2015.

686. Holden AR: Polycythaemia vera in a dog, *Vet Rec* 120:473–475, 1987.

687. McGrath CJ: Polycythemia vera in dogs, *J Am Vet Med Assoc* 164:1117–1122, 1974.

688. Meyer HP, Slappendel RJ, Greydanus-van der Putten SW: Polycythaemia vera in a dog treated by repeated phlebotomies, *Vet Q* 15:108–111, 1993.

689. Miller RM: Polycythemia vera in a dog, *Vet Med Small Anim Clin* 63:222–223, 1968.

690. Peterson ME, Randolph JF: Diagnosis of canine primary polycythemia and management with hydroxyurea, *J Am Vet Med Assoc* 180:415–418, 1982.

691. Quesnel AD, Kruth SA: Polycythemia vera and glomerulonephritis in a dog, *Can Vet J* 33:671–672, 1992.

692. Wysoke JM, Van Heerden J: Polycythaemia vera in a dog, *J S Afr Vet Assoc* 61:182–183, 1990.

693. Dunn JKJA, Evans RJ, et al.: Chronic granulocytic leukaemia in a dog with assoicated bacterial endocarditis, thrombocytopenia and preretinal and retinal hemorrhages, *J Small Anim Pract* 28:1079–1086, 1987.

694. Fine DM, Tvedten HW: Chronic granulocytic leukemia in a dog, *J Am Vet Med Assoc* 214:1809–1812, 1791, 1999.

695. Grindem CB, Stevens JB, Brost DR, et al.: Chronic myelogenous leukaemia with meningeal infiltration in a dog, *Comp Haematol Int* 2:170–174, 1992.

696. Leifer CE, Matus RE, Patnaik AK, et al.: Chronic myelogenous leukemia in the dog, *J Am Vet Med Assoc* 183:686–689, 1983.

697. Jain NC: *The leukemia complex. Schalm's veterinary hematology*, ed 4, Philadelphia, 1986, Lea & Febiger.

698. Pollet L, Van Hove W, Mattheeuws D: Blastic crisis in chronic myelogenous leukaemia in a dog, *J Small Anim Pract* 19:469–475, 1978.

699. Liesveld JLLM: Chronic myelogenous leukemia and related disorders. In Lichtman MA, Kaushansky K, Seligsohn U, et al.: *Williams hemtology*, ed 8, New York, 2010, McGraw Hill.

700. Marino CL, Tran J, Stokol T: Atypical chronic myeloid leukemia in a German Shepherd Dog, *J Vet Diagn Invest* 29:338–345, 2017.

701. Perez ML, Culver S, Owen JL, et al.: Partial cytogenetic response with toceranib and prednisone treatment in a young dog with chronic monocytic leukemia, *Anticancer Drugs* 24:1098–1103, 2013.

702. Cruz Cardona JA, Milner R, Alleman AR, et al.: BCR-ABL translocation in a dog with chronic monocytic leukemia, *Vet Clin Pathol* 40:40–47, 2011.

703. Hiraoka H, Hisasue M, Nagashima N, et al.: A dog with myelodysplastic syndrome: chronic myelomonocytic leukemia, *J Vet Med Sci* 69:665–668, 2007.

704. Rossi G, Gelain ME, Foroni S, et al.: Extreme monocytosis in a dog with chronic monocytic leukaemia, *Vet Rec* 165:54–56, 2009.

705. MacEwen EG, Drazner FH, McClelland AJ, et al.: Treatment of basophilic leukemia in a dog, *J Am Vet Med Assoc* 166:376–380, 1975.

706. Mahaffey EA, Brown TP, Duncan JR, et al.: Basophilic leukaemia in a dog, *J Comp Pathol* 97:393–399, 1987.

707. Mears EA, Raskin RE, Legendre AM: Basophilic leukemia in a dog, *J Vet Intern Med* 11:92–94, 1997.

708. Jensen ALNO: Eosinophilic leukemoid reaction in a dog, *J Small Anim Pract* 33:337–340, 1992.

709. Ndikuwera JSD, Obwolo MJ, et al.: Chronic granulocytic leukaemia/eosinophilic leukaemia in a dog, *J Small Anim Pract* 33:553–557, 1992.

710. Beer PAGA: Essential thrombocythemia. In Lichtman MA Kaushansky K, Seligsohn U, et al.: *Williams hematology*, ed 8, New York, 2010, McGraw-Hill.

711. Bass MCSA: Essential thrombocythemia in a dog: case report and literature review, *J Am Anim Hosp Assoc* 34:197–203, 1998.

712. Dunn JK, Heath MF, Jefferies AR, et al.: Diagnostic and hematologic features of probable essential thrombocythemia in two dogs, *Vet Clin Pathol* 28:131–138, 1999.

713. Hopper PE, Mandell CP, Turrel JM, et al.: Probable essential thrombocythemia in a dog, *J Vet Intern Med* 3:79–85, 1989.

714. Simpson JWER, Honeyman P: Successful treatment of suspected essential thrombocythemia in the dog, *J Small Anim Pract* 31:345–348, 1990.

715. Reagan WJ: A review of myelofibrosis in dogs, *Toxicol Pathol* 21:164–169, 1993.

716. Weiss DJ: A retrospective study of the incidence and the classification of bone marrow disorders in the dog at a veterinary teaching hospital (1996-2004), *J Vet Intern Med* 20:955–961, 2006.

717. Castro-Malaspina, Berk PD: Pathogenesis of myelofibrosis: role of ineffective megakaryopoiesis and megakaryocyte components. In Castro-Malaspina H, Wasserman LR, editors: *Myelofibrosis and the biology of connective tissue*, New York, 1984, Alan R. Liss.

718. Dungworth DL, Goldman M, Switzer J, et al.: Development of a myeloproliferative disorder in beagles continuously exposed to 90Sr, *Blood* 34:610–632, 1969.

719. Prasse KW, Crouser D, Beutler E, et al.: Pyruvate kinase deficiency anemia with terminal myelofibrosis and osteosclerosis in a beagle, *J Am Vet Med Assoc* 166:1170–1175, 1975.

720. Rudolph RHC: Megakaryozytenleukose beim hund, *Kleintier-Praxis* 17:9–13, 1972.

721. Thompson JCJA: Myelofibrosis in the dog: three case reports, *J Small Anim Pract* 24:589–601, 1983.

722. McManus PM: Classification of myeloid neoplasms: a comparative review, *Vet Clin Pathol* 34:189–212, 2005.

723. Thomsen MK, Jensen AL, Skak-Nielsen T, et al.: Enhanced granulocyte function in a case of chronic granulocytic leukemia in a dog, *Vet Immunol Immunopathol* 28:143–156, 1991.

724. Facklam NR, Kociba GJ: Cytochemical characterization of leukemic cells from 20 dogs, *Vet Pathol* 22:363–369, 1985.

725. Grindem CB, Stevens JB, Perman V: Cytochemical reactions in cells from leukemic dogs, *Vet Pathol* 23:103–109, 1986.

726. Mochizuki H, Goto-Koshino Y, Takahashi M, et al.: Demonstration of the cell clonality in canine hematopoietic tumors by X-chromosome inactivation pattern analysis, *Vet Pathol* 52:61–69, 2015.

727. Goldman EEGJ: Clinical diagnosis and management of acute nonlymphoid leukemias and chronic myeloproliferative disorders. In Feldman BF Zinkel J, Jain NC, editors: *Schalm's veterinary hematology*, ed 5, Philadelphia, 2000, Lippincott Williams & Wilkins.

728. Stokol T, Schaefer DM, Shuman M, et al.: Alkaline phosphatase is a useful cytochemical marker for the diagnosis of acute myelomonocytic and monocytic leukemia in the dog, *Vet Clin Pathol* 44:79–93, 2015.

729. Cobbold S, Metcalfe S: Monoclonal antibodies that define canine homologues of human CD antigens: summary of the First International Canine Leukocyte Antigen Workshop (CLAW), *Tissue Antigens* 43:137–154, 1994.

730. Comazzi S, Gelain ME, Spagnolo V, et al.: Flow cytometric patterns in blood from dogs with non-neoplastic and neoplastic hematologic diseases using double labeling for CD18 and CD45, *Vet Clin Pathol* 35:47–54, 2006.

731. Tasca S, Carli E, Caldin M, et al.: Hematologic abnormalities and flow cytometric immunophenotyping results in dogs with hematopoietic neoplasia: 210 cases (2002-2006), *Vet Clin Pathol* 38:2–12, 2009.

732. Villiers E, Baines S, Law AM, et al.: Identification of acute myeloid leukemia in dogs using flow cytometry with myeloperoxidase, MAC387, and a canine neutrophil-specific antibody, *Vet Clin Pathol* 35:55–71, 2006.

733. Peterson ME, Zanjani ED: Inappropriate erythropoietin production from a renal carcinoma in a dog with polycythemia, *J Am Vet Med Assoc* 179:995–996, 1981.

734. Scott RCPA: Renal carcinoma associated with secondary polycythemia in a dog, *J Am Anim Hosp Assoc* 8:275–283, 1972.

735. Waters DJPJ: Secondary polycythemia associated with renal disease in the dog: two case reports and review of literature, *J Am Anim Hosp Assoc* 24:109–114, 1988.

736. Cook SM, Lothrop Jr CD: Serum erythropoietin concentrations measured by radioimmunoassay in normal, polycythemic, and anemic dogs and cats, *J Vet Intern Med* 8:18–25, 1994.

737. Giger U: Serum erythropoietin concentrations in polycythemic and anemic dogs, *Proc 9th Annual Vet Med Forum (ACVIM)* 143–145, 1991.

738. Reimann KA, Knowlen GG, Tvedten HW: Factitious hyperkalemia in dogs with thrombocytosis. The effect of platelets on serum potassium concentration, *J Vet Intern Med* 3:47–52, 1989.

739. Weiss DJ, Aird B: Cytologic evaluation of primary and secondary myelodysplastic syndromes in the dog, *Vet Clin Pathol* 30:67–75, 2001.

740. Friedrichs KRYK: How to collect diagnostic bone marrow samples, *Vet Med* 8:578–588, 2005.

741. Feeney DA, Sharkey LC, Steward SM, et al.: Applicability of 3T body MRI in assessment of nonfocal bone marrow involvement of hematopoietic neoplasia in dogs, *J Vet Intern Med* 27:1165–1171, 2013.

742. Feeney DA, Sharkey LC, Steward SM, et al.: Parenchymal signal intensity in 3-T body MRI of dogs with hematopoietic neoplasia, *Comp Med* 63:174–182, 2013.

743. Schmidt JM, North SM, Freeman KP, et al.: Feline paediatric oncology: retrospective assessment of 233 tumours from cats up to one year (1993 to 2008), *J Small Anim Pract* 51:306–311, 2010.

744. Gorman NT, Evans RJ: Myeloproliferative disease in the dog and cat: clinical presentations, diagnosis and treatment, *Vet Rec* 121:490–496, 1987.

745. Hamlin RH, Duncan RC: Acute nonlymphocytic leukemia in a dog, *J Am Vet Med Assoc* 196:110–112, 1990.

746. Theilen GH MB, Gardner MB: Hematopoietic neoplasms, sarcomas and related conditions. In Theilen GH, Madewell, editors: *Veterinary cancer medicine*, ed 2, Philadelphia, 1987, Lea & Febiger.

747. Lawless S, McMullin MF, Cuthbert R, et al.: (32)P in the treatment of myeloproliferative disorders, *Ulster Med J* 85:83–85, 2016.

748. Smith M, Turrel JM: Radiophosphorus (32P) treatment of bone marrow disorders in dogs: 11 cases (1970-1987), *J Am Vet Med Assoc* 194:98–102, 1989.

749. Lyss AP: Enzymes and random synthetics. In Perry MC, editor: *The chemotherapy source book*, Baltimore, 1992, Williams & Wilkins, pp 398–412.

750. Bolin RW, Robinson WA, Sutherland J, et al.: Busulfan versus hydroxyurea in long-term therapy of chronic myelogenous leukemia, *Cancer* 50:1683–1686, 1982.

751. Rosenthal S, Canellos GP, Whang-Peng J, et al.: Blast crisis of chronic granulocytic leukemia. Morphologic variants and therapeutic implications, *Am J Med* 63:542–547, 1977.

752. Ganser A, Hoelzer D: Treatment of myelodysplastic syndromes with hematopoietic growth factors, *Hematol Oncol Clin North Am* 6:633–653, 1992.

753. Liesveld JL, Lichtman MA: Myelodysplastic syndromes (clonal cytopenias and oligoblastic myelogenous leukemia). In Lichtman MA, Kaushansky K, Seligsohn U, et al.: *Williams hematology*, ed 8, New York, 2010, McGraw-Hill.

754. Jacobs A: Treatment for the myelodysplastic syndromes, *Haematologica* 72:477–480, 1987.

755. Kelsey SM, Newland AC, Cunningham J, et al.: Sustained haematological response to high-dose oral alfacalcidol in patients with myelodysplastic syndromes, *Lancet* 340:316–317, 1992.

756. Ohno R, Naoe T, Hirano M, et al.: Treatment of myelodysplastic syndromes with all-trans retinoic acid. Leukemia Study Group of the Ministry of Health and Welfare, *Blood* 81:1152–1154, 1993.

757. Matus RE, Leifer CE, MacEwen EG, et al.: Prognostic factors for multiple myeloma in the dog, *J Am Vet Med Assoc* 188:1288–1292, 1986.

758. Liu S, Dorfman HD, Hurvitz AI, et al.: Primary and secondary bone tumors in the dog, *J Small Anim Pract* 18:313–326, 1977.

759. Weiss DJ: A retrospective study of the incidence and the classification of bone marrow disorders in the dog at a veterinary teaching hospital (1996-2004), *J Vet Intern Med* 20:955–961, 2006.

760. Tappin SW, Taylor SS, Tasker S, et al.: Serum protein electrophoresis in 147 dogs, *Vet Rec* 168:456, 2011.

761. Fernandez R, Chon E: Comparison of two melphalan protocols and evaluation of outcome and prognostic factors in multiple myeloma in dogs, *J Vet Intern Med* 32:1060–1069, 2018.

762. Thamm DH, Vail DM, Kurzman ID, et al.: GS–9219/VDC-1101-a prodrug of the acyclic nucleotide PMEG has antitumor activity in spontaneous canine multiple myeloma, *BMC Vet Res* 10(30), 2014.

763. Osborne CA, Perman V, Sautter JH, et al.: Multiple myeloma in the dog, *J Am Vet Med Assoc* 153:1300–1319, 1968.

764. MacEwen EG, Hurvitz AI: Diagnosis and management of monoclonal gammopathies, *Vet Clin North Am* 7:119–132, 1977.

765. Carpenter J, Andrews LK, Holzworth J: Tumors and tumor like lesions. In Holzworth J, editor: *Diseases of the cat: medicine and surgery*, Philadelphia, 1987, WB Saunders.

766. Engle G, Brodey RS: A retrospective study of 395 feline neoplasms, *J Am Anim Hosp Assoc* 5:21–31, 1969.

767. Patel RT, Caceres A, French AF, et al.: Multiple myeloma in 16 cats: a retrospective study, *Vet Clin Pathol* 34:341–352, 2005.

768. Taylor SS, Tappin SW, Dodkin SJ, et al.: Serum protein electrophoresis in 155 cats, *J Feline Med Surg* 12:643–653, 2010.

769. Cannon CM, Knudson C, Borgatti A: Clinical signs, treatment, and outcome in cats with myeloma–related disorder receiving systemic therapy, *J Am Anim Hosp Assoc* 51:239–248, 2015.

770. Hanna F: Multiple myelomas in cats, *J Feline Med Surg* 7:275–287, 2005.

771. Mellor PJ, Haugland S, Murphy S, et al.: Myeloma-related disorders in cats commonly present as extramedullary neoplasms in contrast to myeloma in human patients: 24 cases with clinical follow-up, *J Vet Intern Med* 20:1376–1383, 2006.

772. Qurollo BA, Balakrishnan N, Cannon CZ, et al.: Co-infection with Anaplasma platys, Bartonella henselae, Bartonella koehlerae and 'Candidatus Mycoplasma haemominutum' in a cat diagnosed with splenic plasmacytosis and multiple myeloma, *J Feline Med Surg* 16:713–720, 2014.

773. Geigy C, Riond B, Bley CR, et al.: Multiple myeloma in a dog with multiple concurrent infectious diseases and persistent polyclonal gammopathy, *Vet Clin Pathol* 42:47–54, 2013.

774. Cangul IT, Wijnen M, Van Garderen E, et al.: Clinico–pathological aspects of canine cutaneous and mucocutaneous plasmacytomas, *J Vet Med A Physiol Pathol Clin Med* 49:307–312, 2002.

775. Imahori S, Moore GE: Multiple myeloma and prolonged stimulation of reticuloendothelial system, *N Y State J Med* 72:1625–1628, 1972.

776. London CA, Hannah AL, Zadovoskaya R, et al.: Phase I dose-escalating study of SU11654, a small molecule receptor tyrosine kinase inhibitor, in dogs with spontaneous malignancies, *Clin Cancer Res* 9:2755–2768, 2003.

777. Porter DD, Dixon FJ, Larsen AE: The development of a myeloma-like condition in mink with Aleutian disease, *Blood* 25:736–742, 1965.

778. Potter M: A resume of the current status of the development of plasma-cell tumors in mice, *Cancer Res* 28:1891–1896, 1968.

779. Potter M, Morrison S, Miller F: Induction of plasmacytomas in genetically susceptible mice with silicone gels, *Curr Top Microbiol Immunol* 194:83–91, 1995.

780. Bourguet CC, Grufferman S, Delzell E, et al.: Multiple myeloma and family history of cancer. A case–control study, *Cancer* 56:2133–2139, 1985.

781. Cuzick J, De Stavola B: Multiple myeloma-a case-control study, *Br J Cancer* 57:516–520, 1988.

782. Linet MS, Harlow SD, McLaughlin JK: A case-control study of multiple myeloma in whites: chronic antigenic stimulation, occupation, and drug use, *Cancer Res* 47:2978–2981, 1987.

783. Ehrensing G, Craig LE: Intravascular neoplastic cells in canine cutaneous plasmacytomas, *J Vet Diagn Invest* 30:329–332, 2018.

784. Burnett RC, Blake MK, Thompson LJ, et al.: Evolution of a B-cell lymphoma to multiple myeloma after chemotherapy, *J Vet Intern Med* 18:768–771, 2004.

785. Radhakrishnan A, Risbon RE, Patel RT, et al.: Progression of a solitary, malignant cutaneous plasma-cell tumour to multiple myeloma in a cat, *Vet Comp Oncol* 2:36–42, 2004.

786. Mellor PJ, Haugland S, Smith KC, et al.: Histopathologic, immunohistochemical, and cytologic analysis of feline myeloma–related disorders: further evidence for primary extramedullary development in the cat, *Vet Pathol* 45:159–173, 2008.

787. Valli VEJR, Parodi AL, et al.: *Histological classification of hematopoietic tumors of domestic animals*, Washington, DC, 2002, Armed Forces Institute of Pathology and The World health Organization.

788. Drazner F: Multiple myeloma in the cat, *Comp Cont Ed Pract Vet* 4:206–216, 1982.

789. Igase M, Shimokawa Miyama T, Kambayashi S, et al.: Bimodal immunoglobulin A gammopathy in a cat with feline myeloma–related disorders, *J Vet Med Sci* 78:691–695, 2016.

790. Bienzle D, Silverstein DC, Chaffin K: Multiple myeloma in cats: variable presentation with different immunoglobulin isotypes in two cats, *Vet Pathol* 37:364–369, 2000.

791. Facchini RV, Bertazzolo W, Zuliani D, et al.: Detection of biclonal gammopathy by capillary zone electrophoresis in a cat and a dog with plasma cell neoplasia, *Vet Clin Pathol* 39:440–446, 2010.

792. Giraudel JPJ, Guelfi JF: Monoclonal gammopathie in the dog: a retrospective study of 18 cases (1986–1999) and literature review, *J Am Anim Hosp Assoc* 38:135–147, 2002.

793. Jacobs RM, Couto CG, Wellman ML: Biclonal gammopathy in a dog with myeloma and cutaneous lymphoma, *Vet Pathol* 23:211–213, 1986.

794. Peterson EN, Meininger AC: Immunoglobulin A and immunoglobulin G biclonal gammopathy in a dog with multiple myeloma, *J Am Anim Hosp Assoc* 33:45–47, 1997.

795. Ramaiah SK, Seguin MA, Carwile HF, et al.: Biclonal gammopathy associated with immunoglobulin A in a dog with multiple myeloma, *Vet Clin Pathol* 31:83–89, 2002.

796. Souchon F, Koch A, Sohns A: Multiple myeloma with significant multifocal osteolysis in a dog without a detectible gammopathy, *Tierarztl Prax Ausg K Kleintiere Heimtiere* 41:413–420, 2013.

797. MacEwen EG, Patnaik AK, Hurvitz AI, et al.: Nonsecretory multiple myeloma in two dogs, *J Am Vet Med Assoc* 184:1283–1286, 1984.

798. Seelig DM, Perry JA, Avery AC, et al.: Monoclonal gammopathy without hyperglobulinemia in 2 dogs with IgA secretory neoplasms, *Vet Clin Pathol* 39:447–453, 2010.

799. Braund KG, Everett RM, Bartels JE, et al.: Neurologic complications of IgA multiple myeloma associated with cryoglobulinemia in a dog, *J Am Vet Med Assoc* 174:1321–1325, 1979.

800. Hickford FH, Stokol T, vanGessel YA, et al.: Monoclonal immunoglobulin G cryoglobulinemia and multiple myeloma in a domestic shorthair cat, *J Am Vet Med Assoc* 217:1029–1033, 1007–1028, 2000.

801. Hurvitz AI, MacEwen EG, Middaugh CR, et al.: Monoclonal cryoglobulinemia with macroglobulinemia in a dog, *J Am Vet Med Assoc* 170:511–513, 1977.

802. Cowgill ES, Neel JA, Ruslander D: Light-chain myeloma in a dog, *J Vet Intern Med* 18:119–121, 2004.

803. Yamada O, Tamura K, Yagihara H, et al.: Light-chain multiple myeloma in a cat, *J Vet Diagn Invest* 19:443–447, 2007.

804. Gentilini F, Calzolari C, Buonacucina A, et al.: Different biological behaviour of Waldenstrom macroglobulinemia in two dogs, *Vet Comp Oncol* 3:87–97, 2005.

805. Hurvitz AI, Haskins SC, Fischer CA: Macroglobulinemia with hyperviscosity syndrome in a dog, *J Am Vet Med Assoc* 157:455–460, 1970.

806. Hill RR, Clatworthy RH: Macroglobulinaemia in the dog, the canine analogue of gamma M monoclonal gammopathy, *J S Afr Vet Med Assoc* 42:309–313, 1971.

807. Anderson K: Plasma cell tumors. In Holland J, Frei E, Bast RC, et al.: *Cancer medicine*, ed 3, Philadelphia, 1993, Lea & Febiger.

808. Salon W, Cassady JF: Plasma cell neoplasms. In DeVita V, Hellman S, Rosenberg SA, editors: *Cancer: principles and practice of oncology*, ed 5, Philadelphia, 1997, Lippincott.

809. Shull RM: Serum hyperviscosity syndrome associated with IgA multiple myeloma in two dogs, *J Am Anim Hosp Assoc* 14:58–70, 1978.

810. Center SA, Smith JF: Ocular lesions in a dog with serum hyperviscosity secondary to an IgA myeloma, *J Am Vet Med Assoc* 181:811–813, 1982.

811. Hendrix DV, Gelatt KN, Smith PJ, et al.: Ophthalmic disease as the presenting complaint in five dogs with multiple myeloma, *J Am Anim Hosp Assoc* 34:121–128, 1998.

812. Kirschner SE, Niyo Y, Hill BL, et al.: Blindness in a dog with IgA-forming myeloma, *J Am Vet Med Assoc* 193:349–350, 1988.

813. Violette NP, Ledbetter EC: Punctate retinal hemorrhage and its relation to ocular and systemic disease in dogs: 83 cases, *Vet Ophthalmol* 21:233–239, 2018.

814. Boyle T, Holowaychuk MK, Adams AK, et al.: Treatment of three cats with hyperviscosity syndrome and congestive heart failure using plasmapheresis, *J Am Anim Hosp Assoc* 47:50–55, 2011.

815. Forrester SD, Greco DS, Relford RL: Serum hyperviscosity syndrome associated with multiple myeloma in two cats, *J Am Vet Med Assoc* 200:79–82, 1992.

816. Hawkins EC, Feldman BF, Blanchard PC: Immunoglobulin A myeloma in a cat with pleural effusion and serum hyperviscosity, *J Am Vet Med Assoc* 188:876–878, 1986.

817. Hribernik TN, Barta O, Gaunt SD, et al.: Serum hyperviscosity syndrome associated with IgG myeloma in a cat, *J Am Vet Med Assoc* 181:169–170, 1982.

818. Williams D, Goldschmidt MH: Hyperviscosity syndrome with IgM monoclonal gammopathy and hepatic plasmcytoid lymphosarcoma in a cat, *J Small Anim Pract* 23:311–323, 1982.

819. Mundy GR, Bertolini DR: Bone destruction and hypercalcemia in plasma cell myeloma, *Semin Oncol* 13:291–299, 1986.

820. Rosol TJ, Nagode LA, Couto CG, et al.: Parathyroid hormone (PTH)-related protein, PTH, and 1,25-dihydroxyvitamin D in dogs with cancer–associated hypercalcemia, *Endocrinology* 131:1157–1164, 1992.

821. Sheafor SE, Gamblin RM, Couto CG: Hypercalcemia in two cats with multiple myeloma, *J Am Anim Hosp Assoc* 32:503–508, 1996.

822. Twomey JJ: Infections complicating multiple myeloma and chronic lymphocytic leukemia, *Arch Intern Med* 132:562–565, 1973.

823. Dunbar MD, Lyles S: Hemophagocytic syndrome in a cat with multiple myeloma, *Vet Clin Pathol* 42:55–60, 2013.

824. Webb J, Chary P, Northrup N, et al.: Erythrophagocytic multiple myeloma in a cat, *Vet Clin Pathol* 37:302–307, 2008.

825. Yearley JH, Stanton C, Olivry T, et al.: Phagocytic plasmacytoma in a dog, *Vet Clin Pathol* 36:293–296, 2007.

826. Dewhirst MW, Stamp GL, Hurvitz AI: Idiopathic monoclonal (IgA) gammopathy in a dog, *J Am Vet Med Assoc* 170:1313–1316, 1977.

827. Hoenig M, O'Brien JA: A benign hypergammaglobulinemia mimicking plasma cell myeloma, *J Am Anim Hosp Assoc* 24:688–690, 1988.

828. Rusbridge C, Wheeler SJ, Lamb CR, et al.: Vertebral plasma cell tumors in 8 dogs, *J Vet Intern Med* 13:126–133, 1999.

829. Van Bree H, Pollet L, Cousemont W, et al.: Cervical cord compression as a neurologic complication in an IgG multiple myeloma in a dog, *J Am Anim Hosp Assoc* 19:317–323, 1983.

830. DiBartola SP, Reynolds HA: Hypoglycemia and polyclonal gammopathy in a dog with plasma cell dyscrasia, *J Am Vet Med Assoc* 180:1345–1349, 1982.

831. Villiers E, Dobson J: Multiple myeloma with associated polyneuropathy in a German shepherd dog, *J Small Anim Pract* 39:249–251, 1998.

832. Mitcham SA, McGillivray SR, Haines DM: Plasma cell sarcoma in a cat, *Can Vet J* 26:98–100, 1985.

833. O'Keefe DA, Couto CG: Fine–needle aspiration of the spleen as an aid in the diagnosis of splenomegaly, *J Vet Intern Med* 1:102–109, 1987.

834. Werner JA, Woo JC, Vernau W, et al.: Characterization of feline immunoglobulin heavy chain variable region genes for the molecular diagnosis of B–cell neoplasia, *Vet Pathol* 42:596–607, 2005.

835. Munshi N, Anderon KC: Plasma cell neoplasms. In DeVita V, Hellman S, Rosenberg SA, editors: *Cancer: principles and practice of oncology*, ed 7, Philadelphia, 2005, Lippincott Williams & Wilkins.

836. Breitschwerdt EB, Woody BJ, Zerbe CA, et al.: Monoclonal gammopathy associated with naturally occurring canine ehrlichiosis, *J Vet Intern Med* 1:2–9, 1987.

837. Font A, Closa JM, Mascort J: Monoclonal gammopathy in a dog with visceral leishmaniasis, *J Vet Intern Med* 8:233–235, 1994.

838. MacEwen EG, Hurvitz AI, Hayes A: Hyperviscosity syndrome associated with lymphocytic leukemia in three dogs, *J Am Vet Med Assoc* 170:1309–1312, 1977.

839. Matus RE, Leifer CE, Hurvitz AI: Use of plasmapheresis and chemotherapy for treatment of monoclonal gammopathy associated with *Ehrlichia canis* infection in a dog, *J Am Vet Med Assoc* 190:1302–1304, 1987.

840. Fan TM, Kitchell BE, Dhaliwal RS, et al.: Hematological toxicity and therapeutic efficacy of lomustine in 20 tumor–bearing cats: critical assessment of a practical dosing regimen, *J Am Anim Hosp Assoc* 38:357–363, 2002.

841. Farhangi M, Osserman EF: The treatment of multiple myeloma, *Semin Hematol* 10:149–161, 1973.

842. Lippi I, Perondi F, Ross SJ, et al.: Double filtration plasmapheresis in a dog with multiple myeloma and hyperviscosity syndrome, *Open Vet J* 5:108–112, 2015.

843. Bartges JW: Therapeutic plasmapheresis, *Semin Vet Med Surg (Small Anim)* 12:170–177, 1997.

844. Farrow BR, Penny R: Multiple myeloma in a cat, *J Am Vet Med Assoc* 158:606–611, 1971.

845. Anderson K, Ismaila N, Flynn PJ, et al.: Role of bone-modifying agents in multiple myeloma: american society of clinical oncology clinical practice guideline update, *J Clin Oncol* 36:812–818, 2018.

846. Mhaskar R, Kumar A, Miladinovic B, et al.: Bisphosphonates in multiple myeloma: an updated network meta–analysis, *Cochrane Database Syst Rev* 12:CD003188, 2017.

847. Kisseberth WC, MacEwen EG, Helfand SC, et al.: Response to liposome–encapsulated doxorubicin (TLC D-99) in a dog with myeloma, *J Vet Intern Med* 9:425–428, 1995.

848. Ito K, Kobayashi M, Kuroki S, et al.: The proteasome inhibitor bortezomib inhibits the growth of canine malignant melanoma cells in vitro and in vivo, *Vet J* 198:577–582, 2013.

849. Araujo KP, Bonuccelli G, Duarte CN, et al.: Bortezomib (PS-341) treatment decreases inflammation and partially rescues the expression of the dystrophin–glycoprotein complex in GRMD dogs, *PLoS One* 8:e61367, 2013.

850. Boostrom BO, Moore AS, DeRegis CJ, et al.: Canine cutaneous plasmacytosis: 21 cases (2005-2015), *J Vet Intern Med* 31:1074–1080, 2017.

851. McHale B, Blas–Machado U, Oliveira FN, et al.: A divergent pseudoglandular configuration of cutaneous plasmacytoma in dogs, *J Vet Diagn Invest* 30:260–262, 2018.

852. Mikiewicz M, Otrocka–Domagala I, Pazdzior–Czapula K, et al.: Morphology and immunoreactivity of canine and feline extramedullary plasmacytomas, *Pol J Vet Sci* 19:345–352, 2016.

853. Stilwell JM, Rissi DR: Immunohistochemical labeling of multiple myeloma oncogene 1/interferon regulatory factor 4 (MUM1/IRF-4) in canine cutaneous histiocytoma, *Vet Pathol* 55:517–520, 2018.

854. Baer KE, Patnaik AK, Gilbertson SR, et al.: Cutaneous plasmacytomas in dogs: a morphologic and immunohistochemical study, *Vet Pathol* 26:216–221, 1989.

855. Clark G, Berg J, Engler SJ, et al.: Extramedullary plasmacytomas in dogs: results of surgical excision in 131 cases, *J Am Anim Hosp Assoc* 28:105–111, 1992.

856. Kyriazidou A, Brown PJ, Lucke VM: An immunohistochemical study of canine extramedullary plasma cell tumours, *J Comp Pathol* 100:259–266, 1989.

857. Lucke V: Primary cutaneous plasmacytomas in the dog and cat, *J Small Anim Pract* 28:49–55, 1987.

858. Platz SJ, Breuer W, Pfleghaar S, et al.: Prognostic value of histopathological grading in canine extramedullary plasmacytomas, *Vet Pathol* 36:23–27, 1999.

859. Rakich PM, Latimer KS, Weiss R, et al.: Mucocutaneous plasmacytomas in dogs: 75 cases (1980–1987), *J Am Vet Med Assoc* 194:803–810, 1989.

860. Rowland PH, Valentine BA, Stebbins KE, et al.: Cutaneous plasmacytomas with amyloid in six dogs, *Vet Pathol* 28:125–130, 1991.

861. Culp WT, Ehrhart N, Withrow SJ, et al.: Results of surgical excision and evaluation of factors associated with survival time in dogs with lingual neoplasia: 97 cases (1995–2008), *J Am Vet Med Assoc* 242:1392–1397, 2013.

862. Sykes SE, Byfield V, Sullivan L, et al.: Feline respiratory extramedullary plasmacytoma with lymph node metastasis and intrahistiocytic amyloid, *J Comp Pathol* 156:173–177, 2017.

863. Aoki M, Kim T, Shimada T, et al.: A primary hepatic plasma cell tumor in a dog, *J Vet Med Sci* 66:445–447, 2004.

864. Chaffin K, Cross AR, Allen SW, et al.: Extramedullary plasmacytoma in the trachea of a dog, *J Am Vet Med Assoc* 212:1579–1581, 1998.

865. Choi YK, Lee JY, Kim DY, et al.: Uterine extramedullary plasmacytoma in a dog, *Vet Rec* 154:699–700, 2004.

866. Hayes A, Gregory SP, Murphy S, et al.: Solitary extramedullary plasmacytoma of the canine larynx, *J Small Anim Pract* 48:288–291, 2007.

867. Perlmann E, Dagli ML, Martins MC, et al.: Extramedullary plasmacytoma of the third eyelid gland in a dog, *Vet Ophthalmol* 12:102–105, 2009.

868. Schoniger S, Bridger N, Allenspach K, et al.: Sinonasal plasmacytoma in a cat, *J Vet Diagn Invest* 19:573–577, 2007.

869. Van Wettere AJ, Linder KE, Suter SE, et al.: Solitary intracerebral plasmacytoma in a dog: microscopic, immunohistochemical, and molecular features, *Vet Pathol* 46:949–951, 2009.

870. Witham AI, French AF, Hill KE: Extramedullary laryngeal plasmacytoma in a dog, *N Z Vet J* 60:61–64, 2012.

871. Smithson CW, Smith MM, Tappe J, et al.: Multicentric oral plasmacytoma in 3 dogs, *J Vet Dent* 29:96–110, 2012.

872. Fukumoto S, Hanazono K, Kawasaki N, et al.: Anaplastic atypical myeloma with extensive cutaneous involvement in a dog, *J Vet Med Sci* 74:111–115, 2012.

873. Mayer MN, Kerr ME, Grier CK, et al.: Immunoglobulin A multiple myeloma with cutaneous involvement in a dog, *Can Vet J* 49:694–702, 2008.

874. Atherton MJ, Vazquez–Sanmartin S, Sharpe S, et al.: A metastatic secretory gastric plasmacytoma with aberrant CD3 expression in a dog, *Vet Clin Pathol* 46:520–525, 2017.

875. Hamilton TA, Carpenter JL: Esophageal plasmacytoma in a dog, *J Am Vet Med Assoc* 204:1210–1211, 1994.
876. MacEwen EG, Patnaik AK, Johnson GF, et al.: Extramedullary plasmacytoma of the gastrointestinal tract in two dogs, *J Am Vet Med Assoc* 184:1396–1398, 1984.
877. Jackson MW, Helfand SC, Smedes SL, et al.: Primary IgG secreting plasma cell tumor in the gastrointestinal tract of a dog, *J Am Vet Med Assoc* 204:404–406, 1994.
878. Bellezza E, Bianchini E, Pettinelli S, et al.: Intestinal plasmacytoma causing colocolic double intussusception in an adult dog, *J Small Anim Pract* 57:718, 2016.
879. kupanoff P, Popovitch CA, Goldschmidt MH: Colorectal plasmacytomas: a retrospective study of nine dogs, *J Am Anim Hosp Assoc* 42:37–43, 2006.
880. Trevor PB, Saunders GK, Waldron DR, et al.: Metastatic extramedullary plasmacytoma of the colon and rectum in a dog, *J Am Vet Med Assoc* 203:406–409, 1993.
881. Meis JM, Butler JJ, Osborne BM, et al.: Solitary plasmacytomas of bone and extramedullary plasmacytomas. A clinicopathologic and immunohistochemical study, *Cancer* 59:1475–1485, 1987.
882. Breuer W, Colbatzky F, Platz S, et al.: Immunoglobulin-producing tumours in dogs and cats, *J Comp Pathol* 109:203–216, 1993.
883. Kyriazidou A, Brown PJ, Lucke VM: Immunohistochemical staining of neoplastic and inflammatory plasma cell lesions in feline tissues, *J Comp Pathol* 100:337–341, 1989.
884. Majzoub M, Breuer W, Platz SJ, et al.: Histopathologic and immunophenotypic characterization of extramedullary plasmacytomas in nine cats, *Vet Pathol* 40:249–253, 2003.
885. Michau TM, Proulx DR, Rushton SD, et al.: Intraocular extramedullary plasmacytoma in a cat, *Vet Ophthalmol* 6:177–181, 2003.
886. Carothers MA, Johnson GC, DiBartola SP, et al.: Extramedullary plasmacytoma and immunoglobulin-associated amyloidosis in a cat, *J Am Vet Med Assoc* 195:1593–1597, 1989.
887. Brunnert SR, Altman NH: Identification of immunoglobulin light chains in canine extramedullary plasmacytomas by thioflavine T and immunohistochemistry, *J Vet Diagn Invest* 3:245–251, 1991.
888. Fernandez NJ, West KH, Jackson ML, et al.: Immunohistochemical and histochemical stains for differentiating canine cutaneous round cell tumors, *Vet Pathol* 42:437–445, 2005.
889. Ramos–Vara JA, Miller MA, Valli VE: Immunohistochemical detection of multiple myeloma 1/interferon regulatory factor 4 (MUM1/IRF-4) in canine plasmacytoma: comparison with CD79a and CD20, *Vet Pathol* 44:875–884, 2007.
890. Marcos R, Canadas A, Leite-Martins L, et al.: What is your diagnosis? Cutaneous nodules and atypical blood cells in a dog, *Vet Clin Pathol*, 2018.
891. Rout ED, Shank AM, Waite AH, et al.: Progression of cutaneous plasmacytoma to plasma cell leukemia in a dog, *Vet Clin Pathol* 46:77–84, 2017.
892. Lee AR, Lee MS, Jung IS, et al.: Imaging diagnosis-FDG-PET/CT of a canine splenic plasma cell tumor, *Vet Radiol Ultrasound* 51:145–147, 2010.
893. Wright ZM, Rogers KS, Mansell J: Survival data for canine oral extramedullary plasmacytoma: a retrospectve analysis (1996–2006), *J Am Anim Hosp Assoc* 44:75–81, 2008.
894. Ware K, Gieger T: Use of strontium-90 plesiotherapy for the treatment of a lingual plasmacytoma in a dog, *J Small Anim Pract* 52:220–223, 2011.
895. Mellor PJ, Polton GA, Brearley M, et al.: Solitary plasmacytoma of bone in two successfully treated cats, *J Feline Med Surg* 9:72–77, 2007.
896. Zikes CD, Spielman B, Shapiro W, et al.: Gastric extramedullary plasmacytoma in a cat, *J Vet Intern Med* 12:381–383, 1998.
897. Frazier KS, Hines 2nd ME, Hurvitz AI, et al.: Analysis of DNA aneuploidy and c-myc oncoprotein content of canine plasma cell tumors using flow cytometry, *Vet Pathol* 30:505–511, 1993.

34

Miscellaneous Tumors

CHRISTINE MULLIN AND CRAIG A. CLIFFORD

Incidence and Risk Factors

Hemangiosarcoma (HSA), also known as *malignant hemangio-endothelioma* or *angiosarcoma* (AS), is a malignant tumor composed of neoplastic endothelial cells. HSA occurs more frequently in dogs than in any other species[1–4] and represents about 2% of all canine tumors in general and 45% to 51% of canine splenic malignancies.[1–5] HSA is much less common in the cat, occurring in approximately 0.5% of cats examined at necropsy and accounting for 2% of all feline neoplasms in general.[6]

HSA is seen mostly in middle-aged to older animals, although there are rare reports of HSA occurring in dogs less than 3 years of age.[2,3,6,7] Any breed is potentially at risk, but German shepherds, golden retrievers, Labrador retrievers, and other large-breed dogs are overrepresented in several case series.[2,3,6,8,9] There may be a slight male predisposition in dogs.[3,6,10] In cats, older domestic shorthairs are most commonly affected,[11] although there is no clear sex predisposition.

In dogs, cutaneous HSA develops more frequently in the skin along the ventral abdomen and conjunctiva in short-haired and lightly pigmented breeds, reflecting the causal association with ultraviolet light exposure that has also been documented in research beagles.[12–14] Some reports suggest a hormonal association with canine HSA development, specifically with regard to neutering, given the findings that HSA appears more common in spayed females versus intact females and late neutered females versus intact or early neutered females.[2,15,16] The significance of these findings in the general population of client-owned dogs is unclear, because no large and well-controlled studies have been performed to assess the effect of neutering on the risk of dogs developing HSA.

Although traditionally considered to develop from malignant transformation of mature peripheral endothelial cells, recent molecular data suggest that HSA may arise from bone marrow progenitor cells that undergo dysregulated maturation and subsequently move to peripheral vascular sites to form tumors.[17–19] Furthermore, genomic profiling studies have identified distinct molecular subtypes of HSA that suggest a probable heterogeneity within this tumor type.[19–21] Mutations in tumor suppressor genes such as *p53* and *Ras* have been implicated in the pathogenesis of

AS in murine and human studies[22–24]; although it appears that *p53* and *Ras* mutations are infrequent in canine HSA,[25,26] *PTEN* inactivation was demonstrated in more than 50% of evaluated canine HSA samples.[27] Key growth- and apoptosis-regulating proteins such as pRB, cyclin D1, Bcl2, and survivin are overexpressed in HSA when compared with hemangiomas or normal tissues.[26,28]

There is growing evidence that dysregulation of angiogenic pathways may be important in the pathogenesis of HSA. Several studies have demonstrated abundant expression of angiogenic markers such as vascular endothelial growth factor (VEGF), basic fibroblast growth factor (bFGF), platelet-derived growth factor (PDGF), and angiopoetin-2, with concomitant expression of their corresponding cellular receptors in HSA cells and tissues.[18,29–31] An increased level of VEGF was documented in the plasma of dogs with HSA as compared with healthy controls,[32] whereas serum endothelin-1, a proangiogenic vasoactive peptide, was higher in dogs with splenic HSA as compared with healthy dogs and those with other splenic diseases.[33] These findings suggest the potential role for overstimulation of proangiogenic pathways as a promoter of tumor cell proliferation and survival.

Pathology and Natural Behavior

In the dog, the most common primary site for HSA is the spleen.[1,3,5,6,8,34] Other frequent anatomic sites include the heart, skin and subcutis, and liver.[3,12,15,35–39] Primary HSA has also been reported in the lung, kidney, retroperitoneal space, muscle, bone, oral and nasal cavities, eyelid and conjunctiva, urinary bladder, digit, and mediastinum.[7,40–48] Although HSA is the most common splenic neoplasm encountered in the dog, it is by no means the only differential for splenomegaly or splenic masses in dogs[1,5,10,34] Two large pathologic studies reported that approximately 50% of dogs with splenic tumors had malignant disease and 50% to 74% of these malignancies were HSA,[1,34] whereas other studies evaluating dogs presenting with a nontraumatic hemoabdomen found that 63% to 70% of all dogs had HSA.[49–51] It is important to note that several other splenic masses may have a similar gross and ultrasonographic appearance to HSA, and the differential diagnosis list for a dog with a splenic tumor includes other neoplasms (e.g., lymphoma, nonangiomatous/nonlymphomatous sarcomas) and nonneoplastic etiologies (e.g., nodular hyperplasia, extramedullary hematopoiesis, hematoma).[1,5,34] Interestingly, in one study larger splenic masses and heavier spleens were more likely to be benign.[52]

The heart is the second most common primary site for canine HSA and is the most common cardiac neoplasm in dogs. HSA most commonly originates from the right atrium or auricle; however, other cardiac sites have been reported.[15,35–37] Although previously thought to be a rather frequent occurrence based on necropsy studies, one study showed the presence of concurrent splenic and cardiac HSA to be uncommon (8.7%).[53]

Although typically aggressive, the biologic behavior of HSA can vary depending on primary tumor location, as certain primary HSA sites, specifically the skin, can be associated with a less aggressive disease course.[14] The more common visceral forms are characterized by local infiltration and metastatic dissemination early in the course of disease. Metastasis occurs either hematogenously or via intracavitary implantation after tumor rupture. Metastasis can occur at any site; however, the liver, omentum, peritoneum, and lungs are the most frequent sites of dissemination.[2–4] In dogs, HSA is the most common tumor to metastasize to the brain.[54]

In the cat, cutaneous and visceral (e.g., spleen, liver, intestine) locations are the most commonly reported primary sites for HSA.[11,55–60] Other reported sites in the cat include the heart, thoracic cavity, eyelid or conjunctiva, digit, and nasal cavity.[39,55,61–63] The biologic behavior of feline HSA is not as well described as in dogs, but is likely similar. Feline cutaneous and subcutaneous HSA are associated with the same clinical problems as other soft tissue sarcomas, specifically local invasiveness and postoperative tumor recurrence.[11,56,58] As in dogs, feline visceral HSA has a high metastatic rate, with the most common metastatic sites being the liver, omentum, and lungs.[15,55,59]

Grossly, HSA lesions may be of variable size, pale gray to dark red or purple, soft to gelatinous and friable, and typically contain blood-filled or necrotic areas that can ooze or overtly bleed (Fig. 34.1). Histologically, HSA is composed of markedly pleomorphic and mitotically active spindloid endothelial cells that form irregular anastomosing vascular spaces and channels that contain variable amounts of blood and/or thrombi.[1–3,5,6,10,12,13,34,36,38] Immunohistochemistry for von Willebrand's factor (factor VIII–related antigen) or CD31/platelet endothelial cell-adhesion molecule can be used to demonstrate endothelial derivation and support the diagnosis of HSA and rule out other sarcomas.[10,56,64,65]

History and Clinical Signs

Historical findings are largely dictated by tumor location and may vary from vague, nonspecific signs of illness to acute collapse and death secondary to hemorrhagic shock. The majority of patients with visceral HSA will present in an emergent scenario secondary to tumor rupture and subsequent internal hemorrhage. Associated clinical signs include acute lethargy, weakness, and collapse secondary to blood loss. Other common historical findings include weight loss, hyporexia, abdominal distension, vomiting, exercise intolerance, and dyspnea.[37,49–51] Dogs with renal HSA may have a history of hematuria.[40] Possible physical examination findings in the emergency setting include tachycardia with poor pulse quality, pale mucous membranes, and palpable abdominal fluid wave or abdominal mass effect.[49–51] Patients with cardiac tamponade secondary to rupture of a right atrial HSA are typically critical on presentation and may have muffled heart sounds, pulsus paradoxus, ascites (secondary to right heart failure from tamponade), or circulatory collapse.[36,37] HSA presentations involving the skin or subcutis differ in that they are generally not seen on an emergent basis and further vary based on whether the lesion is primarily

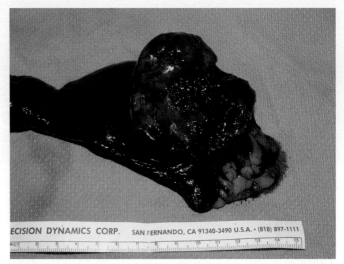

• **Fig. 34.1** Postoperative image of splenic hemangiosarcoma from a dog, illustrating the multilobulated and friable nature of this tumor. (Photo courtesy Julius Liptak, BVSc, MVetClinStud, FACVSc, DACVS, DECVS, Alta Vista Animal Hospital, Ottawa, Canada.)

dermal, subcutaneous, or intramuscular. Tumors may range from small, discrete, blood blisterlike lesions to much larger, deeply seated, painful, bruised and/or bleeding masses.[12–14,38,66–68]

In the cat, clinical signs depend on location and extent of the tumor. Cats with visceral HSA usually have a history of lethargy, anorexia, vomiting, collapse, dyspnea, or distended abdomen.[11,55,57,59,69] On physical examination, pallor, pleural or peritoneal fluid, and a palpable abdominal mass may be detected. Feline cutaneous and subcutaneous HSAs appear clinically similar to those seen in dogs.[11,55–58]

Diagnostic Techniques and Workup

Complete staging for a confirmed or suspected HSA patient typically includes hematology and serum biochemistry profile, coagulation profile, three-view thoracic radiographs, abdominal ultrasound, and in some cases, echocardiography. In both dogs and cats, regenerative and nonregenerative anemias are common and typically characterized by the presence of schistocytes, acanthocytes, and nucleated red blood cells, which are associated with microangiopathic-related damage, vasculitis, and acute hemorrhage.[70–73] Blood typing and/or cross matching may be indicated if surgery is planned in a severely anemic patient. Neutrophilic leukocytosis is common and may be secondary to a paraneoplastic syndrome or tumor necrosis. Thrombocytopenia, likely secondary to acute hemorrhage, intratumoral destruction, and coagulopathic consumption, is also quite common and observed in 75% to 97% of cases.[37,72,73] Alterations in secondary coagulation parameters (prothrombin time [PT], partial thromboplastin time [PTT], fibrin degradation product [FDP], fibrinogen, d-dimers), consistent with disseminated intravascular coagulation, are present in nearly 50% of patients with visceral HSA.[72,73] Serum biochemistry changes are typically nonspecific and may include hypoalbuminemia, azotemia, and elevations in liver enzymes.[37] In one study, more than 50% of cats with visceral HSA had increased aspartate transaminase activity.[69]

A clinical staging system for HSA is presented in Table 34.1. Because most patients present with primary visceral disease, abdominal ultrasound is frequently employed as part of the initial

TABLE 34.1	Clinical Staging System for Canine Hemangiosarcoma
Primary Tumor (T)	
T0	No evidence of tumor
T1	Tumor less than 5 cm diameter and confined to primary tissues
T2	Tumor 5 cm or greater or ruptured, invading subcutaneous tissues
T3	Tumor invading adjacent structures, including muscle
Regional Lymph Nodes (N)	
N0	No regional lymph node involvement
N1	Regional lymph node involvement
N2	Distant lymph node involvement
Distant Metastasis (M)	
M0	No evidence of distant metastasis
M1	Distant metastasis
Stages	
I	T0 or T1, N0, M0
II	T1 or T2, N0 or N1, M0
III	T2 or T3, N0, N1 or N2, M1

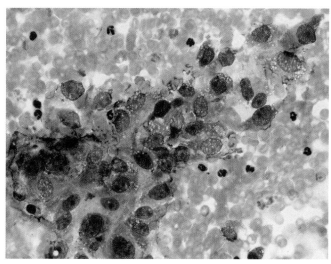

• **Fig. 34.2** Lung mass aspirate from an 11-year-old Catahoula leopard hound with multiple masses throughout the liver and lungs. The figure depicts an aggregate of spindle to irregularly shaped cells with moderately basophilic, vacuolated cytoplasm and large oval nuclei exhibiting coarsely stippled chromatin and multiple prominent nucleoli of variable size. (Image courtesy Casey LeBlanc, DVM, PhD, DACVP, Eastern VetPath, Bethesda, MD.)

investigation. Ultrasonographically, lesions typically have a heterogeneous appearance ranging from hypoechoic to targetoid to mixed echogenicity with areas of cavitation, often accompanied by a peritoneal effusion.[74,75] Although preliminary data suggest that the more advanced technique of contrast harmonic ultrasonography may hold promise in identifying HSA and differentiating it from benign etiologies, it is still not a widely used technique in clinical practice.[76,77] Three-view thoracic radiographs are essential as part of routine screening for pulmonary metastatic disease. The radiographic appearance of HSA varies but is often described as a nodular to interstitial coalescing miliary pattern. One study reported a sensitivity of 78% for detecting metastatic pulmonary HSA with radiography and that the false-negative rate was significantly decreased when three views (vs. one or two) were obtained.[78] In dogs with pericardial effusion secondary to cardiac HSA, radiographs will typically reveal a globoid cardiac silhouette, with or without distension of the caudal vena cava.[79]

For dogs with cardiac HSA, echocardiography is the main modality for identifying the primary tumor, and the presence of pericardial effusion tends to improve the detection of such masses.[80] Echocardiography can also be used to assess cardiac function before doxorubicin (DOX) chemotherapy in breeds at risk for dilated cardiomyopathy.[81] For dogs with cardiac HSA that has ruptured, electrocardiographic (ECG) signs consistent with pericardial effusion (decreased amplitude QRS complex and electrical alternans) may be noted during cardiac evaluation. In addition, ventricular arrhythmias are common in dogs with splenic and cardiac HSA.[35,82]

Advanced imaging modalities including computed tomography (CT) and magnetic resonance imaging (MRI) can be used for all forms of HSA, and their integration into routine metastasis screening, surgical planning, and serial restaging may improve prognostication and patient selection for therapy. Specifically, CT and MRI may aid in defining the anatomic origin and extent of disease for surgical and radiation therapy (RT) planning,[83] in discriminating between benign and malignant splenic and hepatic lesions, and in early detection of pulmonary metastasis.[84–86]

Recently, there has been interest in the assessment of biomarkers for cancer screening and diagnosis, particularly with respect to HSA. Plasma cardiac troponin I, a highly specific and sensitive marker for myocardiocyte damage, was shown to be significantly elevated in dogs with cardiac HSA versus dogs with HSA at other sites, dogs with other neoplasms, and dogs with non-HSA pericardial effusions.[87,88] In addition, plasma concentrations of VEGF and urine concentrations of bFGF were shown to be elevated in dogs with HSA versus normal controls[32,89]; however, neither was found to correlate with remission status, disease stage, or outcome. Thymidine kinase, a marker of DNA synthesis expressed only in proliferating cells, was significantly higher in the serum of dogs with HSA compared with that of healthy dogs.[90] Another biomarker, serum collagen XXVII, whose peptide components are associated with invasion and angiogenesis, was significantly higher in dogs with large HSA metastatic burdens compared with healthy dogs and interestingly, reductions in collagen XXVII peptide levels were noted after surgical resection of HSA lesions.[91] Conversely, these levels became elevated again on tumor recurrence, thus showing potential utility for this peptide as a serial biomarker for HSA.[91]

Ultimately, a definitive diagnosis of HSA usually requires histopathology. Fine-needle aspirate (FNA) cytology of suspected HSA lesions is often of low diagnostic yield due to hemodilution.[92] Similarly, cytology of HSA-associated effusions is rarely diagnostic; although tumor cells are likely present, they are heavily diluted with peripheral blood. In the infrequent scenario in which cytology is diagnostic, samples typically consist of large, pleomorphic spindle cells that display multiple criteria of malignancy (Fig. 34.2).

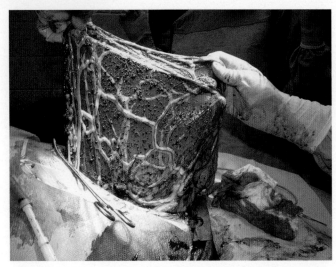

• **Fig. 34.3** Intraoperative image of multifocal omental metastasis in a dog with splenic hemangiosarcoma. Note the multifocal raised, red lesions along the surface of the omentum. (Photo courtesy Julius Liptak, BVSc, MVetClinStud, FACVSc, DACVS, DECVS, Alta Vista Animal Hospital, Ottawa, Canada.)

Treatment

Surgery

Surgery remains the primary method of treatment for almost all dogs and cats with localized, nonmetastatic HSA. For cutaneous or subcutaneous HSA, surgical considerations are similar to those for malignant skin tumors and soft-tissue sarcomas (see Chapter 22). Dermal HSA is typically discrete, and surgical margins of 1 to 2 cm and a fascial plane deep are often adequate. For some subcutaneous and almost all intramuscular HSA, the tumor will be very locally invasive and may have associated edema and bleeding. Wide margins can be difficult to achieve and amputation may be required if the tumor is located on a limb.

For splenic HSA, splenectomy is indicated and can be performed with sutures, staples, or electrothermal vessel sealant devices. At the time of splenectomy, the abdomen should be thoroughly explored and any suspicious lesions in the liver and/ or omentum (Fig. 34.3) should be excised and submitted for histopathology. A recent study showed that although hepatic lesions that were multiple and/or dark red or black were more likely to be HSA, only 50% of grossly abnormal livers were confirmed to contain HSA metastasis. Furthermore, almost 60% of histologically benign lesions were obtained from grossly abnormal livers.[93] For solitary hepatic and renal HSA, liver lobectomy and nephrectomy are indicated, respectively.

Surgical tumor removal is rarely performed for primary cardiac HSA; however, right atrial appendage masses can be resected with a stapling device or hand suturing via thoracotomy or thoracoscopy.[35,94,95] A small number of case reports and series describe reconstructive procedures with pericardial patch grafts where extensive tumor resection was performed.[96,97] Aside from tumor removal, an open or thoracoscopic pericardiectomy can be performed as a palliative procedure.[98]

Chemotherapy

Given the very high metastatic rate of canine HSA, adjuvant chemotherapy is indicated in essentially all cases, with the exception of most purely dermal HSAs. The literature suggests that DOX, which has been evaluated in both the adjuvant and neoadjuvant settings, is the most active agent against HSA. Protocols reported include single-agent DOX and DOX-containing combination protocols such as DOX and cyclophosphamide (CYC) (AC); DOX and minocycline; vincristine, DOX, and CYC (VAC); vincristine, DOX, and methotrexate; dacarbazine, DOX, and vincristine (DAV); DOX and ifosfamide; DOX and dacarbazine; and DOX and deracoxib.[3,99–107] Other chemotherapy agents with apparent single agent activity against HSA include ifosfamide, liposome-encapsulated DOX (Doxil, Caelyx), which has been evaluated both as an intravenous and intraperitoneal treatment, and epirubicin, which is a noncardiotoxic stereoisomer of DOX.[108–111]

Owing to the vascular nature of the disease, therapy directed against angiogenesis is a logical avenue of exploration. There has been growing interest in the use of metronomic chemotherapy (low-dose chemotherapy with or without nonsteroidal antiinflammatory drugs and other potentially antiangiogenic agents) in HSA patients.[112] One study reported a similar outcome for dogs with stage II splenic HSA treated with a combination of splenectomy, piroxicam, and metronomic chemotherapy (alternating courses of CYC and etoposide) compared with that of dogs receiving conventional DOX-based chemotherapy.[113] Two subsequent studies assessing metronomic chemotherapy and DOX in canine HSA produced divergent results. In the first study, slightly more than half the dogs received DOX alone and the rest received DOX followed by metronomic chemotherapy with CYC and thalidomide. The median time to metastasis and median survival time (MST) were significantly longer for dogs receiving DOX plus metronomic therapy.[114] In the other study, dogs were treated with splenectomy and DOX with or without subsequent metronomic CYC and there was no significant difference in outcome noted in the group receiving metronomic therapy.[115] It is worth pointing out that in the latter study, several dogs had stage III disease and there were a number of patients with macroscopic HSA remaining after surgery, whereas dogs with measurable metastasis were not included in the first study. Furthermore, a third study documented significantly improved outcomes in dogs receiving adjuvant single-agent thalidomide postsplenectomy, suggesting that the discrepant survival benefit noted between the two previously mentioned studies may be due to the inclusion of thalidomide along with CYC.[116] Lomustine and chlorambucil have also been evaluated in the metronomic setting for dogs with HSA, but patient numbers were too small and presentations too variable to derive a meaningful interpretation of the associated outcomes.[117,118]

In cats, similar DOX-based protocols may be employed for patients considered to be at high risk of metastasis or for those with advanced disease,[11,58,59] although systematic evaluations are lacking. Metronomic chemotherapy may also be considered for cats with HSA, although agent dosing and scheduling are empiric. Some antitumor activity of carboplatin has been reported in feline HSA.[119]

Immunotherapy

Very few studies have been conducted to evaluate biologic therapy for HSA. One early study evaluating the postoperative use of a mixed killed bacterial vaccine with DOX chemotherapy and reported some improvement in survival time in dogs with splenic HSA as compared with that seen with splenectomy alone.[3] Another study evaluated the combination of an allogeneic tumor cell lysate vaccine and DOX for various forms of canine HSA and showed that although dogs mounted an HSA-specific immunity, there was no significant improvement in survival.[120] Dogs receiving adjuvant AC chemotherapy combined with liposome-encapsulated muramyl tripeptide-phosphatidylethanolamine (L-MTP-PE), an immunomodulator derived from mycobacterial cell walls that increases monocyte tumoricidal activity, had a significantly better MST (9.1 months) than dogs receiving AC alone (5.7 months).[121] Although approved for the treatment of osteosarcoma in humans in the European Union, L-MTP-PE is not commercially available in the United States and thus no further formal investigations have been performed.

Radiation Therapy

RT is uncommonly used for HSA because of the predilection for this tumor in visceral sites as well as the high metastatic rate. One study evaluating hypofractionated (palliative) RT for nonsplenic HSA reported a high response rate, but no significant effect on overall survival.[122] Hypofractionated RT has been evaluated for dogs with cardiac HSA and in a pilot study appeared to reduce the frequency of cardiac tamponade, leading to an MST of 2.5 months.[123]

Targeted Therapies

Given the marginal improvement in survival achieved with conventional therapy for dogs with visceral HSA, the potential application of more targeted therapies is certainly warranted. Expression of receptor tyrosine kinase family members including PDGF receptor (PDGFR), VEGF receptor (VEGFR), and stem cell factor receptor (KIT), among others, has been documented in canine HSA.[29-31] Although in vitro assessments of targeted small molecule inhibitors such as masitinib (inhibitor of PDGF and KIT), imatinib (inhibitor of KIT and PDGFR), and dasatinib (inhibitor of KIT, PDGFR, and SRC) have demonstrated growth inhibition and induction of apoptosis in canine HSA cell lines, the drug concentrations required for this effect in vivo may be difficult to achieve without significant toxicity.[30,124] Toceranib phosphate (TOC, Palladia), which blocks signaling of KIT, PDGFR, and VEGFR family members, has demonstrated in vivo activity against multiple tumor types.[125] Although there is some interest in the use of toceranib phosphate for HSA given the high expression of VEGF and VEGFR, the administration of TOC in dogs with stage I or II HSA after splenectomy and DOX therapy resulted in no apparent improvement in median disease-free interval or MST.[126] eBAT, a bispecific epidermal growth factor (EGF)-urokinase angiotoxin, was evaluated in a small group of dogs before standard DOX chemotherapy, leading to an MST of 8.5 months and a 6-month survival rate of 70.6%, both of which were significantly improved compared with a historical control group receiving DOX only.[127]

Alternative Therapies

Yunnan Baiyao (YB), a Chinese herbal medicine that has long been used for its antiinflammatory, hemostatic, pro-wound healing, and analgesic properties in people, has also been anecdotally used to control bleeding in dogs with both nonmalignant and malignant conditions, including HSA. In a preliminary in vitro study, YB led to dose- and time-dependent cell death via caspase-mediated apoptosis in three canine HSA cell lines[128]; however, two laboratory studies demonstrated no modulation of coagulation

parameters in normal dogs receiving oral YB[129,130] and a recent retrospective study evaluating a combination of YB and epsilon-aminocaproic acid in dogs with presumed cardiac HSA suggested no benefit in terms of time to recurrence of hemopericardium or overall survival time.[131] Polysaccharopeptide (PSP), the bioactive agent from the mushroom *Coriolus versicolor*, was recently evaluated in a small pilot study in dogs with splenic HSA. A modest numerical improvement in MST was noted in the high dose cohort (*n* = 5) in comparison to historical controls receiving DOX-based therapy, although a true positive effect of PSP on time to metastasis and overall survival was not clearly evident based on statistical analysis.[132]

Prognosis

Canine

The prognosis for canine HSA is highly dependent on tumor location, stage of disease, and therapy pursued. A summary of the results of several reports on the treatment of splenic HSA is presented in Table 34.2. Overall, the prognosis for dogs with splenic HSA treated with surgery alone is extremely poor, with MSTs ranging from 19 to 86 days, largely due to the high metastatic rate.[1-3,5] Therefore the generally accepted treatment approach for splenic HSA includes DOX-based chemotherapy after surgery. Even with the addition of chemotherapy, MSTs increase only to 5 to 7 months[99-103,107] and the 12-month survival percentage remains 10% or less. Stage plays a role in prognosis, where stage I (nonruptured, nonmetastatic) splenic HSA may have a more favorable outcome (MST 239–355 days) than stage II (ruptured) splenic HSA (MST 120–148 days) when postoperative chemotherapy is used.[107,121] One study incorporated a histologic grading scheme into survival analysis and demonstrated that dogs with low-grade tumors had a better prognosis than dogs with intermediate- or high-grade tumors.[99] Primary renal HSA may be associated with a more favorable outcome than other visceral HSA, with an MST of 9 months in one small study.[40] Conversely, retroperitoneal HSA typically carries a poorer prognosis, with a reported MST of 37.5 days.[41] For true cutaneous HSA, which includes superficial tumors involving the dermis only, surgical removal can often be curative and MSTs of 780 to 987 days have been reported for dogs treated with surgery alone.[14,38] In one study, dogs undergoing surgical removal of dermal HSA were noted to have increased overall survival (MST 1570 days), particularly dogs with ventral tumor location (MST 1085 days), and those with evidence of solar-induced changes on histopathology (MST 1549 days).[14] Conversely, dogs whose cutaneous tumors displayed subcutaneous invasion had a higher chance of developing metastasis (relative risk 2.04) and a subsequently poorer longterm survival (MST 539 days).[14] HSAs originating in the subcutaneous and intramuscular tissues are typically more aggressive than dermal HSA, with higher metastatic rates and shorter MSTs.[6,38,66,68] Therefore adjuvant chemotherapy is typically part of recommended therapy for dogs with subcutaneous and intramuscular HSA.[66,68] Two studies reported divergent results, where one study reported an MST of more than 3 years for dogs receiving adjuvant DOX after surgical removal of subcutaneous HSA, and 9 months for dogs undergoing the same treatment for intramuscular HSA.[66] The other study reported an overall MST of 8 months for dogs with nonmetastatic subcutaneous or intramuscular HSA treated similarly.[68] For dogs with apparently inoperable subcutaneous or intramuscular tumors, DOX-based chemotherapy may offer some palliation and, in one study, some

TABLE 34.2 **Outcomes for Dogs Treated for Splenic Hemangiosarcoma**

Treatment	MST[a] (days)	Reference
Splenectomy	19–86	2,3,8
Splenectomy + MBV	91	3
Splenectomy + MBV + VMC	117	3
Splenectomy + A	172–210[b]	100,109
Splenectomy + AC	140[c]–180%	101,121
Splenectomy + AC + L-MTP-PE	277	121
Splenectomy + A + VAX	182	120
Splenectomy + A/DER	150	107
Splenectomy + A/IFOS	123	105
Splenectomy + A/DTIC	>550[d]	106
Splenectomy + A + TOC	172	126
Splenectomy + VAC	140–145	8,103,133
Splenectomy + MET$_1$	178	113
Splenectomy + DOX + MET$_2$	NR	114
Splenectomy + DOX + MET$_3$	134	115
Splenectomy + EPI	144	111
Splenectomy + DOXIL (IV)	166	109
Splenectomy + DOXIL (IP)	131	110
Splenectomy + IFOS	147	108
Splenectomy + PSP	117–199	3
Splenectomy + eBAT + DOX	258	127

[a]Not separated by stage of disease.
[b]Data for stage II splenic HSA only.
[c]15/18 had splenic HSA.
[d]5/9 had splenic HSA.

A, Adriamycin (doxorubicin); *C*, cyclophoshamide; *DER*, deracoxib; *DOXIL*, pegylated liposomal encapsulated doxorubicin; *DTIC*, dacarbazine; *eBAT*, bispecific *Egf*-urokinase angiotoxin; *EPI*, epirubicin; *HSA*, hemangiosarcoma; *IFOS*, ifosfamide; *L-MTP-PE*, liposome muramyl tripeptide phosphatidylethanolamine; *M*, methotrexate; *MBV*, mixed bacterial vaccine; *MET$_1$*, metronomic cyclophosphamide/etoposide + piroxicam; *MET$_2$*, metronomic cyclophosphamide + thalidomide; *MET$_3$*, metronomic cyclophosphamide +/– nonsteroidal antiinflammatory; *MST*, median survival time; *PSP*, polysaccharopeptide (*Coriolus versicolor*); *TOC*, toceranib phosphate; *V*, vincristine; *VAX*, tumor lysate vaccine.

tumors responded sufficiently to allow for complete resection.[67] Traditionally, the prognosis for cardiac HSA is considered poor. Without treatment, most dogs succumb to the disease within 2 weeks.[37] In the rare case where surgical removal of cardiac HSA is possible, survival times generally range from 1 to 3 months.[25,94,95] In a small group of dogs receiving adjuvant chemotherapy after surgical tumor removal, an increased MST (175 days) was reported.[94] Although pericardiectomy (via thoracotomy or thoracoscopy) can be considered as a palliative measure, it does not appear to improve survival by itself, with reported MSTs of 2.7 to 4 months.[98] Chemotherapy appears to offer some benefit, as a retrospective study evaluating the use of DOX chemotherapy for dogs with presumptive cardiac HSA documented a 41% objective response rate and

MST of almost 4 months.[37] There is also some evidence to suggest that systemic therapy may offer some benefit to patients with other forms of advanced and inoperable HSA. One study evaluating the combination of DOX and deracoxib reported an MST of 149 days for dogs with stage III splenic HSA, which was similar to the MST of 150 days for dogs of all stages combined.[107] Dogs with advanced stage HSA treated with a DAV protocol had a response rate of 47% and median time to progression of 101 days.[104] Similarly, dogs with stage III HSA treated with a VAC protocol had an MST (195 days) that was similar to that of dogs receiving the same treatment for stage I/II disease (MST 189 days).[133]

Feline

In cats, the prognosis for visceral HSA is poor. Most cats die from recurrence of the primary tumor or metastasis, and MSTs are generally short (77–197 days), owing to metastasis.[59,134] On the other hand, cats with cutaneous and subcutaneous HSAs that are treated with aggressive surgery have reported MSTs of approximately 9 months to 4 years.[11,58] Similar to those in dogs, feline HSAs with subcutaneous involvement are associated with higher rates of incomplete excision (50%–94%) and local recurrence (50%–80%).[11,55,56,58]

Conclusion

In summary, HSA remains one of the most aggressive cancers in dogs and cats and the longterm prognosis for most forms is generally poor. Surgery still offers the best approach to treat HSA even though it is typically only palliative; standard DOX-based chemotherapy has led to incremental improvement in prognosis. New approaches to treatment using combinations of surgery, conventional chemotherapy, metronomic and antiangiogenic therapy, immunotherapy, and targeted agents are needed to improve the outlook for this disease.

Comparative Aspects

In humans, a spectrum of endothelial tumors, including hemangioma, hemangioblastoma, Kaposi's sarcoma, hemangioendothelioma, and AS, is seen. AS is extremely rare in humans and can be a late sequela to RT in women treated for breast cancer.[135] With this exception, it has a lesion distribution and behavior similar to canine HSA. As in dogs, metastasis is frequent and adjuvant chemotherapy provides minimal benefit.

SECTION B: THYMOMA

CARLOS H. DE MELLO SOUZA

Incidence and Risk Factors

Thymoma is an uncommon cranial mediastinal tumor in dogs and cats, but is the second most common cranial mediastinal tumor in both species. Thymomas can occur at any age, but they usually affect older patients. The mean age at presentation in dogs and cats is 9 and 10 years, respectively.[136,137] A breed predisposition has not been clearly identified, but in a recent retrospective multiinstitutional study, 38% of 116 dogs with thymoma were Labrador retrievers and golden retrievers.[138] A sex predisposition has not been identified.[136–138] Risk factors predisposing animals to thymoma have not been identified.

Pathology and Natural Behavior

Thymomas are neoplasms of thymic epithelial cells, but they commonly include other cell populations such as mast cells and mature lymphocytes.[136,139–141] Different histologic types of thymoma have been described, including epithelial, lymphocyte-rich, and clear cell. In cats, cystic thymomas seem to be the most common form, but squamous cell carcinomas and thymolipoma have also been reported.[136,140–144] Thymomas are carcinomas and thus should be considered malignant tumors. The terms benign or malignant thymoma are commonly used and are based on clinical evidence of invasiveness rather than on histologic features of malignancy. Metastasis is rare in both species, [141,145–147] but reported metastatic rate has been as high as 20% in cats with cystic thymomas.[142] The differential diagnoses for mediastinal masses include lymphoma, ectopic thyroid tumor, branchial cysts, and, rarely, sarcomas and metastatic neoplasms. It is important to note that tumors extending from the ribs or sternum into the cranial mediastinum may sometimes resemble a mediastinal mass.[148]

History and Clinical Signs

Clinical signs related to organ displacement due to the presence of a mediastinal mass include lethargy, regurgitation, vomiting, anorexia, weight loss, coughing, tachypnea, and dyspnea. Less commonly, cranial vena cava (CVC) syndrome (edema of the head, neck, and thoracic limbs) may occur and is caused by obstruction of CVC draining the cranial part of the body.[138–143,146–148] Paraneoplastic syndromes are common in dogs and cats and may occur in as many as 67% of dogs with thymoma.[139,140] Reported paraneoplastic syndromes include myasthenia gravis (MG), exfoliative dermatitis, erythema multiforme, hypercalcemia, T-cell lymphocytosis, anemia, myocarditis, and polymyositis. MG and megaesophagus in dogs and exfoliative dermatitis in cats are the most commonly described paraneoplastic syndromes. MG may occur in up to 40% of dogs with thymoma and has also been reported in cats.[138,139,146,147] Concurrent megaesophagus and aspiration pneumonia have been reported in as many as 40% of dogs with thymoma.[139] Paraneoplastic syndromes may occur at presentation, later in the course of the disease, or after tumor removal.[139,141,146,147,149–157] In addition to paraneoplastic syndromes, up to 27% of dogs will have a concurrent second tumor.[138]

Diagnostic Techniques and Workup

Physical examination findings may include edema of the head, cervical area, and/or thoracic limbs secondary to CVC syndrome. The jugular veins may be dilated and tortuous. Auscultation of the thoracic cavity may reveal decreased or absent lung sounds in the cranial thorax because of lung displacement by the mass or pleural effusion. Cardiac displacement may also occur and the heart sounds may be heard either more dorsally, caudally, or both. In small dogs and cats, decreased compressibility of the cranial thorax may also be detected.[138–141,145–146,157]

Complete blood count is often normal, but anemia and thrombocytopenia (secondary to immune-mediated destruction), neutrophilia, and lymphocytosis may occur.[138] Hypercalcemia has been reported in 34% of 116 dogs with thymomas, but is also relatively common finding in cats and dogs with mediastinal lymphoma.[138,141,147,158] Thus the presence of hypercalcemia in an animal with a mediastinal mass cannot be used as the sole

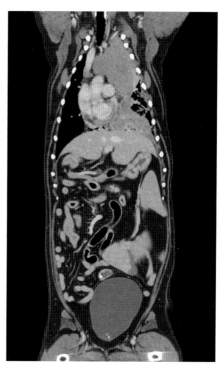

• **Fig. 34.4** Computed tomography of a dog with thymoma (dorsal view). A large cranial mediastinal mass that extends to most of the left side of the chest is depicted.

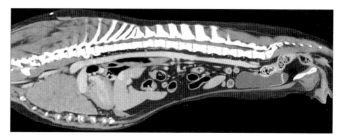

• **Fig. 34.5** Computed tomography of the same patient (sagittal view). The large cranial mediastinal mass compresses the cranial vena cava dorsally and the heart caudally.

means to differentiate thymoma from lymphoma. In both species, hypercalcemia is the result of excessive production of parathyroid hormone–related peptide (PTHrp).[158–162]

Thoracic radiographs may reveal a cranial mediastinal mass, pleural effusion, and/or displacement of the cardiac silhouette (Figs. 34.4 and 34.5). In cats and dogs with MG, megaesophagus and an increase in alveolar or interstitial lung pattern suggestive of aspiration pneumonia may also be detected. In cases with pleural effusion, cytologic analysis of the pleural fluid usually reveals a modified transudate with numerous small mature lymphocytes or a mixed lymphocyte population.[139–141,146,159] Thoracic ultrasonography is useful in the diagnosis and workup of cats and dogs with a cranial mediastinal mass. Cranial mediastinal masses with a cystic appearance and heterogeneous echogenicity were significantly more likely to be thymomas than lymphomas in one study.[163] In addition, ultrasound can be used for guided aspirates or needle-core biopsies of cranial mediastinal masses.[164,165] Endoscopic thoracic ultrasound has been described in dogs, and the reported advantage of this modality is a decrease in artifacts caused by the lungs.[166]

The cytologic diagnosis of thymoma is confirmed with the presence of neoplastic epithelial cells. These are often accompanied by mast cells and variable numbers of small mature lymphocytes.[141,166,167] Unfortunately, nondiagnostic samples are common because of a small percentage of neoplastic epithelial cells resulting in the presence of only small mature lymphocytes or because of the presence of cysts within the mass. In one study, neoplastic epithelial cells were cytologically evident in only 61% of cases.[3] The diagnosis is further complicated because of the fact that both lymphoma and thymoma may be composed mainly of small lymphocytes. In three studies, a presumptive diagnosis of thymoma was made in approximately 20%, 40%, and 77% of mediastinal masses after FNA cytology. A unique feature of thymoma, Hassal's corpuscles, are cytoplasmic structures present in thymocytes that can be used to aid on cytologic diagnosis. Unfortunately, these corpuscles are not usually visualized in Wright's Giemsa preparations in comparison to hematoxylin–eosin used for formalin-fixed samples.[139,146,167,168]

Flow cytometry may be used to aid in the specific diagnosis of mediastinal tumors. Using flow cytometry, thymic lymphocytes can be differentiated from peripheral lymphocytes by their simultaneous expression of CD4 and CD8. In one study, all cases of thymoma included 10% or more of lymphocytes coexpressing CD4 and CD8, whereas six of seven lymphomas contained fewer than 2% of CD4+CD8+ lymphocytes. The one case of lymphoma expressing more than 2% of CD4+CD8+ lymphocytes was readily differentiated from thymomas by flow cytometric scatterplot analysis.[169]

CT is recommended to determine the extent of disease, whether the thymoma is invasive or noninvasive, and to help the surgeon evaluate the feasibility of resection. The definition of surgical resectability will depend on the experience and ability of the surgeon. Vascular invasion, although more challenging, does not necessarily preclude surgery as a treatment option. Tumor thrombi have been successfully removed from within the CVC,[138] and the CVC has been reconstructed with a jugular vein autograft after excision of an invasive thymoma in a dog.[170] If the tumor is deemed inoperable, CT will still be crucial for planning RT. Furthermore, CT-guided biopsies can be obtained during the process. Despite these advantages, nonangiographic CT has been shown to have limitations, including significantly underestimating vascular invasion when compared with surgical exploration. These limitations can be potentially overcome by the use of CT angiography.[171–174]

Therapy

A variety of different modalities have been described for the treatment of thymomas in dogs and cats, including surgery, RT, chemotherapy, and multimodality treatments. Unfortunately, there are no available studies comparing the survival times (STs) of animals treated by these different modalities. In addition, in many studies, animals were treated with a combination of different methods.[139–142,146,150,157,173] In a retrospective study of 11 dogs and 9 cats with invasive and noninvasive thymomas treated with surgery alone, the MST was 790 days and 1825 days for dogs and cats, respectively. One- and 3-year survival rates were 64% and 42% and 89% and 74% for dogs and cats, respectively.[139] In another study, the MST for dogs treated surgically was 635 days, which was significantly better than the MST for dogs not treated surgically (76 days).[138] The successful resection of noninvasive thymomas in dogs by video-assisted thoracoscopy has also been reported.[175]

Two retrospective studies have evaluated RT for the treatment of thymomas. Seventeen dogs and seven cats with thymoma were treated with RT alone or as adjunctive therapy. Twenty cases were available for followup with a 75% response rate (11 partial responses and 4 complete responses). The MSTs for dogs and cats were 248 days and 720 days, respectively. In this study, the total radiation dose (15–54 Gy) and treatment interval (from daily to once weekly) varied markedly and may have affected the response rate and duration of responses. To additionally confound the effects of RT, only five dogs received RT alone. The remaining patients were treated with adjuvant RT after surgery, prednisone, and/or chemotherapy.[176] The second study evaluated eight dogs treated hypofractionated RT alone (48–49 Gy total dose, once weekly, for 6–7 weeks). The overall response rate was 50% and the 1-year survival rate was 75%.[177]

The role of chemotherapy in the management of thymomas has not been defined in cats and dogs. In a recent report, a cat with thymoma achieved a partial response after treatment with DOX, vincristine, and L-asparaginase.[178] Progressive disease was observed in 9 dogs treated with a variety of chemotherapy agents (carboplatin, DOX, vincristine and cyclophosphamide, etc).[138] Chemotherapy and RT can result in a reduction in the size of thymomas, but this effect may be the result of reduction in the nonneoplastic lymphocyte population in the thymus rather than a true anticancer effect.[139–141,146,178,179]

Prognosis

The prognosis is good for dogs and cats with noninvasive thymomas treated with surgery. Perioperative mortality rates range from 20% to 27% in dogs and 11% to 22% in cats,[139,179] but no independent risk factors were identified for perioperative mortality.[180] Prognostic factors in dogs include preoperative MG[139–142,147] and a low percentage of intratumoral lymphocytes.[139] The presence of MG, which was earlier thought to influence survival, did not do so in the most recent and largest retrospective study in dogs. The authors hypothesized that the lack of difference in survival despite these serious conditions likely reflects an improvement in both perioperative and postoperative care that has occurred in recent years.[138]

The prognostic effect of percentage of lymphocytes in the tumor was evaluated; results showed that a high percentage of lymphocytes was associated with longer STs. Age, invasiveness of the tumor, and mitotic index had no effect on prognosis.[139] One veterinary study evaluated the Masaoka–Koga staging system for thymomas in dogs. They showed that dogs classified as lower Masaoga–Koga stage (I or II) had significantly longer STs than dogs with stages II or higher.[138] In cats, cystic thymomas are commonly reported and they have been associated with a better prognosis, although no other possible prognostic factors, such as surgical resectability, were critically evaluated.[139,180,181]

In conclusion, long-term STs should be expected for dogs and cats with thymomas that can be completely resected. Tumor recurrence may occur after excision and a second surgery can be successfully performed. Vascular invasion may increase surgical complexity, but not necessarily deny surgery as an option.[138] RT appears to offer acceptable control rates for those tumors that are unresectable or recur.

Comparative Aspects

Thymic neoplasms constitute 30% of anterior mediastinal masses in adults and fewer than 15% in children. The majority are diagnosed in elderly patients (60 years or older) and a gender or race predilection has not been identified.[182,183] A clinicopathologic classification adopted by the World Health Organization (WHO) correlates well with biologic behavior of thymomas. In the WHO system, cells are classified as spindle (predominant in the medulla), oval and epithelioid (predominant in the cortex), or dendritic. The tumors are then further divided into medullary, mixed, predominantly cortical and cortical thymomas, and well-differentiated and high-grade thymic carcinoma. Medullary and mixed thymomas are considered benign tumors and, even in the face of capsular invasion, will not recur. Predominantly cortical and cortical thymomas display intermediate aggressiveness and have a low risk of relapse independent of their invasiveness. Well-differentiated and high-grade thymomas are highly invasive and associated with a high frequency of relapse and death. The staging system created by Masaoka uses both surgical and histologic signs of invasiveness to describe five different stages that correlate well with prognosis[182,183]:

Stage I: Tumor is grossly encapsulated and no capsular invasion is noted microscopically.
Stage II: Gross invasion occurs to surrounding fatty tissue or mediastinal pleura. Microscopic invasion of the capsule is noted.
Stage III: Gross invasion into neighboring organs (pericardium, great vessels, lungs)
Stage IVa: Pleural or pericardial dissemination
Stage IVb: Lymphatic or hematogenous metastasis

MG is the most common paraneoplastic syndrome associated with thymomas, occurring in 30% to 50% of patients. Red cell aplasia and hypogammaglobulinemia occur in 5% to 10% of patients.

Surgery is the standard-of-care in people with resectable tumors and complete surgical resection is the best predictor for longterm survival in people with thymomas. RT is most commonly indicated for people with extensive or recurrent disease. A variety of chemotherapy drugs have been used to treat inoperable thymomas or in cases in which gross residual disease is present after surgery. Cisplatin, ifosfamide, and prednisone are considered the most effective agents. In addition, neoadjuvant chemotherapy has been shown to influence longterm survival for thymomas in patients with Masaoka stages II and IVa.[182,184,185]

SECTION C: CANINE TRANSMISSIBLE VENEREAL TUMOR

J. PAUL WOODS

Incidence and Risk Factors

Canine transmissible venereal tumor (TVT), also known as transmissible venereal sarcoma and Sticker's sarcoma, infectious sarcoma, venereal granuloma, canine condyloma, transmissible sarcoma, and transmissible lymphosarcoma,[186,187–189] is a naturally occurring, horizontally transmitted infectious histiocytic tumor of dogs usually spread by coitus, but it may also be spread by licking, biting, and sniffing tumor-affected areas.[186,187,190–192] It has been observed occasionally in other canids, such as foxes, coyotes, and jackals.[186,190]

Although TVT has a worldwide distribution, its prevalence is highest in tropical and subtropical areas, particularly in the southern United States, Central and South America, southeast Europe,

Ireland, Japan, China, the Far East, the Middle East, and parts of Africa.[186,190] In enzootic areas, where breeding is poorly controlled and there are high numbers of free-roaming sexually active dogs, TVT is the most common canine tumor.[186,190,191,193] In North America, the prevalence of TVT is correlated with increased rainfall and mean annual temperature.[193] Occasional cases occur in regions otherwise free of TVT after travel to endemic areas as a result of tourism.[194] Pets traveling abroad can be exposed to TVT and carry it back to nonendemic areas; therefore veterinarians may act as the first line of defense against the introduction of TVT as an emerging disease in nonendemic areas.

Because TVT is primarily spread by coitus, free-roaming, sexually intact mature dogs are at greatest risk.[186] Dogs of any breed, age, or sex are susceptible.[186,190,189] No heritable breed-related predisposition has been found.[186,189] In endemic areas, although dogs older than 1 year of age are at high risk, TVT is most common in dogs 2 to 5 years of age.[186] The physical exertions associated with coitus in the dog with extensive abrasions and bleeding make both sexes susceptible to injury to the genital mucosa, which facilitates the exfoliation and implantation of tumor cells.[186,189] Transmission can occur efficiently in either direction between the male dog and the bitch. The most common sites of involvement are the external genitalia, but other sites that can be affected through licking or sniffing include the nasal and oral cavities, subcutaneous tissues, and the eyes.[186–192,195–200]

TVT is a transmissible allograft spread directly from dog to dog across major histocompatibility complex (MHC) barriers, through transplantation of viable tumor cells.[201] TVT and Tasmanian devil facial tumor disease (DFTD) are the only known naturally occurring clonally transmissible cancers that behave like an infectious parasitic neoplastic tissue graft.[202,203] Similar to host–parasite interactions, the successful transmission of TVT requires a confluence of multiple tumor and host traits including environment and behavior to facilitate transfer of tumor cells between hosts, tumor tissue that promotes shedding of large number of cancer cells, tumor cell plasticity to survive transmission and grow in the new host, and permissible host tissue involving angiogenesis.[204,205]

These cancers have evolved into a unique niche by overcoming the limitations of existing within the single host that gave rise to the tumors by gaining the ability to spread between individuals and thus survive long after the original hosts have died.

Pathology and Natural Behavior

TVT was initially recognized in 1876 and was used for the first successful experimental transmission of a tumor.[188,189] A number of characteristics of TVT suggest that the tumor originated in inbred wolves or dogs about 10,000 to 15,000 years ago, around the time that the dog was domesticated. Subsequently, the tumor spread worldwide.[206] TVT has evolved into a transmissible parasite representing the oldest known colony of cloned somatic mammalian cells in continuous propagation.

Tumor growth generally appears on the external genitalia or nasal or oral mucosa within 2 to 6 months of mating and can either grow slowly and unpredictably for years or grow invasively and eventually become malignant and metastasize.[186–190] Extragenital lesions can occur both alone (in isolation) and in association with genital lesions; however, it has been suggested that in most cases neoplastic foci can be detected on the genitalia.

TVT usually remains localized, but metastasis occurs in up to 5% to 17% of cases to regional lymph nodes (LNs), subcutaneous tissue, skin, eyes, oral mucosa, liver, spleen, peritoneum, hypophysis, brain, and bone marrow.[186,195,207,208,209] Because TVT is also transmitted by licking, sniffing, and biting, many cases of reported metastases may instead actually be spread by mechanical extension, autotransplantation, or heterotransplantation.

TVT is commonly described as a round (or discrete) cell tumor and suggested to be of histiocytic origin.[187–189] This is supported by immunohistochemical (IHC) expression of vimentin, lysozyme, alpha-1-antitrypsin (AAT), and macrophage-specific ACM1, as well as negative IHC staining specific for other cell types.[187–189,192,210–212] TVT also expresses p53, proliferating cell nuclear antigen (PCNA), Ki67, MYC, retinoblastoma (Rb), cyclin D1, matrix metalloproteases (MMPs) -2 and -9, and variably expresses S-100.[212–214] IHC has been helpful in confirming metastatic TVT in various anatomic locations.[207,208,209] Furthermore, there have been reports describing TVT cells with intracellular *Leishmania* organisms, also suggesting a histiocytic origin.[200,215]

Cytogenetic and genetic analyses have provided robust evidence of clonality. Whereas normal canine chromosomes consist of 76 acrocentric autosomes plus submetacentric X and Y sex chromosomes, TVT cells have a vastly rearranged karyotype consisting of 57 to 59 chromosomes, including 15 to 17 submetacentric chromosomes as a result of multiple centric fusions.[187,188,192,207] However, the total number of chromosome arms in TVT is grossly comparable to that in the normal dog, so it appears that the karyotypic rearrangement is not associated with significant change in DNA content.[201,206] Although TVT cells are aneuploid, they exhibit remarkably stable and similar karyotypes in samples obtained from widely separate geographic regions (i.e., different continents).[201] Likewise, molecular genetic studies of globally distributed TVT tumors provide evidence of a monophyletic origin, which has diverged into subclades.[201,216,217]

In addition, TVT cells all share an insertion of a long interspersed nuclear element (LINE-1) upstream of the c-*myc* oncogene that is not found in normal dog genomes.[218–220] This insertion has the potential to disrupt transcriptional regulation of downstream genes, possibly initiating oncogenic activity, and may have been causally involved in the origin of the tumor.[221] This unique rearranged LINE-c-*myc* gene sequence has been used with polymerase chain reaction (PCR) as a diagnostic marker of TVT to confirm diagnosis.[222,223] TVT cells have also demonstrated point mutations in the tumor suppressor gene *p53*, which is responsible for protecting the integrity of the DNA.[219,224,225] Mutations of such a key regulator of the cell cycle, apoptosis, and senescence may be another factor in the oncogenesis of TVT.

TVT is an immunogenic tumor and the immunologic response of the host appears to play a critical role in determining the natural behavior of the disease. The course of disease is divided into three distinct phases of growth: a progressive phase (P) in which the tumor grows for 3 to 6 months, then a stationary phase (S) that can last for months to years, which is followed by a regressive phase (R) unless the dog is elderly, in poor general condition, or immunologically compromised, in which case metastasis may occur.[189,226–233] Spontaneous regressions have been associated with immune responses against the tumor; therefore immunosuppression from any cause may be a risk factor for the development and maintenance of TVT and may predispose to widespread dissemination. When spontaneous regression occurs, it usually starts within 3 months after implantation but rarely if the tumor is present for more than 9 months.[186]

Initially, in the P phase, the tumor downregulates MHC class I β_2-microglobulin and class II expression, which allows it to evade the host's histocompatibility barrier, particularly T-cell cytotoxicity.[234] Some cell-surface MHC class I expression remains, likely to prevent recognition and killing by natural killer (NK) cells. This immunoevasion is partly due to the high concentration of tumor-secreted transforming growth factor-beta$_1$ (TGF-β_1), which inhibits tumor MHC antigen expression and NK cell activity.[230] TVT also targets and damages dendritic cells (DCs).[234] It has been suggested that TVT has evolved under survival pressures to escape host immunosurveillance.[235]

Tumor-infiltrating lymphocytes (TILs) produce interferon-gamma (IFN-γ) but fail to promote tumor MHC expression due to inhibition of IFN-γ effects by tumor-derived TGF-β_1, which also suppresses the cytotoxicity of the NK cells that migrate to the tumor site because of low tumor-antigen expression.[227,229,230] However, late in the P phase, a marked increase in immune cell infiltration occurs and TILs produce high concentrations of the proinflammatory cytokine interleukin-6 (IL-6), which acts synergistically with host-derived IFN-γ to antagonize the immunoinhibitory activity of TGF-β_1 and results in MHC expression in up to 40% of tumor cells and restores NK cytotoxicity.[228,236,237] A critical threshold level of IL-6 secreted by TILs has to be reached to trigger TVT into R phase.[230,236] Therefore after progressive growth for 3 to 4 months, the tumor spontaneously regresses with upregulation of MHC antigen expression, possibly under epigenetic control.[235] Regression has been correlated with upregulation of genes involved with inflammation and chemotactic cytokines.[238,239]

In addition to cell-mediated immunity, TVT also elicits a humoral immune response demonstrable by antibodies against TVT antigens.[226,240,241] Dogs recovered from TVT have serum-transferable immunity to reinfection and puppies born to bitches exposed to TVT are less susceptible to the disease.[242] In addition to the host immune response, during TVT regression stromal cells and extracellular matrix (ECM) react comparably to wound repair with collapse of the tumor parenchyma and replacement by fibrous stroma.[233]

History and Clinical Signs

The archetypical TVT patient is a sexually intact young adult dog either living in or having traveled to an area endemic for TVT, with a history of contact (coitus, sniffing, licking, or biting) with dogs of similar signalment.[186,189,190] The primary lesions are usually on the external genitalia. In the male, the tumor is usually located on the caudal part of the penis, requiring caudal retraction of the penile sheath for visualization (Fig. 34.6).[186–189] Occasionally, it is on the prepuce. In the bitch, the tumor is usually in the posterior vagina or vestibule.[186–189] Tumors appear initially as small 1 to 3 mm hyperemic papules that progress by fusing together into nodular, papillary, multilobulated cauliflowerlike or pedunculated proliferations up to 10 to 15 cm in diameter. The mass is firm but friable, with an ulcerated inflamed surface. The tumor often oozes a serosanguineous or hemorrhagic fluid. Examples of extragenital sites are illustrated in Fig. 34.7.

Clinical signs vary according to the location of the lesions. Genital lesions often manifest with chronic signs of discomfort or hemorrhagic discharge from the penile sheath or vulva for weeks to months before diagnosis, which can result in anemia.[186,189] Lesions can predispose to ascending bacterial urinary tract infections but rarely interfere with micturition.[243] Extragenital lesions cause a variety of signs, depending on anatomic location, such as sneezing, epistaxis, epiphora, halitosis, tooth loss, exophthalmos, skin masses, facial deformation, and regional LN enlargement.

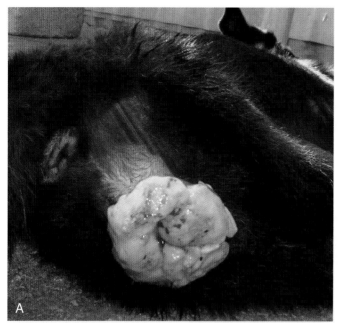

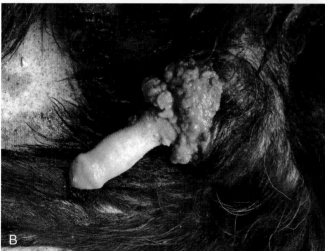

• **Fig. 34.6** Typical appearance of external genitalia affected by canine transmissible venereal tumor. **(A)** Female: irregular, friable, bleeding cauliflowerlike mass on the vagina. **(B)** Male: multinodular, friable cauliflowerlike mass at the base of the penis. (Reprinted with permission from Ostrander EA, Davis BW, Ostrander GK. Transmissible tumors: breaking the cancer paradigm. *Trends Genet.* 2016;32:1–15.)

Diagnostic Techniques and Workup

A presumptive diagnosis of TVT can be obtained based on history (including travel), signalment, clinical signs, and physical findings in dogs with the classic presentation. Definitive diagnosis is based on cytologic examination of cells obtained by swabs, FNAs or imprints of the tumors or histologic examination of a biopsy from the mass. TVT is described as a discrete (or round) cell tumor. TVT has a characteristic morphologic appearance on cytopathology and is often diagnosed without the need for histopathology (see Fig. 7.37). Exfoliative cytology demonstrates uniform discrete round to polyhedral-shaped cells with moderately abundant pale blue cytoplasm and an eccentrically located nucleus, with occasional binucleation and mitotic figures.[187–189,192] Single or multiple nucleoli are often observed, surrounded by clumped

chromatin. The most characteristic feature is the presence of numerous discrete clear cytoplasmic vacuoles, often referred to as a "string of pearls." In R phase, TVTs contain a higher number of infiltrating lymphocytes. Other round cell tumors, including lymphomas, mast cell tumors, plasma cell tumors, histiocytomas, and amelanotic melanomas, are important differential diagnoses but are generally not confused with TVT on cytopathology.

Histopathology of TVT reveals compact masses of round or polyhedral cells with slightly granular, vacuolated, eosinophilic cytoplasm.[187–189,192] The neoplastic cells are arranged in a diffuse pattern and supported by a thin trabecula of fibrovascular tissue. Regressing tumors are infiltrated by lymphocytes, plasma cells, and macrophages.[189] For atypical TVTs, if there is doubt about the diagnosis, specific molecular techniques can be used (e.g., in situ PCR of the rearranged LINE–c-*myc* gene sequence).[222,223]

The incidence of metastatic spread of TVT has been reported as less than 15%. However, in most cases of TVT, tumor staging is not performed. Therefore the actual metastatic rate might be higher. Regional LNs should always be evaluated for metastasis by palpation and cytopathology. A thorough physical examination is essential to rule out other possible sites of involvement (i.e., skin, subcutis, nasal and oral cavities, eye, orbit). Diagnostic imaging is usually not required except with invasive TVT of the nasal cavity, orbit, or unusual locations. However, abdominal ultrasound may be used to image regional LNs. Complete blood count (CBC), serum biochemistry profile, and urinalysis do not reveal specific changes. Dogs bearing a large tumor burden of TVT have been associated with a paraneoplastic erythrocytosis that may require temporary symptomatic therapy.[189]

Therapy

TVTs will respond to many forms of therapy; however, chemotherapy is the most effective. Single-agent vincristine (0.5–0.7 mg/m² or 0.025 mg/kg intravenously [IV], once weekly for 3–6 treatments) results in a complete and durable response in 90% to 95% of treated dogs.[186,190,196,197,200,232,238,241,244–248] Other single-agent and combination multiagent protocols employing cyclophosphamide, vinblastine, methotrexate, L-asparginase, and prednisolone have not demonstrated superiority to vincristine alone.[244,245] Resistant cases can be treated with DOX (25–30 mg/m² IV, every 21 days for three treatments).[190,195] Theoretically, if/when immune checkpoint inhibitors become available in veterinary medicine, they may be effective against TVT because it is an immunogenic tumor with regression correlated with immune cells and inflammation. The immune modulators might be used to treat chemotherapy resistant TVT or to reduce the dose of chemotherapy needed to achieve remission.

RT has demonstrated efficacy against TVT. In a study using orthovoltage RT at total doses of 1000 to 3000 cGy, all 18 dogs treated responded with a complete and durable response, with seven dogs requiring a single fraction of 1000 cGy and 11 dogs requiring two or three fractions.[249] Another study using megavoltage radiation (Co60) reported all 15 dogs achieving complete and durable responses with three fractions administered over 1 week, for an average total dose of 1500 cGy.[196] Therefore RT can be considered an effective treatment for TVT, particularly for lesions showing resistance to chemotherapy or located in sanctuary sites from chemotherapy (i.e., brain, testicle, eye).

Surgery can be an effective treatment for small localized TVT; however, surgery has an overall recurrence rate of 30% to 75%.[248,250,251] Marginal surgical excision is not effective, and it

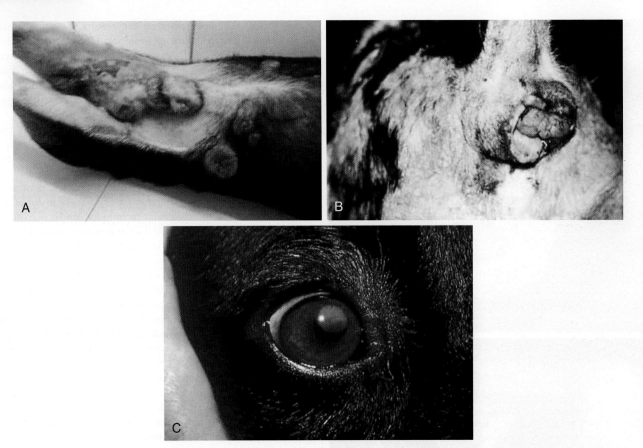

• **Fig. 34.7** Other primary tumor sites. (A) Male dog with cutaneous dissemination of transmissible venereal tumor (TVT) on the ventral abdomen. (B) Mucocutaneous TVT of the anal area in a dog. (C) Corneal involvement with TVT in a dog. (Courtesy Pr. Noeme S. Rocha.)

can be difficult to obtain wide surgical margins in the areas in which TVT typically appears. [248,250,251] In addition, tumor transplantation into the surgical wound by contamination from instruments or gloves may also cause postoperative tumor recurrence.

Other therapies described in spontaneous and experimentally induced cases include biologic-response modifiers (IL-2), piroxicam, cryosurgery, radiofrequency ablation, laser ablation, and electrochemotherapy. [252–257]

Reduction of the incidence of TVT is possible by having dog owners and breeders carefully examine all males and females before mating to avoid breeding affected animals. [186] In addition, stray dogs can act as a TVT reservoir; therefore the mingling of breeding dogs with strays should be prevented. In some areas, the control of ownerless, free-roaming dogs can drastically reduce the incidence of TVT. TVT can enter the wild canid population through physical contact, and it is not known whether TVT may pose a threat to endangered wild canids. [205]

Prognosis

In most cases, TVT remains localized and rarely becomes disseminated, with some dogs having spontaneous regression. For those dogs requiring treatment with vincristine or RT, the prognosis for complete and durable clinical remission is excellent. Therefore the overall prognosis of canine TVT is generally very good to excellent.

SECTION D: MESOTHELIOMA

LAURA D. GARRETT

Incidence and Risk Factors

Mesothelioma is a rare neoplasm of dogs and cats affecting the cells lining the coelomic cavities of the body. In 1962, Gerb et al cited reports of one case of mesothelioma in 1000 dogs and three cases in 5315 dogs. [258] In dogs, primary mesothelial tumors affecting the thoracic cavity, abdominal cavity, pericardial sac, and vaginal tunics of the scrotum have been reported. [259–264] In the cat, primary mesotheliomas have been reported in the pericardium, pleura, and peritoneum, as well as throughout the abdomen, with lung and mediastinal lymph node metastases. [265–270] Exposure to asbestos may be an important contributory factor to mesothelioma development in pet dog populations. Affected dogs often have owners who have jobs or hobbies for which exposure to asbestos is a known risk. [271] The level of asbestos in lung tissues of affected dogs has been documented to be greater than in controls. [271,272] Asbestos refers to a family of silicate minerals that crystallize into long, flexible fibers. The fibers are categorized into two groups: thin rodlike amphiboles, and long curly serpentine, the main type being chrysotile. In humans, much

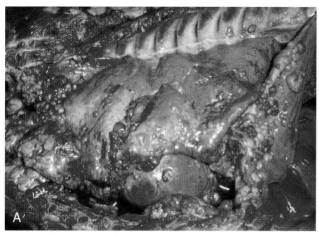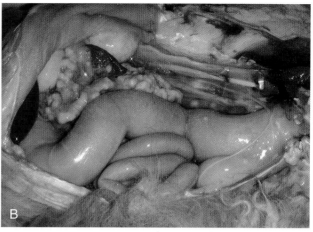

• **Fig. 34.8** (A) Pleural, parietal, and pericardial surfaces of a dog at necropsy illustrating nodular lesions histologically confirmed as mesothelioma. (B) Mesothelioma involving the peritoneal surfaces of a cat at necropsy.

greater risk has been related to amphibole asbestos compared with chrysotile exposure.[273] Chrysotile now accounts for 90% of asbestos used worldwide.[273]

The underlying mechanisms of the neoplastic transformation of mesothelial cells relates to the direct and indirect interaction of asbestos with mesothelial cells and the chronic inflammatory response initiated by activated macrophages attempting to engulf the asbestos fibers. The chronic inflammatory response also creates a distinct immunosuppressive tumor microenvironment, leading to infiltration with myeloid-derived suppressor cells, tumor-associated macrophages, and regulatory T cells, which likely contributes to tumor progression.[274] Although a wide array of mutations have been identified in mesotheliomas, the most frequent mutational events involve inactivation of tumor suppressor genes, including cyclin-dependent kinase inhibitor 2A (CDKN2A), BRCA1 association protein 1 (BAP1), and neurofibromin 2 (NF2).[275,276] Numerous cytokines including platelet-derived growth factor and vascular endothelial growth factor (VEGF) produced by stimulated macrophages or mesothelial cells are likely important in the pathogenesis of mesothelioma.[277] A report of five golden retrievers that developed pericardial mesothelioma after a long (30–54 months) history of idiopathic hemorrhagic pericardial effusion supports the concept that chronic inflammation may lead to neoplastic transformation in canine mesothelial cells. [278]

Mesothelial tumors occur most often in older animals; however, in cattle and sheep, newborn or young animals may be affected. Juvenile mesothelioma has been reported in two mixed-breed dogs under 1 year of age; no underlying etiology was identified.[279,280] A report of a 7-week-old puppy with mesothelioma suggests a congenital form may exist.[281]

Pathology and Natural Behavior

The normal mesothelium is a monolayer of flattened mesothelial cells. These cells are distinguished by the presence of microvilli, desmosomes, and phagocytic potential. Disease conditions associated with inflammation or irritation of the lining of body cavities commonly result in a marked proliferation of the mesothelial cells. Fluid accumulation in a body cavity promotes exfoliation and implantation of mesothelial cells. Mesotheliomas are considered

malignant because of their ability to seed the body cavity, but distant metastasis is rare.

Mesothelial cells appear morphologically as epithelial cells; however, their derivation is from mesoderm. Mesothelioma can appear histologically as epithelial, mesenchymal, or biphasic, which is a combination of the two.[282] The epithelial form, which resembles carcinoma or adenocarcinoma, is by far the most common form in small animals. There are also several reports of a variation of the mesenchymal form, which resembles sarcoma and is referred to as *sclerosing mesothelioma*.[261,283–285] The biphasic form of mesothelioma has been reported in two dogs and a cat. [286–288] A cystic peritoneal mesothelioma has also been reported in a dog.[289] This is a rare, benign, slowly progressive form of mesothelioma in humans, which is treated with surgical excision when the disease is localized.

History and Clinical Signs

Mesotheliomas occur as a diffuse nodular mass or multifocal masses covering the surfaces of the body cavity (Fig. 34.8). Extensive effusions occur as a result of exudation from the tumor surface or from tumor-obstructed lymphatics; therefore the most common presenting sign is dyspnea from pleural effusion or a distended abdomen from peritoneal effusion. Dogs with pericardial or heart-base mesotheliomas can present with tamponade and right-sided heart failure.[290–292]

Sclerosing mesothelioma is a variation of mesothelial tumor seen primarily in male dogs, with German shepherd dogs overrepresented.[261,283,284,293] These tumors present as thick fibrous linings in the abdominal and/or pleural cavities. Restriction occurs around organs in the affected area, and in the abdomen such changes can impinge on organs and lead to vomiting and urinary tract signs.

Diagnostic Techniques and Workup

Mesothelioma should be suspected in adult dogs presenting with a history of chronic, nonspecific clinical signs and fluid accumulation in any body cavity. Routine echocardiography and abdominal ultrasound are not typically helpful because the tumor cells cling to epithelial surfaces and a mass lesion is uncommonly noted.[294]

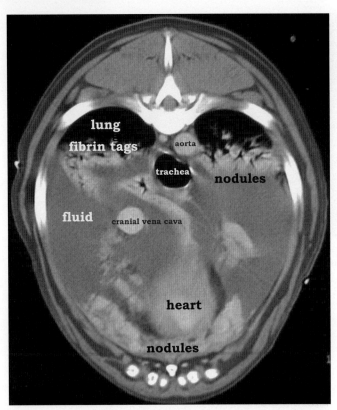

• **Fig. 34.9** A thoracic computed tomography image (with contrast) from a dog with histologically diagnosed mesothelioma. The effusion resolved after the first of five doxorubicin chemotherapy (30 mg/m², q3wk, IV) treatments.

In a study of echocardiography of dogs with pericardial effusion, a discrete cardiac mass was identified in only 5 of 15 dogs with effusion due to mesothelioma.[292] Thoracic CT may be of benefit to identify nodular lesions and to assess lung parenchyma in the presence of pleural effusion[295,296] (Fig. 34.9). Dogs with neoplastic pleural effusion are more likely to be older and on CT have thickening only of the parietal pleura compared with dogs with inflammatory effusion.[297] Although noted in only 3 of 20 dogs with malignant effusion, CT evidence of chest wall invasion was specific for neoplasia.

Cytologic evaluation of fluid can be diagnostic for other disease processes such as infection or lymphoma but will not conclusively diagnose mesothelioma. Mesothelial cells proliferate and exfoliate under any circumstance associated with fluid accumulation in a body cavity. Reactive mesothelial cells display many cytologic features of malignancy, making a definitive diagnosis of neoplasia via cytology impossible in most cases. Although one study found pericardial fluid pH analysis to be a discriminatory test to differentiate benign from malignant effusions, subsequent studies found too much overlap for the test to be of benefit.[298,299] Elevation in pleural effusion fibronectin concentrations in dogs and cats is a sensitive but nonspecific test for malignancy; mesothelioma can be ruled out if fibronectin levels are not increased.[300]

Establishing a definitive diagnosis of malignant mesothelioma may be difficult, particularly early in the disease. The diagnosis of mesothelioma requires adequate tissue sampling, preferably from an open, visually directed biopsy. Increasing availability of thoracoscopy and laparoscopy for small animals provides a less invasive way to evaluate these cases.[301] In either procedure, the clinician is encouraged to biopsy any body cavity lining and any regional lymph nodes when an obvious cause for fluid accumulation is not found. Sclerosing mesothelioma must be distinguished from chronic inflammatory diseases of the body cavity, such as chronic peritonitis, and histologic examination of biopsy material is essential to establish the diagnosis. Embolized, nonneoplastic mesothelial cells within lymph nodes is a rare finding in humans with cavity effusions and has been reported in dogs affected with idiopathic hemorrhagic pericardial effusion; care must be taken to not overinterpret these cells as indicative of metastasis.[302]

The most useful criteria in establishing a diagnosis of mesothelioma are that the tumor is primarily a neoplasm of the coelomic cavity lining and that the method of tumor spread is by transcoelomic implantation. Therefore mesothelioma should be considered when the bulk of the neoplastic tissue exists on the coelomic surface. Histologically, mesotheliomas need to be differentiated from carcinomas, adenocarcinomas, or sarcomas, depending on the morphologic type of the mesothelioma. Unfortunately, there are no cellular markers that conclusively define the mesothelial cell, and the diagnosis of mesothelioma remains a challenge in human medicine despite advances in IHC staining and molecular testing. Histologic diagnosis is based on morphologic assessment supported by clinical and imaging findings, with IHC and molecular testing adding further details.[303] Currently, the most useful mesothelial markers to support a diagnosis of malignant pleural mesothelioma in humans are calretinin, Wilms' tumor gene (WT1), cytokeratin 5/6 (CK5/6), and D2-40. However, 30% of mesotheliomas are a "null" phenotype and will be negative for these markers.[303]

Treatment and Prognosis

No satisfactory treatment exists for mesothelioma. Radical excision may benefit some animals, but usually the tumors are too advanced locally and have spread by implantation early in the course of disease. In one case report, a 2-year-old Siberian husky with a solitary sclerosing mesothelioma affecting the left thoracic diaphragmatic surface with pericardial and mediastinal adhesions was treated with aggressive surgical resection and diaphragmatic reconstruction using the transversus abdominis muscle.[304] The dog recovered well, but subcutaneous masses at the surgery site, as well as hepatic and renal masses, were noted 54 days postoperatively, leading to euthanasia. Pericardiectomy may palliate mesothelioma patients that present with cardiac tamponade; two dogs treated with surgery alone survived 4 and 9 months in one report.[305] In another report, the MST in five dogs treated with pericardiectomy was 13.6 months; three of these dogs received adjuvant IV chemotherapy (two DOX, one mitoxantrone).[306] A dog treated with pericardiectomy, intrathoracic and IV cisplatin, and IV DOX remained free of disease at 27 months.[307] In a report of eight dogs with pericardial mesothelioma, the MST was 60 days (range 15–300 days) after partial pericardiectomy. The one dog that survived 300 days was treated with DOX and intracavitary cisplatin for the 4 months preceding death.[294] Thoracoscopic partial pericardiectomy is a less invasive procedure than open thoracic surgical pericardiectomy and has been successfully performed in dogs with malignant pericardial effusions, including four dogs with mesotheliomas.[308] Although reported only in one dog, thoracoscopy portal site seeding from contamination with mesothelioma cells on instruments or cannulas or via leakage of malignant effusion is a potential complication.[309] Short-term complications and longterm outcomes of thoracoscopic pericardial window to treat pericardial effusion, idiopathic (10) or neoplastic (5), were reported in 15 dogs, one of which had mesothelioma.[310] The procedure had a complication rate of 25%, low mortality (7%), and short hospitalization stay (1 day). The meso-thelioma case lived the longest of the neoplastic cases, at 107 days. In another study, 58 dogs with idiopathic or malignant pericardial effusion (at least 10 of which were mesotheliomas) treated with thoracoscopic pericardial window or thoracotomy and subtotal pericardectomy were evaluated. The median disease-free interval and MST for dogs with malignant effusions, although short at approximately 3 to 4 months, did not significantly differ between the two surgical techniques.[311] Thus the less invasive procedure can be considered for palliation of malignant pericardial effusions. For palliative management of pleural effusion, a permanent port can be placed that allows for both ease of effusion removal and administration of intracavitary chemotherapy.[312] The MST for animals with untreated mesotheliomas in any location is difficult to assess from reports, as the tumors are rare and animals frequently are euthanized at the time of diagnosis.

Intracavitary cisplatin has shown palliative potential in the dog; it was well tolerated and greatly decreased mesothelioma-associated thoracic fluid accumulation in three dogs in one study.[313] The treatments also appeared to arrest tumor growth for a limited time. Two doses of intracavitary carboplatin was safely administered to a cat with suspected pleural mesothelioma and resulted in transient resolution of clinical signs for a total of 54 days, at which point the owners discontinued therapy.[314] Unfortunately, local penetration of intracavitary chemotherapy occurs only to a limited depth (2–3 mm), and thus large masses will not be affected significantly, other than from ultimate exposure to the systemically absorbed intracavitary drug. In such cases, combining debulking surgery or systemic chemotherapy such as DOX or mitoxantrone with intracavitary cisplatin may be beneficial. For peritoneal mesothelioma, four doses of intracavitary cisplatin in two dogs and carboplatin in one cat, combined with piroxicam administration, resolved the effusion in all cases.[315] One of the dogs had debulking surgery first; this dog was still in remission at 2 years, whereas the other dog and the cat lived 8 and 6 months, respectively. IV chemotherapy may provide benefit in some patients; single-agent IV cisplatin administered every 3 weeks was reported to improve clinical signs in a dog with bicavitary epithelial mesothelioma, until sudden death occurred 5 months after treatment initiation.[316]

Comparative Aspects

In humans, approximately 70% to 80% of mesotheliomas are linked to occupational exposure to aerosolized asbestos fibers, with the type of employment, such as construction work, ship building, heating trades, and insulation work significantly increasing relative risk.[317] There is a long latency period from time of exposure to tumor development, ranging from 12 to 50 years. Less often, several naturally occurring minerals with elongated structures, termed naturally occurring asbestos (NOA), are associated with mesothelioma development. These cases are seen in regional populations in many sites worldwide, affect men and women equally, and have a younger age at onset compared with occupational exposure cases.[318]

In humans with mesothelioma, the median survival is approximately 1 year from symptom onset. Prognosis is associated with the histologic subtype, and multiple other factors have been assessed to refine prognosis, stratify patients for clinical trials, and guide targeted therapies.[274,319,320] Chemotherapy, specifically pemetrexed or raltitrexed, combined with cisplatin or carboplatin, is the standard of care firstline therapy.[321] There is ongoing controversy regarding the therapeutic role of surgery

and/or RT, as nonrandomized observational studies have shown improved survival with multimodal treatment but randomized studies have not.[321,322] With the tremendous growth in understanding of the genetic alterations found in mesotheliomas, a wide array of other novel therapies are under investigation in randomized clinical trials in humans.[274] Overall, mesothelioma still carries a poor prognosis. Improved ability to assess an individual's tumor's markers and mutations will help guide therapy, including novel agents, and will hopefully improve survival time in the future.

SECTION E: NEOPLASIA OF THE HEART

JENNA H. BURTON AND JOSHUA A. STERN

Incidence and Risk Factors

Cardiac and pericardial neoplasms are rare in both dogs and cats. The frequency at which dogs were diagnosed with cardiac tumors in a Veterinary Medical Data Base (VMDB) search over a 14-year time frame was 0.19%, with 84% of tumors identified as primary cardiac neoplasia.[323] In two canine necropsy series, the frequency at which primary or metastatic neoplasia was detected ranged from 2.7% to 3.1% of all cases examined and represented 11.7% to 28.3% of all cancers diagnosed in these dogs at necropsy.[324,325] Reports are conflicting as to whether primary or metastatic tumors predominate in dogs as the reported frequency of secondary cardiac tumors ranges from 16% to 86%.[323–326] Cardiac metastases may be common in dogs with advanced stage cancer, but remain clinically silent and challenging to diagnosis antemortem, leading to likely underreporting of these events except when necropsy is performed.[326–328]

Cardiac tumors generally occur in middle-aged to older dogs.[323–326] Hemangiosarcoma (HSA) is the most common primary heart tumor in dogs, followed by aortic body tumors (ABTs) such as chemodectomas and paragangliomas. HSA and ABT represent 40% to 69% and 8% to 28% of all primary cardiac tumors in VMDB and necropsy studies, respectively.[323,325,326,329] Breeds potentially at increased risk for cardiac HSA include golden retrievers and German shepherds; boxers, Labrador retrievers, and cocker spaniels are commonly reported to develop cardiac HSA as well.[323,324,330–332] ABTs occur most frequently in older brachycephalic breeds, such as bulldogs, boxers, and Boston terriers, and it has been suggested that chronic hypoxia may stimulate development of these tumors in brachycephalic breeds;[323,333–335] however, nonbrachycephalic breeds such as German shepherds, Labrador retrievers, and golden retrievers also develop ABT at increased frequency and not all brachycephalic breeds develop ABT, which suggests other factors likely contribute to its pathogenesis.[323,336,337]

Cardiac tumors are even less common in cats, with an overall incidence of 0.0275% in a VMDB search.[338] Cardiac lymphoma, both primary and secondary, predominates.[326,339,340] As with other forms of lymphoma, feline leukemia virus (FeLV) infection likely plays a role in cardiac lymphomagenesis in cats.[326,339] Several case reports of ABT in cats exist and cardiac HSA is rare.[326,341–346]

Pathology and Natural Behavior

Tumors of the heart may occur at the heart base or in pericardial, intracavitary, or intramural locations. Primary tumors may be benign or malignant, with the latter predominating, and most occur in the right atrium and auricle in the dog.[323,329] Cardiac HSA is frequently associated with hemorrhagic pericardial effusion and cardiac tamponade and tends to have high rates of metastasis.[330,332,347] ABTs are the second most common primary neoplasm of the heart in dogs, and lymphoma and ectopic thyroid carcinoma are observed with some frequency as well.[323–326,329,348–359] Reported but rare malignant tumors include mesothelioma, myxosarcoma, chondrosarcoma, fibrosarcoma, osteosarcoma, rhabdomyosarcoma, undifferentiated sarcoma, leiomyosarcoma, thyroid carcinosarcoma, peripheral nerve sheath tumor, granular cell tumor, malignant mesenchymoma, and anaplastic carcinoma.[360–385] Histologically benign cardiac tumors have been reported and may cause lifethreatening clinical signs because of their location despite their biologically benign behavior. Reported benign cardiac tumors include myxoma, lipoma, thyroid adenoma, hamartoma, Schwannoma, leiomyoma, and fibroma.[359,386–399] In contrast to those in humans, metastatic cardiac tumors are diagnosed with less frequency than primary tumors in dogs, likely due to the high incidence of cardiac HSA in this species and absence of cardiac specific clinical signs for many secondary tumors.[323,326,328] Tumors reported to metastasize to the heart in dogs include HSA, lymphoma, mammary gland carcinoma, melanoma, pheochromocytoma, histiocytic sarcoma, gastric adenocarcinoma, liposarcoma, malignant mesenchymoma, rhabdomyosarcoma, extraskeletal osteosarcoma, fibrosarcoma, and pulmonary carcinoma.[326,328,400–412]

Cardiac tumors in cats tend to be malignant although benign intrapericardial cysts have been reported.[413,414] In addition to lymphoma, ABT, and HSA, single case reports of primary cardiac ganglioneuroma, rhabdomyosarcoma, and myxoma exist.[415–417] Metastatic lesions have been reported to arise from squamous cell carcinoma, mammary gland carcinoma, and pulmonary carcinoma.[326,418]

History and Clinical Signs

Tumors of the heart generally cause clinical signs secondary to alterations of cardiac function and may result from a mass obstructing blood flow to and from the heart, external cardiac compression that impedes filling such as pericardial effusion, and/or arrhythmias or decreased contractility resulting from myocardial infiltration or ischemia of the myocardium. Clinical signs are influenced more by the tumor location, tumor size, and presence of pericardial effusion than the specific histology of the tumor. Sudden death may occur secondary to cardiac arrhythmias or tumor rupture and subsequent blood loss, with or without cardiac tamponade. Tumors, particularly cardiac HSA, arising in the right side of the heart often cause signs of right-sided congestive heart failure due to inflow obstruction or the presence of cardiac tamponade secondary to pericardial effusion. Signs of right heart failure often result from the presence of bi- or tricavitary effusion and may present as abdominal distention, dyspnea, exercise intolerance, and/or acute collapse. Clinical signs commonly reported for dogs with confirmed or suspected HSA of the heart are often nonspecific in nature and are described in Table 34.3.

Clinical signs associated with ABT may include abdominal distension, weight loss, dyspnea, anorexia or inappetence, signs of gastrointestinal tract disease, lethargy, cough, and collapse. Although many dogs with ABT may have clinical signs that persist for weeks to months before diagnosis, some will present acutely as well.[336,419,420] Clinical signs for cats with cardiac neoplasia most frequently include tachypnea, dyspnea, hyporexia, weight loss, and lethargy; acute collapse appears to occur less frequently than in dogs.[339,345,421]

Diagnostic Techniques and Workup

Differential diagnosis of a cardiac tumor is often made based on clinical history, physical examination, and radiographic findings. Diagnosis requires imaging, which is routinely achieved by echocardiography and sometimes through additional advanced modalities such as CT or MRI. Incidental diagnosis of subclinical cardiac tumors may be encountered at necropsy. In the majority of cases, antemortem cytologic or histologic confirmation of neoplasia is not obtained; however, in cases where technically feasible and with acceptable clinical risk, FNA or biopsy may provide importance guidance on therapeutic options.[422]

Much like clinical signs, physical exam findings vary widely depending on location and hemodynamic consequences of the cardiac tumor. Patients with incidentally identified cardiac tumors may have apparently normal physical examinations. Auscultatory abnormalities are common secondary to pericardial effusion and include muffled heart sounds, pericardial friction rubs, or tumor plops (intermittent diastolic sounds secondary to tumor motion). In addition, arrhythmias may be auscultated, particularly in patients with myocardial involvement. Pulmonary auscultation may reveal abnormalities consistent with left-sided congestive heart failure, such as increased bronchovesicular sounds and/or soft crackles. Pulse quality derangements are common in patients in low-output states, such as cardiac tamponade. Jugular venous distention and pulsation may also be observed secondary to elevated right heart pressure with pericardial effusion or obstructive lesions.

Many components of the diagnostic evaluation are related to the common concomitant condition of pericardial effusion. An electrocardiogram may be normal in patients with cardiac tumors or may show a wide variety of cardiac arrhythmias, which are frequently related to the site of the cardiac tumor and infiltration of the myocardium.[423] Conduction disturbances, such as atrioventricular blocks or bundle branch blocks, may be observed with myocardial infiltration and may be as severe as complete atrioventricular block as previously reported with cardiac lymphoma.[349] Supraventricular or ventricular arrhythmias may be observed in cases of cardiac tumors with or without pericardial effusion. ST segment changes may be observed secondary to myocardial ischemia with or without pericardial effusion.[424] Sinus tachycardia is common with cardiac tamponade or in cases with heart failure acquired secondary to obstructive cardiac tumors.

TABLE 34.3	Frequency of Commonly Reported Clinical Signs for Dogs with Suspected or Confirmed Cardiac Hemangiosarcoma	
Clinical Sign	**Reported Frequency (%)[331,332,458,459,462]**
Lethargy	35–93
Anorexia or inappetence	19–46
Acute collapse	13–54
Coughing/respiratory difficulty	13–42
Vomiting	11–38
Weakness	0–56

Radiographs are insensitive in the diagnosis of cardiac tumors, with a reported sensitivity of only 47% for cardiac HSA.[425] Many radiographic findings are associated with the presence of pericardial effusions. Animals with a large-volume pericardial effusion may have a globoid cardiac silhouette with crisp margins owing to reduced cardiac motion (Fig. 34.10). Smaller fluid accumulations may allow visualization of chamber contours and atrial/tumor shadows.[338] In the setting of cardiac tamponade, animals may have diminutive pulmonary arteries and veins with distention of the caudal vena cava. In cardiac tamponade or in the setting of obstructive mass lesions, fluid accumulations such as pleural effusion, ascites, or pulmonary edema may be observed.[423] Mass lesions, if seen, are most common in the areas of the right atrium and heart base and may elevate the intrathoracic trachea.[338] Lung metastases may also be observed.

Echocardiography is the most widely used imaging tool for identifying tumors of the heart in cats and dogs.[426—428] In a study of 107 dogs with pericardial effusion, the sensitivity and specificity of echocardiography were 82% and 100%, respectively, for detection of a cardiac mass; with detection of right atrial/auricular masses being slightly higher (82% sensitivity and 99% specificity) than that of heart base tumors (74% sensitivity and 98% specificity).[429] The positive and negative predictive values of echocardiography were 100% and 75%, respectively, for detection of a cardiac mass.[429] In a small study of histologically-confirmed HSA of the right atrium and/or auricle, echocardiography had a positive predictive value of 92% (11/12) and a negative predictive value of 64% (9/14) in dogs.[428] Tumor location (extrapericardial, noncavitary pericardial, and small auricular masses) and size appeared to be the most important factors leading to false-negative results via echocardiography.[428] This finding was supported by a larger recent study of 51 dogs with histologically confirmed HSA of the right atrium (Fig. 34.11a) or right auricle (Fig. 34.11b), where right atrial tumors were more readily diagnosed (95% detection rate) than right auricular tumors (60% detection rate).[331] Additionally, tumor location is shown to be only moderately predictive for correctly identifying underlying tumor type (i.e., HSA vs. chemodectoma, etc.).[430] Pericardial effusions are commonly associated with cardiac tumors in both cats and dogs,[385,428,429,431] being present in 42% (10 of 24) of patients with echocardiographically diagnosed cardiac tumors in a recent study.[430] Pericardial effusion is more commonly identified in patients with cardiac HSA, occurring in 82% of cases in a recent study.[331] Echocardiographic diagnosis of mesothelioma is challenging, as many small lesions are below the resolution echocardiography and a single, larger mass lesion is uncommon in this tumor type. Echocardiography is particularly useful to evaluate for acquired pulmonary or aortic stenosis (Fig. 34.12) and may aid in identifying the extent of the tumor and possible myocardial or vascular invasion. Additional advanced imaging modalities, including CT, MRI, positron emission

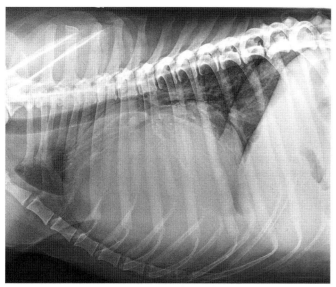

• **Fig. 34.10** A right lateral thoracic radiograph of a dog with pericardial effusion and cardiac tamponade secondary to cardiac hemangiosarcoma. The globoid cardiomegaly with crisp margins and diminutive pulmonary vasculature are characteristic of pericardial effusion. There is small volume pleural effusion and reduced abdominal detail, which were secondary to concomitant right heart failure.

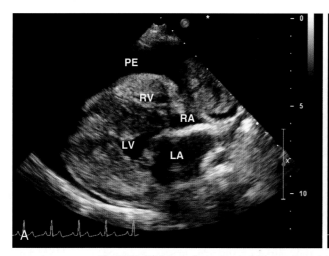
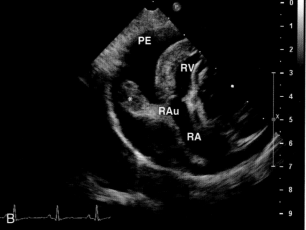

• **Fig. 34.11** (A) A two-dimensional, right parasternal, long-axis, echocardiographic image from a dog with a suspected cardiac hemangiosarcoma (HSA). The top of the image shows the right side of the heart and a large right atrial, heterogenous mass lesion *(asterisk)* consistent with cardiac HSA is observed along with pericardial effusion *(PE)*. The collapsed right atrium *(RA)*, right ventricle *(RV)*, left atrium *(LA)*, and left ventricle *(LV)* are labeled. (B) A cranial, left apical, echocardiographic image from a dog with PE is shown allowing visualization of the collapsed RA and right auricle *(RAu)*. A small heterogeneous lesion *(asterisk)* consistent with cardiac HSA is seen at the tip of the right auricle.

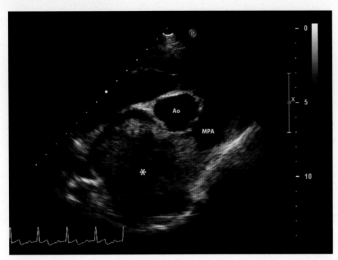

• **Fig. 34.12** A right parasternal, short-axis, basilar view, echocardiographic image from a dog with a suspected aortic body tumor. A large mass lesion *(asterisk)* consistent with an aortic body tumor is seen adjacent to the cross-sectional aorta *(Ao)* and compressing the region of the main pulmonary artery branches. The right branch of the main pulmonary artery has extraluminal compression secondary to the heart base tumor, which is creating a pressure overload on the right ventricle and subsequent right-sided congestive heart failure in this patient.

tomography (PET), and PET/CT, may be useful for selected cases, particularly in preparation for possible surgical or radiation-based therapies.[432–436]

Other clinical diagnostic methods for the evaluation of cardiac or pericardial masses include pneumopericardiography, selective and nonselective angiography, gated radionuclide imaging, and endomyocardial biopsy.[338,401,437] These techniques are infrequently used in favor of accessible imaging by echocardiography, cardiac MRI, and CT/angiography. Cytologic evaluation of pericardial fluid and pericardial fluid pH has been shown in multiple studies to be of limited utility in discriminating between neoplastic and nonneoplastic causes of pericardial effusion[438–440]; however, in the setting of a patient with pericardial effusion and no obvious cardiac tumor by echocardiography, pericardial fluid cytology may offer a diagnosis in approximately 8% of cases.[441] Improved diagnostic yield (20%) of pericardial fluid cytology was identified in cases where the pericardial effusion had a hematocrit of less than 10%.[441]

Cardiac troponin I (cTnI) appears to be useful for diagnosing cardiac HSA in dogs.[442,443] cTnI is a sensitive and specific marker for myocardial ischemia and necrosis. Dogs with cardiac HSA had significantly higher concentrations of cTnI than did dogs with idiopathic pericardial effusion.[442] In another study, the median plasma cTnI concentration was higher in dogs with cardiac HSA compared with dogs with HSA at other sites, dogs with other neoplasms, and dogs with pericardial effusion not caused by HSA. Furthermore, dogs with cTnI concentrations higher than 0.25 ng/mL were likely to have cardiac HSA, and a plasma cTnI higher than 2.45 ng/mL indicated that cardiac involvement is likely in dogs with confirmed HSA.[443] In practice, the measurement of cTnI may aid in reducing the number of false-negative results by echocardiogram. The authors routinely measure cTnI in patients with pericardial effusion and no obvious tumor on echocardiogram, using the published cutoff value of greater than 0.25 ng/mL as a likely indication of cardiac HSA.[443]

For dogs and cats with a cardiac mass and suspected neoplasia, every effort should be made to determine the extent of disease and the existence of primary or metastatic sites elsewhere in the patient. In addition to echocardiography and/or other advanced imaging modalities, a minimum database is recommended, including a CBC, serum biochemical profile, urinalysis, coagulation profile, thoracic radiographs, and abdominal ultrasound. Concurrent splenic masses have been reported in 9 of 31 (29%) dogs with suspected primary cardiac HSA with 42% of dogs having metastases to other sites such as the liver, mesentery, omentum, and lungs.[444] Conversely, this same retrospective study identified concurrent right atrial lesion in 2 of 23 (8.7%) dogs with primary splenic HSA whereas a previous necropsy study reported that 6 of 25 (24%) dogs with splenic HSA had a concurrent right atrial lesion.[444,445]

In a minority of cases, a diagnosis may be obtained by FNA cytology, endomyocardial biopsy, or open surgical or thoracoscopic biopsy. A recent small case series of 6 dogs reported 100% success of obtaining a diagnostic cytology sample by FNA. This technique resulted in minor complication in two of six dogs and required general anesthesia for four of six aspiration attempts.[446] Despite this recent publication, the majority of cases remain treated based on anatomic location of the mass (e.g., right auricle assumed to be HSA) owing to the risks of obtaining a definitive diagnosis in the setting of limited therapeutic options.

Therapy

Initial treatment for patients with cardiac tumors consists of therapies directed at the secondary complications to improve cardiac output and hemodynamic function; however, interventions to manage complications such as arrhythmias and congestive heart failure will have limited efficacy unless management of the primary tumor is initiated. The use of endovascular stents as palliation has been described in two dogs with cardiac masses obstructing venous return to the right atrium.[447] Surgical resection of primary cardiac masses may be considered, but is generally limited to tumors arising from the right auricle (see Fig. 34.11b).[330,332,448–452] Successful resection of intracardiac masses has been reported, but requires specialized anesthetic intervention and surgical equipment not readily available in many veterinary hospitals, and preferably subspecialty training in cardiovascular surgery.[351,352,365,451,453]

Subtotal pericardiectomy for dogs with heart base masses has been shown to improve survival in dogs with ABTs and mesothelioma, regardless of whether pericardial effusion is present at the time of diagnosis.[336,337] However, pericardiectomy alone does not improve outcomes for dogs with cardiac HSA.[454] As dogs with pericardial effusion treated with thoracoscopic pericardial window are more likely to have recurrence of pericardial effusion than dogs treated with open thoracotomy and subtotal pericardiectomy, the latter is preferable for dogs expected to have prolonged survival (i.e., ABT or mesothelioma).[455] Thoracoscopic approaches for subtotal pericardiectomy and resection of cardiac masses are being performed more frequently as surgeons become more experienced in minimally invasive surgical techniques.[452,456,457] Resection of right atrial or auricular masses suspected to be HSA should be considered palliative owing to the high metastatic rate and adjuvant chemotherapy is recommended to prolong survival.[332]

DOX-based chemotherapy protocols are commonly used for the treatment of dogs with cardiac HSA, either as primary therapy or after surgery. Protocols described for cardiac HSA include DOX alone or in combination with cyclophosphamide (CYC), vincristine (VCR), VCR/CYC, metronomic chemotherapy, ifosfamide, dacarbazine, or toceranib phosphate (TOC).[458–461] The use of Yunnan Baiyao and epsilon-aminocaproic acid has been evaluated for dogs with right atrial masses and pericardial effusion; however, patient outcomes were similar to pericardiocentesis alone.[462] Preliminary evidence exists that TOC may mitigate clinical signs for dogs with heart base tumors, and further investigation into this treatment option is warranted.[463] The role of TOC in the management of heart base tumors in cats is unknown at this time.[341,342] Chemotherapy protocols for cats with cardiac or pericardial lymphoma have not been well described, but multiagent protocols such as CHOP (combinations of cyclophosphamide [C], doxorubicin [H, hydroxydaunorubicin], vincristine [O, Oncovin], and prednisone [P]) or COP (CHOP without the addition of doxorubicin) should be considered.[339,412]

The role of RT in the management of cardiac tumors has not yet been well studied. Administration of a single 12 Gy fraction to dogs with right atrial masses and concurrent pericardial effusion appears to be safe and decreased the frequency of palliative pericardiocentesis.[436] Full-course fractionated RT appears feasible and may be beneficial for dogs with heart base masses alone or postoperatively; however, reports are limited to a few cases at this time.[420,464,465]

Prognosis

The prognosis for cardiac HSA is poor. MSTs for dogs with cardiac HSA treated with surgical resection alone range from 16 days to 4 months.[330,332,448,454,457] The addition of DOX-based chemotherapy after surgical resection significantly improves survival for dogs with cardiac HSA, with an MST of 175 days when treated with surgery and adjuvant chemotherapy compared with 42 days when treated with surgery alone.[332] Dogs with presumptive cardiac HSA treated with DOX-based protocols have a response rate of 41%, progression-free survival time of 66 days, and MST of 116 to 140 days.[458,459] Although surgical resection is often not feasible for dogs with ABT, the prognosis for dogs with ABT is improved when pericardiectomy is performed with MSTs ranging from 661 to 730 days.[336,337] Dogs with ABT that do not undergo pericardiectomy have significantly worse outcomes, with reported MSTs ranging from 42 to 129 days.[336,337] Outcomes for other primary cardiac tumors in dogs have not been well studied; however, a number of case reports suggest primary resection of the mass can result in prolonged survival times.[351,354,364,365]

The prognosis for cats with primary cardiac tumors is generally poor. One study evaluating pericardial lymphoma in cats reported an MST of only 9 days; however, one cat treated with a CHOP-based chemotherapy protocol had a survival time of more than 750 days.[339]

Comparative Aspects

Primary tumors of the heart and pericardium are rare in humans; the majority of cardiac neoplasms are metastatic lesions. Reported incidence of primary cardiac tumors in people range from 0.02% to 0.056%.[466,467] About 75% of cardiac tumors in humans are benign with myxomas comprising about half of benign tumors in adults; lipoma, papillary fibroelastoma, and hemangioma occur less commonly.[468] Cardiac myxomas are generally solitary, arise from the left ventricle, and surgical resection is the treatment of choice.[469] Rhabdomyoma is the most frequent primary cardiac

tumor in infants and children.[468] Familial cardiac rhabdomyomas frequently occur in association with tuberous sclerosis complex, an autosomal dominant disorder caused by mutations in predominantly the *TSC2* gene and less frequently the *TSC1* gene.[470] Infants with cardiac rhabdomyoma often have multifocal lesions that arise predominantly in the ventricles; surgical intervention is rarely required as the majority of these lesions will partially or completely regress with time.[470,471]

Sarcomas are the most common malignant cardiac tumor, with approximately one-third of malignant tumors diagnosed as angiosarcoma, one-fifth as rhabdomyosarcoma, and with lymphoma being infrequent.[468] More recent reports based on Surveillance, Epidemiology, and End Results registry data suggest that angiosarcomas and non-Hodgkin lymphoma (NHL) currently have a similar incidence rate of 0.108 and 0.107 per 10^6 person-years, respectively, with the incidence of NHL steadily increasing over the study time period (2000–2014).[472] Similar to those in dogs, most sarcomas arise from the atria, with the right atrium being more commonly affected than the left.[468,473] Surgical resection is commonly performed; however, the prognosis for primary cardiac sarcomas treated with surgery alone is poor, with in-hospital postoperative mortality of 22% and MSTs ranging from 9.6 to 20 months.[473,474] The benefit of chemotherapy and RT is not well defined; however, a small study demonstrated that neoadjuvant DOX/ifosfamide may improve survival of patients with right-sided sarcoma.[475,476]

Secondary cardiac tumors predominate in humans, with incidence rates ranging from 2.3% to 18.3% in autopsy studies.[477] Pericardial metastases are most common, followed by epicardial and myocardial metastases. Tumors with the highest rate of cardiac metastasis include mesothelioma, melanoma, pulmonary adenocarcinoma, undifferentiated carcinoma, and pulmonary squamous cell carcinoma, and breast carcinoma.[477] Tumors that have preferential cardiac metastasis compared with other sites include melanoma, bronchoalveolar carcinoma, and renal carcinoma.[477]

SECTION F: HISTIOCYTIC DISEASES

CRAIG A. CLIFFORD, KATHERINE A. SKORUPSKI AND PETER F. MOORE

Background

Several well-defined histiocytic proliferative diseases have been recognized in dogs and cats (Table 34.4).[478] The clinical presentation, behavior, and responsiveness to therapy vary tremendously between the syndromes observed. The challenge in some instances is to differentiate them from granulomatous or reactive inflammatory diseases, or from lymphoma, through examination of regular paraffin sections. Fortunately, there has been considerable progress in identifying markers that can be used to further characterize cell lineages in complex leukocytic infiltrates.

Histiocytic Differentiation

The development of canine specific markers for differentiation molecules of macrophages and dendritic cells (DCs) has enabled the identification of the cell lineages involved in canine histiocytic diseases.[479–483] The majority of canine histiocytic diseases involve proliferations of cells of various DC lineages. The term histiocyte has been used to generically describe cells of DC or macrophage

TABLE 34.4	Recognized Histiocytic Proliferative Diseases in Dogs and Cats				
Disease	Species	Cell of Origin	Key Morphologic Features		Immunophenotype
Histiocytoma	Dog	LC	Lesions have an epidermal focus ("top-heavy") and intraepidermal foci are common. Histiocytes have diverse nuclear morphology (round, ovoid, indented, or complex nuclear contours. Multi-nucleated cells and cytologic atypia are rare.		CD1a, CD11c/CD18, E-cadherin, Iba-1, CD204 (neg.)
Cutaneous Langerhans cell histiocytosis	Dog	LC	Multiple cutaneous lesions are observed. Metastasis to lymph nodes and internal sites is possible. Lesions are otherwise identical to histiocytoma, but may have a higher frequency of multinucleated cells and cytologic atypia.		Identical to histiocytoma
Pulmonary Langerhans cell histiocytosis	Cat	LC	There is multinodular to diffuse involvement of all lung lobes. Lesions consist of cohesive histiocytic infiltrates, which obliterate terminal airways and extend to pleural surfaces. Birbeck's granules observed by TEM.		CD1a#, CD11c*/CD18, E-cadherin, Iba-1*, CD204*
Cutaneous histiocytosis	Dog	iDC– activated	Vasocentric lesions are focused on mid-dermis to subcutis ("bottom heavy"). Lesions are pleocellular but are dominated by histiocytes and lympho-cytes. Lympho-histiocytic vasculitis is commonly observed. Histiocytes lack cytologic atypia, and multinucleated giant cells are rare. Skin draining lymph nodes may be infiltrated.		CD1a, CD4, CD11c/CD18, CD90, Iba-1, CD204*
Systemic histiocytosis	Dog	iDC– activated	Lesions are identical to cutaneous histiocytosis in skin. Lesions extend to lymph nodes, ocular and nasal mucosa, and internal organs.		CD1a, CD4, CD11c/CD18, CD90, Iba-1*, CD204*
Histiocytic sarcoma	Dog, Cat	iDC	Mass lesions are observed in spleen, lung, lymph node, periarticular and other primary tissue sites. Histiocytes are pleomorphic, mononuclear and multinucleated giant cells with marked cytologic atypia.		CD1a, CD11c/CD18, Iba-1, CD204 (variable)
Histiocytic sarcoma—hemophagocytic	Dogs Cat	Macrophage	Mass lesions are lacking. Diffuse splenomegaly and insidious infiltration of liver lung and bone marrow are consistently observed. Splenic red pulp is expanded by erythrophagocytic histiocytes. Mononuclear and multinucleated giant cells, with cytologic atypia are common. Alternatively, histio-cytes may have little cytologic atypia.		CD1a (low), CD11d/CD18 (dog), iba-1, CD204
Feline progressive histiocytosis	Cat	iDC	Skin nodules and plaques are observed. Lesions occupy the dermis with an epidermal focus. Intra-epidermal foci (40%) occur. In early lesions, histiocytes have minimal cytologic atypia. In later lesions, histiocytes manifest cytologic atypia as described for histiocytic sarcoma.		CD1a, CD11c*/CD18, CD5 (50%), Iba-1, CD204 (vari-able)
Dendritic cell leukemia	Dog	iDC	Predominant blood and bone marrow involvement is observed. There is diffuse infiltration of spleen, lung, and liver. Histiocytes manifest moderate cytologic atypia in blood and tissues.		CD1a, CD11c/CD18, Iba-1*, CD204*

CD1a* expected, not assessed to date.
CD11c* expected but not currently assessable in cats.
CD204* not reported.
Iba-1* not reported.

iDC, Interstitial dendritic cell; *LC,* Langerhans cell; *TEM,* transmission electron microscopy.

lineage. Histiocytes differentiate from CD34+ stem cell precursors into macrophages and several DC lineages. Intraepithelial DCs are also known as Langerhans cells (LCs). Interstitial DCs occur in perivascular locations in many organs except the brain, although they do occur in the meninges. Perhaps the most studied interstitial

DCs are the dermal DCs of skin. Dendritic cells that occur in T cell domains in peripheral lymphoid organs (lymph node [LN] and spleen) are known as interdigitating DCs. Interdigitating DCs in LNs are composed of resident DCs and migratory DCs. The migra-tory DCs arrive in lymphatics from tissues and consist of LCs and interstitial DCs.[484] Cytokines and growth factors that influence DC development include FLT3 ligand, granulocyte-macrophage colony stimulating factor (GM-CSF), tumor necrosis factor-alpha (TNF-α), interleukin-4 (IL-4), and transforming growth factor-beta (TGF-β).[484,485] Macrophage development from CD34+ precursors is influenced by GM-CSF and macrophage colony stimulating factor (M-CSF). Blood monocytes can differentiate into either macrophages under the influence of M-CSF, or into DCs under the influence of GM-CSF and IL-4.[484,486,487]

Dendritic cells are the most potent antigen presenting cells (APC) for induction of immune responses in naïve T cells. The development of canine specific monoclonal antibodies for functionally important molecules of DCs and macrophages has enabled their identification in canine tissues, especially skin.[481,488] Dendritic cells occur in two major locations: within the epidermis (LCs), and within the dermis, especially adjacent to postcapillary venules (dermal interstitial DCs).[489] Canine DCs abundantly express CD1a molecules which, together with MHC class I and MHC class II molecules, are responsible for presentation of peptides, lipids, and glycolipids to T cells.[481,482,490] Hence, DCs are best defined by their abundant expression of molecules essential to their function as APC. Of these, the family of CD1 proteins is largely restricted in expression to DCs in skin, whereas MHC class I and II are more broadly expressed.

The beta-2 integrins (CD11/CD18) are critically important adhesion molecules, which are differentially expressed by all leukocytes. CD11/CD18 expression is highly regulated in normal canine macrophages and DCs. CD11c is expressed by LCs and interstitial DCs, whereas macrophages predominately express CD11b (or CD11d in the splenic red pulp and bone marrow). A subset of dermal interstitial DCs also express CD11b.[491-493] In diseased tissues, these beta-2 integrin expression patterns may be broadened. Langerhans cells and dermal interstitial DCs are also distinguishable by their differential expression of E-cadherin (LCs+) and Thy-1 (CD90) (dermal interstitial DCs+). Langerhans cells localize within epithelial tissue via E-cadherin homotypic adhesion with E-cadherin expressed by epithelial cells.[485]

Migration of DCs (as veiled cells) beyond the skin to the paracortex of LNs, where they join forces with interdigitating DCs, occurs after contact with antigen. Successful interaction of DCs and T cells in response to antigenic challenge also involves the orderly appearance of costimulatory molecules (B7 family—CD80 and CD86) on DCs and their ligands (CD28 and CTLA-4) on T cells.[494-496] In situ DCs have low expression of MHC class II and costimulatory molecules and are more receptive to antigen uptake. Migratory DCs upregulate MHC class II and B7 family members and become more adept at antigen presentation to T cells.[495,496]

Aspects of the developmental and migratory program of DCs are recapitulated in canine histiocytic diseases. Defective interaction of DCs and T cells appears to contribute to the development of reactive histiocytoses (cutaneous histiocytosis [CH] and systemic histiocytosis [SH]), which are related interstitial DC disorders arising out of disordered immune regulation. The distant migratory potential of DCs is of immense clinical significance in the adverse prognosis of histiocytic sarcomas (HSs), which largely originate in interstitial DCs and rapidly disseminate.

Immunophenotyping

To classify hematopoietic neoplasia according to the WHO system as applied to the dog, it is important to have access to markers for IHC analysis.[497,498] Determination of lineages of histiocytes (macrophages, interstitial type DCs, and Langerhans cells) is best

performed in unfixed cytologic smears or snap frozen tissues, or by flow cytometry. Important markers for the dissection of the histiocytic lineage that are only detectable in fresh smears or snap frozen tissues include CD1a, CD11b, CD11c, CD80, and CD86. It is possible to presumptively identify histiocytes in formalin fixed paraffin embedded (FFPE) tissues by using combinations of lymphoid markers coupled with CD18 and CD11d staining (Table 34.4) in an appropriate morphological context. Additional useful markers of histiocytic lineage in FFPE tissues include Iba-1 (ionized calcium binding molecule-1), the macrophage class A scavenger receptors (CD163 and CD204), and E-cadherin. Iba-1 identifies macrophages and DCs, whereas the class A scavenger receptors are largely expressed by macrophages in normal tissues.[499] However, the scavenger receptors, CD163 and CD204, are also expressed by DC subsets in some species.[500,501] The potential exists for coexpression of class A scavenger receptors on DCs in diseased tissue. Alternatively, there is some evidence for mixed lineages in HS, particularly in the central nervous system of dogs.[502]

Cutaneous Histiocytoma

Cutaneous histiocytoma is a benign tumor of Langerhans cells that often occurs as a single lesion in young dogs (<3 years of age), although histiocytomas do occur in dogs of all ages. In a retrospective review from the United Kingdom of histopathologic diagnoses of neoplasia in dogs less than 1 year, CH was the most common diagnosis, representing 89% of 20,280 submissions.[503] These tumors typically present as a solitary raised pink skin mass, often in the cranial portion of the body. The growth of the lesion can be quite rapid (1–4 weeks), but tumors usually spontaneously regress within 1 to 2 months of presentation.[503-509] IHC is rarely necessary to diagnose histiocytomas; however, expression of E-cadherin is unique to histiocytomas and can help differentiate histiocytomas from reactive histiocytosis (CH, SH).[479,482,510,511] When necessary, this differentiation can be made based on IHC or flow cytometry. The factors that determine the onset of regression in canine histiocytomas are unknown. Regression may be rapid or delayed for many months. Regression is mediated by CD8+ αβT lymphocytes.[478,482] Migration of tumor histiocytes and/or tumor infiltrating reactive interstitial DC to draining LNs likely activates CD4+ T cells, which would assist in CD8+ cytotoxic T-cell recruitment. Because massive CD8+ T-cell infiltration is observed with histiocytoma regression, immunosuppression should be avoided once a definitive diagnosis of histiocytoma has been reached to avoid interference with cytotoxic T-cell function. E-cadherin expression has been found to be associated with lymphoid infiltrate and stage of regression of histiocytomas.[512] Cases of multiple or metastatic histiocytomas are rare and may require IHC to differentiate from lymphoma or other round cell tumors if cells are poorly differentiated. These cases are usually classified as cutaneous Langerhans cell histiocytosis (LCH).[478]

Cutaneous Langerhans Cell Histiocytosis

Cutaneous LCH is a disease comprising multiple or diffuse cutaneous tumors of LC origin with or without metastasis to LNs or internal organs.[478,513,514] Lesions are identical morphologically and immunohistochemically to histiocytomas, but may have more cytologic atypia. Cutaneous LCH limited to skin appears to be more common in Shar Pei dogs, but can occur in any breed. Delayed regression of cutaneous LCH can occur, even in cases with widespread disease, and may be delayed for up to 10 months before onset of regression. In the authors' experience, lesions do not regress in about half of cases and dogs are euthanized due to complications related to extensive ulcerated skin lesions. Attempts to treat diffuse cutaneous LCH are rarely reported, but there is one report of a complete but temporary response to lomustine (CCNU) in a dog with diffuse cutaneous LCH.[515] In addition, there is one report of a complete response to griseofulvin treatment in an 8-month-old puppy with diffuse cutaneous LCH.[516] Dogs with solitary lesions, but with metastasis to an LN, may have a better prognosis. A study reported on eight dogs with a solitary cutaneous histiocytoma and LN metastasis treated with surgery alone. Outcomes were excellent, with most alive 1 to 4 years after diagnosis.[517] Cases of diffuse LCH with rapid progression to LN and internal organ involvement appear to have a poorer prognosis in the authors' experience.

Reactive Histiocytosis

The reactive histiocytosis can be separated into CH and SH. Cutaneous histiocytosis represents a benign, diffuse aggregation of histiocytes that grows rapidly into infiltrating nodules, plaques, and crusts within the skin and subcutaneous tissue.[478,479,481,509,518,519] This disease tends to occur in younger dogs; however, one study noted a range of 2 to 11 years. A breed predisposition has yet to be identified; however, in one study, golden retrievers, great Danes, and Bouvier des Flanders were more common.[519] One study suggested a male predilection; however, in a second larger study, no sex predilection was identified.[479,519] Forty-four percent of dogs in one study had a previous history of dermatologic disease, with allergic dermatitis being most common. The median duration of time from appearance of lesions to diagnosis via biopsy in this study was 1.75 months (range 0–30 months).[519]

CH is limited to the skin and subcutis, but can be multifocal. The head, pinnae, limbs, and scrotum are the commonly reported sites.[479,518,519] Lesions may also be found on the nasal planum and within nasal mucosa, the gross appearance of which has been described as a "clown nose." In one study, 10 of 32 dogs had nasal planum/nares involvement, which presented as swelling, erythema, depigmentation, and stertorous respiration.[519] Histologically, lesions contain a pleocellular histiocytic infiltrate, often perivascular within the dermis and subcutaneous tissue. Lymphoid infiltrates and some neutrophils are common and vascular invasion may be present. These histiocytic cells express CD1a, CD1b, CD1c, CD11c, MHC class II molecules, Thy-1 and CD4 but are negative for E-cadherin.[478,479,481] The expression of Thy-1 and CD4 aids in identification of cell of origin, which appears to be the activated interstitial DC.

CH usually follows a benign course and responds to immunosuppressive therapy, although spontaneous regressions have also been reported. Local therapies are not often successful, as lesions typically recur in other locations. Systemic corticosteroids are usually the firstline therapy and partial responses are seen in the majority of dogs.[479,509,518,519] Many dogs require continuous therapy to prevent recurrence. In one study of 32 dogs, all had complete resolution of lesions within a median of 45 days (range, 10–162 days) from initial therapy.[518] In this study, initial therapy included prednisone alone or in combination with antibiotics (*n* = 12), prednisone with tetracycline/doxycycline and niacinamide (*n* = 4), prednisone and azathioprine (*n* = 3), and tetracycline/niacinamide either alone or in combination with vitamin E and essential fatty acids (*n* = 6). Of the 19 dogs receiving prednisone, daily dosages ranged from 0.5 mg/kg to 2 mg/kg.[518]

Longterm maintenance therapies may be warranted to prevent recurrence; however, affected dogs may have a prolonged survival time. In 32 dogs with complete resolution of their lesions, 17 were maintained on a variety of medications including 12 with tetracycline/niacinamide either alone (*n* = 7) or in various combinations with safflower oil, essential fatty, or vitamin E.[518] Other maintenance therapies included cyclosporine/ketoconazole, azathioprine alone, prednisone and azathioprine, or prednisone alone. Immunosuppressive agents such as leflunomide and cyclosporine A/ketoconazole and azathioprine may demonstrate efficacy in steroid refractory cases.

SH is similar to cutaneous histiocytosis in its IHC staining pattern and cell of origin, the activated interstitial DC. The distinguishing feature is involvement of nonskin organs. The Bernese mountain dog (BMD), Rottweiler, golden retriever, and Irish wolfhound are overrepresented and the disease appears to be familial in the BMD.[479,509,520–524] Dermal lesions manifest in the skin with similar site predilection as CHS; however, other sites including the subcutis, eyes, nasal epithelium, LNs, bone marrow, spleen, liver, lung, or mucous membranes are also affected. Clinical signs vary depending on the affected tissue and severity of disease; however, depression, anorexia, weight loss, conjunctivitis, and harsh respiration are common. Clinicopathologic features of SH are varied; however, anemia, monocytosis, and lymphopenia are consistently reported, and hypercalcemia is occasionally reported.[479,509,520–524]

Lesions may have a waxing and waning presentation, but generally do not spontaneously resolve. Corticosteroids alone appear ineffective in controlling this disease in the long term.[479,508,516] The use of azathioprine, cyclosporine A, or leflunomide has yielded longterm control in some cases. Some have suggested a significant role of T cells in this disease via inappropriate DC and T-cell interactions due to abnormal regulation of accessory ligands on both cell types.[479,481] The clinical course of this disease is often prolonged but rarely results in death. Generally, there are episodes of response to therapy followed by recrudescence, and many dogs are euthanized as a result of repeated relapses or failure to respond to therapy.[479,509,520–524]

Histiocytic Sarcoma

Genetics and Biologic Behavior

HS was first reported in the dog in the late 1970s and a predisposition in BMDs was discovered in 1986.[525,526] HS has since been identified in many breeds, and flat-coated retrievers (FCR), Rottweilers, and miniature schnauzers also appear to be overrepresented.[525–527] In Japan, the Pembroke Welsh Corgi also appears to be overrepresented.[528] Dogs are commonly middle aged or older, but HS has been reported in dogs as young as 3 years of age.

Genetic and epidemiologic studies in the BMD have revealed clues about the etiology of HS. A Swiss inheritance study found the genetic predisposition for HS in BMD to be so widespread within the breed that selective breeding was deemed impossible.[529] One genetic study evaluating copy number aberrations in the BMD and FCR found deletions of the tumor suppressor genes CDKN2A/B, RB1, and PTEN.[530] In a genome-wide association study, a haplotype spanning MTAP and part of CDKN2A was found in 96% of BMD with HS.[531] A gain-of-function mutation in PTPN11 was recently identified in canine HS, and 37% of BMDs with HS studied had the mutation compared with 9% of HS in other dog breeds.[532] Two studies have also found a correlation between prior joint disease and risk of periarticular HS (PAHS) in the BMD.[533,534]

Breed differences have also been studied. Two studies have found that FCR are more likely to have HS of the limbs and BMD have more diffuse visceral disease.[530,535] Localized HS is seven times more frequent in the FCR than in the BMD and disseminated HS is two times more frequent in the BMD than the FCR. FCR with HS were also older at diagnosis than BMDs with HS in one study (mean 8.6 vs 7.7 years).[530] Differences in histopathology between these breeds have also been described.[536]

HS may present with either localized or loco-regional organ involvement or with a disseminated/multiorgan involvement. HS is the preferred term identifying malignant tumors of histiocytic origin, and the older term "malignant histiocytosis" refers specifically to the disseminated form of the disease. Reported anatomic sites include lung, LN, liver, spleen, stomach, pancreas, mediastinum, skin, skeletal muscle, central nervous system, bone, bone marrow, nasal cavity, and eyes[537–546] (Fig. 34.13). It was reported that 5% of primary brain tumors were HS, as were 4.5% of secondary brain tumors in a necropsy population.[547,548] In a series of 26 dogs with ocular HS, ocular involvement was usually found in association with disseminated disease.[543] HS is the most common periarticular tumor in dogs, and IHC staining is required to differentiate them from "true" synovial cell sarcoma.[538] In periarticular tumors, IHC for CD18, cytokeratin, and smooth muscle actin can aid in differentiation of PAHS and synovial cell sarcoma.[538]

Hemophagocytic HS (HHS) is a subtype of HS that arises from macrophages rather than DC and is described in more detail later in this section.[483] The HHS variant can be definitively differentiated only through confirmation of an IHC staining pattern consistent with macrophages, though clinical factors such as visceral location or hematologic and biochemical abnormalities may raise suspicion.[483] Clinically, this form behaves more aggressively due, at least in part, to its cellular ability to phagocytose material including host blood cells.

History and Clinical Signs

Presenting complaints and clinical signs vary widely depending on site(s) of tumor involvement, but nonspecific symptoms such as lethargy, inappetence, and weight loss are common in dogs with disseminated HS. Other common signs include a visible mass, lameness, cough, vomiting, and lymphadenomegaly.[528] Lymphadenomegaly is sometimes the only clinical sign and can appear at a site distant to other tumor lesions. Patients may also present with clinical signs related to severe anemia or thrombocytopenia, especially in dogs with the HHS variant.[483,540–542]

Diagnosis and Staging

A diagnosis of HS can be obtained via cytologic or histologic examination of tumor tissue; however, definitive diagnosis can be challenging in pleomorphic tumors that have morphologic characteristics similar to carcinomas or round cell tumors. HS cells are large, discrete, mononuclear cells that often display marked anisocytosis and anisokaryosis. Nuclei are round, oval, or reniform with prominent nucleoli and cytoplasm is moderate to abundant, lightly basophilic, and vacuolated. Mitotic figures are common and some tumor cells may display erythrophagocytosis and/or multinucleated giant cells (Figs. 34.14 and 34.15).[478,480,547] Evidence to support a diagnosis of HS may be acquired through immunocytochemistry or IHC on formalin fixed tissues using antibodies to CD18.[480] The class A macrophage scavenger receptor CD204 also serves as a useful marker of canine HS and has been used

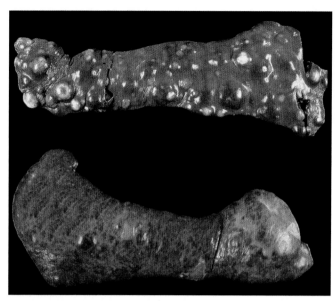

• **Fig. 34.13** Canine histiocytic sarcoma (HS) in the spleen. **Top.** Discrete mass formation is characteristic of HS of interstitial dendritic cell origin. **Bottom.** Diffuse splenomegaly with ill-defined mass formation is characteristic of hemophagocytic HS of macrophage origin. (Image courtesy PF Moore.)

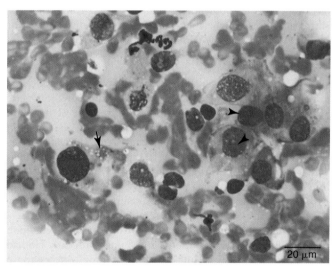

• **Fig. 34.14** Cytology of histiocytic sarcoma in the liver of a dog. Note individualized and loosely cohesive moderately pleomorphic spindle cells with prominent nucleoli (*arrowheads*). Some demonstrate phagocytic activity (*arrow*). (Wright-Giemsa, 100× objective.) (Courtesy Elizabeth Little, VMD, DACVP, IDEXX Laboratories, Langhorne, PA.)

to evaluate both formalin-fixed, paraffin-embedded samples and air-dried cytology.[499,548] The pan-macrophage marker ionized calcium-binding adapter molecule 1 (Iba1) also appears to have utility as a marker of cells of monocyte and macrophage lineage, though it cannot differentiate the various histiocytic disorders.[549] If fresh or frozen tissue is available, further confirmation and subclassification of the cell of origin can be performed using antibody staining for CD1 or the CD11 α subunits.[478,480] Recently, the CADET[f] histiocytic malignancy assay has become commercially available. Using this assay, tumor biopsy or cytology samples are evaluated for copy number aberrations consistent with those found in cases of confirmed HS. The sensitivity and specificity of the assay have been estimated to be 78% and 95%, respectively.[530,550]

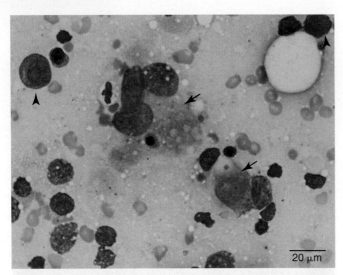

• **Fig. 34.15** Cytology of histiocytic sarcoma in the bone marrow of a dog. Neoplastic cells (arrows) and erythroid progenitors (arrowheads) are visible. Note phagocytic activity of neoplastic cells. (Wright-Giemsa, 100× objective.) (Courtesy Elizabeth Little, VMD, DACVP, IDEXX Laboratories, Langhorne, PA.)

Because HS is multifocal or disseminated in most dogs, complete staging is recommended. Complete blood count and biochemical screens may be abnormal in dogs with disseminated or HHS.[480,483,542] Anemia is common and usually regenerative when caused by erythrophagocytosis by neoplastic cells. Leukocytosis, thrombocytopenia, increased liver enzymes, hypoalbuminemia, and hypocholesterolemia are frequent findings, and hypercalcemia occurs occasionally.[542] HS was the second most common cause of pancytopenia in dogs in a retrospective study of 51 dogs at a veterinary teaching hospital.[551] Hyperferritinemia has also been documented in dogs with HS and is theorized to be result of ferritin production by tumor cells.[552,553] Eighty-nine percent of dogs with HS had hyperferritinemia in one study, although IMHA, liver disease, and lymphoma were also associated with high rates of hyperferritinemia.[553] A recent study attempting to screen healthy BMDs for early HS found that serum ferritin may serve as a potential marker of the disease. High ferritin levels were common in dogs with clinical HS, but only 2 of 5 dogs with early HS had high ferritin levels, suggesting that further study is necessary to explore the utility of ferritin as a screening test for BMDs.[554]

Thoracic radiography and abdominal ultrasonography commonly reveal abnormalities.[542] Pulmonary involvement may appear as a diffuse interstitial infiltrate, patchy consolidated areas, or focal or multifocal mass lesions. The right middle lung lobe is the most common pulmonary location for HS and internal air bronchograms are commonly seen.[555,556] Radiographic evidence of sternal, cranial mediastinal, and/or tracheobronchial lymphadenopathy may also be noted. Hepatosplenomegaly, splenic or hepatic mottling, or discrete nodules or masses in these organs are the most common abdominal ultrasonographic abnormalities.[557]

Bone marrow aspiration cytology may reveal tumor infiltrate, especially in patients with cytopenias. In addition, flow cytometry has been used to differentiate etiology of hemophagocytosis in bone marrow samples containing more than 5% macrophages and cytologic evidence of hemophagocytosis.[558] Results suggested that cellular distribution in scatter plots and number of histiocytes may help differentiate neoplastic from nonneoplastic causes of hemophagocytosis.

Treatment and Prognosis

The clinical course of disseminated HS, if left untreated, is rapid and usually fatal, whereas the localized form may be more slowly progressive.[480] Few reports documenting survival duration after surgical excision of localized HS exist. However, in a series of 18 PAHS confirmed with CD18 staining, the MST for dogs undergoing amputation was 6 months and the metastatic rate was 91%.[538] Interestingly, the periarticular form of HS may be associated with a better prognosis than that at other locations. In one study, dogs with PAHS lived significantly longer than did dogs with non-PAHS, with overall MSTs of 391 and 128 days, respectively,[559] despite the presence of suspected metastasis at diagnosis in 13 of 19 dogs with PAHS. Still, dogs with PAHS with no evidence of metastasis at diagnosis (MST 980 days) lived significantly longer than those with evidence of metastasis (MST 253 days).[559] Prolonged survival has also been reported in dogs with localized HS in other anatomic sites treated with local and systemic therapy, however.[560] Thus it is not clear whether PAHS has a better prognosis owing to its more localized nature or due to an inherent difference in clinical behavior.

CCNU appears to be the most effective chemotherapy agent against HS in dogs. One study reported a 46% response rate to CCNU in 56 dogs with gross measurable disease with a median remission duration of 85 days. The MST of responders was 172 days compared with 60 days in nonresponders.[542] In this study, anemia, thrombocytopenia, hypoalbuminemia, and splenic involvement, all factors associated with the hemophagocytic subtype of HS, were associated with a grave prognosis. Corticosteroids did not improve response to therapy in this study. In a prospective study of 21 dogs with HS treated with 90 mg/m² of CCNU, the response rate was lower at 29%, though 67% of dogs received only one dose of CCNU.[561] The median response duration was 96 days. CCNU therapy used as an adjuvant to surgery and/or RT RT may result in lengthy survival times in dogs with localized HS. One retrospective study documented an MST of 19 months in 16 dogs with localized HS treated with aggressive combination therapy.[560]

CCNU has also been studied in combination with DOX to treat HS, and when administered in an alternating fashion every 2 weeks, the response rate was 58% with a median time to progression of 185 days.[562] Dacarbazine has been studied in the rescue setting for HS and was associated with a response rate of 18%, with an event-free survival time in responders of 70 days.[563] The efficacy of epirubicin against HS has also been studied and was associated with a response rate of 29%.[564]

Individual reports of responses to liposomal DOX and paclitaxel chemotherapy also exist.[565,566] In addition, a case report of a dog with cutaneous disseminated HS described temporary remissions resulting from multiple treatments including cyclophosphamide, vincristine, prednisone, mitoxantrone, dacarbazine, and etoposide.[567] Studies of metronomic chemotherapy targeting angiogenesis and the immune environment have also included dogs with HS. Responses to metronomic lomustine and chlorambucil have both been reported.[568,569] The bisphosphonate clodronate has been studied in histiocytic cell lines and in five dogs with HS.[570] Two of the five dogs treated with a liposomal formulation of clodronate experienced tumor regression and further study is warranted.

The efficacy of RT against HS has not been fully studied; however, preliminary evidence suggests that HS is radioresponsive. In a report of 37 FCR with mostly PAHS, dogs undergoing RT lived longer than those not having RT with an MST of 182 days.[571] Dogs treated with a set combined protocol of a palliative RT and CCNU had an MST of 208 days. Further study into the optimal RT protocol for HS is necessary.

Hemophagocytic Histiocytic Sarcoma

Hemophagocytic HS is a variant of HS that originates from the tissue macrophage, not the DC.[483] This more aggressive form of HS invariably involves the spleen, but dogs may also have liver, bone marrow, LN, and/or lung involvement. Splenic involvement is usually diffuse, resulting in gross enlargement with diffuse nodular infiltrates. In one study, common hematologic findings in dogs with HHS included a regenerative anemia (94%), thrombocytopenia (88%), hypoalbuminemia (94%), and hypocholesterolemia (69%).[483] A presumptive diagnosis of HHS may be obtained through splenic cytology, which shows infiltration with atypical to highly pleomorphic macrophages displaying phagocytosis of red blood cells, splenic origin red cell precursors, and white blood cells. However, definitive diagnosis and differentiation from nonhemophagocytic HS requires immunophenotyping. To date, effective treatment of HHS has not been described. Reported survival times are extremely short, ranging from days to 1 to 2 months, regardless of therapy.[483,542]

Feline Histiocytic Diseases

Histiocytic neoplasms are much rarer in cats than dogs, but three distinct forms have been documented to date. These include HS, with features similar to those of the canine disease; feline progressive histiocytosis (FPH), a cutaneous form of histiocytic neoplasia with indolent, but progressive behavior; and LCH, with disease localized primarily to the lungs.

Feline Histiocytic Sarcoma

HS of DC origin and hemophagocytic HS of macrophage origin have both been documented in cats.[572–580] With both variants, cats usually present with multifocal or disseminated disease. Spleen, liver, and bone marrow involvement are most common, but LN, lung, trachea, mediastinum, kidney, bladder, and CNS involvement is also reported. Bone marrow involvement appears commonly in cats.[573] Severe anemia and thrombocytopenia are also common findings and may indicate bone marrow involvement and/or hemophagocytic HS, which can be confirmed though immunophenotyping of tumor tissue samples.[571–573] The localized form of HS is rare in cats, but has been reported in the tarsus of three cats, on the nasal bridge or planum in three cats, and in the stomach of one cat.[580,581] An aggressive clinical course is typical of HS in cats, particularly in those with anemia and suspected hemophagocytic HS. Effective treatment options for feline HS have not been well studied, though reports of responses to CCNU, masinitib, and RT exist.[574,581]

Feline Progressive Histiocytosis

FPH is a neoplasm of DC that occurs initially on the skin and progresses over time to involve multiple organs.[581,582] Lesions appear on the skin as multiple firm, haired or hairless, dermal papules or nodules with a predilection for the head, feet, and legs. The lesions may enlarge gradually and coalesce into plaques, and can become ulcerated and painful over time. An example of a cat

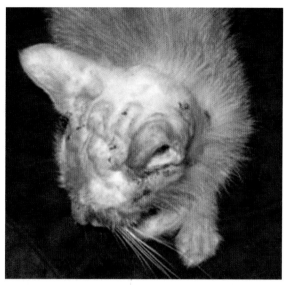

• **Fig. 34.16** A cat with advanced feline progressive histiocytosis. The lesions consist of multiple coalescing hairless dermal nodules on the head, some of which have become ulcerated. (Courtesy Emily Rothstein, DVM, DACVD, Animal Allergy and Dermatology Service of Connecticut, Plantsville, CT.)

with advanced lesions in shown in Fig. 34.16. The disease is usually progressive over months or years (median 13.4 months) with late spread to LNs, lungs, and abdominal visceral organs. Females appear to be overrepresented.

A diagnosis of FPH is made through biopsy and histopathologic evaluation of skin lesions. Lesions appear histologically as poorly circumscribed multinodular aggregates or masses of round cells with or without epitheliotropism in the dermis and, occasionally, invading subcutis. Cells have mild to moderate anisocytosis and anisokaryosis, and mitotic figures are rare. IHC may be necessary to confirm the diagnosis and rule out other round cell tumors.[582] Staging test results are usually negative for internal organ involvement early in the course of disease, but tumor may be found in LNs, lung, and/or abdominal viscera as the disease progresses. Surgical excision may control solitary, superficial skin lesions early in the course of disease, but development of additional skin lesions is expected. Skin lesions do not appear to respond to corticosteroid therapy, and effective medical treatment of diffuse skin or visceral lesions has not yet been described.[581] In a recent study, one cat with FPH experienced a spontaneous regression, another achieved a complete response to masitinib therapy, and yet another had a partial response to CCNU.[582]

Pulmonary Langerhans Cell Histiocytosis

A single case series exists describing an aggressive neoplasm arising from Langerhans cells in three cats.[583] All three cats presented for respiratory compromise or distress with symptom duration ranging from 5 days to 7 months. Thoracic radiographs showed a diffuse, severe bronchointerstitial lung pattern with diffuse military to nodular opacities in all lung fields. Symptomatic therapy was unsuccessful in all cats and the diagnosis of LCH was made on necropsy through the use of extensive immunostaining and electron microscopy confirming the presence of Birbeck's granules. At necropsy, metastasis to pancreas, kidneys, liver, and/or visceral LNs was noted in all three cats.

Comparative Aspects

Histiocytic neoplasia is extremely rare in people, and many purported cases were reclassified as lymphomas with the advent of IHC and advanced molecular testing.[584] More recently, the disease has been better described and classified into HS, Langerhans cell sarcoma, LCH, follicular dendritic cell sarcoma, interdigitating cell sarcoma, and indeterminate dendritic cell sarcoma.[585] HS in humans presents in the LN in one-third of patients, in the skin in one-third of patients, and in extranodal sites in the remaining patients. The intestinal tract is the most common extranodal site and hepatosplenomegaly is common. Some patients may also present with multiple anatomic sites of involvement and 70% of patients present with advanced stage (III or IV) disease.[584] HS in humans is an aggressive neoplasm that is often refractory to therapy and results in death in most patients. Similar to that in dogs, hypoalbuminemia is associated with a poorer prognosis in people with histiocytic neoplasia.[585] Braf and MEK mutations have been found in some cases of HS and other histiocytic neoplasia types.[585,586]

The results of a recent study using genome-wide array comparative genomic hybridization to evaluate copy number alternations suggest that canine HS may offer a valuable model for the human counterpart.[530] Extrapolation of data derived from canine histiocytic disorders to human histiocytic proliferation may help further our understanding of the disease to promote the development of new and effective therapeutic modalities for both species. Because many of the recurrent genetic changes are evolutionarily conserved with those reported in human histiocytic proliferations, this further points to a shared conserved pathogenesis.

References

1. Spangler WL, Culbertson MR: Prevalence, type, and importance of splenic diseases in dogs: 1,480 cases (1985-1989), *J Am Vet Med Assoc* 200:829–834, 1992.
2. Prymak C, McKee LJ, Goldschmidt MH, et al.: Epidemiologic, clinical, pathologic, and prognostic characteristics of splenic hemangiosarcoma and splenic hematoma in dogs: 217 cases (1985), *J Am Vet Med Assoc* 193:706–712, 1988.
3. Brown NO, Patnaik AK, MacEwen EG: Canine hemangiosarcoma: retrospective analysis of 104 cases, *J Am Vet Med Assoc* 186:56–58, 1985.
4. Clifford CA, de Lorimier LP: Hemangiosarcoma. In Ettinger SJ, Feldman EC, Cote E, editors: *Textbook of veterinary internal medicine*, ed 8, St. Louis, 2017, Elsevier, pp 2093–2102.
5. Spangler WL, Kass PH: Pathologic factors affecting postsplenectomy survival in dogs, *J Vet Intern Med* 11:166–171, 1997.
6. Schultheiss PC: A retrospective study of visceral and nonvisceral hemangiosarcoma and hemangiomas in domestic animals, *J Vet Diagn Invest* 16:522–526, 2004.
7. Yoon HY, Kang HM, Lee MY: Primary cranial mediastinal hemangiosarcoma in a young dog, *Ir Vet J* 67(15), 2014.
8. KA Powers BE, Withrow SJ, et al.: Splenomegaly in dogs: predictors of neoplasia and survival after splenectomy, *J Vet Intern Med* 3:160–166, 1989.
9. Tamburini BA, Trapp S, Phang TL, et al.: Gene expression profiles of sporadic canine hemangiosarcoma are uniquely associated with breed, *PLoS One* 4:e5549, 2009.
10. Gamlem H, Nordstoga K, Arnesen K: Canine vascular neoplasia–a population-based clinicopathologic study of 439 tumours and tumour-like lesions in 420 dogs, *APMIS* (Suppl)41–54, 2008.
11. Johannes CM, Henry CJ, Turnquist SE, et al.: Hemangiosarcoma in cats: 53 cases (1992-2002), *J Am Vet Med Assoc* 231:1851–1856, 2007.
12. Hargis AM, Ihrke PJ, Spangler QL, et al.: A retrospective clinicopathologic study of 212 dogs with cutaneous hemangiomas and hemangiosarcomas, *Vet Pathol* 29:316–328, 1992.
13. Nikula KJ, Benjamin SA, Angleton GM, et al.: Ultraviolet radiation, solar dermatosis, and cutaneous neoplasia in Beagle dogs, *Radiat Res* 129:11–18, 1992.
14. Szivek A, Burns RE, Gericota B, et al.: Clinical outcome in 94 cases of dermal haemangiosarcoma in dogs treated with surgical excision: 1993-2007, *Vet Comp Oncol* 10:65–73, 2012.
15. Ware WA, Hopper DL: Cardiac tumors in dogs: 1982-1995, *J Vet Intern Med* 13:95–103, 1999.
16. Torres de la Riva G, Hart BL, Farver TB, et al.: Neutering dogs: effects on joint disorders and cancers in golden retrievers, *PLOS One* 8:e55937, 2013.
17. Lamerato-Kozicki AR, Helm KM, Jubala CM, et al.: Canine hemangiosarcoma originates from hematopoietic precursors with potential for endothelial differentiation, *Exp Hematol* 34:870–878, 2006.
18. Fosmire SP, Dickerson EB, Scott AM, et al.: Canine malignant hemangiosarcoma as a model of primitive angiogenic endothelium, *Lab Invest* 84:562–572, 2004.
19. Gorden BH, Kim JH, Sarber AL, et al.: Identification of three molecular and functional subtypes in canine hemangiosarcoma through gene expression profiling and progenitor cell characterization, *Am J Pathol* 184:985–995, 2014.
20. Tamburini BA, Phang TL, Fosmire SP, et al.: Gene expression profiling identifies inflammation and angiogenesis as distinguishing features of canine hemangiosarcoma, *BMC Canc* 10:619, 2010.
21. Thomas R, Borst L, Rotroff D, et al.: Genomic profiling reveals extensive heterogeneity in somatic DNA copy number aberrations of canine hemangiosarcoma, *Chrom Res* 22:305–319, 2014.
22. Naka N, Tomita Y, Nakanashi H, et al.: Mutations of p53 tumor-suppressor gene in angiosarcoma, *Int J Cancer* 71:952–955, 1997.
23. Arbiser JL, Moses MA, Fernandez CA, et al.: Oncogenic H-ras stimulates tumor angiogenesis by two distinct pathways, *Proc Natl Acad Sci USA* 94:861–866, 1997.
24. Garcia JM, Gonzalez R, Silva JM, et al.: Mutational status of K-ras and TP53 genes in primary sarcomas of the heart, *Br J Cancer* 82:1183–1185, 2000.
25. Mayr B, Zwetkoff S, Schaffner G, et al.: Tumour suppressor gene p53 mutation in a case of haemangiosarcoma of a dog, *Acta Vet Hung* 50:157–160, 2002.
26. Yonemaru K, Sakai H, Murakami M, et al.: The significance of p53 and retinoblastoma pathways in canine hemangiosarcoma, *J Vet Med Sci* 69:271–278, 2007.
27. Dickerson EB, Thomas R, Fosmire P, et al.: Mutations of phosphatase and tensin homolog deleted from chromosome 10 in canine hemangiosarcoma, *Vet Pathol* 42:618–632, 2005.
28. Murakami M, Sakai H, Kodama A, et al.: Expression of the anti-apoptotic factors Bcl-2 and survivin in canine vascular tumours, *J Comp Pathol* 139:1–7, 2008.
29. Yonemaru K, Sakai H, Murakami M, et al.: Expression of vascular endothelial growth factor, basic fibroblast growth factor, and their receptors (flt-1, flk-1, and flg-1) in canine vascular tumors, *Vet Pathol* 43:971–980, 2006.
30. Dickerson EB, Marley K, Edris W, et al.: Imatinib and dasatinib inhibit hemangiosarcoma and implicate PDGFR-β and Src in tumor growth, *Transl Oncol* 6:158–168, 2013.
31. Kodama A, Sakai H, Matsuura S, et al.: Establishment of canine hemangiosarcoma xenograft models expressing endothelial growth factors, their receptors, and angiogenesis-associated homeobox genes, *BMC Cancer* 14:363, 2009.
32. Clifford CA, Hughes D, Beal MW, et al.: Plasma vascular endothelial growth factor concentrations in healthy dogs and dogs with hemangiosarcoma, *J Vet Intern Med* 15:131–135, 2001.
33. Fukumoto S, Miyasho T, Hanazono K, et al.: Big endothelin-1 as a tumour marker for canine hemangiosarcoma, *Vet J* 204:269–274, 2015.

34. Eberle N, von Babo V, Nolte I, et al.: Splenic masses in dogs. Part 1: epidemiologic, clinical characteristics as well as histopathologic diagnosis in 249 cases (2000-2011), *Tierarztl Prax Ausg K Kleintiere Heimtiere* 40:250–260, 2012.

35. Aronsohn M: Cardiac hemangiosarcoma in the dog: a review of 38 cases, *J Am Vet Med Assoc* 187:922–926, 1985.

36. Yamamoto S, Hoshi K, Hirakawa A: Epidemiological, clinical and pathological features of primary cardiac hemangiosarcoma in dogs: a review of 51 cases, *J Vet Med Sci* 75:1433–1441, 2013.

37. Mullin CM, Arkans MA, Sammarco CD, et al.: Doxorubicin chemotherapy for presumptive cardiac hemangiosarcoma in dogs, *Vet Comp Oncol* 14:e171–e183, 2016.

38. Ward H, Fox LE, Calderwood-Mays MB, et al.: Cutaneous hemangiosarcoma in 25 dogs: a retrospective study, *J Vet Intern Med* 8:345–348, 1994.

39. Aupperle H, Marz I, Ellenberger C, et al.: Primary and secondary heart tumours in dogs and cats, *J Comp Pathol* 136:18–26, 2007.

40. Locke JE, Barber LG: Comparative aspects and clinical outcomes of canine renal hemangiosarcoma, *J Vet Intern Med* 20:962–967, 2006.

41. Liptak JM, Dernell WS, Ehrhart EJ, et al.: Retroperitoneal sarcomas in dogs: 14 cases (1992-2002), *J Am Vet Med Assoc* 224:1471–1477, 2004.

42. Giuffrida MA, Bacon NJ, Kamstock DA: Use of routine histopathology and factor VIII-related antigen/von Willebrand factor immunohistochemistry to differentiate primary hemangiosarcoma of bone from telangiectatic osteosarcoma in 54 dogs, *Vet Comp Oncol* 15:1232–1239, 2017.

43. Deleted in proof.

44. Dennis MM, Ehrhart N, Duncan CG, et al.: Frequency of and risk factors associated with lingual lesions in dogs: 1,196 cases (1995-2004), *J Am Vet Med Assoc* 228:1533–1537, 2006.

45. Fujita M, Takaishi Y, Yasuda D, et al.: Intranasal hemangiosarcoma in a dog, *J Vet Med Sci* 70:525–528, 2008.

46. Pirie CG, Knollinger AM, Thomas CB, et al.: Canine conjunctival hemangioma and hemangiosarcoma: a retrospective evaluation of 108 cases (1989-2004), *Vet Ophthalmol* 9:215–226, 2006.

47. Liptak JM, Dernell WS, Withrow SJ: Haemangiosarcoma of the urinary bladder in a dog, *Aust Vet J* 82:215–217, 2004.

48. Wobeser BK, Kidney BA, Powers BE, et al.: Diagnoses and clinical outcomes associated with surgically amputated canine digits submitted to multiple veterinary diagnostic laboratories, *Vet Pathol* 44:355–361, 2007.

49. Pintar J, Breitschwerdt EB, Hardie EM, et al.: Acute nontraumatic hemoabdomen in the dog: a retrospective analysis of 39 cases (1987-2001), *J Am Anim Hosp Assoc* 39:518–522, 2003.

50. Hammond TN, Pesillo-Crosby SA: Prevalence of hemangiosarcoma in anemic dogs with a splenic mass and hemoperitoneum requiring a transfusion: 71 cases (2003-2005), *J Am Vet Med Assoc* 232:553–558, 2008.

51. Aronsohn MG, Dubiel B, Roberts B, et al.: Prognosis for acute nontraumatic hemoperitoneum in the dog: a retrospective analysis of 60 cases (2003-2006), *J Am Anim Hosp Assoc* 45:72–77, 2009.

52. Mallinckrodt MJ, Gottfried SD: Mass-to-splenic volume ratio and splenic weight as a percentage of body weight in dogs with malignant and benign splenic masses: 65 cases (2007-2008), *J Am Vet Med Assoc* 239:1325–1327, 2011.

53. Boston SE, Higginson G, Monteith G: Concurrent splenic and right atrial mass at presentation in dogs with HSA: a retrospective study, *J Am Anim Hosp Assoc* 47:336–341, 2011.

54. Snyder JM, Lipitz L, Skorupski KA, et al.: Secondary intracranial neoplasia in the dog: 177 cases (1986-2003), *J Vet Intern Med* 22:172–177, 2008.

55. Scavelli TD, Patnaik AK, Mehlhaff CJ, et al.: Hemangiosarcoma in the cat: retrospective evaluation of 31 surgical cases, *J Am Vet Med Assoc* 187:817–819, 1985.

56. Miller MA, Ramos JA, Kreeger JM: Cutaneous vascular neoplasia in 15 cats: clinical, morphologic, and immunohistochemical studies, *Vet Pathol* 29:329–336, 1992.

57. Kraje AC, Mears EA, Hahn KA, et al.: Unusual metastatic behavior and clinicopathologic findings in eight cats with cutaneous or visceral hemangiosarcoma, *J Am Vet Med Assoc* 214:670–672, 1999.

58. McAbee KP, Ludwig LL, Bergman PJ, et al.: Feline cutaneous hemangiosarcoma: a retrospective study of 18 cases (1998-2003), *J Am Anim Hosp Assoc* 41:110–116, 2005.

59. Culp WT, Drobatz KJ, Glassman MM, et al.: Feline visceral hemangiosarcoma, *J Vet Intern Med* 22:148–152, 2008.

60. Sharpe A, Cannon MJ, Lucke VM, et al.: Intestinal haemangiosarcoma in the cat: clinical and pathological features of four cases, *J Small Anim Pract* 41:411–415, 2000.

61. Pirie CG, Dubielzig RR: Feline conjunctival hemangioma and hemangiosarcoma: a retrospective evaluation of eight cases (1993-2004), *Vet Ophthalmol* 9:227–231, 2006.

62. Wobeser BK, Kidney BA, Powers BE, et al.: Diagnoses and clinical outcomes associated with surgically amputated feline digits submitted to multiple veterinary diagnostic laboratories, *Vet Pathol* 44:362–365, 2007.

63. Newkirk KM, Rohrbach BW: A retrospective study of eyelid tumors from 43 cats, *Vet Pathol* 46:916–927, 2009.

64. von Beust BR, Suter MM, Summers BA: Factor VIII-related antigen in canine endothelial neoplasms: an immunohistochemical study, *Vet Pathol* 25:251–255, 1988.

65. Ferrer L, Fondevila D, Rabanal RM, et al.: Immunohistochemical detection of CD31 antigen in normal and neoplastic canine endothelial cells, *J Comp Pathol* 112:319–326, 1995.

66. Bulakowski EJ, Philibert JC, Siegal S, et al.: Evaluation of outcome associated with subcutaneous and intramuscular hemangiosarcoma treated with adjuvant doxorubicin in dogs: 21 cases (2001-2006), *J Am Vet Med Assoc* 233:122–128, 2008.

67. Wiley JL, Rook KA, Clifford CA, et al.: Efficacy of doxorubicin-based chemotherapy for non-resectable canine subcutaneous haemangiosarcoma, *Vet Comp Oncol* 8:221–233, 2010.

68. Shiu KB, Flory AB, Anderson CL, et al.: Predictors of outcome in dogs with subcutaneous or intramuscular hemangiosarcoma, *J Am Vet Med Assoc* 238:472–479, 2011.

69. Culp WT, Weisse C, Kellogg ME, et al.: Spontaneous hemoperitoneum in cats: 65 cases (1994-2006), *J Am Med Assoc* 236:978–982, 2010.

70. Childress MO: Hematologic abnormalities in the small animal cancer patient, *Vet Clin North Am Small Anim Pract* 42:123–155, 2012.

71. Warry E, Bohn A, Emanuelli, et al.: Disease distribution in canine patients with acanthocytosis: 123 cases, *Vet Clin Pathol* 42:465–470, 2013.

72. Hargis AM, Feldman BF: Evaluation of hemostatic defects secondary to vascular tumors in dogs: 11 cases (1983-1988), *J Am Vet Med Assoc* 198:891–894, 1991.

73. Maruyama H, Miura T, Sakai M, et al.: The incidence of disseminated intravascular coagulation in dogs with malignant tumor, *J Vet Med Sci* 66:573–575, 2004.

74. Wrigley RH, Park RD, Konde LJ, et al.: Ultrasonographic features of splenic hemangiosarcoma in dogs: 18 cases (1980-1986), *J Am Vet Med Assoc* 192:1113–1117, 1988.

75. Cuccovillo A, Lamb CR: Cellular features of sonographic target lesions of the liver and spleen in 21 dogs and a cat, *Vet Radiol Ultrasound* 43:275–278, 2002.

76. O'Brien RT: Improved detection of metastatic hepatic hemangiosarcoma nodules with contrast ultrasound in three dogs, *Vet Rad Ultrasound* 48:146–148, 2007.

77. Ohlerth S, Dennler M, Ruefli E, et al.: Contrast harmonic imaging characterization of canine splenic lesions, *J Vet Intern Med* 22:1095–1102, 2008.

78. Holt D, Van Winkle T, Schelling C, et al.: Correlation between thoracic radiographs and postmortem findings in dogs with hemangiosarcoma: 77 cases (1984-1989), *J Am Vet Med Assoc* 200:1535–1539, 1992.

79. Stafford Johnson M, Martin M, Binns S, et al.: A retrospective study of clinical findings, treatment, and outcome in 143 dogs with pericardial effusion, *J Small Anim Pract* 45:546–552, 2004.

80. MacDonald KA, Cagney O, Magne ML: Echocardiographic and clinicopathologic characterization of pericardial effusion in dogs: 107 cases (1995-2006), *J Am Vet Med Assoc* 235:1456–1461, 2009.

81. Ratterree W, Gieger T, Pariaut R, et al.: Value of echocardiography and electrocardiography as screening tools prior to doxorubicin administration, *J Am Anim Hosp Assoc* 48:89–96, 2012.

82. Wendelburg KM, O'Toole TE, McCobb E, et al.: Risk factors for perioperative death in dogs undergoing splenectomy for splenic masses: 539 cases (2001-2012), *J Am Vet Med Assoc* 245:1382–1390, 2014.

83. LeBlanc AK, Daniel GB: Advanced imaging for veterinary cancer patients, *Vet Clin Small Anim* 37:1059–1077, 2007.

84. Clifford CA, Pretorius ES, Weisse C, et al.: Magnetic resonance imaging of focal splenic and hepatic lesions in the dog, *J Vet Intern Med* 18:330–338, 2004.

85. Fife WD, Samii VF, Drost WT, et al.: Comparison between malignant and nonmalignant splenic masses in dogs using contrast-enhanced computed tomography, *Vet Radiol Ultrasound* 45:289–297, 2004.

86. Armbrust LJ, Biller DS, Bamford A, et al.: Comparison of three-view thoracic radiography and computed tomography for detection of pulmonary nodules in dogs with neoplasia, *J Am Vet Med Assoc* 240:1088–1094, 2012.

87. Shaw SP, Rozanski EA, Rush JE: Cardiac troponins I and T in dogs with pericardial effusion, *J Vet Intern Med* 18:322–324, 2004.

88. Chun R, Kellihan HB, Henik RA, et al.: Comparison of plasma cardiac troponin I concentrations among dogs with cardiac hemangiosarcoma, noncardiac hemangiosarcoma, other neoplasms, and pericardial effusion of nonhemangiosarcoma origin, *J Am Vet Med Assoc* 237:806–811, 2010.

89. Duda LE, Sorenmo KU: Urine basic fibroblast growth factor in canine hemangiosarcoma. In *Proceedings of the Veterinary Cancer Society Annual Conference*, 73, 1997, Chicago.

90. Thamm DH, Kamstock DA, Sharp CR, et al.: Elevated serum thymidine kinase activity in canine splenic hemangiosarcoma, *Vet Comp Oncol* 10:292–302, 2012.

91. Kirby GM, Mackay A, Grant A, et al.: Concentration of lipocalin region of collagen XXVII alpha I in the serum of dogs with hemangiosarcoma, *J Vet Intern Med* 25:497–503, 2011.

92. Bertazzolo W, Dell'Orco M, Bonfanti U, et al.: Canine angiosarcoma: cytologic, histologic, and immunohistochemical correlations, *Vet Clin Pathol* 34:28–34, 2005.

93. Clendaniel DC, Sivacolundhu RK, Sorenmo KU, et al.: Association between macroscopic appearance of liver lesions and liver histology in dogs with splenic hemangiosarcoma: 70 cases (2004-2009), *J Am Anim Hosp* 50:e6–e10, 2014.

94. Weisse C, Soares N, Beal MW, et al.: Survival times in dogs with right atrial hemangiosarcoma treated by means of surgical resection with or without adjuvant chemotherapy: 23 cases (1986-2000), *J Am Vet Med Assoc* 226:575–579, 2005.

95. Ployart S, Libermann S, Doran I, et al.: Thoracoscopic resection of right auricular masses in dogs: 9 cases (2003–2011), *J Am Vet Med Assoc* 242:237–241, 2013.

96. Morges M, Worley DR, Withrow SJ, et al.: Pericardial free patch grafting as a rescue technique in surgical management of right atrial HSA, *J Am Anim Hosp Assoc* 47:224–228, 2011.

97. Verbeke F, Binst D, Stegen L: Total venous inflow occlusion and pericardial auto-graft reconstruction for right atrial hemangiosarcoma resection in a dog, *Can Vet J* 53:1114–1118, 2012.

98. Case BL, Maxwell M, Aman A, et al.: Outcome evaluation of a thoracoscopic pericardial window procedure or subtotal pericardectomy via thoracotomy for the treatment of pericardial effusion in dogs, *J Am Vet Med Assoc* 242:493–498, 2013.

99. Ogilvie GK, Powers BE, Mallinckrodt CH, et al.: Surgery and doxorubicin in dogs with hemangiosarcoma, *J Vet Intern Med* 10:379–384, 1996.

100. Sorenmo KU, Baez JL, Clifford CA, et al.: Efficacy and toxicity of a dose-intensified doxorubicin protocol in canine hemangiosarcoma, *J Vet Intern Med* 18:209–213, 2004.

101. Sorenmo KU, Jeglum KA, Helfand SC: Chemotherapy of canine hemangiosarcoma with doxorubicin and cyclophosphamide, *J Vet Intern Med* 7:370–376, 1993.

102. Sorenmo K, Duda L, Barber L, et al.: Canine hemangiosarcoma treated with standard chemotherapy and minocycline, *J Vet Intern Med* 14:395–398, 2000.

103. Hammer AS, Couto CG, Filppi J, et al.: Efficacy and toxicity of VAC chemotherapy (vincristine, doxorubicin, and cyclophosphamide) in dogs with hemangiosarcoma, *J Vet Intern Med* 5:160–166, 1991.

104. Dervisis NG, Dominguez PA, Newman RG, et al.: Treatment with DAV for advanced-stage hemangiosarcoma in dogs, *J Am Anim Hosp Assoc* 46:170–178, 2011.

105. Payne SE, Rassnick KM, Northrup NC, et al.: Treatment of vascular and soft-tissue sarcomas in dogs using an alternating protocol of ifosfamide and doxorubicin, *Vet Comp Oncol* 1:171–179, 2003.

106. Finotello R, Stefanello D, Zini E, et al.: Comparison of doxorubicin-cyclophosphamide with doxorubicin-dacarbazine for the adjuvant treatment of canine hemangiosarcoma, *Vet Comp Oncol* 15:25–35, 2017.

107. Kahn SA, Mullin CM, de Lorimier LP, et al.: Doxorubicin and deracoxib adjuvant therapy for canine splenic hemangiosarcoma: a pilot study, *Can Vet J* 54:237–242, 2013.

108. Rassnick KM, Frimberger AE, Wood CA, et al.: Evaluation of ifosfamide for treatment of various canine neoplasms, *J Vet Intern Med* 14:271–276, 2000.

109. Teske E, Rutteman GR, Kirpenstein J, et al.: A randomized controlled study into the efficacy and toxicity of pegylated liposome encapsulated doxorubicin as an adjuvant therapy in dogs with splenic haemangiosarcoma, *Vet Comp Oncol* 9:283–289, 2011.

110. Sorenmo K, Samluk M, Clifford C, et al.: Clinical and pharmacokinetic characteristics of intracavitary administration of pegylated liposomal encapsulated doxorubicin in dogs with splenic hemangiosarcoma, *J Vet Intern Med* 21:1347–1354, 2007.

111. Kim SE, Liptak JM, Gall TT, et al.: Epirubicin in the adjuvant treatment of splenic hemangiosarcoma in dogs: 59 cases (1997-2004), *J Am Vet Med Assoc* 231:1550–1557, 2007.

112. Biller B: Metronomic chemotherapy in veterinary patients with cancer: rethinking the targets and strategies of chemotherapy, *Vet Clin North Am Small Anim Pract* 44:17–829, 2014.

113. Lana S, U'Ren L, Plaza S, et al.: Continuous low-dose oral chemotherapy for adjuvant therapy of splenic hemangiosarcoma in dogs, *J Vet Intern Med* 21:764–769, 2007.

114. Finotello R, Henriques J, Sabattini S, et al.: A retrospective analysis of chemotherapy switch suggests improved outcome in surgically removed, biologically aggressive canine hemangiosarcoma, *Vet Comp Oncol* 15:493–503, 2017.

115. Matsuyama A, Poirier VJ, Mantovani F, et al.: Adjuvant doxorubicin with or without metronomic cyclophosphamide for canine splenic hemangiosarcoma, *J Am Anim Hosp Assoc* 53:304–312, 2017.

116. Bray, et al.: Thalidomide prolongs survival in dogs with splenic hemangiosarcoma, *J Small Anim Pract* 59:85–91, 2017.

117. Tripp CD, Fidel J, Anderson CL, et al.: Tolerability of metronomic administration of lomustine in dogs with cancer, *J Vet Intern Med* 25:278–284, 2011.

118. Leach TN, Childress MO, Greene SN, et al.: Prospective trial of metronomic chlorambucil chemotherapy in dogs with naturally occurring cancer, *Vet Comp Oncol* 10:102–112, 2011.

119. Kisseberth WC, Vail DM, Yaissle J, et al.: Phase I clinical evaluation of carboplatin in tumor-bearing cats: a Veterinary Cooperative Oncology Group study, *J Vet Intern Med* 22:83–88, 2008.

120. U'Ren LW, Biller BJ, Elmslie RE, et al.: Evaluation of a novel tumor vaccine in dogs with hemangiosarcoma, *J Vet Intern Med* 21:113–120, 2007.

121. Vail DM, MacEwen EG, Kurzman ID, et al.: Liposome-encapsulated muramyl tripeptide phosphatidylethanolamine adjuvant immunotherapy for splenic hemangiosarcoma in the dog: a randomized multi-institutional clinical trial, *Clin Cancer Res* 1:1165–1170, 1995.

122. Hillers KR, Lana SE, Fuller CR, et al.: Effects of palliative radiation therapy on nonsplenic hemangiosarcoma in dogs, *J Am Anim Hosp Assoc* 43:187–192, 2007.

123. Nolan MW, Arkans MM, LaVine, et al.: Pilot study to determine the feasibility of radiation therapy for dogs with right atrial masses and hemorrhagic pericardial effusion, *J Vet Cardiol* 19:132–143, 2017.

124. Lyles SE, Milner RJ, Kow K, et al.: In vitro effects of the tyrosine kinase inhibitor, masitinib mesylate, on canine hemangiosarcoma cell lines, *Vet Comp Oncol* 10:223–235, 2012.

125. London C, Mathie T, Stingle N, et al.: Preliminary evidence for biologic activity of toceranib phosphate (Palladia(®)) in solid tumours, *Vet Comp Oncol* 10:194–205, 2012.

126. Gardner HL, London CA, Portela RA, et al.: Maintenance therapy with toceranib following doxorubicin-based chemotherapy for canine splenic hemangiosarcoma, *BMC Vet Res* 11:131, 2015.

127. Borgatti A, Koopmeiners JS, Sarver AL, et al.: Safe and effective sarcoma therapy through bispecific targeting of EGFR and uPAR, *Mol Cancer Ther* 16:956–965, 2017.

128. Wirth KA, Kow K, Salute ME, et al.: In vitro effects of Yunnan Baiyao on canine hemangiosarcoma cell lines, *Vet Comp Oncol* 14:281–294, 2016.

129. Egger C, Gibbs D, Wheeler J, et al.: Effect of oral administration of Yunnan Baiyao on periprocedural hemorrhage in dogs undergoing nasal biopsy: a prospective, randomized, double-blinded controlled study, *Am Jour Trad Chin Vet Med* 11:27–36, 2016.

130. Frederick J, Boysen S, Wagg C, Chalhoub S: The effects of oral administration of Yunnan Baiyao on blood coagulation in beagle dogs as measured by kaolin-activated thromboelastography and buccal mucosal bleeding times, *Can J Vet Res* 81:41–45, 2017.

131. Murphy LA, Panek CM, Bianco D, Nakamura RK: Use of yunnan baiyao and epsilon aminocaproic acid in dogs with right atrial masses and pericardial effusion, *J Vet Emerg Crit Care* 27:121–126, 2017.

132. Brown DC, Reetz J: Single agent polysaccharopeptide delays metastases and improves survival in naturally occurring hemangiosarcoma, *Evid Based Comp Alt Med* 2012, 2012. 3284301.

133. Alvarez FJ, Hosoya K, Lara-Garcia A, et al.: VAC protocol for treatment of dogs with stage III hemangiosarcoma, *J Am Anim Hosp Assoc* 49:370–377, 2013.

134. Gordon SS, McClaran JK, Bergman PJ, et al.: Outcome following splenectomy in cats, *J Fel Med Surg* 12:256–261, 2010.

135. Simonart T, Heenen M: Radiation-induced angiosarcomas, *Dermatology* 209:175–176, 2004.

136. Parker GA, Casey HW: Thymomas in domestic animals, *Vet Pathol* 13:353–364, 1976.

137. Aronsohn M: Canine thymomas, *Vet Clin North Am* 15:755–776, 1985.

138. Robat CS, Cesario L, Gaeta R, et al.: Clinical features, treatment options, and outcome in dogs with thymoma: 116 cases (1990-2010), *J Am Vet Med Assoc* 243:1448–1454, 2013.

139. Zitz JC, Birchard SJ, Couto GC, et al.: Results of excision of thymomas in cats and dogs: 20 cases (1984-2005), *J Am Vet Med Assoc* 232:1186–1192, 2008.

140. Aronsohn MG, Schunk KL, Carpenter JL, et al.: Clinical and pathologic features of thymomas in 15 dogs, *J Am Vet Med Assoc* 184:1355–1362, 1984.

141. Atwater SW, Powers BE, Park RD, et al.: Canine thymomas: 23 cases (1980-1991), *J Am Vet Med Assoc* 205:1007–1013, 1994.

142. Patnaik AK, Lieberman PH, Erlandson RA, et al.: Feline cystic thymomas: a clinicopathologic, immunohistologic, and electron microscopic study of 14 cases, *J Feline Med Surg* 5:27–35, 2003.

143. Carpenter JL, Valentine BA: Brief communications and case reports: squamous cell carcinoma arising in two feline thymomas, *Vet Pathol* 29:541–543, 1992.

144. Vilafranca M, Font A: Thymolipoma in a cat, *J Feline Med and Surg* 7:125–127, 2005.

145. Robinson WC, Cantwell HD, Crawley RR, et al.: Invasive thymoma in a dog: a case report, *J Am Anim Hosp Assoc* 13:95–97, 1977.

146. Bella JR, Stiff ME, Russel RG: Thymoma in the dog: two case reports and review of 20 additional cases, *J Am Vet Med Assoc* 183:306–311, 1983.

147. Day MJ: Review of thymic pathology in 30 cats and 36 dogs, *J Sm Anim Pract* 38:393–403, 1997.

148. Bell FW: Neoplastic diseases of the thorax, *Vet Clin of North Am Sm Anim Pract* 17:387–409, 1987.

149. Darke PG: Myasthenia gravis, thymoma, and myositis in a dog, *Vet Rec* 97:392–395, 1975.

150. Carpenter JL, Holzworth J: Thymoma in 11 cats, *J Am Vet Med Assoc* 181:248–251, 1982.

151. Turek MM: Cutaneous paraneoplastic syndromes in dogs and cats: a review of the literature, *Vet Dermatol* 14:279–296, 2003.

152. Rottenberg S, von Tscharner C, Roosje PJ: Thymoma-associated exfoliative dermatitis in cats, *Vet Pathol* 41:429–433, 2004.

153. Uchida K, Awamura Y, Nakamura T, et al.: Thymoma and multiple thymic cysts in a dog with acquired myasthenia gravis, *J Vet Med Sci* 64:637–640, 2002.

154. Stenner VJ, Parry BW, Holloway SA: Acquired myasthenia gravis associated with a non-invasive thymic carcinoma in a dog, *Aust Vet J* 81:543–546, 2003.

155. Paciello O, Maiolino P, Navas L, et al.: Acquired canine myasthenia gravis associated with thymoma: histological features and immuno-localization of HLA type II and IgG, *Vet Res Commun* 27(Suppl 1):715–718, 2003.

156. Moffet AC: Metastatic thymomas and acquired generalized myasthenia gravis in a beagle, *Can Vet J* 48:91–93, 2007.

157. Singh A, Boston SE, Poma R: Thymoma-associated exfoliative dermatitis with post-thymectomy myasthenia gravis in a cat, *Can Vet J* 51:757–760, 2010.

158. Foley P, Shaw D, Runyon C: Serum parathyroid hormone-related protein concentration in a dog with thymomas and persistent hypercalcemia, *Can Vet J* 41:867–870, 2000.

159. Theilen GH, Madewell BR: Tumors of the respiratory tract and thorax, ed 1, *Veterinary cancer medicine*, Philadelphia, 1979, Lea & Febiger, pp 535–566.

160. Harris CL, Klausner JS, Caywood DD, et al.: Hypercalcemia in a dog with thymomas, *J Am Anim Hosp Assoc* 27:281–284, 1991.

161. Bolliger AP, Graham PA, Richard V, et al.: Detection of parathyroid hormone-related protein in cats with humoral hypercalcemia of malignancy, *Vet Clin Pathol* 31:3–8, 2002.

162. Marconato L, Stefanello D, Valenti P, et al.: Predictors of long-term survival in dogs with high-grade multicentric lymphoma, *J Am Vet Med Assoc* 238:480–485, 2011.

163. Patterson MME, Marolf A: Sonographic characteristics of thymoma compared with mediastinal lymphoma, *J Am Anim Hosp Assoc* 50:409–413, 2014.

164. Reickle JK, Wisner ER: Non-cardiac thoracic ultrasound in 75 feline and canine patients, *Vet Radiol and Ultrasound* 41:154–162, 2000.

165. Larson MM: Ultrasound of the thorax (non-cardiac), *Vet Clin of North Am* 39:733–745, 2009.

166. Gashen L, Kircher P, Hoffman G, et al.: Endoscopic ultrasound for the diagnosis of intrathoracic lesions in two dogs, *Vet Radiol Ultrasound* 44:292–299, 2003.

167. Rae CA, Jacobs RM, Couto CG: A comparison between the cytological and histological characteristics in thirteen canine and feline thymomas, *Can Vet J* 30:497–500, 1989.

168. Cowell RL, Tyler RD, Meinkoth JH: The lung parenchyma. In *Diagnostic cytology of the dog and cat*, ed 2, St Louis, 1999, Mosby.

169. Lana S, Plaza S, Hampe K, Burnett R, et al.: Diagnosis of mediastinal masses in dogs by flow cytometry, *J Vet Intern Med* 20:1161–1165, 2006.

170. Holsworth IG, Kyles AE, Bailiff NL: Use of a jugular vein autograft for reconstruction of the vena cava in a dog with invasive thymoma and cranial vena cava syndrome, *J Am Vet Med Assoc* 225:1205–1210, 2004.

171. Yoon J, Feeney DA, Cronk DE, et al.: Computed tomographic evaluation of canine and feline mediastinal masses in 14 patients, *Vet Radiol Ultrasound* 45:524–526, 2004.

172. Zekas LJ, Crawford JT, O'Brien RT: Computed tomographic-guided biopsy of intrathoracic lesions in 50 dogs and cats, *Vet Radiol Ultrasound* 46:200–204, 2005.

173. Hylands R: Veterinary diagnostic imaging, *Thymoma, Can Vet J* 47:593–596, 2006.

174. Scherrer W, Kyles A, Samii V, et al.: Computed tomographic assessment of vascular invasion and resectability of mediastinal masses in dogs and cats, *NZ Vet J* 56:330–333, 2008.

175. Maciver MA, Case JB, Monnet EL, et al.: Video-assisted extirpation of cranial mediastinal masses in dogs: 18 cases (2009-2014), *J Am Vet Med Assoc* 250:1283–1290, 2017.

176. Smith AN, Wright JC, Brawner Jr WR, et al.: Radiation therapy in the treatment of canine and feline thymomas: a retrospective study (1985-1999), *J Am Anim Hosp Assoc* 37:489–496, 2001.

177. Goto S, Murakami M, Kawabe M, et al.: Hypofractionated radiation therapy in the treatment of canine thymoma: retrospective study of eight cases, *Vet Radiol Ultrasound* 58:613–620, 2017.

178. Tong LJ, Hosgood G, Labruyere J, et al.: Marked cytoreduction of a lymphocyte-rich mediastinal thymoma with neoadjuvant chemotherapy in a cat, *JFMS Open Rep* 1:2055116915585024, 2015.

179. Moore AS: Chemotherapy for intrathoracic cancer in dogs and cats, *Probl Vet Med* 4:351–364, 1992.

180. Garneau MS, Price LL, Withrow SJ, et al.: Perioperative mortality and long-term survival in 80 dogs and 32 cats undergoing excision of thymic epithelial tumors, *Vet Surg* 44:557–564, 2015.

181. Gores BR, Berg J, Carpenter JL: Surgical treatment of thymomas in cats: 12 cases (1987-1992), *J Am Vet Med Assoc* 204:1782–1785, 1994.

182. Tomaszek S, Wigle DA, Keshavjee S, et al.: Thymomas: review of current clinical practice, *Ann Thorac Surg* 87:1973–1980, 2009.

183. Masaoka A, Monden W, Nakahara K, et al.: Follow-up study of thymomas with special reference to their clinical stages, *Cancer* 48:2485–2492, 1981.

184. Ried M, Guth H, Potzger T, et al.: Surgical resection of thymomas still represents the first choice of treatment, *Thorac Cardiovasc Surg* 60:145–149, 2012.

185. Cardillo G, Carleo F, Giunti R, et al.: Predictors of survival in patients with locally advanced thymomas and thymic carcinoma (Masaoka stages III and IVa), *Eur J Cardiothorac Surg* 37:819–823, 2010.

186. Ganguly B, Das U, Das AK: Canine transmissible venereal tumour: a review, *Vet Comp Onc* 14:1–12, 2013.

187. Agnew DW, MacLachlan NJ: Tumors of the genital systems. In Meuten DJ, editor: *Tumors in domestic animals*, ed 5, Ames, 2017, Wiley Blackwell, pp 689–722.

188. Schlafer DH, Foster RA: Female genital system. Male genital system. In ed 6, Maxie G, editor: *Pathology of domestic animals*, vol. 3. St. Louis, 2016, Elsevier, pp 358–464, 465–510.

189. Cohen D: The canine transmissible venereal tumor: a unique result of tumor progression, *Adv Cancer Res* 43:75–112, 1985.

190. Birhan G, Chanie M: A review on canine transmissible venereal tumor: from morphologic to biochemical and molecular diagnosis, *Acad J Anim Dis* 4(3):185–195, 2015.

191. Lima CRO, Rabelo RE, Vulcani VAS, et al.: Morphological patterns and malignancy criteria of transmissible venereal tumor in cytopathological and histopathological exams, *Braz J Vet Res Anim Sci* 50(3):238–246, 2013.

192. Mukaratirwa S, Gruys E: Canine transmissible venereal tumour: cytogenetic origin, immunophenotype, and immunobiology: a review, *Vet Q* 25:101–111, 2003.

193. Hayes HM, Biggar RJ, Pickle LW, et al.: Canine transmissible venereal tumor: a model for Kaposi's sarcoma? *Am J Epidemiol* 117:108–109, 1983.

194. Mikaelian I, Girard C, Ivascu I: Transmissible venereal tumor: a consequence of sex tourism in a dog, *Can Vet J* 39:591, 1998.

195. Rogers KS, Walker MA, Dillon HB: Transmissible venereal tumor: a retrospective study of 29 cases, *J Am Anim Hosp Assoc* 34:463–470, 1998.

196. Ojeda J, Mieres M, Soto F, et al.: Computer tomographic imaging in 4 dogs with primary nasal canine transmissible venereal tumor and differing cellular phenotype, *J Vet Intern Med* 32:1172–1177, 2018.

197. Rezaei M, Azizi S, Shahheidaripour S, et al.: Primary oral and nasal transmissible venereal tumor in a mix-breed dog, *Asian Pac J Trop Biomed* 6(5):443–445, 2016.

198. Filgueira K, Peixoto G, Fonseca Z: Canine transmissible venereal tumor with multiple extragenital locations, *Acta Sci Vet* 41:1–6, 2013.

199. Strakova A, Murchison EP: The changing global distribution and prevalence of canine transmissible venereal tumour, *BMC Vet Res* 10, 2014. 168–168.

200. Albanese E, Poli A, Millanta F, et al.: Primary cutaneous extragenital canine transmissible venereal tumor with Leishmania-laden neoplastic cells: a further suggestion of histiocytic origin? *Vet Dermatol* 13:243–246, 2002.

201. Ostrander EA, Davis BW, Ostrander GK: Transmissible tumors: breaking the cancer paradigm, *Trends Genet* 32(1):1–15, 2016.

202. Belov K: Contagious cancer: lessons from the devil and the dog, *Bioessays* 34:285–292, 2012.

203. Murchison EP, Wedge DC, Alexandrov LB, et al.: Transmissible dog cancer genome reveals the origin and history of an ancient cell lineage, *Science* 343:437–440, 2014.

204. Belov K: The role of the major histocompatibility complex in the spread of contagious cancers, *Mamm Genome* 22:83–90, 2011.

205. Ujvari B, Papenfuss AT, Belov K: Transmissible cancers in an evolutionary context, *Bioessays* 38:S14–S23, 2016.

206. Rebbeck CA, Thomas R, Breen M, et al.: Origins and evolution of a transmissible cancer, *Evolution* 63(9):2340–2349, 2009.

207. Pereira JS, Silva AB, Martins AL, et al.: Immunohistochemical characterization of intraocular metastasis of a canine transmissible venereal tumor, *Vet Ophthalmol* 3:43–47, 2000.

208. Lopes PD, dos Santos ACAA, Silva JES: Canine transmissible venereal tumor in the genital area with subcutaneous metastases in the head - case report, *RPCV* 110:120–123, 2015.

209. Alkan H, Satilmis F, Alcigir ME, et al.: Clinicopathological evaluation of disseminated metastases of transmissible venereal tumor in a spayed bitch, *Acta Scientiae Veterinariae* 45:1–6, 2017.

210. Mozos E, Méndez A, Gómez-Villamandos JC, et al.: Immunohistochemical characterization of canine transmissible venereal tumor, *Vet Path* 33:257–263, 1996.

211. Mascarenhas MB, Peixoto PV, Ramadinha RR, et al.: Immunohistochemical study of genital and extragenital forms of canine transmissible venereal tumor in Brazil, *Pesq Vet Bras* 34(3):250–254, 2014.

212. Ajayi OL, Oluwabi M, Ajadi RA, et al.: Cytomorphological, histopathological and immunohistochemical observations on the histiocytic origin of canine transmissible venereal tumour, *Sokoto J Vet Sci* 16(2):10–20, 2018.

213. Gupta K, Sood NK: Pathological and immunohistochemical studies on rare cases of primary extra-genital transmissible venereal tumours in the mammary gland, *Vet Med* 57(4):198–206, 2012.

214. Akkoc A, Nak D, Demirer A, et al.: Immunocharacterization of matrix metalloproteinase-2 and matrix metalloproteinase-9 in canine transmissible venereal tumors, *Biotech Histochem* 92(2):100–106, 2017.

215. Kegler K, Habierski A, Hahn K, et al.: Vaginal canine transmissible venereal tumour associated with intra-tumoural Leishmania spp. Amastigotes in an asymptomatic female dog, *J Comp Path* 149:156–161, 2013.

216. Decker B, Dais BW, Rimbault M, et al.: Comparison against 186 canid whole-genome sequences reveals survival strategies of an ancient clonally transmissible canine tumor, *Genome Res* 25:1646–1655, 2015.

217. Strakova A, Leathlobhair MN, Wang G-D: Mitochondrial genetic diversity, selection and recombination in a canine transmissible cancer, *eLife* 5:e14552, 2016.

218. Katzir N, Rechavi G, Cohen JB, et al.: "Retroposon" insertion into the cellular oncogene c-myc in canine transmissible venereal tumor, *Proc Natl Acad Sci USA* 82:1054–1058, 1985.

219. Choi YK, Kim CJ: Sequence analysis of canine LINE-l elements and p53 gene in canine transmissible venereal tumor, *J Vet Sci* 3:285–292, 2002.

220. Fonseca LS, Mota LSLS, Colodel MM, et al.: Spontaneous canine transmissible venereal tumor: association between different phenotypes and the insertion LINE−1/c−myc, *Rev Colomb Cienc Pec* 25:402–408, 2012.

221. Strakova A, Murchison EP: The cancer which survived: insights from the genome of an 11 000 year−old cancer, *Curr Opin Genet Dev* 30:49–55, 2015.

222. Liao KW, Lin ZY, Pao HN, et al.: Identification of canine transmissible venereal tumor cells using in situ polymerase chain reaction and the stable sequence of the long interspersed nuclear element, *J Vet Diagn Invest* 15:399–406, 2003.

223. Castro KF, Strakova A, Tinucci-Costa M, et al.: Evaluation of a genetic assay for canine transmissible venereal tumour diagnosis in Brazil, *Vet Comp Oncol* 15(2):615–618, 2017.

224. Sánchez-Servín A, Martínez S, Cárdova-Alarcon E, et al.: TP53 polymorphisms allow for genetic sub-grouping of the canine transmissible venereal tumor, *J Vet Sci* 10(4):353–355, 2009.

225. Stockman D, Ferrari HF, Andrade AL, et al.: Detection of the tumour suppressor gene TP53 and expression of p53, Bcl-2 and p63 proteins in canine transmissible venereal tumour, *Vet Comp Oncol* 9(4):251–259, 2011.

226. Fenton MA, Yang TJ: Role of humoral immunity in progressive and regressive and metastatic growth of the canine transmissible venereal sarcoma, *Oncology* 45:210–213, 1988.

227. Perez J, Day MJ, Mozos E: Immunohistochemical study of the local inflammatory infiltrate in spontaneous canine transmissible venereal tumour at different stages of growth, *Vet Immunol Immunopathol* 64:133–147, 1998.

228. Hsiao YW, Liao KW, Hung SW, et al.: Effect of tumor infiltrating lymphocytes on the expression of MHC molecules in canine transmissible venereal tumor cells, *Vet Immunol Immunopathol* 87:19–27, 2002.

229. Liao KW, Hung SW, Hsiao YW, et al.: Canine transmissible venereal tumor cell depletion of B lymphocytes: molecule(s) specifically toxic for B cells, *Vet Immunol Immunopathol* 92:149–162, 2003.

230. Hsiao YW, Liao KW, Hung SW, et al.: Tumor-infiltrating lymphocyte secretion of IL-6 antagonizes tumor-derived TGF-βl and restores the lymphokine-activated killing activity, *J Immunol* 172:1508–1514, 2004.

231. Siddle HV, Kaufman J: Immunology of naturally transmissible tumours, *Immunology* 144(1):11–20, 2015.

232. Gonzalez CM, Griffey SM, Naydan DK, et al.: Canine transmissible venereal tumour: a morphological and immunohistochemical study of 11 tumours in growth phase and during regression after chemotherapy, *J Comp Path* 122:241–248, 2000.

233. Mukaratirwa S, Chimonyo M, Obwolo M, et al.: Stromal cells and extracellular matrix components in spontaneous canine transmissible venereal tumour at different stages of growth, *Histol Histopathol* 9:1117–1123, 2004.

234. Liu CC, Wang YS, Lin CY, et al.: Transient downregulation of monocyte-derived dendritic-cell differentiation, function, and survival during tumoral progression and regression in an *in vivo* canine model of transmissible venereal tumor, *Cancer Immunol Immunother* 57:479–491, 2008.

235. Fassati A, Mitchison NA: Testing the theory of immune selection in cancers that break the rules of transplantation, *Cancer Immunol Immunother* 59:643–651, 2010.

236. Hsiao YW, Liao KW, Chung TF, et al.: Interactions of host IL-6 and IFN-γ and cancer-derived TGF-ß1 on MHC molecule expression during tumor spontaneous regression, *Cancer Immunol Immunother* 57:1091–1104, 2008.

237. Ballestero Fêo H, Montoya Flórez L, Yamatogi RS, et al.: Does the tumour microenvironment alter tumorigenesis and clinical response in transmissible venereal tumour in dogs? *Vet Comp Oncol* 16:370–378, 2018.

238. Chiang HC, Liao AT, Jan TR, et al.: Gene-expression profiling to identify genes related to spontaneous tumor regression in a canine cancer model, *Vet Immunol Immunopathol* 151:207–216, 2013.

239. Frampton D, Schwenzer H, Marino G, et al.: Molecular signatures of regression of the canine transmissible venereal tumor, *Cancer Cell* 33:620–633, 2018.

240. Cohen D: Detection of humoral antibody to the transmissible venereal tumour of the dog, *Int J Cancer* 10:207–212, 1972.

241. Calvert CA, Leifer CE, MacEwen EG: Vincristine for treatment of transmissible venereal tumor in the dog, *J Am Vet Med Assoc* 181:163–164, 1982.

242. Yang TJ, Palker TJ, Harding MW: Tumor size, leukocyte adherence inhibition and serum level of tumor antigen in dogs with the canine transmissible venereal sarcoma, *Cancer Immunol Immunother* 33:255–262, 1991.

243. Batamuzi EK, Kristensen F: Urinary tract infection: the role of canine transmissible venereal tumour, *J Small Anim Pract* 37:276–279, 1996.

244. Amber EI, Henderson RA, Adeyanju JB, et al.: Single-drug chemotherapy of canine transmissible venereal tumor with cyclophosphamide, methotrexate, or vincristine, *J Vet Intern Med* 4:144–147, 1990.

245. Singh J, Rana JS, Sood N, et al.: Clinico-pathological studies on the effect of different anti-neoplastic chemotherapy regimens on transmissible venereal tumours in dogs, *Vet Res Comm* 20:71–81, 1996.

246. Nak D, Nak Y, Cangul IT, et al.: A clinico-pathological study on the effect of vincristine on transmissible venereal tumour in dogs, *J Vet Med A* 52:366–370, 2005.

247. Scarpelli KC, Valladão ML, Metze K: Predictive factors for the regression of canine transmissible venereal tumor during vincristine therapy, *Vet J* 183:362–363, 2010.

248. Fathi M, Ashry M, Ali KM, et al.: Clinico-pathological evaluation and treatment outcomes of canine transmissible venereal tumor using three different protocols, *Pak Vet J* 38(2):204–208, 2018.

249. Thrall DE: Orthovoltage radiotherapy of canine transmissible venereal tumors, *Vet Radiol* 23:217–219, 1982.

250. Idowu AL: A retrospective evaluation of four surgical methods of treating canine transmissible venereal tumour, *J Small Anim Pract* 25:193–198, 1984.

251. Amber EI, Henderson RA: Canine transmissible venereal tumor evaluation of surgical excision of primary and metastatic lesions in Zaria-Nigeria, *J Am Anim Hosp Assoc* 18:350–352, 1982.

252. Knapp DW, Richardson RC, Bottoms GD, et al.: Phase I trial of piroxicam in 62 dogs bearing naturally occurring tumors, *Chemother Pharmacol* 29:214–218, 1992.

253. Ahmed M, Liu Z, Afzal KS, et al.: Radiofrequency ablation: effect of surrounding tissue composition on coagulation necrosis in a canine tumor model, *Radiology* 230:761–767, 2004.

254. Suzuki DOH, Berkenbrock JA, de Olveira KD, et al.: Novel application for electrochemotherapy: immersion of nasal cavity in dog, *Artif Organs* 41(8):767–784, 2017.

255. Chou PC, Chuang TF, Jan TR, et al.: Effects of immunotherapy of IL-6 and IL-15 plasmids on transmissible venereal tumor in beagles, *Vet Immunol Immunopathol* 130:25–34, 2009.

256. Pai CC, Kuo TF, Mao SJT, et al.: Immunopathogenic behaviors of canine transmissible venereal tumor in dogs following an immunotherapy using dendritic/tumor cell hybrid, *Vet Immunol Immunopathol* 139:187–199, 2011.

257. Den Otter W, Hack M, Jacobs JJ, et al.: Effective treatment of transmissible venereal tumors in dogs with vincristine and IL2, *Anticancer Res* 35(6):3385–3391, 2015.

258. Geib LW, DeNarvaez F, Eby CH: Pleural mesothelioma in a dog, *J Am Vet Med Assoc* 140:1317–1319, 1962.

259. Cihak RW, Roen DR, Klaassen J: Malignant mesothelioma of the tunica vaginalis in a dog, *J Comp Pathol* 96:459–462, 1986.

260. Vascellari M, Carminato A, Camali G, et al.: Malignant mesothelioma of the tunica vaginalis testis in a dog: Histological and immunohistochemical characterization, *J Vet Diagn Invest* 23:135–139, 2011.

261. Dubielzig RR: Sclerosing mesothelioma in five dogs, *J Am Anim Hosp Assoc* 15:745–748, 1979.

262. Thrall DE, Goldschmidt MH: Mesothelioma in the dog: six case reports, *J Am Vet Radiol Soc* 19:107–115, 1978.

263. Morini M, Bettini G, Morandi F, et al.: Deciduoid peritoneal mesothelioma in a dog, *Vet Pathol* 43:198–201, 2006.

264. Son NV, Chambers JK, Shiga T, et al.: Sarcomatoid mesothelioma of tunica vaginalis testis in the right scrotum of a dog, *J Vet Med Sci*, 2018. https://doi.org/10.1292/jvms.18-0186. epub ahead of print.

265. Kobayashi Y, Usuda H, Ochiai K, et al.: Malignant mesothelioma with metastases and mast cell leukaemia in a cat, *J Comp Path* 111:453–458, 1994.

266. Tilley LP, Owens JM, Wilkins RJ, et al.: Pericardial mesothelioma with effusion in a cat, *J Am Anim Hosp Assoc* 60– 65, 1975.

267. Umphlet RC, Bertoy RW: Abdominal mesothelioma in a cat, *Mod Vet Pract* 69:71–73, 1988.

268. Bacci B, Morandi F, De Meo M, et al.: Ten cases of feline mesothelioma: an immunohistochemical and ultrastructural study, *J Comp Pathol* 134:347–354, 2006.

269. Heerkens TM, Smith JD, Fox L, et al.: Peritoneal fibrosarcomatous mesothelioma in a cat, *J Vet Diagn Invest* 23:593–597, 2011.

270. Schaer M, Meyer D: Benign peritoneal mesothelioma, hyperthyroidism, nonsuppurative hepatitis, and chronic disseminated intravascular coagulation in a cat: a case report, *J Am Anim Hosp Assoc* 24:195–202, 1988.

271. Glickman LT, Domanski LM, Maguire TG, et al.: Mesothelioma in pet dogs associated with exposure of their owners to asbestos, *Environ Res* 32:305–313, 1983.

272. Harbison ML, Godleski JJ: Malignant mesothelioma in urban dogs, *Vet Pathol* 20:531–540, 1983.

273. Hughes RS: Malignant pleural mesothelioma, *Am J Med Sci* 329:29–44, 2005.

274. Yap TA, Aerts JG, Popat S, et al.: Novel insights into mesothelioma biology and implications for therapy, *Nat Rev Cancer* 17:475–488, 2017.

275. Bueno R, Stawiski EW, Goldstein LD, et al.: Comprehensive genomic analysis of malignant pleural mesothelioma identifies recurrent mutations, gene fusions and splicing alterations, *Nat Genet* 48:407–416, 2016.

276. Ugurluer G, Chang K, Gamez ME, et al.: Genome-based mutational analysis by next generation sequencing in patients with malignant pleural and peritoneal mesothelioma, *Anticancer Res* 36:2331–2338, 2016.

277. Belli C, Anand S, Tassi G, et al.: Translational therapies for malignant pleural mesothelioma, *Expert Rev Respir Med* 4:249–260, 2010.

278. Machida N, Tanaka R, Takemura N, et al.: Development of pericardial mesothelioma in golden retrievers with a long-term history of idiopathic haemorrhagic pericardial effusion, *J Comp Pathol* 131:166–175, 2004.

279. Kim JH, Choi YK, Yoon HY, et al.: Juvenile malignant mesothelioma in a dog, *J Vet Med Sci* 64:269–271, 2002.

280. Vural SA, Ozyildiz Z, Ozsoy SY: Pleural mesothelioma in a nine-month-old dog, *Ir Vet J* 60:30–33, 2007.

281. Leisewitz AL, Nesbit JW: Malignant mesothelioma in a seven-week-old puppy, *J S Afr Vet Assoc* 63:70–73, 1992.

282. Corson JM: Pathology of mesothelioma, *Thorac Surg Clin* 14:447–460, 2004.

283. Geninet C, Bernex F, Rakotovao F, et al.: Sclerosing peritoneal mesothelioma in a dog - a case report, *J Vet Med A Physiol Pathol Clin Med* 50:402–405, 2003.

284. Schoning P, Layton CE, Fortney WD, et al.: Sclerosing peritoneal mesothelioma in a dog evaluated by electron microscopy and immunoperoxidase techniques, *J Vet Diagn Invest* 4:217–220, 1992.

285. D'Angelo AR, Di Francesco G: Sclerosing peritoneal mesothelioma in a dog: Histopathological, histochemical and immunohistochemical investigations, *Vet Ital* 50:301–305, 2014.

286. Dias Pereira P, Azevedo M, Gartner F: Case of malignant biphasic mesothelioma in a dog, *Vet Rec* 149:680–681, 2001.

287. Sato T, Miyoshi T, Shibuya H, et al.: Peritoneal biphasic mesothelioma in a dog, *J Vet Med A Physiol Pathol Clin Med* 52:22–25, 2005.

288. Al-Dissi AN, Philibert H: A case of biphasic mesothelioma with osseous and chondromatous differentiation in a cat, *Can Vet J* 52:534–536, 2011.

289. DiPinto MN, Dunstan RW, Lee C: Cystic, peritoneal mesothelioma in a dog, *J Am Anim Hosp Assoc* 31:385–389, 1995.

290. Cobb MA, Brownlie SE: Intrapericardial neoplasia in 14 dogs, *J Small Anim Pract* 33:309–316, 1992.

291. McDonough SP, MacLachlan NJ, Tobias AH: Canine pericardial mesothelioma, *Vet Pathol* 29:256–260, 1992.

292. MacDonald KA, Cagney O, Magne ML: Echocardiographic and clinicopathologic characterization of pericardial effusion in dogs: 107 cases (1985-2006), *J Am Vet Med Assoc* 235:1456–1461, 2009.

293. Gumber S, Fowlkes N, Cho DY: Disseminated sclerosing peritoneal mesothelioma in a dog, *J Vet Diagn Invest* 23:1046–1050, 2011.

294. Stepien RL, Whitley NT, Dubielzig RR: Idiopathic or mesothelioma-related pericardial effusion: clinical findings and survival in 17 dogs studied retrospectively, *J Small Anim Pract* 41:342–347, 2000.

295. Echandi RL, Morandi F, Newman SJ, et al.: Imaging diagnosis-canine thoracic mesothelioma, *Vet Radiol Ultrasound* 48:243–245, 2007.

296. Reetz JA, Buza EL, Krick EL: Ct features of pleural masses and nodules, *Vet Radiol Ultrasound* 53:121–127, 2012.

297. Watton TC, Lara-Garcia A, Lamb CR: Can malignant and inflammatory pleural effusions in dogs be distinguished using computed tomography? *Vet Radiol Ultrasound* 58:535–541, 2017.

298. Fine DM, Tobias AH, Jacob KA: Use of pericardial fluid ph to distinguish between idiopathic and neoplastic effusions, *J Vet Intern Med* 17:525–529, 2003.

299. de Laforcade AM, Freeman LM, Rozanski EA, et al.: Biochemical analysis of pericardial fluid and whole blood in dogs with pericardial effusion, *J Vet Intern Med* 19:833–836, 2005.

300. Hirschberger J, Pusch S: Fibronectin concentrations in pleural and abdominal effusions in dogs and cats, *J Vet Intern Med* 10:321–325, 1996.

301. Reggeti F, Brisson B, Ruotsalo K, et al.: Invasive epithelial mesothelioma in a dog, *Vet Pathol* 42:77–81, 2005.

302. Peters M, Tenhundfeld J, Stephan I, et al.: Embolized mesothelial cells within mediastinal lymph nodes of three dogs with idiopathic haemorrhagic pericardial effusion, *J Comp Pathol* 128:107–112, 2003.

303. Ali G, Bruno R, Fontanini G: The pathological and molecular diagnosis of malignant pleural mesothelioma: a literature review, *J Thorac Dis* 10:S276–S284, 2018.

304. Liptak JM, Brebner NS: Hemidiaphragmatic reconstruction with a transversus abdominis muscle flap after resection of a solitary diaphragmatic mesothelioma in a dog, *J Am Vet Med Assoc* 228:1204–1208, 2006.

305. Kerstetter KK, Krahwinkel DJ, Millis DL, et al.: Pericardiectomy in dogs: 22 cases (1978-1994), *J Am Vet Med Assoc* 211:736–740, 1997.

306. Dunning D, Monnet E, Orton EC, et al.: Analysis of prognostic indicators for dogs with pericardial effusion: 46 cases (1985-1996), *J Am Vet Med Assoc* 212:1276–1280, 1998.

307. Closa JM, Font A, Mascort J: Pericardial mesothelioma in a dog: long-term survival after pericardiectomy in combination with chemotherapy, *J Small Anim Pract* 40:383–386, 1999.

308. Jackson J, Richter K, Launer D: Thoracoscopic partial pericardiectomy in 13 dogs, *J Vet Intern Med* 13:529–533, 1999.

309. Brisson BA, Reggeti F, Bienzle D: Portal site metastasis of invasive mesothelioma after diagnostic thoracoscopy in a dog, *J Am Vet Med Assoc* 229:980–983, 2006.

310. Atencia S, Doyle RS, Whitley NT: Thoracoscopic pericardial window for management of pericardial effusion in 15 dogs, *J Small Anim Pract* 54:564–569, 2013.

311. Case JB, Maxwell M, Aman A, et al.: Outcome evaluation of a thoracoscopic pericardial window procedure or subtotal pericardectomy via thoracotomy for the treatment of pericardial effusion in dogs, *J Am Vet Med Assoc* 242:493–498, 2013.

312. Brooks AC, Hardie RJ: Use of the PleuralPort device for management of pleural effusion in six dogs and four cats, *Vet Surg* 40:935–941, 2011.

313. Moore AS, Kirk C, Cardona A: Intracavitary cisplatin chemotherapy experience with six dogs, *J Vet Intern Med* 5:227–231, 1991.

314. Sparkes A, Murphy S, McConnell F, et al.: Palliative intracavitary carboplatin therapy in a cat with suspected pleural mesothelioma, *J Feline Med Surg* 7:313–316, 2005.

315. Spugnini EP, Crispi S, Scarabello A, et al.: Piroxicam and intracavitary platinum-based chemotherapy for the treatment of advanced mesothelioma in pets: preliminary observations, *J Exp Clin Cancer Res* 27(6), 2008.

316. Seo KW, Choi US, Jung YC, et al.: Palliative intravenous cisplatin treatment for concurrent peritoneal and pleural mesothelioma in a dog, *J Vet Med Sci* 69:201–204, 2007.

317. Campbell NP, Kindler HL: Update on malignant pleural mesothelioma, *Semin Respir Crit Care Med* 32:102–110, 2011.

318. Noonan CW: Environmental asbestos exposure and risk of mesothelioma, *Ann Transl Med* 5:234, 2017.

319. Wang S, Ma K, Wang Q, et al.: The revised staging system for malignant pleural mesothelioma based on surveillance, epidemiology, and end results database, *Int J Surg* 48:92–98, 2017.

320. Pass HI, Goparaju C, Espin-Garcia O, et al.: Plasma biomarker enrichment of clinical prognostic indices in malignant pleural mesothelioma, *J Thorac Oncol* 11:900–909, 2016.

321. Katzman D, Sterman DH: Updates in the diagnosis and treatment of malignant pleural mesothelioma, *Curr Opin Pulm Med*, 2018. https://doi.org/10.1097/MCP.0000000000000489. epub ahead of print.

322. Kapeles M, Gensheimer MF, Mart DA, et al.: Trimodality treatment of malignant pleural mesothelioma: an institutional review, *Am J Clin Oncol* 41:30–35, 2018.

323. Ware WA, Hopper DL: Cardiac tumors in dogs: 1982–1995, *J Vet Intern Med* 13:95–103, 1999.

324. Walter JH, Rudolph R: Systemic, metastatic, eu- and heterotope tumours of the heart in necropsied dogs, *Zentralbl Veterinarmed A* 43:31–45, 1996.

325. Girard C, Hélie P, Odin M: Intrapericardial neoplasia in dogs, *J Diagn Invest* 11:73–78, 1999.

326. Aupperle H, März I, Ellenberger C, et al.: Primary and secondary heart tumours in dogs and cats, *J Comp Pathol* 136:18–26, 2007.

327. Treggiari E, Pedro B, Dukes-McEwan J, et al.: A descriptive review of cardiac tumours in dogs and cats, *Vet Comp Oncol* 15:273–288, 2017.

328. Massimo V, Rossella T, Federica R, et al.: Whole body computed tomographic characteristics of skeletal and cardiac muscular metastatic neoplasia in dogs and cats, *Vet Radiol Ultrasound* 54:223–230, 2013.

329. Janus I, Nowak M, Noszczyk-Nowak A, et al.: Epidemiological and pathological features of primary cardiac tumours in dogs from Poland in 1970-2014, *Acta Vet Hung* 64:90–102, 2016.

330. Aronsohn M: Cardiac hemangiosarcoma in the dog: a review of 38 cases, *J Am Vet Med Assoc* 187:922–926, 1985.

331. Yamamoto S, Hoshi K, Hirakawa A, et al.: Epidemiological, clinical and pathological features of primary cardiac hemangiosarcoma in dogs: a review of 51 cases, *J Vet Med Sci* 75:1433–1441, 2013.

332. Weisse C, Soares N, Beal MW, et al.: Survival times in dogs with right atrial hemangiosarcoma treated by means of surgical resection with or without adjuvant chemotherapy: 23 cases (1986–2000), *J Am Vet Med Assoc* 226:575–579, 2005.

333. Hayes HM: An hypothesis for the aetiology of canine chemoreceptor system neoplasms, based upon an epidemiological study of 73 cases among hospital patients, *J Small Anim Pract* 16:337–343, 1975.

334. Patnaik AK, Liu S-K, Hurvitz AI, et al.: Canine chemodectoma (extra-adrenal paragangliomas)-a comparative study, *J Small Anim Pract* 16:785–801, 1975.

335. Noszczyk-Nowak A, Nowak M, Paslawska U, et al.: Cases with manifestation of chemodectoma diagnosed in dogs in Department of Internal Diseases with Horses, Dogs and Cats Clinic, Veterinary Medicine Faculty, University of Environmental and Life Sciences, Wroclaw, Poland, *Acta Vet Scand* 52, 2010.

336. Vicari ED, Brown DC, Holt DE, et al.: Survival times of and prognostic indicators for dogs with heart base masses: 25 cases (1986–1999), *J Am Vet Med Assoc* 219:485–487, 2001.

337. Ehrhart N, Ehrhart EJ, Willis J, et al.: Analysis of factors affecting survival in dogs with aortic body tumors, *Vet Surg* 31:44–48, 2002.

338. Ware WA: Cardiac neoplasia. In Kirk RW, Bonagura JD, editors: *Kirk's current veterinary therapy XII*, Philadelphia, 1995, WB Saunders, pp 873–876.

339. Amati M, Venco L, Roccabianca P, et al.: Pericardial lymphoma in seven cats, *J Feline Med Surg* 16:507–512, 2014.

340. Carter TD, Pariaut R, Snook E, et al.: Multicentric lymphoma mimicking decompensated hypertrophic cardiomyopathy in a cat, *J Vet Intern Med* 22:1345–1347, 2008.

341. Hansen Sonya C, Smith Annette N, Kuo Kendon W, et al.: Metastatic neuroendocrine carcinoma of aortic body origin in a cat, *Vet Clin Pathol* 45:490–494, 2016.

342. Willis R, Williams AE, Schwarz T, et al.: Aortic body chemodectoma causing pulmonary oedema in a cat, *J Small Anim Pract* 42:20–23, 2008.

343. Paltrinieri S, Riccaboni P, Rondena M, et al.: Pathologic and immunohistochemical findings in a feline aortic body tumor, *Vet Pathol* 41:195–198, 2004.

344. Tilley LP, Bond B, Patnaik AK, et al.: Cardiovascular tumors in the cat, *J Am Anim Hosp Assoc* 17:1009–1021, 1981.

345. Merlo M, Bo S, Ratto A: Primary right atrium haemangiosarcoma in a cat, *J Feline Med Surg* 4:61–64, 2002.

346. George C, Steinberg H: An aortic body carcinoma with multifocal thoracic metastases in a cat, *J Comp Pathol* 101:467–469, 1989.

347. Berg J: Pericardial disease and cardiac neoplasia, *Semin Vet Med Surg (Small Anim)* 9:185–191, 1994.

348. MacGregor JM, Faria MLE, Moore AS, et al.: Cardiac lymphoma and pericardial effusion in dogs: 12 cases (1994–2004), *J Am Vet Med Assoc* 227:1449–1453, 2005.

349. Stern JA, Tobias JR, Keene BW: Complete atrioventricular block secondary to cardiac lymphoma in a dog, *J Vet Cardiol* 14:537–539, 2012.

350. Sims CS, Tobias AH, Hayden DW, et al.: Pericardial effusion due to primary cardiac lymphosarcoma in a dog, *J Vet Intern Med* 17:923–927, 2003.

351. Bracha S, Caron I, Holmberg DL, et al.: Ectopic thyroid carcinoma causing right ventricular outflow tract obstruction in a dog, *J Am Anim Hosp Assoc* 45:138–141, 2009.

352. Boes K, Messick J, Green H, et al.: What is your diagnosis? Impression smear from an intracardiac mass in a dog, *Vet Clin Pathol* 39:119–120, 2010.

353. Kang M-H, Kim D-Y, Park H-M: Ectopic thyroid carcinoma infiltrating the right atrium of the heart in a dog, *Can Vet J* 53:177–181, 2012.

354. Rioja E, Beaulieu K, Holmberg DL: Anesthetic management of an off-pump open-heart surgery in a dog, *Vet Anaesth Analg* 36:361–368, 2009.

355. Ridge L, Swinney G: Angiotrophic intravascular lymphosarcoma presenting as bi–cavity effusion in a dog, *Aust Vet J* 82:616–618, 2004.

356. Karlin ET, Yang VK, Prabhakar M, et al.: Extracardiac intrapericardial myxosarcoma causing right ventricular outflow tract obstruction in a dog, *J Vet Cardiol* 20:129–135, 2018.

357. Yamamoto S, Fukushima R, Kobayashi M, et al.: Mixed form of pericardial mesothelioma with osseous differentiation in a dog, *J Comp Pathol* 149:229–232, 2013.

358. Southerland EM, Miller RT, Jones CL: Primary right atrial chondrosarcoma in a dog, *J Am Vet Med Assoc* 203:1697–1698, 1993.

359. Bright JM, Toal RL, Blackford LM: Right ventricular outflow obstruction caused by primary cardiac neoplasia, *J Vet Intern Med* 4:12–16, 1990.

360. Brower A, Herold LV, Kirby BM: Canine cardiac mesothelioma with granular cell morphology, *Vet Pathol* 43:384–387, 2006.

361. Adissu HA, Hayes G, Wood GA, et al.: Cardiac myxosarcoma with adrenal adenoma and pituitary hyperplasia resembling carney complex in a dog, *Vet Pathol* 47:354–357, 2010.

362. Beal MW, McGuire LD, Langohr IM: Axillary artery tumor embolism secondary to mitral valve myxosarcoma in a dog, *J Vet Emerg Crit Care* 24:751–758, 2014.

363. Hsieh BM, Cohen M, Levitzke B, et al.: What is your diagnosis? Low-grade myxosarcoma arising from the heart valve, *J Am Vet Med Assoc* 242:1067–1068, 2013.

364. Briggs OM, Kirberger RM, Goldberg NB: Right atrial myxosarcoma in a dog, *J S Afr Vet Assoc* 68:144–146, 1997.

365. Foale RD, White RAS, Harley R, et al.: Left ventricular myxosarcoma in a dog, *J Small Anim Pract* 44:503–507, 2006.

366. Worley DR, Orton EC, Kroner KT: Inflow venous occlusion for intracardiac resection of an occluding right ventricular tumor, *J Am Anim Hosp Assoc* 52:259–264, 2016.

367. Dupuy-Mateos A, Wotton PR, Blunden AS, et al.: Primary cardiac chondrosarcoma in a paced dog, *Vet Rec* 163:272, 2008.

368. Caro-Vadillo A, Pizarro-Díaz M, Martínez-Merlo E, et al.: Clinical and pathological features of a cardiac chondrosarcoma in a dog, *Vet Rec* 155:678, 2004.

369. Asakawa MG, Ames MK, Kim Y: Primary cardiac spindle cell tumor in a dog, *Can Vet J* 54:672–674, 2013.

370. Speltz MC, Manivel JC, Tobias AH, et al.: Primary cardiac fibrosarcoma with pulmonary metastasis in a Labrador retriever, *Vet Pathol* 44:403–407, 2007.

371. Madarame H, Sato K, Ogihara K, et al.: Primary cardiac fibrosarcoma in a dog, *J Vet Med Sci* 66:979–982, 2004.

372. Wohlsein P, Cichowski S, Baumgärtner W: Primary endocardial malignant spindle-cell sarcoma in the right atrium of a dog resembling a malignant peripheral nerve sheath tumour, *J Comp Pathol* 132:340–345, 2005.

373. Fries R, Achen S, O'Brien MT, et al.: Primary cardiac tumor presenting as left ventricular outflow obstruction and complex arrhythmia, *J Vet Cardiol* 19:441–447, 2017.

374. Gómez-Laguna J, Barranco I, Rodríguez-Gómez IM, et al.: Malignant mesenchymoma of the heart base in a dog with infiltration of the pericardium and metastasis to the lung, *J Comp Pathol* 147:195–198, 2012.

375. Machida N, Kobayashi M, Tanaka R, et al.: Primary malignant mixed mesenchymal tumour of the heart in a dog, *J Comp Pathol* 128:71–74, 2003.

376. Timian J, Yoshimoto SK, Bruyette DS: Extraskeletal osteosarcoma of the heart presenting as infective endocarditis, *J Am Anim Hosp Assoc* 47:129–132, 2011.

377. Sato T, Shibuya H, Suzuki K, et al.: Extraskeletal osteosarcoma in the pericardium of a dog, *Vet Rec* 155:780, 2004.

378. LaRock RG, Ginn PE, Burrows CF, et al.: Primary mesenchymal chondrosarcoma in the pericardium of a dog, *J Vet Diagn Invest* 9:410–413, 1997.

379. Perez J, Perez-Rivero A, Montoya A, et al.: Right-sided heart failure in a dog with primary cardiac rhabdomyosarcoma, *J Am Anim Hosp Assoc* 34:208–211, 1998.

380. Sanford SE, Hoover DM, Miller RB: Primary cardiac granular cell tumor in a dog, *Vet Pathol* 21:489–494, 1984.

381. Krotje LJ, Ware WA, Niyo Y: Intracardiac rhabdomyosarcoma in a dog, *J Am Vet Med Assoc* 197:368–371, 1990.

382. Vicini DS, Didier PJ, Ogilvie GK: Cardiac fibrosarcoma in a dog, *J Am Vet Med Assoc* 189:1486–1488, 1986.

383. Almes KM, Heaney AM, Andrews GA: Intracardiac ectopic thyroid carcinosarcoma in a dog, *Vet Pathol* 45:500–504, 2008.

384. Fews D, Scase TJ, Battersby IA: Leiomyosarcoma of the pericardium, with epicardial metastases and peripheral eosinophilia in a dog, *J Comp Pathol* 138:224–228, 2008.

385. Cobb MA, Brownlie SE: Intrapericardial neoplasia in 14 dogs, *J Small Anim Pract* 33:309–316, 1992.

386. de Nijs MI, Vink A, Bergmann W, et al.: Left ventricular cardiac myxoma and sudden death in a dog, *Acta Vet Scand* 58:41, 2016.

387. Fernandez-del Palacio MJ, Sanchez J, Talavera J, et al.: Left ventricular inflow tract obstruction secondary to a myxoma in a dog, *J Am Anim Hosp Assoc* 47:217–223, 2011.

388. Akkoc A, Ozyigit MO, Cangul IT: Valvular cardiac myxoma in a dog, *J Vet Med A Physiol Pathol Clin Med* 54:356–358, 2007.

389. Machida N, Hoshi K, Kobayashi M, et al.: Cardiac myxoma of the tricuspid valve in a dog, *J Comp Pathol* 129:320–324, 2003.

390. Brambilla Paola G, Roccabianca P, Locatelli C, et al.: Primary cardiac lipoma in a dog, *J Vet Intern Med* 20:691–693, 2008.

391. Ben–Amotz R, Ellison GW, Thompson MS, et al.: Pericardial lipoma in a geriatric dog with an incidentally discovered thoracic mass, *J Small Anim Pract* 48:596–599, 2007.

392. Kolm US, Kleiter M, Kosztolich A, et al.: Benign intrapericardial lipoma in a dog, *J Vet Cardiol* 4:25–29, 2002.

393. Simpson DJ, Hunt GB, Church DB, et al.: Benign masses in the pericardium of two dogs, *Aust Vet J* 77:225–229, 1999.

394. Di Palma S, Lombard C, Kappeler A, et al.: Intracardiac ectopic thyroid adenoma in a dog, *Vet Rec* 167:709, 2010.

395. Machida N, Katsuda S, Yamamura H, et al.: Myocardial hamartoma of the right atrium in a dog, *J Comp Pathol* 127:297–300, 2002.

396. Tjostheim SS, Kellihan HB, Csomos RA, et al.: Vascular hamartoma in the right ventricle of a dog: Diagnosis and treatment, *J Vet Cardiol* 17:321–328, 2015.

397. Thomason JD, Rapoport G, Fallaw T, et al.: Pulmonary edema secondary to a cardiac schwannoma in a dog, *J Vet Cardiol* 17:149–153, 2015.

398. Gallay J, Bélanger MC, Hélie P, et al.: Cardiac leiomyoma associated with advanced atrioventricular block in a young dog, *J Vet Cardiol* 3:71–77, 2011.

399. Lombard CW, Goldschmidt MH: Primary fibroma in the right atrium of a dog, *J Small Anim Pract* 21:439–448, 1980.

400. Hilbe M, Hauser B, Zlinszky K, et al.: Haemangiosarcoma with a metastasis of a malignant mixed mammary gland tumour in a dog, *J Vet Med A Physiol Pathol Clin Med* 49:443–444, 2002.

401. Ogilvie GK, Brunkow CS, Daniel GB, et al.: Malignant lymphoma with cardiac and bone involvement in a dog, *J Am Vet Med Assoc* 194:793–796, 1989.

402. Lowe AD: Alimentary lymphosarcoma in a 4-year-old Labrador retriever, *Can Vet J* 45:610–612, 2004.

403. Wilkerson MJ, Dolce K, DeBey BM, et al.: Metastatic balloon cell melanoma in a dog, *Vet Clin Pathol* 32:31–36, 2003.

404. Sabocanec R, Culjak K, Vrbanac L, et al.: A case of metastasizing ovarian granulosa cell tumour in the myocardium of a bitch, *Acta Vet Hung* 44:189–194, 1996.

405. Uno Y, Momoi Y, Watari T, et al.: Malignant histiocytosis with multiple skin lesions in a dog, *J Vet Med Sci* 55:1059–1061, 1993.

406. Sako T, Kitamura N, Kagawa Y, et al.: Immunohistochemical evaluation of a malignant pheochromocytoma in a wolfdog, *Vet Pathol* 38:447–450, 2001.

407. Guglielmini C, Civitella C, Malatesta D, et al.: Metastatic pericardial tumors in a dog with equivocal pericardial cytological findings, *J Am Anim Hosp Assoc* 43:284–287, 2007.

408. Weishaar KM, Edmondson EF, Thamm DH, et al.: Malignant mesenchymoma with widespread metastasis including bone marrow involvement in a dog, *Vet Clin Pathol* 43:447–452, 2014.

409. Akkoc A, Ozyigit MO, Yilmaz R, et al.: Cardiac metastasising rhabdomyosarcoma in a great Dane, *Vet Rec* 158:803, 2006.

410. Ramoo S: Hypertrophic osteopathy associated with two pulmonary tumours and myocardial metastases in a dog: a case report, *N Z Vet J* 61:45–48, 2013.

411. Wang FI, Liang SL, Eng HL, et al.: Disseminated liposarcoma in a dog, *J Vet Diagn Invest* 17:291–294, 2005.

412. Shih JL, Brenn S, Schrope DP: Cardiac involvement secondary to mediastinal lymphoma in a cat: regression with chemotherapy, *J Vet Cardiol* 16:115–120, 2014.

413. Less R, Bright J, Orton E: Intrapericardial cyst causing cardiac tamponade in a cat, *J Am Anim Hosp Assoc* 36:115–119, 2000.

414. Sarah MS, Janice MB: Chronic cardiac tamponade in a cat caused by an intrapericardial biliary cyst, *J Feline Med Surg* 12:338–340, 2010.

415. Kobayashi R, Ohsaki Y, Yasuno K, et al.: A malignant and metastasizing feline cardiac ganglioneuroma, *J Vet Diagn Invest* 24:412–417, 2012.

416. Venco L, Kramer L, Sola LB, et al.: Primary cardiac rhabdomyosarcoma in a cat, *J Am Anim Hosp Assoc* 37:159–163, 2001.

417. Campbell MD, Gelberg HB: Endocardial ossifying myxoma of the right atrium in a cat, *Vet Pathol* 37:460–462, 2000.

418. Klausner JS, Bell FW, Hayden DW, et al.: Hypercalcemia in two cats with squamous cell carcinomas, *J Am Vet Med Assoc* 196:103–105, 1990.

419. Shaw TE, Harkin KR, Nietfeld J, et al.: Aortic body tumor in full-sibling English bulldogs, *J Am Anim Hosp Assoc* 46:366–370, 2010.

420. Rancilio NJ, Higuchi T, Gagnon J, et al.: Use of three-dimensional conformal radiation therapy for treatment of a heart base chemodectoma in a dog, *J Am Vet Med Assoc* 241:472–476, 2012.

421. Cote E, MacDonald KA, Meurs KM, et al.: Cardiac neoplasia. In Cote E, MacDonald KA, Meurs KM, et al., editors: *Feline cardiology*, ed 1, West Sussex, UK, 2011, John Wiley & Sons, pp 201–204.

422. Pedro B, Linney C, Navarro-Cubas X, et al.: Cytological diagnosis of cardiac masses with ultrasound guided fine needle aspirates, *J Vet Cardiol* 18:47–56, 2016.

423. Nelson OL, Ware WA: Pericardial effusion. In Bonagura JD, Twedt DC, editors: *Kirk's current veterinary therapy XV*, Philadelphia, 2014, WB Saunders, pp 816–823.

424. Im M, Stern JA: ECG of the month, *J Am Vet Med Assoc* 248:497–500, 2016.

425. Holt D, Van Winkle T, Schelling C, et al.: Correlation between thoracic radiographs and postmortem findings in dogs with hemangiosarcoma: 77 cases (1984-1989), *J Am Vet Med Assoc* 200:1535–1539, 1992.

426. Gidlewski J, Petrie JP: Pericardiocentesis and principles of echocardiographic imaging in the patient with cardiac neoplasia, *Clin Tech Small Anim Pract* 18:131–134, 2003.

427. Thomas WP, Sisson D, Bauer TG, et al.: Detection of cardiac masses in dogs by two-dimensional echocardiography, *Vet Radiol* 25:65–72, 1984.

428. Fruchter AM, Miller CW, O'Grady MR: Echocardiographic results and clinical considerations in dogs with right atrial/auricular masses, *Can Vet J* 33:171–174, 1992.

429. MacDonald KA, Cagney O, Magne ML: Echocardiographic and clinicopathologic characterization of pericardial effusion in dogs: 107 cases (1985-2006), *J Am Vet Med Assoc* 235:1456–1461, 2009.

430. Rajagopalan V, Jesty SA, Craig LE, et al.: Comparison of presumptive echocardiographic and definitive diagnoses of cardiac tumors in dogs, *J Vet Intern Med* 27:1092–1096, 2013.

431. Rush JE, Keene BW, Fox PR: Pericardial disease in the cat: a retrospective evaluation of 66 cases, *J Am Anim Hosp Assoc* 26:39–46, 1990.

432. De Rycke LM, Gielen IM, Simoens PJ, et al.: Computed tomography and cross-sectional anatomy of the thorax in clinically normal dogs, *Am J Vet Res* 66:512–524, 2005.

433. Mai W, Weisse C, Sleeper Meg M: Cardiac magnetic resonance imaging in normal dogs and two dogs with heart base tumor, *Vet Radiol Ultrasound* 51:428–435, 2010.

434. Hansen AE, McEvoy F, Engelholm SA, et al.: FDG PET/CT imaging in canine cancer patients, *Vet Radiol Ultrasound* 52:201–206, 2011.

435. Naude SH, Miller DB: Magnetic resonance imaging findings of a metastatic chemodectoma in a dog, *J S Afr Vet Assoc* 77:155–159, 2006.

436. Nolan MW, Arkans MM, LaVine D, et al.: Pilot study to determine the feasibility of radiation therapy for dogs with right atrial masses and hemorrhagic pericardial effusion, *J Vet Cardiol* 19:132–143, 2017.

437. Keene BW, Rush JE, Cooley AJ, et al.: Primary left ventricular hemangiosarcoma diagnosed by endomyocardial biopsy in a dog, *J Am Vet Med Assoc* 197:1501–1503, 1990.

438. Sisson D, Thomas WP, Ruehl WW, et al.: Diagnostic value of pericardial fluid analysis in the dog, *J Am Vet Med Assoc* 184:51–55, 1984.

439. Fine DM, Tobias AH, Jacob KA: Use of pericardial fluid pH to distinguish between idiopathic and neoplastic effusions, *J Vet Intern Med* 17:525–529, 2003.

440. de Laforcade AM, Freeman LM, Rozanski EA, et al.: Biochemical analysis of pericardial fluid and whole blood in dogs with pericardial effusion, *J Vet Intern Med* 19:833–836, 2005.

441. Cagle LA, Epstein SE, Owens SD, et al.: Diagnostic yield of cytologic analysis of pericardial effusion in dogs, *J Vet Intern Med* 28:66–71, 2014.

442. Shaw SP, Rozanski EA, Rush JE: Cardiac troponins I and T in dogs with pericardial effusion, *J Vet Intern Med* 18:322–324, 2004.

443. Chun R, Kellihan HB, Henik RA, et al.: Comparison of plasma cardiac troponin I concentrations among dogs with cardiac hemangiosarcoma, noncardiac hemangiosarcoma, other neoplasms, and pericardial effusion of nonhemangiosarcoma origin, *J Am Vet Med Assoc* 237:806–811, 2010.

444. Boston SE, Higginson G, Monteith G: Concurrent splenic and right atrial mass at presentation in dogs with hemangiosarcoma: a retrospective study, *J Am An Hosp Assoc* 47:336–341, 2011.

445. Waters DJ, Caywood DD, Hayden DW, et al.: Metastatic pattern in dogs with splenic haemangiosarcoma: clinical implications, *J Small Anim Pract* 29:805–814, 1988.

446. Chow N-H, Chan S-H, Tzai T-S, et al.: Expression profiles of ErbB family receptors and prognosis in primary transitional cell carcinoma of the urinary bladder, *Clin Cancer Research* 7:1957–1962, 2001.

447. Taylor S, Rozanski E, Sato AF, et al.: Vascular stent placement for palliation of mass-associated chylothorax in two dogs, *J Am Vet Med Assoc* 251:696–701, 2017.

448. Wykes PM, Rouse GP, Orton EC: Removal of five canine cardiac tumors using a stapling instrument, *Vet Surg* 15:103–106, 1986.

449. Ogilvie GK, Powers BE, Mallinckrodt CH, et al.: Surgery and doxorubicin in dogs with hemangiosarcoma, *J Vet Intern Med* 10:379–384, 1996.

450. Verbeke F, Binst D, Stegen L, et al.: Total venous inflow occlusion and pericardial auto-graft reconstruction for right atrial hemangiosarcoma resection in a dog, *Can Vet J* 53:1114–1118, 2012.

451. Morges M, Worley DR, Withrow SJ, et al.: Pericardial free patch grafting as a rescue technique in surgical management of right atrial HSA, *J Am Anim Hosp Assoc* 47:224–228, 2011.

452. Crumbaker DM, Rooney MB, Case JB: Thoracoscopic subtotal pericardiectomy and right atrial mass resection in a dog, *J Am Vet Med Assoc* 237:551–554, 2010.

453. Buchanan JW, Boggs LS, Dewan S, et al.: Left atrial paraganglioma in a dog: echocardiography, surgery, and scintigraphy, *J Vet Intern Med* 12:109–115, 1998.

454. Dunning D, Monnet E, Orton EC, et al.: Analysis of prognostic indicators for dogs with pericardial effusion: 46 cases (1985-1996), *J Am Vet Med Assoc* 212:1276–1280, 1998.

455. Case JB, Maxwell M, Aman A, et al.: Outcome evaluation of a thoracoscopic pericardial window procedure or subtotal pericardectomy via thoracotomy for the treatment of pericardial effusion in dogs, *J Am Vet Med Assoc* 242:493–498, 2013.

456. Atencia S, Doyle RS, Whitley NT: Thoracoscopic pericardial window for management of pericardial effusion in 15 dogs, *J Small Anim Pract* 54:564–569, 2013.

457. Ployart S, Libermann S, Doran I, et al.: Thoracoscopic resection of right auricular masses in dogs: 9 cases (2003–2011), *J Am Vet Med Assoc* 242:237–241, 2012.

458. Mullin CM, Arkans MA, Sammarco CD, et al.: Doxorubicin chemotherapy for presumptive cardiac hemangiosarcoma in dogs, *Vet Comp Oncol* 14:e171–e183, 2016.

459. Ghaffari S, Pelio DC, Lange AJ, et al.: A retrospective evaluation of doxorubicin-based chemotherapy for dogs with right atrial masses and pericardial effusion, *J Small Anim Pract* 55:254–257, 2014.

460. Pellin MA, Wouda RM, Robinson K, et al.: Safety evaluation of combination doxorubicin and toceranib phosphate (Palladia®) in tumour bearing dogs: a phase I dose–finding study, *Vet Comp Oncol* 15:919–931, 2016.

461. de Madron E, Helfand SC, Stebbins KE: Use of chemotherapy for treatment of cardiac hemangiosarcoma in a dog, *J Am Vet Med Assoc* 190:887–891, 1987.

462. Murphy LA, Panek CM, Bianco D, et al.: Use of Yunnan Baiyao and epsilon aminocaproic acid in dogs with right atrial masses and pericardial effusion, *J Vet Emerg Crit Care* 27:121–126, 2017.

463. McQuown B, Arteaga T, Cunningham S, et al.: Palladia (toceranib phosphate) in the treatment of heart base tumors, *Vet Cancer Soc Ann Conf*, 2014.

464. Obradovich JE, Withrow SJ, Powers BE, et al.: Carotid body tumors in the dog eleven cases (1978–1988), *J Vet Intern Med* 6:96–101, 1992.

465. Kelsey KL, Kubicek LN, Bacon NJ, et al.: Neuromuscular blockade and inspiratory breath hold during stereotactic body radiation therapy for treatment of heart base tumors in four dogs, *J Am Vet Med Assoc* 250:199–204, 2017.

466. Reynen K: Frequency of primary tumors of the heart, *Am J Cardiol* 77:107, 1996.

467. Lam KY, Dickens P, Chan AC: Tumors of the heart. A 20-year experience with a review of 12,485 consecutive autopsies, *Arch Pathol Lab Med* 117:1027–1031, 1993.

468. McAllister HA, Hall RJ, Cooley DA: Tumors of the heart and pericardium, *Curr Probl Cardiol* 24:59–116, 1999.

469. Shapiro LM: Cardiac tumours: diagnosis and management, *Heart* 85:218–222, 2001.

470. Jóźwiak S, Kotulska K, Kasprzyk-Obara J, et al.: Clinical and genotype studies of cardiac tumors in 154 patients with tuberous sclerosis complex, *Pediatrics* 118:e1146–e1151, 2006.

471. Sciacca P, Giacchi V, Mattia C, et al.: Rhabdomyomas and tuberous sclerosis complex: our experience in 33 cases, *BMC Cardiovasc Disord* 14, 66–66, 2014.

472. Saad AM, Abushouk AI, Al-Husseini MJ, et al.: Characteristics, survival and incidence rates and trends of primary cardiac malignancies in the United States, *Cardiovasc Pathol* 33:27–31, 2018.

473. Ramlawi B, Leja MJ, Abu Saleh WK, et al.: Surgical treatment of primary cardiac sarcomas: review of a single-institution experience, *Ann Thorac Surg* 101:698–702, 2016.

474. Bakaeen FG, Reardon MJ, Coselli JS, et al.: Surgical outcome in 85 patients with primary cardiac tumors, *Am J Surg* 186:641–647, 2003.

475. Llombart-Cussac A, Pivot X, Contesso G, et al.: Adjuvant chemotherapy for primary cardiac sarcomas: the IGR experience, *Br J Cancer* 78:1624–1628, 1998.

476. Abu Saleh WK, Ramlawi B, Shapira OM, et al.: Improved outcomes with the evolution of a neoadjuvant chemotherapy approach to right heart sarcoma, *Ann Thorac Surg* 104:90–96, 2017.

477. Bussani R, De–Giorgio F, Abbate A, et al.: Cardiac metastases, *J Clin Pathol* 60:27–34, 2007.

478. Moore PF: A review of histiocytic diseases in dogs and cats, *Vet Pathol* 51:167–184, 2014.

479. Affolter VK, Moore PF: Canine cutaneous and systemic histiocytosis of dermal and dendritic origin, *Am J Dermatopathol* 22:40–48, 2000.

480. Affolter VK, Moore PF: Localized and disseminated histiocytic sarcoma of dendritic cell origin in dogs, *Vet Pathol* 39:74–83, 2002.

481. Moore PF, Affolter V, Olivry T, et al.: The use of immunological reagents in defining the pathogenesis of canine skin disease involving proliferation of leukocytes. In Kwochka KW, Wilemse T, von Tscharner C, editors: *Advances in veterinary dermatology*, Oxford, 1998, Butterworth-Heinemann, pp 77–94.

482. Moore PF, Schrenzel MD, Affolter VK, et al.: Canine cutaneous histiocytoma is an epidermotropic Langerhans cell histiocytosis that expresses CD1 and specific beta 2-integrin molecules, *Am J Pathol* 148:1699–1708, 1996.

483. Moore PF, Affolter VK, Vernau W, et al.: Canine hemophagocytic histiocytic sarcoma: a proliferative disorder of CD11d+ macrophages, *Vet Pathol* 43:632–645, 2006.

484. Shortman K, Naik SH: Steady-state and inflammatory dendritic-cell development, *Nat Rev Immunol* 7:19–30, 2007.

485. Larregina at, Morelli AE, Spencer LA, et al.: Dermal-resident CD14+ cells differentiate into Langerhans cells, *Nat Immunol* 2:1151–1158, 2001.

486. Shortman K, Caux C: Dendritic cell development: multiple pathways to nature's adjuvants, *Stem Cells* 15:409–419, 1997.

487. Shortman K, Liu YJ: Mouse and human dendritic cell subtypes, *Nat Rev Immunol* 2:151–161, 2002.

488. Ricklin ME, Roosje P, Summerfield A: Characterization of canine dendritic cells in healthy, atopic, and non-allergic inflamed skin, *J Clin Immunol* 30:845–854, 2010.

489. Zaba LC, Krueger JG, Lowes MA: Resident and "inflammatory" dendritic cells in human skin, *J Invest Dermatol* 129:302–308, 2009.

490. Looringh van Beeck FA, Zajonc DM, Moore PF, et al.: Two canine CD1a proteins are differentially expressed in skin, *Immunogenetics* 60:315–324, 2008.

491. Danilenko DM, Moore PF, Rossitto PV: Canine leukocyte cell adhesion molecules (LeuCAMS): characterization of the CD11/CD18 family, *Tiss Antig* 40:13–21, 1992.

492. Danilenko DM, Rossitti PV, Van der Vieren M, et al.: A novel canine leukointegrin, alpha d beta 2, is expressed by specific macrophage subpopulations in tissue and a minor CD8+ lymphocyte subpopulation in peripheral blood, *J Immunol* 155:35–44, 1995.

493. Ricklin ME, Roosje P, Summerfield A: Characterization of canine dendritic cells in healthy, atopic, and non-allergic inflamed skin, *J Clin Immunol* 30:845–854, 2010.

494. Scalapino KJ, Daikh DI: CTLA-4: a key regulatory point in the control of autoimmune disease, *Immunol Rev* 223:143–155, 2008.

495. Banchereau J, Steinman RM: Dendritic cells and the control of immunity, *Nature* 392:245–252, 1998.

496. Banchereau J, Briere F, Caux C, et al.: Immunology of dendritic cells, *Ann Rev Immunol* 18:767–811, 2000.

497. Swerdlow SH, Campo E, et al.: *WHO classification of tumors of the haematopoietic and lymphoid tissues*, Lyon, 2008, International Agency for Research on Cancer (IARC).

498. Valli VEO: Histological classification of hematopoietic tumors of domestic animals. In Valli VEO, R Jacobs RM, et al.: *World health organization international histological classification of tumors of domestic animals*, Washington, D.C., 2002, Armed Forces Institute of Pathology, American Registry of Pathology.

499. Kato Y, Murakami M, Hoshino Y, et al.: The class A macrophage scavenger receptor CD204 is a useful immunohistochemical marker of canine histiocytic sarcoma, *J Comp Pathol* 148:188–196, 2013.

500. Marquet FM, Bonneau F, Pascale C, et al.: Characterization of dendritic cells subpopulations in skin and afferent lymph in the swine model, *PLoS One* 6:e16320, 2011.

501. Yi H, Guo C, Yu X, et al.: Targeting the immunoregulator SRA/CD204 potentiates specific dendritic cell vaccine-induced T-cell response and antitumor immunity, *Cancer Res* 71:6611–6620, 2011.

502. Ide T, Uchida K, Kagawa Y, et al.: Pathological and immunohistochemical features of subdural histiocytic sarcomas in 15 dogs, *J Vet Diagn Invest* 23:127–132, 2011.

503. Schmidt JM, North SM, Freeman KP, et al.: Canine paediatric oncology: retrospective assessment of 9522 tumours in dogs up to 12 months (1993-2008), *Vet Comp Oncol* 8:283–292, 2010.

504. Glick AD, Holscher M, Campbell GR: Canine cutaneous histiocytoma: ultrastructural and cytochemical observations, *Vet Pathol* 13:374–380, 1976.

505. Kelly DF: Canine cutaneous histiocytoma. A light and microscopic study, *Vet Pathol* 7:12–27, 1970.

506. Bostock DE: Neoplasms of the skin and subcutaneous tissues in dogs and cats, *Br Vet J* 142:1–19, 1986.

507. Rothwell TLW, Howlett CR, Middleton DJ, et al.: Skin neoplasms of dogs in Sydney, *Aust Vet J* 64:161–164, 1987.

508. Gross TL, Affolter VK: Advances in skin oncology. In Kwochka KW, Willemse T, von Tscharner C, editors: *Advances in veterinary dermatology*, Oxford, UK, 1998, Butterworth-Heinmann, pp 382–385.

509. Angus JC, de Lorimier LP: Lymphohistiocytic neoplasms. In Campbell KL, editor: *Small animal dermatology secrets*, Philadelphia, 2004, Hanley and Belfus, pp 425–442.

510. Ramos-Vara JA, Miller MA: Immunohistochemical expression of E-cadherin does not distinguish canine cutaneous histiocytoma from other canine round cell tumors, *Vet Pathol* 48:758–763, 2011.

511. Baines SJ, McInnes EF, McConnell I: E-cadherin expression in canine cutaneous histiocytomas, *Vet Rec* 162:509–513, 2008.

512. Pires I, Queiroga FL, Alves A, Silva F, et al.: Decrease of E-cadherin expression in canine cutaneous histiocytoma appears to be related to its spontaneous regression, *Anticancer Res* 29:2713–2717, 2009.

513. Schmitz L, Favara BE: Nosology and pathology of Langerhans cell histiocytosis, *Hematol Oncol Clin North Am* 12:221–246, 1998.

514. Munn S, Chu AC: Langerhans cell histiocytosis of the skin, *Hematol Oncol Clin North Am* 12:269–286, 1998.

515. Maina E, Colombo S, Stefanello D: Multiple cutaneous histiocytomas treated with lomustine in a dog, *Vet Dermatol* 25:559–599, 2014.

516. Nagata M, Hirata M, Ishida T, et al.: Progressive Langerhans' cell histiocytosis in a puppy, *Vet Dermatol* 11:241–246, 2000.

517. Faller M, Lamm C, Affolter VK, et al.: Retrospective characterisation of solitary cutaneous histiocytoma with lymph node metastasis in eight dogs, *J Small Anim Pract* 57:548–552, 2016.

518. Mays MB, Bergeron JA: Cutaneous histiocytosis in dogs, *J Am Vet Med Assoc* 188:377–381, 1986.

519. Palmeiro BS, Morris DO, Goldschmidt MH, et al.: Cutaneous reactive histiocytosis in dogs: a retrospective evaluation of 32 cases, *Vet Dermatol* 18:332–340, 2007.

520. Scott DW, Angurano DK, Suter MM: Systemic histiocytosis in 2 dogs, *Canine Pract* 14:7–12, 1987.

521. Moore PF: Systemic histiocytosis of Bernese mountain dogs, *Vet Pathol* 21:554–563, 1984.

522. Scott DW, Miller WH, Griffin CE: *Lymphohistiocytic neoplasms. Muller and Kirk's small animal dermatology*, Philadelphia, 2000, WB Saunders, pp 1130–1357.

523. Scherlie PH, Smedes SL, Feltz T, et al.: Ocular manifestations of systemic histiocytosis in a dog, *J Am Vet Med Assoc* 201:1229, 1992.

524. DeHeer HL, Grindem CB: Histiocytic disorders. In Jaim NC, editor: *Schalm's veterinary hematology*, ed 4, Philadelphia, 1986, Lea & Febiger, pp 696–702.

525. Moore PF: Malignant histiocytosis of Bernese mountain dogs, *Vet Pathol* 23:1–10, 1986.

526. Rosin A, Moore P, Dubielzig R: Malignant histiocytosis in Bernese mountain dogs, *J Am Vet Med Assoc* 188:1041–1045, 1986.

527. Lenz JA, Furrow E, Craig LE, et al.: Histiocytic sarcoma in 14 miniature schnauzers-a new breed predisposition? *J Small Anim Pract* 58:461–467, 2017.

528. Takahashi M, Tomiyasu H, Hotta E, et al.: Clinical characteristics and prognostic factors in dogs with histiocytic sarcomas in Japan, *J Vet Med Sci* 76:661–666, 2014.

529. Voegeli E, Welle M, Hauser B, et al.: Histiocytic sarcoma in the Swiss population of Bernese mountain dogs: a retrospective study of its genetic predisposition, *Schweiz Arch Tierheilkd* 148:281–288, 2006.

530. Hedan B, Thomas R, Motsinger-Reif A, et al.: Molecular cytogenetic characterization of canine histiocytic sarcoma: a spontaneous model for human histiocytic cancer identifies deletion of tumor suppressor genes and highlights influence of genetic background on tumor behaviour, *BMC Cancer* 11:201, 2011.

531. Shearin AL, Hedan B, Cadieu E, et al.: The MTAP-CDKN2A locus confers susceptibility to a naturally occurring canine cancer, *Cancer Epidemiol Biomarkers Prev* 21:1019–1027, 2012.

532. Thaiwong T, Sirivisoot S, Takada M, et al.: Gain-of-function mutation in PTPN11 in histiocytic sarcomas of Bernese mountain dogs, *Vet Comp Oncol* 16:220–228, 2018.

533. Manor EK, Craig LE, Sun X, et al.: Prior joint disease is associated with increased risk of periarticular histiocytic sarcoma in dogs, *Vet Comp Oncol* 16:E83–E88, 2018.

534. van Kuijk L, van Ginkel K, de Vos JP, et al.: Peri-articular histiocytic sarcoma and previous joint disease in Bernese mountain dogs, *J Vet Intern Med* 27:293–299, 2013.

535. Constantino-Casas F, Mayhew D, Hoather TM, et al.: The clinical presentation and histopathologic–immunohistochemical classification of histiocytic sarcomas in the flat coated retriever, *Vet Pathol* 48:764–771, 2011.

536. Erich SA, Constantino-Casas F, Dobson JM, et al.: Morphological distinction of histiocytic sarcoma from other tumor types in Bernese mountain dogs and flatcoated retrievers, *Vivo* 32:7–17, 2018.

537. Dobson J, Hoather T, McKinley TJ, et al.: Mortality in a cohort of flat-coated retrievers in the UK, *Vet Comp Oncol* 7:115–121, 2009.

538. Craig LE, Julian ME, Ferracone JD: The diagnosis and prognosis of synovial tumors in dogs: 35 cases, *Vet Pathol* 39:66–73, 2002.

539. Hayden DW, Waters DJ, Burke BA, et al.: Disseminated malignant histiocytosis in a golden retriever: clinicopathologic, ultrastructural, and immunohistochemical findings, *Vet Pathol* 30:256–264, 1993.

540. Kohn B, Arnold P, Kaser-Hotz B, et al.: Malignant histiocytosis of the dog: 26 cases (1989-1992), *Kleintierpraxis* 38:409–424, 1993.

541. Fant P, Caldin M, Furlanello T, et al.: Primary gastric histiocytic sarcoma in a dog—a case report, *J Vet Med* 51:358–362, 2004.

542. Skorupski K, Clifford C, Paoloni M, et al.: CCNU for the treatment of dogs with histiocytic sarcoma, *J Vet Int Med* 21:121–126, 2007.

543. Naranjo C, Dubielzig R, Friedrichs K: Canine ocular histiocytic sarcoma, *Vet Ophthalmol* 10:179–185, 2007.

544. Vernau KM, Higgins RJ, Bollen AW, et al.: Primary canine and feline nervous system tumors: intraoperative diagnosis using the smear technique, *Vet Pathol* 38:47–57, 2001.

545. Snyder J, Lipitz L, Skorupski K, et al.: Secondary intracranial neoplasia in the dog: 177 cases (1986-2003), *J Vet Intern Med* 22:172–177, 2008.

546. Mariani CL, Jennings MK, Olby NJ, et al.: Histiocytic sarcoma with central nervous system involvement in dogs: 19 Cases (2006–2012), *J Vet Intern Med* 29:607–613, 2015.

547. Brown DE, Thrall MA, Getzy DM, et al.: Cytology of canine malignant histiocytosis, *Vet Clin Pathol* 23:118–123, 1994.

548. Kato Y, Funato R, Hirata A, et al.: Immunocytochemical detection of the class A macrophage scavenger receptor CD204 using air-dried cytologic smears of canine histiocytic sarcoma, *Vet Clin Pathol* 43:589–593, 2014.

549. Pierezan F, Mansell J, Ambrus A, et al.: Immunohistochemical expression of ionized calcium binding adapter molecule 1 in cutaneous histiocytic proliferative, neoplastic, and inflammatory disorders of dogs and cats, *J Comp Pathol* 151:347–351, 2014.

550. *The CADETSM HM assay*. 2018. Retrieved from: https://www.sentinelbiomedical.com/cadet-hm-for-vets/

551. Weiss DJ, Evanson OA, Sykes J: A retrospective study of canine pancytopenia, *Vet Clin Pathol* 28:83–88, 1999.

552. Newlands CE, Houston DM, Vasconcelos DY: Hyperferritinemia associated with malignant histiocytosis in a dog, *J Am Vet Med Assoc* 205:849–851, 1994.

553. Friedrichs K, Thomas C, Plier M, et al.: Evaluation of serum ferritin as a tumor marker for canine histiocytic sarcoma, *J Vet Intern Med* 24:904–911, 2010.

554. Nielsen LN, McEvoy F, Jessen LR, et al.: Investigation of a screening programme and the possible identification of biomarkers for early disseminated histiocytic sarcoma in Bernese mountain dogs, *Vet Comp Oncol* 10:124–134, 2012.

555. Tsai S, Sutherland-Smith J, Burgess K, et al.: Imaging characteristics of intrathoracic histiocytic sarcoma in dogs, *Vet Radiol Ultrasound* 53:21–27, 2012.

556. Barrett LE, Pollard RE, Zwingenberger A, et al.: Radiographic characterization of primary lung tumors in 74 dogs, *Vet Radiol Ultrasound* 55:480–487, 2014.

557. Cruz-Arambulo R, Wrigley R, Powers B: Sonographic features of histiocytic neoplasms in the canine abdomen, *Vet Radiol Ultrasound* 45:554–558, 2004.

558. Weiss DJ: Flow cytometric evaluation of hemophagocytic disorders in canine, *Vet Clin Pathol* 31:36–41, 2001.

559. Klahn SL, Kitchell B, Dervisis N: Evaluation and comparison of outcomes in dogs with periarticular and nonperiarticular histiocytic sarcoma, *J Am Vet Met Assoc* 239:90–96, 2001.

560. Skorupski K, Rodriguez C, Krick E, et al.: Long-term survival in dogs with localized histiocytic sarcoma treated with CCNU as an adjuvant to local therapy, *Vet Comp Oncol* 7:139–144, 2009.

561. Rassnick K, Moore A, Russell D, et al.: Phase II, open-label trial of single-agent CCNU in dogs with previously untreated histiocytic sarcoma, *J Vet Intern Med* 24:1528–1531, 2010.

562. Cannon C, Borgatti A, Henson M, et al.: Evaluation of a combination chemotherapy protocol including lomustine and doxorubicin in canine histiocytic sarcoma, *J Sm Anim Pract* 56:425–429, 2015.

563. Kezer KA, Barber LG, Jennings SH: Efficacy of dacarbazine as a rescue agent for histiocytic sarcoma in dogs, *Vet Comp Oncol* 16:77–80, 2018.

564. Mason SL, Finotello R, Blackwood L: Epirubicin in the treatment of canine histiocytic sarcoma: sequential, alternating and rescue chemotherapy, *Vet Comp Oncol* 16:E30–E37, 2018.

565. Vail DM, Kravis LD, Cooley AJ, et al.: Preclinical trial of doxorubicin entrapped in sterically stabilized liposomes in dogs with spontaneously arising malignant tumors, *Cancer Chemother Pharmacol* 39:410–416, 1997.

566. Poirier VJ, Hershey AE, Burgess KE, et al.: Efficacy and toxicity of paclitaxel (Taxol) for the treatment of canine malignant tumors, *J Vet Intern Med* 18:219–222, 2004.

567. Uno Y, Momio Y, Watari T, et al.: Malignant histiocytosis with multiple skin lesions in a dog, *J Vet Med Sci* 55:1059–1061, 1993.

568. Tripp CD, Fidel J, Anderson CL, et al.: Tolerability of metronomic administration of lomustine in dogs with cancer, *J Vet Intern Med* 25:278–284, 2011.

569. Leach TN, Childress MO, Greene SN, et al.: Prospective trial of metronomic chlorambucil chemotherapy in dogs with naturally occurring cancer, *Vet Comp Oncol* 10:102–112, 2011.

570. Hafeman S, London C, Elmslie R, et al.: Evaluation of liposomal clodronate for treatment of malignant histiocytosis in dogs, *Cancer Immunol Immunother* 59:441–452, 2010.

571. Fidel J, Schiller I, Hauser Y, et al.: Histiocytic sarcomas in flat-coated retrievers: a summary of 37 cases (November 1998-March 2005), *Vet Comp Oncol* 4:63–74, 2006.

572. Friedrichs K, Young K: Histiocytic sarcoma of macrophage origin in a cat: case report with a literature review of feline histiocytic malignancies and comparison with canine hemophagocytic histiocytic sarcoma, *Vet Clin Pathol* 37:121–128, 2008.

573. Walton RM, Brown DE, Burkhard MJ, et al.: Malignant histiocytosis in a domestic cat: cytomorphologic and immunohistochemical features, *Vet Clin Pathol* 26:56–60, 1997.

574. Kraje AC, Patton CS, Edwards DF: Malignant histiocytosis in 3 cats, *J Vet Intern Med* 15:252–256, 2001.

575. Smoliga J, Schatzberg S, Peters J, et al.: Myelopathy caused by a histiocytic sarcoma in a cat, *J Small Anim Pract* 46:34–38, 2005.

576. Bell R, Philbey A, Martineau H, et al.: Dynamic tracheal collapse associated with disseminated histiocytic sarcoma in a cat, *J Small Anim Pract* 47: 461-464, 2006.

577. Court E, Earnest-Koons K, Barr S, et al.: Malignant histiocytosis in a cat, *J Am Vet Med Assoc* 203:1300–1302, 1993.

578. Ide T, Uchida K, Tamura S, et al.: Histiocytic sarcoma in the brain of a cat, *J Vet Med Sci* 72:99–102, 2010.

579. Ide K, Setoguchi-Mukai A, Nakagawa T, et al.: Disseminated histiocytic sarcoma with excessive hemophagocytosis in a cat, *J Vet Med Sci* 71:817–820, 2009.

580. Pinard J, Wagg C, Girard C, et al.: Histiocytic sarcoma in the tarsus of a cat, *Vet Pathol* 43:1014–1017, 2006.

581. Treggiari E, Ressel L, Polton GA, et al.: Clinical outcome, PDGFRB and KIT expression in feline histiocytic disorders: a multicentre study, *Vet Comp Oncol* 15:65–77, 2017.

582. Affolter V, Moore P: Feline progressive histiocytosis, *Vet Pathol* 43:646–655, 2006.

583. Busch M, Reilly C, Luff J, et al.: Feline pulmonary Langerhans cell histiocytosis with multiorgan involvement, *Vet Pathol* 45:816–824, 2008.

584. Jaffe ES: Histiocytic and dendritic cell neoplasms. In Jaffe ES, Harris HL, Stein H, et al.: *World Health Organization classification of tumors: pathology and genetics of tumors of haematopoietic and lymphoid tissues*, 2001, pp 275–288.

585. Shimono J, Miyoshi H, Arakawa F, et al.: Prognostic factors for histiocytic and dendritic cell neoplasms, *Oncotarget* 19:98723–98732, 2017.

586. Ozkaya N, Dogan A, Abdel-Wahab O: Identification and targeting of kinase alterations in histiocytic neoplasms, *Hematol Oncol Clin North Am* 31:705–719, 2017.

Index

Note: Page numbers followed by "f" indicate figures, "t" indicate tables and "b" indicate boxes.

Brain tumor *(Continued)*
  clinical signs of, 658–660, 659f
  diagnosis of, 660–662
    biopsy and pathology of, 661–662
    cerebrospinal fluid analysis, 662
    diagnostic imaging, 660–661, 660f–661f
    minimum database, 660
  in dogs, 657–658, 658t
  epidemiology of, 657
  history of, 658–660
  incidence of, 657
  pathophysiology of, 658–660
  prognosis for, 662–665
  treatment of, 662–665
    chemotherapy, 662–663
    novel therapeutics, 665
    palliative care, 662, 663f
    radiation therapy, 664–665
    surgery, 663–664
BRCA1/2 mutation, breast cancer and, 605
Breakpoint cluster region, 148
Breast cancer
  oncogenic mutations in, 347
  sex hormones and, 92
BRM. *see* Biologic-response modifier
Bromocriptine, for canine pituitary-dependent
  hypercortisolism, 567
BSA. *see* Body surface area
Buffy coat smear, 389
Buprenorphine
  dose and effects of, 293t–294t
  efficacy of, 295
Burkitt lymphoma, 26
Butorphanol, dose and effects of, 293t–294t

C
Cabergoline, for canine pituitary-dependent
  hypercortisolism, 567
Cadherin, 53
Calcium, 100
Calcium supplementation, for
  hypoparathyroidism, 581
Calgary-Cambridge Guide, 313
California Animal Neoplasm Registry
  (CANR)
  cancer incidence/prevalence and cases of, 83t
  goal of, 82–83
CAM. *see* Cell adhesion molecule
Canarypox virus, 240
Cancer
  aneuploidy theory of, 6–7
  angiogenesis and, 6–7
  apoptosis, resisting of, 6
  body size and, 3–4, 3f
  cytoplasmic pathways and, 258
  definition of, 62
  diagnosis of, 70–74
    electron microscopy, 74
    flow cytometry/polymerase chain
      reaction, 74
    histochemical stain, 71
    immunohistochemistry, 71–74

Cancer *(Continued)*
  dietary substrate for, 301
  early diagnosis of, 55
  enabling characteristics, 48–49
    genome instability, 49
    tumor-promoting inflammation, 49
  energy metabolism adjustment and, 48
  epigenetic events and, 10
  etiology of, 1–35
  feline immunodeficiency virus and, 93
  feline leukemia virus and, 23
  gastrointestinal manifestations of
    cancer cachexia and anorexia, 98
    gastrointestinal ulceration, 98–100
  genetic basis of, 1
  genomic changes and, 40–45
  genomic dysregulation in, 146–147
  growth suppressors, evading, 5–6
  hallmarks of, 4, 44f, 45–48
    antigrowth signal, insensitivity to, 46
    deregulating cellular energetics, 8–9
    evading growth suppressors, 5–6
    genomic instability, 7
    proliferative signaling, 4–9
    replicative capacity, 46–47
    self-sufficiency of growth signals, 45–46
    therapeutic targeting of, 5f
    tumor-promoting inflammation, 7–8
    Warburg effect, 8–9
  heritable *versus* sporadic (nonheritable), 1
  imaging modalities for, 113–121
    computed tomography, 115–117
    magnetic resonance image, 117–118
    nuclear scintigraphy, 118
    PET/CT and/or PET/MR, 118–121
    radiography, 113
    ultrasonography, 113–115
  immortalization of, 6
  immune surveillance of, 231
  incidence of, 82–83
    in canines, 82–83
  invasion and metastasis of, 7, 8f
  manifestations of, 99b
    fever, 107
    hypertrophic osteopathy, 99b, 106–107
  neutering/spaying and, 92
  nutritional management for, 300
  occurrence of
    information sources on, 85
    proportional morbidity ratio and, 83
  pain level from, 288–289
  paraneoplastic syndromes and, 99b
  personalized medicine in, 154–155
  prevalence of
    in cats, 83
    in dogs, 83
    proportional measures, 83–84
  prevention of, 170–171
  risk factors for, 85–93, 87t
    nutritional, 301–302
  risk of, 1–3, 2f
  signal transduction and, 257

Cancer *(Continued)*
  stochastic model and, 10–11
  surgical resection of, as cure, 164–168, 167f
  treatment of
    all natural cure for, 330
    antiangiogenic therapy, 6–7
    antibody therapy for, 240–241
    gene therapy, 251
    molecular/targeted therapy, 251–285
    personalized medicine, 347–348
  waste sites and, 92
Cancer anorexia
  effects of, 98, 300–301
  evaluation for, 98
Cancer-associated fibroblast, 51
Cancer cachexia
  effects of, 98, 300–301
  evaluation for, 98
  occurrence of, 98
Cancer-causing virus, 19
Cancer cell
  destruction of, 255
  evolution of, 51
  pathways to, 49
  rescue of, 254
  signaling and, 45–46
Cancer gene, 41
Cancer immunosurveillance, 9
Cancer immunotherapy. *see* Immunotherapy
Cancer metabolism, 300
Cancer organ system, parts of, cancer cells and
  stem cells, 50
Cancer progenitor, 10–11
Cancer registry, 82
  cancer incidence/prevalence and cases of,
    83t
Cancer stem cell (CSC), 10–11
  colony formation and, 50
  sites for, 50
  spheres of, 11f
  tumor growth/metastasis and, 50
Cancer therapy
  pharmacologic principles in, 188–190
  population pharmacokinetics and, 198
  response to, 184t
  safety concerns for, 188
Canine acute myeloid leukemia,
    myeloproliferative neoplasms, and
    myelodysplasia, 730–739, 730b
  acute myeloid leukemia, 732–734, 733f,
    734t
    treatment, 738
  incidence and risk factors, 730–731
  myeloproliferative neoplasms, 734–735
    basophilic and eosinophilic leukemia,
      735
    chronic myelogenous leukemia, 734–735
    essential thrombocythemia, 735
    polycythemia vera, 734
  other bone marrow disorders, 735–739
    diagnostic techniques and workup,
      736–738, 737f